Textbook of
Perinatal
Medicine

Textbook of
Perinatal
Medicine

THIRD EDITION

Volume 1

Editors

ASIM KURJAK MD
Professor
Department of Obstetrics and Gynecology
Rector of DIU Libertas International University
Croatia

FRANK A CHERVENAK MD
Given Foundation Professor and Chairman
Department of Obstetrics and Gynecology
Weill Medical College of Cornell University
New York Presbyterian Hospital
USA

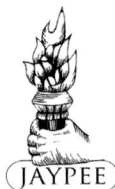

JAYPEE *The Health Sciences Publisher*

New Delhi | London | Philadelphia | Panama

Jaypee Brothers Medical Publishers (P) Ltd

Headquarters

Jaypee Brothers Medical Publishers (P) Ltd
4838/24, Ansari Road, Daryaganj
New Delhi 110 002, India
Phone: +91-11-43574357
Fax: +91-11-43574314
Email: jaypee@jaypeebrothers.com

Overseas Offices

J.P. Medical Ltd
83 Victoria Street, London
SW1H 0HW (UK)
Phone: +44 20 3170 8910
Fax: +44 (0)20 3008 6180
Email: info@jpmedpub.com

Jaypee Medical Inc
The Bourse
111 South Independence Mall East
Suite 835, Philadelphia, PA 19106, USA
Phone: +1 267-519-9789
Email: jpmed.us@gmail.com

Jaypee Brothers Medical Publishers (P) Ltd
Bhotahity, Kathmandu, Nepal
Phone: +977-9741283608
Email: kathmandu@jaypeebrothers.com

Jaypee-Highlights Medical Publishers Inc
City of Knowledge, Bld. 237, Clayton
Panama City, Panama
Phone: +1 507-301-0496
Fax: +1 507-301-0499
Email: cservice@jphmedical.com

Jaypee Brothers Medical Publishers (P) Ltd
17/1-B Babar Road, Block-B, Shaymali
Mohammadpur, Dhaka-1207
Bangladesh
Mobile: +08801912003485
Email: jaypeedhaka@gmail.com

Website: www.jaypeebrothers.com
Website: www.jaypeedigital.com

Inquiries for bulk sales may be solicited at: jaypee@jaypeebrothers.com

Textbook of Perinatal Medicine (Volume 1)

First Edition: 1998

Second Edition: 2006

Third Edition: **2015**

ISBN 978-93-5152-085-6

Printed at Replika Press Pvt. Ltd.

Dedicated to

Biserka, Alan and Igor
and
Judy, Francis and Joseph
With Love and Gratitude

—Asim and Frank

CONTRIBUTORS

A Adra
Department of Obstetrics and Gynecology
American University of Beirut Medical Center
Beirut, Lebanon

JL Alcazar
Department of Obstetrics and Gynecology
Clinica Universitaria de Navarra
Pamplona, Spain

Z Alfirevic
Department of Obstetrics and Gynecology
Liverpool Women's Hospital
Liverpool, UK

MM Anceschi
Institute of Gynecology, Perinatology and Child Health
University of Rome La Sapienza
Rome, Italy

A Antsaklis
Department of Fetal-Maternal Medicine
Alexandra Maternity Hospital
Athens, Greece

Z Appelman
Institute of Genetics, Kaplan Medical Center
Rehovot, Israel

B Arabin
Department of Perinatology
Isala Clinics
Zwolle, The Netherlands

J Babnik
Department of Obstetrics and Gynecology
University Medical Center
Ljubljana, Slovenia

JM Bajo Arenas
Department of Obstetrics and Gynecology
Getafe University Hospital
Madrid, Spain

LS Bakketeig
Department of Epidemiology
University of Southern Denmark
Odense, Denmark

R Baraibar
Department of Pediatrics
Institute Universitari Dexeus
Barcelona, Spain

Y Baytur
Department of Obstetrics and Gynecology
Bayar University, Medical School
Manisa, Turkey

A Beke
Department of Obstetrics and Gynecology
Semmelweis University Medical School
Budapest, Hungary

G Benagiano
Department of Gynecological Sciences
Perinatology and Child Care, University "La Sapienza"
Rome, Italy

K Benirschke
University of California
San Diego, USA

K Biedermann
Department of Obstetrics and Gynecology
Kantonales Frauenspital
Chur, Switzerland

DJ Birnbach
Department of Anesthesiology
University of Miami School of Medicine
Miami, USA

I Blickstein
Department of Obstetrics and Gynecology
Kaplan Medical Center
Rehovot, Israel

F Bonilla-Musoles
Department of Obstetrics and Gynecology
Valencia School of Medicine
Valencia, Spain

R Bracci
Institute of Preventive Pediatrics and Neonatology
University of Siena
Siena, Italy

B Brambati
Center of Prenatal Diagnosis
Milan, Italy

VNA Breeveld-Dwarkasing
Department of Pathobiology
Division of Veterinary Anatomy and Physiology
Faculty of Veterinary Medicine, Utrecht University
Utrecht, The Netherlands

B Breyer
University of Zagreb
Faculty of Electrical Engineering and Computing
Zagreb, Croatia

H Budge
Centre for Reproduction and Early Life
Institute of Clinical Research, University Hospital
Nottingham, UK

P Buekens
School of Public Health and Tropical Medicine
Tulane University
New Orleans, USA

F Carmona
Institut Clinic de Ginecologis, Obstetricia I Neonatologia
Hospital Clinic, University of Barcelona
Barcelona, Spain

MRG Carrapato
Department of Pediatrics and Neonatology
Hospital de Sao Sebastiao
Santa Maria da Feira, Portugal

JM Carrera
Fetal Medicine Service
Departamento de Obstetricia y Ginecologia
Instituto Universitario Dexeus
Barcelona, Spain

R Chaoui
Center for Prenatal Diagnosis and Human Genetics
Berlin, Germany

ST Chasen
Weill College of Cornell University
New York, USA

FA Chervenak
Weill Medical College of Cornell University
New York Presbyterian Hospital
New York, USA

S Cicero
Fetal Medicine Foundation
London, UK

WR Cohen
Department of Obstetrics and Gynecology
Weill Medical College of Cornell University
New York, USA

C Comas
Fetal Medicine Unit, Department of Obstetrics and Gynecology
Instituto Universitario Dexeus
Barcelona, Spain

L Cornette
The Peter Congdon Neonatal Unit
Leeds General Infirmary
Leeds, UK

L de Crespigny
Murdoch Children's Research Institute
Royal Children's Hospital, University of Melbourne
Victoria, Australia

A Csaba
Department of Obstetrics and Gynecology
Semmelweis University Medical School
Budapes, Hungary

V D'Addario
Fetal Medicine Unit
Department of Obstetrics and Gynecology
University of Bari
Bari, Italy

F Daffos
Departement de Diagnostic Prenatal et de Foetologie
Institute de Puericulture de Paris
Paris, France

M Dan
Unit of Infectious Diseases, Wolfson Medical Center
Holon, Israel

JE Deaver
Women's Health Research
Jamaica Hospital Medical Center
New York, USA

R Derom
Association de Soutien a la Recherche Scientifique au Profit des Naissances Multiples
Destelbergen, Belgium

GC di Renzo
Center of Perinatal and Reproductive Medicine
University of Perugia
Perugia, Italy

E Doménech
Department of Pediatrics, Faculty of Medicine of La Laguna
University Hospital of the Canary Islands
Tenerife, Spain

SM Donn
Division of Neonatal-Perinatal Medicine
CS Mott Children's Hospital
University Michigan Health System
Ann Arbor, USA

† A Drazancic
Department of Obstetrics and Gynecology
Medical School University of Zagreb
Zagreb, Croatia

JW Dudenhausen
Department of Obstetrics
Charite Campus Virchow Klinikum
Berlin, Germany

SJ English
The Peter Congdon Neonatal Unit
Clarendon Wing, Leeds General Infirmary
Leeds, UK

AK Ertan
Department of Obstetrics and Gynecology
Saarland University Medical School
Homburg, Germany

J Espinoza
Perinatology Research Branch, National Institute of Child Health and Human Development, NH, DHHS, Bethesda, Maryland, and Department of Obstetrics and Gynecology
Wayne State University School of Medicine
Detroit, Michigan, USA

MI Evans
Institute for Genetics
Mt Sinai School of Medicine
New York, USA

E Fabre
Department of Obstetrics and Gynecology
Hospital Clinico Universitario
Zaragoza, Spain

SJ Fasouliotis
Department of Obstetrics and Gynecology
Hebrew University Ein-Kerem, Hadassah Medical Center
Jerusalem, Israel

R Floyd
Department of Obstetrics, Gynecology and Women's Health
University of Missouri-Columbia, School of Medicine
Columbia, Missouri, USA

M Foley
Department of Obstetrics and Gynecology
National Maternity Hospital
Dublin, Ireland

JA Fortney
Heilbrunn Department of Population and Family Health
Columbia University
New York, USA

EA Friedman
Department of Obstetrics and Gynecology
Albert Einstein College of Medicine
New York, USA

K Fukushima
Department of Obstetrics and Gynecology
Graduate School of Medical Sciences
Kyushu University, Higashi-Ku
Fukuoka, Japan

K Ghebremeskel
Institute of Brain Chemistry and Human Nutrition
London Metropolitan University
London, UK

F Goffinet
Research Epidemiology Unit for Prenatal and Women's Health
Port Royal Maternity Hospital
Paris, France

LF Gonçalves
Perinatology Research Branch, National Institute of Child Health
and Human Development, NIH, DHHS, Bethesda, Maryland, and
Department of Obstetrics and Gynecology
Wayne State University School of Medicine
Detroit, Michigan, USA

C Gordon
Department of Rheumatology
City Hospital
Birmingham, UK

JL Graf
Department of Pediatric Surgery
University of California
San Francisco, USA

BE Grand
Department of Fetal Medicine
Juan A Fernandez Hospital of Buenos Aires
Argentina

A Grunebaum
Weill Cornell Medical Center
New York, USA

B Hargitai
First Department of Obstetrics and Gynecology
Semmelweis University Medical School
Budapest, Hungary

MR Harrison
Department of Pediatric Surgery
University of California
California, USA

L Hellström-Westas
Department of Pediatrics
University Hospital Lund
Lund, Sweden

J Herczeg
Teaching Hospital of the
University of Szeged
Szeged, Hungary

P Hilton
Women's Services, Royal Victoria Infirmary
Newcastle upon Tyne, UK

W Holzgreve
Women's University Hospital Basel
Basel, Switzerland

H Hopp
Charity Clinic for Obstetrics
Campus Benjamin Franklin
Berlin, Germany

T Hosono
Department of Medical Engineering
Osaka Electro-communication University
Shijonawate, Osaka, Japan

T Ikeda
Department of Obstetrics and Gynecology
Miyazaki Medical College, University of Miyazaki
Kihara, Kiyotake-Cho
Miyazaki, Japan

S Iniesta
Santa Cristina University Hospital
Universidad Autonoma de Madrid
Madrid, Spain

I Kassis
Ichilov Hospital, University of Tel Aviv
Tel Aviv, Israel

A Khurana
The Ultrasound Laboratory
New Delhi, India

DA Krantz
NTD Laboratories Inc
East Meadow, New York, USA

I Krause
Department of Pediatrics
Schneider Children's Medical Center of Israel
Sackler School of Medicine, Tel Aviv University
Tel Aviv, Israel

S Kupesic
Paul L Foster School of Medicine
Texas Tech University Health Sciences Center at El Paso
El Paso, Texas, USA

A Kurjak
DIU Libertas International University
Zagreb, Croatia

ML Kush
Department of Obstetrics, Gynecology and Reproductive Sciences
University of Maryland School of Medicine
Baltimore, Maryland, USA

HJ Landy
Division of Maternal-Fetal Medicine
Department of Obstetrics and Gynecology
Georgetown University Hospital
Washington, DC, USA

O Lapaire
Women's University Hospital Basel
Basel, Switzerland

L Lewi
Department of Obstetrics and Gynecology
University Hospital Gasthuisberg
Leuven, Belgium

G Lindmark
Department of Women's and Children's Health
Uppsala University
Uppsala, Sweden

GA Little
Dartmouth-Hitchcock Medical Center
Neonatology, Lebanon

JA Low
Department of Obstetrics and Gynecology
Queen's University, Kingston
Ontario, Canada

R Luzietti
Center of Perinatal and Reproductive Medicine
University of Perugia
Perugia, Italy

IZ MacKenzie
Department of Obstetrics and Gynecology
John Radcliffe Hospital
Oxford, UK

K Maeda
Department of Obstetrics and Gynecology
Tottori University, Nadamachi
Yonago, Japan

S Maheshwari
Department of Pediatric Cardiology
Narayana Hrudayalaya, Anekal Taluk
Bengaluru, Karnataka, India

GP Mandruzzato
Department of Obstetrics and Gynecology
Istituto per l'infanzia IRCCS "Burlo Garofolo"
Trieste, Italy

T Marton
Department of Histopathology
Birmingham Women's Hospital
Birmingham, UK

G Maso
Department of Obstetrics and Gynecology
Istituto per l'infanzia IRCCS "Burlo Garofolo"
Trieste, Italy

A Matias
Department of Obstetrics and Gynecology
Faculty of Medicine, University Hospital of S Joao
Porto, Portugal

† LT Merce
Assisted Reproduction Unit
International Ruber Hospital
Madrid, Spain

E Merz
Department of Obstetrics and Gynecology
Krankenhaus Nordwest
Frankfurt/Main, Germany

D Miron
Pediatric Department A, Ha'Emek Medical Center
Afula, Israel

G Monni
Department of Obstetrics and Gynecology
Prenatal and Preimplantation Genetic Diagnosis
Fetal Therapy, Ospedale Microcitemico
Cagliari, Italy

N Montenegro
Department of Obstetrics and Gynecology
Faculty of Medicine
University Hospital S Joao
Porto, Portugal

A Morag
Clinical Virology Unit
Hadassah University Hospitals
Jerusalem, Israel

C Mortera
Diagnostico Prenatal y Perinatal
Institut Dexeus, Cardio-hemodinamica
Hospital Sant J de Deu
Barcelona, Spain

A Mulic-Lutvica
Department of Women's and Children's Health
Uppsala University
Uppsala, Sweden

MF Murphy
Department of Hematology
Oxford Radcliffe Hospitals NHS Trust
Oxford, UK

LJ Nelson
Department of Philosophy
Santa Clara University
Santa Clara, California, USA

C Nelson-Piercy
Department of Obstetrics
St Thomas's Hospital
London, UK

KH Nicolaides
Fetal Medicine Foundation
London, UK

JG Nijhuis
Department of Obstetrics
Academisch Ziekenhuis Maastricht
The Netherlands

J Nizard
Department of Obstetrics and Gynecology
Hopital de Poissy-Saint-Germain en Laye
Poissy, France

Z Novak-Antolic
Department of Obstetrics and Gynecology
University Medical Center
Ljubljana, Slovenia

K Olshtain-Pops
Department of Clinical Microbiology and Infectious Diseases
Hadassah University Hospital
Jerusalem, Israel

KM Paarlberg
Department of Obstetrics and Gynecology
University Hospital Vrije Universiteit
Amsterdam, The Netherlands

M Pajntar
Department of Obstetrics and Gynecology
University Medical Center
Ljubljana, Slovenia

A Papageorgiou
Department of Neonatology
Jewish General Hospital, Montreal
Quebec, Canada

E Papiernik
University Rene Descartes
Maternite de Port Royal Hospital Cochin
Paris, France

C Paul
Department of Obstetrics and Gynecology
King's College Hospital
London, UK

L Pereira
Maternal Fetal Medicine
Oregon Health and Science University
Portland, Oregon, USA

POD Pharoah
FSID Unit of Perinatal and Pediatric Epidemiology
Department of Public Health
University of Liverpool
Liverpool, UK

T Podymow
Division of Nephrology and Hypertension
Weill Medical College of Cornel University
New York, USA

RK Pooh
CRIFM Clinical Research Institute of Fetal Medicine PMC
Osaka, Japan

P Prats
Prenatal Diagnosis Unit
Department of Obstetrics and Gynecology
Institut Universitari Dexeus
Barcelona, Spain

E Quarello
Department of Obstetrics and Gynecology
CHI Poissy St Germain, Universite Paris-Ouest
Poissy, France

R Romero
Perinatology Research Branch
National Institute of Child Health and Human Development
National Institute of Health, DHHS
Bethesda, Maryland, USA

G Rosner
Genetic Institute
Tel Aviv Sourasky Medical Center
Israel

P Rozenberg
Department of Obstetrics and Gynecology
Poissy-Saint Germain Hospital
Versailles-Saint Quentin University
Poissy Cedex, France

FF Rubaltelli
Department of Neonatology
Ospedale Careggi Reparto
Florence, Italy

E Rubinstein
Section of Infectious Diseases
University of Manitoba
Winnipeg, Manitoba, Canada

RM Sabatel Lopez
Department of Obstetrics and Gynecology
University of Grenada
Spain

N Sagawa
Department of Obstetrics and Gynecology
Mie University Graduate School of Medicine
Tsu, Mie, Japan

S Saito
Department of Obstetrics and Gynecology
Toyama Medical and Pharmaceutical University
Toyama-shi, Toyama, Japan

E Saling
Institut fuer Perinatale Medizin
Berlin, Germany

OD Saugstad
Department of Pediatric Research
The National Hospital
Oslo, Norway

JG Schenker
Department of Obstetrics and Gynecology
Hadassah University Hospital
Jerusalem, Israel

S Scherjon
Department of Obstetrics
Leiden University Medical Center
Leiden, The Netherlands

BS Schifrin
Department of Obstetrics and Gynecology
Loma Linda University School of Medicine
Loma Linda, California, USA

Y Schlesinger
Division of Infectious Diseases
Shaare Zedek Medical Center
Jerusalem, Israel

NJ Sebire
Department of Histopathology
Camelia Botnar Laboratories
Great Ormond Street Hospital
London, UK

C Sen
Department of Obstetrics and Gynecology
Cerrahpasa Medical School
Istanbul, Turkey

M Seoud
Department of Obstetrics and Gynecology
American University of Beirut Medical Center
Beirut, Lebanon

B Serra
Department of Obstetrics and Gynecology
Instituto Universitario Dexeus
Barcelona, Spain

F Sethna
Fetal Medicine Unit
Department of Obstetrics and Gynecology
St George's Hospital NHS Trust
London, UK

M Shapiro
Department of Clinical Microbiology and Infectious Diseases
Hadassah University Hospital
Jerusalem, Israel

DT Spira
Department of Parasitology
Hebrew University, Hadassah Medical School
Jerusalem, Israel

M Stanojevic
Department of Obstetrics and Gynecology
Neonatal Unit, Sveti Duh Hospital
Zagreb, Croatia

Z Stembera
WHO Collaborating Center for Perinatal Medicine and
Human Reproduction
Institute for the Care of Mother and Child
Prague, Czech Republic

GM Stirrat
Centre for Ethics in Medicine
University of Bristol
Bristol, UK

KNS Subramanian
Georgetown University Hospital
Washington, DC, USA

G Sylvestre
The New York Presbyterian Hospital
Weill Medical College of Cornell University
New York, USA

A Tabor
Copenhagen University Hospital
Department of Obstetrics and Gynecology
Hvidovre Hospital
Hvidovre, Denmark

HA Tanriverdi
Department of Obstetrics and Gynecology
Karaelmas University Medical School
Kozlu/Zonguldak, Turkey

S Tercanli
University Women's Hospital
Basel, Switzerland

JM Thomas
National Collaborating Center for Women and Children's Health
London, UK

JM Troyano
Division of US and Fetal Medicine
University Hospital of the Canary Islands
La Laguna, Tenerife, Spain

K Tsukimori
Department of Obstetrics and Gynecology
Graduate School of Medical Sciences
Kyushu University, Higashi-Ku
Fukuoka, Japan

FA van Assche
Department of Gynecology
Catholic University of Leuven
Leuve, Belgium

PP van den Berg
Department of Obstetrics and Gynecology
University Hospital Nijmegen
Nijmegen, The Netherlands

J van Eyck
Department of Perinatology
Isala Clinics
Zwolle, The Netherlands

HP van Geijn
Department of Obstetrics and Gynecology
University Hospital Vrije Universiteit
Amsterdam, The Netherlands

WJ van Wijngaarden
Department of Obstetrics and Gynecology
Ziekenhuis Bronovo
Den Haag, The Netherlands

Y Ville
Department of Obstetrics and Gynecology
Poissy-Saint Germain Hospital
Versailles-Saint Quentil University
Poissy Cedex, France

LS Voto
Fundacion Miguel Margulies
Buenos Aires, Argentina

N Wake
Department of Molecular Genetics
Medical Institute of Bioregulation
Kyushu University, Beppu
Oita, Japan

J Walker
Department of Obstetrics and Gynecology
St James University Hospital
Leeds, UK

CP Weiner
Department of Obstetrics, Gynecology and
Reproductive Sciences
University of Maryland School of Medicine
Baltimore, Maryland, USA

DJ Williams
Institute of Women's Health, University College London
Elizabeth Garrett Anderson Obstetric Hospital
London, UK

MSI Wingate
Department of Maternal and Child Health
University of Alabama at Birmingham
Birmingham, Alabama, USA

DC Wood Jr
Fetal Cardiology, Maternal Fetal Medicine
Department of Obstetrics and Gynecology
Thomas Jefferson University, Philadelphia
Pennsylvania, USA

Y Yaron
Prenatal Genetic Diagnosis Division
Genetic Institute, Tel Aviv Sourasky Medical Center
Tel Aviv, Israel

L Yeo
Department of Obstetrics
Gynecology and Reproductive Sciences
Division of Maternal Fetal Medicine
UMDNJ – Robert Woods Johnson Medical School
New Brunswick, New Jersey, USA

KA Yunis
Department of Pediatrics
American University of Beirut Medical Center
Beirut, Lebanon

P Zalloua
Department of Obstetrics and Gynecology
American University of Beirut Medical Center
Beirut, Lebanon

MA Zoppi
Department of Obstetrics and Gynecology
Prenatal and Preimplantation Genetic Diagnosis
Fetal Therapy, Ospedale Microcitemico
Cagliari, Italy

PREFACE

Perinatal medicine is among the most challenging and beautiful areas of study and practice. It deals with events before birth, when the fetus is a patient and during the immediate neonatal period. The World Association of Perinatal Medicine is dedicated to the study of all aspects of perinatal biology, physiology, screening, diagnosis, management and ethics, with the goal of continuous quality improvement in the care of maternal, fetal and neonatal patients.

This textbook is based on a previous work that was produced by the European Association of Perinatal Medicine in 1998. Because perinatal medicine is now a global area of study, it is appropriate that the current textbook is a product of the World Association of Perinatal Medicine. The bonds that link perinatologists together transcend geographic, political, religious and lingual differences, resulting in a globalization that optimizes clinical care.

This textbook consists of over 200 chapters divided into 20 sections which span the depth and breadth of the field. This book reproduces in large part of the previous edition, with some modifications.

We are grateful to the authors of the 201 chapters and the editors of the 20 sections who have worked so diligently with us to produce this textbook that we believe bears testament to the importance and success of international collaboration in perinatal medicine.

Asim Kurjak

Frank A Chervenak

CONTENTS

Volume 1

Section 3: Evidence-based Medicine and Epidemiology
Z Alfirevic, L Cabero-Roura

Section 4: Ultrasound
A Kurjak, Y Ville

Section 5: Doppler Ultrasound
S Weiner, AK Ertan

Section 6: Basic Science
H Nakano, Y Murata

Section 7: Fetal Diagnosis and Therapy
W Holzgreve, M Evans

Section 8: Screening and Risk Assessment
G Monni, S Chasen

Volume 2

Section 12: Prenatal Diagnosis and Therapy
K Nicolaides, A Antsaklis

Section 13: Intrauterine Growth
JM Carrera, GP Mandruzzato

Section 14: Preterm Delivery
GC di Renzo, R Romero

Section 19: Maternal Disease
A Grunebaum, LS Voto

Section 20: The Challenge Facing Developing Countries
JJ Sciarra, A Adra

SECTION 1

Neonatology

M Levene, MRG Carrapato

1

Transition at Birth

OD Saugstad

INTRODUCTION

The transition from fetal to postnatal life is characterized by a number of dramatic changes in physiological, biochemical, immunologic and hormonal functions. The fetus is fully dependent on the maternal supply not only of oxygen and nutrients but also of a number of hormones and other important substances. The thermal control of the fetus is also taken care of by the mother. Intestinal and breathing movements as well as nonshivering thermogenesis are partially inhibited. Large organs as the lungs and liver are not very active. The fetus is also asleep most of the time. These are some important reasons the oxygen requirements and metabolism are low in fetal life. Cardiac output is low with a low systemic blood pressure. A relatively low blood glucose level and oxygen supply is, therefore, sufficient to ensure substrate for energy metabolism at this stage.

During the last trimester the fetus prepares itself to meet the extrauterine milieu; energy stores are established, minerals and trace elements are deposited, both white and brown fat accumulate, the lungs mature both structurally and biochemically. The latter means that the surfactant system matures and the antioxidative defense develops in order for the fetus to breathe and to be able to withstand the sudden increased oxidative stress induced by the high oxygen concentration in ambient air. Many epithelial transport functions of different organs mature in late fetal and early neonatal life.

After birth, the newly born infant is responsible for its own oxygenation and ventilation. The partially inhibited status of the fetus is immediately reversed at birth. It is awake, aroused, breathing and crying. Metabolism increases with a subsequent increased oxygen demand, and the newborn can initiate lipolysis and mobilize glucose. The higher oxygen consumption of the brain is one reason the newborn brain is more vulnerable to hypoxia than in fetal life. The sharp increase in oxygen exposure makes it necessary for the newborn infant to protect itself from oxygen toxicity. Transition to birth is, therefore, not only a matter of redistribution of the circulation, maturation of the lungs and the surfactant system with alveolar gas exchange, it is much more complex and probably only a small part of this is understood. In the following some of these aspects will be discussed.

GROWTH

General Principles

The greatest growth rate in human life occurs in the fetal period. The increase from a fertilized egg to a term newborn infant is in weight 6×10^{12}, in length 5,000 fold, and in surface area 61×10^6. After birth, growth slows down still the greatest postnatal growth rate occurs immediately after birth.

Prenatal growth is dependent on maternal, placental and fetal factors. In the first trimester growth occurs by increase in cell number, in the second trimester there is an increase both in number and in cellular size. In the third trimester growth is mainly by cellular growth since the rate of mitosis slows down. During the first two trimesters the fetus has reached approximately 1/3rd of its term weight. In this period only 50 grams fat are accumulated by contrast to approximately 500 grams deposited the last trimester. Of the approximately 95 kcal/kg/day needed by the fetus 40 kcal are spent for growth. Prenatal growth is dependent on autocrine and paracrine growth factors as insulin like factors 1 and 2; however, insulin as well plays a major role in prenatal growth. Macrosomia is a well-known effect of fetal hyperinsulinism and these children have increased body fat at 1 year of age. Abnormal patterns in insulin like growth factor 2 gene expression may lead to the Beckwith Wiedemann syndrome. These infants are large with elevated insulin levels.

Postnatal growth is mainly regulated through pituitary growth hormones, thyroid hormone and other hormones. In fetal life growth hormone (GH) is high in the fetus; however, the number of GH receptors is low. That GH plays some role in fetal growth is reflected in poor growth of children with GH deficiency or GH receptor deficiency (Laron syndrome) and its action is mediated by insulin like growth factors. During the first weeks of extrauterine life GH falls and already the first day of life a pulsatile release of GH has been detected with a pulse periodicity of 73 minutes, with higher peaks and more frequent pulses found in small for gestational age (SGA) than in appropriate for gestation age (AGA) infants. This pulsatility is controlled by the stimulatory GH-releasing hormone and the inhibitory somatostatin both of these produced in the hypothalamus. Thyroid hormone is a major factor in postnatal growth and an acute elevation with a peak in TSH is found immediately after birth with a decline the first 5–6 days after birth. Leptin is produced in adipose tissue and also regulates growth. Its role in fetal life is unknown, but high concentrations are found in the umbilical cord with a gradual decrease over the next 3 months. Androgens decrease leptin values so that girls have higher concentrations than boys from birth, the significance of this seem not to be understood.

The changes in body composition the fetus undergo with the advancement of gestation is a progressive decrease in total water, extracellular water, sodium and chloride and an increase in intracellular water, potassium, calcium and magnesium. The postnatal body composition changes are characterized by increase in adipose tissue with a peak around 4–6 months, a progressive decrease in body water with a relative increase of intracellular water.[1-6]

Fluid Shift

In early fetal life approximately 95% of the fetus is water which gradually decreases throughout gestation being 80% at 8 months and 75% at term. Mode of delivery does not seem to influence this. Simultaneously with this decline in body water, there is a drastic decrease in extracellular and a gradual increase in intracellular water. This tendency continues until 9 months of age when body water constitutes 62%. However, the total body water related to surface area does not change very much in this period. Maximal intracellular water of 43% of body weight is reached at 2 months of age at the same time extracellular water is 30%. The term newborn loses 5–10% of its body weight and the preterm more. This is mainly due to loss of water; however, it is not clear whether this loss is predominantly from the extra or intracellular space or perhaps both.

In the newborn the first day of life the blood volume is to a large extent dependent on placental transfusion at the time of delivery which can be up to 25–50 mL/kg within 3 minutes. Whether or not this increase in blood volume of 50% is harmful is not clear. A delayed cord clamping may lead to a gradual increase in hematocrit within a couple of hours. This is caused by plasma loss of 30 mL/kg the following 4 hours due to a shift of fluid from the plasma into the interstitial space in addition to an increased urinary output.[7,8]

Recently, it has become clear that specific water channels Aquaporines play an important role in water transport and water balance. Aquaporine 1 and 4 have been found in the brain, 9 in the skin, 2 in the kidney, etc. The newborn kidneys reduced ability to concentrate the urine is probably due to lack of aquaporines. Aquaporines are active also in the perinatal period and probably are important for removing fluid from the lung and in so-called transitory tachypnea of the newborn.

Carbohydrates

Glucose is the major source of energy in fetal life and the fetus is entirely dependent on glucose delivery from the mother. It seems that the human fetus does not produce glucose until the end of the gestation, and the brain requires a continuous glucose supply that is received from the mother—at term at a rate of 4–7 mg/kg/min. This equals 6–10 g glucose/kg/day and represents approximately 60% of the calories needed by the fetus. Glucose is transported by facilitated carrier-mediated placental diffusion. Several facilitated glucose transporters have been identified and recently cloned. They comprise a family of structurally related families and are designated GLUT. The primary function of these is to mediate the exchange of glucose between blood and the cytoplasm of the cell. Several of these GLUT are present in early fetal life.

Blood glucose is lower in the fetus compared with the mother but there is a significant correlation between maternal and fetal levels at least if the maternal levels are not too low (< 4.4 mmol/L) under which fetal concentrations are independent of maternal levels. At birth, the transplacental supply of nutrients is abruptly interrupted. The newborn infant, therefore, has to produce glucose from its own endogenous stores until feeding is started. At birth blood glucose is 60–75% of maternal levels and then falls over the next 1–2 hours stabilizing at 2.5—3.3 mmol/L (45–60 mg/dL) in healthy term infants within 24 hours. Maternal glucose supplementation during labor and delivery seems to blunt this decrease. With the initiation of feeding it increases and after 24 hours is between 45 and 90 mg/dL.

Glucose can be metabolized to either lactate which occurs in anaerobic conditions or acetyl-CoA (Ac-CoA) under aerobic conditions. Pyruvate can be metabolized to either lactate or Ac-CoA, this is partly regulated by the relative amounts of the isoenzymes of lactate dehydrogenase (LDH). In adult brain the LDH isoenzyme composition favors aerobic oxidation of glucose, but in the fetal and newborn brain the LDH composition allows anaerobic glycolysis. The placenta is impermeable to both insulin and glucagon which are produced by the fetus at least from the 10th week of gestation. Glucose stimulates insulin in the third trimester only.

In late gestation approximately 50% of the glucose is converted to glycogen in the liver and muscle, and to fat in the liver and adipose tissue. Glucose storage is regulated primarily by insulin but also by glucocorticoids. Glycogen is low until approximately 36 weeks of gestation; however, triples in the liver until term when it reaches a maximum both in the liver and skeletal muscles. In other organs as myocardium and lungs, the peak is reached somewhat earlier declining toward term. Glycogen is the initial substrate for glucose but only for a few hours. Within 24 hours after birth the glycogen stores are more or less exhausted. Gluconeogenesis from fat and protein is, therefore, necessary to meet the metabolic demands and this is in principle a postnatal event. Fat is, therefore, an important substrate for glucose production in the early newborn period. Although key enzymes for gluconeogenesis are present in the liver from early fetal life gluconeogenetic activity is not expressed in utero at least not until near term. In late gestation fetal gluconeogenes is, therefore, occurs and may contribute to fetal glucose levels especially if the glucose supply from the mother is reduced for instance during maternal fasting or by intrauterine growth retardation. Initiation of lipolysis and gluconeogenesis is promoted by hormonal and enzymatic changes occurring the first day of life. The insulin/glucagon ratio is rapidly decreasing after birth and the high postnatal concentrations of catecholamines, cortisone, and TSH contribute to this. In the newborn infant glycerol can be converted to glucose contributing up to 20% of the hepatic glucose production. It has been shown that preterm infants less than 28 weeks of gestation have the capability of gluconeogenesis from glycerol.[9-13]

Proteins

In the second and third trimester, protein synthesis is especially high, however, with a reduced rate toward term. The term newborn infant has about 0.5 kg of protein after a many-fold linear increase in the last half of the gestation. Protein synthesis slows down toward term but is still high, approximately fivefold higher compared with adult levels. In fact, not only synthesis is high in fetal life, but breakdown of proteins is also increased giving a high protein turnover in the fetus. There is a substantial organ difference with the highest rate of protein synthesis in the placenta, heart and liver (half-life 1 day) compared with half-life of 1 week in muscle. A number of growth factors may be responsible for this as the Insulin-like growth factor (IGF-1). For this reason the amino acid concentration in fetal plasma is higher than later in life and the fetal/maternal amino acid ratio in plasma is high with a peak in the second trimester when it is approximately 3:1 falling to 1.5:1 toward term. Intrauterine growth retardation is characterized by a falling fetal/maternal plasma amino acid ratio mainly due to an augmentation in the maternal levels.

Amino acids are transported across the placenta both by a direct active transfer of essential amino acids and placental cytosolic synthesis of nonessential amino acids. A number of amino acid transporters – at least twelve have recently been identified. The rate of amino acid utilization is about 4 g/kg/day similar to the estimated intake of very premature infants. A protein intake in the postnatal period of 2.8 g/kg/day is close to the minimal intake needed to ensure weight gain and nitrogen retention equal to intrauterine rates and a protein intake of 3–4.3 g/kg/day is recommended. Some amino acids which are nonessential in postnatal life are essential in fetal life due to inadequate maturation of enzyme systems. One example of this is the absence of cystathionase making the fetus completely dependent on the mothers cystine supply. During the first hour postnatally, there is a rapid fall in plasma amino acid levels.[14,15]

Lipids

The fetus requires both essential and nonessential fatty acids from the mother and fat represents 1/6th of body weight at term.

Free fatty acid supply to the fetus may occur through a process of facilitated membrane translocation involving a plasma membrane protein, placental synthesis and release into the umbilical circulation, or lipolysis of triglycerides, lipoproteins or phospholipids from either the maternal or fetal side. The free fatty acid concentration and composition in the fetus reflect maternal values. It is well-known that maternal manipulation with diet may change the growth and development of the fetus. For instance, mothers fed a diet high in Docosahexenoic acid (DHA) deliver babies with higher birth weight. These children seem to mature earlier and have a higher IQ at the age of 4. Triglycerides are hydrolyzed to fatty acids by lipoprotein lipases which are secreted by capillary endothelium. Lipoprotein lipase is stimulated by insulin and is present in fetal life with low activities in muscle and heart but higher in the lungs. This may be of importance for surfactant synthesis and maturation. After birth the activity of this enzyme increases both in preterm and term infants. However, in preterm infants the clearance of circulating triglycerides is reduced due to a lower enzyme activity than in the term infants and this activity seems to be directly related to the degree of prematurity. In the human fetus, the enzymes for cholesterol and liopoprotein metabolism develop early in gestation. As LDL receptor expression also increases in gestation serum cholesterol and LDL decrease to levels lower than observed in early postnatal life. In breastfed infants, these metabolites increase rapidly and are doubled from day 1 to day 7 of life but still only half of adult levels.

In the last 8 weeks of gestation subcutaneous fat increases rapidly from approximately 20–350 g, and deep body fat 10–80 g. The total fat content increases from 6 gram at 22 weeks to 500 g at term.

Fatty acid catabolism is an important energy source in postnatal life. High concentrations of free fatty acids and glycerol soon after birth indicate the onset of lipolysis and lipid oxidation. Free fatty acids and glycerol increase sharply and peak around 120 minutes after birth. Beta-oxidation of fatty acids occurs in the mitochondria. Ac-CoA is transesterified to carnitine by carnitine acyltransferase located on the inner mitochondrial membrane. Fatty acid oxidation is limited in the fetal myocardium because of a low concentration of carnitine and a limited number of mitochondria. Liver, brain, placenta and lung also have limited capacity to oxidize fatty acids. After birth, however, fatty acid oxidation increases substantially and remains high until the time of weaning.

Lipogenesis is found in fetal tissue from 12 weeks of gestation and is stimulated by insulin and inhibited by glucagon or cAMP. Fatty acid synthesis declines after birth when the diet is milk which is rich in fat. Placental transfer of ketone body by contrast to glycerol has been described. The fetus uses ketone bodies as substrates for oxidation and lipogenesis.[10,16-19]

MINERAL METABOLISM

The placenta actively transports calcium to the fetus to allow rapid fetal skeletal mineralization. From 20 to 26 weeks of gestation fetal levels are maintained about 0.25 mmol/L (1 mg/dL) above the maternal level. The last trimester calcium stores quadruples. In humans 2/3rd of the mean 30 g calcium in healthy term fetus is transported the last trimester. At birth the constant calcium supply is interrupted and there is a normal fall in serum calcium in the first hour after birth reaching a stable level after 24–48 hours of age of about 2–2.25 mmol/L. During the next days there is a subsequent gradual increase reaching serum calcium of about 2.5 mmol/L at 1 week of age. In one study serum ionized calcium concentrations decreased from in mean 1.45 mmol/L at birth to 1.33 mmol/L at 2 hours and 1.23 mmol/L at 24 hours of age.

At birth parathyroid hormone is low increasing 2–4 fold during the first 2 days of life giving an efficient response after 3–4 days. By contrast, calcitonin levels are high in the newborn thereby inhibiting calcium mobilization from bone. Magnesium, zinc and phosphorus are also transported actively across the placenta from the mother to the fetus. During the first week of life magnesium levels show small variations, correlating directly with serum calcium and inversely with phosphorous. Adequate Zinc levels are needed for normal fetal growth and postnatally the requirements are approximately 2 mg/day. Zinc deficiency in infancy may lead to failure to thrive, and reduced immunological function. Globally Zinc deficiency represents a major health problem in infancy.[20-23]

HORMONES

The endocrine system is involved in growth, reproduction, cellular nutrition, as well as energy, thermal, cardiovascular and fluid homeostasis. Many hormones do not cross the placenta but are found in the fetus around 10–12 weeks of gestation. This is true for GH, insulin, prolactin and thyroxin.

Prolactin may play an important role in regulating fluid balance in fetal life. At term its levels are 20 fold higher than adult levels and decline rapidly in the first week after birth. This reduction may be linked to the decline in total body water after birth. Prolactin may also have a maturational effect on the pulmonary surfactant system in combination with glucocorticoids and thyroidea hormones. Thyrotropin releasing factor regulates TSH and prolactin secretion. As early as 12 weeks of gestation, it is clear that the fetus produces thyroxin and around 13 weeks of gestation TSH producing cells have been identified. TSH both stimulates growth as well as contributes to differentiation of the thyroid gland. TSH does not cross the placenta and T3 and T4 do not cross in sufficient quantity for the fetus. The fetus is, therefore, dependent on its own pituitary and thyroid hormones in addition to supply from the mother. By contrast, thyrotropin releasing factor crosses the placenta and stimulates fetal TSH. Fetal total and free T4 as well as thyroxin binding globulin values increase during the gestation and reach the level of the mean adult values around 36 weeks. In umbilical cord blood TSH is low and increases rapidly within the first 10–15 minutes after birth, and T4 reaches a peak after 48 hours as a response to the high TSH concentration. TSH remains high the first day of life before it reaches its low normal adult levels. The half time of T4 is much shorter in the neonatal period compared with adult life making the thyroxin requirements many times higher than in the adult period.

From the 8th week of gestation the fetal adrenal converts pregnenolone to dehydroepiandrosterone sulfate which in the fetal liver and other tissues is hydroxylated to 16-hydroxy-dehydroepiandrosterone which passes to the placenta and forms estriol. Since estrogen is important in maintaining pregnancy the fetus, therefore, contributes to this itself.

The fetal adrenal cortex promotes fetal organ enzyme maturation and in the last part of the gestation ACTH and cortisol levels increase in the fetus influencing maturation of enzyme systems in the lung, gastrointestinal tract and possibly other organs. After birth cortisol levels decrease reaching adult levels by the age of 2–3 months.[2,22,24-27]

STRESS AT BIRTH

There is a dramatic activation of the adrenal, the sympathetic, and the parasympathetic systems toward term. The sympathoadrenal system develops in fetal life and the newborn infant has large adrenals and extrachromaffin tissue in the paraganglia. The adrenal cortex matures toward term and releases substantial amounts of epinephrine and norepinephrine near term. Corticosteroids around birth mature the surfactant system by inducing its synthesis, as well as antioxyenzymes in the lung and further play a role in the labor process. Corticosteroids also induce the expression of phenylethanolamine-N-methyl-transferase which converts norepinephrine to epinephrine. The transition at birth is characterized by high levels of catecholamines, angiotensin and vasopressin. The catecholamine levels are higher than in any other period of life under physiological circumstances. Norepinephrine constitutes approximately 85% of total catecholamines and in plasma is normally increased 20 fold or more during the first stage of labor. Also in the newborn infant the catecholamine levels are very high continuing to rise immediately after birth then decreasing to the prelabor levels during the first 24 hours or so (Fig. 1.1). This is vital for the successful postnatal adaptation.

The newly born infant is normally awake and alert. In these few hours, before it falls asleep, it is supersensitive to sensory stimulation. This arousal might be caused by the catecholamine surge at birth. An activation of catecholamines in the brain especially in the locus ceruleus in the brainstem finds place, and the turnover of norepinephrine increases several fold before birth. The high concentration of catecholamines also increases myocardial contractility, increases peripheral vascular resistance, promotes surfactant secretion, reduces production and increases absorption of lung water, mobilizes glucose and free fatty acids as energy substrates, and initiates nonshivering thermogenesis. The increase in circulating catecholamines at birth, therefore, probably is vital for cardiovascular adaptation at birth. Rhythmic lung inflation also increases plasma catecholamine levels as does cooling and umbilical cord clamping.

Sympathetic nervous activity especially of the baroreceptors and chemoreceptors increases during gestation and the influence of the parasympathetic system on the resting heart rate increases with maturation. In fetal life sympathetic tone is high and is important in maintaining fetal arterial blood pressure. The basal sympathetic

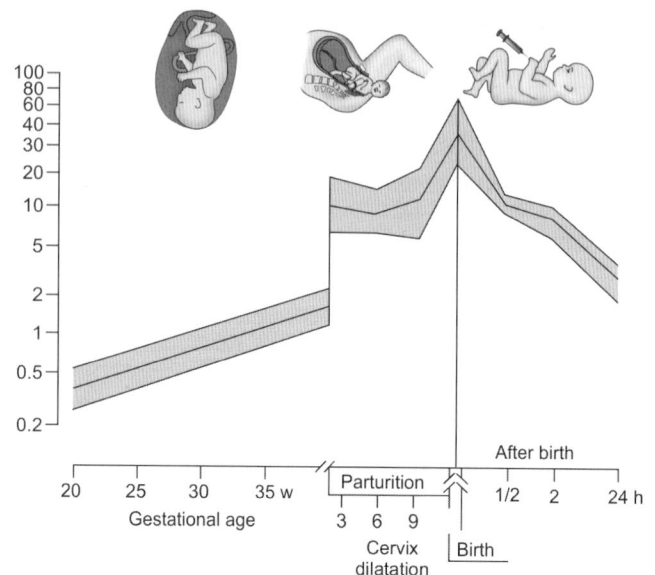

Fig. 1.1: Norepinephrine concentration before, during and after birth
Source: Reference 28

tone fluctuates in the normal state and this is more important in fetal than in newborn life to generate blood pressure variability and is related to change in behavioral state of the fetus. At birth the activity increases further for instance in renal sympathetic nerves 3–4 fold, this is, however, observed only in full term and not preterm animals. This effect is also blunted by antenatal dexamethasone.[28,29]

DEVELOPMENT OF BREATHING

In the fetus spontaneous and rhythmic activity of the diaphragm and respiratory muscles occur already from weeks 10–11 of gestation. The fetal breathing is, by contrast to postnatal breathing, not continuous and with advancing gestational age fetal breathing movements become more sporadic and occur only during electrophysiological activity comparable to rapid eye movement (REM) states. From about 30 weeks of gestation the breathing seems to be more strongly influenced by the behavioral state and a powerful central inhibitory mechanism is functioning during non-REM activity. Near term the human fetus performs breathing movements approximately 25–30% of the time. By contrast to the adult in whom hypoxemia stimulates breathing, in the fetus it causes a rapid depression independently of the physiological state this is also regulated centrally possibly via some metabolites such as adenosine.

The first breath occurs normally at 10–30 seconds of life but is delayed in birth asphyxia and also in those given pure oxygen compared with room air. Immediately after birth breathing is irregular and deep but within minutes a regular breathing rhythm is established, and such a continuous breathing rhythm is activated by a number of stimulants. Separation of the placenta in itself stimulates respiration perhaps by decrease of inhibitory substances such as adenosine and PGE_2 which are produced there. Since, the concentration of, for instance PGI_2 decreases relatively slowly after birth, other factors must be responsible for the rapid initiation of respiration. Oxygenation of the lungs itself seems to stimulate respiration and may contribute to this establishment.

It is clear that respiratory control in the postnatal period is multifactorial. Important are airway mechanoreflexes, thermoregulation, chemoreflexes and behavioral states. The influence of the behavioral states on newborn breathing patterns is important especially since the newborn spends so much time asleep. During wakefulness and REM sleep breathing is irregular; in quiet sleep breathing is slower and more regular.

Immediately after birth thermal inputs play a major role in regulating the respiration. A cool environment stimulates breathing and it has been suggested that the increased metabolic drive this initiates in order to keep the infant in the thermoneutral zone stimulates breathing. After a few weeks the thermoneutral zone widens and this mechanism seems to be less influential. Instead vagal stimuli become more important and stretch receptors in the airways and lung parenchyma and chest wall determine both breathing depth and frequency. Lung inflation inhibits respiration; this phenomenon is known as the Hering-Breuer reflex and is more active in the newborn than in the adult and more active in the term than in the preterm infant. Further, it is more active during quiet sleep than in active sleep (REM sleep). The importance of mechanosensory receptors in the airways in regulating the respiration plays only a minor role immediately after birth and increases in the first week after birth.

The chemoreceptors in the carotid body respond both to pCO_2 and pO_2. In fetal life the set point for pO_2 is much lower than in postnatal life which means they are silenced immediately after birth. The sensitivity of the chemoreceptors both in the carotid body and in the aorta then slowly shifts toward adult levels during the next few days. In fetal life the chemoreceptors are increasing their activity when paO_2 decreases below 2.7–3.3 kPa (20–25 mm Hg). After birth resetting of the chemoreceptors increases their activity if paO_2 decreases below 12–13.3 kPa (90–100 mm Hg). The mechanism for this resetting is not fully understood and it has been suggested that the level of catecholamines such as dopamine in the carotid body may play a role. Four to seven weeks postnatally chemo regulation is established as the most important regulator of the respiration.

Hypercapnia affects the fetal breathing movements in REM-like sleep only; however, much more weakly than after birth when resistance to hypercapnic respiratory stimulation disappears during quiet sleep state. Sensitivity to CO_2 increases with increasing gestational age and is therefore, less developed in the preterm than in the term infant. Hypoxia in the term newborn infant results in hyperventilation for some minutes followed by normalization or reduced ventilation due to a fall in respiratory frequency. This second phase of ventilatory depression is more marked in the preterm infant who often will not go through the initial hyperventilation when exposed to hypoxia and thus has a response to hypoxia similar to the fetus.[30-33]

PERINATAL TRANSITION OF THE LUNGS

The lung development goes through several stages: the embryonic (3–7 weeks postconception), pseudoglandular (5–17 weeks), canalicular (16–26 weeks), saccular (24–38 weeks), alveolar (36 weeks to 2 years postnatally). A detailed description of these is found in several textbooks. Suffice here to mention that in the canalicular stage the appearance of vascular canals multiply to form the alveolar-capillary respiratory membrane which is the air-blood barrier and the future gas exchange surface. The epithelium is thinner and gas exchange may find place at the end of this stage. The saccular stage is characterized by dilatation of terminal respiratory units into alveolar saccules and ducts with a reduction in the interstitial tissue. The alveolar stage is characterized by formation of secondary alveolar septa that partition the terminal ducts and saccules into mature alveoli. The alveolar septa are becoming thinner during this stage which also increases the surface area of the lungs significantly. Most alveoli, 80%, are formed after birth.[31,34]

Inflation

In fetal life the lungs are fluid-filled and a normal fluid volume is a major determinant of normal lung growth. Lung liquid is actively secreted by epithelial cells but the formation and volume decrease toward term. At birth an abrupt stop is needed. It seems that labor itself more than mechanical squeezing of lung fluid clears the lung of its liquid. The secretary process in fetal life is abruptly switched to allow absorption from the lung lumen into the fetal circulation. Two hours after birth the lung liquid normally is cleared. Epinephrine but not norepinephrine, seems to be important to induce Na^+ transport out of the lumen. Epithelial sodium (Natrium) channels (ENaC) are important regulators of lung liquid clearance and parallels the rise of cortisol in late gestation of guinea pigs. Recently, the role of water channels, so-called Aquaporines, for clearing lung water after birth has been focused on (see the section "Fluid Shift"). Transitory tachypnea of the newborn is by many considered as a condition in which an inadequate lung liquid clearance is found due to a low stress at birth (exemplified by C-section). At birth the infant must inflate its lungs to provide a large enough area for gas exchange in the course of a few minutes. The first respiratory effort must be large enough to overcome the great resistance caused by the surface tension of the lung liquid. Pulmonary surfactant lowers the surface tension and therefore, facilitates the expansion of the lung. In the absence of surfactant a positive end expiratory pressure of about 28 cm H_2O to avoid lung collapse and maintain an adequate functional residual capacity is necessary.

Inflation of the lung of a normal infant at birth is probably nearly accomplished with the first cry if it is vigorous. Karlberg and coworkers recorded the first breath in a series of 11 normal term infants to occur at the age of 6–93 seconds. Opening of alveoli occurs serially, each unit going to full inflation before the next one opens. Lung inflation is extremely rapid and after only 1/3rd of a second the lungs look inflated as assessed by chest X-ray. Pleural pressures vary from 10 to 70 cm H_2O subatmospheric during the first breath. Others have registered opening pressures around 30 cm H_2O. This large pressure is applied for only 0.5–1 second and during the first expiration there is a high positive pleural pressure of 20–30 cm H_2O. The pressure difference from inspiration to expiration in one single breath may, therefore, be formidable, up to 100 cm H_2O. Still, most children need an intrathoracic pressure of less than 10 cm H_2O to open their lungs versus 4 cm H_2O in normal breathing. The tidal volumes of the first breath in term infants were found by Karlberg and coworkers to vary between 12–67 mL.

Functional residual capacity increases quickly from about 17 mL/kg at 10 minutes of age to 25–35 mL/kg at 30 minutes, the same as 4 days of age. Lung compliance increases gradually during

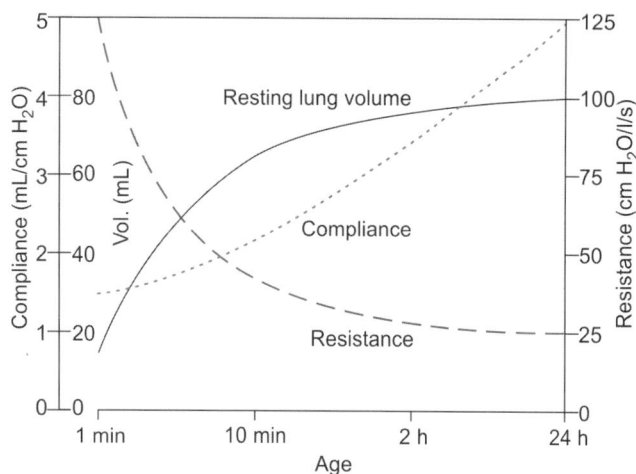

Fig. 1.2: Change in lung mechanics the first 24 hour of life
Source: Reference 36

the first week of life and by 1–2 days of life the compliance is 4–5 fold greater than it was during the first few breaths. Simultaneously, resistance to airflow is decreased by 1/2 to 1/4th of the first registered values (Fig. 1.2).

Following the initial inflation of the lung, the intra-alveolar lung fluid moves into the interstitium and is partially absorbed by the capillaries. Cold, light, noise, increased force of gravity and falling pO_2 and pH all contribute to the initial gasping and subsequent breathing. The intrathoracic pressure an infant can generate is also dependent on the stability of the chest wall and the strength of the respiratory muscles. Following aeration of the lungs the pulmonary vascular resistance decreases and pulmonary blood flow increases, left atrial pressure increases and the foramen ovale closes (see the section "Transition of the Circulation").[35-38]

Gas Exchange

pH in the umbilical vein blood is in mean 7.33 in normal term infants and in arterial umbilical blood reaches a minimum of about 7.20–7.25 a few minutes after birth and then is normally between 7.33 and 7.36 at 20 minutes of age. In some investigations pH already at 1 hour reaches 7.40–7.42. pCO_2 in umbilical vein cord blood has a mean of 5.7 kPa (43 mm Hg) and $paCO_2$ peaks around 8–9.3 kPa (60–70 mm Hg) immediately after birth and then quickly normalizes to around 5.3 kPa (40 mm Hg) or even a little lower than this by 20–60 minutes after birth. paO_2 in umbilical vein cord blood has a mean of 3.7 kPa (28 mm Hg) and quickly rises to 6.7–8 kPa (50–60 mm Hg) within the first 20–60 minutes after birth and then gradually increases toward adult levels over the next days, depending on how quickly the foramen ovale and the ductus arteriosus close.[39]

Surfactant

Pulmonary surfactant is synthesized, stored, secreted, and cleared in the type II cells in the alveoli. There are almost twice as many type II cells than the flat type I cells but they cover only 5–10% of the alveolar surface. In addition to surfactant, they synthesize and secrete many other bioactive components such as coagulation factors, cytokines, growth factors, and lysozyme and lysosomal enzymes. Active synthesis of surfactant begins in the second

trimester and around 35–36 weeks adult pool size is obtained. At term, only a fraction of normal amount of surfactant is present in the alveoli. With lung inflation at birth a dramatic secretion of surfactant occurs and a normal pool of surfactant is established in the alveoli after a few hours.

Maturation of surfactant is delayed by 1–2 weeks in males compared with females and is not only dependent on the amount of surfactant produced but also on the surfactant composition. It has been shown in several mammalian species that considerable changes take place in the composition of surfactant as maturation of the fetus occurs. One of these is the increase of phosphatidylcholine and dipalmitoylphosphatidylcholine with a concomitant decrease in phosphatidylethanolamine. This is reflected by an increasing lecithin/sphingomyelin ratio in amniotic fluid during the maturation process. The percentage of disaturated lecithin increases and reaches about 50% around 34 weeks of gestation. The acidic phospholipids of surfactant follow a different pattern. At around 34–35 weeks phosphatidylglycerol becomes present and increases, simultaneously phosphatidylinositol peaks before it decreases toward term.[40]

Surfactant Proteins

Experiments with several animal species have shown that the production of surfactant proteins in the fetal lung increases toward term. In humans mRNA for surfactant proteins A, B and C were detected as early as 13 weeks of gestation and by 24 weeks their levels were 50% and 15% of adult levels of mRNA for surfactant protein B and C respectively. In contrast, mRNA for surfactant protein A is very low before 24 weeks of gestation. In rat lung surfactant protein A increases substantially during the last 3–4 days of gestation, reaching a peak at the first day of life. In adult lungs its level doubles compared with the neonatal level. In humans surfactant protein A normally appears in amniotic fluid around 30–32 weeks of gestation and increases with surfactant lipids toward term. Surfactant protein B increases more gradually during gestation and continues to do so the first day after birth with a slight decrease in the adult glucocorticoids seem to increase the production of surfactant proteins A, B, C, and D. The hydrophilic surfactant proteins A and D are important for host defense and the hydrophobic proteins B and C for stabilization and rapid adsorption and spreading of the surfactant film. Surfactant protein B deficiency is a rare autosomal recessive disorder leading to lethal respiratory distress even in term infants. Recently, mutations in the transport of surfactant protein B from the lamellar bodies in type 2 cells to the surface have been detected giving a similar clinical picture as surfactant protein B deficiency. Surfactant protein C deficiency is an autosomal recessive disease and clinically not as dramatic as surfactant protein B deficiency but may lead to interstitial inflammation and pulmonary fibrosis.[41-43]

TRANSITION OF THE CIRCULATION
Vascular Changes

In fetal life the pulmonary and systemic vascular systems are coupled in parallel by contrast to the postnatal period when the blood circulation is coupled in series through the right side of the heart to the lungs and then through the left side of the heart to the systemic circulation to return to the right side of the heart through the systemic and the pulmonary vasculature (Fig. 1.3). The fetal

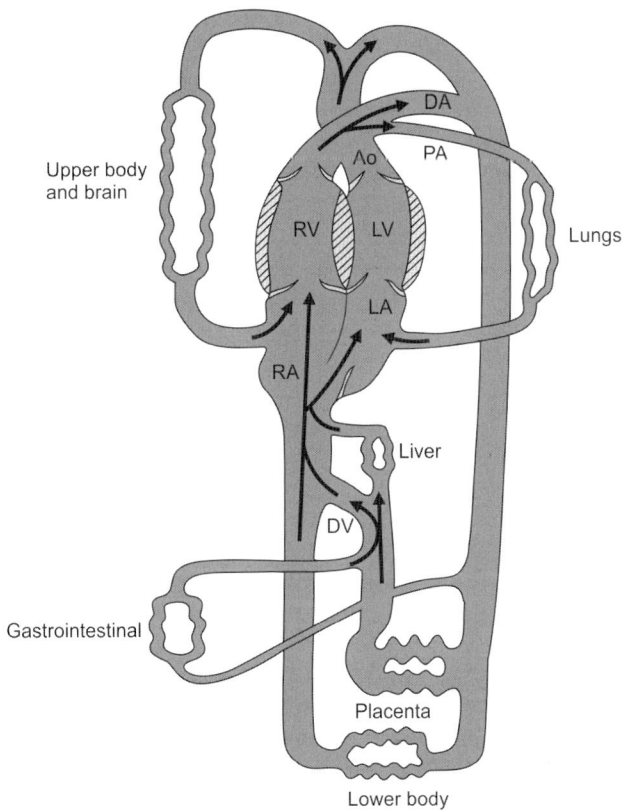

Fig. 1.3: The fetal circulation

Abbreviations: DA: ductus arteriosus, DV: ductus venosus, LA: left atrium, LV: left ventricle, PA: pulmonary artery, RA: right atrium, RV: right ventricle.
Source: Reference 44

circulation is characterized by a low systemic and a high pulmonary vascular resistance, the opposite situation of postnatal life. The fetal circulation is designed to provide a large blood flow to the placenta and supply less to the lungs since the fetal lung has no gas exchange until birth. Due to the large surface of the placenta the fetal circulation has a low resistance, and the blood pressure, therefore, needs not to be high. The fetal circulation is further characterized by the presence of three shunts which facilitate venous return from the placenta. These are the ductus venosus and the two right to left shunts reducing blood flow through the lungs (foramen ovale and ductus arteriosus). Through the foramen ovale (the opening between the right and left atrium), and the ductus arteriosus (the connection between the pulmonary trunk and the aorta), blood is bypassed away from lung tissue into the systemic circulation. The three shunts mentioned above, therefore, contribute to a separation between blood rich in oxygen and nutrients supplied from the placenta via the umbilical vein; this blood supplies the brain and myocardium.

During fetal life, blood is oxygenated in the placenta and returns to the fetal body via the umbilical vein, which joins the portal vein in the hepatic sinus. About 40% of the combined ventricular output goes through the placenta. This volume of blood, approximately 200 mL/kg fetal weight per minute, can be distributed through the ductus venosus directly into the inferior cava vein bypassing the hepatic microcirculation, or it can pass via the portal veins through the hepatic circulation and then enter the inferior caval vein through the hepatic veins. In the fetal sheep about 70% of the venous return is derived from the lower portion of the body, and 20% from the superior vena cava. Of the remaining 10% approximately 7% comes from the pulmonary circulation—a fraction increasing toward term and 3% from the myocardium. About 55% of the umbilical venous return passes through the ductus venosus and the rest mainly through to the right lobe of the liver.

The fetal liver is a highly compliant organ able to regulate the distribution of umbilical blood flow during fetal stress. Umbilical blood flow does not change significantly from normal values when fetal hypoxemia is induced by maternal hypoxia; however, the intrahepatic circulation is redistributed so that flow through the ductus venosus is increased. This increased flow is distributed to favor the brain, myocardium and placenta in order to secure more oxygenated blood to these vital organs during hypoxemia. After traversal through the ductus venosus and entry into the inferior caval vein oxygenated blood from the placenta does not mix with deoxygenated blood from the lower body. This blood when entering the inferior caval vein streams in parallel with blood from the lower body. When entering the right atrium the blood from placenta and the blood from the lower body are split by *Crista Dividens* and blood originating from the ductus venosus preferentially crosses the foramen ovale into the left side of the heart and therefore, the myocardium and the head are supplied with oxygen enriched blood. Blood from the lower body and right liver lobe preferentially passes through the tricuspid valve into the right ventricle together with blood from the superior vena cava. Thus blood with lower oxygen content is pumped out of the right ventricle and reaches the lower parts of the body.

Doppler studies in humans have demonstrated that the ductus venosus is a narrow vessel projecting a high-velocity jet posteriorly to reach the foramen ovale. The high peak velocity in the ductus venosus may give the blood sufficient momentum to reach the foramen ovale without extensive mixing with deoxygenated and nutrient poor blood. Blood streaming, therefore, not only occurs in parallel, but also side by side at different velocities when entering the right atrium.

Umbilical venous blood has a pO_2 of 4–4.7 kPa (30–35 mm Hg). After mixing with portal venous and inferior caval blood, the pO_2 is about 3.5 –3.7 kPa (26–28 mm Hg). Venous blood returning from the superior cava vein has a pO_2 of 1.6 –1.9 kPa (12–14 mm Hg) and this combines with the inferior caval vein stream passing through the tricuspid valve giving a pO_2 in the right ventricle of 2.4–2.5 kPa (18–19 mm Hg). The pO_2 of the blood entering the left ventricle and the ascending aorta is about 3.1–3.3 kPa (23–25 mm Hg), slightly less than in the proximal part of inferior caval vein due to mixing with blood from the pulmonary veins in the left atrium. The descending aortic blood which is a mixture of blood passing through the ductus arteriosus and the aortic isthmus has a pO_2 of 2.7–2.9 kPa (20–22 mm Hg). Postnatally, there is essentially no mixing of blood oxygenated in the lungs and systemic venous blood.

Fetal pulmonary vascular resistance falls with advancing gestational age primarily due to the great increase in the number of pulmonary vessels, expanding the total cross sectional area of the vascular bed. Pulmonary blood flow and pulmonary artery pressure increase substantially in the fetal sheep from mid-gestation toward term.[44-49]

Establishment of the Postnatal Lung

The most dramatic changes in the circulation occur at birth when gas exchange through the lungs is established. Immediately after birth the umbilical placental blood flow is stopped and the pulmonary circulation is established adequately. Neither in the placenta nor the umbilical cord vessels adrenergic or cholinergic nerve fibers is detected. So the regulation of cord flow is probably mainly due to vasoactive factors. Within a minute after birth umbilical blood flow is less than 1/5th of the fetal level. Simultaneously a significant decrease in umbilical artery and vein diameters are observed within another minute. The mechanisms behind this are not fully understood but both cooling, increased oxygen tension and stretching of the cord may play a role. Locally produced mediators such as serotonin are powerful constrictors of umbilical vessels. The umbilical vessels also constrict by mechanical stimulation, particularly stretching, and the constriction is upheld by the immediate increase in systemic oxygen tension. Simultaneously, venous return through the inferior cava vein is reduced by removal of the placental circulation. Cessation of venous return reduces flow through the ductus venosus and this vessel, therefore, closes passively within 3–7 days after birth.

After birth ventilation of the lungs with air results in a fourfold to tenfold increase in pulmonary blood flow which is associated with a relatively rapid fall in pulmonary vascular resistance (Fig. 1.4). These effects are mediated both by mechanical lung changes, lowering of pCO_2 and increase in pO_2, each factor accounting for the pulmonary vasodilator effects seen after birth.

In addition to the structural adaptation of the pulmonary circulation after birth there are a number of vasoactive substances participating in the regulation of the pulmonary vascular tone in the perinatal period. The pulmonary vascular endothelium is central in the regulation of vascular tone. By stimulation the endothelial cells may release vasoactive substances into the circulation, or release

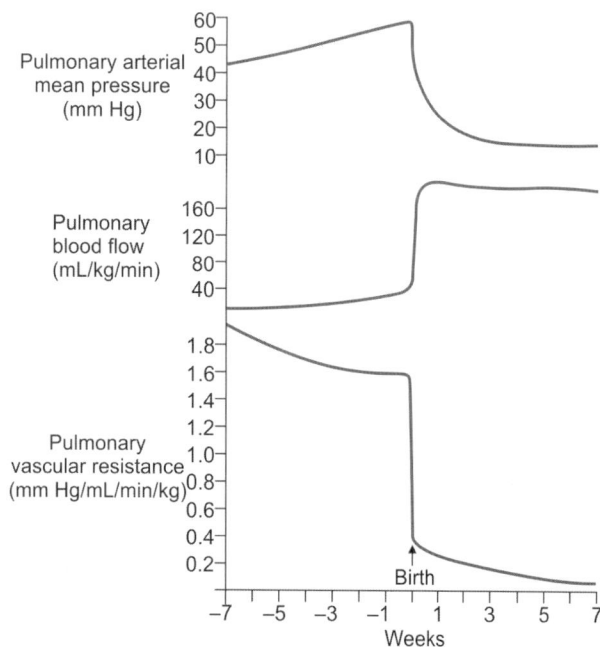

Fig. 1.4: Changes in fetal pulmonary arterial pressure, pulmonary blood flow, and vascular resistance in the perinatal period

Source: Reference 46

lung tissue enzymes involved in the activation or inactivation of vasoactive mediators.

In recent years endothelium derived relaxing factors such as nitric oxide (NO) have been identified and together with PGI_2 may be responsible for the rapid decrease in pulmonary vascular resistance that occurs at the onset of normal ventilation after birth. In fetal circulation there is an increased production of NO compared with adult levels is found. This NO contributes to the low vascular resistance and increased flow for instance in the gastrointestinal tract. Increased fetal oxygen tension increases release of NO. The increase in pulmonary blood flow in response to the high oxygen concentration at birth as well as distention of the lung seems to be mediated, at least partly by NO. This system seems to be especially potent near term; the reaction of the preterm is diminished. Endogenous NO production is augmented due to induction of especially endothelial nitric oxide synthase (e NOS). In the baboon both inducible and e NOS activities increase during gestation falling toward term. However, the total NOS activity seems to be preserved. Both hypoxemia and diaphragmatic hernia decrease NOS expression. A lack of neuronal NO synthetase has been found in neonatal hypertrophic pyloric stenosis. Arachidonic acid metabolites are involved in the physiological regulation of the perinatal circulation. PGI_2 is a strong pulmonary vasodilatator. Mechanical stimulation of the lungs leads to PGI_2 production and ventilation of the fetal lung itself increases concentration of PGI_2 in pulmonary venous blood. The release of this metabolite is also stimulated by histamine, bradykinin, reactive oxygen species (ROS), and adenosine triphosphate (ATP), as well as angiotensin II which is high immediately after birth.

Bradykinin is a potent vasoconstrictor in the umbilicoplacental circulation but otherwise is usually a vasodilator. Bradykinin is released in fetal lungs during ventilation with air or during hyperbaric oxygenation. It is, therefore, possible that bradykinin could play a role in postnatal pulmonary circulatory changes. Endothelium dependent vasoconstriction can also be stimulated by substances and factors such as acetylcholine, thrombin, serotonin, physical forces and hypoxia. There are also endothelium derived vascular constricting factors such as metabolites of arachidonic acid (Thromboxane A_2 and PGH_2) as well as endothelin and free radicals. In animal studies it has been shown that ROS are able to potently constrict the pulmonary vasculature and to dilate the ductus arteriosus. It has been shown both in the lungs and in the isolated ductus arteriosus that ROS stimulate the production of prostaglandins. In the lungs there seems to be a balance between dilating and constricting prostaglandins. The constrictor tromboxane A_2 (TXA_2) is elevated first followed by the dilator PGI_2 when the pulmonary circulation is exposed to free oxygen radical generating systems. These substances, therefore, can have both constrictory and dilatory effects on the pulmonary circulation dependent on the balance between TXA_2 and PGI_2. Superoxide radicals for instance can act by inactivating NO and also by activation of endothelial cyclooxygenase products. In addition, endothelin and angiotensin II have a prolonged effect on tone and structure of blood vessels.

Remodeling of the pulmonary vasculature occurs immediately after birth contributing to the decrease in pulmonary vascular resistance. In the precapillary arteries the endothelial cells shortly after birth become slimmer, the surface/volume ratio increases so the vessel wall becomes thinner, and the lumen diameter increases. Further, small unopened muscular arteries are recruited to the pulmonary circulation during the first day after birth. Thus, a structural adaptation to extrauterine life consists of changes in cell shape and position. The structural remodeling during the first 2 weeks of life in the pig lungs contributes to the reduction in mean pulmonary artery pressure from 55 to 14 mm Hg.

The baroreflex setting of heart rate mediated by baroreceptor fibers in the carotic body and aortic arch is active in both fetal and newborn life, however, with different sensitivity and shifts toward higher pressures during development.[46,50,51]

Ductus Arteriosus

The open ductus arteriosus in fetal life diverts blood away from the lungs toward the descending aorta. The patent ductus is regulated both by dilating and contracting factors. Prostaglandins play an important role in maintaining the patency and the ductus is especially sensitive to the dilating action of PGE_2. Oxygen is a potent constrictor of the ductus and becomes more effective the more mature the fetus is. This is due to the fact that in early fetal life the ductus has decreased muscular development causing less contractile ability. In fetal lambs the ductus arteriosus is also more sensitive to the dilating effect of PGE_2 in the preterm than near term. This is due to a developmental alteration in sensitivity of the vessels to prostaglandins. It is circulating PGE_2 probably produced in the placenta, which probably controls the ductus arteriosus in utero. After birth when the oxygen tension increases the ductal wall is itself capable to produce PGE_2. Reactive oxygen metabolites (ROS) may stimulate PGE_2 synthesis in the isolated ductal wall from fetal lambs. In the ductus arteriosus ROS can, therefore, contribute to dilatation by turning on prostaglandin synthesis in the ductal wall. The functional closure of the ductus, therefore, is promoted by increase in oxygen tension and a p450 hemoprotein located in the smooth muscle plasma membrane is a receptor of the oxygen induced events. Further, a decrease in blood pressure within the ductus itself, a decrease in circulating PGE_2 (due to loss of placental prostaglandin synthesis and increase in prostaglandin removal by the lungs), and finally a decrease in PGE_2 receptors in the ductus wall also contribute to constriction of the ductus. In full-term infants closure of the ductus arteriosus occurs in two phases with a functional closure within the first hour after birth due to smooth muscle constriction, and the anatomic closure due to closure of the lumen due to thickening of the intima and loss of smooth muscle cells. This is caused by progressive thickening of the intima so it eventually occludes the constricted lumen. Smooth muscles migrate from media into the intima layer. Vascular endothelial growth factor (VEGF) plays an important role in this intimal "cushion".[52-54]

Myocardium

At the end of gestation right and left ventricular systolic pressures are equal, 65–70 mm Hg. The cardiac output of the right ventricle is, however, in fetal life 50% higher than the left ventricle mainly due to the fact that the left ventricle has a high afterload caused by the high vascular resistance of the head, neck and forelimbs, while the right ventricles afterload is lower because of the low umbilical-placental resistance. The removal of the low resistance placental circulation results in an increase in systemic vascular resistance. The combined ventricular output in the fetal lamb is about 500 mL/kg/min; however, after birth there is an increase in total cardiac output and during the first day each ventricle ejects approximately

350 mL/kg/min. During the next weeks in the newborn lamb, there is a rapid decrease in cardiac output to a level of about 150 mL/kg/min and then it falls slowly to the adult level of 70–80 mL/kg/min. Cardiac output changes parallels changes in oxygen consumption.

O_2 consumption is almost identical in the adult and fetal hearts; however, the fuel used by them are different since the adult heart uses fatty acids and the fetal heart is an obligatory user of carbohydrates as substrate for oxidative phosphorylation. In the fetal lamb 60% of these carbohydrates are lactate, 35% glucose and 5% pyruvate. This can explain why a fall in circulating glucose concentrations result in myocardial depression in fetal and neonatal life but not later in life. In fact, it has been shown that fatty acids are detrimental to fetal cardiac function. In order to use fatty acids as fuel they must be transformed to Ac-CoA which is transesterified with carnitine and in this form transported across the mitochondrial membrane by the transport enzyme carnitine-palmitoyltransferase (CPT). CPT is inhibited by malonyl-CoA which is high in fetal life. Malonyl-CoA is regulated by glucagon and during the delivery glucagon concentration increases sharply thereby reducing the concentration of malonyl-CoA and releasing CPT inhibition allowing fatty acid oxidation to proceed.

The contractile properties of the myocyte also differ in fetal and adult life. Only about 30% of fetal cardiac muscle consists of contractile elements compared with approximately 60% in the adult. The velocity of shortening of the myocyte is also lower in fetal life. Especially preterm infants and to some degree also the term infants have, therefore, a much reduced ability to tolerate an increase in afterload. The change from fetal to adult performance seems, however, to occur quickly after birth.

At birth, cardiac output increases considerably and left ventricular level is doubled compared with fetal levels. This higher left ventricular inotropy and performance is due to sympathethicoadrenal stimulation after birth and triiodothyronine seems to be important in maturation of the fetal myocardial response. After birth myocardial contractility is greatly increased but because of the high demands on the circulation to provide the increased oxygen requirements for metabolism, there is also little reserve available, and thus volume loading results in only a small rise in cardiac output. In a fetus an increase in heart rate gives a fall in end diastolic volume and stroke volume unless ventricular diastolic filling is maintained. The rearrangement of the circulation after birth leads to an increased end diastolic left ventricular volume which leads to an increased stroke volume. The days after birth, a gradual decrease in cardiac output/kg is observed returning to the fetal levels.

Fetuses at mid gestation have individualized heart rates that are stable. The control of heart rate variability seems to develop later and fetal heart rate variability is predictive of neonatal heart rate variability not until 30 weeks. With increasing gestation there is a reduced fetal heart rate variability and this demonstrates development of the autonomic nerve system during the gestation. Heart rate at birth is around 160–180 beats per minute and decreases to 120 beats per minute in sleeping newborn infants and to 140–160 beats per minute in awake newborn infants. The postnatal situation compared with the fetal is characterized by decrease in heart rate, postextrasystolic potentiation increases, and inotropic responses to catecholamine elevation suggesting that the postnatal heart has a greater potential reserves than in fetal life.[45,46,49]

SHIFT IN OXYGEN TRANSPORT

The newborn infant has a higher oxygen demand than the fetus and the oxygen consumption typically is increased between twofold and threefold the first day of life. O_2 consumption per kg body weight is higher in the newborn than in the adult and the fetus. In adult life, it is about half that in the immediate newborn period; however, when compared with body surface area this age difference seems to disappear. The delivery of oxygen to the tissues depends on (1) the oxygen content of the blood, (2) the cardiac output, (3) the distribution of the circulation and (4) the affinity of oxygen to hemoglobin. In fetal blood there is a high affinity to oxygen. The postnatal decrease in hemoglobin O_2 affinity is caused by an increase in adult hemoglobin at the expense of fetal hemoglobin, and an increase from birth in the concentration of 2,3-diphosphoglycerate (DPG). During gestation until 34 weeks, fetal hemoglobin comprises about 90% of the total hemoglobin falling to 80% at term and from birth to 8 months of age there is a gradual decline in fetal hemoglobin to less than 2%. Fetal red cells have a higher oxygen affinity than adult ones which is achieved by a reduced interaction between fetal hemoglobin with 2,3-DPG than in adult hemoglobin. The concentration of 2,3-DPG in fetal and adult cells is almost the same. 2,3-DPG present in the erythrocytes decreases the affinity to O_2 through an allosteric action with the hemoglobin molecule. DPG does not bind as strongly to fetal hemoglobin as the adult hemoglobin, in addition it is low immediately after birth making a high O_2 affinity immediately after birth with a p50 of approximately 2.7 kPa (20 mm Hg) versus 4 kPa (30 mm Hg) at 8 months of age. Therefore, in the newborn period and early infancy when the fetal hemoglobin concentration is high, intraerythrocyte change in 2,3-DPG has little effect on p50, however, later in life the modulating effect of 2,3-DPG on oxygen affinity plays a more important role. In the fetal period the high oxygen carrying capacity and greater oxygen affinity of fetal blood in fact compensate for the 1/5th to 1/4th oxygen tension of adult blood ending up with a rather similar oxygen saturation at term and in adult life. Fetal blood also is slightly hypercarbic and acidotic whereas the maternal blood is hypocarbic and alkalotic. The Bohr effect, that is the shift in the oxygen equilibrium curve to the right by increased pCO_2 or decreased pH, giving a higher oxygen tension, is more pronounced with a lower pH and more efficient in the fetus. In addition, a higher temperature of the fetus contributes to a shift in the fetal dissociation curve to the right.[55-57]

TISSUE INJURY

Energy Metabolism

Most of the oxygen taken into the body is used in cell energy metabolism. The metabolic process is a redox process where energy is released in a stepwise fashion and stored as ATP. Energy metabolism can schematically be divided into three parts. In step 1 glucose, amino acids and fatty acids are broken down to acetyl coenzyme A (Ac-CoA). In the second step Ac-CoA enters the tricarboxylic acid (Krebs) cycle, a final common pathway of all fuel substrates in aerobic cells. Here acetyl groups are metabolized to form carbon dioxide and hydrogen ions. In step 3, the hydrogen ions enter the respiratory chain of the cell, a series of electron carriers linked to oxidative phosphorylation, with ATP formed in a stepwise

manner. Oxygen is the final electron acceptor and is necessary for a continuous oxidation of reduced coenzymes in the respiratory chain. Oxygen, therefore, can be considered as the "garbage cleaner" of energy metabolism taking care of its waste products, the electrons after having traversed through the respiratory chain.

The energy metabolism tends to keep the energy charge, EC $\{EC = 0.5 [(ATP) + (ADP) / (ATP) + (ADP) + (AMP)]\}$ of the cell at an optimal level which is around 0.85. This can be achieved in two ways; either by increasing the ATP concentration or to increase the catabolism of AMP. In hypoxia with lack of energy the cell might be forced to choose the latter alternative. An accelerated breakdown of adenosine monophosphate (AMP) occurs. This is a hazardous compensation since the cells might loose its purine pool irreversibly. One of the intermediate breakdown products is, however, adenosine. This metabolite has important control feedback functions in brain hypoxia, partly because it is an active vasodilatator and thus contributes to a higher oxygen supply to hypoxic tissues and partly because adenosine in itself cuts down brain metabolism. When adenosine accumulates because of energy deficiency, this metabolite fights back by contributing to an increased oxygen supply and a decreased energy need. This is important also because a breakdown product from adenosine is hypoxanthine. This metabolite accumulates in tissues and body fluids during hypoxia and its extracellular concentration reflects the intracellular energy charge. However, hypoxanthine is also a potential oxygen radical generator during reoxygenation and it is, therefore, probably advantageous for the organism to try to keep the hypoxanthine concentration as low as possible.

Before the cell's energy charge falls markedly, several biochemical compensatory mechanisms are activated. First, glycolysis is accelerated many fold. Pyruvate is reduced to lactate, while nicotinamide adenine nucleotide (NADH) is oxidized to NAD^+. This is the basis for the use of lactate as a clinical marker of hypoxia. Lactate augmentation merely reflects the compensation mechanism. Although hypoxanthine and lactate parallels each other in many clinical settings, hypoxanthine nevertheless more correctly reflects the intracellular energy status of the cells.

As soon as oxygen delivery to the cells decline the mitochondria also change their metabolism to utilize available oxygen more efficiently. The compensation takes place 30–60 minutes after a reduction in oxygen supply. In the fetus or in the immediate newborn period mitochondrial adaptation already is maximal. A fetus has a respiratory capacity of about 300% of the adult, but by 10–14 days after birth the newborn and adult levels equate in this respect. What does this mean for the fetus and newborn? First, they are able to utilize the limited oxygen supply very efficiently. On the other hand, the fetus is unable to make cellular respiratory adaptations if hypoxia occurs. From this point of view, the fetus and newborn are more vulnerable to hypoxia than older patients.

Hypoxic Injury to the Perinatal Brain

It has been known since Boyle's classical experiment in 1670 that newborn animals can resist hypoxia longer than adult ones. In the 1960s and 1970s, it was shown that the preterm monkey can withstand hypoxia longer than the term one. In fact, in the fetal monkey there was an exponential relation between duration of hypoxia and gestational age when the outcome measure was neurologic brain injury (cerebral palsy). The younger the animal the longer it could resist hypoxia before brain injury occured. Thus, mature fetal rats survive in pure nitrogen more than 25 times longer and 1 day old rats about 10 times longer than adult rats. One part of the explanation for this seems to be that newborn animals can preserve cerebral circulation and thus ensure supply of substrates for energy metabolism better than in the adult. Further, it is known that oxygen demand of the brain is lower in fetal life and inceases with gestation. The immature brain has smaller neurons which are less branched with fewer synapses. The energy requirement is, therefore, lower and the cerebral metabolic rate of oxygen is lower in the immature brain compared with the adult. The fetal brain is also able to use alternative sources such as ketone bodies as fuel for energy metabolism. Further, the glycolytic capacity allows the immature brain to regenerate ATP at a higher rate than in the adult brain.

The perinatal period is also accompanied by dramatic neurochemical changes. The concentration of excitatory aminoacids such as glutamate peaks around term and may contribute to a higher sensitivity to hypoxia in the term compared with the preterm infant.[58,59]

Apoptosis and Necrosis

Apoptosis is an important part of development and homeostasis. For instance in the developing brain perhaps up to half of the cells undergo apoptosis, in spite of the fact that the distinction between apoptotic and necrotic death is considered less clear than previously. These two modes of cell death are by many considered as a continuum running from apoptosis to necrosis more than two different entities. Infants who have undergone secondary energy failure after for instance birth asphyxia have a tendency to loose their neurons by necrosis, while those dying in utero have experienced more apoptotic death. The same injury may induce apoptosis in the fetus or newborn and necrosis in the adult organism. To make it more complex the same cell may undergo apoptosis if the injury is mild and necrosis if it is severe. Oxidative stress plays an important role for initiating apoptosis for instance through opening up the mitochondrial permeability transition pore. This reduces the mitochondrial membrane potential and release of substances that are involved in apoptosis for instance cytochrome C and Apaf-1, both of these activate caspase-3 that is specifically involved in the apoptotic execution. As mentioned already the fetus is more susceptible to oxidative stress than the term newborn and therefore also perhaps more susceptible to this mechanism.[60]

Development of Antioxidants

In fetal life paO_2 is around 3.3 kPa (25 mm Hg) and after birth rises quickly to 8 kPa (60 mm Hg) over the next 30 minutes. In order to survive in an oxygen rich atmosphere antioxidant systems must be well developed at birth. A number of defense systems have been described. In the lung and kidney a maturation of anti-oxyenzymes as superoxide dismutases, glutathione peroxidase and catalase seem to occur near term in animal fetuses. In fact the maturation of these systems occurs in parallel with the maturation of the surfactant system. Furthermore, preterm infants with gestational age of 24–29 weeks have only 50% activity of Cu/Zn superoxide dismutase in cord erythrocytes compared with term infants. Glutathione is a major intracellular antioxidant and is found in high concentrations (millimolar) in eukaryotic cells. Glutathione is the substrate for glutathione peroxidase which catalyses oxidation of reduced to oxidized glutathione at the expense of hydrogen peroxide. The rate of glutathione synthesis from methionine is strongly reduced in preterm infants compared with term ones. These data, therefore, suggest that at least the intracellular defense against free radicals is low in many organs in fetal life and probably also in the human fetus. A preterm infant is, therefore, more vulnerable to increased oxidative stress and attacks of free radicals than a term one. By contrast to the intracellular defense, extracellular antioxidants seem to be adequately developed at term, and the concentration of several extracellular antioxidants as ascorbate is very high in umbilical cord (see Chapter 7).[61-64]

THERMAL REGULATION

In fetal life the body temperature is efficiently regulated to be 0.5°C higher than the maternal. The tight linkage between fetal and maternal body temperature is called a "heat clamp" that prevents the fetus from independent regulation of its temperature. At birth a dramatic change in the thermal environment occurs. During the first hour of life core body temperature can fall to less than 36°C if the newborn is not taken care of optimally. After 8 hours body temperature has usually returned to the normal adult range. Since the newborn infant has a relatively large body surface area and limited thermal insulation it is necessary to wrap the newborn infant adequately. The newborn infant in fact has the capability to regulate the temperature by sweating and can also respond to a cool environment by increasing metabolic rate. This takes place without shivering, is activated by catecholamines, and the heat is generated mainly from brown fat which is present in large amounts in the full term infant. Although the fetus may mobilize brown fat the thermogenic responses still are very low. These require increased oxygen and substrate consumption. The combination of hypoxia and hypothermia, therefore, is dangerous.[25,65]

SKIN

The transition from intrauterine to extrauterine life is dramatic for the skin, perhaps the largest organ of the body. It immediately must be a barrier to water loss, it takes part in thermoregulation, is protecting against infections, has an antioxidant function, and protects against UV light. The skin is a barrier to chemicals and is needed for tactile discrimination as well as being an important emotional and psychological link between the child and its caregivers. The skin of the term by contrast to the preterm infant also has a highly developed immunological system. In utero the skin is in a sterile environment but already in the birth canal, it is colonized and specific cells in the epidermal layer take part in host defense.

Prenatally, lipid synthesis is necessary for production of vernix caseosa forming a barrier which is needed for a successful adaptation to postnatal life. The vernix also may function as an endogenous skin cleanser removing for instance carbon particles. Of interest is that both the stratum corneum of epidermis and the brain contain very high concentrations of ceramides. The close embryological relation between these two organs both derived ectodermally makes this an interesting observation. At birth the epidermis is pH neutral but rapidly over the first postnatal week, develops an "acid mantle" which is characteristic of human skin. This acidic surface can be destroyed by using alkaline soaps for infant bathing and is delayed in very low birth weight infants. The acid mantle is believed to be important in antimicrobial defense as well as keeping the integrity of the epidermal barrier. Postnatally transepidermal water loss that increases after birth is an important regulator of DNA and lipid synthesis in the epidermis.[66]

CIRCADIAN RHYTHMS

The clock for the circadian rhythms is set by the suprachiasmatic nucleus. It is fascinating that the neurons in this area of the brain in vitro oscillate with a period close to 24 hours. This is regulated by light which in a complex way affects gene expression of transcription factors. Efferent pathways from the suprachiasmatic nerve control the pineal function, and regulate the rhythms of endocrine, cardiovascular, temperature and even behavioral circadian variations.

From mid-gestation the suprachiasmatic nucleus is present in the fetus and diurnal rhythms are found in the human fetus after 20 weeks. Whether or not they are intrinsically regulated or due to maternal control for instance via maternal melatonin rhythms is unclear. However, in fetal life the maternal rhythms are mainly followed by the rhythm of the mother exemplified by cortisol fluctuations. By contrast, fetal autonomic activity that controls the heart rate follows a 12-hour cycle and not the mother's 24 hour rhythm. This 12-hour rhythm disappears immediately after birth and around 2–4 weeks the 24-hour rhythm is established. It takes 8–12 weeks before postnatal circadian rhythms in sleep and wakefulness as well as plasma cortisol and melatonin are established.[25,67]

GENE ACTIVATION AT BIRTH

In the near future the transition at birth will be described by shift in different gene activity and not only by physiological and biochemical changes. Labor affects the mRNA encoding for a number of enzymes such as tyrosine hydroxylase, dopamine-beta-hydroxylase. mRNA encoding for substance P increases many folds in the nucleus tractus solitarius the first day of life. Substance P probably plays a role for the central respiratory control by promoting the hypoxic drive from peripheral chemoreceptors. Depression of genes is also described at birth and in some circumstances there is a shift from one isoform to the other. One example is the expression of genes that encode the muscle-specific and nonmuscle-specific isoforms of cytochrom oxidase subunit VIa during prenatal and postnatal life of striated muscle in the mouse. The nonmuscle form is the predominant isoform in fetal life and is gradually at the end of gestation and early neonatal life replaced by the muscle-specific isoform both in cardiac and skeletal muscle.[68]

CONCLUSION

In order to understand both normal development as well as disease processes in the newborn infant it is necessary to have insight into the complex changes which occur in relation to birth. Previously the physiological processes have been emphasized giving us valuable knowledge in the perinatal transition of the cardiovascular and pulmonary systems. Recently, biochemical changes in relation to birth have been understood more in full as for instance the maturation of the surfactant system and antioxidative systems. Presently more and more data will accumulate, teaching us how the transition at birth is regulated at the gene level. In this way, it could hopefully be possible to modulate the disease processes in relation to the birth processes in a much more efficient and powerful way than we understand today.

REFERENCES

1. Ambler GR, Gluckman PD. Postnatal growth. In: Gluckman PD, Heymann MA (Eds). Perinatal and Pediatric Pathophysiology. London: Edward Arnold; 1993. pp. 170-90.
2. Girard J, Ferre P. Metabolic and hormonal changes around birth. In: Jones CT (Ed). Biochemical Development of the Fetus and Neonate. Amsterdam: Elsevier Biomedical Press; 1982. pp. 517-51.
3. Gospodarowicz D. The role of growth factors in organ growth and differentiation. In: Jones CT (Ed). The Biochemical Development of the Fetus and Neonate. Amsterdam: Elsevier Biomedical Press; 1982. pp. 101-25.
4. Milner RDG. Prenatal growth control. In: Gluckman PD, Heymann MA (Eds). Perinatal and Pediatric Pathophysiology. London: Edward Arnold; 1993. pp. 162-9.
5. Parkes MJ. The transition between growth-homone independent and growth-hormone dependent growth. In: Jones CT, Nathanielsz PW (Eds). The Physiological Development of the Fetus and the Newborn. London: Academic Press; 1985. pp. 55-8.
6. Styne DM. Endocrine factors affecting neonatal growth. In: Polin RA, Fox WW, Abman SH (Eds). Fetal and Neonatal Physiology, 3rd edition. Philadelphia: Saunders; 2004. pp. 266-75.
7. Friis-Hansen B. Water and electrolyte balance before and after birth. In: Rooth G, Saugstad OD (Eds). The Roots of Perinatal Medicine. New York: Thieme-Stratton Inc; 1985. pp. 39-47.
8. Brace RA. Fluid distribution in the fetus and neonate. In: Polin RA, Fox WW, Abman SH (Eds). Fetal and Neonatal Physiology, 3rd edition. Philadelphia: Saunders; 2004. pp. 1341-50.
9. Khalan SC. Metabolism of glucose and methods of investigation in the fetus and newborn. In: Polin RA, Fox WW, Abman SH (Eds). Fetal and Neonatal Physiology, 3rd edition. Philadelphia: Saunders; 2004. pp. 449-64.
10. Milner RDG. Fat and carbohydrate metabolism. In: Gluckman PD, Heymann MA (Eds). Perinatal and Pediatric Pathophysiology. London: Edward Arnold; 1993. pp. 84-102.
11. Philips AF. Oxygen consumption and general carbohydrate metabolism of the fetus. In: Polin RA, Fox WW, Abman SH (Eds). Fetal and Neonatal Physiology, 3rd edition. Philadelphia: Saunders; 2004. pp. 465-78.
12. Simmons RA. Cell glucose transport and glucose handling during fetal and neonatal development. In: Polin RA, Fox WW, Abman SH (Eds). Fetal and Neonatal Physiology, 3rd edition. Philadelphia: Saunders; 2004. pp. 487-93.
13. Sunehag A, Ewald U, Gustafsson J. Extremely preterm infants (< 28 weeks) are capable of gluconeogenesis from glycerol on their first day of life. Pediatr Res. 1996;40:553-7.

14. Hay WW, Regnault TRH. Fetal requirements and placental transfer of nitrogenous compounds. In: Polin RA, Fox WW, Abman SH (Eds). Fetal and Neonatal Physiology, 3rd edition. Philadelphia: Saunders; 2004. pp. 509-27.
15. Milner RDG. Protein and amino acid metabolism. In: Gluckman PD, Heymann MA (Eds). Perinatal and Pediatric Pathophysiology. London: Edward Arnold; 1993. pp. 71-8.
16. Herrera E, Lascuncion MA. Maternal-fetal transfer of lipid metabolites. In: Polin RA, Fox WW, Abman SH (Eds). Fetal and Neonatal Physiology, 3rd edition. Philadelphia: Saunders; 2004. pp. 375-88.
17. Van Arde JE, Wilke S, Feldman M, et al. Accretion of lipid in fetus and newborn. In: Polin RA, Fox WW, Abman SH (Eds). Fetal and Neonatal Physiology, 3rd edition. Philadelphia: Saunders; 2004. pp. 388-404.
18. Persson B. Lipid metabolism. Acta Obst Gynecol Scand. 1969;48(Suppl 3):92-6.
19. Helland IB, Smith L, Saarem K, et al. Maternal supplementation with very-long-chain n-3 fatty acids during pregnancy and lactation augments children's IQ at 4 years of age. Pediatrics. 2003;111:e39-44.
20. Husain SM, Mughal MZ, Tsang RC. Calcium, phosporous and magnesium transport across the placenta. In: Polin RA, Fox WW, Abman SH (Eds). Fetal and Neonatal Physiology, 3rd edition. Philadelphia: Saunders; 2004. pp. 314-22.
21. Loughead JL, Mimouni F, Tsang RC. Serum ionized calcium concentrations in normal neonates. Am J Dis Child. 1988;142:516-8.
22. Prada JA. Calcium regulating hormones. In: Polin RA, Fox WW, Abman SH (Eds). Fetal and Neonatal Physiology, 3rd edition. Philadelphia: Saunders; 2004. pp. 303-14.
23. Hambridge KM, Krebs NF. Zink in the fetus and neonate. In: Polin RA, Fox WW, Abman SH (Eds). Fetal and Neonatal Physiology, 3rd edition. Philadelphia: Saunders; 2004. pp. 342-47.
24. Gluckman PD. The onset and organization of hypothalamic control in the fetus. In: Jones CT, Nathanielsz PW (Eds). The Physiological Development of the Fetus and the Newborn. London: Academic Press; 1985. pp. 103-11.
25. Grimberg A, Kutikov JK. Hypothalamus. Neuroendometabolic Center. In: Polin RA, Fox WW, Abman SH (Eds). Fetal and Neonatal Physiology, 3rd edition. Philadelphia: Saunders; 2004. pp. 1871-80.
26. Sack J. The hypothalamic-pituitary-thyroid axis. In: Gluckman PD, Heymann MA (Eds). Perinatal and Pediatric Pathophysiology. London: Edward Arnold; 1993. pp. 302-10.
27. Thorpe-Beeston JG, Nicolaides KH, Felton CV, et al. Maturation of the secretion of the thyroid hormone and thyroid stimulating hormone in the fetus. N Engl J Medicine. 1991;324:532-6.
28. Lagercrantz H. Stress, arousal, and gene activation at birth. News Physiol Sci. 1996;11:214-8.
29. Segar JL. Neural regulation of blood pressure during fetal and newborn life. In: Polin RA, Fox WW, Abman SH (Eds). Fetal and Neonatal Physiology, 3rd edition. Philadelphia: Saunders; 2004. pp. 715-26.
30. Johnson P. The development of breathing. In: Jones CT, Nathanielsz PW (Eds). The Physiological Development of the Fetus and the Newborn. London: Academic Press; 1985. pp. 201-10.
31. Avery ME, Fletcher BD, Williams RG. The Lung and Its Disorders in the Newborn Infant. Philadelphia: WB Saunders Co; 1981.
32. Saugstad OD. Physiology of resuscitation. In: Polin RA, Fox WW, Abman SH (Eds). Fetal and Neonatal Physiology, 3rd edition. Philadelphia: Saunders; 2004. pp. 763-72.
33. Saugstad OD, Rootwelt T, Aalen O. Resuscitation of asphyxiated newborn infants with room air or oxygen: an international controlled trial: the Resair 2 study. Pediatrics. 1998;102(1):e1.
34. Wert SE. Normal and abnormal structural development of the lung. In: Polin RA, Fox WW, Abman SH (Eds). Fetal and neonatal physiology, 3rd edition. Philadelphia: Saunders; 2004. pp. 783-801.
35. Barker PM, Southern KW. Regulation of liquid secretion and absorption by the fetal and neonatal lung. In: Polin RA, Fox WW, Abman SH (Eds). Fetal and neonatal physiology, 3rd edition. Philadelphia: Saunders; 2004. pp. 822-34.
36. Godfrey S. Growth and development of the respiratory system: Functional development. In: Davis JA, Dopping J (Eds). Scientific Foundations of Paediatrics, 2nd edition. London: Heineman; 1981. pp. 432-50.
37. Karlberg P, Cherry RB, Escardo FE, et al. Respiratory studies in newborn infants. II. Pulmonary ventilation and mechanics of breathing in the first minutes of life, including the onset of respiration. Acta Paediatrica. 1962;51:121-36.
38. Vyas H, Milner AD, Hopkins IE. Intrathoracic pressure and volume changes during the spontaneous onset of respiration in babies born by caesarean section and by vaginal delivery. J Pediatr. 1981;99:787-91.
39. Sjostedt S, Rooth G, Caligara F. The oxygen tension in the cord blood after normal delivery. Acta Obstet Gynecol Scand. 1960;39:34-8.
40. Kulovich MV, Hallman MB, Gluck L. The lung profile. Am J Obstet Gynecol. 1979;135:57-63.
41. Hamvas A, Nogee LM, White FV, et al. Progressive lung disease and surfactant dysfunction with a deletion in surfactant protein C gene. Am J Respir Cell Mol Biol. 2004;30:771-6.
42. Nogee LM. Genetic mechanisms of surfactant deficiency. Biol Neonate. 2004;85(4):314-8.
43. Whitsett JA. Composition of pulmonary surfactant lipids and proteins. In: Polin RA, Fox WW, Abman SH (Eds). Fetal and Neonatal Physiology, 3rd edition. Philadelphia: Saunders; 2004. pp. 1005-13.
44. Rudolph AM. Congenital Diseases of the Heart. Chicago: Year Book Medical Publishers, Inc; 1974.
45. Rudolph AM. Organization and control of the fetal circulation. In: Jones CT, Nathanielsz PW (Eds). The Physiological Development of the Fetus and the Newborn. London: Academic Press; 1985. pp. 343-53.
46. Rudolph AM. Fetal circulation and cardiovascular adjustment at birth. In: Rudolph AM (Ed). Pediatrics. Norwalk: Appleton & Lange; 1987. pp. 1219-23.
47. Soifer SJ, Fineman JR, Heyman MA. Cardiovascular system: the pulmonary circulation. In: Gluckman PD, Heymann MA (Eds). Perinatal and Pediatric Pathophysiology. London: Edward Arnold; 1993. pp. 519-25.
48. Kiserud T, Eik-Nes SH, Hellevik LR, et al. Ductus venosus—longitudinal Doppler velocimeter study of the human fetus. J Maternal Fetal Invest. 1992;2:5-11.
49. Anderson PAW, Kleinman CS, Lister G, et al. Cardiovascular function during development and the response to hypoxia. In: Polin RA, Fox WW, Abman SH (Eds). Fetal and Neonatal Physiology, 3rd edition. Philadelphia: Saunders; 2004. pp. 635-69.
50. Kinsella JP, Shaul PW. Physiology of nitric oxide in the developing lung. In: Polin RA, Fox WW, Abman SH (Eds). Fetal and Neonatal Physiology, 3rd edition. Philadelphia: Saunders; 2004. pp. 731-43.
51. Ignarro LJ, Buga GM. Cardiovascular system: vascular smooth muscle and endothelial function. In: Gluckman PD, Heymann MA (Eds). Perinatal and Pediatric Pathophysiology. London: Edward Arnold; 1993. pp. 462-71.
52. Clyman RI. Cardiovascular system: ductus arteriosus. In: Gluckman PD, Heymann MA (Eds). Perinatal and Pediatric Pathophysiology. London: Edward Arnold; 1993. pp. 525-9.
53. Clyman RI. Mechanisms regulating closure of the ductus arteriosus. In: Polin RA, Fox WW, Abman SH (Eds). Fetal and Neonatal Physiology, 3rd edition. Philadelphia: Saunders; 2004. pp. 743-8.

54. Clyman RI, Saugstad OD, Mauray F. Reactive oxygen metabolites relax the lamb ductus arteriosus by stimulating prostaglandin production. Circulat Res. 1989;64:1-8.
55. Lister G Cardiovascular system: oxygen transport. In: Gluckman PD, Heymann MA (Eds). Perinatal and Pediatric Pathophysiology. London: Edward Arnold; 1993. pp. 547-55.
56. Delivoria-Papadopolous M, McGowan JE. Oxygen transport and delivery. In: Polin RA, Fox WW, Abman SH (Eds). Fetal and Neonatal Physiology, 3rd edition. Philadelphia: Saunders; 2004. pp. 880-9.
57. Wood WG. Erythropoiesis and haemoglobin production during development. In: Jones CT (Ed). Biochemical Development of the Fetus and Neonate. Amsterdam: Elsevier Biomedical Press; 1982. pp. 127-62.
58. Myers RE. Experimental models of perinatal brain damage: relevance to human pathology. In: Gluck L (Ed). Intrauterine Asphyxia and the Developing Brain. Chicago: Year Book Publishers, Inc; 1977. pp. 37-97.
59. Levene MI, Anthony MY. Perinatal asphyxia and neonatal seizures. In: Gluckman PD, Heymann MA (Eds). Perinatal and Pediatric Pathophysiology. London: Edward Arnold; 1993. pp. 274-9.
60. Mehmet H, Bessley J, Edwards D. Apoptosis and necrosis. In: Polin RA, Fox WW, Abman SH (Eds). Fetal and Neonatal Physiology, 3rd edition. Philadelphia: Saunders; 2004. pp. 72-9.
61. Frank L, Sosenko IRS. Prenatal development of lung antioxidant in four species. J Pediatr. 1987;110:106-10.
62. Frank L. Development of the antioxidant defences in fetal life. Semin Neonatol. 1988;3:173-82.
63. Berger HM, Molicki JS, Moison RMW, et al. Extracellular defence against oxidative stress in the newborn. Semin Neonatol. 1998;3:183-90.
64. Pallardo FV, Sastre J, Asensi M, et al. Physiological changes in glutathione metabolism in fetal and newborn rat liver. Biochem J. 1991;274:891-3.
65. Power GG, Blood AB, Hunter CJ. Perinatal thermal physiology. In: Polin RA, Fox WW, Abman SH (Eds). Fetal and Neonatal Physiology, 3rd edition. Philadelphia: Saunders; 2004. pp. 541-8.
66. Hoath SB. Physiologic development of the skin. In: Polin RA, Fox WW, Abman SH (Eds). Fetal and Neonatal Physiology, 3rd edition. Philadelphia: Saunders; 2004. pp. 595-611.
67. McMillen C. Biological rhythms. In: Gluckman PD, Heymann MA (Eds). Perinatal and Pediatric Pathophysiology. London: Edward Arnold; 1993. pp. 254-6.
68. Parssons WJ, Williams RS, Shelton JM, et al. Developmental regulation of cytochrome oxidase subunit VIa isoforms in cardiac and skeletal muscle. Am J Physiol. 1996;270:H567-74.

2 Neonatal Jaundice

F Rubaltelli, C Dani

INTRODUCTION

Neonatal jaundice is one of the most common conditions of the newborn. Neonatologists are concerned about this problem, not only for the risk of bilirubin encephalopathy in very low birthweight infants and in full-term infants with hemolysis due to different causes [rhesus and ABO hemolytic disease, glucose-6-phosphate dehydrogenase (G-6-PD) deficiency, etc.], but also because of the anxiety that jaundice in the full-term neonate gives to parents.

In neonates, jaundice becomes apparent at higher bilirubin serum concentrations in comparison to adults (5–7 mg/dL or 85–120 mmol/L in comparison to 2–3 mg/dL or 35–50 mmol/L). If we take into account clinically evident jaundice, we can say that almost 60–70% of term infants and almost all prematures present with jaundice. But, if we consider a cut-off of > 12.9 mg/dL (220 mmol/L), which in full-term infants is the most accepted limit to consider jaundice as deserving attention, only 5% or less present with a bilirubin serum concentration higher than that.[1,2]

Neonatal jaundice is principally the result of transient deficiency of bilirubin conjugation, some deficiency of hepatic uptake and intracellular transport, and an increased enterohepatic circulation of the pigment. It is notable that bilirubin production in the newborn is two or more times greater than that in the adult per kilogram of body weight.[2] The serum bilirubin level at any point in time is dependent upon the rate of bilirubin production minus the rate of bilirubin excretion.

The largest portion of bilirubin derives from heme breakdown of hemoglobin, myoglobin, mitochondrial and microsomal cytochromes, catalase and peroxidase. Heme degradation probably occurs by auto-oxidation after reduction of ferric (Fe^{3+}) heme to the ferrous state (Fe^{2+}) by the action of heme oxygenase and NADPH cytochrome c (P450) reductase.[3,4] The methane bridge carbon of the heme is eliminated as carbon monoxide (CO). At the end of this process biliverdin is formed, and is subsequently reduced to bilirubin through the activity of biliverdin reductase. For each molecule of bilirubin formed, a molecule of CO is produced, which constitutes the basis for measuring bilirubin production by determination of the CO concentration in the expired air, or the carboxyhemoglobin content of the blood.[2]

Three isoforms of HO have been isolated, inducible heme oxygenase (HO-1), constitutive heme oxygenase (HO-2), and the more recently discovered and less active heme oxygenase isoform (HO-3).[5] HO-1 is a known stress response protein, whose transcription can be induced by a whole array of stresses, including endotoxin, transition-metals, heme, hemoglobin and other heme proteins.[6] Indeed, it has been suggested that HO-1 induction might represent a generalized response to oxidative stress[5,7,8] and that it could confer cellular protection against oxidant stress. However,

recent studies suggest that HO-1 induction might not always be beneficial and that the release of redox-active iron from heme might induce an increase of oxidative stress.[9,10] Moreover, in vitro studies[11,12] suggested that the possible protective antioxidant action of HO-1 could occur within a narrow range, as occurs when HO-1 is over-expressed and free iron release may obviate any cytoprotective effect against oxidative stress.[13]

BILIRUBIN SOLUBILITY

Bilirubin is derived from heme by separation from methyne-bridge. The configuration on the C-5 and C-14 bridges is very important, and bilirubin preferentially takes the Z form. Moreover, (Z,Z) bilirubin IXa has a configuration that makes the formation of intramolecular hydrogen bridge linkages possible. For this reason, it is almost insoluble in aqueous media (1–10 nmol/L at pH 7.4), but dissolves readily in a number of nonpolar solvents. The degree to which bilirubin (B) ionizes with the propionic acid residue depends on the pH, and this is decisive both for the distribution of the molecule and for its toxicity:

$$B^{2-} + H \leftrightarrow BH^-; BH^- + H+ \rightarrow BH_2$$

The dissociation constants cannot be determined with absolute precision owing to the problem of solubility, but they are found to be approximately $pK_1 = 4.4$ and $pK_2 = 6.5$.[14]

All modifications of the molecule which prevent the formation of hydrogen bridges cause an increase in water solubility. In the human, this takes the form of an esterification of the residue of propionic acid with glucuronic acid, which makes excretion in the bile possible. Obviously, monoconjugated bilirubin is less soluble than diconjugated bilirubin, and can thus precipitate in the biliary tract forming stones. Alkalinization (salt formation) or the addition of nonpolar solvents, such as chloroform, methanol, ethanol, etc. also result in better solubility, and this is the key mechanism used in the laboratory to differentiate between direct-reacting (mostly the conjugated form) and indirect-reacting (unconjugated) bilirubin.

DISTRIBUTION OF BILIRUBIN IN THE BODY

The distribution of bilirubin in the body is essentially determined by its firm binding to albumin. However, the presence of a visible jaundice seems due, at least in part, to the presence of bilirubin in the skin. Therefore, there is a dynamic competition between tissue binding sites and albumin binding sites. In fact, albumin binds bilirubin according to the law of mass action:

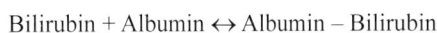

$$\text{Bilirubin} + \text{Albumin} \leftrightarrow \text{Albumin} - \text{Bilirubin}$$

$$\frac{(\text{Albumin} - \text{Bilirubin})}{\text{Albumin} \times \text{Bilirubin}} = KA$$

Two classes of binding sites have been observed: a primary binding site with an extremely high affinity for bilirubin ($KA_1 = 7 \times 7 \times 10^7$ L/mol at 37°C), and one or two other binding sites with a lesser affinity ($KA_2 = 5 \times 5 \times 10^5$ L/mol). The concentration of free bilirubin is mostly determined by the molar relationship between bilirubin and albumin. However, bilirubin can be displaced from its binding site by certain drugs, such as sulfisoxazole, benzoate, salicylate, etc. Nowadays, every drug intended for use in newborns must be accompanied by evidence that it has no effect on bilirubin-albumin binding.[15]

At the hepatic level, bilirubin is taken up at the sinusoidal membrane level, but about 40% is then regurgitated into the plasma again. The albumin-bilirubin complex seems to bind to specific receptors located on the basolateral surface of the sinusoidal plasmatic membrane of the hepatocyte much better than bilirubin alone.[16] In the hepatocyte, bilirubin reacts with binding proteins, the most important being glutathione S-transferase, thus preventing its regurgitation into the plasma. Bilirubin has a low solubility in water due to the fact that its hydrophilic groups are masked by hydrogen bonds; however, it is made hydrosoluble by esterification in the endoplasmic reticulum, with one or both propionic acid side-chains reacting with a sugar residue to form mono- or diesters; in this way the formation of hydrogen bonds is prevented.[17]

The formation of bilirubin glycosides is catalyzed by uridine diphosphate (UDP) glycosyltransferase, an enzyme system that utilizes bilirubin as an acceptor substrate, and UDP sugars (especially glucuronic acid) that act as donor substrates. Transfer from binding proteins to the enzyme system does not necessarily require a higher affinity for the enzyme binding site, because bilirubin is far more soluble in membranes than in the aqueous cytoplasm, and the reaction could, therefore, take place simply by means of a favorable partitioning. Furthermore, the bilirubin monoglucuronide could be converted into diglucuronide by the same enzyme system, following a 180° rotation of the monoglucuronide molecule, or it could even be excreted without modification in the bile.

OXIDATIVE STRESS AND NEONATAL HYPERBILIRUBINEMIA

Several reports emphasized the antioxidant role of bilirubin, which in human neonatal plasma seems to have a greater antioxidant potency than urates, α-tochoferol, or ascorbates.[18] In particular, unconjugated bilirubin is able to scavenge singlet oxygen with high efficiency, to react with superoxide anions and peroxyl radicals, and to serve as reducing substrate for peroxidases in the presence of hydrogen peroxide or organic hydroperoxides. Nevertheless, although the antioxidant effect of bilirubin as a scavenger of reactive oxygen species (ROS) is well documented in vitro[19-22] as well as in animal studies,[23] its role in vivo has not been definitively cleared in preterm infants.[22-27]

Recently, two studies investigated the possible relationship between bilirubin plasma levels and oxidative stress in newborn infants[28,29] excluding that bilirubin acts as antioxidant agent "in vivo". It was demonstrated that the decrease of bilirubin plasma level (probably induced by phototherapy) was associated with the concurrent increase of HO-1 activity in blood and the decrease of oxidative stress, suggesting an antioxidant effect of HO-1 exerted "in vivo" by mechanisms other than bilirubin formation. These protective mechanisms could involve the removal of the pro-oxidant heme, the removal of hydrogen superoxide during the degradation of heme, the induction of ferritin synthesis, which sequesters redox-active iron, and the regulation of superoxide anion production. Other possible mechanisms could involve the multiple ways by which CO modulates inflammatory processes, such as the reduction of neutrophil adhesion and extravasation,[30] the reduction of histamine release from mast cells and human basophils,[31,32] inhibition of the expression of proinflammatory cytokines such as TNFα and IL-1β and an increase of anti-inflammatory cytokine IL-10.[33]

These studies confirmed the findings of Yigit et al.[34] who found no correlation between oxidative stress and total bilirubin in preterm infants with nonhemolytic hyperbilirubinemia, and Gopinathan et al.[35] who observed no correlation between bilirubin plasma level and total plasma antioxidant capacity in preterm infants. On the other hand, Belanger et al.[36] found an association between reduction of the antioxidant capacity of plasma after exchange transfusion, and the ensuing decrease of bilirubinemia. This result, however, as indicated by the authors, could be explained by factors other than bilirubin decrease, such as oxidative stress induced by a large amount of transfused blood and the consequent overload of iron through transfusion. Hammerman et al.[37] found a correlation between Btot and plasmatic antioxidant capacity, but the bilirubinemia of their patients was lower than that reported in other studies. To explain these conflicting results, it may be considered that the correlation between bilirubin plasma level and the antioxidant capacity of plasma could change at low and high values, and could be affected by phototherapy through its lowering effect on bilirubin, which, moreover, could also explain the lack of correlation between bilirubin and HO-activity.

CAUSES OF NEONATAL JAUNDICE

Physiological Jaundice

So-called physiological or developmental jaundice (which could be especially harmful for the small preterm infant) is due to an imbalance between increased pigment load and reduced hepatic handling. The latter seems mainly determined by the low activity of bilirubin UDP glucuronosyltransferase, the hepatic microsomal enzyme which conjugates bilirubin with one or two sugar moieties. It is now accepted that, even in the absence of impaired biliary secretion, a fraction of the esterified bilirubins formed in the liver normally refluxes from hepatocyte to plasma. Measuring the esterified bilirubins in the plasma of newborn infants has made it possible to demonstrate definitively that neonatal jaundice is mainly due to an increased bilirubin production with subnormal conjugation.[38] On the other hand, infants with the lowest plasma concentration of total bilirubin exhibited the highest fraction of conjugates. The percentage of diconjugates relative to total conjugates is 15% on the first day of life. This value tends to increase slightly with age.[38] In premature infants, serum monoconjugates paralleled the course of total and unconjugated bilirubin, but the values were significantly lower than those found in full-term infants.[17,38]

From the practical point of view, we can rule out the diagnosis of physiological jaundice if plasma or serum bilirubin concentration exceeds at any time 12.9 mg/dL (220 mmol/L) in full-term infants or 5–8 mg/dL (85–138 mmol/L) in preterm infants,[39] if jaundice becomes evident in the first 24 hour of life, if bilirubin concentration increases more than 5 mg/dL (85 mmol/L) per day, and if direct reacting plasma bilirubin exceeds 1.5–2 mg/dL (25–35 mmol/L) (it is important to determine conjugated bilirubin by a chromatographic method.[17,38]

Jaundice in Breastfed Neonates

An increased incidence of early-onset jaundice has been reported in breastfed infants, both full-term and preterm.[40,41] However, an increased bilirubin synthesis, demonstrated by an increased CO production, possibly secondary to caloric deprivation, has not been proven.[42] The process of bilirubin conjugation, investigated in breastfed and formula-fed infants by means of the determination of serum concentrations of unconjugated and esterified bilirubin, and the proportion of diesterified (as percentage of esterified bilirubin) pigment, appeared not to be different between the two groups of infants, showing that bilirubin production and conjugation were not different.[43] In addition, a recent study comparing the incidence of neonatal jaundice in 605 infants exclusively breastfed on demand, in 623 who received both breastfeeding and formula feeding, and in 226 exclusively formula-fed, demonstrates that the incidence of neonatal hyperbilirubinemia (> 12.9 mg/dL or 220 mmol/L) in full-term infants is both insignificant (< 5%) and not correlated with demand breastfeeding.[1] These results were recently confirmed in a population of 2,174 infants with gestational age more than or equal to 37 weeks where hyperbilirubinemia was not found to be correlated with breastfeeding, but rather with an increased weight loss, dehydration, and caloric deprivation which could enhance the enterohepatic circulation of bilirubin.[44]

Hemolytic Jaundice

Fetomaternal blood group incompatibility, particularly ABO and rhesus hemolytic disease, are the most common causes of severe jaundice. Nowadays, rhesus hemolytic disease is infrequent due to maternal prophylaxis with anti-rhesus immunoglobulins. However, ABO hemolytic disease still remains an important cause of indirect hyperbilirubinemia and anemia in full-term as well as preterm neonates. Suspicion of ABO or rhesus hemolytic disease must be confirmed by a direct Coombs test carried out on the newborn blood.

Glucose-6-Phosphate Dehydrogenase Deficiency

Glucose-6-phosphate dehydrogenase (G-6-PD) deficiency is frequently associated with neonatal jaundice and sometimes kernicterus. The pathogenesis of this jaundice remains in part unclear, because increased erythrocyte breakdown is not always a major factor in its development.[45] In some patients overt hemolysis, due to different substances, is detected, and in others no signs of hemolysis are detectable (normal level of carboxyhemoglobin). In this group of patients it has been shown that a deficiency in bilirubin conjugation does exist.[45] It is possible that G-6-PD is also involved in some steps (possibly UDP glucuronic acid synthesis) of bilirubin conjugation.

Congenital Nonobstructive, Nonhemolytic Jaundice

Crigler–Najjar disease is a rare disorder of bilirubin metabolism caused by a deficiency of hepatic UDP glucuronyl transferase, and characterized by high serum levels of unconjugated bilirubin

that appear in the first day after birth and continue through life. Based on the responsiveness of the serum bilirubin concentration to phenobarbital, this disease can be distinguished as either type 1, which does not respond to phenobarbital, or type 2, which responds to barbiturates and other drugs that induce enzyme synthesis. Type 2 is probably caused by a partial enzymatic deficiency. In type 1 and type 2 Crigler–Najjar disease, it is possible to detect traces of monoconjugated but not diconjugated bilirubin both in serum and in bile.[46]

BILIRUBIN ENTRY INTO THE BRAIN

Some clinical observations suggest that several mechanisms may be involved with the entry of bilirubin pigment into the brain. In fact, bilirubin seems to enter into the brain both as free bilirubin acid and as bilirubin-albumin complex, by passage through a disrupted blood-brain barrier that is often caused by hyperosmolality and hypercarbia. It seems that even during physiological jaundice there is a steady passage of unbound bilirubin across this barrier. Furthermore, these low levels of bilirubin do not seem to be harmful; in fact, it is also possible that cerebral stores of bilirubin oxidase are able to metabolize bilirubin in loco. Obviously, the entry of bilirubin into the brain can be significantly increased in the presence of high plasma bilirubin concentrations, particularly if the albumin binding capacity is exceeded.[47] Ahlfors et al. reported that in term newborns unbound bilirubin levels between 0.9 and 2 μg/dL produce subtle and reversible changes in auditory brainstem response latency, and described the case of an infant who developed a kernicterus at a total bilirubin concentration of 31.7 mg/dL and unbound bilirubin concentration of 7.7 μg/dL.[48] However, in preterm infants bilirubin-induced changes in auditory brainstem response can begin at unbound bilirubin level of 0.5 μg/dL and kernicterus becomes likely at 1–1.5 μg/dL.[49]

Effects of Bilirubin on Neurologic Functions

It is well known that bilirubin acts to uncouple oxidative phosphorylation and, consequently, inhibits the respiratory chain by causing certain toxic effects.[50] However, a number of studies carried out on experimental animals show no difference in bilirubin binding between different brain regions, nor in the rate of bilirubin disappearance from the cerebral tissues.[51] Moreover, it is still unclear as to why bilirubin has a preferential localization at the level of the basal ganglia. One proposed explanation relies on the possibility that bilirubin may be metabolized locally at different rates.[51] In fact, the typical findings of kernicterus are a yellow staining of the subthalamic, dentate and inferior olivary nuclei and the globus pallidus. Cellculture models suggest that bilirubin initially interacts with cellular membranes, affects ion channels and neurotransmitters, and ultimately leads to deranged metabolism and cell death.[52] The clinical picture of kernicterus is also fairly uniform in these children, with convulsions and opisthotonus followed by hypotonia, high-pitched crying and fever. The sequelae in the survivors consist of neurogenic hearing disorders, choreoathetosis with asymmetrical spasticity and paralysis of upward gaze, together with other neurologic manifestations. Ambulation, despite severe athetosis, is generally reached by the age of 5 years.[53]

Brainstem auditory-evoked potentials are altered by bilirubin in various ways.[54,55] In some studies it has been observed to change the conduction latencies, in others it lowered the conduction wave amplitude, both of which fit with the follow-up observation of deafness in kernicteric babies. Some studies note reversibility of these altered potentials through lowering of high bilirubin levels.[56,57]

Bilirubin-induced membrane potential-lowering may impair nerve conduction along the auditory pathway, which may be reversible if each cell endures only temporary malfunction or if a sufficient number of neurons in the nerve survive the toxicity to maintain function.

It is commonly accepted that (1) bilirubin may be toxic for cells; (2) kernicterus can occur when unconjugated bilirubin levels are high and (3) the mechanism of bilirubin toxicity is mostly unknown.

MEASUREMENT OF BILIRUBINEMIA

The majority of published studies on bilirubin in infants were made measuring its level on capillary blood with spectrophotometric methods. Some studies compared capillary and venous measurement of bilirubinemia, but their results were conflicting.[58,59] Therefore, to confirm a high value of bilirubin plasma level in a venous sample is not recommended. Recently, new devices have permitted an easier and more reliable transcutaneous measurement of bilirubin. The Chromatics Colormate III™ (Chromatics Color Science International Inc., New York, NY, USA) is still based on the color of the skin, estimating serum bilirubin from skin-reflectance (skin color) whereas the BiliCheck™ (Respironics, Murrysville, Pennsylvania, USA measures transcutaneous bilirubin by utilizing the entire spectrum of visible light (380 to 760 nm) reflected by the skin. Data obtained using Bili-Check™ suggest that this device provides measurements within 2–3 mg/dL (34–51 µmol/L) of the bilirubin serum concentration.[60] These devices could be used as screening tools but, in some circumstances, also as substitutes for serum bilirubin measurements, in particular when its value is lower than 15 mg/dL (257 µmol/L).

TREATMENT OF NEONATAL HYPERBILIRUBINEMIA

Bilirubin is bound to albumin in the blood, and when its concentration exceeds the binding capacity of the carrier, unbound or free bilirubin concentration increases and results in its redistribution between the tissues (brain) and the vascular space ('free' bilirubin theory). Thus, not only is the serum bilirubin concentration important in judging whether an infant is at risk of bilirubin toxicity, but the albumin concentration and the bilirubin/albumin ratio are also of critical importance. In fact, Ahlfors suggests that when the bilirubin/albumin ratio is < 8 mg/g (136 mmol/g) and the neonate appears well, exchange transfusion is probably not necessary.[61]

Exchange transfusion, first performed in 1925 by Alfred Purvis Hart and then implemented by LK Diamond in 1947 using the umbilical vein to withdraw and to perfuse blood, was the only treatment available until 1958 when Cremer and colleagues[62] showed that both sunlight and blue light were able to reduce jaundice in newborns. In fact, phototherapy is now the most widely used method worldwide for the treatment of jaundiced babies.

The mechanisms by which light renders the insoluble bilirubin molecule (bilirubin IX-alpha Z,Z), at physiologic pH, soluble and rapidly excretable in the biliary tract are the transformation of the Z,Z configuration at the C4–C5 and C15–C16 double bonds to

the E configuration in one or both double bonds, thus forming the configurational isomers E,Z or Z,E or E,E.[63-65] Of these isomers, the predominant one is the Z,E form. However, the Z,E change is reversible, and after phototherapy it reconverts in the bile or in the intestines to the Z,Z isomer. In addition, intramolecular cyclization of bilirubin can occur as a result of phototherapy, to form a structural isomer called lumirubin, which cannot be reconverted to native bilirubin. Moreover, lumirubin, which is formed at a lower rate in comparison to the configurational isomers, seems to be excreted more rapidly in the bile than the other isomers.

There is a striking regional selectivity that causes isomerization to take place at the double bond of the CH-bridges. Because of the specific preference evidenced by one-half of the bilirubin molecule in binding to human albumin, the E configuration in position 15 is the main isomer formed. This selectivity is lacking to a large extent in a number of the animals used in experimental studies. Finally, the available data suggest that bilirubin is bound to albumin at the site of the light effect, namely in the skin.

The extent to which isomerization, cyclization or oxidation exert the therapeutic effect of light is determined mainly by the quantum yield of the photochemical reactions and the speed of the transport processes up to the excretory phase.

The quantum yield of configurational isomerization is probably very high; isomers are formed very quickly, and they can be detected within a few minutes after light treatment. On the other hand, photocyclization proceeds more slowly, and depends on the wavelength employed. Moreover, the quantum yield of bilirubin oxidation is very low, and it is most probable that the excretion of catabolites formed in the process takes place rapidly. Since the excretion rate of lumirubin is very high, it is conceivable that, in phototherapy for neonatal jaundice, bilirubin photocyclization is the most effective mechanism of bilirubin photometabolism, followed by configurational isomerization and, finally, photooxidation.

THE BRONZE BABY SYNDROME

The bronze baby syndrome (BBS) is a rare pathological condition that appears during phototherapy. The typical characteristic is a grayish-brown discoloration of the skin, serum, and urine. This condition was first described by Kopelman and colleagues,[66] who observed the typical discoloration in the skin of a newborn following phototherapy. They found that the onset of the syndrome was linked to an increase in conjugated bilirubin, implying a cholestatic disorder; moreover, they also related it to hemolytic anemia. Since then, various authors have attempted to explain the biochemical mechanism responsible for the onset of this syndrome.[67,68] In this connection, Kopelman and colleagues noted a reduced bilirubin binding capacity in newborns suffering from BBS. They suspected that bilirubin photoproducts might be responsible both for the bronze discoloration and for the change in binding capacity ascertained by the salicylate method". Autopsy evidence later showed that this peculiar discoloration was also present in the kidneys, liver, and peritoneum. Clark and associates[67] and Rubaltelli and colleagues,[68] in particular, found anatomical signs of kernicterus in two newborns who died with this syndrome. They considered this observation to be confirmation that the pigments responsible for BBS increase the risk of bilirubin neurotoxicity, as suggested by the reported decline in the albumin binding capacity.[66,69]

In 1982 a notably higher concentration of porphyrins was found in the serum of patients with BBS.[70] Two cases of this syndrome, with very high serum porphyrins, probably due to some degree of cholestasis, were described.[71,72] The porphyrins were identified as Cu^{2+}-uroporphyrin, Cu^{2+}-coproporphyrin-, and Cu^{2+}-protoporphyrin. In fact, the absorption spectrum of serum specimens from infants with BBS showed spectral features typical of bilirubin (peak absorption around 460 nm), as well as an intense band with a peak at about 400 nm and broad absorbance in the near-UV and the 600–700 nm region. The latter two features were not confirmed by the absorption spectra of control sera. The sera of bronze babies also exhibited a wide range of fluorescence emission spectra, with peaks at 585, 619 and 670 nm. This finding indicates that absorption in the 400 nm band does not reflect the presence of residual hemoglobin in the serum because hemoproteins are known to be devoid of any appreciable fluorescence in the red region. Instead, the emission spectra observed are characteristic of porphyrin compounds.

Chromatographic separation led to the conclusion that the main component is Cu^+-protoporphyrin IX, although small amounts of Cu^+-coproporphyrin II and Cu^+-uroporphyrin III are also present. These porphyrins do not seem to have an appreciable photosensitizing effect. Furthermore, there was no evidence of significant alterations in the UV spectrum of irradiated serum from infants with BBS or in cord blood serum with added synthetic Cu^+-porphyrins. This is due to the well-known shortening of the half-life of excited porphyrin as a consequence of the binding of the Cu^+ ion on the tetrapyrrolic ring.[73]

These investigations show that the grayish-brown skin color is a result of the photolability of the Cu^{2+}porphyrins. Indeed, Cu^+-porphyrins in the serum of infants with BBS or in aqueous solutions are converted under irradiation with visible light into brown photoproducts with a higher absorption in near-UV and red spectral regions. Moreover, the presence of bilirubin increases the photodegradation rate of Cu^+-porphyrins, suggesting that bilirubin acts as a photosensitizer in this process.

GUIDELINES FOR THE TREATMENT OF UNCONJUGATED HYPERBILIRUBINEMIA

Full-Term Newborn Infants

Neonatal jaundice (total bilirubin serum concentration > 12.9 mg/dL) (220 mmol/L) occurs in around 5% of normal neonates.[1] In the majority of cases, it is a physiologic or developmental jaundice,[1,74] which does not need any treatment. However, it is important to exclude the presence of a rhesus or ABO hemolytic disease, and the possibility that the jaundice could be an early sign of an inborn error of metabolism, or sepsis, etc.

It is suggested that a direct Coombs test plus blood group and rhesus determination should be carried out on the cord blood of every neonate, and, when jaundice is present, the neonatologist should evaluate the appropriateness of a serum bilirubin determination in relation to the day of appearance and intensity of the jaundice, etc. A bilirubin serum level of 20 mg/dL (340 mmol/L) in a normal full-term newborn infant is no longer considered an indication for exchange transfusion.[74] In the absence of a hemolytic disorder, and with a bilirubin level in the range 20–25 mg/dL (340–425 mmol/L) exchange transfusion might be considered, but this decision must be based on a careful evaluation of the risk/benefit ratio.

Following Wennberg's suggestions,[47] one should take into consideration not only the serum bilirubin level but also the albumin serum concentration: that is, by multiplying the albumin value in grams by seven, a value is obtained which corresponds to the level when an exchange transfusion is indicated.

It is recommended that phototherapy be started during the first 24 hour of life if the serum bilirubin level exceeds 4–7 mg/dL (70–120 mmol/L), or during the second 24 hour of life if it exceeds 11–15 mg/dL (190–260 mmol/L), and in all cases whenever it exceeds 15 mg/dL (260 mmol/L). Phototherapy should be carried out for at least 24 hour, and should be interrupted when bilirubin serum concentration is decreased by more than or equal to 2 mg/dL ($\geq$ 35 mmol/L).

However, the American Academy of Pediatrics has recently published guidelines for the management of hyperbilirubinemia in the newborn infant of 35 or more weeks of gestation, which report in depth on current recommendations for prevention, diagnosis, and treatment of neonatal jaundice.[75] The approach to jaundice in preterm infants appears more difficult because there are no specific evidence-based guidelines for the use of phototherapy and exchange transfusion in these infants. Different authors have reported a range of bilirubin plasma level for intervention in various circumstances, but none of these indications has greater validity than another.[39] However, considering that in preterm infants kernicterus has almost disappeared probably due to aggressive phototherapy, it is probable that the current management of jaundice in these infants is correct.

Other possible therapeutic interventions are immunoglobulin therapy in immune hemolytic jaundice and administration of the heme oxygenase inhibitor Sn-mesoporphyrin. Alcock et al., in a metaanalytical study on term and preterm infants with rhesus and ABO incompatibility, found that the rate of exchange transfusion decreased significantly in the immunoglobulin treated group. The mean number of exchange transfusions per infant was also significantly lower in the immunoglobulin treated group.[76] As for Sn-mesoporphyrin, its use is very promising both for the prevention and the treatment of neonatal jaundice. However, this drug is as yet under research and is not commercially available.[77]

Premature Newborn Infants

In the last few years, a number of studies have shown that currently neither kernicterus nor clinical signs of bilirubin encephalopathy are found in premature babies (see the important review of Conolly and Volpe).[78] These findings were reported despite the fact that higher bilirubin serum concentrations were allowed compared with studies reported in the 1960s and 1970s, when kernicterus was not a rare occurrence.[79,80] It is possible that the improved quality of health care has reduced the appearance of preterm kernicterus, the pathogenesis of which is still not completely understood.[80-85]

The definition of prematurity (< 37 weeks of gestational age) includes neonates of very different gestational ages. Moreover, a generous use of phototherapy has allowed a reduction of high bilirubin serum concentrations, and as a result exchange transfusion is no longer used very often. However, it seems rational to initiate light treatment independently of the age of the premature infant, whenever the bilirubin serum concentration is more than or equal to 8 mg/dL (135 mmol/L), provided that no hemolysis is present. In fact, exchange transfusion must be considered when bilirubin reaches the level of 18 mg/dL (305 mmol/L). Furthermore, for the premature newborn one can use Wennberg's formula[47] to identify infants needing exchange transfusion: multiplying by six the value of serum albumin concentration (in grams) one obtains the threshold value for exchange transfusion.

REFERENCES

1. Rubaltelli FF. Unconjugated and conjugated bilirubin pigments during perinatal development. IV. The influence of breast-feeding on neonatal hyperbilirubinemia. Biol Neonate. 1993;64:104-9.
2. Maisels MJ, Pathak A, Nelson NM, et al. Endogenous production of carbon monoxide in normal and erythroblastotic newborn infants. J Clin Invest. 1971;50:1-8.
3. Yoshinaga T, Sassa S, Kappas A. The occurrence of molecular interactions among NADPH-cytochrome-c reductase, heme oxygenase, and biliverdin reductase in heme degradation. J Biol Chem. 1982;257:7786-93.
4. Yoshinaga T, Sassa S, Kappas A. A comparative study of heme degradation by NADPH-cytochrome-c reductase alone and by the complete heme oxygenase system. J Biol Chem. 1982;257:7794-802.
5. Keyse SM, Applegate LA, Tromvoukis Y, et al. Oxidant stress leads to transcriptional activation of the human heme oxygenase gene in cultured skin fibroblast. Mol Cell Biol. 1990;10:4967-9.
6. Lamb NJ, Quinlan GJ, Mumby S, et al. Haem oxygenase shows prooxidant activity in microsomal and cellular systems: implication for the release of low-molecular-mass iron. J Biochem. 1999;344:153-8.
7. Vile GF, Basu-Modak S, Waltner C, et al. Heme Oxygenase 1 mediates an adaptive response to oxidative stress in human skin fibroblasts. Proc Natl Acad Sci USA. 1994;91:2607-10.
8. Lautier D, Luscher P, Tyrrell RM. Endogenous glutathione levels, modulate both constitutive and UVA radiation/hydrogen peroxide inducible expression of the human heme oxygenase gene. Carcinogenesis. 1992;13:227-32.
9. Gutteridge JMC. Fate of oxygen free radicals in extracellular fluids. Biochem Soc Trans. 1982;10:72-3.
10. Dennery PA, Spitz DR, Yang G, et al. Oxygen toxicity and iron accumulation in the lungs of mice lacking heme oxygenase-2. J Clin Invest. 1998;101:1001-11.
11. Dennery PA, Sridhar KJ, Lee CS, et al. Heme oxygenase-mediated resistance to oxygen toxicity in hamster fibroblasts. J Biol Chem. 1997;272:14937-42.
12. Suttner DM, Sridhar K, Le CS, et al. Protective effects of transient HO-1 overexpression on susceptibility to oxygen toxicity. Am J Physiol. 1999;276:L443-51.
13. Dennery PA. Regulation and role of heme oxygenase in oxidative injury. Curr Top Cell Regul. 2000;36:181-99.
14. Jährig K, Jährig D, Meisel P. Phototherapy. Treating Neonatal Jaundice with Visible Light. München: Quintessenz-Verlags-GmbH; 1993.
15. Brodersen R. Binding of bilirubin to albumin. CRC Crit Rev Clin Lab Sci. 1979;11:305-99.
16. Berk PD, Potter BJ, Stremmel W. Role of plasma ligand binding proteins in the hepatocellular uptake of albumin bound organic anion. Hepatology. 1987;7:165-76.
17. Rubaltelli FF. Bilirubin metabolism in the newborn (editorial). Biol Neonate. 1993;63:133-8.
18. Halliwell B, Gutteridge JM. Role of free radicals and catalytic metal ions in human disease: an overview. Methods Enzymol. 1990;186:1-85.
19. Kentaro H, Satoshi Y, Akio F, et al. Oxidative stress in newborn infants with and without asphyxia as measured by plasma antioxidants and free fatty acids. Biochem and Biophisic Res Comm. 1999;257:244-8.
20. Hardy P, Peri KG, Lahaie I, et al. Increased nitric oxide synthase and action preclude choroidal vasoconstriction to hyperoxia in newborn pig. Circ Res. 1996;79:504-11.
21. Abran D, Varma DR, Chemtob S. Increased thromboxane-mediated contractions of retinal vessels of newborn pig to peroxides. Am J Physiol. 1995;268: H628-32.
22. Chemtob S, Abran D, Hardy P. Peroxide-cyclooxygenase interactions in postasphyxial changes in retinal and choroidal hemodinamics. J Appl Physiol. 1995;78:2039-46.
23. James L, Greenough A, Naik S. The effect of blood transfusion on oxygenation in premature ventilated neonates. Eur J Pediatr. 1997;156:139-41.
24. Cooke RWI, Clark D, Nickel-Dwyer M, et al. The apparent role of blood transfusion in the development of retinopathy of prematurity. Eur J Pediatr. 1993;152:833-6.
25. Shaw JCL. Iron absorption by the premature infants: the effect of transfusion and iron supplementation on the serum ferritin levels. Acta Paediatr Scand. 1982;299:S83-9.
26. Lackman GM, Schnieder C, Bohner J. Gestational age-dependent reference values for iron and selected proteins of iron metabolism in serum premature human neonates. Biol Neonate. 1998;74:208-13.
27. Siimes MA, Addiego JE, Dallman PR. Ferritn in serum, diagnosi of iron deficiency and overload in infants and children. Blood. 1974;43:581-90.
28. Dani C, Martelli E, Bertini G, et al. Bilirubin plasma level and oxidative stress in preterm infants. Arch Dis Child Fetal Neonatal Ed. 2003;88:F119-23.
29. Dani C, Masini E, Bertini G, et al. Pediatr Res (in press).
30. Ndisang JF, Masini E, Mannaioni PF, et al. Carbon monoxide and cardiovascular inflammation. In: Wong R (Ed). Boca Raton, FL, USA: CRC Press; 2002. pp. 165-80.
31. Mirabella C, Baronti R, Berni LA, et al. Hemin and carbon monoxide modulate the immunological response of human basophils. Int Arch Allergy Immunol. 1999;118:259-60.
32. Di Bello MG, Berni L, Gai P, et al. A regulatory role of carbon monoxide in mast cells function. Inflamm Res. 1998;1:S7-8.
33. Otterberin LE, Bach FH, Alam J, et al. Carbon monoxide has anti-inflammatory effects involving the mitogen-activated protein kinase pathway. Nat Med. 2000;6:422-8.
34. Yiğit S, Yurdakök M, Kilin K, et al. Serum malondialdehyde concentrations in babies with hyperbilirubinemia. Arch Dis Child Fetal Neonatal Ed. 1999;80:F235-7.
35. Gopinathan V, Miller NJ, Milner AD, et al. Bilirubin and ascorbate antioxidant activity in neonatal plasma. FEBS Lett. 1994;349:197-200.
36. Bellanger S, Lavole JC, Chessex P. Influence of bilirubin on the antioxidant capacity of plasma in newborn infants. Biol Neonate. 1997;71:233-8.
37. Hammerman C, Goldstein R, Kaplan M, et al. Bilirubin in the premature: toxic waste or natural defense? Clin Chem. 1998;44:2551-3.
38. Muraca M, Blanckaert N, Rubaltelli FF, et al. Unconjugated and conjugated bilirubin pigments during perinatal development. I. Studies on rat serum and intestine. Biol Neonate. 1986;49:90-5.
39. Maisels MJ, Watchko JF. Treatment of jaundice in low birthweight infants. Arch Dis Child Fetal Neonatal Ed. 2003;88:F459-63.

40. Maisels MJ, Gifford K, Antle CE, et al. Jaundice in the healthy newborn infant: a new approach to an old problem. Pediatrics. 1988;81:505-11.

41. Lucas A, Baker BA. Breast milk jaundice in premature infants. Arch Dis Child. 1986;61:1063-7.

42. Stevenson DK, Bartoletti AL, Ostrander CR, et al. Pulmonary excretion of carbon monoxide in human infant as an index of bilirubin production. IV. Effects of breast-feeding and caloric intake in the first postnatal week. Pediatrics. 1980;65:1170-2.

43. Rubaltelli FF, Muraca M, Vilei MT, et al. Unconjugated and conjugated bilirubin pigments during perinatal development. III. Studies on serum of breast-fed and formula-fed neonates. Biol Neonate. 1991;60:144-7.

44. Bertini G, Dani C, Tronchin M, et al. Is breastfeeding really favoring early neonatal jaundice? Pediatrics. 2001;107:E41.

45. Kaplan M, Rubaltelli FF, Hammerman C, et al. Conjugated bilirubin in neonates with glucose-6-phosphate deficiency. J Pediatr. 1996;128:695-7.

46. Rubaltelli FF, Novello A, Zancan L, et al. Serum and bile bilirubin pigments in the differential diagnosis of Crigler–Najjar disease. Pediatrics. 1994;94:553-6.

47. Wennberg RP. Cellular basis of bilirubin toxicity. NY State J Med. 1991;91:493-6.

48. Ahlfors CE. Unbound bilirubin in a term newborn with kernicterus. Pediatrics. 2003;111:1110-2.

49. Amin SB, Ahlfors C, Orlando MS, et al. Bilirubin and serial auditory brainstem response in premature infants. Pediatrics. 2001;107:664-70.

50. Zetterstrom R, Ernster L. Bilirubin, an uncoupler of oxidative phosphorylation in isolated mitochondria. Nature. 1956;178:1335-7.

51. Hansen WR. Bilirubin in the brain. Distribution and effects on neurophysiological and neurochemical processes. Clin Pediatr. 1994;33:452-9.

52. Ochoa EL, Wennberg RP, An Y, et al. Interaction of bilirubin with isolated presynaptic nerve terminals: functional effects on the uptake and release of neurotransmitters. Cell Mol Neurobiol. 1993;13:69-86.

53. Rubaltelli FF, Griffith PF. Management of neonatal hyperbilirubinemia and prevention of kernicterus. Drugs. 1992;43:864-72.

54. Karplus N, Lee C, Cashore WJ, et al. The effect of brain bilirubin deposition on auditory brainstem evoked responses in rats. Early Hum Dev. 1988;16:185-94.

55. Vohr BR, Lester B, Rapisardi G, et al. Abnormal brainstem function correlates with acoustic cry features in term infants with hyperbilirubinemia. J Pediatr. 1989;115:303-8.

56. Nakamura H, Takada S, Shimabaku R, et al. Auditory nerve and brainstem responses in newborn infants with hyperbilirubinemia. Pediatrics. 1985;75:703-8.

57. Wennberg RP, Ahlfors CE, Bickers R, et al. Abnormal auditory brainstem response in a newborn infant with hyperbilirubinemia: improvement with exchange transfusion. J Pediatr. 1982;100:624-6.

58. Leslie GI, Philips JB, Cassady G. Capillary and venous bilirubin values: are they really different? Am J Dis Child. 1987;141:1199-200.

59. Eidelman AI, Schimmel MS, Algur N, et al. Capillary and venous bilirubin values: they are different—and how! Am J Dis Child. 1989;143:642.

60. Bertini G, Rubaltelli FF. Non-invasive bilirubinometry in neonatal jaundice. Semin Neonatol. 2002;7:129-33.

61. Ahlfors CE. Criteria for exchange transfusion in jaundiced newborns. Pediatrics. 1994;93:488-94.

62. Cremer RJ, Perryman PW, Richards DH. Influence of light on the hyperbilirubinemia of infants. Lancet. 1958;1:1994-7.

63. Cohen A, Ostrow J. New concepts in phototherapy: photoisomerization of bilirubin IX-alpha and the potential toxic effect of light. Pediatrics. 1980;65:740-50.

64. Lightner D, Wooldridge T, McDonagh A. Configurational isomerization of bilirubin and the mechanisms of jaundice phototherapy. Biochim Biophys Res Comm. 1979;86:235-43.

65. Lightner D, Woolridge T, McDonagh A. Photobilirubin: an early bilirubin photoproduct detected by absorbance difference spectroscopy. Proc Natl Acad Sci. 1979;76:29-32.

66. Kopelman AE, Brown RS, Odel GB. The bronze baby syndrome: a complication of phototherapy. J Pediatr. 1972;81:446-50.

67. Clark CF, Torii S, Hamamoto Y, et al. The 'bronze baby' syndrome: postmortem data. J Pediatr. 1976;88:461-4.

68. Rubaltelli FF, Da Riol R, D'Amore ESG, et al. The bronze baby syndrome: evidence of increased tissue concentration of copper porphyrins. Acta Paediatr. 1996;85:381-4.

69. Ebbesen F. Low reserve albumin for binding of bilirubin in neonates with deficiency of bilirubin excretion and bronze baby syndrome. Acta Paediatr Scand. 1982;71:415-20.

70. Jori G, Reddi E, Rubaltelli FF. Bronze baby syndrome: evidence for an increased serum porphyrin concentration. Lancet. 1982;1:1073.

71. Jori G, Reddi E, Rubaltelli FF. Porphyrin metabolism in the bronze baby syndrome. In: Stern L, Bard H, Friis Hansen B (Eds). Intensive Care in the Newborn. New York: Masson Publ Co.; 1993. pp. 41-5.

72. Rubaltelli FF, Jori G, Reddi E. Bronze baby syndrome: a new porphyrin-related disorder. Pediatr Res. 1983;17:327-30.

73. Cauzzo G, Gennari G, Jori G, et al. The effect of the chemical structure on the photosensitizing efficiency of porphyrins. Photochem Photobiol. 1977;25:389-95.

74. Newman TB, Maisels MJ. Evaluation and treatment of jaundice in the term newborn: a kinder, gentler approach. Pediatrics. 1992;89:809-18.

75. American Academy of Pediatrics. Management of hyperbilirubinemia in the newborn infant 35 or more weeks of gestation. Pediatrics. 2004;114:297-316.

76. Alcock GS, Liley H. Immunoglobulin infusion for isoimmune haemolytic jaundice in neonates. Cochrane Database Syst Rev. 2002;(3):CD003313.

77. Kappas A. A method for interdicting the development of severe jaundice in newborns by inhibiting the production of bilirubin. Pediatrics. 2004;113:119-23.

78. Connolly AM, Volpe JJ. Clinical features of bilirubin encephalopathy. Clin Perinatol. 1988;17:371-9.

79. Harris RC, Lucey JF, MacLean RJ. Kernicterus in premature infants associated with low concentration of bilirubin in the plasma. Pediatrics. 1958;21:875-83.

80. Gartner LM, Snyder RN, Chabon RS. Kernicterus: high incidence in premature infants with low serum bilirubin concentrations. Pediatrics. 1970;45:906-17.

81. Jardine DS, Rogers K. Relationship of benzyl alcohol to kernicterus, intraventricular hemorrhage, and mortality in preterm infants. Pediatrics. 1989;83:153-60.

82. Seidman DS, Paz I, Stevenson DK, et al. Neonatal hyperbilirubinemia and physical and cognitive performance at 17 years of age. Pediatrics. 1991;88:828-33.

83. Van de Bor M, Ens-Dokkum M, Schreuder AM, et al. Hyperbilirubinemia in low-birthweight infants and outcome at 5 years of age. Pediatrics. 1992;89:359-64.

84. O'Shea TM, Dillard RG, Klinepeter KL, et al. Serum bilirubin levels, intracranial hemorrhage, and the risk of developmental problems in very-low-birthweight neonates. Pediatrics. 1992;90:888-92.

85. Bergman I, Hirsch RP, Fria TJ, et al. Cause of hearing loss in the high-risk premature infant. J Pediatr. 1985;106:95-101.

3

Management of Hypotension in the Neonatal Period

SJ English

INTRODUCTION

Hypotension is a commonly encountered problem in the neonatal intensive care unit. It occurs in up to 40% of very low birth weight (VLBW) (<1,500 g) infants, and is almost universally seen in the extreme preterm baby, most commonly in the first 48 hours after birth. Its importance lies in its possible causal link with brain injury in these infants.[1-4]

There are numerous controversies surrounding the management of hypotension in the preterm infant. As more extremely preterm babies are surviving, our accepted definitions of hypotension are being challenged. The level of blood pressure required to maintain tissue perfusion in these babies is unknown, and the effects of standard therapy are relatively under-researched. As a result, the level of hypotension at which treatment is instigated, and the treatment chosen, largely remain subject to personal preference.

DEFINITION

Normal blood pressure has proven difficult to define in preterm babies, partly because it varies with gestational and postnatal age,[5,6] but also because the range of blood pressure, that will ensure adequate organ perfusion, is not known. There have been a number of studies attempting to define the normal range of blood pressure in the neonate. These have resulted in two widely accepted definitions of hypotension:

1. Mean arterial blood pressure less than the 10th centile for gestation/birth weight and postnatal age.[1]

2. Mean arterial blood pressure less than gestational age in weeks. This is derived from the first definition, following the observation that the 10th centile for mean blood pressure is roughly equal to the gestational age.[5] It is worth remembering, however, that this is only valid in the first 48 hours of life, and that blood pressure rises steeply over the first five postnatal days.

Most neonatal units use the gestational age as a guide when instituting treatment for hypotension. It is important, however, to assess other markers of tissue perfusion, such as capillary refill time, the presence of metabolic acidosis, and urine output when deciding whether to treat.

PATHOGENESIS

Hypovolemia

Hypovolemia causes hypotension by decreasing the preload, leading to reduced cardiac output. In neonates hypovolemia may result from acute hemorrhage (antenatal or postnatal), or from fluid loss due to capillary leak, as seen in septicemia or acute abdominal pathology. It is generally accepted that hypovolemia is an uncommon primary cause of hypotension in the sick preterm infant.[7] It may, however, be implicated in a small number of babies, and should always be considered.

Myocardial Dysfunction

There is good evidence that myocardial dysfunction plays an important role in the development of hypotension in preterm infants in the first few hours of life.[8] There are several factors which contribute to myocardial dysfunction, the foremost of which is immaturity of the myocardium. Hypoxic damage to the heart muscle, acidosis, sepsis, and the presence of a ductal shunt will all adversely affect myocardial function, leading to decreased cardiac output and hypotension. Congenital structural heart defects may also present with hypotension secondary to reduced cardiac output.

Downregulation of Adrenergic Receptors

There is growing evidence that a proportion of sick preterm infants have relative adrenal insufficiency, demonstrating a low cortisol response to human corticotropin releasing hormone.[9-12] Because glucocorticoids have a role in regulating the expression of cardiovascular adrenergic receptors, these infants may be incapable of responding to endogenous or exogenous sympathomimetic agents.[13]

MEASUREMENT

Intra-arterial blood pressure monitoring through an umbilical or peripheral arterial catheter is widely accepted as the gold standard. Studies comparing oscillometric with invasive measurement demonstrate that, providing cuff size is standardized, oscillometric measurement seems to be accurate within the normal range.[14,15] However, concern has been expressed that at the lower levels it consistently overestimates the blood pressure, providing false reassurance to the clinician.[16] In situations where intra-arterial monitoring is not possible, it is also important to assess other markers of tissue perfusion.

CLINICAL RELEVANCE

Tissue Perfusion

In neonatology blood pressure is regularly used as a marker of systemic organ perfusion, and our efforts to maintain a normal blood pressure are based on the belief that we are preserving tissue perfusion. Unfortunately, there are little data to support this. In preterm infants there is only a weak correlation between blood pressure and cardiac output.[17] Furthermore, since blood pressure is the function of blood flow and systemic vascular resistance, blood pressure may not reflect the blood flow in end organs, as the vascular resistance will vary. Several methods that may be useful for assessing systemic blood flow and tissue perfusion in neonates are being evaluated.

Left ventricular output is often used in adults to assess systemic blood flow. Measurements of ventricular outputs in neonates may be confounded by shunts through a patent ductus or foramen ovale. Systemic blood flow in the superior vena cava of newborn infants has been successfully measured, using Doppler echocardiography. Flow in the superior vena cava is thought to reflect blood flow in the upper body, particularly the brain, and appears to correlate well with left ventricular output in babies with a closed duct.[18]

Near infrared spectroscopy (NIRS) has been used to measure hemoglobin flow and venous saturation in the forearm of hypotensive preterm babies.[19] Using this technique, it has been demonstrated that peripheral oxygen delivery and consumption are lower in hypotensive babies, but that oxygen extraction is similar to normotensive controls, with no rise in lactate concentration. This suggests that in hypotensive babies, peripheral oxygen delivery is still adequate for tissue demands, challenging the need to routinely correct hypotension. NIRS has also been used to monitor cerebral circulation in sick premature infants. Unfortunately, it has not clearly demonstrated whether there is a direct relationship between mean arterial blood pressure and cerebral intravascular oxygenation.[20,21]

As NIRS and cardiac output measurements are not continuous, their role in the decision to treat a blood pressure level remains unclear. They do, however, question our present practice of using a single value below which treatment should be started. Further research in this area is obviously needed before techniques such as this have direct relevance to the management of hypotension.

Cerebral Injury

Sick VLBW infants have reduced cerebral vascular autoregulation compared with term infant, with the postulated effect that significant hypotension may lead to cerebral hypoperfusion.[22,23] Episodes of systemic hypotension have been linked to cerebral hemorrhage, ischemia, and to an increased risk of long-term neurological sequelae.[1,3,4] Hypotension is thought to lead to intraventricular hemorrhage by causing ischemic damage to the germinal matrix, which bleeds on re-perfusion. It is unlikely that overenthusiastic correction of hypotension is involved, as episodes of hypertension are not associated with the occurrence of intraventricular hemorrhage. There is no clear evidence that systemic hypotension, in itself, leads to periventricular leukomalacia,[3] although it may be a factor in babies who are also septic. Interestingly, there is little evidence to support the view that treating hypotension prevents any of these sequelae.

MANAGEMENT

The aim of treating hypotension is to preserve adequate organ perfusion and thus to prevent complications such as cerebral injury. However, a cause for hypotension should always be sought before treatment is instituted. Important conditions to exclude include:

- Blood loss
- Pneumothorax
- Sepsis
- Patent ductus arteriosus

- High positive intrathoracic pressure (secondary to mechanical ventilation)
- Heart failure.

If one of the above causes is identified the primary treatment of the hypotension is to institute the specific treatment for the underlying condition. In most instances, a cause for hypotension in the neonatal period will not be determined, although myocardial dysfunction has been identified as a common factor, and treatment will be initiated on the basis of unit protocols. These normally follow a stepwise approach beginning with volume support followed by inotropes and in some the use of steroids.

Volume Support

As previously discussed, hypovolemia is an infrequent cause of hypotension in the sick preterm infant.[7] It is also difficult to diagnose in the immediate postnatal period, as indicators such as urine output and capillary refill time are unreliable. However, because it does occasionally occur, and it is relatively easy to treat, most units adopt a policy of moderate volume replacement prior to the institution of inotropes.

Fluids available for volume replacement may be either crystalloid or colloid. The main difference between the two is the oncotic pressure effect, according to Starling's law, and the theoretical difference in the length of time they remain in the intravascular space. However, the volume administered appears to be more important than protein content in producing a sustained increase in blood pressure in preterm infants,[24] and isotonic saline has been shown to be as effective as 5% albumin for treating hypotension in this population.[25] Crystalloids are also significantly cheaper than colloids, and do not carry the same infection risk.

As colloid and crystalloid are equally effective in treating hypotension in the neonatal period, and considering the other advantages of using isotonic saline, it would seem that the safest approach to volume replacement would be to use 10–20 mL/kg 0.9% saline given over 30 minutes in the first instance. Albumin (4.5%) should be reserved for babies who are likely to be hypovolemic secondary to protein losing conditions, such as babies who have undergone gastrointestinal surgery.

Dopamine and Dobutamine

Since myocardial dysfunction plays an important role in the development of hypotension in preterm infants in the first few hours of life,[8] it is clear that inotropic agents should be of some benefit in the management of hypotension in these babies. The use of inotropes is, however, historically based rather than evidence based, and there are few data relating to associated mortality and morbidity.

Unsurprisingly, dopamine is more effective than volume expansion in restoring normal blood pressure in preterm infants.[26] Dopamine is an exogenous sympathomimetic amine which exerts its cardiovascular effects by the dose dependent stimulation of dopaminergic and α- and β-adrenergic receptors. In the preterm population dopamine causes a dose dependent increase in mean arterial blood pressure in doses of 5–20 μg/kg/min.[27-29]

The main hemodynamic effects of dopamine are to increase myocardial contractility and peripheral vascular tone. The increase in myocardial contractility is due both to a direct stimulation of α- and β-adrenoceptors, and indirectly through its action on β$_2$-adrenoceptors, stimulating the release of endogenous noradrenaline.[30] In adults, the vasotonic effects of dopamine are dose dependent. At doses less than 5 μg/kg/min dopamine stimulates peripheral dopaminergic receptors resulting in the selective dilatation of renal, mesenteric and coronary arteries. At higher doses more than 10 μg/kg/min it causes vasoconstriction by stimulation of α-adrenergic receptors. The dose dependent effects of dopamine on vascular tone in the preterm neonate are less clear,[29,30] although there are emerging concerns that it may have a potent vasoconstrictive effect on the pulmonary vasculature.[31]

Studies in adults suggest that, in sick hypotensive patients, there is a downregulation of adrenergic receptors, requiring much higher doses of dopamine to maintain blood pressure.[13] However, there have been no such studies in neonates. The fact that some preterm infants may also have relative adrenal insufficiency[9] may explain the occurrence of pressor resistance. Further research is clearly required in order to define a maximum dose for dopamine as the use of high doses (> 25 μg/kg/min) has not been studied.

Dobutamine is a relatively cardioselective sympathomimetic amine which exerts its positive inotropic action by direct stimulation of cardiac α- and β-adrenoceptors. It has several theoretical advantages over dopamine: (1) it has limited chronotropic effect, (2) its use is not associated with an increase in systemic vascular resistance[27] and (3) it does not rely on release of endogenous catecholamines for any part of its action.

There is relatively little research into the use of dobutamine in preterm neonates, and it is generally used as a second-line drug, in patients unresponsive to dopamine. It is infused at rates of 5–20 μg/kg/min,[27,32-35] and has been shown to increase left ventricular performance in these doses.[36] The use of high doses (> 25 μg/kg/min) has not been studied. Dobutamine can cause hypercontractile heart failure in the presence of left ventricular hypertrophy, resulting in paradoxical hypotension.[37] It should, therefore, be used with caution in babies with existing cardiac disease.

In the preterm infant dopamine is significantly more effective than dobutamine in the treatment of systemic hypotension, with no differences in short-term complications such as intraventricular hemorrhage and necrotizing enterocolitis.[38] No data are available on long-term outcome for either drug.

Other Agents

Most neonatal units advocate the use of adrenaline or noradrenaline in cases where dopamine and dobutamine have failed to maintain "normal" blood pressure. However, very few studies have looked at the use of these agents in preterm infants, most of the data originating from animal studies. Both adrenaline and noradrenaline, when used in addition to dopamine, do restore normal blood pressure in sick, hypotensive neonates without causing significant cerebral, myocardial or renal vasoconstriction.[39,40] The use of these agents is, however, associated with a high mortality rate of over 50%.

Dopexamine, a relatively new synthetic catecholamine, with predominant β$_2$-adrenergic and dopaminergic activity, has been shown to be effective in raising blood pressure, and improving arterial pH and urine output.[41] In neonates who are hypotensive secondary to septic shock, methylene blue, an inhibitor of soluble guanylate cyclase, has been shown to be effective in increasing blood pressure.[42]

Further research is clearly needed in this area before the routine use of any of these agents can be recommended.

Steroids

Antenatal steroids are now commonly given to mothers in preterm labor. They have been shown to have an independent effect (from the effect on respiratory distress syndrome) on reducing the incidence of hypotension in the preterm infant.[43]

In neonates with hypotension who are unresponsive to volume or pressor administration, there is growing evidence that steroids may be of some value. The theory is that infants with refractory hypotension may have relative adrenal insufficiency.[9-12] The resulting low levels of circulating cortisol in these babies may be insufficient to counteract any downregulation of cardiovascular adrenergic receptors which occurs in critical illness,[13] rendering them resistant to treatment with sympathomimetic agents.

In infants with severe hypotension refractory to both volume expansion and inotropes, treatment with either single dose dexamethasone or a 5-day course of hydrocortisone has been shown to be successful, with discontinuation of inotropes within 54 hours. This effect is sustained for many days following the administration of steroids.[12,44-46] Although the effect may not be evident for up to 6 hours, in my experience it is usually seen within 2 hours of treatment.

There are some groups who have advocated the use of hydrocortisone in smaller doses as prophylaxis against hypotension in at risk VLBW infants.[47] Side effects from postnatal steroids, including the long-term risk of adverse neurological outcome, are well documented and probably prohibit prophylactic use.[48]

Based on the available evidence the use of steroids in the treatment of severe, intractable hypotension, resistant to inotropes, is probably justified. This may be in the form of a single dose of 250 μg/kg dexamethasone or a 5-day tapering course of hydrocortisone starting at 2.5 mg/kg qds. Obviously, there is a balance of risks against benefits, but the short-term benefit of preventing death must outweigh the long-term risks, which are anyway unproven. Further research is obviously needed to determine the optimum dose and course.

CONCLUSION

The management of hypotension in preterm infants remains a controversial area in current neonatal practice. Research in this area is relatively limited, which in part is probably due to the difficulty in obtaining continuous measures of tissue perfusion. There is no consensus on either the definition of hypotension or the level at which treatment should be initiated. The effects of aggressive correction are relatively under-researched, and there are few data on morbidity and mortality in relation to the use of volume support and inotropes. The aim of management must be to attain adequate tissue perfusion and oxygenation, but there may be little or no relation between blood pressure and organ perfusion. Further research is required into methods of assessing tissue perfusion, which can be used alongside monitoring of blood pressure to guide the neonatologist in deciding when to intervene.

Continuous invasive arterial blood monitoring remains the preferred method of recording blood pressure. Decisions to treat hypotension should be based on the general condition of the infant, not on the mean arterial blood pressure alone. On the basis of the available evidence, Figure 3.1 outlines a suggested guideline for the management of hypotension in the neonatal period.

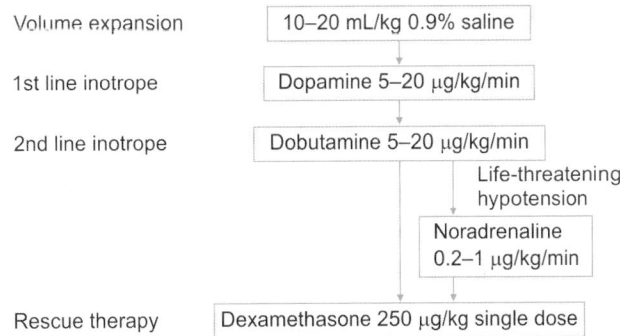

Fig. 3.1: Management of hypotension in neonates
Source: Reference 49

REFERENCES

1. Watkins AMC, West CR, Cooke RWI. Blood pressure and cerebral haemorrhage and ischaemia in VLBW infants. Early Hum Dev. 1989;19:103-10.
2. Miall-Allen VM, De Vries LS, Whitelaw AGL. Mean arterial BP and neonatal cerebral lesions. Arch Dis Child. 1987;62:1068-9.
3. Dammann O, Allred EN, Kuban KC, et al. Systemic hypotension and white-matter damage in preterm infants. Dev Med Child Neurol. 2002;44(2):82-90.
4. Low JA, Froese AB, Galbraith RS, et al. The association between newborn hypotension and hypoxemia and outcome during the first year. Acta Paediatr. 1993;82(5):433-7.
5. Nuntnarumit P, Yang W, Bada-Ellzey HS. Blood pressure measurements in the newborn. Clin Perinatol. 1999;26:981-96.
6. Lee J, Rajadurai VS, Tan KW. Blood pressure standards for very low birthweight infants during the first day of life. Arch Dis Child Fetal Neonatal Ed. 1999;81:F168-70.
7. Dimitriou G, Greenough A, Mantagos J, et al. Metabolic acidosis, core-peripheral temperature difference and blood pressure response to albumin infusion in hypotensive, very premature infants. J Perinat Med. 2001;29(5):442-5.
8. Gill AB, Weindling AM. Cardiac function in the shocked very low birthweight infant. Arch Dis Child. 1993;6817-21.
9. Scott SM; Watterberg KL. Effect of gestational age, postnatal age, and illness on plasma cortisol concentrations in premature infants. Pediatr Res. 1995;37(1):112-6.
10. Tantivit P, Subramanian N, Garg M, et al. Low serum cortisol in term newborns with refractory hypotension. J Perinatol. 1999;19(5): 352-7.
11. Heckmann M, Wudy SA, Haack D, et al. Serum cortisol concentrations in ill preterm infants less than 30 weeks gestational age. Acta Paediatr. 2000;89(9);1098-103.
12. Ng PC, Lam CWK, Fok TF, et al. Refractory hypotension in preterm infants with adrenocortical insufficiency. Arch Dis Child Fetal Neonatal Ed. 2001;84:F122-4.
13. Hausdorff WP, Caron MG, Lefkowitz RJ. Turning off the signal: desensitization of b-adrenergic receptors. FASEB J. 1990;4:33-40.
14. Kimble Kj, Darnall RA, Yelderman MD. An automated technique for estimating mean arterial pressure in critically ill newborns. Anesthesiology. 1981;54:423-5.
15. Dellagramaticas HD, Wilson AJ. Clinical evaluation of the Dinamap non-invasive blood pressure monitor in preterm neonates. Clin Phys Physiol Meas. 1981;2:271-6.
16. Diprose GK, Evans DH, Archer LNJ, et al. Dinamap fails to detect hypotension in very low birthweight infants. Arch Dis Child. 1986;61:771-3.
17. Kluckow M, Evans N. Relationship between blood pressure and cardiac output in preterm infants requiring mechanical ventilation. J Pediatr. 1996;129(4):506-12.
18. Kluckow M, Evans N. Superior vena cava flow in newborn infants: a novel marker of systemic blood flow. Arch Dis Child Fetal Neonatal Ed. 2000;82:F182-7.
19. Wardle SP, Yoxall CW, Weindling AM. Peripheral oxygenation in hypotensive preterm babies. Pediatr Res. 1999;45(3):343-9.
20. Tsuji M, Saul JP, du Plessis A, et al. Cerebral intravascular oxygenation correlates with mean arterial pressure in critically ill premature infants. Pediatrics. 2000;106(4):625-32.
21. Wardle SP, Yoxall CW, Weindling AM. Determinants of cerebral fractional oxygen extraction using near infrared spectroscopy in preterm neonates. J Cereb Blood Flow Metab. 2000;20(2):272-9.
22. Panerai RB, Kelsall AWR, Rennie JM, et al. Cerebral autoregulation dynamics in premature newborns. Stroke. 1995;26:74-80.
23. Pryds O, Edwards AD. Cerebral blood flow in the newborn infant. Arch Dis Child Fetal Neonatal Ed. 1996;74:F63-9.
24. Emery EF, Greenough A, Gamsu HR. Randomized controlled trial of colloid infusions in hypotensive preterm infants. Arch Dis Child. 1992;67:1185-8.
25. King W So, Tai F Fok, Pak C Ng, et al. Randomized controlled trial of colloid or crystalloid in hypotensive preterm infants. Arch Dis Child Fetal Neonatal Ed. 1997;76:F43-6.
26. Gill AB, Weindling AM. Randomized controlled trial of plasma protein fraction versus dopamine in hypotensive very low birth weight infants. Arch Dis Child. 1993;69:284-7.
27. Roze JC, Tohier C, Maingueneau C, et al. Response to dobutamine and dopamine in the hypotensive very preterm infant. Arch Dis Child. 1993;69:59-63.
28. Padbury JF, Agata Y, Baylen BG, et al. Dopamine pharmacokinetics in critically ill newborn infants. J Pediatr. 1986;110:293-8.
29. Seri I, Abbasi S, Wood D, et al. Regional hemodynamic effects of dopamine in the sick preterm neonate. J Pediatr. 1998:133:728-34.
30. Seri I. Cardiovascular, renal, and endocrine actions of dopamine in neonates and children. J Pediatr. 1995;126:333-44.
31. Liet J-M, Boscher C, Gras-Leguen C, et al. Dopamine effects on pulmonary artery pressure in hypotensive preterm infants with patent ductus arteriosus. J Pediatr. 2002;140:373-5.

32. Klarr JM, Faix RG, Pryce CJE, et al. Randomized, blind trial of dopamine versus dobutamine for treatment of hypotension in preterm infants with respiratory distress syndrome. J Pediatr. 1994;125:117-22.

33. Greenough A, Emery EF. Randomized trial comparing dopamine and dobutamine in preterm infants. Eur J Pediatr. 1993;152(2):164-5.

34. Hentschel R, Hensel D, Brune T, et al. Impact on blood pressure and intestinal perfusion of dobutamine or dopamine in hypotensive preterm infants. Biol Neonate. 1995;68(5):318-24.

35. Miall-Allen VM, Whitelaw AGL. Response to dopamine and dobutamine in the preterm infant less than 30 weeks gestation. Crit Care Med. 1989;17:1166-9.

36. Stopfkuchen H, Queisser-Luft A, Vogel K. Cardiovascular response to dobutamine determined by systolic time intervals in preterm infants. Crit Care Med. 1990;18(7):722-4.

37. Germanakis I, Bender C, Hentscel R, et al. Hyper-contractile heart failure caused by catecholamine therapy in premature neonates. Acta Paediatr. 2003;92:836-8.

38. Subedhar NV, Shaw NJ. Dopamine versus dobutamine for hypotensive preterm neonates. Cochrane Database Systemat Rev. 2000;2:CD001242.

39. Seri I, Evans J. Addition of epinephrine to dopamine increases blood pressure and urine output in critically ill extremely low birthweight neonates with uncompensated shock. Pediatr Res. 1998;43:194.

40. Derleth DP. Clinical experience with norepinephrine infusions in critically ill newborns. Pediatr Res. 1997;41:145.

41. Kawczynski P, Piotrowski A. Circulatory and diuretic effects of dopexamine infusion in low-birth-weight infants with respiratory failure. Intensive Care Med. 1996;22(1):65-70.

42. Driscoll W, Thurin S, Carrion V, et al. Effect of methylene blue on refractory neonatal hypotension. J Pediatr. 1996;129:904-8.

43. Moise AA, Wearden ME, Kozinetz CA, et al. Antenatal steroids are associated with less need for blood pressure support in extremely preterm infants. Paediatrics. 1995;95(6):845-50.

44. Bourchier D, Weston PJ. Randomised trial of dopamine compared with hydrocortisone for the treatment of hypotensive very low birth weight infants. Arch Dis Child Fetal Neonatal Ed. 1997;76:F174-8.

45. Seri I, Tan R, Evans J. Cardiovascular effects of hydrocortisone in preterm infants with pressor-resistant hypotension. Pediatrics. 2001;107(5):1070-4.

46. Gaissmaier RE, Pohlandt F. Single-dose dexamethasone treatment of hypotension in preterm infants. J Pediatr. 1999;134:701-5.

47. Rajah V. Treatment of hypotension in very low birthweight infants (letter). Arch Dis Child Fetal Neonatal Ed. 1998;78:F156.

48. Sweet DG, Halliday HL. A risk-benefit assessment of drugs used for neonatal chronic lung disease. Drug Safety. 2000;22:389-404.

49. Dasgupta SJ, Gill AB. Hypotension in the very low birthweight infant: the old, the new, and the uncertain. Arch Dis Child Fetal Neonatal Ed. 2003;88:F450-4.

4 Cytokines and Neonatal Disease

L Cornette, H Logghe

FETAL AND NEONATAL INFLAMMATORY RESPONSES

This review is designed to guide the reader through the framework given in Figure 4.1, summarizing the concept of perinatal inflammation/infection and current factors that may influence the overall outcome under study. Several diseases in the newborn, such as sepsis, chronic lung disease and bronchopulmonary dysplasia (CLD/BPD) and necrotizing enterocolitis (NEC), are characterized by the presence of inflammation. Given mounting evidence suggests a continuum between antenatal and postnatal inflammations, and adverse neonatal outcome,[1,2] we will first study the fetal inflammatory response, prior to expanding on inflammatory responses emerging in the neonatal period.

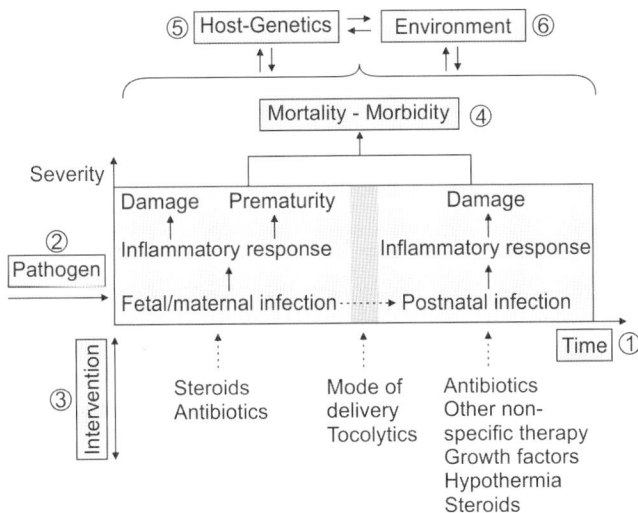

Fig. 4.1: The fetal/neonatal inflammatory response

By definition, an inflammatory response is a protective response to an infection or an injury, mediated by pro-inflammatory cytokines, i.e. low-molecular-weight glycoproteins, predominantly produced by the monocyte-macrophage cell line at the inflammatory site. Pro-inflammatory cytokines (e.g. IL-1β, IL-18, IFN-γ, TNF-α) are primarily responsible for initiating an effective defense (i.e. acute phase response) against exogenous pathogens, whereas anti-inflammatory cytokines (e.g. IL-4, IL-10) are involved in the downregulation of exacerbated inflammatory processes and maintenance of homeostasis for proper functioning of the vital organs.[3]

Fetal Inflammatory Response Syndrome

The majority of women delivering before 28 weeks with or without preterm premature rupture of membranes (PrePROM), show evidence of intrauterine infection. A mechanism postulated is microbial invasion of the uterine cavity resulting in a fetal systemic cytokine or inflammatory response through aspiration, otitis, conjunctivitis or omphalitis.[4] However, only a small proportion of these women will have a positive amniotic fluid culture.[5] Intra-amniotic *inflammation* would, therefore, appear to be a better predictor for imminent preterm delivery rather than intra-amniotic *infection.*[6]

Such active participation of the fetus in a systemic antenatal inflammatory response is, therefore, commonly studied using cordocentesis techniques. Indeed, the fetal inflammatory response syndrome (FIRS) was originally defined by relating increased fetal cord plasma IL-6 to the onset of spontaneous preterm labor (through increased fetal adrenal cortisol production and subsequent prostaglandin release).[7] More recent studies have revealed that the FIRS involves the synergistic action of different cytokines and several complex host defense mechanisms.[8] In addition, through the study of differential placental versus fetal immune cytokine responses within animal models, we now know that a FIRS, rather than the maternal infection, causes fetal multiorgan injury.[9]

Fetal Brain/Fetal Neurotoxicity

The fetal brain has been extensively studied within the context of intrauterine inflammation.[10,11] Funisitis, i.e. infection of the umbilical cord, and chronic chorioamnionitis have been associated with an increased risk for intraventricular hemorrhage.[12,13] Fetal vasculitis has been linked with an elevenfold increased risk for development of periventricular echolucencies.[14] Histopathological examination of infant brain specimens shows overexpression of TNF-α in the microglia cells of periventricular leukomalacia (PVL) lesions with cytokine production being highest in infected infants.[15]

However, a clear link between intrauterine infection/inflammation and neurologic outcome in preterm babies is not confirmed in all studies, as much of the confusion arises from different timings of blood sampling across different studies. Cytokine levels in neonatal blood (day 2 or 3) are likely to be influenced by respiratory or infectious complications, as well as different levels of intensive care, and thus may be different from umbilical cord blood levels.[16] In order to establish a causal link between antenatal infection and neonatal brain disease in individual cases, one needs to provide evidence of placental infection, elevated inflammatory mediators in both umbilical cord and postnatal infant blood, presence of moderate to severe encephalopathy and/or neuroradiological confirmation of brain injury.

Proposed mechanisms for neurotoxicity associated with pro-inflammatory cytokines comprise (1) a direct cytolytic effect on neurons and oligodendrocyte precursors (either through in situ cytokine production or through systemic cytokines crossing the blood-brain barrier), (2) induction of excitatory amino acid release, (3) increased caspase activity resulting in amplified apoptosis, (4) abnormalities in the coagulation cascade or (5) fetal hypotension.[10,14,15,17] Further clarification of these and other mechanisms will increase the likelihood of successful therapeutic interventions.

Many studies focus on the interaction between cytokine and excitatory amino acid release (e.g. glutamate). It is now recognized that an antenatal inflammation-related insult to the central nervous system comprises both infection (pro-inflammatory cytokine release) and hypoxia-ischemia (excessive excitatory neurotransmitter release). The interaction between both entities is, however, complex. Firstly, injury to the brain during antenatal infection may be secondary either to cytokinemia, i.e. cytokines crossing the blood-brain barrier, or to the interruption of placental blood flow resulting in asphyxia.[17] Secondly, animal work indicates that administration of a low dose of bacterial endotoxin (lipopolysaccharides) dramatically sensitizes the immature brain to injury and induces cerebral infarction in response to short episodes of hypoxia-ischemia that by themselves cause no or little injury.[18] Thirdly, increased levels of IL-1 and TNF-α, and neutrophil invasion into infarcted areas have been reported following hypoxia-ischemia in the absence of infection.[18-20] Fourthly, complex interaction effects between both inflammation and excitotoxicity exist, as for example IL-1β perpetuates excitotoxic brain damage in vivo, whereas it ameliorates neuronal death in vitro.[20] Others have reported similar dual neurotrophic and detrimental effects exerted by cytokines following ischemia.[21] Finally, a complex interaction between hypoxia-ischemia and inflammation is also reflected in the neuropathology of white matter abnormalities observed in infants born to mothers with chorioamnionitis.[22] Careful review of animal work suggests that cytokines can be neurotoxic through a process of "sensitizing" the immature brain, i.e. lowering the threshold at which a hypoxic-ischemic insult triggers apoptosis.[23] Further clinical studies investigating the relationship between fetal infection/inflammation, feto-placental thrombosis and subsequent adverse neurological outcome will therefore be challenging.[24]

Other Fetal Morbidity

Fetal exposure to infection/inflammation, similar to antenatal administration of glucocorticoids can, on the one hand, result in maturation of the *lungs*. However, antenatal chorioamnionitis can also prime the fetal lung to respond differently to postnatal events, increasing the risk of CLD/BPD.[25]

Histological chorioamnionitis has been associated with a noticeable reduction of volume and corticomedullary differentiation of the *thymus*, a reduced number of thymocytes, and infiltration of macrophages into the parenchyma.[26]

Finally, a FIRS can result in preterm delivery (and, hence, possible neonatal morbidity), as increased fetal and not maternal serum IL-6 is one of several cytokines that precedes imminent preterm delivery.[8]

Neonatal Inflammatory Responses

Sepsis

The progression to septic shock in infants born to mothers with acute chorioamnionitis is rarely seen in the immediate neonatal period. However, a significant association between funisitis and congenital sepsis has been described.[2]

Neonatal sepsis in the absence of chorioamnionitis is predominantly mediated by IL-1, IL-6 and TNF-α. Sepsis-related mortality is well correlated with multiple organ failure (MOF) caused by uncontrolled inflammation, immunodeficiency (prolonged neutropenia, lymphopenia, hypogammaglobulinemia) and endothelial injury with thrombotic microangiopathy. Septic newborns have low von Willebrand factor (vWF) cleaving metalloprotease activity (ADAMTS-13), resulting in high amounts of circulating ultra-large vWF multimers that lead to microvascular platelet thrombosis and MOF.[27]

Little is known about the profile of pro- and anti-inflammatory cytokines in septic preterm infants, in whom the immune system may be considered as immature. An exaggerated pro-inflammatory response together with an inadequate anti-inflammatory compensation may result in an adverse clinical outcome, as a persistent high IL-6/IL-10 ratio implies a poor prognosis in very low-birth-weight patients.[1] Alternatively, a persistently high IL-10 concentration can be an early indicator of a poor prognosis in preterm neonates with sepsis.[28]

Necrotizing Enterocolitis

Necrotizing enterocolitis is a devastating intestinal disease that primarily occurs in low-birth-weight premature infants. Its etiology is not well-known and may consist of intestinal immaturity, intestinal ischemia, changes in microbiological environment related to enteral feeding practices with an increased inflammatory response as the final common pathway. The evidence suggesting a causal association between chorioamnionitis and subsequent NEC is very sparse, although some retrospective case-control studies suggest a significantly higher frequency of PrePROM and chorioamnionitis in infants with NEC.[29]

Inflammatory mediators involved in NEC are tissue and circulating pro-inflammatory cytokines (IL-1, IL-6, IL-8, TNF-α), platelet-activating factor, leukotriene C4, iNOS, endothelin-1 and thromboxane. These mediators are believed to stimulate signal transduction and gene transcription, leading to apoptosis or programmed cell death, secondary inflammation, increased intestinal wall permeability and, ultimately, necrosis. Conversely, IL-10, IL-11, IL-12, erythropoietin and epidermal growth factor have been shown to play an important role in the prevention of intestinal injury. Using a neonatal rat model, the protective effect of maternal milk has been associated with increased ileal production of anti-inflammatory IL-10.[30] Also, enteric organisms such as nonvirulent *Salmonella* strains are capable of attenuating intestinal inflammatory responses.[31]

Chronic Lung Disease/Bronchopulmonary Dysplasia

Many aspects of the inflammatory response in the context of CLD/BPD remain to be elucidated.

On the one hand, artificially induced lung inflammation through intra-amniotic injection of pro-inflammatory cytokines in rabbits results in increased lung volumes, increased surfactant production and improved gas exchange.[32] Likewise, fetal exposure to chorioamnionitis can lead to enhanced lung maturation similar to the effect yielded by antenatal glucocorticoids.[25] This is in line with the findings from the UK EPICure study, indicating that infants born below 26 weeks gestation are more likely to die in the absence of chorioamnionitis and antenatal administration of glucocorticoids.[33]

Alternatively, as previously mentioned, antenatal inflammation can disrupt the process of alveolarization, resulting in alveolar simplification and priming of the fetal lung, rendering it vulnerable for further injury postnatally.[25,34] Indeed, prolonged postnatal mechanical ventilation (>7 days) of lungs that are primed in this way, together with postnatal infection (sepsis or pneumonia) may result in a secondary inflammatory response and the development of CLD/BPD.[35,36] Support for this hypothesis stems from the observation that predominantly, memory cells from the immune system, i.e. lymphocytes and monocytes, are observed in bronchoalveolar lavage fluids obtained from ventilated and antenatally inflamed animal lungs.[37]

Ongoing lung damage in the premature infant may also be caused by failure to downregulate inflammatory responses.[38] Data suggest that preterm newborns with lung inflammation may be unable to activate the anti-inflammatory cytokine IL-10. Comparing preterm infants with term infants in respiratory failure, the ability of lung macrophages to produce TNF-α is nearly identical, whereas a trend toward diminished levels of IL-10 expression exists in the preterm group.[39] Such data suggest an imbalance between pro- and anti-inflammatory responses leading to CLD/BPD.

The role of transforming growth factor-β (TGF-β), i.e. a cytokine participating in adult chronic inflammatory diseases, is still to be elucidated in neonatal inflammatory processes.[40]

Retinopathy of Prematurity

Retinopathy of prematurity (ROP) is an ischemia-induced proliferative retinopathy, affecting premature infants with low birth weight. The process of retinal neovascularization in ROP is complex, involving several angiogenic factors, such as vascular endothelial growth factor. Potential medical therapies for ROP not only include modulators of such angiogenic factors but also endogenous inhibitors and anti-inflammatory drugs. The latter drugs have shown to be efficacious against neovascularization in several animal models of oxygen-induced retinopathy and are currently already trialed for adult diabetic retinopathy and age-related macular degeneration.[41]

PERINATAL INFLAMMATORY RESPONSES, NEONATAL DISEASE AND NEUROMORBIDITY

Both animal and clinical data suggest that intrauterine infection can be linked to adverse neurological outcome either via infection/inflammation induced white matter damage or via infection/inflammation induced preterm birth.[42,43] A recent meta-analysis (23 studies) revealed a significant association between clinical chorioamnionitis, cystic PVL (RR 3.0; 95% CI, 2.2–4.0) and cerebral palsy (RR 1.9; 95% CI, 1.4-2.5), whereas histologic chorioamnionitis was associated with cystic PVL (RR 1.6; 95% CI, 1.5–2.9) but less with cerebral palsy (RR 1.6, 95% CI, 0.9–2.7).[12] The same group recently described an increased risk for neurological sequelae in term infants with funisitis.[44]

It is also likely that postnatal infection/inflammation contributes to a long-term adverse neurodevelopment, as a recent UK trial indicated a four times higher risk of cerebral palsy amongst infants

with neonatal sepsis compared to those without.[45] A significant association between increased levels of inflammatory cytokines in the newborn and the development of spastic di-, quadri- and hemiplegia has been demonstrated[24] with increased concentrations of cytokines (TNF-α, IL-1β, IL-6 and the anti-inflammatory IL-10) correlating with cerebral lesions detected by MRI.[46]

However, several variables account for the observation that not all studies suggest such association between infection/inflammation and adverse outcome in newborn infants (see Fig. 4.1), i.e. (1) timing issues, (2) nature of the infectious/inflammatory process, (3) established and new anti-insult strategies, (4) morbidity in organs other than the brain, (5) genetic influences and (6) environmental factors.

Timing Issues

Clinical chorioamnionitis is based on the acute presence of two or more of the following clinical signs: maternal temperature, maternal tachycardia, fetal tachycardia, maternal leukocytosis, uterine tenderness and foul smelling amniotic fluid. However, intrauterine infection may also remain undetected for months as a chronic indolent inflammatory process. Also, bacterial vaginosis can result in intrauterine colonization present at conception; if the organisms are not cleared within 4–8 weeks after the expanding membranes seal the endometrial cavity, the infection may result in preterm delivery. Hence, in the absence of clear criteria to identify the severity and duration of in utero infection, it is not surprising that the clinical outcome is unpredictable, ranging from normal fetal development with histologic chorioamnionitis as an incidental finding to severe chorioamnionitis leading to in or ex utero death with long-term neurological sequelae.[25]

Type and Presence of Pathogen

Not only timing but also the nature of the infection may determine the outcome.[43] For example, administration of a low dose of *Escherichia coli* 055:B5 endotoxin to rats, prior to short periods of hypoxia-ischemia, increases the overall brain injury.[18] However, the opposite effect is observed using a different bacterial toxin (lipoteichoic acid) in a similar rat model.[47] Amniotic fluid contaminated with *E. coli* but not with *Ureaplasma urealyticum* and *Mycoplasma* increases the risk of CLD/BPD,[48] although one could criticize that the latter two species are more difficult to grow in vitro.

Evidence suggests that preterm delivery and neonatal morbidity may be better predicted by the degree and nature of the FIRS to infection (i.e. the host response) than by the presence of (a combination of) pathogens (i.e. positive amniotic cultures).[8,49] It is within this context that functional polymorphisms of the different cytokines may play a role as they may determine each individual's genetic susceptibility and response to infection.

Anti-insult Strategies

As perinatal infection/inflammation seems to be an important risk factor for adverse neonatal outcome, the development of appropriately designed (brain) protective strategies will, to a great extent, become indispensable within neonatal care over the next decade.[50] However, the difficulties experienced hereto are at least threefold: (1) we are currently unable to prospectively identify those infants at greatest risk for developing (neuro)morbidity; (2) the presence of both beneficial and detrimental physiologic effects by cytokines complicates any targeted intervention; (3) the origin of perinatally acquired brain damage is currently thought to be multifactorial, possibly including hypoxia/perfusion failure, thyroid hormone deficiency, genetic factors, thrombotic processes, growth factor deficiency, excess free reactive oxygen production and antenatal infection.[51]

Antenatal Strategies

Steroids: Endogenous glucocorticoids, released by the fetal adrenal cortex, downregulate the expression and action of cytokines both in the periphery and in the brain.[52] Likewise, antenatal administration of exogenous steroids can result in a reduced FIRS.[53] Antenatal steroids administered to women at risk for preterm delivery decrease the risk of death, respiratory distress[54] and protect very-low-birth-weight infants against the risk of neuromorbidity.[55] However, antenatal steroids do not reduce the incidence of CLD/BPD, as the drug induces alveolar simplification and hence primes the lungs for postnatal ventilation-mediated injury.[25] In addition, whereas betamethasone yields an initial suppressive effect on inflammation, it may ultimately result in "late inflammation".[56]

It, thus seems that the exposure to infection/inflammation together with antenatal administration of glucocorticoids can both "mature and injure" the fetus. The "net effect" in terms of adverse neonatal outcome may depend on exposure to postnatal noxious interventions such as ventilation, high concentration of oxygen, etc. These time-dependent interactions between steroids and inflammation warrant further investigation.

Antibiotics: The administration of antibiotics following PrePROM results in a significant reduction in chorioamnionitis, a delay in delivery and reduced neonatal morbidity (e.g. neonatal infection, use of surfactant, oxygen need, abnormal findings on cranial ultrasound).[57] Due to an increased risk of NEC, co-amoxiclav should be avoided, whilst erythromycin seems a better choice, possibly because of a smaller endotoxin release by damaged bacteria.[58] The current treatment for clinical chorioamnionitis is delivery of the fetus and subsequent treatment with antibiotics. Maternal treatment in such cases is ineffective because the amniotic cavity is largely a sequestered site inaccessible to antibiotics.

Mode of delivery: Normal labor is always associated with some form of hypoxic stress, which may be detrimental if the fetal brain is more vulnerable to hypoxia in the presence of antenatal infection/inflammation. However, there is no clear evidence that suggests an elective caesarean section is more neuroprotective than normal labor in the case of (chronic or acute) chorioamnionitis.

Postnatal Strategies

Nonspecific therapy for severe sepsis comprises antibiotics, aggressive fluid resuscitation, inotropes and ventilatory support. More specific strategies are aimed at tapering of sepsis-related immunodeficiency syndromes by using recombinant growth factors, such as G-CSF, GM-CSF and interferon. Recombinant activated protein C is an anti-inflammatory, antithrombotic and fibrinolytic agent that has been successfully used in severe sepsis in adults. However, its use is not approved in infants or children.[59]

Treatment of *NEC* currently consists of antibiotics and hemodynamic stabilization, within some cases the need to proceed to surgery. However, a better understanding of the mechanisms underlying its pathogenesis is needed. For example, understanding the protective effects of maternal milk could be beneficial either in the prevention of NEC or in the development of future therapeutic strategies to cure NEC.[30]

Postnatal steroids are commonly administered in severe CLD/BPD, as data suggest that preterm newborns with lung inflammation may be unable to activate anti-inflammatory cytokine pathways.[39] Dose-related inhibition of cytokine synthesis is indeed observed when treating monocytes with dexamethasone in vitro.[60] Although early postnatal anti-inflammatory therapy could help in preventing CLD/BPD, prophylactic dexamethasone cannot be recommended as there are a number of potential interactions between surfactant and cytokine effects on the preterm lung which have not been fully evaluated.[38] In addition, postnatal administration of steroids has been associated with neurodevelopmental impairment warranting further randomized controlled evaluation of its risks versus benefits.[61]

It is to be hoped that we will see multicenter clinical trials over *the next decade*, evaluating inflammatory protection and inflammatory response modification in the newborn infant. Such requires further detailed animal work of immune modulatory drugs and their kinetics within the newborn age group.[62] Inflammatory protection can be achieved by exogenous administration of IL-10, although complex differential effects between its central and peripheral effects need further exploration.[63] The exogenous administration of response modifiers/receptor antagonists currently evaluated in animal models (e.g. IL-1β receptor antagonist or soluble TNF-receptor) may not be without risk, as many of the pro-inflammatory cytokines exhibit fragile equilibria of biological activity.[64] As an example, the presence of TNF-α can have beneficial effects, whereas blocking TNF-α in adults with septic shock results in increased mortality.[65] Future strategies, therefore, must aim to "redress the optimal cytokine balance" rather than "preventing the inflammatory response".

Morbidity in Organs other than the Brain

Is there any evidence that a neonatal inflammatory response (e.g. sepsis, NEC) involves an increased risk for neuromorbidity?

Sepsis/NEC

The role of pro-inflammatory cytokines during sepsis/NEC in the etiology of cerebral palsy remains controversial. However, preliminary reports suggest a significant association between TNF-α, IL-8, and an abnormal cognitive and psychomotor outcome at the age of 24–28 months.[66]

Lung Inflammation

A complex interaction exists between lung and brain inflammatory processes. Lung disease has been mimicked in transgenic mice that overexpress human IL-1β in the respiratory epithelium.[67] The expression of a number of genes participating in inflammation was also increased in their brains, although no major histological differences were detected compared to control animals. Ventilation of inflamed preterm lungs may also result in more lung inflammation, creating an excess of cytokines in the systemic circulation, which in turn may promote the development of CLD/BPD, and, in addition, may result in remote (brain) damage.[37]

Host–Genetics

Single-nucleotide polymorphisms (SNPs) consist of single base substitutions in a DNA sequence. Almost all genes contain SNPs, but only a minority of SNPs result in amino acid variation in protein products. In addition, many of the functional SNPs occur in the promoter region rather than the gene itself and affect protein levels through altered transcription. Polymorphism-association studies compare the prevalence of a genetic marker in persons with a given condition to the prevalence in controls.[68] Gene polymorphisms that may influence perinatal outcome through alteration of the response to infection, have been reported for the IL-1 receptor antagonist,[69] IL-6,[70] Interferon-γ[71] and TNF-α.[72] Likewise, cytokine gene polymorphisms may modify the risk for brain injury and hence act as an endogenous inflammatory response modification mechanism.[22] As an example, the IL-6 -174G|C genotype has been associated with impaired neurological outcome in preterm children.[73]

Cytokines are able to mediate intravascular cell adhesion, coagulation and/or thrombosis, and vasoconstriction. In the presence of an existing thrombophilia or a cytokine polymorphism resulting in increased susceptibility to infection, the actions of these cytokines in the fetal brain may be enough to result in adverse neurological outcome.[74]

Such outcome-related research is complicated by the fact that (1) one needs to examine the frequencies of several cytokine genotypes, (2) in infants as well as in mothers, (3) whilst taking into account demographics, newborn illness severity and several other risk factors. The ultimate goal is to use identified SNPs as a biologic guide to target new anti-inflammatory strategies toward the most genetically vulnerable premature infants (i.e. pharmacogenomics).

Environment

Impaired neurodevelopment after a fetal/neonatal inflammatory response most likely occurs via a complex interaction between genetic and environmental processes, such as home environment, maternal education, socioeconomic and ethnic backgrounds.

CONCLUSION

We investigated the available evidence suggesting a link between inflammatory responses and adverse neonatal outcome. Currently there is no silver bullet to prevent an impaired neurodevelopmental outcome in the event of a fetal and/or neonatal inflammatory response. Future research needs to focus on (1) the relation between fetal, maternal and neonatal inflammatory processes, i.e. CLD/BPD and NEC; (2) the interaction between inflammatory responses and genetic or environmental factors; (3) the use of advanced techniques for laboratory research and neuroimaging; (4) large and well-designed observational studies that use well-defined outcome variables for transparent logistic regression analyses in large samples of patients, with sufficiently long periods of follow-up.[64] Although such research will be complex, only then we may become successful in the identification of prenatal and postnatal risk profiles that permit the introduction of new anti-inflammatory interventions in the newborn.

REFERENCES

1. Yoon BH, Romero R, Park JS, et al. The relationship among inflammatory lesions of the umbilical cord (funisitis), umbilical cord plasma interleukin 6 concentration, amniotic fluid infection, and neonatal sepsis. AJOG. 2000;183:1124-9.

2. Watterberg KL, Demers LM, Scott SM, et al. Chorioamnionitis and early lung inflammation in infants in whom bronchopulmonary dysplasia develops. Pediatrics. 1996;97:210-5.

3. Ng PC, Li K, Wong RP, et al. Proinflammatory and anti-inflammatory cytokine responses in preterm infants with systemic infections. Arch Dis Child Fetal Neonatal Ed. 2003;88: F209-13.

4. Goldenberg RL, Hauth JC, Andrews WW. Intrauterine infection and preterm delivery. N Engl J Med. 2000;18;342:1500-7.

5. Jacobsson B, Mattsby-Baltzer I, Andersch B, et al. Microbial invasion and cytokine response in amniotic fluid in a Swedish population of women with preterm prelabor rupture of membranes. Acta Obstet Gynecol Scand. 2003;82:423-31.

6. Romero R, Yoon BH, Mazor M, et al. A comparative study of the diagnostic performance of amniotic fluid glucose, white blood cell count, interleukin-6 and gram stain in the detection of microbial invasion in patients with preterm premature rupture of membranes. AJOG. 1993;169:839-51.

7. Gomez R, Romero R, Ghezzi F, et al. The fetal inflammatory response syndrome. Am J Obstet Gynecol. 1998;179:194-202.

8. Romero R, Gomez R, Ghezzi F, et al. A fetal systemic inflammatory response is followed by the spontaneous onset of preterm parturition. AJOG. 1998;179:186-93.

9. Bell MJ, Hallenbeck JM, Gallo V. Determining the fetal inflammatory response in an experimental model of intrauterine inflammation in rats. Pediatr Res. 2004;56(4):541-6.

10. Yoon BH, Kim CJ, Romero R, et al. Experimentally induced intrauterine infection causes fetal brain white matter lesions in rabbits. AJOG. 1997;177:797-802.

11. Yoon BH, Jun JK, Romero R, et al. Amniotic fluid inflammatory cytokines (interleukin-6, interleukin-1β, and tumor necrosis factor-α), neonatal brain white matter lesions, and cerebral palsy. AJOG. 1997;177:19-26.

12. Wu YW, Colford JM. Chorioamnionitis as a risk factor for cerebral palsy: A meta-analysis. JAMA. 2000;284:1417-24.

13. Hitti J, Krohn MA, Patton DL, et al. Amniotic fluid tumor necrosis factor-alpha and the risk of respiratory distress syndrome among preterm infants. AJOG. 1997;177:50-6.

14. Leviton A, Paneth N, Reuss ML, et al. Maternal infection, fetal inflammatory response, and brain damage in very low birth weight infants. Developmental Epidemiology Network Investigators. Pediatr Res. 1999a;46:566-75.

15. Kadhim H, Tabarki B, Verellen G, et al. Inflammatory cytokines in the pathogenesis of periventricular leukomalacia. Neurology. 2001;56:1278-84.

16. Hagberg H. No correlation between cerebral palsy and cytokines in postnatal blood of preterms: commentary on the article by Nelson et al. on page 600. Pediatr Res. 2003;53:544-5.

17. Shalak LF, Laptook AR, Jafri HS, et al. Clinical chorioamnionitis, elevated cytokines, and brain injury in term infants. Pediatrics. 2002;110:673-80.

18. Eklind S, Mallard C, Leverin AL, et al. Bacterial endotoxin sensitizes the immature brain to hypoxicischemic injury. Eur J Neurosci. 2001;13:1101-6.

19. Bona E, Andersson AL, Blomgren K, et al. Chemokine and inflammatory cell response to hypoxia-ischemia in immature rats. Pediatr Res. 1999;45:500-9.

20. Loddick SA, Rothwell NJ. Mechanisms of tumor necrosis factor alpha action on neurodegeneration: interaction with insulin-like growth factor-1. Proc Natl Acad Sci USA. 1999;96:9449-51.

21. Hagan P, Barks JD, Yabut M, et al. Adenovirus-mediated over-expression of interleukin-1 receptor antagonist reduces susceptibility to excitotoxic brain injury in perinatal rats. Neuroscience. 1996;75:1033-45.

22. Dammann O, Durum SK, Leviton A. Modification of infection-associated risks of preterm birth and white matter damage in the preterm newborn by polymorphisms in the tumor necrosis factor locus? Pathogenesis. 1999;1:171-7.

23. Hagberg H, Wennerholm UB, Sävman K. Sequelae of chorio-amnionitis. Current Opinion Inf Dis. 2002;15:301-6.

24. Nelson KB, Dambrosia JM, Grether JK, et al. Neonatal cytokines and coagulation factors in children with cerebral palsy. Ann Neurol. 1998;44:665-75.

25. Jobe AH. Antenatal factors and the development of bronchopulmonary dysplasia. Sem Neonatol. 2003;8:9-17.

26. Toti P, De Felice C, Stumpo M, et al. Acute thymic involution in fetuses and neonates with chorioamnionitis. Hum Pathol. 2000;31:1121-8.

27. Levy GG, Nichols WC, Lian EC. et al. Mutations in a member of the ADAMTS gene family cause thrombotic thrombocytopenic purpura. Nature. 2001;413:488-94.

28. Romagnoli C, Frezza S, Cingolani A, et al. Plasma levels of interleukin-6 and interleukin-10 in preterm neonates evaluated for sepsis. Eur J Pediatr. 2001;160:345-50.

29. Martinez-Tallo E, Claure N, Bancalari E. Necrotizing enterocolitis in full-term or near-term infants: Risk factors. Biol Neonate. 1997;71:292-8.

30. Dvorak B, Halpern MD, Holubec H. et al. Maternal milk reduces severity of necrotizing enterocolitis and increases intestinal IL-10 in a neonatal rat model. Ped Research. 2003;53:426-33.

31. Neish AS, Gewirtz AT, Zeng H, et al. Prokaryotic regulation of epithelial responses by inhibition of IkappaB-alpha ubiquitination. Science. 2000;289:1560-3.

32. Bry K, Lappalainen U, Hallman M. Intraamniotic interleukin-1 accelerates surfactant protein synthesis in fetal rabbits and improves lung stability after premature birth. J Clin Invest. 1997;99:2992-9.

33. Costeloe K, Hennessy E, Gibson AT, et al. The EPICure study: Outcomes to discharge from hospital for infants born at the threshold of viability. Pediatrics. 2000;106:659-71.

34. Willet KE, Kramer BW, Kallapur SG, et al. Intra-amniotic injection of IL-1 induces inflammation and maturation in fetal sheep lung. Am J Physiol Lung Cell Mol Physiol. 2002;282: 411-20.

35. Speer CP. New insights into the pathogenesis of pulmonary inflammation in preterm infants. Biol Neonate. 2001;79:205-9.

36. Van Marter LJ, Dammann O, Allred EN, et al. Chorioamnionitis, mechanical ventilation, and postnatal sepsis as modulators of chronic lung disease in preterm infants. J Pediatr. 2002;140:171-6.

37. Kramer BW, Ikegami M, Jobe AH. Intratracheal endotoxin causes systemic inflammation in ventilated preterm lambs. Am J Respir Crit Care Med. 2002;165: 463-9.

38. De Dooy JJ, Mahieu LM, Van Bever HP. The role of inflammation in the development of chronic lung disease in neonates. Eur J Pediatr. 2001;160:457-63.

39. Blahnik MJ, Ramanathan R, Riley CR, et al. Lipopolysaccharide-induced tumor necrosis factor-alpha and IL-10 production by lung macrophages from preterm and term neonates. Pediatr Res. 2001;50:726-31.

40. Marek A, Brodzicki J, Liberek A, et al. TGF-β (transforming growth factor-β) in chronic inflammatory conditions – a new diagnostic prognostic marker? Med Sci Monit. 2002;8(7): RA145-51.

41. Mechoulam H, Pierce EA. Retinopathy of prematurity: molecular pathology and therapeutic strategies. Am J Pharmacogenomics. 2003;3:261-77.

42. Dantzer R, Wollman EE, Vitkovic L, et al. Cytokines, stress, and depression. Conclusions and perspectives. Adv Exp Med Biol. 1999;46:317-29.

43. Dammann O, Kuban K, Leviton A. Perinatal infection, fetal inflammatory response, white matter damage, and cognitive limitations in children born preterm. Ment Ret Dev Disab Res Rev. 2002;8:46-50.

44. Wu YW, Malin BT, Johnson LL, et al. Funisitis and neurologic abnormalities in term infants. Ped Research. 2003;53:545A.

45. Wheater M, Rennie JM. Perinatal infection is an important risk factor for cerebral palsy in very-low-birthweight infants. Dev Med Child Neurol. 2000;42:364-7.

46. Duggan PJ, Maalouf EF, Watts TL, et al. Intrauterine T-cell activation and increased proinflammatory cytokine concentrations in preterm infants with cerebral lesions. Lancet. 2001;358:1699-700.

47. Palmer C, Roberts RL, Towfighi J, et al. Endotoxin pretreatment protects neonatal rats from hypoxic ischemic brain injury. Pediatr Res. 2001;49:122A.

48. Mittendorf R, Covert R, Montag A, et al. Association between fetal inflammatory response syndrome and bronchopulmonary dysplasia. Ped Research. 2003;53: 387A.

49. Yoon BH, Romero R, Moon JB, et al. Clinical significance of intraamniotic inflammation in patients with preterm labor and intact membranes. AJOG. 2001;185:1130-6.

50. Perlman JM. Markers of asphyxia and neonatal brain injury. N Engl J Med. 1999;341:364-5.

51. Gressens P, Rogido M, Paindaveine B, et al. The impact of neonatal intensive care practices on the developing brain. J Pediatr. 2002;140:646-53.

52. Goujon E, Parnet P, Aubert A, et al. Corticosterone regulates behavioral effects of zlipopolysaccharide and interleukin-1 beta in mice. Am J Physiol. 1995;269:154-9.

53. Crowley PA. Antenatal corticosteroid therapy: A meta-analysis of the randomized trials, 1972 to 1994. AJOG. 1995;173:322-35.

54. Shimoya K, Taniguchi T, Matsuzaki N, et al. Chorioamnionitis decreased incidence of respiratory distress syndrome by elevating fetal interleukin-6 serum concentration. Hum Reprod. 2000;15:2234-40.

55. Leviton A, Dammann O, Allred EN, et al. Antenatal corticosteroids and cranial ultrasonographic abnormalities. AJOG. 1999;181: 1007-17.

56. Kallapur SG, Kramer BW, Moss TJ, et al. Maternal glucocorticoids increase endotoxin-induced lung inflammation in preterm lambs. Am J Physiol Lung Cell Mol Physiol. 2003;284:633-42.

57. Kenyon SL, Taylor DJ, Tarnow-Mordi W, et al. Broad-spectrum antibiotics for preterm, prelabour rupture of fetal membranes: The ORACLE I randomized trial. ORACLE Collaborative Group. Lancet. 2001;357:979-88.

58. Kenyon SL, Taylor DJ, Tarnow-Mordi W, et al. Broad-spectrum antibiotics for spontaneous preterm labour: The ORACLE II randomized trial. ORACLE Collaborative Group. Lancet. 2001;357:989-94.

59. Matthay MA. Severe sepsis—a new treatment with both anticoagulant and anti-inflammatory properties. N Engl J Med. 2001;344:759-62.

60. Schultz C, Rott C, Temming P, et al. Enhanced interleukin-6 and interleukin-8 synthesis in term and preterm infants. Pediatr Res. 2002;51:317-22.

61. Barrington KJ. The adverse neuro-developmental effects of postnatal steroids in the preterm infant: a systematic review of RCTs. BMC Pediatrics. 2001;1:1.

62. Dembinski J, Behrendt D, Martini R, et al. Modulation of pro- and anti-inflammatory cytokine production in very preterm infants. Cytokine. 2003;21:200-6.

63. Mesples B, Plaisant F, Gressens P. Effects of interleukin10 on neonatal excitotoxic brain lesions in mice. Brain Res Dev Brain Res. 2003;141:25-32.

64. Dammann O, Leviton A. Brain damage in preterm newborns: Biological response modification as a strategy to reduce disabilities. J Pediatr. 2000;136: 433-8.

65. Fisher CJ, Agosti JM, Opal SM, et al. Treatment of septic shock with the tumor necrosis factor receptor: Fc fusion protein. The Soluble TNF Receptor Sepsis Study Group. N Engl J Med. 1996;334: 1697-702.

66. Lodha AK, Asztalos E, Moore AM. Elevated cytokines and poor neurodevelopmental outcome in prematurity and NEC. Ped Research. 2003;53:386A.

67. Lappalainen U, Bry K. Lung disease in newborn mice overexpressing IL-1 in the lung. Ped Research. 2003; 53:461A.

68. Peters RG, Boekholdt SM. Gene polymorphisms and the risk of myocardial infarction—an emerging relation. N Engl J Med. 2002; 347:1963-5.

69. Witkin SS, Gerber S, Ledger WJ. Influence of interleukin-1 receptor antagonist gene polymorphism on disease. Clin Infect Dis. 2002;34:204-9.

70. Terry CF, Loukaci V, Green FR. Cooperative influence of genetic polymorphisms on interleukin 6 transcriptional regulation. J Biol Chem. 2000;275:18138-44.

71. Orsi N, Logghe H, Lynch K, et al. Carriage of the high secreting interferon gamma polymorphism is associated with an increased risk of preterm delivery and premature rupture of membranes. AJOG. 2002;187:S120.

72. Hajeer AH, Hutchinson IV. Influence of TNF-α gene polymorphisms on TNF-α production and disease. Hum Immunol. 2001;62:1191-9.

73. Harding D, Dhamrait S, Humphries SE, et al. Is Interleukin-6 genotype associated with outcome after preterm birth? Ped Research. 2003;53:540A.

74. Gibson C, MacLennan A, Goldwater P, et al. Antenatal causes of cerebral palsy: associations between inherited thrombophilias, viral and bacterial infection, and inherited susceptibility to infection. Obstetrical and Gynecological Survey. 2003;58:209-20.

CHAPTER 5

Neonatal Sepsis

A Papageorgiou, E Pelausa, L Kovacs

INTRODUCTION

Globally, neonatal infection results in half a million deaths each year, the vast majority of which occur in developing countries, and is the third most common cause of death in the first 28 days of life.[1] Although recent advances in medical care have resulted in improved survival rates of the smallest and sickest infants, they have also inadvertently resulted in increased rates of serious infection with organisms previously considered noninvasive, such as coagulase-negative staphylococci (CoNS). This is particularly true in the presence of extreme prematurity, exposure to invasive procedures, indwelling catheters, and prolonged use of broad-spectrum antibiotics.

Neonatal sepsis is a clinical syndrome characterized by systemic signs of infection, accompanied by a positive blood culture. However, this ideal definition is not met in a significant number of cases. The fact that sepsis is part of every differential list of neonatal symptomatology underlines the wide variety in which it may manifest. To "rule out sepsis" is the most common diagnostic dilemma in neonatology. When clinical signs of sepsis are present, the appropriate therapeutic measures should be undertaken, including the initiation of empiric antibiotic therapy, even in the absence of a positive blood culture or of supporting laboratory evidence. The rationale for this approach is the appreciable mortality and morbidity associated with neonatal sepsis. The frequent absence of a positive blood culture can be explained by many factors, such as the small blood volumes sent for culture, suboptimal processing of specimens, previous exposure to intrapartum antibiotics, and the intermittent nature of the bacteremia. Therefore, in the presence of clinical signs compatible with sepsis, laboratory tests are generally helpful not to "rule out", but rather to confirm the presence of sepsis.

Neonatal sepsis can be categorized according to age at the time of presentation. Early-onset sepsis (EOS) refers to cases presenting within the first 72 hours of life, and late-onset sepsis (LOS) presents at four or more days of life. These two subcategories may have different origins, bacteriologic profiles, and clinical presentation (Table 5.1).

Whereas EOS reflects exposure and risks around birth, LOS denotes neonatal care practices that impact on the infant. In the Western world, group B streptococcus (GBS) and *Escherichia coli* (*E. coli*) are the predominant pathogens, whereas in developing countries, *Staphylococcus (S. aureus)*, Klebsiella species and *E. coli* account for 55% of cases[1-3] (Table 5.2).

Neonatal sepsis occurs in 2–8 infants per thousand live births, and the incidence increases 50-fold in low birth weight infants.[4] It is also estimated that a quarter of infected neonates may develop meningitis. Mortality ranges from 10% to 20% and serious sequelae, particularly in the presence of meningitis, may occur in up to 20–30% of cases.

The neonate is at particular risk of infection for three main reasons: (1) immaturity of the immune system, (2) ineffective structural barriers (e.g. skin, mucous membranes), and (3) absence or paucity of protective flora. The limited microbial defense arises from a lack of antigenic memory, low concentrations of T and B cells and passage from a sterile intrauterine environment to the postnatal environment. Pro- and anti-inflammatory cytokines and other mediators are involved in the continued persistence of systemic signs of sepsis, even after bacterial killing. The effect of specific cytokines on cell tissues and organs provide insight into the inflammatory response.[5] Currently, there are no specific early diagnostic markers to distinguish sepsis from a noninfectious process known as the "systemic inflammatory response syndrome". However, there is mounting evidence of a link between infection-inflammation and organ damage to the fetus and the newborn. Inflammation may induce both teratogenic and destructive effects. Hence, the extensive use of empiric broad spectrum antenatal or postnatal antibiotics is not surprising. On the other hand, this approach also carries the risk of increasing the prevalence of microbial flora resistant to commonly used antibiotics.

Chorioamnionitis is an acute inflammation of the fetal membranes due to ascending microbial infection. It is more common following prolonged rupture of the membranes, but may also occur despite intact membranes, as is the case with *Ureaplasma* species and *Mycoplasma hominis*, which are present in the lower genital tract of about 70% of women.[6] Chorioamnionitis is a common cause of preterm labor and

Table 5.1: Comparison of early-onset and late-onset sepsis

Characteristics	Early-onset sepsis	Late-onset sepsis
Age at presentation	≤ 72 hours	≥ 4 days
Source of organism	Mother's genital tract	Mother NICU environment
Clinical presentation	Rapid, multiorgan, frequent pneumonia	Slow progression, focal, frequent meningitis
Mortality rate	10–40%	5–20%

Table 5.2: Principal pathogens implicated in neonatal sepsis

Early-onset sepsis	Late-onset sepsis
Group B streptococcus	Coagulase-negative staphylococci
Escherichia coli	*Staphylococcus aureus*
Other Gram-negatives	*Escherichia coli*
Other Gram-positives	Klebsiella species
Listeria monocytogenes	Pseudomonas species

its incidence rises with decreasing gestational age (GA).[7] Although nearly 80% of infants born prior to 28 completed weeks of gestation are exposed to chorioamnionitis, the incidence of neonatal infection does not exceed one-third of those exposed. Premature infants exhibit the highest sepsis-related mortality and morbidity, claiming the lives of approximately 3,000 neonates worldwide every day. The fetal inflammatory response to sepsis (FIRS) is also responsible for a significant rate of neonatal mortality and morbidity.[8] Morbidity from FIRS includes multiorgan effects, particularly on the brain and lungs, but also on the thymus, the adrenal glands, the gastrointestinal (GI) tract, the cardiovascular system, and the eyes.[9] The clinical diagnosis of chorioamnionitis is often difficult, and many cases remain clinically silent. Only histological examination of the placenta can truly correlate the diagnosis of the fetal inflammatory response to chorioamnionitis.[7]

EARLY-ONSET SEPSIS

Most infants with EOS demonstrate clinical illness within 24 hours after birth, with respiratory distress and subtle clinical signs of instability. Pathogens are usually acquired from the mother's genitourinary tract. The portal of entry is the upper airway mucosa, respiratory system, digestive tract or via trauma to the skin and soft tissues, with invasion and infection reflecting the infant's diminished immunocompetence and the virulence of the pathogen.

The incidence in the United States has remained stable at about 0.8 cases per 1,000 live births, with an estimated annual burden of 3,320 cases and 390 deaths. GBS and *E. coli* are the most common pathogens. In one study, the rate of EOS from GBS was 0.41 per 1,000 live births and from *E. coli* was 0.28 per 1,000 live births. The majority of infants with invasive GBS infection are born at term (73%). *E. coli* and other Gram-negative organisms are identified more often in septic premature infants. Epidemiological trends show a decreasing incidence of GBS disease, mainly attributable to the prenatal screening and intrapartum prophylactic antibiotic protocol.[10-13]

Group B Streptococcus

Group B Streptococcus (*Streptococcus agalactiae*) remains the most common cause of EOS in neonates, resulting in significant morbidity and mortality. It is a Gram-positive aerobic diplococcus, culturing in pairs or short chains, and is classified into ten subtypes based on its capsular polysaccharides. Type Ia, Ib, II, III and V account for 95% of cases in the US. Type III is responsible for the majority of cases of early-onset meningitis and of late-onset GBS disease. GBS is part of the normal vaginal flora, with the natural reservoir being the GI tract.[14] Colonization of the lower genital tract occurs in 10–30% of women, is variable and transient, such that colonization early in pregnancy does not predict colonization at delivery.[15] GBS bacteriuria occurs in 2–7% of pregnancies, is evidence of heavy colonization and is associated with increased risk of neonatal disease.[16] Diabetes in pregnancy is associated with higher rates of GBS colonization.[17] Heavy colonization with GBS is associated with preterm labor and premature rupture of membranes.[18] Risk factors for neonatal infection include prematurity (GA <37 weeks), prolonged rupture of membranes (>12–18 hours), fever in labor, intra-amniotic infection, young maternal age, black race, Hispanic ethnicity, low levels of maternal GBS-specific anticapsular antibody and previous delivery of an infant with invasive GBS disease.[2]

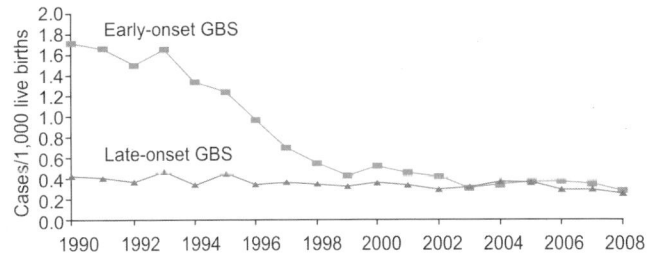

Fig. 5.1: Rates of early- and late-onset Group B Streptococcur (GBS) sepsis, 1990–2008

Prior to intrapartum antibiotic prophylaxis (IAP), EOS from GBS had an incidence of approximately 2 per 1,000 live births (Fig. 5.1).[12] With IAP, the incidence of neonatal disease has decreased (0.34–0.37 per 1,000 live births) and death from EOS GBS is now uncommon, although mortality is higher among preterm infants, with case fatality rates up to 20%, compared to 2–3% among term infants.[19] GBS infection is acquired vertically, with exposure to GBS in the vagina of a colonized mother, through ascending infection to the amniotic fluid, invasion of intact membranes or rarely hematogenous spread. EOS GBS presents as bacteremia (74%), meningitis (14%) and pneumonia (12%).[20] A high index of suspicion and aggressive neonatal care has contributed to the observed decline in mortality.

In 2001–2002, the Center for Disease Control (CDC) in the US, the Haute Autorité de Santé in France and many health boards recommended universal, culture-based screening at 35–37 weeks, with IAP when results were positive for GBS or there were risk factors for neonatal sepsis during labor. In 2010, this was expanded to accept positive identification of GBS colonization from new technologies such as chromogenic agar media and nucleic acid amplification tests (NAATs).[12] IAP is recommended when screening is positive for GBS and where there are risk factors of neonatal infection. Optimal IAP is treatment with penicillin, ampicillin or cefazolin. At least 4 hours of IAP with one of these beta-lactam antibiotics has been shown to be effective in preventing neonatal early-onset GBS sepsis. The efficacy of other antibiotics when the mother has serious penicillin allergy, including clindamycin, vancomycin and erythromycin, has not been demonstrated.[10-12]

The efficacy of a proactive strategy and IAP in reducing rates of EOS from GBS is significant. However, debate remains about whether this culture-based strategy is the optimal use of current resources: 22% of mothers in labor at term will receive IAP to prevent disease in 0.2% of infants and prevent mortality in 0.01% of infants.[21] Another potential negative effect of this strategy is the development of bacterial resistance; thus far, there has not been a rise in non-GBS pathogens, particularly ampicillin-resistant *E. coli*, though close surveillance is warranted.[22] Furthermore, IAP does not prevent LOS from GBS.

Escherichia coli

E. coli are Gram-negative bacilli. Strains with K1 capsular polysaccharide antigen cause 40% of cases of Gram-negative septicemia and 80% of cases of meningitis and are associated with greater invasiveness and severity of infection.[23] Other virulence factors include pili or fimbriae which are filamentous surface appendages that assist with adhesion to epithelial cells, the presence of flagella which are necessary for motility, production of hemolysin which induces formation of pores in cell membranes, production of aerobactin which increase iron uptake and antibiotic resistance with beta-lactamases.

E. coli is the most common cause of urinary tract infection (UTI) in the neonatal period, accounting for 80% in several large series. Prior to the 1970s and the appearance of GBS, *E. coli* was the leading cause of neonatal sepsis. At the present time, with widespread use of IAP and a decrease in the incidence of GBS infections, *E. coli* is re-emerging, with some concern regarding ampicillin-resistant *E. coli* infections. Although the incidence of *E. coli* infections has remained stable for term infants, there has been an increase in premature infants. Risk factors for *E. coli* infection include prematurity, birth weight less than 1,500 grams, intrapartum fever, IAP and prolonged premature rupture of the membranes. No effective prophylactic strategy has been identified. *E. coli* sepsis and meningitis are associated with high mortality and morbidity rates.

Other Pathogens

Gram-negative bacteria that cause neonatal infection include *Klebsiella, Enterobacter, Proteus, Citrobacter, Pseudomonas, Serratia, Salmonella species* and rarely *Haemophilus influenzae* and anaerobic Gram-negative bacilli. Most often acquired from the mother's genital tract, horizontal spread from personnel and environmental sites, such as sinks, respiratory therapy equipment and countertops, can occur. Predisposing factors have been identified, such as metabolic abnormalities (e.g. galactosemia), fetal hypoxia, acidosis, prematurity, prolonged rupture of membranes, maternal intrapartum antibiotics, invasive procedures, and indwelling catheters. Multiple mechanisms of resistance in Gram-negative bacilli include overproduction of chromosomal or plasmid-derived AmpC beta-lactamase and plasmid-mediated extended-spectrum beta-lactamases (ESBL), with resistance to penicillins, cephalosporins and monobactams. Empiric treatment should begin with ampicillin and gentamicin until the susceptibility pattern is known and antibiotic choice can be tailored to the specific pathogen.

Listeria monocytogenes are aerobic, Gram-positive bacilli that cause primarily food borne diseases from contaminated foods, such as unpasteurized milk, soft cheeses, undercooked meats and unwashed raw vegetables. Maternal illness can present as malaise, headache, GI symptoms, fever and back pain, with prodromal illness identified in 65% prior to delivery of an infected fetus.[24] Fetal infection results from transplacental transmission following maternal bacteremia and ascending spread from vaginal colonization. Neonatal illnesses present as early-onset (usually pneumonia and septicemia) and late-onset (usually meningitis) diseases, similar to GBS. In severe infection, an erythematous rash with small papules termed "granulomatosis infantisepticum" can occur. Treatment consists of ampicillin and gentamicin for 10–14 days.

LATE-ONSET SEPSIS

Whereas the incidence of EOS has decreased over the last decade, the incidence of late-onset sepsis LOS has remained stable at approximately 0.35 cases per 1,000 live births (Fig. 5.1).[12] In a recent paper describing a prospective population-based French regional data, Didier described three major types of LOS: CoNS

among preterm infants, *E. coli*-induced UTI in term infants and GBS with severe infection.[25] The median age of presentation is reported to be 20 days. Preterm infants have higher rates of LOS and higher mortality. Very-low-birth weight (VLBW) infants had an LOS rate of 21–24% and more than 50% of infants weighing less than 750 grams at birth have at least one episode of LOS.[67] Stoll et al found LOS in 36% of extremely premature infants (22–28 weeks). Predominant organisms were Gram-positive (70%), CoNS (48%), Gram-negative (18%) and fungi (12%).[2]

Coagulase-Negative Staphylococci

As a result of the great advances in neonatal care, coagulase-negative staphylococci are responsible for the majority of LOS in hospitalized infants. Coagulase-negative staphylococci (CoNS) are the most common cause of bacteremia and septicemia in preterm infants, particularly in the VLBW (<1500 grams) and indeed, episodes of health-care related bacteremia in all age groups. Of 16 CoNS species, *Staphylococcus epidermidis* (*S. epidermidis*), *S. hemolyticus*, *S. saprophyticus*, *S. scheleiferi* and *S. lugdunensis* are often associated with human infections. CoNS inhabit the skin and mucous membranes. By 2–4 days of age, most infants are colonized by CoNS in multiple sites. Inoculation can be at the time of placement of central venous devices and skin breaks, through mucous membranes and the gut, and less frequently via the hands of health care personnel. CoNS produce an exopolysaccharide slime biofilm that promotes binding of the CoNS to medical devices such as central venous catheters, peritoneal and ventricular shunts, which make the organisms relatively inaccessible to host defenses particularly to phagocytosis by macrophages, and to antibiotics. The incubation period can be variable, with a long delay between acquisition and disease. Risk factors for CoNS are diminished immunocompetence and presence of indwelling devices. Thus, there is an inverse relationship between gestation and birth weight versus risk of CoNS sepsis. Of interest, the number of central lines, and central line duration, are associated with increased risk for neonatal sepsis.[26]

Staphylococcus aureus

Staphylococci are catalase-positive, Gram-positive cocci that appear like grape clusters under the microscope. They are ubiquitous and survive extreme conditions of dryness, heat, low-oxygen and high salt. *S. aureus* are the only species of staphylococci that produce coagulase. Colonies are golden and strongly hemolytic on blood agar. They produce a range of toxins, including alpha-toxin, beta-toxin, gamma-toxin, delta-toxin, exfoliatin, enterotoxins, Panton-Valentine leukocidin (PVL), and toxic shock syndrome toxin-1 (TSST-1). *S. aureus* has many surface proteins that allow the organism to bind to tissues and foreign bodies, thus permitting the organism to adhere to catheters, prosthetic and other devices. *S. aureus* colonizes the skin, nasopharynx, GI tract and umbilical area in most neonates. *S. aureus* colonization varies from 20% to 90% after the first week of life.[27] In a more recent study, *S. aureus* neonatal intensive care unit (NICU) colonization rates were 6.4–13.5 cases per 1,000 patient days.[28] The sources of most colonizing isolates are initially the nursery staff or the immediate environment.[29]

Although *S. aureus* colonization is common in neonates, the development of an infection is relatively rare. Infection developed in 2.3% of *S. aureus* colonized neonates in one study.[30] The risk factors for *S. aureus* sepsis is related to increased host susceptibility from multiple factors such as immature immunity, presence of foreign bodies (e.g. central lines, endotracheal and GI tubes), poor nutrition and prolonged hospitalization. Other factors include disruption of skin integrity due to procedures and tape removal and exposure to broad-spectrum antibiotics. Infection can be mild to severe with abscess formation. *S. aureus* pneumonias are characterized by the development of pneumatoceles. Premature infants are at an even greater risk for morbidity and mortality.[31]

Group B Streptococcus

Population data show an incidence rate of GBS LOS from 0.1 to 0.24 per 1,000 live births, with preterms having a higher rate (1.4 per 1,000 live births) than term infants (0.24/1,000 live births). Mothers remain an important source of infection. One recent study found that at the time of LOS diagnosis, 64% of mothers had positive GBS rectovaginal carriage and 3% had GBS mastitis.[32] The latter is consistent with previous suggestions of GBS mastitis as a possible means of GBS transmission via infected breast milk, resulting in heavy infant colonization and subsequent infection. IAP was associated with delayed presentation and milder disease. Classifications of infection were sepsis (57%), meningitis (36%) and focal disease such as septic arthritis or cellulitis (7%).[32] Severe disease, with need for catecholamine support, mechanical ventilation, seizures, meningitis, brain lesions or death, was seen in 45%; mild disease was seen in 22%. Earlier presentation of LOS (from 7 to 30 days) and the presence of neonatal meningitis, was associated with a higher incidence of neonatal brain injury and death.

Pseudomonas Species

Pseudomonas are opportunistic pathogens that most commonly affect the immunocompromised. Strictly aerobic, these Gram-negative bacilli are of relatively low virulence. They are ubiquitous, with a predilection to moist, humid environments, and are primarily waterborne organisms. *Pseudomonas aeruginosa* is the most common species. Infections are serious and often life-threatening, typically targeting the respiratory tract and causing pneumonia. Other infections include endocarditis, peritonitis, meningitis, ecthyma gangrenosum, bacteremia, and overwhelming septicemia. Treatment can be difficult due to innate resistance to many antibiotics and the ability to develop new resistance after exposure to antimicrobial agents. Their resistance to most antibiotics is attributed to efflux pumps, which pump out the antibiotics before the antibiotics are able to act. Some bacteria also produce exopolysaccharides which are associated with biofilm formation, making phagocytosis by macrophages difficult. *Pseudomonas* has been cultured in unexpected places, such as antiseptic solutions, quaternary ammonium compounds, bottled mineral water, sinks and ventilators. Like other Gram-negative bacteria, most *Pseudomonas* species are resistant to penicillin and related beta-lactam antibiotics, but a number are sensitive to piperacillin, ticarcillin and tobramycin.[23]

CLINICAL PRESENTATION OF NEONATAL SEPSIS

The possibility of sepsis must be considered in the differential diagnosis of any unstable infant or any infant having a change in his or her clinical condition and tolerance of handling. Changes in clinical signs overtime are important clues to the presence and evolution of sepsis.

Early-onset sepsis often mimics the progression of noninfectious diagnoses such as respiratory distress syndrome (RDS) and metabolic disorders. Presentation in most infants is within 24 hours and can be fulminant, with a devastating scenario of shock, metabolic acidosis, cardiorespiratory collapse and death.

Late-onset sepsis in the modern era of IAP may be changing. The presentation of LOS occurs later in the current era, with a mean age of 19 ± 7 days.[33] An association between IAP administration, delayed LOS presentation, and milder disease has also been described.

For both EOS and LOS, the clinical presentation of neonatal sepsis may be subtle. Presenting signs include changes in respiratory status with nasal flaring, grunting, tachypnea, irregular respiratory patterns, costal retractions, increased respiratory effort, cyanosis, worsening apnea and overt respiratory failure. Cardiac signs pointing to pulmonary hypertension, decreased cardiac output, hypoxemia may progress to overt cardiogenic shock, hypotension, pallor, poor capillary perfusion and bradycardia, signs that are highly associated with mortality. Metabolic signs include hyperthermia and hyperglycemia, hypothermia and hyperthermia, secondary jaundice, metabolic acidosis. Neurologic signs are observed in only 30% with culture-proven meningitis, such as irritability, stupor, coma, seizures, bulging anterior fontanelle, extensor rigidity. Cutaneous signs include bruising, petechiae, cutis marmorata and the harlequin sign signifying vascular instability. Abdominal distension signifying ileus and hepatosplenomegaly are common abdominal findings.

DIAGNOSTIC EVALUATION

Evaluation for neonatal sepsis begins with a complete history and thorough physical examination. There should be review of the antenatal, intrapartum and postnatal course to identify risk factors for neonatal sepsis. The physical examination is important to gage the stability of the infant, the need for immediate supportive care, to determine focal findings suggesting the diagnosis, and to identify targeted investigations.

Laboratory studies to "rule out sepsis" usually begin with tests for stability such as serum glucose, blood gas and a complete blood count. Hyperglycemia is common and points to a non-specific response to stress. Respiratory acidosis heralds respiratory instability. The presence of metabolic acidosis should raise caution about circulatory stability and worsening status. Changes in the white blood cell count (WBC) and differential, platelets and platelet indices, and infection markers such as C-reactive protein (CRP) through serial measurements may facilitate the diagnosis of sepsis. Severe leukopenia (WBC $< 5 \times 10^9$/L), severe neutropenia ($< 0.5 \times 10^9$/L), an elevated immature-to-total (I/T) neutrophil ratio (> 0.2) and thrombocytopenia are associated with infection. Acute phase reactants such as CRP (measured 8–24 hours after infection) and procalcitonin (measured 2–12 hours after infection), and changes in their values overtime with serial testing can give supportive information. CRP has good negative predictive value: if CRP remains persistently normal, then bacterial sepsis is highly unlikely. Other markers of infection and inflammation include Immunoglobulin M (IgM), CD11b, CD64, IL-6, IL-8. and could give addition supportive evidence of infection.[34]

The gold standard remains blood or sterile site culture. Single-site blood culture (with ideally ≥1 mL of blood and preferably prior to the start of antibiotics) can be effective in isolating the organism within 12–24 hours. If the blood culture is positive, a repeat culture within 24–48 hours after starting antibiotics will demonstrate clearing and assist in the decision about duration of treatment.

The incidence of meningitis is relatively low in EOS and most clinicians elect to perform a lumbar puncture (LP) only in the presence of a positive blood culture. However, large studies have demonstrated up to a 38% rate of culture-proven meningitis in neonates with suspected sepsis and negative blood cultures. This underlines the importance of exercising best clinical judgment about obtaining an LP whenever an infant is suspected to have neonatal sepsis, particularly with LOS. If the infant is unstable, the LP should be deferred until stability, while ensuring that the empiric treatment also covers for potential meningitis until a definitive diagnosis can be made. If the cerebrospinal fluid (CSF) culture is positive, the LP should be repeated, ideally 24 to 48 hours later, in order to demonstrate clearing of the infection and to assist in the decision about duration of treatment. In many cases, the LP is performed after recent IAP in the mother or initiation of empiric antibiotic therapy in the neonate, and the culture results are thus expected to be negative. In those cases, the diagnosis of meningitis can be supported by findings of pathogens on Gram-stain and via cell count analysis. In atraumatic samples, the WBC count is usually less than 10–20 cells/mm³. The median number of WBC in infants with meningitis who were more than or equal to 35 weeks was 477/mm³ whereas the count was less at 110/mm³ in infants less than 34 weeks gestation.[35] CSF protein in term infants is usually less than 100 mg/dL; severe elevations of CSF protein point to fungal infection. CSF glucose is 70–80% of serum glucose taken contemporaneously; severely low CSF glucose points to bacterial meningitis. Many of these CSF abnormalities may persist for several days.[36]

Urinary culture is not indicated in EOS but is imperative in the evaluation of LOS. The ideal sample is obtained by sterile suprapubic aspiration.[37] Sterile urinary bladder catheterization is also a common method to obtain urine for culture. "Clean catch" and sterile bag samples are seen as less invasive techniques but are really only helpful if they show no growth.

Tracheal aspirate culture from the endotracheal tube in intubated infants will demonstrate colonization. Though there is poor correlation between tracheal colonization and actual invading pathogens in pneumonia, the choice of antibiotics for empiric treatment can be directed by these results until definitive tests are available. In our NICU, we send tracheal aspirates for culture once a week in babies who are intubated for intervals longer than 1 week. In this way, our NICU tracks the potential pathogens present in our environment and their susceptibilities.

Other investigations should be directed by the clinical presentation. In the face of thrombocytopenia or bleeding, coagulation studies may be indicated to diagnose disseminated intravascular coagulation (DIC) and the need of blood product treatment. Diagnostic imaging should be based on presentation: chest radiography for respiratory distress may demonstrate pneumonia, pleural effusions; CT and MRI of the brain may demonstrate abscesses, infarctions or obstruction to CSF flow when there are neurologic signs.

MANAGEMENT

Prompt treatment is the standard of care when neonatal sepsis is suspected, with empiric intravenous antibiotics given even as diagnostic tests are completed. The first steps are to insure overall stability with attention to the ABCs of acute care: airway, breathing, circulation, and particularly for preterm infants, temperature and glucose control. Monitoring of the vital signs should be continuous and noninvasive, including blood pressure, O_2 saturation and transcutaneous PCO_2. The baby should be placed in an incubator or radiant bed for easy access for care and continuous observation. Intensive care may warrant ventilatory support for respiratory failure, circulatory support for hypotension and poor cardiac output with fluid boluses and inotropic/chronotropic agents, systemic steroids for inadequate adrenal response particularly in premature infants, and blood products such as fresh frozen plasma (FFP), cryoprecipitate and platelets for DIC. After stabilization, nutrition will be the mainstay of recovery and should be given equal importance. Very unstable infants should be transferred to a Level III/IV neonatal center.

Empiric intravenous antibiotics for EOS consist of the combination of an expanded-spectrum penicillin and an aminoglycoside, thus providing coverage for both Gram-positive and Gram-negative organisms. Ampicillin and gentamicin have been the mainstay of therapy over the past three decades in many developed countries and have been recommended by the World Health Organization for developing countries, although their effectiveness may not be as good in the latter.[38] The added advantage of the combination of ampicillin and gentamicin is their synergistic activity against GBS and *L. monocytogenes*. Empiric use of the third generation cephalosporins, such as cefotaxime, instead of gentamicin is discouraged, as recent studies have shown no added benefit, and the potential risk of antimicrobial resistance and invasive candidiasis.[34] Again, the choice of empiric antibiotics should be tailored to the prevalent local pathogens and to their antibiotic sensitivities.

Most infants will show an improvement within 1–2 days of initiating treatment. If cultures are negative after 2–3 days, the clinician is faced with the dilemma: is this a true negative and no infection is present, in which case antibiotics should be stopped, or is this a false negative result, a situation which may be more likely with the use of IAP. The decision to continue treatment for a therapeutic interval should be based on review of the clinical course, diagnostic data and maternal and intrapartum risk factors. If the cultures are positive, definitive diagnosis is confirmed and the best therapeutic duration must be determined based on clinical course, complications and negative results on repeat blood, LP or other invasive testing. The usual treatment courses are 7–10 days for uncomplicated bacteremia without focus. Shorter intervals are being evaluated and may be the direction for the future. Optimal treatment duration for clinical sepsis with negative cultures is unclear.[2]

A diagnosis of meningitis necessitates changes in antibiotics to insure CSF penetration. A third-generation cephalosporin, such as cefotaxime, or a carbapenem should be added and the ampicillin increased to "meningitic" doses. Therapy is tailored to the pathogen and its antibiotic susceptibilities. A repeat LP is recommended within 24–48 hours after initiation of antibiotic therapy. Antibiotics are administered for 2 weeks after sterilization of the CSF or a minimum of 2 weeks for Gram-positive meningitis and three weeks for Gram-negative meningitis.[2]

For LOS, the choice of empiric antibiotics should be directed by the suspected infection and pathogen. Premature infants, particularly with indwelling catheters, should be covered for CoNS. With the high prevalence of cloxacillin-resistant staphylococci, vancomycin has been in favor, such that, the empiric antibiotic combination for LOS most widely used in premature and surgical infants is gentamicin and vancomycin. This combination has increased risks for ototoxicity, nephrotoxicity and selection for vancomycin-resistant organisms. On the other hand, there is evidence that the administration of high-dose cloxacillin in synergistic combination with gentamicin, may provide an equally good clinical response, even in the presence of organisms deemed cloxacillin-resistant in vitro.[39] In our NICU, we have successfully used this combination of antibiotics (cloxacillin 200 mg/kg/day divided into two doses plus gentamicin) for many years. We limit the administration of vancomycin to infants with persistent positive cultures or those with an extreme clinical presentation.

Infants with necrotizing enterocolitis may be initially treated with ampicillin and gentamicin. Additional coverage for anaerobic organisms, with clindamycin or metronidazole, should be considered in more severe cases. Previous exposure to broad-spectrum antibiotics may point to resistant pathogens, and more potent antibiotics such as third-generation cephalosporins or carbapenems may be considered. Knowledge of an infant's microbial colonization status and current sensitivities may also help to determine the choice of antibiotics.

LOS meningitis requires the same aggressive care and support as EOS meningitis, with cefotaxime as part of the antibiotic regimen. Definitive antibiotics should be chosen when the pathogen and its sensitivities have been identified, and duration of therapy should be based on results of repeat cultures, clinical diagnosis and clinical response.

Additional adjunctive therapies that have been forwarded but remain unproven in efficacy include granulocyte transfusion, intravenous immunoglobulin (IVIG), exchange transfusion, recombinant cytokines, granulocyte-macrophage colony-stimulating factors and glutamine, and cannot yet be recommended.[2]

SPECIFIC CONSIDERATIONS

The following section highlights important issues that deserve special review.

Central Line-associated Bloodstream Infections

Central line-associated bloodstream infections (CLABSI) are an undesired consequence of the success of modern neonatology, with improved survival of the smallest and sickest infants and the use of central venous devices, particularly percutaneously-inserted central catheters (PICC). Between 8.3% and 33% of neonates admitted to the NICU have PICC. CLABSI is associated with higher mortality and long-term sequelae.

Prevalent use of these central catheters led to the advent of the most common source of neonatal infections, with an incidence of about 11 per 1,000 catheter days in neonates weighing less than 1,000 grams, versus 4 per 1,000 catheter days in babies weighing

more than 2,500 grams. The highest rates of infection occur in those with PICC (13 per 1,000 catheter days) and surgical newborns with central venous catheters whose infection rate is 24%.[40] For the past 20 years, there have been vigorous efforts to combat the rise of CLABSI, which at one point seemed inevitable in the very premature and the surgical infants. Research efforts have reaffirmed the importance of rigorous hand washing, and of strict aseptic technique during the insertion and maintenance of these catheters.

The diagnosis of CLABSI is problematic in neonates. As most cases of CLASBI are caused by CoNS, which are usually noninvasive skin commensals and which are also readily grown in contaminated culture specimens, the criteria for definitive diagnosis remain contentious. In an infant with a central venous catheter, CLABSI must be considered when there are clinical changes or signs of instability. Two positive blood cultures, taken at two different times are required to make a definitive diagnosis of CLABSI in an infant with a central venous device if the pathogen is CoNS or other usually noninvasive organism. Other definitions of CLABSI include one positive blood culture and one positive sterile site culture and finally, one positive blood culture in an infant with the picture of severe clinical sepsis.[2]

The primary pathogen is CoNS followed by *S. aureus*, Candida species and Enterococcus species.[41] The clinical presentation of CLABSI ranges from mild signs to a severe process with cardiorespiratory failure. Meningitis is uncommon, even with repeated positive blood cultures, such that most clinicians do not perform LPs for these septic episodes. Infants often show rapid recovery with antibiotics and supportive therapy. For candidal CLABSI, most experts recommend the prompt removal of the central venous device. For bacterial CLABSI, the guidelines are less specific, recognizing that alternative venous access may be difficult in these infants. Thus the central venous device may be kept in situ unless the infant fails to clear the bacteremia.

Ventilator-Associated Pneumonia

Ventilator-associated pneumonia (VAP) is defined as a pulmonary infection occurring 48 hours or more after the institution of mechanical ventilation. Although ventilator-associated pneumonia is now a well-recognized entity in older children and adults, this condition is often underdiagnosed or overdiagnosed in the newborn population. This is particularly true in premature infants, who frequently demonstrate diffuse, chronic parenchymal opacification on chest radiography as a result of bronchopulmonary dysplasia. As opposed to older populations, VAP in newborns is rarely lobar in distribution, but is rather a diffuse bilateral process. Furthermore, antibiotics administered for suspected or proven sepsis will generally treat any concurrent pneumonia, without the latter necessarily being diagnosed. The most common organisms implicated include Pseudomonas species, *S. aureus*, Enterobacter species, and Klebsiella species.[41]

Infants with VAP generally present with a deterioration of ventilatory status and with copious, thick, yellow-green respiratory secretions. In addition to antibiotic therapy, the use of chest physiotherapy, bronchodilators, more frequent suctioning, and mucolytic agents may be helpful. Improvement in ventilatory status usually ensues within a few days of the onset of treatment.

Much effort is recently being made to reduce the incidence of this condition through evidence-based changes in practice. These include elevation of the head of the bed, in-line suctioning, avoiding the use of H_2 blockers, use of proper hand hygiene, and ensuring regular cleaning or changing of ventilator-related hardware.[42,43]

Invasive Candidiasis

Invasive candidiasis refers to a systemic infection of vital organs and normally sterile body fluids with Candida species. In VLBW infants, it accounts for 2.5% of bloodstream infections.[44] The organism is notoriously difficult to grow from blood, with a sensitivity of only 29% in adults.[45] Given the very small volume of blood sent for culture in neonates, *Candida* infections are likely underdiagnosed. Diagnosis of central nervous system (CNS) candidiasis is even more problematic, and the indications for performing an LP become more critical.

Multiple sites of colonization are associated with an increased risk of invasive disease.[46] Other risk factors are displayed in Table 5.3. It is interesting that the incidence of candidiasis varies greatly by center, from 2.4% to 20.4%.[47] Positive urine cultures in a premature infant obtained optimally through sterile catheterization or suprapubic aspiration should be viewed as equivalent to a positive blood culture, with the need for systemic evaluation and treatment. Although fluconazole is commonly used as first-line therapy, each NICU should identify its predominant candidal pathogen and sensitivities. It is important to appreciate that *C. glabrata* is often resistant to fluconazole, and thus empiric treatment with amphotericin B deoxycholate or micafungin would be more appropriate.

Mortality from invasive candidiasis may be as high as 19%.[48] Early antifungal treatment and removal of infected indwelling catheters have been shown to improve survival.[49]

Multiple trials in VLBW infants have demonstrated that fluconazole prophylaxis during the first 6 weeks of life have reduced fungal colonization and invasive disease without resistance or other drug adverse effects. Such a practice in VLBW infants could potentially prevent 2,000–3,000 cases of invasive candidiasis, 200–300 deaths, and could result in 400–500 fewer infants with adverse neurodevelopmental outcomes per year in the US.[44] The Infectious Disease Society of America, the American Academy of Pediatrics (AAP) and the Cochrane Collaboration support the benefit of antifungal prophylaxis in preterm infants, particularly for units with a high prevalence of invasive candidiasis.[46,50] Of interest, prophylactic oral nystatin may be as effective as fluconazole in

Table 5.3: Risk factors for invasive candidiasis in premature infants

- Broad-spectrum antibiotics
- Use of multiple antibiotics
- Prolonged duration of antibiotic administration
- Delayed enteral feeding
- Duration of parenteral duration > 5 days
- Intravenous lipid infusion > 7days
- Indwelling catheters
- Endotracheal intubation
- Use of histamine 2 receptor blockers
- Length of hospitalization > 7 days
- Male gender

preventing fungal colonization, although the elevated osmolarity of the former may increase the risk of developing NEC. Further research is required to demonstrate specific benefit of this strategy.[51]

Viruses and Other Pathogens

Viruses and other pathogens are ubiquitous and may mimic bacterial infections. The possible presence of these organisms should be considered whenever the clinical course is not evolving as expected, despite appropriate empiric antibiotic therapy, and particularly in the presence of persistent thrombocytopenia, conjugated jaundice, skin rashes, or hepatosplenomegaly. Of particular note here are systemic *Herpes simplex* virus infections, which may result in mortality or severe sequelae if left untreated. Enteroviral infections may also result in severe multiorgan involvement but, unfortunately, no effective antiviral treatment is available at this time. Hepatitis and HIV infections must be considered, particularly in endemic areas.

The role of infections with Ureaplasma and *Mycoplasma* species in the evolution of bronchopulmonary dysplasia (BPD) has been debated for decades, with renewed interest following recent publications demonstrating elevated colonization rates of the maternal urogenital tract.[52,53] Thus, although these organisms do not cause neonatal sepsis per se, it may still be of use to screen premature infants requiring prolonged ventilation and to consider treatment with erythromycin or azithromycin.[54]

OUTCOME AND LONG-TERM SEQUELAE

Neonatal sepsis, particularly with Gram-negative organisms, is associated with significant mortality and morbidity. Mortality is predominantly associated with a birth weight less than 2,500 grams, an absolute neutrophil count less than 1.5×10^9/L, hypotension, apnea and presence of a pleural effusion.[55] Mortality is higher for very premature infants for both EOS and LOS.

Particular attention should be paid to infants surviving after neonatal meningitis, who may have devastating outcomes, with 20% of survivors having severe disability, such as cerebral palsy and serious neurodevelopmental impairment.[56,57] Development, vision and hearing should be followed after hospital discharge and throughout childhood.

Multiple confounding factors complicate the analysis of the impact of neonatal sepsis on the outcomes of premature infants. Volpe et al. describe cerebral white matter injury, particularly periventricular leukomalacia, with a multifactorial process involving the production of proinflammatory cytokines, increased blood-brain barrier permeability, hypotension, impaired autoregulation of cerebral blood flow and hypoxic ischemic events.[58] Extremely premature infants with bacterial or fungal culture-proven sepsis have been found to have a higher risk of cerebral palsy, neurodevelopmental impairment (NDI), microcephaly, deafness, and blindness.[59-61] Thus, there is a clear need for long-term follow-up in this population.

PREVENTION

Prevention of infection is of paramount importance, requiring a comprehensive, multidisciplinary strategy, including rigorous hand-washing, strict sterile or aseptic techniques, and continuous surveillance. Many promising prophylactic approaches have failed to show effectiveness in large, multicenter trials, including the administration of glutamine and immunoglobulins (pooled, specific or monoclonal), and their use cannot be recommended at this time. The following care practices have been demonstrated to reduce the incidence of neonatal infections.

Human Milk Feeding

Human milk feeding has been demonstrated to have many beneficial effects in decreasing the incidence of infections during the neonatal period and beyond. Human milk contains substances with direct and indirect anti-infective actions such as lactoferrin (LF), lactoperoxidase, lysozyme, IgA, IgM, cytokines, interferon, oligosaccharides, bifidogenic factors, platelet-activating factor acetylhydrolase, vitamin E, beta carotene and ascorbic acid. It has a trophic effect on the gut mucosa, impacting on gut-permeability and maturation of the intestinal epithelium, which may result in less translocation of pathogens.[62-64] Promotion of normal commensal intestinal flora with lactobacilli could protect against colonization from more invasive pathogens and directly promote normal intestinal epithelium maturation. Of interest, the protective effect of milk feedings require average intakes higher than 50 mL/kg/day and fresh milk, rather than pasteurized donor milk. Better long-term neurodevelopment and a higher intelligence quotient are additional incentives to promotion of breast milk feedings.[65,66]

Management of Central Venous Devices

The use of central venous devices (CVD) is prevalent in the care of the sickest infants but has been associated with the rise in CLABSIs. Multiple studies have shown the effectiveness in prevention and reduction of such infections through "proactive" policies, that describe adherence to stringent asepsis techniques and a dedicated CVD team that inserts, cares for and oversees all line-related issues including on-going education and surveillance.[67] Kime et al. reported reduction of CLABSI from 15.6 per 1,000 catheter days to zero.[68] In our own NICU, we instituted a comprehensive CVD care bundle and observed an 84% decrease in our infection rate from 6.6 per 1,000 catheter days to 1.04 per 1,000 catheter days. Ongoing research is needed to optimize CVD care and to explore the benefits from promising approaches such as "in-line filters", "intra-removal" prophylaxis strategy (administration of two doses of cefazolin during CVD removal) and of controversial strategies such as scheduled removal and reinsertion of the CVD, e.g. after 15 days when the odds of developing a bloodstream infection increases abruptly.[69-71]

Probiotics

Probiotics promote healthy gut colonization and maturation. How this is effected remains to be better understood. There is immunomodulation, anti-infective activities with production of bacteriostatic and bactericidal substances (e.g. the antibiotic peptide reutercyclin) and effects on gut permeability. A recent Cochrane review supports the use of probiotics to decrease NEC, decrease sepsis and mortality.[72] Despite its many purported benefits, the use of probiotics remains limited because of lack of availability of pharmacological-grade products, lack of data on long-term outcomes and paucity of guidelines for use.[73]

Restriction of H$_2$ Blockers

In addition to potential harms in premature infants from H$_2$ blockers, these agents are also associated with increased rates of infections. The mechanism of action is most probably interference with gastric acidity and altered gut flora.[74] Bianconi et al. reported that the use of ranitidine was associated with an increase in the incidence of LOS, with an odds ratio (OR) 6.98 (95% CI 3.78–12.94, p < 0.0001).[75] Current best practice is to limit or avoid the use of H$_2$ blockers in neonates.

CONCLUSION AND FUTURE DIRECTIONS

Neonatal infections remain a challenge whose prevention, prompt diagnosis and optimal therapy should result in significant improvements in survival and long-term outcome. Optimal neonatal practices to decrease infection include judicious and shortened use of antibiotics, establishment of the neonatal gut microbiome with early human milk feeding, stringent hand hygiene, proactive care bundles for indwelling devices, microbial stewardship, and vigilant surveillance by each NICU of their predominant infectious pathogens and their susceptibilities. Many countries have established developed prospective infection surveillance networks in an effort to identify problem areas and to monitor the impact of various interventions.[76]

Innovative research, particularly in immunology and microbiology, may discover new therapies such as anticytokines, immunoglobulins, vaccines, lactoferrin and rapid diagnostic tests to effect treatment with less delay, to protect infected infants from brain injury and the other sequelae of infection, and best of all to prevent infection.

REFERENCES

1. Black RE, Cousens S, Johnson HL, et al. Global, regional and national causes of child mortality in 2008: a systematic analysis. Lancet. 2010;375:1969-87.
2. Shane AL, Stoll BJ. Recent developments and current issues in the epidemiology, diagnosis, and management of bacterial and fungal neonatal sepsis. Am J Perinatol. 2013;30(2):131-42.
3. Anderson-Berry AL. Neonatal Sepsis. emedicine.medscape.com, July 2012.
4. Fanaroff AA, Stoll BJ, Wright LL, et al. Trends in neonatal morbidity and mortality for very low birth weight infants. Am J Obstet Gynecol. 2007;196(2):147e1-8.
5. Buhimschi CS, Bhandari V, Han YW, et al. Using proteomics in perinatal and neonatal sepsis: hopes and challenges for the future. Curr Opin Infect Dis. 2009;22:235-43.
6. Kasper DC, Mechtler TP, Reischer GH, et al. The bacterial load of Ureaplasma parvum in amniotic fluid is correlated with an increased intrauterine inflammatory response. Diagn Microbiol Infect Dis. 2010;67:117-21.
7. Holzman C, Lin X, Senagore P, et al. Histologic chorioamnionitis and preterm delivery. Am J Epidemiol. 2007;166:786-94.
8. Gotsch F, Romero R, Kusanovic JP, et al. The fetal inflammatory response syndrome. Clin Obstet Gynecol. 2007;50(3):652-83.

9. Gantert M, Been JV, Gavilanes AW, et al. Chorioamnionitis: a multiorgan disease of the fetus? J Perinatol. 2010;30 (Suppl):S21-30.

10. American Academy of Pediatrics policy statement: recommendations for the prevention of perinatal group B streptococcal (GBS) disease. Pediatrics. 2011;128(3):611-6.

11. Canadian Pediatric Society Position Statement: Management of the infant at increased risk for sepsis. Paediatr Child Health. 2007;12(10):893-905.

12. Verani JR, McGee L, Schrag SJ. Prevention of perinatal group B streptococcal disease—revised guidelines from CDC, 2010. MMWR Recomm Rep. 2010;59(RR-10):1-36.

13. Money DM, Dobson S. The prevention of early-onset neonatal group B streptococcal disease. J Obstet Gynaecol Can. 2004;26(9):826-40.

14. Schuchat A, Wenger JD. Epidemiology of group B streptococcal disease: risk factors, prevention strategies, and vaccine development. Epidemiol Rev. 1994;16:374-402.

15. Hansen SM, Uldbjerg N, Kilian M, et al. Dynamics of *Streptococcus agalactiae* colonization in women during and after pregnancy and in their infants. J Clin Microbiol. 2004;42:83-9.

16. McKenna DS, Matson S, Northern I. Maternal group B streptococcal (GBS) genital colonization at term in women who have asymptomatic GBS bacteriuria. Infect Dis Obstet Gynecol. 2003;11(4):203-7.

17. Ramos E, Gaudier FL, Hearing LR, et al. Group B streptococcus colonization in pregnant diabetic women. Obstet Gynecol. 1997;89:257-60.

18. Regan JA, Klebanoff MA, Nugent RP, et al. Colonization with group B streptococci in pregnancy and adverse outcome. VIP Study Group. Am J Obstet Gynecol. 1996;174(4):1354-60.

19. Phares CR, Lynfield R, Farley MM, et al. Epidemiology of invasive group B streptococcal disease in the United States, 1999-2005. JAMA. 2008;299:2056-65.

20. Davies HD, Raj S, Adair C, et al. Population-based active surveillance for neonatal group B streptococcal infections in Alberta, Canada: implications for vaccine formulation. Pediatr Infect Dis J. 2001;20(9):879-84.

21. Embleton N, Wariyar U, Hey E. Mortality from early onset group B streptococcal infection in the United Kingdom. Arch Dis Child Fetal Neonatal Ed. 1999;80:F139-41.

22. Moore MR, Schrag SJ, Schuchat A. Effects of intrapartum antimicrobial prophylaxis for prevention of group-B-streptococcal disease on the incidence and ecology of early-onset neonatal sepsis. Lancet Infect Dis. 2003;3:201-13.

23. Pickering LK. Red Book: 2009 Report of the Committee on Infectious Diseases, 28th edition. Elk Grove Village, IL: American Academy of Pediatrics; 2009. p. 292.

24. Pickering LK. Red Book: 2009 Report of the Committee on Infectious Diseases, 28th edition. Elk Grove Village, IL: American Academy of Pediatrics; 2009. p. 428.

25. Didier C, Streicher MP, Chognot D, et al. Late-onset neonatal infections: incidences and pathogens in the era of antenatal antibiotics. Eur J Pediatr. 2012;171(4):681-7.

26. Pickering LK. Red Book: 2009 Report of the Committee on Infectious Diseases, 28th edition. Elk Grove Village, IL: American Academy of Pediatrics; 2009. pp. 600-15.

27. Cimolai N. *Staphylococcus aureus* outbreaks among newborns: new frontiers in an old dilemma. Am J Perinatol. 2003;20:125-36.

28. Gooch JJ, Britt EM. *Staphylococcus aureus* colonization and infection in newborn nursery patients. Am J Dis Child. 1978;132:893-6.

29. Boubaker K, Diebold P, Blanc DS, et al. Panton-valentine leukocidin and staphylococcal skin infections in schoolchildren. Emerg Infect Dis. 2004;10:121-4.

30. Healy CM, Hulten KG, Palazzi DL, et al. Emergence of new strains of methicillin-resistant *Staphylococcus aureus* in a neonatal intensive care unit. Clin Infect Dis. 2004;1239:1460-6.

31. McAdams RM, Mazuchowski E, Ellis MW, et al. Necrotizing staphylococcal pneumonia in a neonate. J Perinatol. 2005;25:677-9.

32. Berardi A, Rossi C, Lugli L, et al. Group B streptococcus late-onset disease: 2003-2010. Pediatrics. 2013;131(2):e361-8.

33. Ecker KL, Donohue PK, Kim KS, et al. The impact of group B streptococcus prophylaxis on late-onset neonatal infections. J Perinatol. 2013;33:206-11.

34. Polin RA and the Committee on Fetus and Newborn. Management of neonates with suspected or proven early-onset bacterial sepsis. Pediatrics. 2012;129:1006-15.

35. Garges HP, Moody MA, Cotton CM, et al. Neonatal meningitis: What is the correlation among cerebrospinal fluid cultures, blood cultures and cerebrospinal fluid parameters? Pediatrics 2006;117(4):1094–100.

36. Srinivasan L, Harris MC, Shah SS. Lumbar puncture in the neonate: challenges in decision making and interpretation. Semin Perinatol. 2012;36(6):445-53.

37. Bonadio WA. Urine culturing technique in febrile infants. Pediatr Emerg Care. 1987;3:75-8.

38. Downie L, Armiento R, Subhi R, et al. Community-acquired neonatal and infant sepsis in developing countries: efficacy of WHO's currently recommended antibiotics—systematic review and metaanalysis. Arch Dis Child. 2013;98:146-54.

39. Blayney MP, Al Madani M. Coagulase-negative staphylococcal infections in a neonatal intensive care unit: in vivo response to cloxacillin. Paediatr Child Health. 2006;11(10):659-63.

40. Njere I, Islam S, Parish D, et al. Outcome of peripherally inserted central venous catheters in surgical and medical neonates. J Pediatr Surg. 2011;46:946-50.

41. Hocevar SN, Edwards JR, Horan TC, et al. Device-associated infections among neonatal intensive care unit patients: incidence and associated pathogens reported to the National Healthcare Safety Network, 2006–2008. Infect Control Hosp Epidemiol. 2012;33(12):1200-6.

42. Foglia E, Meier MD, Elward A. Ventilator-associated pneumonia in neonatal and pediatric intensive care unit patients. Clin Microbiol Reviews. 2007;20(3):409-25.

43. Garland JS. Strategies to prevent ventilator-associated pneumonia in neonates. Clin Perinatol. 2010;37:629-43.

44. Kaufman DA. Challenging issues in neonatal candidiasis. Curr Med Res Opin. 2010;26:1769-78.

45. Hsieh E, Smith PB, Jacqz-Aigrain E, et al. Neonatal fungal infections: When to treat? Early Hum Dev. 2012;88(Suppl 2):S6-10.

46. Leibovitz E. Strategies for the prevention of neonatal candidiasis. Pediatr Neonatol. 2012;53:83-9.

47. Benjamin DK Jr, Stoll BJ, Gantz MG, et al. Neonatal candidiasis: epidemiology, risk factors and clinical judgement. Pediatrics 2010;126:e865-73.

48. Ascher SB, Smith PB, Watt K, et al. Antifungal therapy and outcomes in infants with invasive Candida infections. Pediatr Infect Dis J. 2012;31:439-43.

49. Benjamin DK Jr, Stoll BJ, Fanaroff AA, et al. Neonatal candidiasis among extremely low birth weight infants: risk factors, mortality rates, and neurodevelopmental outcomes at 18 to 22 months. Pediatrics. 2006;117:84-92.

50. Manzoni P, Mostert M, Jacqz-Aigrain E, et al. The use of fluconazole in neonatal intensive care -units. Arch Dis Child. 2009;94:983-7.

51. Aydemir C, Oguz SS, Dizdar EA, et al. Randomized controlled trial of prophylactic fluconazole versus nystatin for the prevention of fungal colonization and invasive fungal infection in very low birth weight infants. Arch Dis Child Fetal Neonatal Ed. 2011;96:F164-8.

52. Goldenberg RL, Andrews WW, Goepfert AR, et al. The Alabama Preterm Birth Study: Umbilical cord blood *Ureaplasma urealyticum* and *Mycoplasma hominis* cultures in very preterm newborn infants. Am J Obstet Gynecol. 2008;198(1): 43e1-5.

53. Viscardi RM, Hasday JD. Role of Ureaplasma species in neonatal chronic lung disease: epidemiologic and experimental evidence. Pediatr Res. 2009;65(5 Pt 2):84R-90R.

54. Speer CP. Inflammation and bronchopulmonary dysplasia: a continuing story. Semin Fetal Neonatal Med. 2006;11:354-62.

55. Payne NR, Burke BA, Day DL, et al. Correlation of clinical and pathologic findings in early onset neonatal group B streptococcal infection with disease severity and prediction of outcome. Pediatr Infect Dis J. 1988;7(12):836-47.

56. De Louvois J, Halket S, Harvey D. Neonatal meningitis in England and Wales: sequelae at 5 years of age. Eur J Pediatr. 2005;164:730-4.

57. Adams-Chapman I, Stoll BJ. Neonatal infection and long-term neurodevelopmental outcome in the preterm infant. Curr Opin Infect Dis. 2006;19:290-7.

58. Volpe JJ. Postnatal sepsis, necrotizing enterocolitis, and the critical role of systemic inflammation in white matter injury in premature infants. J Pediatr. 2008;153(2):160-3.

59. Schlapbach LJ, Aebischer M, Adams M, et al. Impact of sepsis on neurodevelopmental outcome in a Swiss National Cohort of extremely premature infants. Pediatrics. 2011;128:e348-56.

60. Alshaikh B, Yusuf K, Sauve R. Neurodevelopmental outcomes of very low birth weight infants with neonatal sepsis: systematic review and meta-analysis. J Perinatol. 2013;33(7):558-64.

61. Stoll BJ, Hansen NI, Adams-Chapman I, et al. Neurodevelopmental and growth impairment among extremely low-birth-weight infants with neonatal infection. JAMA. 2004;292(19):2357-65.

62. Manzoni P, De Luca D, Stronati M, et al. Prevention of nosocomial infections in neonatal intensive care units. Am J Perinatol. 2013; 30(2):81-8.

63. Shulman RJ, Schanler RJ, Lau C, et al. Early feeding, antenatal glucocorticoids, and human milk decrease intestinal permeability in preterm infants. Pediatr Res. 1998;44:519-23.

64. Schanler RJ, Shulman RJ, Lau C. Feeding strategies for premature infants: beneficial outcomes of feeding fortified human milk versus preterm formula. Pediatrics. 1999;103 (6 Pt 1):1150-7.

65. Schanler RJ, Lau C, Hurst NM, et al. Randomised trial of donor human milk versus preterm formula as substitutes for mothers' own milk in the feeding of extremely premature infants. Pediatrics. 2005;116:400-6.

66. Lucas A, Morley R, Cole TJ, et al. Breastmilk and subsequent intelligence quotient in children born preterm. Lancet. 1992; 339(8788):261-4.

67. Golombek SG, Rohan AJ, Parvez B, et al. "Proactive" management of percutaneously inserted central catheters results in decreased incidence of infection in the ELBW population. J Perinatol. 2002; 22:209-13.

68. Kime T, Mohsini K, Nwankwo MU, et al. Central line "attention" is their best prevention. Adv Neonatal Care. 2011;11(4):242-8.

69. Jack T, Boehne M, Brent BE, et al. In-line filtration reduces severe complications and length of stay on pediatric intensive care unit: a prospective, randomized, controlled trial. Intensive Care Med. 2012;38:1008-16.

70. Hemels MA, van den Hoogen A, Verboon-Maciolek MA, et al. Prevention of neonatal late-onset sepsis associated with the removal of percutaneously inserted central venous catheters in preterm infants. Pediatr Crit Care Med. 2011;12:445-8.

71. Advani S, Reich NG, Sengupta A, et al. Central line-associated bloodstream infection in hospitalized children with peripherally inserted central venous catheters: extending risk analyses outside the intensive care unit. Clin Infect Dis. 2011;52:1108-15.

72. Alfaleh K, Anabrees J, Bassler D, et al. Probiotics for prevention of necrotizing enterocolitis in preterm infants. Cochrane Database Syst Rev. 2011;(3):CD005496.

73. Murquia-Peniche T, Mihatsch WA, Zegarra J, et al. Intestinal mucosal defense system, part 2. Probiotics and prebiotics. J Pediatr. 2013;162 (3 Suppl):S64-71.

74. Malcolm WF, Cotten CM. Metoclopramide, H2 blockers and proton pump inhibitors: pharmacotherapy for gastroesophageal reflux in neonates. Clin Perinatol. 2012;39(1):99-109.

75. Bianconi S, Gudavalli M, Sutija VG, et al. Ranitidine and late-onset sepsis in the neonatal intensive care unit. J Perinat Med. 2007; 35:147-50.

76. Vergnano S, Menson E, Kennea N, et al. Neonatal infections in England: the NeonIN surveillance network. Arch Dis Child Fetal Neonatal. 2011;96:F9-14.

6 Advances in Neonatal Ventilation

SM Donn, SK Sinha

INTRODUCTION

Ever since Hippocrates first described the use of intubation and positive pressure ventilation to support respiration approximately 2,400 years ago, the goals of mechanical ventilation have remained essentially unchanged. We continue to attempt to achieve and maintain adequate pulmonary gas exchange, minimize the risk of lung injury, reduce the patient work of breathing, and optimize patient comfort. The introduction of surfactant replacement therapy, antenatal corticosteroid treatment, and the deployment of state-of-the-art mechanical ventilators have all changed the demographics of the "old bronchopulmonary dysplasia (BPD)" and presented new challenges in neonatal intensive care. Although, we have made a start, the evidence as to how to best approach the problem is as yet insufficient upon which to draw specific therapeutic conclusions or make clinical recommendations. Until we have created a sufficient evidence base, it seems prudent, therefore, to rely on the basic tenet of medicine, "Primum Non Nocere: First, Do No Harm". Therapy, in this case mechanical respiratory support, should be directed at avoiding the potentially damaging effects of oxygen therapy, the trauma from excessive pressure and/or volume; the adverse consequences of atelectasis; and the role of inflammation and infection in the pulmonary injury sequence, which is now well established. In addition, the new technology has given us the opportunity to observe the potentially deleterious effects of inappropriate airway flow, referred to as "rheotrauma".[1] The challenge is to identify the most appropriate device, technique and strategies especially as philosophies of respiratory management differ so widely amongst the individual clinicians and institutions.[2]

THE PAST

The last three decades brought tremendous advances in the management of newborns with respiratory failure. The use of continuous distending pressure, first introduced by Gregory et al.,[3] was a remarkable step in maintaining alveolar stability and improving survival in premature infants with respiratory distress syndrome (RDS). Mechanical ventilation of newborns resulted in the first report of a new disorder, BPD (also referred to as chronic lung disease, CLD), described by Northway et al. in 1967,[4] in which infants developed chronic parenchymal lung and airway injury characterized by inflammation and squamous metaplasia of the respiratory epithelium.

The 1970s brought the widespread practice of mechanical ventilation to neonatal intensive care, utilizing primarily continuous flow, time-cycled, pressure limited ventilators. It dramatically extended the limits of viability, although the incidence of BPD continued to rise. In 1975 Philip attributed the pathogenesis of BPD to the combined effects of exposure to oxygen and positive pressure ventilation overtime.[5]

The technological revolution accelerated in the 1980s with the advent of high-frequency ventilation (HFV). This new form of mechanical ventilation utilized delivered gas volumes that were smaller than the anatomical dead space at very high rates in an attempt to lower airway pressure and achieve more uniform gas distribution within the lung. Continuous noninvasive monitoring was introduced, with transcutaneous gas monitoring and pulse oximetry becoming readily available. Toward the end of the decade, surfactant replacement therapy became a reality, overcoming the biochemical effects of the premature lung. Yet, CLD persisted.

The 1990s were characterized by the continued proliferation of technology. Real-time breath-to-breath pulmonary monitoring became feasible, and with it a host of new ventilator modes and modalities were introduced into clinical practice, such as synchronized intermittent mandatory ventilation (SIMV), assist-control (patient-triggered) ventilation, pressure control ventilation (PCV), pressure support ventilation (PSV) and volume-targeted ventilation. This decade also saw a dramatic change in the demographics and the nature of CLD. Infants surviving RDS were even smaller and more premature. Chronic lung changes (the "new BPD")[6,7] were now characterized by a decrease in alveolarization of the lung, with less inflammation and scarring, but with diminished surface area and functional lung units. The incidence of CLD approached 30–40%, depending upon how one chose to define it.

THE PRESENT

Management strategies in the new millennium represent a broad spectrum with little consensus, ranging from "noninvasive" techniques to the highly invasive extracorporeal membrane oxygenation (ECMO). Almost all of the clinical trials conducted to date, which have utilized CLD as the primary outcome measure have failed to demonstrate a benefit in lowering its incidence.

Continuous Distending Pressure

Continuous positive airway pressure (CPAP) is a form of distending pressure applied to the airways of a spontaneously breathing infant. It works by abolishing the upper airway occlusion and preventing atelectasis of the lungs, thus maintaining adequate Functional Residual Capacity (FRC). CPAP as a primary strategy was popularized by the work of Wung and colleagues beginning in the early 1970s.[8] This approach was based on a dependence on spontaneous breathing, the avoidance of sedative and paralytic drugs, and acceptance of "abnormal" blood gases. The approach did result in a dramatic reduction in CLD, but it was never subjected to a randomized clinical trial. Moreover, only pulmonary and not long-term neurodevelopmental outcomes have been reported. In recent years, there has been a resurgence in the use of CPAP because it is a noninvasive technique and easy to apply. Several different devices and ways to administer CPAP are now available including the Infant Flow Driver® and Bubble CPAP®.[9,10]

The infant CPAP system™ (Electro Medical Equipment Ltd., Sussex, England) uses a dedicated flow driver and gas generator with fluid-flip, variable flow, continuous positive airway pressure. The Bernoulli effect directs gas flow toward each nostril, and the Coanda effect causes the inspiratory flow to flip and leave the generator chamber via the expiratory limb. This is supposed to assist spontaneous breathing and reduce the work of breathing by decreasing expiratory resistance and maintaining stable airway pressure throughout the respiratory cycle.

In the Bubble CPAP system (Fisher and Paykel, Auckland, New Zealand), the blended gas is heated and humidified and then delivered to the infant through a secured nasal prong cannula. The distal end of the expiratory tubing is immersed underwater, and at 4 liters per minute of gas flow the CPAP pressure generated is equal to the level of the CPAP probe. Varying the depth of the underwater expiratory tube can vary the CPAP pressure. It has also been proposed that chest vibrations produced with bubble CPAP may contribute to gas exchange. Bubble CPAP appears to be an effective and inexpensive option for providing respiratory support to premature infants.

There are as yet no controlled trials to compare the efficacy or superiority of one system over another. Many questions are as yet unanswered. Is there a "best" way to provide CPAP? Does primary CPAP therapy delay or alter the benefit of surfactant replacement therapy in babies who ultimately require it? Is caloric expenditure higher than with mechanical ventilation? Does "bubble CPAP" confer any physiologic advantages?

Conventional Mechanical Ventilation

Conventional mechanical ventilation (CMV) attempts to deliver physiologic tidal volumes to the patient with the lung at or near FRC. In doing so, we are utilizing the steepest portion of the pressure-volume relationship, where pulmonary compliance is the best and where the change in delivered volume occurs at the lowest increment in driving pressure. The concept is demonstrated nicely in Figure 6.1, a schematic pressure-volume graph. Ventilation at normal FRC, the middle loop, results in the best hysteresis and compliance axis, compared to either ventilating at high FRC, the upper loop, which leads to overexpansion and the risk of barotrauma and volutrauma, or compared to ventilating at low FRC, the lower loop, which leads to atelectasis and the risk of atelectotrauma.[11-14]

The principles of mechanical ventilation are based on pulmonary physiology.[15] Oxygenation is a function of mean airway pressure. Mean airway pressure is usually adjusted by increasing the peak inspiratory pressure (PIP), the positive end expiratory pressure (PEEP), and/or the inspiratory time. Ventilation refers to carbon dioxide removal and is the product of tidal volume and frequency (rate). The tidal volume is proportional to the difference between the PIP and the PEEP, a value referred to as the amplitude. It is crucial that clinicians understand that there are significant differences among the various neonatal respiratory disorders and that differing pathophysiologic conditions call for different strategies. For instance, a preterm baby with RDS (low lung volume, homogeneous disease) is very different than a term baby with meconium aspiration syndrome (high lung volume, heterogeneous disease).

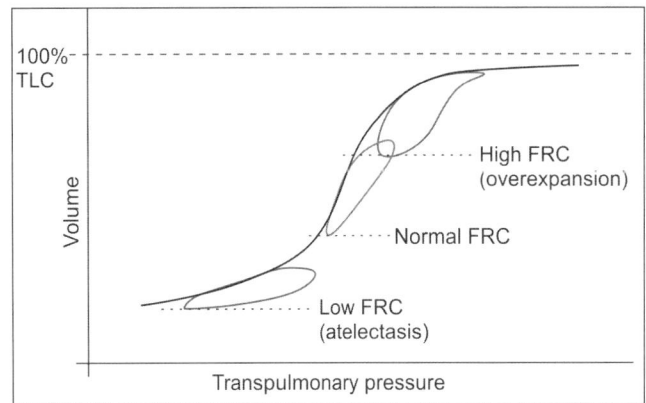

Fig. 6.1: Static pressure-volume relationship. Optimal ventilation occurs at normal FRC, where compliance is best and incremental volume changes occur at the least pressure change. Ventilating above FRC results in overexpansion of the lung and increases the risks of barotrauma and volutrauma; ventilating below FRC may result in atelectasis and its attendant consequences

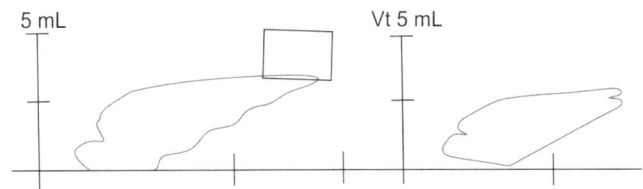

Fig. 6.2: Left: Real-time pressure volume loop demonstrating overinflation. Note the flattened portion at high pressure, where no additional volume is recruited. **Right:** A normal pressure-volume loop, showing satisfactory hysteresis

Mechanical ventilation is as much an art as a science. Great care must be taken to balance the life-saving benefit and the potentially injurious effects of positive pressure ventilation. Excessive inspiratory pressure can be detected by real-time pulmonary graphic monitoring.[16] This is shown in Figure 6.2. On the left, the pressure-volume relationship demonstrates hyperinflation, with exaggerated hysteresis and an upper inflection point on the inspiratory limb. A more normal pressure-volume relationship is shown on the graph on the right.

Until recently, the effects of airway flow on pulmonary mechanics have only been conceptual. Airway flow, which is the time rate of volume delivery, must be appropriately controlled. Rheotrauma refers to injury caused by inappropriate flow. If flow is excessive, it may result in turbulence, gas trapping, and inadvertent PEEP, leading to overdistension and the potential for thoracic airleaks.

If flow is inadequate, it may create "air hunger" or "flow starvation" and increase the patient's work of breathing.

Turbulence, or nonlaminar flow, can be created by excessive circuit flow. This can decrease the efficiency of gas exchange. If inspiratory airway flow exceeds expiratory airway flow, gas trapping and inadvertent PEEP may develop, increasing the risk of airleaks and contributing to elevated pulmonary vascular resistance. Paying close attention to respiratory time constants, the product of resistance and compliance, may help to avoid this.

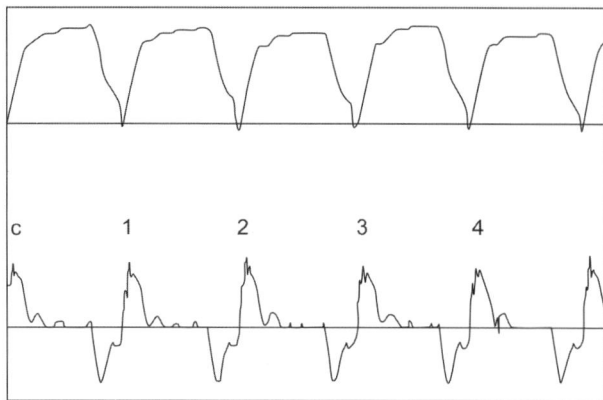

Fig. 6.3: Real-time pressure (top) and flow (bottom) waveforms. The flow waveform demonstrates gas trapping. The expiratory portion (below baseline) does not return to a zero flow state (baseline) before the initiation of the subsequent breath, which prevents complete emptying of the lung

Gas trapping can also be detected by real-time monitoring. Figure 6.3 demonstrates an abnormality in the expiratory flow waveform, which does not return to the zero flow baselines prior to the initiation of the next breath. This pattern calls for immediate adjustments in ventilator parameters, such as a reduction in flow, a decrease in the inspiratory time, or a slowing of the ventilator rate if mandatory ventilation is being used.

For more than 30 years, neonatal ventilation has been accomplished using time-cycled, pressure-limited devices. This form of ventilation is easy-to-use and leaves all parameters to the discretion of the clinician. The baby may breathe spontaneously between the mechanical breaths from continuous flow in the ventilator circuit. These spontaneous breaths receive ventilatory support by PEEP only. Recent technological advances have introduced a variety of newer modes of ventilation, which were not available to neonatal populations before. They are also based on sound physiological principles but often cause confusion. It is important that clinicians make themselves aware of the commonly used nomenclature. This can be best understood by using a hierarchical organization of ventilator modes:[17]

1. Parent mode—Determined by the control variable. This can be pressure, volume, or flow, and at any one time the mechanical breath can be controlled by only one of these.
2. The daughter mode—Determined by the breath type which has four phases (phase variables):
   a. Initiation of inspiration (trigger)
   b. Inspiration (limit)
   c. The change from inspiration to expiration (cycle)
   d. Termination or expiration (baseline variable).

Pressure, volume, flow and time are used as phase variables and determine the parameters of each ventilatory cycle. For example, in time-cycled, pressure-limited ventilation, the ventilator controls the airway pressure and the inspiratory phase lasts according to the time set by the clinician. On the other hand, in volume controlled ventilation, the ventilator controls and measures the tidal volume generated by the machine irrespective of lung compliance. A ventilator is a flow controlled if the gas delivery is limited by flow.

This type of ventilator also controls the tidal volume even though it does not measure it directly.

Pressure-Targeted Ventilation

Modalities of ventilation that target pressure as the dependent or "limit" variable include time-cycled, pressure-limited ventilation (TCPLV); flow-cycled, pressure limited ventilation (FCPLV); PCV, and PSV. What all of these have in common is a fixed pressure limit that the ventilator will not exceed. Thus, delivery of tidal volume depends primarily on the patient's lung mechanics, of which compliance is the most contributory. TCPLV has a fixed inspiratory time and flow rate, FCPLV has a variable inspiratory time (set by the patient) and a fixed flow rate, and PCV has a fixed inspiratory time and variable inspiratory flow rate, which is proportional to patient effort. PSV is a spontaneous mode, used to support spontaneous breathing, generally during weaning. It can be used alone (if there is reliable respiratory drive) or in combination with SIMV. Pressure support breaths are flow-cycled, so there is variable inspiratory time, and offer variable inspiratory flow proportional to patient effort. Pressure support breaths are pressure-limited and may also be time-limited.

Pressure-targeted modalities may be used in several modes. Intermittent mandatory ventilation (IMV) involves the delivery of mechanical breaths at a fixed rate, selected by the clinician, with the patient able to breathe spontaneously between mechanical breaths. SIMV also involves a fixed mechanical rate, but the ventilator "looks" for spontaneous effort during a timing window in order to synchronize the start of a mechanical breath with the start of a spontaneous breath (see Triggered Ventilation on next page). Assist-control ventilation provides a mechanical breath each time the patient breathes spontaneously, provided the trigger threshold is met, and also has a set control rate in case of patient apnea or inability to exceed the trigger threshold.

Volume-Targeted Ventilation

More recent technological advances have also enabled measurement of delivered tidal volumes and made possible the reintroduction of volume-targeted ventilation to newborn infants.[18] This form of CMV allows the clinician to select a specific tidal volume to be delivered to the patient. Pressure is permitted to fluctuate, creating a "self-weaning" style of ventilation. Volume cannot truly be used as a cycling mechanism in the newborn because of gas leaks around the uncuffed endotracheal tubes used in clinical practice, so it is better to refer to this form of CMV as volume-targeted, volume-limited, or volume-controlled ventilation. One of the advantages, it offers over pressure-limited ventilation is that it responds to changes in pulmonary compliance. If compliance improves (e.g. following the administration of surfactant), pressure is decreased. Conversely, if compliance decreases (e.g. with pulmonary edema), pressure is increased to provide the desired tidal volume. Earlier technological limitations of volume-targeted ventilation included high trigger sensitivity and asynchrony, slow response times (long trigger delays), highly compliant circuits (leading to increased compressible volume loss), and the inability to both provide and measure the small tidal volumes required by premature infants. These have all been overcome (although not all of the devices providing volume-targeted ventilation can accurately measure tidal volume at the proximal airway).

Few studies to date have examined the effects of volume-targeted ventilation on neonatal outcomes. The investigation of Sinha et al.,[19] randomized larger preterm infants to receive volume-targeted or pressure-targeted ventilation, with tidal volume delivery tightly controlled. Infants assigned to the volume group had a shorter duration of ventilation, a strong trend to less CLD, and fewer severe neuroimaging abnormalities than the pressure group. Since this study, advances in the technology have enabled delivery of even smaller tidal volumes and extended the capability to provide volume-targeted ventilation to the smallest premature infants. A large clinical trial is presently underway.

Hybrid Forms of Ventilation

Attempts have been made to combine the best features of both pressure-targeted and volume-targeted ventilation, resulting in a number of hybrid modalities.[18,20-22] Volume-guarantee® and pressure-regulated volume control® ventilation utilize a breath averaging technique to constantly adjust delivered tidal volume in response to changing patient lung mechanics. Volume-assured pressure support (VAPS)® adjusts the delivery of gas during a single breath to provide a minimum tidal volume by extending inspiratory time and slightly ramping inspiratory pressure until the desired volume has been provided.[23] All three of these modalities appear promising but are in need of further investigation.

Proportional assist ventilation (PAV)[24] is an adaptive form of mechanical ventilation in which the inspiratory pressure is determined by the elastic and resistive properties of the patient. In the only published clinical trial, PAV was noted to be associated with lower mean airway and transpulmonary pressure at an equivalent fraction of inspired oxygen and similar carbon dioxide removal rate. Again, preliminary results are encouraging and ongoing evaluations may help to define the role of this modality.

Mandatory minute ventilation is a modality, which combines SIMV and PSV. A desired minute ventilation (the product of tidal volume and frequency per minute) is set by the clinician, and as long as the patient is able to meet this target spontaneously, all of the breaths are pressure-supported. If the minute ventilation falls below the desired level, the ventilator will provide additional "catch-up" SIMV breaths, using a breath averaging technique. This form of ventilation is also being actively investigated.

Permissive Hypercapnia

A recent lung-protective strategy that has been evaluated is permissive hypercapnia. This approach was based on an observation by Kraybill et al. in 1989,[25] in which infants displaying the highest carbon dioxide levels had the lowest incidence of BPD. The rationale behind permissive hypercapnia is that it decreases volutrauma, reduces the duration of ventilation, decreases the complications associated with hypocapnia, and increases oxygen unloading at the tissues by the Bohr effect. Two prospective controlled trials[26,27] did demonstrate a reduction in the duration of ventilation but failed to show a decrease in the incidence of CLD. Although the strategy is attractive, further work is necessary to determine its place in the management of neonatal respiratory failure.

Triggered Ventilation

Although IMV was the major ventilatory mode utilized for newborns for more than 25 years (Fig. 6.4, left panel), it was not

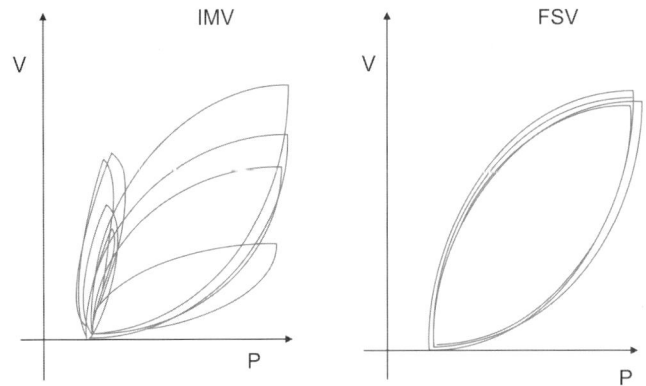

Fig. 6.4: Graphic comparison of IMV (left) and flow synchronized ventilation (FSV; assist-control) (right). Note the wide variability of delivered tidal volumes in IMV, depending on whether the baby and ventilator are in or out of phase. In FSV, every breath is the same, since baby and ventilator are always 100% synchronous

without hazard. One of its major drawbacks is the development of asynchrony, where the ventilator cycles at a programmed rate and the patient breathes independently, sometimes with and sometimes against the mechanical breath. Asynchrony has been shown to have adverse physiological consequences. "Fighting the ventilator" may lead to inconsistent tidal volume delivery, increased work of breathing (and the need for higher mechanical support), inefficient gas exchange, and airleaks. Other organ systems may also be affected. Nearly 20 years ago, Perlman and Volpe[28] demonstrated the adverse effects of asynchrony on cerebral blood flow velocity and its high association with intraventricular hemorrhage.

Figure 6.4 is a graphic comparison of IMV (left) and flow synchronized assist/control ventilation (right) and the difference is striking. In addition to the relatively feeble spontaneous breaths, supported only be PEEP, pressure-targeted IMV can result in widely variable tidal volumes, depending upon whether the baby and ventilator are in or out of phase with one another. Synchronization results in a consistently reproducible pattern of gas delivery with nearly identical pulmonary mechanics with each breath.

Synchronized or patient-triggered ventilation utilizes a patient-derived signal to initiate a mechanical breath. The signal is a surrogate of spontaneous breathing and may be a change in airway flow or pressure, abdominal movement, or thoracic impedance. One of the keys to successful triggered ventilation is a short response time or trigger delay. This is the interval between reaching the trigger threshold and the delivery of gas to the proximal airway. Long trigger delays mean that the baby may be considerably into the inspiratory cycle before receiving mechanical support, thus increasing the work of breathing and decreasing synchrony.[29]

Flow signals may also be used to terminate a breath, thus fully synchronizing the baby and the ventilator in both inspiration and expiration. This is referred to as flow-cycling. Flow-cycling is advantageous during assist-control ventilation as a safeguard against gas trapping and inversion of the inspiratory:expiratory ratio. If a baby becomes tachypneic during time-cycled assist-control, the fixed inspiratory time means that the expiratory time will become shorter and shorter as the baby breathes faster and faster. With flow-cycling, the inspiratory time will become shorter, since the breath terminates at a percentage of peak inspiratory flow

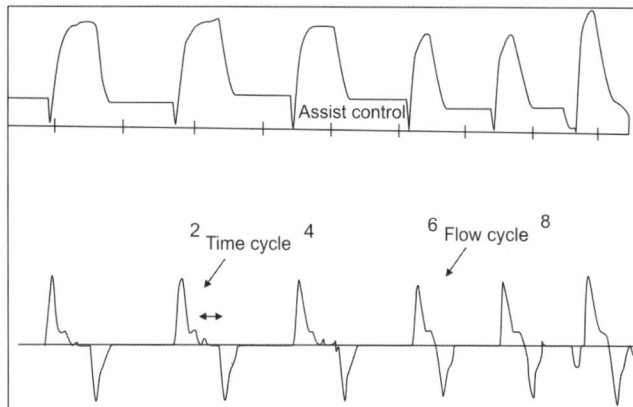

Fig. 6.5: Pressure (top) and flow (bottom) waveforms demonstrating the differences between time-cycling and flow-cycling. In time-cycling, the inspiratory phase continues for a fixed period; expiration does not begin until the exhalation valve opens. This results in a plateau pressure. In flow-cycling, inspiration ends as a percentage of peak inspiratory flow. Thus, inspiration cycles directly into expiration and results in a more spiked pressure waveform

rather than at a fixed time. Flow-cycling is also incorporated in PSV, where an inspiratory pressure "boost" is applied to spontaneous breaths to help overcome the work of breathing imposed by the narrow lumen endotracheal tube, ventilator circuit, and demand valve. PSV is primarily a weaning mode, but is also a form of synchronized ventilation[30] (Fig. 6.5). Unfortunately, the evidence base for synchronized ventilation is also variable, and its role in the prevention of BPD still needs to be determined.[31-33]

High-Frequency Ventilation

High-frequency ventilation (HFV) is generally divided into two subcategories. High-frequency jet ventilation (HFJV) uses a jet injector and pulsed or interrupted flow, usually in the range of 240–600 breaths per minute. It involves passive exhalation and is thus dependent on the elastic recoil of the lungs for emptying. It is used in tandem with a conventional ventilator, which provides PEEP and conventional or sigh breaths. High-frequency oscillatory ventilation (HFOV) is different from HFJV and involves the use of distending pressure to inflate the lung to a static volume, and usually piston-driven displacement during inspiration and active exhalation. Typical rates for HFOV are 8–15 Hz. The delivered gas volumes are even smaller than those during HFJV. Management is relatively straight forward, with oxygenation controlled by adjusting mean airway (distending) pressure and ventilation controlled by adjusting the amplitude of the oscillations.

High-frequency jet ventilation was shown to be more effective than rapid rate CMV in the management of preterm infants with pulmonary interstitial emphysema, but few studies have examined its effect on CLD as a primary outcome measure. One study by Keszler et al.[34] did show a reduced incidence of CLD and a decreased need for home oxygen, but the comparison group was ventilated with IMV and the results of this study may not be applicable today.

High-frequency oscillatory ventilation has been more intensively studied but the investigations have yielded conflicting results. In 1996, Gerstmann et al.[35] demonstrated increased survival

without CLD, but Rettwitz-Volk et al.[36-37] found no differences in a 1998 report. Thome et al. showed a shorter time to extubation in an earlier trial, but a later study in 1999[38] found no differences in the incidence of death, CLD, or intraventricular hemorrhage. The two most recent studies, both published in 2002, also had discrepant results. The Neonatal Ventilation Study of Courtney et al.[37] found a small reduction in the incidence of CLD, whereas the UKOS study of Johnson et al. found no reduction.[39] The Courtney study utilized SIMV with inspiratory times of 0.25–0.4 seconds in the comparison group; the Johnson study utilized IMV with inspiratory times set at 0.4 seconds. Perhaps the work of breathing was higher in the former study and may explain some of the differences in the results.

At present, the use of HFOV as a primary treatment strategy does not appear to be supported by the available evidence. The latest recommendation of the Cochrane Library[40] is consistent with this.

Extracorporeal Membrane Oxygenation

Extracorporeal membrane oxygenation (ECMO) is a form of extracorporeal life support in which the circulation is diverted from the body to an artificial lung for gas exchange. ECMO was originally done through catheters placed in the right common carotid artery and right internal jugular vein (venoarterial), but this necessitated permanent ligation of these vessels. Venoarterial ECMO has now been largely replaced by veno-venous ECMO, using a double-lumen catheter in the right interval jugular vein. It has been shown to be efficacious in infants more than 34 weeks or more than 2,000 gram who have reversible respiratory failure, unresponsive to "conventional" treatment, and with a more than 80% probability of death. Although ECMO is technically feasible in infants as small as 800 gram, it requires systemic anticoagulation, and thus the risk of severe cerebral hemorrhage precludes its use in smaller newborns.

Neonatal ECMO utilization for respiratory failure has declined substantially as newer treatments such as inhaled nitric oxide (iNO) and HFV have evolved. However, it remains as the penultimate rescue technique in infants with suitable indications.[41]

Inhaled Nitric Oxide Therapy

Nitric oxide in conjunction with appropriate ventilatory support is currently indicated in the management of newborns of term and near term gestation with hypoxemic respiratory failure associated with evidence of pulmonary hypertension. Its use in the management of hypoxemic respiratory failure in the preterm infant, however, has not yet been established and any such use remains investigational.

The physiologic rationale for the clinical use of iNO in hypoxemic respiratory failure is based on its ability to achieve sustained and potent pulmonary vasodilation without causing systemic hypotension. Persistent pulmonary hypertension of the newborn is a disorder associated with diverse underlying pathologies, which is characterized by high pulmonary vascular resistance causing extrapulmonary right-to-left shunting of blood across the patent ductus arteriosus, foramen ovale or both, leading to severe hypoxemia. iNO abolishes or decreases this shunt by lowering the pulmonary arterial pressure, often producing the immediate improvement in oxygenation seen in infants with PPHN.

The neonatal inhaled nitric oxide study group (NINOS)[42] and the clinical inhaled nitric oxide research group (CINRGI) are the pivotal multicenter randomized trials that have demonstrated that iNO therapy improved oxygenation and reduced the need for ECMO treatment in term and near-term (= 34 weeks of gestation) infants with hypoxemic respiratory failure and persistent pulmonary hypertension by 15–24%.

Finer recently reviewed the role of nitric oxide for respiratory failure in infants born at or near term.[43] Twelve eligible randomized controlled trials were included in the analysis. iNO therapy was shown to reduce the incidence of combined outcome of death or need for ECMO. The reduction was purely in the need for ECMO; mortality was not reduced. This finding is primarily results from the efficacy of rescue ECMO for these infants.

The role of iNO in preterm infants with hypoxemic respiratory failure is controversial. Unblinded clinical studies and case reports have shown that iNO acutely improves oxygenation in preterm infants.[44]

In a recent controlled trial, Schreiber et al.[45] showed a reduction in the combined outcome of survival without chronic lung disease in preterm infants given iNO early compared to those given placebo. The effect was only seen in infants who had less severe respiratory failure (OI < 7) at entry and not in more sick babies. Another study, the INNOVO trial from the UK failed to demonstrate any benefit,[46] but it recruited babies who had more severe respiratory failure. Additional trials are underway and until we know more, the role of iNO in preterm infants remains uncertain.

Monitoring

Continuous monitoring of the mechanically ventilated newborn has also been a major technological advance. In the earlier era of mechanical ventilation, monitoring was intermittent and inferential. Assessments were made on the basis of a daily chest radiograph to crudely estimate lung volumes, and occasional blood gas measurements to evaluate gas exchange. Transcutaneous oxygen monitoring demonstrated the foibles of this approach. The development of pulse oximetry and continuous invasive therapy has enabled tighter control of oxygenation and ventilation, and the introduction of real-time pulmonary graphic monitoring[16] has finally given the clinician breath-to-breath feedback about the interaction of the ventilator and the patient. It allows for the customization or "fine tuning" of ventilation for the individual baby and the evaluation of treatments which have a narrow therapeutic index. Monitoring is not a substitute for close clinical observation, but it can serve to augment the bedside care of ventilated newborns.

Weaning from Mechanical Ventilation

Weaning refers to the process in which the work of breathing is shifted from the mechanical ventilator to the patient. In order for the baby to be successfully weaned and extubated, there are a number of physiologic essentials. The baby must have reliable respiratory drive and be capable of sustaining alveolar ventilation once support is lessened, then removed. This requires neuromuscular competence. Adequate calories must be provided to fuel the work of breathing (but too many non-nitrogen calories can also increase carbon dioxide production). Factors known to impede the weaning process should be avoided or at least considered. They include electrolyte imbalance and metabolic alkalosis, anemia, infection, patent ductus arteriosus and/or congestive heart failure, neurologic

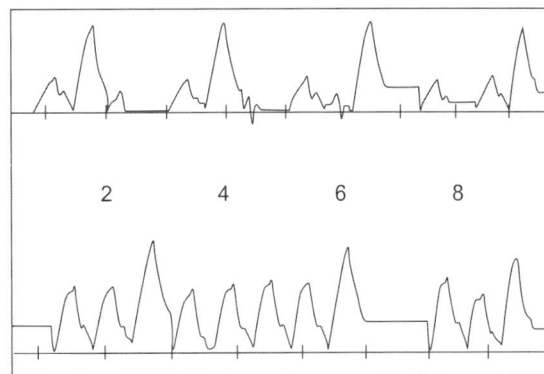

Fig. 6.6: Top: Larger breaths are mechanical SIMV breaths, smaller breaths are spontaneous, supported only by PEEP. **Bottom:** Pressure support has been added to spontaneous breaths. These partially supported breaths are not quite as robust as the SIMV breaths (by choice), but are far better than the unsupported spontaneous breaths in the upper panel

dysfunction, and the effects of pharmacologic agents, such as analgesics and sedatives.

In general, the most harmful parameters should be decreased first. If the fraction of inspired oxygen is high, it should be weaned to less than 0.4 as oxygenation permits. If PIP or PEEP is high, it should likewise be decreased. The advent of triggered ventilation has altered weaning strategy, since reduction in the ventilator rate during assist-control does little if the patient is breathing above the control rate. Most studies to date have demonstrated that any form of triggered ventilation is superior to IMV in decreasing the time of ventilation.[47] Care should be taken to avoid fatiguing the baby by decreasing the ventilator rate during (S)IMV, since there is no support for spontaneous breathing other than PEEP. Perhaps augmenting this with PSV will be the solution (Fig. 6.6).

Controversies still abound regarding adjunctive treatments during the weaning process. Although studies do support the use of methylxanthines, concerns exist regarding long-term safety. Similarly, diuretics and bronchodilators have been used with varying success, but some measure of efficacy should be assessed if treatment is to be continued. Corticosteroids have received a great deal of attention, primarily related to their use in the prevention and treatment of BPD. Neurodevelopmental concerns appear justified,[48,49] and the use of corticosteroids in the weaning/extubation process should be limited to short-term treatment of infants who have failed extubation because of upper airway edema.

Prior prospective indices to determine readiness for extubation have not been helpful. However, the ability to measure pulmonary mechanics, tidal volume and minute ventilation has been shown to have a high positive predictive value in determining when to extubate a preterm infant recovering from RDS.[50] Alternatively, in the larger infant, one might consider extubation when the degree of support appears to equal the imposed work of breathing. This is another area ripe for investigation.

Optimizing Mechanical Ventilation

How can we optimize conventional ventilation? First, we need to ask good clinical questions. Second, we need to design the right tools to answer them. Third, we need to accurately and succinctly define our terminology and our outcome measures. A significant example of this is how we choose to define "BPD". There can be an enormous variation in the incidence of BPD within the same population, depending on how one chooses to define BPD. We need to find a better way to do this, and the work of Walsh and colleagues on determining a functional or physiological definition of CLD is an encouraging beginning.[51]

We clearly need to develop a better evidence base with respect to the multiple ways we can now ventilate babies. From this, we should be able to ask even better questions. It is possible that we have relied too heavily on meta-analysis, and we need to understand its limitations. Again, as an example, although the focus of most analyses has been on ventilation practices, which very well may be the most important variable affecting pulmonary outcomes, are the cited studies adequately controlled for other clinical parameters which can and do impact the pathogenesis of BPD, including nutritional practices; management of blood pressure and fluids; the approach to the PDA; the use of analgesics and sedatives, and respiratory drugs; antibiotic practices; ancillary care; and very importantly, the variability in the host response?

THE FUTURE

As we ask the important questions, other outcomes besides just CLD need to be considered. CLD is an intermediate outcome variable, but it may not be as important as looking at longer range assessments, of which neurodevelopmental outcome is probably the most important. Similarly, short-term measures may also be significant. For instance, if there are no differences in either CLD or neurodevelopmental outcomes between two styles of ventilation, we should pay close attention to the short-term measures, such as patient comfort, cost effectiveness and acute complications, such as pneumothorax and days of ventilation.

What is the ideal mode of ventilation? It is one which delivers a breath that synchronizes with patient's own spontaneous respiratory effort. It maintains adequate and consistent tidal volume delivery and minute ventilation at low airway pressures. It is able to respond to sudden or unpredictable changes in pulmonary mechanics or patient demand. It provides the lowest possible work of breathing for the baby.

What is the ideal ventilator? It is one that achieves all of the important goals of mechanical ventilation. It provides a variety of modes and modalities that can ventilate even the most challenging pulmonary diseases. It has monitoring capabilities to adequately assess ventilator and patient's performance. It has safety features and alarms that offer lung protective strategies. Most importantly, perhaps, it is used by a clinician willing to investigate its optimal uses and clinical applications.

Where do we go from here? The technology is only going to become more complex, the choices more numerous, and the decisions more perplexing. It will be imperative for us to harness the technology appropriately and, most importantly, safely.

ACKNOWLEDGMENT

We acknowledge the useful contribution from Dr Samir Gupta, Senior Clinical Fellow and Mrs Victoria Hall, PA, in preparing this manuscript.

REFERENCES

1. Attar MA, Donn SM. Mechanism of ventilator-induced lung injury in premature infants. Semin Neonatol. 2002;7(5):353-60.
2. Donn SM, Sinha SK. Newer techniques of mechanical ventilation: an overview. Semin Neonatol. 2002;7(5):401-8.
3. Gregory G, Kitterman J, Phibbs R. Treatment of the idiopathic respiratory distress syndrome with continuous positive airway pressure. N Engl J Med. 1971;284:1333-40.
4. Northway WH Jr, Rosan RC, Porter DY. Pulmonary disease following respiratory-therapy of hyaline-membrane disease. Bronchopulmonary dysplasia. N Engl J Med. 1967;276(7):357-68.
5. Philips AGS. Oxygen plus pressure plus time. The aetiology of bronchopulmonary dysplasia. Pediatrics. 1975;55:44-50.
6. Jobe AH, Bancalari E. Bronchopulmonary dysplasia. A J of Resp and Crit Care Med. 2001;163(7):1723-9.
7. Jobe A. The new BPD: an arrest of lung development. Pediatr Res. 1999;1999(46):641-3.
8. Wung JT, James LS, Kilchevsky E, et al. Management of infants with severe respiratory failure and persistence of fetal circulation without hyperventilation. Pediatrics. 1985;76:488-92.
9. Morley C. Continuous distending pressure. Arch Dis Child Fetal Neonatal Ed. 1999;81:F152-6.
10. De Paoli AG, Davis PG, Faber B, et al. Devices and pressure sources for administration of nasal continuous positive airway pressure (NCPAP) in preterm neonates. Cochrane Database of Syst Rev. 2002;(4):CD002977.
11. McCulloch PR, Forkert PG, Froese AB. Lung volume maintenance prevents lung injury during high frequency oscillatory ventilation in surfactant-deficient rabbits. Am Rev Respir Dis. 1988;137(5):1185-92.
12. Dos Santos CC, Slutsky AS. Invited review: mechanisms of ventilator-induced lung injury: a perspective. J Appl Physiol. 2000;89(4):1645-55.
13. Bond DM, Froese AB. Volume recruitment maneuvers are less deleterious than persistent low lung volumes in the atelectasis-prone rabbit lung during high-frequency oscillation. Critical Care Medicine. 1993;21(3):402-12.
14. Froese AB. Role of lung volume in lung injury: HFO in the atelectasis-prone lung. Acta Anaesthesiol Scand Suppl. 1989;90:126-30.
15. Harris T, Wood B. Physiologic Principals in Assisted Ventilation of the Neonate. In: Goldsmith J, Karotkin E (Eds). Philadelphia: WB Saunders Company; 1996. pp. 21-68.
16. Sinha SK, Nicks JJ, Donn SM. Graphic analysis of pulmonary mechanics in neonates receiving assisted ventilation. Archives of Disease in Childhood Fetal and Neonatal Edition. 1996;75(3):F213-8.
17. Carlo WA, Ambalavanan N, Chatburn RL. Classification of mechanical ventilation devices. In: Sinha SK, Donn SM (Eds). Manual of Neonatal Respiratory Care. Armonk, NY: Futura Publishing Co. Inc.; 2000. pp. 122-7.
18. Sinha S, Donn S. Volume-controlled ventilation: variations on a theme. Clinics in Perinatology. 2001;28(3):547-60.

19. Sinha SK, Donn SM, Gavey J, et al. Randomised trial of volume controlled versus time cycled, pressure limited ventilation in preterm infants with respiratory distress syndrome. Arch Dis Child Fetal Neonatal Ed. 1997;77(3):F202-5.

20. Cheema IU, Ahluwalia JS. Feasibility of tidal volume-guided ventilation in newborn infants: a randomized, crossover trial using the volume guarantee modality. Pediatrics. 2001;107(6):1323-8.

21. Donn SM, Sinha SK. Newer modes of mechanical ventilation for the neonate. Current Opinion in Pediatrics. 2001;13(2):99-103.

22. Dekeon M. Pressure control ventilation and pressure-regulated-volume-controlled ventilation. In: Sinha SK, Donn S (Eds). Manual of Neonatal Respiratory Care. Armonk, NY: Futura Publishing Company, Inc; 2000. pp. 161-2.

23. Sinha SK, Donn SM. Volume controlled ventilation. In: Goldsmith JP, Karotkin EH (Eds). Assisted Ventilation of the Neonate, 4th edition. Philadelphia: Elsevier; 2003.

24. Schulze A, Bancalari E. Proportional assist ventilation in infants. Clinics in Perinatology. 2001;28(3):561-78.

25. Kraybill EN, Runyan DK, Bose CL, et al. Risk factors for chronic lung disease in infants with birth weights of 750 to 1000 grams. J Pediatr. 1989;115:115-20.

26. Amato MB, Barbas CS, Medeiros DM, et al. Effect of a protective-ventilation strategy on mortality in the acute respiratory distress syndrome. N Engl J Med. 1998;338(6):347-54.

27. Carlo WA, Stark AR, Wright LL, et al. Minimal ventilation to prevent bronchopulmonary dysplasia in extremely-low-birthweight infants. J Pediatr. 2002;141(3):370-4.

28. Perlman JM, Volpe JJ. Cerebral blood flow velocity in relation to intraventricular hemorrhage in the premature newborn infant. J Pediatr. 1982;100(6):956-9.

29. Donn SM, Sinha SK. Controversies in patient-triggered ventilation. Clin Perinatol. 1998;25(1):49-61.

30. Sinha SK, Donn SM. Pressure support ventilation. In: Sinha SK, Donn SM (Eds). Manual of Neonatal Respiratory Care. Armonk, NY: Futura Publishing Co Inc.; 2000. pp. 157-60.

31. Greenough A. Update on patient triggered ventilation. Clin Perinatol. 2001;28(3):533-46.

32. Baumer JH. International randomised controlled trial of patient-triggered ventilation in neonatal respiratory distress syndrome. Arch Dis Child Fetal Neonatal Ed. 2000;82(1):F5-10.

33. Donn SM, Greenough A, Sinha SK. Patient triggered ventilation. Arch Dis Child Fetal Neonatal Ed. 2000;83(3):F225-6.

34. Keszler M, Modanlou HD, Brudno DS, et al. Multicenter controlled clinical trial of high-frequency jet ventilation in preterm infants with uncomplicated respiratory distress syndrome. Pediatrics. 1997;100(4):593-9.

35. Gerstmann DR, Minton SD, Stoddard RA, et al. The Provo multicenter early high-frequency oscillatory ventilation trial: improved pulmonary and clinical outcome in respiratory distress syndrome. Pediatrics. 1996;98(6 Pt 1):1044-57.

36. Rettwitz-Volk W, Veldman A, Roth B, et al. A prospective, randomized, multicenter trial of high-frequency oscillatory ventilation compared with conventional ventilation in preterm infants with respiratory distress syndrome receiving surfactant. J Pediatr. 1998;132(2):249-54.

37. Courtney SE, Durand DJ, Asselin JM, et al. High frequency oscillatory ventilation versus conventional mechanical ventilation for very-low-birth-weight infants. N Engl J Med. 2002;347(9):643-52.

38. Thome U, Kössel H, Lipowsky G, et al. Randomized comparison of high-frequency ventilation with high-rate intermittent positive pressure ventilation in preterm infants with respiratory failure. J Pediatr. 1999;135(1):39-46.

39. Johnson AH, Peacock JL, Greenough A, et al. High-frequency oscillatory ventilation for the prevention of chronic lung disease of prematurity. N Engl J Med. 2002;347(9):633-42.

40. Henderson-Smart DJ, et al. Elective high frequency oscillatory ventilation versus conventional ventilation for acute pulmonary dysfunction in preterm infants. Cochrane Database of Systematic Reviews (Computer File). 2004;(2):CD000104.

41. Schumacher RE, Baumgart S. Extracorporeal membrane oxygenation, 2001: the odyssey continues. Clin Perinatol. 2001;28(3):629-53.

42. Neonatal Inhaled Nitric Oxide Study Group. Inhaled nitric oxide in full-term and nearly full-term infants with hypoxic respiratory failure. N Engl J Med. 1997;336(9):597-604.

43. Finer NN, Barrington KJ. Nitric oxide for respiratory failure in infants born at or near term. (update of Cochrane Database Syst Rev. 2000;(2): CD000399; PMID: 10796358). Cochrane Database of Systematic Reviews. 2001;(2):CD000399.

44. Kinsella JP, Walsh WF, Bose CL, et al. Inhaled nitric oxide in premature neonates with severe hypoxaemic respiratory failure: a randomised controlled trial. Lancet. 1999;354(9184):1061-5.

45. Schreiber M, Gin-Mestan K, Marks JD, et al. Inhaled nitric oxide in premature infants with the respiratory distress syndrome. N Engl J Med. 2003;349:2099-107.

46. Field D. The Innovo Trial: Preliminary results for NO use in preterm infants. Arch Dis Child. 2003;88:A1.

47. Sinha SK, Donn SM. Weaning babies from mechanical ventilation. Seminars in Neonatology. 2002;7:421-8.

48. Yeh T, Lin YJ, Lin HC, et al. Outcomes at school age after postnatal dexamethasone therapy for lung disease of prematurity. N Engl J Med. 2004;350:1304-13.

49. Finer N, Craft A, Vaucher YE, et al. Postnatal steroids: short term gain, long term pain? J Pediatr. 2000;137:9-13.

50. Gillespie L, Whyte S, Sinha SK, et al. Usefulness of the minute ventilation test in predicting successful extubation in newborn infants: a randomized controlled trial. J Perinat. 2003;23:205-7.

51. Walsh MC, Wilson-Costello D, Zadell A, et al. Safety, reliability, and validity of a physiologic definition of bronchopulmonary dysplasia. J Perinatol. 2003;23:451-6.

7

Clinical Care of the Very Preterm Infant

L Hellström-Westas, LJ Bjorklund, M Lindroth

REGIONALIZATION OF CARE

The concept of regionalization of perinatal care was introduced in the late 1960s in Canada,[1] and during the 1970s perinatal centers were established in developed countries. The goal was to identify the high-risk pregnancies and to transfer mothers to tertiary hospitals, which were organized, staffed and equipped for the multidisciplinary task of providing optimal maternal and neonatal care. In Europe, the regionalization of preterm infants in the late 1990s was evaluated in a survey (EUROPET) showing that there were great variations in the regionalization programs between different countries.[2,3] In some countries, governmental policies exist; in others national scientific societies issue guidelines, usually stressing intrauterine transfers and delivery in level III centers for very preterm infants. The size of the delivery units varies considerably, the average number of births per maternity unit being 500–3,000. Large maternity units usually have adjacent level III neonatal intensive care units (NICUs), although the organization of them varies.[4]

In USA, a trend toward deregionalization has occurred since the late 1980s, referring to a process of moving away from transfers to referral centers providing the highest quality of care to promote competing hospitals with less expertise. The difference in functioning level is not clear to the public, and thus decisions on which caring centers to choose may be taken on nonmedical grounds, such as convenient location.[5] Deregionalization may also be a result of too small tertiary neonatal units without possibility to admit all newborn patients requiring intensive care. As a result of the remarkable increase in survival of the very preterm infants during the last decades, the patient load in tertiary NICUs often exceeds their capacities. Thus, the criteria used for defining high-risk pregnancies tend to be stricter, i.e. only the most immature infants are transferred to level III units and less immature preterm infants with considerable morbidity risks are increasingly treated in level II units. This development is unfortunate, since the way that perinatal care is organized may have a substantial impact on clinical outcomes, such as mortality and disability rates. Birth at a hospital with a regional NICU is associated with a lower risk-adjusted mortality than birth at a hospital with no NICU, intermediate NICU of any size, or small community hospitals.[6]

The size of the NICU has an impact on the outcome, as example was reported in a Finnish national study where the lowest mortality and disability rates were reported in the largest academic NICU.[7] In a California study on preterm infants with a birth weight less than 2,000 gram, risk-adjusted neonatal mortality was significantly lower for births that occurred in hospitals with level III NICUs with an average census of more than 15 patients per day.[8] No evidence-based recommendations are available on the optimal size of a NICU. However, a reasonable sized NICU is mandatory for running a neonatal service with all necessary functions: Neonatologists

available around the clock, experienced staff, full range of medical intensive care with cardiology and surgical services including bedside operations, and capacities to expand the facilities during high demand periods due to preterm multiple births. Regional units should have an academic function, providing high quality specialist training and performing research on their preterm cohorts as well as repeated quality assessments of treatment strategies. Further, tertiary academic units should participate in national and international networks, e.g. for collaborative use of quality improvement techniques, and translation of research into practice, which may result in accelerated and effective practice changes and implementation of evidence-based interventions.[9]

The rapid development of technology in newborn medicine, e.g. ventilators and incubators for preterm infants, leads to a continuous need for new investments in intensive care equipments. Centralization of neonatal care decreases the need for overlapping functions in level III and level II centers, especially investments in expensive technology. Regional resources for expensive frontline equipments should be allocated to the regional center, which should have responsibility for evaluating them scientifically and keep them in continuous use thus providing a high-level of technical know-how in the staff. The performance of intensive care could be facilitated by a computerized clinical information system, which ensures precision in physician orders, improves medication management, facilitates reporting, and provides detailed documentation of care and continuous monitoring of parameters from technical equipments. Implementing of computerized physician order, entry has been shown to reduce medication turn-around times and medication errors.[10]

The limited health resources can be efficiently used with a well-organized tiered network with regionalization of highly specialized intensive care and several level II units for the intermediate care.[11] This organization model aims at a balance between efficiency and accessibility to services and requires transfer of the preterm infant after the intensive care period to the next level unit.

TRANSPORT

Regionalization of perinatal care requires a well-organized transfer service as well as presents an opportunity to establish a safe and efficient transfer network.[12] The goal should be that all high-risk pregnancies are identified antenatally and the transfer to the perinatal center with level III NICU should take place in utero. However, there will be a small group of preterm infants acutely delivered outside the tertiary perinatal center, as well as newborn infants with unexpected complications and postnatal disorders, who need to be transferred postnatally to the regional center.

Neonatal transport service requires an appropriate referral system, trained personnel and management structures.[13] Depending on the population base and the geography different solutions can be applied. For emergency postnatal transports of very preterm infants to the level III units, it is crucial that the transport team is trained in neonatal intensive care of this patient group. Prior to the transfer the infant should be stabilized and the intensive care should be continued and monitored during the transport. According to the EUROPET survey in 1996 on large NICUs in Europe, the average national inborn rate of preterm infants less than 30–32 weeks of gestation exceeded 75% in the majority of countries.[14] Thus, the need for postnatal transports of very preterm infants is fortunately an uncommon situation, which however, is a highly demanding task in order to avoid transport related complications.

THE NEONATAL INTENSIVE CARE UNIT

The goal should be to deliver all very preterm infants in a tertiary perinatal center with a neonatal unit well-experienced in all aspects of intensive care. Active management has contributed to the improved prognosis for very preterm infants during the last decade[15,16] in addition to other factors, such as level of antenatal care and socio-economic factors, and administration of antenatal steroids. Ideally, the NICU should be located close to the delivery unit and to the operating theatre, so that intrahospital transports can be avoided after delivery. It is necessary for neonatal units who treat very preterm infants to develop clinical routines for the care of these infants. Such routines should include guidelines for minimal handling and strategies for keeping the number of invasive procedures to a minimum. The noise level in the NICUs is often high, and consequently measures should be taken to reduce noise and light, and include environmental guidelines.

IMMEDIATE CARE AT BIRTH

The initial clinical care of the very preterm infants differs from the care of more mature infants in several aspects. In this context we will emphasize the initial care of extremely preterm infants born before 28 weeks of gestation. The very preterm infants have higher mortality and are more likely to develop intraventricular hemorrhages (IVH), symptomatic persistent ductus arteriosus (PDA), sepsis, necrotizing enterocolitis (NEC) and bronchopulmonary dysplasia (BPD) as compared to more mature infants.[7,17] They are also at higher risk for developing cerebral palsy and disturbances in attention and cognition. Close perinatal collaboration between obstetricians and neonatologists is essential for healthy survival of these infants.

Prior to delivery, the parents should be informed by the neonatal staff about expectations for survival and morbidity, based on recent statistics. The parents should always be allowed to express their own expectations, and if time allows also have the possibility of a visit to the NICU before the delivery. This goal can sometimes be difficult to achieve, not least with an expecting mother in active labor or with preeclampsia, nevertheless it should always be attempted. In vaginal deliveries, immediate postnatal stabilization of the very preterm infant can preferably take place in the delivery room, close to the parents.

The initial care of the very preterm infants should be very carefully planned.[18] Evaporative heat loss during the first minute of life can cause severe cooling of these infants, and a low temperature on admission to the NICU is an independent risk factor of death.[17] Radiant heater open beds designed for resuscitation should be used. In addition, hypothermia can be prevented by wrapping the wet body of the infant in a plastic bag as soon as possible after birth.[19,20] After rapid stabilization, the infant can be placed directly in a preheated incubator. This transfer can be avoided by initial use of combination incubators with both radiant heater open bed and double wall incubator alternatives. The incubator is then moved to the NICU and used for the continuing care of the infant. In order to minimize the disturbance of the very preterm infant, all later procedures, e.g. insertion of umbilical lines, should be done without moving the infant from the incubator.

It is of vital importance that adequate equipment for resuscitation is available in the delivery room or operating theater. For this purpose, mobile resuscitation beds are very useful. Modern pulse oximeters can give correct values for oxygen saturation and heart rate within a few minutes after birth,[21] and it is no longer acceptable to rely on intermittent heart rate auscultation and visual assessment of skin color. The pulse oximeter probe should preferably be placed on the right hand to assess preductal saturation.[22] The more common placement on one foot may result in lower readings early in life, with a risk for unnecessary oxygen treatment. Although current guidelines still recommend that 100% oxygen should be used for resuscitation,[23] there is increasing evidence suggesting that lower oxygen exposure is beneficial for newborn infants.[24,25] Healthy, full term infants are not expected to reach preductal oxygen saturation above 90% until 10 minutes after birth,[25] and there is no reason to strive for higher levels in premature infants. The resuscitation bed must be equipped with an inspired gas blender for precise oxygen administration.[22] If oxygen saturation rises above 93%, oxygen supply should be rapidly reduced or discontinued.[26]

The initial ventilatory management of the very preterm infant is currently much debated.[27] In general, previous studies recommended that premature infants should be intubated and given prophylactic surfactant early after birth, but it has been questioned whether this is applicable to current babies.[28] These babies are often more immature, but may paradoxically both have an accelerated lung maturation at birth and a highly vulnerable lung with a disposition to develop BPD.[29] Animal studies indicate that the immature lung may be particularly sensitive to ventilation-induced injury very early after birth,[30] and epidemiological studies imply that an aggressive initial respiratory management including early intubation and surfactant may be associated with an increased risk for BPD.[31] In many centers, there is now a trend against routine delivery room intubation in favor of early application of continuous positive airway pressure (CPAP).[32] A recent trial showed that delivery room intubation could be avoided in 53% of infants born at 24–25 weeks of gestation.[33] Another approach, aiming to avoid mechanical ventilation early in life, is to perform endotracheal intubation immediately after birth and give prophylactic surfactant, followed by rapid extubation to nasal CPAP. However, preliminary results from one study showed that, in infants born at 27–29 weeks of gestation, there was no added benefit from prophylactic surfactant when early CPAP was used.[34] It is not known if the same is true also for more immature infants. Ongoing multicenter trials on delivery room management of preterm infants may provide new evidence on treatment strategies.[27]

Although the preterm infant may appear severely depressed at birth, immediate intubation is usually not indicated. Even if a prophylactic surfactant strategy is chosen, there is no proven benefit from giving surfactant before the first breath.[35] Bag and mask ventilation of preterm infants may be difficult, and gas exchange will probably be very inefficient unless the baby contributes by making gasps.[36] Even so, the vast majority of small infants will respond to bag and mask ventilation with a rapid increase in heart rate. Once the baby starts breathing spontaneously, its efforts can be supported if adequate equipment is available. Unfortunately, the commonly used self-inflating resuscitation bags have severe limitations.[37] The oxygen supply is difficult to regulate, and the bags have a poorly working pressure limitation. Consequently, high pressures (> 40 cm H_2O) are easily generated, especially at high ventilatory rates. Tidal volumes are unknown and can potentially become very large. Moreover, there is usually no way of obtaining CPAP or positive end-expiratory pressure (PEEP), and therefore no way to effectively support the baby's spontaneous breathing.

The Neopuff® Infant Resuscitator (Fisher and Paykel, Auckland, NZ) is a commonly used T-piece system with adjustable PEEP and peak pressure that can be attached to a face mask or an endotracheal tube. It can easily be used to apply nasal or face mask CPAP immediately after birth (Fig. 7.1). It has been suggested that a relatively high distending pressure (up to 8 cm H_2O) should be used in this situation.[37] If the baby responds well, CPAP with the same device can be continued during transportation to the NICU. In an experimental setting, the Neopuff®device produced reliable and reproducible peak inspiratory pressures and PEEP.[38,39] However, there are at present no published clinical trials evaluating this method against other systems.

At all very preterm deliveries, surfactant should be immediately available. According to Scandinavian tradition, infants are not intubated for the sole purpose of giving surfactant. However, if the very preterm infant needs intubation for resuscitation, surfactant should be given as soon as the endotracheal tube is presumed to be in a correct position. Many infants respond rapidly and may soon be breathing room air on endotracheal tube-CPAP, in which case early extubation can be considered.

Even if the infant is intubated and surfactant is administered in the delivery room, there is usually sufficient time to allow the parents to see their baby before transportation to the NICU. The father can usually take part in this transport, and photographs can be taken as a first memory. After arrival to the NICU and within the first hour of life, venous and arterial catheters are inserted for blood sampling, infusion of glucose, and for arterial blood pressure monitoring.

NUTRITION

The beneficial effects of early enteral feeding on the development of the gut of the preterm infant are well-recognized.[40,41] Recent data indicate improved short-term and long-term outcome in preterm infants fed human milk as compared to formula-fed infants.[42-44] Enteral feedings with small amounts of human milk (1–2 mL every 3 h) can usually be started within the first hour of life in very preterm infants.[45] The primary feed should be the infant's own mother's milk, but until it is available, heat-treated donor milk is used.

In order to reduce the number of invasive procedures, indwelling central venous catheters (CVCs) for fluid and drug administration can be used. Although the risks for example thrombosis, with umbilical venous catheters are well known, this is for the very preterm infants an easy and rapid way of gaining venous access. Before use, the position should always be checked with X-ray and the catheter should always allow withdrawal of blood. An umbilical venous catheter, in correct position with the tip of the catheter in the inferior vena cava, is suitable for supplementary parenteral nutrition during the first day of life. Double lumen catheters are useful, since they allow a steady infusion in one lumen while intermittent injections can be given in the other lumen without the need for additional peripheral intravenous lines during the first day. After 3–4 days the umbilical venous catheter can be replaced by a peripherally inserted central venous catheter (PICC). When the tip of a PICC is optimally located in the upper vena cava (as checked by X-ray) it can often be used also for blood sampling.[46]

Initially, an infusion of glucose is given, replaced as soon as possible by a glucose-amino acid solution providing glucose at a rate of 4–6 mg/kg/min.[47] Before the third day of life, there is usually no need to add electrolytes except calcium. To reduce the risk of hyperchloremic metabolic acidosis, sodium acetate should be used instead of sodium chloride in the intravenous solutions. Providing adequate nutrition and sufficient caloric intake is a problem during the first week of life in very preterm infants.[47] For this reason, intravenous lipids should usually be started already in the second day of life, with close supervision of serum triglycerides. A multivitamin preparation is included in the lipid solution to reduce the risk of peroxidation. The initial daily dose of lipids is usually 0.5 g/kg, which, if tolerated without hyperlipidemia, is increased stepwise to 2 g/kg during the first week of life, only rarely increased to 3 g/kg.[48]

The enteral milk feedings are gradually increased on a day-to-day basis. When the very preterm infant can tolerate 75–80% of the total volume intake by the enteral route, i.e. 130–160 mL/kg of a total daily volume intake of 170–200 mL/kg, the supplementary parenteral nutrition can be omitted. The infant's own mother's milk is the preferred source of the enteral nutrition. All mothers should be encouraged to express their milk during the preterm period and to breast-feed their infants after discharge from the neonatal unit. If the mother cannot supply her infant with milk, pasteurized banked donor milk is used, or a preterm formula. Administered human milk can be analyzed for macronutrient content (protein, energy)[49,50] and thus the fortification can be individually planned, aiming at a daily protein and energy intake of 3.5 (-4.0) g/kg and

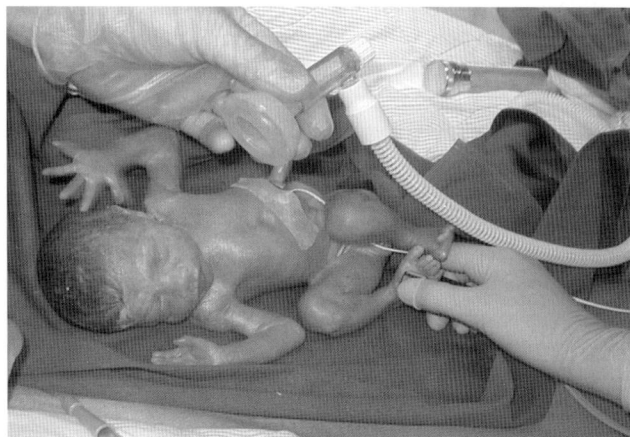

Fig. 7.1: Immediate care after delivery. This vigorous and spontaneously breathing infant is just about to be assisted with face mask continuous positive airway pressure (CPAP) by the Neopuff®. An oxygen saturation probe is applied to the right foot (*Courtesy:* Mats Blennow)

120 kcal/kg, respectively. Higher energy intakes are often required in infants with BPD. Weekly biochemical monitoring of protein status should be performed in the very preterm infants by, e.g. measuring serum levels of urea and transthyretin (prealbumin).[51] Calcium and particularly phosphorus supplementation is needed for adequate bone mineralization in human milk-fed infants.[44]

CLINICAL MONITORING

Respiratory and hemodynamic instability is common in very preterm infants. Close surveillance is essential, both during the early acute phase, characterized by postnatal adaptation and respiratory distress, and at later stages when nosocomial infections and recurrent apneas are common. Initial clinical signs of infection may be subtle, but often precede deterioration in vital parameters. The clinical monitoring includes regular observations of vitality, color, heart rate, respiration, body temperature, bowel movements and diuresis.

Fluid and electrolyte balance are closely related to evaporation and heat loss from the immature skin.[52] The insensible water loss from the immature skin is highest during the first 2 days of life, and then decreases during the first week.[53] The skin of the most immature infants often becomes dry and cracked during the first week of life. Various methods for preventing this, e.g. by applying prophylactic ointment have been evaluated, but shown that this strategy may be associated with an increased risk for nosocomial sepsis.[54] Double-walled incubators with a high humidity, starting at 80%, should be used in these infants to diminish the inevitable water losses (Fig. 7.2). The daily fluid requirements average 85–100 mL/kg. However, the most immature infants may require more during the first day of life. Serum levels of electrolytes (sodium, potassium and ionized calcium) should be measured and monitored daily during the initial course. Hypocalcemia can usually be corrected by IV administration of calcium, either as bolus or added to the intravenous infusion. Hypernatremia (serum sodium above 150 mmol/L) is usually caused by too low fluid intakes, or by too large

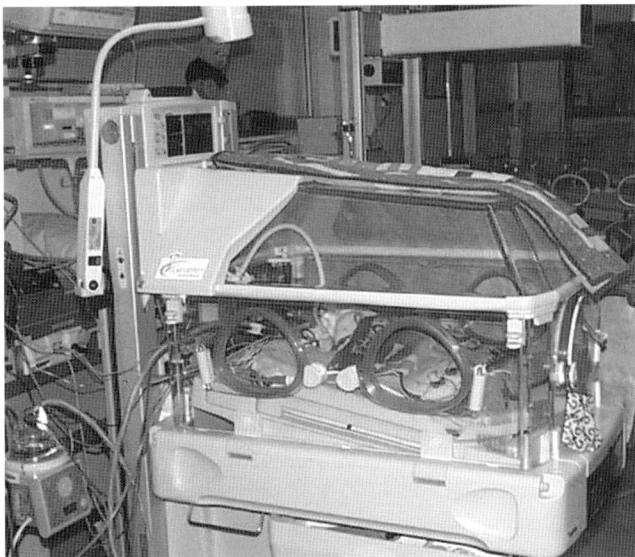

Fig. 7.2: Double-walled incubators are used for optimal thermal management of very preterm infants. When the infants are stable an incubator cover can be used in order to reduce noise and light

insensible water loss, or by adding sodium too early to intravenous infusions. Nonoliguric hyperkalemia sometimes occurs during the first day of life in the most immature infants and does not seem to be related to kidney function.[55] Kidney function is difficult to evaluate in the very preterm infants during the first day of life. The serum creatinine levels are often affected by the maternal creatinine level, although very high serum creatinine and urea levels, and oliguria may be seen in infants with poor kidney function. Urinary output mainly reflects the fluid balance and is also a sign that the arterial blood pressure is sufficient. A diuresis of 1–2 mL/kg/h after 24 h of age is usually adequate. Blood transfusions are often needed in the initial care of very preterm infants. In many hospitals, diuretics are given as routine after blood transfusions. This strategy has no support by controlled studies, and a frequent use of diuretics may increase the risk for nephrocalcinosis.[56] Blood and urinary glucose levels should be checked regularly, particularly during the first week of life, in order to avoid both hypoglycemia and hyperglycemia. Almost all very preterm infants need phototherapy for hyper-bilirubinemia, and initially serum bilirubin should be checked daily.[57] In computerized clinical information systems, algorithms for insensible water loss can be included providing continuous water-balance monitoring. Thus, dehydration and hypernatremia can be avoided. Continuous glucose infusion, without interruption, is important for stable blood glucose values. The most immature infants may need insulin infusion for adequate glucose intake.

Continuous monitoring of vital parameters is necessary in the care of very preterm infants. These infants often need monitoring of electrocardiogram or heart rate, respiration and oxygen saturation at least until they have reached 32–33 weeks of gestation. In the initial phase, blood pressure is preferably monitored through an indwelling umbilical or peripheral artery catheter, since non-invasive blood pressure monitoring is less reliable. Continuous transcutaneous measurement of blood gases, i.e. partial pressures of oxygen and carbon dioxide, is often very useful although the fragile skin during the first day of life sometimes limits the time when electrodes can be applied. Transcutaneous monitoring of PCO_2 levels can reduce the need for blood gas samples and give early indications of hypocarbia, which indicates that ventilator settings should be promptly reduced. Monitoring PCO_2 is important since low $PaCO_2$ values are associated with decreased cerebral blood flow and development of periventricular leukomalacia, and also with development of BPD.[58] Continuous monitoring of oxygen saturation is a standard procedure in all NICUs, and most units have guidelines for oxygen saturation limits in very preterm infants, often with a wide range between 85% and 95%. However, more research is needed in order to obtain evidence on whether the lower or higher values of this range would be preferable.[59] High, or unstable oxygen saturation is a risk factor for retinopathy of prematurity (ROP), and very preterm infants should be regularly examined by ophthalmologists from around 32 weeks of gestation until full-term for early detection and treatment of ROP. Continuous monitoring of electrocortical activity with amplitude-integrated electroencephalography (aEEG), a simplified method utilizing one or two channels of filtered and time-compressed EEG, is increasingly being used in neonatal units. The method shows changes overtime in cerebroelectrical background activity and can be used also in preterm infants. Degree of electrocortical background depression in aEEG activity shows good correlation with grade of IVH and outcome.[60-62] The method also reveals subclinical seizure activity. Normal data for very preterm infants have been published recently.[63]

INFECTIONS

Perinatal infections [bacterial vaginosis, premature rupture of membranes (PROM), chorioamnionitis] are important causes of very preterm birth. In contrast, early-onset bacterial infections (positive culture before 72 h of age) in the offspring are uncommon, and blood cultures drawn at the time of arterial line insertion are usually negative. An increasing use of antibiotics before and during labor has led to a substantial decrease in early group B streptococcal infections, but simultaneously there has been an increase in prevalence of *E. coli* sepsis.[64] These infections may have a rapidly progressive course with severe hypoxic respiratory failure and early demise.

Late-onset nosocomial bloodstream infections are much more common, occurring in between 10% and 30% of very low birth weight infants.[65] They are usually less severe than early infections, but are still associated with a significant morbidity. Coagulase negative staphylococci (CoNS) are by far the most common pathogens, being implicated in around 50% of cases.[66] CoNS infections often occur at around 10–14 days of age. The source of bacteremia is usually a CVC that has been colonized with CoNS, either by skin contamination during insertion or through the catheter hub during later manipulations.[67] Symptoms are unspecific and include apneas, increased oxygen requirement, respiratory insufficiency, and sometimes also arterial hypotension. Serum level of C-reactive protein is increased, but this may not be seen until after 12–24 hours. Treatment with vancomycin is often started already when an infection is first suspected, leading to a substantial overuse of this drug. It is not known how long one can safely wait before starting vancomycin treatment,[67] but in relatively stable infants it is usually possible to wait until there is an increase in serum levels of C-reactive protein. If an adequate amount of blood (1 mL) is taken for culture, vancomycin can be discontinued after 48 hour if blood culture and ancillary tests are still negative.[67] Antibiotic treatment of CoNS bacteremia is often started without removal of the CVC, but if the baby has a delayed clinical response and if bacteremia persists, the line must be withdrawn.[68,69] CoNS bloodstream infections are not associated with an increased mortality,[70] but these infections often herald the start of a period of clinical deterioration with need for mechanical ventilation, opening of the ductus arteriosus, development of BPD,[71,72] and an increased length-of-stay. There is also a concern that sepsis increases the likelihood of having an adverse neurodevelopmental outcome.

Candida infections occur particularly in extremely preterm infants. Colonization of mucoepithelial surfaces with *Candida* appears to be a prerequisite for systemic infection,[73] and invasive disease usually results from a colonizing *Candida* strain, rather than from some different isolate.[74] Colonization is most often vertical from the mother at birth, usually with *Candida albicans*, but horizontal colonization from care providers in the NICU also occurs, and is thought to be the primary mode of transmission for *Candida parapsilosis*.[74] Congenital cutaneous candidiasis is relatively uncommon, presenting with diffuse skin rash, in some cases burn-like desquamations, and sometimes pulmonary involvement in the first day of life.[69,75] There is usually no fungemia, but systemic treatment is definitely indicated in the very preterm infants. There is an association between the presence of intrauterine contraceptive devices or cerclage during pregnancy and congenital candidiasis.

Some very immature infants (mean gestational age 24 weeks) have invasive fungal dermatitis. Erosive skin lesions with crusting develop during the first 2 weeks of life. Blood culture is often positive, and the port of entry into the bloodstream is probably through dermal vessels.[75] One outbreak of systemic candidiasis was associated with the use of a petrolatum ointment, emphasizing the risk that skin care product may damage the delicate dermal barrier in immature infants.[76] However, the intestinal epithelium is considered the primary portal of entry for most systemic *Candida* infections.[74] Such infections often occur in the second week or life or later, often in the aftermath of a CoNS infection treated with vancomycin, but sometimes as the first nosocomial infection in an extremely preterm infant. Other risk factors are mechanical ventilation, CVC, and treatment with broad-spectrum antibiotics, corticosteroids, or H_2 blockers. Symptoms are often unspecific. Abdominal distension and discoloration, and especially spontaneous intestinal perforation, should raise suspicion of invasive candidiasis.[75] Though *Candida* is known to cause end-organ invasion (meningitis, renal candidiasis, endocarditis, endophthalmitis), this is rarely evident at the time of first symptoms. Serum level of C-reactive protein is usually moderately elevated. Thrombocytopenia is probably more pronounced in invasive candidiasis than in other nosocomial infections.[66] The diagnosis of invasive candidiasis is difficult because blood cultures are often negative, but other diagnostic tests are currently under evaluation. Measurement of urinary D-arabinitol/L-arabinitol ratio may be used in neonates.[77,78]

Central venous catheters are extremely important in the pathogenesis of neonatal candidiasis. These catheters are usually not the primary port of entry, but once in the bloodstream, *Candida* organisms can adhere and even penetrate into the catheter wall[78], which becomes the source of end-organ damage, at the same time making the organisms inaccessible to antimicrobial drugs. It has been stated that removal or replacement of the CVC should be completed within 24 hours of notification of a positive blood culture for *Candida*.[78] A recent review stated that if a *Candida* infection is suspected and the patient is clinically stable and has not had previous antifungal therapy, fluconazole is suitable empiric therapy.[79] Amphotericin B should be considered in severe or life-threatening infections pending results of cultures.

Infections with Gram-negative bacteria are relatively uncommon, but often present with a more rapid clinical deterioration and may be associated with shock, coagulation problems and increased mortality.[66,70] In many neonatal units, there has recently been a substantial increase in infection with *Enterobacter*, usually resistant to cephalosporins.[80] An empiric antibiotic policy including ampicillin and cefotaxime was shown to be associated with an increased prevalence of resistant Gram-negative bacteria, especially *Enterobacter*, as compared with a policy including penicillin and an aminoglycoside.[81] Spread of *Enterobacter* between patients is well documented, and outbreaks have been contained by simple hygienic measures and restrictions in the use of cephalosporins.[82,83]

In view of the relative immune deficiency of premature infants and the necessary invasive care with multiple broken barriers, a high prevalence of nosocomial infections may seem inevitable. However, there is great variation among centers in the incidence of such infections which is not explained by different case mix.[65] It follows that these infections should to a large extent be seen as preventable complications of treatment. A recent survey showed that the staff of units with a particularly low rate of nosocomial sepsis tended to see such infections as a breakdown in care that could have been prevented.[65]

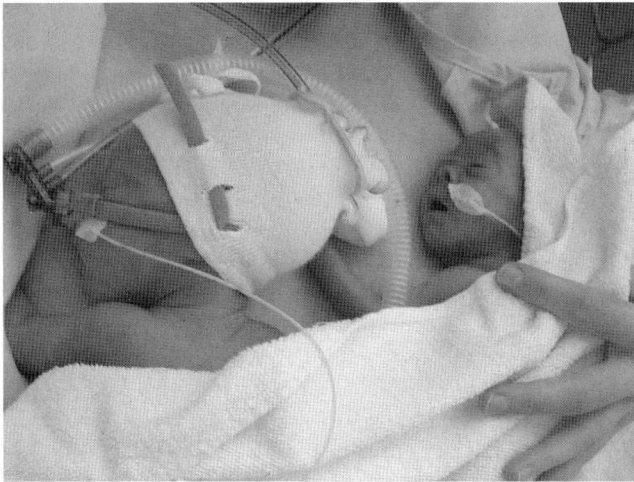

Fig. 7.3: Kangaroo care of twins. The twin to the left is treated with nasal continuous positive airway pressure (CPAP) and fed mother's milk through a nasogastric tube (*Courtesy*: Ann-Cathrine Berg)

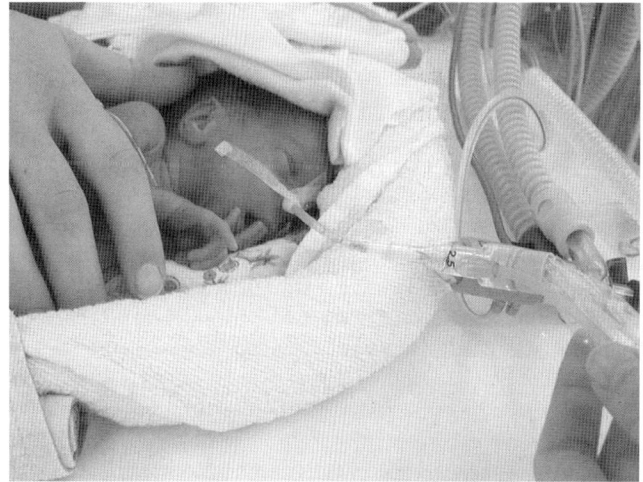

Fig. 7.4: Giving support to an infant during care procedures is an important part of developmental care. This infant is supported by the hand of a parent during endotracheal suctioning (*Courtesy*: Ann-Cathrine Berg)

Hand hygiene is of great importance in preventing the spread of bacteria and fungi between patients. The availability of waterless alcohol hand rubs in close proximity to the incubators makes compliance more likely. In adult wards, the education of patients about the importance of hand washing and asking that they remind their caregivers to wash has been very successful,[84] and perhaps we should teach the parents of preemies to do the same. Good nutrition with an emphasis on enteral feeding with human milk probably diminishes the risk of infection. Indwelling venous catheters and intravenous lipids are important risk factors for CoNS bloodstream infection. Strategies for maximal barrier precautions and aseptic techniques during catheter placement are important, as well as strict guidelines for blood sampling through catheters and for hub manipulations. The use of "antibiotic locks" to prevent catheter-related bloodstream infections seems to be a promising technique, but it remains to be evaluated in clinical trials.[85] The use of fluconazole prophylaxis to prevent neonatal candidiasis is probably safe and can be considered in high-risk patients, but larger studies are needed.[86]

DEVELOPMENTALLY SUPPORTIVE CARE

Behavioral problems, including attention deficit and hyperactivity disorders, are common among surviving children who were born very preterm.[87,88] The reasons for this are not known, but it is believed that environmental influence from the extrauterine environment negatively affects the development of the immature central nervous system.[89,90]

One of the most important parts in the care of preterm infants is to promote emotional attachment between the infant and its parents. Family-focused neonatal care has been increasingly practiced during the last two decades. Systematic strategies for this include free visiting hours and early involvement of parents in care procedures, e.g. diaper changes and feeding, creation of good family memories with hand- and footprints, photographs and diaries, etc. Kangaroo care promotes attachment between the infant and its parents, and development of preterm infants.[91,92] Kangaroo care can often start already during the first week of life (Fig. 7.3).[93]

It was previously shown that reduced light, and day and night light promoted sleep in preterm infants, and this effect persisted several months after discharge.[94] Incubator covers are increasingly being used in order to reduce light and noise. However, as a single procedure in neonatal care their effect has only been investigated in a few studies. In a small observational study there were only minor effects on quiet sleep from the incubator covers in stable preterm infants.[95] Neonatal individualized developmental care and assessment program (NIDCAP) is based on formal observations of the preterm infants during a care procedure. The observations are made by medical personnel, often neonatal nurses, who have received special training in this method. Individual recommendations for the nursing care are made from the results of these observations, (Fig. 7.4). Treatment with NIDCAP is associated with shorter need for respiratory support and shorter duration of stay in the NICU.[96,97] Recently, it was shown that NIDCAP is associated with structural changes of the brain, as shown by magnetic resonance imaging and diffusion tensor imaging techniques, and with increased neurophysiological maturation, as shown by EEG.[98]

PAIN AND ITS TREATMENT

Pain is defined by the international association for the study of pain as an unpleasant sensory and emotional experience associated with actual or potential tissue damage or described in terms of such damage.[99] According to this definition, pain is always a subjective phenomenon with subjective reporting.

Thus individuals, as preterm infants, not capable of reporting pain would not experience such. However, based on empirical evidence it has been proposed that physiological and behavioral responses are valid indicators of pain.[100]

Whether the fetus feels pain, and if so, from which gestational age has been a controversial issue. The thalamocortical fibers, which are considered crucial for nociception, are present between the 20th week and 34th week of gestation. The afferent fibers grow into the cortical plate after the 26th week of gestation, but already between 20 weeks and 26 weeks synaptic circuits occur between the subplate and the cortical plate indicating neuroanatomical basis for the fetus to feel pain.[101] Evoked potentials suggest that thalamic inputs reach the cortex at 29 weeks.[102] Pain threshold is lower in preterm infants than in term infants and later in life.[103] Even in full term infants, the threshold remains low after injury.[104] This suggests that the exposure to multiple procedures in the neonatal period increases pain awareness. Newborn infants undergoing intensive care are subjected to repeated daily procedures. Very preterm infants are likely to experience a large number of invasive procedures during the neonatal care period.[105,106] The most immature infants may be exposed to several hundreds of potentially painful procedures, including, blood sampling and endotracheal intubation.[105] Neonatal pain experiences may alter later pain responses in children.[89] The gentle care of very preterm infants also includes some aspects of standard care procedures, e.g. painful stimuli from venous or arterial punctures for blood sampling. Painful stimuli can cause fluctuation in arterial blood pressure that may affect cerebral blood flow. This could contribute to cerebral hemorrhages or ischemia.[107] However, it has also been shown that blood sampling from umbilical artery catheters can affect cerebral blood volume in preterm infants. This can be avoided by very slow withdrawal of blood from the catheter.[108] Other care procedures associated with changes in cerebral blood volume in very preterm infants include endotracheal suctioning and surfactant administration.[109,110] Because on the many procedures and long-lasting mechanical ventilation, routine opioid infusion or bolus injections were introduced during the early 1990s in many NICUs as a pain relief during the first day of life to preterm infants undergoing assisted ventilation and repeated procedures. Several behavioral pain scales have been developed for preterm infants, but are however not widely used in clinical routine.[111-113] In order to administer optimal analgesia, repeated assessments using pain scales are recommended.

Controversies still exist regarding the severity of pain and need for pain relief for preterm infants undergoing intensive care. With the development of synchronized ventilation, preference of nasal CPAP, and indwelling lines to minimize procedures, the liberal use of opioids has recently been questioned. In the neurologic outcomes and pre-emptive analgesia in neonates (NEOPAIN) study[113] infants were randomized to receive either morphine or placebo infusion. The results showed that opioid treated infants did not have a more beneficial outcome than infants in the placebo group and in some cases even worse outcome. Referring to this study, the goal would be a priori to reduce the amount of distress and pain by the use of non-pharmacological means, including individualized care. Only when obvious pain is present, such as procedural or postoperative pain, a routine administration would be advisable. Otherwise, the use of potentially hazardous analgesics should only be given if a pain scale assessment or behavioral observations indicate the presence of distress and pain despite nonpharmacological intervention to minimize it. This approach would produce a more focused pain treatment, probably with fewer side effects.

ETHICAL ASPECTS

During the last 20 years, there has been a growing concern about the ethical issues surrounding the most preterm infants who are at the limits of viability and intact survival. The majority of deaths, around 80%, in very premature infants occur in the first 3 days of life in spite of full intensive care.[114] Neonatologists caring for these infants need to address the question whether to continue care or to withdraw ongoing intensive care. Such discussion may arise when the patient suffers from severe brain or pulmonary injury and the

chance of survival is low and the possibility of healthy survival is extremely low.[115] The first principle of treatment is always to act in the best interest of the patient and the family according to the Hippocratic rules, i.e. never to hurt or harm, if possible to relieve, sometimes to cure, and always to console.

When evaluating the question on withdrawal of intensive care, the situation should be analyzed using the traditional ethical principles of (1) benefit, (2) harm, (3) autonomy and (4) justice. This analysis should be performed in a two dimensional model taking into account the different interest groups, i.e. the infant, parents, caretakers and even the society.[116]

For the evaluation, a summary of all medical facts is needed, from which an estimated probable prognosis is derived. Sometimes the decision is not difficult or controversial, such as in babies with Potter syndrome (absence of kidneys) or hydranencephaly. However, when outcome is not inevitably fatal or the interest of the parents and the infants diverge, the decision-making needs a thorough discussion. In these instances, nonmedical factors such as social or economic factors may influence the decision. A decision to withdraw treatment should always be taken by a senior consultant, and usually by a team of them, after careful discussions with all involved staff. The medical course and prognosis should be carefully and repeatedly explained to the parents, and their opinion should be taken into consideration. If parents cannot accept the recommendation to withdraw treatment, the discussions should be repeated. A special situation is prolonged delivery-room resuscitation of extremely premature infants at the limits of viability, where urgent decisions usually are needed in the interest of the infant. On such occasions, thorough discussion with the parents before delivery is of greatest importance for the decision-making.[117]

There is usually time to arrange for death to be filled with dignity also for the most immature infants.

Good psychological care of the parents is essential since they will continue to live with strong and sad memories of this time. A professional, warm, and empathic care by experienced staff will assist them in this difficult situation. The parents' wishes regarding social or cultural ceremonies, e.g. baptism, or for information to or presence of relatives or friends should be fulfilled. Rituals connected to death are important for coping with the loss and sorrow after the death. The terminal care of the dying baby should be carefully planned and performed, including sufficient sedation and analgesia, in order to omit further suffering. A dying infant should be cared for in a single room together with the parents. One or two experienced staff members should participate and assist the parents in this situation.

THE OUTCOME OF VERY PRETERM INFANTS

The outcome of very preterm infants has significantly improved during the last two decades, and especially of those with a gestational age below 28 weeks.[118,119] Most follow-up studies of preterm cohorts are defined by birth weight, either including extremely low birth weight infants (ELBWI, < 1,000 g) or very low birth weight infants (VLBWI, < 1,500 g). The mortality rate is correlated to immaturity, the more preterm the infant the higher the mortality.[7] The limit of viability seems to be about 23 weeks of gestation, since survival after 22 weeks of gestation is very rare, but after 23 weeks about 10% according to regionalized long-term follow-up studies from the postsurfactant era, i.e. from the 1990s.[120-122] In a national cohort, the stillborn rate was 60% in infants delivered after 22 gestational weeks, 35% after 23 weeks, and 25% after 24 weeks,[7] suggesting that there may be a less active care during birth in the very immature infants resulting in intrapartal death or classification as dead if there is bradycardia at birth. In this cohort, the long-term survival of live-born infants born after 24 weeks of gestation was 40%, but less than half of them were classified as completely normally developed at 1.5 years of age.[120]

Despite increasing survival, the rate of neurodevelopmental impairment has remained similar, which results in an increased absolute number of infants with abnormalities.[122,123] Severe handicap, such as cerebral palsy, deafness, blindness, and mental retardation have in recent studies been reported to occur in 15% to 25%.[118,123] Even more common are cognitive dysfunction and

learning disabilities. In a large VLBWI birth cohort study in the Netherlands, assessment at the age of 9 years showed that 56% of children in mainstream education needed special assistance at school or were below the age-appropriate level.[123] Similar results have been reported from other countries.[124] Most of the learning difficulties seem to be related to low overall IQ.[88]

Several perinatal risk factors have been associated with poor school performance, such as low birth weight, need for assisted ventilation, and IVH.[125] Intrauterine growth restriction in preterm infants is associated with increased morbidity, and low postnatal growth resulting in smaller size at school age, and poorer school performance as compared to appropriately grown siblings.[126] The high incidence of sequelae in very preterm infants warrants long-term follow-up of regional cohorts for quality control of the demanding perinatal care and long-lasting neonatal intensive care.

REFERENCES

1. Swyer PR. The regional organization of special care for the neonate. Pediatr Clin North Am. 1970;17:761-76.
2. Debauche C, Van Reempts P, Kollée L, et al. Maternal and neonatal transfer policies in Europe. Prenat Neonat Med. 1999;4(Suppl 1): 5-14.
3. Kollée L, Chabernaud J, Van Reempts P, et al. Perinatal transport practices: a survey of inborn versus outborn very preterm infants admitted to European neonatal intensive care units. Prenat Neonat Med. 1999;4 (Suppl 1):61-72.
4. Papiernik E, Zeitlin J, Milligan D, et al. Variations in the organization of obstetric and neonatal intensive care in Europe. Prenat Neonat Med. 1999;4(Suppl 1):73-87.
5. Hein HA. Regionalized perinatal care in North America. Semin Neonatol. 2004;9:111-6.
6. Cifuentes J, Bronstein J, Phibbs CS, et al. Mortality in low birth weight infants according to level of neonatal care at hospital of birth. Pediatrics. 2002;109:745-51.
7. Tommiska V, Heinonen K, Ikonen S, et al. A national short-term follow-up study of extremely low birth weight infants born in Finland in 1996-1997. Pediatrics. 2001;107:1-9e.
8. Phibbs CS, Bronstein JM, Buxton E, et al. The effects of patient volume and level of care at the hospital of birth on neonatal mortality. JAMA. 1996;276:1054-9.
9. Sharek PJ, Baker R, Litman F, et al. Evaluation and development of potentially better practices to prevent chronic lung disease and reduce lung injury in neonates. Pediatrics. 2003;111:e426-31.
10. Cordero L, Kuehn L, Kumar RR, et al. Impact of computerized physician order entry on clinical practice in a newborn intensive care unit. J Perinatol. 2004;24:88-95.
11. Tucker J, Parry G, Fowlie PW, et al. ABC of preterm birth. Organization and delivery of perinatal services. BMJ. 2004;329:730-2.
12. Cornette L. Contemporary neonatal transport: problems and solutions. Arch Dis Child Fetal Neonatal Ed. 2004;89:F212-4.
13. Lupton BA, Pendray MR. Regionalized neonatal emergency transport. Semin Neonatol. 2004;9:125-31.
14. Zeitlin J, Papiernik E, Bréart G, EUROPET group. Regionalization of perinatal care in Europe Semin Neonatol. 2004;9:99-110.
15. Shankaran S, Fanaroff A, Wright L, et al. Risk factors for early death among extremely low birth weight infants. Am J Obstet Gynecol. 2002;186:796-802.
16. Hakansson S, Farooqi A, Holmgren PA, et al. Proactive management promotes outcome in extremely preterm infants: a population-based comparison of two perinatal management strategies. Pediatrics. 2004;114:58-64.
17. Costeloe K, Hennessy E, Gibson AT, et al. The EPICure study: outcomes to discharge from hospital for infants born at the threshold of viability. Pediatrics. 2000;106:659-71.
18. Fowlie PW, McGuire WM. ABC of preterm birth. Immediate care of the preterm infant. BMJ. 2004;329:845-8.
19. Vohra S, Frent G, Campbell V, et al. Effect of polyethylene occlusive skin wrapping on heat loss in very low birth weight infants at delivery: a randomized trial. J Pediatr. 1999;134:547-51.
20. Björklund LJ, Hellström-Westas L. Reducing heat loss at birth in very preterm infants. J Pediatr. 2000;137:739-40.
21. Kopotic RJ, Lindner W. Assessing high-risk infants in the delivery room with pulse oximetry. Anesth Analg. 2002;94(1 Suppl):S31-S36.
22. Finer NN, Rich WD. Neonatal resuscitation: raising the bar. Curr Opin Pediatr. 2004;16:157-62.
23. International guidelines for neonatal resuscitation: an excerpt from the guidelines 2000 for cardiopulmonary resuscitation and emergency cardiovascular care: International consensus on science. Pediatrics. 2000;106:e29.
24. Lundstrom KE, Pryds O, Greisen G. Oxygen at birth and prolonged cerebral vasoconstriction in preterm infants. Arch Dis Child Fetal Neonatal Ed. 1995;73:F81-6.
25. Saugstad OD. The role of oxygen in neonatal resuscitation. Clin Perinatol. 2004;31:431-43.
26. Chow LC, Wright KW, Sola A, et al. Can changes in clinical practice decrease the incidence of severe retinopathy of prematurity in very low birth weight infants? Pediatrics. 2003;111:339-45.
27. Dunn MS, Reilly MC. Approaches to the initial respiratory management of preterm neonates. Paediatr Respir Rev. 2003;4: 2-8.
28. Morley C, Davis P. Surfactant treatment for premature lung disorders: a review of best practices in 2002. Paediatr Respir Rev. 2004;5(Suppl A):S299-304.
29. Van Marter LJ, Dammann O, Allred EN, et al. Chorioamnionitis, mechanical ventilation, and postnatal sepsis as modulators of chronic lung disease in preterm infants. J Pediatr. 2002;140:171-6.
30. Ingimarsson J, Björklund LJ, Curstedt T, et al. Incomplete protection by prophylactic surfactant against the adverse effects of large lung inflations at birth in immature lambs. Intensive Care Med. 2004; 30:1446-53.
31. Van Marter LJ, Allred EN, Pagano M, et al. Do clinical markers of barotrauma and oxygen toxicity explain interhospital variation in rates of chronic lung disease? Pediatrics. 2000;105:1194-201.
32. Narendran V, Donovan EF, Hoath SB, et al. Early bubble CPAP and outcomes in ELBW preterm infants. J Perinatol. 2003;23:195-9.

33. Finer NN, Carlo WA, Duara S, et al. The National Institute of Child Health and Human Development Neonatal Research Network. Delivery room continuous positive airway pressure/positive end-expiratory pressure in extremely low birth weight infants: a feasibility trial. Pediatrics. 2004;114:651-7.

34. Thomson MA. Continuous positive airway pressure and surfactant; combined data from animal experiments and clinical trials. Biol Neonate. 2002;81(Suppl 1):16-9.

35. Kendig JW, Ryan RM, Sinkin RA, et al. Comparison of two strategies for surfactant prophylaxis in very premature infants: a multicenter randomized trial. Pediatrics. 1998;101:1006-12.

36. Palme-Kilander C, Tunell R. Pulmonary gas exchange during face mask ventilation immediately after birth. Arch Dis Child. 1993;68:11-6.

37. O´Donnell CPF, Davis PG, Morley CJ. Resuscitation of premature infants: What are we doing wrong and can we do better? Biol Neonate. 2003;84:76-82.

38. Finer NN, Rich W, Craft A, et al. Comparison of methods of bag and mask ventilation for neonatal resuscitation. Resuscitation. 2001;49:299-305.

39. Hussey SG, Ryan CA, Murphy BP. Comparison of three manual ventilation devices using an intubated mannequin. Arch Dis Child Fetal Neonatal Ed. 2004;89:F490-3.

40. Lucas A, Bloom SR, Aynsley-Green A. Gut hormones and "minimal enteral feeding". Acta Paediatr Scand. 1986;75:719-23.

41. McClure RJ, Newell SJ. Randomised controlled study of clinical outcome following trophic feeding. Arch Dis Child Fetal Neonatal Ed. 2002;82:F29-33.

42. Lucas A, Morley R, Cole TJ, et al. Breast milk and subsequent intelligence quotient in children born preterm. Lancet. 1992;339:261-4.

43. Schanler RJ. The use of human milk for premature infants. Pediatr Clin North Am. 2001;48:207-19.

44. Hylander MA, Strobino DM, Pezzullo JC, et al. Association of human milk feedings with a reduction in retinopathy among very low birth weight infants. J Perinatol. 2001;21:356-62.

45. Bellander M, Ley D, Polberger S, et al. Tolerance to early human milk feeding is not compromised by indomethacin in preterm infants with persistent ductus arteriosus. Acta Paediatr. 2003;92:107-48.

46. Polberger S, Jirwe M, Svenningsen NW. Silastic central venous catheters for blood sampling and infusions in newborn infants. Prenat Neonat Med. 1998;3:340-5.

47. Ziegler EE, Thureen PJ, Carlson SJ. Aggressive nutrition of the very low birth weight infant. Clin Perinatol. 2002;29:225-44.

48. Putet G. Lipid metabolism of the micropremie. Clin Perinatol. 2000;27:57-69.

49. Michaelsen KF, Skafte L, Badsberg JH, et al. Variation in macronutrients in human bank milk: influencing factors and implications for human milk banking. J Pediatr Gastroenterol Nutr. 1990;11:229-39.

50. Polberger S, Räihä NCR, Juvonen P, et al. Individualized protein fortification of human milk for preterm infants: comparison of ultrafiltrated human milk protein and a bovine whey fortifier. J Pediatr Gastroenterol Nutr. 1999;29:332-8.

51. Moro GE, Minoli I, Ostrom M, et al. Fortification of human milk: evaluation of a novel fortification scheme and of a new fortifier. J Pediatr Gastroenterol Nutr. 1995;20:162-72.

52. Modi N. Management of fluid balance in the very immature neonate. Arch Dis Child Fetal Neonatal Ed. 2004;89:F108-11.

53. Agren J, Sjors G, Sedin G. Transepidermal water loss in infants born at 24 and 25 weeks gestation. Acta Paediatr. 1998;87:1185-90.

54. Edwards WH, Conner JM, Soll RF. Vermont oxford network neonatal skin care study group. The effect of prophylactic ointment therapy on nosocomial sepsis rates and skin integrity in infants with birth weights of 501 to 1000 g. Pediatrics. 2004;113:1195-203.

55. Gruskay J, Costarino AT, Polin RA, et al. Nonoliguric hyperkalemia in the premature infant weighing less than 1000 grams. J Pediatr. 1988;113:381-6.

56. Betremieux P, Hartnoll G, Modi N. Should frusemide be prescribed after packed cell transfusions in the newborn? Eur J Pediatr. 1997;156:88-9.

57. Maisels MJ, Watchko JF. Treatment of jaundice in low birth weight infants. Arch Dis Child Fetal Neonatal Ed. 2003;88: F459-63.

58. Collins MP, Lorenz JM, Jetton JR, et al. Hypocapnia and other ventilation-related risk factors for cerebral palsy in low birth weight infants. Pediatr Res. 2001;50:712-9.

59. Cole CH, Wright KW, Tarnow-Mordi W, et al. Resolving our uncertainty about oxygen therapy. Pediatrics. 2003;112; 1415-9.

60. Greisen G, Hellstrom-Westas L, Lou H, et al. EEG depression and germinal layer hemorrhage in the newborn. Acta Paediatr Scand. 1987;76:519-25.

61. Hellström-Westas L, Rosén I, Svenningsen NW. Cerebral function monitoring during the first week of life in extremely small low birth weight infants. Neuropediatrics. 1991;22:27-32.

62. Hellström-Westas L, Klette H, Thorngren-Jerneck K, et al. Early prediction of outcome with aEEG in premature infants with large IVH. Neuropediatrics. 2001;32:319-24.

63. Olischar M, Klebermass K, Kuhle S, et al. Reference values for amplitude-integrated electroencephalographic activity in preterm infants younger than 30 weeks' gestational age. Pediatrics. 2004;113:e61-6.

64. Stoll BJ, Hansen N, Fanaroff AA, et al. Changes in pathogens causing early-onset sepsis in very-low-birth weight infants. N Engl J Med. 2002;347:240-7.

65. Edwards WH. Preventing nosocomial bloodstream infection in very low birth weight infants. Semin Neonatol. 2002;7:325-33.

66. Clark R, Powers R, White R, et al. Nosocomial infection in the NICU: a medical complication or unavoidable problem? J Perinatol. 2004;24:382-8.

67. Clark R, Powers R, White R, et al. Prevention and treatment of nosocomial sepsis in the NICU. J Perinatol. 2004;24:446-53.

68. Benjamin Jr DK, Miller W, Garges H, et al. Bacteremia, central catheters, and neonates: when to pull the line. Pediatrics. 2001;107:1272-6.

69. Nistala K, Nicholl R. Should preterm neonates with a central venous catheter and coagulase negative staphylococcal bacteremia be treated without removal of the catheter? Arch Dis Child. 2003;88:458-9.

70. Benjamin Jr DK, DeLong E, Cotton CM, et al. Mortality following blood culture in premature infants: increased with Gram-negative bacteremia and candidemia, but not Gram-positive bacteremia. J Perinatol. 2004;24:175-80.

71. Gonzalez A, Sosenko IR, Chandar J, et al. Influence of infection on patent ductus arteriosus and chronic lung disease in premature infants weighing 1000 grams or less. J Pediatr. 1996;128:470-8.

72. Liljedahl M, Bodin L, Schollin J. Coagulas negative staphylococcal sepsis as a predictor of bronchopulmonary dysplasia. Acta Paediatr. 2004;93:211-5.

73. Chapman RL. Candida infections in the neonate. Curr Opin Pediatr. 2003;15:97-102.

74. Bendel CM. Colonization and epithelial adhesion in the pathogenesis of neonatal candidiasis. Semin Perinatol. 2003; 27:357-64.

75. Rowen JL. Mucocutaneous candidiasis. Semin Perinatol 2003;27:406-13.

76. Campbell JR, Zaccaria E, Baker CJ. Systemic candidiasis in extremely low birth weight infants receiving topical petrolatum ointment for skin care: a case-control study. Pediatrics. 2000;105:1041-5.

77. Sigmundsdóttir G, Christensson B, Björklund LJ, et al. Urine Darabinitol/L-arabinitol ratio in the diagnosis of invasive candidiasis in newborn infants. J Clin Microbiol. 2000;38:3039-42.

78. Benjamin Jr DK, Garges H, Steinbach WJ. Candida bloodstream infection in neonates. Semin Perinatol. 2003;27:375-83.

79. Bliss JM, Wellington M, Gigliotti F. Antifungal pharmacotherapy for neonatal candidiasis. Semin Perinatol. 2003;27:365-74.

80. Hervas JA, Ballesteros F, Alomar A, et al. Increase of Enterobacter in neonatal sepsis: a twenty-two year study. Pediatr Infect Dis J. 2001;20:134-40.

81. de Man P, Verhoeven BAN, Verbrugh HA, et al. An antibiotic policy to prevent emergence of resistant bacilli. Lancet. 2000;355:973-8.

82. v Dijk Y, Bik EM, Hochstenbach-Vernooij S, et al. Management of an outbreak of enterobacter cloacae in a neonatal unit using simple preventive measures. J Hosp Infect. 2002;51:21-6.

83. Calil R, Marba STM, von Nowakonski A, et al. Reduction in colonization and nosocomial infection by multiresistant bacteria in a neonatal unit after institution of educational measures and restriction in the use of cephalosporins. Am J Infect Control. 2001;29:133-8.

84. McGuckin M, Waterman R, Storr J, et al. Evaluation of a patient-empowering hand hygiene programme in the UK. J Hosp Infect. 2001;48:222-7.

85. Garland J, Alex C, Henrickson K, et al. A randomized pilot trial of a vancomycin-heparin lock solution (VHLS) for prevention of catheter-related bloodstream infection (CRBSI) in neonates. Pediatr Res. 2002;51:298A.

86. Kaufman D. Strategies for prevention of neonatal invasive candidiasis. Semin Perinatol. 2003;27:414-24.

87. Stjernqvist K, Svenningsen NW. Ten-year follow-up of children born before 29 gestational weeks: health, cognitive development, behavior and school achievement. Acta Paediatr. 1999;88:557-62.

88. Marlow N. Neurocognitive outcome after very preterm birth. Arch Dis Child Fetal Neonatal Ed. 2004;89:F224-8.

89. Anand KJ, Scalzo FM. Can adverse neonatal experiences alter brain development and subsequent behavior? Biol Neonate. 2000;77: 69-82.

90. Nagy Z, Westerberg H, Skare S, et al. Preterm children have disturbances of white matter at 11 years of age as shown by diffusion tensor imaging. Pediatr Res. 2003;54:672-9.

91. Charpak N, Ruiz-Pelaez JG, Figueroa de CZ, et al. A randomized, controlled trial of kangaroo mother care: results of follow-up at 1 year of corrected age. Pediatrics. 2001;108:1072-9.

92. Feldman R, Eidelman AI, Sirota L, et al. Comparison of skin-to-skin (kangaroo) and traditional care: parenting outcomes and preterm infant development. Pediatrics. 2002;110:16-26.

93. Tornhage CJ, Stuge E, Lindberg T, et al. First week kangaroo care in sick very preterm infants. Acta Paediatr. 1999;88:1402-4.

94. Mann NP, Haddow R, Stokes L, et al. Effect of night and day on preterm infants in a newborn nursery: randomised trial. BMJ. 1986;293:1265-7.

95. Hellström-Westas L, Inghammar M, Isaksson K, et al. Short-term effects of incubator covers on quiet sleep in stable preterm infants. Acta Paediatr. 2001;90:1004-8.

96. Als H, Lawhorn G, Duffy FH, et al. Individualized developmental care for the very low birth weight preterm infant. JAMA. 1994;272: 853-8.

97. Westrup B, Kleberg A, Stjernqvist K, et al. A randomized controlled trial to evaluate the effects of NIDCAP in a Swedish setting. Pediatrics. 2000;105:66-72.

98. Als H, Duffy FH, McAnulty GB, et al. Early experience alters brain function and structure. Pediatrics. 2004;113:846-57.

99. Merskey H, Albe-Fessard DG, Bonica JJ, et al. Pain terms: a list with definitions and notes on usage. Recommended by the IASP Subcommittee on Taxonomy. Pain. 1997;6:249.

100. Anand KJ, Craig KD. New perspectives on the definition of pain. Pain. 1996;67:209-11.

101. Mrzljak L, Uylings HB, Kostovic I, et al. Prenatal development of neurons in the human prefrontal cortex: IA qualitative Golgi study. J Comp Neurol. 1988;271:355-86.

102. Klimach VJ, Cooke RWI. Maturation of the neonatal somatosensory evoked response in preterm infants. Dev Med Child Neurol. 1988;30:208-14.

103. Fitzgerald M, Anand KJ. Developmental neuroanatomy and neurophysiology of pain. In: Schechter NL, Berde CB, Yaster M (Eds). Pain in Infants, Children and Adolescents. Baltimore: Williams and Wilkins; 1993. pp. 11-31.

104. Andrews K, Fitzgerald M. Cutaneous flexion reflex in human neonates: a quantitative study of the threshold and stimulus-response characteristics after single and repeated stimuli. Dev Med Child Neurol. 1999;41:696-703.

105. Barker DP, Rutter N. Exposure to invasive procedures in neonatal intensive care unit admissions. Arch Dis Child Fetal Neonatal Ed. 1995;72:F47-8.

106. Holsti L, Grunau RE, Oberlander TF, et al. Specific Newborn Individualized Developmental Care and Assessment Program movements are associated with acute pain in preterm infants in the neonatal intensive care unit. Pediatrics. 2004;114:65-72.

107. Wells JT, Ment LR. Prevention of intraventricular hemorrhage in preterm infants. Early Hum Dev. 1995;42:209-33.

108. Schulz G, Keller E, Haensse D, et al. Slow blood sampling from an umbilical artery catheter prevents a decrease in cerebral oxygenation in the preterm newborn. Pediatrics. 2003;111:e73-6.

109. Skov L, Ryding J, Pryds O, et al. Changes in cerebral oxygenation and cerebral blood volume during endotracheal suctioning in ventilated neonates. Acta Paediatr. 1992;81:389-93.

110. Skov L, Hellstrom-Westas L, Jacobsen T, et al. Acute changes in cerebral oxygenation and cerebral blood volume in preterm infants during surfactant treatment. Neuropediatrics. 1992; 23:126-30.

111. Stevens B, Johnston C, Petryshen P, et al. Premature Infant Pain Profile: development and initial validation. Clin J Pain. 1996;12:13-22.

112. Debillon T, Zupan V, Ravault N, et al. Development and initial validation of the EDIN scale, a new tool for assessing prolonged pain in preterm infants. Arch Dis Child Fetal Neonatal Ed. 2001;85:F36-41.

113. Anand KJ, Hall RW, Desai N, et al. NEOPAIN Trial Investigators Group. Effects of morphine analgesia in ventilated preterm neonates: primary outcomes from the NEOPAIN randomised trial. Lancet. 2004; 363:1673-82.

114. Meadow W, Reimshisel T, Lantos J. Birth weight-specific mortality for extremely low birth weight infants vanishes by four days of life: epidemiology and ethics in the neonatal intensive care unit. Pediatrics. 1996;97:636-46.

115. Whitelaw A. Death as an option in neonatal intensivecare. Lancet 1986;2:328-31.

116. Doyal L. The moral foundation of the clinical duties of care: needs, duties and human rights. Bioethics. 2001;15:520-35.

117. Goldschmidt JP, Ginsburg HG, McGettigan MC. Ethical decisions in the delivery room. Clin Perinatol. 1996;23: 529-50.

118. Tin W, Wariyar U, Hey E. Changing prognosis for babies of less than 28 weeks' gestation in the north of England between 1983 and 1994. Northern Neonatal Network. BMJ. 1997;314:107-11.

119. Darlow BA, Cust AE. Australian and New Zealand Neonatal Network Improved outcomes for very low birth weight infants: evidence from New Zealand national population based data. Arch Dis Child Fetal Neonatal Ed. 2003;88:F23-8.

120. Tommiska V, Heinonen K, Kero P, et al. A national 2 year follow up study of extremely low birth weight infants born in 1996-1997. Arch Dis Child Fetal Neonatal Ed. 2003;88:F29-35.

121. Doyle LW, Victorian Infant Collaborative Study Group. Outcome at 5 years of age of children 23 to 27 weeks gestation, refining the prognosis. Pediatrics. 2001;108:134-41.

122. Yu VYH, Doyle LW. Regionalized long-term follow-up. Semin Neonatol. 2004;9:135-44.

123. Hille ET, den Ouden AL, Bauer L, et al. School performance at nine years of age in very premature and very low birth weight infants: perinatal risk factors and predictor sat five years of age. Collaborative project on preterm and small for gestational age (POPS) infants in the netherlands. J Pediatr. 1994;125:426-34.

124. Saigal S, Hoult LA, Streiner DL, et al. School difficulties at adolescence in aregional cohort of children who were extremely low birth weight. Pediatrics. 2000;105:325-31.

125. Bylund B, Cervin T, Finnstrom O, et al. Very low birth weight children at 9 years: school performance and behavior in relation to risk factors. Perinat Neonat Med. 2000;5:124-33.

126. Monset-Couchard M, de Bethmann O, Relier J-P. Long-term outcome of small versus appropriate size for gestational age cotwins/triplets. Arch Dis Child Fetal Neonatal Ed. 2004;89:F310-4.

8

Can We Establish a Universal Lower Limit of Viability?

What are the medical and ethical implications?

MRG Carrapato

INTRODUCTION

Over the last few decades, perinatal mortality has been greatly reduced and in most western countries now stands in single figures, albeit with many geographical asymmetries. The overall good results achieved are primarily the consequence of National Health Policies toward rationalization of human and financial resources with modern technology playing a subsidiary role for the high-risk pregnancy and neonate. The development of neonatal intensive care has been shown to be effective in the survival of preterm infants without a significant increase in later morbidity, at least for the larger, more mature neonates.

The World Health Organization places 22 weeks of gestational age or 500 g birth weight as the lower limit, at least for the purpose of perinatal statistics, and the International Classification of Diseases describes the perinatal period as starting at 22 completed weeks. The European Association of Perinatal Medicine (EAPM) defines the perinatal period: "... from 22 completed weeks (154 days) gestation and ends seven complete days after birth"[1] which is to imply that the lower limit of viability stands at 22 weeks of gestation. The question, with all its medical, legal, social and financial implications, is how close are we, as a whole, in this pursuit?

LOWER LIMIT OF VIABILITY—FACT OR NOT QUITE?

Biological survival will depend on not just the presence of a given organ but on its functional maturation, a sequential evolution often referred to as the "developmental windows". Alveolarization, essential for survival, is a process that includes anatomical, physiological and biochemical differentiation starting from about 24 weeks of gestation, progressing until term and continuing throughout the postnatal period and childhood. "Viability", therefore, would be around 24 weeks. To lower this limit, strategies ranging from antenatal steroids, postnatal surfactant and different ventilatory modes have been attempted with some success, but as an example, after 30 years of clinical practise, antenatal steroids show quite disappointing results at below 24 weeks of gestation,[2,3] and they might also delay and alter postnatal alveolarization.[4-6] Nevertheless, in recent years, an increased survival of very immature infants has been reported ranging from 2% to 35% at 23 weeks and in some perinatal centers in the USA, these figures approach 50% amongst live-born infants, between 17% and 58% at 24 weeks and vary from 35% to 85% at 25 weeks.[7-21]

Survival and outcome data on extremely preterm infants, between 22 weeks and 26 weeks, has been widely reported and reviewed.[7,10-12,15-18,22,23] Allen, in a retrospective study of infants born between 22 weeks and 25 weeks, showed that mortality at 6 months corrected age was 75% for neonates born at less than 24 weeks gestation, with no survivors at 22 weeks whilst at 25 completed weeks, survival was in the region of 80%.[23] Hack and Kilpatrick showed similar survival rates of around 40% and 80% respectively for 24 weeks and 26 weeks of gestational age, especially after the introduction of steroids and surfactant.[12-15] Cooke has reported an increasing survival rate of extremely preterm infants from the early 1980s to the 1990s: in the early period, from 1982 to 1985, there were no survivors at 23 weeks of gestational age whilst in the later part of the study, between 1990 to 1993, 35% of these infants survived to discharge.[7] Tin et al. in a prospective, population-based regional survey, also showed that the survival of very immature infants has improved progressively since the early 1980s, particularly after the introduction of surfactant in clinical practise, although the impact of surfactant was only evident in those babies of 25 or more gestational weeks.[9] A national population-based study carried out in the UK and Ireland in the mid-1990s, of all infants born between 22 weeks and 25 weeks of gestation, revealed two survivors to discharge at 22 weeks, with increasing survival rates from 11% at 23 weeks to 44% at 25 weeks of gestation.[17] However, in the last decade, survival among live births even at 22 weeks has been reported as being from 14% to 19%.[24-26] In a survey of 21 European countries registered with the EAPM, representing a wide spectrum of different regions from Scandinavia to Southern, Central and Eastern European countries, the mortality rate for infants weighing between 500 g and 749 g at birth, stands at 54.4% but showed very wide variations within countries, approaching a 90% mortality rate in the less-affluent countries as opposed to 26% in the more developed regions.[27] It is quite obvious from the findings of this survey that obstetric and neonatal practises, as well as available resources and facilities, are playing a major role in the survival of these very immature infants, but, both human and financial resources apart, why should there be such a discrepancy for reported survival rates at the threshold of viability?

There can be several reasons and explanations. First of all, many of the earlier studies referred to birth weight rather than to gestational age, and therefore included more mature babies who were growth retarded [although intrauterine growth restriction (IUGR) babies of the same gestational age usually have a poor prognosis].[22,28-31] Then, again, with some of the earlier reports referring to gestational age, how accurate was dating based on menstrual estimates in the absence of scanning in early pregnancy? Even in recent data, gestational age is often inferred from the first day of the last menstrual period with scanning only prevailing if it differs more than 2 weeks from the menstrual dates.[32-36] At this "threshold for viability", a few days or a couple of hundred grams will make all the difference when reporting survival rates. On the other hand, many studies are regional/population-based[7,9,14,17,35,36] whilst others refer either to individual perinatal tertiary centers with very few numbers as a whole, or to multicenter collaborative studies[13,15,23,33,34,37-41] with quite different outcomes. Some studies refer to the outcome of pregnancy from the beginning of labor, including still and live births, others include only live births, whilst others only survival rates for infants admitted to the neonatal intensive care units. This selection bias may overestimate survival rates by as much as 100% at 23 weeks and even up to 50% at 24 weeks of gestation.[42] Also, in some perinatal centers, both obstetricians and neonatologists may invest aggressively at these lower gestational ages whilst in others, no active management will be contemplated because both the fetuses and babies are considered nonviable or because of the very poor overall outcome in the event of survival.[43-48] Whether the mode of delivery at this very low gestational age will make any appreciable difference for survival is very debatable, and cesarean section has not been proved to be better.[24,27,49-53] Indeed, the increasing morbidity for the mother and the future consequences of a vertical incision at this stage of pregnancy should perhaps preclude a cesarean in favor of a vaginal delivery, at least for fetal reasons. Further to all the aforementioned explanations for such discrepancies in survival reporting, other confounding data related to pregnancy will also influence survival and, therefore the outcome, namely, IUGR, preeclampsia, PPRM/oligohydramnios, antepartum hemorrhage, infection/chorioamnionitis, etc.[15,24,49,54,55] Gender and ethnicity, especially, meet with conflicting results at these very low gestational ages.[56-60]

WHAT IS THE OUTCOME FOR THE SURVIVORS

Survival is not (and should not be) the only goal in perinatal medicine when attempting to establish a "lower limit of viability". Outcome and quality of life should, at the beginning of a new century, be a major priority. Although several follow-up studies on these very immature babies have shown that increasing survival has not been mirrored by an increase in cerebral palsy, the fact is that a proportionally higher number of infants are now survivors of very low gestational age and birth weight. Furthermore, the major neuromotor, psychomotor, neurosensory and cognitive dysfunctions are found especially in the most immature infants, below 25 gestational weeks.[10-14,17] Over a period of 12 years, between 1983 and 1984 in the North of England, although the survival rate at gestational age greater than 24 weeks had improved (whilst at gestational age below 24 weeks, the overall survivor rate remained unchanged at 4%) the proportion of survivors with severe disability stayed unaltered at around 25%, with 10% being so profoundly disabled as to have to live a completely dependent life.[9] From the results of the European survey, based either on regional or national data, it was also shown that chronic lung disease ranged from 16.7% to 60% at 36 weeks corrected age, retinopathy of prematurity (ROP) from 5.5% to 40%, intraventricular hemorrhage Grade III from 15% to 35%, necrotizing enterocolitis from 3% to 23% and nosocomial infection from 23% to 50%. All these complications were common to all countries and were directly related to either the degree of prematurity or the survival rate, being especially prevalent at 26 weeks of gestation or less. As expected, the picture was somewhat reversed, the countries with the better survival rates showing a higher incidence of sequelae, especially in visual impairment and chronic lung disease. At the time of the survey in 1998, almost everyone in Europe was using antenatal steroids, particularly between 26 weeks and 32 weeks of gestation, and postnatal surfactant, either prophylactically or as a rescue. In those days, there were no criteria for the use of postnatal steroids. Seven countries out of 21 would never use them whilst, of the remaining 14, 6 would apply them early—mostly systemically, with the remainder only contemplating their use late in the course of respiratory distress syndrome (RDS), if ventilatory dependent.[27] [These figures might be somewhat distorted and not reflect usual medical practise in Europe since some neonatal units were, at the time, enrolled in a controlled trial of postnatal steroid studies—an open study of early corticosteroid treatment (OSECT).]

On this basis, it could be argued that as recently as the last decade, these very immature infants were receiving quite different treatment across the globe even from center to center within the same area. However, Vohr et al. reporting on the long-term outcome of a collaborative study of babies on the threshold of viability in the 1990s in the USA, and Wood et al. from a population-based cohort in the UK and Ireland, reporting on behalf of the EPICure study group, both showed that of the surviving children with birth weights less than 750 g or gestational ages below 25 weeks, between 30% to 50% had moderate or severe neuromotor or neurosensorial disabilities and very often had multiple handicaps.[17,61] In a review of the world literature, Hack and Fanaroff estimated that of the survivors of 23 weeks of gestation, over a third had a severe disability from cerebral palsy to blindness and/or deafness with subnormal cognitive function. At 24 weeks of gestation, the range of severe disability was from 22% to 45% and at 25 weeks, from 12% to 35% and, in general, these rates overlapped those of children born before the 1990s.[62]

It is quite plausible that some of the adverse outcome in survivors at these low gestational ages may not be just the direct effect of prematurity and/or low birth weight per se, but also the result of the hostile intrauterine milieu leading to preterm delivery from inflammatory mediators, to IUGR, hypoxic-ischemic insults, metabolic imbalances, etc.

These would perhaps explain the somewhat better, and paradoxical, reported outcome of multiple pregnancies at these very low gestational ages in contrast to the general outcome of multiples at the later stages of pregnancy, presumably because the reasons for preterm delivery would rest with multiplicity alone, in the absence of the adverse factors for singletons' preterm deliveries.[60]

Postnatal events, from nosocomial infection to anemia and hemodynamic instability, metabolic derangements of hyper/hypoglycemia and electrolytic disturbances, etc. may also play an adjuvant role in the overall picture of survival with multiple handicaps. But one area in particular should call for special caution: the possible role of iatrogenically-induced disability. Many of these tiny babies are, from the very early start, often subjected to a whole panoply of maneuvers and medications known to alter hemodynamics, blood flow and perfusion, from xantines to nonsteroidal anti-inflammatory drugs, namely indomethacin, diuretics, volume expanders, antimicrobials with known toxic side effects, paralyzing agents and sedatives, etc. In recent years, two "old" tools in perinatal care have been submitted to re-evaluation and reappraisal, with growing concern as to their use and misuse.

Antenatal corticosteroids (ANC) have been shown to be associated with a significant reduction of RDS, neonatal death and intra/periventricular hemorrhage[63-65] with a possible synergistic effect with postnatal surfactant therapy.[66] A single course of ANC results in benefits without significant adverse effects with long-term follow-up studies up to adulthood showing no adverse neurological or cognitive outcome.[67] Betamethasone has shown a reduced risk of cystic periventricular leukomalacia and, therefore has become the recommended steroid for enhanced lung maturation.[68] The available evidence of ANC in multiple pregnancies is somewhat conflicting regarding both use and outcome,[69] whilst the use of ANC in diabetic pregnancies is also controversial for the reduction of RDS, as the adverse steroid-induced hyperglycemia on fetal lung maturation may offset any beneficial effects.[70]

From animal data and observational human studies, there is increasing concern that repeated courses of ANC may lead to immediate and long-term harmful effects upon growth, lung and brain development delay[71-76] and at the present, only a single course is advocated with subsequent courses reserved for randomized control trials.[77] How much the widespread use of repeated courses of steroids in the 1990s may be playing a subsidiary role in the adverse outcome of some of these tiny survivors, in addition to prematurity and low birth weight, remains an open question.

Postnatal steroids have been shown to promote early extubation in ventilatory-dependent extremely low birth weight infants, but randomized control studies fail to demonstrate any significant reduction in death rates or in the development of chronic lung disease.[78,79] Furthermore, in addition to the immediate effects of hyperglycemia, hypertension, gastrointestinal tract bleeding and perforation, there is growing concern that they may also be responsible for adverse outcome on growth, cerebral palsy and neurosensory impairment.[79-86] For these reasons, at the present time, postnatal steroids should only be considered for the extubation of ventilatory-dependent babies and only upon informed consent of the parents.

More than 60 years after the initial report of retinal blindness in preterm babies subjected to excess O_2 supplementation, a high proportion of these tiny babies still survive these days with more or less severe ROP. The "optimal" level (and "correct" monitoring) for O_2 supplementation remains as yet unknown. A few years ago an observational study of the case notes of surviving infants delivered before 28 weeks of gestation showed a significant decrease of ROP (6% vs 27.2%) if they were maintained at SaO_2 levels between 70% and 90%. Furthermore, it was also shown that there was much less time on ventilation, less oxygen dependency at 36 weeks corrected age, a better weight gain and, especially, no increase in mortality or cerebral palsy.[87] Not surprisingly, this publication caused considerable polemic[88-93] and ongoing debate.[94-98] Understandably, SaO_2 monitoring has become common practise in most neonatal intensive care units with considerable benefit, i.e. comfort, over repeated arterial punctures and complications from invasive procedures. However, there is very little correlation between PaO_2 levels and SaO_2, both below 84% and above 94% for SaO_2 to keep an ideal PaO_2 between 50 mm Hg and 70 mm Hg.[99] Also, SaO_2 monitoring is dependent upon the methodology used[100,101] and other variables will have to be considered, namely, hemoglobin levels and associated medications that may interfere with cerebral and retinal blood flow and perfusion and not just SaO_2/PaO_2 levels. Nevertheless, ROP is a significant handicap, especially at the lower limit of viability, and caution should reappraise the "physiological" saturations inferred from the more mature infants and extrapolated to these extremely preterm babies, especially in the first few days of life.

Over and above the immediate and short-term sequelae, how are these tiny survivors performing at a later stage? The available long-term evidence—school age and above—generally shows that besides neuromotor and neurosensorial impairments, a high proportion of these children reveal significant learning difficulties and behavioral and educational problems, only adding further to the burden and placing an enormous responsibility upon society as a whole, particularly for the allocation of financial and human resources to provide the necessary collateral help.[102-108] Furthermore, these children will grow to adulthood into a competitive world of "perfection". How sensitive are we to handle their multitude of needs and how prepared are we to integrate them into society with fairness and equity?

WHAT ARE THE ETHICAL IMPLICATIONS?

Ethics, the study of ideal conduct, classed as a branch of philosophy,[109] should be above cultural barriers, be universal and should center upon respect for mankind: easily said, often not practised. Deontology, the science of duty, the branch of knowledge, which deals with moral obligations,[110] the science of professional duties and etiquette,[111] is often referred to as being synonymous with ethics. Laws vary from country to country and sometimes between states within the same country.

It would, thus appear to be quite unrealistic to argue the attainability of a common denominator derived from such widespread philosophical, religious and moral views, to frame it within the various legal requirements, to dictate the codes of rules and to expect it to be internationally accepted, yet that is the essence of ethics.

In perinatal medicine, the overall ethical principles of autonomy, beneficence and non-maleficence are even more difficult to apply than in most branches of medicine due to the often conflicting interests of the mother (and partner) and the fetus. The fetus, regardless of its semantic definitions, its rights, its independent moral status and so forth[112,113] is an entity representing human life. The question is, of course, when does human life begin from the biological, moral, religious, legal and social perspectives. Perhaps the concept of "a fetus as a patient, if not a person", might be the pragmatic answer, at least, for the immediate implications of medical and ethical decisions.[114,115] For similar reasons, we approach the subject of neonatal ethics from a practising angle focusing on medical management and decisions at the threshold of viability. Far from guidelines, these thoughts, hopefully unbiased, express our concern, and independent views on the complexities of universal medical ethics.

Reports in the last 10 years of survival at 22 weeks of gestation[24-26] and less than 400 g birth weight[116] have led to a change in legislation[117] and to a redefinition of the "perinatal period"[1] and the aim for the survival of the most immature of babies became only natural and pressing. Accepting the (theoretical) concept of 22 weeks of gestation as the lower limit of viability, what then is the evidence to support this claim and what is the outcome? The answer to the first question is the proverbial case that confirms the exception and as for the quality of survival, none of the reported survivors was free from neurological sequelae.[24-26,117-118]

And what about at 23 weeks (or 23 weeks and a couple of days)? From here on, it is an open game and the stakes are high, with survival rates from 2% to 35% at 23 weeks to 35–85% at 25 weeks.[7,10-14] It is quite clear that there are enormous geographical asymmetries even within countries with similar demographics, and it is, thus, not surprising that some countries will place their lower limit of viability at 24–25 weeks of gestation.[27]

The ethical questions to practising neonatologists are whether they should accept their own reality of survival and try to improve on quality rather than quantity, or whether they should try to compete with the more advanced countries and aim for the threshold of viability? Who should decide on that? Should it be an individual (local) decision or a matter of national (regional) policy? What are the ethics and moral implications of these decisions? Could it possibly be that in practise, new technologies would change matters? What would be the financial resources needed, could they be afforded, and again, what would be the ethical implications of discrimination on financial grounds?

Of the general ethical principles of autonomy, beneficence and non-maleficence, the first does not apply to the neonate for obvious reasons. However, as a person with independent moral status, the newborn is entitled to the full demands and obligations of beneficence and of *primum non nocere*. In everyday practise, the concept of "in the best interest of the patient" has also gained access to neonatal medicine in order to surmount the subtleties of definition from "sustained life" to "quality of life".[119-121] However, this begs the question, in the best interests of whom—the baby, the parents or society, and who should decide? Handicap is a notion often defined by healthy, normal people, which may or may not be shared by the affected individuals themselves. Perhaps, it is a question of degree: what is more acceptable, the survival of a severely physically handicapped but intellectually sound child or, on the contrary, an individual who is completely mentally dependent but who has no physical impairment? And who will be the judge? With the present low birth rate in most western societies, "perfection" is understandably always the goal. However, it is not also a sign of moral perfection when a society is prepared to accept the difference, showing compassion and solidarity with its less fortunate members? On one issue at least, everyone would agree that whatever the dilemmas and however difficult, decisions must never be taken upon account of sex, eugenics, religious or economic prejudice and never based on a doctor's own cultural or religious beliefs.[122-123]

Futile treatment is currently used in medicine to mean that any treatment beyond a certain point would be unjustifiable. Neonatologists, often young, are frequently faced in the middle of the night with the crucial decision (based very often upon inaccurate information on gestational age) of whether or not to initiate active, aggressive management of the extremely immature infant at the threshold of viability.

In doubt, active resuscitative measures should be started in the labor ward.[124] The decision to further continue intensive care can always be reversed after revaluation and counseling to the parents, but this does not imply that decisions to continue or withdraw treatment should rest upon them. Decisions to withdraw or withhold treatment should always be the responsibility of the most senior physician after discussion with all the staff, including the nurses, and upon informing the parents. The "phantom of the law" is often used as an argument for the continuation of futile intensive care. In fact, in most places what is unlawful is the preservation of life at all costs, against the dignity of the human being. As for the ethics of treatment withdrawal, once again, what

is morally wrong is to prolong useless and hopeless treatments, contradicting the Hippocratic rules of "not to harm, if possible to cure, but always to relieve and console". Yet, the same European survey revealed that a considerable number of countries had no policies or consensus for DNR/withdrawal of life support therapies (67% and 48% respectively).[27] Advancing technologies can often cause procrastination over medical decisions which, when based on a particularly sophisticated tool, may be mistaken for good medical practise.

Neuroimaging is often quoted in this context: but how reliable and infallible is neuroimaging for the prediction of function? It might assist but does not replace clinical judgment of when to withdraw or withhold life-supporting therapies that would be quite unethical and unacceptable.

Most importantly, once the medical decision has been reached to withdraw advanced life-support treatment, the baby should be allowed to die in privacy, with dignity, surrounded by the warmth, care and love of his parents with the full support of the medical and nursing staff. Fortunately, in most cases, parents accept medical judgments based on sound clinical evidence, knowledge and good faith and are almost always relieved that the decision has been taken out of their hands. Occasionally, medical decisions to withdraw or withhold treatment do not meet with the parents' agreement or approval because of their particular philosophical, cultural or religious beliefs. Frustrating as this may be, professionals must understand and accept these feelings and must continue medical treatment until such time as further counseling may reverse the parents' decision. In the last resort, if consensual agreement cannot be reached in the best interest of human dignity for the baby, the question of treatment withdrawal may be addressed to the courts.[124]

CAN A UNIVERSAL LOWER LIMIT OF VIABILITY BE ESTABLISHED?

It is quite obvious from the world literature and from individual realities that a threshold exists for each and everyone, whatever it might be. However, commendable the pursuit and quest to emulate the best results, for the meantime, individual thresholds must be recognized. It is within this reality that decisions can be made when faced with the extremely preterm infant, and that an educated prognosis can be discussed with parents. Improvements can then be pursued based upon continuous self-auditing, in strict adherence to the moral conduct of good medical practise toward the most vulnerable of all patients, the sick and extremely preterm infant.

ACKNOWLEDGMENTS

Grateful thanks are due to the collaborators from the participating European countries for their invaluable assistance: van Reempts P, Belgium; Polak-Babic J, Croatia; Hadjidemetriou, Cyprus; Zoban P, Czech Republic; Marlow N, England; Varrendi H, Estonia; Jarvenpaa AL, Finland; Fetter WE, Kollee L, Holland; Temesvari P, Hungary; Dagbjartsson A, Iceland; Bevilacqua G, Italy; Halliday H, Northern Ireland; Meberg A, Norway; Gadzinowski J, Poland; Peixoto JC, Portugal; Mulutina K, Serbia; Pajntar M, Slovenia; Domenech E, Spain; Sedin G, Sweden; Moessinger A, Switzerland; Can G, Turkey. Also thanks to my departmental colleagues Catarina Prior and Susana Tavares for their help with literature searching.

REFERENCES

1. Dunn PM, McIlwaine G. Perinatal Audit. A Report Produced for the European Association of Perinatal Medicine. London: The Parthenon Publishing Group; 1996. p 39.

2. Chapman SJ, Hauth JC, Bottoms SF, et al. Benefits of maternal corticosteroid therapy in infants weighing less or equal to 1000 g at birth after preterm rupture of the amnion. MJ Obstets Gyneco. 1999;180:677-82.

3. Elimian A, Verma U, Canterino J, et al. Effectiveness of antenatal steroids in obstetric sub groups. Obstet Gynecol. 1999;93:174-9.

4. Massaro D. Postnatal development of alveoli. Regulation and evidence for a critical period in rats. J Clin Invest. 1985;76: 1294-9.

5. Stewart JD, Sienko AE, Gonzalez CL, et al. Placebo-controlled comparison between a single dose and a multidose of betamethasone in accelerating lung maturation of mice offspring. Am J Obstet Gynecol. 1998;179:1241-7.

6. Ikegami M, Gobe AH, Newnham J, et al. Repetitive prenatal glucocorticoids improve lung function and increase growth in preterm lambs. Am J Respir Crit Care Med. 1987;156:178-84.

7. Cooke RWI. Improved outcome for infants at the limits of viability. Eur J Pediatr. 1996;155:665-7.

8. Synnes AR, Ling EW, Whitfield MF, et al. Perinatal outcomes of a large cohort of extremely low gestational age infants (twenty-three to twenty-eight completed weeks of gestation). J Pediatr. 1994;125(6 pt 1):952-60.

9. Tin W, Wariyar U, Hey E. Changing prognosis for babies of less than 28 weeks gestation in the north of England between 1983 and 1994. Br Med J. 1997;314 (7074):107-11.

10. Emsley HC, Wardle SP, Sims DG, et al. Increased survival and deteriorating developmental outcome in 23–25 week-old gestation infants 1990–4 compared with 1984-9. Arch Dis Child Fetal Neonatal. 1998;78(2):F99-104.

11. Hack M, Friedman H, Fanaroff AA. Outcomes of extremely low birth weight infants. Pediatrics. 1996;98(5):931-7.

12. Hack M, Fanaroff AA. Outcome of children of extremely low birth weight and gestational age in the 1990s. Early Hum Dev. 1999; 53(3):193-218.

13. Lefebvre F, Glorieux J, St-Laurent-Gagnon T. Neonatal survival and disability rate at age 18 months for infants born between 23 and 28 weeks of gestation. Am J Obstet Gynecol. 1996;174(3):833-8.

14. Finnström O, Otterblad Olausson P, Sedin G, et al. Neurosensory outcome and growth at three years in extremely low birth weight infants: Follow up results from the Swedish national prospective study. Acta Paediatr. 1998;87(10):1055-60.

15. Kilpatrick SJ, Schlueter MA, Piecuch R, et al. Outcome of infants born at 24–26 weeks gestation: I. Survival and Cost. Obstet Gynecol. 1997;90(5):803-8.

16. Lorenz JM. Survival of extremely preterm infants in North America in the 1990s. Clin Perinatol. 2000;27: 255-62.

17. Wood NS, Marlow N, Costeloe K, et al. Neurologic and developmental disability after extremely preterm birth. EPICure Study Group. New Engl J Med. 2000;343:378-84.

18. Batton DJ, DeWitte DB, Espinosa R, et al. The impact of fetal compromise on outcome at the border of viability. Am J Obstet Gynecol. 1998;178:909-15.

19. Bahado-Singh RO, Dash J, Deren O. Prenatal prediction of neonatal outcome in the extremely low birth weight infant. Am J Obstet Gynecol. 1998;178:900-15.

20. El-Metwally D, Vohr B, Tucker R. Survival and neonatal morbidity at the limits of viability in 1990s; 22-25 weeks. J Pediatr. 2000;137: 616-22.

21. McElrath TF, Robinson JN, Ecker JF. Outcome of infants born at 23 weeks gestation. Obstet Gynecol. 2001;97:49-52.

22. Stevenson DK, Wright LL, Lemons JA, et al. Very low birth weight outcomes of the National Institute of Child Health and Human Development Neonatal Research Network, January 1993 through December 1994. Am J Obstet Gynecol. 1998,179.1632-9.

23. Allen MC, Donohue PK, Dusman AE. The limit of viability—neonatal outcome of infants born at 22–25 weeks' gestation. N Eng J Med. 1993;329(22):1597-601.

24. Bottoms SF, Paul RH, Iams JD. Obstetric determinants of neonatal survival: Influence of willingness to perform cesarean delivery on survival of extremely low birth weight infants. Am J Obstet Gynecol. 1997;176: 960-6.

25. Lemons JA, Bauer CR, Oh W, et al. Very low birth weight outcomes of the National Institute of Child Health and Human Development Neonatal Research Networks, January 1995 through December 1996. NICHD Neonatal Research Network. Pediatrics. 2001;107: E1.

26. Chan K, Ohlsson A, Synnes A, et al. Canadian Neonatal Network. Survival, morbidity and resource of infants of 25 weeks' gestational age or less. Am J Obstet Gynecol. 2001;185:220-6.

27. Carrapato MRG, Costa R. The lower limit of viability in Europe. Proceedings III International Conference on Perinatal Medicine of Romanian Association of Perinatal Medicine. 1999;33-9.

28. Reiss I, Landmann E, Heckman M, et al. Increased risk of bronchopulmonary displasia and increased mortality in very preterm infants being small for gestational age. Arch Gynecol Obstet. 2003;269:40-4.

29. Bardin C, Zelkowitz P, Papageorgiou A. Outcome of small for gestational age and appropriate for gestational age infants born before 27 weeks gestation. Pediatrics. 1997;100(2):E4.

30. Cooke RWI. Factors affecting survival and development in extremely tiny babies. Sem Neonatol. 1996;1:267-76.

31. Spinillo A, Capuzzo E, Piazzi G, et al. Significance of low birth weight for gestational age among very preterm infants. Br J Obstet Gynecol. 1997;104:668-73.

32. MacDonald H; American Academy of Pediatrics. Committee on fetus and newborn. Perinatal care at the threshold of viability. Pediatrics. 2002;110(5):1024-7.

33. The Vermont-Oxford Trials Network: very low birth weight outcomes for 1990. Investigators of the Vermont-Oxford Trials Network Database Project. Pediatrics. 1993;91:540-5.

34. O'Shea TM, Klinepeter KL, Goldstein DJ, et al. Survival and development disability in infants with birth weight of 501–800 grams, born between 1979 and 1994. Pediatrics. 1997;100:982-6.

35. Bohin S, Draper ES, Field DJ. Impact of extremely immature infants on neonatal services. Arch Dis Child. 1996;74F:110-13.

36. Cartlidge PHT, Stewart JH. Survival of very low birth weight and very preterm infants in a geographically defined population. Acta Paediat. 1997;86:105-110.

37. Robertson C, Sauve RS, Christianson HE. Province-based study of neurologic disability amongst survivors weighing 500 through 1249 grams at birth. Pediatrics. 1994;93:636-40.

38. Casiro O, Bingham W, MacMurray B, et al. One-year follow-up of 89 infants with birth weights of 500–749 grams and respiratory distress syndrome randomized to two rescue doses of synthetic surfactant or air placebo. J Pediatr. 1995;26:853-60.

39. Ferrara TB, Hoekstra RE, Couser RJ, et al. Survival and follow-up of infants born at 23 to 26 weeks of gestational age: Effects of surfactant therapy. J Pediatr. 1994;124:119-24.

40. Piecuch RE, Leonard CH, Cooper BA, et al. Outcome of infants born at 24 to 26 weeks gestation. II Neurodevelopmental outcome. Obstet Gynecol. 1997;90:809-14.

41. Nishida H. Perinatal Health Care in Japan. J Perinatol. 1997;17:70-4.

42. Evans DJ, Levene MI. Evidence of selection bias in preterm survival studies: A systematic review. Arch Dis Child Fetal Neonatal Ed. 2001;84:F79-84.

43. Oei J, Askie LM, Tobienski R, et al. Attitudes of neonatal clinicians towards resuscitation of the extremely premature infant: An exploratory survey. J Paediatric Child Health. 2000;36:357-62.

44. Munro M, Yu VY, Partridge JC, et al. Antenatal counselling, resuscitation practices and attitudes among Australian neonatologists towards life support in extreme prematurity. Aust NZ Obstet Gynecol. 2001;41:275-80.

45. Campbell D, Fleischman AR. Limits of viability: dilemmas, decisions and decision-makers. Am J Perinatol. 2001;18:117-28.

46. Molholm HB, Greisen G. Preterm delivery and calculation of survival rate below 28 weeks of gestation. Acta Paediat. 2003;92:1335-8.

47. Rhoden NK. Treating baby Doe: The ethics of uncertainty. Hastings Cent Rep. 1986;16:34-42.

48. Lorenz JM, Paneth N, Getton JR. Comparison of management strategies for extreme prematurity in the USA and Netherlands: Outcomes and resource expenditure. Pediatrics. 2001;108:1269-74.

49. Hagen R, Benninger H, Cliffings D, et al. Very preterm birth – A regional study. Part I: Maternal and obstetric factors. Brit J Obstet Gynecol. 1996;103:230-8.

50. Amon E, Steigerwald J, Winn H. Obstetric factors associated with survival of the borderline viable liveborn infant (500–750 gm). Am J Obstet Gynecol. 1995;418 (Abstract).

51. Jones HA, Lumley JM. The effects of the mode of delivery on neonatal mortality in very low birth weight infants born in Victoria, Australia: Cesarean section is associated with increased survival in breech-presenting, but not vertex-presenting infants. Paediatric Perinat Epidemiol. 1997;1:181-99.

52. Grant A, Penn ZJ, Steer PJ. Elective or selective caesarean delivery of the small baby? A systematic review of the control trials. Brit J Obstet Gynecol. 1996;103:1197-200.

53. Bauer J, Hentschel R, Zahradnik H, et al. Vaginal delivery and neonatal outcome in extremely low birth weight infants below 26 weeks of gestational age. Am J Perinatol. 2003;20:181-8.

54. Gascon G, Skoll A, Lefevbre F, et al. The influence of maternal factors on the outcome at 18 months of babies born at 23 to 28 weeks gestation. Am J Obstet Gynecol. 1995;172:418.

55. Iannuci TA, Tomich PG, Gianopoulos JG. Etiology and outcome of extremely low birth weight infants. Am J Obstet Gynecol. 1996;174:1896-902.

56. Verloove-Vanhorick P, Veen S, Ens-dochum MH, et al. Sex difference in disability and handicap at 5 years of age in children born at very short gestation. Pediatrics. 1994;93:576-9.

57. Alexander GR, Kogan M, Bader G, et al. US birth weight/gestational age-specific neonatal mortality: 1995–1997 rates for whites, hispanics and blacks. Pediatrics. 2003;111:61-6.

58. Allen MC, Alexander GR, Tompkins ME, et al. Racial differences in temporal changes in newborn viability and survival by gestational age. Paediatr Perinat Epidemiol. 2000;14:152-8.

59. Petrova A, Mehta R, Anwar M, et al. Impact of race and ethnicity on the outcome of preterm infants below 32 weeks' gestation. J Perinat. 2003;23:404-8.

60. Draper ES, Manktelow B, Field DJ, et al. Prediction of survival for preterm births by weight and gestation age: retrospective population based study. BMJ. 1999;319:1093-7.

61. Vohr BR, Wright LL, Dusick AM. Neurodevelopment and functional outcomes of extremly low birth weight infants in the National Institute of Health and Human Development Neonatal Research Network. 1993-1994. Pediatrics. 2000;105: 1216-26.

62. Hack M, Fanaroff AA. Outcomes of children of extremely low birth weight and gestational age in the 1990s. Sem Neonatal. 2000;5:89-106.

63. Wright LL, Harbar JD, Gunkel H, et al. Evidence from multi-centre networks on the current use and effectiveness of antenatal corticosteroids in low birth weight infants. Am J Obstet Gynecol. 1995;173:263-9.

64. National Institute of Health. Effect of corticosteroids for fetal maturation on perinatal outcomes. NIH Consensus Statement. National Institute of Health. 1994;12:1-24.

65. Crowley P. Prophylactic corticosteroids for preterm birth. Cochrane Database Syst Ref. 2002;4:CD000065.

66. Jobe AH, Mitchell BR, Gunkel JH. Beneficial effects of the combined use of prenatal corticosteroids and postnatal surfactant in preterm infants. Am J Obstet Gynecol. 1993;168:508-13.

67. Vermillion ST, Soper DE, Chasedunn-Roark J. Neonatal sepsis after betamethazone administration to patients with preterm premature rupture of membranes. Am J Obstet Gynecol. 1999;181: 320-7.

68. Baud O, Foix-L'Hellas L, Kaminski M, et al. Antenatal glucocorticoid treatment and cystic periventricular leucomalacia in very premature infants. N Eng J Med. 1999;34:1190-6.

69. Hashimoto LN, Hornung RW, Linsell CJ, et al. Effects of antenatal glucocorticoid on outcome of very low birth weight multifetal gestations. Am J Obstet Gynecol. 2002;187:804-10.

70. Carlson KS, Smith BT, Post M. Insulin acts on the fibroblast to inhibit glucocorticoid stimulation of lung maturation. J Appl Physiol. 1984;57:1577-9.

71. Walfisch A, Hallak M, Mazor M. Multiple courses of antenatal steroids: Risks and benefits. Obstet Gynecol. 2001;98:491-7.

72. Kay HH, Bird IM, Coe CL, et al. Antenatal steroids treatment and adverse fetal effects: What is the evidence? J Soc Gynecol. Investig. 2000;7:269-78.

73. Goldenberg RI, Wright LL. Repeated courses of antenatal corticosteroids. Obstet Gynecol. 2001;97: 316-7.

74. Newnham JP. Is prenatal glucocorticoid administration another origin of adult disease. Clin Exp Pharmacol Physiol. 2001;28: 957-61.

75. Vermillion ST, Soper DE, Newman RB. Neonatal sepsis and death after multiple courses of antenatal beta-methasone therapy. Am J Obstet Gynecol. 2000;183:810-14.

76. Aghajfari E, Murphy K, Matthews S, et al. Repeated doses of antenatal corticosteroids in animals: A systematic review. Am J Obstet Gynecol. 2002;186:843-9.

77. National Institutes of Health Consensus Development Panel. Antenatal corticosteroids revisited: Repeat courses. National Institutes of Health Consensus Development Conference Statement, August 17-18, 2000. Obstet Gynecol. 2001;98:144-50.

78. Halliday HL, Patterson CC, Halahakoon CW. A multicentre, randomized, open study of early corticosteroid treatment (OSECT) in preterm infants with respiratory illness: Comparison of early and late treatment and of dexamethasone and inhaled budesonide. Pediatrics 2001;107:232-40.

79. Vermont Oxford Network Steroid Study Group. Early postnatal dexamethasone therapy for the prevention of chronic lung disease. Pediatrics. 2001;108:741-8.

80. Nicholl RM, Greenough A, King M, et al. Growth effects of systemic versus inhaled steroids in chronic lung disease. Arch Dis Child Fetal Neonatal Ed. 2002;87:F59-61.

81. Stark AR, Carlo WA, Tyson JE, et al. National Institute of Child Health and Human Development Neonatal Research Network. Adverse effects of early dexamethasone in extremely low birth weight infants. N Eng J Med. 2001;344:95-101.

82. French NP, Hagan R, Evans SF, et al. Size at birth and subsequent developments. Am J Obstet Gynecol. 1999;180:114-21.

83. Yeh TF, Lin YJ, Lin CH, et al. Early postnatal (>12 hr) dexamethasone (D) therapy for prevention of BPD in preterm infants with RDS – a two-year follow-up study. Pediatrics. 1998;101(5):e7.

84. Oshea TM, Kothadia JM, Klinepeter KL, et al. Randomized placebo-controlled trial in very low birth weight infants to reduce the duration of ventilation dependency: outcome of study participants at one year adjusted age. Pediatrics. 1999;104:15-21.

85. Shinwell ES, Karplus M, Reich D, et al. Early postnatal dexamethasone treatment and increased incidence of cerebral palsy. Arch Dis Child Fetal Neonatal Ed. 2000;83:F177-81.

86. The Royal Women's Hospital, The Mercy Hospital for Women, Monash Medical Center, The Royal Children's Hospital, The Newborn Emergency Transport Service and The Victorian Perinatal Data Collection Unit, Melbourne, Australia. Postnatal corticosteroids and sensorial neural outcome at 5 years of age. J Paediatr Child Health. 2000;36:256-61.

87. Tin W, Milligan DWA, Pennfather P, et al. Pulse oximetry, severe retinopathy, and outcome at one year in babies of less than 28 weeks' gestation. Arch Dis Child Fetal Neonatal Ed. 2001;F106-10.

88. Primhak R. Oxygen saturation and retinopathy of prematurity. Letters to the Editor. Arch Dis Child Fetal Neonatal Ed. 2001;85: F75-8.

89. Tin W, Milligan DWA, Pennfather P. Oxygen saturation and retinopathy of prematurity. Authors' response. Arch Dis Child Fetal Neonatal Ed. 2001;85:F75-8.

90. Roberton NRC. Two sacred cows of neonatal intensive care. Letters to the Editor. Arch Dis Child Fetal Neonatal Ed. 2001;85:F75-8.

91. Hey E. Two sacred cows of neonatal intensive care. Authors' response. Arch Dis Child Fetal Neonatal Ed. 2001;85:F75-8.

92. McIntosh N. High or low oxygen saturation for the preterm baby. Arch Dis Child Fetal Neonatal Ed. 2001;84:F149-50.

93. Marlow N. High or low oxygen saturation for the preterm baby. Arch Dis Child Fetal Neonatal Ed. 2001;84:F149-50.

94. Tin W, Walker S, Lacamp C. Oxygen monitoring in preterm babies: Too high, too low? Paediatr Respir Rev. 2003;4:9-14.

95. Sinha SK, Tin W. The controversies surrounding oxygen therapy in neonatal intensive care units. Curr Opin Pediatr. 2003;15:161-5.

96. Tin W, Wariyar U. Giving small babies oxygen: 50 years of uncertainty. Semin Neonatol. 2002;7:361-7.

97. Tin W. Optimal oxygen saturation for preterm babies. Do we really know? Biol Neonate. 2004;85:319-25.

98. Tin W. Oxygen therapy: 50 years of uncertainty. Pediatrics. 2002;110:615-16.

99. Wasunna A, Whitelaw AGI. Pulse oximetry in preterm infants. Arch Dis Child. 1987;62:957-61.

100. Gibson LY. Pulse oximeter in the neonate intensive care unit: A co-relational analysis. Pediatric Nursing. 1996;21:511-15.

101. Grieve SH, McIntosh N, Laing IA. Comparison of two different pulse oximeters in monitoring preterm infants. Crit Care Med. 1997; 25:2051-4.

102. Nadeau L, Boivin M, Tessier R, et al. Mediators of behavioural problems in 7-year-old children born after 24–28 weeks of gestation. J Dev Behav Pediatr. 2001;22:1-10.

103. Anderson P, Doyle LW. Victorian Infant Collaborative Study Group. Neural behavioural outcomes of school-age children born extremely low birth weight or very preterm in the 1990s. JAMA. 2003;289:3264-72.

104. Harding L, Walker LG, Lloyd D, et al. A controlled study of children born at gestation 28 weeks or less: Psychological characteristics at seven to ten years of age. Health Bull (Edinb). 2001;59:81-90.

105. Darlow BA, Horwood LJ, Mogridge N, et al. Survival and disability at 7– 8 years of age in New Zealand infants less than 28 weeks' gestation. NZ Med J. 1998;111:204-7.

106. Petrou S, Mehta Z, Hockley C, et al. The impact of preterm birth on hospital in-patient admissions and costs during the first five years of life. Pediatrics. 2003;192:1290-7.

107. Bowen JR, Gibson FL, Hand PJ. Educational outcome at 8 years for children who were born extremely prematurely: A controlled study. J Paediatr Child Health. 2002;38:438-44.

108. Taylor HG, Klein N, Hack M. School-age consequences of birth weight less than 750 g: A review and update. Dev Neuro Psychol. 2000;17:289-321.

109. Sebastian A. Dictionary of the History of Medicine. London: The Parthenon Publishing Group; 1999.

110. Simpson J, Weiner E. The Oxford English Dictionary. London: Oxford University Press; 1989.

111. Dorland WAN. Dorland's Illustrated Medical Dictionary. 30th edition. New York: Saunders; 2003.

112. McCullough LB, Chervenak FA. Ethics in Obstetrics and Gynecology, New York: Oxford University Press; 1994.

113. Elias S, Annas GJ. Reproductive Genetics and the Law. Chicago: Year Book Medical Publishers; 1987.

114. Chervenak FA, McCullough LB. The Fetus as a Patient : Implications for directive versus non-directive counselling for fetal benefits. Fetal Diagn Ther. 1991;6:93-100.

115. Chervenak FA, McCullough LB. Ethics in Perinatal Medicine: Textbook of Perinatal Medicine. Ed. Kurjak. London: The Parthenon Publishing Group; 2000.

116. Ginsberg HG, Goldsmith JP, Stedman CM. Hospital caretechniques resulting in intact survival of a 380 g infant. Acta Paediatr. 1998;101(5):e7.

117. Nishida H, Ishizuka Y. Survival rate of extremely low birth weight infants and its effect on the amendment of the Eugenic Protection Act in Japan. Acta Paediat Jpn. 1992;34(6):612-6.

118. Nishida H. Outcome of infants born preterm with special emphasis on extremely low birth weight infants. Baillieres Clin Obstet Gynaecol. 1993;7(3):611-31.

119. Hull D. The viable child. J Royal Col Phys London. 1988;22: 169-75.

120. Rennie JM. Perinatal management at the lower margin of viability. 1996;74:F214-18.

121. Dunn PM, Stirrat GM. Capable of being born alive? Lancet. 1984;i:553-55.

122. Recommendations on ethical issues in Obstetrics and Gynecology by the FIGO Committee for the study of ethical aspects of human reproduction: Ethical aspectsin the management of severely malformed infants. London: FIGO;1994.

123. Schenker JG. Codes of perinatal ethics. An international perspective. Clin Perinatol. 2003;30:45-65.

124. Recommendations on ethical issues in Obstetrics and Gynecology by the FIGO Committee for the study of ethical aspects of human reproduction: Ethical aspects in the management of newborn infants at the threshold of viability. London: FIGO; 1994.

CHAPTER

9

The Offspring of Maternal Diabetes

Perinatal events and future outcome

MRG Carrapato, S Tavares, C Prior

INTRODUCTION

The 1989 St Vincent's Declaration stated, as a 5-year goal, "...that the outcome of the diabetic pregnancy should approach that of non-diabetic pregnancies"[1] and indeed, over the last 25 years significant reductions in spontaneous abortions, stillbirths, congenital malformations and perinatal mortality have been achieved at least in centers with a special interest in diabetic pregnancy and in selected populations.[2-9] However, reports have shown that even in western countries, spontaneous abortions may be as high as 17%, the stillbirth rate to be five times greater, congenital malformations to range from four to ten times the usual rate, perinatal mortality to be fivefold, neonatal mortality fifteen times greater, and that infant mortality might be trebled as the result of diabetic pregnancies.[10-13] Although population-based studies from Norway have reported considerably better outcomes,[14] data from other countries have continued to show bad results. In a cross-sectional study conducted in twelve perinatal centers in France between 2000–2001 involving 435 diabetic pregnancies, both type 1 and 2, perinatal mortality was six times greater than the national rate, severe congenital malformations were double and preterm delivery eight times the national level. Cesarean rates at 59%, shoulder dystocia at 7.6% and macrosomia at 17.3% added to the burden. Preconceptional care was provided in only 48.5% and 24% of women with type 1 and 2 diabetes respectively, even though women with type 1 diabetes were being followed at least biannually in diabetic centers.[15] Unplanned pregnancies, therefore, remained at similar levels to those observed in the 1990s[16] and close to the reported rates in a recent survey in the USA.[17] In a nationwide prospective study from the Netherlands between 1999–2000, although planned pregnancies were observed in 84% of women with type 1 diabetes and glycemic control was considered good (HbA$_1$C < 7.0%), in about 75% of subjects the outcome was considerably worse than the general population with preeclampsia twelve times greater, cesarean sections 43%, perinatal mortality 2.8%, congenital malformations 8.8%, macrosomia 45.1% with 27.4% of shoulder dystocia, and neonatal hypoglycemia in approximately two-thirds of neonates.[18] These poor results have also been reported for type 2 diabetics and range from congenital malformations eleven times greater, a twofold risk of stillbirth, perinatal mortality 2.5 times higher, risk of neonatal deaths 3.5 times greater and a sixfold risk of death in the first year of life.[19,20]

It would, therefore, appear that nearly 15 years on from the St Vincent's Declaration the goal of a similar outcome for diabetic and non-diabetic pregnancies has yet to be attained.

When addressing diabetic embryofetopathy several issues are necessarily raised: What are the problems? Why does it happen? What is the outcome? Can it be avoided?

PERI(NEO)NATAL PROBLEMS OF THE INFANT OF THE DIABETIC MOTHER (IDM)

Pregestational Diabetes Mellitus (preDM)

The potential complications affecting the conceptus of the diabetic woman have been identified for centuries[21] and range from an increased incidence of fetal demise to congenital malformations and a multitude of immediate neonatal problems including: macrosomia/IUGR, RDS, hypoglycemia, polycythemia, hypocalcemia, hyperbilirubinemia, heart failure and cardiomyopathy, renal vein thrombosis and small left colon. Although these clinical manifestations are seen especially in uncontrolled diabetic mothers, some of the morbidities, namely macrosomia, hypoglycemia, jaundice and RDS, are still more common in the IDM despite good metabolic control and, in general, these neonates still require a higher rate of neonatal intensive care unit admission than the control population.

Congenital Malformations

Although a whole range of congenital malformations involving multiple organ systems, without specific syndromes, have been observed in preDM, both type 1 and 2, some dysmorphies and malformations are more common, including the association of dysplastic external ears and oculoauriculovertebral spectrum (OAVS).[22] Caudal regression anomalies, in particular sacral agenesis (with a 200–600 fold risk ratio), neural tube and CNS defects (relative risk ranging from 3 for anencephaly to a 40–400 fold risk for holoprosencephaly), cardiac malformations, from ASD, VSD to TGV and truncus arteriosus (four to six times greater) to renal defects, from agenesis to ureter duplication with a risk ratio from six to twenty-three times respectively have all been repeatedly observed in diabetic pregnancies.[18,23-26] Most of these congenital malformations occur particularly in the offspring of uncontrolled diabetic women with very poor, or no, preconceptional care. They appear to be directly related to HbA1C levels, ranging from similar levels to those of the general population, with "excellent metabolic control" (HbA$_1$C < 6.9%), to 5.1% (with "good metabolic control", HbA1C 7.0% to 8.5%) to 22.4% incidence with a greater than 8.6% HbA$_1$C.[27] Reid and Ylinen have also shown similar results and correlation with HbA$_1$C suggesting that a good metabolic control could greatly reduce the impact of congenital malformations in the outcome of diabetic pregnancies.[28,29] By enrolling diabetic women to intensive metabolic control before conception, Furhmann showed that major congenital malformations could be reduced to 1.1%, rising to high uncorrected rates for those presenting later in pregnancy.[30,31] Since then, many other authors have shown similar good results from preconceptional care aimed at good metabolic glycemic control.[4,5,7-9,32,33] From the available evidence, it would seem that tight metabolic control for at least 6–12 months prior to conception would greatly reduce the burden of congenital malformations to almost normal rates. Nevertheless, even in the best series, corrected rates for diabetes-related malformations are considerably higher than those for the rest of the population, despite good metabolic control, i.e. preconceptional care and HbA$_1$C levels.[4,5,7,18] This raises several points, from the evaluation of good metabolic control and the best parameters, to the question of compliance and whether hyperglycemia is the only teratogenic fuel per se or additional to other predisposing or adjuvant factors, as outlined in the etiopathogeny of diabetic embryo-fetopathy.

Macrosomia

Ranging from 17% to 50% in the offspring of preDM[15, 18,34-36] macrosomia poses a major problem for both Obstetricians and Neonatologists. In an attempt to diagnose fetal macrosomia, many different ultrasound parameters have been proposed with differing results, from estimated fetal weight (EFW) to abdominal circumference, to the more sophisticated evaluation of fetal subcutaneous fat tissue thickness (SCFTT) of various body segments (mid-arm and mid-thigh fat and lean mass, abdominal and subscapular fat mass, cheek fat) to fetal fat layer, intraventricular septal thickness, etc.[37-39] How reliably can it be diagnosed by the practicing obstetrician, outside major research institutes if, in effect, he is referring to a large-for-gestational-age (LGA) fetus based on the estimated weight and abdominal circumference?[40,41] This is an important question. Whilst both share common characteristics, the true macrosomic fetus will have other peculiarities due to its abnormal fat distribution, especially affecting the shoulder girdle, leading to dystocia and its complications. Should, therefore, all (true) macrosomic fetus be delivered by cesarean section? Perhaps not, but in practice they are. As for the pediatrician, the term macrosomia is also often used to describe a large baby and, again, although sharing common problems of hypoglycemia, polycythemia, hypocalcemia and hyperbilirubinemia, the true macrosomic baby will also be a candidate for birth (intrapartum) asphyxia, brachial palsy and cardiomyopathy.

Moreover, rather than mentioning any given weight or babies weight/gestational age, as is traditionally done for macrosomia, it would be more appropriate to refer to ponderal indices (PI = fetal weight in grams/fetal height in cm^3 × 100) against the estimated centile for gestational age.[42-44] This approach, besides differentiating the normal large-for-gestational age (LGA) from the true macrosomic neonate, may also have other implications, particularly with regard to long-term outcome.

Hypoglycemia

Another issue relates to neonatal hypoglycemia and its never-ending controversies. What in fact is neonatal hypoglycemia and does it matter? Methodological problems of glucose measurements-capillary to venous blood, whole blood to plasma values, sample containers and transport, etc. all account for the different definitions of hypoglycemia. Glucose concentration in whole blood is about 10–15% lower than in plasma and due to the usually high hematocrit of the IDM, plasma, rather than whole blood, should be used for the definition of hypoglycemia. Moreover, what low blood sugar level might be harmful? Will a (given) low blood sugar in the absence of symptoms be less damaging than when

coupled to clinical manifestations? And if, at the follow-up, these children are found to be performing below par, is it because of neonatal hypoglycemia or is it due to poor antenatal metabolic control? Conversely, could it possibly be that in order to overcome hypoglycemia, the neonate is able to utilize other substrates as an alternative to glucose for brain metabolism? The answer is a partial 'yes' for lactate in the immediate neonatal period but quite unlikely for other, more important fuels, namely ketone bodies, given the sustained hyperinsulinism-inhibiting lipolysis. For these reasons, it would therefore be recommended to keep blood levels in the range of more than or equal to 2.6 mmol/L regardless of gestational and postnatal age, by promoting early enteral feeds. If oral feeds are not being tolerated or are contraindicated, IV glucose should be started at 5–6 mg/kg/min and may be subsequently increased accordingly to the lack of response to 8–10 mg/kg/min. If the neonate has symptomatic hypoglycemia, especially related to neuroglycopenia, a bolus IV glucose administration of 0.25–0.05 g/kg should be given followed by glucose infusion at the required rate to maintain normal glycemia. As soon as possible, enteral feeds with either breast milk or formula should be promoted and gradually increased to avoid reactive hypoglycemia if glucose infusion is decreased too rapidly. Glucagon administration of 200–300 µg/kg may occasionally be required to enhance glucose release from glycogen storages and to increase hepatic acids oxidation.

Respiratory Distress Syndrome

Premature delivery remains a hazard due to either maternal or fetal well-being, mostly in poorly-controlled women or with associated pregnancy complications or due to underlying disorders secondary to diabetes itself. Hyaline membrane disease (HMD) is more common in infants of diabetic mothers at any gestational age due to either inhibition or decreased surfactant synthesis, consequence of fetal hyperinsulinism.[45-50] In general, both in vivo and in vitro, insulin opposes the glucocorticoid stimulating effect upon lung maturation[51-53] by a complex cascade of impaired mechanisms, from blockade of fibroblasts—pneumocyte—factor (FBF) release and directly inhibiting phospholipid synthesis by type 2 cells[54] to reducing surface protein synthesis[55] or both.

Antenatal corticosteroids have been shown to promote fetal lung maturation in normal pregnancies. Their use in diabetic pregnancy remains controversial as the adverse steroid-induced hyperglycemia on fetal lung maturation may offset any beneficial effects.[54] In addition, the acute rise of severe hyperglycemia in the mother needs to be taken into account and caution demands close monitoring during antenatal corticosteroid administration and several schemes have been proposed for supplementary insulin to counteract the unbalanced hyperglycemic status.[56,57]

Whether the routine assessment of fetal lung maturation by lamella bodies counts, or lecithin/sphingomyelin ratios should be performed in reliably-dated pregnancies, at term, is doubtful and lately is becoming less advocated.[58-62]

If HMD remains a common neonatal problem, RDS in the offspring of diabetic mothers is further aggravated not only by the concomitant polycythemia and hyperviscocity, hypoxia and pulmonary hypertension, occasionally heart failure, but especially by the high rate of cesarean sections, often without previous labor.

Hypocalcemia

Calcium homeostasis depends upon the equilibrium between intestinal absorption and renal excretion under hormonal regulation. Parathormone mobilizes calcium from bone, promotes its renal tubular reabsorption and stimulates 1,25 hydroxy vitamin D production. Vitamin D increases calcium and phosphate intestinal absorption and regulates bone metabolism mediated by parathormone. Hypocalcemia, on the other hand, stimulates parathormone release. In pregnancy, calcium is actively transferred across the placenta from maternal circulation under the influence of the parathyroid hormone-related peptide (PTHrP) with maternal parathormone and vitamin D having very little influence due to their inability to cross the placenta. Fetal plasma calcium is higher than maternal levels, especially with advancing pregnancy (total and ionized calcium 10–11 mg/dL and 6 mg/dL respectively) and consequently the parathyroid glands show reduced activity.[63-65] At birth, following the suppression of maternal-fetal transferral of calcium, the plasma levels fall within the first 24 hours of life, leading to parathormone release and the normalization of calcium levels by 2 weeks of life.[63,64] Total calcium concentrations in the neonate are dependent upon gestational age, albumin levels and pH.

Hypocalcemia occurs in up to 50% of IDM, usually on the first 3 days of age, often associated to hyperphosphatemia and hypomagnesemia[63-65] probably due to delayed parathyroid response and correlated to the duration and severity of maternal diabetes although the mechanisms remain elusive.[63-65] Pulmonary disease and/or asphyxia worsening the hypocalcemia.[63-65]

In the absence of clinical manifestation, it is debatable whether calcium determination should be performed routinely. On the contrary, with preterm delivery, respiratory compromise, asphyxia, sepsis, etc. calcium levels should be performed and corrected. Prolonged QTc (QT corrected for heart rate over 0.4 sec) on the ECG requires special attention but with the possibility of heart block, refractory bradycardia and hypotension, calcium administration should be carefully monitored.

Persistent hypocalcemia may be the result of the concomitant hypomagnesemia and is unlikely to be corrected if magnesium levels are not adjusted. With significant hyperphosphatemia ($Ca_2 \times PO_4 > 80$) calcium administration may lead to calcification of the soft tissues if the high phosphate levels are not lowered primarily.[63,64,66]

Polycythemia

The definition of polycythemia may include infants with or without symptoms having hematocrits greater than 65%. The reported incidence of polycythemia ranges from 0.4% to 12% in newborns, but it affects up to 30% of infants of poorly controlled diabetic mothers.

Fetal red cells have a larger mean cell volume and are less deformable then more mature cells, leading to increased viscosity. Low fetal oxygenation and tissue hypoxia increase erythropoietin levels stimulating erythropoiesis and leading to high fetal hemoglobin. Some authors speculate that fetal plasma erythropoietin concentration is significantly correlated to maternal high affinity HgA_1C[67-69] whilst others suggest that the increased erythropoiesis in fetus of diabetic pregnancies may be subsequent to fetal hypoxemia, the result of hyperglycemia, hyperinsulinemia and hyperketonemia, in line with Freinkel's concept of "pregnancy as a tissue culture experience".[70,71] The chronic hypoxemic state in utero may thus explain some cases of fetal death. In the neonate, symptomatic polycythemia may present with RDS, congestive heart failure and, occasionally, pulmonary hypertension. Neurological signs include jitteriness, irritability, seizures and apnea. Potential sequelae of polycythemia may be thrombosis, gangrene and stroke. The treatment of polycythemia, especially if symptomatic, is the standard partial exchange transfusion.

Jaundice

Physiological jaundice is a common neonatal problem due to transient glucoronyl transferase deficiency, immature hepatic intra cellular uptake and transport, increased enterohepatic circulation and occurring in 60–70% of newborns. However, clinically significant jaundice (total bilirubin greater than 12.9 mg/dL at term) affects only 5% of these babies.[72]

In the IDM, the risk of clinically important jaundice is up to 30% and is due to multifactorial causes from prematurity, to polycythemia and increased hemolysis, and macrosomia, with ponderal indices, rather than weight/gestational age showing a better correlation with bilirubin levels.[69,73-75]

Gestational Diabetes Mellitus (GDM)

Gestational diabetes mellitus usually develops in the second half of pregnancy. With advancing pregnancy considerable demands are placed upon insulin to meet increasing maternal metabolism. If the threshold is surpassed maternal hyperglycemia may supervene. Although some studies also point to a higher incidence of congenital malformations in association with GDM, most cases are probably pre GDM diagnosed in pregnancy especially type 2, with pre-pregnancy BMI and advanced maternal age playing a very conspicuous role.[76-80] Congenital malformations aside, the whole spectrum of peri(neo)natal problems overlap those of pre GDM and contribute to the high maternal fetal and neonatal morbidities.

The incidence of GDM varies from 3% to 5% depending upon whether screening is universal or only for women at risk.

In our Institution over the 2 year period from 1 January 2002 to 31 December 2003, from an unselected population of 5,930 women, after universal 1 hour 50 grams glucose screening, followed by 3 hour 100 grams OGTT, 211 women were confirmed as having GDM. Seven women, diagnosed in the first week as having had possible preGDM detected only in pregnancy (mean BMI 32.5, mean age 32.4 years) were eliminated from the study.

Among the multigest and multipara, 7.2% had had previous GDM, with 24% miscarriage and 4.3% late fetal death.

In the present pregnancy, the average gestational age at the time of diagnosis was 27 weeks and the mean HbA_1C was 4.3% (range 3.4–5.7%). All women (20.4%) required insulin treatment to maintain good metabolic control.

Complications of pregnancy included pregnancy-induced hypertension (8:3.8%), preeclampsia (3:1.4%), HELLP (3:1.4%), placenta abruption (3:1.4%), thrombocytopenia (4:1.9%), oligohydramnios (2:0.9%), ACIU (2:0.9%). There were no maternal or perinatal deaths.

Delivery was by cesarean section in 43.9% and by instrument delivery in 8.8% whilst for a control group of macrosomic babies of non-diabetic mothers these figures were 36.4% and 9.2% respectively. The average birth weight at 38 weeks was 3,121 grams (SD 424 gr) and length 48.55 cm (SD 1.77 cm).

Table 9.1: Comparative neonatal morbidities of IDM and LGA

Morbidity	IDM (n)	IDM (%)	LGA (n)	LGA (%)	X² (p)
Fractured clavicles	4	2	9	5.4	0.79
Brachial plexus palsy	1	0.5	2	1.2	0.47
Congenital malformations	9*	4.3	9**	4.7	0.582
Prematurity	21	10.2	11	6.6	0.959
Hypoglycemia	6	3.1	4	2.4	0.663
RDS	8	4.1	4	2.4	0.342
Jaundice	63	32.6	28	16.8	<0.001
Polycythemia	7	3.6	9	5.4	0.437
Hypocalcemia	9	4.7	2	1.2	0.054

*Hypospadias 2, Hydronephrosis 2, Hypoplasia of distal phalanx 1, CHD 4 (3 VSD; 1 ASD) **Epispadias 1, Hypospadias 1, Hydronephrosis 1, CHD 5 (2 VSD; 3 ASD); craniofacial dysmorphy 1

Neonatal morbidities expressed in Table 9.1, compared to large- for-gestational age (LGA) neonates of non-diabetic mothers, were considerably better than in many series. Several points, though, need to be considered. The incidence of macrosomia (BW/GA > 90th centile) was identified in only 6 (2.9%) a figure that is just above that of our unselected population (2.8%). However, if ponderal indices (PI) are applied instead of BW/GA, the incidence rises to 31 (16.1%) of babies with PI more than 90th centile, especially with advancing gestational age (22% and 25% at 39 and 40 weeks respectively), suggesting a population of short obese babies within our population of gestational diabetes in contrast to LGA neonates of non-diabetic mothers which are large and long (Table 9.2). We would, therefore, consider PI to be a more accurate and true reflection of macrosomia than just birth weight/

gestational age. Another area for concern is the high incidence of cesarean sections which suggests labor induced failure, because even correcting for PI, only 16.1% were macrosomic newborns, questioning the current practice of elective induction at 38 weeks of gestation. The proportion of small-for-gestational age (SGA) within our diabetic population (10.3% vs 13.64% in our general population), suggests an adequate metabolic control.

Although there were very few cases of RDS in our neonates, mostly due to the paucity of very small, extremely preterm infants, we observed that of those with respiratory problems, more than half were pulmonary adaptation syndromes in neonates delivered by cesarean section at 37 weeks of gestation.

In summary, even within perinatal centers, although maternal and peri(neo)natal adverse results can be greatly improved, GDM remains a public health problem of considerable proportions.

WHY DOES IT HAPPEN?

In a theoretical model, according to Freinkel's concept of "pregnancy as a tissue culture experience", the whole pathogenesis and spectrum of fetal and neonatal mortality and morbidity could primarily be attributed to the excessive transferral of glucose from mother to fetus, inducing fetal hyperglycemia, leading to fetal pancreatic islet hypertrophy and B cell hyperplasia with a consequent rise in insulin secretion.[81] Chronic fetal hyperinsulinism results in raised metabolic rates and oxygen consumption causing fetal hypoxemia which, in turn, would be responsible for the increased rate of stillbirths and birth asphyxia as well as for the excessive erythropoietin production and polycythemia.[68-70,82,83] In addition, fetal hyperinsulinism would be responsible for increased fetal substrate intake, leading to fat synthesis, with the resulting adiposity, macrosomia and visceromegaly. Furthermore, fetal hyperinsulinism may also be responsible for the development of respiratory distress syndrome at

Table 9.2: Body proportions of IDM and LGA per gestational age

GA (Weeks)	IDM (207/5930) Weight (± SD)	IDM (207/5930) Length (± SD)	IDM (207/5930) PI (± SD)	LGA (167/5930) Weight (± SD)	LGA (167/5930) Length (± SD)	LGA (167/5930) PI (± SD)	Sig
41				4650 (167.19)	54.8 (1.85)	3.3 (0.35)	
40	3389 (231.90)	49.0 (1.79)	2.9 (0.39)	4328 (211.08)	52.1 (1.27)	3.1 (0.22)	>0.005
39	3332 (341.51)	49.1 (1.73)	2.8 (0.29)	4208 (263.40)	51.87 (1.63)	3.1 (0.22)	<0.005
38	3121 (424.14)	48.5 (1.77)	2.7 (0.26)	3989 (137.89)	50.9 (1.57)	3.0 (0.31)	<0.005
37	2900 (337.07)	47.8 (1.80)	2.6 (0.21)	3751 (204.07)	51.0 (1.24)	2.8 (0.21)	<0.005
36	2645 (220.76)	46.5 (1.62)	2.6 (0.22)	3495 (111.13)	49.8 (2.68)	2.9 (0.47)	>0.005
35	2343 (82.14)	44.0 (2.74)	2.8 (0.45)	3233 (101.16)	47.0 (2.60)	3.1 (0.49)	>0.005
Total	3074.3 (432.87)	48.4 (1.94)	2.7 (0.27)	4133.6 (351.98)	51.55 (1.81)	3.0 (0.28)	<0.005

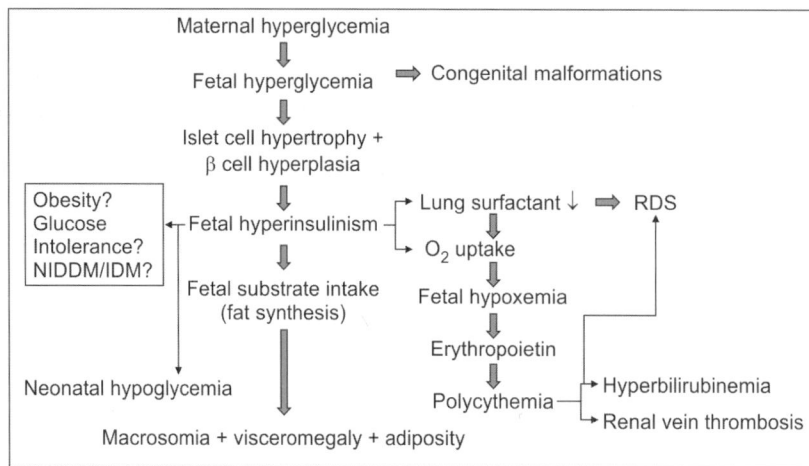

Fig. 9.1: Diabetic embryofetopathy

birth by either inhibiting or decreasing lung surfactant synthesis.[45-50] Neonatal hypoglycemia may be a combination of several factors including sustained hyperinsulinism and lack of counter-regulatory hormonal responses impairing hepatic glucose production, deficient lipolysis and increasing peripheral glucose uptake.[84-86] It would seem, therefore, that uncontrolled maternal hyperglycemia could start the whole spectrum of diabetic embryofetopathy (Fig. 9.1). It is quite possible, however, that other metabolic fuels, either besides or in association with glucose, from lipids to amino acids, may also cross the placenta in a concentration gradient inversely proportional to insulin availability, further contributing to the abnormal fetal milieu.[70,71,87] Depending upon the timing of gestation, during critical developmental stages, the same metabolic fuels would have different effects upon the fetus. Over the last 15 years there has been increasing evidence from animal and human studies to support the theory that in addition to sugars (glucose, galactose and mannose) other metabolic fuels, from ketones to deranged lipid peroxidation, may be responsible for the pathomechanisms of congenital malformations providing that they are present at certain (high) levels for a reasonable amount of time and especially at crucial "developmental windows".[88-91] Dietary supplementation of deficient substrates (arachidonic acid and myoinositol), free oxygen radical scavenging enzymes and antioxidants have been shown in vivo and in vitro to reduce the rate of malformation in the offspring of diabetic animals.[92-95] Whether such strategies might be applicable to clinical practice remain a promising but open question.

Similarly, the same general principles of multifactorial pathomechanisms have been postulated for macrosomia including and ranging from ketone bodies to free fatty acids, "selected" amino acids and with a conspicuous role for IGF1 and IGF2 at local level. Maternal insulin antibodies and insulin counter-regulatory hormones may, in addition, further contribute to the resulting macrosomia.[96-101]

Toward the end of the second trimester, at a time of increasing cerebral cortical differentiation and maturation, it is quite conceivable that a metabolic insult may result in altered neurological or intellectual behavior[102-106] and, during the third trimester, proliferation of fetal adipocytes, muscle cells and pancreatic β cells may then be responsible for "programming" the later development of several adult disorders.[107-111]

WHAT IS THE OUTCOME?

Neonatal complications of the IDM in spite of the high morbidities involved are now quite well managed with intensive neonatal care. It is questionable whether these babies are more prone to developing neurological, behavioral and learning disabilities and, if so, whether they are due to an unfavorable intrauterine metabolic environment or to other perinatal and early life events operating on different fetal determinants. Most of the early reports of severe brain damage are, reassuringly, now of historical interest.[112,113] Nevertheless, well-documented evidence points to mild to moderate psychomotor and psychosocial impairment in the offspring of these mothers. Whilst it is quite possible that early neonatal events may play a role, available data also places a suspicious emphasis on intrauterine life.[102-105]

The long-term outcome, on the other hand, poses several questions. Some studies point to a higher incidence of childhood obesity in the offspring of these mothers whilst others fail to find such correlations. Conflicting results might be the result of the different methodologies involved, including different definitions and very often small numbers, without adequate control populations.[114-116]

Finally, a major issue is whether some adult diseases of metabolic and vascular disorders may have had a fetal origin. In recent years, there has been accumulating evidence, both from animal studies and epidemiological data, to suggest that fetal β cell hyperplasia and hyperinsulinism may induce irreversible changes leading to obesity, glucose intolerance and even overt non-insulin-dependent diabetes and, perhaps, a protective effect against type 1 diabetes later in life—a model very much in line with the "Barker Hypothesis" of the fetal origins of adult disease.[107-111,117,118] What might be the relative weight of genetics versus intrauterine events remains to be confirmed[119,120] but it is quite interesting that at least in experimental models, the prevention of hyperglycemia in pregnancy significantly reduces the prevalence of diabetes in the next generations.[111]

WHAT CAN BE DONE?

Based on the assumption that poor maternal homeostasis is at the core of the problem and that tight metabolic control might change the outcome of a diabetic pregnancy to normal, why then are such poor results being reported even in developed countries? Admittedly, most of these bad performances are for preDM. But, even allowing for different data collection, lack of uniform criteria in definitions and case identification,[121-123] the fact remains that overall results are far from satisfactory. It can be argued that they are due to poor medical and social care and they most probably are. It can also be argued that poor metabolic control has not been achieved or that "good" is not necessarily "optimal". Alternatively, it can be put forward that there might be an abnormal genetic background contribution (evidence is pretty scanty) or that there might be other metabolic fuels besides glucose operating at different developmental stages of pregnancy thus accounting for the etiopathogenesis of the whole syndrome. It is quite possible that some, or all, of these metabolic fuels may, per se or in synergie, play a significant role in the whole metabolic disturbance and it is quite conceivable that besides the classical approach to strict glucose control, other dietary manipulations with supplementation or replacement of deficient substracts might hold a promise for the near future. For the moment, however, priority should focus on intensive prenatal care for diabetic women and the identification of women for the development of GDM and, once diagnosed, placing them on a strict glycemic control throughout pregnancy. The cost efficiency of screening all women for GDM is often discussed and likewise, whether many of these women are over-treated unnecessarily. Argument, however, should concentrate not just on the immediate effects of GDM but on the long-term consequences for both the mother and her offspring.

ACKNOWLEDGMENT

The authors gratefully acknowledge the antenatal data on Diabetic Mothers supplied by Dr Célia Araújo.

REFERENCES

1. Diabetes Care and Research in Europe: The St Vincent Declaration. WHO/IDF Europe. Diabetic Med. 1990;7:360.
2. Teramo K, Kuusisto AN, Raivio KO. Perinatal outcome of insulin-dependent diabetic pregnancies. Ann Clin Res. 1979;11:146-55.
3. Jervell J, Bjerkedal T, Moe N. Outcome of pregnancies in diabetic mothers in Norway 1967-76. Diabetologia. 1980;8:131-4.
4. Molsted-Pedersen L, Pedersen J. Congenital malformations in diabetic pregnancies. Clinical viewpoints. Acta Paediatr Scand Suppl. 1985;320:79-84.
5. Hanson U, Persson B, Thunnel S. Relationship between haemoglobin A1c in early Type I (insulin-dependent) diabetic pregnancy and the occurrence of spontaneous abortion and fetal malformation in Sweden. Diabetologia. 1990;33:100-4.
6. Roberts AB, Pattison NS. Pregnancy in women with diabetes mellitus, twenty years experience: 1968-1987. N Z Med J. 1990;103:211-3.
7. Kitzmiller JL, Gavin LA, Gin GD, et al. Preconception care of diabetes. Glycemic control prevents congenital abnomalies. JAMA. 1991;265:731-6.
8. McElvy SS, Miodovnik M, Rosenn B, et al. A focused preconceptional and early pregnancy program in women with type I diabetes reduces perinatal mortality and malformation rates to general population levels. J Matern Fetal Med. 2000;9:14-20.
9. Diabetes Control and Complications Trial Research Group. The effects of intensive treatment of diabetes on the development and progression of long-term complications in insulin-dependent diabetes mellitus. N Eng J Med. 1993;329:977-86.
10. Hawthorne G, Robson S, Ryall EA, et al. Prospective population-based survey of outcome of pregnancy in diabetic women: results of the Northern Diabetic Pregnancy Audit, 1994. BMJ. 1997;315:279-81.
11. Casson IF, Clarke CA, Howard CV, et al. Outcomes of pregnancy in insulin-dependent diabetic women: results of a five year population cohort study. BMJ. 1997;315:275-8.
12. Penney GC, Mair G, Pearson DW, et al. Outcome of pregnancies in women with type 1 diabetes in Scotland: a national population-based study. Br J Obstet Gynaecol. 2003;110:315-8.
13. Hadden DR, McCance D, Traub AI. Ten-year outcome of diabetic pregnancy in Northern Ireland: the case for centralization. Diabetic Med. 1998;15(Suppl 1):S16.
14. Hawthorne G, Irgens LM, Lie RT. Outcome of pregnancy in diabetic women in Northern England and Norway, 1994-7. BMJ. 2000;321:730-1.
15. Diabetic and Pregnancy Group, France. French multicentric survey of outcome of pregnancy in women with pregestational diabetes. Diabetes Care. 2003;26:2990-93.
16. Gestation and Diabetes in France Study Group. Multicenter survey of diabetic pregnancy in France. Diabetes Care. 1991;14:994-1000.
17. American Diabetes Association. Preconceptional care of women with diabetes. Diabetes Care. 2003;26(Suppl 1):S91-3.
18. Evers IM, de Valk HW, Visser GH. Risk of complications of pregnancy in women with type I diabetes: nationwide prospective study in the Netherlands. BMJ. 2004;328(7445):915-20.
19. Dunne F, Brydon P, Smith K, et al. Pregnancy in women with type 2 diabetes: Twelve-years outcome data 1990-2002. Diabetic Med. 2003;20:734-8.
20. Hadden DR, Cull CA, Croft DJ, et al. Poor pregnancy outcome for women with type 2 diabetes. Diabetic Med. 2003;20:506-7.
21. Le Corche E. Du diabetic dans ses rapports avec la vie intrauterine menstruation et la grossesse. Ann Gynecol. 1885;24:25-7.
22. Wang R, Martinez-Frias ML, Graham JM Jr. Infants of diabetic mothers are at increased risk for the oculoauriculo-vertebral sequence: a case-based and case-control approach. J Pediatr. 2002;141:611-7.
23. Kucera J. Rate and type of congenital anomalies among offspring of diabetic women. J Reprod Med. 1971;7:73-82.
24. Mills JL, Baker L, Goldman AS. Malformations in infants of diabetic mothers occur before the seventh gestational week. Diabetes. 1979;28:292-3.
25. Barr M Jr, Hanson JW, Currey K, et al. Holoprosencephaly in infants of diabetic mothers. J Pediatr. 1983;102:565-8.
26. Wren C, Birrel G, Hawthorne G. Cardiovascular malformations in infants of diabetic mothers. Heart. 2003;89:1217-20.
27. Miller EM, Hare JW, Cloherty JP, et al. Major congenital anomalies and elevated hemoglobin A1c in early weeks of diabetic pregnancy. N Engl J Med. 1981;304:1331-4.
28. Reid M, Hadden D, Harley JM, et al. Fetal malformations in diabetics with high haemoglobin A1c in early pregnancy (letter). BMJ (Clin Res Ed). 1984;289:001.
29. Ylinen K, Aula P, Stenman UH, et al. Risk of minor and major fetal malformations in diabetics with haemoglobin A1c values in early pregnancy. BMJ. 1984;289:345-6.
30. Furhmann K, Reiher H, Semmler K, et al. Prevention of congenital malformations in infants of insulin-dependent diabetic mothers. Diabetes Care. 1983;6:219-23.

31. Furhmann K, Reiher H, Semmler K, et al. The effect of intensified conventional insulin therapy before and during pregnancy on the malformation rate in offspring of diabetic mothers. Exp Clin Endocrinol. 1984;83:173-7.

32. Steel JM. Prepregnancy counseling and contraception in the insulin-dependent diabetic patient. Clin Obstet Gynecol. 1985;28:553-66.

33. DCCT 1996. The Diabetes Control and Complications Trial Research Group. Pregnancy outcomes in the diabetes control and complications trial. Am J Obstet Gynaecol. 1996;174:1343-53.

34. Martin Carballo G, Fernandez Cano G, Grande Aragon C, et al. Infants of diabetic mothers (IDM) I—Macrosomia and growth factors. An Esp Pediatr. 1997;47:295-301.

35. Cordero L, Landon MB. Infant of diabetic mother. Clin Perinatol. 1993;20:635-48.

36. Carvalheiro M. Diabetes in pregnancy: state of the art in Mediterranean countries, Portugal. Ann 1st Super Sanita. 1997;33:303-6.

37. Larciprete G, Valensise H, Vasapollo B, et al. Fetal subcutaneous tissue thickness (SCTT) in healthy and gestational diabetic pregnancies. Ultrasound Obstet Gynecol. 2003;22:591-7.

38. Bethune M, Bell R. Evaluation of the measurement of the fetal fat layer, interventricular septum and abdominal circumference percentile in the prediction of macrosomia in pregnancies affected by gestational diabetes. Ultrasound Obstet Gynecol. 2003;22:586-90.

39. Greco P, Vimercati A, Hyett J, et al. The ultrasound assessment of adipose tissue deposition in fetuses of "well controlled" insulin-dependent diabetic pregnancies. Diabet Med. 2003;20:858-62.

40. Buchanan TA, Kjos SL, Montoro MN, et al. Use of fetal ultrasound to select metabolic therapy for pregnancies complicated by mild gestational diabetes. Diabetes Care. 1994;17:275-83.

41. Gilby JR, Williams MC, Spellacy WN. Fetal abdominal circumference measurements of 35 and 38 cm as predictors of macrosomia. A risk factor for shoulder dystocia. J Reprod Med. 2000;45:936-8.

42. Roje D, Ivo B, Ivica T, et al. Gestational age—the most important factor of Neonatal Ponderal Index. Yonsei Med J. 2004;45:273-80.

43. Patterson RM, Pouliot MR. Neonatal morphometrics and perinatal outcome: who is growth retarded? Am J Obstet Gynecol. 1987;157:691-3.

44. Dombrowski MB, Stanley MB, Johnson MP, et al. Birth weight—length ratios, ponderal indexes, placental weights, and birth weight—placenta ratios in a large population. Arch Pediatr Adolesc Med. 1994;148:508-12.

45. Bourbon JR, Farrell PM. Fetal lung development in the diabetic pregnancy. Pediatr Res. 1985;19:253-67.

46. Tyden O, Berne C, Eriksson U. Lung maturation in fetuses of diabetic rats. Pediatr Res. 1980;14:1192-5.

47. Warburton D. Chronic hyperglycaemia with secondary hyperinsulinemia inhibits the maturational response of fetal lamb lungs to cortisol. J Clin Invest. 1983;72:433-40.

48. Warburton D, Parton L, Buckley S, et al. Effects of glucose infusion on surfactant and glycogen regulation in fetal lamb lung. J Appl Physiol. 1987;63:175-06.

49. Levine DH. Hyperinsulinemia and decreased surfactant in fetal rabbits. Dev Pharmacol Ther. 1985;8:284-91.

50. Rooney SA, Ingleson LD, Wilson CM, et al. Insulin antagonism of dexamethasone-induced stimulation of cholinephosphate cytidyltransferase in fetal rat lung in organ culture. Lung. 1980;158:151-5.

51. Gross I, Smith GJ, Wilson CM, et al. The influence of hormones of the biochemical development in fetal rat lung in organ culture. II. Insulin. Pediatr Res. 1980;14:834-8.

52. Smith BT, Girout CJ, Robert M, et al. Insulin antagonism of cortisol action on lechithin synthesis by cultured fetal lung cells. J Pediatr. 1975;87:953-5.

53. Pignol B, Bourbon J, Ktorza A, et al. Lung maturation in the hiperinsulinemic rat fetus. Pediatr Res. 1987;21:436-41.

54. Carlson KS, Smith BT, Post M. Insulin acts on the fibroblasts to inhibit glucocorticoid stimulation of lung maturation. J Appl Physiol. 1984;57:1577-9.

55. Snyder JM, Kwun JE, O'Brien JA, et al. The concentration of 35-kDa surfactant apoprotein in amniotic fluids from normal and diabetic pregnancies. Pediatr Res. 1988;24:728-34.

56. Kaushal K, Gibson JM, Railton A, et al. A protocol for improved glycemic control following corticosteroid therapy in diabetic pregnancies. Diabet Med. 2003;20:73-5.

57. Mathiesen ER, Christensen AB, Hellmuth E, et al. Insulin dose during glucocorticoid treatment for fetal lung maturation in diabetic pregnancy: test of an algorithm. Acta Obstet Gynecol Scand. 2002;81:835-9.

58. Kjos SL, Berkowitz KM, Kung B. Prospective delivery of reliably dated term infants of diabetic mothers without determination of fetal lung maturity: comparison to historical control. J Matern Fetal Neonatal Med. 2002;12:433-7.

59. Langer O. The controversy surrounding fetal lung maturity in diabetes in pregnancy: a re-evaluation. J Matern Fetal Neonatal Med. 2002;12:428-32.

60. DeRoche ME, Ingardia CJ, Guerette PJ, et al. The use of lamellar body counts to predict fetal lung maturity in pregnancies complicated by diabetes mellitus. Am J Obstet Gynecol. 2002;187:908-12.

61. Piper JM. Lung maturation in diabetes in pregnancy: if and when to test. Semin Perinatol. 2002;26:206-9.

62. Moore TR. A comparison of amniotic fluid fetal pulmonary phospholipids in normal and diabetic pregnancy. Am J Obstet Gynecol. 2002;186:641-50.

63. Abrams SA. Neonatal hypocalcemia. In: Rose BD (Ed). UpToDate 2004. Wellesley, MA.

64. Nold JL, Georgieff MK. Infants of diabetic mothers (review). Pediatr Clin North Am. 2004;51:619-37.

65. Riskin A, Haney PM. Infant of a diabetic mother. In: Rose BD (Ed). UpToDate 2004. Wellesley, MA.

66. Choukair MK. The Harriet Lane Handbook. Johns Hopkins Hospital; Mosby; 2000.

67. Salvesen DR, Brudenell JM, Snijders RJ, et al. Fetal plasma erythropoietin in pregnancies complicated by maternal diabetes mellitus. Am J Obstet Gynecol. 1993;168:88-94.

68. Salvesen DR, Brudenell MJ, Nicolaides KH. Fetal polycythemia and thrombocytopenia in pregnancies complicated by maternal diabetes mellitus. Am J Obstet Gynecol. 1992;166:1287-93.

69. Mimouni F, Miodovnik M, Siddiqi TA, et al. Neonatal polycythemia in infants of insulin-dependent diabetic mothers. Obstet Gynaecol. 1986;68:370-2.

70. Freinkel N, Metzger BE. Pregnancy as a tissue culture experience: the critical implications of maternal metabolism for fetal development. Ciba Foundation Symposium. 1978;63:3-28.

71. Freinkel N, Metzger BE. Emerging challenges in diabetes and pregnancy: diabetic embryopathy and gestational diabetes. In: Alberti KGMM, Krall LP (Eds). The Diabetes Annual. Amsterdam: Elsevier Science Publishers; 1988. pp. 179-201.

72. Rubaltelli FF. Unconjugated and conjugated bilirubin pigments during perinatal development. IV. The influence of breastfeeding on neonatal hyperbilirubinemia. Biol Neonate. 1993;64:104-9.

73. Peevy KJ, Landaw SA, Gross SJ. Hyperbilirubinemia in infants of diabetic mothers. Pediatrics. 1980;66(3):417-19.

74. Jahrig D, Jahrig K, Stiete S, et al. Neonatal jaundice in infants of diabetic mothers. Acta Paediatr Scand Suppl. 1989;360:101-7.

75. Ballard JL, Rosenn B, Khoury JC, et al. Diabetic fetal macrosomia: significance of disproportionate growth. J Pediatr. 1993;122:115-9.

76. Garcia-Patterson A, Erdozain L, Ginovart J, et al. In human gestational diabetes mellitus congenital malformations are related to pre-pregnancy body mass index and to severity of diabetes. Diabetologia. 2004;47:509-14.

77. Cedergren MI, Kallen BA. Maternal obesity and infant heart defects. Obes Res. 2003;11:1065-71.

78. atkins ML, Rasmussnen SA, Honein MA, et al. Maternal obesity and risk for birth defects. Pediatrics. 2003;111:1152-8.

79. Sheffield JS, Butler-Koster EL, Casey BM, et al. Maternal diabetes mellitus and infant malformations. Obstet Gynecol. 2002;100:925-30.

80. Mikhail LN, Walker CK, Mittendorf R. Association between maternal obesity and fetal cardiac malformations in African-Americans. J Natl Med Assoc. 2002;94:695-700.

81. Pedersen J. Hyperglycaemia-hyperinsulinism theory and birthweight. In: Pedersen J (Ed). The Pregnant Diabetic and Her Newborn. Baltimore: Williams and Wilkins; 1977.

82. Carson BS, Phillipps AS, Simmons MA, et al. Effects of a sustained insulin infusion upon glucose uptake and oxygenation of the ovine fetus. Pediatr Res. 1980;14:147-52.

83. Widness JA, Susa JB, Garcia JF, et al. Increased erythropoiesis and elevated erythropoietin in infants born to diabetic mothers and in hyperinsulinic rhesus fetuses. J Clin Invest. 1981;67:637-42.

84. Artal R, Platt LD, Kammula RK, et al. Sympathoadrenal activity in infants of diabetic mothers. Am J Obstet Gynecol. 1982;142:436-9.

85. Bloom SR, Johnston DI. Failure of glucagon release in infants of diabetic mothers. BMJ. 1972;4:453-4.

86. Stern L, Ramos A, Leduc J. Urinary catecholamine excretion in infants of diabetic mothers. Pediatrics. 1968;42:598-605.

87. Milner RDG. Amino acids and beta cell growth in structure and function. In: Merkatz IR, Adam PAJ (Eds). The Diabetic Pregnancy: A Perinatal Perspective. New York: Grune and Stratton; 1979.

88. Reece EA, Homko C, Wiznitzer A. Metabolic changes in diabetic and nondiabetic subjects during pregnancy. Obstet Gynecol Surv. 1994;49:64-71.

89. Hod M, Star S, Passonneau JV, et al. Effect of hyperglycemia on sorbitol and myo-inositol content of cultured rat conceptus: failure of aldose reductase inhibitors to modify myo-inositol depletion and dysmorphogenesis. Biochem Biophys Res Commun. 1986;140:974-80.

90. Reece EA, Homko CJ, Wu YK. Multifactorial basis of the syndrome of diabetic embryopathy. Teratology. 1996;54:171-82.

91. Eriksson UJ, Borg LA. Diabetes and embryonic malformations. Role of substrate-induced free-oxygen radical production for dysmorphogenesis in cultured rat embryos. Diabetes. 1993;42:411-9.

92. Hagay ZJ, Weiss Y, Zusman I, et al. Prevention of diabetes-associated embryopathy by overexpression of the free radical scavenger copper zinc superoxide dismutase in transgenic mouse embryos. Am J Obstet Gynecol. 1995;173:1036-41.

93. Goldman AS, Baker L, Piddington R, et al. Hyperglycemia-induced teratogenesis is mediated by a functional deficiency of arachidonic acid. Proc Natl Acad Sci USA. 1985;2:8227-31.

94. Khandelwal M, Wu YK, Borenstein M, et al. Dietary phospholipid therapy, hyperglycaemia-induced membrane changes and associated diabetic embryopathy. Am J Obstet Gynecol. 1995;172:265-71.

95. Khandelwal M, Reece EA, Wu YK, et al. Dietary myo-inositol in hyperglycemia-induced embryopathy. Teratology. 1998,57.79-84.

96. Menon RK, Cohen RM, Sperling MA, et al. Transplacental passage of insulin in pregnant women with insulin-dependent diabetes mellitus. Its role in fetal macrosomia. N Engl J Med. 1990;323:309-15.

97. Reece EA, Homko C, Wiznitzer A. Metabolic changes in diabetic and nondiabetic subjects during pregnancy. Obstet Gynecol Surv. 1994;49:64-71.

98. Rosenn BM, Miodovnik M, Khoury JC, et al. Deficient counter regulation: a possible risk factor for excessive fetal growth in IDDM pregnancies. Diabetes Care. 1997;20:872-4.

99. Schwartz R, Gruppuso PA, Petzold K, et al. Hyperinsulinemia and macrosomia in the fetus of the diabetic mother. Diabetes Care. 1994;17:640-8.

100. Yan-Jun L, Tsushimo T, Minei S, et al. Insulin-like factors (IGFs) and IGF-binding proteins (IGFBP-1, -2, -3) in diabetic pregnancy: relationship to macrosomia. Endocr J. 1996;43:221-31.

101. Roth S, Abernathy MP, Lee WH, et al. Insulin-like growth factors I and II peptide and messenger RNA levels in macrosomic infants of diabetic pregnancies. J Soc Gynecol Investig. 1996;3:78-84.

102. Ornay A, Ratzon N, Greenbaum G, et al. Neurobehaviour of school age children born to diabetic mothers. Arch Dis Child Fetal Neonatal Ed. 1998;79(2):F94-9.

103. Ornay A, Wolf A, Ratzon N, et al. Neurodevelopmental outcome at early school age of children born to mothers with gestational diabetes. Arch Dis Child Fetal Neonatal Ed. 1999;81(1):F10-4.

104. Rizzo TA, Dooley SL, Metzger BE, et al. Prenatal and perinatal influences on long-term psychomotor development in offspring of diabetic mothers. Am J Obstet Gynecol. 1995;173:1753-8.

105. Rizzo TA, Metzger BE, Dooley SL, et al. Early malnutrition and child neurobehavioural development: insight from the study of children of diabetic mothers. Child Dev. 1997;68:26-38.

106. Silverman BL, Rizzo TA, Cho NH, et al. Long-term effects of the intrauterine environment. The Northwestern University Diabetes in Pregnancy Centre. Diabetes Care. 1998;21(Suppl 2):B142-9.

107. Dorner G, Plagemann A, Reinagel H. Familial diabetes aggregation in type I diabetics: gestational diabetes an apparent risk factor for increased diabetes susceptibility in the offspring. Exp Clin Endocrinol. 1987;89:84-90.

108. Dorner G, Steindel E, Thoelke H, et al. Evidence for decreasing prevalence of diabetes mellitus in childhood apparently produced by prevention of hyperinsulinism in the foetus and newborn. Exp Clin Endocrinol. 1984;84:134-42.

109. Martin AO, Simpson JL, Ober C, et al. Frequency of diabetes mellitus in mothers of probands with gestational diabetes: possible maternal influence on the predisposition to gestational diabetes. Am J Obstet Gynecol. 1985;151:471-5.

110. Pettitt DJ, Aleck KA, Baird HR, et al. Congenital susceptibility to NIDDM. Role of intrauterine environments. Diabetes. 1988;37:622-8.

111. Van Assche FA, Holemans K, Aerts L. Fetal growth and consequences for later life. J Perinat Med. 1998;26:337-46.

112. Howarth JC, McRae KN, Dilling LA. Prognosis of infants of diabetic mothers in relation to neonatal hypoglycaemia. Dev Med Child Neurol. 1976;18:471-9.

113. Persson B, Gentz J. Follow-up of children of insulin-dependent and gestational diabetic mothers: neuropsychological outcome. Acta Pediatr Scand. 1984;73:349-58.

114. Vohr BR, Lipsitt LP, Oh W. Somatic growth of children of diabetic mothers with reference to birth size. J Pediatr. 1980;97:196-9.

115. Vohr BR, McGarvey ST, Tucker R. Effects of maternal gestational diabetes on offspring obesity at 4–7 years of age. Diabetes Care. 1999;22:1284-91.

116. Whitaker RC, Pepe MS, Seidel KD, et al. Gestational diabetes and the risk of offspring obesity. Pediatrics. 1998;101:E9.

117. Van Assche FA, Aerts L, Holemans K, et al. Fetal consequences of maternal diabetes. In: Andreani D, Bompiani G, Di Mario U, Faulk WP, Galluzo A (Eds). Immunobiology of Normal and Diabetic Pregnancy. New York: John Wiley; 1990.

118. Warram JH, Martin BC, Krolewski AJ. Possible mechanisms for the diminished risk of IDDM in the children of diabetic mothers. In: Andreani D, Bompiani G, Di Mario U, Faulk WP, Galluzo A (Eds). Immunobiology of normal and diabetic pregnancy. New York: John Wiley; 1990.

119. Hales CN, Barker DJ. Type 2 (non-insulin-dependent) diabetes mellitus: the thrifty phenotype hypothesis. Diabetologia. 1992;35:595-601.

120. Phillips DI, Barker DJ, Hales CN, et al. Thinness at birth and insulin resistance in adult life. Diabetologia. 1994;37:150-4.

121. Johnston F. Outcome of pregnancy in diabetic women. Authors did not define criterion for case selection (author reply). BMJ. 2001;322:614.

122. Golding J, ALSPAC (Avon Longitudinal Study of Parents and Childen) Study Team. Outcome of pregnancy in diabetic women. More investigation is needed into whether control of diabetes is really poorer in England than Norway. BMJ. 2001;322(7286):614-5.

123. Hawthorne G, Irgens LM, Tie RT, et al. Retraction of paper on maternal diabetes (letter). BMJ. 2003;327:929.

10 Neonatal Seizures

A Beke, Z Papp

DEFINITION

Seizures have been defined as abnormal, paroxysmal, stereotypical clinical events that are initiated by the hypersynchronous activity of neurons in the brain.[1] They represent rapid alteration in the function of the nervous system by which the motor, behavioral or autonomic functions (or all of these) are clinically affected. Seizures are far commoner in the first month of life than at any other time. Neonatal seizures have been described in both clinical and electrical terms. Clinical seizures have been described as occurring in close association with electroencephalograph (EEG) seizure activity (epileptic in origin), and without accompanying EEG seizure activity (presumably non-epileptic in origin). All the clinical seizures described indicate the presence of significant central nervous system dysfunction. In this regard, the findings of EEG monitoring studies do not change a fundamental concept concerning seizures of the newborn: each newly diagnosed neonatal seizure represents a neurological emergency.[2]

INCIDENCE

Conventionally, the neonatal period is limited to the first 4 weeks of life. However, some authors[3,4] define neonatal seizures as those that occur up to 44 weeks of postmenstrual age, to take into account premature birth. Although convulsive phenomena are the most frequent among the major neurological disorders in the neonatal period, their precise frequency is unknown because many of the subtle manifestations of neonatal convulsions may escape recognition. Conversely, jittery and tremulous movements, common at this period, are often mistaken for convulsive seizures, although their significance is completely different. The true incidence of neonatal seizures varies in different series from 0.15% to 1.4%.[5–10] Scher et al.[11] found that the incidence of seizures among all neonates admitted to the intensive care unit was 2.3%, and the group of preterm neonates of less than 30 weeks of gestational age had a seizure frequency of 3.9%, which was significantly higher than that of older preterm or full-term neonates. The very high incidence (up to 22.7%) reported in premature infants by Bergman et al.[6] is probably due to the frequency of non-epileptic events in this group.[1] Seay and Bray[12] reported seizures in 20% of infants admitted to the intensive care unit, weighing 2,500 g or below. In general, an incidence of neonatal seizures of between 4 and 6 per 1,000 infants seems to be a realistic figure. This figure is much higher among the most immature infants. Neonatal seizures appear to be associated with major morbidities and surgical interventions in very low birth weight infants. Continuous electroencephalographic monitoring could be warranted in infants following surgical treatment.[13]

PATHOPHYSIOLOGY

The site of paroxysmal activity may arise from previously normal neurons. This fire due to a trigger and abnormal conduction occurs through neighboring neurons. Alternatively, the neuronal focus may be inherently abnormal and fires repetitively. Seizures in infants and children may be due to either or both mechanisms. Ten seizures indicate the presence of a central nervous system dysfunction and may contribute to additional brain injury.[14–16]

Brain maturation progresses rapidly during the last weeks of gestation and in the postnatal period. Structural and functional development of the central nervous system is reflected in the rapidly changing bioelectrical activity and behavior of the brain. This has been extensively documented during the past decades in studies of various mammalian species[17,18] and human preterm and newborn infants.[19–21] In the term newborn, the archicortex (i.e. diencephalon and brainstem) is at a relatively more advanced stage of development than is the neocortex. A significant percentage of paroxysmal electrical discharges in the newborn brain, which arise from subcortical gray matter, might not be identified by EEG scalp recordings. Two possible explanations exist for clinical seizures without an electrographic signature:[22]

1. Tonic posturing and motor automatism are epileptic but are generated in the brainstem, and the paroxysmal electrical epileptic activity is not manifested at the scalp and not recorded by surface EEG electrodes.

2. Tonic posturing and motor automatisms are generated and elaborated at a brainstem level by a non-epileptic mechanism.

It has been suggested that the latter explanation is more plausible.[23,24] Although the lack of a close association to EEG seizure activity would only suggest that tonic posturing and motor automatisms are not epileptic in origin, it is these clinical characteristics of the behaviors that provide the evidence for a non-epileptic mechanism. Tonic posturing and motor automatism may be evoked by tactile stimulation; a graded increase occurs in the magnitude of the response proportional to an increase in the intensity of the stimulus at a single site (temporal summation) or an increase in the number of sites of stimulation (spatial summation). The response may spread to muscle groups other than those originally stimulated (irradiation of the response). Both provoked and spontaneous tonic posturing and motor automatism may be suppressed by restraint or repositioning of the body or affected limbs. All of these features are typical of reflex behaviors[25–27] and are not characteristic of epileptic seizures. On this basis, it has been proposed that tonic posturing and motor automatisms result from depression of forebrain function and the consequent disinhibition of the brainstem centers that facilitate primitive reflex behaviors.[23,24] This hypothesis is based not only on clinical observations but also on the correlation of these findings with experimental studies of reflex physiology in animals.[24,28] Primitive reflex behaviors are normally mediated by spinal mechanisms and facilitated by centers within the brainstem. These centers are tonically inhibited by the forebrain and may be stimulated by proprioceptive and entroceptive pathways activated by limb and truncal manipulation. When the forebrain is depressed, brainstem centers are disinhibited, and primitive reflexes may occur spontaneously or be evoked by stimulation. It has been proposed that these behaviors, as a group, be designated "brainstem release phenomena" rather than epileptic seizures.[26,29] Although neurons are in place by the time of birth, their axonal and dentritic ramifications and synaptic connections are still incompletely developed in the neonatal human brain,[30,31] and myelination is limited to a few pathways not including the main hemispheric commissures.[32] The hyperexcitability of the immature cortex is explained by the underdevelopment of the myelinization and the characteristic phenomena;[33–35] the modification of the shapes of spikes depends on the developmental stage of dendrites; the propagation of discharges is determined by the state of maturity of the cortical and subcortical and interhemispherial connections.[36]

Kolmodin and Meyerson[37] found the age-related variations of the potential stable and others observed the role of the enzymatic reactions.[38,39] In addition, synaptic connection and transport across synaptic membranes are much less efficient in the immature brain.[40] Both inhibitory [γ-amino butyric acid (GABA)-ergic] and excitatory receptors are present in the human newborn but are not fully developed or are not completely functional because of the incomplete development of the appropriate circuitry.[41,42] There is evidence that the inhibitory dopamine transmitters have a predominant effect over excitatory transmitters in the developing brain.[43] The neonatal brain appears uniquely susceptible to seizure because neonatal GABA receptors are excitatory, and are functionally more active than N-methyl-D-aspartate (NMDA) receptors at this time of life.[44] The absence of generalized tonic-clonic seizures probably reflects both the lack of a sufficient degree of cortical organization (which is necessary to propagate and sustain the electrical discharge) and the failure of interhemispheric transmission, resulting from commissural immaturity. Experimental data suggest that neonatal seizures may have a deleterious effect on the developing brain, depleting cerebral glucose, which may interfere with DNA synthesis, glial proliferation and differentiation and myelinization.[45–47] Younkin et al.[48] using nuclear resonance spectroscopy, showed a marked depletion of brain phosphocreatine and adenosine triphosphate during a subtle seizure, which was reversed following phenobarbital therapy and seizure cessation. Animal studies have shown that seizures impair neurogenesis and derange neuronal structure, function and connectivity (cells that fire together). The hippocampus has been well studied because it is particularly susceptible to seizure-induced injury. Seizures cause synaptic reorganization with aberrant growth (sprouting) of the dentate granule cell (DGC) axons (i.e. the mossy fibers).[49] There is also apoptosis in the inner granule cell layer of the dentate hilus, and bilateral hippocampal sclerosis has been found at autopsy in human babies who suffered prolonged seizures. Seizures lead to a mismatch between energy supply and demand, and although there is a rise in cerebral flow this may not be sufficient to meet the requirement.[50] Neonates have a low cerebral metabolic rate and a fragmentary neuronal network, making them less vulnerable to neuronal damage and cell loss than adults and more resistant to the toxic effects of glutamate. However, seizures undoubtedly can inhibit brain growth, modify neuronal circuits and increase neuronal

excitability. Recurrent seizures during early development have been shown to result in impairment of visual-spatial learning and memory.[51,52] Status epilepticus and recurrent seizures have also been shown to predispose the brain to seizures in later life.[53] Magnetic resonance spectroscopy studies show areas of cerebral metabolic dysfunction in babies with seizures.[54] Status epilepticus can result in eighty Neonatal seizures Kurjak-09.qxd 11/16/2005 7:22 PM Page 80 necrotic damage to the thalamus in immature rats.[55] The response of the developing brain to epileptic seizures and to status epilepticus is highly age specific. Neonates with their low cerebral metabolic rate and fragmentary neuronal networks can tolerate relatively prolonged seizures without suffering massive cell death, but severe seizures in experimental animals inhibit brain growth, modify neuronal circuits and can lead to behavioral deficits and to increase in neuronal excitability. Past infancy, the developing brain is characterized by a high metabolic rate, exuberant neuronal and synaptic networks and overexpression of receptors and enzymes involved in excitotoxic mechanisms. The outcome of seizures is highly modeled dependent. Status epilepticus may produce massive neuronal death, behavioral deficits, synaptic reorganization or chronic epilepsy in some models, and little damage in others. We now have some models that reliably lead to spontaneous seizures and chronic epilepsy in the vast majority of animals, demonstrating that seizure-induced epileptogenesis can occur in the developing brain. The mode of cell death from status epilepticus is largely (but not exclusively) necrotic in adult, while the incidence of apoptosis increases at younger ages. Seizure-induced necrosis has many of the biochemical features of apoptosis, with early cytochrome release from mitochondria and capsase activation. Wasterlain et al. speculate that this form of necrosis is associated with seizure-induced energy failure.[56] A recent finding is that neonatal seizures can permanently disrupt neuronal development, induce synaptic reorganization, alter plasticity and "prime" the brain to increased damage from seizure later in life. This finding has led to a renewal of interest in the topic of neonatal seizures, particularly regarding treatment.[57]

Edwards et al. found that prenatal stress alters the seizure threshold and the development of kindled seizures in infant and adult rats. Their findings indicate that stress, particularly during the latter half of pregnancy, may play an important role in increasing vulnerability to seizures in the unborn offspring.[58] The idea that stem cells may play a role in the pathophysiology or potential treatment of specific epilepsy syndromes is relatively new.[59] Knowledge of the normal neurogenesis pathways in the mature brain has led to recent studies of neurogenesis in rodent models of acute seizures or epileptogenesis. Current evidence indicates that single brief or prolonged seizures, as well as repeated kindled seizures, increase DGC neurogenesis. Recent work also suggests that pilocarpine-induced status epilepticus increases rostral forebrain subventricular zone (SVZ) neurogenesis and caudal SVZ gliogenesis. These abnormalities include aberrant mossy fiber reorganization, persistence of immature DCG structure (e.g. basal dendrites) and abnormal migration of newborn neurons to ectopic sites in the dentate gyrus. Taken together, these findings suggest a proepileptogenic role of seizure- or injury-induced neurogenesis in the epileptic hippocampal formation. However, the induction of forebrain SVZ neurogenesis and directed migration to injury after seizures and other brain insults underscores the potential therapeutic use of neural stem cells as a source for neuronal replacement after injury.

THE CLASSIFICATION OF NEONATAL SEIZURES

Recently, neonatal seizures have been characterized and classified according to their presumed pathophysiology, with the suggestion that some neonatal seizures are epileptic in origin and others are not (Table 10.1).[2,60,61] Seizure recognition, characterization and classification create the foundation of care of the neonate who may be at risk for central nervous system dysfunction. For classification of neonatal seizures and for making a guide to clinical recognition, a workshop was formed in the USA [participants: Subcommission on Classification and Terminology of Pediatric Epilepsy, Commission on Classification and Terminology, International League against Epilepsy (ILAE) and the Clinical Research Centers for Neonatal Seizures, National Institute of Neurological Disorders and Stroke, National Institute of Health (NIH)]. The report of the newest classification was published by Mizrahi this year.[62] The classification system and the infants presented in the workshop are based on a prospective, clinical study of infants with seizures that have been documented by bedside, video-EEG monitoring. Each seizure was examined by all the investigators together, characterized and then classified by consensus.

Approximately, 65% of neonatal seizures are not clearly associated with apparent cortical electrographic seizure activity on the basis of EEG recordings from surface electrodes.[24,63] Neonatal seizure types differ considerably from seizures observed commonly in older children, principally because the newborn infant is less able to sustain organized, generalized epileptiform discharges. The most widely accepted and most often clinically applied classification scheme is that proposed and recently updated by Mizrahi and Kellaway (Table 10.2). Some clinical seizures are characterized by just one type of movement. However, other seizures are more complex. They may begin with one type of movement, which is then followed by others in a sequence typical for that specific seizure. The most effective application of this classification is to use it as a basis to identify the individual components of a single seizure, rather than to classify an entire complex event.

Several seizure types frequently occur together in the same infant; subtle seizures are frequently associated with other types in the severely ill neonate.[5] In addition, various seizure types may be generated by different mechanisms—either epileptic or non-epileptic. The clinical characteristics of a specific seizure may

Table 10.1: Electroclinical classification of neonatal seizures

Clinical seizures with a consistent electrocortical signature

A. Focal clonic
   Unifocal
   Multifocal
      Alternating
      Migrating
   Hemiconvulsive
   Axial
B. Myoclonic
   Generalized
   Focal
C. Focal tonic
   Asymmetric truncal
   Eye deviation

Clinical seizures with no electrocortical signature

A. Motor automatisms
   Oral-buccal-lingual movements
   Ocular movements
   Progression movements
      Pedaling
      Stepping
      Rotary arm movements
   Complex purposeless movements
B. Generalized tonic
   Extensor
   Flexor
   Mixed extensor/flexor
C. Myoclonic
   Generalized
   Focal

(*Source:* Adapted from Younkin[2] with permission)

Table 10.2: Classification of neonatal seizures

I. Clonic
   A. Unifocal : 1. limb, 2. facial and 3. hemiconvulsive
   B. Multifocal: 1. alternating and 2. bilateral, asynchronous
   C. Axial: 1. abdominal and 2. diaphragm
II. Tonic
   1. Focal: 1. ocular (sustained eye deviation), 2. limb posturing and 3. asymmetric
   2. Generalized: 1. symmetric—a. flexion, b. extension and c. mixed flexion-extension and 2. asymmetric
III. Myoclonic
   1. Generalized
   2. Focal
   3. Multifocal (fragmentary)
IV. Spasm (generalized)
   1. Flexion
   2. Extension
   3. Mixed extension-flexion
V. Motor automatisms
   A. Oral-buccal-lingual movements: 1. chewing and 2. sucking
   B. Ocular signs: 1. random eye movements and 2. blinking, rhythmic eye opening
   C. Limb (movements of progression): 1. pedaling and 2. swimming
   D. Complex purposeless movements
VI. Autonomic nervous system signs
   A. Respiratory: 1. tachypnea and 2. respiratory pause
   B. Cardiac: 1. tachycardia and 2. bradycardia
   C. Cardiovascular: 1. hypertension and 2. hypotension
   D. Vasomotor: 1. flushing and 2. pallor
   E. Pupillary dilatation
   F. Salivation
   G. Other
VII. No clinical signs—electrical seizure only
VIII. Unclassified
ILAE–NIH classification of neonatal seizures

(*Source:* Modified from Mizrahi[62])

designate its pathophysiology. Thus, the classification of a seizure may suggest a specific mechanism of generation, leading eventually to considerations of therapy and long-term prognosis.

Clonic Seizures

Clonic seizures consist of rhythmic muscle jerking that can involve any part of the body and are often associated with simultaneous epileptiform activity on EEG.[64] Two subtypes are recognized, focal and multifocal clonic.

Focal clonic seizures have limited, usually unilateral, involvement of the face, limbs or axial muscles and are often not associated with alterations of the level of consciousness. In many instances, there is an underlying focal lesion, e.g. focal cerebral infarction. However, it is important to realize that metabolic derangements, e.g. hypoglycemia, may present as focal seizures in the newborn.[16] Cockburn et al.[65] reported clonic seizures with late hypocalcemia.

Multifocal clonic seizures are observed more frequently in the term newborn, and are a relatively benign form. They involve non-synchronized clonic movements of the extremities, which differ from multifocal clonic seizures in older infants in that abnormal movements in newborns usually migrate in an unordered, non-Jacksonian fashion. For example, clonic movements of one hand may be followed by jerking of the opposite leg.[66] This particular seizure type may be explained by the immature stage of development of the cerebral cortex of the term infant. Thus, although there is sufficient interneuronal communication to permit sustained seizure activity, the immaturity of synaptic development and axonal myelination may prevent the organized spread of electrical impulses. Because of this, generalized tonic-clonic seizures, which are symmetric and synchronous, occur infrequently in the term newborn.[30]

Tonic Seizures

Tonic seizures are most often generalized, featuring tonic extension of all limbs (which resembles "decerebrate" posturing), or, occasionally, flexion of the upper limb with the extension of the legs (which resembles "decorticate" posturing). Eye signs such as opening or closing movements of eyelids, staring, gaze deviation or the occurrence of a few clonic jerks may be a clue to their epileptic mechanism. Volpe[30] found tonic seizures to be particularly common among premature infants, and they accounted for 70% of fits seen in infants weighing 2,500 g or less. This form of seizure occurs in infants with significant cerebral injury [e.g. massive intraventricular hemorrhage (IVH)] and is associated with a bad prognosis. In approximately 85% of cases, the abnormal posturing is accompanied by electrical seizure activity or autonomic phenomena and the response to anticonvulsant therapy is poor.[12,30] This observation gives rise to the possibility that such posturing represents abnormal brainstem release phenomena as opposed to true epileptic seizures.[23,30,67] In these instances, although there is no corresponding electrical seizure activity, the interictal EEG is usually severely abnormal with marked voltage suppression.[29]

Myoclonic Seizures

Myoclonic seizures, which may be focal, multifocal or generalized, are rare in the neonatal period. They may occur in infants of any gestational age and are associated with time-synchronized EEG discharges only in a minority of cases.[24] They are characterized by rapid, unilateral or bilateral, single or multiple flexion jerks of the upper extremities, but to a lesser extent. Myoclonic seizures often signify severe structural or metabolic cerebral disturbance. They often persist into infancy as more or less atypical infantile spasms.[68,69] A benign variety of neonatal myoclonus has been described, which occurs characteristically only during sleep. Focal and multifocal myoclonic activity may be observed, which is difficult to distinguish clinically from epileptic seizures. However, the correlation with the sleep state and the absence of associated EEG abnormalities may be helpful in this. It typically resolves spontaneously before 6 months of age.[70–72]

Spasms

Spasms may be flexor, extensor or mixed extensor and flexor, and may occur in clusters. Spasms cannot be provoked by stimulation or suppressed by restraint. Pathophysiology is epileptic.

Motor Automatisms (Subtle Seizures)

Subtle seizures may be the most common type and are present to some degree in most term newborns with seizures. This category includes all paroxysmal steps of behavior in newborns that may be sustained, and that cannot be readily classified as myoclonic seizures. Subtle or minimal seizures are also termed "motor automatisms" by some investigators.[73] The most common clinical manifestation is a variety of ocular movements, e.g. eye opening, tonic horizontal deviation of the eyes; orofacial movements, such as repetitive chewing, swallowing, drooling; rotatory limb movements or complex patterns, like pedaling, boxing, swimming or stepping, and autonomic disturbances, such as hyperpnea, vasomotor abnormalities, salivation or modification of the heart rate. Abnormal eye movements, especially in the horizontal plane are of special diagnostic value.[74,75] Unlike sustained eye deviation is typical of focal tonic seizure of epileptic origin; the ocular signs of motor automatisms are less well defined. They include random eye movements, eye opening and blinking.[62] Motor automatisms and generalized tonic posturing may coexist, since their pathophysiologic mechanisms are the same.

Autonomic nervous system signs are often combined with motor automatisms apneic seizures are common, sometimes in isolation,[76,77] but more often in association with ocular or other autonomic signs. Fenichel et al.[78] found that apneic seizures were not[3] accompanied by bradycardia, as opposed to the much more frequent non-epileptic apneas of the premature infant, which last 20s or more. Other studies involving simultaneous video-EEG investigations demonstrated that subtle clinical phenomena are frequently accompanied by simultaneous electrical discharges in premature infants.[79] The EEG signs that are associated with subtle seizures occur commonly in the temporal leads,[64] which is not surprising as similar clinical features are frequently observed in older children in complex partial seizures, which originate in the temporal lobes. Alterations in the autonomic function as a seizure manifestation raise particular diagnostic problems. Thus, although apneic episodes in the premature infant may rarely be a manifestation of seizure activity,[79] they are much more likely to be related to other mechanisms. In contrast, apnea in the term newborn appears to be associated more commonly with electrical seizure activity. Recently, the apneic episodes have been observed and differentiated in newborns and especially in prematures with a new polygraphic computerized method (SLEEP Labor). We can also determine the type of apnea exactly: central, obstructive or mixed. Figure 10.1 shows a polygraphic investigation demonstrating a central apnea (cenA-) following the electrical activity change on the FP1 channel. There is no significant change in ECG (examination of the author). Infantile spasms and episodic apnea (associated with electroencephalographic seizure activity) may also occur as neonatal seizures, but they are rare and currently do not warrant major classifications.[3]

Isolated seizures are relatively uncommon in the neonatal period. The occurrence of at least a few attacks is the rule. However, neonatal seizures tend to be self-limited and to last 24–96 hour,[80–82] which complicates the assessment of therapy further.

Neonatal status epilepticus has been defined by Dreyfus-Brisac and Monod[83,84] as the repetition of clinical and/or purely electrical seizures with the interictal persistence of an abnormal neurological status. Cukier et al.[82] redefined the term with greater precision as the occurrence of electrical seizure discharges, each lasting at least 10s and repeated for several hours, in association with an abnormal neurological state and unconsciousness. Clinical seizures may or may not be present. The latter definition does not include repeated clinical seizures without ictal EEG concomitants such as those that may occur in neonates who have been convulsing for many hours.[85] The term serial seizures is perhaps preferable to that of status epilepticus in the neonatal period because it does not refer to an abnormal interictal neurological state, which may be impossible to assess reliably on account of the interference of drug treatment.[3] With prolonged convulsive episodes, there is a tendency for individual seizures to change from well-marked to poorly organized attacks, clinically as well as electrically.

ETIOLOGY

Although the etiology of neonatal seizures is extremely diverse, most of them can be attributed to hypoxic-ischemic encephalopathy (about 65% of neonatal seizures), intracranial hemorrhage (about 15%), metabolic disturbances (hypoglycemia, hypocalcemia), intracranial infection and cerebral cortical dysgenesis. (Table 10.3).

Hypoxic-ischemic encephalopathy is the most important cause of neonatal seizures in infants and in all gestational ages.[30] It has been estimated to account for approximately two-thirds of all cases. Seizures area major manifestation of moderate or severe intrapartum hypoxic-ischemia encephalopathy in approximately 50% of affected term newborns and are associated with long-term neurological sequelae in at least 20–40% of cases.[30,86]

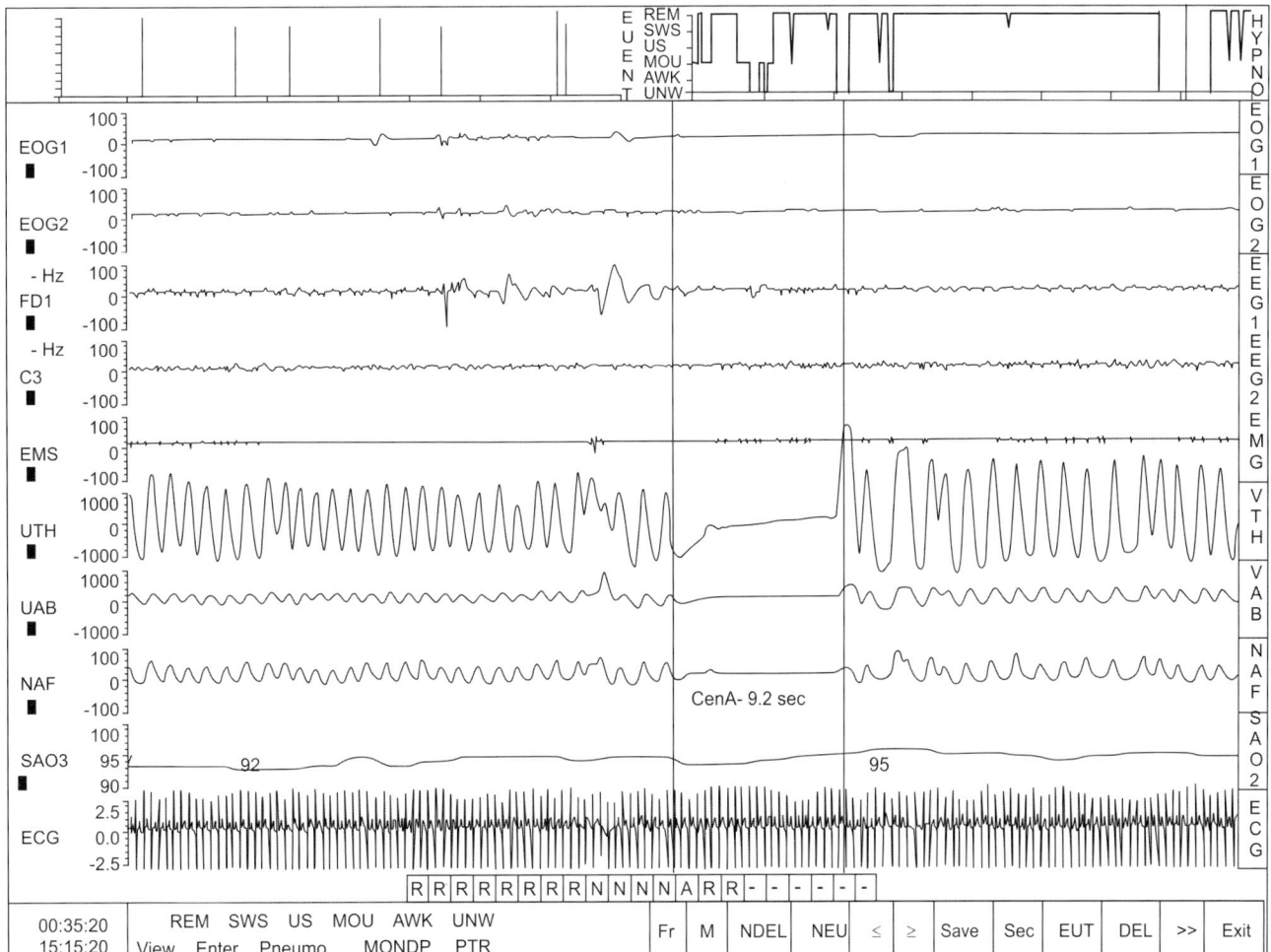

Fig. 10.1: Central apnea demonstrated by polygraph

Table 10.3: Correlation of time of onset of seizures and etiology

Most frequent time of onset	Etiology of seizures
<48 hours	Hypoxic-ischemic encephalopathy
	Intracranial hemorrhage
	Hypoglycemia
	Sepsis-meningitis
	Congenital viral infection
	Drug withdrawal
	Local anesthetic intoxication
	Pyridoxine dependency
	Nonketotic hyperglycinemia
	Urea cycle disorders
48–72 Hours	Cerebral dysgenesis
	Cerebral infarction
	Ketotic hyperglycinemia
	Urea cycle disorders
>7 Days	cerebral dysgenesis
	Organic acidopathies
	Amino acidopathies
	Urea cycle disorders
	Bacterial meningitis

(*Source:* Adapted from Hill and Volpe[73] with permission)

Many cases are probably of prenatal origin, so a low weight for date and other signs of dysmaturity are common findings.[66] Postnatal respiratory insufficiency causes less than 10% of cases of hypoxic encephalopathy.[30] Ischemia is secondary to intrauterine asphyxia with cardiac insufficiency. Seizures begin most frequently during the first day of life,[87–89] and 60% of the patients with this condition have already had fits by 12 hour.[30] The seizures are often isolated at the start. Of the cases of neonatal status epilepticus 75–85% have been attributed to hypoxic insult.[30] Seizures may be of any type and are often prolonged and refractory to anticonvulsant therapy. Brown[90] has pointed out that the seizures usually occur when infants show a transition in muscle tone. The interictal EEG is of the "tracé paroxystique" or inactive tracing type in severe cases.[91] The convulsions may be extremely difficult to control by drugs. Levene et al.[92] have reported neonatal convulsions due to asphyxia to occur in 2 per 1,000 full-term infants. Delivoria-Papadopoulos and Mishra studied the mechanism of cerebral hypoxia in the fetus and newborn that results in neonatal morbidity and mortality as well a long-term sequelae such as mental retardation, seizure disorders and cerebral palsy. Using electron spin resonance (ESR) spectroscopy they demonstrated that tissue hypoxia results in increased free-radical generation in the cortex of fetal guinea pigs and newborn piglets.[93] Normally, more than 80% of the oxygen consumed by the cell is completely reduced by cytochrome oxidase to reactions with the cytoplasm and mitochondria that produce a superoxide anion radical. To protect cells from the deleterious effects of free radicals, a number of enzymatic and non-enzymatic defenses such as catalase, superoxide dismutase, glutathione peroxidase, ascorbic acid and vitamin E are present in cells.

The hypoxia-induced increase in lipid peroxidation products was shown to be also associated with a decrease in cell membrane Na^+, K^+-ATPase activity. The direct demonstration of production of free radicals during hypoxia was documented by measuring the signal of spin adducts using ESR, which allows direct identification and characterization of free radicals.[94] The brain tissue hypoxia modified the NMDA receptor ion channel recognition and modulation sites. A higher increase in NMDA receptor agonist-dependent Ca^{2+} in synaptosomes was demonstrated. The increase in intracellular Ca^{2+} may activate several enzymatic pathways such as phospholipase A and metabolism of arachidonic acid by cyclooxygenase and lipoxygenase, conversion of xanthine dehydrogenase to xanthine oxidase by proteases and activation of nitric oxide synthase. In summary, studies demonstrated that cerebral tissue hypoxia results in increased free-radical generation that may lead to the oxidation of brain cell membrane lipids, membrane enzymes, receptor proteins as well as the nuclear DNA precipitating the hypoxic neuronal injury in the fetus and newborn.

Intracranial Hemorrhage

This condition is often difficult to establish conclusively as a primary cause of seizure distinct from hypoxic-ischemic encephalopathy or traumatic injury, because of the frequent association of these conditions. There are three important types of hemorrhage according to localization.

Intraventricular hemorrhage is a very common lesion in extremely premature infants, but germinal matrix/IVH is associated relatively rarely with seizures. However, large IVHs, especially if there is associated intraparenchymal hemorrhagic infarction (which accounts for approximately 15% of all examples of IVH), may occur together with generalized tonic seizures, most often as part of a catastrophic deterioration evolving to coma and respiratory arrest. This clinical setting and type of seizure signify an ominous prognosis.[30]

Subdural hemorrhage is most commonly associated with traumatic delivery or non-accidental shaking injury. The associated cerebral contusion frequently results in focal clonic and subtle seizures. Such seizures most commonly begin during the first 48 hour of life.[95] Subdural hemorrhage occurring as a result of tentorial tears is not necessarily fatal and may have a relatively good prognosis. Primary subarachnoid hemorrhage, especially of a minor degree, is a very common occurrence in newborns and is usually not of major clinical significance. When seizures occur secondary to the subarachnoid hemorrhage in the full-term infant, they occur most commonly on the second day of life.[96] During the interictal period, affected infants often appear remarkably healthy, leading to the descriptive term "well baby with seizures". Spanish authors have reported neonatal convulsions and subarachnoid hemorrhage after paroxetine treatment in the third trimester of pregnancy.[97]

Neonatal Stroke

Billard et al.[98] reported eight infants presenting focal seizures between the age of 8 hours and 72 hours and all had evidence of cerebral infarction on the computed tomography (CT) scan. Only three of these infants showed evidences of subsequent handicap. Venkataraman et al. studied 11 full-term babies with neonatal troke. Seizure was the most common presenting sign, with paucity of other focal neurological deficits.[99]

The few days before and after birth are a time of special risk for stroke in both mother and infant, probably related to activation of coagulation mechanisms in this critical period. Arterial ischemic stroke around the time of birth is recognized in about 1 in 4,000 full-term infants, and may present with neurological and systemic signs in the newborn.[100] Neonatal seizures are most commonly the clinical finding that triggers assessment. In other children, prenatal stroke is recognized only retrospectively, with emerging hemiparesis or seizure after the early month of life. Risk factors for perinatal stroke include hereditary or acquired thrombophilias and environmental factors. Perinatal stroke underlies an important share of congenital hemiplegic cerebral palsy, and probably some spastic quadriplegic cerebral palsy and seizure disorders. There is much to be learned about the natural history of perinatal stroke, and there are as yet no evidence-based strategies for prevention or treatment.

Intracranial Infection

Both the bacterial and the non-bacterial types of intracranial infection are common causes of neonatal seizures. Seizures secondary to bacterial meningitis are most likely to occur after the first week of life. Like the common metabolic disturbances, they are of particular concern because definitive therapy is of primary importance. Of the bacterial infections, meningitides secondary to group B streptococci, *Listeria monocytogenes* and *Escherichia coli* are the most common. In addition to bacterial meningitis, meningo-encephalitis may occur due to herpes simplex, Coxsackie and toxoplasmosis. In the latter case, toxoplasmosis may be acquired in early pregnancy and extensive brain damage may have occurred by the time of delivery. Cytomegalovirus and rubella infections acquired in early pregnancy may also present with neonatal fits, without any signs of other infections. Septicemic infants, without meningitis, may also develop seizures. The cause of this can be the complication associated with infection and hypoglycemia or hypotension. Diarrhea due to infection may cause disturbances in the sodium balance, which may also cause seizures. Herpes simplex virus type 1 (HSV-1) encephalitis is the most common cause of acquired epilepsy in human. Chen et al. studied in vitro HSV-1-infected organotypic hippocampal slice culture to elucidate the underlying mechanisms of HSV-1-associated acute seizure activity. The results suggest that a direct change in excitability of the hippocampal CA3 neuronal network and HSV-1-induced neuron loss resulting in subsequent mossy fiber reorganization may play an important role in the generation of epileptiform activity.[101]

Metabolic Disturbances

Although different kinds of metabolic derangement and certain intoxications are associated with convulsive phenomena in newborn infants, abnormalities of glucose and divalent cation homeostasis are the most frequent.

Hypoglycemia is most common in infants who are small for their gestational age and in infants of mothers with diabetes or gestational diabetes.[102] The brain can use few sources of energy, glucose being the most important. Hypoglycemia may cause devastating neurological damage when the brain's energy reserves are exhausted. The most important determinant of the occurrence of neurological signs in neonatal hypoglycemia appears to be the duration of this. Monod et al.[103] observed that among the prematures, hypoglycemia may be very low, without any seizures. Neurological symptoms consist most commonly of jitteriness, stupor, hypotonia and apnea, as well as seizures. The onset of the seizures is usually early, often on the second postnatal day. In many instances hypoglycemia occurs in the context of hypoxic-ischemic encephalopathy, IVH or infection. Secondary transient hypoglycemia may occur in association with meningitis or following exchange transfusion. Persistent hypoglycemia may be observed in certain inborn errors of metabolism, e.g. galactosemia, fructosemia, leucin sensitivity, glucos-6-phosphatase deficiency, etc. Other rare disorders that must be considered include the Beckwith–Wiedemann syndrome, pancreatic islet cell tumors and anterior pituitary hypoplasia. The importance of early diagnosis and treatment of hypoglycemia has become more critical. Recent data suggest that even moderate hypoglycemia in the premature newborn may be associated with poor outcome.[104]

Electrolyte Disturbances

Divalent cations are regulators of the ion fluxes associated with membrane depolarization. Because of this, abnormalities in their homeostasis are more likely to result in electrical seizures than in the homeostasis in monovalent cations. However, both hyponatremia and hypernatremia have been associated with seizures because of derangements in cell volume. The most common cause of these disturbances is inappropriate fluid therapy. In infants with serious neurological or pulmonary disease, the syndrome of inappropriate secretion of antidiuretic hormone may result in severe hyponatremia and seizures.[30]

Hypocalcemia/Hypomagnesemia

Infants with seizures due to hypocalcemia are usually alert between seizures and the seizures are often multifocal and migratory. Hypocalcemia occurs at two peak times in the newborn period. Early hypocalcemia, which occurs in the first 2–3 days of life, seems to be in association with other potential etiologic factors that appear to play a major role in the origin of the convulsions. The definition of hypocalcemia is taken to be serum calcium below 1.75 mmol/L (7 mg/dL). The ionized calcium is a more important predictor; unfortunately, this is a difficult measurement in clinical practice. Ionized calcium is responsible in part for axonal conduction as well as neuromuscular function. In addition, magnesium is an important comineral for the function of the neuromuscular junction.[10] Functional hypocalcemia can be diagnosed by assessing cardiac neuromuscular conduction on the electrocardiograph. Early-onset-hypocalcemia is often observed in the context of hypoxic-ischemic encephalopathy, in newborns with low birthweight, in prematures with hyaline membrane disease and in infants of diabetic mothers. In rare cases, early severe hypocalcemia is due to parathyroid hypoplasia or aplasia. The commonest condition associated with absent parathyroid is Di George syndrome. An infusion of intravenous calcium may be useful for determining whether seizures are caused directly by the low calcium level. Late-onset hypocalcemia is relatively uncommon and presents as an isolated condition without other associated or underlying diseases. Classically, such hypocalcemic infants are large, term infants who have avidly consumed a milk preparation with a suboptimal ratio of phosphorus to calcium and phosphorus to magnesium, e.g. cow's milk. The neurological syndrome is consistent and distinctive, and it consists primarily of hyperactive tendon reflexes. Hypocalcemia fits are treated with intravenous 10% calcium gluconate and the seizures should stop soon after administration. Hypomagnesemia often coexists with hypocalcemia and convulsions are likely to occur at serum levels below 0.3 mmol/L. Giving magnesium alone to hypocalcemic infants caused both serum magnesium and calcium to rise.[65] Manzar mentioned a case of a newborn with late-onset seizure with hypocalcemia, hyperphosphatemia and raised parathyroid hormone. The infant did not have any stigmata of pseudohypoparathyroidism. The hypocalcemia was initially resistant to calcium therapy but responded to vitamin D analog therapy. Transient pseudohypoparathyroidism was entertained.[105]

Congenital Abnormalities

Tables 10.4 and 10.5 list inborn errors of metabolism and neuronal storage diseases that may cause neonatal fits.[10]

Pyridoxine dependency is a rare, autosomal recessive disorder of the pyridoxine metabolism. Pyridoxine is a cofactor necessary for the synthesis of the inhibitory neurotransmitter GABA, a deficiency that may presumably produce severe neonatal seizures recalcitrant to all treatment except the administration of large doses of pyridoxine.[106] Fewer than 100 patients have been reported, and only four reports have included examples of brain imaging findings.

Gospe et al. found in their patient progressive magnetic resonance changes—dilatation of the ventricular system, cortical and white matter atrophy. The abnormalities may be due to chronic excitotoxicity caused by an imbalance of cerebral levels of GABA and glutamic acid.[107]

Kernicterus

Bilirubin is a neurotoxic substance that may cause a clinical syndrome in severely jaundiced infants, referred to as kernicterus. The most severe form of this condition includes opisthotonus, sunsetting and neonatal tonic seizures.

Any abnormality in the cerebral development may cause neonatal seizures but disorders of neuronal migration are particularly likely to be associated with abnormal neurological behavior and fits. Seizures in these infants are usually very difficult to control. Genetically determined disorders such as Sturge–Weber syndrome, tuberose sclerosis and incontinentia pigmenti may also rarely cause neonatal convulsion.[10] Hennel et al. found in their

Table 10.4: Inborn errors of metabolism which may cause neonatal seizures

- Maple syrup urine disease
- Urea cycle defects
- Tyrosinemia
- Nonketotic hyperglycinemia
- Proprionic acidemia
- Methyl malonic acidemia
- Other organic acidemias

(*Source:* Adapted from Levene[10] with permission).

Table 10.5: Neonatal storage diseases which may cause neonatal fits

- Adrenoleukodystrophy
- Alexander's disease
- Alper's disease
- Gaucher's disease
- Krabbe's leukodystrophy
- Niemann Pick disease
- Tay Sachs disease
- Zellweger's syndrome

(*Source:* Adapted from Levene[10] with permission.)

case with incontinentia pigmenti evolution of acute microvascular hemorrhagic infarcts in the periventricular white matter in the first week of life. The associated magnetic resonance angiogram findings consisted of decreased branching and poor filling of intracerebral vessels.[108] Table 10.6 lists some congenital cerebral abnormalities that may be associated with neonatal convulsion.[10] Wada et al. show a female patient who has enlargement of lateral ventricles and atrophy of the brain associated with infantile spasms. The ventriculomegaly was documented in utero at as early as the 28th week of gestation with lactic acidosis due to deficiency of the pyruvate dehydrogenase E1 (alpha) subunit, demonstrating that the changes characteristic of this disease can occur antenatally. The mechanism of infantile spasms in this disease may be linked to mosaicism of the brain cells involving the normal enzyme and the mutant enzyme.[109]

Intoxications

Local Anesthetics

Seizure may occur when local anesthetics are administered to the mother for episiotomy, or for other types of maternal analgesia. The major clinical features of toxicity include a very low Apgar score, apnea or severe hypoventilation, severe bradycardia and hypotonia and severe bradycardia. Seizures occur early and are commonly tonic in nature. These features are also seen in hypoxic-ischemic encephalopathy. There are two distinguishing features that aid in its differentiation from perinatal hypoxia: the absence of the pupillary response to light and the absence of eye movement with the oculocephalic (doll's eye) maneuver. The absence of these signs is unusual in hypoxic encephalopathy during the first 12 hours of life. Management depends on prompt recognition. The half-life of the drug in the blood is approximately 8–10 hours.

Methylxanthine

Both theophyllin and caffeine overdosage have resulted in seizures in the neonatal period.[8]

Drug Withdrawal

Passive addiction of the newborn and drug withdrawal may be related to maternal ingestion of cocaine, narcotic-analgesics and sedative hypnotics. Many findings demonstrate that exposure to alcohol during brain development can permanently alter the physiology of the hippocampal formation, thus promoting epileptic activity, enhancing kindling and facilitating spreading depression.

Table 10.6: Congenital cerebral abnormalities which may be associated with neonatal convulsions

- Neurofibromatosis
- Pachygyria
- Sturge–Weber syndrome
- Micropolygyria
- Incontinentia pigmenti
- Congenital porencephaly
- Tuberose sclerosis
- Hydrocephalus
- Hydranencephaly
- Holoprosencephaly

(*Source:* Adapted from Levene[10] with permission.)

Epileptic Syndromes in the Neonatal Period

Subgroups can be recognized among the neonatal convulsions on the basis of the age at onset and/or characteristics of fits and associated neurological manifestations. Although there is some relationship between the age at the onset of seizures and the associated clinical manifestations on the one hand, and etiology and prognosis on the other, it is difficult to isolate well-defined "epileptic syndromes" during the neonatal period. Most groupings are rather loose, and only familial seizures and a few rare syndromes such as neonatal myoclonic encephalopathy[110,111] stand out clearly.

Neonatal myoclonic encephalopathy[30] is a syndrome characterized clinically by the occurrence of erratic, fragmentary myoclonus of early onset, usually in association with other types of seizures and, from the EEG viewpoint, by a stable suppression–burst pattern persisting after 2 weeks of age.[110,112,113] Seizures associated with the myoclonus include partial motor seizures, massive myoclonias and tonic spasms that are not usually observed before 4–5 months of age. The onset is in the neonatal period and all affected infants have severe neurological impairment; half of them die before the age of 6 months.[112] Familial cases are frequent; a recessive inheritance is probable in some of the cases. The syndrome may result from undetermined metabolic defects or from brain malformations.[114] The relationship of neonatal myoclonic encephalopathy with early infantile epileptic encephalopathy (Ohtahara disease) is not entirely clear. The two conditions have several clinical and EEG characteristics in common, including the occurrence of tonic spasms and a suppression-burst pattern. Lombroso[115] accepts that early myoclonic encephalopathy is distinct from the Ohtahara syndrome but considers the latter only as a variant of infantile spasms.

Benign Familial Epilepsy

An autosomal dominant syndrome of neonatal seizures unrelated to recognized etiologies has been described.[116] The gene for this transient, primary epilepsy of infancy has been recently assigned to chromosome 20q.[117] The onset of the seizures is usually on the second or third postnatal day, and in the interictal period, the infants appear remarkably well. Seizures may occur at a frequency of 10–20 per day or even more. The disorder is usually self-limiting. Neurological development is normal. Because of the benign course yet striking clinical presentation, the history of affected family members might easily be missed unless specifically sought.[118]

The '*fifth-day fits*' syndrome is characterized by repeated seizures that occur between the third and the seventh days of life in full-term neonates without any abnormal gestational and obstetric antecedent and without any neurological abnormality during the first day of life. According to Dehan et al.,[119] the attacks are of two main types: (1) clonic focal or multifocal convulsions and (2) apneic spells. They last on an average 20 hours. The interictal EEG shows preserved rhythms and a normal organization of sleep. Bursts of alternating delta-rhythms or "theta pointu alternant" are observed in three-quarters of the patients. Dehan et al. and other authors have underlined the benignity of fifth day fits when all the criteria of the syndrome were present.[119–121]

Intrauterine seizures have been suspected in several reports.[122,123] Movements identified by mothers as probably convulsive in nature occur mainly in the last days or weeks of gestation. Pyridoxine dependency is a possible cause of intrauterine convulsions,[122,124] but other causes, especially brain dysplasia, can be suspected.

Mulley et al. in their review, describe the significant number of new gene associations with epilepsy syndromes that have emerged during the past year, together with additional mutations and new electrophysiological data relating to previously known gene associations. Idiopathic epilepsies are predominantly a family of channelopathies. The corresponding ion channel mutations show measurable in vitro abnormalities that are likely to affect transmission between neurons. In their paper autosomal dominant juvenile myoclonic epilepsy was demonstrated to be a channelopathy associated with a GABAa receptor, (alpha) 1 subunit mutation. Benign familial neonatal infantile seizures were delineated as another channelopathy of infancy, by molecular characterization of sodium channel, (alpha) 2 subunit defects. A sodium channel, (alpha) 2 subunit defect was previously found to be associated with generalized epilepsy with febrile seizure plus (GEFS+). Similarly, the clinical spectrum associated with potassium channel, KQT-like mutations was extended to include the channelopathy, myokymia and neonatal epilepsy. Mutations in the non-ion channel genes, leucin-rich, glioma inactivated 1 gene and Aristaless related homebox gene (causative gene in X-linked infantile spasms) have emerged as important causes of their specific syndromes, with mutations in the last gene frequently underlying X-linked mental retardation with epilepsy.

There are now nine ion channel subunit genes implicated in ten syndromes of idiopathic epilepsy.

The boundaries between clinically defined "idiopathic" and "cryptogenic" epilepsies are being blurred by the demonstration of sodium channel mutation in the infantile syndrome of severe myoclonic epilepsy in infancy. Genetic heterogeneity has been so far proven for three of the syndromes: autosomal dominant frontal lobe epilepsy, benign familial neonatal seizure and GEFS+. Considerable phenotypic heterogeneity occurs in association with mutations in four of the genes described in GEFS+: sodium channel, (beta) 1 subunit (SCN1B); sodium channel, (alpha) 1 subunit (SCN1A); sodium channel, (alpha) 2 subunit (SCN2A) and GABAa receptor, (gamma) 2 subunit (GABRG2).

Whether progress toward understanding the genetic basis for the rare epilepsies will relate to the development of therapies for the common epilepsies remains to be established, but progress to date has provided remarkable insights into the neurobiology of the epilepsies.[125]

DIAGNOSIS

First- and second-line investigations in infants with seizures are listed in Table 10.7.[10]

Diagnostic evaluation must begin with a careful history and physical examination. From the maternal history, it is important to determine the possibility of drug abuse, intrauterine infection and genetic or metabolic disorders. Laboratory investigations should focus initially on treatable causes, such as metabolic disorders and infection. Lumbar puncture or treatment with meningitic doses of antibiotics and acyclovir may be indicated. Rapid diagnosis of the underlying etiology is of major importance to enable the institution of specific and definitive therapy as well as for accurate prediction of the outcome. However, in such instances the diagnosis of a specific underlying disease may have important genetic implications for the family. The time of the onset of seizures may assist in determining an underlying etiology. If the initial screening investigations fail to confirm the etiology, additional studies may be obtained, e.g. CT,

Table 10.7: First- and second-line investigations in infants with seizures

In all infants immediately:
- Clinical history
- Blood sugar
- Sodium
- Calcium
- Magnesium
- Ultrasound brain scan
- Lumbar puncture
- Blood culture

If the above are negative and the infant is still fitting:
- Prenatal viral screen
- Urine for amino acid chromatogram
- Urine for organic acid profile
- Sugar chromatography for galactose
- Pyridoxine infusion
- Computer tomography or magnetic resonance scan

(*Source:* Adapted from Levene[10] with permission.)

Table 10.8: Clinical characteristics which distinguish jitteriness from seizures

Clinical features	Jitteriness	Seizures
Stimulus-sensitive movements	+	–
Movements cease with restraint	+	–
Associated abnormal eye movements	–	+
Quality of movement	Tremor	Clonic jerking

–, absent; +, present.
(*Source:* Adapted from Hill and Volpe[73] with permission.)

cranial ultrasonography, magnetic resonance imaging, serum amino acids, blood pyruvate and lactate, urine amino acids and organic acids, maternal and fetal titer of TORCH [toxoplasma, others, rubella, cytomegalovirus, herpes (hepatitis)] group and syphilis, and urinary drug screen.[30,126]

Differential Diagnosis

Jitteriness is a common movement disorder of the newborn, which may be misinterpreted as epileptic seizures. The major features that distinguish jitteriness from seizures are summarized in Table 10.8.[118] The distinction between jitteriness and seizures may be difficult at times because both may occur in a similar context, e.g. hypoxic-ischemic encephalopathy, hypoglycemia, hypocalcemia. Drug withdrawal is another common cause of jitteriness.[127]

EEG in Diagnosis

Despite advances in neuroimaging techniques over the past decades that have helped identifying structural lesions of the central nervous system, EEG continues to provide valuable insight into brain function by demonstrating focal or diffuse background abnormalities and epileptiform abnormalities. It is an extremely valuable test in patients suspected of epilepsy and in patients with altered mental status and coma. Patterns in the EEG make it possible to clarify the seizure type; it is indispensable for the diagnosis of non-convulsive status epilepticus and for separating epileptic from other paroxysmal (nonepileptic) episodes. There are EEG patterns predictive of the cause of the encephalopathy (i.e. triphasic waves in metabolic encephalopathy) or the location of the lesion (i.e. focal polymorphic delta activity in lesions of the subcortical white matter). An EEG is most helpful in assessing normal or abnormal brain functioning in a newborn because of the serious limitation in performing an adequate neurological examination on the neonate who is intubated or paralyzed for ventilatory control. Under such circumstances, the EEG may be the only tool available to detect an encephalopathic process or the occurrence of epileptic seizures.[128] Neonatal EEG abnormalities may be transient and of benign significance, or may be persistent and severe, indicating neurological morbidity. The clinical usefulness of the EEG is enhanced by recording as soon as possible after the onset of symptoms of the suspected insult, although during the first day of life the stress of birth and the effect of anesthesia may complicate the interpretation of the tracing. If an EEG appears abnormal, recordings may be repeated in 48–72 hours, and at weekly or biweekly intervals until discharge or normal patterns appear. Continuous EEG monitoring may be of value for the diagnosis of seizures in newborns that are treated with muscular paralysis to improve assisted ventilation.[129]

The major EEG correlates of neonatal seizures include focal or multifocal spikes or sharp waves and focal monorhythmic discharges. Care must be taken not to confuse epileptiform activity and normal sharp transients in recordings of premature newborns or "tracé alternant" patterns of quiet sleep in term newborns with seizures. Abnormal motor activity is associated with EEG abnormalities on routine surface recordings in only approximately one-third of the recordings.[126] Several modifications of electroencephalographic techniques have been developed recently to improve the quantification of the frequency and the duration of the seizure activity. These include serial or continuous EEG recordings, and simultaneous video-EEG recordings. Cerebral function monitoring (CFM) is widely used to detect neonatal seizure but comparing with video recording, the observer usually detects generalized seizures but approximately half of all focal neonatal seizures may be missed using CFM only. The CFM may thus be useful for long-term monitoring alone. The digital EEG technology can improve the accuracy of EEG interpretation and lead to more accurate recognition of electroencephalographic features and thereby improve the diagnostic utility of EEG.[130] Clinical interpretation of the EEG during this age-period is difficult because of its rapidly changing morphology. The main characteristics of EEG maturation in preterm infants were a progressive spatiotemporal differentiation, with an increase of rhythmic activities and a decrease of discontinuity. A strong relationship was found between the postmenstrual age of the infants and EEG maturity, but there were exceptions to this rule. A longer duration of extrauterine life had a small accelerating influence on EEG maturation. The relationship between EEG pattern types and behavioral states becomes more stable with increasing age.[131]

Clinically significant and common EEG abnormalities noted in the neonatal period are the next:[132]

Isoelectric pattern in the absence of hypothermia or acute systemic disorders indicates severe and diffuse cerebral dysfunction and is associated with a high incidence of neurological sequelae in survivors.

The paroxysmal pattern, which is characterized by suppression-burst activity, must be distinguished from the discontinuous pattern of the normal preterm, and consists of irregular bursts of abnormal activity on an isoelectric or markedly attenuated ground. The paroxysmal pattern is usually associated with neurological sequelae.

Excessively slow background pattern occurs most commonly in abnormal term newborns, who lack the usual spectrum of beta, delta and transients, are poorly reactive and are not associated with normal wake-sleep cycles; the incidence of neurological sequelae is high.

Persistent asymmetry of the background (reduced by 50%) is sometimes associated with underlying structural lesions, including intracranial hemorrhage.

Excessive interhemispheric asynchrony is commonly noted in association with other EEG abnormalities.

Positive rolandic sharp waves may occur in association with IVH in the newborn, and the positive component is of high amplitude, may be broad in configuration and may be followed by a lower-amplitude negative wave, as well as with other separate focal abnormalities. Positive rolandic sharp waves have also been recorded in neonatal infants with nonhemorrhagic disorders and in apparently normal preterm infants.

Electroencephalographic seizures in preterm and term newborns are associated with a combined mortality and neurological morbidity of approximately 30%; they appear as ictal, repetitive focal or generalized spiking, rhythmic focal or generalized delta and occasionally rhythmic alpha or theta-like activities. There are few specific pathologic EEG patterns associated with specific illnesses (neonatal herpes encephalitis, congenital malformations or Aicardi syndrome).

Patrizi et al. observed the characteristics of EEG ictal activity in preterm and full-term infants.[133] They investigated the trend for a closer relationship between behavioral changes during the electroencephalographic seizure when the background activity was normal or moderately abnormal than when background activity was severely abnormal. In both, preterm and full-term infants, the most common site of seizure origin was the temporal lobe. Full-term infants commonly had sharp waves, spikes, sharp and slow waves and spike and slow waves at the onset of the ictus while rhythmic delta activity was most common in the preterm infants. Preterm infants typically had a regional onset to the ictus whereas full-term infants most frequently had a focal onset. There was no clear relationship between onset, morphology, frequency or propagation of the ictal discharge in both age groups. The results demonstrate that while the type of ictal discharge is related to gestational age, there is a rich variety in the onset, morphology and frequency of the ictal discharges in both groups. Generally, neonatal ictal patterns lack a close correlation with the underlying pathology.

Therapy

The newborn exhibiting seizure activity should be treated on an urgent basis with adequate support ventilation and perfusion, correction of any underlying metabolic derangements and the use of anticonvulsant-medication.

Treatment of neonatal seizures is directed toward minimizing physiological and metabolic derangements that are associated with the epileptic process and to prevent recurrence of seizures. The choice of anticonvulsants in the treatment of neonatal seizures should consider the unique characteristics of neonatal seizures and the efficacy, toxicity and pharmacologic appropriateness of the drug. All aspects of toxicity are to be considered, but two factors of immediate concern in neonates are changes in heart rate and effects on brain growth.[132] The generally used order of antiepileptic drugs and their doses are indicated in Table 10.9.

Phenobarbital continues to be the first-line drug for the treatment of neonatal seizures. A loading dose of up to 40 mg/kg achieves therapeutic levels in the serum within a short time. Therapeutic levels are 20–40 mg/L (80–160 μmol/L). Babies who are not artificially ventilated can be rendered apneic by a single loading dose of 40 mg/kg, and it is usual to give two separate doses of 20 mg/kg in this situation. If clinical and EEG-revealed seizures persist despite a phenobarbital concentration greater than 40 μ/mL, phenytoin should be added; approximately one-third to half the babies with seizure respond to phenobarbital, about 90% respond to a combination of phenobarbital and phenytoin. The dose of phenytoin is 15 mg/kg given as an intravenous "push" at a rate no greater than 1 mg/kg/min. Phenytoin is probably the best choice as second-line treatment in babies who fail to respond to phenobarbital, but problems with hypotension and arrhythmias have been reported when there is hidden myocardial damage accompanying hypoxic-ischemic encephalopathy.

Most of the benzodiazepines have been tried in the newborn. The use of diazepam is controversial. Diazepam has a very long half-life in babies, of approximately 30–75 hours, and because of the respiratory depressant effects that occur when the levels accumulate this drug is not suitable for prolonged infusion. Lorazepam and clonazepam are also given; the latter is traditionally given intravenously or as an infusion. Hypersalivation and increased bronchial secretion are frequent side effects. Midazolam is a newer benzodiazepine that has proved effective in treating status epilepticus. Midazolam has been reported to cause myoclonic jerking and dystonic posturing in preterm babies when it was used for sedation. The neurodevelopment outcome was better in a group of preterms sedated with morphine, than it was when midazolam was used.

There is very little published experience with any other antiepileptic drug in the newborn. Paraldehyde was popular during the 1970s and 1980s, but it is now difficult to obtain. Sodium valproate has hepatotoxicity. Vigabatrin is not available in an intravenous form, and there is a risk of incurring visual field effects, which cannot be monitored precisely in babies. There is virtually no neonatal experience with lamotrigine or carbamazepine, or with other, new antiepileptic drugs, like oxcarbazepine, gabapentin, topiramate. In animal models, the acute and chronic effects of hypoxia can be prevented by pretreatment with topiramate. Topiramate was administered before the hypoxic insult and prevented the expression of the hypoxia-induced seizure.[134] Anticonvulsant therapy must be tailored to the individual needs of the child. Most neonatal seizures are secondary to an acute cerebral insult and thus tend to resolve within 2–4 days. If there has been status epilepticus or if seizures have not been controlled with phenobarbital alone, we continue anticonvulsants for at least 3 months.[2]

Table 10.9: Treatment of neonatal seizures

Initial therapy

1. Phenobarbital 20 mg/kg IV; if seizures continue, phenobarbital 10 mg/kg IV every 15–30 minutus to a total of 40 mg/kg or to a serum level of 40 µg/mL

2. Phenytoin 20 mg/kg IV; if seizures continue, phenytoin 10 mg/kg intravenously to a serum level of 20 µg/mL. If seizures continue

3. Diazepam   0.1–0.3 mg/kg IV repeated as necessary, or 0.7–2.75 mg/h continuous intravenous infusion
   Lorazepam   0.05–0.10 mg/kg IV repeated as necessary
   Paraldehyde   200–400 mg/kg IV over first hour, then 16 mg/kg/h; adjust infusion rate based on EEG response

Since clinical detection of seizures is frequently inaccurate, it is helpful to have continuous and video-EEG monitoring during the initiation of therapy. The EEG is especially helpful in making decisions regarding additional diazepam or lorazepam, or in adjusting the rate of paraldehyde infusion

Maintenance therapy

1. Phenobarbital 3–4 mg/kg/day IV, IM or orally, starting 12 h after the loading dose

2. Phenytoin 3–4 mg/kg/day IV starting after the loading dose

3. Primidone 12–20 mg/kg/day

(*Source:* Adapted from Younkin[2] with permission.)

Specifics of the Pharmacology of Antiepileptic Drugs in Neonates

Binding Profile

Painter et al.[135] found that there is significant correlation between phenobarbital and phenytoin in vitro binding and the total protein and albumin concentration. Phenobarbital is exclusively but weakly albumin bound. The finding that in vivo phenobarbital binding was not significantly correlated with total protein or albumin may explained by the influence of other factors known to affect albumin binding, such as bilirubin concentration, pH changes, the elevations of free fatty acid concentration and drugs administered to critically ill neonates.

Half-life

Morselli et al.[136] studied the influence of age on the half-life of diazepam. The metabolic pathway of diazepam develops only some time after birth, so premature babies show a significantly longer half-life than full-term infants. Carbamazepine autoinduces its own biotransformation, usually during the first 4–6 weeks of treatment. Beginning at a relatively low dose and progressively increasing the dose can avoid the fall in drug concentration.

Toxicity

Phenytoin toxicity is known to cause cardiac arrhythmias and exacerbate seizures. Elevated free concentrations of phenobarbital are known to cause hypotension and respiratory depression. Phenytoin has less of a sedative effect than phenobarbital and clonazepam, thus allowing a more reliable clinical assessment of improvement.[137] Interpatient variability of the various antiepileptic drugs is extensive in newborns, and intraindividual variation occurs in all premature and full-term newborns during the neonatal period. The extensive variability means that the therapy should begin with a relatively small dose, which is increased stepwise until either seizures are controlled or side effects occur.[138]

The Effect of Antiepileptic Drugs on the EEG

Bell et al.[139] show a marked depressant effect of phenobarbitone and diazepam on the EEG in newborn babies. The effect of sedation on the maximum interburst interval was greater than expected, particularly when compared to reports on adults.[140] The authors suppose that the drugs are acting on subcortical generators, such as the thalamus and reticular formation, which play a major role in maintaining the background EEG in newborns. Determination of effectiveness of therapy is important in the management of neonatal seizures. With the antiepileptic treatment the clinical control of the convulsions was obtained in more than 80% of the cases, while control of the electrical convulsions was obtained only in 62.5%. There was a highly significant association between favorable response to treatment and normal neurological examination at hospital discharge and at 1 year of age. It is necessary to confirm by means of EEG record the neonatal clinical convulsion before and after having established the anticonvulsive treatment, as the control of electrical convulsion improves the neurological outcome.[141]

Long-Term Treatment

There is little agreement on how long to continue anticonvulsant therapy in the neonate. We agree with the opinion of Levene, who stops all drugs when the infant has had no seizure for 7 days as long as they show no neurological abnormality.[10] In those in whom seizures recur or who are neurologically abnormal, medication is continued for 3 months, when they are reviewed. Drugs are stopped if the infant appears to be neurologically normal.

PROGNOSIS

Several factors may influence the neurological outcome of neonates who have clinical seizures. These include the nature and degree of the underlying neuropathologic process, the possible adverse effects of epileptic activity on the developing brain, the secondary effects of the seizures (for example, hypoventilation or hypoperfusion) and the potential adverse effects of antiepileptic drugs. Several studies, however, suggest that seizures associated with certain etiologic factors have a worse prognosis than others (Table 10.10). Normal outcomes occur with increasing frequency in each of the following: hypoxic-ischemic encephalopathy, intracranial hemorrhage, hypoglycemia, unknown cause, hypocalcemia.[23] In monitored infants in whom outcome was assessed only at hospital discharge, the highest morbidity and mortality were associated with seizures due to hypoxic-ischemic encephalopathy and the lowest in infants with

Table 10.10: Prognosis of neonatal seizures-relation to neurological disease

Neurological disease	Normal development (%)*
Hypoxic-ischemic encephalopathy	50
Intraventricular hemorrhage**	10
Primer subarachnoid hemorrhage	90
Hypocalcemia:	
• Early onset	50**
• Late onset	100
Hypoglycemia	50
Bacterial meningitis	50
Development defect	0

*Prognosis is for those cases with the stated neurological disease when seizures are a manifestation (thus, value usually will differ from overall prognosis for the disease) ;+values are rounded off to nearest 5%; ^usually serves intraventricular hemorrhage associated with major periventricular hemorrhagic infarcion; **represents primarily the prognosis approaches that later onset hypocalcemia if no or only minor neurological illness present.
(*Source:* Adapted from Volpe[30] with permission.)

subarachnoid hemorrhage, hypoglycemia and hypocalcemia.[24,28] The outcome of neonatal seizures is mainly dependent on their cause. Newborns with seizure were three times more likely (16%) to develop cerebral palsy than were controls (6%). The adverse outcomes observed after neonatal encephalopathy included both cerebral palsy and global developmental delay without motor deficit. For years, it has been held that intellectual difficulties can only accompany motor problems in the postasphyxia syndrome, and are not seen in isolation, but this view is now beginning to be challenged. Over the years, the reported outcome of neonatal encephalopathy with seizures has been remarkably consistent, with about 25% adverse outcomes in babies with moderate encephalopathy and 66% adverse outcomes (33% dead, 33% disabled) in those with severe encephalopathy, usually defined as coma. The background electroencephalogram abnormality consistently performs best as an outcome predictor; babies with burst suppression or a markedly attenuated background pattern that persists for longer than 12 hours after birth have an adverse outcome.[57]

The Role of EEG and the Clinical Neurological Status

The extreme ends of the spectrum of clinical neurological status during the newborn period are useful indicators of the outcome. Thus, infants with flaccid coma and seizures generally have an unfavorable outcome, whereas infants with consistently preserved consciousness, activity, reflexes and tone have a more favorable outcome.[96] Infants, who had non-epileptic seizures consisting of tonic posturing and motor automatism, most often had hypoxic-ischemic encephalopathy, interictal lethargy or obtundation, the nature of the abnormal EEG, and poor short-term outcome. In the infants who had epileptic seizures (focal-clonic or focal-tonic), an association was noted with focal structural lesions, subarachnoid hemorrhage and metabolic abnormalities; and with interictal alertness, normal background EEG activity and a relatively good shortterm outcome. These clinical and electrographic features suggest a delimited process rather than diffuse injury, which is

probably the important factor in the relatively good short-term outcome of these infants. Abnormal neurological examination on discharge was a good predictor of an unfavorable outcome and abnormal polysomnographic recording a moderate predictor.[142] Several investigators have demonstrated that the interictal EEG is a useful prognostic indicator in the term infants. In one large series, a normal interictal EEG was associated with an 86% chance of normal development at the age of 4 years.[96] In contrast, infants with flat, periodic or multifocal EEGs had only an 8% probability of a normal outcome. The burst-suppression pattern, which is included in this group of EEGs with a poor prognosis has a superficial resemblance to the tracé alternant pattern seen in quiet sleep in the normal term newborn. Moreover, 25–35% of term newborns with seizures will have EEGs that are borderline, or demonstrate less marked abnormalities associated with an uncertain prognosis. Bergman et al.[6] demonstrated that the outcome of neonates who had manifested seizures for more than 3 days was associated with moderate or severe neurological injury. Babies with normal clinical examination, cranial ultrasound, CT and EEG results at 7–14 days usually have a good prognosis. Estimates of the incidence of epilepsy in children with neonatal seizures vary from 15% to 20%.[96]

MATERNAL EPILEPSY

Risk of Maternal Seizure

Pregnancy in women with epilepsy is accompanied by increased maternal and fetal risk. During pregnancy, seizure can cause maternal and fetal hypoxia and acidosis. The increase in seizure has been reported to occur mostly during the first trimester[31] or evenly throughout pregnancy.[25,26] In animal studies, estrogen is generally proconvulsant; conversely, progesterone generally has an anticonvulsant effect.[46] Status epilepticus is an uncommon complication of pregnancy, but when it occurs it carries high maternal and fetal mortality rates (31% and 48%, respectively).[26] The effects of non-convulsive seizures on the developing fetus are not clear.

Antiepileptic Drug Pharmacokinetics during Pregnancy and Lactation

The ideal management of women with epilepsy during pregnancy and the postpartum period involves achieving an optimal balance between minimizing fetal and neonatal exposure to the deleterious influences both of antiepileptic drugs and of seizures.[143] During the past decade, consensus guidelines have emphasized minimizing the associated risk by optimizing a woman's antiepileptic drug regimen and initiating supplemental folic acid before conception, and high-dose folate supplementation prior to conception and during organogenesis. However, there are no current guidelines regarding the best management once a woman with epilepsy becomes pregnant. Because of large intraindividual and interindividual variability, some authors recommend at least monthly monitoring of antiepileptic drug concentration.[144] During mothers taking the most of antiepileptic drugs indicate extensive transplacental transfer and low to moderate excretion into breast milk, the breast milk/maternal plasma concentration ratios less than 1.

In the newborn, special care should be given to congenital malformations, vitamin K supplementation and symptoms of neonatal withdrawal. Breastfeeding should be allowed for the most anticonvulsive drugs unless the infant becomes symptomatic.[145]

Fetal Anticonvulsant Syndrome

The cause of this syndrome is probably multifactorial, but recent studies have indicated that antiepileptic drugs are a major offending factor.[15,20,21] If women with epilepsy are in need of antiepileptic drugs for seizure control, then monotherapy at the lowest effective dose should be employed. Offspring are at increased risk of major congenital malformation, a rate of 4–7% (2–3% in normal population), including congenital heart disease, cleft lip/palate, neural tube defects and urogenital defects. The risk of malformations increases with the number of antiepileptic drugs to which the fetus is exposed during pregnancy[10,11] and possibly with the daily amount or peak concentration of individual drugs. Data for valproic acid are suggestive of a dose-response effect for the risk of neural tube defects.[9,12,14,15]

Results of studies investigating cognitive outcome report an increased risk of mental deficiency in 1.4–6% of children of women with epilepsy (including both seizures[17] and in utero exposure to antiepileptic drugs[18]), compared with 1% of controls. Unlike major malformations, exposure to antiepileptic drugs during the last trimester may actually be the most detrimental for cognitive outcome.[19]

REFERENCES

1. Mizrahi EM. Consensus and controversy in the clinical management of neonatal seizures. In: Volpe JJ (Ed). Clinics in Perinatology-Neonatal Neurology. Philadelphia, PA: W.B. Saunders Company; 1989. pp. 16.
2. Younkin D. Neonatal seizures. In: Nelson NM (Ed). Current Therapy in Neonatal-Perinatal Medicine. Philadelphia, PA: BC Decker Inc.; 1990. pp. 321-7.
3. Aicardi J. Epilepsy in Children, 2nd edition. New York: Raven Press; 1994.
4. Giovanardi RP, Santucci M, Gobbi G, et al. Long-term follow-up of severe myoclonic epilepsy of infants. In: Fukuyama Y, Kamoshita S, Ohtsuka C, Susuki Y (Eds). Modern Perspectives of Child Neurology. Tokyo: Japanese Society of Child Neurology; 1991. pp. 205-13.
5. Aicardi J. Neonatal seizures. In: Dam M, Gram L (Eds). Comprehensive Epileptology. New York: Raven Press; 1991.
6. Bergman I, Painter MJ, Hirsch RP, et al. Outcome in neonates with convulsions treated in an intensive care unit. Ann Neurol. 1983;14:642-7.
7. Goldberg HJ. Neonatal convulsions: a 10 year review. Arch Dis Child. 1983;58:976-8.
8. Legido A, Clancy, RR, Berman HP. Neurologic outcome after electroencephalographically proven neonatal seizures. Pediatrics. 1991;88(3):538-96.
9. Erikson M, Zetterstrom R. Neonatal convulsions. Incidence and causes in the Stockholm area. Acta Paediatr Scand. 1979;68: 807-11.
10. Levene MI. Neonatal seizures. In: Levene M (Ed). Neonatal Neurology. New York: Churchill Livingstone; 1987. pp. 201-35.
11. Scher MS, Kosaburo A, Beggarly MM, et al. Electrographic seizures in preterm and full-term neonates; clinical correlates, associated brain lesions, and risk for neurologic sequalae. Pediatrics. 1993;91(1):128-34.
12. Seay R, Bray PF. Significance of seizures in infants weighing less than 2500 grams. Arch Neurol. 1977;34:381-2.
13. Kohelet D, Shochat R, Lusky A, et al. Risk factors for neonatal seizures in very low birthweight infants: population based survey. J Child Neurol. 2004;19(2):123-8.
14. Fenichel GM. Neonatal Neurology. New York: Churchill Livingstone; 1980.
15. Freeman JM. Neonatal seizures. In: Dreyfuss FE (Ed). Pediatric Epileptology. Boston: John Wright, PSAG Inc.; 1983. pp. 159-72.
16. Volpe JJ. Neonatal seizures; current concepts and classification. Pediatrics. 1989;84:422-8.
17. Purpura DP. Synaptogenesis in mammalian cortex; problems and perspectives. In: Sterman MB, McGinty D, Adinolfy M (Eds). Brain Development and Behaviour. London: Academic Press; 1971. pp. 23-40.
18. Shapiro S. Hormonal and environmental influences on rat brain development and behavior. In: Sterman MB, McGinty D, Adinolfy M (Eds). Brain Development and Behaviour. London: Academic Press; 1971. pp. 307-23.
19. Dreyfus-Brisac C. The electroencephalogram of full term newborns and premature infants. In: Remond A, Lairy GC (Eds). Handbook of Electroencephalography and Clinical Neurophysiology. Amsterdam: Elsevier; 1962. pp. 6-23.
20. Nolte R, Schulte FJ, Michaelis R, et al. Power spectral analysis of the EEG of newborn twins in active and quiet sleep. In: Kellaway P, Petersen I (Eds). Clinical Electroencephalography in Children. Stockholm: Almquist and Wiksell; 1968. pp. 89-96.
21. Watanabe K, Iwase K, Hara K. Development of slow-wave sleep in low birthweight infants. Dev Med Child Neurol. 1974;16:23-31.
22. Bergey GK, Swaiman KF, Schrier BK. Adverse effects of phenobarbital on morphological and biochemical development of fetal mouse spinal cord neurons in culture. Ann Neurol. 1981;1:584-8.
23. Kellaway P, Mizrahi EM. Neonatal seizures. In: Lüders H, Lesser RP (Eds). Epilepsy: Electroclinical Syndromes. London: Springer Verlag; 1987. pp. 13-47.
24. Mizrahi EM, Kellaway P. Characterization and classification of neonatal seizures. Neurology. 1987;37:1837-44.
25. Lindsley DB, Schreiner LH, Magoun HW. An electomyographic study of spasticity. J Neurophysiol. 1949;12:197-203.
26. Mori S, Nishimura H, Aoki M. Brain stem activation of the spinal cord stepping generator. In: Hobson JA, Brazier MAB (Eds). The Reticular Formation Revisited. New York: Raven Press; 1980. pp. 241-65.
27. Sherrington CS, Creed RS, Denny-Brown DE. Reflex Activity of the Spinal Cord. London: Oxford University Press; 1932.
28. Kellaway P, Mizrahi EM. Electroencephalographic, therapeutic, and pathophysiologic studies of neonatal seizures. In: Wasterlain CG, Vert P (Eds). Neonatal Seizures: Pathophysiology and Pharmacologic Management. New York: Raven Press; 1990. pp. 1-13.
29. Kellawey P, Hrachovy RA. Status epilepticus in newborn. A perspective on neonatal seizures. In: Deldago-Escueta AV, Wasterlain CG, Treiman, DM (Eds). Advances in Neurology. Status Epilepticus. New York: Raven Press; 1983. pp. 93-9.
30. Volpe JJ. Neurology of the Newborn, 2nd edition. Philadelphia, PA: Saunders; 1987. pp. 129-58.
31. Yakovlev PI, Lecours AR. The myelogenetic cycles of regional maturation of the brain. In: Minkowski A (Ed). Regional Development of the Brain in Early Life. Philadelphia, PA: F. A. Davies; 1967. pp. 3-70.
32. Yamamoto N, Watanabe K, Negoro T. Partial seizures evolving to infantile spasms. Epilepsia. 1988;29:34-40.

33. Yakovlev PI. Maturation of cortical substrata of epileptic events. World Neurol. 1962;3:299-304.

34. Purpura DP. Relationship of seizure susceptibility to morphologic and physiologic properties of normal and abnormal immature cortex. In: Kellaway P, Petersen I (Eds). Neurologic and Electroencephalographic Studies in Infancy. New York: Grune and Stratton; 1964.

35. Purpura DP, Shoffer RJ, Scraff J. Intracellular study of spike potentials synaptic activities of neurons in immature neocortex. In: Minkowski (Ed). Regional Development of the Brain in Early Life. New York: Grune D. Stratton; 1967. pp. 117-21.

36. Wright FS, Bradley WE. Maturation of epileptiform activity. Electroencephalogr Clin Neurophysiol. 1968;25:259-69.

37. Kolmodin GM, Meyerson BA. Ontogenesis of paroxysmal cortical activity in fetal sheep. Electroencephalogr Clin Neurophysiol. 1952;21:589-600.

38. Bonasera N, Smorto M, Bonavita V. Izoniacid seizures in the developing rat and the content of pyridoxal-5-phosphat in the brain. Brain Res. 1967;4:383-6.

39. Millichap JG. Development of seizure pattern in newborn animals. Significance of brain carbonic anhydrase. Proc Soc Exp Biol Med. 1957;96(1):125-9.

40. Kato M, Malamut BL, Caveness WF, et al. Local cerebral glucose utilization in newborn and pubescent monkeys during focal motor seizures. Ann Neurol. 1980;7:204-12.

41. Ricci GF, Mecaelli O, De Feo MR. Ontogenesis of GABAergic and glutamergic receptors in the developing brain. In: Wasterlain CG, Vert P (Eds). Neonatal Seizures. New York: Raven Press; 1990. pp. 209-20.

42. Rondouin G. GABAergic inhibition and convulsive seizures. In: Wasterlain CG, Vert P (Eds). Neonatal Seizures. New York: Raven Press; 1990. pp. 221-30.

43. Johnston MV, Singer HS. Brain neurotransmitters and neuromodulators in pediatrics. Pediatrics. 1982;70:57-68.

44. Holmes GL, Khazipov R, Ben-Ari Y. New concept in neonatal seizures. Neuro Report. 2002;13:3-8.

45. Vannucci RC, Vasta F. Energy state of the brain in experimental neonatal status epilepticus. Pediatr Res. 1985;19:396-9.

46. Wasterlain CG, Dwyer B. Brain metabolism during prolonged seizures in neonates. Adv Neurol. 1983;34:241-60.

47. Wasterlain CG, Vert P (Eds). Neonatal Seizures. New York: Raven Press; 1990.

48. Younkin DP, Delivoria-Papadopoulos M, Maris J, et al. Cerebral metabolic effects of neonatal seizures measured with in vivo 31P NMR spectroscopy. Ann Neurol. 1986;20:513-9.

49. McCabe BK, Silvera DC, Cilio MR, et al. Reduced neurogenesis after neonatal seizures. J Neurosci. 2001;6:2094-103.

50. Boylan GB, Panerai RB, Rennie JM, et al. Cerebral blood flow velocity during neonatal seizures. Arch Dis Child. 1999;80:105-10.

51. Sogawa Y, Monokoshi M, Silveira DC, et al. Timing of cognitive deficits following neonatal seizures: relationship to histological changes in the hippocampus. Dev Brain Res. 2001;131:73-83.

52. Rogalski Landrot I, Minokoshi M, Silveira DC, et al. Recurrent neonatal seizures: relationship of pathology to the electroencephalogram and cognition. Dev Brain Res. 2001;129:27-8.

53. Koh S, Storey TW, Santos TC, et al. Early-life seizures in rats increase susceptibility to seizure-induced brain injury in adulthood. Neurology. 1999;53:912-21.

54. Miller SP, Weiss J, Barnwell, et al. Seizure-associated brain injury in term newborn in perinatal asphyxia. Neurology. 2001;58:542-8.

55. Kubova H, Druga R, Lukasiuk K, et al. Status epilepticus causes necrotic damage in the mediodorsal nucleus of the thalamus in immature rats. J Neurosci. 2001;21:3593-9.

56. Wasterlain CG, Niquet J, Thompson KW, et al. Seizure-induced neuronal death in immature brain. Prog Brain Res. 2002;135: 335-53.

57. Rennie JM, Boylan GB. Neonatal seizures and their treatment. Curr Opin Neurol. 2003;16(2):177-81.

58. Edwards HE, Dortok D, Tam J, et al. Prenatal stress alters seizure thresholds and the development of kindled seizures in infant and adult rats. Horm Behav. 2002;42(4):437-47.

59. Parent JM, Lowenstein DH. Seizure-induced neurogenesis: are more new neurons good for an adult brain? Prog Brain Res. 2002;135:121-31.

60. Aicardi J. Complex partial seizures in childhood. In: Parsonage M, Grant RHE, Craig AG, Ward AA Jr (Eds). Advances in Epileptology: XIVth Epilepsy International Symposium. New York: Raven Press; 1983. pp. 237-42.

61. Aicardi J. Diseases of the Nervous System in Childhood. London: Mac Keith Press; 1992.

62. Mizrahi EM. Classification on neonatal seizures. A guide to clinical recognition. ILEA Workshop on Neonatal Seizures Classification-Script, Houston, TX; 2004.

63. Roos RAC, Van Dijk JG. Reflex-epilepsy induced by immersion in hot water; case report and review of the literature. Eur Neurol. 1988;28:6-10.

64. Mizrahi EM. Neonatal seizures: problems in diagnosis and classification. Epilepsia. 1987;28:546-55.

65. Cockburn F, Brown JK, Belton NR, et al. Neonatal convulsions associated with primary disturbance of calcium, phosphorus and magnesium metabolism. Arch Dis Child. 1973;48:99-108.

66. Lombroso CT. Prognosis in neonatal seizures. In: Deldago-Escueta AV, Wasterlain CG, Freiman DM, Orter RJ (Eds). Advances in Neurology. Status Epilepticus. New York: Raven Press; 1983. pp. 101-13.

67. Sarnat HB. Pathogenesis of decerebrate seizures in the premature with intraventricular haemorrhage. J Pediatr. 1975;87:154-5.

68. Lombroso CT. Seizures in the newborn period. In: Vinken PJ, Bruyn GW (Eds). Handbook of Clinical Neurology. The Epilepsies. Amsterdam: North-Holland; 1974. pp. 189-218.

69. Lombroso CT. Neonatal seizures. In: Resor SR, Kutt H (Eds). The Medical Treatment of Epilepsy. New York: Marcel Dekker; 1992. pp. 115-25.

70. Coulter DL, Allen RJ. Benign neonatal sleep myoclonus. Arch Neurol. 1982;39:191-2.

71. Resnik T, Mosh S, Perotta L, et al. Benign neonatal sleep myoclonus. Arch Neurol. 1986;43:266-8.

72. Daoust-Roy J, Seshia SS. Benign neonatal sleep myoclonus. Am J Dis Child. 1992;146:1236-41.

73. Hill A, Volpe JJ. Neonatal seizures. In: Roberton NRC (Ed). Textbook of Neonatology, 2nd edition. New York: Churchill Livingstone; 1992. pp. 1043-55.

74. Blume WT. Clinical and electroencephalographic correlates of the multiple independent spike foci pattern in children. Ann Neurol. 1978;4:541-7.

75. Watanwbe K, Hara K, Miyazaki S, et al. Apneic seizures in the newborn. Am J Dis Child. 1982;15:584-96.

76. Navelet Y, Wood RC, Robieux C, et al. Seizures presenting as apnea. Arch Dis Child. 1989;64:357-9.

77. Fenichel GM. Seizure in newborns. In: Fenichel GM (Ed). Neonatal Neurology. Edinburgh: Churchill Livingstone; 1985. pp. 25-52.

78. Fenichel GM, Olson BJ, Fitzpatrick JE. Heart rate changes inconvulsive and nonconvulsive neonatal apnea. Ann Neurol. 1980;7:577-82.

79. Radvanyi-Bouvet MF, Vallecalle MH, Morel-Kahn F, et al. Seizures and electrical discharges in premature infants. Neuropediatrics. 1985;16:143-8.

80. Bour F, Plouin P, Jalin C, et al. Les états de mal unilatéraux au cours de la période neonatale. Rev EEG Neurophysiol Clin. 1983;13: 162-7.

81. Camfield PR, Camfield CS. Neonatal seizures: a commentary on selected aspects. J Child Neurol. 1987;2:244-51.

82. Cukier F, Sfaello Z, Dreyfus-Brisac C. Lés états de mal du nouveau-né terme et du prématuré dans un centre de réanimation néonatale. Aspects cliniques, électroencephalographiques et évolution. Gaslini. 1976;8:100-6.

83. Dreyfus-Brisac C, Monod N. Neonatal status epilepticus. In: Remond A (Ed). Handbook of Electroencephalography and Clinical Neurophysiology. Amsterdam: Elsevier; 1977. pp. 39-52.

84. Monod N, Dreyfus-Brisac C, Sfaello Z. Presentation et prognosticde l'état de mal épileptique néonatal: Étude clinique et EEG de 150 cas. Arch Fr Pédiatr. 1969;26:1085.

85. Dreyfus-Brisac C, Peschanski N, Radvanyi MF, et al. Convulsions du noveau-né. Aspects clinique, électroencéphalographique, étiopathogenique et prognostique. Rev EEG Neurophysiol. 1981;11:367-78.

86. Sarnat HB, Sarnat MS. Neonatal encephalopathy following fetal distress. Arch Neurol. 1976;33:696-705.

87. Fenichel GM. Hypoxic-ischemic encephalopathy in the newborn. Arch Neurol. 1983;40:261-6.

88. Hill A, Volpe JJ. Seizures, hypoxic-ischaemic brain injury and intraventricular hemorrhage in the newborn. Ann Neurol. 1981;10:109-21.

89. Minchon P, Niswandeer K, Chalmers I. Antecedents and outcome of very early neonatal seizures in infants born at or near term. Br J Obstet Gynecol. 1987;94:431-5.

90. Brown JK. Convulsions in the newborn period. Dev Med Child Neurol. 1974;15:823-46.

91. Dreyfus-Brisac C. Neonatal electroencephalography. In: Scarpelli EM, Cosmi EV (Eds). Reviews of Perinatal Medicine. New York: Raven Press; 1979. p. 3.

92. Levene MI, Kornberg J, Williams THC. The incidence and severity of post-asphyxial encephalopathy in full-term infants. Early Hum Dev. 1985;11:21-6.

93. Delivoria-Papadopoulos M, Mishra OP. Mechanisms of perinatal cerebral injury in fetus and newborn. Ann N Y Acad Sci. 2000;900:159-68.

94. Maulik D, Zanelli SA, Numagami Y, et al. Oxygen free radical generation during in utero hypoxia in the fetal guinea pig brain. Brain Res. 1999;817:117-22.

95. Craig WS. Convulsive movements occurring in the first ten days of life. Arch Dis Child. 1960;35:336-44.

96. Rose AL, Lombroso CT. Neonatal seizure states. Pediatrics. 1970;45:404-25.

97. Salvia-Roiges MD, Garcia LI, Gonce-Mellgren A, et al. Neonatal convulsion and subarachnoid hemorrhage after in utero exposure to paroxetine. Rev Neurol. 2003;36(8):724-6.

98. Billard C, Dulac O, Diebler C. Ramollissement cerebral ischemique du noveau-né. Une etiologie possible des états de mal convulsifs neonatals. Arch Fr Pédiatr. 1982;39:677-83.

99. Venkataraman A, Kingsley PB, Kalina P, et al. Newborn brain infarction: clinical aspects and magnetic resonance imaging. CNS Spectr. 2004;9(6):436-44.

100. Nelson KB, Lynch JK. Stroke in newborn infants. Lancet Neurol. 2004;3(3):150-8.

101. Chen SF, Huang CC, Wu HM, et al. Seizure, neuron loss, and mossy fiber sprouting in herpes simplex virus type 1-infected organotypic hippocampal cultures. Epilepsia. 2004;45(4):322-32.

102. Pagliara AS, Karl IE, Haymond M. Hypoglycemia in infancy and childhood. J Pediatr. 1973;8:365-79.

103. Monod N, Dreyfus-Brisac C, Scafello Z, et al. Depistage et prognostic de l'état de mal néonatal. Arch Fr Pédiatr. 1969;26:1085-102.

104. Lucas A, Morley R, Cole T. Adverse neurodevelopmental outcome of moderate hypoglycaemia. Br Med J. 1988;297:1304-8.

105. Manzar S. Transient pseudohypoparathyroidism and neonatalseizure. J Trop Pediatr. 2001;47(2):113-4.

106. Johnson GM. Powdered goat's milk: pyridoxyne deficiency andstatus epilepticus. Clin Pediatr. 1982;21:494-5.

107. Gospe SM Jr, Hecht ST. Longitudinal MRI findings in pyridoxine dependent seizures. Neurology. 1998;51(81):74-8.

108. Hennel SJ, Ekert PG, Volpe JJ, et al. Insight into the pathogenesis of cerebral lesions in incontinentia pigmenti. Pediatr Neurol. 2003;29(2):148-50.

109. Wada N, Matsuishi T, Nonaka M, et al. Pyruvate dehydrogenase E 1a subunit deficiency in a female patient. Brain Dev. 2004;26(1):57-60.

110. Aicardi J, Goutieres F. Encéphalopathie myoclonique néonatale. Rev EEG Neurophysiol Clin. 1978;8:99-101.

111. Schlumberger E, Dulac O, Plouin P. Early infantile epileptic syndrome(s) with suppression—burst; nosological considerations. In: Roger J, Bureay M, Dravet C, Dreifuss FE, Perret A, Wolf P (Eds). Epileptic Syndromes in Infancy, Childhood and Adolescence, 2nd edition. London: John Libbey; 1992. pp. 35-42.

112. Aicardi J. Epileptic syndromes in childhood. Overview and classification. In: Ross E, Reynolds E (Eds). Paediatric Perspectives on Epilepsy. Chichester: J. Wiley; 1985. pp. 65-71.

113. Dalla Bernardina B, Fontana E, Sgro V, et al. Generalised or partial atonic seizures—inhibitory seizures—in children with partial epilepsy. Electroencephalogr Clin Neurophysiol. 1990;75:S31-2.

114. Aicardi J. Myoclonic epilepsies of infancy and childhood. In: Fahn S, Marsden CD, Van Woert MH (Eds). Advances in Neurology. Myoclonus. New York: Raven Press; 1986. p. 43.

115. Lombroso CT. Early myoclonic encephalopathy, early infantile epileptic encephalopathy and benign and severe infantile myoclonic epilepsies: a critical review and personal contributions. J Clin Neurophysiol. 1990;7:380-408.

116. Zonana J, Silvey K, Strimling B. Familial neonatal and infantile seizures: an autosomal dominant disorder. Am J Med Gen. 1984;18:455-9.

117. Leppert M, Anderson VE, Quattlebaum T, et al. Benign familial neonatal convulsions linked to genetic markers on chromosome 20. Nature, 1989;337:647-8.

118. Mellits ED, Holden KR, Freeman JM. Neonatal seizures. II. Multivariate analysis of factors associated with outcome. Pediatrics. 1981;70:177-85.

119. Dehan M, Quilleron D, Navelet Y, et al. Les convulsions du cinquieme jour de la vie: une nouveau syndrome. Arch Fr Pédiatr. 1977;34:730-42.

120. Levy SR, Abroms IF, Marshall PC, et al. Seizures and cerebral infarction in the full-term newborn. Ann Neurol. 1985;17:366-70.

121. Pryor DS, Don N, Macourt DC. Fifth day fits: a syndrome of neonatal convulsions. Arch Dis Child. 1981;56:753-8.

122. Bejsovec M, Kulenda Z, Ponca E. Familial intrauterine convulsions in pyridoxine dependency. Arch Dis Child. 1967;42:201-7.

123. Holmes GL. Neonatal seizures. In: Pedley TA, Meldrum BS (Eds). Recent Advances in Epilepsy. Edinburgh: Churchill Livingstone; 1985. pp. 207-37.

124. Miikati MA, Travathan E, Krishnamoorthy K, et al. Pyridoxine-dependent epilepsy: EEG investigations and long-term follow-up. Electroencephalogr Clin Neurophysiol. 1991;78:215-21.

125. Mulley JC, Scheffer IE, Petrou S, et al. Channelopathies as a genetic cause of epilepsy. Curr Opin Neurol. 2003;16(2):171-6.

126. Legido A, Clancy RR, Behrman PH. Recent advances in the diagnosis, treatment and prognosis of neonatal seizures. Pediatr Neurol. 1988;4:79-86.

127. Hill A, Volpe JJ. Neonatal seizures. In: Avery GB, Fletcher MA, Macdonald MG (Eds). Neonatology: Pathophysiology and Management for the Newborn, 4th edition. Philadelphia, PA: JB Lippincott Company; 1994. pp. 1118-34.

128. Markand ON. Pearls, perils, and pitfalls in the use of the electroencephalogram. Semin Neurol. 2003;23(1):7-46.

129. Eyre JA, Oozeer RC, Wilkinson AR. Diagnosis of neonatal seizures by continuous recording and rapid analysis of the electroencephalogram. Arch Dis Child. 1983;58:785-90.

130. Levy SR, Berg AT, Testa FM, et al. Comparison of digital and conventional EEG interpretation. J Clin Neurophysiol. 1998;15(6):476-80.
131. Nolte R, Haas G. A polygraphic study of bioelectrical brain maturation in preterm infants. Dev Med Child Neurol. 1978;20: 167-82.
132. Streletz LJ, Graziani LJ. Electroenchephalography and evoked potentials in neonates. In: Nelson NM (Ed). Current Therapy in Neonatal-Perinatal Medicine. Philadelphia, PA: BC. Decker Inc.; London: The C.V. Mosby Company; 1986. pp. 329-32.
133. Patrizi S, Holmes GL, Orzalesi M, et al. Neonatal seizures: characteristics of EEG ictal activity in preterm and fullterm infants. Brain Dev. 2003;25(6):427-37.
134. Koh S, Jensen FE. Topiramate blocks perinatal hypoxia-induced seizures in rat pups. Ann Neurol. 2001;50:366-72.
135. Painter MJ, Minnigh MB, Gaus L, et al. Neonatal phenobarbital and phenytoin binding profiles. J Clin Pharmacol. 1994;34:312-7.
136. Morselli PL, Pippenger CE, Penry JK. Antiepileptic Drug Therapy in Pediatrics. New York: Raven Press; 1983.
137. Albani M. Phenytoin in infancy and childhood. Adv Neurol. 1983;34:457-64.
138. Dodson WE. Aspects of antiepileptic treatment in children. Epilepsia. 1988;29(Suppl 3):S10-4.
139. Bell AH, Greisen G, Pryds O. Comparison of the effects of phenobarbitone and morphine administration on EEG activity in preterm babies. Acta Paediatr. 19934;82:35-9.
140. Jorgensen EP. The EEG during severe barbiturate intoxication. Acta Neurol Scand. 1970;46(Suppl 43):281.
141. Domenech Martinez E, Castro-Conde JR, Herraiz-Culebras T, et al. Neonatal convulsion: influence of the electroencephalographic pattern and the response to treatment on the outcome. Rev Neurol. 2003;37(5):413-20.
142. Garcias Da Silva LF, Nunes ML, Da Costa JC. Risk factors for developing epilepsy after neonatal seizures. Pediatr Neurol. 2004;30(4):271-7.
143. Penell PB. Antiepileptic drug pharmacokinetics during pregnancy and lactation. Neurology. 2003;61(69):35-42.
144. Yerby MS. Quality of life, epilepsy advances, and the evolving role of anticonvulsants in women with epilepsy. Neurology. 2000;55:S21-31.
145. Baumeister FAM. Epilepsy and pregnancy from the neuropaediatric perspective. Gynaekol Prax. 2003;27(3):425-31.
146. Gal P, Roop C, Robinson H, et al. Theophyllin induced seizures in accidentally overdosed neonates. Pediatrics. 1980;65:547-9.
147. Aicardi J. Epilepsy in brain-injured children. Dev Med Child Neurol. 1990;32:191-202.

11 Oxygen Toxicity

R Bracci

INTRODUCTION

Although the toxic effects of oxygen have been known since the end of the 19th century,[1] the first evidence of a relationship between oxygen toxicity and neonatal diseases emerged in the early 1950s when retinopathy was observed in premature infants breathing high concentrations of oxygen.[2] At about the same time, the red cells of newborns were demonstrated to have increased susceptibility to oxygen damage.[3] This made it clear that oxygen species were particularly toxic to neonatal red cells which were damaged by exposure to H_2O_2 and substances producing H_2O_2.

Great advances in our understanding of toxic effects of oxygen were made in the years that followed, when oxygen toxicity was recognized to be due to the development of reactive oxygen species (ROS). The main ROS are the superoxide anion (O_2^{-}), H_2O_2, lipid peroxide (LOOH), peroxyl radicals $RO_2^{\cdot-}$ and the hydroxyl radical (OH·). Other important radicals are the highly reactive electron delocalized phenoxyl radical ($C_6H_5O\cdot$) and nitric oxide radicals (NO·).[4-8]

The term ROS includes free radicals, which are atoms or molecules with one or more unpaired electrons. Free radicals may react with other radicals, the unpaired electrons forming a covalent bond. The resulting molecule may decompose other molecules into toxic products. Free radicals may react with nonradical molecules in free radical chain reactions, which are stopped by antioxidant enzymes or protein reactions. $O_2^{\cdot-}$ is the precursor of most ROS and a mediator in oxidative chain reactions. Dismutation of $O_2^{\cdot-}$ by superoxide dismutase (SOD) produces H_2O_2 which in turn may be fully reduced to water by glutathione peroxidase (GSH-Px) and catalase (Cat) or partially reduced to OH·. The latter reaction is called the Fenton-Haber Weiss reaction and is catalyzed by reduced transition metals.[4-9] ROS are involved in the following reactions:

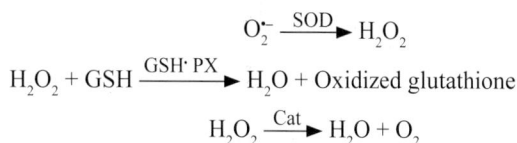

$$O_2^{\cdot-} \xrightarrow{\text{SOD}} H_2O_2$$

$$H_2O_2 + GSH \xrightarrow{\text{GSH· PX}} H_2O + \text{Oxidized glutathione}$$

$$H_2O_2 \xrightarrow{\text{Cat}} H_2O + O_2$$

A deficiency of scavenging reduces the detoxification of H_2O_2 and $O_2^{\cdot-}$ and increases the formation of OH· by metal activation following the Fenton reaction:[4-9]

$$Fe^{2+} + H_2O_2 \longrightarrow Fe^{3+} + OH\cdot + OH^-$$

There is no specific scavenger for this radical: once released, OH reacts with lipoproteins, cell membranes, lipids, proteins, DNA, amino acids and other molecules. OH· is one of the strongest oxidants in nature and may damage tissues.

Oxidative tissue damage may be mediated by reactive nitroxide species.[9-11] The reaction product of NO^{-} and $O_2^{\cdot-}$ is the unstable molecule peroxynitrite ($ONOO^-$) which is regarded as highly reactive and hence destructive, although it seems to be trapped by cellular antioxidants and other factors at low concentration.[12-14]

It is important to remember that free radical reactions are a normal occurrence in living organisms and ROS are not necessarily toxic. Vascular tone appears to be modulated by the contrasting effects of NO· and $O_2^{\cdot-}$.[15] Production of $O_2^{\cdot-}$ by phagocytes is an important defense mechanism, but extracellular release of free radicals by activated phagocytes is itself a mechanism of tissue damage during inflammation.[5,16] Oxidative balance, therefore, is an intriguing question, and much recent research has increased our knowledge of the relations between ROS and human diseases.

OXIDATIVE STRESS

An excess of ROS, as well as reactive nitrogen species (RNS), in relation to detoxification capacity is called *oxidative stress*, a term used to describe imbalance between oxidants and antioxidants that is a potential cause of damage. If oxidative stress is mild, cell defenses may increase by a complex mechanism which generally involves enhanced gene expression of ROS scavenging activities.[6,17,18] Severe oxidative stress is generally followed by cell injury which may proceed to necrosis or apoptosis.[4-6] The involvement of oxidative stress in the mechanism of apoptosis has been extensively studied.[19-22]

The pathological conditions leading to oxidative stress are extremely complex. It is, therefore, necessary to identify the biochemical basis of oxidative stress in order to prevent or treat oxygen toxicity.[4-7,9,23]

Reactive Oxygen Species Production

Two main sites have been recognized as sources of ROS: the extracellular compartment with phagocyte activation and the endogenous source with mitochondrial function.[13] Both these sites are important in the pathogenesis of fetal and neonatal diseases.

Intracellular and extracellular production of ROS is provided by activated phagocytes.[24] ROS released inside phagocytes during infection and cytokine production can also alter the extracellular oxidative balance and harm tissues since the cells undergo an efflux of $O_2^{\cdot-}$.[25] However, opsonization and activation of phagocytes is also known to occur during the hypoxanthine-xanthine oxidase reaction and, therefore during hypoxia-reoxygenation.[26]

Mitochondria are the primary source of superoxide, and it has been demonstrated that mitochondrial dysfunction is responsible for increased superoxide release. The mitochondrial electron transport chain contains redox centers which may leak electrons to oxygen, constituting the primary source of $O_2^{\cdot-}$ in most tissues.[9] Research into myocardial physiology has demonstrated that under normal conditions, mitochondrial electron transport reduces 95% of oxygen to H_2O by tetravalent reduction without any free radical intermediates and the remaining 5% is reduced by the univalent pathway in which free radicals are produced.[27,28]

During acidosis and hypoxia ischemia, mitochondrial dysfunction occurs and ROS production increases while antioxidant defenses are depleted and metal ions may play a role in generating $OH^{\cdot}$.[29] ROS production by mitochondria may increase during hypoxia ischemia as a result of dramatic increases in cytosolic calcium concentrations. Since mitochondrial enzymes, such as pyruvate dehydrogenase and α-oxyglutarate dehydrogenase, are normally regulated by Ca cycling across the inner mitochondrial membrane, when intracellular Ca increases, cycling may become excessive and lead to increased ROS production, while structural alterations to the inner mitochondrial membrane may be followed by mitochondrial respiratory chain disorganization with further increases in ROS.[30-33] During asphyxia, $OH^{\cdot}$ production also increases as a result of release of iron from safe sites.[27] Acidosis may, therefore, enhance $OH^{\cdot}$ mediated tissue injury.[34]

When oxygen is restored to ischemic tissue, free radical reperfusion injury occurs by several mechanisms including the xanthine-xanthine oxidase reaction.[27,35] Reperfusion injury is considered a major source of oxidative stress and has been reported in heart, kidney, liver lung and intestine, particularly in necrotizing enterocolitis (NEC).[27,36]

Hyperoxia has been demonstrated to be associated with increased mitochondrial production of $O_2^{\cdot-}$.[9] The rate of mitochondrial $O_2^{\cdot-}$ production increases linearly with increasing oxygen concentration.[37] Under normobaric hyperoxic conditions, the only organs affected by ROS formation are the lungs since they are the only ones in direct contact with atmospheric oxygen.[9] However, under hyperbaric conditions other tissues become exposed to a hyperoxic environment and increased ROS formation has been found in other organs.[9] Other sources of ROS include catecholamines, prostaglandins and xenobiotics previously reduced by certain enzymes.[4-6]

Endothelial dysfunction caused by oxidative stress and leading to vascular disease has been extensively investigated.[38-41] The endothelium is normally protected against ROS; however, overproduction may occur via mitochondrial reactions, xanthine-xanthine oxidase reaction, vascular as well as phagocytic NAD(P)H oxidases and toxin-induced reactions. There is also growing body of evidence linking blood cell and endothelial cell interactions in enhanced production of ROS.[38-42] Oxidative stress to endothelium may be due to ROS or reactive NO mediated peroxynitrite.[11] $O_2^{\cdot-}$ therefore, promotes tissue damage by reacting with NO, reducing NO bioavailability and producing toxic $ONOO^-$.[38-41] The presence of nonprotein-bound iron (NPBI) during acidosis, hypoxia and infections causes $OH^{\cdot}$ release and may exacerbate ROS mediated tissue injury.[10,19,41,43] The resulting vascular endothelial dysfunction elicits a number of maladaptive phenomena that impair normal healthy blood vessels. The normal vascular environment is lost, exposing the lumen to the possibility of thrombosis, while the decrease in NO production and enhanced endothelin 1 production lead to vasoconstriction[38] which also seems to be enhanced by inhibition of PGI.[43] Endothelial injury due to oxidative stress has been demonstrated to play a key role in coagulation disorders by enhancing procoagulant activity.[44,45]

Antioxidants

The antioxidant system can be classified in two major groups: (1) enzyme activities and (2) low-molecular-weight antioxidants.[13] The enzyme group is represented in the reactions mentioned above. Other important antioxidant enzymes are thioredoxin reductase and glutathione transferase (GSH-T). It is important that $O_2^{\cdot-}$ dismutation be associated with balanced H_2O_2 detoxification. It has been suggested that overexpression of SOD may lead to deleterious effects if not balanced by GSH-Px.[46,47] This observation underlines the key role of GSH in protecting against oxidative stress.[48] The enzyme-based antioxidant system includes extracellular SOD, the only extracellular scavenger of $O_2^{\cdot-}$ which also plays a key role in scavenging $O_2^{\cdot-}$ produced in the extracellular compartment by phagocytes, endothelium and other mechanisms.[49]

The low-molecular-weight antioxidant group contains a large number of compounds which are capable of preventing oxidative damage by direct or indirect interactions with ROS. The effects of these molecules are complex, since the same molecule may have prooxidant or antioxidant effects depending on bioavailability, metabolism and tissue properties as well as interactions between enzymatic and nonenzymatic antioxidants. Ascorbic acid may have prooxidant and antioxidant properties.[50] Coenzyme Q is a source of $O_2^{\cdot-}$ when partially reduced and an antioxidant when fully reduced.[51] One of the most studied antioxidants is α-tocopherol, but competition between different forms and their uptake and the synergistic or inhibitory role of other compounds are not yet understood. Furthermore, non-antioxidant effects of α-tocopherol have been demonstrated.[52] Iron binding proteins have major antioxidant activity, protecting against metal induced $OH^{\cdot}$ production.[53]

REACTIVE OXYGEN SPECIES IN FETUS AND NEONATE

Excessive oxidative stress and particularly $OH^{\cdot}$ can impair cell function, and induce apoptosis in rapidly growing structures. An oxidized state can also be beneficial since ROS may activate transcription factors and promote fetal development, but both of which are sensitive to uncontrolled oxidative stress.[54] The effects of ROS are secondary to its direct toxicity and indirect effects, such as vasoconstriction in the lung or systemic circulation.[55,56] Another important condition of oxidative stress produced by $O_2^{\cdot-}$ and NO derived free radicals is impaired placental function, which may lead to fetal growth retardation.[57]

Oxidative stress in the fetus and newborn may result from decreased antioxidants, increased ROS or both. The fetus has a lower antioxidant capacity than older babies and adults. Free radical scavenger enzyme activities and many other components of the antioxidant system are low. Studies in various animals have shown that the main ROS detoxifying enzymes, GSH-Px, Cat and SOD, increase during intrauterine life.[58,59] At least in the lungs and liver, detoxifying reactions ruled by SOD, GSH-Px, and catalase are fully expressed only after birth.[58,59] Scavenger activities involving glutathione transferase have been studied in the fetus and newborn and seem to vary widely in different animal species.[60]

In the human newborn, the scavenger enzyme activities were first investigated in erythrocytes: Cat and GSH-Px were found deficient in most of infants, and SOD only in some.[46,61,63] SOD activity is reported to increase in the lungs of the human fetus during intrauterine life.[64,65] Normal values of GSH-Px have been reported in leukocytes of full-term newborns.[66]

Nonenzyme antioxidant factors are reported to be lower in the fetus and newborn than in adults and older babies,[67-69] partially because of deficient placental transfer of some antioxidants.[54] However, antioxidant capacity of neonatal plasma is controversial since peroxy radical trapping capacity and chain-breaking antioxidants, the same or higher than in adults, have been observed.[70,71] These differences can be ascribed to the study methods, the components of antioxidant capacity tested and the timing of blood sampling. Infant condition also plays a role since asphyxia and acidosis may reduce certain components of antioxidant power.[72] Plasma antioxidant capacity is not correlated with any neonatal pathology. On the contrary, other markers suggest ROS toxicity in neonates.[71,73-75] Irrespective of total antioxidant capacity, a deficiency in particular antioxidant factors, such as ceruloplasmin and transferrin, may play an important role in neonatal susceptibility to oxidative stress and particularly to metal-induced OH⁻ production.[76,77] Low concentrations of transferrin have been found in neonates, especially premature ones, and high plasma levels of ascorbic acid may create a condition of risk due to the prooxidant effect of iron. The finding of increased bleomycin-detectable iron in premature and some full-term infants is evidence of the real risk of increased prooxidant effects of iron in neonates.[78] High saturation of transferrin is, therefore, probably a risk factor for oxidative stress. It is generally accepted that non-transferrin bound iron (NTBI) is a pathological manifestation, and it is extremely rare in adults, in whom even the presence of NPBI in iron overload is uncommon.[79] Levels of NPBI in plasma of newborns are correlated with other markers of oxidative stress and high plasma NPBI has been found in hypoxic newborns with poor outcome.[80] Compensatory protection against oxidative stress in neonates is demonstrated by high activity of glutathione reductase (GR) and high recycling of glutathione (GSH) in red cells.[81] However, several observations have shown that preterm infants have lower and age-related plasma concentrations of GSH and higher concentrations of GSSG than adults.[82] This is interesting since a low GSH/GSSG ratio is a reliable index of generalized oxidative stress.[83] Reliable markers such as F2-isoprostanes, allantoin and the oxidized form of Coenzyme Q provide further evidence of oxidative stress in neonates.[72,84,85] Oxidative stress in neonates has also been demonstrated by higher values of Coenzyme Q120 in those born by vaginal delivery than by elective caesarean section.[86]

Oxidative stress is involved in tissue damage induced by infection and sepsis. Although there is general agreement that neonatal phagocytes, and especially those of premature infants have abnormalities of various functions,[87] active neonatal secretion of proinflammatory cytokines suggests a very complex situation in which oxidative stress following infection may be more dangerous in newborns, especially if premature, than in adults.[88]

The high levels of peroxides found in cord blood of fetuses with asphyxia are in line with the hypothesis of high ROS production in the placenta and umbilical structures during hypoxia.[89-91] However, it should be remembered that the oxidative balance of the fetus is not the same as that of the neonate because of the peroxidase content of the placenta.[92,93]

The first condition suspected to be responsible for increased oxygen toxicity, namely hyperoxia, has recently been demonstrated to cause the oxidative stress responsible for lung injury and possibly generalized tissue damage.[94] The definition of hyperoxia

in newborns is closely related to oxygen requirements during the first hours of life, when the baby is suddenly exposed to higher oxygen tension than in the uterus. The oxidative stress recorded in animal experiments with hyperoxia could occur in neonates with oxygen tensions lower than previously considered.[94]

Endothelial injury by ROS following asphyxia or infection may lead to vasoconstriction and coagulation disorders, which are particularly harmful to newborns, due to the procoagulative state of fetus and neonate.[45]

Links between ROS and endothelial cell injury seem to play a role in the development of preeclampsia since increased oxidative stress has been demonstrated in preeclamptic woman.[95,96] Although the pathogenesis of preeclampsia is poorly understood, it seems that oxidative stress plays an important role.[97]

ROS are involved in many diseases of newborns and adults such as necrotizing enterocolitis, renal failure and septic shock. Neonatal conditions of particular interest concern red cells, lung, retina and brain.

RED CELLS

Several observations in animal and human erythrocytes have demonstrated that release of free radicals inside red cells may affect membrane structure during oxidation of hemoglobin.[98,99] Membrane structure may also be damaged by ROS uptake from the extracellular medium where they may arise from ischemia-reperfusion, phagocyte activation, endothelial metabolism, hyperoxia, lipoprotein peroxidation and other sources.[100-101] Uptake of free radicals by red cells can be regarded as a mechanism protecting the tissues from oxidative injury, since the high antioxidant enzyme activities of erythrocytes can scavenge extracellular ROS. However, excessive oxidative stress leads to hemolysis followed by free iron and free radical release, and possible tissue damage.[102] In newborns, antioxidant activities are generally lower than in adults, and seem to be even lower in premature infants.[61-63,103-105] Activities such as GSH-Px increase rapidly in the first days, presumably as a result of increased exposure to ROS.[106,107] Exposure of red cells to ROS after birth is also demonstrated by a decrease in GSH-T in the first days of life in response to ROS production.[108] Very active GSH recycling occurs in normal newborns, but asphyxia and acidosis have been reported to depress it, as well as ATP.[81] GSH recycling also seems deficient in infants with RDS and chronic lung disease (CLD).[109] Chemiluminescence assays have demonstrated higher ROS production in newborns than adults.[110] This observation is in line with the demonstration of high lipid peroxidation and decreased Coenzyme Q10.[111] The red cells of newborns appear to be more susceptible to the toxic effects of oxidative stress than those of adults.[112] Besides low scavenger enzyme activities, newborn red cells have other characteristics, such as lipid content and composition, which predispose them to oxidative stress.[112] Vitamin E levels are not only much lower in the neonatal than the adult red cell, but requirements of the vitamin are also higher, as shown by increased recycling.[113] ROS are generated in red cells not only under pathological but also under normal conditions.[114,115] Animal studies have demonstrated the key role of oxidative stress caused by intraerythrocyte iron release in a reactive form and hydroxyl radical production in the development of membrane protein damage.[102] Oxidative cross-linking of membrane proteins can produce clustering of the major erythrocyte membrane spanning protein band 3.[116,117] The clusters provide recognition sites for antibodies against senescent cells and trigger their removal from circulation. In the absence of efficient protection by antioxidant factors, oxidative stress, therefore, appears to be responsible for release of iron in a reactive form, predisposing red cells to hemolysis through the formation of senescence antigen.[117] Paradoxically, recent observations show that autoxidation of hemoglobin may occur in vitro at low oxygen tension.[118]

Studies in newborns have shown interesting analogies between experimental and clinical observations. The free iron content of red cells of newborns is higher than that of adults and is significantly correlated with pH and base deficit as well as with plasma lipid peroxide products, expressed by malondialdehyde (MDA) concentrations.[119] Incubation of newborn and adult red cells in vitro showed higher iron release in the former under aerobic and anaerobic conditions. It is interesting that during anaerobic incubation, increased O_2 production, free iron release and senescence antigen production showed the highest significant differences between adults and neonates.[110,120] In vitro studies show that incubated neonatal red cells release iron in reactive form. This iron is recovered in the incubation medium at the end of incubation, apparently irrespective of hemolysis, demonstrating that reactive iron may be released by stressed red cells and diffuses outside the cell.[121] This finding suggests that oxidative stress in erythrocytes may be involved in the increase in NPBI in plasma of asphyxiated neonates. In conclusion, several reports suggest that acidosis and hypoxia may generate red cell damage via ROS.

PULMONARY OXYGEN TOXICITY

Oxygen toxicity is particularly harmful for the lungs. The mechanism of damage is complex. Lung injury may be caused directly by ROS production in response to hyperoxia or indirectly by ROS due to phagocyte activation and inflammation. The two mechanisms seem to be integrated.

Chronic lung disease, a severe complication of prematurity, was long thought to be due to high concentrations of oxygen in inspired air and barotrauma. ROS are now generally accepted to be largely responsible for lung injury in preterm infants since several studies using different methods have demonstrated products of ROS reactions in premature infants with CDL.[122-127] The particular toxicity of ROS in the immature lung is due to the low antioxidant capacity of premature infants, which does not increase rapidly as in the full-term lung, as well as to the possibly high toxicity of ROS in rapidly developing tissues.[128] Increased production of ROS under certain conditions may also play a role. The main sources of ROS production in the immature lung are ischemia-reperfusion, phagocytosis and increased mitochondrial activity mainly due to hyperoxia. Mitochondrial oxidative stress following hyperoxia has been demonstrated by a decrease of intramitochondrial GSH/GSSG redox status.[129] High inspired oxygen fraction (FiO_2) may be responsible for lung injury and high lipid peroxidation, as demonstrated by high F2-isoprostane levels in the lungs of animals exposed to high oxygen concentrations.[130] Effects of hyperoxia in the lung and a close relationship between oxidative stress and inflammation have been demonstrated. Magnetic resonance studies have confirmed the previously reported experimental data on the consequences of hyperoxia in the lungs of premature newborn

animals, namely edema, congestion, immune cell infiltration and decreased number of alveoli per square meter.[131,132] Prolonged moderate hyperoxia induces airway hyperresponsiveness and histological changes similar to those of CLD.[133] Increased type IV collagenase in bronchoalveolar lavage suggests a role of this factor in lung damage and particularly in disruption of the extracellular matrix. It is interesting that injury produced by oxidative stress involves matrix metalloproteinases (MMP) and tissue inhibitor of matrix metalloproteinase (TIMP) which are also involved in infections.[134] Increased MMP-8 and MMP9 associated with decreased TIMP have been reported in amniotic fluid during infection and chorioamnionitis, a condition frequently associated with development of CLD.[88] These findings are in line with reports of phagocyte activation and increased cytokine production. The finding of a large number of neutrophils and high concentrations of interleukin-8 and leukotrienes in bronchopulmonary lavage of infants with severe CLD demonstrates the role of inflammatory reactions and ROS production in the development of this disease.[135,136]

The toxic effects of ROS on the lungs appear to be due to iron-mediated OH· release.[125] This radical alters surfactant composition and causes decreased surfactant production by injuring type II pneumocytes.[125,137] Peroxynitrite formation from O_2 and NO· can also cause lung injury.[138] ROS can modify production of vasoactive substances by the endothelium, and this might be important in CLD since increased endothelin-1 has been demonstrated to be associated with inflammation and lung disease.[139] Oxidative stress has been studied in the lungs of premature rats and a complex orchestra of genes involved in inflammation, coagulation, fibrinolysis, extracellular matrix turnover, cell cycle, signal transduction and alveolar enlargement have been found to be affected by oxidative stress.[140] The combined effect of oxygen and inflammation on the origin of CLD also emerges from studies of bronchopulmonary lavage and tracheal aspirate in which increased levels of markers of oxidative stress, such as protein carbonyls and myeloperoxidase activity in neutrophils of premature infants who developed CLD, have been found.[141,142] Increased lipid peroxidation in plasma of premature infants with CLD and periventricular leukomalacia has been reported.[78] Conditions of oxidative stress possibly responsible for CLD and retinopathy have also been reported.[143] These observations suggest a combined effect of oxidative stress in the pathogenesis of CLD, brain damage and retinopathy.

RETINOPATHY

Although the origins of retinopathy of prematurity (ROP) are multifactorial, the role of oxygen toxicity, which was first detected half a century ago, has been confirmed by experimental and clinical studies. ROS have been recognized to play an important role, particularly in the first stage of eye injury when hyperoxia seems to affect the vascular endothelium arresting normal blood vessel development.[144] Hyperoxia also seems to inhibit vascular endothelium growth factor and involvement of oxidative stress in vascular obliteration caused by apoptotic vascular endothelial cells has also been suggested.[144] The hypothesis of a complex mechanism of oxidative stress in the development of ROS is also suggested by the observation of a role of iron intake,[145] decreased GSH/GSSG ratio[146] and NPBI[147] in patients with ROP. Morphological abnormalities of ROP, such as "gap junctions", are an expression of lipoperoxidation, which has been demonstrated in the retina as a result of free radical release.[148]

A relationship between free radical release, induced retinal injury and cyclooxygenase pathway activity has been reported.[149] Abnormalities of retinal vasculature have demonstrated that reversal vasoconstriction by dilator prostaglandin during oxidative stress in newborns may facilitate neovascularization of the retina of premature animals.[150] The role of peroxides in inducing abnormal retinal vasculature has also been demonstrated by the marked vasoconstriction which these molecules produce in the retinal vasculature of premature animals.[151]

BRAIN INJURY

Reactive oxygen species may affect the brain by different interacting systems involving membrane damage, astrocyte dysfunction, abnormalities of n-methyl-D-aspartate, receptors and particularly increased intracellular calcium and mitochondrial dysfunction.[152,153] ROS may also cause indirect injury by inducing cerebrovascular spasms.[154] Iron-induced OH production may occur during brain injury because the low transferrin content of cerebrospinal fluid (CSF) is saturated by iron released from cells with a high iron content, and free and unbound iron becomes available for the Fenton reaction.[152]

The brain is low in catalase and has moderate amounts of SOD and GSH-Px; its membrane lipids are rich in polyunsaturated fatty acids which are sensitive to oxidative stress.[152] In the fetus and newborn, protection against ROS seems to be even poorer than in adults, especially in the glia, and sensitivity to oxidative stress seems particularly high in the first hours of life.[152-157] The first mechanism of brain damage due to ROS to be investigated was that of ischemia-reperfusion and hypoxanthine xanthine oxidase reaction.[158] The importance of this mechanism emerged from the finding of high concentrations of hypoxanthine in blood and CSF during hypoxia, and from experimental data demonstrating inhibition of ROS release by allopurinol, an inhibitor of xanthine oxidase.[159] However, Delivoria et al.[160] demonstrated that hypoxia results in brain cell membrane damage as shown by increased membrane lipid peroxidation and decreased Na^+/K^+-ATPase activity, irrespective of reoxygenation. High levels of isoprostane-8, another marker of oxidative stress, also suggest responsibility of ROS in brain damage during asphyxia,[161] while electron spin resonance spectroscopy has shown that tissue hypoxia results in increased free radical generation in the cerebral cortex.[162] Levels of conjugated dienes and fluorescent compounds, markers of lipid peroxidation, have also been detected in the brain of newborn animals with asphyxia, particularly during recovery from single or repeated episodes.[163] Histochemical studies of brains of neonatal rats after hypoxic ischemic injury demonstrated that iron increases rapidly in the first 24 hours in regions of ischemic injury, suggesting oxidative stress induced by OH produced via the Fenton reaction.[164] The effects of ROS are also due to brain hypoxia-induced generation of NO free radicals; peroxynitrite is formed when O_2 predominate over scavenger system and NO increases as an effects of increased nitric oxide synthase.[153]

However, during ischemia, a number of metabolic changes occur and prostaglandin metabolism and dopamine oxidation have been found to have a role in the release of ROS.[165] The recent availability of reliable markers of oxidative stress, such as isoprostanes and particularly F2-isoprostane and 8-isoprostane,

has provided evidence of involvement of oxidative stress in the development of cerebral white matter injury, since these compounds were detected in the CSF of premature infants with white matter damage.[161] Further confirmation of this involvement was the finding of increased carbonyls, a marker of protein oxidation in CSF of these neonates.[161] It is interesting that none of the observed infants had infections and their CSF, unlike in meningitis, did not contain chlorotyrosine, a marker of leukocyte oxidant activity.[166] Indirect evidence of the responsibility of ROS in brain damage of asphyxiated infants comes from the observation of NPBI in CSF.[167] Increased NPBI resulting from asphyxia or hemorrhage has an important role in the development of brain injury, one reason being that early differentiating oligodendroglia is poor in ROS detoxification systems and enables a peroxide accumulation and OH generation by the Fenton reaction.[152,168]

Several observations also suggest ROS involvement in brain injury during hyperoxia.[169,170] Decreases in cerebral blood flow in response to O_2 administration have been detected in human studies[170] and reduced blood flow was observed in premature newborns treated with high O_2 concentrations.[171] However, animals kept in hyperoxia showed a reduction in blood flow which was not statistically significant.[172]

Considering the interaction between ROS and inflammatory mediators, oxidative stress to the endothelium may play an important role in the development of brain damage.[173]

Relationships between ROS and brain damage are suggested by the link between increased markers of oxidative stress and clinical observations.

Oxidative stress in premature and full-term newborns with asphyxia is demonstrated by high plasma levels of lipid hydroperoxides and evidence of the MDA reaction.[174,175] Markers of oxidative stress, such as high-performance liquid chromatography (HPLC) determinations of MDA, 4-hydroxynonenal, total hydroperoxide and carbonyl groups, are significantly higher in asphyxiated babies.[174-177] It is interesting that markers of oxidative stress, such as total hydroperoxides, remain high for weeks in sick babies.[177] Isoprostanes, a reliable marker of oxidative stress, have been reported to be higher in cases of fetal distress.[178]

High levels of NPBI in plasma of asphyxiated newborn are evidence of a role of ROS in the development of brain injury in hypoxia-ischemia. The reports of Dorrepal et al.[179] indicated that this occurrence, which is peculiar to neonates, is associated with severe brain damage. Buonocore et al.[180] recently tested the predictivity of traditional indicators of brain damage in relation to neurodevelopmental outcome. They demonstrated that plasma NPBI is the most reliable marker of severe outcome in asphyxiated newborns.[180]

MARKERS OF OXIDATIVE STRESS

If oxidative damage contributes significantly to neonatal pathology, it is essential to be able to accurately measure oxidative stress. Two basic approaches have been suggested: (1) attempting to trap ROS and measure levels of trapped molecules; (2) measuring the oxidative damage done by ROS.[181] Other frequently used approaches are inaccurate.[181] Erythrocyte enzyme activities, which were the first indication of the low antioxidant resistance of newborns, are not fully reliable since the enzyme activities of red cells are age dependent and values may be expression of young or old red cell populations.[181] Measurement of total antioxidants usually involves major contributions from urate, ascorbate, bilirubin and albumin-SH groups which are variable and may not accurately reflect antioxidant power.[181] However, plasma antioxidants, if measured in conjunction with other parameters, may be useful in the detection of imbalance between free radicals and antioxidants. Chromatographic profiles of antioxidants in human plasma can provide indications of single component deficiencies which may be useful to distinguish particular deficiencies or increased consumption of a factor involved in a particular disease.[182]

Lipid oxidation is a complex process and commonly used methods, such as thiobarbituric acid (TBA), are questionable. The TBA test should not be used because most TBA-reactive material in the human body is not related to lipid peroxidation.[181] Measurement of MDA by HPLC is more indicative of lipid peroxidation, although MDA is only one of the many aldehydes formed during this process.[181] It is more logical to measure 4-hydroxynonenal.[181] The best biomarker of lipid peroxidation is isoprostanes which are specific end-products of peroxidation of polyunsaturated fatty acids.[181,183] Most work has been done with F2-isoprostane which arises from arachidonic acid peroxidation. Neuroprostane or F4-isoprostane has also been measured.[183] They are best measured by mass spectrometry.[184] It is important to remember that isoprostanes are rapidly metabolized so that increased values may indicate slower metabolism and not increased production.[181]

Measurement of ethane and pentane in expired air were among the first methods of detecting of oxidative stress in asphyxiated neonates.[185] These assays have the advantage of being noninvasive and independent of the complex matrix of blood.[186] However, variations in the methods make it difficult to compare populations.[187] Simultaneous measurement of pentane and MDA has been carried out to asses oxidative stress. In studies on human hyperoxia, increased values of both markers were found but no correlation between pentane and MDA was observed, probably because they are metabolized differently.[188]

Profiles of aldehydes pentanal, hexanal, 2-hexanal, heptanal, 2-heptanal, 2-octenal, 2-nonenal and 4-hydroxynonenal formed during autoxidation of fatty acids, such as oleic, linoleic, α-linoleic, α-linoleic and arachidonic, seem to improve the sensitivity of detection.[189]

Determination of protein carbonyl concentrations provides information regarding protein involvement in ROS reactions. The carbonyl assay as applied to tissues and body fluids measures the average extent of protein modification.[181] The use of proteomics to identify specifically oxidized proteins appears to be a promising method.[190] Research on plasma of newborns has shown interesting selectively oxidized proteins during asphyxia.[191]

Total hydroperoxides represents a measure of overall oxidative stress, given that they are the intermediate oxidative products of lipids, peptides and amino acids.[176]

Percentages of oxidized forms of coenzyme Q-10 have also been used to demonstrate oxidative stress in asphyxiated newborns.[72]

A major marker of oxidative stress is the GSH/GSSG ratio, which directly reflects alteration of intracellular redox status.[192] GSH is a cofactor of GSH-Px and also has the antioxidant effect of binding Cu^{2+}, contributing to delivery of copper to the apoprotein of copper enzymes and decreasing free metal available for the Fenton reaction. Filomeni et al.[192] showed a relationship between intracellular GSH levels and mitochondrial-dependent apoptotic

pathways. Under oxidative stress, GSSG may be produced at a high rate and extruded from cells into the extracellular milieu.[192] Since blood glutathione may reflect GSH status in other less accessible tissues, measurement of GSH and GSSG in blood has been considered an essential index of overall oxidative status and a useful indicator of risk of disease.

The GSH/GSSG ratio has been used as a measure of oxidative stress in neonates. Decreased ratios were observed in premature infants with severe RDS and newborns resuscitated with 100% O_2.[193,194] Lower GSH/GSSG ratios were found in very low birth weight infants even when they were breathing room air.[195]

Levels of nitrotyrosine have been reported to be a marker of $ONOO^-$ production resulting from phagocyte activation in inflammatory processes.[196] Therefore, nitrotyrosine can also be used as a marker of oxidative stress since total nitration is consistent with amplified cell levels of O_2 in the presence of NO and CO_2.[197]

Allantoin can be measured in body fluids, and its plasma levels are high under conditions of oxidative stress.[198] Assays in urine give reliable results.[199]

8-Hydroxydeoxyguanosine (8-OHdG) has been reported to be a reliable a marker of oxidative stress. This molecule can be assayed in urine and has been done in newborns. While no differences in relation to gestational age have been reported by some authors,[200] others[201] observed a negative correlation between 8-OHdG and gestational age, confirming that premature infants are more subject to oxidative stress.

Plasma levels of NPBI appear to be a reliable marker of oxidative stress and close relationships between these levels and plasma carbonyls have been reported.[197] At least in neonates, both assays can be regarded as markers of potential risk of pathology due to oxygen toxicity.

Isolevuglandins (structural isomers and stereoisomers of cyclooxygenase-generated levoglandins) may be formed via free radical-mediated pathways and have been proposed as a sensor of lipid peroxidation initiated by myeloperoxidase.[202]

PREVENTION AND THERAPY
Avoiding Oxidative Stress

Reactive oxygen species are normally produced in living organisms. Their properties and complex role in the development of diseases make prevention and antioxidant therapy very difficult in newborns as well as in adults. Obviously, avoidance of conditions such as asphyxia, hyperoxia and retinal light exposure, under which excessive free radical release occurs, are the best defense against development of imbalances in prooxidant and antioxidant factors in the neonate. It is also important to remember that infections and particularly sepsis may be a severe source of oxidative stress. Frequent reports of NPBI in plasma of neonates suggest that indiscriminate iron supplementation should be avoided.

The concept of optimal oxygenation of newborns has recently been revised in order to clarify whether the optimal oxygen saturation unanimously accepted for normal infants and adults is also the best for sick neonates especially if premature. The relationship between hemoglobin oxygen saturation, risk of oxidative stress and oxygen toxicity is still a problem. Even a recent Cochrane review failed to define the target range for maintaining blood oxygen levels in preterm/low birth weight infants.[203] This is presumably due to the complex mechanism of oxygen toxicity which may be expressed at different percentages of O_2 saturation under different conditions. Conventional indications suggest that optimal oxygen tension should be maintained between 50 mm Hg and 70 mm Hg.[204] High O_2 saturation seems to be necessary for infants with CLD and infants with prethreshold retinopathy.[205] However, in view of susceptibility of some neonates to oxidative stress, it has been suggested that oxygen saturation maintained within physiological limits could result in moderate hyperoxia that could generate an excess of ROS. Experimental studies in animals in the first 24 hours of life demonstrated a threshold of oxygen-restricted metabolism at $PaO_2 = 40$ Torr.[206] Shulze et al.[207] did not observe signs of mismatch between systemic oxygen delivery and demand in low birth weight infants kept at O_2 93–96% and 89–92% saturation. A significant decrease in CLD and ROP without any differences in mortality were observed in extremely low birth weight infants kept at less than 95% O_2 saturation compared to those kept at more than 95%.[208] Important indications on the use of oxygen were recently reported by Cow et al.[209] in a 5-year study in a tertiary neonatal center where oxygen therapy was adjusted to optimize neonatal care and decrease the incidence of ROP. They recommended avoidance of repeated increase and decrease in FiO$_2$ in response to the oxygen saturation monitor and maintenance of oxygen saturation within "acceptable" limits. They also recommended an alarm setting for oxygen saturation below 85% and above 93% for newborns under 32 weeks of age. More recently, comparison of two populations of high risk newborns kept at O_2 saturations of 88–98% and 70–90% showed a significant reduction in ROP in the group at lower O_2 saturation but no differences in mortality or poor outcome.[210,211]

Hyperoxia and oxidative stress may occur during neonatal resuscitation. In an attempt to avoid the risk of tissue damage caused by ROS in the first hours of life, when susceptibility to oxidative stress is particularly high, the effects of reduction of O_2 were investigated. Some animal studies demonstrated identical outcome variables, including blood pressure, lung hemodynamics, acid-base status, cerebral blood flow and brain oxygenation whether resuscitation was done with room air or 100% oxygen.[212] In other experiments with animals subjected to ischemia and hypoxia, reoxygenation with 100% oxygen was followed by better restoration of microcirculation but no difference in biochemical markers of brain injury.[213] Comparison of short and long duration of oxygen treatment after cerebral asphyxia in newborn piglets confirmed the efficacy of reoxygenation with room air.[214] Potential risks associated with resuscitation with 100% oxygen are suggested by the observation of increased production of ROS with respect to room air.[215,216] Clinical studies have demonstrated no differences in short-term outcome between newborns resuscitated with room air and 100% oxygen.[217,218] The same results were observed in a follow-up at 18 months and 24 months.[219] Vento et al.[194] demonstrated that room air resuscitation was associated with significantly less oxidative stress. It is important to note that they demonstrated increased oxidative stress following resuscitation with 100% oxygen was demonstrated by the sensitive GSH/GSSG ratio which is a marker of generalized oxidative stress.[192] The satisfactory results of room air resuscitation in terms of outcome and avoidance of oxidative stress were recently confirmed by the same authors.[220] A reduction in mortality and no evidence of harm were described

in a Cochrane review.[221] However, the authors concluded that there is insufficient evidence on which to recommend a policy of using room air over 100% oxygen or vice versa for resuscitation of newborns.[221] Although the guidelines do not discourage high FiO$_2$, it seems reasonable to conclude that 100% oxygen should not be used routinely.

Antioxidants

Much research has recently been carried out to find substances with antioxidant activity.[222] These substances can be divided into those decompartmentalizing metal complexes, those limiting ROS production, those modifying antiradical defenses and enhancing intracellular or extracellular antioxidant levels, those incorporating lipophilic antioxidant into membranes and those scavenging superoxide.[222]

Substances inhibiting phagocyte activation or xanthine oxidase and arachidonic acid metabolism, or decompartmentalizing free iron and making it available for the Fenton reaction, have also been investigated, together with those scavenging ROS directly or repairing ROS-induced membrane injury, like calcium antagonists and beta-blockers.

On the whole, the results obtained in newborns have been uncertain. Although substances such as ascorbate are considered to be antioxidants in vitro and in vivo, they may act as prooxidant factors by causing metal-induced release of ROS.[223] Several other antioxidant substances have been used in newborn animals and humans in an attempt to improve the worst prognosis of damage presumed to be due to ROS. Many, such as SOD, showed the same disadvantages in newborns as in adults.[224] Other drugs, such as allopurinol, have shown good results in animals,[225] but no advantages in human newborns, especially those with hypoxic ischemic encephalopathy.[226] Indomethacin, which has been shown to have antioxidant effects in humans, reduces the incidence and severity of intraventricular hemorrhage but, it is not known whether this effect is due to antioxidant activity.[227] Involvement of metal-induced ROS in brain damage suggested treatment with chelating agents. Desferrioxamine seemed to have a protective effect in animals which has not yet been demonstrated in humans.[228] No definite results have been obtained by retinol supplementation.[229] Among the antioxidants, melatonin has a special place since it has been reported to have several interesting effects such as enhancement of antioxidant enzyme activities and neutralization of H_2O_2 singlet oxygen and peroxynitrite.[230] Melatonin also appears to scavenge OH˙.[231] Administration of melatonin to neonates with RDS has been reported to lower concentrations of proinflammatory cytokines.[232] In septic newborns melatonin also lowers levels of oxidative markers such as MDA and 4-hydroxylalkenals and improves prognosis.[233]

Some drugs commonly used in neonatology, such as aminophylline, are reported to have antioxidant properties.[234] Vitamin E is a powerful, widely tested antioxidant and although no definite agreement has been reached on its use, interesting results have been reported even in human newborns. Analysis of nine randomized controlled trials of prophylactic use of vitamin E supplementation in very low birth weight infants showed no statistically significant reduction in the incidence of retinopathy and hemorrhage confined to the germinal matrix, although a significant reduction in the incidence of intraventricular hemorrhage was found.[235] Some formulations of vitamin E are poorly absorbed[236] and the metabolism and membrane distribution of the vitamin is uncertain; apart from this, there is no doubt about the effectiveness of α-tocopherol in protecting membranes and plasma lipoproteins from lipoperoxidation. In view of the potential activity of α-tocopherol and its proven deficiency in newborns, administration of vitamin E at the commonly recommended doses should be considered in any high risk neonates.[237,238] Doses from 10 mg/kg/day to 25 mg/kg/day in the first 3 days of life should protect premature infants in the first weeks[239] Serum levels should be monitored in order to avoid levels exceeding 3 mg/dL. Subsequently, human milk or formula should be sufficient to maintain adequate vitamin levels.[239] Conclusions of a recent Cochrane review are that vitamin E supplementation to preterm infants reduces the risk of intracranial hemorrhage but increases the risk of sepsis; in very low birth weight infants it seems to reduce the risk of retinopathy and blindness.[240] There is no evidence to support the use of vitamin E at high doses or the aim of keeping serum tocopherol levels above 3.5 mg/dL.[240]

Peroxidation products in stored lipid emulsions have been shown to increase lipid peroxidation in vivo in newborns and adults.[241] Since parenteral nutrition has been associated with increased formation of ROS, it is necessary to protect intralipid from light and add vitamins.[242] However, adaptation to factors responsible for oxidative stress has been demonstrated by Pitkanen et al.[242] who found attenuated lipid peroxidation in preterm infants after repeated doses of intravenous lipids.

Micronutrients also play a role in protection against oxidative stress. Selenium is part of the GSH-Px molecule, and a close correlation exists between selenium and GSH-Px.[243] Very severe RDS has been reported in selenium-deficient human babies.[244] However, while the deficiency of GSH-Px has been demonstrated in premature infants deficient in selenium,[245] the quantity of selenium supplementation to premature infants has yet to be established.[246]

Finally, the protective effects of bilirubin against ROS have been conclusively proved.[247,248] Although hyperbilirubinemia can be regarded as a natural antioxidant factor, the risk of brain damage due to high plasma levels of this molecule, particularly in premature babies, should not be underestimated.

REFERENCES

1. Smith JL. The pathological effects due to increase of oxygen tension in the air breathed. J Physiol (London). 1899;24:19-35.
2. Patz A, Hoeck I, de la Cruz E. Studies on the effect of high oxygen administration in retrolental fibroplasia. Am J Ophthalmol. 1952;35:1248-53.
3. Gordon HH, Nitowsky HM, Cornblath M. Studies of tocopherol deficiency in infants and children. Hemolysis of erythrocytes in hydrogen peroxide. Am J Dis Child. 1955;90:669-81.
4. Halliwell B, Gutteridge JMC. Free Radical Biology and Medicine, 2nd edition. Oxford: Clarendon Press; 1989.
5. Halliwell B, Gutteridge JMC, Cross CE. Free radicals, antioxidants, and human disease: where are we now? J Lab Clin Med. 1992;19:598-620.
6. Halliwell B. Free radicals, antioxidants, and human disease: curiosity, cause, or consequence? Lancet. 1994;344:721-4.
7. Gutteridge JMC. Lipid peroxidation and antioxidants as biomarkers of tissue damage. Clin Chem. 1995;41:1819-28.
8. Fridovich I. Superoxide dismutase: an adaptation to a paramagnetic gas. J Biol Chem. 1989;264:7761-4.
9. Turrens JF. Mitochondrial formation of reactive oxygen species. J Physiol. 2003;552:335-44.
10. Radi R, Cassina A, Hodara R, et al. Peroxynitrite reactions and formation in mitochondria. Free Rad Biol Med. 2002;33:1451-64.
11. Wink DA, Miranda KM, Effey MG. Effects of oxidative and nitrosatide stress in cytotoxicity. Semin Perinatol. 2000;24:20-3.
12. Beckman JS, Viera L, Estevez A, et al. Nitric oxide and peroxynitrite in the perinatal period. Semin Perinatol. 2000;24:37-41.
13. Granot E, Kohen R. Oxidative stress in childhood in health and disease states. Clin Nutr. 2004;23:3-11.
14. Balavoine GG, Geletii YV. Peroxynitrite scavenging by different antioxidants. I. Convenient assay. Nitric Oxide. 1999;3:40-54.
15. Halliwell B. Superoxide, iron, vascular endothelium and reperfusion injury. Free Rad Res Commun. 1989;5:315-8.
16. Weiss SJ. Tissue destruction by neutrophils. N Engl J Med. 1989;320:365-76.
17. Wiese AG, Pacifici RE, Davies KJA. Transient adaptation to oxidative stress in mammalian cells. Arch Biochem Biophys. 1995;318:231-40.
18. Jaiswal AK. Antioxidant response element. Biochem Pharmacol. 1994;48:439-44.
19. Warren MC, Bump EA, Medeiros D, et al. Oxidative stress-induced apoptosis of endothelial cells. Free Radic Biol Med. 2000;29:537-47.
20. Clutton S. The importance of oxidative stress in apoptosis. Br Med Bull. 1997;53:662-8.
21. Takahashi A, Masuda A, Sun M, et al. Oxidative stress-induced apoptosis is associated with alterations in mitochondrial caspase activity and Bcl-2-dependent alterations in mitochondrial pH. Brain Res Bull. 2004;62:497-504.
22. Salvayre R, Auge N, Benoisi H, et al. Oxidized low-density lipoprotein-induced apoptosis. BBA. 2002;1585:213-21.
23. Azzi A, Davies KJA, Kelly F. Free radical biology—terminology and critical thinking. FEBS Lett. 2004;558:3-6.
24. Grisham MB. Reactive oxygen species in immune responses. Free Radic Biol Medicine. 2004;36:1479-80.
25. Ginsburg I, Kohen R. Cell damage in inflammatory and infectious sites might involve a coordinated "crosstalk"among oxidants, microbial haemolysis and ampiphiles, cationic proteins, phospholipases, fatty acids, proteinases and cytokines (an Overview). Free Rad Res. 1995;22:489-517.
26. Grisham MB, Hernandez LA, Granger DN. Xanthine oxidase and neutrophil infiltration in intestinal ischemia. Am J Physiol. 1986;251:G567-74.
27. Becker LB. New concepts in reactive oxygen species and cardiovascular reperfusion physiology. Cardiovasc Res. 2004;61:461-70.
28. Ferrari R, Ceconi C, Curello S, et al. Role of oxygen free radicals in ischemic and reperfused myocardium. Am J Clin Nutr. 1991;53:215S-22S.
29. Hess ML, Manson NH. Molecular oxygen: friend and foe. The role of the oxygen free radical system in the calcium paradox, the oxygen paradox and ischemia/reperfusion iniury. J Mol Cell Cardiol. 1984;16:969-85.
30. Buonocore G, Perrone S, Bracci R. Free radicals and brain damage in the newborn. Biol Neonate. 2001;79:180-6.
31. Turrens JF. Superoxide production by the mitochondrial respiratory chain. Biosci Rep. 1997;17:3-8.
32. Taylor DL, Edward D, Mehmet H. Oxidative metabolism, apoptosis and perinatal brain injury. Brain Pathol. 1999;9:93-117.

33. Kroemer G, Dallaporta B, Reshe-Rigon M. The mitochondrial death/life regulator in apoptosis and necrosis. Annu Rev Physiol. 1998;60:619-42.

34. Schafer FQ, Buettner GR. Acidic pH amplifies iron-mediated lipid peroxidation in cells. Free Radic Biol Med. 2000;28:1175-81.

35. Saugstad OD. Hypoxanthine as an indicator of hypoxia: its role in health and disease through free radical production. Pediatr Res. 1998;23:143-50.

36. Ikeda H, Suzuki Y, Suzuki M, et al. Apoptosis is a major mode of cell death caused by ischaemia and ischaemia/reperfusion injury to the rat intestinal epithelium. Gut. 1998;42:530-7.

37. Turrens JF, Freeman BA, Levitt JG, et al. The effect of hyperoxia on superoxide production by lung submitochondrial particles. Arch Biochem Biophys. 1982;217:401-10.

38. Fenster BE, Tsao PS, Rockson SG. Endothelial dysfunction: clinical strategies for treating oxidant stress. Am Heart J. 2003;146:218-26.

39. Channon KM, Guzik TJ. Mechanisms of superoxide production in human blood vessels: relationship to endothelial dysfunction, clinical and genetic risk factors. J Physiol Pharmacol. 2002;53:515-24.

40. Yokoyama M. Oxidant stress and atherosclerosis. Curr Opin Pharmacol. 2004;4:110-5.

41. Ullrich V, Bachschmid M. Superoxide as a messenger of endothelial function. Biochem Biophys Res Commun. 2000;278:1-8.

42. Loscalzo J. Oxidant stress: a key determinant of atherothrombosis. Biochem Soc Trans. 2003;31:1059-61.

43. Zou M, Jendral M, Ulrich V. Prostaglandin endoperoxide-dependent vasospasm in bovine coronary arteries after nitration of prostacyclin synthase. Br J Pharmacol. 1999;126:1283-92.

44. Salvemini D, Cuzzocrea S. Oxidative stress in septic shock and disseminated intravascular coagulation. Free Radic Biol Med. 2002;33:1173-85.

45. Kreuz WM, Veldmann AM, Fisher D, et al. Neonatal sepsis: a challenge in hemostaseology. Semin Thromb Hemost. 1999;25:531-5.

46. Rotilio G, Rigo A, Bracci R, et al. Determination of red blood cell superoxide dismutase and glutathione peroxidase in newborns in relation to neonatal hemolysis. Clin Chim Acta. 1997;81:131-4.

47. Gardner R, Salvador A, Moradas-Ferreira P. Why does SOD overexpression sometimes enhance, sometimes decrease, hydrogen peroxide production? A minimalist explanation. Free Radic Biol Med. 2002;32:1351-7.

48. Wu G, Fang YZ, Yang S, et al. Glutathione metabolism and its implications for health. J Nutr. 2004;134:489-92.

49. Nozik-Grayck E, Dieterle CS, Piantadosi CA, et al. Secretion of extracellular superoxide dismutase in neonatal lungs. Am J Physiol Lung Cell Mol Physiol. 2000;279:L977-84.

50. Abudu N, Miller JJ, Attaelmannan M, et al. Vitamins in human arteriosclerosis with emphasis on vitamin C and vitamin E. Clin Chim Acta. 2004;339:1125.

51. Beyer RE. The participation of coenzyme Q in free radical production and antioxidation. Free Radic Biol Med. 1990;8:545-65.

52. Ricciarelli R, Zingg JM, Azzi A. The 80th anniversary of vitamin E: beyond its antioxidant properties. Biol Chem. 2002;383(3-4):457-65.

53. Halliwell B, Gutteridge JMC. The antioxidants of human extracellular fluids. Arch Biochem Biophys. 1990;280:1-8.

54. Dennery PA. Role of redox in fetal development and neonatal diseases. Antioxid Redox Signal. 2004;6:147-53.

55. Weinberger D, Laskin DL, Heck DE, et al. Oxygen toxicity in premature infants. Toxicol Appl Pharmacol. 2002;181:60-7.

56. Hooper SB, Coulter CL, Deayton JM, et al. Fetal endocrine responses to prolonged hypoxemia in sheep. Am J Physiol. 1990;259:R703-8.

57. Khullar S, Greenwood SL, McCord N, et al. Nitric oxide and superoxide impair human placental amino acid uptake and increase Na+ permeability: implications for fetal growth. Free Radic Biol Med. 2004;36:271-7.

58. Frank L, Sosenko IRS. Prenatal development of lung antioxidant enzymes in four species. J Pediatr. 1987;110:106-10.

59. de Haan JB, Tymms MJ, Cristiano F, et al. Expression of copper/zinc superoxide dismutase and glutathione peroxidase in organs of developing mouse embryos, fetuses, and neonates. Pediatr Res. 1994;35:188-96.

60. Jung K, Henke W. Developmental changes of antioxidant enzymes in kidney and liver from rats. Free Radic Biol Med. 1996;20:613-7.

61. Jones PEH, McCance RA. Enzyme activities in the blood of infants and adults. Biochem J. 1949;45:464-7.

62. Gross RT, Bracci R, Rudolph N, et al. Hydrogen peroxide toxicity and detoxification in the erythrocytes of newborn infants. Blood. 1967;29:481-93.

63. Ochoa JJ, Ramirez-Tortosa MC, Quilez JL, et al. Oxidative stress in erythrocytes from premature and full term infants during the first 72 h of life. Free Rad Res. 2003;37:317-22.

64. Dobashi K, Asayamat K, Hayashibe H, et al. Immunohistochemical study of copper-zinc and manganese superoxide dismutases in the lungs of human fetuses and newborn infants: developmental profile and alterations in hyaline membrane disease and bronchopulmonary dysplasia. Virchows Arch. 1993;423:177-84.

65. Strange RC, Cotton W, Fryer AA, et al. Studies on the expression of Cu, Zn superoxide dismutase in human tissues during development. Biochem Biophys Acta. 1988;964:260-5.

66. Bracci R, Calabri G, Bettini F, et al. Glutathione peroxidase in human leukocytes. Clin Chim Acta. 1970;29:345-8.

67. Sullivan JL, Newton RB. Serum antioxidant activity in neonates. Arch Dis Child. 1988;63:748-57.

68. Gopinathan V, Miller NJ, Milner AD, et al. Bilirubin and ascorbate antioxidant activity in neonatal plasma. FEBS Lett. 1994;349:197-200.

69. Rogers S, Witz G, Anwar M, et al. Antioxidant capacity and oxigen radical diseases in the preterm newborn. Arch Pediatr Adolesc. 2000;154:544-8.

70. Luukkainen P, Aejmelaeus R, Alho H, et al. Plasma chain-breaking antioxidants in preterm infant with good and poor short-term outcome. Free Rad Res. 1999;30:189-97.

71. Lindeman JH, van Zoeren-Grobben D, Schrijver J, et al. The total free radical trapping ability of cord blood plasma in preterm amd term babies. Pediatr Res. 1989;26:20-4.

72. Hara K, Yamashita S, Fujisawa A, et al. Oxidative stress in newborn infants with and without asphyxia as measured by plasma antioxidants and free fatty acids. Biochem Biophys Res Commun. 1999;257:244-8.

73. Pitkanen OM, Hallman M, Andersson SM. Correlation of free radical-induced lipid peroxidation with outcome in very low birth weight infants. J Pediatr. 1990;116:760-4.

74. Ahola T, Fellman V, Kjellmer I, et al. Plasma 8-isoprostane is increased in preterm infants who develop bronchopulmonary dysplasia or periventricular leukomalacia. Pediatr Res. 2004;56:88-93.

75. Goil S, Truog W, Brnes C. Eight-epi-PGF2á: a possible marker of lipid peroxidation in term infants with severe pulmonary disease. J Pediatr. 1998;132:349-51.

76. Lindeman JH, Houdkamp E, Lentjes EG, et al. Limited protection against iron-induced lipid peroxidation by cord blood plasma. Free Radic Biol Med. 1992;16:285-94.

77. Lindeman JHN, Lentjes EG, van Zoeren-Grobben D, et al. Postnatal changes in plasma ceruloplasmin and transferrin antioxidant activies in preterm babies. Biol Neonate. 2000;78:73-6.

78. Evans PJ, Evans P, Kovar IZ, et al. Bleomycin-detectable iron in the plasma of premature and full-term neonates. FEBS Lett. 1992;303:210-2.

79. Breuer W, Hershko C, Cabantchik ZI. The importance of non-transferrin bound iron in disorders of iron metabolism. Transfus Sci. 2000;23:185-92.

80. Berger HM, Mumby S, Gutteridge JMC. Ferrous ions detected in iron-overloaded cord blood plasma from preterm and term babies: implications for oxidative stress. Free Rad Res. 1995;22:555-9.

81. Clahsen PC, Moison RMW, Holtzer CAJ, et al. Recycling of glutathione during oxidative stress in erythrocytes of the newborn. Pediatr Res. 1992;32:399-402.

82. Smith CV, Hansen TN, Martin NE, et al. Oxidant stress responses in premature infants during exposure to hyperoxia. Pediatr Res. 1993;34:360-5.

83. Donough J, O'Donovan, Fernandes CJ. Mitochondrial glutathione and oxidative stress: implications for pulmonary oxygen toxicity in premature infants. Mol Genet Metabo. 2000;71:352-8.

84. Berger MT, Polidori MC, Dabbag A, et al. Antioxidant activity of vitamin C in iron-overloaded human plasma. J Biol Chem. 1997;272:15656-60.

85. Moison RM, de Beaufort A, Haasnoot AA. Uric acid and ascorbic acid redox ratio in plasma and tracheal aspirate of preterm babies with acute and chronic lung disease. Free Radic Biol Med. 1997;23:226-34.

86. Compagnoni G, Lista G, Giuffrè B, et al. Coenzyme q(10) levels in maternal plasma: correlation with mode of delivery. Biol Neonate. 2004;86:104-7.

87. Johnston RB Jr. Function and cell biology of neutrophil and mononuclear phagocytes in the newborn infant. Vaccine. 1998;16:1363-8.

88. Bracci R, Buonocore G. Chorioamnionitis: a risk factor for fetal and neonatal morbidity. Biol Neonate. 2003;83:85-96.

89. Arnould T, Michiels C, Remacle J. Hypoxic human umbilical vein endothelial cells induce activation of adherent polymorphonuclear leukocytes. Blood. 1994;83:3705-16.

90. Wang W, Pang CCP, Rogers MS, et al. Lipid peroxidation in cord blood at birth. Am J Obstet Gynecol. 1996;174:62-5.

91. Holcberg G, Kossenjans W, Miodovnik M, et al. The interaction of nitric oxide and superoxide in the human fetal-placental vasculature. Am J Obstet Gynecol. 1995;173:528-33.

92. Toh N, Inoue T, Kuraya M, et al. Antioxidative activities of a reductant in the ultrafiltrate of human placental homogenate. Biol Res Pregnancy. 1987;8:47-52.

93. Murth KR, Joseph P, Kulkarni AP. 2-Aminofluorene bioactivation by human term placental peroxidase. Teratog Carcinog Mutagen. 1995;15:115-26.

94. Saugstad OD. Is oxygen more toxic than currently believed? Pediatrics. 2001;108:1203-5.

95. Wang Y, Walsh SW, Kay HH. Placental lipid peroxides and thromboxane are increased and prostacyclin is decreased in women with preeclampsia. Am J Obstet Gynecol. 1992;167:946-9.

96. Walsh SW, Vaughan JE, Wang YP, et al. Placental isoprostane is significantly increased in preeclampsia. FASEB. 2001;15:79-81.

97. Moretti M, Phillips M, Abouzeid A, et al. Increased breath markers of oxidative stress in normal pregnancy and in preeclampsia. Am J Obstet Gynecol. 2004;190:1184-90.

98. Goldberg B, Stern A, Peisach J. The mechanism of superoxide anion generation by its interaction of phenylhydrazine with hemoglobin. J Biol Chem. 1976;251:3045-51.

99. Lync RE, Fridovich I. Permeation of the erythrocyte stroma by superoxide radical. J Biol Chem. 1978;253:4697-9.

100. Winterbourn CC, Stern A. Human red cells scavenge extracellular hydrogen peroxide and inhibit formation of hypochlorous acid and hydroxyl radical. J Clin Invest. 1987;80:1486-91.

101. Weiss SJ. Neutrophil-mediated methemoglobin formation in the erythrocyte. The role of superoxide and hydrogen peroxide. J Biol Chem. 1982;257:2947-53.

102. Ferrali M, Signorini C, Ciccoli L. Iron release and membrane damage in erythrocytes exposed to oxidizing agents, phenylhydrazine, divicine and isuramil. Biochem J. 1992;285:295-301.

103. Ripalda MJ, Rudolph N, Wong SL. Developmental patterns of antioxidant defense mechanisms in human erythrocytes. Pediatr Res. 1989;26:366-9.

104. Phylactos AC, Leaf AA, Costeloe K, et al. Erythrocyte cupric/zinc superoxide dismutase exhibits reduced activity in preterin and low-birthweight infants at birth. Acta Paediair. 1995;84:1421-5.

105. Bracci R, Bagnoli F, De Donno ML, et al. Red cell superoxide dismutase and other erythrocyte enzyme activities in the newborn infants with hyperbilirubinemia. Ital J Biochem. 1979;28:73-5.

106. Bracci R, Buonocore G, Talluri B, et al. Neonatal hyperbilirubinemia. Evidence for a role of the erythrocyte enzyme activities involved in the detoxification of oxygen radicals. Acta Paediatr Scand. 1988;77:349-56.

107. Vives Corrons JL, Pujades MA, Colomer D. Increase of enzyme activities following the in vitro peroxidation of normal human red blood cells. Enzyme. 1988;39:1-7.

108. Neefjes VME, Evelo CTA, Daars LGM, et al. Erythrocyte glutathione S transferase as a marker of oxidative stress at birth. Arch Dis Child Fetal Neonatal Ed. 1999;81:F130-3.

109. Moison RMW, Haasnoot AA, van Zoeren-Grobben D, et al. Red blood cell glutathione and plasma sulfhydryls in chronic lung disease of the newborn. Acta Paediatr. 1997;86:1363-9.

110. Ciccoli L, Rossi V, Leoncini S, et al. Iron release, superoxide production and binding of autologous IgG to band 3 dimers in newborn and adult erythrocytes exposed to hypoxia and hypoxia-reoxygenation. Biochim Biophys Acta. 2004;1672:203-13.

111. Robles R, Palomino N, Robles A. Oxidative stress in the neonate. Early Hum Dev. 2001;65(Suppl):S75-81.

112. Jain SK. The neonatal erythrocyte and its oxidative susceptibility. Semin Hematol. 1989;26:286-300.

113. Jain SK, Wise R, Bocchini JJ. Vitamin E and vitamin equinone levels in red blood cells and plasma of newborn infants and their mothers. J Am Coll Nutr. 1996;15:44-8.

114. Kondo M, Itoh S, Kusaka T, et al. The ability of neonatal and maternal erythrocytes to produce reactive oxygen species in response to oxidative stress. Early Human Development. 2002;66:81-8.

115. Bracci R, Benedetti PA, Ciambellotti V. Hydrogen peroxide generation in the erythrocytes of newborn infants. Biol Neonate. 1970;15:135-41.

116. Signorini C, Ferrali M, Ciccoli L. Iron release, membrane protein oxidation and erythrocyte aging. FEBS Lett. 1995;362:165-70.

117. Kay MM. Mechanism of removal of senescent cell by human macrophages in situ. Proc Natl Acad Sci USA. 1975;72:3521-5.

118. Rifkind JM, Zhang L, Levy A, et al. The hypoxic stress on erythrocytes associated with superoxide formation. Free Radic Res Commun. 1991;12-13:645-52.

119. Buonocore G, Zani S, Perrone S, et al. Intraerythrocyte nonprotein bound iron and plasma malondialdehyde in the hypoxic newborn. Free Radic Biol Med. 1998;25:766-70.

120. Ciccoli L, Rossi V, Leoncini S, et al. Iron release in erythrocytes and plasma nonprotein-bound iron in hypoxic and nonhypoxic newborns. Free Radical Research. 2003;37:51-8.

121. Bracci R, Perrone S, Buonocore G. Oxidant iniury in neonatal erythrocytes during the perinatal period. Acta Paediatr Suppl. 2002;438:130-4.

122. Saugstad OD. Mechanisms of tissue injury by oxygen radicals: implications for neonatal disease. Acta Paediatr. 1996;85:1-4.

123. Bancalari E, Gerhardt T. Bronchopulmonary dysplasia. Pediatr Clin N Am. 1986;33:1-23.

124. Mirro R, Armstead W, Leffler C. Increased airway leukotriene levels in infants with severe bron chopulmonary dysplasia. Am J Dis Child. 1990;144:160-1.

125. Moison RMW, Palinckx JJS, Roest M, et al. Induction of lipid peroxidation of pulmonary surfactant by plasma of preterm babies. Lancet. 1993;341:79-82.

126. Ogihara T, Okamoto R, Kim HS, et al. New evidence for the involvement of oxygen radicals in triggering neonatal chronic lung disease. Pediair Res. 1996;39:117-9.

127. Varsila E, Pitkanen O, Hallman M, et al. Immaturity-dependent free radical activity in premature infants. Pediatr Res. 1994;36:55-9.

128. Frank L. Developmental aspects of experimental pulmonary oxygen toxicity. Free Radic Biol Med. 1991;11:463-94.

129. O'Donovan DJ, Rogers LK, Kelley DK, et al. CoASH and CoASSG Levels in lung of hyperoxic rats as potential biomarkers of intramitochondrial oxidant stresses. Pediatr Res. 2002;51:346-53.

130. Vacchiano CA, Tempel GE. Role of nonenzymatically generated prostanoid, 8-iso-PGF(2-alpha), in pulmonary oxygen toxicity. J Appl Physiol. 1994;77:2912-7.

131. Wilson WL, Mullen M, Olley PM, et al. Hyperoxia induced pulmonary vascular and lung abnormalities in young rats and potential for recovery. Pediatr Res. 1985;19:1059-67.

132. Appleby C, Towner RA. Magnetic resonance imaging of pulmonary damage in the term and premature rat neonate exposed to hyperoxia. Pediatr Res. 2001;50:502-7.

133. Denis D, Fayon MJ, Berger P, et al. Prolonged moderate hyperoxia induced hyperresponsiveness and airway inflammation in newborn rats. Pediatr Res. 2001;50:515-9.

134. Schock BC, Swett DG, Ennis M, et al. Oxidative stress and increased type-IV collagenase levels in bronchoalveolar lavage fluid from newborn babies. Pediatr Res. 2001;50:29-33.

135. Grigg J, Arnon S, Chase A, et al. Inflammatory cells in the lungs of premature infants on the first day of life: perinatal risk factors and origin of cells. Arch Dis Child. 1993;69:40-3.

136. Kotecha S, Chan B, Azam N, et al. Increase in interleukin 8 and soluble intercellular adhesion molecule 1 in bronchoalveolar lavage fluid from premature infants who develop chronic lung disease. Arch Dis Child. 1995;72:F90-6.

137. Crim J, Longmore WJ. Sublethal hydrogen peroxide inhibits alveolar type II cell surfactant phospholipid biosynthetic enzymes. Am Physiol. 1995;12:L129-35.

138. Ischiropoulos H, Almehdi AB, Fisher AB. Reactive species in ischemic rat lung injury: contribution of peroxynitrite. Am Physiol. 1995;13:L158-64.

139. Kojima T, Hattori K, Hirata Y, et al. Endothelin-1 has a priming effect on production of superoxide anion by alveolar macrophages: its possible correlation with bronchopulmonary dysplasia. Pediatr Res. 1996;39:112-6.

140. Wagenaar GT, Horst SA, van Gastelen MA, et al. Gene expression profile and histopathology of experimental bronchopulmonary dysplasia induced by prolonged oxidative stress. Free Radic Biol Med. 2004;36(6):782-801.

141. Buss ICH, Darlow BH, Winterbourn CC. Elevated protein carbonyls and lipid peroxidation products correlating with myeloperoxidase in tracheal aspirates from premature infants. Pediatr Res. 2000;47:640-5.

142. Schock BC, Sweet DG, Halliday HL, et al. Oxidative stress in lavage fluid of preterm infants at risk of chronic lung disease. Am J Physiol Lung Cell Mol Physiol. 2001;281:L1386-91.

143. Winterbourn C, Chan T, Buss H, et al. Protein carbonyls and lipid peroxidation products as oxidation markers in preterm infant plasma: association with chronic lung disease and retinopathy and effects of selenium supplementation. Pediatr Res. 2000;48:84-90.

144. Smith LEH. Pathogenesis of retinopathy of prematurity. Growth Horm IGF Res. 2004;14:S140-4.

145. Dani C, Reali MF, Bertini G, et al. The role of blood transfusions and iron intake on retinopathy of prematurity. Early Hum Dev. 2001;62:57-63.

146. Papp A, Nemeth I, Karge E, et al. Glutathione status in retinopathy of prematurity. Free Radic Biol Med. 1999;27:738-43.

147. Hairano K, Morinobu T, Kim H, et al. Blood transfusion increased radical promoting nontransferrin bound iron in preterm infants. Arch Dis Child Fetal Neontal. 2001;84:F188-93.

148. Armstrong D, Hiramitsu T, Gutteridge Nilsson SE. Studies on experimentally induced retinal degeneration I. Effect of lipid peroxides on electroretinographic activity in the albino rabbit. Exp Eye Res. 1982;35:157-71.

149. Chemtob S, Roy MS, Abran D, et al. Prevention of postasphyxial increase in lipid peroxides and retinal function deterioration in the newborn pig by inhibition of cyclooxygenase activity and free radical generation. Pediatr Res. 1993;33:336-40.

150. Abran D, Hardy P, Varma DR, et al. Mechanisms of the biphasic effects of peroxides on the retinal vasculature of newborn and adult pigs. Exp Eye Res. 1995;61:285-92.

151. Abran D, Varma DR, Chemtob S. Increased thromboxane-mediated contractions of retinal vessels of newborn pigs to peroxides. Am J Physiol. 1995;37:H628-32.

152. Halliwell B. Reactive oxygen species and the central ervous system. J Neurochem. 1992;59:1609-23.

153. Delivoria-Papadopoulos M, Mishra OP. Mechanism of perinatal cerebral injury in fetus and newborns. Ann N Y Acad Sci. 2000;900:159-68.

154. Cook DA, Vollrath B. Free radicals and intracellular events associated with cerebrovascular spasm. Cardiovasc Res. 1995;30:493-500.

155. Oka A, Belliveau MJ, Rosenberg PA, et al. Vulnerability of oligodendroglia to glutamate: pharmacology, mechanisms, and prevention. J Ncurosci. 1993;13:1441-53.

156. Abdelrahman A, Parks JK, Devereaux MW, et al. Developmental changes in newborn lamb brain mitochondrial activity and postasphyxial lipid peroxidation. Proc Soc Exp Biol Med. 1995;209:170-7.

157. Volpe JJ. Neurobiology of periventricular leukomalacia in the premature infant. Pediatr Res. 2001;50:553-6.

158. Poulsen JP, Oyasaeter S, Sanderud J, et al. Hypoxanthine, xanthine, and uric acid concentrations in the cerebrospinal fluid, plasma, and urine of hypoxemic pigs. Pediatr Res. 1990;28:477-81.

159. Palmer C, Vannucci RC, Towfighi J. Reduction of perinatal hypoxic-ischemic brain damage with allopurinol. Pediatr Res. 1990;27:332-6.

160. Goplerud JM, Mishra OP, Delivoria-Papadopoulos M. Brain cell membrane dysfunction following acute asphyxia in newborn piglets. Biol Neonate. 1992;61:33-41.

161. Inder T, Mocatta T, Darlow B, et al. Elevated free radical products in the cerebrospinal fluid of VLBW infants with cerebral white matter injury. Pediatr Res. 2002;52:213-8.

162. Maulik D, Numagami Y, Osnishi ST, et al. Direct measurement of oxygen free radicals during in utero hypoxia in the fetal guinea pig brain. Brain Res. 1998;798:166-72.

163. DiGiacomo JE, Pane CR, Gwiazdowski S, et al. Effects of graded hypoxia on brain cell membrane injury in newborn piglets. Biol Neonate. 1992;61:25-32.

164. Palmer C, Menzies SL, Roberts RL, et al. Changes in iron histochemistry after hypoxic-ischemic brain injury in the neonatal rat. J Neurosci Res. 1999;56:60-71.

165. Olano M, Song DK, Murphy S, et al. Relationship of dopamine, cortical oxygen pressure, and hydroxyl radicals in brain of newborn piglets during hypoxia and posthypoxic recovery. J Neurochem. 1995;65:1205-12.

166. Inder T, Mocatta T, Darlow B, et al. Markers of oxidative injury in the cerebrospinal fluid of premature infant with meningitis and periventricular leukomalacia. J Pediatr. 2002;140:617-21.

167. Savman K, Nilsson UA, Blennow M, et al. Non-proteinbound iron is elevated in cerebrospinal fluid from preterm infants with posthemorrhagic ventricular dilatation. Pediatr Res. 2001;49:208-12.

168. Back SA, Gan X, Li Y, et al. Maturation-dependent vulnerability of oligodentrocytes to oxidative stress induced death caused by glutathione depletion. J Neurosci. 1998;18:6241-53.

169. Jamieson DD. Lipid peroxidation in brain and lungs from mice exposed to hyperoxia. Biochem Pharmacol. 1991;41:749-56.

170. Watson NA, Beard SC, Ataf N, et al. The effect of hyperoxia on cerebral blood flow: a study in healthy volunteers using magnetic resonance phase-contrast angiography. Eur J Anaesthesiol. 2000;17(3):152-9.

171. Niijima S, Shortland DB, Levene MI, et al. Transient hyperoxia and cerebral blood flow velocity in infants born prematurely at full term. Arch Dis Child. 1998;63(10):1126-30.

172. Fumagalli M, Mosca F, Knudsen GM, et al. Transient hyperoxia and residual cerebrovascular effects in the newborn rat. Pediatric Research. 2004;55:380-4.

173. Leviton A, Dammann O. Coagulation, inflammation and risk of neonatal white matter damage. Pediatr Res. 2004;55:541-5.

174. Supnet MC, David-Cu R, Walther FJ. Plasma xanthine oxidase activity and lipid hydroperoxide levels in preterm infants. Pediatr Res. 1994;36:283-7.

175. Schmidt H, Grune T, Muller R, et al. Increased levels of lipid peroxidation products malondialdehyde and 4 hydroxynonenal after perinatal hypoxia. Pediatr Res. 1996;40:15-20.

176. Buonocore G, Perrone S, Longini M, et al. Total hydroperoxide and advanced oxidation protein products in preterm hypoxic babies. Pediatr Res. 2000;47:221-4.

177. Buonocore G, Perrone S, Longini M, et al. Oxidative stress in preterm neonates at birth and on the seventh day of life. Pediatr Res. 2002;52:46-9.

178. Qin Y, Wang CC, Kuhn H, et al. Determinants of umbilical cord arterial 8-iso-prostaglandin F2alpha concentration. BJOG. 2000;107(8):973-81.

179. Dorrepal CA, Berger HM, Benders MJN, et al. Nonprotein-bound iron in postasphyxial reperfusion injury in the newborn. Pediatrics. 1996;98:883-9.

180. Buonocore G, Perrone S, Longini M, et al. Nonprotein bound iron as early predictive marker of neonatal brain damage. Brain. 2003;126:1224-30.

181. Halliwell B, Whiteman M. Measuring reactive species and oxidative damage in vivo and in cell culture: how should you do it and what do result mean? British Journal of Pharmacology. 2004;142:231-55.

182. Polidori MC, Stahl W, Eichler O, et al. Profiles of antioxidants in human plasma. Free Radical Biology and Medicine. 2001;30:456-62.

183. Roberts Lj 2nd, Morrow JD. Products of the isoprostane pathway: unique bioactive compound and markers of lipid peroxidation. Clle Mol Life Sci. 2002;59:808-20.

184. Lawson JA, Rokach J, Fitzgerald GA. Isoprostanes: formation, analysis and use as indices of lipid peroxidation in vivo. J Biol Chem. 1999;264:24441-4.

185. Varsila E, Hallman M, Andersson S. Free-radical-induced lipid peroxidation during the early neonatal period. Acta Paediatr. 1994;83:692-5.

186. Nycyk JA, Drury JA, Cooke RWI. Breath pentane as a marker for lipid peroxidation and adverse outcome in preterm infants. Arch Dis Child Fetal Neonatal Ed. 1998;79:F67-9.

187. Springfield JR, Levitt MD. Pitfalls in the use of breath pentane measurements to assess lipid peroxidation. J Lipid Res. 1994;35:1497-504.

188. Loiseaux-Meunier MN, Bedu M, Gentou C, et al. Oxygen toxicity: simultaneous measure of pentane and malondialdehyde in humans exposed to hyperoxia. Biomed Pharmacother. 2001;55:163-9.

189. Ogihara T, Hirano K, Morinobu T, et al. Raised concentrations of aldehyde lipid peroxidation products in premature infants with chronic lung disease. Arch Dis Child Fetal Neonatal Ed. 1999;80:F21-5.

190. Butterfield DA. Proteomics: a new approach to investigate oxidative stress in Alzheimer's disease brain. Brain Res. 2004;1000(1-2):1-7.

191. Marzocchi B, Perrone S, Paffetti P, et al. Nonprotein bound and plasma protein oxidant stress at birth. Pediatr Res. 2004,55:291A.

192. Filomeni G, Rotilio G, Ciriolo MR. Cell signaling and the glutathione redox system. Biochem Pharmacol. 2002;64:1057-64.

193. Nemeth I, Boda D. Blood glutathione redox ratio as a parameter of oxidative stress in premature infants with RDS. Free Radic Biol Med. 1994;16(3):347-53.

194. Vento M, Asensi M, Sastre J, et al. Resuscitation with room air instead of 100% oxygen prevents oxidative stress in moderately asphyxiated term neonates. Pediatrics. 2001;107:642-7.

195. Smith CV, Hansen TN, Martin NE, et al. Oxidant stress responses in premature infants during exposure to hyperoxia. Pediatr Res. 1993;34:360-5.

196. Eiserich JP, Hristova M, Cross CE, et al. Formation of nitric oxide-derived inflammatory oxidants by myeloperoxidase in neutrophils. Nature. 1998;391:393-7.

197. Koeck T, Fu X, Hazen SL, et al. Rapid and selective oxygen regulated protein tyrosine "Denitration" and nitration in mitochondria. J Biol Chem. 2004;279:27257-62.

198. Grootveld M, Ehalliwell B. Measurement of allantoin and uric acid in human body fluids. A potential index of free radical reactions in vivo? Biochem J. 1987;243:803-8.

199. Mikami T, Kita K, Tomita S, et al. Is allantoin in serum and urine a useful indicator of exercise-induced oxidative stress in humans? Free Rad Res. 2000;32:235-44.

200. Drury JA, Jeffers G, Cooke RW. Urinary 8-hydroxy-deoxyguanosine in infants and children. Free Radic Res. 1998;28:423-8.

201. Matsubasa T, Uchino T, Karashima S, et al. Oxidative stress in very low birth weight infants as measured by urinary 8-OHdG. Free Radic Res. 2002;36(2):189-93.

202. Poliakov E, Brennan ML, Macpherson J, et al. Isolevuglandins, a novel class of isoprostenoid derivatives, function as integrated sensors of oxidant stress and are generated by myeloperoxidase in vivo. FASEB J. 2003;17:2209-20.

203. Askie LM, Henderson-Smart DJ. Restricted versus liberal oxygen exposure for preventing morbidity and mortality in preterm or low birth weight infants (Cochrane Review). Cochrane Database Syst Rev. 2004;4:CD001077.

204. Wolkoff LI, Narula P. Issue in neonatal and pediatric oxygen therapy. Respir Care Clin N Am. 2000;6:675-91.

205. Askie L. Appropriate levels of oxygen saturation for preterm infants. Acta Paediatr Suppl. 2004;444:26-8.

206. Torrance SM, Wittnich C. Blood lactate and acid-base balance in graded neonatal hypoxia: evidence for oxygen restricted metabolism. J Appl Physiol. 1994;77(5):2318-24.

207. Schulze A, White K, Way RC, et al. Effect of the arterial oxygenation level on cardiac output, oxygen extraction, and oxygen consumption in low birth weight infants receiving mechanical ventilation. J Pediatr. 1995;126:777-84.

208. Sun SC. Relation of target SpO2 levels and clinical outcome in ELBW infants on supplemental oxygen. Pediatr Res. 2002;51:350A.

209. Chow LC, Wright KW, Sola A, et al. Can changes in clinical practice decrease the incidence of severe retinopathy of prematurity in very low birth weight infants? Pediatrics. 2003;111:339-45.

210. Tin W, Milligan DWA, Pennefather P, et al. Pulse oximetry, severe retinopathy, and outcome at one year in babies of less than 28 weeks gestation. Arch Dis Child Fetal Neonatal Ed. 2001;84:F106-10.

211. Tin W. Optimal oxygen saturation for preterm babies. Biol Neonate. 2004;85:319-25.

212. Rootwelt T, Loberg M, Moen A, et al. Hypoxemia and reoxination with 21% or 100% oxygen in newborn pigs. Changes in blood pressure, base deficit, and hypoxanthine and brain morphology. Pediatr Res. 1992;32:107-13.

213. Solas AB, Kalous P, Saugstad OD. Reoxygenation with 100 or 21% oxygen after cerebral hypoxia ischemia hypercapnia in newborn piglets. Biol Neonate. 2004;85:105-11.

214. Solas AB, Munkeby BH, Saugstad OD. Comparison of short- and long-duration oxygen treatment after cerebral asphyxia in newborn piglets. Pediatr Res. 2004;54:125-31.

215. Kondo M, Itoh S, Isobe K, et al. Chemiluminescence because of the production of reactive oxygen species in the lungs of newborn piglets during resuscitation periods after asphyxiation load. Pediatr Res. 2000;47:524-7.

216. Kutzsche S, Ilves P, Kirkeby OJ, et al. Hydrogen peroxide production in leukocytes during cerebral hypoxia and reoxygenation with 100% or 21% oxygen in newborn piglets. Pediatr Res. 2001;49: 834-42.

217. Ramij S, Abuja S, Thirupuram S, et al. Resuscitation of asphyxic newborn infants with room air or 100% oxygen. Pediatr Res. 1993;34:809-12.

218. Saugstad OD, Rootwelt T, Aalen O. Resuscitation of asphyxiated newborn infants with room air or oxygen: an international controlled trial: the resair 2 study. Pediatrics. 1998;102:e1.

219. Saugstad OD, Ramji S, Irani SF, et al. Resuscitation of newborn infants with 21% or 100% oxygen: Follow-up at 18 to 24 months. Pediatrics. 2003;112:296-300.

220. Vento M, Asensi M, Sastre J, et al. Oxidative stress in asphyxiated term infants resuscitated with 100% oxygen. J Pediatr. 2003;142:240-6.

221. Tan A, Schulze A, O'Donnell CPF, et al. Air versus oxygen for resuscitation of infants at birth (Cochrane Review). The Cochrane Database Syst Rev. 2004;3:CD002273.

222. Rice-Evans CA, Diplock AT. Current status of antioxidant therapy. Free Rad Biol Med. 1993;15:77-96.

223. Powers HJ, Loban A, Silvers K, et al. Vitamin C at concentrations observed in premature babies inhibits the ferroxidase activity of caeruloplasmin. Free Radic Res. 1995;22(1):57-65.

224. Greenwald RA. Superoxide dismutase and catalase as therapeutic agents for human diseases. A critical review. Free Rad Biol Med. 1990;8:201-9.

225. Palmer C, Vannucci RC, Towfighi J. Reduction of perinatal hypoxic-ischemic brain damage with allopurinol. Pediatr Res. 1990;27: 332-6.

226. Russell GAB, Cooke RWI. Randomised controlled trial of allopurinol prophylaxis in very preterm infants. Arch Dis Child. 1995;73: F27-31.

227. Bada HS, Green RS, Pourcvrous M, et al. Indomethacin reduces the risk of severe intraventricular hemorrhage. J Pediatr. 1989;115: 631-7.

228. Peeters Sholte C, Braun K, Koster J, et al. Effects of allopurinol and deferroxamine on reperfusion injury of the brain in newborn piglets after neonatal hypoxia ischemia. Pediatr Res. 2003;54: 516-22.

229. Mupanemunda RH, Lee DSC, Fraher IJ, et al. Postnatal changes in serum retinol status in very-low-birth-weight infants. Early Hum Dev. 1994;38L:45-54.

230. Pieri C, Marra M, Moroni F, et al. Melatonin, a peroxyl radical scavenger more efficient than vitamin E. Life Sci. 1994;55:PL271-6.

231. Tan DX, Chen LD, Poeggeler B, et al. Melatonin: a potent, endogenous hydroxyl radical scavenger. Endocrine J. 1993;1: 57-66.

232. Gitto E, Reiter RJ, Cordaro SP, et al. Oxidative and inflammatory parameters in respiratory distress syndrome of preterm newborns: beneficial effects of melatonin. Am J Perinatol. 2004;21:209-16.

233. Gitto E, Karbownik M, Reiter RJ, et al. Effects of melatonin treatment in septic newborns. Pediatric Research. 2001;50:756-60.

234. Lapenna D, Degioia S, Mezzetti A, et al. Aminophylline: could it act as an antioxidant in vivo? Eur J Clin Invest. 1995;25:464-70.

235. Law MR, Wijewardene K, Wald NJ. Is routine vitamin E administration justified in very-low-birthweight infants? Dev Med Child Nenrol. 1990;32:442-50.

236. Italian Collaborative Group on Preterm Delivery. Absorption of intramuscular vitamin E in premature babies. Dev Pharmacol Ther. 1991;16:13-21.

237. Marx MM, Cronin JH. Medications used in the newborn. In: Clothery JP, Stark AR (Eds). Manual of Neonatal Care. Boston: Little, Brown and Company; 1992. pp. 619-33.

238. Holland BM, Wardrop CAJ. Oxygen transport by the blood, haematinics and blood cell component therapy in the neonate. In: Rylance G, Harvey D, Aranda JV (Eds). Neonatal Clinical Pharmacology and Therapeutics. Oxford: Butterworth Heinemann; 1991. pp. 211-23.

239. Tanaka H, Mino M, Takeuchi T. A nutritional evaluation of vitamin E status in very-low-birthweight infants with respect to changes in plasma and red blood cell tocopherol levels. J Nutr Sci Vitaminol. 1988;34:293-7.

240. Brion LP, Bell EF, Raghuveer TS. Vitamin E supple mentation for prevention of morbidity and mortality in preterm infants. Cochrane Database Syst Rev. 2003;(3):CD003665.

241. Silvers KM, Sluis KB, Darlow BA, et al. Limiting light-induced lipid peroxidation and vitamin loss in infant parenteral nutrition by adding multivitamin preparations to Intralipid. Acta Pediatr. 2001;90:242-9.

242. Pitkanen OM, Luukkainen P, Andersson S. Attenuated lipid peroxidation in preterm infants during subsequent doses of intravenous lipids. Biol Neonate. 2004;85(3):184-7.

243. Van Callie-Bertrand M, Degenhart HJ, Fernandes J. Selenium status of infants on nutritional support. Acta Paediatr Scand. 1984;73: 816-9.

244. Darlow BA, Inder TE, Graham PI. The relationship of selenium status to respiratory outcome in the very-lowbirthweight infant. Pediatrics. 1995;96:314-9.

245. Tubman TR, Halliday HL, McMaster D. Glutathione peroxidase and selenium levels in the preterm infant. Biol Neonate. 1990;58: 305-10.

246. Daniels L, Gibso R, Simmer K. Randomised clinical trial of parenteral selenium supplementation in preterm infants. Arch Dis Child. 1996;74:F158-64.

247. Dennery PA, McDonagh AF, Spitz DR, et al. Hyper-bilirubinemia results in reduced oxidative injury in neonatal Gunn rats exposed to hyperoxia. Free Read Biol Med. 1995;19:395-404.

248. Nakamura H, Uetani Y, Komura M, et al. Inhibitory action of bilirubin on superoxide production by polymorphonuclear leukocytes. Biol Neonate. 1987;52:273-8.

12

Pathology of the Neonate

B Hargitai, T Marton, Z Papp

INTRODUCTION

Obstetrical care of high standard and regular ultrasound scanning usually leads to prenatal diagnosis of developmental abnormalities and often prevents perinatal pathologists to encounter those in term or near-term neonates. Therefore, dysmorphology and congenital abnormalities are more and more the subject of the fetopathology whilst growth abnormalities, hypoxic injuries, preterm birth, infection remains a major problem in neonatal medicine. Congenital tumor and genetic metabolic disease is rare in general, but may have a great impact on the life of the family especially when it is part of a syndrome and has a high recurrence risk. Stillbirth and early neonatal death rate, due to birth-related events, have significantly decreased in the last 40 years (from 7.9 to 0.5 per 1,000 total births) in the United Kingdom[1] and similar trend can be observed in many other European countries. The number of litigation cases following intrapartum neonatal death is increasing, and thus potentially the postmortem report has medicolegal importance. It is highly recommended for obstetricians to ask for a postmortem examination and to encourage the parents to give permission for a full autopsy. It is a good practice to have regular discussions with the perinatal pathologist and to provide the pathologist with detailed clinical information prior postmortem examination.

GROWTH ABNORMALITIES AND INTRAUTERINE GROWTH RESTRICTION. ASSESSMENT OF IUGR DURING PERINATAL POSTMORTEM EXAMINATION

Massive cell division and differentiation takes place in the developing fetus and result in a linear growth until the thirty-eighth week of gestation. Any failure of the complicated biochemical routes and control system, shortfall in nutritional agents or oxygen supply may lead to growth abnormalities. In obstetric practice ultrasonographic assessment of biparietal diameter (BPD), femur length and other fetal measurements were found to be useful to date the pregnancy.[2] To estimate the duration of the pregnancy, the most frequently used method is to count the gestational weeks from the first day of the mother's menstrual period. Although many charts of fetal and neonatal measurements are available in textbooks, most of these have been created decades ago.[3-5] Perinatal pathology centers have to update these data, especially to reflect characteristics of a given geographical and ethnical population.

During perinatal necropsy the appropriate measurements of the body (weight, crown-rump length, crown-heel length, foot length, head circumference) and organ weight always have to be taken and should be compared with the normal values, apt for the counted gestational age. Neonates, born between the thirty-seventh and

forty-first gestational weeks are term neonates and those born before the thirty-seventh week are preterm neonates, expressing signs of prematurity. Both term and preterm babies can be of appropriate weight for the gestational age or may weigh less than the expected normal value. Babies who weigh 2,500 g or less are called low birthweight neonates and those under 1,500 g are designated as very low birthweight. Small-for-date or small-for-gestational-age (SGA) infants measure less than third, fifth, or tenth centile or less than two standard deviations below the mean. Small-for-dates infants are not necessarily growth restricted and babies suffering from intrauterine growth restriction are not always small-for-date!

Intrauterine growth restriction (IUGR) is usually detected during the third trimester of pregnancy. In case of an early onset growth restriction the fetal organs are smaller but proportionally developed. The serial BPD measurements are lower and parallel with the normal values from the early pregnancy. This type of IUGR is usually associated with intrauterine infections, chromosome abnormalities, e.g. Down's syndrome, triploidy (Fig. 12.1) and many other malformation syndromes. Late onset of IUGR is usually caused by environmental factors such as malnutrition due to placental dysfunction or maternal under-nutrition, reduced uteroplacental perfusion related to maternal hypertension, preeclampsia, diabetes mellitus or maternal smoking. In late onset of IUGR the infant's body is disproportional, the head circumference is relatively large, and the brain weight/liver weight ratio is elevated.

Pathological and histological assessment of IUGR requires accurate measurement of body weight, crown-heal length, crown-rump length, head circumference, foot length, organ weights, and

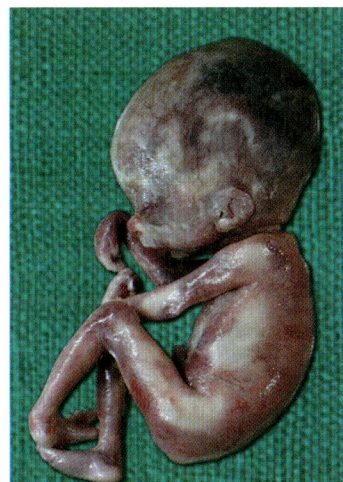

Fig. 12.1: Triploidy: Note the relatively large head and atrophic body, small jaw and low set ear of this fetus

microscopic examination of the parenchymal organs. Elevated brain weight/liver weight ratio [Mean 2.8 (range 1.7–4.1)],[6,7] lower crown-rump length than head circumference, immature brain gyral pattern,[8] decreased nephron counts and presence of nephrogenic zone of the kidney after the thirty-sixth week of gestation,[9] bone growth plate abnormalities and specific placental findings are sensitive markers of IUGR.[10]

Infants, who weigh more than the normal value for a particular gestational age, are called heavy-for-dates babies. This condition can be constitutional and usually is associated with high maternal body weight or higher parity. Maternal diabetes mellitus and gestational diabetes are often complicated with increased somatic size (macrosomia) when the diabetes of the mother is not sufficiently controlled. Macrosomia, unilateral hyperplasia, or single organ overgrowth can be seen in so-called overgrowth syndromes. This group includes Beckwith-Wiedemann syndrome, characterized by hemihyperplasia, macroglossia, omphalocele, and increased risk of pediatric neoplasms, most frequently Wilm's tumor. Simpson-Golabi-Bernel syndrome, an X-chromosome linked disorder, is associated with macrosomia, congenital heart defects among other abnormalities.[11] Perlman syndrome, autosomal recessive, is characterized by macrosomia at birth, cardiac malformation, hypertrophy of the islets of Langerhans, bilateral renal hamartomas and sometimes nephroblastomatosis.[12] Weaver syndrome is characterized by accelerated growth and osseous maturation, bears considerable overlap with Soto's syndrome, both of them associated with congenital heart defects and higher risk of malignancy.[13]

PATHOLOGICAL SEQUELS OF INTRAUTERINE ASPHYXIA

Intrauterine asphyxia is a common cause of fetal death and may lead to severe organ failure such as long-term neurodevelopmental injuries in the surviving infant. During the last two decades, it has become evident that only a minority of cerebral palsy and severe neurological damage begins at labor. In contrast, chronic or subacute intrauterine asphyxia is responsible for about 80% of cases.[14,15] In case of acute intrauterine asphyxia, pathological events lead to fetal demise or major damage within 24 hours, while in chronic intrauterine asphyxia the estimated time course is 3 weeks or more. Specific causes of intrauterine asphyxia and associated pathological events can be identified in 50–80% of stillbirth cases.[16] Clinical data and pathological examination may help to clarify the mechanism of damage and reveal maternal, placental or fetal causes such as maternal disease, hemorrhage, placental malfunction, fetal malformation, second trimester loss of a twin in monochorionic pregnancy, or infection.

During the course of the postmortem of a fetus or a neonate who underwent intrauterine asphyxia, a combination of features associated with the predisposing causes as well as symptoms related to intrauterine hypoxic stress can be seen.

Acute intrauterine asphyxia is characterized by petechial hemorrhages on the epicardium along coronary arteries and at base of aorta and pulmonary trunk, visceral pleura, meconium in the airways, massive intrapulmonary hemorrhage, subcapsular hemorrhage of the liver, interstitial corticomedullary hemorrhage of the kidney and subcapsular hematoma of the adrenal glands. Microscopic examination reveals aspirated meconium, squames in the airways (Fig. 12.2), myocardial contraction band changes, cortical

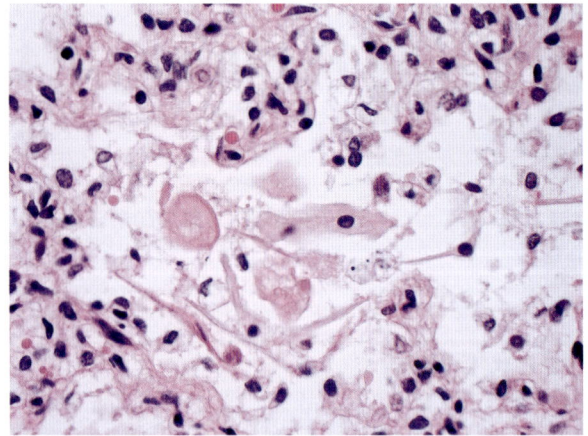

Fig. 12.2: Squamous cells in the alveoli of a stillborn fetus

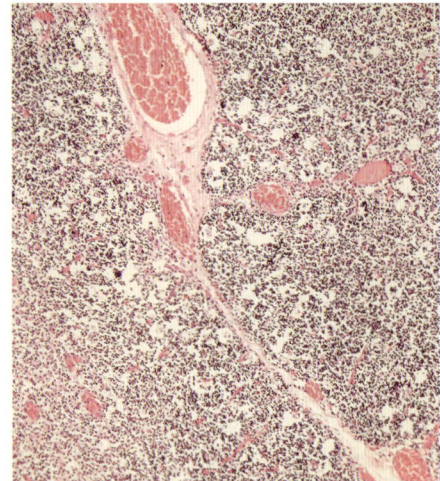

Fig. 12.3: Starry sky reaction in the thymus of a neonate. The whitish small areas represent missing thymocytes as a result of subacute stress

histiocytosis in the thymus and cystic degeneration of the adult cortical zone in the adrenals.

There are usually no petechial hemorrhages in subacute asphyxia/hypoxia. Microscopically, shrinking of the cortex, prominent Hassal's corpuscles and histiocytosis can be observed in the thymus, with lymphocytolysis, the depletion of lymphocytes results in a typical "starry sky" pattern (Fig. 12.3). In the adrenals lipid depletion and reaccumulation is present in the middle fetal cortex (Fig. 12.4). Chronic intrauterine hypoxia leads to fetal growth retardation with asymmetric or disproportionate pattern, reduced muscle and subcutaneous fat. Microscopically, reaccumulation of lipid and fatty change in the outer fetal cortex of the adrenal gland is characteristic. The thymus shows severe involutional changes with thin or diminished cortex and crowding of the Hassal's corpuscles (Fig. 12.5). In the enchondral growth plate of the bones irregular costochondral junction can be observed.

Intrauterine hypoxia leads to congestion in the central nervous system. Grossly, flattening of the gyri and compression of lateral ventricles can be seen. Microscopically, different stages of neuronal degeneration, necrosis and apoptosis are typical for hypoxic

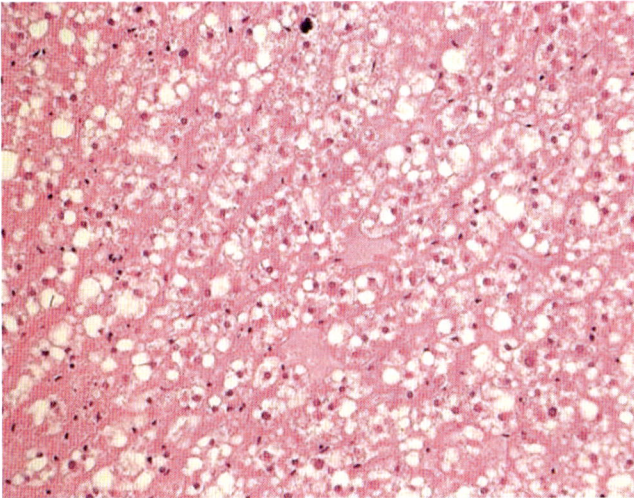

Fig. 12.4: Severe lipid reaccumulation in the adrenal cortex

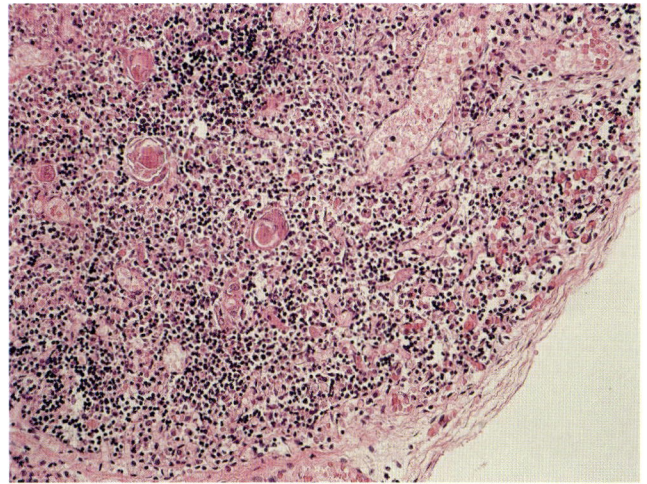

Fig. 12.5: Atrophic cortex of the thymus, prominent Hassal's corpuscles

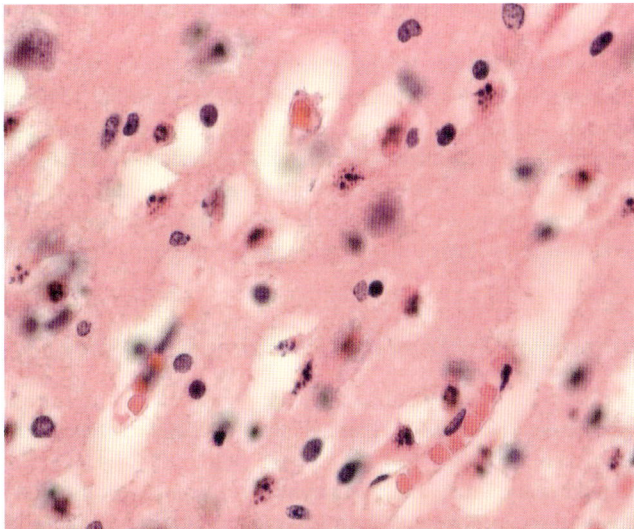

Fig. 12.6: High number of apoptotic figures in the hippocampus of a neonate with hypoxic ischemic encephalopathy

ischemic changes in thalamus, midbrain, pons, and basal ganglia. Angulation of the neurons, karyorrhexis, and karyopicnosis are characteristic signs of neuronal apoptosis (Fig. 12.6). Late consequences of hypoxic ischemic brain damage may include massive loss of brain tissue causing porencephaly, hydrocephaly, cystic changes, and subsequent microcephaly.

PREMATURITY OR IMMATURITY

Neonates, delivering before 37 completed weeks of gestation are called preterm neonates. The direct causes of preterm labor are not entirely understood although many associated pathological events have been studied such as maternal diseases, socioeconomic factors, previous reproductive events, effect of twinning and fetal factors. Structural and functional immaturity of preterm babies causes major problems in postnatal life during adaptation. Hypoglycemia, hypothermia, high blood potassium level, and anemia are frequent complications. Pathological appearance of organ specific alterations

has been changed due to technical development of neonatal intensive care and new therapeutic methods.

Pathology of the Respiratory System in Premature Infants

Infantile Respiratory Distress Syndrome and Hyaline Membrane Disease

Infantile respiratory distress syndrome (IRDS) is a frequent condition in preterm infants and is characterized by a well-defined clinical picture: rapid increase in oxygen requirement and demand for ventilation, cyanosis, tachypnea, intercostal and sternal recession, increasing expiratory pressure and a typical grunting noise at expiration. Radiological staging is possible but not always consistence with the degree of respiratory failure. In an advanced stage, the picture of "white lungs" appears on X-ray.

The underlying cause behind the acute respiratory failure of preterm neonates is the functional and structural immaturity of the lung. The reduced number and incomplete formation of airways, inefficient production of surfactant factor, lack of antioxidant defence lead to a number of immunopathological processes similarly to diffuse alveolar damage syndromes. The exact mechanism of the initial epithelial injury is not known but ischemia, volu- and baro-trauma, oxygen toxicity are likely to play major role.[17] Most babies survive IRDS and in about 50% of cases there are no significant complications in the respiratory system. The outcome is less favorable with younger gestational age. The incidence is higher in males, and symptoms can be more severe in infants of diabetic mothers, in multiple pregnancies and after intrauterine asphyxia.[18]

In preterm babies who die in the first week of life with symptoms of IRDS, the lungs are heavy, purple colored and have a liver-like texture due to atelectasia. Microscopically, most airways are collapsed, but terminal airways are distended, the bronchial epithelial lining is necrotic. As soon as at an hour after birth, hyaline membrane starts to develop lining the primitive airways that consists of nuclear debris of epithelial cells as well as necrotic cell mass and exudates from inflammatory cells. A few hour later polymorphonuclears, macrophages migrate into the septa and after

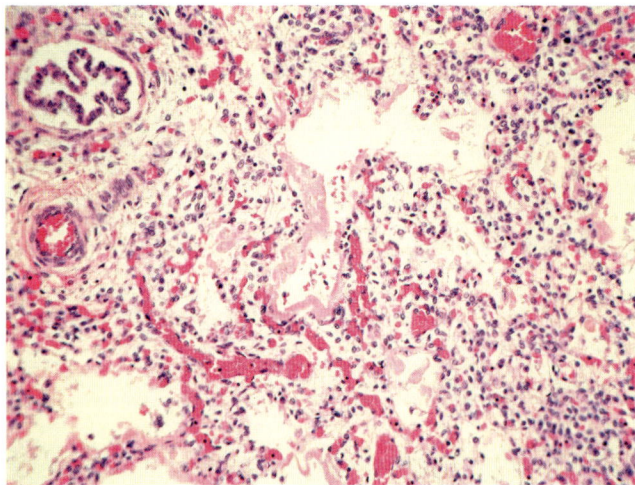

Fig. 12.7: Eosinophilic membrane lines the inner surface of the airway

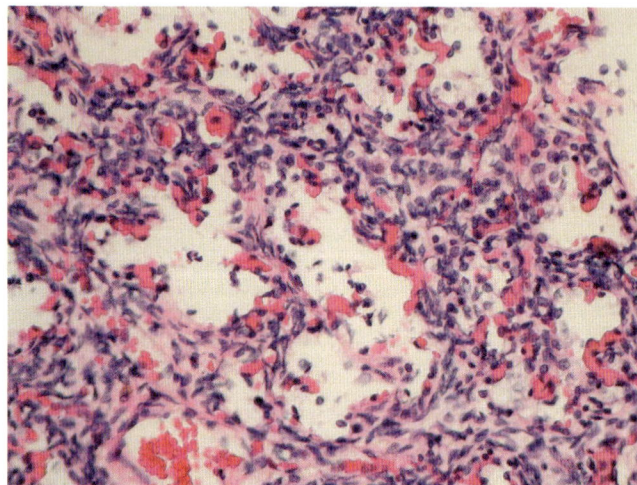

Fig. 12.8: Simplified airways, widened interalveolar septa are present in chronic lung disease

2 days regenerative changes in the epithelium become visible. Hyaline membrane (Fig. 12.7) is strongly associated with IRDS, but can be present in acute asphyxia, in some infections (e.g. group B streptococcus infection) and in pulmonary hemorrhage.

The incidence of IRDS and hyaline membrane disease (HMD) has been significantly reduced with surfactant administration and especially the preventive use of natural surfactant is proved to be useful. Steroid administration before preterm labor is a common practice, the benefits and complications of which are still investigated.[19,20]

Changing Morphology of Chronic Lung Disease

Clinical definition of chronic lung disease (CLD) requires demand for assisted or supported ventilation after 28 days of life, radiological signs, and previous acute respiratory failure of the infant, most frequently IRDS-HMD. The classical morphology of chronic lung injury has changed and is rarely seen today. Therefore, the term "bronchopulmonary dysplasia" is not appropriate for the majority of the cases and "chronic lung disease" is preferred currently.

Traditionally, three stages could be distinguished in BPD based on histology of the lung.

- In acute exudative early reparative stage (1–9 days) persisting hyaline membrane, lack of type III, pneumocytes, bronchiolar epithelial necrosis, obliterative bronchiolitis, interstitial edema, congestion, and initial septal fibrosis can be seen.
- In subacute fibroproliferative stage (10–30 days) increasing interstitial and perialveolar fibrosis, necrotizing tracheobronchitis, smooth muscle proliferation, dilated bronchiole and terminal airways are present.
- In the late stage (after 1 month) prominent septal fibrosis, reduced number and anatomical distortion of terminal airways, metaplastic changes in bronchial epithelium, pulmonary hypertensive changes in pulmonary arterioles are typical findings.

The changing morphology of chronic lung disease might be a result of the longer survival time of the very immature, very low birth-weight preterm infants and the technical improvement of intensive care, especially ventilation. Characteristic morphological changes include less exudative fibroproliferative signs but a dramatic

fall in the number of airways' and gas exchange surface (Fig. 12.8). The proximal airways are collapsed and in contrast, the terminal structures are dilated. Patchy fibrosis may be present but is not dominant. Inflammatory morphological changes are not common, although, significant inflammatory response is associated with CLD and there is an increased level of inflammatory cytokines. It is suggested that the current morphology of chronic lung disease might be the consequence of an alveolar developmental abnormality due to the lack of physiological signal during lung remodeling in the highly immature infants.[21,22]

Pulmonary Air Leak and Pulmonary Hemorrhage

Positive pressure ventilation may result in alveolar overdistension and rupture. The air can be pressed into the pleural cavities leading to pneumothorax. Air leakage into the pulmonary tissues results in pulmonary interstitial emphysema. Pneumopericardium is usually associated with other air leaks and is a severe complication threatening with pericardial tamponade. Systemic air embolism is a very rare complication of ventilation and may lead to sudden death.

Intraalveolar and interstitial hemorrhage is frequently associated with HMD. Massive hemorrhage is occasionally a terminal event while alveolar and subpleural hemorrhage are rather associated with acute asphyxia.

Pathology of the Central Nervous System in Premature Infants (Germinal Matrix Hemorrhage, Intraventricular Hemorrhage and Periventricular Leukomalacia)

A reasonable improved prognosis has been documented in the last decade, the incidence of intracerebral hemorrhage and ischemic white matter damage in preterm infants is still high and may be responsible for long-term neurodevelopmental sequels such as hydrocephalus, spastic diplegia, hemiplegia, quadriplegia, learning difficulties, and behavioral problems.[23,24]

The pattern of neuropathological changes in preterm brain differs from those that can be found in term neonates. Most frequent pathological findings in preterms are germinal matrix/intraventricular hemorrhage and periventricular leukomalacia, and in contrast with the term brain tissue, the most vulnerable areas are the periventricular germinal matrix and white matter. Although basal ganglia are far more frequently affected in term babies, pontosubicular necrosis has been observed in a high ratio of preterm infants.[25] The fetal brain is characterized by an active neurogenesis, dense aggregation of precursor cells in the subependymal germinal layer, and a paucity of myelin. Neuronal precursors migrate from the germinal layer into the cortex, where later also glial cells are produced, and by the thirty-sixth week of gestation only residual foci of the germinal matrix can be seen. The germinal matrix bears a delicate vascular pattern, consisting of vulnerable capillaries, having no muscular wall. Sudden changes in the blood pressure, disturbed autoregulation, higher fibrinolytic activity, increased permeability of vessel walls, caused by hypoxia contribute in pathogenesis of germinal matrix hemorrhage. Bleeding may occur in one focus but can be multiple, unilateral or bilateral. According to Papile's grading system, bleeding restricted to the germinal matrix represent grade 1; hemorrhage, breaking into the lateral ventricle is regarded as grade 2; in more severe cases dilatation of ventricles follows the hemorrhage (grade 3) and parenchymal damage (grade 4) can be observed in about 10% of the cases.[26] Germinal matrix and intraventricular hemorrhage usually develop in the first 3 days of life. High-grade intraventricular hemorrhage, associated with respiratory distress syndrome, is a leading cause of death, and grade 1–4 hemorrhage is present in as many as 83% of very low birthweight preterm infants in our postmortem examinations. On histology, extravasation of red blood cells, tissue damage, a few days later many hemosiderin laden macrophages and petrified neurons can be seen.

Periventricular leukomalacia is related to sudden drop of the blood pressure and the most vulnerable sites are the vascular watershed areas, where the decreased perfusion leads to ischemia.[27] Recent studies have revealed relationship between intrauterine infection, acute high-grade chorioamnionitis, funisitis and white matter injuries.[28,29] On macroscopical examination, whitish-yellowish foci can be seen with a chalk white rim, usually within the paraventricular white matter, in the temporal lobe and in the tapetum. The lesion tends to be multifocal and bilateral. Histologically, signs of coagulative necrosis, microglial and astrocytic reaction, groups of macrophages and mineralized neurons can be present. In later stage, cystic changes develop in the injured sites leading to the typical picture of multicystic periventricular leukomalacia (Fig. 12.9).

Necrotizing Enterocolitis (NEC)

The onset of the NEC is usually during the first 2 weeks for preterm infants. Although the exact initial cause is not known, alimentary and iatrogenic aspects are investigated. Immaturity is strongly associated with this condition but the etiological role of early enteral feeding is now challenged.[30,31] In contrast, perinatal asphyxia, and respiratory distress syndrome were not among the risk factors in the study of Kanto,[32] but umbilical cord catheterization increased the chance of NEC.[33] An infectious component has also been suspected by many investigators but no pathogenic organism has been found yet.[34,35] Breast milk proved to have a protective role.[36]

The clinical picture of NEC is characterized by lethargy, pale skin tone, abdominal distension, bloody stool and vomits. Radiology shows distended, gas-containing bowels and occasionally gas perforation into the abdominal cavity. The outcome is less favorable

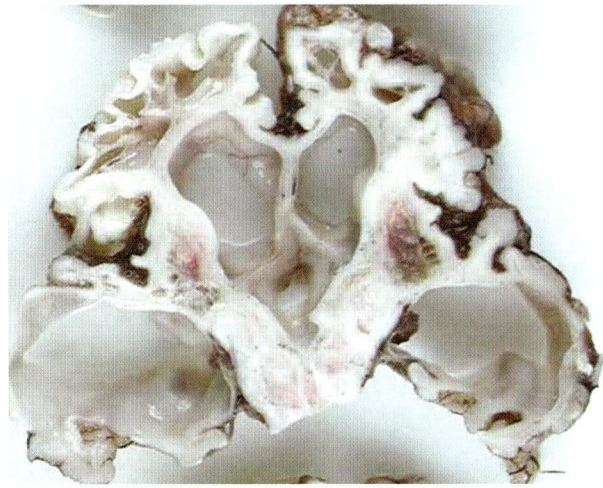

Fig. 12.9: Postischemic change in the brain. The ventricles are dilated, and there are multiple cysts in the white matter (postnecrotic porencephaly)

for very low birthweight infants, and for cases complicated with perforation, peritonitis, sepsis and intravascular coagulopathy.

Postmortem or postoperative examination of the bowels reveals distended, thin or paper like bowel wall, sites of perforation, greenish-brownish exudate on the visceral peritoneum. The number of the villi of the small intestine is diminished and the wall is showing different degree of edema, hemorrhagic necrosis and gangrenous inflammation. The picture can be similar in the lower part of the intestinal tract.

Retinopathy of Prematurity (RoP) and Other Pathological Conditions Associated with Prematurity

Retinopathy of preterm infants was described in the early 40s, and was regarded as retrolental fibroplasia (Terry 1942). The frequency dropped when the adverse effect of concentrated oxygen was recognized, but rose again with the increasing survival time of very low birthweight infants. According to the current practice, high-risk babies (less than 1,500 g and/or born before thirty-second week of gestation) are monitored in order to prevent retinal detachment and blindness, as total retinal detachment being the most severe stage of this condition.[37] The site of the changes is the junction of the vascularized and avascular retina, where demarcation, fibro-vascularization and neovascularization develops as a pathological reaction of the immature tissue for angiogenetic signals. The detailed pathway of this procedure is not yet entirely understood.

There are other, clinically important consequences of the altered metabolic functions, which do not have characteristic morphological appearance, such as hypothermia, hypoglycemia, and higher blood potassium level. Anemia of preterm infants presents with extensive extramedullary hemopoesis and occasionally fatty changes of the adrenal cortex.

The risk of sudden infant death syndrome is higher for preterm babies.

Preterm birth is very frequently complicated with perinatal infections, which are discussed under a separate subtitle.

PERINATAL INFECTIONS

Frequent Pathological Sequels of Intrauterine Infections

The incidence of the intrauterine infection reaches a peak in the second trimester. The two most frequent mechanisms are the ascending genital tract infections and the transplacental hematogenous spread. The pathogenesis of intraamniotic infections and the most common pathogenic agent are summarized in Table 12.1.

The consequences of intrauterine infection include early, spontaneous, preterm labor and premature rupture of membranes,[38] and occasionally generalized fetal infection. Developmental abnormalities and other clinical features related to particular intrauterine infections are well described in pediatric pathology.[4] CMV infection is known to be associated with severe central nervous system damage, microcephaly with multifocal calcification, chorioretinitis, hearing loss, neonatal hepatitis, while Rubella infection may lead to cardiac malformation, deafness, and eye defects. The incidence of Syphilis infection is very low and the vertical transmission rate for HIV showed a decreasing trend in the industrialized countries during the recent years.[39,40] The statistics is less favorable in the developing countries.[41]

The pathomorphological signs of intrauterine infection have to be carefully looked for in case of stillbirth or neonatal death. Symmetric type of IUGR is a common association. Frequent macroscopic and microscopic features of viral and bacterial infections are summarized in Table 12.2.

Neonatal Infection

Neonatal infection is frequent in preterm infants, with a higher risk and worse prognosis for low birthweight infants.

Sepsis occurring in the first 3 days of life, is called early-onset neonatal sepsis, can be a devastating neonatal problem, with high mortality rate. Although neonatal sepsis is not very frequent (2–4 per 1,000 live births) in developed countries, the rate increases for preterm infants and those born to mothers with infections or prolonged rupture of the fetal membranes. Group B streptococci and enterobacteriaceae are the main causes of early-onset sepsis in more developed countries.[42]

Late-onset neonatal sepsis (> 72 hours) is usually caused by Gram-positive agents, especially coagulase-negative staphylococci.[43,44]

Rarely, other Streptococci, *Haemophilus influenzae, Serratia marcescens, Malassezia furfur, Salmonella, Pseudomonas aeruginosa, Campylobacter* and *Listeria monocytogenes* leads to neonatal infection. *Candida albicans* is the most common among fungal infections, which often colonizes the baby from birth, and sometimes causes pneumonia in infants treated with antibiotics.

The costs and benefits of intrapartum antibiotic prophylaxis therapy should be carefully evaluated and the therapeutic policies reconsidered in the light of the new data on increasing frequency of nosocomial infections.[45,46]

The most severe complications of early and late-onset infections are pneumonia and meningitis, but enteral and urogenital infections, conjunctivitis and skin rushes may be also present. Pathological signs are frequently poor and non-specific. Macro-

Table 12.1: Mechanism and common pathogens of intrauterine infections

	Virus	Bacteria	Fungi	Protozoa
Transcervical	Herpes simplex or genitalis, HIV-1 (infection during labor)	Group B *Streptococcus*, *E. coli* and *H. influenzae*	*C. albicans*	
Transplacental	CMV, parvovirus, rubella and HIV-1	Group B *Streptococcus* and *L. monocytogenes*		*Toxoplasma, Chlamydia psittaci, Treponema pallidum* and *Borrelia*

Table 12.2: Typical macroscopic and microscopic features of intrauterine infections in the fetus and in the placenta

	Macroscopic signs	Microscopic signs
Bacterial Infection Placenta	• Opaque or greenish–brownish membranes in transcervical infection • Placental abscesses in case of transplacental spreading	• Transcervical infection • Acute, high-grade chorioamnionitis, • Fetal chorionic vessel vasculitis, and funisitis • Transplacental infection • Acute villitis, deciduitis • Microabscesses, microgranulomas, e.g. in listeriosis
Fetus	• Macroscopic features of septic shock Leptomeningeal purulent exudate and congestion in meningitis • Occasionally periventricular leukomalacia	• Intrauterine pneumonia infiltration with polymorphonuclear leukocytes in the airways, interstitial inflammatory reaction • Microabscesses of the parenchymal organs
Viral Infection Placenta		• Subacute or chronic villitis, specific virus inclusions, e.g. parvovirus B19, CMV
Fetus	• Hepatosplenomegaly • Icterus, petechiae • Hydrops • IUGR • Developmental malformation	• Specific virus inclusions, e.g. parvovirus B19, CMV, HSV • Hemolysis-hemosiderin deposition • Focal necrosis, dystrophic calcification, e.g. HSV

scopically, skin rushes, congestion of the parenchymal organs, petechiae, adrenal hemorrhage, rarely leptomeningeal purulent exudate can be observed. Microscopically, inflammatory infiltrate of the airways is present in the congested, edematous lung tissue, with interstitial reaction. Special stains may help to visualize fungi. Samples for microbiological laboratory test should be taken during postmortem examination.

CONGENITAL TUMORS AND TUMOR-LIKE LESIONS

Epidemiology, Biological Behavior and Etiology of Congenital Tumors

Neonatal tumors, (including congenital tumors) occurring within the first 28 days of life, represent an age-specific group of neoplastic lesions. The reported incidence (2003) ranged between 1 per 12,500 and 27,500 live births in the United Kingdom and United States of America and varied from 17 to 121 per million births worldwide.[47]

Abnormal tissue swellings and masses present at birth are often regarded as congenital tumors, although many types of them do not fulfil the criteria of true neoplasias. These tumor-like lesions, traditionally called hamartomas and choristomas, are probably due to tissue developmental abnormalities, differentiation and migration defects off cells resulting in a pathological architecture.

Benign and tumor-like lesions are reasonably frequent and usually harmless–such as infantile hemangioma, most small congenital nevi—but occasionally bear more clinical significance and complications, e.g. Kaposiform hemangioendothelioma associated with Kasabach-Merritt syndrome and fetal hydrops.[48] The biological behavior of neonatal tumors can not always be predicted based on their morphological appearance. Benign congenital lesions may have a risk of malignant transformation, e.g. malignant melanoma can develop in giant congenital nevus.[49-51] Infantile hemangioma may show spontaneous regression, however lesions of large size may cause cardiac failure or consumptional coagulopathy. The histologically benign cardiac fibroma or cardiac rhabdomyoma may represent poor prognosis for its unfavorable location. In contrast, some tumors of malignant histological appearance tend to show significantly better prognosis in early life, e.g. neuroblastoma, hereditary retinoblastoma and congenital fibrosarcoma.

A unique group of true congenital neoplasias are regarded as embryonal tumors. These are characterized by a uniformly primitive histological picture resembling embryonal-fetal appearance of the organ in which they arise. This group include neuroblastoma, nephroblastoma (Wilm's tumor), hepatoblastoma, retinoblastoma, embryonal rhabdomyosarcoma and medulloblastoma. Some embryonal tumors are familial, such as 40% of retinoblastomas and familial Wilm's tumors, while others associate with inherited syndromes, e.g. glycogenosis type I and hepatocellular carcinoma, or α-1 antitripsin deficiency and hepatoblastoma. In a few sporadic malformation syndromes there is a higher risk of neonatal tumors, for example in Beckwith-Wiedemann syndrome, a higher risk of nephroblastoma, hepatoblastoma and adrenal cancer can be observed, or in Hirschsprung's disease, which is occasionally associated with neuroblastoma. There is a long list of many other inherited syndromes including metabolic disorders, phacomatoses, DNA repair defects, immune deficiency syndromes, carrying a higher risk of different malignant tumors, but most of these develop only in later childhood.

Neonates with structural chromosomal anomalies may present with congenital tumors, trisomy 18 and 13 can be associated with teratomas, trisomy 18 with nephroblastoma and hepatoblastoma.[52] Acute megakaryocytic leukemia is a well-known complication of Down's syndrome in early neonatal age.[53]

On the other hand, frequency of congenital abnormalities—spina bifida, abnormalities of ribs, eyes—was higher in children with solid tumors (Wilm's tumor, Ewing sarcoma, hepatoblastoma) than in population based controls. This observation directs future studies in underlying gene disorders.[54]

Enviromental factors including ionizing radiation, particular drugs taken during pregnancy, and maternal CMV, varicella, influenza and HIV virus infections have been implicated in the etiology of neonatal (and pediatric) tumors.[55-57]

Common Types of Solid Neonatal Tumors

The incidence of neonatal tumors is similar in different reports, teratoma and neuroblastoma being the most common, followed by soft tissue tumors, renal and CNS tumors and leukemias.[47]

Congenital and Neonatal Teratoma

Fetal and neonatal germ cells tumors have different clinical course and morphology from those occurring in older children or adults. Congenital teratoma has been described in numerous sites, most frequently in sacrococcygeal location, but ovarial, testicular, mediastinal, cervicofacial, retroperitoneal, abdominal and intracranial location has also been documented (Figs 12.10A to D). There are published cases of teratoma developing in the placenta or umbilical cord. Prenatal diagnosis, recognition of risk factors, and intrauterine therapeutic interventions improved the outcome, although maternal complications, polyhydramnios, fetal cardiac failure, fetal hydrops, tumor rupture are not uncommon.[58-60]

Macroscopically, teratoma presents as a solid and cystic mass, potentially containing well-formed organoid structures. The traditional histological definition requires presence of tissues from all three germ layers and most teratomas fulfil these criteria. Immature tissue is usually present in 20–50% of cases[4,61] and the histological grading is based on the amount of immature tissue,[62] however, immature neural elements do not indicate malignancy in this age group. True malignant tumors, most frequently yolk-sac tumor, was present in 5.8% of teratomas with the highest incidence (10%) in sacrococcygeal teratoma and a tumor recurrence rate of 5% was reported in a recent review.[61]

Presacral sacrococcygeal teratoma has a worse prognosis than those in postsacral location, gastric teratoma has a good prognosis, while the outcome of the intracranial teratomas is poor, with few exceptions.[63-66] The main prognostic factors of fetal and neonatal teratoma are the size and location, the completeness of surgical excision, and presence of malignant tumor (yolk-sac tumor).

Congenital Neuroblastoma

The incidence of congenital neuroblastoma is similar to the teratoma thus it is the most frequent malignant tumor of the neonatal period. Ultrasonographic features of the tumor have been described and prenatal diagnosis gives opportunity for appropriate planning and management.[67,68]

Congenital neuroblastoma usually presents with an abdominal or adrenal mass but extraadrenal location, disseminated form,

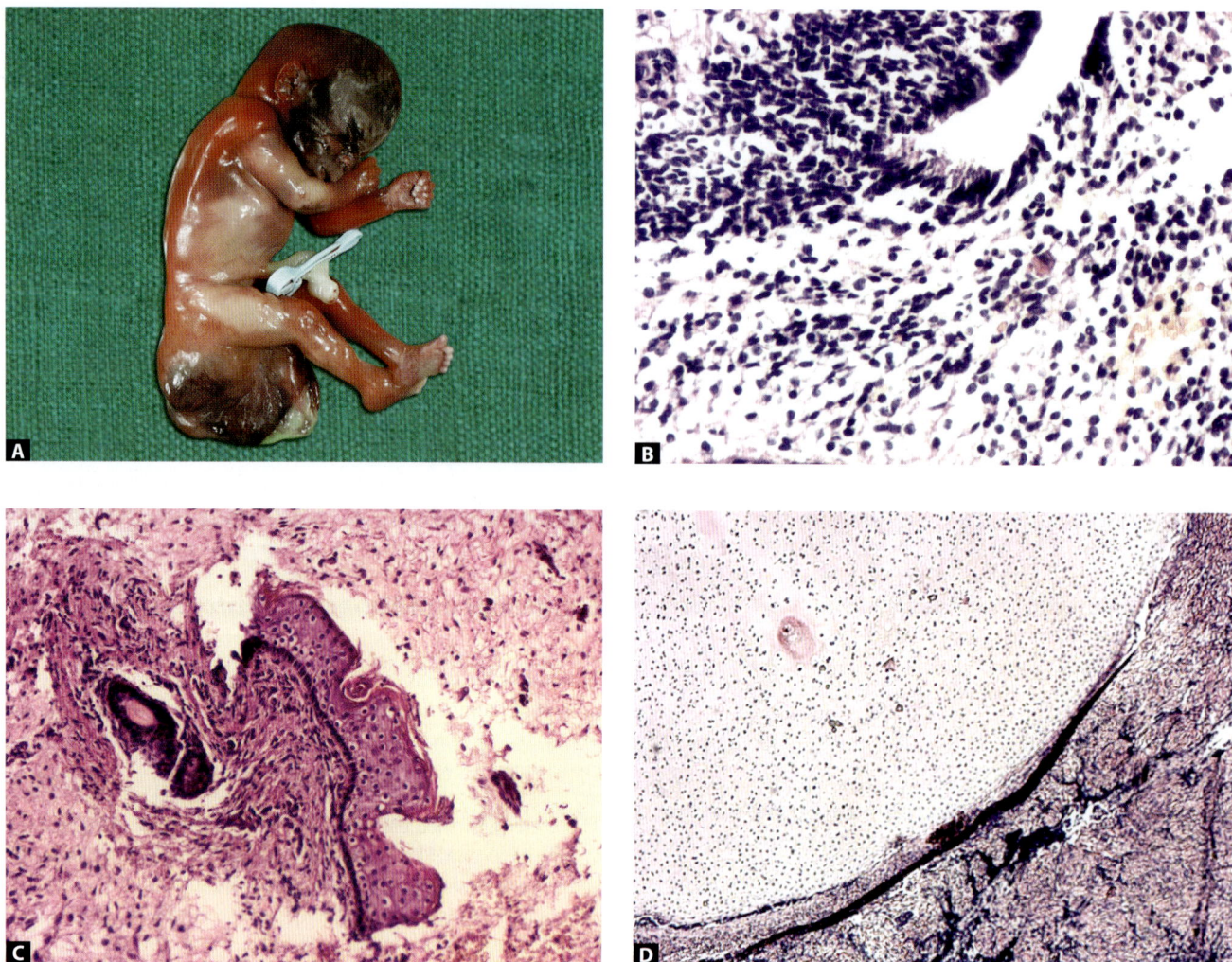

Figs 12.10A to D: Sacrococcygeal teratoma in a fetus of twenty-third weeks of gestation. (A) Macroscopic picture of the large, mainly presacral tumor; (B to D) Microscopic examination reveals immature neural elements, squamous epithelium with a hair follicle, and hyaline cartilage tissue

massive liver involvement, and metastasis of the skin and placenta can occur.[67-72]

The morphological features are not different from those in older children, and the same histological criteria are used for classification.[73] Immunohistochemistry and electron microscopy confirm the histological diagnosis. Molecular genetics is a useful aid to detect prognostic factors. N-myc amplification, expression of bcl-2, an apoptosis suppressing protein, are associated with unfavorable histology and bad prognosis.[74] The outcome of congenital neuroblastoma is generally favorable. A special pattern, characterized by small primary tumor, disseminated spreading, and low N-myc copy numbers is termed as Stage IV-S neuroblastoma. Spontaneous regression is not an uncommon finding in this stage.[75-77] Only a small proportion of congenital neuroblastomas require aggressive therapy. Life-threatening respiratory complication might be related to massive hepatomegaly.

Soft Tissue Tumors

Fibromatosis: This is a unique group of tumors with diverse clinicopathologic features.

The histological picture varies according to the specific types, but shares common features, like presence of intersecting bands of spindle cells in variably collagenized stroma. The lesions might be more cellular than the similar adult type alterations and show an aggressive growth. In contrast with the occasionally formidable picture the outlook is favorable. Spontaneous regression is not uncommon, although local recurrence may occur.[78]

Congenital myofibromatosis may present as a solitary lump and show spontaneous regression, while in its generalized form carries a poor prognosis due to visceral involvement (Figs 12.11A and B). Fibromatosis colli is a palpable mass in the sternocleidomastoid muscle, occurs in young infants, while infantile digital fibromatosis may present on the fingers and toes. Cranial fasciitis and fibrous hamartoma of infancy are both rapidly growing lesions of the subcutaneous soft tissue, the former localized on the skull.

Sarcoma: Congenital infantile fibrosarcoma is a fibroblastic-myofibroblastic proliferation, a rapidly growing lesion resulting in massive tumor. The histological appearance is sarcoma-like but the prognosis is good, with 5-year survival of more than 90% and metastases are very rare.[78] Some cases have a characteristic

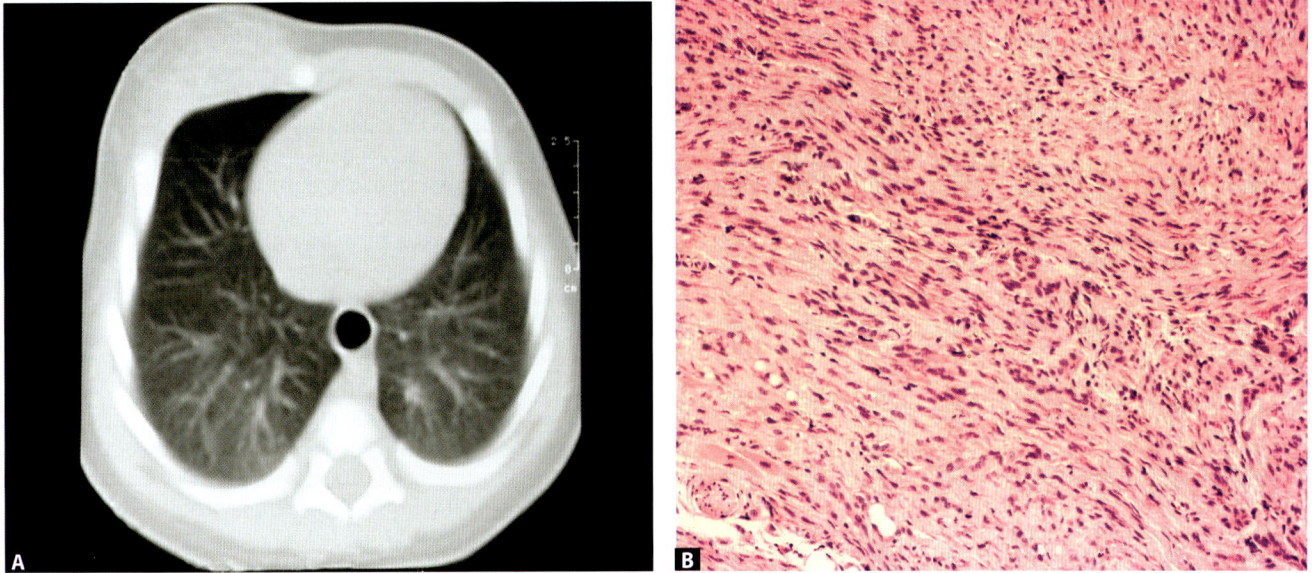

Figs 12.11A and B: Soliter infantile myofibromatosis in a term baby. (A) CT scan shows soft tissue swelling around the second rib, on the right, suggesting infiltrative growth; (B) Characteristic microscopic appearance, with bindles of spindle cells, and small round primitive looking cells. The soliter lesion bears an excellent prognosis

chromosomal translocation with t(12;15)(p13;q25) and an *ETV6-NTRK3* gene fusion or *ETV6* gene rearrangement.[79] Embryonal rhabdomyosarcoma shares similar features in young infants and children, having a 5-year survival of 66%. Embryonal rhabdomyosarcoma displays loss of heterozygosity on chromosome 11p15.5, a tumor related locus at 11q, numerical abnormalities, trisomy 8 and other abnormalities. However, these findings do not, as yet, have diagnostic or prognostic significance.[80,81]

Neural/Neuroectodermal Tumors

Neural tumors in young infants are usually associated with neurofibromatosis type 1 (NF1). Plexiform neurofibromas are histologically benign lesions with premalignant potential as in about 10% of the NF 1 patient malignant peripheral nerve-sheath tumor (MPNST) develops from it. Congenital peripheral/primitive neuroectodermal tumor (PNET) have been reported in several sites.[82-84] PNET and Ewing sarcoma are now considered the same entity, based on their shared genetic abnormalities, being consistently associated with chromosomal translocation and functional fusion of the *EWS* gene to any of several structurally related transcription factor genes (*EWS-FLI-1, EWS-ERG, EWS-ETV1, EWS-E1AF*, etc.).[85]

Adipose Tumors of the Neonate

Lipoblastoma, a typical benign tumor of fat tissue of the early childhood, occasionally may be present at birth. The circumscribed type is more common, with superficial location, while the diffuse type (lipoblastomatosis) originates from deep soft tissue, has an infiltrative growth pattern and recurs more frequently. Characteristic clonal karyotypic changes can be demonstrated and

help to distinguish from childhood and adult lipomas as well as from myxoid liposarcoma.[86]

Intracranial Tumors

Most frequently diagnosed intracranial tumor is teratoma, primitive neuroectodermal tumor, medulloblastoma, astrocytoma, glioblastoma multiforme and ependymoma. Plexus choroideus papilloma, ganglioglioma and low-grade astrocytoma have the best prognosis, but the overall survival rate of perinatal brain tumors was only 28% in a recent review. Stillbirth is frequent and hydrocephalusmacrocephaly is often diagnosed prenatally.[87-90]

Congenital Tumors of the Kidney

Congenital mesoblastic nephroma is a benign tumor, occasionally leads to fetal hydrops and polyhydramnios. Although, the tumor mass can be huge and extend beyond the kidney, surgical treatment is usually curative. Histologically, the tumor consists of spindle cells of myofibroblastic origin. A more cellular variant is known which carries the same t(12;15)(p13;q25) and *ETV6-NTRK3* gene fusion as infantile fibrosarcoma.[91]

Rhabdoid tumor of the kidney is an aggressive tumor with bad prognosis and distinct morphological features. It is characterized by deletion of the *hSNF5/INI1* gene, which links it to other rhabdoid tumors of infancy that arise in the soft tissue and brain.[92]

Congenital and infantile Wilm's tumor is rare and shows a strong association with presence of nephrogenic rests (persistent metanephric blastema) in the kidney.[93] Recent molecular genetic findings suggest a multistep model of the pathogenesis in Wilm's tumor and supports the precursor role of nephrogenic rests.[94] Nephrogenic rest as well as nephroblastoma may present in bilateral location. Nephroblastoma of the early infancy has a good prognosis.[95,96]

REFERENCES

1. Members of the CESDI Organization (2001). Confidential Enquiry into Stillbirths and Deaths in Infancy 8th Annual Report. London: Maternal and Child Health Research Consortium. [online] Available from http://www.cmace.org.uk/Publications.aspx [Accessed September, 2014].
2. Degani S. Fetal biometry: Clinical, pathological, and technical considerations. Obstet Gynecol Surv. 2001;56(3):159-67.
3. Gilbert-Barness E. Potter's Pathology of the Fetus and Infant. St. Louis, Baltimore, Boston, Carlsbad, Naples, New York, Philadelphia, Portland, Madrid, Mexico City, Singapore, Sydney, Tokyo, Wiesbaden: Mosby; 1997.
4. Keeling JW. Fetal and Neonatal Pathology. 2nd edition. London, Berlin, Heidelberg, New York, Paris, Tokyo, Hong Kong, Barcelona, Budapest: Springer-Verlag; 2001.
5. Wigglesworth JS, Singer DB. Textbook of Fetal and Perinatal Pathology. Boston, Oxford, London, Edinburgh, Melbourne, Paris, Berlin, Vienna: Blackwell Scientific Publications; 1991.
6. Anderson JM. Increased brain weight-liver weight ratio as a necropsy sign of intrauterine undernutrition. J Clin Pathol. 1972;25(10):867-71.
7. Mitchell ML. Fetal brain to liver weight ratio as a measure of intrauterine growth retardation: Analysis of 182 stillborn autopsies. Mod Pathol. 2001;14(1):14-9.
8. Dorovini-Zis K, Dolman CL. Gestational development of brain. Arch Pathol Lab Med. 1977;101(4):192-5.
9. Hinchliffe SA, Lynch MR, Sargent PH, et al. The effect of intrauterine growth retardation on the development of renal nephrons. Br J Obstet Gynaecol. 1992;99(4):296-301.
10. Khong TY, Yee KT. Pathology of intrauterine growth retardation. Am J Reprod Immunol. 1989;21(3-4):132-6.
11. Terespolsky D, Farrell SA, Siegel-Bartelt J, et al. Infantile lethal variant of Simpson-Golabi-Behmel syndrome associated with hydrops fetalis. Am J Med Genet. 1995;59(3):329-33.
12. Perlman M, Levin M, Wittels B. Syndrome of fetal gigantism, renal hamartomas, and nephroblastomatosis with Wilms' tumor. Cancer. 1975;35(4):1212-7.
13. Douglas J, Hanks S, Temple IK, et al. NSD1 mutations are the major cause of Sotos syndrome and occur in some cases of Weaver syndrome but are rare in other overgrowth phenotypes. Am J Hum Genet. 2003;72(1):132-43.
14. Jacobsson B, Hagberg G. Antenatal risk factors for cerebral palsy. Best Pract Res Clin Obstet Gynaecol. 2004;18(3):425-36.
15. MacLennan A. A template for defining a causal relation between acute intrapartum events and cerebral palsy: International consensus statement. BMJ. 1999;319(7216):1054-9.
16. Magee JF. Investigation of stillbirth. Pediatr Dev Pathol. 2001;4(1):1-22.
17. Krauss AN. New methods advance treatment for respiratory distress syndrome. Pediatr Ann. 2003;(329):585-91.
18. Weisman LE. Populations at risk for developing respiratory syncytial virus and risk factors for respiratory syncytial virus severity: Infants with predisposing conditions. Pediatr Infect Dis J. 2003;22(2 Suppl):S33-7.
19. Garland JS, Alex CP, Pauly TH, et al. A three-day course of dexamethasone therapy to prevent chronic lung disease in ventilated neonates: A randomized trial. Pediatrics. 1999;104(1 Pt1):91-9.
20. Shah PS. Current perspectives on the prevention and management of chronic lung disease in preterm infants. Paediatr Drugs. 2003;5(7):463-80.
21. Bhandari A, Bhandari V. Pathogenesis, pathology and pathophysiology of pulmonary sequelae of bronchopulmonary dysplasia in premature infants. Front Biosci. 2003;8:e370-80.
22. Coalson JJ. Pathology of new bronchopulmonary dysplasia. Semin Neonatol. 2003;8(1):73-81.
23. Hoekstra RE, Ferrara TB, Couser RJ, et al. Survival and long-term neurodevelopmental outcome of extremely premature infants born at 23–26 weeks' gestational age at a tertiary center. Pediatrics. 2004;113(1 Pt1):e1-6.
24. Vollmer B, Roth S, Baudin J, et al. Predictors of long-term outcome in very preterm infants: Gestational age versus neonatal cranial ultrasound. Pediatrics. 2003;112(5):1108-14.
25. Skullerud K, Westre B. Frequency and prognostic significance of germinal matrix hemorrhage, periventricular leukomalacia, and pontosubicular necrosis in preterm neonates. Acta Neuropathol (Berl). 1986;70(34):257-61.
26. Papile LA, Burstein J, Burstein R, et al. Incidence and evolution of subependymal and intraventricular hemorrhage: A study of infants with birth weights less than 1,500 gm. J Pediatr. 1978;92(4):529-34.
27. Takashima S, Tanaka K. Development of cerebrovascular architecture and its relationship to periventricular leukomalacia. Arch Neurol. 1978;35(1):11-6.
28. Wu YW, Colford JM Jr. Chorioamnionitis as a risk factor for cerebral palsy: A meta-analysis. JAMA. 2000;284(11):1417-24.
29. Yoon BH, Kim CJ, Romero R, et al. Experimentally induced intrauterine infection causes fetal brain white matter lesions in rabbits. Am J Obstet Gynecol. 1997;177(4):797-802.
30. Flidel-Rimon O, Friedman S, Lev E, et al. Early enteral feeding and nosocomial sepsis in very low birthweight infants. Arch Dis Child Fetal Neonatal Ed. 2004;89(4):F289-92.
31. Stoll BJ. Epidemiology of necrotizing enterocolitis. Clin Perinatol. 1994;21(2):205-18.
32. Kanto WP Jr, Wilson R, Breart GL, et al. Perinatal events and necrotizing enterocolitis in premature infants. Am J Dis Child. 1987;141(2):167-9.
33. Rand T, Weninger M, Kohlhauser C, et al. Effects of umbilical arterial catheterization on mesenteric hemodynamics. Pediatr Radiol. 1996;26(7):435-8.
34. Faustini A, Forastiere F, Giorgi Rossi P, et al. An epidemic of gastroenteritis and mild necrotizing enterocolitis in two neonatal units of a University Hospital in Rome, Italy. Epidemiol Infect. 2004;132(3):455-65.
35. Sharma R, Garrison RD, Tepas JJ, et al. Rotavirus-associated necrotizing enterocolitis: An insight into a potentially preventable disease? J Pediatr Surg. 2004;39(3):453-7.
36. McGuire W, Anthony MY. Donor human milk versus formula for preventing necrotizing enterocolitis in preterm infants: Systematic review. Arch Dis Child Fetal Neonatal Ed. 2003;88(1):F11-4.
37. Ells A, Hicks M, Fielden M, et al. Severe retinopathy of prematurity: Longitudinal observation of disease and screening implications. Eye. 2004.
38. Goldenberg RL, Culhane JF. Infection as a cause of preterm birth. Clin Perinatol. 2003;30(4):677-700.
39. Duong T, Ades AE, Gibb DM, et al. Vertical transmission rates for HIV in the British Isles: Estimates based on surveillance data. BMJ. 1999;319(7219):1227-9.
40. Gibb DM. Reduction of mother-to-child transmission of HIV infection: Non-pharmaceutical interventions and their implementation. Int J STD AIDS. 1998;9(Suppl 1):1921.

41. Lepage P, Van de Perre P, Msellati P, et al. Mother-to-child transmission of human immunodeficiency virus type 1 (HIV-1) and its determinants: A cohort study in Kigali, Rwanda. Am J Epidemiol. 1993;137(6):589-99.

42. Moore MR, Schrag SJ, Schuchat A. Effects of intrapartum antimicrobial prophylaxIs for prevention of group-B-streptococcal disease on the incidence and ecology of early-onset neonatal sepsis. Lancet Infect Dis. 2003;3(4):201-13.

43. Isaacs D, Barfield C, Clothier T, et al. Late-onset infections of infants in neonatal units. J Paediatr Child Health. 1996;32(2):158-161.

44. Stoll BJ, Hansen N. Infections in VLBW infants: Studies from the NICHD Neonatal Research Network. Semin Perinatol. 2003;27(4):293-301.

45. Baltimore RS. Neonatal sepsis: Epidemiology and management. Paediatr Drugs. 2003;5(11):723-40.

46. Clark R, Powers R, White R, et al. Nosocomial Infection in the NICU: A Medical Complication or Unavoidable Problem? J Perinatol. 2004;24(6):382-8.

47. Moore SW, Satge D, Sasco AJ, et al. The epidemiology of neonatal tumors. Report of an international working group. Pediatr Surg Int. 2003;19(7):509-19.

48. Martinez AE, Robinson MJ, Alexis JB. Kaposiform hemangioendothelioma associated with nonimmune fetal hydrops. Arch Pathol Lab Med. 2004;128(6):678-81.

49. Hoss DM, Grant-Kels JM. Significant melanocytic lesions in infancy, childhood, and adolescence. Dermatol Clin. 1986;4(1):29-44.

50. Leech SN, Bell H, Leonard N, et al. Neonatal giant congenital nevi with proliferative nodules: A clinicopathologic study and literature review of neonatal melanoma. Arch Dermatol. 2004;140(1):83-8.

51. Richardson SK, Tannous ZS, Mihm MC Jr. Congenital and infantile melanoma: Review of the literature and report of an uncommon variant, pigment-synthesizing melanoma. J Am Acad Dermatol. 2002;47(1):77-90.

52. Satge D, Van Den Berghe H. Aspects of the neoplasms observed in patients with constitutional autosomal trisomy. Cancer Genet Cytogenet. 1996;87(1):63-70.

53. Al-Kasim F, Doyle JJ, Massey GV, et al. Incidence and treatment of potentially lethal diseases in transient leukemia of Down syndrome: Pediatric Oncology Group Study. J Pediatr Hematol Oncol. 2002;24(1):9-13.

54. Narod SA, Hawkins MM, Robertson CM, et al. Congenital anomalies and childhood cancer in Great Britain. Am J Hum Genet. 1997;60(3):474-85.

55. Leotta N, Alvaro F, Dalla-Pozza L, et al. Concurrent HIV infection and neuroblastoma. J Paediatr Child Health. 2003;39(3):236-8.

56. Marias BJ, Peinaar J, Gie RP. Kaposi sarcoma with upper airway obstruction and bilateral chylothoraces. Pediatr Infect Dis J. 2003;22(10):926-8.

57. Reyes C, Abuzaitoun O, De Jong A, et al. Epstein-Barr virus-associated smooth muscle tumors in ataxia-telangiectasia: A case report and review. Hum Pathol. 2002;33(1):133-6.

58. Chisholm CA, Heider AL, Kuller JA, et al. Prenatal diagnosis and perinatal management of fetal sacrococcygeal teratoma. Am J Perinatol. 1999;16(2):89-92.

59. Chisholm CA, Heider AL, Kuller JA, et al. Prenatal diagnosis and perinatal management of fetal sacrococcygeal teratoma. Am J Perinatol. 1999;16(1):47-50.

60. Hedrick HL, Flake AW, Crombleholme TM, et al. Sacrococcygeal teratoma: Prenatal assessment, fetal intervention, and outcome. J Pediatr Surg. 2004;39(3):430-8.

61. Isaacs H Jr. Perinatal (fetal and neonatal) germ cell tumors. J Pediatr Surg. 2004;39(7):1003-13.

62. Gonzalez-Crussi F, Winkler RF, Mirkin DL. Sacrococcygeal teratomas in infants and children: Relationship of histology and prognosis in 40 cases. Arch Pathol Lab Med. 1978;102(8):420-5.

63. Canan A, Gulsevin T, Nejat A, et al. Neonatal intracranial teratoma. Brain Dev. 2000;22(5):340-2.

64. Chien YH, Tsao PN, Lee WT, et al. Congenital intracranial teratoma. Pediatr Neurol. 2000;22(1):72-4.

65. Hunt SJ, Johnson PC, Coons SW, et al. Neonatal intracranial teratomas. Surg Neurol. 1990;34(5):336-42.

66. Saleem SM, Hussain S, Nazir Z. Gastric teratoma—a rare benign tumour of neonates. Ann Trop Paediatr. 2003;23(4):305-8.

67. Granata C, Fagnani AM, Gambini C, et al. Features and outcome of neuroblastoma detected before birth. J Pediatr Surg. 2000;35(1):88-91.

68. Kurjak A, Zalud I, Jurkovic D, et al. Ultrasound diagnosis and evaluation of fetal tumors. J Perinat Med. 1989;17(3):173-93.

69. Millman GC, Lodha AK, Moore AM, et al. Disseminated congenital neuroblastoma presenting at birth. Arch Dis Child. 2003;88(3):191.

70. Smith R, Chan HS, deSa DJ. Placental involvement in congenital neuroblastoma. J Clin Pathol. 1981;34(7):78-9.

71. Nguyen TQ, Fisher GB Jr, Tabbarrah SO, et al. Stage IV-S metastatic neuroblastoma presenting as skin nodules at birth. Int J Dermatol. 1988;27(10):712-3.

72. Yamashina M, Kayan H, Katayama I, et al. Congenital neuroblastoma presenting as a paratesticular tumor. J Urol. 1988;139(4):796-7.

73. Shimada H, Ambros IM, Dehner LP, et al. The International Neuroblastoma Pathology Classification (the Shimada system). Cancer. 1999;86(2):364-72.

74. Goto S, Umehara S, Gerbing RB, et al. Histopathology (International Neuroblastoma Pathology Classification) and MYCN status in patients with peripheral neuroblastic tumors: A report from the Children's Cancer Group. Cancer. 2001;92(10):2699-708.

75. Haas D, Ablin AR, Miller C, et al. Complete pathologic maturation and regression of stage IVS neuroblastoma without treatment. Cancer. 1988;62(4):818-25.

76. Hachitanda Y, Hata J. Stage IVS neuroblastoma: A clinical, histological, and biological analysis of 45 cases. Hum Pathol. 1996;27(11):1135-8.

77. Stokes SH, Thomas PR, Perez CA, et al. Stage IV-S neuroblastoma. Results with definitive therapy. Cancer. 1984;53(10):2083-6.

78. Coffin CM, Dehner LP. Fibroblastic-myofibroblastic tumors in children and adolescents: A clinicopathologic study of 108 examples in 103 patients. Pediatr Pathol. 1991;11(4):569-88.

79. Knezevich SR, McFadden DE, Tao W, et al. A novel ETV6-NTRK3 gene fusion in congenital fibrosarcoma. Nat Genet. 1998;18(2):184-7.

80. Coffin CM, Dehner LP. Soft tissue tumors in first year of life: A report of 190 cases. Pediatr Pathol. 1990;10(4):509-26.

81. Chen Z, Coffin CM, Smith LM, et al. Cytogenetic-clinicopathologic correlations in rhabdomyosarcoma: A report of five cases. Cancer Genet Cytogenet. 2001;131(1):31-6.

82. Daw JL, Wiedrich TA, Bauer BS. Congenital primitive neuroectodermal tumor of the hand: A case report. J Hand Surg Am. 1997;22(4):743-6.

83. Smith LM, Adams RH, Brothman AR, et al. Peripheral primitive neuroectodermal tumor presenting with diffuse cutaneous involvement and 7;22 translocation. Med Pediatr Oncol. 1998;30(6):357-63.

84. Yamada T, Takeuchi K, Masuda Y, et al. Prenatal imaging of congenital cerebral primitive neuroectodermal tumor. Fetal Diagn Ther. 2003;18(3):137-9.

85. de Alava E, Gerald WL. Molecular biology of the Ewing's sarcoma/primitive neuroectodermal tumor family. J Clin Oncol. 2000;18(1):204-13.

86. Chen Z, Coffin CM, Scott S, et al. Evidence by spectral karyotyping that 8q11.2 is nonrandomly involved in lipoblastoma. J Mol Diagn. 2000;2(2):73-7.

87. Buetow PC, Smirniotopoulos JG, Done S. Congenital brain tumors: A review of 45 cases. AJNR Am J Neuroradiol. 1990;11(4):793-9.

88. Buetow PC, Smirniotopoulos JG, Done S. Congenital brain tumors: A review of 45 cases. AJR Am J Roentgenol. 1990;155(3):587-93.

89. Isaacs H Jr. I. Perinatal brain tumors: A review of 250 cases. Pediatr Neurol. 2002;27(4):249-61.

90. Isaacs H Jr. II. Perinatal brain tumors: A review of 250 cases. Pediatr Neurol. 2002;27(5):333-42.

91. Argani P, Fritsch M, Kadkol SS, et al. Detection of the ETV6-NTRK3 chimeric RNA of infantile fibrosarcoma/cellular congenital mesoblastic nephroma in paraffin-embedded tissue: application to challenging pediatric renal stromal tumors. Mod Pathol. 2000;13(1):29-36.

92. Argani P, Ladanyi M. Recent advances in pediatric renal neoplasia. Adv Anat Pathol. 2003;10(5):243-60.

93. Beckwith JB, Kiviat NB, Bonadio JF. Nephrogenic rests, nephroblastomatosis, and the pathogenesis of Wilms' tumor. Pediatr Pathol. 1990;10(1-2):1-36.

94. Charles AK, Brown KW, Berry PJ. Microdissecting the genetic events in nephrogenic rests and Wilms' tumor development. Am J Pathol. 1998;153(3):991-1000.

95. Kullendorff CM, Wiebe T. Wilms' tumour in infancy. Acta Paediatr. 1998;87(7):747-50.

96. Ritchey ML, Azizkhan RG, Beckwith JB, et al. Neonatal Wilms tumor. J Pediatr Surg. 1995;30(6):856-9.

13

Medical Management of Newborn with Severe Malformations—Ethical Aspects

M Stanojevic

INTRODUCTION

Neonatology is relatively new field of medicine developed as a separate subspecialty in the last several decades due to the need to address the high mortality rates of newborns compared with other age groups of children.[1] In most newborns, adaptation to extrauterine life is uneventful, while on rare occasions it could be even life-threatening. Hopefully, many adaptation disorders are transient and self-limiting, although in some situations they can affect development of the infant or even cause death in the first minute or day of life.

Development of medical technology in the second half of the 20th century enabled:[2]

Better thermal care for newborns

- Application of mechanical ventilation in critically ill neonates
- Management of congenital malformations using new surgical methods especially in the field of cardio- and neurosurgery
- Development of new diagnostic methods like neuro- and cardio-imaging,
- Genetic and metabolic diagnostics
- Administration of recently developed new medications.

All these technological achievements have become milestones of the new medical field of medicine called neonatology.

This leap in technology not only allowed the survival of many newborns during dangerous period of adaptation without health damage, but also significantly decreased gestational age and birthweight of infants with increasing chances of survival.[1] Not so long ago, infants below 34 weeks of gestation had limited chances to survive, while nowadays even infants at 25 weeks of gestation have over 50% chance to survive.

However, this triumph of technology over nature has its dark side. In addition to hundreds of thousands of newborns, who thanks to modern medicine have chances of unimpaired development, there is also a group of severely damaged children who survived for the same reason.[1] Many of them are incapable of independent living with a lot of pain and other problems of low quality of life. At that point, modern medicine is facing the problem of the possibility to extend the life of many newborns with virtually lethal congenital malformations or other rare diseases. So, the potential of modern medicine to preserve life of the sickest newborns should not be overestimated, because it raises many ethical issues, which are compared to technical possibilities, still waiting to be solved.

Confronting the moral dilemmas that have arisen with the development of medical science, with existing bioethical concepts a long conflict between two different ethical options traditional Christian, and pragmatic ethics has become more evident.[1-4] This conflict is so important that advantage of one of these concepts over the other can severely influence the course and dynamics of the development of biomedical sciences for many years.[1-4] The essential question is whether these two concepts are proposing solutions for neonatologists faced with challenging ethical situations in daily medical practice in the current cultural context.[1-4] It seems that the problem could be more understandable if the answers to some substantial questions could be answered:[1-4]

- Is the value of human life dependent on its quality?
- it possible not to undertake life-saving procedures in some severely malformed or extremely premature newborns? In other words, who deserves access to neonatal intensive care?
- some babies too sick or too premature for newborn intensive care? Is it possible to abandon life-saving procedure in newborns if it is futile?
- Who decides whether an infant receives care and how are these decisions made?
- How can this care be assured and equitably distributed?
- Who pays for this care?

Too many questions, hardly any answers.

DEFINITIONS OF CONGENITAL MALFORMATIONS AND RARE DISEASES

Congenital malformations and rare diseases can sometimes be detected in neonatal period. As in both groups of diseases life threat could happen, and on some occasions quality of life is questionable, many ethical questions can arise.

The terms "congenital anomalies", "birth defects", and "congenital malformations" are all used to describe developmental defects that are present at birth.[2] The term anomaly is commonly used for all types of structural defects, chromosomal abnormalities, genetic syndromes, metabolic defects, functional and behavioral defects.[2,3] Congenital malformations can be at least classified according to the type, cause and pathogenesis.[3] The concept of teratology has been introduced in order to define maldevelopment and to introduce taxonomic innovations.[4] Classifications of structural defects have been proposed which define the term congenital malformations in a stricter sense as "morphological defects of an organ, part of an organ, or larger part of the body as a result of an intrinsically abnormal developmental process".[5] Malformations are distinguished in this classification from other structural defects, disruptions, deformations, and dysplasia, by their "intrinsic nature of defect", meaning that the development of the organ was abnormal from the start, or near the start of its development.[3,5] Human congenital abnormalities can be divided and defined as follows: Malformation, a primary structural defect, distinguished from deformation, an alteration in a previously normally formed part; anomalad, a malformation together with its subsequently derived structural changes; syndrome, a recognized pattern of malformations with a given etiology; and association, a pattern of malformations, not a syndrome or anomalad.[3] Teratology, which is more extended term than dysmorphology, has numerous applications and modes of study like clinical, experimental, behavioral, ecological, epidemiological, toxicological, and molecular.[4]

There is no single, widely accepted definition for rare diseases and criteria for the disease to be rare. This is why many criteria are used to define rare disease like the number of people living with a disease, the existence of adequate treatments or the severity of the disease.[6,7] The definitions used in the medical literature are based on the prevalence of rare diseases ranging from 1/1,000 to 1/200,000 persons. In the US, the Rare Disease Act of 2002 defines rare disease strictly according to prevalence, as "any disease or condition that affects less than 200,000 persons in the US," or about 1 in 1,500 people.[6] In Japan, the legal definition of a rare disease is one that affects fewer than 50,000 patients in Japan, or about 1 in 2,500 people. The European Commission on Public Health defines rare diseases as "life-threatening or chronically debilitating diseases which are of such low prevalence that special combined efforts are needed to address them".[7] The term low prevalence is defined as less than 1 in 2,000 people. Diseases that are statistically rare, but not also life-threatening, chronically debilitating, or adequately treated, are excluded from the definition. Sometimes, rare diseases are diagnosed in neonatal period and some of them might be life-threatening without adequate treatment. Therefore, for some infants suffering from "rare disease" the same ethical problem can arise like in children with life-threatening congenital malformations.

EPIDEMIOLOGY AND OUTCOME OF CONGENITAL MALFORMATIONS

Estimates of the prevalence of congenital anomalies vary between 2% and 6% of births.[5] The prevalence may vary considerably depending on the definition and criteria used to include or exclude minor malformations, the time period of follow-up after birth and ethnicity.[8] Major structural congenital anomalies are commonly reported to be present in 2–3% of births.[9] In European Network of Congenital Anomaly Registries (EUROCAT) centers, the prevalence of congenital anomalies (including major structural defects, chromosomal abnormalities, some inborn errors of metabolism, and genetic syndromes) was 2.3% between 1990 and 1994, varying from 0.99 to 3.61 in individual centers.[9]

According to the World Health Organization (WHO) data from 36 countries in the period of 44 years (1950 to 1994), infant mortality rate decreased on average 68.8%, while infant mortality attributable to congenital malformations decreased only 33.4%.[10] Overall, about one-quarter of early neonatal deaths are due to congenital anomalies ranging from 21% to 42%. About 15–20% of fetal deaths are attributed to congenital anomalies in most countries. Some of these variations may be due to differences in policies for antenatal screening and terminations of pregnancy for congenital anomalies. If anomalies are detected and terminated before 22 weeks of pregnancy, this should reduce fetal and neonatal deaths due to congenital anomalies. In countries which allow terminations after 22 weeks of gestation, this policy may increase the percentage of fetal deaths due to congenital anomalies.

Causes of neonatal deaths vary between the early and the late neonatal periods, with deaths caused by preterm birth, asphyxia,

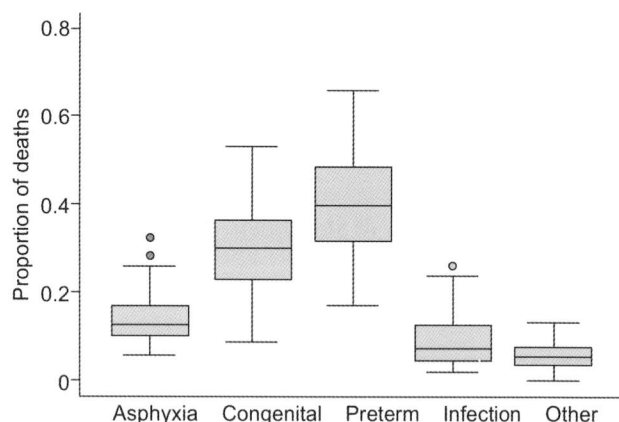

Fig. 13.1: Box plots showing the proportional distribution of causes of neonatal mortality for the vital registration data (44 countries)[11]

and congenital defects occurring predominantly during the first week of life and infection being the major cause of neonatal deaths thereafter.[11] Congenital anomalies are among the leading causes of infant mortality and important contributor to childhood and adult morbidity. It is estimated that about 20–30% of neonatal deaths could be attributed to major congenital malformations (Fig. 13.1).[11] Major congenital anomalies are abnormalities which are severe enough to reduce life expectancy or compromise normal function.[10] If major malformations cause stillbirth or infant death in more than 50% of cases, they are considered lethal.[10] If newborn infant with major congenital malformation cannot survive without medical intervention, than malformation is considered severe.[10]

The etiology of congenital anomalies is unknown in 30–45% of affected babies.[10] A genetic cause was considered to be responsible for 10–30% of all birth defects, environmental factors for 5–10%, multifactorial inheritance for 20–35%.[10]

CARE FOR INFANTS WITH SEVERE AND LIFE-THREATENING MAJOR CONGENITAL MALFORMATIONS

During pregnancy the prospective parents anticipate a normal child, although many have lingering fear that the infant may be malformed. In many cases diagnosis of severe congenital malformation is made prenatally. It would be much easier for the infant, parents and health-care provider to begin communication before birth. The aim of this communication between parents and health care provider is:[12]

- To make parents understand the condition of the child
- To inform them about the possibilities of the treatment
- To provide them with the information about the prognosis and outcome.

All the information should be as accurate as possible and related to the condition of their child, although most of given information will be based on statistical data from the literature and investigations, and will not describe the real situation of the infant's condition. The parents should be informed about the ability of the physicians to give the accurate information about the infant's health.[13] The family should be kept fully informed of the infant's evolving status and prognosis. Expression of empathy is of utmost importance for the communication between physician and parents. In some circumstances, like labor, it is better to delay informing parents about the infant's health situation, because it could affect adversely the course of labor.[14]

When parents are informed that fetus is malformed or otherwise damaged their initial response is often denial together with the fillings of guilt, anxiety, self-pity and sadness which in fact are grief responses to the loss of the anticipated normal child.[13,14] It is very important that the physician has enough knowledge to make a correct diagnosis, prognosis, management plan and genetic counseling. In communication with parents, physician should talk to both parents indicating as accurate as possible the consequences of the situation for the infant and for the family. After such treatment, the parents are ready to make vast majority of very important decisions in very delicate situation.[13]

Fetuses and neonates with congenital anomalies can be divided into six groups:[12]

1. Those who have the potential for total recovery
2. Those with anomalies that would allow for a nearly normal life
3. Those with malformations requiring permanent supervision and/or medical care
4. Those with somatic rest defect and subnormal mental development
5. Those with serious somatic and mental damage
6. Those with anomalies that are incompatible with life.

The physician should lower the anxiety of the parents, should follow the morals of a civilized society, should act according to the law, and finally, should convince himself to be a solution to a problem and not to be a cause of any.[12]

According to the American Academy of Pediatrics, there are three possibilities concerning the treatment with intensive care in decision-making process based on the infant's prognosis:[13]

1. The intensive care is indicated if survival is likely and the risk of severe morbidity is low.
2. The intensive care is not indicated if the survival is not likely and would be accompanied by severe unacceptable morbidity and suffering.
3. In some cases, the situation could be in between those two situations and prognosis is not certain, but very likely to be very poor. In that situation, parental desires should determine the treatment approach.

In the first situation of "normality", where child affected with deformation is interpreted as "normal child", which means that the disorder is curable and the infant can lead a normal life thereafter.[12-14] This group of infants includes those with single defects such as cleft lip, some congenital heart defects (CHD), pyloric stenosis, hexodactyly, etc. Parents should be informed that the child is normal, with a small problem which is curable and can be easily and adequately solved. The statement that the infant is normal is very important as well as the information that the condition is correctable.[12,14] Such approach to the counseling can help parents with realistic acceptance of the problem. In case when physicians fail to make acceptance of infant's condition, than relations between parents and their child may develop in two undesirable directions: rejection or overprotection.[12-14]

In the second group when dealing with severely malformed infant, like anencephaly, severe neural tube defects, hydranencephaly, holoprosencephaly, the trisomy 18 and 13 syndrome, the 4p-syndrome, the Meckel-Gruber or Potter syndrome, the physician must give parents the option of no medical intervention.[14] All mentioned disorders are severely limiting infant's capacity to survive and function even with full medical support including intensive care.[12-15] The doctor should say that even if the life will be preserved for some time, the baby has no capacity for continued survival. In the case of intervention the functional capability of the baby will be very limited. The physician should state that the kindest approach to the infant is that of no medical intervention, and ask for the permission for such an approach. In such way parents are informed about the basic course of the problem, helped to interpret the situation, and given the option of no medical intervention in the best interest of the child.[12-15] They should be aware that the baby will be provided with compassionate care and that suffering will be minimal.[12-15] Sometimes when parents are faced with end-of-life decisions, they will need psychological or social worker help to overcome their problem.[15] Parental complaints are more likely to occur due to misunderstanding, confusion and tension among staff and parents as a result of a failure to have in place or to implement agreed protocols.[16]

When dealing with intermediate situation, the counseling of the parents is very complicated and individualized, depending on the nature and the severity of the handicap. The accurate information is again very important, including facts relative to the cause of the problem, the usual range of functional and other limitations, and what can be done in order to help the child to adapt to the problem.[14] In this situation, the parents should be helped to accept their child with the problem, informing them that there are other families with the same or similar problems.[12-14]

Generally, this counseling process is very hardworking and time-consuming. Any medical professional who is counseling parents of malformed newborns should be aware that parents may need several meetings to accept the situation and to understand it.[14] Sometimes, the same information rephrased is well-accepted, and on another occasion the parents do not even notice the problem. Some parents are almost incapable of accepting a handicapping disorder of their child, while the others can develop deep parental love for a malformed and handicapped child.[12,14]

Is Treatment of Neonates with Severe Congenital Anomalies Always Justified?

It is always the question what is late outcome of children treated for severe congenital anomalies. The meanings of "late" and "outcomes" have historically been from the perspective of the physician and rarely from the perspective of the patient or parent.[17] Usually "late" outcome studies in the literature for severe congenital malformations span a decade or less, certainly not how a parent (or a child) would envision a truly long-term result.[17] Parents of children with severe congenital malformations are asking for predictions that span a lifetime and exactly how long that lifetime will be. For most of the severe congenital malformations these data are very rarely available. In addition, "outcome" studies most commonly deal with early functional or surgical outcome, mortality and, occasionally, long-term treatment or late neurodevelopmental outcomes.[17] Patients' perspectives and interests are frequently quite different and include ability to live normal life or to determine possible limitations, self-image, and the ability to work in a normal job, the ability to obtain health and life insurance, and other important health-related quality of life issues.[17] From the medical point of view as well as from the general believe and expectation

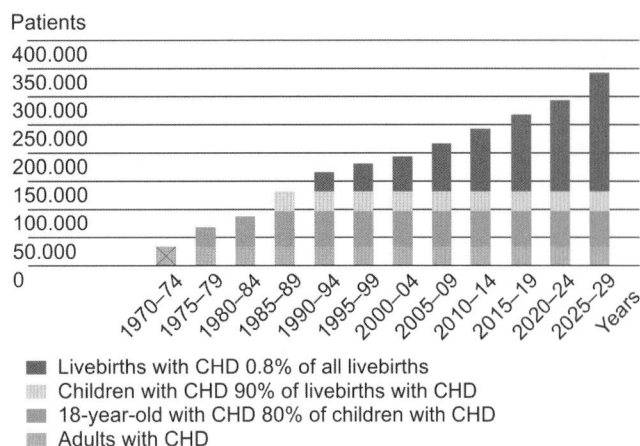

Fig. 13.2: Estimated clinical relevance of CHD in the upcoming years in Germany[18]

Livebirths with CHD 0.8% of all livebirths
Children with CHD 90% of livebirths with CHD
18-year-old with CHD 80% of children with CHD
Adults with CHD

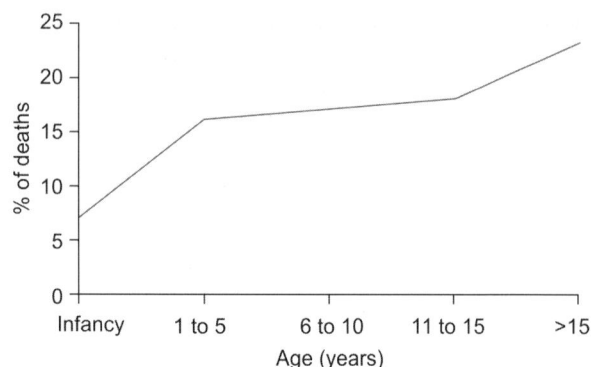

Fig. 13.3: Continuous increase in death rate of children after myelomeningocele repair[19]

Table 13.1: Summary of major late morbidities after surgery for congenital heart disease applicable to many lesions[17]

Congenital heart defect	Major late morbidity
Applicable to many lesions (Tetralogy of Fallot, D-TGA, HLHS)	• Late death • Reintervention • Heart failure/ventricular dysfunction • Rhythm disturbances and need for pacemaker • Endocarditis • Coronary occlusion • Stroke • Thrombosis • Protein-losing enteropathy • Exercise limitations and restrictions • Neurocognitive impairment • Decreased ability to tolerate pregnancy • Difficulty obtaining insurance • Need for chronic medications • Impaired functional status and health-related QOL

Abbreviations: D-TGA, D-transposition of the great arteries; HLHS, hypoplastic left heart syndrome; QOL, quality of life

that medicine is capable of performing miracles, it is expected that children with severe congenital malformations will become adults with surgically corrected disease, which is shown on the example of children with CHD (Fig. 13.2).[17] Number of children with CHD surviving infancy is increasing, reaching 90%, most of them (80%) are surviving till adolescence and percentage of those survivors who are reaching adulthood is increasing as presented in Figure 13.2.[18]

This progress was possible thanks to progress in pediatric cardiology, heart surgery and anesthetics. As patients with CHD grow older, they are likely to encounter many health problems, social and other difficulties remaining chronically ill for the rest of their lives.[17] Surgical operations are often followed by secondary diseases, which limit the patient's quality of life and ability to lead a normal life, and can even be life-threatening.[17] The number of, in that way affected children, adolescents and adults is steadily

increasing, since there is no cure as such for this particular condition.[17] Extrapolations indicate that the clinical relevance of CHD can be expected to rise dramatically in the coming years in Germany.[18] Summary of different morbidities after surgery for CHD is shown in the Table 13.1.[17]

It cannot be determined if the increased risk of late mortality in CHD is due to the intrinsic CHD, its management in an earlier era, or a combination of factors.[17]

Severe congenital anomaly associated with questionable outcome is spina bifida. This is due to the high mortality rate reaching 24% to the early adulthood, as shown in Figure 13.3.[19]

In the large series of 71 children followed up after treatment due to spina bifida, the following data were collected: motor level, ventriculoperitoneal shunt status, education/employment, seizure history, mobility, bladder/bowel continence, tethered cord, scoliosis, latex allergy, posterior cervical decompression, tracheostomy and/or gastrostomy tube.[19] Out of 71 children from the cohort, 86% had cerebrospinal fluid diversion, with 95% having undergone at least one shunt revision.[19] Two revisions was the commonest occurrence (21%).[14] About 41% of the shunted study population had 2–3 shunt revisions.[19] 4 patients had more than 10 shunt revisions; 1 patient has had 31 revisions.[19] 32% of patients had undergone a tethered cord release, with 97% having an improvement or stabilization in their preoperative symptoms.[19] 49% had scoliosis, with 43% eventually requiring a spinal fusion.[19] 16 patients (23%) had at least one seizure.[19] About 85% were attending or had graduated from high school and/or college.[19] More than 80% of young adults had social bladder continence.[19] Approximately, 1/3rd of patients were allergic to latex, with 6 patients having experienced a life-threatening reaction.[19] At least 75% of children born with a myelomeningocele can be expected to reach their early adult years.[19] As previously demonstrated, mobility decreases from early childhood to the early teen years. Fortunately, the patients who remain mobile in their teens continue to ambulate a majority of the time (75–100%) in their young adulthood.[19] About 46% of young adults (33/71) continue to ambulate, and 9 patients (13%) ambulate 25–50% of the time.[19] 29 (41%) out of 71 young adults rely solely upon their wheelchairs for locomotion.[19] One of the greatest challenges in medicine today is establishing a network of care for these adults with spina bifida.

Congenital hydrocephalus is one of severe congenital anomalies always connected with strong concerns of parents and health-care professionals. A cohort of 155 hydrocephalic children who underwent first-time ventriculoperitoneal shunt insertion between the years 1978 and 1983 was followed up on an annual outpatient basis for a period of 10 years or until death.[20] Their academic records and the surgical morbidity and mortality encountered over the 10-year study period were used as the main outcome measures.[20] For those children surviving until school-age, 59% were able to attend a normal school.[20] Only 29% of children with congenital hydrocephalus required special schooling compared to children with hydrocephalus secondary to infection (postmeningitic) or intraventricular hemorrhage of whom 60% required special schooling.[20] Shunt revision was not needed in 44% of patients in this cohort. The commonest reasons for shunt revision were blockage (49%) and infection (19%) which predominantly occurred within the first year of their original shunt procedure.[20] Overall the infection rate was 12% (44/380 procedures).[20] Furthermore, an increased incidence of shunt infection was noted in those under 6 months old.[20] There was 11% mortality during the 10-year follow-up period for those with nontumor-related hydrocephalus.[20]

In the recent study, mortality caused by hydrocephalus and its treatments was between 0% and 3% depending on the duration of follow-up.[21] Shunt event-free survival (EFS) was about 70% at 1 year and 40% at 10 years.[21] The EFS after endoscopic third ventriculostomy appears better but likely benefits from selection bias and long-term figures are not available.[21] Shunt infection affects between 5% and 8% of surgeries, and 15% and 30% of patients according to the duration of follow-up.[21] Shunt independence can be achieved in 3–9% of patients, but the definition of this varies.[21] Broad variations in the prevalence of cognitive sequel, affecting 12–50% of children, and difficulties at school, affecting between 20% and 60%, attest of disparities among studies in their clinical evaluation.[21] Epilepsy, affecting 6–30% of patients, has a serious impact on outcome.[21] In adulthood, social integration is poor in a substantial number of patients but data are sparse.[21]

More optimistic results could be found in the studies dealing with the patients operated due to abdominal wall defects in the neonatal period. In the two studies, the results of long-term morbidity and quality of life in patients with gastroschisis and giant omphalocele born between the periods 1948 and 1980 and 1975–1984 were presented.[22,23] Both studies concluded that most patients (median follow-up was 26.5 years; range 17–48 years, and 14.2 years; range 10–20 years) with abdominal wall defects were healthy adults with few or no factors restricting their activities or decreasing their quality of life.[22,23] In the third study presenting patients treated from 1971 through 2004 general agreement with these two studies was shown.[24] Educational level of the study group was comparable with the national population.[24] After a high level of medical intervention in early life, minor and giant omphalocele patients report similar long-term results except for the cosmetic problems more serious in giant omphalocele.[24] However, this did not influence quality of life in either group and is comparable to that of healthy young adults.[24] With the latter positive prospect in mind, expectant parents with fetal diagnosis of omphalocele and parents of newborns with omphalocele should be informed that the high burden of surgical interventions their child will need to undergo, will likely yield a good health status in the long-term, especially when there are no associated anomalies.[24]

On the example of few severe surgically correctable congenital malformations, the diversity of short and long-term outcomes has been shown. Before making decision to treat the patient many facts should be taken under consideration and parents should be thoroughly counseled. It could be learned from the example of CHD that with better medical and specifically surgical care better results could be obtained. However, when treating child with severe congenital malformation doctors and the parents should be aware that the future is unpredictable concerning long-term outcome, which is important issue to deal with for the family and for the medical professionals. Sometimes, treatment of incurable congenital malformation and compassionate care afterward is enabling parents to provide infant with loving care throughout the duration of infant's life which also should be discussed with parents.[25]

Euthanasia

The important issue which should be raised is the euthanasia in sick newborns with hopeless prognosis in Netherlands known as Groningen protocol published by Verhagen et al.[26-29]. They provided medical and general community with information concerning end-of-life decision-making process in newborns with incurable conditions.[26-29] They also informed medical community with detailed information about how and when the implementation of end-of-life decisions based on quality of life considerations took place.[26-29] This approach has received considerable criticism from the media and from the public. Some of the defenders of such approach claimed that criticisms that have been leveled against the protocol were based on genuine moral disagreements; others seem to rest on misinterpretations, mistranslations, or other misreading.[28,29]

As opponents to this practice said that neonatal euthanasia cannot be supported because primary duty of physicians is to never harm the patients.[30] The main argument for such statement is that even if one accepts the justification of voluntary active euthanasia in adults, neonatal euthanasia cannot be supported, because physicians and parents can never accurately assess the suffering of the children.[30] Therefore, any such system would condemn to death some children whose suffering is not unbearable.[30] The ethical backbone of end-of-life decision-making for adults and adolescents is patient autonomy.[31] For children unable to express their desires, such decisions have traditionally involved the withdrawal of care for treatment futility.[30-32] According to some opinions, the protocol violates the traditional ethical codes of physicians and the moral values of the overwhelming majority of the citizens of the world.[33] The scope and limits of euthanasia approach has been extensively explored ethically and legally.[31,34,35]

Legal Issues of Care for Newborns with Incurable Diseases

According to some investigations, the law concerning the management of newborns with serious incurable diseases is different in various European countries ranging from compassionate care to euthanasia. In most countries existing laws are based on the principle of respect for human life based on the two ethical principles: *Primum Non Nocere,* and *Salus Aegroti Suprema Lex.* The Hippocratic Oath, The Declaration of Geneva and the International Code of Medical Ethics all state that the duty of doctors is to put the welfare of their patients first.[36,37] The parents have the authority to make decisions on behalf of their children, and their consent should be sought to treatment, except in cases of emergency. If parental decisions are contrary to the best interest of the child, doctors should apply to the courts for permission to overrule parental decision.[36,37]

There are no specific law regulations concerning withholding or withdrawing care for critically sick or malformed neonates in Croatia, like in many developing countries. We miss discussions on those bioethical issues in professional societies and there are no guidelines or articles in existing codes directed to the neonatal population. Although ethical committees do exist in the hospitals, neonatal issues are rarely in the scope of their interest. There are several laws which are regulating the issues of dying patient, euthanasia, and other bioethical problems which are not specific only for the neonatal population. It should be pointed out that some bioethical problems are specific for the neonatal period and should be addressed separately from the adult population in the existing law regulations in Croatia. According to Croatian law, euthanasia is not allowed in any situation, so it is forbidden for malformed or neonates at the limits of viability. All those newborns should get compassionate care, to enable dying with dignity.

It is argued that there is typically no emergency when infants are delivered with incurable congenital malformation, and parents should be asked for informed consent before resuscitation in the delivery room.[36]

The Born-Alive Infants Protection Act passed in the US Congress in 2002.[37] At the beginning considered as an antiabortion act, the things changed after US Department of Health and Human Services stated: "As a matter of law and policy, US Department of Health and Human Services will investigate all circumstances where individuals and entities are reported to be withholding medical care from an infant born alive in potential violation of federal statutes".[37] Indeed, under a straightforward reading of the instruction, a family member could conceivably trigger an investigation after observing a delivery of 20-week fetus who maintains a heartbeat for an hour before its death.[37] Most physicians would not consider this an emergency medical condition and, rather than perform a screening examination, would provide comfort care for the newborn and support for the family.[37] The guideline, however, does not state that professional acumen trumps the layperson's observations in these instances; thus, physicians are left unclear about whether screening examinations are required for all newborns regardless of a priori, reasoned considerations of survivability.[37] At that point, decisions about withholding or discontinuing medical treatment that is considered futile may be considered by providers in conjunction with the parents acting in the best interest of their child.[37] However, most pediatricians skilled in screening and resuscitation are not currently called on to perform this function when the gestational age of a nonviable fetus is reasonably certain before delivery.[37] If under the law screening is now required at any gestational age, professional procedure immediately after previable births may need modification.[37] These regulations are not in concordance with current medical and ethical principles of the treatment of infants with lethal major congenital malformations.[37]

Care for the Parents after the Death of the Infant with Congenital Malformation

The EUROCAT 17 registries reported that from 4,366 cases diagnosed with the 11 severe structural malformations 53% (2300) were live births, 4% (183) fetal deaths and 43% (1863) terminations of pregnancy.[38] The gestational age at which malformation was

detected prenatally in 68 (range, 36–88%) of cases was 24 weeks.[38] The highest prenatal detection rate was 94% for anencephaly, and lowest for transposition of great arteries (27%).[38] Termination of pregnancy was performed in more than half of the prenatally diagnosed cases, except for those with transposition of the great arteries, diaphragmatic hernia and gastroschisis, in which 30–40% of the pregnancies with a prenatal diagnosis were terminated.[38]

In another study during the 10-year period, 380 deaths (0.8%) of a total of 47.820 live births occurred in the hospital.[39] Care was not initiated or was withdrawn in close to 72% of those deaths; total care until death occurred in 28%.[40] The majority of deaths of infants born in the hospital occurred as the result of selected no initiating of care or as a result of withdrawing care in infants not responding or considered to have a futile outcome.[39] Only slightly more than one quarter of the infants received total care until the time of death.[39] Type of care according to general categories of causes of death from the same study is shown in Figure 13.4.[39] It is clearly indicated that congenital malformations account for the same percentage (between 30% and 40%) in all three types of care: noninitiation of care, care withdrawal and total care.[39]

The procedure during palliative care should be thoroughly explained to the parents.[40] The plan for palliative care can contain the following procedures:[14]

- Dry and warm baby, provide warm blankets
- Provide heat
- Allow mothers to room in
- Minimize disruptions within medically safe practice for mother
- Lower lights if desired
- Allow presence of parents and extended family as much as possible without disrupting the work flow in the unit
- Make siblings comfortable; they may wish to write letters or draw for the baby

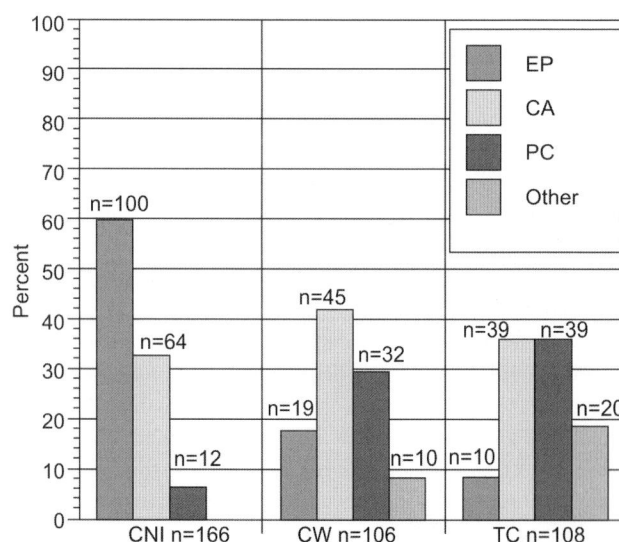

Fig. 13.4: Type of care according to general categories of causes of death[39]

Abbreviations: EP, extreme prematurity; CA, congenital anomaly; PC, prematurity and complications; other, asphyxia, hydrops, and rare conditions that did not fit into other categories; CNI, care not initiated; CW, care withdrawn; TC, total care

- Begin bereavement preparation and memory building, if indicated, to include hand and footprints, pictures, videos, locks of hair
- Encourage parent-child bonding and interaction: bathe, dress baby, feeds, diaper change.

Medical interventions, spiritual needs and funeral details should be discussed with parents and the proposed list of procedures could be:

Selected Medical Interventions

- Humidified oxygen
- Nasal cannula oxygen
- Suction
- Morphine sublingual 0.15 mg/kg or IV 0.05 mg/kg as needed
- Buccal midazolam or oral clonazepam as needed
- Artificial hydration or nutrition
- Natural hydration or nutrition.

Spiritual Care

- Religious preference
- Identified religious leader
- Religious ritual desired at or near time of death.

In the Event of Child's Death in Hospital

- Diagnostic procedures
- Autopsy preference
- Tissue/organ procurement preferences
- Funeral home chosen by family
- Rituals required for body care.

After infant's death, the grieving process will begin and physician communication with parents is crucial.[41] The physician should express condolences for parental loss and sincere sympathy with them, offering generous help to the parents who are dealing with difficult situation, and patiently answering all their questions.[14] This approach will help the parents to cope with the feelings of guilt, loss and desperation.[42] During the conversation, the parents should be informed to come for any kind of help in the future, which in fact is giving them the hope for family planning. Parents should be informed about the causes of death and possibilities of reoccurrence of the disease as well as the possibilities for the prevention, if appropriate. Sometimes attending the memorial or funeral service by the attending physician may be appropriate.[14] This will let the family know that the concern they perceived was real and sincere. On the other hand, it may also allow some healing for the practitioner, who otherwise may "burn out" from the emotional exhaustion of the investment in children who die and their families.[14] Giving oneself permission to love and let go is important, and societal rituals may assist in the resolution of the professionals' grief as well.[14] Families are generally overcome with appreciation when the physician attends the memorial or funeral.[14]

CONCLUSION

Parents are always expecting healthy child and dealing with difficult situation of having malformed infant with incurable state is distressing and emotionally exhausting either the diagnosis is made pre- or postnatally. In the situations when the infant is severely malformed, there is a difficulty to distinguish between parents' and babies' interests, and medical professionals are faced with the responsibility to prolong a life with the prospective of severe disability.[43] Appropriate management plan for the child and sincere care for the family and counseling are the most important for the parents and the family, which has been often very exhausting for the medical staff. Appropriate medical knowledge and effective, empathic communication is an essential skill of medical staff caring for infants with life-threatening congenital malformations and their families. The future guidelines for newborn end-of-life decisions should follow at least the same moral criteria used for older patients.[43]

REFERENCES

1. Gadzinowski J, Jopek A. Neonatologia - między etyką a pragmatyzmem. Nauka. 2007;3:21-30.
2. Available from http://www.eurocat.ulster.ac.uk/pdf/Landfill-Sites-Chapters-1-to-5.pdf. [Acessed May 2009]
3. Kalter H. Congenital malformations: An iquiry into classification and nomanclature. J Med Genet. 1998;35:661-5.
4. Kalter H. Origin and meaning of 'teratology'. Teratology. 2002;65: 3-4.
5. Moore KL, Persaud TVN. The Developing Human: Clinically Oriented Embryology, 7th edition. Philadelphia: WB Saunders Co; 2003.
6. Available from http://frwebgate.access.gpo.gov/cgi-bin/getdoc. cgi?dbname=107_cong_bills&docid=f:h4013rh.txt.pdf. [Accessed June 2009].
7. Available from http://www.eurordis.org/IMG/pdf/princeps_document-EN.pdf. pdf. [Accessed May 2009].
8. Terry PB, Bissenden JG, Condie RG, et al. Ethnic differences in congenital malformations. Arch Dis Child. 1985;60:866-79.
9. Available from http://www.bio-medical.co.uk/eurocatlive/search2. cgi. [Accessed July 2009].
10. Kumar P, Burton BK. Congenital Malformations: Evidence-based evaluation and management. New York: McGraw-Hill Medical; 2008.
11. Lawn JE, Wilczynska-Ketende K, Cousens SN. Estimating the causes of 4 million neonatal deaths in the year 2000. Int J Epidemiol. 2006;35:706-18.
12. Pinter AB. End-of-life decision before and after birth: changing ethical considerations. J Pediatr Surg. 2008;43:430-6.
13. Committee on Fetus and Newborn. Noninitiation or withdrawal of intensive care for high-risk newborns. Pediatrics. 2007;119;401-3.
14. Levetown M, Committee on Bioethics. Communicating with children and families: from everyday interactions to skill in conveying distressing information. Pediatrics. 2008;121:e1441-60.
15. Provoost V, Cools F, Deconinck P, et al. Consultation of parents in actual end-of-life decision-making in neonates and infants. Eur J Pediatr. 2006;165:859-66.

16. Chiswick M. Infants of borderline viability: ethical and clinical considerations. Semin Fetal Neonatal Med. 2008;13:8-15.

17. Schulz AH, Wernowsky G. Outcomes in pediatric cardiac surgery. Late outcomes in patients with surgically treated congenital heart diseases. Semin Thorac Cardiovasc Surg Pediatr Card Surg Ann. 2005;8:145-56.

18. Competence network for congenital heart defects. [online] Available from. www. kompetenznetz-ahf.de/.

19. Bowman RM, McLone DG, Grant JA, et al. Spina bifida outcome: a 25-year prospective. Pediatr Neurosurg. 2001;34:114-20.

20. Casey ATH, Kimmings EJ, Kleinlugtebeld AD, et al. The long-term outlook for hydrocephalus in childhood. Pediatr Neurosurg. 1997;27:63-70.

21. Vinchon M, Rekate H, Kulkarni AV. Pediatric hydrocephalus outcomes: a review. Fluids Barriers CNS. 2012;9:18.

22. Tunell WP, Puffinbarger NK, Tuggle DW, et al. Abdominal wall defects in infants. Survival and implications for adult life. Ann Surg. 1995; 221:525-8.

23. Koivusalo A, Lindahl H, Rintala RJ. Morbidity and quality of life in adult patients with a congenital abdominal wall defect: a questionnaire survey. J Pediatr Surg. 2002;37:1594-01.

24. van Eijck FC, Hoogeveevn YL, van Weel C, et al. Minor and giant omphalocele: long-term outcomes and quality of life. J Ped Surg. 2009;44:1355-9.

25. Milstein JM, Kovar LB, Kovar LJ, et al. Piece of my mind. A path to wholeness. JAMA 2012;308:985-6.

26. Verhagen E, Sauer PJJ. The Groningen protocol—euthanasia in severely ill newborns. N Engl J Med. 2005;352:959-62.

27. Verhagen AAE, Sauer PJJ. End-of-life decisions in newborns: an approach from the Netherlands. Pediatrics. 2005;116:736-9.

28. Verhagen AA, van der Hoeven MA, van Meerveld RC, et al. Physician medical decision-making at the end of life in newborns: insight into implementation at 2 Dutch centers. Pediatrics. 2007;120:e20-8.

29. Moratti S. End-of-life decisions in dutch neonatology. Med Law Rev. 2010;18:471-96.

30. Lindemann H, Verkerk M. Ending the life of a newborn: the Groningen Protocol. Hastings Cent Rep. 2008;38:42-51.

31. Kon AA. Neonatal euthanasia is unsupportable: the Groningen protocol should be abandoned. Theor Med Bioethics. 2007;28:453-63.

32. Bondi SA, Gries D, Faucette K. Neonatal euthanasia? Pediatrics. 2006;117:983.

33. Jotkowitz A, Glick S, Gesundheit B. A case against justified nonvoluntary active euthanasia (the Groningen Protocol). Am J Bioeth. 2008;8:23-6.

34. Chervenak FA, McCullough LB, Arabin B. The Groningen Protocol: Is it necessary? Is it scientific? Is it ethical? J Perinat Med. 2009;37:199-205.

35. Barry S. Quality of life and myelomeningocele: an ethical and evidence-based analysis of the Groningen Protocol. Pediatr Neurosurg. 2010;46:409-14.

36. Krug EF 3rd. Law and ethics at the border of viability. J Perinatol. 2006;26:321-4.

37. Sayeed SA. Baby doe redux? The Department of Health and Human Services and the Born-Alive Infants Protection Act of 2002: a cautionary note on normative neonatal practice. Pediatrics. 2005;116:e576-85.

38. Garne E, Loane M, Dolk H, et al. Prenatal diagnosis of severe structural congenital malformations in Europe. Ultrasound Obstet Gynecol. 2005;25:6-11.

39. Barton L, Hodgman JE. The contribution of withholding or withdrawing care to newborn mortality. Pediatrics. 2005;116:1487-91.

40. Saugstad OD. When newborn infants are bound to die. Acta Paediatr. 2005;94:1535-7.

41. Walther FJ. Withholding treatment, withdrawing treatment, and palliative care in the neonatal intensive care unit. Early Hum Dev. 2005;81:965-72.

42. Provoost V, Cools F, Mortier F, et al. Medical end-of-life decisions in neonates and infants in Flanders. Lancet. 2005;365:1315-20.

43. Bellieni CV, Tei M, Coccina F, et al. Why do we treat the newborn differently? J Matern Fetal Neonatal Med. 2012;25 Suppl 1:73-5.

SECTION 2

Ethical and Legal Dimensions

FA Chervenak, LB McCullough

14 Ethics: An Essential Dimension of Perinatal Medicine

FA Chervenak, LB McCullough

INTRODUCTION

Ethics is an essential dimension of perinatal medicine.[1-3] In this chapter, we develop a framework for clinical judgment and decision-making about the ethical dimensions of perinatal medicine. We will emphasize a preventive ethics approach that anticipates the potential for ethical conflict and adopts ethically justified strategies to prevent those conflicts from occurring. Preventive ethics in perinatal medicine helps to build and sustain a strong physician-patient relationship.

This chapter has five parts. First, we define ethics, medical ethics, and the fundamental ethical principles of medical ethics; beneficence and respect for autonomy. Second, we show how these two principles should interact in perinatal medicine, with emphasis on the clinical ethical concept of the fetus as a patient. Third, we describe different concepts of the ethical principles of justice. Fourth, we examine ethical issues in managed care, with particular attention to the virtues of the physician as a professional. Fifth, we describe a new formal tool for critically appraising the literature of medical ethics, including perinatal ethics.

ETHICS AND MEDICAL ETHICS

Ethics is understood to be the disciplined study of morality. Medical ethics is, therefore, the disciplined study of morality in medicine, and concerns the obligations of physicians and health care organizations to patients, as well as the obligations of patients.[4] Medical ethics should be distinguished from the many sources of morality in pluralistic societies. These include law, our political heritage as a free people, the world's religions, ethnic and cultural traditions, families, the traditions and practices of medicine (including medical education and training), and personal experience. Medical ethics since the eighteenth century European and American enlightenments has been secular.[5] It makes no reference to God or revealed tradition, but to what rational philosophical discourse produces. Therefore, ethical principles and virtues should be understood to apply to all physicians, regardless of their personal religious and spiritual beliefs.[6]

The traditions and practices of medicine constitute an important source of morality for physicians, because they are based on the obligation to protect and promote the health-related interests of the patient. This obligation tells physicians what morality in medicine ought to be in very general, abstract terms. Providing a detailed, clinically applicable account of that obligation is the central task of medical ethics, using ethical principles.[4]

Ethical Principles

The Principle of Beneficence

The ethical principle of beneficence requires one to act in a way that is expected reliably to produce the greater balance of benefits over harms in the lives of others.[6] To put this principle into clinical practice requires a reliable account of the benefits and harms relevant to the care of the patient and of how those goods and harms should be reasonably balanced against each other when not all of them can be achieved in a particular clinical situation. In medicine, the principle of beneficence requires the physician to act in a way that is reliably expected to produce the greater balance of clinical benefits over clinical harms for the patient.[4]

Beneficence-based clinical judgment has an ancient pedigree, with its first expression found in the Hippocratic Oath and accompanying texts.[7] Beneficence-based clinical judgment aims to interpret reliably the health-related interests of the patient from a rigorous clinical perspective which is provided by accumulated scientific research, clinical experience, and reasoned responses to uncertainty. Such a rigorous clinical perspective is thus not the function of the individual clinical perspective of any particular physician and therefore, should not be based merely on the clinical impression or intuition of an individual physician. On the basis of this rigorous clinical perspective, which should be based on the best available evidence, beneficence-based clinical judgment identifies the clinical benefits that can be achieved for the based on the competencies of medicine. The benefits that medicine is competent to seek for patients are the prevention and management of disease, injury, handicap, and unnecessary pain and suffering and the prevention of premature or unnecessary death. Pain and suffering become unnecessary when they do not result in achieving the other goods of medical care, e.g. allowing a woman to labor without effective analgesia.[4] Non-maleficence means that the physician should not, on balance, cause harm, and is best understood as expressing the limits of beneficence. This is also known as "Primum non nocere" or "first do no harm". This commonly invoked dogma is really a Latinized misinterpretation of the Hippocratic texts which emphasized beneficence while avoiding harm when approaching the limits of medicine.[4]

There is an inherent risk of paternalism in beneficence-based clinical judgment. By this we mean that beneficence-based clinical judgment, if it is mistakenly taken by the physician to be the sole source of moral responsibility, and therefore moral authority in medical care, invites the unwary physician to conclude that beneficence-based judgments can be imposed on the patient irrespective of her autonomy. Paternalism is a dehumanizing response to the patient and, therefore, should be avoided in the practice of perinatal medicine.

The preventive ethics response to paternalism is for the physician to explain the diagnostic, therapeutic and prognostic reasoning that leads to his or her clinical judgment about what is in the interest of the patient and her pregnancy so that the patient can assess that clinical judgment for herself. The physician should first explain to the patient the major factors of this reasoning process, including matters of uncertainty. In neither medical law nor medical ethics does this require that the patient be provided with a complete medical education.[8] The physician should then explain how and why other clinicians might reasonably differ from his or her clinical judgment. The physician should then present a well-reasoned response to this critique. The outcome of this process should be that beneficence-based clinical judgments take on a rigor that they sometimes lack, and the process of their formulation includes explaining them to the patient. In complex areas, such as perinatal medicine, beneficence-based clinical judgment will frequently result in the identification of a continuum of clinical strategies that protect and promote health-related interests. Awareness of this feature of beneficence-based clinical judgment provides an important preventive ethics antidote to paternalism by increasing the likelihood that one or more of these medically reasonable, evidence-based alternatives will be acceptable to the patient. This feature of beneficence-based clinical judgment also provides a preventive ethics antidote to "gag" rules that restrict physician's communications with the managed care patient.[9] All beneficence-based alternatives must be identified and explained to all patients, regardless of how the physician is paid, especially those that are well established in evidence-based perinatal medicine.

One advantage for the physician in carrying out this approach to communicating with the patient would be, we believe, to increase the likelihood of compliance.[10] This is an especially pertinent consideration in perinatal medicine, e.g. self-observation for unusual weight gain, bleeding, or signs of premature labor. Another advantage would be to provide the patient with a better-informed opportunity to make a decision about whether to seek a second opinion. The approach outlined above should make such a decision less threatening to her physician, who has already shared with the patient the limitations on clinical judgment.

The Principle of Respect for Autonomy

To complement the principle of beneficence, there is emphasis in the literature of medical ethics on the principle of respect for autonomy.[6] This principle requires one always to acknowledge and carry out the value-based preferences of the adult, competent patient, unless there is compelling ethical justification for not doing so, e.g. prescribing antibiotics for viral respiratory infections. The pregnant patient increasingly brings to her medical care her own perspective on what is in her and her pregnancy's interest. The principle of respect for autonomy translates this into autonomy-based clinical judgment. Because each patient's perspective on her interests is a function of her values and beliefs, it is impossible to specify in advance the benefits and harms of the patient's autonomy-based clinical judgment. Indeed, it would be inappropriate for the physician to do so, because the definition of her benefits and harms

and their balancing are the prerogative of the patient. Autonomy-based clinical judgment is strongly antipaternalistic in nature.[4]

The responsible practice of perinatal medicine depends on an operationalized concept of autonomy to make it relevant to clinical practice. We, therefore, identify three sequential autonomy-based behaviors on the part of the patient:

1. Absorbing and retaining information about her condition and alternative diagnostic and therapeutic responses to it.
2. Understanding that information (i.e. evaluating and rank-ordering those responses and appreciating that she could experience the risks of treatment).
3. Expressing a value-based preference. The physician has a role to play in each of these. They are, respectively:
    i. To recognize the capacity of each pregnant patient to deal with medical information (and not to underestimate that capacity), provide information (i.e. disclose and explain all medically reasonable alternatives, i.e. supported in beneficence-based clinical judgment), and recognize the validity of the values and beliefs of the patient,
    ii. Not to interfere with but, when necessary, to assist the patient in her evaluation and ranking of diagnostic and therapeutic alternatives for managing her condition, and
    iii. To elicit and implement the patient's value-based preference.[4]

Beneficence and Respect for Autonomy in Perinatal Practice

The ethical principles of beneficence and respect for autonomy play a central role in perinatal practice. There are obviously beneficence-based and autonomy-based obligations to the pregnant patient: the physician's perspective on the pregnant woman's health-related interests provides the basis for the physician's beneficence-based obligations to her. Her own perspective on those interests provides the basis for the physician's autonomy-based obligations to her. Because of an insufficiently developed central nervous system, the fetus cannot meaningfully be said to possess values and beliefs. Thus, there is no basis for saying that a fetus has a perspective on its interests. Hence, there can be no autonomy-based obligations to any fetus. The language of fetal rights has no meaning, and therefore, no application to the fetus in perinatal clinical judgment and practice, despite its popularity in public and political discourse in the United States and other countries. The physician does have a perspective on the fetus's health-related interests, and the physician can have beneficence-based obligations to the fetus, *but only when the fetus is a patient*.[4]

Clinical Ethical Concept of the Fetus as a Patient

The clinical ethical concept of the fetus as a patient is essential to perinatal clinical judgment and practice. Developments in fetal diagnosis and perinatal management strategies to optimize fetal outcome have become widely accepted, encouraging the development of this concept. This concept has considerable clinical significance, because when the fetus is a patient, directive counseling, that is recommending clinical management for fetal benefit, is appropriate, and when the fetus is not a patient, nondirective counseling, that is offering, but not recommending, a form of management for fetal benefit, is appropriate. However, these seemingly straightforward roles for directive and nondirective counseling are often difficult to apply in actual perinatal practice, because of uncertainty about when the fetus is a patient. This concerns moral status, i.e. whether others have an ethical obligation to the fetus to protect and promote its interests.

One prominent approach for establishing whether or not the fetus has the moral status of being a patient has involved attempts to show whether or not the fetus has independent moral status. Independent moral status for the fetus means that one or more characteristics that the fetus possesses in and of itself, and therefore, independently of the pregnant woman or any other factor, generate and therefore ground clinical obligations to the fetus on the part of the pregnant woman and her physician.

Many fetal characteristics have been proposed as the basis for such independent moral status, including moment of conception, implantation, central nervous system development, quickening, and the moment of birth. It should come as no surprise that there is considerable variation among ethical arguments about when the fetus acquires independent moral status. Some take the view that the fetus has independent moral status from the moment of conception or implantation. Others believe that independent moral status is acquired in degrees, thus resulting in "graded" moral status. Still others hold, at least by implication, that the fetus never has independent moral status so long as it is in utero.[11,12]

Despite an enormous amount of theological and philosophical literature on this subject, there has been no closure on a single authoritative account of the independent moral status of the fetus. This outcome should be expected, because, given the absence of a single method that would be authoritative for all of the markedly diverse theological and philosophical schools of thought involved in this sometimes acrimonious debate, closure is impossible. For closure ever to be possible, debates about such a final authority within and between theological and philosophical traditions would have to be resolved in a way satisfactory to all, an inconceivable intellectual and cultural event. Claims about the independent moral status of the fetus as the basis for claims about the fetus as a patient have no stable or clinically applicable meaning. We, therefore abandon these futile attempts to understand the fetus as a patient in terms of independent moral status of the fetus and turn to an alternative approach.

Our analysis of the clinical ethical concept of the fetus as a patient starts with the recognition that being a patient does not require that one possess independent moral status. Rather, being a patient means that one can benefit from the applications of the clinical skills of the physician. More precisely stated, a human being is properly regarded as a patient when two conditions are met: that a human being (1) is presented to the physician and (2) there exist clinical interventions that are reliably expected to be efficacious, in that they are reliably expected to result in a greater balance of clinical benefits over harms for the human being in question.[13] We call this the dependent moral status of the fetus as a patient.

The authors have argued elsewhere that beneficence-based obligations to the fetus exist when the fetus is reliably expected later to achieve independent moral status as a child and person. The fetus is a patient when the fetus is presented for medical interventions, whether diagnostic or therapeutic, that reasonably can be expected to result in a greater balance of goods over harms for the child and person the fetus can later become during early childhood.[4] The clinical ethical significance of the concept of the fetus as a patient, therefore, depends on links that can be established between the fetus and its later achieving independent moral status.

The Viable Fetus as a Patient

One such link is viability. Viability is not an intrinsic property of the fetus because viability should be understood in terms of both biological and technological factors. It is only by virtue of both factors that a viable fetus can exist ex utero and thus achieve independent moral status. It is important to appreciate that these two factors do not exist as a function of the autonomy of the pregnant woman. When a fetus is viable, that is, when it is of sufficient maturity so that it can survive into the neonatal period and achieve independent moral status given the availability of the requisite technological support, and when it is presented to the physician, the fetus is a patient.

Viability exists as a function of biomedical and technological capacities. These differ in different parts of the world. As a consequence, there is no worldwide, uniform gestational age to define viability. In the United States, we believe viability presently occurs at approximately 24 weeks of gestational age.[14]

When the fetus is a patient, directive counseling for fetal benefit is ethically justified. In perinatal practice, directive counseling for fetal benefit involves recommending against termination of pregnancy, recommending against non-aggressive management, or recommending aggressive management. Aggressive obstetric management includes interventions such as fetal surveillance, tocolysis, cesarean delivery, or delivery in a tertiary care center when indicated. Non-aggressive obstetric management excludes such interventions. Directive counseling for fetal benefit, however, must always take account of the presence and severity of fetal anomalies, extreme prematurity, and obligations to the pregnant woman.

The strength of directive counseling for fetal benefit justifiably varies according to the presence and severity of anomalies. As a rule, the more severe the fetal anomaly, the less directive counseling should be for fetal benefit. In particular, when lethal anomalies, such as anencephaly, can be diagnosed with certainty, there are no beneficence-based obligations to provide aggressive management. Such fetuses are dying patients, and the counseling, therefore, should be nondirective in recommending between non-aggressive management and termination of pregnancy, but directive in recommending against aggressive management for the sake of maternal benefit.[15] By contrast, third-trimester abortion for Down syndrome or achondroplasia is not ethically justifiable, because the future child with high probability will have the capacity to grow and develop as a human being.[16,17]

Directive counseling for fetal benefit in cases of extreme prematurity of viable fetuses is appropriate. In particular, this is the case for what we term just-viable fetuses, those with a gestational age of 24–26 weeks, for which there are significant rates of survival but high rates of mortality and morbidity. These rates of morbidity and mortality can be increased by non-aggressive obstetric management, whereas aggressive obstetric management may favorably influence outcome. Thus, it appears that there are substantial beneficence-based obligations to just-viable fetuses to provide aggressive obstetric management. This is all the more the case in pregnancies beyond 26 weeks of gestational age. Directive counseling for fetal benefit is, therefore, justified in all cases of extreme prematurity of viable fetuses. Of course, such directive counseling is appropriate only when it is based on documented efficacy of aggressive obstetric management for each fetal indication. For example, such efficacy has not been demonstrated for routine cesarean delivery to manage extreme prematurity.

All directive counseling for fetal benefit must occur in the context of balancing beneficence-based obligations to the fetal patient against beneficence-based and autonomy-based obligations to the pregnant woman. Any such balancing must recognize that a pregnant woman is obligated only to take reasonable risks of perinatal interventions that are reliably expected to benefit the viable fetus or child later. A unique feature of perinatal ethics is that the pregnant woman's autonomy influences whether, in a particular case, the viable fetus ought to be regarded as presented to the physician.

Obviously, any strategy for directive counseling for fetal benefit that takes account of obligations to the pregnant woman must anticipate the possibility of conflict between the physician's recommendation and a pregnant woman's autonomous decision to the contrary. Such conflict should be managed preventively through the use of the informed consent process as an ongoing dialogue throughout a woman's pregnancy, augmented as necessary by negotiation and respectful persuasion.[18]

The Previable Fetus as a Patient

The only possible link between the previable fetus and the child it can become is the pregnant woman's autonomy, because technological factors cannot result in the previable fetus becoming a child. The link, therefore, between a previable fetus and the child is established only by the pregnant woman's decision to confer the status of being a patient on her previable fetus. The previable fetus has no claim to the status of being a patient independently of the pregnant woman's autonomy. The pregnant woman is, therefore, free to withhold, confer, or, having once conferred, withdraw the status of being a patient on or from her previable fetus according to her own values and beliefs. The previable fetus is presented to the physician as a function of the pregnant woman's autonomy.[4]

Counseling the pregnant woman regarding the management of her pregnancy when the fetus is previable should be nondirective in terms of continuing the pregnancy or having an abortion if she refuses to confer the status of being a patient on her fetus. If she does confer such status in a settled way, at that point beneficence-based obligations to her fetus come into existence, and directive counseling for fetal benefit becomes appropriate for these previable fetuses. Just as for viable fetuses, such counseling must take account of the presence and severity of fetal anomalies, extreme prematurity, and beneficence-based and autonomy-based obligations to the pregnant woman.

For pregnancies in which the woman is uncertain about whether to confer such status, the authors propose that the fetus be *provisionally* regarded as a patient. This justifies directive counseling against behavior that can harm a fetus in significant and irreversible ways, e.g. substance abuse, especially alcohol, until the woman settles on whether to confer the status of being a patient on the fetus.

In particular, nondirective counseling is appropriate in cases of what we term near-viable fetuses, that is, those that are 22–23 weeks of gestational age, for which there are anecdotal reports of survival. In our view, aggressive obstetric and neonatal management

should be regarded as clinical investigation (i.e. a form of medical experimentation), not a standard of care.[14] There is no clinical obligation on the part of any pregnant woman to confer the status of being a patient on a near-viable fetus because the efficacy of aggressive obstetric and neonatal management has yet to be proven.

The In Vitro Embryo as a Patient

A subset of previable fetuses as patients concerns the in vitro embryo.[19] It might seem that the in vitro embryo is a patient because such an embryo is presented to the physician. However, for beneficence-based obligations to a human being to exist, it must also be the case that medical interventions are reliably expected to be efficacious.

Whether the fetus is a patient depends on links that can be established between the fetus and its eventual independent moral status. Therefore, whether medical interventions on the in vitro embryo should be reliably expected to be efficacious for the child later depends on whether that embryo later becomes viable. Otherwise, no benefit of such intervention can meaningfully be said to result. An in vitro embryo becomes viable only when it survives in vitro cell division, transfer, implantation, and subsequent gestation to such a time that it becomes viable. The process of achieving viability occurs only in vivo and is, therefore, entirely dependent on the woman's decision regarding the status of the fetus(es) as a patient, should assisted conception successfully result in the gestation of the previable fetus(es). Whether an in vitro embryo will become a viable fetus, and whether medical intervention on such an embryo will benefit the fetus and future child, are both functions of the pregnant woman's autonomous decision to withhold, confer, or, having once conferred, withdraw the moral status of being a patient on the previable fetus(es) that might result from assisted conception.

It, therefore, is appropriate to regard the in vitro embryo as a previable fetus rather than as a viable fetus. As a consequence, any in vitro embryo(s) should be regarded as a patient only when the woman into whose reproductive tract the embryo(s) will be transferred confers that status. Thus, counseling about preimplantation diagnosis should, therefore, be nondirective, just as it should be for previability counseling. One additional justification is that the woman may elect not to implant abnormal embryos. These embryos will not become patients, and so there is no basis for directive counseling regarding them. Information should be presented about prognosis for a successful pregnancy and the possibility of confronting a decision about selective reduction, depending on the number of embryos transferred. Counseling about how many in vitro embryos should be transferred should be rigorously evidence based.[20]

JUSTICE AND PERINATAL MEDICINE

Ethical concerns about justice arise when economic, clinical, or other resources are scarce. Justice requires that in the distribution of resources, each should receive what is due to him or her. Different concepts of justice define "due" in different ways. Each strives to result in a fair distribution of benefits, i.e. access to resources, and burdens, the risks that could follow from lack of such access.

Utilitarianism is a theory of justice that makes central the obligation to produce the greatest good for the greatest number in the management of scarce resources. To be successful in guiding practical, day-to-day decisions about the allocation of resources, utilitarianism requires an account of the greatest good. For society overall, it has been difficult, if not impossible, to define what the greatest good is. The value of utilitarianism is the balance it seeks to achieve among benefits and burdens of scarce resources, so that inequalities do not become inequities, i.e. unfair. Critics of utilitarians have pointed out that sometimes utilitarianism results in inequities, i.e. shared distributions of benefits and burdens.[21]

Two other concepts of justice have been developed to address this problem. The first of these is a libertarian concept of justice. This concept of justice was developed to correct for tyrannical burdens that pure utilitarianism could create. In particular, libertarianism was developed to give priority to individual freedom and property rights, as correctives to the potential excesses of utilitarianism and, in the political realm, of state power. Libertarians argue that in a market that places different values on different services and products, and in which there is an equal opportunity to develop one's talents, those who provide more highly valued services rightly earn more than those who provide less valued (though not necessarily less intrinsically valuable) services. Everyone should get to keep what he or she earns through these marketplace exchanges, reflecting the strong emphasis of the libertarian concept of justice on property rights. Libertarian theories emphasize fairness of process, rather than equality of outcomes.

The other concept of justice that has been developed is an egalitarian concept of justice. This concept was developed to protect vulnerable and disadvantaged members of society, who may lose out in a utilitarian distribution of scarce resources. This concept of justice corrects for unfair outcomes in the form of undue burdens on those least able to protect themselves.

These three and other concepts of justice remain in unresolved competition in ethics generally, in medical ethics,[22] and in perinatal ethics. It is fair to say that the medical ethics literature is strongly influenced by a concept of justice that calls for fair equality of opportunity (an element of libertarian justice) and protection of the least well off (an element of egalitarian justice). However, it is also fair to say that no single concept of justice shapes health care policy in the United States. This lack of a conceptually coherent health care policy is a long-standing feature of American health care policy. In particular, unlike many other developed countries, the United States has yet to create a universal right to health care, though there are selective entitlements.

MANAGED CARE AND THE PROFESSIONAL VIRTUES

The practice of perinatal medicine is coming under managed care, which involves a set of strategies used by both private and public payers to control the cost of medical care. Two main business tools are used to achieve this goal:

1. Creating conflicts of interests in how physicians are paid, diplomatically called "sharing economic risk".
2. Increasingly strict control of clinical judgment and practice through such means as practice guidelines, critical pathways, physician report cards and retrospective chart review. These business tools generate ethical challenges to perinatologists that seriously threaten the virtues that define the fiduciary character of medicine as a profession.[23]

In medicine, the physician is the patient's fiduciary. The physician should be competent and use clinical competence as a matter of routine and habit primarily to protect and promote patients' interests rather than pursue his or her own interests. Virtues are those traits and habits of character that routinely focus the concern and behavior of an individual on the interests of others and thereby habitually blunt the motivation to act on self-interest one's primary consideration. We believe that four virtues constitute the physician-patient relationship based on the physician as fiduciary.[4]

The first virtue is *self-effacement*. This professional virtue requires the physician not to act on the basis of potential differences between the patient and the physician such as race, religion, national origin, gender, sexual orientation, manners, socioeconomic status, or proficiency in speaking English. Self-effacement prevents biases and prejudices arising from these differences that could adversely impact on the plan of care for the patient.

The second professional virtue is *self-sacrifice*. This requires physicians to accept reasonable risks to themselves. As one example, perinatologists manifest this virtue in their willingness to perform a cesarean delivery for an HIV+ patient, following accepted standards. In both fee-for-service and managed care, the professional virtue of self-sacrifice obligates the physician to blunt economic self-interest and focus on the patient's need for relief when the two are in conflict.

The third professional virtue, *compassion*, motivates the physician to recognize and seek to alleviate the stress, discomfort, pain, and suffering associated with the patient's disease and illness. Self-effacement, self-sacrifice and compassion provide the basis for a powerful ethical response to the business tool of conflicts of interest by the physician.

This response is strengthened by the fourth professional virtue, *integrity*. This virtue imposes an intellectual discipline on the physician's clinical judgments about the patient's problems and how to address them. Integrity prescribes rigor in the formation of clinical judgment. Clinical judgment is rigorous when it is based on the best available scientific information or, when such information is lacking, consensus clinical judgment and on careful thought processes of an individual physician that can withstand peer review. Integrity is thus an antidote to the pitfalls of bias, subjective clinical impressions, and unexamined clinical "common sense" that can undermine evidence-based practice. Integrity provides the basis for the physician's ethical response to the business tool of control of clinical judgment and practice.

None of these four virtues is absolute in its ethical demands. The task of medical ethics is to identify both the application and the limits of these four virtues. The concept of legitimate self-interest provides the basis for these limits. Legitimate self-interest includes protecting the conditions for practicing medicine well, fulfilling obligations to persons in the physician's life other than the patient, and protecting activities outside the practice of medicine that the physician finds deeply fulfilling.

Managed Care and the Physician as Fiduciary

The fee-for-service practice of medicine unconstrained by fiduciary obligations could and did in the past lead to harm to patients from nonindicated over-utilization of resources. It is a violation of the standard of care to subject patients to unnecessary active intervention in order to achieve personal economic gain. Managed care unconstrained by fiduciary obligations puts patients at risk of harm by denying access to the standard of care. This will occur if patients are subjected to unnecessary risk from withholding appropriate care and intervention in order to achieve reduced cost.[23,24]

Financial incentives to the physician and supervision of clinician decision-making with strict controls over utilization are the business tools managed care uses. Forms of payment by managed care plans, such as capitation and withhold, deliberately impose an economic conflict of interest on the physician.[25] Every time the physician uses a resource, e.g. consultation, diagnostic testing, or surgical procedures, the physician pays an economic penalty. The ethical challenge occurs when the patient's interests are subordinated to the pursuit of financial rewards and thereby harmed by this underutilization.

The professional virtue of self-sacrifice prohibits the physician from making the avoidance of such financial risk the *primary* consideration. Avoiding financial risk as one's *primary* consideration involves an ethically pathologic process that leads naturally and quickly to the abandonment of self-effacement (economically driven managed care for some patients but not for others), compassion (patients' health-related concerns do not matter but are only a means to maximize revenues), and integrity (the standard of care is sacrificed to maximize revenues). Importantly, physicians are not sanctioned by society to engage in the destruction of medicine as a fiduciary profession, because it is a public trust, not a private fiefdom.

Physicians should not assume that managed care organizations (MCOs) are unwilling to negotiate contracts to reduce the severity of economic conflicts of interest. Physicians should, therefore, make a good faith effort to negotiate these matters. If the MCO refuses to negotiate and the economic risk of not signing the contract is very significant, then the physician should voluntarily accept the ethical responsibility to be alert to and manage these conflicts of interest well. First, integrity requires that the physician avoid the self-deception of underestimating any potential influence on clinical judgment and practice by the conflict of interest. Second, once these contracts are signed, the professional virtues add an important dimension to total quality management: diligent monitoring of conflicts of interest to prevent them from resulting in substandard care should be among the physician's "accountabilities". Third, the realities of managed care mean that, for the near term at least, increasing financial sacrifice may be required to protect the integrity of medicine as a fiduciary profession. Fourth, in group practice, there should be a fair sharing of economic self-sacrifice. In particular, individual efforts to tune the system to one's economic advantage in a group, for example, avoiding the care of high-risk pregnancies, and to the disadvantage of colleagues should be avoided.

The second business tool of managed care, increasingly strict control of clinical judgment and practice, is a heterogeneous phenomenon. Some managed care plans are poorly capitalized and poorly managed. They compete by price, with little or no attention given to the quality of their services. A "bottom line" mentality dominates, with economic savings and net revenue maximization the overriding values. These poorly managed companies have little or no understanding of or interest in the fiduciary nature of medicine, and so their controls of clinical judgment and practice are driven almost entirely by economic considerations.

Physicians subject to management controls by such companies face the very difficult challenge of trying to get such companies to constrain their economic interests by their fiduciary obligations, a daunting task but not, we believe, an impossible task. The concerns of ethics, especially to protect the integrity of the fiduciary enterprise, may frequently be swept aside when they are not ignored altogether. However, as the fiduciaries of patients, physicians in such managed care organizations are the ultimate bulwark on which patients and society must be able to rely at the present time to protect patients from management's unbridled pursuit of economic self-interest. Physicians, therefore, should strenuously resist and seek to change management controls driven solely by economic considerations. Adhering to evidence-based medicine of perinatal practice becomes a powerful tool for achieving this goal. If physicians refused to cooperate with such poorly managed companies, systematic dissociation would result in a loss of market share or, more optimistically, better management.

Being a physician-controlled, managed care organization provides no immunization against the ethical challenges of the business tools of managed care. These new physician-owned provider entities will not provide a solution in and of themselves to the ethical threats of conflict of interest and control of clinical judgment and practice. The virtue-based arguments we made will apply to these new entities without exception.

There is no conclusive evidence that preserving medicine as a fiduciary profession is impossible, even given the enormous economic power of managed care organizations. Ethics teaches us that business and economic power are not absolute and should always be called to account for their consequences. Society has not given MCOs the moral authority or permission to destroy the fiduciary character of medicine as a consequence of the pursuit of economic interest and power. Nor has society given physicians moral authority or permission to cooperate willfully with this destruction. Quite the opposite, society counts on physicians because ultimately society can count on no one else to preserve and advocate for the fiduciary character of the medical profession.

Argument-based Ethics

Before turning to the presentation of a formal tool,[26] for critically appraising the ethics literature, it is important to distinguish descriptive from normative medical ethics. The proposed formal tool is designed to be applied to the latter. Descriptive medical ethics uses empirical methods to obtain data that describe the actual ethical judgments, practices, and policies of physicians and health care organizations, of patient and their families, and of the larger society. These articles also report the results of ethically justified interventions for their clinical effects. Descriptive ethics articles use accepted methods of empirical research, such as interviews analyzed with qualitative methods and questionnaire research analyzed with quantitative methods.[27,28] Such empirical studies are common in the medical literature and should be critically appraised using appropriate methodology that has already been well described.[29-37]

The literature of normative medical ethics is argument-based. It, therefore, uses the tools of ethical analysis and argument to explore the implications of ethical concepts for what clinical practice and organizational and health care policy ought to be, as we did above with respect to the clinical ethical concept of the fetus as a patient. Normative ethics scholarship offers reasoned conclusions about what clinical judgment, decision-making, and behavior ought to be, rather than empirically based descriptions of what these are.

Formal Assessment Tool

The new critical appraisal tool presented here is adapted from recent work on critical appraisal of the medical literature reporting the results of qualitative research (Table. 14.1).[26]

Does the Article Address a Focused Ethics Question?

Normative ethics articles in perinatal medicine should have a clear, well-defined focus. This focus should be reflected in the title and made explicit in the introductory section of the paper. There are a number of possible domains for the focus of normative ethics literature, including theoretical issues (such as whether the fetus is a patient or a person), clinical issues for a specific patient population (the management of pregnancy in a diabetic patient), research issues for a specific population (surgical management of fetal spina bifida), organizational management issues (quality improvement and cost control of IVF services), and public policy issues (partial-birth abortion).

The importance of the issue should be explained, which can be theoretical or clinical. The issue may be important for research or for organizational and public policy. The importance of the issue should be justified. It is important that the article should identify the perspective from which importance of the issue is claimed, whether that of physicians, scientific investigators, patients, patient's families and other support networks, payers, health care organization leadership, and scholars and public officials concerned with health policy. The target audience for the article should be made clear.

Table 14.1: Formal assessment tool

1. Does the article address a focused ethics question?
   a. Does the article address a clearly stated and focused ethical issue or problem?
   b. Is the issue important and why?
   c. Is justification for the importance presented?
   d. From whose perspective is importance claimed?
2. Are the arguments that support the results of the article valid?
   a. Is the literature search complete?
   b. Are the analysis and argument of cited papers reported clearly and accurately?
   c. What is the quality of the paper's ethical analysis and argument?
3. What are the results?
   a. What are the conclusions of the paper's ethical analysis and argument?
4. Will the results help me in clinical practice?
   a. Will the help be practical?
   b. Will the help be theoretical?
   c. How should the reader change his or her thinking, attitudes, practices or policies?

Are the Arguments that Support the Results of the Article Valid?

This question concerns whether the results of the article, i.e. the conclusions that it draws about what morality in medicine ought to be, are supported by high quality ethical analysis and argument. The literature of normative ethics in perinatal medicine is now quite extensive, making it increasingly unlikely that there is no prior relevant literature that should be considered. Relevant literature should be cited and analysis and arguments from this literature should be presented clearly and accurately. In the basic and clinical science literature investigators are increasingly expected to elucidate the search strategies, including key words, databases, bibliographies, and other sources used. The same standard should begin to be met by the normative ethics literature. In assessing the search of an article, the critical reader should first ask, how adequate is the article's search strategy? Inasmuch as all are major forms of scholarship in bioethics, are articles, book chapters, and books cited?

Is the literature carefully reviewed? By this we mean that major positions on the issue should be presented in a clear and unbiased fashion. How these positions have developed and their critical interaction should be explained, so that the reader is provided with a reliable account of the best thinking on the subject. Major positions should be critically appraised for their strengths and weaknesses and how well they have responded to criticisms that advanced against them.

What is the quality of the paper's analysis and argument? Quality turns on both validity and soundness. Validity concerns the formal qualities of ethical analysis and argument. Are relevant clinical and other facts clearly identified and supported? Are key concepts and ethical appeals clearly stated and reasonably related to clinical information? Are these concepts and appeals used with consistent meaning throughout the argument? Do the reasons given for the position, the premises of the argument, fit together into a coherent whole? Is the conclusion that follows from those premises clearly stated? Normative ethics in perinatal medicine is not an "ivory tower" enterprise; it concerns issues of vital importance in clinical practice and research and in organizational management and health policy. Physician readers are, therefore, entitled to expect authors of normative medical ethics scholarship to take a clinically relevant and applicable stand that is supported by the argument presented.[4,38]

Soundness concerns the substance of the ethical analysis and argument, including especially whether the conclusion should be regarded as reliable, i.e. one on which the physician can act with confidence that patient care will be improved as a result. Reliable arguments are those in which a clear warrant of defense is given for each premise or reason offered in support of the conclusion.

In preventing readers' bias,[39] it is helpful to identify the disciplines represented among the authors. The normative medical ethics literature is distinctive in that work of high quality by nonclinicians should influence the clinical judgment and decision-making of physicians, just a work on infectious diseases of the reproductive tract by microbiologists or on pharmacokinetics of gynecologic cancer chemotherapy by pharmacologists rightly influences clinical judgment and practice. Normative ethics work, therefore, should not be dismissed when only some or even none of the authors are physicians.

At the same time, the reader should beware positive or negative bias toward an article, based on the reputation of the author(s) or of the journal. Just as in the basic and clinical sciences, the standing of authors in journals in obstetrics and gynecology or in the field of bioethics is no guarantee of quality in normative medical ethics.

What are the Results?

The results of normative ethics are the conclusions of ethical analysis and argument. These conclusions should be clearly stated and easy to find in the article.

Will the Results Help Me in Clinical Practice?

The results of normative ethics articles and books can be helpful in at least three ways. First, they may have important practical implications, especially if the paper incorporates evidence to support the clinical utility of acting on the conclusions of the paper. The quality of the empirical evidence cited should be assessed in the same way as evidence should be assessed in any medical or scientific article.[29-37] The results for clinical practice, research, organizational management, or policy should be assessed as well. Second, they may have important theoretical implications, which do not depend on whether an intervention was performed and evaluated. Identifying such theoretical implications results in critical assessment and revision of ethical frameworks and appeals based on them. Finally, readers of the normative ethics literature should ask themselves how they should change their thinking (clinical judgment and reasoning), attitudes (toward patients, their families, and legal institutions), clinical practice, or organizational policies. This is a crucial step in the literature on evidence-based medicine and is similarly crucial here.

CONCLUSION

In this chapter, we have provided a general ethical framework for perinatal clinical judgment and practice. Implementing this framework on a daily basis is essential to creating and sustaining a professional physician-patient relationship in perinatal medicine. This framework emphasizes preventive ethics, i.e. the recognition that the potential for ethical conflict is built into clinical practice and the use of such clinical tools as informed consent and negotiation to prevent such conflict from occurring. This framework comprehensively appeals to the ethical principles of beneficence, respect for autonomy, and justice, and the professional virtues of self-effacement, self-sacrifice, compassion and integrity. Finally, a formal tool can now be used to critically evaluate the literature of ethics in perinatal medicine.

REFERENCES

1. American College of Obstetricians and Gynecologists. Ethics in Obstetrics and Gynecology. Washington, DC: American College of Obstetricians and Gynecologists; 2002.
2. Association of Professors of Gynecology and Obstetrics. Exploring medical-legal issues in obstetrics and gynecology. Washington, DC; APGO Medical Education Foundation; 1994.
3. FIGO Committee for the Study of Ethical Aspects of Human Reproduction. Recommendations of Ethical Issues in Obstetrics and Gynecology. London: International Federation of Gynecology and Obstetrics; 1997.
4. McCullough LB, Chervenak FA. Ethics in Obstetrics and Gynecology. New York: Oxford University Press; 1994.
5. Engelhardt HT Jr. The Foundations of Bioethics, 2nd edition. New York: Oxford University Press; 1995.
6. Beauchamp TL, Childress JF. Principles of Biomedical Ethics, 5th edition. New York: Oxford University Press; 2001.
7. Hippocrates. Oath of hippocrates. In: Temkin O, Temkin CL (Eds). Ancient Medicine: Selected Papers of Ludwig Edelstein. Baltimore: Johns Hopkins University Press; 1976. p. 6.
8. Faden RR, Beauchamp TL. A History and Theory of Informed Consent. New York: Oxford University Press; 1986.
9. Brody H, Bonham VL Jr. Gag rules and trade secrets in managed care contracts: ethical and legal concerns. Arch Intern Med. 1997;157:2037-43.
10. Wear S. Informed Consent: Patient Autonomy and Clinician Beneficence within Health Care, 2nd edition. Washington, DC: Georgetown University Press; 1998.
11. Callahan S, Callahan D (Eds). Abortion: Understanding Differences. New York: Plenum Press; 1984.
12. Annas GJ. Protecting the liberty of pregnant patient. N Engl J Med. 1988;316:1213-4.
13. Chervenak FA, McCullough LB. Ethics in obstetrics and gynecology: an overview. Euro J Obstet Gynecol Reprod Med. 1997;75:91-4.
14. Chervenak FA, McCullough LB. The limits of viability. J Perinat Med. 1997;25:418-20.
15. Chervenak FA, McCullough LB. An ethically justified, clinically comprehensive management strategy for third-trimester pregnancies complicated by fetal anomalies. Obstet Gynecol. 1990;75:311-6.
16. Chervenak FA, McCullough LB. Campbell S. Is third trimester abortion justified? Brit J Obstet Gynaecol. 1995;102:434-5.
17. Chervenak FA, McCullough LB. Campbell S. Third trimester abortion: is compassion enough? Brit J Obstet Gynaecol. 1999;106:293-6.
18. Chervenak FA, McCullough LB. Clinical guides to preventing ethical conflicts between pregnant women and their physicians. Am J Obstet Gynecol. 1990;162:303-7.
19. Chervenak FA, McCullough LB, Rosenwaks Z. Ethical considerations in newer reproductive technologies. Seminars in Perinatol. 2003;27:427-34.
20. Chervenak FA, McCullough LB, Rosenwaks Z. Ethical dimensions of the number of embryos to be transferred in vitro fertilization. J Assist Reprod Genet. 2001;18:583-7.
21. Sterba JF, Justice. In: Reich WT (Ed). Encyclopedia of Bioethics, 2nd edition. New York: Macmillan; 1995. pp. 1308-15.
22. Chervenak FA, McCullough LB. Professionalism and justice in the leadership of academic medical centers. Acad Med. 2002;77:45-7.
23. Chervenak FA, McCullough LB, Chez R. Responding to the ethical challenges posed by the business tools of managed care in the practice of obstetrics and gynecology. Am J Obstet Gynecol. 1996;175:524-7.
24. Council on Ethical and Judicial Affairs of the American Medical Association. Ethical issues in managed care. JAMA. 1995;273:330-5.
25. Spece RG, Shimm DS, Buchanan AE (Eds). Conflicts of Interest in Clinical Practice and Research. New York: Oxford University Press; 1996.

26. McCullough LB, Coverdale JH, Chervenak FA. Argument-based medical ethics: a formal tool for critically appraising the normative medical ethics literature. Am J Obstet Gynecol. 2004;191:1097-102.

27. Sulmasy DP, Sugarman J. The many methods of medical ethics (or thirteen ways of looking at a blackbird). In: Sugarman J, Sulmasy DP (Eds). Methods in Medical Ethics. Washington, DC: Georgetown University Press; 2001. p. 318.

28. Sugarman J, Faden R, Weinstein J. A decade of empirical research in medical ethics. In: Sugarman J. Sulmasy DP (Eds). Methods in Medical Ethics. Washington, DC: Georgetown University Press; 2001. pp. 19-28.

29. Oxman AD, Cook DJ. Guyatt GH. Users' guides to the medical literature. VI. How to use an overview. JAMA. 1994;272:1367-71.

30. Guyatt GH. Sackett DL. Cook DJ. Users' guides to the medical literature. II. How to use an article about therapy or prevention. A. Are the results of the study valid? JAMA. 1993;270:2598-601.

31. Guyatt GH, Sackett DL, Cook DJ. Users' guides to the medical literature. II. How to use an article about therapy or prevention. B. What were the results and will they help me in caring for my patients? JAMA. 1994;271:59-63.

32. Wilson MC, Hayward RS, Tunis SR, et al. Users' guides to the medical literature. VIII. How to use clinical practice guidelines. A. Are the recommendations valid? JAMA. 1995;274:570-4.

33. Wilson MC, Hayward RS, Tunis SR, et al. Users' guides to the medical literature. VIII. How to use clinical practice guidelines. A. What are the recommendations and will they help you in caring for your patients? JAMA. 1995;274:1630-2.

34. Giacomini MK, Cook DJ. Users' guides to the medical literature. XXIII. Qualitative research in health care. A. Are the results of the study valid? Evidence-Based Medicine Working Group. JAMA. 2000;284:357-62.

35. Giacomini MK, Cook DJ. Users' guides to the medical literature. XXIII. Qualitative research in health care. B. What are the results and how do they help me care for my patients? Evidence-based Medicine Working Group. JAMA. 2000;284:478-82.

36. Drummond MF, Richardson WS, O'Brien BJ, et al. Users' guides to the medical literature. XIII. How to use an article on economic analysis of clinical practice. A. Are the results of the study valid? Evidence-Based Medicine Working Group. JAMA. 1997;277:1552-7.

37. O'Brien BJ, Heyland D, Richardson WS, et al. Users' guides to the medical literature. XIII. How to use an article on economic analysis of clinical practice. B. What are the results and how do they help me in caring for my patients? Evidence-Based Medicine Working Group. JAMA. 1997;277:1802-6.

38. Chervenak FA, McCullough LB. What is obstetric ethics? J Perinat Med. 1995;23:331-41.

39. Owen R. Reader bias. JAMA. 1982;247:2533-4.

15 Ethical Committees

JG Schenker

INTRODUCTION

In the last two decades, ethical issues in medicine have come to the forefront of public consciousness, with concern focusing on several important areas. Advances in scientific and technological knowledge have created ethical dilemmas about what is right and wrong, about life and death issues, as well as issues of equality, justice and personal preferences. Biomedical ethics also raised issues on patients' rights, which required steps to be taken to protect patient's welfare and to promote patients' autonomy.

Society's concern for ethical issues in medical practice has led to a growing need for the medical profession to become fully aware of the public view not only on individual patient-physician relationships, but also on how medical developments affect social structure and health policies. Health policy makers as well must examine the ethical basis of decision-making, prioritization, and conflicts of interest as they influence health care locally, nationally and internationally.

Biomedical ethical issues, guidelines, principles and regulations cut across national boundaries and often have universal implications. Although cultures differ, certain values are common to all. In this context, the most important is respect for human dignity, and this should not be negotiable. The establishment of international and interdisciplinary forums in which scientists and lay people can exchange views on topics of immediate concern, unhampered by administrative, political, or other considerations was needed. They are intended especially for the discussion of the scientific and technical bases of advances in biology and medicine and other related areas and their social, economic, ethical, administrative and legal implications forums in which scientists and lay people can exchange views on topics of immediate concern, unhampered by administrative, political or other considerations was needed.

The range of ethical questions raised by new scientific achievements in the life science and methods of taking care of women's health, especially assisted reproduction, have been debated by international political and professional bodies. Within international committees, diverse geographic, ethnic, cultural, linguistic and religious backgrounds are represented.

NUREMBERG CODE

The first international code of ethics for research involving human subjects—the Nuremberg Code—was a response to the atrocities committed by Nazi research physicians that were revealed at the Nuremberg War Crimes Trials. Many of their experiments had entailed the deliberate killing of, or infliction of grievous injuries on, prisoners whose rights to consent or refuse were ignored. Thus, it was to prevent repetition by physicians of such attacks on the rights and welfare of human beings that human-research ethics came into being. The Nuremberg Code, issued in 1947[1] laid down the standards for carrying out human experimentation, emphasizing the subject's voluntary consent.

a. The voluntary consent of the human subject is essential. This means that the person involved should have legal capacity to give consent; should be so situated as to be able to exercise free power of choice without the intervention of any element of force, fraud, deceit, duress, over-reaching, or other ulterior form of constraint or coercion; and should have sufficient knowledge and comprehension of the elements of the subject matter involved as to enable him to make an understanding and enlightened decision. This latter element requires that before the acceptance of an affirmative decision by the experimental subject there should be made known to him the nature, duration and purpose of the experiment; the method and means by which it is to be conducted; all inconveniences and hazards reasonably to be expected; and the effects upon his health or person that may possibly come from his participation in the experiment. The duty and responsibility for ascertaining the quality of the consent rests upon each individual who initiates, directs or engages in the experiment. It is a personal duty and responsibility that may not be delegated to another with impunity.

b. The experiment should be such as to yield fruitful results for the good of society, unprocurable by other methods or means of study, and not random and unnecessary in nature.

c. The experiment should be so designed and based on the results of animal experimentation and knowledge of the natural history of the disease or other problem under study that the anticipated results will justify the performance of the experiment.

d. The experiment should be so conducted as to avoid all unnecessary physical and mental suffering and injury.

e. No experiment should be conducted where there is an a priori reason to believe that death or disabling injury will occur, except, perhaps, in experiments where the experimental physicians also serve as subjects.

f. The degree of risk to be taken should never exceed that determined by the humanitarian importance of the problem to be solved by the experiment.

g. Proper preparations should be made and adequate facilities provided to protect the experimental subject against even remote possibilities of injury, disability or death.

h. The experiment should be conducted only by scientifically qualified persons. The highest degree of skill and care should be required through all stages of the experiment of those who conduct or engage in the experiment.

i. During the course of the experiment, the human subject should be at liberty to bring the experiment to an end if he has reached the physical or mental state where continuation of the experiment seems to him to be impossible.

j. During the course of the experiment, the scientist in charge must be prepared to terminate the experiment at any stage if he has probable cause to believe, in the exercise of the good faith, superior skill, and careful judgment required of him, that a continuation of the experiment is likely to result in injury or death to the experimental subject. All research involving human subjects should be conducted in accordance with three basic ethical principles, namely: respect for persons, beneficence and justice.

The Nuremberg Code document was criticized because it does not distinguish between different types of biomedical experimentation. The Nuremberg Code makes the subject's legal capacity to consent a prerequisite to experimentation, thus excluding from participating in research many people who might benefit from the results obtained, including children, the mentally ill, and others who are unable to give legal consent.

UNESCO—THE UNITED NATIONS EDUCATIONAL, SCIENTIFIC AND CULTURAL ORGANIZATION

The United Nations Educational, Scientific and Cultural Organization (UNESCO) was established on November 16, 1945.[2] The main objective of UNESCO is to contribute to peace and security in the world by promoting collaboration among nations through education, science, culture, and communication to further universal respect for justice, for the rule of law, and for the human rights and fundamental freedoms that are affirmed for the peoples of the world without distinction of race, sex, language or religion. At the international level, UNESCO has been one of the principal promoters of the reflection on ethics of living. In 1993, UNESCO created the International Bioethics Committee (IBC). The IBC[3] is a forum for debate and reflection and for the elaboration of UNESCO's normative actions, particularly with regard to the implementation of the Universal Declaration on the Human Genome and Human Rights. It is up to the IBC to keep up with progress in genetics while taking care to ensure respect for the values of human dignity and freedom in view of the potential risks of irresponsible attitudes in biomedical research. The IBC has drafted statutes and published reports on the ethical aspects of human embryonic stem cell research and its use in therapeutic research; ethical issues on genetic screening and the testing, treatment, storage, and use of genetic data on genetic screening; and human gene therapy.

WHO—WORLD HEALTH ORGANIZATION

The Health Organization of the League of Nations was setup in Geneva in 1919. In 1945, the United Nations Conference on International Organization established a new, autonomous, international health organization—the World Health Organization (WHO). The objective of the WHO is the attainment by all peoples of the highest possible level of health.[4]

The WHO's constitution affirms fundamental ethical principles, such as the equality of rights and the unalienable dignity of all human beings. The WHO has set technical standards and proposed guidelines and codes of good practice in virtually all its fields of activity, including the widely publicized areas of organ transplantation, breast-milk substitutes, essential drugs, the marketing of pharmaceuticals, and, more recently, reproductive health, environmental health, and emerging diseases. The WHO also contributes to harmonizing legislation and terminology and fosters the dissemination and exchange of information on these subjects. Ethics continues to provide the basis for the WHO's activities and functions. Several WHO programs have their own ethical review committees; additional activities are carried by consultation on ethics and health at global level.

DECLARATION OF HELSINKI

The Declaration of Helsinki, promulgated in 1964 by the World Medical Association, is the fundamental document in the field of ethics in biomedical research and has had considerable influence on the formulation of international, regional, and national legislation and codes of conduct. The Declaration, revised in Tokyo in 1975, in Venice in 1983, and again in Hong Kong in 1989,[5] is a comprehensive international statement of the ethics of research involving human subjects. It is the mission of the physician to safeguard the health of the people. The physician's knowledge and conscience are dedicated to the fulfillment of this mission. Medical progress is based on research that ultimately must rest in part on experimentation involving human subjects. In current medical practice, most diagnostic, therapeutic, or prophylactic procedures involve hazards.

The purpose of biomedical research involving human subjects must be to improve diagnostic, therapeutic, and prophylactic procedures and the understanding of the etiology and pathogenesis of disease. In the field of biomedical research, a fundamental distinction must be recognized between medical research in which the aim is essentially diagnostic or therapeutic for a patient and medical research, the essential object of which is purely scientific and without implying direct diagnostic or therapeutic value to the person subjected to the research.

In 1992, International Ethical Guidelines for Biomedical Research Involving Human Subjects were introduced by The Council for International Organizations of Medical Sciences and WHO based on ethical principles.[6] All research involving human subjects should be conducted in accordance with three basic ethical principles: respect for persons, beneficence and justice. Respect for persons incorporates at least two fundamental ethical considerations:

i. Respect for autonomy, which requires that those who are capable of deliberation about their personal choices should be treated with respect for their capacity for self-determination.

ii. Protection of persons with impaired or diminished autonomy, which requires that those who are dependent or vulnerable be afforded security against harm or abuse.

For all biomedical and clinical research involving human subjects, the investigator must obtain the informed consent of the prospective subject. Informed consent is based on the principle that competent individuals are entitled to choose freely whether to participate in research. Informed consent protects the individual's freedom of choice and respects the individual's autonomy. In the case of an individual who is not capable of giving informed consent (e.g. a fetus, a newborn, or a small child), the proxy consent of a properly authorized representative should be obtained. In all human research, ethical guidelines have differentiated between beneficial (therapeutic) and non-beneficial (non-therapeutic) research. The therapeutic research subject stands to gain as much from the research, whether it be a procedure or a drug, as to lose from it. In the non-therapeutic research, the subject cannot possibly benefit himself, and any benefits can, therefore, only add to others. The risks of a non-beneficial research fall solely on the research subject, whereas the benefits may extend beyond the research subject to the population as a whole.

The spirit of the Declaration of Helsinki is that, in medical research, the interests of science and society should never take precedence over considerations related to the well-being of the subject. Only a minimal level of risk may be allowed for volunteers to subject themselves for the benefit of others. However, it remains a problem to decide what sorts of levels of risk are acceptable in the case of pregnant women and where the subjects of non-therapeutic research are not autonomous (e.g. premature and newborn babies).

It is generally accepted that pregnant and nursing women are not suitable subjects of clinical trials other than those that are designed to respond to the health needs of such women or their fetuses or nursing infants. Clinical trials for conditions associated with or aggravated by pregnancy and to test the safety and efficacy of drugs, methods, and devices for detecting fetal abnormalities and well-being are of primary importance in the medical field of perinatology. The justification for the participation of pregnant women in clinical trials is that they should not be deprived arbitrarily of the opportunity to benefit from investigational drugs, vaccines, or other agents that promise therapeutic or preventive benefit. In all cases, risks to pregnant women, fetuses and newborns should be minimized, as far as sound research design permits. As a general rule, pregnant or nursing women should not be the subjects of clinical trials except when such trials as are designed to protect or advance the health of pregnant or nursing women or fetuses or nursing infants and for which women who are not pregnant or nursing would not be suitable subjects. Such research may have a differential impact on the pregnant woman and the fetus, with one benefiting while the other does not. At the extreme, the research that is beneficial to the one may actually be harmful to the other.

Some therapeutic research on fetuses in utero must be allowed. It contributes to the discovery of new methods for treating fetal health problems. There is a consensus that research on fetuses in utero should be treated as human subjects research, and governed by the policies for human subjects research. Because fetuses in utero and pregnant women are linked to each other, research on one may affect the other. Such research may have a differential impact on the pregnant woman and the fetus, with one benefiting while the other does not, and may be harmful to the other. The fundamental presupposition of all ethical policies is that the independent review process for human subjects research must consider the interests and rights of both parties in reviewing research protocols. Most guidelines have also imposed additional requirements on the acceptable level of risk to the fetuses involved in the research protocol. It is assumed that fetuses have some moral standing so that some concern must be devoted to their interests and rights.

Sir John Peel's report, published in 1972,[7] presented governmental guidelines concerning the ethics of fetal research. The recommendations were as follows:

- Viable fetuses should not be subjected to non-beneficial research.
- Research is permitted on the whole alive previable fetus, dead fetus, or its organs.
- Dead fetuses or tissues may be used in accordance with the provisions of the Human Tissue Act, which governs the postmortem use of human tissue.
- Parental informed consent should be obtained.
- The validity of the research should be assured.

The National Commission for the Protection of Human Subjects in Biomedical and Behavioral Research was established in July 1974[8] and issued its recommendations. The guidelines have certain things in common the British guidelines but differ on some grounds. They have in common that dead fetuses and their tissues are to be afforded the respect of other dead human bodies and tissues. Fetuses with a chance of survival are to be treated like children. Willful damage to the fetus in utero may not be caused, presumably lest a mother change her mind about abortion. Significant differences are that in the United States, regulations fathers can veto the research, whereas in the British guidelines there is no such specific provision. In Britain, it is proposed that non-beneficial research is to be done on the fetus in utero or the viable fetus, whereas in United States it may be done if there is minimal risk.

COUNCIL OF EUROPE

In 1985, the Council of Europe created a multidisciplinary body with experts appointed by each member country. This committee has already produced documents on reproduction research on human subjects, prenatal diagnosis and screening, and genetic testing. Once the Committee of Ministers approves these documents, they become recommendations for the national parliaments, which may or may not decide to follow them. The European assembly and other committees have also issued reports related to bioethical problems. The Council of Europe, which represents all the democratic countries of Europe, has organized a European Convention on Bioethics. The Committee published protocols regarding human experiments and organ transplantation.[9]

FIGO COMMITTEE FOR THE STUDY OF ETHICAL ASPECTS OF HUMAN REPRODUCTION

In 1985, the FIGO Committee for the Study of Ethical Aspects of Human Reproduction was established.[10] Its main objectives were the recording and study of general ethical problems emanating from the research and practice of human reproductive medicine, with the aim of providing guidelines to the attention of physicians and the public in developed and developing countries.

From its inception this committee was not intended to solve these ethical dilemmas, but rather to raise discussion by suggesting perspectives that this group of health professionals, lawyers, and ethicists came to in carefully crafted analysis and debate over these issues. Given the rich field of ethical issues in women's health that derive from not only the reproductive life cycle, but the economic and political status of women internationally—this committee will always confront new issues and even new aspects of old issues that challenge ethical perspectives and practice. There are continual variations on themes the committee has raised in the past through new medical developments. The social status of women, the constraints on health care dollars, and the health status of women have also increased the need for the committee to address the broader set of rights and economic issues that directly influence the health of women and the ethical setting of their care.

The committee was composed of a range of international members who represented developing and developed countries and had a significant interest and expertise in medical ethics. The members of the FIGO Committee are obstetricians, gynecologists, oncologists, lawyers, and public health workers, all of whom represent diverse geographic, ethnic, cultural, linguistic, and religious backgrounds. Among the 14 members, 13 were chairs of leading obstetric and gynecologic departments.

The initial task of the FIGO Committee for the Study of Ethical Aspects of Human Reproduction was to identify and study the important ethical problems confronting health care practitioners in human reproduction. The identified ethical problems were to be brought to the attention of physicians and the public in the developed and developing countries to provide ethical guidelines where appropriate. This task has assumed greater importance with the continuing challenge of ensuring that women are granted human and reproductive rights worldwide. Furthermore, the complexity of incorporating the many ethical aspects of reproductive issues in differing societies for issues such as cloning, or patenting of the human genome, argue for the need for such a consensus body.

There is no other body internationally that confronts these issues with a view toward the impact on the health care of women. Because of this, the opinions of the committee are used by women's health practitioners internationally to assist them in setting national or local standards, to expand the depth of discussion of these issues locally, and to support their advocacy for improvements in the health and status of women internationally. In the face of rapid cultural and scientific change, this is a critical role of ever-greater need. Women are clearly vulnerable in countries where their health care rights are either nonexistent or threatened, and thus, these guidelines can be a powerful force to support the rights of women.

The work of the Committee: In its first Congress as a standing committee, the Ethics Committee presented three seminars: medical ethics and medically assisted reproduction, AIDS with emphasis on ethical aspects, and refusal of obstetrical care (maternal health, fetal health, and neonatal health), which were published in the proceedings of the Rio Congress.

The early focus of the Committee, from 1985 to 1991, was clearly in areas central to obstetrics and gynecology practice, with a focus on such areas as sterilization, research on pre-embryo, and elective reduction of multiple pregnancies. In that same time period, however, the committee began to explore what the ethical responsibilities of societies of gynecology and obstetrics were for the broader issues of provision of reproductive health care and women's health in general. This led to a seminar during the FIGO Singapore Congress focusing on issues such as:

- How much are mothers worth?
- Distribution of resources between primary and tertiary reproductive care.
- Availability of resources for newborn care.
- Macro-ethical issues in obstetrics and gynecology.

This key seminar was chaired by Professor Sureau and Schenker, and marked an important expansion of the thinking of the Committee beyond that of the common bioethical analysis of the time, which focused on principals such as benefit (beneficence), harm (maleficence), and patient autonomy in the area of human rights and justice. During this time, the Committee also began to align its meetings with regional meetings that paralleled the focus of the committee on ethical aspects of human reproduction. The first of these took place in Cairo in 1991 and focused on bioethics in human reproduction research in the Muslim World. The committee meeting foreshadowed an area of ongoing controversy in medicine—that of transplantation. At that time the group considered whether research on pre-embryos was required in order to broaden our knowledge of the developmental process, to improve the treatment of infertility and the control of reproduction, and to permit genetic screening with its potential for the prevention and treatment of birth defects. The Committee recognized and tried to incorporate the diverse spectrum of ethical, cultural and religious values regarding the status of the pre-embryo. However, agreement was reached on some key areas even with these divergent views:

a. First, research on pre-embryos was only ethically acceptable when its purpose is for the benefit of human health and only if animal models would not suffice.

b. The committee felt that no developing human pre-embryo might be kept alive beyond 14 days after fertilization (not including any time during which the embryo had been frozen).

c. Research projects on pre-embryos should be authorized by ethical and/or other appropriate bodies in the country and, if allowed, appropriate informed consent must be obtained before undertaking research on pre-embryos, normally both gamete donors. Furthermore, provision of gametes and pre-embryos should not be subject of commercial profit.

d. The committee was unable to reach a consensus as to whether research should be limited to surplus pre-embryos or should also include preembryos specifically generated for research, a debate that continues worldwide. The discussion over this issue established the precedent that committee statements required consensus, and where that was not possible, debates were either not included or included with the caveat that there was no consensus.

The deliberations are made public through committee statements published in scientific journals and in specific reports. The FIGO committee has discussed and provided guidelines on general issues in women's health and advocacy, issues on genetics, embryo research, contraception, abortion, and reproductive endocrinology issues regarding pregnancy, maternal-fetal health, and neonates. The first bound publication of the collated Issues and Guidelines appeared in 1994, 1997, and 2000, and by 2003 had grown to a body of work that encompassed such that with the translations into Spanish and French, covers 232 pages.[11]

The method of analysis adopted by the committee evolved early on and consisted of position papers on a topic identified by the committee that were circulated prior to committee meetings in the working language of the committee, English.

These research papers explicated the problem, the present status of knowledge, and the various ethical stances or issues that were identified in the literature. At times, the committee invited outside experts in areas where there was not felt to be adequate depth of expertise or where there were other FIGO Committees working on the medical or rights aspects of the same issue. The papers were presented at the meeting and a consensus about the important background and ethical issues was identified.

Depending on the issues, further work on synthesizing these into a set of reflections or guidelines might take place at the meeting or over several meetings, until every word of each document was reviewed, read, and revised by all the members of the committee. Proposed statements were read line by line and edited by the entire committee to assure that not only the content was acceptable to the committee, but that the translations to French and Spanish would not contain errors because of the likely translation from English.

The committee statements, opinion are independent from FIGO member societies or executive board. The documents represent the result of that carefully researched and considered discussion. This independence has been particularly helpful to FIGO in providing ethical guidance regarding the relationship of the federation to industry, initially formulated as internal "Guidelines for Relations between Industry and FIGO" in 1991. The committee collaborates with international organizations such as the World Health Organization on various aspects of women's health to ensure that the ethical aspects are fully covered.

The committee members represent a wide spectrum of religions and countries, and numerous members have co-coordinated with multiple international committees to encourage and ensure inclusion of these ethical aspects in regular and extraordinary meetings.

WAPM—WORLD ASSOCIATION OF PERINATAL MEDICINE

In 1999, the World Association of Perinatal Medicine established an Ethical Committee. The main objectives of the committee are:[12]

- To study the ethical problems that emanate from practice and research in perinatal medicine.
- To provide guidelines for the practice of obstetrics and neonatology.
- To bring the ethical issues to the attention of physicians, nurses, paramedical staff and the public.

NATIONAL ETHICS COMMITTEES

National ethics committees are setup by governments to advice on regulations or proposed legislation concerning moral bioethical programs that raise controversy among professionals and the public. National committees were originally created due to an increasing demand among doctors and researchers for some authoritative guidance as to what was permissible in issues where no law exists. The nature of the membership of such committees is of even greater importance. The chairman must be unrelated to the medical or research profession. The members of national ethics committees must represent a broad range of values and professional expertise in the fields of medicine, law, administration, media, economics, public policy and moral philosophy. Within committees dealing with reproductive health, for example, at least 50% of the members must be women. Governmental or non-governmental bodies have issued reports on ethical and legal aspects, especially in the fields

of perinatal care, assisted reproduction technologies and human experimentation. Scientific progress is ahead of what society is willing to accept, and the reports of the bioethical committees protect the public by monitoring and, when necessary, regulating scientific practice. There is no single solution to a moral problem. A committee must incorporate a number of different moral ideals and reach a workable compromise. The law that these committees create must be in step with moral beliefs, or it will not be implemented. It is the task of the ethics committee to try to produce some consensus, based on all considerations, and to recommend it for practice. Several problems arise in the setup of the committees. Who should make moral decisions in controversial public issues? How is the committee's membership to be determined? In a pluralistic, mainly secular society there are no moral experts per se. Committees who serve public morality must conform to certain specifications of expertise. The committee members must be capable of understanding the scientific background of the subject matter of the issue. They must be acquainted with moral philosophy and understand the nature of ethics. The members must be intelligent and creative and not dogmatic. It is imperative that people who hold particular moral or religious views that make them impervious to the language of consensus are not included in the committee's team. They may be incapable of sympathy and flexibility and thus not be of use. The members must also be readily available to perform this extremely time-consuming task. One major disadvantage of these committees is that sometimes the advent of new technologies is ahead of committee deliberations. If a previous committee decision was opposed to specific new advances, their use may be delayed until the committee changes its original decision. It is imperative that people who hold particular moral or religious views that make them impervious to the language of consensus are not included in the committee's team. In most western countries, committees are setup ad hoc to address specific subjects of public bioethical concern.

The Warnock Committee on Human Fertilization and Embryology (1984) had a great influence on subsequent legislation in the United Kingdom.[13] In the United States, legislation that seems to reinforce ethical conduct may actually replace the exercise of ethical judgment with unreflective obedience to law. They may be incapable of sympathy and flexibility. The Belmont Report (1979) identified the basic ethical principles that should emphasize the conduct of biomedical and behavioral research involving human subjects and developed guidelines that should be followed to assure that such research is conducted in accordance with those principles.[14] The guidelines provided by national committees are usually converted into laws by legislation that introduces criminal punishment for violation. Legislation that seems to reinforce ethical conduct may actually replace the exercise of ethical judgment with unreflective obedience to law. The experience of Assisted Reproductive Technology (ART) practice demonstrated that countries with voluntary guidelines seem to enjoy public confidence, and public pressure for a change seems minimal. Countries with legislative surveillance seem to agree that it works well, although there are understandable complaints about the slowness of the legislative process and the difficulty of having regulations changed once they are in place, and thus, not be of use.

CONCLUSION

The range of ethical questions raised by new scientific achievements in the life science, and methods of taking care of women's health especially, has been debated by international political and professional bodies. Biomedical ethical issues, guidelines, principles, and regulations cut across national boundaries and often have universal implications. Although cultures differ, certain values are common to all. In this context, the most important value is respect for human dignity, and this should not be negotiable. The establishment of international and interdisciplinary forums in which scientists and lay people can exchange views on topics of immediate concern, unhampered by administrative, political, or other considerations, was needed. They are intended especially for the discussion of the scientific and technical bases of advances in biology and medicine and other related areas and their social, economic, ethical, administrative, and legal implications. Commissions appointed by institutions, governments, and international bodies serve to alleviate the medical profession from making ethical decisions and to protect human subjects from any harm. The deliberations of these committees are usually followed by guidelines of operation, which in many cases have become abiding law. For these committees to be of full advantage, they must convene promptly as issues arise so as not to delay medical advances from being implemented.

REFERENCES

1. The Nuremberg Code. In: Anna GJ, Grodin MA (Eds). The Nazi doctors and the Nuremberg Code: human rights in human experimentation. New York: Oxford University Press; 1992.
2. Constitution. London: UNESCO; 1945.
3. International Bioethics Committee. Statutes of the International Bioethics Committee. London: UNESCO; 1998.
4. WHO. From small beginnings. World Health Forum. 1988;9:29-34.
5. World Medical Association. Declaration of Helsinki. In: Anna GJ, Grodin MA (Eds). The Nazi doctors and the Nuremberg Code: human rights in human experimentation. New York: Oxford University Press; 1992. pp. 311-43.
6. International ethical guidelines for biomedical research involving human subjects. In: Bankowski Z, Levine RJ (Eds). Proceedings of the 26th CIOMS Conference, Geneva, Switzerland 5-7 February 1992. Geneva: CIOMS; 1993. pp. 1-36.
7. Department of Health and Social Security, Scottish Home and Health Department, Welsh Office. The use of fetuses and fetal material for research: report of the advisory group. London: Her Majesty's Stationery Office; 1972.
8. US Department of Health, Education, and Welfare, Office of the Secretary. Protection of human subjects: proposed amendments concerning fetuses, pregnant women, and in vitro fertilization. Federal Register 42, no. 9. January 13, 1977. pp. 2792-3.
9. The Council of Europe. Principles concerning medical research on human beings. WHO Int Digest Health Legislation. 1990;41:3-6.
10. Schenker JG (Ed). Recommendations on ethical issues in obstetrics and gynecology by the FIGO Committee for the Study of Ethical Aspects of Human Reproduction. London: FIGO; 1994. pp. 7-8.
11. Recommendations on ethical issues in obstetrics and gynecology by the FIGO Committee for the Study of Ethical Aspects of Human Reproduction. London: FIGO; 1994, 1997, 2000, 2003.
12. Schenker JG. Report from the Ethical Committee of the World Association of Perinatal Medicine. J Perinat Med. 2000;28:3-6.
13. Warnock DM. Report of the Committee of Inquiry into Human Fertilization and Embryology. London: HMSO; 1984.
14. National Commission for the Protection of Human Subjects of Biomedical and Behavioral Research. The Belmont Report: ethical principles and guidelines for the protection of human subjects of research. United States: Office for Protection from Research Risks; 1979. pp. 1-8.

16 Education in Perinatal Ethics

GM Stirrat

INTRODUCTION

Amazing advances, in for example, genetics, reproductive technologies, and perinatal medicine, occurred in the latter part of the 20th century. As Radcliffe-Richards[1] has said "Science keeps on throwing up new situations which, in some ways resemble familiar ones but in others are utterly unlike them; and we try to solve the resulting problems by stretching our old familiar categories to fit, but with ever increasing strains and cracks appearing everywhere." Those of us who practice perinatal medicine are required to consider a wide range of ethical questions, sometimes on a daily basis. Some of them relate to our specialty while others are generic (e.g. consent, confidentiality, and resource allocation). The problems can be complex and true dilemmas where the choices are between equally undesirable alternatives. Over 30 years ago, Campbell[2] wrote, "moral dilemmas will continue to occur in medicine as long as choices have to be made which involve putting one set of values against another." Unfortunately ready-made answers cannot be found in textbooks (not even this one!), because the situations in which the problems arise and the stories of the people involved are all different from any other. The desired goals may also be different. For example, the prevention of disease and health promotion tend to raise different issues and require different solutions than the relief of symptoms, pain and suffering, or the cure of disease.

The 21st century will bring further advances in what can be done, but the prevailing ethical climate suggests that there will continue to be much less critical consideration of what "ought" to be done. How then can we as individuals and as a community of physicians reduce the risk of Radcliffe-Richards's "strains and cracks" from causing the edifice of our professional practice from crumbling around us? If you ask an architect, builder or constructional engineer that question, their answer will be "Get the foundations right!"[3] Would it not, therefore, seem prudent that those training to perinatal physicians be properly grounded in the theories and principles behind the increasingly complex ethical decisions in which they will inevitably be closely involved in their subsequent career?

This chapter is based on several fundamental premises:

1. Each one of us is required to think ethically and act morally (i.e. we are all moral agents).
2. Ethics is about individuals living and working in community.[4] It is not just about "me" and "mine". As Campbell[5] states "there can be no possibility of freedom for anyone individual if that person acts without reference to all other moral agents."
3. Medical ethics is not solely a matter of moral theory, it is "an ethics of relation and practice."[4] Thus ethics is for something and must be translatable into moral action. It has to work in real life.
4. The dominant individualistic version of autonomous choice is fundamentally (and, in the long-run, potentially fatal) flawed.[6,7] Stirrat and Gill,[7] among others, have suggested a principled version of patient autonomy that involves the provision of sufficient and understandable information and space for a patient, who has the capacity to make a settled choice about medical interventions on herself and to do so responsibly in a manner considerate to others. A lifetime in clinical practice strongly suggests that this model best fits the optimal patient-doctor relationship in which there is a mutual, unspoken agreement between the parties that recognizes the duties and obligations each to the other with bilateral trust at the heart of this relationship. This is discussed further below.
5. The discipline of medical ethics is not qualitatively different from ethics in general. The fundamental ethical principles underpinning medical practice should be shared by society in general. However, by virtue of being a profession, we clearly have special obligations to the patients we serve. In the United Kingdom, the "Duties of a Doctor" are clearly laid down by the General Medical Council (GMC)[8] whose primary roles are "To protect the public by setting standards for professional practice, overseeing medical education, keeping a register of qualified doctors and taking action when a doctor's fitness to practice is in doubt." Table 16.1 outlines the duties of a doctor as set down by the GMC.[8]

   The code of medical ethics of the American Medical Association (AMA)[9] states, "a physician must recognize responsibility not only to patients, but also to society, to other health professionals, and to self." The two main items on the agenda of the first meeting of the Association in 1847 were the establishment of a code of ethics and the creation of minimum requirements for medical education and training. Table 16.2 shows the principles adopted by the AMA as "standards of conduct which define the essentials of honorable behavior for the physician."
6. Ethics is a necessary part of good clinical practice. Ethical judgments must take full account of all the circumstances of the case and be based on sound principles. Decisions must be consistent, free from contradiction, and clinically relevant. Exercise by physicians of their clinical judgment is frequently attacked as paternalism. While, in some instances, this can be so, it may also be the doctor fulfilling his or her duty to the patient by exercising his or her own autonomy, and as such, may be entirely justified. Indeed, there will be some occasions, particularly in perinatal medicine, in which acquiescence to a requested intervention against one's clinical or ethical judgment will be abrogation of one's duty as a doctor!

7. The patient-physician covenant relationship depends totally on the trust of the former that the latter will act at all times with the highest ethical standards. Indeed, not only is trust "the fundamental virtue at the heart of being a good doctor," it also allows us all to function socially as individuals in a complex society,[11] and "every genuine moral community is built on the trust that its members will look beyond personal interests and individual concerns toward a truly common good."[12] The words "trust" or "trustworthy" can be found on several occasions in the GMC's "Duties of a Doctor" (Table 16.1) and it is implicit in the AMA's Code of Ethics (Table 16.2). Among other authors, Draper and Sorell[10] argue that the patient has reciprocal duties but it is not appropriate to discuss this further here.

The relationship between ethics and morals has been compared to that between DNA and cell proteins.[13] Within the DNA (ethics) lies the fundamental information for the cell to function. The proteins (morals) produced by the cell interpreting and following that information do two things—they express both the nature and character of the cell and also perform its specific function. In addition, cells must work together within and among bodily structures and organs. The cell that expresses its individuality at the expense of its neighbors is "neoplastic" and may become malignant, ultimately causing the demise of the body. What this might suggest about the long-term consequences of the dominance of the primacy of the individual—"I," "me," and "mine"—in today's society are among the factors that lead to my concern about the potentially fatal flaw in this view of autonomy.

BASIS FOR ETHICS

Since at least the time of Socrates (470–399 BC) people have asked questions like, "How do we know what is good?" "How should I live?" "How can we know which decision is right?" and "What is justice?" Ethics or moral philosophy addresses these fundamental questions in order to establish a basis for moral judgments. Morals are the specific judgments, codes, or beliefs of particular groups or societies and the actions that follow from these.

DIVERSITY OF MORAL THEORY

In 1972 Campbell[2] wrote, "The essence of morality is that there is uncertainty." As a young obstetrician wrestling with a whole series of ethical dilemmas at that time, I found this very threatening. I was like Montaigne who said, "Tell me of your certainties; I have doubts enough of my own." Indeed, I venture to suggest that we all find uncertainty difficult to deal with. We would much prefer "meanings that are completely clear" and "truths that are completely certain."[14]

Table 16.1: Duties of a doctor (UK General Medical Council)[7]

"Patients must be able to trust doctors with their lives and well-being. To justify that trust, we as a profession have a duty to maintain a good standard of practice and care and to show respect for human life."
As a doctor you must:

- Make the care of your patient your first concern
- Treat every patient politely and considerately
- Respect patients' dignity and privacy
- Listen to patients and respect their views

- Recognize the limits of your professional competence
- Be honest and trustworthy
- Respect and protect confidential information
- Make sure that your personal beliefs do not prejudice your patients' care. Act quickly to protect patients from risk if you have good reason to believe that you or a colleague may not be fit to practice

- Give patients information in a way they can understand
- Respect the rights of patients to be fully informed in decisions about their care
- Keep your professional knowledge up-to-date

- Avoid abusing your position as a doctor
- Work with colleagues in the ways that best serve patients' interests

In all these matters you must never discriminate unfairly against your patients or colleagues. And you must always be prepared to justify your actions to them

Table 16.2: American Medical Association principles of medical ethics[8]

The medical profession has long subscribed to a body of ethical statements developed primarily for the benefit of the patient. As a member of this profession, a physician must recognize responsibility not only to patients, but also to society, to other health professionals, and to self. The following principles adopted by the American Medical Association are not laws, but standards of conduct which define the essentials of honorable behavior for the physician:

I. A physician shall be dedicated to providing competent medical service with compassion and respect for human dignity
II. A physician shall deal honestly with patients and colleagues, and strive to expose those physicians deficient in character or competence, or who engage in fraud or deception
III. A physician shall respect the law and also recognize a responsibility to seek changes in those requirements which are contrary to the best interests of the patient
IV. A physician shall respect the rights of patients, of colleagues, and of other health professionals, and shall safeguard patient confidences within the constraints of the law
V. A physician shall continue to study, apply and advance scientific knowledge, make relevant information available to patients, colleagues, and the public, obtain consultation, and use the talents of other health professionals when indicated
VI. A physician shall, in the provision of appropriate patient care, except in emergencies, be free to choose whom to serve, with whom to associate, and the environment in which to provide medical services
VII. A physician shall recognize a responsibility to participate in activities contributing to an improved community

Campbell[2] stated, "Many people seek to handle situations of uncertainty by elevating their personal convictions to the status of inherent and all-embracing rules, which must apply to every situation, whatever its complexities and ambiguities. Others try to reduce all moral dilemmas to questions of technical skill." He considered that both of these reactions were commonly found among physicians and nurses, "many of whom may feel that there is little to be argued about in medical ethics, either because they do not themselves see any moral ambiguities in their professional practice or because they consider all the decisions taken to be purely matters of clinical judgment." Personal experience suggests that, although such individuals still exist, the vast majority of health-care professionals are anxious to learn how to make more reflective and consistent ethical judgments in the face of the problems that they face day by day.

Of course, "moral philosophy does not attempt to "solve" moral dilemmas."[2] Rather, "it attempts to provide a rational framework for understanding the complexities of moral judgment."[2] It is entirely appropriate that we try to make sense out of uncertainty, and we do so by classification and codification of what we think we know. We need frameworks as reference points to allow us to progress through our lives as individuals in society, much as a ship traveling across the ocean. Indeed, Jonsen[15] suggests that "moral principles are not unlike the sky-marks used in celestial navigation: a position is determined and a course marked by continual reference to fixed points—sun, stars, and planets. At the same time, the navigator must look not only to the sky-marks but also to any visible landmarks and to the wind and waves. Thus while principles provide an indispensable general guiding direction, other features of the problem must be taken into consideration as the passage from moral question to moral answer is navigated."

It is, perhaps, not only inevitable, but also appropriate that a multiplicity of theoretical approaches to ethics should have arisen. Campbell has suggested, "The diversity of ethical theories is about as wide as the diversity of ways of understanding the relationship between man and his environment."[2]

The first of the two main theories is *deontology* or "duties in action." The best example is found in the writing of the philosopher Immanuel Kant in the 18th century. The essence of Kant's ethics is:

- Certain kinds of acts are intrinsically right and others intrinsically wrong determined by a set of rules.
- The rules must be universally applicable, coherent (i.e. not contradictory) within what Kant called "a rational system of nature" and capable of being freely adopted by "a community of rational beings."
- Among the rules are "do not kill, cause pain, disable, deprive of freedom or pleasure;" and "do not deceive, break promises, cheat, break laws, or neglect one's duty."
- Each of us has a set of duties to our fellow men and women. One of the most important duty is to "act so that you treat humanity, whether in your own person or in that of any other, always as an end, and never as a means only." It is this maxim that has, for example, contributed to concerns about so-called "savior sibling" procedures in which a child is conceived with the primary intention of being a source of compatible tissue for a seriously ill sibling.
- An action should not be judged to have been right or wrong by its consequences in individual situations.

No theory is without problems, and the main difficulties with this theory are defining the meaning of "rational" and agreeing on universally applicable rules.

The second main theory, developed in the 19th century by Jeremy Bentham and John Stuart Mill, is *consequentialism*, in which the rightness or wrongness of an action is based solely on consequences.[16] They named their theory *Utilitarianism*, and argued that the maximization of pleasure or happiness was what made acts right. This has been summarized as "The greatest happiness of the greatest number." Consequentialist theories can be further divided—*act consequentialism* states that the right action is the one that produces the most good. In *rule consequentialism*, the test is whether an action accords with a set of rules whose general acceptance would result in the most good. In each case "good" is determined solely by the beneficial consequences. The problem with consequentialism is that, although consequences are undoubtedly important in moral judgments and actions, happiness is highly subjective, and what is good (let alone the greatest good) is not always easy to determine. Moreover, benefiting the majority could result in ignoring vulnerable minorities. Where do the seriously disadvantaged in our society, such as the very preterm infant, the severely disabled child, the terminally ill, or the elderly with dementia, fit with this philosophy? A rule to protect the vulnerable could be set aside if it did not promote general happiness.

Clearly these theories are not, of themselves, sufficient for the resolution of clinical problems in real life and several other views have been developed to try to deal with their inherent problems. The *Four Principle Approach*, otherwise known as "Principlism," shown in Table 16.3 (and see Beauchamp[17]) was formulated as a basis for working out practical solutions for problems in medical ethics.

Critics say, with some justification, that these are merely a checklist without an underlying theory, are often in conflict with one another (with no internal resolution), and do not deal with emotional aspects or relationships. In particular, as has already been noted, the concept of autonomy is widely misunderstood. It does not necessarily mean doing what someone requests or demands at one point in time. It implies a settled view of the individual reached by deliberation as to what is in his or her own long-term best interests. It is also to be balanced with the autonomy of others, including, in this context, medical staff. Regrettably, the four principles are all too often used as a mantra to be applied by the lazy to every ethical issue without thought or discrimination.

Table 16.3: The four principles (Principlism)[17]

Principle	The obligation/duty
Beneficence	• To do what is in the patient's best interests • To provide benefits balanced against risks
Nonmaleficence	• Not to cause harm and, indeed, seek to prevent it
Autonomy (self-rule)	• To respect the right of the individual to make choices about her own life in the context of equal respect for everyone else involved
Justice	• To treat patients fairly and without unfair discrimination • Fairness in the distribution of benefits and risks

If, however, one recognizes their shortcomings and incorporates some other insights such as those discussed below, the four principles can provide a useful framework for analyzing ethical problems (Table 16.4A).

Other useful perspectives can be found in:

Narrative ethics:[18] This takes account of the patient's and the physician's context, emotions and relationships. Indeed, whatever one's approach, the patient's story must be part of the ethical relationship and one's own feelings are relevant to the moral choices. It is important that the latter be recognized, if only to ensure that one's feelings do not inappropriately influence the choice of the patient.

Virtue ethics: Instead of asking, "How should I act?" this asks "How should I live?"[19] This system tried to define excellence of character or behavior to which individuals or groups should aspire. One aspect is caring about someone, rather than just caring for him or her, and it can provide a useful perspective in, for example, those faced with chronic and/or serious illness or disability.

Feminist approaches to ethics:[20] One form of feminist ethics attempts to balance the dominant masculine ethos of traditional ethics with a more feminine perspective. The ethics is one of caring for individuals and, although caring resolutions may be different in their outcomes, they are linked by personal regard and respect given to individuals.

However, "formal frameworks, for all their value, need to be supplemented with other ethical approaches, based more on interpretation and judgment than on formal deduction or algorithm"[18] and "Any particular theory, when applied deductively, is shown to be inadequate sooner or later."[21]

Sherwin[22] suggests, "No moral theory can do the work normally expected of it, because none provides reliable grounds for resolving all moral complexities through deductive application of its central principles" and "Doing bioethics well requires appeal to the insights provided by multiple theories." Ethical reflection depends on having a set of core ethical beliefs that describe clear cases of morally objectionable or praiseworthy behavior which contribute the prototypes of ethical deliberation." Rather than trying to force us to choose a single, comprehensive theory to apply to all cases, she finds it preferable to view different theoretical perspectives as providing alternative "frameworks" or "templates" for different sorts of approaches to problems. She suggests that we use competing theories as a set of lenses through which we can get a clearer view of complex moral problems. Some lenses will provide clearer understanding than others.

Dunstan's[4] criteria for the practice of ethics in medicine are: good moral theories, the elucidation of principles to which implicit or explicit appeal can be made, the discipline of logic for the framing of good arguments and the exposure of bad ones, learning the "art of moral reasoning," discipline in the use of words without clichés, and "wisdom above all."

MAKING ETHICAL JUDGMENTS

There are two main ways in which ethical issues arise. The first is while dealing with patients and their clinical problems. The second is when faced with an issue in abstract (e.g. "what do you think of cloning?"). Dealing with the former tends to inform one's approach to the latter and, incidentally, provides valuable insights not given to the nonclinician.

How then do we go about making ethical judgments in the clinical context? McCullough and Chervenak[21] advocate five

Table 16.4A: Making ethical judgments—1. Analysis

Analyze the problem(s)
- What are its elements?: For example, medical, ethical, legal, etc.
- What parties are involved?: Such as the patient, her family, one or more fetus, statutory authorities (e.g. social workers, police), health-care professionals, etc.
  - Who is the appropriate advocate for the fetus?
- How do their perspectives fit together or conflict and, if the latter, what are the appropriate mechanisms for resolution?
- What is its context?: For example, social, ethnic, economic (within this may be issues about rationing).

Consider the underlying principles involved
- It may be useful to start with the four principles (beneficence, do no harm, autonomy and justice)[17]
  - What is in the patient's best interests?
  - How can I balance this with the avoidance of harm?
  - Is the patient competent? If so:
    - Is she expressing her settled view on what she wants?
    - Am I respecting her right to make choices about her own life?
    - Does this conflict with the autonomy of others and, if so, how is this to be resolved?
  - If she is not competent (e.g. a minor or an unconscious adult), or if this is open to question (e.g. a child aged 12–13), how is this to be dealt with?
  - Are there any issues of justice? e.g.
    - Is the patient being unfairly discriminated against?
    - Is there any conflict between what I consider to be in the patient's best interest and what can be provided?
    - What other perspectives could assist in resolution?
  - Have the patient's social context, emotions and relationships been adequately considered?
  - Am I sure that I am treating the patient as a person?
  - Are we both caring for and caring about the patient?

individually necessary and jointly sufficient criteria for rigorous analysis. These are:

- Clarity: Terms and concepts must have precise meaning.
- Consistency: Those terms must always be used with that precise meaning and reasoning must be free of contradiction.
- Coherence: Ethical deliberations must be internally consistent and noncontradictory.
- Applicability: The results of ethical deliberations can be applied in the clinical and research settings.
- Adequacy: The judgments allow ethical conflicts to be identified, managed, or, preferably, prevented.

It has to be emphasized that there is no magic formula, and indeed, Dan Callahan has suggested (personal communication, 2002) that "ethical theory ultimately does not matter very much—90% is educated common sense."

My own approach to making ethical judgments involves consideration of a series of questions under five task-orientated headings as outlined in Tables 16.4B that move from ethical analysis to clinical action.

THE PURPOSE AND PROCESS OF EDUCATION IN ETHICS

If Callahan is correct that 90% of ethics is educated common sense, why should anyone need training in ethics? The key is in the qualifying adjective, "educated." I once bought a wooden plaque on Cape Cod that read, "The one thing about common sense is that it is not so common!" Josh Billings (the pen name of Henry Wheeler Shaw), the renowned 19th century humorist, said two wise things on the subject: "Common sense is the knack of seeing things as they are, and doing things as they ought to be done" and "Learning is the art of knowing how to use common sense to advantage." Thomas Huxley's aphorism that "Science is nothing but trained and organized

Table 16.4B: Making ethical judgments—2. Action

Move toward recommending actions that best meet the criteria given in Table 16.4A
- What are the proposed objectives? For example, cure, relief of symptoms (e.g. pain and suffering), or prevention of disease?
  - Which objectives are essential and which desirable?
  - What alternatives are available (including doing nothing)?
  - What are the risks of acting (or failing to act) and what is their probability and severity?
  - Do the expected benefits outweigh the potential risks?
    - Has the patient been properly informed of the available options?
  - Is she competent to give consent?
    - If so, has the consent being obtained properly?
    - If yes, put chosen option into effect.
  - If she is not competent whom, if anyone, can legally give consent?

Dealing with potential or actual conflict:
This difficult area cannot be dealt with comprehensively here, but examples include:
- The patient refuses to accept the recommended interventions.
  - If competent, she has the right to do so, even if it leads to harm of herself (or unborn child). Do not coerce her. Among the things to do are:
    - If junior, inform more senior colleagues. If senior, seek advice through clinical governance channels
    - Make sure that full contemporaneous notes are made
- She requests intervention that informed medical opinion suggests is not justified or in her best interests
  - You are not bound to do as she asks, particularly if it is contrary to your principles
  - Offer referral for another opinion or, if needs be, transfer care to another team (In the UK, if the patient is requesting termination of pregnancy you are obliged to refer to another practitioner)
  - (Then as above)
- Another party tries to intervene inappropriately, e.g.
  - The family or another third party asks for confidential information
    - The presumption is that confidentiality must be kept
    - Any breach can only be justified in exceptional circumstances
  - It is preferable that this be with the knowledge of the patient
  - However, if, e.g. it is judged that the patient would be seriously harmed by knowing that her illness is terminal, but that it would be in her best interests that a close relative should know about it, information may be divulged without consent
- The family asks that the patient be not told the truth of her illness
  - The assumption (possibly rebuttable with good grounds—see example above) must be to tell the truth at all times
  - Not to do so can have regrettable consequences, e.g. who is she to trust when she discovers any deception?
  - Remember that your primary duty of care is to your patient and not her family

Good communication skills in general, and knowing how to impart bad news in particular, are central to being a good doctor

Review the outcome
- Ethical issues do not lend themselves easily to audit, but it may be useful to record and review major cases from time to time
- In individual cases, remember that a good or bad outcome does not necessarily mean that the intervention was right or wrong

common sense."[23] applies equally to ethics. He suggests that the former differs from common sense "only as a veteran may differ from a raw recruit: and its methods differ from those of common sense only as far as the guardsman's cut and thrust differ from the manner in which a savage wields his club." To change the metaphor, no one expects the child with an innate musical ability to sit down at the piano and immediately play Beethoven sonatas. The talent needs to be developed both by understanding the theory underpinning the music and also by practicing increasingly complex compositions. It must also be rewarding for the student! Thus, it is with ethics.

I believe that far more is achieved if a teacher starts from where the students are and builds on their inherent abilities, rather than start from where the teacher is and expect the students to soak up facts and opinions that do not necessarily relate to their own experiences. In the United Kingdom, the majority of students come to medical school from high school at about 18 years of age. Teaching in ethics in medicine in the University of Bristol begins shortly after the students commence their course and follow several weeks working with family practitioners meeting patients, learning about their problems and discerning the ethical issues involved. It subsequently runs as a vertical theme through all 5 years of the course. We never cease to be amazed at the maturity with which these talented young people address complex ethical issues often from their own experiences. This develops as the course progresses. They have the talent; it is our task to let it flourish.

Not long ago, I had one of the most rewarding teaching experiences of my life at the other end of the age spectrum. I was asked to speak to an older women's group on a reproductive ethics topic. Instead of lecturing them on the subject (on which, if truth be told, I was not an expert) I had prepared four hypothetical cases of increasing ethical complexity. Members of the group presented each case, the facts of the matter were discussed and questions addressed. We then began to consider the ethics of each case. In a very short time, the key ethical issues had been raised and debated, and by the time the fourth case had been completed, we had discussed a range of issues that would not have disgraced a textbook of ethics. Of course we did not come up with many firm answers, but these women not only discovered that they could think (something their families had probably told them implicitly or explicitly that they could no longer do), but also that their opinions were meaningful. What is more, they were not only thinking ethics on that day, but had been doing so all their lives! They also learned that there were few absolute answers, but had derived the principles to address the dilemmas by their own efforts. It was gratifying to see their self-esteem rise as the session progressed, and they left rejoicing in the experience. Henry Brook Adams, the historian, wrote in 1907 "a teacher affects eternity: he can never tell where his influence stops." Our objective in education in ethics is no less!

PHASES OF EDUCATION IN ETHICS

The most effective way to achieve proper education in ethics is to begin early and build on it through school, college, medical school, and continuing professional development.

1. Education in human relationships: This should begin early in school days and become a more formal study of ethics for all students in high school and college, where it should be part of the examined curriculum. The objective is for the student to learn how to think, not what to think.

2. Introduction to bioethics: This should commence in medical school, concentrating on a patient-centered approach to medicine, and be part of the examined curriculum. This has been emphasized by the GMC in "Tomorrow's Doctors—recommendations on undergraduate medical education."[24] The focus should not only be on knowledge, but also skills and attitudes as shown in Table 16.5. Both clinical and research governance should be included. There is increasing emphasis on this course being interprofessional, involving students from a variety of health-care professions. The confrontation of some issues will be traumatic for some students. Teachers must be sensitive to it. Earlier this is recognized and dealt with, the better. In addition, having been Dean of a medical faculty, I realize that the problem of the failing student is more often a problem in attitude rather than ability. This too must be recognized early for remedial action to be instituted and, if necessary, the student encouraged to join an alternative course of study for which he or she is more suited. It is too late for this to be recognized for the first time after qualification, perhaps as a result of an event that resulted in harm to a patient.

3. A core generic course for health-care professionals: It is suggested that these practice-based modular courses be designed for doctors working in hospitals, family practice, and public health, nurses, midwives, allied health professionals, and health-care managers. The courses would be an integral part of their continuous professional development. The design would have to recognize that not all participants are starting from the same point in their understanding of basic bioethics. A "core and options" design would allow this to be the first part of a specialty specific program (in our case Perinatal Medicine). Among the proposed objectives of these courses would be:

- To provide an introduction to (or revision of) basic theory in bioethics and to the relationship between ethics and the law.
- To develop consistent, critical, and reflective attitudes to ethical decision-making in the health-care setting.
- To increase awareness of ethical dilemmas faced in different health-care settings.
- To understand better the ethical problems facing colleagues in different disciplines.
- To reinforce best practices in clinical and research governance.
- The desired learning outcomes would include:
- A working knowledge of basic concepts and theories in clinical ethics.
- A greater confidence in confronting ethical issues encountered in clinical practice.
- A more consistent approach to dealing with similar ethical issues as they affect individual patients.
- A better understanding of the social and institutional context of decision-making in health care.
- Improved interprofessional communication, learning, and decision-making.
- Improved communication of ethical issues with the patients and their families.

Table 16.5: Introduction to bioethics in medical school

Objective	Key issues

Increasing knowledge	• In ethics there are very few cut and dry solutions to problems. In part this is because the problems themselves are so varied
	• As a practical discipline, ethics involves fitting general principles to specific circumstances in a way that respects these variations, but this does not mean deciding arbitrarily or with prejudice
	• The course should cover the main principles of ethics in medicine (e.g. respect for autonomy, beneficence, justice) and ethical concepts to be used in making morally reasonable judgments (e.g. duty, rights, virtue, consequences)
	• The students should learn:
	  ▪ The relevant law and professional codes of conduct that determine specific obligations owed by doctors to patients, society and each other
	  ▪ How best to determine what is morally important and relevant in a given medical situation; without this moral understanding it is impossible to apply rules or concepts in a sensitive and constructive way
	  ▪ The centrality of the patient's narrative in determining what is important for her and her medical care

Developing skills	The course should aim to develop skills of analysis, judgment and rational argument about moral issues in medicine. The context should always be their relevance to the practice of medicine and good patient care
Improving attitudes	The student should become aware of the wide variety of patients' attitudes to health, illness, doctors and society, the ways in which these impact on the medical relationship, and the ways in which their own attitudes play a part in this relationship The ways in which ethical issues in medicine are not only about hard decisions for doctors, but about making decisions with patients in personal, social, and institutional contexts should be explored This approach to patients' attitudes will inevitably involve the students confronting and rethinking their own, and this can be threatening for some. Problematic attitudes should be identified, acknowledged by the student and, if possible, remedied

Source: Based on the Ethics and Law in Medicine Vertical Theme Course in the University of Bristol Medical School, 2003/4

Table 16.6A outlines some suggested modules for such a course in basic bioethics. Formative and summary assessments would be incorporated and candidates could gain credits toward, e.g. a master's degree in bioethics.

4. Specific course in perinatal medicine: In this model, participants would have completed and gained credits in the generic course. This too could benefit from being interdisciplinary. Table 16.6B is a guide to the possible subjects to be included in the curriculum for such a course. Tables 16.7A and B lists some suggested texts relevant to both the generic and specific curriculum. It is for the users to adapt these suggestions to their requirements.

DOES EDUCATION IN ETHICS MAKE ANY DIFFERENCE?

It is not sufficient to assert that education in ethics is a good thing. Evaluation is required in support of the program to justify the commitment and expense, and to provide an evidence-base for future work. But what outcomes can be used? Among those suggested are ethical sensitivity, attitudes, reasoning ability, and decision-making. There is some literature on promoting ethical sensitivity in modern medical practice,[25-30] but the main focus has been on medical students.[31-32] Although some attempts have been made to measure the general effectiveness of ethics training,[33-36] the work lacks substantial investigation and discussion of different methods of moral education. One study has attempted to evaluate the effects of an intensive ethics course on health-care professionals, including physicians and nurses.[37] It was carried out during an open conference. Only about half of the participants provided direct patient care, and there were no data on the proportions of health-care professionals taking part, so no real conclusions can be drawn from it. More rigorous work is required.

SUMMARY

Ethics is the system of thought that analyzes and provides a rational framework for moral judgments. Among the key features of ethics are:

• It must be translatable into moral action.

• It is a public system rather than a private activity, and no one can act morally without reference to other individuals.

• The fundamental ethical principles underpinning medical ethics are those of society in general.

• Ethical analysis must be clear, consistent, internally consistent, and free of contradiction.

• The judgments made must allow ethical conflicts to be identified, managed or preferably, prevented.

The most effective way to achieve proper education in ethics is to begin early and build on it through school, college, medical school, and continuing professional development. Among the purposes of education in ethics are the development of consistent, critical and reflective attitudes to ethical decision-making, increasing awareness of ethical dilemmas in one's own practice and that of others, and reinforcement of best practices in clinical and research governance.

Table 16.6A: Suggested basic bioethics modules for a core generic curse for health-care professionals

Module 1:   Overview of bioethics—"What ought I do?" Dealing with uncertainty, etc.
Module 2:   Competing theories, e.g. duties versus consequences
Module 3:   Other important concepts, e.g. principlism, virtue and narrative ethics, autonomy, paternalism
Module 4:   Ethics and the law
Module 5:   Ethics and the professions: For example, confidentiality, informed consent, and the vulnerable and failing doctor
Module 6:   Making ethical judgments
Module 7:   Methods of ethics support in practice

Among the suggested core topics might be:

- Patients' rights, expectations and reality
- Consent, confidentiality, communication
- Legal framework in relevant countries
- Economics, to include resource allocation and prioritization

- Refusal of treatment
- Conflicts of interest
  - For example, commercial enterprises in medical practice
- Clinical governance
  - Managing and reducing risk, clinical error: poor performance, support structures
  - Clinical ethics committees

- Quality of life issues
- Decision-making, to include:
  - Partnerships in decision-making, e.g. interdisciplinary career perspectives; patient/parental perspectives
  - Dealing with uncertainty
  - "Futile" treatment
  - Withdrawing or withholding treatment
  - Religious and secular influences on decision-making
- Generic issues at the beginning and end of life
- Research governance
  - Evidence-based medicine
  - Properly informed consent
  - Innovative interventions
  - Fraud and misconduct
  - Research ethics committees

Table 16.6B: Indicative curriculum for a specific course in perinatal medicine

- Human genetics
- Conception and birth
- New reproductive technologies; pre-embryo research; stem cells and cloning
- The law and perinatal medicine

- The fetus as person and patient
- Patient choice and the maternal-fetal relationship
- Obstetric interventions "on demand"

- Prematurity (particularly the very preterm infant at or near the threshold of viability)

- Screening, antenatal diagnosis and counseling
- Sex selection for medical and nonmedical reasons
- Termination of pregnancy

- Feticide
- Nonselective embryo reduction
- Antepartum management of fetal anomalies
- Drug dependency in pregnancy
- Critical care obstetrics
- HIV infection in pregnancy
- Ethical aspects of the care of the newborn

- Ethical aspects of the care of the malformed or brain damaged infant

Table 16.7A: A guide to a bibliography for core ethical subjects

Medical Ethics Today	The BMA's handbook of ethics and law	BMJ Publishing Group, London, 2004	A comprehensive, concise and authoritative guide to medical ethics
Medical Ethics, 2nd edition	Campbell A, Charlesworth M, Gillett G, Jones G	Oxford University Press, New York/Oxford, 1997	An invaluable primer for the subject accessible to the nonexpert
Clinical Ethics, 5th edition	Jonsen AR, Siegler M, Winslade WJ	McGraw-Hill, New York, 2002	A "must read" in this context "Facilitates solutions to everyday ethical problems"
Principles of Health Care Ethics	Edited by Gillon R	John Wiley, Chichester/ New York, 1994	A detailed in depth analysis of the field
Principles of Biomedical Ethics, 5th edition	Beauchamp TL, Childress JF	Oxford University Press, New York/Oxford, 2001	Another excellent source book
Bioethics—An Introduction to the History, Methods and Practice	Jecker NS, Jonsen AR, Pearlman RA	Jones & Bartlett Publishers, Boston, 997	It does as it says

Contd...

Contd...

Medical Ethics—A Case-based Approach	Schwartz L, Preece PE, Hendry RA	Saunders, Edinburgh/ New York, 2002	A useful guide
Medicine, Patients and the Law, 3rd edition	Brazier M	Penguin Books, London, 2003	A scholarly work by an eminent legal authority
Medical Ethics and the Law— The Core Curriculum	Hope T, Savulescu J, Hendrick J	Churchill Livingstone, Edinburgh/New York, 2003	A useful guide
Autonomy and Trust in Bioethics	O'Neill O	Cambridge University Press, Cambridge, England, 2002	A must for anyone who wishes to understand the true nature of autonomy
Three Methods of Ethics	Baron MW, Pettit P, Slote M	Blackwell Publishers, Oxford/ Malden/Mass, 1997	For those who wish to consider more deeply and contrast Kantian ethics, consequentialism and virtue ethics
The Health Care Professional as Friend and Healer	Edited by Thomasma DC and Kissell JL	Georgetown University Press, Washington DC, 2000	This book builds on the work of Edmund Pellegrino. A "must read" in this context

Table 16.7B: A guide to a bibliography for perinatal ethics

Ethics and Perinatology	Editors Goldworth A, Silverman W, Stevenson DK, Young EWD	Oxford University Press, New York/Oxford, 1995	A required text for this field
Ethics in Obstetrics and Gynecology	McCullough LB, Chervenak FA	Oxford University Press, New York/Oxford, 1994	Another valuable reference for this field
Ethics in Obstetrics and Gynecology	American College of Obstetricians and Gynecologists	ACOG, Washington DC, 2002	A compilation of the subjects considered by the ACOG Ethics Committee and another invaluable source of material
Recommendations on Ethical Issues in Obstetrics and Gynecology	The FIGO Committee for the Ethical Aspects of Human Reproduction and Women's Health	FIGO, 2000	A compilation of the subjects considered by the FIGO Ethics Committee and also an invaluable source of material
Ethical Issues in Maternal-Fetal Medicine	Editor Dickenson DL	Cambridge University Press, Cambridge, England, 2002	Contains succinct but deep analyses of many relevant issues
Crucial Decisions at the Beginning of Life	McHaffie H	Radcliffe Medical Press, Oxford, 2001	A descriptive account of parents' experiences of treatment withdrawal from their infants
Should the Baby Live? The Problems of Handicapped Infants	Kuhse H, Singer P	Oxford University Press, New York/Oxford, 1985	A controversial book that discusses issues that must be addressed in this context
Selective Non-treatment of Handicapped Newborns: Moral Dilemmas in Neonatal Medicine	Weir RF	Oxford University Press, New York/Oxford, 1988	A necessary source book in this context for understanding how better to deal with clinical and ethical dilemmas
The Worth of Child	Murray TH	University of California Press, Berkeley, 1996	A deep and compassionate analysis of many of the relevant issues

REFERENCES

1. Radcliffe-Richards J. Maternal-fetal conflict. In: Bewley S, Ward RH (Eds). Ethics in Obstetrics and Gynaecology. London: RCOG Press; 1994. pp. 34-42.
2. Campbell AV. Moral dilemmas and ethical theories. Moral Dilemmas in Medicine. Edinburgh: Churchill Livingstone; 1972. pp. 1-13.
3. Stirrat GM. Education in ethics. Clin Perinatol. 2003;30:1-15.
4. Dunstan G. Should philosophy and medical ethics be left to the experts? In: Bewley S, Ward RH (Eds). Ethics in Obstetrics and Gynaecology. London: RCOG Press; 1994. pp. 3-8.
5. Campbell AV. The freedom that is health. Health as Liberation. Cleveland, Ohio: The Pilgrim Press; 1995. pp. 1-24.

6. O'Neill O. Gaining autonomy and losing trust? Autonomy and Trust in Bioethics. Cambridge: Cambridge University Press; 2002. pp. 1-27.

7. Stirrat GM, Gill R. Autonomy in medical ethics after O'Neill. J Med Ethics. 2004 [in press].

8. General Medical Council. Duties of a Doctor. London: GMC; 1998.

9. American Medical Association. Council on Ethical and Judicial Affairs. Principles of medical ethics. Code of Medical Ethics, 2000-2001 edition. Chicago. p. xii.

10. Draper H, Sorell T. Patient's responsibilities in medical ethics. Bioethics. 2003;16:335-52.

11. O'Donovan LJ. A profession of trust: reflections on a fundamental virtue. In: Thomasma DC, Kissell JL (Eds). The Health Care Professional as Friend and Healer. Washington: Georgetown University Press; 2000. pp. 1-9.

12. Pellegrino ED. Being a physician: does it make a moral difference? Advances in Otolaryngology—Head and Neck Surgery. 1992;6: 1-10.

13. Stirrat GM. How to approach ethical issues. Obstetrician Gynaecol (RCOG). 2003;5:214-7.

14. Westphal M. Post-modern theology. Concise Routledge Encyclopaedia of Philosophy. London, New York: Routledge; 2000. p. 699.

15. Jonsen A. Clinical ethics and the four principles. In: Gillon R (Ed). Principles of Healthcare Ethics. Chichester, New York: John Wiley & Sons; 1994. pp. 13-21.

16. Baron MW, Pettit P, Slote M. The consequentialist perspective. Three Methods of Ethics. Oxford: Blackwell. pp. 92-174.

17. Beauchamp TL. The 'four principles approach'. In: Gillon R (Ed). Principles of Healthcare Ethics. Chichester, New York: John Wiley & Sons; 1994. pp. 3-12.

18. Brody H. The four principles and narrative ethics. In: Gillon R (Ed). Principles of Healthcare Ethics. Chichester, New York: John Wiley & Sons; 1994. pp. 207-15.

19. MacIntyre A. After Virtue: A Study in Moral Theology, 2nd edition. London: Duckworth; 1985.

20. Tong R. Feminist ethics. Concise Routledge Encyclopaedia of Philosophy. London, New York: Routledge; 2000. p. 278.

21. McCullough LB, Chervenak FA. A framework for ethics in a clinical setting. Ethics in Obstetrics and Gynecology. New York, Oxford: Oxford University Press; 1994. pp. 3-81.

22. Sherwin S. Foundations, frameworks and lenses. The Role of Theories in Bioethics. Oxford: Blackwell; 1999. pp. 198-206.

23. Huxley TH. The Method of Zadig. Collected Essays (1893-4). London: Macmillan; 1893.

24. General Medical Council. Tomorrow's Doctors—Recommendations on Undergraduate Medical Education. London: GMC; 1993.

25. Andre J. Learning to see: moral growth during medical training. J Med Ethics. 1992;18:148-52.

26. Herbert P, Mesline EM, Dunn EV, et al. Measuring ethical sensitivity in medical students: using vignettes as an instrument. J Med Ethics. 1990;16:141-45.

27. Herbert PC, Meslin EM, Dunn EV. Measuring the ethical sensitivity of medical students: a study at the University of Toronto. J Med Ethics. 1992;18:142-7.

28. Savulescu J, Crisp R, Fulford KWM, et al. Evaluating ethics competence in medical education. J Med Ethics. 1999;25:367-74.

29. Walker RM, Miles SH, Stocking CB, et al. Physicians and nurses perceptions of ethics problems on general medical-services. J Gen Int Med. 1991;6:424-9.

30. Zalewski Z. What philosophy should be taught to the future medical professionals? Med Health Care Philos. 2000;3:161-7.

31. Goldie J, Schwartz L, McConnachie A, et al. Impact of a new course on students' potential behaviour on encountering ethical dilemmas. Med Educ. 2001;35:295-312.

32. Green B, Miller PD, Routh CP. Teaching ethics in psychiatry: a one-day workshop for clinical students. J Med Ethics. 1995;21:234-8.

33. Bebeau MJ. Designing an outcome-based ethics curriculum for professional-education-strategies and evidence of effectiveness. J Moral Education. 1993;22:313-26.

34. Fischer GS, Arnold RM. Measuring the effectiveness of ethics education. J Gen Int Med. 1994;9:655-6.

35. Holm S, Nielsen GH, Norup M, et al. Changes in moral reasoning and the teaching of medical ethics. Med Educ. 1995;29:420-3.

36. Self DJ, Davenport E. Measurement of moral development in medicine. Camb Q Healthcare Ethics. 1996;5:269-77.

37. Malek JI, Geller G, Sugarman J. Talking about cases in bioethics: the effects of an intensive course on health care professionals. J Med Ethics. 2000;26:131-6.

CHAPTER

17 Words Matter: Nomenclature and Communication in Perinatal Medicine

L de Crespigny

LANGUAGE

The general public now accepts of the importance of using appropriate language. Their acceptance contrasts with to the attitude of many doctors who are quick to dismiss the importance of word choice in treating patients. The goal of this chapter is first to demonstrate that word choice by professionals involved in prenatal diagnosis is important, and second to consider ethically appropriate word choices in our specialty.

Sexist and discriminatory language is now recognized to be unacceptable. This is because we are aware that such language impacts negatively on others. As long ago as 1977, the United States Department of Labor revised 3,000 of its approximately 30,000 titles for occupations. Advertisers are well aware of the importance of language and spend huge resources choosing names for products and developing phrases to describe them. Language is also the tool of trade of politicians. When there was an outcry over the government's harsh treatment of asylum-seekers, the Australian Prime Minister, John Howard, recently declared that his party was endeavoring to govern in the interests of the mainstream of the Australian community. Shortly afterwards, when the majority of Australians believed that he should dismiss the Governor General who had failed to act on child sexual abuse claims, he indicated he would not be succumbing to the clamor of the mob. In other words, when the majority of Australians agreed with him, they represented the "mainstream", but when most disagreed, it was "the mob" talking.[1]

People now take care to avoid sexist and discriminatory language. Racist language, in particular, is acknowledged as being offensive and inappropriate. It is hurtful to, and places stress on, other people. Nobody working in prenatal diagnosis could fail to be aware of the unique stresses placed on a couple who are given bad news following a prenatal test. Despite this, however, there is remarkably little literature analyzing what word choice in prenatal diagnosis leaves couples feeling most comfortable. The importance of language has had very little focus in medicine generally—indeed discussions on word choice may be perceived as trivial.

LANGUAGE, REALITY, AND MORAL JUDGMENT

Language makers and users of language are in a position to influence reality; language is a vehicle for them to construct, reinforce and reproduce their particular bias or view of reality.[2] People's language can influence opinion: for example, a group might be called "freedom fighters" if we support their cause, others may call the same group "terrorists" if they wish to present them as evil.[3]

Doctors practicing in prenatal diagnosis are language makers in their specialist field. By their language, they can subtly influence how their patients perceive a problem. We know that doctors have the potential to influence a patient's decision of what to do when a fetal anomaly is diagnosed. They can do this both by their choice of what information to impart and in the way that they impart it. One group found that the proportion of women choosing pregnancy termination following the diagnosis of a facial cleft was 50%. It dropped to 5% following the introduction of "emergency counseling by the clef team".[4] Women feel vulnerable and are susceptible to influence from their doctor following the diagnosis of fetal abnormality. There are few, if any, areas of medicine in which the language used by doctors is more important than in communicating with women having prenatal testing. Women are feeling stressed and may need to make one of the biggest decisions of their lives—to consider whether to have an abortion if a major abnormality is found.

Loftus and Palmer,[5] who summarized their results as follows, demonstrated the impact of language on memory:

Two experiments are reported in which subjects viewed films of automobile accidents and then answered questions about events occurring in the films. The question, "About how fast were the cars going when they smashed into each other?" elicited higher estimates of speed than questions which used the verbs *collided, bumped, contacted*, or *hit* in place of *smashed*. On a retest 1 week later, those subjects who received the verb *smashed* were more likely to say "yes" to the question, "Did you see any broken glass?" even though broken glass was not present in the film. These results are consistent with the view that the questions asked subsequent to an event can cause a reconstruction in one's memory of that event.

The unique emotive experience suffered by women given a diagnosis of fetal abnormality far exceeds that of people watching a film. It is reasonable to assume that the doctor's language would have at least as much impact on patients as did the wording of questions to watchers of the crash film. In prenatal diagnosis there is the added factor that the doctor is seen as "the expert". Following the diagnosis of fetal abnormality, patients will often ask their doctor what is the best course of action. They will even attempt to read into a doctor's words or manner whether he or she thinks an abortion is warranted. It is not the role of the doctor to make a moral judgment about what is best for any particular patient. However, patients may be highly influenced not only by what the doctor says, but also by inferences from the doctor's word choice. The use of words such as "baby" and "mother" when the doctor means "fetus" and "pregnant woman" may result in the patient thinking that her doctor considers that her fetus has the status of a baby and she is already a mother. It might be expected that such a word choice may influence the patient's decision about abortion. In the crash film the questioner's language influenced the subjects' perception. Following detection of a fetal abnormality, the doctor's language at the time of diagnosis could affect the woman's decision on abortion. If her doctor, either directly or by word choice, infers that the fetus is a baby, this might also impact in the woman's ultimate ability to come to terms with her decision.

MEDICAL LANGUAGE

In a field closely allied to prenatal testing, Bowker[2] explores the level of gender insensitivity in specialist language in the field of infertility. She cites examples demonstrating that the language used for similar problems leading to male and female infertility is often gender insensitive. For example, "sperm antibodies" are described as being present in a male, while a woman whose cervical mucus develops such antibodies is described as having "hostile mucus". She claims that the choices of language are not always innocent and may be determined by belief systems that underlie them. Language may attempt to portray men in a more positive light and women in a negative one. She also notes that the term "expected date of confinement" suggests punishment and imprisonment reflecting the male doctor's control over the place of birth and birthing practices. The terms "expected date of delivery" or "due date" are more gender sensitive. Bowker concludes that even when a doctor claims not to have a bias against women, the language that he uses to communicate to patients may be based on such a bias and may, therefore have a harmful effect, even in the absence of a malicious intent.

A detailed analysis of the terms commonly used in obstetrical ultrasound practice would be valuable. Some language is clearly gender insensitive, such as cervical incompetence and the labeling of a woman as a "recurrent aborter". Some language is simply insensitive, such as intrauterine growth retardation (instead of restriction, to avoid a perceived association with intellectual retardation) or a fetal anomaly scan (instead of a fetal normality scan, to focus on the normal).

Doctors also use terms that could lead to misconceptions in the eyes of colleagues as well as the public. It has been suggested that "myocardial infarction" should be replaced by "coronary occlusion" since the goal of current treatment is to prevent the myocardial death that follows coronary occlusion.[6] The same author also proposed replacing the term "hypertension" which falsely suggests that the condition is related to tension or stress, and replacing "cardiac failure" with "cardiac insufficiency".

The medical profession has been slow to acknowledge the importance of language, dismissing it as being "politically correct". The term "political correctness" is now used as a slogan of opprobrium, referring to someone who is an ideological monster.[7] Doctors dislike linguistic change and find it threatening, suggesting that there is something more acceptable about their own linguistic preference.[7] Why is it that the Right to Life movement long ago learned to use "killing of babies" instead of "abortion," while doctors often still speak as if language is mere political correctness and does not impact on people's opinions?

LANGUAGE IN OBSTETRICS

Although doctors are often dismissive of "politically correct" language, our journals have overtime reduced discriminatory language. The use of "husbands and wives" when the author means "men and women" would no longer be accepted, although these terms are used in a leading journal as recently as 1984.[8] Similarly, one would not now expect to find in a standard medical text a quote

such as "it has been said that bad girls get babies but good girls get myomata".[9] While this may have been presented as a joke, it helps perpetuate sexism by suggesting "good girls comply with the stereotypical portrayal of women as chaste and passive".[10]

The RCOG Study Group on Problems in Early Pregnancy: Advances in Diagnosis in Management[11] has recommended that in early pregnancy loss, the term "abortion" be replaced by "miscarriage". It is recommended that "spontaneous miscarriage" replace "spontaneous abortion", "early embryonic demise" and "fetal demise" replace "blighted ovum" and "missed abortion" respectively, and "incomplete miscarriage" be used instead of "incomplete abortion".[12] The general community has long accepted that our language is important in influencing the way people see reality; this is also starting to be accepted in our specialty.

LANGUAGE IN PRENATAL DIAGNOSIS

Ethical dilemmas pervade the specialty of prenatal diagnosis. However, there has so far been little attempt to review the language we use and the impact it may have on other professionals, and even more importantly on our patients. It is time doctors were more considered and considerate in their word choice. The terms "fetus" and "pregnant woman" are grammatically more correct than "baby" and "mother." The latter names are used by some (including anti-abortionists) euphemistically with a more sinister motivation—namely to blur reality. Anti-abortionists use baby and mother as "linguistic fig leaves" to suggest that abortion must be wrong;[7] while the motivation of doctors using these terms is likely to differ from anti-abortionists, it may be misinterpreted by patients.

How do we determine the most appropriate terminology for the language of our specialty? Should we survey our patients and let them decide terminology? One such survey showed pregnant women had a strong preference to be called "patient" rather than "mother", "client", "consumer", "customer", "lady", "woman" or "pregnant woman".[13] Another study surveyed women in an antenatal clinic in an attempt to decide whether to use the term "mother-to-be", "pregnant woman", "maternant", "patient", "client" or "consumer".[14] The authors concluded, "Simple softer terms like mother-to-be please a vast majority". While we do not know the gestation of these women, given that most women have healthy pregnancies, it must be assumed that most of these women believed they had, and in fact had, healthy pregnancies. How would their answers have changed if, immediately after filling out this questionnaire, their doctor had told them that their fetus had a major abnormality? The softer pleasing term of "mother-to-be" suddenly seems inappropriate—the patient will probably choose not to be a mother this time. Would the doctor using the term "mother-to-be" have an impact on their patient's decision whether or not to continue with the pregnancy? Would the patient think that the doctor is insinuating that since she is a mother-to-be and not a pregnant woman that the doctor, therefore, opposes an abortion? If the woman has an abortion, might her grief be prolonged because of her concern that the doctor had implied that she should have become a mother?

Mothers, and presumably mothers-to-be, do not kill their children/fetuses. Pregnant women, however, do have a right to abortion in some circumstances in most Western societies. We cannot expect patients in an outpatient survey to think through these issues. Sometimes, word choice is better resolved by reflection and discussion, because the appropriate survey cannot be easily carried out. Word choice is not always best resolved by surveying patients—just as medical treatments are not. Doctors have a role in patient and community education.

Another study suggested that some patients preferred the term "baby" to "fetus".[15] Researchers in Canada examined the results of a questionnaire sent to women who had been informed of ultrasound findings of "serious anomalies", soft markers of aneuploidy, or obstetric complications. Approximately 900 patients were seen in the study year, the number who declined to participate was not recorded, but 117 agreed to participate in the survey. Surveys were returned by 65% of the 117. This shows the difficulty in both performing and analyzing the results of such a survey—questionnaires were analyzed from only 76 (8%) of the original approximately 900 eligible women.

More women felt strongly that they preferred to have their health care provider use the word "baby" when giving them bad news. A smaller number felt it important to hear the word "fetus". There was a significant minority who considered the terms used to be unimportant. There was great diversity of opinion among the women.

It is not clear from this paper how many women had chosen pregnancy termination following diagnosis of a serious anomaly. It might be expected that many women who continue their pregnancy, who have made the decision that they are going to have a baby, would prefer the term baby to be used. This would apply particularly to the women in this study who completed the survey up to 9 months after their ultrasound visit, so would by then either have a baby or be very late in pregnancy.

In our use of language in the specialist field of prenatal testing we have a number of goals:

1. To maximize the information provided to pregnant women: the words we use should be descriptive and easily understood by the majority of pregnant women.

2. Be respectful of women's choices. While some have suggested that prenatal diagnosis is a "select and destroy" mission, most support the concept of prenatal diagnosis enhancing autonomous choices of pregnant women. The enhancement of autonomy should apply not only to choice of tests, but also to what information they receive from these tests (does the woman wish to know "everything" including all low risk markers of aneuploidy?), and the decision whether to continue the pregnancy or have an abortion.[16]

3. Reduce risks of long-term psychological maladjustment: Since we have few data on the impact of language on psychological adjustment to adverse pregnancy outcome, we must theorize on its impact. Surveying healthy women at an antenatal clinic does not answer this question.

4. Promote bonding in normal healthy pregnancies: This is not only through our language, but also by the use of technology, for example offering of 3D and 4D ultrasound when available.

At times points 3 and 4 may appear to be in conflict. In showing pregnant women ultrasound images, we may promote bonding only to discover later in the examination that there is a fetal abnormality. The bonding itself is not necessarily a problem if the patient later chooses pregnancy termination. Indeed, counselors go to great lengths to support bonding by offering photographs, footprints, etc. following termination for fetal abnormality, and such a policy is supported by patient groups. We should not shield women from the fact that the fetus they aborted looks human, but we can use language that indicates that even though it looks human, it does not have human characteristics such as a conscious life and an ability to plan. Careful use of language can support this message.

Rothman has coined the phrase "tentative pregnancy"[17] to describe the state of limbo that women are in prior to completion of prenatal testing. Women cannot say with confidence that "I am going to have a baby" until after the completion of prenatal testing. Those of us in prenatal diagnosis know that most women in whom a major fetal abnormality is diagnosed will choose pregnancy termination. Women who have had a previous pregnancy terminated because of fetal abnormality are uniquely aware of their "tentative pregnancy". Their relief and excitement at the completion of a normal mid-trimester ultrasound examination is plainly visible. Women are increasingly aware that a mid-trimester ultrasound examination is primarily for fetal anomaly detection and that a mid-trimester scan is the final prenatal test. Although women anxiously await the results of any prenatal test, the defining moment for pregnant women has become the news of a normal mid-trimester ultrasound examination. It is rare that subsequent events or testing cause a pregnant woman to rethink pregnancy termination.

Our language should support and enhance the autonomy of pregnant women.[18] It is a normal mid-trimester ultrasound examination that indicates to most pregnant women that their fetuses will become babies. They will become mothers after the birth. They are now unlikely to request abortion—a fetal anomaly is now unlikely to be found. Our word choice should acknowledge that our language is focused on the woman, and not on the views of the doctor.

The *Oxford English Dictionary* defines "mother" as a female parent, one who has borne a child. It is, therefore, grammatically incorrect to use the term "mother" for a pregnant woman. Pregnant women and mothers have contrasting rights and responsibilities. Pregnant women have the right to abortion in certain circumstances in most western countries, while it is illegal for a mother to kill or fail to care for her child.

The definitions of "baby" are more variable. The *Oxford English Dictionary* includes both unborn and newly born human beings as a baby while the *Collins Dictionary* defines a baby as a child in the first year or two of life. It is proposed that "fetal patient" (or the lay terms "child" or "baby") should be used when it is unlikely that termination of pregnancy would be requested.[18] For most women, this is after normal results of prenatal testing. An exception is the woman who in early pregnancy clearly indicates that she would not consider termination of pregnancy for fetal abnormality; she has given the status of a fetal patient to her previable fetus. She is free to withdraw that status at any time.[18]

The goal should be to remain as neutral as possible in the choice of words prior to the completion of prenatal testing in an attempt to avoid inadvertent directive counseling. The term "fetus" is neutral in that it does not imply the fetus has the status of a baby; it implies that pregnancy termination is still considered acceptable. Following completion of prenatal testing the term "fetal patient" is advocated with "child" or "baby" as the analogous lay term.[18]

The term "mother" is clearly defined, and should be used when grammatically correct. "Mother" is appropriate when describing a woman who has borne a child and is inappropriate when describing a pregnant woman who has not borne a child. What alternative proposals for word choice might be suggested?

1. In an earlier paper the author argued that the terms "pregnant woman" and "fetus" should replace "mother" and "baby" throughout pregnancy.[19] Such language supports the claim that "a pregnant woman…should have the right to make decisions about her own body up until the time of birth. In a difficult decision, the woman's present right to bodily integrity should prevail over the rights of the potential person".[20]

   The law puts great importance on the moment of birth. Late abortion is legal in many parts of the world, especially in the presence of a major fetal abnormality. In most western countries late abortion is available for lethal abnormalities. Using the term "fetus" throughout pregnancy supports the philosophy that women late in pregnancy may put their rights above those of the fetus in the unusual situation when these are in conflict.

   There are good reasons for reserving the term "baby" for after birth and "fetus" before birth. This word choice is consistent with the definition of baby in at least some dictionaries. It supports the autonomy of the pregnant woman throughout pregnancy.

   On balance, however, the author suggests the use of "baby" is preferred following completion of prenatal testing. A disadvantage of using the term "fetus" late in pregnancy is that it might potentially prolong the "tentative pregnancy" in the eyes of the pregnant woman. Women benefiting from modern obstetrical and neonatal care have good reason for being confident that "they are going to have a baby" after completion of testing; it would be a pity if our language diminished that confidence. Very few women have reason to request abortion after standard tests are completed. There is little reason not to enhance such confidence by using the lay term "baby" late in pregnancy.

2. Those opposing abortion following potential fetal viability may argue that from viability the term "baby" should be used. Given a normal mid-trimester ultrasound examination, few women will have further prenatal tests in the few weeks prior to potential viability. Even fewer women suddenly change their mind at this late stage and decide that their apparently normal pregnancy is unwanted and they wish to have abortion. To propose viability as being decisive in determining word choice would result in the doctor prolonging the tentative pregnancy to support his or her ethical position. For the patient, the completion of prenatal testing is the more critical time.

3. Finally, even after reflection, some doctors may choose to call the fetus a "baby" from conception. This is the position of the Right to Life movement, since it enhances their view that abortion is tantamount to killing babies. These doctors are using word choice to deliberately promote their personal views on the status of the fetus. Others may claim that they use the term "baby" throughout pregnancy because it is more patient-friendly—better understood by some women. However, the term "fetus" is now widely used and understood in the lay context, few adults find this term confusing. Young children and some adults may be more comfortable with "unborn baby" and "mother-to-be"—These are acceptable alternatives to "baby."

   Some might claim that the language proposed contradicts the language used by many pregnant women who prefer to think of their child as a baby. The doctor participating in such baby talk may please some pregnant women and may be preferred by many, or even most, women who will proceed to have a baby. However, the long-term interests of the patient may be better served by more neutral language, particularly if the outcome to the pregnancy is adverse. It would be unfortunate if patients interpreted the doctor's participation in baby talk as the euphemistic language of an anti-abortionist.

   It is important to consider the impact of our language on women continuing the pregnancies. But the life-long distress felt by many women following pregnancy loss means that this group deserves our special attention. These women are at greatest risk and they will not have a baby. The critical issue is how language impacts on women who are considering pregnancy termination. The author's proposition is that by using neutral language, such as "fetus" and "pregnant woman", these terms are not only more accurate, but assist in ensuring that the pregnant woman does not misinterpret the health care provider as having an anti-abortion bias.

   We need to be sensitive that women who give the status of a patient to the fetus, in other words women who have made a prior decision to continue the pregnancy, might prefer the use of "baby" to "fetus". We should use whatever language is most supportive of our patients.

   After a miscarriage or pregnancy termination, some couples like to think of and refer to their fetus as a baby. They may even name the fetus. Even women having a pregnancy termination may wish the fetus to be considered as a baby, and that preterm labor is being induced in the best interests of the baby. It is important that our language is supportive of our patients and flexible, so enhancing their best interests. No rigid framework is correct for all situations. This is not to say, however, that the doctor should support the "baby talk" of a woman early in pregnancy, excited by the first images of her fetus on the ultrasound screen. Not all pregnant women appreciate that prenatal testing may mean that they withdraw the status of a baby from their fetus. We, as professionals need to be aware that we should, in general, support neutral language, even when caring for excited couples early in pregnancy. Doctors would be less tempted to indulge in baby talk if they perceived there was any risk that this could result in more prolonged psychological sequelae for a woman who subsequently chose pregnancy termination in the presence of a fetal abnormality. The principle guiding the physician should be respect for the patient.

   Our respect for the patient also extends to others in the family. The term "father" should be avoided during pregnancy. A male partner or husband becomes an expectant father following normal prenatal test.[18] If the partner is a woman, she becomes the expectant parent at that time.

CONCLUSION

The best interests of our patients are served by using language that supports patient autonomy and is neutral. While it remains a "tentative" pregnancy, i.e. prior to the completion of normal prenatal tests, the term "fetus" should be used. Following normal prenatal testing, only in rare situations will the pregnant woman request an abortion. It is appropriate that the term "fetal patient," or lay terms "child" or "baby," be then used. To be a mother, however, one must have borne a child.

Our language should support the autonomous views of the patient. The language proposed is not intended to be rigidly adhered to in all situations, but rather is an appropriate starting point, after which we as health providers need to be responsive to the position of the pregnant woman. It is important to individualize language to accommodate the views of individual patients. It is, however, time for doctors to acknowledge that their language can influence reality, particularly since they are frequently considered experts, not only in prenatal diagnosis, but also in morality. Doctors' language has a powerful influence not only on the way patients think, but potentially also on the decisions that they make.

REFERENCES

1. Henderson G. When the mainstream becomes a mob, blame the dingo pack. The Age. 2002;11.
2. Bowker L. Terminology and gender sensitivity; a corpus-based study of the LSP of infertility. Language in Society. 2001;30: 589-601.
3. Schulz MR. The semantic derogation of women. In: Thorne B, Henley N (Eds). Language and Sex: Difference and Dominance. 1975. pp. 64-75.
4. Moss A. Controversies in cleft lip and palate management. Ultrasound in Obstetrics and Gynecology. 2001;18:420-1
5. Loftus EF, Palmer JC. Reconstruction of automobile destruction: an example of the interaction between language and memory. J Verbal Learning and Verbal Behaviour. 1974;13:585-9.
6. O'Rourke MF. What's in a name? Would that which we call "cardiac failure," by any other name threaten less? MJA. 1997;166:372-3.
7. Burridge K, Polcor-Big Brother, Bowdler T, et al. Style in context: language at large. In: Peters PH (Ed). Proceedings of Style Councils. 1996, 1997 and 1999.
8. Stray-Pedersen B, Stray-Pedersen S. Etiologic factors and subsequent reproductive performance in 195 couples with a prior history of habitual abortion. Am J Obstet Gynecol. 1984;148:140-4.
9. Llewellyn-Jones D. Fundamentals of Obstetrics and Gynaecology. London: Faber & Faber; 1982.
10. Harres A. The representation of women in three medical texts ARAL Series S number 10. 1993;35-3.
11. Grudzinskas JG, O'Brien PMS. Problems in early pregnancy: Advances in Diagnosis and Management. London: RCOG Press; 1997.
12. Hutchon DJR. Understanding miscarriage or insensitive abortion: time for more defined terminology? Am J Obstet Gynecol. 1998;179:397-8.
13. Denning AS, Tuttle LK, Bryant VJ, et al. Ascertaining women's choice of title during pregnancy and childbirth. Aust N Z J Obstet Gynaecol. 2002;42:1259.
14. Batra N, Lilford RJ. Not clients, not consumers and definitely not maternants. European J Obstet Gynecol and Reproductive Biology. 1996;64:197-9.
15. Alkazaleh F, Thomas M, Grebenyuk J, et al. What women want: Women's preferences of caregiver behavior when prenatal sonography findings are abnormal. Ultrasound Obstet Gynecol. 2004;23:56-62.
16. de Crespigny L, Savulescu J. Is paternalism alive and well in obstetric ultrasound? Helping couples choose their children. Ultrasound Obstet Gynecol. 2002;20:213-6.
17. Rothman BK. A tentative pregnancy: prenatal diagnosis and the future of motherhood. Viking, New York; 1986.
18. de Crespigny L, Chervenak F, McCullough L. Mothers and babies, pregnant women and fetuses. Br J Obstet Gynaecol. 1999;106: 1235-7.
19. de Crespigny L. What's in a name—is the pregnant woman a mother? Is the fetus a baby? Aust NZ J Obstet Gynaecol. 1996;36:435-6.
20. Special project, Legal rights and issues surrounding conception, pregnancy and birth "maternal rights vs fetal rights". Vanderbilt Law Review 819 at 1986;849;39.

18 The Beginning of Human Life—Scientific and Religious Controversies

A Kurjak, JM Carrera

INTRODUCTION

One of the most controversial topics in modern bioethics, science, and philosophy is the beginning of individual human life. In the seemingly endless debate, strongly stimulated by recent technologic advances in human reproduction, a synthesis between scientific data and hypothesis, philosophical thought, and issues of humanities has become necessary to deal with ethical, juridical, and social problems.[1] Furthermore, in this field there is a temptation to ask science to choose between opinions and beliefs that tend to neutralize one another. Indeed, the question of when human life begins requires the essential aid of different forms of knowledge. Here we become involved in the juncture between science and religion, which needs to be carefully explored.[2]

Obviously, the beginning of human life is seen differently by different individuals, groups, cultures and religions. Fundamental to productive debate and reconciliation between minority and majority groups is an understanding of the ill-defined concept of "the beginning of human life".[3]

Entering this field, scientists have been remiss in failing to translate science into the terms that allow mankind to share their excitement of discovering life before birth. Regardless of the remarkable scientific development, curiosity and speculations dating back to Hippocrates, life before birth still remains a big secret. Different kinds of intellectuals involved themselves in trying to contribute to the solution of the human life puzzle. They are led by the idea that each newborn child will only reach its full potential if its development in utero is free from any adverse influence, providing the best possible environment for the embryo/fetus. Considering the embryo/fetus, it should be always kept in mind the amazing aspect of these parts of human life in which the pregnant woman and the embryo/fetus, although locked in the most intimate of relationships, are at all times two separate individuals. Accepting the embryo/fetus as a person opens a new set of questions about its personality and human rights.

THE DEFINITION OF LIFE

Proper answers to the question of how to define human life are complicated. Nowadays, dilemmas consider the respect of human life from the birth to death involving not just biology, but other sciences also. Philosophy, theology, psychology, sociology, law and politics evaluate this topic from different point of views. Integration of all could result in a useful answer.

Some authors say that that life as such does not exist—no one has ever seen it. Szent–Gyorgy says that the noun "life" has no significance because there is no such thing as "life." Le Dantez holds that the expression "to live" is too general, and that it is better to say a dog "dogs" or a fish "fishes" than a dog or a fish lives.[4]

When defining life, it should be considered not just as it is today, but as it might have been in its primordial form and as it will be in the future. All present forms of life appear as something completely new. Life, then, is transferred and not conceived in each new generation. Furthermore, the phenomenon of life has existed on earth for approximately 3.5 billion years. Consequently, although the genome of a new embryo is unique, the make-up of an embryo is not new. If life is observed through the cell, then every life (and human also) is considered as a continuum. Human cells and mankind have existed on earth continuously since the appearance of the first man. However, if the definition refers to a single human being or the present population, the statement that "human life is a continuum" is not acceptable.[5]

Life, in a true sense of the word, begins when the chemical matter gives rise, in a specific way, to an autonomous, self-regulating, and self-reproducing system. Life is connected with a living being, and it creates its own system as an indivisible whole—It forms its individuality. One of the most important characteristics of living beings is reproduction. Reproduction is a means of creating new life by transferring forms of an old one into newly formed human being. Therefore, variability, individual development and harmony characterize human beings. Individuality is the most essential characteristic of human beings consisting of new life, but also all human life forms through evolution, characterized by phenotype, behavior and the capability to recognize and adapt. Human embryo and fetus gradually develop into these characteristics.

"Human life" poses a semantic problem. The placenta is "human life", as is every individual cell or organ of the human body, but "human life" is clearly not equivalent to "human being". It is, therefore, mandatory to differentiate between organic or vegetative human life and "potential personal human life". The latter term allows various groups to identify a point of the continuum between abortion and birth to which they can ascribe appropriate values and rights.[3]

Although we should not forget that in the same way today's research is tomorrow's benefit,[6] concerning human life, conclusions should not be treated one-sidedly from one perspective. This reality should be regarded in all its richness: the embryo gives the biologist and geneticist substance for consideration, but talking about the beginning of a human life requires philosophical/anthropological consideration, as well as theological and social sciences. In its protection, we have to include ethics and law. This approach leads to the conclusion that it is necessary to reject reductionism as well as integrism, and to find a "golden middle" between these two methodologies.[1]

WHAT DOES BIOLOGY SAY?

Biology characterizes human beings by the dynamics of the system and its self-control (homeostasis), excitability (response to stimuli of different nature and origins), self-reproducibility, the heredity of the characters and the evolutionary trend.[1] For biologists, it is important to specify which form of life phenomena we are referring to: cell, organism population or species. The basic level of organization and the simplest form of life is the cell. Biologically speaking, human cellular life never stops or if it did, the extinction of the human species would result and is passed on from one generation to another. Human individual organismic life is defined within its life cycle, which is temporarily limited, i.e. it has a beginning and an end.[7] It is obvious that life is a highly dynamic phenomenon that could be described and explained through the careful study of life processes and interactions by interdisciplinary approach. In human spermatozoa and oocyte are two essential cells involved in creating human life (Figs 18.1 and 18.2). It is clear that biologists are most qualified to render judgment on the structure and function of cells. To quote Scarpelli,[8] the very broad scope of biological science (from molecular to behavioral biology, and from unicellular to multisystem forms) brings with it the justifiable understanding that the biological scientist knows and is able to define the state of being alive or "life". If not, the science fails.

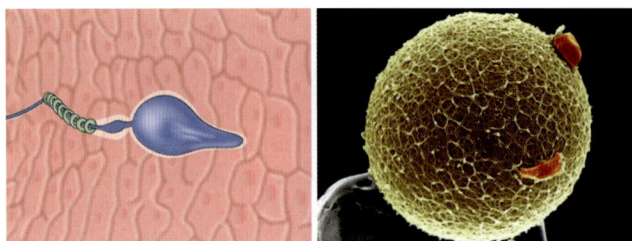

Fig. 18.1: Schematic presentation of spermatozoa and oocyte

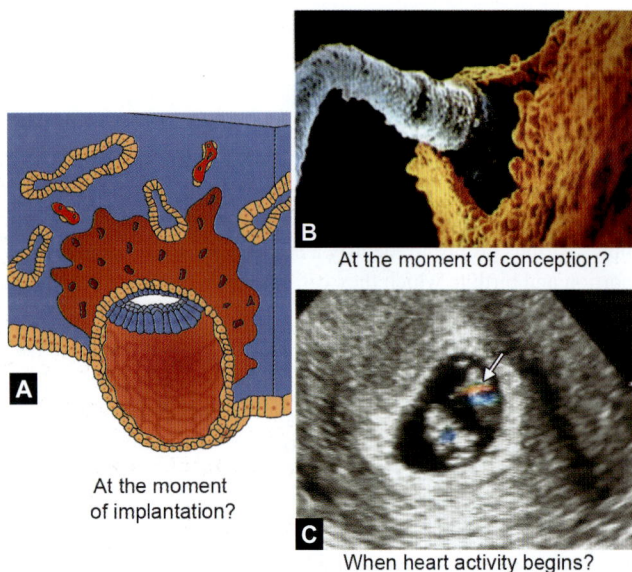

At the moment of conception?

At the moment of implantation?

When heart activity begins?

Figs 18.2A to C: Some possible questions on the beginning of human life

The biological scientist, who may specialize within one or another domain of the broad scope, has particular and definitive knowledge and understanding of the living individual that is his specialty. If not, disorder will rise above failure.

Understanding of the beginning of human life and development of the embryo/fetus could provide definitive resolution. However, with the recent possibility of visualizing early human development virtually from conception, perinatologists should be those who by study, training, practice and research are singularly qualified.[9]

While science provides us data about physical development of the human being, it does not provide information about its personality and personhood. These are philosophical, rather than scientific topics.

HUMAN EMBRYOGENESIS

Only proper understanding of the process of human embryogenesis enables answering scientifically the question of when the life cycle of a human individual starts. Therefore, in the following text the main steps of the human developmental process are going to be briefly described, primarily during the first 15 days following fertilization.

A human being originates from two living cells: the oocyte and the spermatozoon, transmitting the torch of life to the next generation. The oocyte is a cell approximately 120 μm in diameter with a thick membrane, known as the zona pellucida. The spermatozoon moves, using the flagellum or tail, and the total length of the spermatozoon including the tail is 60 μm.[10]

After syngamy, the zygote undergoes mitotic cell division as it moves down the Fallopian tube toward the uterus. A series of mitotic divisions then leads to the development of the pre-embryo. The newly divided cells are called blastomeres. From 1 to 3 days after syngamy, there is a division into two cells, then four cells. Blastomeres form cellular aggregates of distinct, totipotent, undifferentiated cells that, during several early cell divisions, retain the capacity to develop independently into normal pre-embryos. As the blastocyst is in the process of attaching to the uterine wall, the cells increase in number and organize into two layers of cells. Implantation progresses as the outer cell layer of the blastocyst, the trophectoderm, invades the uterine wall and erodes blood vessels and glands. Having begun five or more days after fertilization with the attachment of the blastocyst to the endometrial lining of the uterus, implantation is completed when the blastocyst is fully embedded in the endometrium several days later. Even during these 5–6 days, modern medicine introduces the possibility of making preimplantation genetic diagnosis.

However, at this time, these cells are not yet totally differentiated in terms of their determination to specific cells or organs of the embryo. The term pre-embryo, then, includes the developmental stages from the first cell division of the zygote through the morula and the blastocyst. By approximately the fourteenth day after the end of the process of fertilization, all cells, depending on their position, will have become parts of the placenta and membranes or the embryo. The embryo stage, therefore, begins approximately 16 days after the beginning of the fertilization process and continues until the end of 8 weeks after fertilization, when organogenesis is complete.[11]

The pre-embryo is the structure that exists from the end of the process of fertilization until the appearance of a single primitive streak. Until the completion of implantation, the pre-embryo is capable of dividing into multiple entities, but does not contain enough genetic information to develop into an embryo, it lacks of genetic material from maternal mitochondria and of maternal and parental genetic messages in the form of messenger RNA or proteins. Therefore, during the pre-embryonic period, it has not yet been determined with certainty that a biological individual will result, or would be one or more (identical twins forming), so that the assignment of the full rights of an individual human person is inconsistent with biological reality.

One conclusion from this is that the pre-embryo requires the establishment of special rules in the society: it cannot claim absolute protection based on claims of personhood; although meriting respect, it does not have the same moral value that a human person has. Today, one largely accepted opinion is that until the fourteenth day from fertilization or at least, until implantation—the human embryo may not be considered, from the ontological point of view, as an individual.

Genetic uniqueness and singleness coincide only after implantation and restriction have completed, which is about 3 weeks after fertilization. Until that period, the zygote and its sequelae are in a fluid process, are not physical individual, and therefore, cannot be a person.

It is well-known that high percentages of oocytes which have been penetrated never proceed on to further development, and that many oocytes which do, are thwarted so early in their development that their presence is not even recognized. It is suggested that 30% of conceptions detected by positive reactions to human chorionic gonadotropin (HCG) tests abort spontaneously before these pregnancies are clinically verified.

The newly conceived pre-embryo presents itself as a biologically defined reality. However, the status of the pre-embryo as an individual remains a great mystery. In the present scientific scene especially with the progress of ultrasound technologies, prenatal psychology and therapeutics opened a window into prenatal life of embryo and fetus confirming the evidence that the embryo/fetus is a true subject itself.[12,13]

PERSONALITY

Defining personality is very complex. There is still no clear definition of personality. One dictionary offers "what constitutes an individual as distinct person", but does not define what the "what" is. Another dictionary asserts "the state of existing as a thinking intelligent being". This definition might lead to the inference that personality increases pro rata with intelligence, or that some people may not have a personality at all if we followed Bertrand Russell's dictum that "most people would rather die than think and many, in fact, do!" Kenneth Stallworthy's *Manual of Psychiatry* is more help with the definition that "personality is the individual as a whole with everything about him which makes him different from other people", because we can certainly distinguish fetuses from each other and from other people. With the next sentence—"personality is determined by what is born in the individual in the first place and by everything which subsequently happens to him in the second"—We are really in the field.[1,3]

Viewpoints on the nature of "personhood" and what it means ethically and legally vary widely. In his proposed Life Protection Act, Sass acknowledges that a fetus with formed synapses is not a "person" in the usual sense of the word, connoting consciousness and self-consciousness.[14] Veatch sees the problem as defining the life that has full moral standing,[15] while Knutson[16] has noted that "those who employ spiritual or religious definitions of when life begins tend to place the beginning of life earlier than those who employ psychological, sociological or cultural definitions".

Led by the truism, "No insignificant person was ever born", human beings should be valued from birth to natural death. It is hard to establish proper values and exact definitions. This becomes especially problematic when prenatal life is considered. The above stated truism opens an important question: "Is the person-unborn a person in the first place and, if so, is the person-unborn a 'significant' person?"[1]

Let us evaluate further present controversies. There is no doubt that the embryo and fetus in utero are biologically human individuals prior to birth. The child who is born is the same developing human individual that was in the mother's womb. Birth alone cannot confer natural personhood or human individuality. This is confirmed by preterm deliveries of babies who are as truly human and almost as viable as those whose gestation goes to full term. All the known evidence supports the human fetus being a true ontological human individual and consequently a human person in fact, if not in law. *A human person cannot begin before the appropriate brain structures are developed that are capable of sustaining awareness.* The same applies to a grossly malformed fetus. It would still be a human individual even if its human nature was not perfect or its functions quite normal. Nobody questions the humanity of a Down's syndrome fetus or child. A fetus or child with severe open spina bifida is not less of a human being. The same should be said for the live anencephalic fetus or infant with only brainstem functions. It is a human individual even if it lacks a complete brain and usually survives birth by only a few hours or a day.

"Person" and "personhood" are the legally operational terms in the United States and many other countries. Alternatively, "person" and "personhood" are replaced by terms such as "viable outside the uterus", "a woman's right to privacy," and "a woman's right to choose". In each case, viable, privacy and choice, the life-support provider may legally order transfer of the dependent individual into a morbid environment. For this group, dilemma (which includes the stem cell, abortion and cloning debates) is abated, but not resolved.[3]

Human society created several standards in defining "person" or "human being" based on what is familiar and easy recognizable.[1] For example, a human speaks, understands and laughs. Absence of these characteristics (mutism, autism and stoicism) does not disqualify. To the contrary, the conclusion is that the characteristics we have come to associate with being a person may not be applicable to each individual person. Therefore, it is necessary to establish criteria for a definition of "person" in society and in time (Figs 18.3 and 18.4). Some prominent Italian professors[12] committed themselves to caring for the embryo in such a way; giving the same dignity to every patient, and the human conditions to grow and develop, to educate others inside and outside the specialty, and to carry out research involving all the components of society.

When do we become a person?

When a person is recognized in a society?

Does science know the answer?

Is the answer a matter of religion?

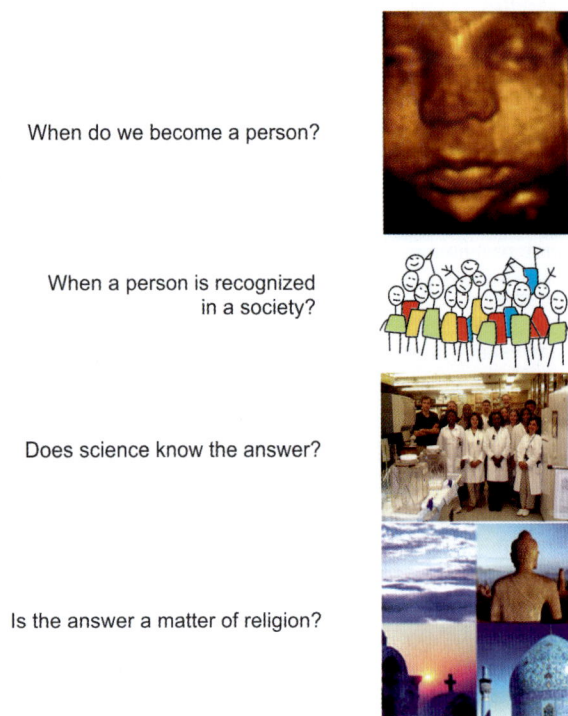

Fig. 18.3: Some questions about the definition of a person

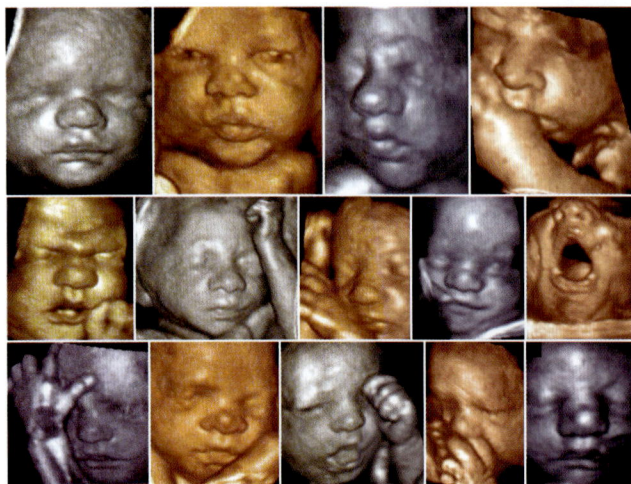

Fig. 18.4: Different behavioral patterns of the fetuses in second half of pregnancy. Are they different personalities?

EMBRYO AS A PATIENT: BIOETHICAL ASPECTS

The idea of the embryo/fetus as a miniaturized infant or adult is true to the extent that the embryonic/fetal physiologist must be able to apply knowledge of every system after birth, yet quite untrue in failing to recognize the many ways in which life before birth differs fundamentally from life after birth.[6] The newly conceived form presents itself as the biologically defined reality: it is an individual that is completely human in development that autonomously, moment by moment without any discontinuity, actualizes its proper form in order to realize through intrinsic activity, a design present

in its own genome (Figs 18.5 to 18.10).[12] The embryo as a patient is best understood as the subset of the concept of the fetus as the patient. These two concepts opened a whole set of questions regarding ethical problems. The embryo as the patient is indivisible from its mother. However, balance is needed in protecting the interests of the embryo/fetus and the mother. One prominent approach to understanding the concept of the embryo/fetus as a patient has involved attempts to show whether or not the embryo/fetus has independent moral status, or personhood.[17-19] Independent moral status for the fetus would mean that one or more of the characteristics possessed either in, or of the embryo/fetus itself, and therefore independently of the pregnant woman or any other factor, generate, and therefore ground obligations to the embryo/fetus on the part of the pregnant woman and her physician.

A wide range of intrinsic characteristics has been considered for this role, e.g. moment of conception, implantation, central nervous system development, quickening, and the moment of birth.[20] Given the variability of proposed characteristics, there are many views about when the embryo/fetus does or does not acquire independent moral status. Some take the view that the embryo/fetus possesses independent moral status from the moment of conception or implantation. Others believe that the embryo/fetus acquires independent moral status in degrees, thus resulting in "graded" moral status. Still others hold, at least implicitly, that the embryo/fetus never has independent moral status so long as it is in utero.[19]

Being a patient does not require that one possesses independent moral status.[21] Being a patient means that one can benefit from the application of the clinical skills of the physician.[22] Put more precisely, a human being without independent moral status is properly regarded as a patient when the following conditions are met: that a human being is presented to the physician for the purpose of applying clinical interventions that are reliably expected to be efficacious, in that they are reliably expected to result in a greater balance of goods over harms in the future of the human being in question.[20] In other words, an individual is considered a patient when a physician has beneficence-based ethical obligations to that individual.

To clarify the concept of the embryo/fetus as the patient, beneficence-based obligation is necessary to be provided. Beneficence-based obligations to the fetus and embryo exist when the fetus can later achieve independent moral status.[22] This leads to the conclusion that ethical significance of the unborn child is in direct link with the child to be born—the child, it can become.

LEGAL STATUS OF THE EMBRYO

When discussing law, it should be always kept in mind that medicine is international, but law is not. Before the era of Aristotle, who taught that human life begins when the fetus is formed, human life was considered to begin at birth. Prior to birth, the fetus was not an independent human being but, like an organ, part of the mother.[23] Thus the birth of a full-term infant has been used in the laws of various countries to signify the beginning of the human life that is to be protected.

Indeed, the status of the human embryo is not juridically defined and relies on the political, social and religious influences in each country. Interestingly, nearly all countries of the Western world use the twelfth week of pregnancy as the limit for legal abortion. It is not the end of the first trimester, which is 13.3 weeks, and there is no other particular biological event to justify this limit.

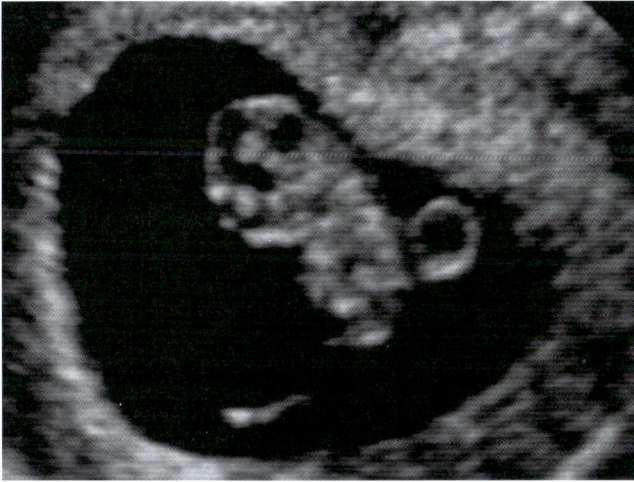

Fig. 18.5: Transvaginal sonography of the 8 weeks embryo with yolk sac

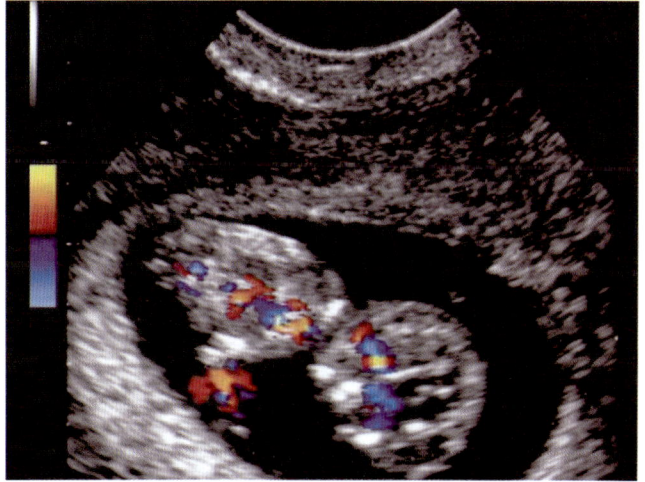

Fig. 18.6: Color Doppler visualization of entire embryonic circulation

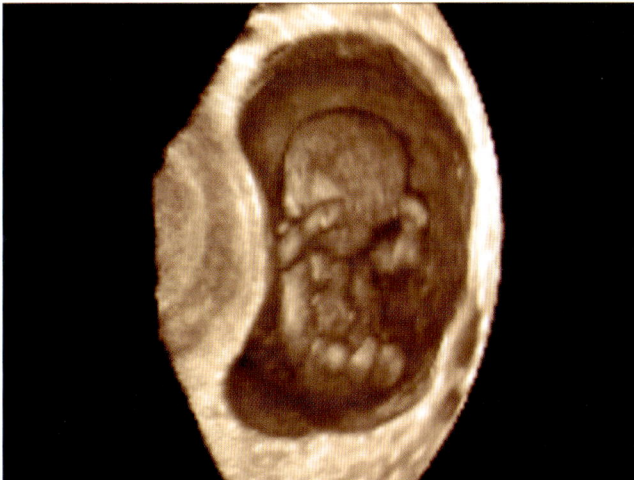

Fig. 18.7: Ten weeks of gestation. Intrauterine content with early fetus. Many anatomical landmarks are visible

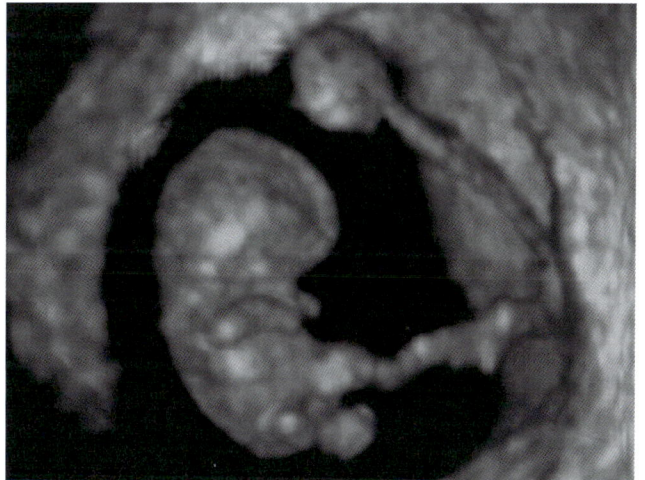

Fig. 18.8: Nine weeks embryo with vitelline duct and yolk sac seen in three dimensions

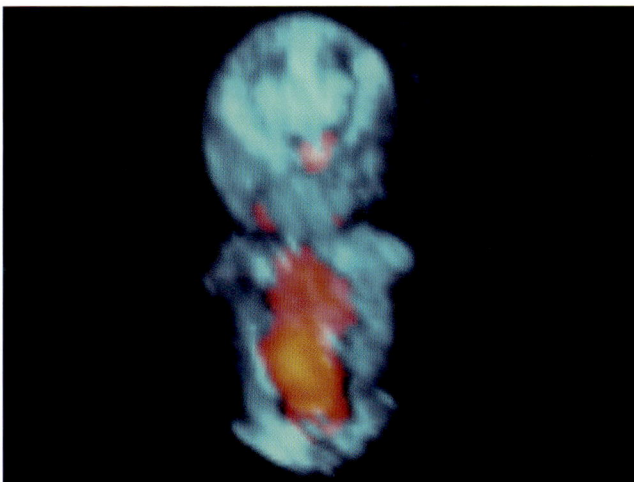

Fig. 18.9: Eleven weeks embryo with entire peripheral and central vascularization visualized by 3D power Doppler

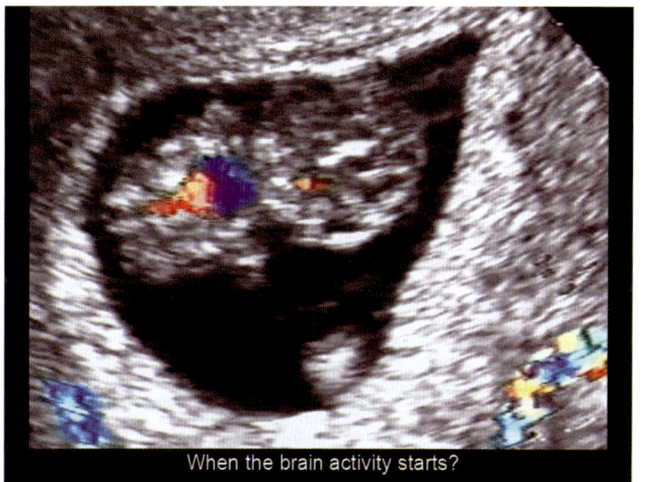

Fig. 18.10: The earliest detection of brain circulation at 7 weeks and 4 days of gestation

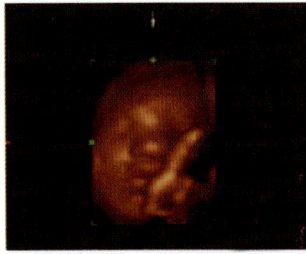

When fetal movement are felt?

At the time of birth?

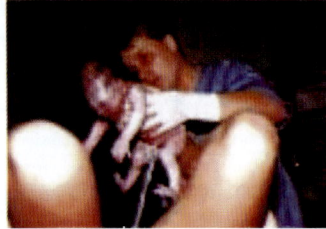

Fig. 18.11: Another possible question about the beginning of check the indentation life

It is hard to answer the question when human life should be legally protected. At the time of conception? At the time of implantation? At the time of birth? (Fig. 18.11). In all countries (except Ireland and Liechtenstein), juridical considerations are based on Roman law. Roman civil law says that the fetus has rights when it is born or if it is born-nasciturus.

Few countries agree with the definition of the beginning of human personality at the time of conception. The majority does not grant legal status to the human embryo in vitro (i.e. during the 14 days after fertilization). Thus, even in the absence of legal rights, there is no denying that the embryo constitutes the beginning of human life, a member of the human family. Therefore, whatever the attitude, every country has to examine which practices are compatible with the respect of that dignity and the security of human genetic material.[24]

ARGUMENTS FOR BEGINNING OF HUMAN LIFE AND HUMAN PERSON AT FERTILIZATION

The fundamental approaches of biomedical and social (secular) practice must begin with the understanding that the subject before birth is a person and that "personhood" is conferred by successful fertilization of the egg. To hide from this in silence or ignorance should be unacceptable to all, as stressed by Scarpelli.[9]

The view that human life begins when sperm and eggs fuse to give rise to a single cell human zygote, whose genetic individuality and uniqueness remain unchanged during normal development, is widely supported. Because the zygote has the capacity to become an adult human individual, it is thought it must be one already. The same zygote organizes itself into an embryo, a fetus, a child and an adult. By this account, the zygote is an actual human individual and not simply a potential one, in much the same way as an infant is an actual human person with potential to develop to maturity and not just a potential person. As Scarpelli pointed out, outside the realm of religious dogma, there has been no one whose existence can be traced back to any entity other than the fertilized egg. The biological line of existence of each individual, without exception, begins precisely when fertilization of the egg is successful.[9]

The process of fertilization actually begins with conditioning of the spermatozoon in the male and female reproductive tracts.

Thereafter, fertilization involves not only the egg itself, but also the various investments which surround the egg at the time it is released from the ovary follicle. Fertilization, therefore, is not an event, but a complex biochemical process requiring a minimum of 24 hours to complete syngamy, that is the formation of a diploid set of chromosomes. During this process, there is no commingling of maternal and paternal chromosomes within a single nuclear membrane (prezygote); after this process, the parental chromosomes material is commingled (zygote).

Among the many other activities of this new cell, most important is the recognition of the new genome, which represents the principal information center for the development of the new human being and for all its further activities. For the better understanding of the very nature of the zygote, two main features are to be at least mentioned here. The first feature is that the zygote exists and operates from syngamy on as a being, ontologically one, and with a precise identity. The second feature is that the zygote is intrinsically oriented and determined to a definite development. Both identity and orientation are due essentially to the genetic information with which it is endowed. That is why many do believe that this cell represents the exact point in time and space where a new human individual organism initiates its own life cycle.[1]

ARGUMENTS AGAINST THE BEGINNING OF HUMAN LIFE AT FERTILIZATION

Today, one largely accepted opinion is that until the fourteenth day from fertilization or at least, until implantation—the human embryo may not be considered, from the ontological point of view, as an individual. There are at least five main reasons in favor of this opinion:

1. Before the formation of the embryonic disk, the embryo is "a mass of cells, genetically human", "a cluster of distinct individual cells", which are each "distinct ontological entities in simple contact with the others".[25] The genetically unique, newly developed DNA, a genome, is not established until 48 hours after sperm penetration. The ovum and sperm lie side by side for more than 48 hours before they finally merge. In biological terms, this renders conception as a process that occurs overtime and not a specific point in time.[3]

2. Until approximately the fourteenth day after fertilization, all that happens is simply a preparation of the protective and nutritional systems required for the future needs of the embryo. Only when the entity called embryonic disk is formed, can the embryo develop into a fetus.[26]

3. The monozygotic twins phenomenon or chimeras can occur. In fact, this seems to be the strongest reason why the embryo is denied the quality of individuality, and as a proof that the zygote cannot be an ontologically human being. In approximately one-third of cases the embryo divides at about the two cells stage, and in the other two-thirds, the inner cell mass divides within the blastocyst from day 38. Occasionally, the division takes place from day 8–12, but usually it is not complete, thereby forming conjoined identical twins or two-headed individuals. The chimera, resulting from the recombination of two individual to become one individuum (and detectable through genetic testing), provides another argument against the equivalence of conception and the beginning of human life: no individuum has died, yet one has ceased to exist.

4. Coexistence of the embryo with its mother is a necessary condition for an embryo belonging to the human species, and this condition can be obtained only at implantation.[19] However, there is evidence that development of a human embryo in vitro can continue well beyond the stage of implantation, and that mouse embryos implanted under the male renal capsule can reach the fetal stage. It is also argued, or at least implied, that so many human embryos die before or after implantation that it would be lacking in realism to accept that the human individual begins before implantation.

It is well-known that high percentages of oocytes which have been penetrated never proceed on to further development, and that many oocytes which do, are thwarted so early in their development that their presence is not even recognized. Up to 50% of ovulated eggs and zygotes recovered after operations were found so grossly abnormal that it would be very unlikely that they would result in viable pregnancies. It is also suggested that 30% of conceptions detected by positive reactions to HCG tests abort spontaneously before these pregnancies are clinically verified. The scientific literature is not unanimous on the incidence of natural wastage prior to, and during, implantation in humans, varying from 15% to as much as 50%. The vast majority of these losses are due to chromosomal defects caused during gametogenesis and fertilization.[27]

Genetic uniqueness and singleness coincide only after implantation and restriction have completed, which is about 3 weeks after fertilization. Until that period, the zygote and its sequelae are in a fluid process and are not a physical individual, and therefore cannot be a person.

Although in a set of twins one individuum can disappear, genetic and individual identities are now more or less equivalent. Many eminent Catholic writers, among them the Australian priest Norman Ford, author of *When Did I Begin?* consider implantation to mark the beginning of human life; they maintain that the pre-embryo has only intrinsic potential and must be protected only from the time of implantation.[28]

5. The product of fertilization may be a tumor, a hydatidiform mole, or chorioepithelioma. Though the mole is alive and of human origin, it is definitely not a human individual or human being. It lacks a true human nature from the start and has no natural potential to begin human development.

A teratoma is another clear instance of cells developing abnormally that results from the product of fertilization, but which could not be considered to be a true human individual with a human nature. It has no potential to develop into an entire fetus or infant. Clearly, the fetus with the teratoma would be a human individual, but not the attached teratoma itself. Obviously, not all the living cells that develop from the conceptus, the early embryo, or the fetus form an integral part of a developing human individual.[1]

DIFFERENT RELIGIOUS TEACHINGS AND HISTORICAL ASPECTS

The Catholic Church's teachings are clearly described in the Introduction Donum Vitae: "A human creature is to be respected and treated as a person from conception and therefore from that same time his (her) rights as a person must be recognized, among which in the first place is the invaluable right to life of each innocent human creature".

In 1997, the Third Assembly of the Pontifical Academy for Life was held in Vatican City. It has been concluded that "at the fusion of two gametes, a new real human individual initiates its own existence, or life cycle, during which—given all the necessary and sufficient conditions—it will autonomously realize all the potentialities with which he is intrinsically endowed". The embryo, therefore, from the time the gametes fuse, is a real human individual, not a potential human individual. It was even added that recent findings of human biological science recognize that in zygotes resulting from fertilization, the biological identity of a new human individual is already constituted.[29,30]

In Western Europe and in North and South America these opinions are mostly based on Judeo-Christian theology, in Arabian Countries, in Africa, and in Asia prevail the influences of the Islamic and Buddhist religions. Although their approach to the beginning of human life is impressively similar, each of these religions has different attitudes to the problem of embryo research, infertility and its therapy. In a fact, while the Jewish attitude toward infertility is expressed in the Talmud sayings and in the Bible (synthesized in the first commandment of God to Adam "Be fruitful and multiply"), the Christian point of view establishes no absolute right to parenthood. According to the Islamic views, attempts to cure infertility are not only permissible, but also a duty.

Islamic teaching is based on prophet Mohammed description: "The creation of each of you in his mother's abdomen assumes a "nutfa" (male and female semen drops) for 40 days, then becomes "alaga" for the same (duration), then a "mudgha" (like a chewed piece of meat) for the same, then God sends an angel to it with instructions. The angel is ordered to write the Sustenance, life span, deeds and whether eventually his lot is happiness or misery, then to blow the Spirit into him" (Human developments as described in Qur'an and Sunnah; Moore, et al. In: Some evidence for the truth of Islam, 1981). The summary of this poetic and sacred description is: Soul breathing "ensoulment" occurs at 120 days of gestation from conception.

To make this religious principle applicable to the practice, the Islamic Jurisprudence Council wrote a *Fatwa* in 1990 that said: "Abortion is allowed in the first 120 days of conception if it is proven beyond doubt that the fetus is affected with a severe malformation that is not amenable to therapy, and if his life, after being born, will be a means of misery to both him and his family, and his parents agree". so that there is no difficulty for either the prenatal diagnosis, or for the possible termination of pregnancy within the exposed limits.

Buddhism has imposed strict ethics on priests, but it has relatively lenient attitudes toward lay people, so if medical treatment for infertility is available, people should make use of it.

For about two thousand years, the opinions of Aristotle, the great Greek philosopher and naturalist, on the beginning of the human being were commonly held. He argued that the male semen had a special power residing in it, pneuma, to transform the menstrual blood, first into a living being with a vegetative soul after seven days, and subsequently into one with a sensitive soul 40 days after contact with the male semen.[31]

Aquinas adopted Aristotle's theory, but specified that rational ensolement took place through the creative act of God to transform the living creature into a human being once it had acquired a sensitive soul. The first conception took place over 7 days, while the second conception, or complete formation of the living individual with a complete human nature, lasted 40 days.[32]

Hippocrates believed that entrance of the soul into the male embryo occurred on the thirtieth day of intrauterine life. It entered into the female embryo on the fortieth day. Actually, this idea was a considerable improvement on the scheme found in the Book of Leviticus, where it is suggested that the soul does not enter the female until 40 days after the conception.[33]

In short, the rational soul enables the matter to become a human being, an animated body, an embodied soul, a human person.

Harvey's experiments with deer in 1633 proved Aristotle's theory of human reproduction wrong, without himself finding a satisfactory explanation of human conception. After modern scientists discovered the process of fertilization, most people took for granted that human beings, complete with a rational soul, began once fertilization had taken place.

It is clear that the answer to the question "When has the human being actually come to life?" could only be given by combining the cognition of different religions, philosophies and various biological scientific disciplines. There is a very fine line between the competence of science and the one of metaphysics, and it greatly depends on the individual's philosophical principles. Those two, more or less autonomous intellectual disciplines have very often tried dominating one another, or ignoring each other. It is only recently that the majority of scientists and some theologians have come to realize that the separate meanings of scientific and religious "truths" complement each other, thus representing methodologically independent entities. Current science is not interested in what Nature is, but in the facts that could be stated regarding it, thus trying to explain the term, rather than inventing it. The main difference between science and religion can be seen in the fact that scientific "truths", unlike religious postulates, can and must be experimentally verified and the methods of scientific cognition can be easily explained and learnt. Whereas religion favors irrationality, science prefers an entirely rational approach to matters of importance. Intellectual cognition, when scientifically expressed, usually is in a form of mathematical formulas and presented quantitatively. Contrarily, religion tends to keep its truths in a form of metaphoric expressions, preferring qualitative. Today, there is a tendency, on a higher level, to reopen the dialogue between the science and religion, which was present at the very beginning of our culture. Religion had existed long before science came to life, but science is not to be thought of as a continuation of the religion. Each discipline should preserve its principles, its separate interpretations and its own conclusions. In the end, both of them represent different components of the one and indivisible culture of mankind.

CLINICAL CONTROVERSIES

There are some clinical controversies pertinent in any discussion of when life begins. Spermatozoa are living cells. They present evidence that they are living by their motility. They are equipped with an effective mechanism for movement in the form of a tail that beats under the control of the cytoplasmic droplets within the head. These living cells, which have been manufactured in the testes, are released into the environment provided by the male reproductive tract. They are not yet capable of fertilization. The spermatozoon must first come under the influence of the male reproductive tract, where it acquires the ability to function in fertilization. Even after ejaculation, it is capable of penetrating the egg, and it is modified further by exposure to the female reproductive tract, taking on the

ability or capacity to fertilize. The decision must be made as to whether the spermatozoon is a being (i.e. living and human with the potential for continued life once fertilization has occurred); albeit in another form, it is entitled to the right of protection as a person. Those who deny right for life to the spermatozoon might argue that it is not a complete human cell chromosomally—it contains only the haploid number of chromosomes. Paradoxically, those who take that point of view would insist that an individual born with fewer or more chromosomes than normal is human and entitled to all the rights of "personhood". As Mastroianni stressed, the decision to base the definition of "human life" solely on the number of chromosomes in a given cell has far-reaching implications.[34]

Furthermore, life has been defined as being terminated when brain activity ends. If we were to say that life begins when brain activity starts, we would be admitting that the definition of the beginning of life is dependent upon technology and not upon ethics or morality.

Some suggested that the beginning of human life requires the neural fusion of the periphery with the center, as well as sufficient development of the brain itself.[35] Brody formulated the so-called symmetry concept: if the death of a human being requires the death of the brain, the beginning of human life shall correspond with the beginning of the life of the brain, considered to be at day 32 pc.[36] However, Sass has correctly pointed out that fusion is not established anatomically without neurons which form synapses, which would be expected from embryological development at 70 days (8 weeks) pc.[37]

In this light, let us take for example the accepted definition of birth, which some years ago was described as the complete expulsion of a fetus of 1,000 g or 28 weeks of pregnancy. With advances in perinatal and neonatal intensive care, the line was drawn at 500 g, or approximately 22 weeks of gestation, some years later. This meant that a 20-week-old fetus was not born by definition, even if it was viable. This concept has changed. The same logic applies to a live fetus being accorded the term "life", if we use such definitions as the beginning of brain activity or ultrasonic proof of heartbeat and movement. The establishment of each of these parameters is shifted to an earlier stage year by year by improving technological refinements in electronic and ultrasonic equipment. This leads us to the conclusion that to follow this line of reasoning means to give life, birth, and viability definitions determined by technology. The more advanced the technology, the earlier life begins.

In any consideration of the beginning of human life, it helps to think about when life ends. Let us consider the following: A 2-week-old newborn is hospitalized with massive brain injury suffered in an automobile accident. Despite all measures, no electrical or other brain activity can be detected during the next 2 days and the child is pronounced dead. Its body parts may survive after its death, as after the death of every person of whatever age. Hair and nails grow for days. Kidneys, heart, liver and other organs may go on living for years if transplanted into another individual. Cells taken soon after death and cultured in a laboratory might live well beyond the 72 years or more years this child might have lived, although the life of the infant has ended. The conclusion reached in this case that death of the brain means the end of life, is generally accepted by physicians, courts and the public.[4]

Returning to the question of when life begins, it is true that the DNA of the fertilized egg has the information necessary to form an individual, but so does virtually every other cell in the body.

Nobody would claim full rights for the living cells of the infant killed in the accident, although each has a complete library of DNA. Nor would they for thousands of living skin cells, we loose every time we wash our hands and faces. Is there some stage in the development of the brain that is critical? Or is it the time at which the fetus can survive outside the womb, with or without the support of medical technology? Should we revert to a criterion used for many years, the time of quickening, when one can feel the fetus moving? These are questions still to be answered.

VISUALIZATION OF EARLY HUMAN DEVELOPMENT

Significant advances have been made in recent years in visualizing and analyzing the earliest human development. Most of them have been done by introduction of three-dimensional static and color Doppler and 4D sonography. Many new parameters about early human development are now studied directly by new ultrasound techniques.

Considerable number of biochemical, morphological and vascular changes occur within the follicle during the process of ovulation and luteinization and most of them can be studied by transvaginal ultrasound with color Doppler and 3D facilities.[38] If the oocyte is fertilized, the embryo is transported into the uterus where under favorable hormonal and environmental conditions, it will implant and develop into a new and unique individual. The introduction of transvaginal color Doppler improved the recognition of blood vessels enabling detailed examination of small vessels such as arteries supplying preovulatory follicle, corpus luteum and endometrium.[26]

Perifollicular vascularization can help in identification of follicles containing high quality oocytes, with a high probability of recuperating, fertilizing, cleaving and implanting, while 3D ultrasound enables accurate morphological inspection and detection of cumulus oophorus. Follicles without visualization of the cumulus by multiplanar imaging are not likely to contain fertilizable oocytes. This information is especially useful in patients undergoing ovulation induction.

Following ovulation, the corpus luteum is formed as the result of many structural, functional and vascular changes in the former follicular wall. Color Doppler studies of the luteal blood flow velocities enable evaluation of the corpus luteum function in second phase of menstrual cycle and early pregnancy. When the placenta takes over the role of production of progesterone, the corpus luteum starts regressing.

After ovulation there is a short period during which the endometrial receptivity is maximal. During these few days, a blastocyst can attach to the endometrium and provoke increased vascular permeability and vasodilatation at the implantation site. Trophoblast-produced proteolytic enzymes cause the penetration of the uterine mucosa and erode adjacent maternal capillaries. This results in formation of the intercommunicating lacunar network—the intervillous space of the placenta. A small intradecidual gestational sac can be visualized by transvaginal sonography between 32 and 34 days.[39]

The secondary yolk sac is the earliest extraembryonic structure normally seen within the gestational sac in the beginning of the 5th gestational week. The yolk sac volume was found to increase from 5 to 10 weeks of gestation. When the yolk sac reaches its maximum volume at around 10 weeks, it has already started to degenerate, which can be indirectly proved by a significant reduction in visualization rates of the yolk sac vascularity.[25] Therefore, a combination of functional and volumetric studies by 3D power Doppler helps to identify some of the most important moments in early human development.

The embryonic heart begins beating on about day 22–23, accepting blood components from the yolk sac and pushing blood into the circulation. The embryonic blood begins circulating at the end of the fourth week of development.

The start of the embryo-chorionic circulation changes the source of nourishment to all intraembryonic tissues. The survival and further development of the embryo become dependent on the circulation of embryonic/fetal blood. If the embryo-chorionic circulation does not develop, or fails, the conceptus is aborted. The embryo cannot survive without the chorion (placenta) and the chorion will not survive without the embryo. Avascular degenerated chorionic villi constitute the hydatidiform mole.

Within the embryo, there are three distinct blood circulatory systems:[10]

1. *Vitelline circulation* (from yolk sac to embryo)
2. *Intraembryonic circulation*
3. Two umbilical arteries (from embryo to placenta—*fetoplacental circulation*).

It is possible to visualize and assess them virtually from conception.[40-44]

At 5 weeks from the maternal side of placenta, it is possible to obtain simultaneous three-dimensional imaging of the developing intervillous circulation during the first trimester of pregnancy. Three-dimensional power Doppler reveals intensive vascular activity surrounding the chorionic shell starting from the first sonographic evidence of the developing pregnancy during the fifth week of gestation.

At 7 weeks, three-dimensional power Doppler images depict aortic and umbilical blood flow. Initial branches of umbilical vessels are visible at the placental umbilical insertion.

During the eighth to ninth week, developing intestine is being herniated into the proximal umbilical cord.

At 9–10 weeks, herniation of the mid-gut is present. The arms with elbow and legs with knee are clearly visible, while feet can be seen approaching the midline.

At 11 weeks, three-dimensional power Doppler imaging allows visualization of the entire fetal and placental circulation (Figs 18.6, 18.9, 18.10 and 18.12).

During the eleventh to twelfth week of pregnancy development of the head and neck continues. Facial details such as nose, orbits, maxilla and mandibles are often visible. Herniated mid-gut returns into the abdominal cavity.

NEW POSSIBILITIES FOR STUDYING EMBRYONIC MOVEMENTS AND BEHAVIOR

The latest development of 3D and 4D sonography enables precise study of embryonic and fetal activity and behavior (Fig. 18.13).[45] With four-dimensional ultrasound, movements of head, body, and all four limbs and extremities can be seen simultaneously in three dimensions.[46] Therefore, the earliest phases of the human anatomical and motor development can be visualized and studied

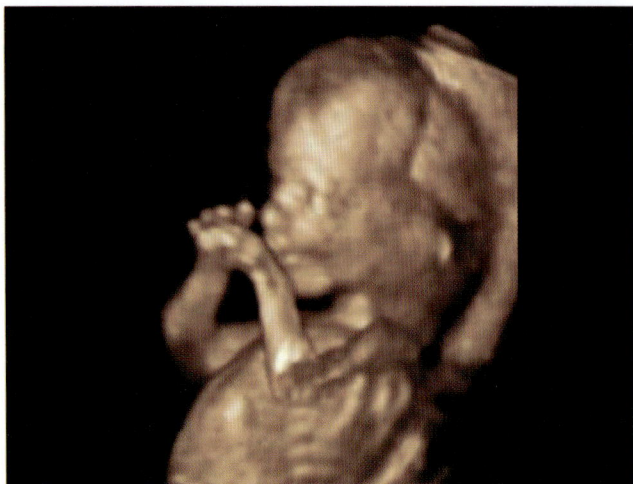

Fig. 18.12: Hand near face movement of the fetus at 16 weeks of gestation, as seen by 3D ultrasound

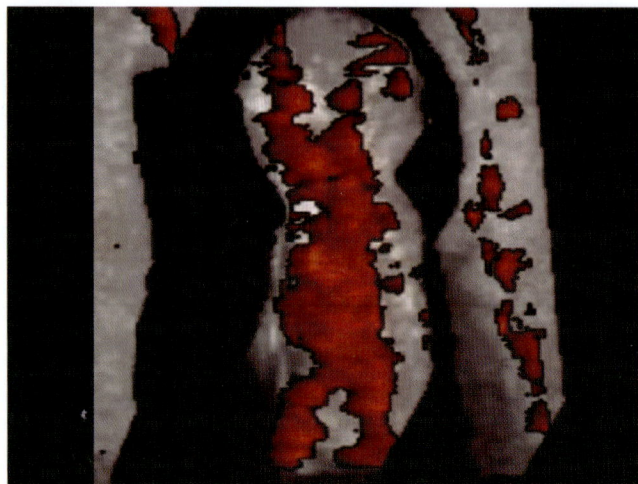

Fig. 18.13: Early triplets clearly visualized by 3D sonography

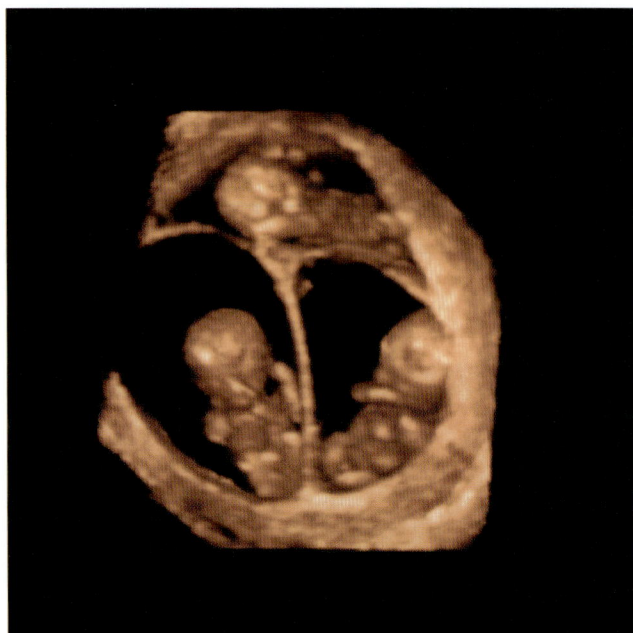

Fig. 18.14: Illustrative example of the complex fetal movements recorded by 4D sonography at 12 weeks of gestation

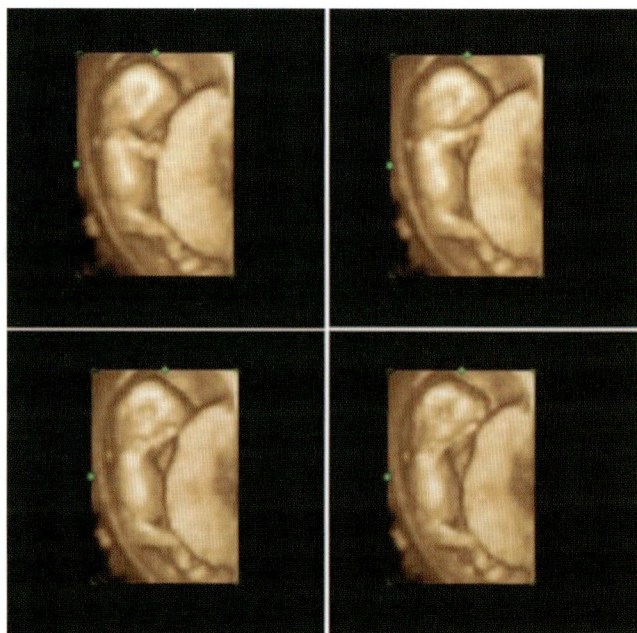

Fig. 18.15: Fourteen-week fetus. Complete vascular anatomy of fetal and placental circulation shown by 3D power Doppler

simultaneously (Figs 18.11, 18.14, 18.18 and 18.19). It is clear that neurologic development—early fetal motor activity and behavior needs to be re-evaluated by this new technique.[47-49] Our group studied the development of the complexity of spontaneous embryonic and fetal movements.[50] With the advancing of the gestational age, the movements become more and more complex. The increase in the number of axodendritic and axosomatic synapses between 8 and 10 weeks, and again between 12 and 15 weeks[51] correlates with the periods of fetal movement differentiation and with the onset of general movements and complex activity patterns, such as swallowing, stretching and yawning, seen easily by 4D technique. By 7–8 weeks of pregnancy, gross body movements appear. They consist of changing the position of the head toward the body. By 9–10 weeks of pregnancy, limb movements appear. They consist of changing the position of the extremities toward the body without the extension or flexion in elbow and knee. At 10–12 weeks of pregnancy, complex limb movements appear. They consist of changes in the position of limb segments toward each other, such as extension and flexion in elbow and knee (Fig. 18.14).

Between 12 and 15 weeks of pregnancy, swallowing, stretching and yawning activities appear. In addition to these activities, it is now feasible to study by 4D ultrasound a full range of facial expression including smiling, crying and eyelid movement (Fig. 18.15).

It is hoped that the new 4D technique will help us have a better understanding of both the somatic and motoric development of the early embryo. It will also enable the reliable study of fetal and even parental behavior.[46]

CONCLUSION

The question of when a human life begins and how to define it, could be answered only through the interconnecting pathways of history, philosophy, medical science and religion (Fig. 18.16 to 18.19). It has not been easy to determine where to draw the fine line between the competence of science and metaphysics in this delicate philosophical field. To a large extent the drawing of this line depends on one's fundamental philosophical outlook. To quote Beller: "The point at which human life begins will always be seen differently by different individuals, groups, cultures and religious faiths. In democracy, there are always at least two sides, and the center holds only when the majority realizes that without a minority, democracy itself is lost. The minority in turn must realize its best chance lies in persuasion by reason and thoughtfulness rather than fanaticism."[3]

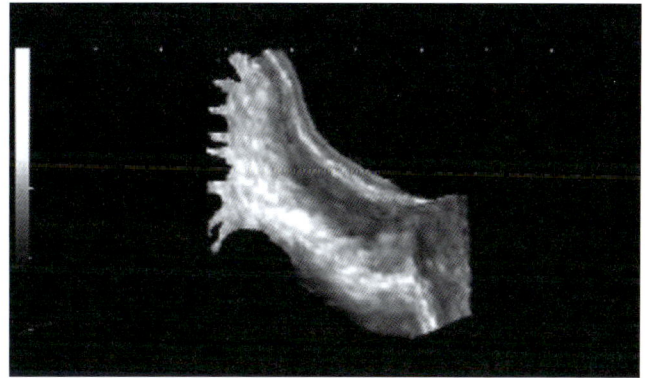

Fig. 18.16: 3D sonography visualization of the part of Fallopian tube

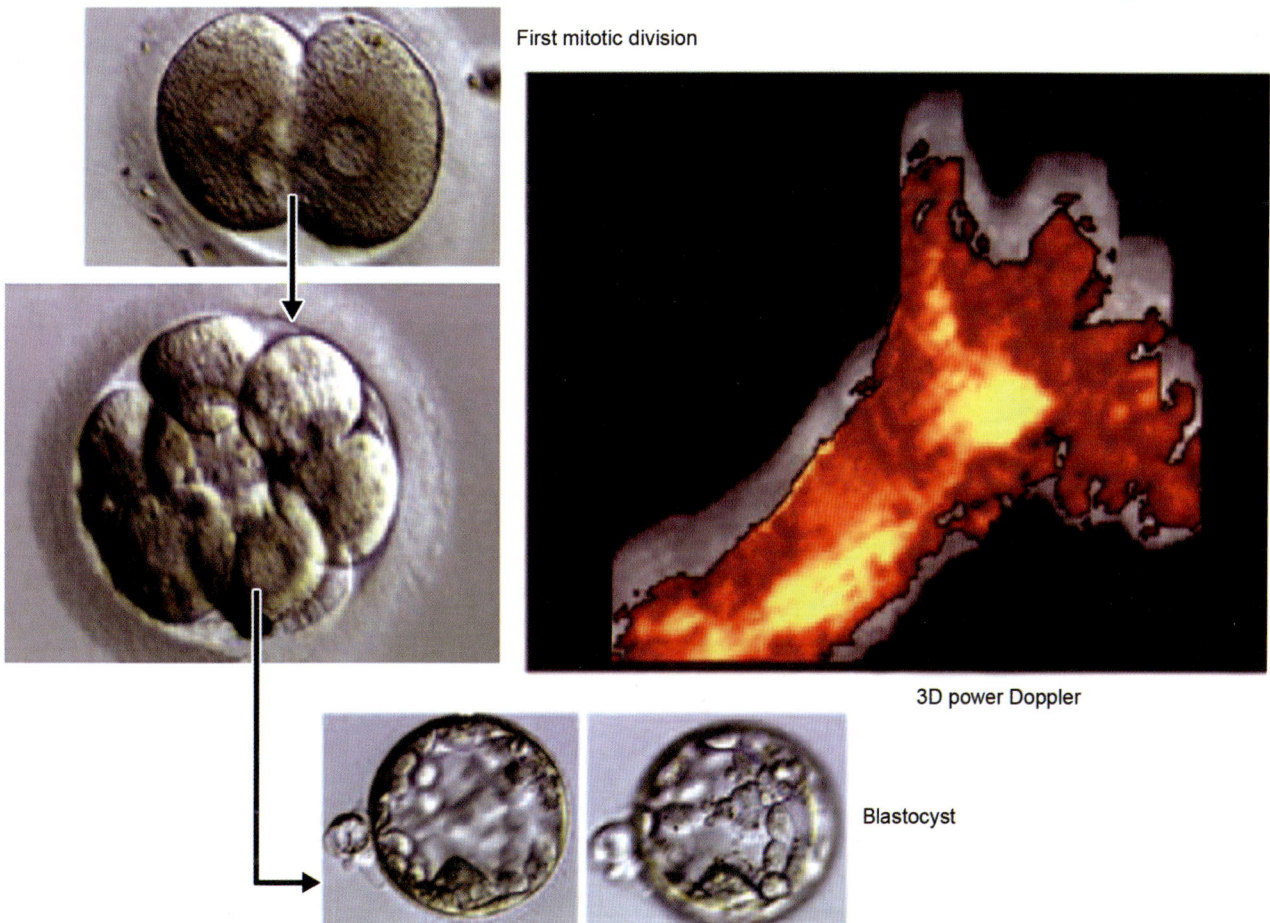

First mitotic division

3D power Doppler

Blastocyst

Fig. 18.17: Visualization of the patency of Fallopian tube by 3D power Doppler sonography, important for successful first mitotic division and transfer of early embryo to uterus

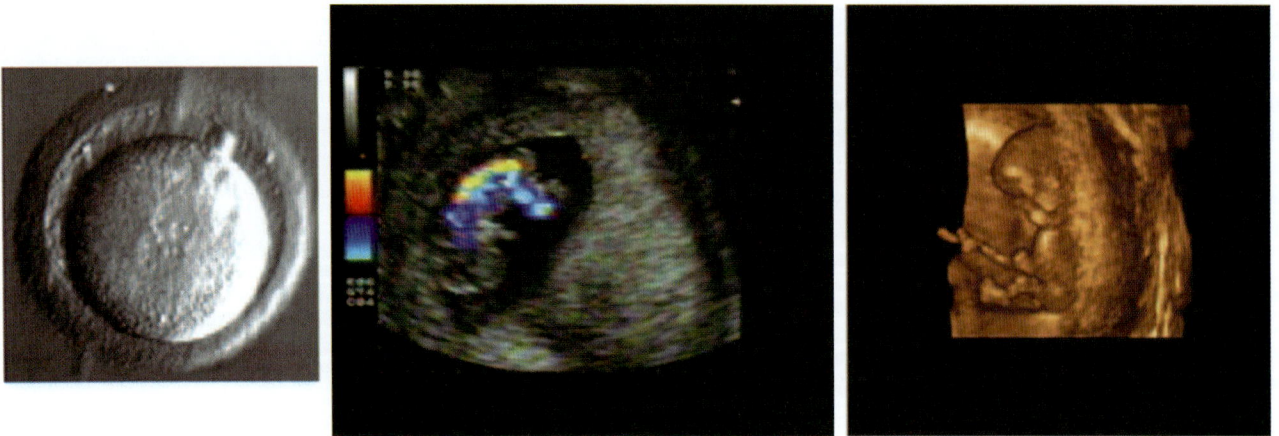

Early human development can now be
visulized virtually from conception

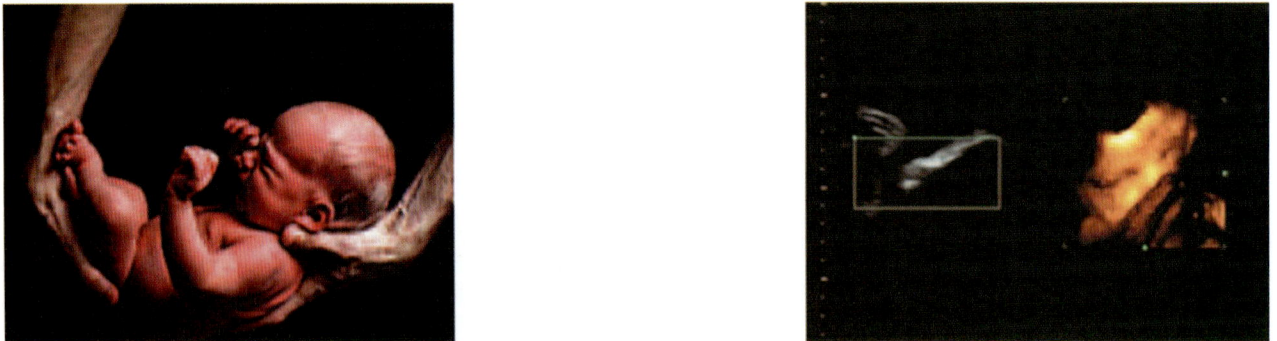

Fig. 18.18: Illustrative example of the use of different medical methods to assess early human development

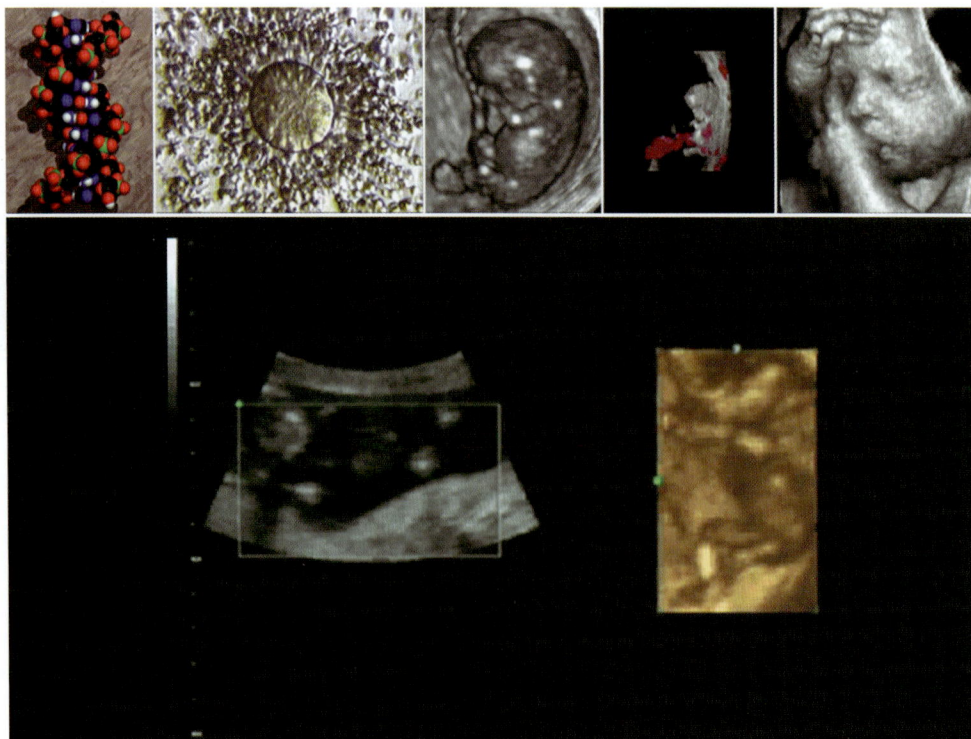

Fig. 18.19: Integrated slide showing continuity of scientific visualization of the beginning of early human development from genetic material to oocyte, morphology of embryo, its vascularization, and fetal behavioral pattern assessed by 4D sonography

REFERENCES

1. Serra A, Colombo R. Identity and status of the human embryo: the contribution of biology. In: de Dios Vial Correa, Sgreccia E (Eds). Identity and Statute of Human Embryo. 1998. p. 128.

2. Kurjak A. The beginning of human life and its modern scientific assessment. Clin Perinatol. 2003;30:27-44.

3. Beller FK, Zlatnik GP. The beginning of human life. Journal of Assisted Reproduction and Genetics. 1995;12(8):477-83.

4. Kurjak A. When does human life begin? Encyclopedia Moderna. 1992. pp. 383-90.

5. Godfrey J. The Pope and the ontogeny of persons (Commentary). Nature. 1995,273:100.

6. Liggins Graham (Mont). Foreword. In: Nathanielsz PW (Ed). Life before Birth and the Time to be Born. New York: Promethean Press Ithaca; 1992.

7. Gilbert SF. Developmental Biology. Sunderland, Mass: Sinauer Associates; 1991. p. 3.

8. Scarpelli EM. Postnatal through adult human life and the scientific deception. In: Atti del I (Ed). Congresso Nazionale della Societa Italiana di Medicina Materno Fetale, Rome, March 17-21, 2003. Medimond (International Proceedings): Bologna, Italy. 2003. pp. 29-36.

9. Scarpelli EM. Personhood: a biological phenomenon. J Perinat Med. 2001;29:417-26.

10. Jirasek JE. An Atlas of the human embryo and fetus. NewYork-London: Parthenon Publishing; 2001.

11. ACOG Committee Opinion: Committee on Ethics: Preembryo research: History scientific background, and ethical considerations. Int J Gynecol Obstet. 1994;45:291-301.

12. Declaration of Professors from Five Faculties of Medicine and Surgery of the universities of Rome, Organizers of the Conference: The Embryo as a Patient.

13. Kurjak A, Azumendi G, Stanojevic M, et al. An attempt to study fetal awareness by four-dimensional ultrasonography (submitted).

14. Sass HM. Brain life and brain death: a proposal for normative agreement. J Med Philos. 1989;14:45-59.

15. Veatch RM. The beginning of full moral standing. In: FK Beller, RF Weir (Eds). The Beginning of Human Life. Dordrecht: Kluwer; 1994. p. 19.

16. Knutson AL. When does human life begin? Viewpoints of public health professionals. Am J Publ Health. 1967;57:2167.

17. Engelhardt HT Jr. The foundation of bioethics. New York: Oxford University Press; 1986.

18. Dunstan GR. The moral status of the human embryo. A tradition recalled. J Med Ethics. 1984;10:38-44.

19. Chervenak FA, McCullough LB, Kurjak A. Ethical implications of the embryo as a patient. In: Kurjak A, Chervenak FA, Carrera JM (Eds). The Embryo as a Patient. New York-London: Parthenon Publishing Group; 2001. pp. 226-30.

20. Curran CE. Abortion: contemporary debate in philosophical and religious ethics. In: Reich WT (Ed). Encyclopedia of Bioethics. New York: Macmillan; 1978. pp. 17-26.

21. Ruddick W, Wilcox W. Operating on the fetus. Hastings Cen Report. 1982;12:10-4.

22. McCullogh LB, Chervenak FA. Ethics in Obstetrics and Gynecology. New York: Oxford University Press; 1994.

23. Connery JR Jr. The ancients and medievals on abortion. In: Horan DJ, Grant ER, Cunningham PC (Eds). Abortion and Constitution. Washington DC: Georgetown University Press; 1987. p. 124.

24. Pierre F, Soutoul JH. Medical and legal complications [Article in French]. J Gynecol Obstet Biol Reprod (Paris). 1994;23(5):516-9.

25. Ford NM. When did I begin? Conception of the Human Individual in History, Philosophy and Science. Cambridge: Cambridge University Press; 1991. pp. 137-46.

26. McLaren A. Prelude to embryogenesis, in the Ciba Foundation, Human Embryo Research, Yes or No? London, New York: Tavistock; 1986. pp. 5-23.

27. Abel F. Nascita e morte dell'uomo: prospective della biologia e della medicina. In: Biolo S (Ed). Nascita e morte dell'uomo. Problemi filosofici e scientifici della bioetica, Genova: Marieti; 1993. pp. 37-53.

28. McCormick KA. Who or what is the preembryo? Kennedy Instit Ethics J. 1991;1:24.

29. Mahoney SJ. Bioethics and belief. London: Sheed and Ward; 1984. p. 80.

30. Johnson M. Delayed hominization. Reflections on some recent catholic claims for delayed hominization. Theological Studies. 1995;56:743-63.

31. Congregation for the Doctrine of the Faith. Instruction on respect for human life in its origin and on the dignity of procreation "Donum Vitae" (February 12, 1987). Acta Apostolicae Sedis. 1988;80:70-102.

32. Ford NM. When did I begin? Cambridge University Press; 1991.

33. Beazley JM. Fetal assessment from conception to birth. In: Kurjak A (Ed). Recent Advances in Ultrasound Diagnosis. Amsterdam: Excerpta Medica; 1980. p. 128.

34. Kurjak A. Kada pocinje zivot. In: Kurjak A (Ed). Ocekujuci Novorodjence, Zagreb: Naprijed; 1987. pp. 18-28.

35. Mastroianni L Jr. Ethical aspects of fetal therapy and experimentation. In: Schenker JG, Weinstein D (Eds). The Intrauterine Life: Management and Therapy. Amsterdam: Excerpta Medica; 1986. pp. 3-10.

36. Beller FK, Reeve J. Brain life and brain death: the anencephalic as an explanatory example. J Med Philos. 1989;14:5-20.

37. Brody B. Abortion and the sanctity of human life: a philosophical view. Cambridge: MIT Press; 1975. p. 109.

38. Sass HM. The moral significance of brain-life-criteria. In: FK Beller, RF Weir RF (Eds). The Beginning of Human Life. Dordrecht: Kluwer; 1994. pp. 57-70.

39. Kupesic S. The first three weeks assessed by transvaginal color Doppler. J Perinat Med. 1996;24:310-7.

40. Kupesic S, Kurjak A, Ivancic-Kosuta M. Volume and vascularity of the yolk sac. J Perinat Med. 1999;27:91-6.

41. Kurjak A, Predanic M, Kupesic S. Transvaginal color Doppler study of middle cerebral artery blood flow in early normal and abnormal pregnancy. Ultrasound Obstet Gynecol. 1992;2:424-8.

42. Kurjak A, Kupesic S. Doppler assessment of the intervillous blood flow in normal and abnormal early pregnancy. Obstet Gynecol. 1997;89:252-6.

43. Kurjak A, Kupesic S, Hafner T. Intervillous blood flow in normal and abnormal early pregnancy. Croatian Med J. 1998;39(1):10.

44. Kurjak A, Kupesic S. Three-dimensional transvaginal ultrasound improves measurement of nuchal translucency. J Perinat Med. 1999;27:97-102.

45. Kurjak A, Kupesic S, Banovic I, et al. The study of morphology and circulation of early embryo by three-dimensional ultrasound and power Doppler. J Perinat Med. 1999;27:145-57.

46. Lee A. Four-dimensional ultrasound in prenatal diagnosis: leading edge in imaging technology. Ultrasound Rev Obstet Gynecol. 2001;1:144-8.

47. Campbell S. 4D, or not 4D: That is the question. Ultrasound Obstet Gynecol. 2002;19:1-4.

48. de Vries JI, Visser GH, Prechtl HF. The emergence of fetal behaviour. I. Qualitative aspects. Early Hum Dev. 1982;7:301-22.

49. de Vries JI, Visser GH, Prechtl HF. The emergence of fetal behaviour. I. Qualitative aspects. Early Hum Dev. 1985;12:99-120.

50. Kurjak A, Vecek N, Hafner T, et al. Prenatal diagnosis: what does four-dimensional ultrasound add? J Perinat Med. 2002;30:57-62.

51. Kurjak A, Azumendi G, Vecek N, et al. Fetal hand movements and facial expression in normal pregnancy studied by four-dimensional sonography. J Perinat Med. 2003;31:496-508.

52. Okado N, Kojima T. Ontogenity of the central nervous system: neurogenesis, fibre connection, synaptogenesis and myelinization in the spinal cord. In: Prechtl HFR (Ed). Continuity of Neural Functions from Prenatal to Postnatal Life. Oxford: Blackwell Scientific; 1984. pp. 46-64.

C H A P T E R

19 Preimplantation Diagnosis

LJ Nelson

INTRODUCTION

Preimplantation genetic diagnosis (PGD) is a technique devised within the last 15 years used primarily to identify genetic disorders or defects in human embryos created by in vitro fertilization (IVF) prior to their implantation for gestation. The two dominant methods of PGD currently in use are polar body biopsy and blastomere biopsy on cleavage stage embryos, though fluorescence in situ hybridization has been used for PGD of common aneuploidies. PGD is an "attractive means of preventing heritable genetic diseases" which, as an alternative to traditional prenatal genetic diagnosis following chorionic villus sampling (CVS) or amniocentesis, can avoid the need for selective abortion of affected fetuses, even though "it is strongly recommended that normality be confirmed by subsequent CVS or amniocentesis."[1] According to the National Society of Genetic Counselors, the primary reason for electing PGD over traditional prenatal diagnosis "is the couple's objection to pregnancy termination."[2]

The PGD is also used to detect aneuploidy (the major cause of inherited diseases) and to select chromosomally normal embryos for implantation mostly in women of advanced maternal age undergoing IVF. The only known risk factor for aneuploidy is maternal age while trisomies appear in 2% of recognized pregnancies of women 25 years old, this number increases up to 19% in women of 40 or more years of age.[3] One study found aneuploidy to be 52% in women aged 40–47.[4] PGD of aneuploidy has been shown to reduce the risk of children with trisomies, increase implantation rates, and decrease spontaneous abortions.[5]

Finally, in cases of parents who have children with bone marrow disorders who are in need of human leukocyte antigen (HLA)-matched stem cell transplantation (e.g. acute lymphoid leukemia) and who wish to conceive another child to serve as a donor of stem cells, PGD can be employed to test embryos for causative gene mutations and simultaneously for HLA alleles with the goal of selecting and transferring only those unaffected embryos which are HLA matched to the sick child. A recent report documents this process as resulting in five singleton pregnancies and the birth of five HLA-matched healthy children.[6]

More than 1,000 unaffected children have been born following PGD; this suggests that the procedure is both accurate and safe.[7] Even thought PGD was described as experimental as recently as 1998,[8] it is now considered "an established technique with specific and expanding applications for standard clinical practice" that is "a viable alternative to postconception diagnosis and pregnancy termination."[1]

This chapter will review and comment upon the central ethical issues raised by PGD. These fall into three major categories:

1. Ethics and the provision of PGD, including the ethics of marketing PGD services, shared risk or refund programs, and disclosure and patient consent.

2. The moral status of the extracorporeal human embryo (those outside a woman's body) and their destruction following embryo selection.

3. The ethically appropriate uses of PGD, including its use to prevent the birth of disabled persons and to select for sex and other traits for nonmedical reasons. The last section examines the importance of each individual clinician making a personal decision, based upon the exercise of an informed conscience, about the ethical propriety of his or her involvement in the provision of PGD services, whether for the prevention of genetic disease and disability or for the selection of sex or some other trait unrelated to health.

ETHICS AND THE PROVISION OF PREIMPLANTATION GENETIC DIAGNOSIS

Marketing

Most of the utilization of IVF and, by implication, PGD, services is not covered by health insurance in the US,[8] and this is likely true elsewhere in the world as well. Consequently, most individuals pay for these services directly out of their own private resources. With the average cost for an IVF cycle in the US being $12,400,[9] the financial commitment for the individuals involved is substantial. Receiving direct payment from patients' appeals to clinicians who are not required to wait weeks or months for insurer reimbursement, or to expend large amounts of time and effort in submitting reimbursement forms, or obtaining pretreatment authorization. These factors make the provision of IVF and PGD an attractive and potentially profitable form of professional practice. The utilization of PGD adds several thousands of dollars in cost over and above those incurred for IVF.

Clinics providing IVF, PGD, and other reproductive health services often advertise in the mass media and make other efforts to attract patients (e.g. free informational seminars, internet sites).

While advertising health-care services is by no means inherently unethical, the traditional professional values of beneficence and loyalty to the patients' interests indicate that the provision of medical services ought not to resemble a common commercial transaction between strangers. Clinicians are in a fiduciary relationship with their patients and are obligated to act so as to deserve and maintain the patient's trust and confidence that their wishes and best interests are being faithfully served. Consequently, the marketing of infertility services ought to place the good of patients above other interests (especially a clinician's or clinic's own economic interests), should not induce patients to accept excessive, unneeded, or unproven services, and should adhere to high standards of honesty and accuracy in the information provided to prospective patients.[10]

For example, one infertility clinic that used advertisements to entice persons to undergo IVF with language suggesting that "the dream of having a child might still come true for you" can be criticized as selling profitable services at the expense of vulnerable people suffering from the anguish and disappointment of childlessness. Another IVF clinic used chemical rather than clinical pregnancies in calculating its "success" rate, a misleading number as only a relatively small portion of chemical pregnancies result in live birth.[10] The "success," that is, healthy live birth, rate of IVF and PGD varies by center, and the staff of each is ethically obligated to be scrupulously careful in calculating and disclosing its rates of success and its rates of error as well. This is particularly important as many PGD centers have not reported their experience, and there currently is no systematic approach to presenting errors. Informal reports suggest an error rate in the range of 1–10%, depending on the disease and assay being evaluated.[1] The European Society for Human Reproduction and Embryology PGD consortium has reported clinical pregnancies in 17% of cases after testing for structural chromosomal abnormalities, 16% after sexing, and 21% after testing for monogenic diseases, while the International Working Group of Preimplantation Genetics has reported a pregnancy rate of about 24%.[11] The former also noted an error rate of 2–3%.

Shared Risk Programs

In addition to traditional fee-for-service pricing, some assisted reproduction programs offer IVF on a shared risk basis by refunding the patient(s) a portion of, or even all, specified fees (pretreatment screening and drug costs are typically excluded from refund) if the patient does not have a live birth or achieve an ongoing pregnancy. However, patients electing shared risk pay a significantly higher initial fee. These alternative payment plans have been criticized as being "exploitative, misleading, and contrary to long-standing professional norms against charging contingent fees for medical services."[12] There is also the objection that shared risk plans create a conflict of interest in which the clinician is induced to take steps to achieve pregnancy regardless of the impact on the patient in order to avoid paying the refund. Assuming fair and adequate disclosure of terms, defenders of the practice point out that it is a legitimate alternative payment plan given the usual absence of insurance coverage which addresses patient concerns about the high cost of many cycles of IVF that fail to achieve pregnancy, a not uncommon outcome.

The claim that all such programs are misleading or exploiting those who are desperate to have a genetically related child by inducing them to purchase a more expensive set of services is not persuasive. While persons contemplating the utilization of expensive IVF services may well suffer greatly from their infertility and may feel some degree of desperation in their efforts to conceive a child, it is wrong to assume that they are inherently unable to determine their own best interests and make decisions with significant economic consequences. The clinicians involved are, of course, obligated to provide patients with sufficient information to make an informed choice of a shared risk plan rather than fee-for-service. The shared risk plans reviewed by the American Society for Reproductive Medicine (ASRM) Ethics Committee were found to meet this standard.[12]

The objection to shared risk plans as an unethical contingency fee is likewise misplaced. The American Medical Association Code of Medical Ethics states that "a physician's fee should not be made contingent on the successful outcome of medical treatment."[13] First, this prohibition is primarily aimed at physicians treating patients who are seeking compensation for their injuries through the legal system. A contingent fee arrangement would strongly tend to bias the physician's opinion in favor of more treatment and more expensive treatment than might be warranted. This concern is absent in assisted reproduction. Second, the prohibition is aimed at dispelling the implication that a good outcome is guaranteed and avoiding unrealistic patient expectations that follow from it. However, shared risks plans are offered precisely because the outcome of the procedure is in serious doubt and the provider is willing to accept some of the financial risk of failure with the patient at the latter's own election.

The final objection based on conflict of interest focuses on the likelihood of a clinician preferring:

- Utilization of egg stimulation procedures that will not only produce more oocytes but also pose more risks to the woman's health.
- Transfer of a larger number of embryos in order to enhance the chances of pregnancy occurring but simultaneously increasing the chances of multiple gestations which pose well-known risks to both offspring and parents. This objection has some merit. These dangers do exist, but they exist equally for IVF services provided on a fee-for-service basis. The solution is not to prohibit shared risk payment plans, but for clinicians both to carefully monitor their own behavior for strict conformance with the patient's best interests and to fully disclose to patients all of the risks and benefits, both to health and wealth, of the different financing arrangements. Also, the ASRM Ethics Committee found no evidence that either danger mentioned here has actually materialized.[12]

Disclosure and Informed Consent

All clinicians should be scrupulous about the accuracy and truthfulness of the methods they use to attract and secure patients who are dependent on professionals for knowledge about the health-care services they receive. Likewise, all information provided by clinicians to patients wanting to utilize PGD should be complete, accurate, and devoid of ambiguity in contrast with typical commercial information which is often deliberately incomplete and ambiguous, and at least sometimes inaccurate. In particular, the risks, burdens, benefits, probabilities of success, and the limits of PGD and IVF should be presented in a matter-of-fact manner and in terms easily accessible to persons unskilled in medical and scientific terminology. In particular, it is "imperative that patients be aware of potential diagnostic errors and the possibility of currently unknown long-term consequences on the fetus (and subsequently born child) of the embryo biopsy procedure."[1]

While the persons seeking PGD will almost certainly be competent adults with an above average amount of education, they are also very likely to be struggling with the reproductive decisions they face and seriously worried about outcomes. Clinicians providing PGD and all other infertility and reproductive services should be especially careful to avoid intentionally exploiting the anxiety and apprehension (or even desperation) of persons who know they are at risk for transmitting a genetic disease to their offspring.

Justice and Ability to Pay

Marked discrepancies in the use of prenatal genetic diagnosis already exist between affluent white women and other women in the US.[8] As PGD becomes more available, this pattern will undoubtedly continue. It is certainly not inherently unethical for clinicians to offer health-care services such as cosmetic surgery, full body scans for detection of abnormalities, Laser-assisted in situ keratomileusis vision correction, or PGD, that are available only to those who can afford to pay for them on their own. But the lack of broad availability of PGD for the less economically advantaged does become ethically problematic to the extent PGD satisfies fundamental human needs but remains unavailable to them (like basic preventive and acute health-care services) or produces "additional social advantages for the well-to-do" by enhancing their offspring to which others cannot get access.[8] Insofar as PGD can be legitimately considered something owed as a matter of social justice to all persons in need, then it is the duty of the society in question to make PGD available to all. Finally, it is worth noting that it is seriously ethically questionable for public funds to be used in the development of PGD services when they are largely available only to persons of high socioeconomic status.

MORAL STATUS OF THE EXTRACORPOREAL EMBRYO

The PGD is intended to result in the selective destruction (or the limbo of indefinite freezing) of extracorporeal human embryos following genetic analysis. Some consider PGD to be morally preferable to traditional prenatal genetic diagnosis because it precludes the need of an abortion to avoid the birth of a genetically abnormal child. This moral advantage to PGD can be understood in one of two ways. First, the woman who would have to undergo the abortion may find it morally preferable from her personal point of view to discard embryos prior to implantation rather than undergoing a surgical or medical abortion with its attendant physical and psychological risks. Second, one could claim that discard is not morally wrong because extracorporeal embryos either lack moral status altogether or have less moral status than gestating embryos or fetuses, either of which makes destroying them in utero via abortion more morally problematic.

For many, the ethical acceptability of the destruction of human embryos turns much more on the inherent moral status or standing of the (gestating or extracorporeal) human embryo than on someone's moral preference for discard over abortion given that both end in the death of the human entity. If, as some contend, all human embryos have the same moral status as live-born persons,[14] then they are entitled to basic rights, including the right not to be killed arbitrarily or for the purpose of advancing the interests of other persons. In this view, PGD that resulted in the destruction of extracorporeal embryos, as well as abortion following traditional prenatal genetic diagnosis, would be seriously morally wrong. The opposing view would hold that embryos lack any moral status whatsoever as they lack any properties, such as sentience or other cognitive traits, that determine moral standing and so can be destroyed at will.

Perhaps the more commonly held and more ethically defensible position is that human embryos deserve some modest moral status because they are alive, have some degree of potential to become human persons, and are in fact valued by moral agents whose views deserve at least some respect and deference from others, but they nevertheless do not possess the full and equal moral standing of persons because they lack interests and other moral claims to personhood. Having a modest level of moral status does not preclude the destruction of embryos for a morally serious reason or purpose, and the informed and conscientious choice of the persons who created the embryos to prevent the birth of a child with a serious genetic disease or abnormality is widely (though by no means universally) considered to be such a reason.

This ethical position roughly parallels that of current American constitutional law which does not recognize embryos or fetuses as legal persons with rights (including the 14th Amendment rights not to be deprived of life, liberty, or property without due process of law and to have the equal protection of the laws), but recognizes considerable value in these entities through the State's substantial interest in preserving potential human life, an interest that becomes particularly compelling at viability.[15] This interpretation of constitutional personhood means that the State may ban postviability abortions (40 states have done so) unless an abortion is necessary to preserve the pregnant woman's life or health, but it may not totally ban previability abortions or otherwise place an undue burden on a woman's right to terminate her pregnancy.[16] In the absence of a state statute prohibiting the practice (and none exist at present), the discarding of embryos following PGD with the informed consent of the gamete sources cannot be considered a violation of the embryo's legal rights or be a form of criminal homicide in the US. Whether the state could constitutionally ban PGD and IVF because they result in embryo discard is uncertain. Such a ban implicates not only the legal status of extracorporeal embryos, but also the constitutionally protected right of the persons whose gametes constitute the embryo to reproduce.[17]

However, the legal status of human embryos is not uniform around the world. Recently, the European Court of Human Rights ruled that the unborn are not human beings entitled to full human rights under applicable human rights conventions and that each national government must settle this legal issue for itself.[18] The legal status of embryos and the legal propriety of PGD vary in Europe. For example, PGD is currently illegal in Germany and Switzerland, although a recent study shows that a majority of Germans think the technique should be permitted for detecting genetic diseases.[19,20] The German Embryo Protection Law protects embryos from "improper use" and forbids genetic analysis of an embryo at the eight-cell stage or before.[21] One Austrian clinician has reported that the legal permissibility of PGD in Austria is unclear.[20] PGD has been authorized in France since 1994, but it is strictly limited to cases in which there is a strong probability of the presence of a severe genetic disorder known to be incurable at the time of diagnosis.[22] The Human Fertilization and Embryology Authority in the United Kingdom has licensed PGD for certain severe or life-threatening disorders at a limited number of clinics.[23] PGD is legally permitted in the Netherlands and Spain as well.[20]

Returning to the ethical analysis, the persons most humanly and ethically connected to human embryos are the individual men and women whose gametes wholly constitute the embryo. Almost all persons care deeply if their gametes or embryos are used for reproduction, and being a genetic parent is linked in profound ways to the individual's identity and the meaning he or she gives to life. Embryos ethically "belong" to the people who created them, even if they are not property like inanimate objects.[24]

Consequently, even though embryos themselves have only modest moral status, it is nonetheless seriously morally wrong to use the extracorporeal embryos of persons for any purpose without their informed consent. A corollary to this view is that the discarding of embryos secondary to PGD with the informed consent of the persons whose gametes created them is morally proper. In other words, the persons who created an embryo have the right of exclusive control over the disposition of those embryos, a right grounded in their interest in making the intimate, personal decision of when and how to reproduce. As no one else has a more significant moral connection to the embryos than the persons who created them, no one else has the moral authority to overrule their decision about the disposition of their embryos. Yet this right of disposition does not render embryos morally insignificant or allow them to be used for a morally trivial purpose; human embryos retain their modest moral status in any event.[24]

ETHICS AND THE CURRENT USES OF PGD

Before considering the ethics of the dominant use of PGD (the prevention of heritable genetic diseases), let us consider the other major uses mentioned previously: the identification (and discard) of chromosomally abnormal embryos in IVF and testing for HLA compatibility with an existing child. A moral objection to the former is actually an objection to the entire IVF process insofar as it results in the discard or indefinite cryopreservation of any human embryos which have the moral status of persons with full and equal basic rights because this status would preclude their destruction or suspended animation. The objection to the intentional destruction of extracorporeal embryos for any purpose rests upon the very controversial conclusion that such immature human entities are entitled to the very same moral respect owed to born persons. Moreover, the objection considers the benefits to the parents of a child born free of a serious, even devastating, genetic disease and to the child herself to be morally irrelevant, a conclusion that seems myopic and incomplete.

The use of PGD for HLA testing and selection of embryos who, when born, can serve as stem cells donors for their seriously ill siblings is certainly more controversial than PGD used for the detection of aneuploidy. The most commonly heard objection here is that the child to be conceived, is being used as a means to benefit the already existing diseased child and her parents and is not being brought into the world for her own sake, a violation of the Kantian principle of respect for persons. For this same reason, the parents' motives for conception of a child are considered ethically improper. Some critics would also claim that the child will be harmed psychologically once she finds out that she was brought into the world for the purpose of saving a sibling.

The moral objection to the child being conceived as a means to an end really has force only if the parents actually have this specific intent and treat the child in a manner consistent with it by, e.g. putting the child up for adoption immediately after stem cell harvesting or abandoning her. No public report could be located that documents such a state of affairs; in fact, the children born in this manner appear to be loved and valuable members of the family just as their ill sibling is. People conceive children for a wide variety of reasons and motives to have help in their old age, to fulfill cultural expectations, to make grandparents of their parents, to honor a command of God, to fulfill their own dreams of parenthood, and so on not all of which are morally admirable or accepted as legitimate by most persons. The real moral test is not the purity of parental motives, but the quality of their behavior during pregnancy and after birth, which should show love, concern, and dedication to their child. Moreover, as existing children can properly serve as bone marrow donors for sick siblings, then it follows by analogy that it is ethically acceptable for parents to make a child who will serve in the same role, assuming all children involved are loved and not subjected to procedures that are clearly contrary to their best interests.[11] Finally, it is implausible to assume that psychological harm will come to children who serve as donors when they are as likely to benefit from knowing, they assisted in preserving their sibling's life.

The most common utilization of PGD is by a particular woman who wishes to avoid bearing a child with a genetic disease or abnormality that she (and commonly a spouse or partner) finds unacceptable. Actually, the risk of bearing such a child is reduced, but not eliminated, because PGD can only detect diseases or conditions with an identified genetic basis (such as certain single gene defects and translocations), and it has an estimated error rate in the range of 1–10%, depending on the particular disease and assay being evaluated.[1] Errors are particularly bothersome when testing autosomal recessive or dominant conditions due to the phenomenon of allele specific dropout.[25]

While the key purpose of traditional, nondirective prenatal diagnosis is to provide persons with information about the genetic constitution of the pregnancy and not to render any opinion on its termination, the same cannot be said of PGD. "The purpose of PGD is not simply to inform couples about the genetic nature of their embryos. The explicit purpose is also to transfer healthy embryos and to discard those destined to be affected. Once a couple has chosen PGD, nondirectiveness is no longer relevant."[8] Therefore, the very purpose of PGD is to avoid the gestation and birth of a child who will have, or is likely to have, an identifiable genetic disease or disability of some sort. Nevertheless, clinicians remain ethically obligated not to impose on the prospective parents the values they bring to the assessment of a given embryo's genetic condition.

As a matter of general principle, prevention of the birth of a (genetically or otherwise) diseased or disabled child (such as one with profound mental retardation) is plainly a morally legitimate goal. If it were not, then it would make no sense to encourage pregnant (or prepregnant) women to avoid smoking tobacco or consuming large amounts of alcohol, to obtain competent prenatal care, or to take folic acid. But the prevention of such births is at least morally permissible, even if it is not morally obligatory.

There are two fundamental moral objections that can be levied at this particular goal:

- The methods taken to avoid the birth—the intentional discarding of embryos in the case of PGD, is morally wrong (this objection, based on the moral status of the embryo, was discussed above).
- The conception of "disease or disability" being utilized by prospective parents and the clinicians assisting their reproduction is morally deficient. In addition, strong moral objections have been made to the use of PGD to determine conditions that cannot plausibly be called "diseases," such as sex and the absence of desirable physical, mental, or social characteristics.

Disease and Disability

Historically, medicine has offered prenatal diagnosis as a means of preventing the birth of children with so-called serious inherited disorders such as Tay Sachs, Trisomy 13, 18 and 21, cystic fibrosis, muscular dystrophy, Huntington, Lesch-Nyhan, and neurofibromatosis. To one degree or another, each of these conditions *may* entail the imposition of pain, suffering, shortened life span, and/or significant inability to engage in typical activities of daily living on the individual with the condition. They also *may* place personal and economic burdens of one degree or another on the individual's parents, family, and even the society in which they live. These considerations lead some individuals to conclude that they would rather not give birth to a child with such a disorder; they then turn to medical professionals such as those who provide PGD—to assist them in effectuating this decision. Embryo selection then prevents disability by avoiding the gestation of individuals who would (or likely) be significantly disabled or diseased if born.

Recently, disability activists have strongly challenged what they deem to be the basic assumption underlying PGD and traditional prenatal diagnosis; reducing the incidence of disease and disability is an obvious and unambiguous good. They rightly criticize certain views that can, and frequently do, support this assumption that the disabled's enjoyment of life is necessarily less than for nondisabled people; that raising a child with a disability is a wholly undesirable thing; and that selective embryo discard or abortion necessarily saves mothers from the heavy burdens of raising disabled children.[26] Not all disabled persons are barred from having a satisfying life by their disability (although the social disadvantages and discrimination they encounter do decrease their quality of life), nor it is the case that raising a disabled child is always terribly burdensome or unrewarding.

However, the ethical critique of the disability activists goes much deeper than this quite proper debunking of broadly drawn and inaccurate assumptions about life with any disability. First, they contend that the medical system tends to exaggerate the "burden" associated with having a disability and underestimates the functional abilities of the disabled. "Conditions receiving priority attention for prenatal (genetic testing) are Down syndrome, spina bifida, cystic fibrosis, and Fragile X, whose clinical outcomes are usually mildly to moderately disabling. Individuals with these conditions can live good lives."[26] The activists also point out how medical language reinforces the negativity associated with disability by using such terms as "deformity" or "defective embryo or fetus."

Second, and more importantly, the disability activists claim that the promotion and use of PGD and traditional prenatal diagnosis "sends a message" to the public that negatively affects existing disabled people and fosters an increase in the oppression and prejudice from which they regularly suffer. The so-called "message" of PGD that the birth of disabled persons who are defective or deformed ought to be prevented—"may have the effect of triggering additional oppression, reinforcing the general public's perception that disability is a tragic mistake (that could and should have been avoided) and that disabled people are, therefore, justifiably marginalized."[26]

Some commentators within the disability community acknowledge that disability itself is not inherently a neutral condition, that it may limit some options and impose real health problems and diminished human capacities. But they also emphasize that "oppressive social conditions have so distorted the public's perceptions (of disability and disabled persons), as well as how disabled individuals themselves might internalize these perceptions, that it is difficult to assess the true impact of disability

on the individual's life experiences."[26] In other words, the real negative impact of disability in and of itself is exceedingly difficult to isolate because of deep and pervasive social discrimination against disabled individuals and widely shared, strongly negative social views on the meaning and personal impact of disability.

Insofar as individual clinicians do, in fact, exaggerate the problems and burdens of living as an individual with a disability or of living with a disabled person as a parent or family member, then they are doing a moral disservice to the people they are duty bound to be helping. Adults who wish to reproduce are ethically obligated to do so in a responsible manner, and this means (insofar as it is possible in a world about which we have imperfect knowledge) gathering and assessing fair and accurate information about what the future might hold for them and the child they might produce. Clinicians (especially genetic counselors) should endeavor to provide this kind of information, supplemented if at all possible by the firsthand information that comes from those who have actually lived with disabilities of various kinds as parents of the disabled or from the disabled individuals themselves. For example, it is certainly true that not all individuals with Down syndrome or their parents live painful, frustrated, or tragically diminished lives. The same is true for individuals with spina bifida, cystic fibrosis, Fragile X, and other genetic disorders.

On the other hand, these conditions are simply not utterly benign or neutral as each may and often does—involve what can fairly be described as an "undesirable event such as pain, repeated hospitalizations and operations, paralysis, a shortened life span, limited educational and job opportunities, limited independence, and so forth."[27] Even though not all instances of such disorders will involve the experience of such problems, a significant risk that an individual may encounter them always exists. A prospective parent who chooses to act on his or her conclusion that it is better for a child not to have, or to be at significant risk to have, such serious disorders is acting reasonably. "We do no one—not disabled individuals, not women, not families—a service by minimizing the physical, mental, and emotional burdens that may result from parenting children with disabilities."[27]

The claim of certain disability advocates that those who utilize PGD as patients or who offer it as clinicians are necessarily "sending a message" to the public that it is ethically right to oppress or discriminate against the disabled, or that the birth of any disabled child is a tragic mistake which ought to have been avoided, is simply untenable. "From the fact, that a couple wants to avoid the birth of a child with a disability, it just does not follow that they value less the lives of existing people with disabilities, any more than taking folic acid to avoid spina bifida indicates a devaluing of the lives of people with spina bifida."[27] The attempt on the part of a prospective parent to avoid the conception and birth of child with a disability through PGD (and it is *always* just an attempt as there are no guarantees) does not mean that he or she would surely reject or fail to love a child born with a disability or show disrespect to an existing disabled person.

While it is morally permissible for a prospective parent to discard an embryo with a genetic disease, it would be seriously wrong for him or her to "discard" or reject a live-born child with the same disease. Adults who reproduce must take moral and legal responsibility for their reproductive decisions, and this necessarily includes accepting the risk that the child born to them may not be "perfect" or not as healthy as they would like. Unlike an embryo that has only modest moral status whose very existence can properly be controlled by the persons who created it, a live-born child is an independent individual with full and equal moral status who has now joined the human community and who cannot be arbitrarily discarded or destroyed by its parents without a serious moral wrong being done. Rejecting or not loving a child solely because he or she has a disability is reasonably considered morally arbitrary and wrong because the child has full and equal moral status while an extracorporeal embryo does not.

Society does not utilize PGD or traditional prenatal diagnosis, whatever "society's" views on disability might be. Individual persons utilize such services with the assistance of individual clinicians, and they do so in order to make deliberate choices about their personal reproduction and about their particular lives rather than leaving these entirely to chance. A choice that each individual makes about his or her own reproduction has no moral implication for how a similar choice ought to be made by another person: a choice not to implant an embryo with the gene for cystic fibrosis, while morally permissible, does not (indeed cannot) mean that the opposite choice by a different person is morally wrong. Nor does such a choice mean that the individual must, therefore, devalue persons living with cystic fibrosis. However, some commentators have argued that under certain circumstances persons have a positive ethical duty not to reproduce.[28]

Suppose PGD reveals the presence of a genetic abnormality, Down syndrome, in an embryo. Someone could say that an individual woman who chooses not to have that embryo transferred into her uterus is rejecting persons with Down syndrome, but there is another, more plausible interpretation as well. "What I would say is 'I do not want my child to be born with Down syndrome,' meaning 'if I have a choice, I want the person who will be my child to be born into a body without such potentially significant limitations'.... That's all [I am expressing]. For a person with a disability to take this as a personal rejection seems unreasonable to me."[29] The claim of the disability activists that the meaning of PGD must be that "people like us will never be born" is unfounded: of course "they will [be born], they just won't have the disability. To me, this objection only really makes sense if people with disabilities are their disabilities" which they are not.[29]

In sum, discrimination against persons with disabilities is just as morally repugnant as discrimination against persons based on race, religion, or sex, but it is not at all clear that PGD reinforces or contributes to this in any manner. Regardless of how society might change (as it surely *ought* to change) its attitudes and practices to decrease or, better, eliminate the socially created disadvantages wrongly placed on the disabled, and regardless of how individual persons might change their views on the prospect of knowingly having a child with a serious disability, other persons "will prefer not to have a child with a serious disability, no matter how wonderful the social services, no matter how inclusive the society. This is a perfectly acceptable attitude, one that does not impugn their ability to be good parents. Nor does this attitude imply a devaluing of the lives of existing people with disabilities, any more than do programs to vaccinate children against polio or ensure that pregnant women get enough folic acid."[27] It is, this individual choice that PGD preserves, although the clinicians who offer PGD have a moral obligation to explore their own and their patients' attitudes about, and understanding of, disability so these individual decisions can be made fairly and responsibly with accurate information about the real world of life with and without disability.

PGD and Selection for Sex and other Desirable Characteristics

Three methods for prepregnancy or prebirth sex selection are available:

1. Prefertilization separation of X-bearing from Y-bearing sperm with selection of the desired sex for artificial insemination or IVF (MicroSort).
2. PGD with transfer of embryos of the desired sex.
3. Traditional prenatal diagnosis and selective abortion. However, given that IVF with PGD is expensive, technologically daunting, and imposes significant burdens on women, it has only limited usefulness as a method for sex selection, though it currently works much better than sperm sorting.[30] This may change as more reports of clinical experience with MicroSort are made publicly available.

Interestingly, the Ethics Committee of the ASRM has opined that "policies to prohibit or condemn as unethical all uses of nonmedically indicated preconception gender selection are not justified,"[1] yet it has also held that "initiation of IVF and PGD solely for sex selection holds even greater risk of unwarranted gender bias, social harm, and the diversion of medical resources from genuine medical need. It should therefore be discouraged."[31] The National Society of Genetic Counselors has flatly stated that couples wanting "sex selection for personal preference are not candidates for PGD."[2] The primary ethical distinction between sperm sorting and PGD rests on the fact that the latter involves the creation and destruction of embryos which have some moral status and are, therefore, entitled to some moral respect, while gametes have no moral status.

The selection of an embryo's sex via PGD is done for two basic reasons:

1. Preventing the transmission of sex-linked genetic disorders such as hemophilia A and B, Lesch-Nyhan syndrome, Duchenne-Becker muscular dystrophy, and Hunter syndrome.
2. Choosing sex to achieve gender balance in a family with more than one child, to achieve a preferred order in the birth of children by sex, or to provide a parent with a child of the sex he or she prefers to raise.[31] While little extended ethical debate exists regarding the former, sex selection for the purpose of preventing the transmission of sex-linked genetic disease, the latter is the subject of heated ethical disagreement.

The ethical objections to sex selection for nonmedical reasons can be grounded both in the very act of deliberately choosing one sex over the other and the untoward consequences of sex selection, particularly if it is performed frequently. Sex selection can be considered inherently ethically objectionable because it makes sex a determinative reason to value one human being over another when it ought to be completely irrelevant; females and males as such always ought to be valued equally and never differentially.

Sex selection can also be ethically criticized for the undesirable consequences it may generate. Choice by sex supports socially created assumptions about the relative value and meaning of "male" and "female," with the latter almost universally being considered seriously inferior to the former. By supporting assumptions that hold femaleness in lower social regard, sex selection enhances the likelihood that females will be the targets of infanticide, unfair discrimination, and damaging stereotypes. The experience in India and China, indicates that sex selection is commonly used to ensure the birth of males over females.[32] At one point in China there were 153 boys for every 100 girls.[30] A more recent report indicates that in parts of China, there are 140 boys for every 100 girls (in contrast to the US and world average of 105 boys for every 100 girls) and suggests that this will likely result in an increase in prostitution and the outright selling of women.[33] A preference for males as first-born could also disadvantage females as research consistently shows that first-born are more aggressive, more achieving, and of higher income and education than later-born children.[30]

Proponents of the ethical acceptability of sex selection would argue that a parent's desire for family balancing can be and typically is morally neutral. The defense of family balancing rests on the view that once a parent has a child of one sex, he or she can properly prefer to have a child of the other sex because the two genders are different and generate different parenting experiences.

To insist (that the experience of parenting a boy is different from that of parenting a girl) is not the case seems breathtakingly simplistic, as if gender played no role either in a person's personality or relationships to others. Gender may be partly cultural (which does not make it less "real"), but it probably is partly biological.... I see nothing wrong with wanting to have both experiences.[30]

Thus, gender differences in fact exist and appear to be both cultural and biological in origin; actual physical and psychological differences exist between male and female children that affect parental child rearing experiences in important ways.[34] Even one noted feminist author has asserted that gender. A similarity and complementarity are morally acceptable reasons for wanting a child of a certain sex.[35]

The defender of sex selection for family balancing can also point out that parents who desire this different experience can do so without believing or acting as if one sex is better than the other and without imposing harmful gender roles (e.g. females are emotional, not rational) upon their children. As persons having such a preference may do without believing that one sex is superior to another and with respect for the equal rights and status of females, proponents would argue that their preference should be respected incident to the exercise of their right to reproduce, especially in the absence of empirical evidence showing that the practice of sex selection actually harms females. Moreover, it can be argued that the modest moral respect due embryos is not offended by a parental choice made on the basis of sex.

It also seems very unlikely that sex selection would significantly skew the male-female balance in the US population or that of other developed Western nations. One US study has shown that among the respondents who would use sex selection, 81% of the women and 94% of the men would want their first-born to be a boy, which would result in more males receiving the advantage of being first-born. But given that this same study found that only 25% of all respondents would use sex selection methods, it appears unlikely that this would dramatically add to the number of first-born males. "Nevertheless, if sex selection became widely available, it might change the American family, making older sisters to younger brothers somewhat less common than they otherwise would be. Whether this change would be harmful enough to justify constraining choice (of sex), however, remains hard to say."[30] Overall, the predictions of potential bad consequences due to sex selection seem too speculative to be determinative of its moral propriety.[31]

An opponent of sex selection for family balancing can argue that good parents—whether prospective or actual—ought never to prefer, favor, or give more love to a child of one sex over the other. For example, a morally good and admirable parent would never love a male child more than a female child, give the male more privileges than a female, or give a female more material things than a male simply because of sex or beliefs about the child's "proper" gender. A virtuous and conscientious parent, then, ought not to think that, or behave as if, a child of one sex is better than the other sex, nor should a good parent believe or act as if, at bottom, girls are really different than boys in the ways that truly matter.

The argument in favor of sex selection for family balancing has to assume that gender and gender roles exist and matter in the lived world. For if they did not, then no reason would exist to differentiate the experience of parenting a male child from that of a female. However, it is precisely the reliance upon this assumption to which the opponent of sex selection objects: accepting and perpetuating gender roles inevitably both harms and wrongs both males and females, although females clearly suffer much more from them than males. While some gender roles or expectations are innocuous (e.g. men don't like asking for directions), the overwhelming majority (e.g. males "are" and "should be" aggressive, women "are" and "should be" self-sacrificing) are not. Consequently, given that sex selection is inevitably gendered and most gender roles and expectations restrict the freedom of persons to be who they wish to be regardless of gender, sex selection is at least strongly ethically suspect, if not outright wrong.

Some would claim that choosing the sex of our children is not the most morally worrisome application of PGD or other forms of medical intervention in reproduction; it is rather the prospect of our ability to choose the characteristics of our offspring. "The real threat comes from the identification of an increasing number of genetic markers associated with conditions that are not life-threatening, but impairing or socially undesirable, such as hyperactivity, homosexuality, and obesity."[36] Botkin notes that the moral reluctance to discard an embryo or abort a fetus for a less than serious medical condition already conflicts with the value of honoring parental autonomy "in this most intimate of enterprises."[8]

This conflict will be "exacerbated by the rapid increase in genetic tests for a wide range of conditions, including late-onset conditions, conditions with a limited impact on health, and, possibly, behavioral or physical characteristics that fall within the normal range."[8] Despite the apparent falsity of strict genetic determinism, "we may only need a popular *perception* of genetic determinism, fueled by creative marketing and weak regulation, to move poorly predictive tests from the laboratory into the clinic... These tests need not be very predictive to be adopted by some couples who want the very best that their sperm, eggs, and money can buy."[8] In this regard, it is also worth recalling the ASRM's characterization of PGD as "an established technique with specific and *expanding* applications for standard clinical practice"[34] (emphasis added).

Sex selection by PGD or traditional prenatal diagnosis is already available, although one recent study shows that a majority of physicians who offer PGD are not willing to do so for sex selection.[37] The existence of genetic tests linked (even tenuously) to certain desirable or undesirable social, psychological, or behavioral characteristics is highly likely to generate at least some demand from people who will pay the going rate for such tests up front in cash and who will be more than capable of giving informed consent to the procedure. The critical ethical question will be: should medical professionals provide any such tests (or sex selection for that matter) on request or, more likely, on demand?

Role of the Individual Clinician's Conscience

It is quite common for bioethicists to call for a "social" resolution of thorny questions like this that arise in medicine.[8,38] One type of social resolution comes from the law. However, an answer to the ethical and practical question of which genetic tests clinicians should offer will almost surely not come from the law which is (at least in the US) a typically politically charged, slow (it is consistently behind developments in science), expensive (for both lobbying and litigation), uncertain, and cumbersome method for regulating what physicians and other clinicians do, especially when it comes to human reproduction. A true social consensus about matters involving embryo destruction is even less likely, as witnessed by the current debate over therapeutic cloning and stem cell research, not to mention abortion. Some semblance of an answer may come from professional medical organizations in the form of "recommendations" or "guidelines," but they probably will be quite general and in need of interpretation and application to specific cases. Professional guidelines may also be intentionally ambiguously worded in order not to create a standard of care that could be legally enforced through civil lawsuits.

What then is a clinician involved in PGD to do? Should she perform PGD for sex selection for nonmedical reasons or for roughly determining, say, IQ (which probably has some genetic basis)? There undoubtedly will be coherent and serious ethical arguments on both sides of the question, as the brief review of the debate over sex selection (above) indicates. Thoughtful and conscientious clinicians will undoubtedly disagree, but this is the same situation with other controversial areas in medicine such as futility, the propriety of treatment in the absence of "medical indications," physician assisted suicide, and physician performed euthanasia.[39]

Little true consensus exists regarding when physicians and other clinicians ought to refuse to do certain interventions because they do not benefit patients, harm patients or others, are inconsistent with the healing nature of medicine, disrespect the value of human life, or are outside the legitimate scope of medicine which should be devoted to promoting human health, not human happiness or simple human preference. As a result of this variability in ethical interpretation, each individual clinician has to make a personal decision, in light of his or her own conscience and understanding of the ethical requirements of responsible professional practice, about which genetic tests he will and will not perform incident to PGD.

Conscience is a form of self-reflection on, and a judgment about, whether a particular act (or omission) is morally right or wrong, good or bad, but it is never self-certifying from the moral point of view.[40] Conscience has to be properly informed by the pertinent moral principles and rules as well as relevant professional values as well. But conscience must, at some point or another, lead the individual to take a stand on pressing ethical issues like which genetic tests of offer incident to PGD. And the stand must at least sometimes be "*this* I will *not* do." The very meaning and integrity of an individual as a moral agent turns on this: the good things any person does can be made complete *only* by the things she *refuses* to do.[39]

When conscientiously refusing to do PGD for sex or a new marker associated with homosexuality or increased height, a clinician is not necessarily adopting the position that it is unethical for any other clinician to act in this manner, although she may believe this to be so and may attempt to persuade others to exercise their consciences in the same manner. An individual clinician who refuses to perform PGD for some specific purpose is primarily acting in way that preserves her *personal* moral integrity and expresses her need to assume *personal* moral responsibility for her actions. Clinicians cannot control the behavior of other professionals in their field, but they can and should choose to conform their own behavior to the ethical standards they personally embrace, even if the field as a whole as not taken a firm stand on the relevant issue.

Each and every clinician involved in assisted reproductive medicine (whether physician, nurse, genetic counselor, or technician) should practice as a responsible individual moral agent who has developed an informed conscience and not as a vending machine of professional services operated on patient demand. Every clinician should recognize that not all of her colleagues may come to the same conclusion as she and that her professional organizations may waffle on certain issues and issue only vague or ambiguous ethical exhortations. But the lack of agreement or consensus on ethical issues does not permit a morally conscientious individual to follow the path of least resistance and simply do whatever can technologically be done and whatever a willing patient will pay for.

CONCLUSION

The PGD is a valuable addition to the repertoire of reproductive medicine as it gives individuals with a documented history of a genetic disorder, the opportunity to begin a wanted pregnancy with little or even possibly no fear that they are transmitting this disorder to their offspring. An outstanding example of this is the recent report of PGD being successfully used to avoid the conception of a child that could have inherited a predisposition to early-onset Alzheimer disease.[41] But if this service becomes embroiled in the detection of conditions having little or nothing to do with health and disease in order to satisfy patient demand or be a profitable business, its practitioners deserve will get and deserve serious ethical criticism.

REFERENCES

1. Practice Committee Report of the American Society for Reproductive Medicine and Society for Assisted Reproductive Technology. Preimplantation genetic diagnosis 2001. [online] Available from www.asrm.org. [Accessed June, 2002].
2. National Society of Genetic Counselors. Preimplantation genetic diagnosis. [online] Available from www.nsgc.org/pr_diagnosis_10_01.asp. [Accessed June, 2002].
3. Bahce M, Escudero T, Sandalinas M, et al. Improvements of preimplantation diagnosis of aneuploidy by using microwave hybridization, cell recycling and monocolour labeling of probes. Mol Hum Reprod. 2000;6:849-54.
4. Marquez C, Sandalinas M, Bahce M, et al. Chromosome abnormalities in 1255 cleavage-stage human embryos. Reprod BioMed Online. 2000;1:17-26.

5. Munne S. Preimplantation genetic diagnosis and human implantation—a review. Placenta. 2003;24:S70-6.

6. Verlinsky Y, Rechitsky S, Sharapova T, et al. Preimplantation HLA testing. JAMA. 2004;29:2079-85.

7. Kuliev A, Verlinsky Y. Thirteen years' experience of preimplantation diagnosis: Report of the Fifth International Symposium on Preimplantation Genetics. Reprod BioMed Online. 2004;8:229-35.

8. Botkin J. Ethical issues and practical problems in preimplantation genetic diagnosis. JLME. 1998;26:17-28.

9. American Society for Reproductive Medicine. [online] Available from www. asrm.org/Patients/FactSheets/invitro.ht-ml. [Accessed July, 2004].

10. Nelson LJ, Clark HW, Goldman RL, et al. Taking the train to a world of strangers: health care marketing and ethics. Hastings Cent Rep. 1989;19:36-43.

11. Sermon K, Van Steirteghem A, Liebaers I. Preimplantation genetic diagnosis. Lancet. 2004;363:1633-41.

12. American Society for Reproductive Medicine Ethics Committee. Shared-risk or refund programs in assisted reproduction. Available at www.asrm.org/Media/Ethics/shared.html. Accessed 8 July 2004.

13. American Medical Association, Council on Ethical and Judicial Affairs. Code of medical ethics. 1997;94-5.

14. President's Council on Bioethics. Human cloning and human dignity: the report of the President's Council on Bioethics. New York: Public Affairs; 2003. pp. 174-5.

15. Nelson LJ, Marshall MF. Ethical and legal analyses of three coercive policies aimed at substance abuse by pregnant women. Report to the Substance Abuse Policy Research Program of the Robert Wood Johnson Foundation, award #030790, 1998.

16. Planned Parenthood of Southeastern Pennsylvania vs Casey, 505 US, 1992;833.

17. Robertson J. Children of choice. Princeton: Princeton University Press; 1994. pp. 22-42.

18. European Court of Human Rights. Case of Vo vs France, 2004. Application no. 53925/00.

19. Preimplantation genetic diagnosis should be allowed in Germany, study reveals. [online] Available from www.medicalnewstoday.com/news.php?newsid=10048. [Accessed July, 2004].

20. Feichtinger W. Preimplantation diagnosis (PGD)—a European clinician's point of view. J Assist Reprod Genet. 2004;21:15-7.

21. Mueller S. Ethics and the regulation of preimplantation diagnosis in Germany. EJAIB. 1997;7:5-6.

22. Comite Consultatif National d'Ethique. Reflections concerning an extension of preimplantation genetic diagnosis. [online] Available from www.ccne-thique.fr/english/pdf/aviso72.pdf. [Accessed July, 2004].

23. Human Fertilisation and Embryology Authority, Advisory Committee on Genetic Testing. Consultation document on preimplantation genetic diagnosis. [online] Available from http://www.publications.doh.gov.uk/pub/docs/doh/preplant.pdf. [Accessed July, 2004].

24. Meyer MJ, Nelson LJ. Respecting what we destroy: reflections on human embryo research. Hastings Cent Rep. 2001;31:16-23.

25. Findlay I, Ray P, Quirke P, et al. Allelic drop-out and preferential amplification in single cells and human blastomeres: Implications for preimplantation diagnosis of sex and cystic fibrosis. Hum Reprod. 1995;10:1609-18.

26. Saxton M. Why members of the disability community oppose prenatal diagnosis and selective abortion. In: Parens E, Asch A (Eds). Prenatal Testing and Disability Rights. Washington DC: Georgetown University Press; 2000. pp. 147-64.

27. Steinbock B. Disability, prenatal testing, and selective abortion. In: Parens E, Asch A (Eds). Prenatal Testing and Disability Rights. Washington DC: Georgetown University Press; 2002. pp. 108-23.

28. Purdy L. Genetics and reproductive risk: can having children be immoral? In: Mappes T, DeGrazia D (Eds). Biomedical Ethics. Boston: McGraw Hill; 2001. pp. 520-7.

29. Baily MA. Why I had amniocentesis. In: Parens E, Asch A (Eds). Prenatal Testing and Disability Rights. Washington DC: Georgetown University Press; 2000. pp. 64-71.

30. Steinbock B. Sex selection: not obviously wrong. Hastings Cent Rep. 2002;32:23-8.

31. Ethics Committee of the American Society for Reproductive Medicine. Sex selection and preimplantation genetic diagnosis. Fertil Steril. 1999;72:595-8.

32. Allahbadia G. The 50 million missing women. J Assist Reprod Genet. 2002;19:411-6.

33. Johnson T. Officials foresee prostitution, selling of women. San Jose Mercury News. 2004; July 8: 1A, 13A.

34. Ethics Committee of the American Society for Reproductive Medicine. Preconception gender selection for nonmedical reasons. Fertil Steril. 2001;75:861-4.

35. Overall C. Ethics and Human Reproduction: A Feminist Analysis. Boston: Allen & Unwin; 1987. p. 27.

36. Wachbroit R, Wasserman D. Patient autonomy and value—neutrality in nondirective genetic counseling. Stanford Law and Policy Review. 1995;6:103-10.

37. Benson K, Udoff L, Escallon C. Physician attitude toward controversial applications of preimplantation genetic diagnosis. J Genet Couns. 2003;12:543-44.

38. Callahan D. Medical futility, medical necessity. Hastings Cent Rep. 1991;21:30-5.

39. Nelson LJ. Medical futility and the clinician's conscience. In: Misbin R, Jennings B, Orentlicher D, Dewar M (Eds). Health Care Crisis? The Search for Answers. University Park: University Publishing Group; 1995. pp. 60-70.

40. Beauchamp TL, Childress JF. Principles of Biomedical Ethics. New York: Oxford University Press; 1994. pp. 475-83.

41. Verlinsky Y, Rechitsky S, Verlinsky O, et al. Preimplantation diagnosis for early-onset Alzheimer disease caused by V717L mutation. JAMA. 2002;287:1018-21.

CHAPTER

20 Genetic Counseling

A Csaba, Z Papp

INTRODUCTION

In the past decades, genetic counseling has assumed an increasingly significant role in medical science. Deep changes in societal expectations coupled with the transforming social structure have led a growing number of married couples to make use of services offered by genetic counseling. Whereas at the time of Semmelweis, the saving of mothers' lives had constituted a breakthrough in obstetrical practice, the 20th century development of neonatology and perinatology leading to improved survival chances in fetuses and newborn babies, brought further significant progress. As birthrates decreased and families tended to be founded at older age, more and more pregnant women chose to take advantage of genetics. It became a more important, if not the most important, objective to enable families burdened with inheritable and accumulating problems to have healthy children. The natural selection process that works on a large scale was no longer acceptable for families desiring to have one or two children; therefore, the demand emerged in developed countries for the safest possible pregnancy care. As part of this development, genetic counseling developed and continues to assume an increasingly significant role. The recent, explosive progress in genetic research has made people believe that now every hereditary disease can be screened in time and prevented, that is, the birth of a sick baby can be avoided with absolute certainty. The requirement of living up to this expectation more comprehensively has led to establishing and launching genetic counseling centers that have become an integral part of the maternity care system. It has become virtually the first priority for families to expect the health care system to prepare and inform them and thus make it possible for them to accept pregnancy as a result of a well-informed and well-considered decision. Society has also recognized that for a number of reasons (healing, psychological, financial, societal, etc.) it is preferable to prevent diseases than treat them after their emergence.

The roots of genetic counseling go back a long time in history. The correction of the undesirable qualities of the human race and the curing of its diseases has preoccupied us since prehistoric times. In one of his works, The State, Plato (427–347 BC) (Fig. 20.1) described the way to improve people in "selective breeding". English scientist Francis Galton was the first to be engaged more thoroughly and more seriously in eugenics. (It was he that introduced the word eugenics in 1883.) In a book written in 1869 (Hereditary Genius), he proposed that outstanding men be married by a plan to well-to-do women in order for a talented race to emerge. In the first half of the 20th century, certain forces disgracefully used the science of genetics and its achievements as a distorted means of eugenics to underpin their racial theories (for the extinction of Jews, blacks and homosexuals) and also in the early 20th century this culminated in political dictatorships ordering sterilization for

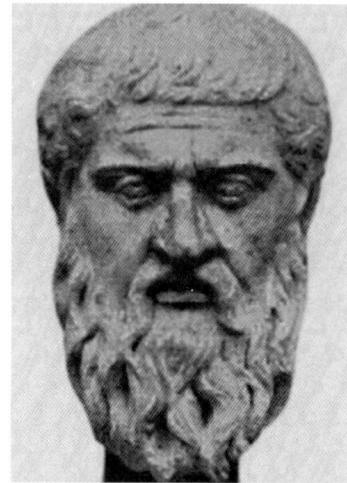

Fig. 20.1: Plato

individuals with high genetic risk. As a result, the application of genetic achievements was long stigmatized and it had a hard time regaining the appreciation it deserves.

Before discovering genetic rules, genetic counseling was based on empirical observations. In this process, it was important to recognize that certain diagnoses were more frequent in certain couples' descendants.

The 20th century witnessed revolutionary progress in the science of genetics that coincided with increasing societal demands and therefore became an integral part of modern genetic counseling. In the beginning, in the age of "classic genetic counseling", our means were quite limited. Genetic diseases were Mendelian disorders or diseases that were inheritable through one gene. Then counseling extended merely to clarifying the genetic, i.e. hereditable nature of a certain disease and informing the patients about the risk or recurrence. This was the time when society's demand for the prevention of diseases emerged, but our scientific and technical possibilities were still rather restricted. Regrettably, we were in no position to offer a reassuring "alternative" to the couples that approached us with their problems. Those asking for advice had to make do with mere information, the rigid percentage numbers of the risk of repetition, on the basis of which they could make their decision on whether to have a child. In many cases, however, the high risk of occurrence and/or recurrence communicated by the physician forever deterred the couple from having another child. To be sure, in other cases, it was useful for the couple to know that with the knowledge about the heredity of the given problem, they could safely have another pregnancy without having to dread the recurrence of the disease that they had feared. In that period, there could occur such a situation (due to a lack of assisted reproduction techniques) when genetic counseling shed light on a disease inherited in a recessive manner, which might have led the couple to the conclusion that their descendants were exposed to a heightened risk. This could, unfortunately, result in the deterioration of the relationship, and even in their divorce, in order that they both could increase their respective chance to have a healthy child. At last, the physician performing genetic counseling was also in a difficult position, since in many cases he was aware that he could not give the assistance that was needed, and he must have sensed the tension generated by the puzzlement in the couple seeking advice. (In certain cases, this feeling has, unfortunately, remained known to physicians providing genetic counseling.)

THEORETICAL AND PRACTICAL MEANS OF GENETIC COUNSELING

Genetic counseling is centered on close interactive communication between those requesting and those giving advice. Genetic counseling centers operate in numerous countries of the world. Their task everywhere is to give information about hereditary diseases, to let patients know about the possible cures, and not least to define the method of heredity. Knowing the type of heredity is indispensable for figuring out the risk of occurrence and/or recurrence, which is the most frequently asked and most important question for pregnant women or couples wanting babies, and therefore seeking counseling.

Thus, genetic counseling can basically be divided into two major branches:

1. Finding out if the disease of a newborn baby, older child or adult is hereditary, making diagnosis, and providing information about the possible treatment.
2. Counseling during pregnancy concerning the occurrence and/or recurrence of hereditary (genetically determined) diseases in a family or those materializing in pregnancy, using prenatal diagnostic tools with the aim of ensuring the birth of a healthy offspring.

Although, the two branches obviously focus on the same diseases, they require different approaches. All over the world, genetic counseling is primarily done by biologists, geneticists, and various medical specialists, mainly pediatricians and obstetricians.[1–3] Pregnant women and their partners facing various genetic problems can base their decision on information and advice made available by these professionals' knowledge and expertise.[4] Counseling can follow two principles: (1) the more widely used *nondirective* genetic counseling and (2) the so-called *directive* genetic counseling.[5] Because the current era is dominated by legal claims against physicians, the nondirective method is more acceptable and more easily defendable, even though in many cases patients expect and demand a decision-shaping process closely guided by the physicians. When applying the nondirective method, the genetic counselor is ready to share information in a nondirective manner without committing to any potential alternative. It is very important that having thoroughly described the disease in question, the consultant should also inform the patient about the risk of occurrence and/or recurrence. After that, diagnostic alternatives should be described and offered if there are any. This has to be done in a fashion, so that the patients seeking counseling can understand the basic facts, and it may vary with the given circumstances. The patient's fear and anxiety must not be worsened by giving an opinion expressed in mystical, complicated sentences that are incomprehensible to ordinary people. By this point, the couples have already started the decision-making process. The physician leaves it to the patients to use the intensive interactive process to arrive at their final decision. Various prenatal screening and diagnostic methods have demonstrated revolutionary progress and have been made indispensable parts and means of modern genetic counseling.

Often screening tests could at least lower the excitement and nervousness, but it was prenatal diagnostics that made the real breakthrough in the practice of genetic counseling. At this point during counseling one has to mention the inevitable necessity to explain the differences between screening tests and diagnostic tests. Society mistakenly confuses the two examinations and attributes to them equal importance. In the daily practice, this can result in erroneous decisions because many regard the reassuring results of the screening tests as a safe diagnosis. Too often we can hear the following statement from a 40-year-old pregnant woman and her 50-year-old husband: "As the biochemical markers (triple-quadro test) are normal, and the genetic ultrasound examination has not detected any visible abnormalities either, we can rest assured, for we cannot have a child with chromosome abnormalities. We do not want amniocentesis". Screening tests are performed to help us detect and "take out" those who face a higher than average risk in certain pathological conditions of concern. Some procedures may serve a screening purpose in some cases while they can have a diagnostic value in association with another disease. Sonography is one of these procedures, but it is only of a screening nature in the case of Down syndrome, while it has a diagnostic value in the case of anencephaly, spina bifida and hydrocephalus.

Among prenatal *diagnostic tools*, we distinguish between *noninvasive* and *invasive* methods. *Sonography*, one of the most frequently and widely used, dynamically developing examination procedure belongs to the first group. In the noninvasive group, we also find the tests using maternal blood, from which tests with fetal cells obtained from maternal circulation deserve more and more attention. The arsenal of invasive prenatal diagnostics is also steadily broadening, but those applied first in the practice of genetic counseling remain its most frequent procedures. These are genetic *amniocentesis* (GAC) and *chorionic villus sampling* (CVS). Invasive procedures, unfortunately, carry certain risks for the fetus and the pregnant woman. Their complications have a considerable influence on the patients' decision, since in many cases they perceive their situation as a choice between bad and worse. In this context, it is understandable that the essential factor on which they base their decision is the intention to opt for the less risky examination if they are given a choice. The pain and tension caused by the examination also appear as a problem in invasive examination, but this does not have a decisive influence when making the final choice. While these procedures are not painless, the pain is not extensive either.

This strong interrelatedness between genetic counseling and prenatal diagnostics is largely determined and driven by ultrasound examinations that, as a result of rapid technological advancements, allow the physician to follow more closely the life of the embryo and the fetus.[6–8] Ultrasound is biologically harmless, so undergoing an ultrasound examination cannot pose a serious dilemma for pregnant women. However, despite the accumulation of an increasingly significant amount of expertise and knowledge, it is often difficult to evaluate and interpret the results of the examination. Modern medical examination equipment with largely improved detection capabilities makes even tiny "suspicious signs" recognizable.[9] Nevertheless, these signs can lead to differing interpretations, thereby causing unwarranted concern among patients. The sonograph can record even tiny divergences from normal conditions that cannot be ignored, because written documents can later serve as legal evidence. Frequently, we are in no position to perform further noninvasive examinations to reassure the patients. This often renders invasive examinations advisable, potentially putting the patients in a difficult decision-making situation. Patients can become anxious or even fearful, because they are apt to treat machine made images virtually as facts, and to interpret them as serious threats to the fetus. It is then a daunting task to dispel anxiety or fear because the patients tend to believe the "objective" computer. Here too, the nondirective method is advisable, and it is important to point out not only the possible pathologic conditions, but also the possibility of a reassuring outcome. For this reason, it is essential to follow closely any abnormalities detected during ultrasound examinations in later stages of the pregnancy and after delivery. This approach can lead us to a stage when images currently interpreted as "suspicious signs" will not result in groundless tension and fears for the pregnant woman.

Practice standards regarding ultrasound examinations during pregnancy vary from country to country. In some countries, one or two examinations are deemed sufficient without providing much detail as to how these should be timed. Nearly a decade ago, we introduced in Hungary a carefully designed system that pays due consideration to the interests of pregnant women and to professional rationality. Our protocol advises four plus one examinations for the pregnant woman, with the first taking place during the first call (usually in the fifth to eighth week), the others after in the tenth to twelfth, the eighteenth to twentieth, the twenty-eighth to thirtieth, and the thirty-sixth to thirty-eighth week. If necessary, we advise an intrauterine examination of the fetus's heart (echocardiography).[10] The pregnant woman must understand that these examinations are part of a series of screening tests meant to check on the intrauterine development of the fetus. Countries advising or performing fewer examinations partly cite high costs and question the efficiency of the examinations. There are also skeptical opinions about whether ultrasound examinations can significantly improve morbidity and mortality indicators.[11] Some others, arguing against ultrasound examinations, also point to the misleading, wrongly reassuring effects of "false negative" diagnoses. Well-elaborated and organized sonographic training can, however, minimize such risks. It is imperative that examinations be carried out and interpreted by trained and experienced professionals.

Such invasive genetic examinations as amniocentesis, chorionic villus sampling, and fetal blood sampling have become indispensable means of prenatal diagnostics and genetic counseling. These examinations allow us to obtain genetic information, leading to major breakthroughs in the development of genetic counseling. Samples obtained during invasive procedures are helpful in performing several examinations, and the number of diseases that can be detected this way is steadily increasing. Beyond detecting chromosome irregularities, these are now important means of diagnosing monogenic inheritable diseases (Mendelian inheritance) as well. From the samples, we can also perform microbiological and serological examinations. The newest molecular genetic techniques are opening a previously unhoped-for dimension in prenatal diagnostics. Beyond dangers arising from the invasive nature of such examinations (due to the higher risk of miscarriage), their more widespread use has raised numerous ethical questions as well. Even when we face increased risks of genetic, inheritable diseases, we must try our best to make sure that no sick children are born, while giving couples a realistic chance to have a healthy newborn. Here, we have a reverse situation: contrary to ultrasound examinations, in this case the interpretation of examination results leaves very few questions owing to diagnostic accuracy from the principle of methods applied. In these cases, however, the examination carries dangers that create significant tension, concern, and complicated decision situations. There can emerge a peculiar and difficult contradiction because the patients would like to have a healthy child, but the examination necessary to make this happen might endanger the further development of the fetus. When the woman makes this decision, the physician must stick with nondirective counseling, which allows him to inform patients about the benefits and drawbacks, but has him answer any further question about what decision to make in a nondirective fashion. The final decision has to come from the woman. The genetic counselor must not assume a "divine role" and cannot be familiar with all relevant aspects of another person's life. Even in cases that seem identical, the final decisions can be different. A 37-year-old couple who already have three healthy children and where the woman can conceive without difficulty is likely to request karyotyping, whereas a couple having tried in vain to conceive a child for 15 years can be very concerned about the threat of miscarriage and may choose not to have such an invasive act performed.

During genetic counseling, certain "semi-invasive" examinations can also be of assistance; these are widely used in screening because of their minimal level of invasiveness. Nevertheless, as a result of their being a screening test, they can produce false positive results, generating serious concern in pregnant women. Biochemical marker tests done from samples of the mother's blood (AFP, BHCG, E2, PAPP-A, Inhibin) constitute one sort of these genetic screening examinations. Besides false positive results, there are some false negative test results as well, which makes it essential to explain to patients that screening examinations do not provide the basis for establishing a diagnosis. In view of the existing risk factors of invasive examinations, one has to aim at putting together as reliable a screening examination protocol as possible. There are ongoing efforts to examine an increasing number of serum markers that can be combined with ultrasound examinations (e.g. nuchal translucency) to improve results. Because of fears of being held accountable and exposed to malpractice claims, the drawing of the point will regrettably increase the number of false positive cases, which, in turn, will demand a larger capacity for intrauterine chromosome analysis.

DECISION-MAKING: RIGHTS AND RESPONSIBILITIES

Physicians who have provided genetic counseling for an anxious married couple have faced their distress and feelings of insecurity. The very uncertainty shadowing the health of their desired offspring puts a considerable burden on the expectant woman and her spouse. Add to that the further risk of various other special circumstances, and the result can be an effectively unbearable load. Those couples seeking genetic counseling almost always carry the "extra burden", that being the very reason why their physician sends them to consult a specialist.

Many decision-making situations crop up during genetic counseling. In certain cases, the first question to answer is whether or not the patient is ready for pregnancy, knowing the genetic risk.

The individual seeking counseling must decide if she wants to have the preferred diagnostic test. Another decision may have to be made with regard to the patient's wish to carry on with or terminate pregnancy in the case of a positive result (indicating disease).[2,12,13]

The diverse nature of genetic problems necessitates separating the following branches in order to better understand decision-making mechanisms:

a. Those cases requiring invasive, high-risk intervention (chromosome defects).
b. Monogenic diseases with a high-risk of occurrence and/or recurrence.
c. Low-risk genetic situations (taking medicine, diagnostic X-ray examinations).
d. Uncertain conditions for which diagnostics are limited (certain infections and anatomical defects detectable by serology or ultrasound where the outcome cannot be predicted).

One important consideration is whether the available means can result in a rock-solid diagnosis, or the problem in hand cannot be diagnosed during pregnancy, although certain results may indicate pathological conditions. The decision-making mechanism seems to be affected by a couple of factors, including risk of recurrence, seriousness of the disease, risk of the procedure, maternal age, previous pathological pregnancies (malformations, miscarriages), number of healthy offspring, level of education, religious faiths, and convictions of conscience.

The kind of genetic counseling, we prefer lets the patients have the final word. Neither the right to make a decision nor the responsibility resulting from that decision can rest with the genetic counselor. This point is important because it makes many legal claims avoidable. The nondirective counseling process can be easily violated, because patients can be manipulated by carefully determining the sequence of sentences. It must be our objective to be as neutral as possible, while providing comprehensive and honest information to patients. Our words ought not to give away which decision we might favor. Although, it is true that we cannot exist without having certain ideals, values, and views, and that we are bound to form an opinion about what we say in a counseling situation, the patients should not sense that we might disagree with their decision or that we might judge them negatively as a result. For the pregnant woman and her partner to accurately feel the weight of their decision, it is necessary to stress that they can choose freely from the alternatives described to them. They have to see clearly the consequences of whatever decision they opt for.

It would be very difficult to conceive of any other counseling mechanism and decision-making process in democratic states where the wide-ranging rights of the individual are safeguarded. In democratic systems, however, one should not forget about obligations and responsibilities. Systems that exclusively emphasize rights, but not the obligations, are moving toward anarchy. This anarchy would obviously apply to the field of genetic counseling as well. For free choice to be preserved, it is crucial that the decision made by the patients in no way influences further pregnancy care, and that the physicians continue to provide the broadest range of services possible.

The weight of the decision requires that pregnant women be given sufficient time to ponder the various dimensions of their choices. In most cases, the pregnant woman finds it reassuring to discuss her situation with her partner or physician and to seek the advice of her family before committing to one of the alternatives. It is highly possible that the patient and the counselor will have to see each other more than once.

During counseling, the physician should be understanding and patient—one cannot overemphasize the role empathy plays in the process. Dramatic statements, gestures, and other forms of nonverbal communication are equally impermissible during nondirective genetic counseling. A written report must be prepared about the counseling session and the patient's decision.

The complex nature of genetic counseling and its relatively short history are bound to raise several moral and ethical questions. Although, there is an emerging consensus on the older problems, the new possibilities and achievements have caused significant rifts among physicians and scientists. These developments are increasingly prevalent in our everyday life, and their divisive effects can be felt in the society as well. When it comes to genetics and our endeavors to influence heredity, society tends to be sharply divided. In these situations, the individual's freedom and need to decide are at play simultaneously.

The counselor is not in an easy situation either. In these complicated and often very difficult decision-making situations, the consultant's room for maneuver is rather limited due to the nondirective principle of counseling. One can feel every now and then that the advice-seeker counts on the consultant's help when making her decision. Limited though the consultant's opportunities may be, he is still able to help by supplying clear and direct information relevant to the case. He is not to use either verbal or metacommunicative means that might suggest he is taking a firm stand on either side of the dilemma. At the same time, the verbal and metacommunicative behavior he does perform must not contradict each other, because that may confuse the other party. He must be patient and compassionate, but focused on the issues in hand, and should not let the advice-seeker's attention wander. He must dissipate fears raised by "rumors" and "horror stories", but must never gloss over or retouch actual facts and dangers. The consultant must always be prepared and set forth possible alternatives along with their advantages, drawbacks and consequences.[14] In many cases, the counselor is aware of the problem's serious and occasionally hopeless prognosis. The recurrence of this mental burden can pose a serious challenge for the physician. In cases of possible abortion, the genetic counselor's role goes beyond merely sharing information. From the moment that patients are confronted with the problem, we have to provide them with support. Besides the bare facts, we also need to point out the potential remedies. We must convey positive messages to the couple so that they can more easily deal with a tragedy. The description of the problem is never meant to deter; therefore, calm, a human voice, and compassion are the most important qualities of a genetic counselor. We stand a much better chance to achieve cooperation if, instead of telling the facts in a cold matter-of-fact manner, we act kindly, and do not conceal the problem. The patients must never sense frustration and exhaustion on the part of the genetic counselor.

It is essential that the decision possibly reflect the common will of the couple, but at a minimum be preceded by a consultation between the partners. The couple frequently wishes to request the advice of the woman's gynecologist before making the final decision. This reinforces the strong bond of confidence that develops between the pregnant woman and her physician. This is especially true when genetic counseling is done by an obstetrician/gynecologist who may also be in charge of the patient's pregnancy.

The woman usually desires the most comprehensive information possible, so she can make an educated final decision. Questions like "How would you decide in my place?" are often put to the genetic counselor. When responding, one has to follow the rules of nondirective counseling and accordingly give information about how the majority of other couples decide in similar situations. It needs to be pointed out to the patients that every individual's and every family's life is different, and therefore, it is impossible to give a generalized answer. The decision is influenced, among other factors, by whether the family already has a healthy child, how many pregnancies the woman has had, how old the couple are, and how long they have been trying to conceive a child. Religion and beliefs certainly also play an important role. After the final decision is made, the couple must be given assistance to be able to deal with the consequences as smoothly as possible. A guilty conscience and the shadow of an irresponsible decision are difficult to dispel in a family, but proficiently executed counseling can prevent them from developing.

ETHICAL AND MORAL ASPECTS OF GENETIC COUNSELING

Diagnostics of Monogenic Diseases (Heterozygote Screening, Human Genome Project, Eugenics)

The molecular genetic research brought to a high stage of development in the last years of the 20th century resulted in an ever more detailed knowledge of the human genetic material. The Human Genome Project (HGP) has established that the sequence of 3.1 billion letters of DNA show that humans are made up of about 30,000 to 40,000 genes.[15,16] This may generate erroneous beliefs in society, because many think that any hereditary gene defect can be detected today, and therefore any given disease can be screened in the embryonic stage. True, more and more monogenic diseases may be diagnosed by polymerase chain reaction (PCR) or other molecular genetic techniques, but science has yet to enable us to detect every genetic defect. These examinations, combined with assisted reproduction techniques, in certain cases make possible the detection of diseases in the pre-embryo conceived by IVF. This doubtlessly important fact can be a strong propaganda factor for the unconditional supporters of this method and can contribute to solidifying it in practice and making its application more widespread by pushing its disadvantages into the background and making use of the media's help. Given that these are costly examinations, it is necessary to bring about a well-established international network of research. If the disease in question is serious, every effort is morally justifiable to organize prenatal diagnostics and make them available. However, HGP and our ever-deepening knowledge also mean that the genetic background of more and more "conditions" can be examined, which conceals ethical dangers. Does humankind not try to implement positive eugenics when unearthing the genetic (hereditary) background of intelligence and physical features? Is there not a strange "preordination", "innate predestination", or "special selection" for those who, because of their financial status, are able to take the opportunity provided by science, however costly, it may be in the beginning? Will it be possible to acquire or

"purchase" favored social status even before childbirth? Will these sayings come true: my child was born to be a banker, a doctor, a lawyer, a teacher or an athlete, an artist? Utopian as this assertion may seem, it is not unimaginable.

Let us play with the idea, and assume that the genetic code of every human disease and human quality, including physical and mental endowments as well as appearance, has become detectable through the HGP. In the present social environment, science and technology provide for the possibility of choosing and creating the socially most "competitive", healthy descendants. If, at the beginning, it is doable through costly procedures, we have already reached the eugenics envisioned by Plato and Sir Francis Galton. Further, there could emerge in society castes firmly embedded for several generations, for with the help of genetic advantages, the descendants of the wealthier would become the leading stratum, while those with no access to these advantages would constitute the stratum of the subordinates and the employees. Would it be "healthy", socially useful, or beneficial if everybody wished to be endowed with Einstein's IQ and Schwarzenegger's or Marylin Monroe's appearance? In our view, this vast acceleration of evolution's long and slow process could lead to unforeseeable tragic consequences.

A more delicate and much more topical aspect of this line of thinking is very much alive today: What are the pathological conditions that justify the induction of premature delivery as they exhaust its scope of indication? Who is to decide on these? If certain conditions (e.g. depression, rheumatoid arthritis, schizophrenia, arteriosclerosis, certain tumors, autoimmune diseases) are proven to be inherited monogenically, is the pregnancy to be terminated if the fetus carries the faulty gene(s) and there is no known therapy? It is of paramount importance that the scope of therapy be extended so that more and more detected diseases can be treated. In order to prevent this, it is urgently necessary to create the proper legal framework of regulations and to introduce rational restrictions instead of outright prohibitions. Historical examples show that whatever can conceivably be done by man will be created sooner or later. We, therefore, cannot lull ourselves into illusions that mere prohibitions can prevent human cloning or that irrational restrictions can prevent the above vision from materializing.

Presymptomatic Diagnostics (Confidentiality of Genetic Data—Relatives, Insurance Companies, Employers, the Family and the Individual)

Presymptomatic diagnostics and so-called "susceptibility testing" are gaining salience with reference to an increasing number of diseases.[17] *Presymptomatic testing* refers to identification of healthy individuals who may have inherited a gene for a late-onset disease, and if so will develop the disorder if they live long enough (e.g. Huntington disease). *Susceptibility (predictive) testing* identifies healthy individuals who may have inherited a genetic predisposition that puts them at increased risk of developing a multifactorial disease (e.g. heart disease, Alzheimer disease or cancer), but who may never develop the disease in question. Do we have the right to inform the patient about the existence of untreatable diseases before symptoms appear? Is it necessary to do so? Are we obliged to do that? Is this individual ill at all? Can or need populations be screened for certain diseases? Indeed, the development of some diseases might be slowed down if changes in lifestyle were implemented.

The knowledge, however, that the development of a serious disease is inevitable in a later stage of one's life could put a heavy burden on his everyday existence and might even change an individual's personality. Surviving in the knowledge that one is to expect to develop a malignant tumor by age 30–40 is difficult. By the same token, possessing the relevant information might result in more careful diagnostic examinations, which should have a substantial effect on the life expectancy.

At the same time, this raises the question of who is entitled to know the information, i.e. confidentiality,[18,19] the individual affected and his relatives? One might think that only the individual affected should, but with the disease in question being a genetic one, are the relatives not affected, too? Do they not have the right to know their risk? Is the parent obliged to tell his or her child? Can the child request the performance of a predictive test? Can the parent make a decision on whether the examination should be performed for her minor child?[20] Presymptomatic and susceptibility testing in the absence of therapeutic options should be available if certain conditions are met. It is important that the individual be provided thorough information about the limits of testing, and the information contribute to enhancing the pathography and informing the family because, in many cases, it is impossible to predict the onset and seriousness of a particular disease and its symptoms. Awareness of susceptibility could induce a change in lifestyle that could prevent or prolong the development of a disease. And if a disease is inevitable, the individual will have a possibility of planning for his or her short life, as in the case of Huntington disease. Such genetic information can influence plans for marriage and having children. Preimplantation genetics could possibly prevent the development of a particular disease in their children. But the basic question remains: Is it good or useful to know what for millennia mankind has had no way of knowing—the ultimate end of life, the number of years, the sequence of probable diseases? Is society prepared for this? Is the human soul strong enough to carry this burden? Do such examinations make sense as long as we lack adequate therapies? Do we have to do everything just because we can? The problem is further complicated by the shortcomings of available predictive genetic tests that still carry a factor of serious uncertainty about whether a disease will develop, and if it does, when exactly and to what extent. Given the onus of this information, if there is no medical advantage concerning prevention or treatment, these examinations had best be postponed until adulthood, when the individual is able to make decisions on crucial aspects of his own life.

Stigmatization, Discrimination

Society tends to single out "other-than-average" individuals, in many cases stigmatizing them. Given the sensitive nature of issues such as reproduction, heredity, child-rearing skills, and the fact that society considers calculable and predictable health defects a serious drawback, exposing information about such issues is unethical. It is for the individual to decide whether or not his genetic profile ought to be made public. Employers, insurance companies, government administrations, and schools are prone to gather the widest possible spectrum of information about their associates.[21-23] The results of presymptomatic and susceptibility tests are beginning to become central issues for these institutions. These organizations would like to have unrestricted access to these data. The individual is essentially interested in the opposite, since the insurance company would surely demand a higher premium if it will be ready to offer insurance at all.

Similarly, an employer would be disinclined to employ someone of whom it is known that in a few years, he or she cannot do his or her job. At the same time, the fear of insurers and employers is also understandable, because the individual can also abuse such genetic information. Those declared "healthy", will not have to reckon with the development of a serious disease in the course of their lives, would not pay for insurance, and even the "ill" would wait almost until the likely development of the disease before they would buy insurance. This could generate unmanageable burdens for insurance companies and could lead to the total collapse of the insurance system. Environmental or occupational (e.g. miners and chemical industry workers, pilots) hazards can play a significant role in the development of certain conditions (e.g. asthma, allergies, heart disease or cancers); therefore, by applying for such jobs, people jeopardize their own health, which can become starting points of future lawsuits. (The employer could propose that the individual should work in a different department, since the desired job could accelerate the development of the disease. If the employee would still choose the job not recommended, which he should have a right to do, then he or she would lose his or her right to sue his company on these grounds.)

Considering the likely rapid dissemination of predictive tests, there is an urgent need to develop a well thought-out, detailed legal framework. Prohibition cannot be allowed, because it would deprive the individual of rather important information. The proper regulation would eliminate the situation of diametrically opposed interests among the parties and would make them interested in wide-ranging examinations. (For instance, at birth everyone should be genetically screened for "susceptibility" and the resulting information should be made available to those concerned, but at the same time, discrimination and the possibility of abuse by the examined individual should be prohibited; emphasis should be placed on prevention, and adequate sets of incentives should be elaborated.) Apparently avoiding stigmatization and discrimination makes a very important goal, but the problem itself is highly complex. It is unacceptable to discriminate against anybody at school, work, or when taking out an insurance policy because of one's genetic background. It must not be allowed either, that individuals misuse this information. Therefore, it is crucial to bring about well-considered, detailed regulation and legislative background. At present, the individual's and the family's personal rights must not suffer damage, and genetic information may be made public only with their consent.

Sex Selection and Sex Determination

Both the prenatal and the preimplantation diagnostic procedures are suitable for the *determination of the sex* of the pre-embryo/embryo or the fetus. The majority of society does not prefer one sex to the other. In certain communities, however, the offspring's sex is very important; therefore, sex determination presents itself as a problem in this controversial moral field. Many civilized societies do not allow carrying out invasive genetic examinations merely to select or determine sex, but loopholes exist in many countries. Where a pregnancy may be terminated at the married couple's request, the decision to do so is often made in the knowledge of the fetus' sex (as a result of karyotyping or an ultrasound examination). In these cases, we speak of sex determination done for nonmedical reasons. Those in favor of this try to rely on demographic/statistical data arguing that in certain cases, it would be favorable to permit it. There are certain research groups and countries where sex determination is permitted if a couple already has a child, and would like to next one to be of the other sex. Some claim that in countries with decreasing populations this could even become an instrument in stopping the declining numbers. In other countries (in Asia), this possibility is seen as one of the factors slowing down population growth.[24,25] They point out previous European experience when the selection of the descendant's sex was possible on the basis of the sperms, and practice showed that this did not change the proportion of the sexes in the population. In 2001, The American Society for Reproductive Medicine ruled that it is proper and ethical to help couples to choose the sex of their babies.[26]

By the same token, sex determination done for nonmedical reasons also has several opponents. The most frequently heard argument against the use of PGD for nonmedical sexing is that a medical method should not be used for non-medical reasons.[27] We are even more concerned that by legalizing this kind of sex determination, we will cross the Rubicon, for it would be classifying the sex of an individual as "abnormality". This would be the first step toward the above described, apparently utopian human interventions that on the surface would be "done for genetic reasons", but in reality would serve a manipulated selection of human qualities. At a later point, this logic could namely have us argue that the decreasing population could be expanded if legal regulations allowed selection on the basis of intelligence or physique, or where the opposite is needed, the "high-quality", "efficient" and "productive" descendants could just as well slow population growth.

In our view, to avoid abusing information about sex revealed by carrying out karyotyping for other reasons, careful regulation is needed that effectively makes it impossible to terminate pregnancy just because the fetus belongs to one or the other sex.[28] Individual (personal) rights must be curtailed, and those uncritically embracing them should not ignore the rights of the fetus. Individualism is not identical to exemption from obeying rules and laws.

Today, sex determination may be justifiably indicated only if a family is affected by a hereditary disease connected to a sex chromosome, and when special molecular diagnostic tools making use of genetic engineering are not yet available. In such a case, if the test reveals that the fetus is male, the couple has the right to ask for the termination of pregnancy so that the disease will be avoided. In this case, we speak of sex determination done for medical reasons. If the preferred method of conception is IVF-ET and the disease in question is an X-determined, recessive one, the so-called preimplantation diagnostics is a possible option, which may ensure that only healthy female pre-embryos get implanted.[29]

Definition of Illness and Health

Differentiating between illness and health presents an increasingly complex problem. According to the WHO's definition, health is a state of complete physical, mental and social well-being, and is not merely the absence of disease or infirmity.[30] Holding the assertion that the absence of disease (an organic, physical decrease in or failure of function) does not in itself *constitute* health makes it difficult to define the conditions that ought to be regarded as healthy. Late-onset diseases, deviations from the statistical norm

and increased susceptibility to cancers are questionable states. These men and women are not ill for a long time, but they are handicapped from a certain point of view. Shall or shall we not treat these states as diseases until we are able to cure already detected genetic predispositions? At the same time, millions of people live happy lives with certain diseases (blindness, absence of fingers, color-blindness, deafness) presuming they are healthy. A number of geniuses would not have been born had they been fallen victim to procured abortion because of conditions considered by society as illnesses.

There is another serious ethical challenge here. Do parents have the right to decide whether or not an obvious infirmity they carry is one that needs screening that might help avoid it in their children? And if they do not, who can decide? If it is left to the parents to make decisions, then strange situations should be expected. A good example is reported by Green.[31] A deaf-mute couple sought genetic counseling their disease's nature being monogenically hereditary. Having been informed about their prospects, they asked for a molecular genetic diagnosis to be made on the 13-week-old fetus. To the pleasure of their consultant, the result was homozygote-recessive, meaning they could expect a healthy offspring. Surprisingly, however, the couple was disappointed by the result, indicating, "We cannot carry on with the pregnancy. How could we bring up a child totally alien to us, able to hear and communicate, while our friends and we live in a different way? We are not capable of establishing the appropriate circumstances".

Terminating Pregnancy Because of Genetic Indications

The most challenging moments of genetic counseling arise when a decision has to be made on the disposition of a pregnancy. From the consultant's point of view, those situations are the most difficult when the problem is so severe and the prognosis is so bad that termination on a genetic basis may be proffered. Even in this case, the goal of nondirective counseling is to inform the patient about this option. The woman is about to resolve one of the most difficult situations of her life. The weight of the decision depends on the gestational age of the pregnancy and other factors. Decisions on serious conditions detected in the first trimester are made easier. Given that most diagnoses are made in the second trimester, when the fetus has already made its first movement, a very close relationship has sometimes developed between fetus and expectant mother by decision-time. She may have seen its face during an ultrasound examination, and she may even know her offspring's sex. Realizing her widening waistline, the people around her may learn about the pregnancy, and this knowledge and having to wait, make it even more difficult for her to cope. The necessity to make a decision presents a major state of crisis, the extent of which depends, among other things, on the obstetrical anamnesis.

In such a case, the task is to give the relevant facts, help the patient to consider them thoughtfully and calmly, and to encourage her to develop positive prospects for the future. It is important to outline the possible short-term and long-term consequences of the decisions, the risk of the defect being recurrent, and the details of its heredity. If the woman opts to continue her pregnancy, she needs to be briefed on what sort of aid she can rely upon from the fields of medicine and social services, as well as family care. Those deciding to terminate the pregnancy must be informed about the procedure to relieve tension and distress. In any case, this should ease the anxiety regarding the operation itself. It must be stressed that if the couple opts to terminate the pregnancy, the procedure must be initiated as early as possible. The methods used for mid-term abortions vary from country to country. Regardless of the method, the objective is to get the procedure over within the shortest possible time and in the least intrusive way. The patient ought to get back to her home as soon as possible to be able to deal with the tragedy with her loved ones. Access must be made available to post-termination counseling.

Woman's and Partner's Freedom of Choice and Representing the Fetus' and the Newborn's Interest: Considerations Relating to Faith and Religion

One basic feature of modern genetic counseling is that the final decision is always made by those seeking assistance.[1] The justification for this appeals to individual rights of freedom and people's right to decide issues affecting their own lives. Obstetrics and genetics, however, are fields where a decision often has to do with another individual (i.e. the embryo, fetus or newborn); therefore, it must not be practiced without limitations and relevant regulation. The problems of fetal life have often been put in the center of debates, not only in professional circles, but also as a political issue. The rigid attitude of the Roman Catholic Church is well-known and stirs a lot of debates even within that faith community. The church turns a deaf ear to the issue of termination and does not accept contraception as a legitimate option (with a few exceptions). Thus, it is difficult to provide the opportunities offered by the achievements of prenatal diagnosis to Catholics. In some liberal circles' view, parents must be assured to have the widest possible sphere of authority. This cannot be readily accepted by a physician or an obstetrician-geneticist. In the United States, it is legally possible that termination be carried out until the twenty-fourth week of pregnancy at the request of the patient and without any medical indication. The test is whether an individual physician accepts the pregnant woman's decision to terminate her pregnancy.

The WHO's position is that after the twenty-fourth week, an end to a pregnancy has to be considered as childbirth and as such, everything has to be done to save the life of the premature infant. Therefore, there are cases where several doctors and nurses make superhuman efforts for weeks to rescue a 490-gram premature baby born after the twenty-fourth week, whereas the life of another baby, perhaps with a little better initial life-expectancy, perhaps even weighing a little more, is taken in minutes because the parents changed their mind "at the last minute". Our era is burdened with lawsuits brought against thousands of doctors, and many tend to give in to patients' request as self-defense. There are cases of minor problems whose long-time prognosis is not known for certain. In such cases, the question is frequently asked, "But surely our child will be healthy? You know we do not want a sick baby". Well, this question is difficult to answer. One must not yield to pressure by irresponsibly allowing termination in such cases. The freedom of choice must be kept in focus, but between reasonable boundaries, too. Regulation established to protect fetal life enables us to do our job, living up to the principles of modern medicine, and actually protect life and health.

Preimplantation Diagnostics; Gene-Therapy

Assisted reproductive techniques are becoming more and more sophisticated, contributing to the expertise that makes it possible to subject the fertilized egg to ever more detailed genetic examinations still outside the mother's body. In the course of the procedure, blastomer, blastocyst and polar-body biopsy take place while the genetic analysis is performed with two major molecular genetic techniques, polymerase chain reaction (PCR) and fluorescence in-situ hybridization (FISH). The high cost of practice and the low pregnancy rate achieved are still considered the two major drawbacks of this new procedure. As our knowledge of the genetic background of diseases expands, the number of those for whom these examinations may be indicated, is also increased. In the future, in vitro fertilization may become more widespread, because it would prevent numerous terminations from happening: pre-embryos carrying disease would not be implanted in the first place. Regulation must not be neglected in this field, because within a short time, society would be confronted with a deluge of unwarranted examinations. The financial and moral burden of this would surely prove unbearable. Positive eugenics must not be allowed to be realized this way.

Currently, the number of gene-therapy procedures is negligible, but intensive research may make some treatments possible soon. This will herald a new age of genetics and, indeed, the whole of medicine. On the one hand, many couples as yet unable to rear children will have the opportunity to do so; on the other hand, one or another of these therapeutic methods might become a way of retrieving health, indeed, a new lease of life for many people.

Financial Considerations

Science is capable of much more today in the fields of genetics and prenatal diagnostics than the health care system is able to offer to society. It is those costly interventions that make the difference. When setting priorities, their social usefulness must always be kept in mind. The needs of the wide social strata must never be sacrificed for the sake of a relatively narrow stratum. This principle will be there to be confronted in the field of genetics and prenatal diagnostics for a long time, because the procedures that have been introduced recently are highly costly. A breakthrough in this field may also be expected, but only if efficient screening/diagnostic methods and treatments are available which are advantageous to the masses of society and for which financial consequences (insurance, work, pensions) are beneficial. The cost-benefit principle may not be accepted without reservation, but it defines what sort of examinations can be routinely carried out in a health care system with a finite budget.

SUMMARY

The basic and clinical science of genetics has made vast progress in a few decades. In accordance with this, genetic counseling has reached the limelight of public attention. Given the fact that the subject of counseling is of momentous consequences and has important effects for both the short and long term, its ethical aspect is paramount. What was inconceivable just half a century ago has become a routine procedure, and for the majority of previously hopeless couples it is now possible to have healthy descendants.

Visions articulated by Plato millennia ago have come close to being realized. While ancient Sparta used exposure of infants on Mount Taigetos as a means of creating a healthy society, today we try to prevent the birth of ill children by examining and improving tiny DNA spirals and base pairs. The question is, indeed whether mankind is ripe enough to use this knowledge for choosing the right way ahead and utilizing the achievements for society's benefit. It is crucial that the relevant regulation be designed. The center of the ethical questions is occupied by the treatment of important personal information and the method of its being made public. The way the problems are dealt with is always changing, just as society is in a constant process of change. It is important, however, that we always be ready to offer proper help to those in need when they need it.

REFERENCES

1. Papp Z. Change in public demand for genetic counselling in the past 25 years. In: Chervenak FA, Kurjak A, Papp Z (Eds). The Fetus as a Patient. The Evolving Challenge. Boca Raton, London, New York, Washington DC; 2002. pp. 130-45.
2. Sjogren B, Uddenberg N. Decision making during the prenatal diagnostic procedure. A questionnaire and interview study of 211 women participating in prenatal diagnosis. Prenat Diagn. 1988;8(4):263-73.
3. Marteau T, Drake H, Bobrow M. Counselling following diagnosis of a fetal abnormality: the differing approaches of obstetricians, clinical geneticists and genetic nurses. J Med Genet. 1994;31: 864-7.
4. Johnson KA, Brensinger JD. Genetic counseling and testing: implications for clinical practice. Nurs Clin North Am. 2000;35: 615-26.
5. Seller MJ. Ethical aspects of genetic counseling. J Med Ethics. 1982;8:185-8.
6. Berkowitz RA. Should every pregnant woman undergo ultrasonography? N Engl J Med. 1993;329:874-5.
7. Chervenak FA, McCullough LB. Ethics and emerging subdiscipline of obstetric ultrasound, and its relevance to the routine obstetric scan. Ultrasound Obstet Gynecol. 1991;1:18-20.
8. Romero R. Routine obstetric ultrasound. Ultrasound Obstet Gynecol. 1993;3:303-7.
9. Egan JF, Malakh L, Turner GW, et al. Role of ultrasound for Down syndrome screening in advanced maternal age. Am J Obstet Gynecol. 2001;185:1028-31.
10. Caughey AB, Lyell DJ, Filly RA, et al. The impact of the use of the isolated echogenic intracardiac focus as a screen for Down syndrome in women under the age of 35 years. Am J Obstet Gynecol. 2001;185:1021-7.
11. Chervenak FA, McCullough LB. Ethical dimensions of ultrasound screening for fetal anomalies. Ann NY Acad Sci. 1998;847:185-90.
12. Hunfield JAM, Wladimiroff JW, Passchier J, et al. Emotional reactions in women in late pregnancy (24 weeks or longer) following the ultrasound diagnosis of a severe or lethal fetal malformation. Prenat Diagn. 1993;13:603-12.
13. Chitty LS, Barnes CA, Berry C. For Debate: continuing with pregnancy after a diagnosis of lethal abnormality: experience of five couples and recommendations for management. BMJ. 1996;313:478-80.
14. Donnai D. The management of the patient having fetal diagnosis. Baillieres Clin Obstet Gynaecol. 1987;1:737-45.
15. Macer D. Whose genome project? Bioethics. 1991;5:183-211.
16. Murray TH, Livny E. The human genome project: ethical and social implications. Bull Med Libr Assoc. 1995;83:14-21.
17. Macer DRJ. Ethics and prenatal diagnosis. In: Milunsky A (Ed). Genetic Disorders and the Fetus: Diagnosis, Prevention and Treatment. Baltimore: John Hopkins University Press; 1998. pp. 999-1024.
18. Grady C. Ethics and genetic testing. Adv Intern Med. 1999;44: 389-411.
19. Rawbone RG. Future impact of genetic screening in occupational and environmental medicine. Occup Environ Med. 1999;56:721-4.
20. Savulescu J. Predictive genetic testing in children. MJA. 2001;175:379-81.
21. Billings PR, Kohn MA, de Cuevas M, et al. Discrimination as a consequence of genetic testing. Am J Hum Genet. 1992;50:476-82.
22. Rothenberg K, Fuller B, Rothstein M, et al. Genetic information and the workplace: legislative approaches and policy challenges. Science. 1997;275:1755-7.
23. Lapham EV, Kozma C, Weiss JO. Genetic discrimination: perspectives of consumers. Science. 1996;274:621-4.
24. Williamson NE. Sex preference and its effect on family size and child welfare. Draper Fund Rep. 1982;11:22-5.
25. Malpani A, Malpani A, Modi D. The use of preimplantation genetic diagnosis in sex selection for family balancing in India. Reprod Biomed Online. 2002;4(1):16-20.
26. Gottlieb S. US doctors say sex selection acceptable for nonmedical reasons. BMJ. 2001;323:82-8.
27. Pennings G. Personal desires of patients and social obligations of geneticists: applying preimplantation genetic diagnosis for non-medical sex selection. Prenat Diagn. 2002;22:1123-9.
28. Sachs BP, Korf B. The human genome project: implications for the practicing obstetrician. Obstet Gynecol. 1993;81:458-62.
29. Botkin JR. Ethical issues and practical problems in preimplantation genetic diagnosis. J Law Med Ethics. 1998;26:17-28.
30. Preamble to the Constitution of the World Health Organization as adopted by the International Health Conference, New York, 19-22 June, 1946. Signed July 22, 1946. Official Records of the World Health Organization. 1948;2:100.
31. Green RM. Prenatal autonomy and the obligation not to harm one's child genetically. J Law Med Ethics. 1997;25:5-15.

CHAPTER

21 Selective Reduction

MI Evans, DW Britt, D Ciorica

INTRODUCTION

Millions of babies have been born benefiting from infertility therapies including more than 1,000,000 in vitro fertilization (IVF) babies over the past 25 years. These fulfilling outcomes, however, have been accompanied with serious side effects. The twin pregnancy rate has doubled to more than 1 in 45. Multiple pregnancies have continually risen. Prematurity and related sequel closely correlate with fetal number (Fig. 21.1) (Table 21.1).[1] Infertility treatments have become so pervasive that more than 70% of all twins and 99% of higher order multiples are initiated by them (Table 21.2). With increasing public and professional attention, some of the very high order multiples have diminished, particularly secondary to lower transfer numbers of embryos in IVF. There are some suggestions that the incidence of triplets and higher is slowly diminishing, but the incidence is still very high.

Perceived pregnancy losses in multiple pregnancies are mostly correlated to how early in pregnancy one establishes the denominator.[2,3] Some perinatal reports are overly optimistic because these physicians do not start counting until they begin to see patients at nearly 20 weeks, at which time most losses have already occurred.[3,4] Many other articles have addressed those issues and will not be repeated here.[4-6]

In the 1980s, about 75% of multifetal pregnancy patients seeking reduction had pregnancies initiated with ovulation induction agents such as Pergonal.[7] However, even with the first month of the lowest dose of Clomid, quintuplets have occurred. Over the years, cases induced by assisted reproductive technologies (ARTs), such as IVF have become increasingly common. Currently, about 70% of patients we see seeking reduction have pregnancies generated by ARTs.[8]

Despite the increased utilization of ARTs,[8] the proportion of cases significantly hyperstimulated, and resulting in quintuplets or more has dramatically decreased to less than 10% of all cases seen by us. Regardless, the 2000 report of the Society of Assisted Reproductive Technologies (SART) suggested that, of all pregnancies achieved by Assisted Reproductive Technologies (ARTs), in the United

RISKS OF PREMATURITY AS A FUNCTION OF FETAL NUMBER

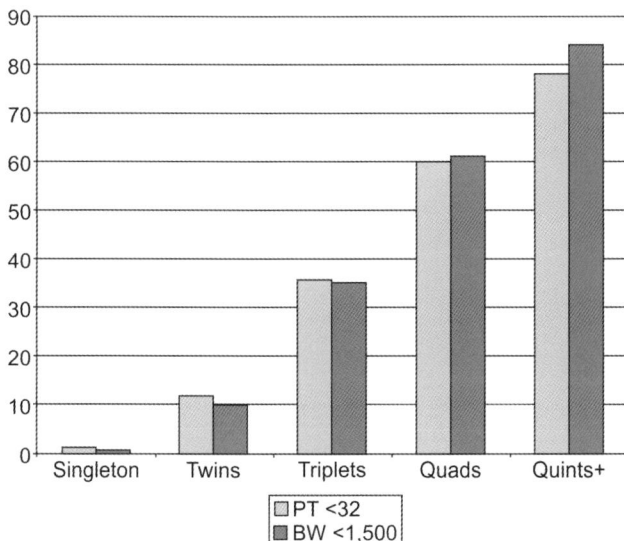

Fig. 21.1: 2002 United States Centers for Disease Control Data. Diagonal lines preterm birth <32 weeks. Shaded area birth weight < 1,500 grams

Table 21.1: Multiple births in the United States

Year	Twins	Triplets	Quadruplets	Quintuplets and higher multiples
2002	125,134	6898	434	69
2001	121,246	6885	501	85
2000	118,916	6742	506	77
1999	114,307	6742	512	67
1998	110,670	6,919	627	79
1997	104,137	6,148	510	79
1996	100,750	5,298	560	81
1995	96,736	4,551	365	57
1994	97,064	4,233	315	46
1993	96,445	3,834	277	57
1992	95,372	3,547	310	26
1991	94,779	3,121	203	22
1990	93,865	2,830	185	13
1989	90,118	2,529	229	40
% Change from				
1989–2002	38.9%	172.8%	89.6%	72.5%

Source: National Vital Statistics Report. 2003, Volume 52, No. 10, p. 22.

Table 21.2: Ratio of observed to expected multiples

Births	Observed	Expected	Ratio
Twins	125,134	44,686	2.80:1
Triplets	6,898	496	13.9:1
Quadruplets	434	6	72.3:1
Quintuplets and higher multiples	69	0.07	985.7:1
Total Births in 2002 — 4,021,726			

States 58.5% are singletons, 28% twins, 7.5% triplets or higher, and 5.9% were unknown. [9,10] In our experience with referred cases of ovulation stimulation, the proportion of cases that are quintuplets or more has likewise fallen but not as remarkably. [11] The vast majority of multifetal cases occur to physicians with the best of equipment and with the best of intentions who have an unfortunate and reasonably unpredictable or unpreventable malloccurrence. Despite this, clearly some cases might have been prevented if increased vigilance had been used. [11-13]

PATIENT ISSUES

The demographics of patients considering multifetal pregnancy reduction (MFPR) have evolved considerably over the past 10–15 years. [11,12] The most dramatic change has been the introduction of donor eggs which has opened the door to "older women". Over 10% of all patients seeking MFPR that we see are over 40 years of age; nearly half of them are using donor eggs. As a consequence of the shift to older patients, many of whom already had previous relationships and children, there is an increased desire by these patients to have only one further child. The number of experienced centers willing to do 2 to 1 reductions is still very limited, but we believe it can be justified in the appropriate circumstances. [11,13] We expect the proportion of all patients with multiples reducing to a singleton to continually rise.

For patients who are "older" particularly using their own eggs, the issue of genetic diagnosis comes into play. By 2001, more than 50% of patients in the United States having ART cycles were over 35 (Table 21.3). [1,9,10,14] In the 80s and early 90s, the most common approach was to offer amniocentesis at 16–17 weeks on the remaining twins. A 1995 paper suggested an 11% loss rate in these cases, which caused considerable concern. [15] However, the issue was settled by a much larger collaborative series in 1998, which showed that loss rates were no higher than comparable controls of MFPR patients who did not have amniocentesis. [16] The collaborative data demonstrate a loss rate of 5%, which was certainly no higher than the group of patients post MFPR who did not have genetic studies.

Since the centers with the most MFPR experience also happened to be the ones who also had the same accomplishments with chorionic villus sampling, combinations of the procedures were very logical. There are two main schools of thought as to the best approach to first trimester genetic diagnosis, i.e. should it be before or after the performance of MFPR? Published data in the early 90s doing the CVS first followed by reductions suggested a 1–2% error rate as to which fetus was which, particularly if the entire karyotype is obtained before going on to reduction. [17] Therefore, for the first 10–15 years, the approach we used was to generally do

the reduction first at approximately 10.5 weeks in patients reducing down to twins or triplets, followed by CVS approximately 1 week later. [11,14] However, in patients going to a singleton pregnancy, essentially putting "all of their eggs in one basket", we believed the best approach was to know what was in the basket before reducing the other embryos. [11,12] In these cases, we performed a CVS on usually all the fetuses or one more than the intended stopping number, and performed a fluorescent in situ hybridization (FISH) analysis with probes for chromosomes 13, 18, 21, X, and Y (Fig. 21.2). Whereas about 30% of overall anomalies seen on karyotype would not be detectable by FISH with these probes, [18] there is always residual risk. [19] The absolute risk given both a normal FISH and a normal ultrasound including nuchal translucency [20] is only about 1/500. We believe that risk is lower than the increased risk from the 2 weeks wait necessary to get the full karyotype. We have now commonly extended this approach to all patients who are appropriate candidates for prenatal diagnosis regardless of the fetal number. Over the past few years, more than half of our patients have combined CVS and MFPR procedures. With data now suggesting increased risks of chromosomal and other anomalies in patients conceiving by IVF and especially with ICSI, the utilization of prenatal diagnosis will likely increase even further. [21-26]

The other approach used by another group was to perform the CVS and complete karyotype first and have the patient come back for the reduction. Although "mistakes" were common 10 years ago, the chance of error has been considerably reduced, and they believed the benefits of the full karyotype justified the wait. The issue as to the better of these two approaches is currently unsettled and would require a very large series to differentiate among small risks.

PROCEDURES

Multifetal pregnancy reduction is a clinical procedure developed in the 1980s when a small number of centers in both the United States and Europe attempted to reduce the usual and tremendously adverse sequel of multifetal pregnancies by selectively terminating or reducing the number of fetuses to a more manageable number. The first European reports by Dumez, [27] and the first American report by Evans, et al. [28] followed by a further report by Berkowitz,

Table 21.3: Maternal age and ART (SART Data – 2001)

All cases	81,915
Fresh non donor	60,780
<35	28,778
35–37	14,416
38–40	11,301
41–42	4,365
42+	2,190

Source: Wright VC, Schieve LA, Reynolds MA, Jeng G: Assisted reproductive technology surveillance Pub Med, MMWR Surveill Summ. 2003, Aug 29;52:1–16.

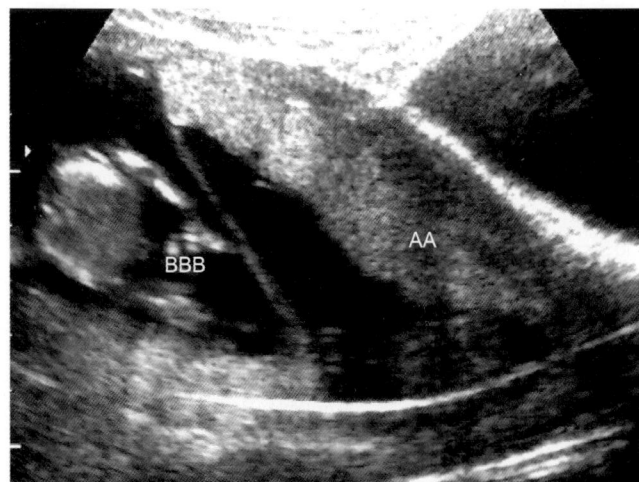

Fig. 21.2: Transcervical CVS being performed on posterior placenta. For this patient, anterior placenta can be reached either transcervically or transabdominally

et al.[29] and later Wapner, et al.[30] described a surgical approach to improve the outcome in such cases.

Even these early reports appreciated the ethical dilemma faced by couples and physicians under such difficult circumstances.[13] In the mid 80s, needles were inserted transabdominally and maneuvered into the thorax for the injection of KCL or mechanical disruption of the fetus by either mechanical destruction, air embolization or potassium chloride injections despite relatively mediocre ultrasound visualization. Transcervical aspirations were also initially tried, but with little success. Some centers also used transvaginal mechanical disruption, but data suggested a significantly higher loss rate than with the transabdominal route.[11,31] Today, virtually all experienced operators perform the procedure inserting needles transabdominally under ultrasound guidance.

OUTCOMES

Several centers with the world's largest experience have, for more than a decade, collaborated to leverage their power of their data. In 1993, the first collaborative report showed a 16% pregnancy loss rate through 24 completed weeks.[17] While by today's standards, that was not a very satisfactory number, it did represent a major improvement for higher order multiple pregnancies. Further collaborative papers have shown continued dramatic improvements in the overall outcomes of such pregnancies (Table 21.4).[11] The 2001 collaborative data demonstrated that the outcome of triplets reduced to twins, and quadruplets reduced to twins now perform essentially as if they started as twins.[11] Even with the tremendous advances in neonatal care for premature babies, the 95% take home baby rate for triplets and the 92% take home baby rate for quadruplets clearly represent dramatic improvements over natural statistics. Not only has the pregnancy loss rate been substantially lowered, but so has the rate of very dangerous early prematurity. Both continue to be correlated with the starting number. Data from the past few years show that the improvements are, not surprisingly, greatest from the higher starting numbers (Fig. 21.3).

The lowest pregnancy loss rates are for those cases reduced to twins with increasing losses for singletons followed by triplets. However, the rate of early premature delivery has been, not surprisingly, highest with triplets followed by twins and lowest with singletons. Mean gestational age at delivery was also lower for higher order cases. Birth weights following MFPR decreased with starting and finishing numbers reflecting increasing prematurity.[32]

While data in the literature are conflicting, our experiences suggest that triplets reduced to twins do much better in terms of loss and prematurity than do unreduced triplets. We believe that if a patient's primary goal is to maximize the chances of surviving children, that reduction of triplets to twins achieves the best live born results. More recent analyses suggest that while mortality is lowest with twins, morbidity is lowest with remaining singletons.

There has continued to be a debate in some circles over whether to reduce triplets or not. Yaron, et al.[33] compared triplets to twins data to unreduced triplets with two large cohorts of twins. The data show substantial improvement of reduced twins as compared to triplets. The data from the most recent collaborative series suggest that pregnancy outcomes for cases starting at triplets or even quadruplets reduced to twins do fundamentally as well as starting as twins. These data, therefore, support some cautious aggressiveness in infertility treatments to achieve pregnancy in difficult clinical situations. However, when higher numbers occur, good outcomes clearly diminish. A 2001 paper suggested that reduced triplets did worse than continuing ones.[34] However, analysis of that series showed a loss rate following MFPR twice that seen in our collaborative series[11] and poorer outcomes in every other category for remaining triplets. Several other recent papers have likewise shown higher risks for "unreduced" triplets than for reduced cases.[35-38] It is clear that one must use extreme caution in choosing comparison groups (Table 21.5). An ever increasing situation involves the inclusion of a monozygotic (MZ) pair of twins in a higher order multiple.[39] Our experience suggests that provided the "singleton" seems healthy, that the best outcomes are achieved by reduction of the MZ twins. Obviously, if the singleton is not healthy, then keeping the twins is the next choice.

Pregnancy loss is only one of the deleterious outcomes. Very early preterm delivery correlates with the starting number. However,

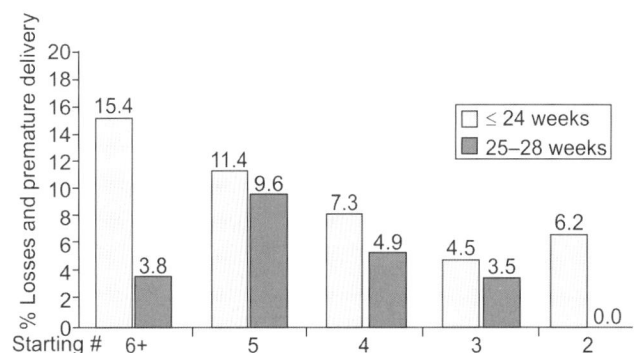

Fig. 21.3: Multifetal pregnancy reduction losses and very prematures by starting number

Source: Evans MI, Berkowitz R, Wapner R, et al. Multifetal pregnancy reduction (MFPR): Improved outcomes with increased experience. A J of Obst and Gynec. 2001;184:97-103.

Table 21.4: Multifetal pregnancy reduction – percentage of losses and deliveries by year

		Losses (weeks)		Deliveries (weeks)			
	Total	% < 24	% > 24	% 25–28	% 29–32	% 33–36	% 37+
1986–90	508	13.2	4.5	10.0	21.1	15.7	35.4
1991–94	724	9.4	0.3	2.8	5.4	21.1	61.0
1995–98	1356	6.4	0.2	4.3	10.2	31.5	47.4

Source: Evans MI, Berkowitz R, Wapner R, et al. Multifetal pregnancy reduction (MFPR): Improved outcomes with increased experience. An J Obstet and Gynecol. 2001;184:97–103.

Table 21.5: Comparison of reduced vs. unreduced triplets

Years	< 24	24–28	MFPR cases (%) Deliveries (weeks) 29–32	33–36	37+
Reduced triplets					
1980s	6.7	6.1	9.1	36.9	47.9
1990–1994	5.7	5.2	9.9	39.2	45.2
1995–1998	4.5	3.2	6.9	28.3	55.1
1998–2002	5.1	4.6	10.8	41.8	37.6
	Mean GA	PMR			
	35.5	10.0/1000			
1998–2002 (3→1)	8.0	4.0	12.0	4.0	72.0
	Mean GA	PMR			
	39.5	0/1000			
Unreduced triplets					
1998 (Leondires)	9.9				
	Mean GA	PMR			
	33.3	55/1000			
1999 (Angel)	8.0				
	Mean GA	PMR			
	32.3	29/1000			
1999 (Lipitz)	25.0				
	Mean GA	PMR			
	33.5	109/1000			
2002 (Francois)	8.3				
	Mean GA	PMR			
	31.0	57.6/1000			

Source: Evans et al. The optimal management of first trimester triplets: Reduce. The Central Association of Obstetricians and Gynecologists Annual Meeting, Las Vegas, Nevada, October 27–30, 2002.

it has not been well appreciated that about 20% of babies born at less than 750 g develop cerebral palsy.[40] In Western Australia, Peterson, et al. showed that the rate of cerebral palsy was 4.6 times higher for twins than singletons per live births, but 8.3 times higher when calculated per pregnancy.[41] Pharoah and Cooke calculated cerebral palsy rates per 1,000 first year survivor at 2.3 for singletons, 12.6 for twins, and 44.8 for triplets.[42]

In the 2001 collaborative report the subset of patients who reduced from two to one (not for fetal anomalies), included 154 patients. These data suggested a loss rate comparable to three to two, but, in about 1/3 of the 2 → 1 cases, there was a medical indication for the procedure, e.g. maternal cardiac disease or prior twin pregnancy with severe prematurity or uterine abnormality.[11]

In recent years, however, the demographics are changing, and the vast majority of such cases are from women in their forties or even fifties, some of whom are using donor eggs and who, more for social than medical reasons, only want a singleton pregnancy.[42,44] New data suggest that twins reduced to a singleton do better than remaining as twins.[13] Consistent with the above, more women are desiring to reduce to a singleton. In a recent series of triplets, we found the average age of outpatients reducing to twins to be 37 years and to a singleton 41 years.[43] While the reduction in pregnancy loss risk for 3–1 is not as much as 3–2 (from 15% to 7% and from 15% to 5% respectively), the gestational age at delivery for the resulting singleton is higher, and the incidence of births < 1,500 g is 10 higher for twins than singletons.[1] These data have made counseling of such patients far more complex than previously (Figs 21.4 and 21.5). Not surprisingly, there are often differences between members of the couple as to the desirability of twins or singleton.[45] There are also profound public health and financial implications to these decisions, as 2000 United States data show that of $10.2 billion spent per year on initial newborn care, 57% of the money is spent on the 9% of babies born at < 37 weeks.[46] This progress is much more likely to rise than fall.

SOCIETAL ISSUES

There will never be a complete societal consensus on MFPR. Opinions have never followed the classic "pro-choice/pro-life" dichotomy.[2,7,11,14.] We believe that the real debate over the next 5–10 years will not be whether or not MFPR should be performed with triplets or more. A serious argument will be put forth over whether or not it will be appropriate to offer MFPR routinely for twins, even natural ones for whom the outcome has commonly been considered "good enough".[43] Our data suggest that reduction, of twins to a singleton actually improves the outcome of the remaining fetus.[43] No consensus on appropriateness of routine two to one reductions, however, is ever likely to emerge. We do, however, expect the proportion of patients reducing to a singleton to steadily increase over the next several years.

The ethical issues surrounding MFPR will also always be controversial. Over the years, much has been written on the subject. Opinions will always vary substantially from outraged condemnation to complete acceptance. No short paragraph could do justice to the subject other than to state that most proponents do not believe this is a frivolous procedure, but see it in terms of the principle of proportionality, i.e. therapy to achieve the most good for the least harm.[13,47-49]

How patients "hear" and internalize data and make decisions with respect to reduction have been a subject of our investigation for several years. Much of the literature on medical decision making has emphasized a rational choice model in which emotions, feelings and values are treated as complications that must be considered as a second stage of an analysis that puts hard data regarding relative risks center stage.[50-51] Even the literature that talks about genuine alternative models of decision-making (systematic versus heuristic, for example), a central assumption is that these are individual differences in style that can be identified through what people say.[52-53]

We have investigated this problem from a different direction, arguing that where controversial, high-anxiety decisions are concerned, patients treat these decisions as an ongoing part of the social reality that they are creating to live in and raise a family.[54] These realities, composed of supportive people and institutions together with complexes of supportive values, norms and attitudes,

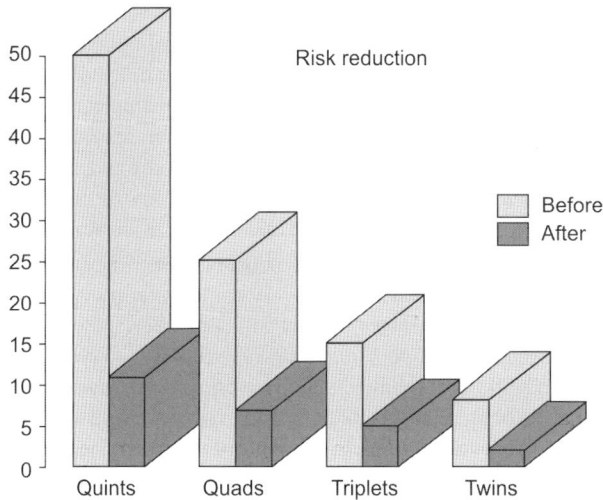

Fig. 21.4: Risk reduction as a function of starting number

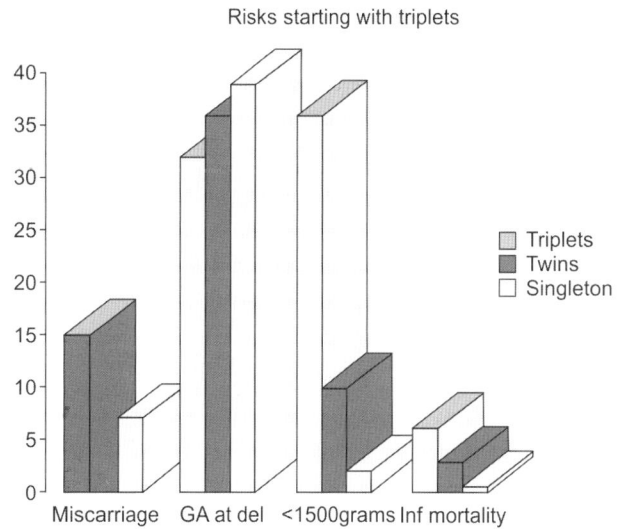

Fig. 21.5: Reduction of triplets to twins has lower loss rates but higher incidence of prematurity, low birth weight and infant mortality than reducing to a singleton

Table 21.6: Frame comparison

	Medical frame	Conceptionalist frame	Lifestyle frame
Intensity of Commitment to having children	High	High	High
Intensity of training in medicine, dentistry, hard sciences and the law	High	Low	Modest
Intensity of commitment to belief that life begins at conception	Modest	High	Modest
Intensity of commitment to career	High	Low	High
Source of moral authority for resolution	Relative survivability of fetuses	Minimization of damage to moral beliefs though a "barely sufficient" reduction	Having a "normal" life in a culture that values both careers and family for women

are the source of frames that the patients use to view the data.[47-49] The decisions they make and how they justify those decisions may help resolve incompatible elements in the realities in which they find themselves enmeshed.

The one thing in common for all such patients is a very strong desire to have a family (Table 21.6). But there does not appear to be a single set of supportive institutions, people and norms that is conducive to going through the pain, stress and resource expenditure of IVF and then consider partial reduction as a pregnancy-management strategy. Rather, we think there are three viable alternative resolutions. The first of these, a rational Medical Model, looks superficially like what one would expect from the rational analysis model. But the commitment to factual analysis comes from their having selected themselves into the hard sciences, medicine, dentistry, engineering or the law—disciplines in which the "facts" are crucial. Such women will want to see the numbers regarding the relative risk associated with different reduction choices and will want to engage in a rigorous discussion of the data and their implications. And they will be likely to choose a final number for reduction that maximizes the chances of a "take-home" baby.

The lens of scientific objectivity is not the only frame through which women who have gone through IVF in order to have a child will examine these data. For those who have immersed themselves in a social reality that has a strong emphasis on norms against abortion and/or reduction—such that they themselves have such normative beliefs and are heavily involved in churches who reinforce similar beliefs—a detached examination of the "facts" is simply not possible. These "facts" hold no special moral authority. Their beliefs and those of the individuals and social institutions in which they have selected themselves have a moral authority as well. The balance that such women will likely seek is one that reduces their relative risk to acceptable limits. So, unless the consequences are dire, they will not reduce or choose to reduce only to three. We labeled such a resolution a conceptionalist frame.

Finally, there are those for whom the demands of career and/or existing children constitute powerful elements in their constructed realities. For such women and this includes many of the older patients we encountered—the essential balance that they seek is a more secular one, a Lifestyle Model, one that emphasizes creating a family situation in which having a family can be balanced with having a career. Such women will more than likely choose reduction to two or even one embryo, depending on the number of other children they have and the level of resources that the family has.

Where women have selected themselves into and/or been trained to accept the legitimacy of rigorously-determined statistics regarding relative risk (a Medical Frame), reduction choices can be straightforward—or at least they can appear to be relatively straightforward. This is usually not the case, however, for women who must forge a resolution amongst potentially incompatible elements, as for women who are struggling to reconcile the potentially oppositional elements of religious beliefs and involvement with risks associated with higher-level pregnancies (Conceptionalist Frame) or those who are struggling to reconcile he potentially-conflicting identities of home and career (Lifestyle Frame). We have been able to examine some of these issues in a few studies to date. In one we were able to trace the extreme fluctuations in anxiety and stress as women progress through IVF and then must confront the painful choice of reduction.[48] In a second, we were able to show that the meaning of detecting a fetal anomaly changes depending on the needs of the patient and her spouse for some confirmation regarding their choice.[47]

CONCLUSION

MFPR has become a well-established and integral part of infertility therapy and the attempts to deal with sequelae of aggressive infertility management. In the mid 1980s, the risks and benefits of the procedure could only be guessed.[10-14] We now have very clear and precise data on the risks and benefits as well as an understanding that the risks increase substantially with the starting and finishing number of fetuses in multifetal pregnancies. The collaborative loss rate numbers, i.e. 4.5% for triplets, 8% for quadruplets, 11% for quintuplets, and 15% for sextuplets or more seem reasonable ones to present to patients for the procedure performed by an experienced operator. Our own experience and anecdotal reports from other groups suggest that less experienced operators have worse outcomes.

Pregnancy loss is not the only poor outcome. The other main issue which is to be concerned is very early preterm delivery and the profound consequences to such infants. Here again, there is an increasing rate of poor outcomes correlated with the starting number. The finishing numbers are also critical, with twins having the best viable pregnancy outcomes for cases starting with three or more. Triplets and singletons do not do as well. However, an emerging appreciation that singletons have prematurity rates less than twins is making the counseling far more complex. We continue to hope, however, that MFPR will become obsolete as better control of ovulation agents and assisted reproductive technologies make multifetal pregnancies uncommon.

REFERENCES

1. Martin JA, Hamilton BE, Ventura SJ, et al. Births: Final Data for 2001. National Vital Statistics Reports volume 51#2. National Center for Health Statistics, Hyattville, MD. 2002.

2. Evans MI, Rodeck CH, Stewart KS, et al. Multiple Gestation: Genetic Issues, Selective Termination, and Fetal Reduction. In: Gleisher N, Buttino L Jr., Elkayam U, Evans MI, Galbraith RM, Gall SA, Sibai BM (Eds). Principles and Practices of Medical Therapy in Pregnancy, 3rd Edition. Norwalk, Connecticut: Appleton and Lange Publishing Co; 1998;pp. 235-42.

3. Evans MI, Ayoub MA, Shalhoub AG, et al. Spontaneous abortions in couples declining multifetal pregnancy reduction. Fetal Diagnosis and Therapy. 2002;17:343-6.

4. Keith LG, Blickstein I (Eds). Triplet Pregnancies. London: Parthenon Press; 2002.

5. Luke B, Brown MB, Nugent C, et al. Risks factors for adverse outcomes in spontaneous versus assisted conception twin pregnancies. Fertil Steril. 2004;81(2):315-9.

6. Anwar HN, Ihab MU, Johnny BR, et al. Pregnancy outcomes in spontaneous twins versus twins who were conceived through in vitro fertilization. Am J Obstet Gynecol. 2003;189(2):513-8.

7. Evans MI, Dommergues M, Wapner RJ, et al. Efficacy of transabdominal multifetal pregnancy reduction: collaborative experience among the world's largest centers. Obstet Gynecol. 1993;82:61-7.

8. Evans MI, Ciorica D, Britt DW, et al. Do reduced multiple pregnancies do better than higher numbers? In: Penna L, Keith L (Guest Eds) Multiple Pregnancy. London: Parthenon Publishers; (In Press).

9. Toner JP. Progress we can be proud of: US trends in assisted reproduction over the first 20 years. Fertil Steril. 2002;78(5):943-50.

10. Wright VC, Schieve LA, Reynolds MA, et al. Assisted reproductive technology surveillance – United States, 2001. MMWR Surveill Summ, 2004;53(1):1-20.

11. Evans MI, Berkowitz R, Wapner R, et al. Multifetal pregnancy reduction (MFPR): Improved outcomes with increased experience. Am J Obst Gynecol. 2001;184:97-103.

12. Adashi EY, Barri PN, Berkowitz R, et al. Infertility therapy-assisted multiple pregnancies (births): An ongoing epidemic. Reprod Med OnLine. 2003;(7):515-42.

13. Evans MI, Fletcher JC. Multifetal pregnancy reduction. In: Reece EA, Hobbins JC, Mahoney MJ, Petrie R (Eds): Medicine of the Fetus and its Mother. Philadelphia: Lippincott Harper Publishing Co; 1992; pp.1345-62.

14. Evans MI, Littman L, St Louis L, et al. Evolving patterns of iatrogenic multifetal pregnancy generation: Implications for aggressiveness of infertility treatments. Am J Obstet Gynecol. 1995;(172):1750-3.

15. Tabsh KM, Theroux NL. Genetic amniocentesis following multifetal pregnancy reduction twins: Assessing the risk. Prenat Diagn. 1995;15:221-3.

16. McLean LK, Evans MI, Carpenter RJ, et al. Genetic amniocentesis (AMN) following multifetal pregnancy reduction (MFPR) does not increase the risk of pregnancy loss. Prenat Diagn. 1998;18:186-8.

17. Brambati B, Tului L, Baldi M, et al. Genetic analysis prior to selective termination in multiple pregnancy: Technical aspects and clinical outcome. Hum Reprod. 1995;10:818-25.

18. Evans MI, Henry GP, Miller WA, et al. International, Collaborative assessment of 146,000 prenatal karyotypes: Expected limitations if only Chromosome-Specific Probes and Fluorescent In Situ hybridization were used. Hum Reprod. 1999;14(5):1213-6.

19. Homer J, Bhatt S, Huang B, et al. Residual risk for cytogenetic abnormalities after prenatal diagnosis by interphase fluorescence in situ hybridizatio (FISH) Prenatal Diagnosis. 2003;23:556-71.

20. Greene RA, Wapner J, Evans MI. Amniocentesis and choironic villus sampling in triplet pregnancy. In: Keith LG, Blickstein I, Oleszcuk JJ (Eds.) Triplet Pregnancy. London: Parthenon Publishing Group; pp. 73-84.

21. Zadori J, Kozinszky Z, Orvos H, et al. The incidence of major birth defects following in vitro fertilization. J Assist Reprod Genet. 2003;20(3):131-2.

22. Pinborg A, Loft A, Schmidt L, et al. Morbidity in a Danish national cohort of 472 IVF/ICSI twins, 1132 non-IVF/ICSI twins and 634 IVF/ICSI singletons: Health-related and social implications for the children and their families. Hum Reprod. 2003;18(6):1234-43.

23. Place I, Englert Y. A prospective longitudinal study of the physical, psychomotor, and intellectual development of singleton children up to 5 years who were conceived by intracytoplasmic sperm injection compared with children conceived spontaneously and by in vitro fertilization. Fertil Steril. 2003;80(6):1388-97.

24. Retzloff MG, Hornstein MD. Is intracytoplasmic sperm injection safe? Fertil Steril. 2003; 80(4):851-9.

25. Kurinczuk JJ. Safety issues in assisted reproduction technology. From theory to reality—just what are the data telling us about ICSI offspring health and future fertility and should we be concerned? Hum Reprod. 2003;18(5):925-31.

26. Tournaye H. ICSI: A technique too far? Int J Androl. 2003;26(2):63-9.

27. Dumez Y, Oury JF. Method for first trimester selective abortion in multiple pregnancy. Contrib Gynecol Obstet. 1986;15:50.

28. Evans MI, Fletcher JC, Zador IE, et al. Selective first trimester termination in octuplet and quadruplet pregnancies: Clinical and ethical issues. Obstet Gynecol. 1988;(71):289-96.

29. Berkowitz RL, Lynch L, Chitkara U, et al. Selective reduction of multiple pregnancies in the first trimester. N Engl J Med. 1988;318:10-43.

30. Wapner RJ, Davis GH, Johnson A. Selective reduction of multifetal pregnancies. Lancet. 1990;335:90-3.

31. Timor-Tritsch IE, Peisner DB, Monteagudo A, et al. Multifetal pregnancy reduction by transvaginal puncture: Evaluation of the technique used in 134 cases. Am J Obstet Gynecol. 1993;168:799-804.

32. Torok O, Lapinski R, Salafia CM, et al. Multifetal pregnancy reduction is not associated with an increased risk of intrauterine growth restriction, except for very high order multiples. Am J Obstet Gynecol. 1998;179:221-5.

33. Yaron Y, Bryant-Greenwood PK, Dave N, et al. Multifetal pregnancy reduction (MFPR) of triplets to twins: Comparison with non-reduced triplets and twins. Am J Obstet Gynecol. 1999;180(5):1268-71.

34. Leondires MP, Ernst SD, Miller BT, et al. Triplets: Outcomes of expectant management versus multifetal reduction for 127 pregnancies. Am J Obstet Gynecol (United States). 1999;72:257-60.

35. Lipitz S, Shulman A, Achiron R, et al. A comparative study of multifetal pregnancy reduction from triplets to twins in the first versus early second trimesters after detailed fetal screening. Ultrasound Obstet Gynecol. 2001;18:35-8.

36. Angel JL, Kalter CS, Morales WJ, et al. Aggressive perinatal care for high-order multiple gestations: Does good perinatal outcome justify aggressive assisted reproductive techniques? AM J Obstet Gynecol. 1999;181:253-9.

37. Sepulveda W, Munoz H, Alcalde JL. Conjoined twins in a triplet pregnancy: Early prenatal diagnosis with three-dimensional ultrasound and review of the literature. Ultrasound Obstet Gynecol. 2003;22(2):199-204.

38. Francois K, Sears C, Wilson R, et al. Twelve year experience of triplet pregnancies at a single institution. Amer J Obstet Gynecol. 2001;185:S112.

39. Yakin K, Kahraman S, Comert S. Three blastocyst stage embryo transfer resulting in a quintuplet pregnancy. Hum Reprod. 2001;16(4):782-4.

40. Neonatal Encephalopathy and Cerebral Palsy: Defining the pathogensis and pathophysiology. Task Force of American College of Obstetricians and Gynecologists, ACOG Washington DC:2003.

41. Petterson B, Nelson K, Watson L, et al. Twins, triplets, and cerebral palsy in births in Western Australia in the 1980s. British Medical Journal. 1993;307:1239-43.

42. Pharoah PO, Cooke T. Cerebral Palsy and Multiple Births. Archives of Disease in Childhood. Fetal and Neonatal edition. 1996;(75):F174-F7.

43. Evans MI, Kaufman MI, Urban AJ, et al. Fetal reduction from twins to a singleton: A reasonable consideration. Obstetrics and Gynecology, (In press). 2004.

44. Templeton A. The multiple gestation epidemic: The role of the assisted reproductive technologies.

45. Kalra SK, Milad MP, Klock SC, et al. Infertility patients and their partners: Differences in the desire for twin gestations. Obstet Gynecol. 2003;102:152-5.

46. St. John EB, Nelson KG, Oliver SP, et al. Cost of Neonatal care according to gestational age at birth and survival status. Am J Obstet Gynecol. 2000;(182):170-5.

47. Britt DW, Risinger ST, Mans M, et al. Devastation and relief: Conflicting meanings in discovering fetal anomalies. Ultrasound in Obstetrics and Gynecology. 2002;20:1-5.

48. Britt DW, Risinger ST, Mans M, et al. Anxiety among women who have undergone fertility therapy and who are considering MFPR: Trends and Scenarios. Journal of Maternal-Fetal and Neonatal Medicine (In press).

49. Britt DW, Evans WJ, Mehta SS, et al. Framing the decision: Determinants of how women considering MFPR as a pregnancy-management strategy frame their moral dilemma. Fetal Diagnosis and Therapy. 2004;19:232-40.

50. Redelmeier DA, Rozin P, Kahneman D. Understanding patients' decisions: cognitive and emotional perspectives. Journal of the American Medical Association. 1993;270: 72-6.

51. Chapman GB, Elstein AS. Cognitive processes and biases in medical decision making. In: Chapman GB, Sonnenberg FA (Eds). Decision Making in Health Care: Theory, Psychology and Applications. New York: Cambridge University Press; 2000. pp. 183-210.

52. Steginga SK, Occhipinti S. The application of the heuristic-systematic processing model to treatment decision making about prostate cancer. Medical Decision Making. 2004;24.

53. Hamm RM. Theory about heuristic strategies based on verbal protocol analysis: The emperor needs a shave. Medical Decision Making. 2004;24:681-6.

54. Britt DW, Campbell EQ. Assessing the Linkage of Norms, Environments and Deviance. Social Forces, (December). 1977. pp.532-49.

22 Neonatal Ethics

KNS Subramanian

BACKGROUND

Neonatal medicine has undergone significant changes over the last four decades. The increasing survival of smaller and younger infants is possible because of medical and technological innovations, such as antenatal steroid administration to a pregnant mother in preterm labor, the availability of surfactant to the premature infants, ventilators of different kinds (conventional, high frequency, etc.), inhaled Nitric Oxide (iNO), and extra corporeal membrane oxygenation (ECMO) to name a few. The mortality rate has improved overtime in USA[1,2] and rest of the world,[3,4] and it has significantly declined in all weight categories. But there also is a need to have uniformity in the denominators we use for defining mortality and morbidity of these infants. Currently, the mortality rates are expressed as deaths per 1,000 live born babies, deaths per all premature infants, by specific weight categories, by admissions to neonatal intensive care units (NICUs), or by deliveries in one hospital, geographic region, or country. The rates vary significantly depending upon which terminology is used. Although rates of significant morbidities or serious handicaps have reduced or have remained steady across many gestational ages or weight groups over the years[5] there is still a high rate of handicaps in lower birth weight or early gestational age groups.[6-8]

With increased survival and an increase in the total number of handicapped infants, society is confronted with the need for special assistance for these children. Decisions regarding resuscitation at the lower ends of gestational age (<24 weeks) and birth weight (<400 g) become increasingly difficult. Decisions regarding the congenitally malformed or infants with chromosomal problems (like trisomy 13 and 18), identified during pregnancy, pose an ethical and moral challenge for the various participants. The pregnant woman and the father of the fetus, along with the family and physicians and other health care providers, struggle with these decisions at times of extreme vulnerability and uncertainty. Numerous publications and guidelines by professional and legal organizations attempt to clarify the issues and guide the parents, health care providers and hospitals. Management of these issues compels the clinicians to make decisions "in the moment of clinical truth".[9]

Significant medical and technological innovations have invaded the NICU. Thoughtful use of such advances might help to save more lives but attention should be paid whether these advances decrease morbidity overtime. Surfactant use from 1990 has significantly increased survival and reduced morbidity. Administration of antenatal steroids to pregnant mothers with preterm labor has increased both pulmonary maturity and survival. Short-term outcomes of those infants appear to be favorable but long-term outcomes are being evaluated. On the other hand, the introduction of ECMO and ventilators occurred without any controlled studies in NICUs. Later, studies suggested limited enefit for some of these therapies. It is critical we evaluate any new medical or surgical therapies before implementing them on a widespread basis in NICUs.

In this chapter some of these issues, such as the lower limit of viability (or how small is too small?), withdrawal and/or withholding life support including nutrition and fluids, economics, role of parents and health care providers, global perspectives, and a common framework for neonatal ethical issues, will be reviewed.

THRESHOLD OF VIABILITY OR HOW SMALL IS TOO SMALL?

The current published statistics about survival and morbidity rates of extremely low birth weight (ELBW) and very low birth weight (VLBW) babies will be presented to assist in addressing the issue of viability. Survivability of infants correlates with gestational age and birth weight. African American infants comprise of 36.8% of the ELBW (<1,000 g) babies born in the USA but account for only 15.5% of all live births. Biomedical and biopsychosocial factors may be contributing to this disproportionate increase in ELBW in African American births, and these dynamics need further investigation.

It is important to know the outcomes of these ELBW and VLBW infants, especially below 25 weeks of gestation, to assist in decision making regarding withholding or withdrawing support. Infants born and admitted to the NICU at or < 23 weeks have a less than 10% chance of survival. Less than 1% survival was reported in ELBW infants with birth weights < 400 g. In a large multicenter review in USA, the survival rate from birth until discharge for infants born between 1996 and 2000 and with birth weights of 401–500 g was 17%. Earlier reports by other investigators were more dismal in terms of survival of infants < 500 g.[10-12]

In a prospective study from England and Ireland[12] the survival rates expressed as a percentage of live births in 1995 for infants at 23, 24, and 25 weeks of gestation were 11%, 26% and 44% respectively. Expressed as a percentage of the admission to NICUs, the survival rates improved to 20%, 34%, and 52% respectively. For the same cohort of infants, the survival rates expressed by birth weight for <500 g, 500–749 g, and 750–999 g infants were 6%, 32%, and 55% respectively.

Birth weight-specific statistics of admissions to NICUs in the USA have shown higher survival rates. The National Institute of Child Health and Human Development (NICHD) network[2] reported survival rates for infants at 23, 24, and 25 weeks of gestation were <20%, 47% and 68% respectively. In the same report, survival rates from birth until discharge for infants born between January 1993 and December 1994 with birth weights of 501–750 g, 751–1,000 g, 1,001–1,250 g, and 1,251–1,500 g were 49%, 85%, 93% and 96% respectively. Among those survivors, chronic lung disease developed in 19%, intra ventricular hemorrhage in 32% (with 11% having severe grades), and periventricular leukomalacia in 6%. The incidence of necrotizing enterocolitis ranged from 3% to 9% and that of late onset sepsis varied from 9% to 34% inversely related to birth weights. Infants in these weight groups stayed in the hospital on an average of 2–4 months. The report also notes that the mortality rate declined by 42% from 1988 to 1994 in all weight groups but with no significant drop in the morbidity rates of infants <750 g (38% in 1988 and 37% in 1994).

In 1997, a report compared the survival and morbidity rates of infants weighing 501–800 g born in North Carolina, USA[5] during three time periods from 1979 to 1984, 1984 to 1989, and 1989 to 1994. Survival rates increased from 20% to 36% to 59% respectively. On the other hand, the major neurosensory impairments at 1 year of age stayed relatively the same, at 25%, 28% and 21%, during the same three periods. Hussain and Rosenkrantz[13] reported, in a 2003 composite of many studies from developed nations, a survival rate of <3.5% at 22 weeks, 21% at 23 weeks, 46% at 24 weeks and 66% at 25 weeks of gestation.

The cohort of infants born in 1995 in England and Ireland at <25 completed weeks were prospectively followed for >6 years. The report in 2005 suggested that the cognitive and neurological deficits were common at school age (21%).[14] A comparison with their classroom peers showed even more impairment (41%). The rates of mild, moderate and severe disabilities were 34%, 24% and 22% respectively in these survivors. 12% had cerebral palsy. Even more sobering were the rates of survival with no disability among this group at 6 years of age: 1%, 3%, and 8% for those born at 23, 24, and 25 weeks of gestation respectively.

While this information will keep changing in the future as mortality and morbidity rates change, one can attempt to address the issue of how small is too small. Biologically, at <22 weeks of gestational age, the physiological and anatomical maturity of the lung will unlikely support extrauterine function and hence survival.[15-17] Over the last 10 years, there seems to be a leveling of improvement in survival in these gestational age groups. This leveling suggests that we may have reached the threshold of viability with the current technology and support. Sharing this information and institutional, regional, national, and global mortality and morbidity reports with parents will be the first step in addressing the issue of viability.

PARENTS ROLE

In USA, parents are generally considered appropriate surrogate decision makers for their children. They are also considered to have the required authority and best interests of the infant in their minds when making decisions about medical care for their children.

Attitudes of parents and health care providers regarding outcomes of ELBW infants, including quality of life have been evaluated in many reports.[18-20] Saigal[18] reported that when presented with hypothetical clinical vignettes, health care providers in NICU were significantly more negative than the parents or the teenaged ELBW children. The parents rated the quality of life as good for their children even though they acknowledged their children have a greater burden than other normal birth weight children. These studies suggest parents are appropriate decision makers in most cases.

It is evident from the available data that the mortality and morbidity rates are high for infants born <24 weeks and/or <500 g. At 23 and 24 weeks even though survival has improved, reported handicaps of survivors should give a pause to those in NICU in pursuing a course of aggressive action in the delivery room and subsequently in the unit. It is important to have the global, national, regional, and institutional data on not only survival but also outcomes of these ELBW infants so that the information can be shared with the parents to assist in decision-making. Because the statistics differ depending upon which denominators are used, one should be clear and consistent in the communication.

The issue of sanctity of life versus quality of life is a running debate in neonatal and obstetric specialties, as well as with the prospective parents. Those who believe in sanctity of life may suggest that it is worth intervening with aggressive support for any live product of conception. Many have difficulty in accepting this notion as necessarily directing anyone to initiate or sustain treatments regardless of the mortality and morbidity. They suggest that it may be preferable to assess intervention after birth so that the decision can be made with more information at hand. On the other hand, the slippery slope argument about the quality of life judgment is well-known. This issue remains a continuing debate in society and adds to the uncertainty in decision-making.

ECONOMICS

As a result of advancing technology hospital bills have increased dramatically, and the total lifetime costs may go up even higher if the infant needs any type of rehabilitation or follow-up care. The cost of care in NICUs in the USA, is now reported as exceeding four billion dollars. A 2003 California study[21] reported an average hospital cost of $224,000 for an infant with birth weight between 500–700 g compared to $4,300 for infants between 2,250 g and 2,500 g and $1,000 for those with birth weights of greater than 3,000 g. In the same study, hospital costs averaged $202,400 for an infant born at 25 weeks compared to $2,600 for an infant born at 36 weeks and $1,100 for 38 week infant. Similarly, another study[22] reported a median cost of $103,600 for infants born between 501 g and 750 g going down to $31,200 for those between 1,251 g and 1,500 g. The hospital costs were highest for infants born at 25–26 weeks of gestation with a median of $101,600 dropping to $18,700 for infants born at >32 weeks. Another 1987 California study[23] calculated that the average cost per first-year survivor in infants in NICUs with birth weights less than 750 g was $273,900; for those who weighed 750–999 g the average cost was $138,800. In a May 16, 1988 article Newsweek quoted the total cost for a surviving fetal infant as $366,480 with additional costs during rehabilitation. However, the aggregate cost of NICU is still far less than the cost of adult intensive care units providing care for those at the end of life.

This brief discussion of the economics of caring for critically ill infants in the NICU is necessary to understand the full impact on families, society and the surviving infant with special needs. The infant's family undergoes severe emotional and financial stress with the birth of an extremely premature infant, and they often are confused, angry and frustrated by resulting issues. This concern needs to be understood by the medical team, and the public and society needs to address it in an open forum.

WITHHOLDING/WITHDRAWAL OF NUTRITION AND FLUIDS

The benefits and burdens of any medical intervention should be assessed so that a determination can be made regarding the withholding/withdrawal (WH/WD) of nutrition and fluids. Most will agree that if the burdens outweigh the benefits, the WH or WD of support to adults, children or neonates is acceptable. Currently, most reports suggest that for adults with terminal conditions it is appropriate for the patient to request WH/WD of nutrition and fluids as well (JAMA 1990).[24,25] Most agree that appropriate family members, especially if authorized to make medical decisions, can request WH/WD of nutrition and fluids for a terminally ill adult patient. Increasingly, pediatric patients are also reported as appropriate candidates for requests for WH/WD in terminal conditions.[26-28] The premise behind such requests is that tube feeding or intravenous alimentation should be considered a medical intervention just like intubation or other treatments. Others would argue that withdrawal of nutrition and fluids, especially from neonates, should not be recommended.

In an excellent review by Carter and Leuthner,[29] the authors hold that WH/WD of nutrition and fluids in newborn infants is also appropriate. They state that the "medical facts such as underlying diagnosis, response to previously given treatments, likely response to appropriate treatments or interventions not yet offered and ultimate prognosis for the infant's condition" should be considered and discussed in detail with the team, parents and extended family. In addition, parents' expectations, culture, religion, traditions and other social values should be brought to bear on this decision for their infant. The health care team should not usurp the authority of the parents without documentation (from independent experts) that they are not capable of making such decisions. The institution's policies and state legal statues should be reviewed and taken in to account. Offering oral feeding in infants should be acceptable as well as pain medications as part of palliative care. Hospice care, if available, for such infants when the WH/WD of care including nutrition and fluids is indicated as a good alternative. More discussion by physicians, the health care community, parental groups, and society is necessary to guide the decision-making about WH/WD of nutrition and fluids in newborn in the future.

GLOBAL PERSPECTIVES

It is clear that ethical decision-making does not take place in the abstract. Societies, nations, cultures and traditions, and religions play an intricate part in such decision making. In developing nations and now in developed nations as well, the economy also plays a role in such decisions at the macro level of national health care policy and micro level in the decision-making of a patient (the principle of justice). In many countries, such as India, Nepal and Sri Lanka,[30] quality of life and economy clearly play a crucial role in parental and societal decisions regarding WH/WD of support. In Singapore[31] using an individualized prognostic strategy, "a consensual decision that respects parental authority and promotes physician beneficence with the best interest of the infant placed in the center of analysis" is being reached. In Israel[32] the maternal birth place and level of religious observance were associated with aggressive intervention in hypothetical cases. In neonatal care, specific guidelines, such as those in Netherlands and Japan[33,34] led to infants at 22 or <25 weeks

of gestation being resuscitated, but resulted in significant mortality and morbidity. Similarly, a study in California, USA requiring resuscitation of all infants >22 weeks of gestation or >450 g resulted in significant mortality and morbidity, leading to a recommendation of providing other than comfort care as exceptional for infants <23 weeks or <500 g. A report from Scotland[35] outlined that eight European countries compared the "legal, ethical and professional settings within which decision-making for neonates took place". Overly aggressive treatment was discouraged and comfort care recommended. Most of the countries prohibited "active intentional ending of life" except Dutch pediatricians. Reports from USA,[36,37] Australia[38,39] and Austria[40] suggest that infants born at tertiary centers with neonatal and perinatal specialties had a better survival rate at these gestational ages. Those transferred in utero to tertiary centers at 23, 24, and 25 or 26 weeks of gestation showed lower morbidity and had a better prognosis. Globally, the viability limit seems to be slowly but steadily converging around 22–24 weeks based on biological and experiential data.

COMMON FRAMEWORK FOR PERINATAL AND NEONATAL ETHICS

Attempting to create a common framework for neonatal and perinatal ethics is a daunting task. We proposed in 1987, a model[41] based on the ethical principles of beneficence and respect for autonomy, incorporating the families, religion, culture and traditions, societies, and nations as part of the fabric of decision-making (Fig. 22.1). With minor modifications, it probably still holds as an anatomical framework for clinicians to work through difficult ethical dilemmas.

The principles of beneficence and respect for autonomy are clearly addressed in the model. The fetus and future neonate along with the pregnant woman are at the center of this schema generating both beneficence and autonomy related obligations. Even though there are ethical obligations generated toward the parent/s, the neonatologist's primary patient is the neonate. The future parent/s is included at the top of the model to reflect the relationship in the neonatal period. The physician is at the base of the model generating ethical obligations to prospective parents, the pregnant woman, and the fetus during the perinatal period and to

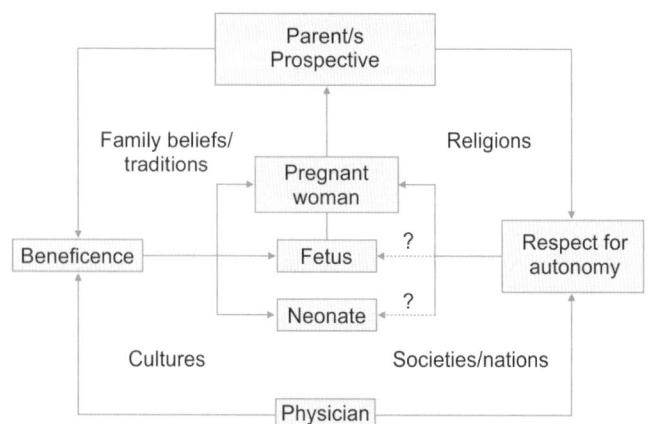

Fig. 22.1: Common framework for perinatal/neonatal ethics, modified from Seminars in Perinatology, 1987, "The Ethics of Perinatal and Neonatal Care".

the neonate and the parents in the postnatal period and beyond. It is recognized that these ethical dilemmas are affected by the context in which they occur and hence the schema recognizes the need to add religious beliefs, traditions, family beliefs and values, cultures, societies, and nations as the very fabric on which this model is built. There are primarily beneficence-based ethical obligations to the fetus and neonate, but the model included autonomy-based obligations as a secondary in the model because some may believe they exist. This structural guidance could be applied to ELBW infants, infants with congenital anomalies such as Trisomy 13, Trisomy 18, anencephalic and other terminally ill infants.

This model extends Pellegrino's proposed framework[9] for clinical ethical dilemmas to the complex perinatal and neonatal areas. This model recommends a collaborative approach to decision-making between the parent/s, physician, and other health care providers acting in the best interest of the baby. Parents should be able to make those decisions for their infant unless they are shown to be incompetent or incapable as assessed by independent specialists such psychiatrists or, of course, the courts. Obtaining the opinion of ethics consult or ethics committee will help the clinician and family in guiding the decision-making. Many families have found the objective view of another expert or group of people helpful in facilitating the discussion and clarification of the facts of the ethical dilemma being faced and the options available.

The four "C"s of clinical ethical decision-making include:

1. Communication
2. Clarification
3. Consistency
4. Caring.

Maintaining a high level of communication between parents and health care providers is necessary in the NICU where issues are extremely complex and highly charged with emotions. Clarification of issues that arise among health care givers and between parents and medical and nursing staff is crucial for problem solving even before a dilemma arises. Providing consistent information available to date by all care givers (provided good communication exist between providers) will allow for trusting environment in which decision-making is encouraged. An attitude of caring from the very beginning provides the necessary environment in which parents feel comfortable in discussing any and all issues about their infants. All four of these facilitate decision-making by the parents and health care providers during difficult times.

GUIDELINES

Currently, there exist guidelines from various organizations including the American Academy of Pediatrics (AAP), AAP Committee on Fetus and Newborn, AAP Committee on Bioethics,[42-44] NICHD consensus conference,[45] American College of Obstetricians and Gynecologists (ACOG), ACOG committee on Obstetric Practice,[46] Canadian Pediatric Society,[47] Thames Regional Perinatal Group,[48] Colorado Collective for Medical Decisions,[49] International Guidelines for Neonatal Resuscitation,[50] NY State Task Force on Life and Law,[51] and from other countries (Table 22.1). At 22 weeks or <23 weeks or <400 g, most guidelines recommend giving only comfort or compassionate care, which is consistent with available data about mortality and morbidity and biological information. Most guidelines will also suggest comfort care at 23 weeks unless parents, after understanding the high risks, want to initiate aggressive attempts. At 24 weeks, resuscitation will depend

upon the assessment of the baby's condition at birth and the parents' understanding of the mortality, morbidity, and prognosis; choosing to intervene to give a trial of life is an appropriate alternative. In some of the recommendations (Italy 2004, New York 1988), 24 weeks or >500 g are used as cutoff points for resuscitation. At 25 weeks and beyond, most guidelines recommend full resuscitation. However, some maintain that a parental request not to resuscitate should be followed even at 25 weeks. Most guidelines base the recommendations on gestational age. Because growth-restricted mature infants are included in the statistics presented by birth weight, a hard birth weight cutoff is more difficult to use in deciding viability.

All guidelines consistently recommend the need for clear communication among physicians, nurses and parents both before delivery and afterwards. Collaborative decision making between parents and physicians, along with other health care providers, is the best way to chart a course that is appropriate for the individual baby and parents, especially in infants expected to be <24 weeks of gestation or <500 g in birth weight. Any strict cutoff by gestational age or birth weight at this edge of viability should be avoided because the prognosis for the individual infant remains uncertain in terms of both mortality and morbidity. Parents who understand the high risks involved in aggressive interventions at the borderline gestational ages should be given the option of assessment at birth and resuscitation. Further action will depend on the infant's condition and NICU course. Even prior to delivery, one should discuss with parents that, if assessment after birth indicates a significantly poor prognosis, withdrawal of support should be an option. There should always be room for individual decision making based on the specifics of the situation, such as a parent with infertility, advanced age, multiple pregnancy losses, etc. Even though ethically there is no difference between WH and WD care, emotionally the latter may be harder for parents or some health care providers. For some, WH may be preferable than WD, but clear communication before and throughout the hospital course will help in making the right decision.

Collaborative or consensus decision-making between the parents, physician and team with careful, clear communication and discussion is the best way to resolve any ethical dilemmas. In situations where disagreement exists between the health care team and parent(s), additional consultations with a colleague and other specialists and/or ethics consults and committee meetings should help clarify the issues and resolve the differences. In those difficult situations where differences remain, one or the other party can seek legal action. Usually courts are not in the best position to resolve these difficult moral and ethical issues except on narrow legal grounds. In many situations law and ethics may not see eye-to-eye in resolving the dilemma.

CONCLUSION

In summary, the tremendous advances made in the last 4 decades in neonatal medicine have also brought difficult ethical dilemmas for health care providers and parents. Over these, years, the lower limit of viability dropped from 28 weeks to 32 weeks to 22 weeks to 23 weeks of gestation. As we reach the physiological and anatomical limits of lung development and extrauterine survival we also reach a natural barrier of lower limit of viability. Of course this can change if there are some additional advances in existing treatments such as liquid ventilation or providing nutrition in a novel way, or new

Table 22.1: Guidelines for care of extremely preterm infants.

Canadian Pediatric Society, 1994

- 22 weeks of gestation: Treatment should be started only at the request of fully informed parents or if it appears that the gestational age was underestimated.

- 23 – 24 weeks of gestation: There is a role for parental wishes, the option of resuscitation, and a need for flexibility in deciding to start or withhold resuscitation, depending on the infant's condition at birth.

- 25 weeks of gestation: Resuscitation should be attempted for all infants who do not have fatal anomalies.

Colorado Collective for Medical Decisions, 2000

- 22 weeks of gestation: Comfort care is the only appropriate choice.

- 23 weeks of gestation: Most participants would advise comfort care, but if parents understood the high risks, they would be willing to initiate a course of intensive care.

- 24 weeks of gestation: Participants are able to support either decision, as long as a collaborative process with good sharing of information occurred.

- 25 weeks of gestation: Most participants were uncomfortable with withholding care, but some were willing to support a parental request for comfort care if there had been good education and an effort at collaboration.

American Academy of Pediatrics/Americal Heart Association Neonatal Resuscitation Program, 2000

- Noninitiation of resuscitation in the delivery room is appropriate for newborns who had confirmed gestation of less than 23 weeks or birth weights of less than 400 g

Thames Regional Perinatal Group, 2000

- Less than or equal to 22 weeks of gestation: Compassionate care only.

- 23 – 24 weeks of gestation: Resuscitation depends on infant's condition at birth.

- 25 – 27 weeks of gestation: Full resuscitation and supportive care.

Source: Boyle RJ, c472 NeoReviews vol.5 No. 11 November 2004.

interventions such as artificial placenta or uterus. But this "medical miracles around the corner" argument or outliers in terms of survival of <23 weeks gestation infants cannot be used for decision making occurring now. Advances in technology and the ability to prolong life should be tempered with the benefits and burdens to the patient. Principles of beneficence and respect for autonomy obligations weigh heavily in neonatal ethical dilemmas in the milieu of principle of justice and cultures, traditions, religions and nations. Weighing the benefits/ burden to the patient should guide everyone in the decision making. The physician has beneficence generated obligations toward the fetus and neonate. The neonatologist has both beneficence and autonomy generated obligations toward the pregnant mother and father during antenatal consultations and subsequently to the parent/s when the neonate comes into the NICUs. Collaborative/consensus/shared decision making with parents, physicians and others, applying the ethical principles outlined in the model, will result in the best practice in NICU for these infants. Judicial uses of the ethics consultant or committee and other experts may facilitate better communication and clarification in difficult circumstances. Providing communication in a clear, consistent and caring way (4 "C"s) and sharing all the information about mortality, morbidity, and prognosis before and after delivery of a high risk infant facilitates decision making.

ACKNOWLEDGMENTS

My thanks to Ms Ninian Kring for preparing the tables and figures and Ramya Sivasubramanian JD for reviewing the manuscript and providing valuable suggestions.

I also thank all the infants that I had the privilege of taking care over the years and their parents for the opportunity to serve and learn from and all the staff, residents, fellows and colleagues at Georgetown University Hospital NICU.

REFERENCES

1. Lemons JA, Bauer CR, Oh W, et al. Very low birth weight outcomes of the National Institute of Child Health and Human Development Neonatal Research Network, January 1995 through December 1996. NICHD Neonatal Research Network. Pediatrics. 2001;107(1):E1.

2. Stevenson DK, Wright LL, Lemons JA, et al. Very low birth weight outcomes of the National Institute of Child Health and Human Development Neonatal Research Network, January 1993 through December 1994. Am J Obstet Gynecol. 1998;179(6, Pt 1): 1632-9.

3. Horbar JD, Badger GJ, Lewit EM, et al. Hospital and patient characteristics associated with variation in 28-day mortality rates for very low birth weight infants. Vermont Oxford Network. Pediatrics. 1997;99(2):149-56.

4. Wood B, Katz V, Bose C, et al. Survival and morbidity of extremely premature infants based on obstetric assessment of gestational age. Obstet Gynecol. 1989;74(6): 889-92.

5. O'Shea TM, Klinepeter KL, Goldstein DJ, et al. Survival and developmental disability in infants with birth weights of 501 to 800 grams, born between 1979 and 1994. Pediatrics. 1997;100(6):982-6.

6. Vohr BR, Wright LL, Dusick AM, et al. Neurodevelopmental and functional outcomes of extremely low birth weight infants in the National Institute of Child Health and Human Development Neonatal Research Network, 1993–1994. Pediatrics. 2000; 105(6):1216-26.

7. Botting N, Powls A, Cooke RW, et al. Cognitive and educational outcome of very-low-birthweight children in early adolescence. Dev Med Child Neurol. 1998;40(10):652-60.

8. Ment LR, Vohr B, Allan W, et al. Change in cognitive function over time in very low-birth-weight infants. J Am Med Assoc. 2003;289(6):705-11.

9. Pellegrino ED. The anatomy of clinical-ethical judgments in perinatology and neonatology: A substantive and procedural framework. Semin Perinatol. 1987;11(3):202-9.

10. Lucey JF, Rowan CA, Shiono P, et al. Fetal infants: The fate of 4172 infants with birth weights of 401 to 500 grams – the Vermont Oxford Network experience (1996–2000). Pediatrics. 2004;113(6):1559-66.

11. Allen MC, Donohue PK, Dusman AE. The limit of viability–neonatal outcome of infants born at 22 to 25 weeks' gestation. N Engl J Med. 1993;329(22):1597-601.

12. Costeloe K, Hennessy E, Gibson AT, et al. The EPICure study: Outcomes to discharge from hospital for infants born at the threshold of viability. Pediatrics. 2000; 106(4):659-71.

13. Hussain N, Rosenkrantz TS. Ethical considerations in the management of infants born at extremely low gestational age. Semin Perinatol. 2003;27(6):458-70.

14. Marlow N, Wolke D, Bracewell MA, et al. Neurologic and developmental disability at six years of age after extremely preterm birth. N Engl J Med. 2005;352(1):9-19.

15. Barbet JP, Houette A, Barres D, et al. Histological assessment of gestational age in human embryos and fetuses. Am J Forensic Med Pathol. 1988;9(1):40-4.

16. DiMaio M, Gil J, Ciurea D, et al. Structural maturation of the human fetal lung: A morphometric study of the development of air–blood barriers. Pediatr Res. 1989;26(2):88-93.

17. deMello DE, Reid LM. Embryonic and early fetal development of human lung vasculature and its functional implications. Pediatr Dev Pathol. 2000;3(5):439-49.

18. Streiner DL, Saigal S, Burrows E, et al. Attitudes of parents and health care professionals toward active treatment of extremely premature infants. Pediatrics. 2001;108(1):152-7.

19. McHaffie HE, Laing IA, Parker M, et al. Deciding for imperilled newborns: Medical authority or parental autonomy? J Med Ethics. 2001;27(2):104-9.

20. Hansen MM, Durbin J, Sinkowitz-Cochran R, et al. Do no harm: Provider perceptions of patient safety. J Nurs Adm. 2003;33(10):507-8.

21. Gilbert WM, Nesbitt TS, Danielsen B. The cost of prematurity: Quantification by gestational age and birth weight. Obstet Gynecol. 2003;102(3):488-92.

22. Rogowski J. Using economic information in a quality improvement collaborative. Pediatrics. 2003;111(4, Pt 2):e411-8.

23. Fischer AF, Stevenson DK. The consequences of uncertainty. An empirical approach to medical decision making in neonatal intensive care. JAMA. 1987;258(14):1929-31.

24. Winter SM. Terminal nutrition: Framing the debate for the withdrawal of nutritional support in terminally ill patients. Am J Med. 2000;109(9):723-6.

25. Hastings Center. Guidelines on the Termination of Life-Sustaining Treatment and Care of the Dying. Briarcliff Manor, NY: The Hastings Center; 1987.

26. Burns JP, Mitchell C, Griffith JL, et al. End-of-life care in the pediatric intensive care unit: Attitudes and practices of pediatric critical care physicians and nurses. Crit Care Med. 2001;29(3): 658-64.

27. Cranford RE. Withdrawing artificial feeding from children with brain damage. Br Med J. 1995;311(7003):464-5.

28. Johnson J, Mitchell C. Responding to parental requests to forego pediatric nutrition and hydration. J Clin Ethics. 2000;11(2): 128-35.

29. Carter BS, Leuthner SR. Decision making in the NICU–strategies, statistics, and "satisficing". Bioethics Forum. 2002;18(3–4):7-15.

30. Subramanian KN, Paul VK. Care of critically ill newborns in India. Legal and ethical issues. J Leg Med. 1995;16(2):263-75.

31. Ho NK. Ethical issues in neonatal paediatrics–the Singapore perspective. Ann Acad Med Singapore. 1995;24(6):910-14.

32. Hammerman C, Kornbluth E, Lavie O, et al. Decision-making in the critically ill neonate: Cultural background v individual life experiences. J Med Ethics. 1997;23(3):164-9.

33. Oishi M, Nishida H, Sasaki T. Japanese experience with micropremies weighing less than 600 grams born between 1984 to 1993. Pediatrics. 1997;99(6):E7.

34. Nishida H, Sakamoto S. Ethical problems in neonatal intensive care unit–medical decision making on the neonate with poor prognosis. Early Hum Dev. 1992;29(1-3):403-6.

35. McHaffie HE, Cuttini M, Brolz-Voit G, et al. Withholding/withdrawing treatment from neonates: Legislation and official guidelines across Europe. J Med Ethics. 1999;25(6):440-6.

36. Yeast JD, Poskin M, Stockbauer JW, et al. Changing patterns in regionalization of perinatal care and the impact on neonatal mortality. Am J Obstet Gynecol 1998;178(1, Pt 1):131-5.

37. Bode MM, O'Shea TM, Metzguer KR, et al. Perinatal regionalization and neonatal mortality in North Carolina, 1968–1994. Am J Obstet Gynecol. 2001;184(6):1302-7.

38. Doyle LW, Casalaz D. Outcome at 14 years of extremely low birthweight infants: A regional study. Arch Dis Child Fetal Neonatal Ed. 2001;85(3):F159-64.

39. Doyle LW, Cheung MM, Ford GW, et al. Birth weight <1501 g and respiratory health at age 14. Arch Dis Child. 2001;84(1):40-4.

40. Hohlagschwandtner M, Husslein P, Klebermass K, et al. Perinatal mortality and morbidity. Comparison between maternal transport, neonatal transport and inpatient antenatal treatment. Arch Gynecol Obstet. 2001;265(3): 113-8.

41. Subramanian KN, McCullough LB. A common framework for perinatal and neonatal medical ethics. Semin Perinatol. 1987;11(3):288-90.

42. American Academy of Pediatrics Committee on Fetus and Newborn. The initiation or withdrawal of treatment for high-risk newborns. Pediatrics. 1995;96(2, Pt 1):362-3.

43. MacDonald H & The Committee on Fetus and Newborn: Perinatal care at the threshold of viability. Pediatrics. 2002;110:1024-7.

44. American Academy of Pediatrics Committee on Bioethics. Ethics and the care of critically ill infants and children. Pediatrics. 1996;98(1):149-52.

45. Higgins RD, Delivoria-Papdopoulos M, Raju NK, et al. Executive summary of the workshop on the border of viability. 2005;1392-6.

46. American Academy of Pediatrics Committee on Fetus and Newborn. Perinatal care at the threshold of viability. American College of Obstetricians and Gynecologists Committee on Obstetric Practice. Pediatrics. 1995;96(5, Pt 1):974-6.

47. Canadian Pediatric Society, Fetus and Newborn Committee. Management of the woman with threatened birth of an infant of extremely low gestational age. Maternal–Fetal Medicine Committee, Society of Obstetricians and Gynaecologists of Canada. Can Med Assoc J. 1994;151(5):547–53.

48. Thames Regional Perinatal Group. Guidelines relating to the birth of extremely immature babies (22–26 weeks gestation). Available from http://www.gapm.org/publication.php. (Accessed March 2000.)

49. Colorado Collective for Medical Decisions. Neonatal Guidelines and Video. Denver, CO.

50. Niermeyer S, Kattwinkel J, Van Reempts P, et al. International guidelines for neonatal resuscitation: An excerpt from the Guidelines 2000 for Cardiopulmonary Resuscitation and Emergency Cardiovascular Care: International Consensus on Science. Contributors and Reviewers for the Neonatal Resuscitation Guidelines. Pediatrics. 2000;106(3):E29.

51. Anonymous. Fetal Extrauterine Survivability. Report of the Committee on Fetal and Extrauterine Survivability to the New York State Task Force on Life and the Law. New York: New York State Task Force on Life and the Law, 1988.

23 Medicolegal Aspects of Perinatal Medicine: European Perspective

J Walker

INTRODUCTION

A pregnant woman has similar rights to any other patient and these are protected by the normal human rights assigned to her by society. Therefore, her informed consent is required before intervention and her right to refuse treatment accepted. However, there is a complication, she carries another potential individual, therefore, her rights and her control over her pregnancy is influenced by the rights assigned to the fetus and how much of these rights are allocated to the mother to hold.

Irrespective of the rights the child has in utero, after birth, its rights are paramount, and although the parents may control these rights to a degree, this is not absolute and their control can be removed in the best interests of the baby. Also in some situations, the rights of the newborn baby can be considered to be present in retrospect, in other words, damage done prior to delivery that results in problems after birth, can give rights of complaint to the baby that were not there at the time of the event. Therefore, potentially, the rights of this one individual, the child, and the rights of others over it, can change at the moment of birth and, in some instances, these change of rights can then be applied retrospectively.

This has caused increasing ethical dilemmas over the years because of the increasing knowledge of pregnancy physiology and, more importantly, the increasing ability to assess and visualize the fetus. This has meant that the fetus is increasingly seen as an individual that has access to medical care and is a factor in medical decision making. This has led to the concept of the "Fetus as a Patient" and by definition, medical rights.[1] Generally, what is good for the baby is good for the mother, so there is no conflict. It is when the mother disagrees with her carers about what is best for the baby that conflict appears.[2,3]

With advances in medical technology and the ability to salvage pregnancies that previously failed, society has begun to believe that medicine can achieve anything. This means that if damage occurs, there has to have been error and negligence. Since the fetus is usually the one that is damaged, it is the baby, or its guardian, that will proceed with litigation, even though the fetus may not have had rights at the time of the event. If a neonatal death occurs, increasingly this may lead to potential criminal proceedings,[4,5] but this can depend on the legal rights of the fetus and whether it is born alive or not. It is in these areas of litigation and fetal rights that there is so much difference between countries.

THE RIGHTS OF THE FETUS

There is no universal truth and that is never more true than for ethical and legal issues. Perinatal doctors in different countries work within different environments. What is acceptable in one country may not be in another, not because it is right or wrong, but because of differences of ethical, legal or social mores.[5] In medicine, we are taught to "first do no harm", but in the case of perinatal medicine, to whom? The problem is that there can be conflict between the concept of the "Fetus as a Patient" and the rights of the mother.

This situation is covered by the term beneficence.[1] Beneficence is the moral principle that one should aim to help and failure to do this when one is in the position to do so is morally wrong. However, one is obligated to act to benefit others when one can do so with minimal risk, inconvenience or expense. In perinatal medicine there is potentially two patients to consider. How much of a conflict this is depends on both legal and moral belief. In general, the life of the mother takes precedent since there is a logic that the health of the mother is important not only to the health of that baby but of any siblings. However, the main governor of the decision making process is the legal rights of the fetus.

If the fetus has the same rights as a newborn baby, decisions can be made on behalf of the baby against the wishes of the mother, so called court ordered care.[2] There is also the potential of the newborn suing for any damage sustained in utero from maternal or other's actions, so called Wrongful Life decisions.[6]

However, where the fetus has no legal rights, the mother's wishes are paramount. It is only variations in law or ethical constraints that will restrict her and her carers' actions. However, this maternal control exists only up to the moment of birth when full neonatal rights exist and the control transfers to the baby or its guardians. This change in legal status occurs in a matter of minutes and can be confusing to the mother, attendant staff and society as a whole. Generally, in European law, the starting point is that a child *en ventre sa mere* is a part of its mother and therefore its rights are held by the mother.[7]

However, in English common law an unborn child has rights to inherit property as follows:

"There is nothing in law to prevent a man from owning property before he is born. His ownership is contingent, for he may never be born at all; but it is nonetheless real and present ownership. A man may settle property on his wife and the children to be born of her. Or he may die intestate and his unborn child will inherit his estate".

This is traditional called "present ownership", that is, a right possessed by the unborn child at that time, but conditional on being born alive. If the child is stillborn, the inheritance (or rights) will revert to someone else. This is referred to as the "born alive rule".[7]

Therefore, any right the fetus has in English common law is dependent on being born alive. This means that actions leading to death of the baby before birth are not subject to the normal crimes against the person but if the baby is born alive and then dies then the baby's existence, and therefore rights exist and action can be taken.

Overall, the legal situation in Europe is somewhat confused and is constantly evolving as will be described. Within the European Community, there is a further complication since the countries are governed by similar European laws on human rights, although there are still differences with the application due to local law in each country.

THE RIGHT TO LIFE

When the European Human Rights Act came into force in 2000, it was felt by many that the "Right to Life" stated in Article 2 could be extended to the unborn fetus. This would protect it from termination of pregnancy and give it equal rights to the mother when considering medical decisions. However, a case based on this belief, has recently been heard in the European Court of Human Rights and it was decided that the rights of the fetus are not covered by Article 2. This is an important landmark decision not based on law but more on lack of consensus of what is right.

The case involved Mrs Vo, one of two women of the same name admitted to the same hospital at the same time, one for a medical examination when 6 months pregnant, the other to have a coil removed. The wrong Mrs Vo went for coil removal. In an attempt to remove the nonexistent coil, Mrs Vo's amniotic sac was pierced and the pregnancy terminated. The doctor was charged with unintentional homicide, the French equivalent of involuntary homicide. He was initially acquitted, but then convicted on appeal and sentenced to 6 months in prison and fined 10,000 francs. He then appealed to the Court of Cassation—France's highest court which overturned the ruling on the grounds that the fetus was not a human being and not entitled to the protection of criminal law.

Mrs Vo then took the case before the Grand Chamber of the European Court (application no. 53924/00). She accused that France's failure to extend the law on unintentional homicide to the unborn violated the State's Article 2-based obligation to respect life. However, the court found in favor of France by 14 votes to 3.

`The Court felt that the decision of when the right to life begins was a question to be decided at national level. They noted that there was no European consensus on the scientific and legal definition of the beginning of life, particular France, where the issue had been the subject of public debate. At best, it could be said that the consensus was that the embryo/fetus belonged to the human race. Its potential and capacity to become a person required some protection in the name of human dignity, without making it a person with the right to life for the purposes of Article 2 or legal status in conflict with the mother. Therefore, the Court was convinced that it was neither desirable, nor even possible as matters stood, to answer the question whether the unborn child was a person for the purposes of Article 2 of the Convention. The main judgment of the Court was to accord each State a degree of autonomy, or a "margin of appreciation" as it is called, to work out the right legal position for itself. So on this view Article 2 did not apply. A minority of the judges felt that there was no issue; since "even if one accepts that life begins before birth, that does not automatically and unconditionally confer on this form of human life a right to life equivalent to the corresponding right of a child after its birth".

Therefore, by a majority of 13–14, the court was in favor of the inapplicability of Article 2, implying a lack of rights for the unborn child and setting a precedent on the legal status of unborn babies that will be applied across European countries.

WRONGFUL LIFE AND WRONGFUL BIRTH

After the baby is born, it has equal rights to the mother and the rest of society. To some extent, these rights can be applied retrospectively and the events that occurred or did not occur prior to birth can, in theory, be litigated against if it adversely affects the baby after birth. There are two particular situations, Wrongful Life and Wrongful Birth, where the plaintiff claims that the baby would rather not have been born, i.e. be terminated. Since this usually involves failure of prenatal diagnosis and termination of pregnancy, this can produce conflict with the various legal and moral arguments.

Definitions

Wrongful life is when the child takes the action against another party for allowing it to be born in a deformed or harmed way caused by actions or inaction prior to birth. In other words, it would rather have been terminated and litigates for damages to help it live as comfortably as possible.

Wrongful birth is when the mother sues other people for being burdened with a disabled child something she could have avoided.

In essence these suits are genetic or prenatal diagnosis litigation cases where termination could have been offered. Again much of the debate has occurred in France but affects all countries.

The Nicholas Perruche Case

In 1982, when Josette Perruche was in early pregnancy, her 4-year-old daughter developed rubella. She told her doctor that, if she had been infected, she wanted a termination rather than risk giving birth to a handicapped child. She had two blood tests, 2 weeks apart, which gave contradictory results. Mrs Perruche was reassured that all was well. However, Nicholas was born with the rubella syndrome and, after investigation, it was discovered that the laboratory had made an error. A case was brought on behalf of Nicholas against the doctors alleging that failure by doctors to diagnose the condition in the womb had prevented a termination of pregnancy and led to Nicholas being born with deformity. The French Court found in his favor stating in its ruling[8] "since mistakes committed by the doctors and the laboratory while carrying out their contract with Mrs Perruche prevented her from exercising her choice to end the pregnancy to avoid the birth of a handicapped child, the latter can ask for compensation for damages resulting from this handicap".

There was great upset to the court ruling. Cathrine Fabre, of the Federation of French Families, said at the time "*we cannot approve the idea of claiming for compensation for being alive*".

Further cases were brought where families argued that if doctors had detected the disabilities prior to birth, they would have had the pregnancies terminated.[9] This case went on appeal to the highest court in France, the Cour de Cassation. The court ruled that disabled children were entitled to compensation if their mothers were not given the chance of an abortion. The court stated that the Perruche precedent remained "*as long as a causal link can be established with an error committed by a doctor*".

Following this doctors and campaigners for the disabled reacted furiously, describing the decision by the court as an incitement to eugenics. The case was widely described as establishing in French law a disabled child's "*right not to be born*". The Collective To Stop Discrimination against the Disabled (CCH), which was set up after the Perruche case, feared that parents would be attacked for giving birth to a handicapped child as a result of the decision. "*This is a real act of phobia. Now parents are going to be attacked and seen as irresponsible because they gave birth to a handicapped child,*" it said. "*The ruling means that the handicapped have no place in our society*", said Yves Richard, a lawyer representing the medical profession. "*There is a real risk of this starting a process that ends with the search for the perfect child*".

Doctors expressed increasing concern that the verdict would push doctors to terminate pregnancies when they were unsure about the normality of the fetus. Some started to refuse to carry out routine antenatal scans as they were worried that they would be sued if a disabled baby was born that they had failed to diagnose. The doctors threatened strike action.

Ethicists and legal specialists also attacked the rulings. "*To allow a child to be born cannot be considered as a mistake—that must be written into law,*" said Laurent Aynes, a professor in civil law at Paris' Sorbonne University. Many called on the government to change the law on the subject. Initially, they held out against legislation, but were forced to act by public pressure and by the decision by some medical staff to stop carrying out prenatal scans. The bill was passed that states that nobody can claim to have been harmed simply by being born. By doing this, the government's ruling brought to an end a year's legal and moral debate.[8]

However, the new parliament bill prohibited Wrongful Life cases only not Wrongful Birth suits. This means that the obstetrician or technician can still be sued, but the parents—not the affected child—will be able to seek damages, but only on the grounds of a "blatant error" by doctors, the argument being that the birth of the disabled child is damaging the life of the mother.

The Dutch Experience

After a court awarded damages to a severely disabled girl for the fact that she was born, MPs called for the Netherlands to follow France and ban damage claims for Wrongful Life. Doctors fear the judgment could lead to a sharp increase in defensive prenatal testing.

The case was of 9-year-old Kelly Molenaar whose parents had informed a midwife at the Leiden University Medical center that a relative of the father was disabled because of a chromosomal abnormality. The midwife reassured them and did not carry out further prenatal diagnostic tests or refer the case to a clinical geneticist. The abnormality was not detected early enough to intervene and Kelly was born with multiple mental and physical disabilities.

She cannot walk, talk or properly recognize her parents; has deformed feet; is believed to be in constant pain; and has had several heart operations. By the age of 21 months, she had been admitted to hospital nine times due to "inconsolable crying".[10]

The court accepted that damage to Kelly resulted from the midwife's error. The appropriate referral would have resulted in a termination and Kelly would not have been born. Damages against the hospital amounting to the cost of Kelly's care and upbringing until her 21st birthday were awarded to her parents. But the court went further, ruling that Kelly herself was liable to damages. The court judged that the damage experienced by Kelly was in a legal sense a predictable consequence of the midwife's mistake. Therefore, the court accepted the possibility of a claim for Wrongful Life. The amount of the damages is still to be decided.

The hospital's lawyers are considering an appeal to the Supreme Court to quash the judgment and MPs are urging the Ministries of Health and Justice to respond to the decision. Boris Dittrich (MP) has called for Dutch law to be changed to prohibit Wrongful Life claims as has happened in France.

Joseph Hubben, Professor of Health Law at the Free University of Amsterdam, said: "*To recognise a disabled life as a source of financial damages gives the wrong signal to society. Disabled people should be fellow citizens not someone who should have been aborted*". He also argued that the decision would increase pressure for more prenatal diagnostic testing not just from parents but also from doctors.

The UK Experience

In 2004, a UK mother was successful in suing her hospital after giving birth to a child with genetic abnormalities. She claimed damages, saying that if she had been informed of the child's disability, she would have had him killed before birth. The baby had extensive scanning but no abnormality was detected. The baby boy was born in 1999 with a genetic abnormality that causes bladder, bowel and genitalia defects. The Hospital, Leeds Teaching Hospitals NHS Trust, had to pay an undisclosed amount of damages to assist the woman in the raising of the child. A spokesman for the Leeds Teaching Hospitals NHS Trust said: "*This was an extremely complex case and one which was defended by the trust because it raised important clinical questions*".

Summary of the European Situation

As can be seen, the European situation is confused, but it would seem that Wrongful Life cases are not being allowed, not only because of the litigation fears it brings, but also the moral aspects deciding that a disabled child is better off not being born. However, Wrongful Birth cases are increasing. These cases, unlike the usual litigation case, which relates to damage sustained, center round the doctor or technician's failure to diagnose a preexisting abnormality and therefore prevented the mother from having the opportunity to terminate the pregnancy. This produces major problems and concern for obstetric units because any scan potential will "miss" an abnormality. Also, which abnormalities "merit" consideration for termination? This is accentuated by a case currently under consideration in the UK where a member of the public has asked for a judicial review on a case of a late termination of pregnancy for a cleft lip and palate.

The upper gestational limit of termination varies from country to country, in France the law allows termination of pregnancy with no upper gestational age limit; in Italy, termination of pregnancy after the time of viability may be legally carried out only when continuation of pregnancy represents, either for physical or psychological reasons a danger to the mother's life. In the UK, the most recent abortion act states that a termination of pregnancy can be carried out for a serious handicap right up until term as long as the baby is born dead.

What, however, is a serious handicap? A paper in 2001, demonstrated that of the 270 children born with cleft lip and/or palate, 23 were positively diagnosed by ultrasound prior to birth.[11] Out of that 23, two ended up having termination of pregnancy, which is just under 10%. The assumption from this and other studies is that, if the diagnosis was available to more couples, then more terminations for cleft lip and palate would be requested. It also implies that there are many causes of fetal abnormality that parents may wish to terminate and which are not currently universally diagnosed or termination offered. In a European survey, only 2% of doctors would offer a termination for cleft lip/palate.[12] Do we need to extend the screening of babies to cover a wider range of abnormalities and offer all termination of pregnancy? If we do not offer them termination and/or the abnormalities are missed, will litigation follow to cover any surgical and other care costs? Who is to decide what a serious handicap is and whether a termination is justified?

LITIGATION—THE EUROPEAN PERSPECTIVE

This problem relating to Wrong Birth cases is adding to the already increasing litigation culture in Europe. There are significant differences between Europe and the US. In Europe:

- The litigation is usually brought by claimants paying for the legal costs. However, this is often supported by government grant (Legal Aid in the UK) although some *"No Win, No Fee"* cases are beginning to appear.
- The cases are heard in front of judges, not juries which mean that the cases are usually less emotive but lead to law of precedent.
- The awards are largely for cost of care required, not suffering. This means that the cost of an award for a child with cerebral palsy may in the region of 4 million UK pounds but if the child dies, the award may only be 20,000.

The cost of litigation is mounting and, at present, the total *potential* payouts for litigation in the UK is more than the total cost of running three London teaching hospitals or providing all maternity care for England for a year. However, this is a misleading statistic, as the total amount *paid out* in *settling* claims each year is only about 1% of the total NHS budget, not a huge sum.[13] In 1998, the rate of litigation was 0.81 closed claims per 1,000 finished consultant episodes. The problem is that 65% of the cost, but not the numbers, are obstetric cases. Because of the rising litigation cost, medical malpractice insurance for obstetricians has escalated. This has led to the UK government bringing in "Crown Indemnity" meaning that the National Health Service (the Crown) will cover the cost of litigation.[14] Therefore, it is the health authority that is sued not the individual doctor. Also, all cases brought against hospitals are defended in England by lawyers working for the National Health Service Litigation Authority (NHSLA), a centralized body. Any costs up to £100,000 are paid by the individual hospitals but above that, the costs are met by the Clinical Negligence Scheme for Trusts (CNST) which was set up in 1995 to indemnify acute NHS Trusts against litigation. CNST grade hospitals according to risk and, when a Trust undergoes this assessment, it can earn a rebate of upto 30% of its indemnity payments, if it can demonstrate significantly good performance in terms of certain risk management processes.[15] This can be a six figure sum.

Therefore, litigation in Europe is becoming an increasing drain on health care resources and governments are stepping in to provide the financial cover in various ways. However, this does not come without strings. Although individuals are no longer targeted for litigation, the government agencies are wielding increasing power to insist on risk management procedures and the appropriate training and supervision of staff. So although individuals are no longer responsible to reduce the litigation threat, the hospitals themselves have financial gains to be made if their staff follows the necessary guidelines and practices. This can be an important driver of improved care.[15]

OBSTETRIC DECISION MAKING

Decision making by doctors is a complex business influenced by training, culture and knowledge of outcome. An good example of this is decision to deliver by CS for the premature fetus. Obstetricians in the different European countries were asked what would be the earliest gestation they would intervene by cesarean section in the fetal interest in three different scenarios:

1. When parents wanted everything possible done to save this baby.
2. When parents were against aggressive management.
3. When it was your child.

In the first situation, the median lowest gestational age at which obstetricians would be willing to perform an emergency cesarean section for fetal indication varied from 24 completed weeks in Sweden and Germany, to 26 in Netherlands, UK, Italy and Spain. Knowledge that parents were against aggressive management would increase this figure by 1 week in Spain, France, Netherlands, Luxembourg and Sweden. Interestingly the most conservative approach, i.e. the latest gestation, was found in scenario 3 where it was your own child.[12] These results imply that if you want to achieve a life birth, then going early can be justified but it is not if the best interests of the parents and the baby are taken into account. The recent Growth Restriction Intervention Trial (GRIT) study would tend to confirm the rightness of that view since delayed delivery reduced long-term disability.[16]

NEONATAL DECISION MAKING

As previously stated, at birth, the baby takes on individual rights which may initially rest with the parents but ultimately can be practiced independently through an appointed guardian. This can cause confusion since before birth, sometimes just minutes before, the maternal rights were paramount, now the baby rights can be in conflict.

Here again, retrospective rights pertain. In English law, termination of pregnancy is allowed right up until term for significant fetal abnormality, however, the baby must be born dead. If the baby is born alive and then dies due to the result of prematurity or of the procedure itself, the doctor who carried out the procedure which led to the baby's death can be charged with manslaughter. This means that late termination usually requires feticide. This adds to the stress and unpleasantness of the procedure for the parents and the staff carrying out the procedure although others feel that it is more humane.[17] The fact that the killing of a handicapped fetus is allowed but it is not minutes later after birth, adds to the confusion.

However, Dr. Eduard Verhagen, of the Groningen Academic Hospital and Dr Louis Kollée of Radboud University Medical Center in the Netherlands, have asserted that euthanasia of infants is occurring worldwide. They called on the Dutch government to regularize the killing of handicapped newborn babies by providing guidelines that will protect physicians from murder charges. They felt that there should be a panel to consider guidelines for euthanasia for people with "no free will", i.e. severely handicapped infants.

The practice varies throughout Europe most commonly in the Netherlands and France but doctors are divided in whether it should be controlled by law.[18] Interestingly, nurses are more in favor that doctors.

An associated problem is when to initiate and/or withdraw care from an infant with a severe abnormality or gross prematurity. This problem was highlighted by the "Baby Messenger" case in the US where a severely ill preterm infant was resuscitated against his parents wishes and was removed by his parents from ventilator support and allowed to die in their arms. The father was initially charged with manslaughter although subsequently acquitted.[19] The approach to the resuscitation of premature babies varies between countries with many producing clear guidelines of when small or abnormal babies should be treated or when treatment should be withdrawn.[20] The different approaches are based on various methodologies including:

- The "statistical" approach whereby treatment is withheld from infants defined as underweight and/or immature.
- The "initiate and reevaluate" approach whereby aggressive treatment is begun and then re-evaluated relative to the infant's progress and parents' wishes.
- A "treat until certainty" approach whereby each infant is treated until death or discharge.

Each of these approaches has advantages and disadvantages. The Danish Council of Ethics produced a protocol that combines a minimum gestational age, maturity and parental wishes. Generally, infants younger than 24 or 25 weeks will not be aggressively treated but this can be modified if the infant looks mature and can be resuscitated using "low technology modalities" and minimal handling.[19] Also the approach can be modified by considerations of parental wishes. The long-term outcome for the baby is greatly influenced by the ability of his parents to provide the care it requires. Therefore, the threshold can be moved down by parents wishing to care for a child that fails to meet the criterion or up by parents requesting to withhold treatment from a newborn that meets the threshold requirement. Under these guidelines, baby messenger would not have been resuscitated. Even had the neonatologist decided that the gestational threshold had been met, the baby's immediate condition following birth did not meet the maturity criterion. This, together with the parent's refusal of ventilator support, should have meant that he should not have been resuscitated. The council's recommendations are based on two main factors: the infant's best interests and economic justice: "*The basis for the (modified threshold) recommendation is that the panel considers the 35% occurrence of severe handicaps in children born after a pregnancy term of 24–25 full weeks to be high in relation to the number of surviving infants; the panel also takes into account the comparison of the expenditure incurred with the possible alternative applications for that amount*".[9] Therefore, the infant's best interests and the cost to society is considered not just survival. A 35% risk of severe impairment may be too high for a parent, physician or policy-maker to accept. However, there is also a chance that the child may lead a relatively normal life. While this may seem a reasonable decision for parents to make, it does result in large numbers of healthy infants being allowed to die to avoid a smaller number of handicapped infants. One benefit of targeting care is to benefit those who would gain most. "*It seems reasonable to exercise reticence in the treatment of extremely preterm infants in order to benefit the slightly less premature, since the prospects of better results increase with age and fewer resources are consumed, allowing more to be helped.*"[10]

In a survey in different European countries, doctors were asked how they would care for a case of extreme prematurity (24 weeks of gestational age, birth weight of 560 g, Apgar score of 1 at 1 minute). Most physicians in every country but the Netherlands would resuscitate this baby and start intensive care.[20] On subsequent deterioration of clinical conditions caused by a severe intraventricular hemorrhage, attitudes diverge: most neonatologists in Germany, Italy, Estonia, and Hungary would favor continuation of intensive care, whereas in other countries some form of limitation of treatment would be the preferred choice. Parental wishes appear to play a role especially in Great Britain and the Netherlands. Interesting, again nurses are more likely than doctors to want to withhold resuscitation in the delivery room and to ask parental opinion regarding subsequent treatment choices. Among doctors who would resuscitate, only in Great Britain and the Netherlands would a substantial percentage change the decision, knowing that parents were against resuscitation. In Estonia, Hungary, Italy, Germany and Spain, most doctors would withhold treatment in case of emergencies, such as cardiac arrest, whereas doctors in Great Britain, the Netherlands, and Sweden would withdraw mechanical ventilation. Only in France and the Netherlands would definitive actions be taken to end life. Therefore, the range of care throughout Europe, in the same clinical situation, varied from active care until there was no hope to positively ending life.

Interestingly, the parents responses to these decisions are varied, partly depending on outcome with 22% of the parents expressing reservations about the length of the dying process. Some reported that this had taken from 3 hours to 36 hours. Deaths that medical teams had predicted would be quick had, according to the parents' recollections, taken from 1.5 hours to 31 hours. When a baby died swiftly, this seemed to confirm the decision to stop but, when babies lingered, doubts were raised.[20]

CONCLUSION

So there is no pan-European perspective, each country has its own approach. The Danes have a varied statistical approach to what should and should not be done, the Dutch similarly have a definite cut of point, with a pragmatic approach toward withdrawal of treatment and even active ending of life, the British wait and see, discuss the case with their colleagues and the parents and largely let nature take its course but will withdraw treatment when clear possibilities of a successful outcome has gone and the Germans will work to save the baby until it dies. This does not appear to be influenced by religious factors but by the social norms of the society that the doctors work.

Similarly the approach toward termination is extremely liberal and uninfluenced by religious prejudice. This is helped by the largely pan-European legal position that the fetus has no rights before birth as this is the main pillar of the right of life battle. The recent findings in the European Courts has ended that fight for the foreseeable future.

However, there is an increasing European problem of litigation with the number and cost of cases increasing. The UK leads the way in this situation and has tried to solve the insurance costs by the government footing the bill. This has just led to spiralling costs. The newer Wrongful Birth cases has opened up what appears to be an endless source of new cases which can be of significant cost. Again Governments have had to intervene to legislate in these situations, not because of the rights or wrongs but for the social good.

REFERENCES

1. Chervenak FA, McCullough LB. The fetus as a patient: An essential concept for the ethics of perinatal medicine. Am J Perinatol. 2003;20(8):399-04.
2. Draper H. Women, forced caesareans and antenatal responsibilities. J Med Ethics. 1996;22(6):327-33.
3. Harris LH. Rethinking maternal-fetal conflict: Gender and equality in perinatal ethics. Obstet Gynecol. 2000;96(5 Pt 1):786-91.
4. Molenaar JC. The legal investigation of a decision not to operate on an infant with Down's syndrome and a duodenal atresia: A report from the Netherlands. Bioethics. 1992;6(1):35-40.
5. McHaffie HE, Cuttini M, Brolz-Voit G, et al. Withholding/withdrawing treatment from neonates: Legislation and official guidelines across Europe. J Med Ethics. 1999;25(6):440-6.
6. Bottis MC. Wrongful birth and wrongful life actions. Eur J Health Law. 2004;11(1):55-9.
7. Wellman C. The concept of fetal rights. Law Philos. 2002;21(1):65-93.
8. Spriggs M, Savulescu J. The Perruche judgment and the "right not to be born". J Med Ethics. 2002;28(2):634.
9. Dorozynski A. Highest French court awards compensation for "being born". BMJ. 2001;323(7326):1384.
10. Sheldon T. Court awards damages to disabled child for having been born. BMJ. 12 2003;326(7393):784.
11. Shaikh D, Mercer NS, Sohan K, et al. Prenatal diagnosis of cleft lip and palate. Br J Plast Surg. 2001;54(4):288-9.
12. Cuttini M. The European Union Collaborative Project on Ethical Decision Making in Neonatal Intensive Care (EURONIC): Findings from 11 countries. J Clin Ethics. 2001;12(3):290-6.
13. Walsh P. Editorial. The AVMA Medical & Legal Journal. 2003;9:108.
14. Palmer RN. United Kingdom 'Crown' indemnity for medical negligence—An overview of the first 18 months of the new scheme. Med Law. 1992;11(7-8):623-7.
15. Wood L. Clinical Negligence Scheme for Trusts and maternity care: Let's redesign services, not patch up outdated systems. Clinical Risk. 2003;9:86-8.
16. Thornton JG, Hornbuckle J, Vail A, et al. Infant well-being at 2 years of age in the Growth Restriction Intervention Trial (GRIT): Multicentred randomised controlled trial. Lancet. 2004;364(9433):513-20.
17. Dommergues M, Cahen F, Garel M, et al. Feticide during second- and third-trimester termination of pregnancy: Opinions of health care professionals. Fetal Diagn Ther. 2003;18(2):91-7.
18. Cuttini M, Casotto V, Kaminski M, et al. Should euthanasia be legal? An international survey of neonatal intensive care units staff. Arch Dis Child Fetal Neonatal Ed. 2004;89(1):F19-24.
19. Gross ML. Avoiding anomalous newborns: Preemptive abortion, treatment thresholds and the case of baby Messenger. J Med Ethics. 2000;26(4):242-8.
20. De Leeuw R, Cuttini M, Nadai M, et al. Treatment choices for extremely preterm infants: an international perspective. J Pediatr. 2000;137(5):608-16.

24 Malpractice Issues in Perinatal Medicine: The United States Perspective

BS Schifrin, MR Lebed, J McCauley

INTRODUCTION

It was probably inevitable that the law and medicine would come into conflict, irrespective of the fact that despite some obviously different approaches, these learned professions share more than they conflict. While medicine is fundamentally inductive and law deductive, both fields are centered in advocacy for the client. When it comes to medicine, the law tries to reconcile a body of science with the art of clinical practice. When it comes to the law, medicine tries to reconcile a body of laws with notions of fault and accountability. The relationship is abetted when the goals of better, more efficient care and prompt and effective methods of dealing with error and adverse outcome are agreed upon. On the other hand, when each profession deems the other side to hold some unscrupulous advantage, when the "playing field is perceived to be not level", and when myth and misdirection are rampant and malpractice premiums have become excessive or insurance coverage unavailable, then the worst of the relationship comes to the fore, and political and legislative resources are recruited to help control the dialogue and the invective, and define or create new rules of engagement. In the end, care is compromised as are notions of justice and access to the law.

HISTORIC PROSPECTIVE OF MALPRACTICE IN THE UNITED STATES

Malpractice suits were unheard of until 1848. Prior to that there was no control over the practice of medicine or its numerous schools of practice. There was no need; patients generally were fatalists, believing that any adverse medical outcome was the will of God. It became an issue after 1848 only because allopathic physicians, to eliminate other "schools of medicine" created objective standards of practice, created national medical societies and national standards, elected to support litigation under tort law rather than contract law, and established the "deep pockets" of malpractice insurance—a profitable industry for attorneys.

But it was only with the beginning of the 1960s that more educated, informed and assertive patients began to question their physicians in the same manner that they evaluated their other goods and services. In general, this was poorly accepted by physicians, who for the most part maintained a traditional authoritarian stance in the care of their patients. The legislative crises of the 1970s and subsequent crises of the 80s, 90s, and present, brought with tort reform Health Maintenance Organizations (HMOs) increasing regulation, decreasing autonomy, strained relations with hospital administrations and allied healthcare providers, and decreased physician and patient satisfaction. Although much has changed from the mid 1800s there is one historic consistency; the major litigen is not outcome, but is physician behavior.

MALPRACTICE LAW

Malpractice law is part of tort, or personal-injury, law that affects large segments of society, including product liability, automobile accidents, airplane crashes, etc. and other examples of unintended harm. As mentioned above, it was the physicians themselves, who determined that due to their superior status, were not subject to contract law with patients, who were not their equal, and set the higher civil law standard of tort law. The objectives of malpractice litigation are straightforward:

1. To resolve disputes fairly with equal opportunity for "justice" on both sides.
2. To compensate persons injured through negligence.
3. To deter unsafe practices, i.e. raise the standard of care,[1] all without resorting to armaments or fisticuffs.

A plaintiff prevails in a lawsuit by proving the 4Ds: that the defendant

1. owed a Duty of care to the plaintiff,
2. that there was a Deviation from an acceptable standard of care,
3. that there was a nontrivial injury to the plaintiff (Damages) that was directly caused by the deviation from the standard of care.[1] A failure to demonstrate anyone of the four means that the requirements, under the law, are not met. To begin the process, a patient approaches a lawyer. The reasons for which patients sue are many.[2-5]

For patients and family members, the physical and emotional devastation of medical error cannot be easily overcome. As a rule, however, this circumstance has been made even more difficult because there was no satisfactory explanation to the patient of the reason for the adverse outcome, there was no admission of negligence, no opportunity for questions, and no consolation for loss.[6,7] In reality, the patients want a forthright explanation of what happened—want to understand if they played a role in it. And if, just if, a mistake had been made, they expect an apology and an offer to compensate for the expense and aggravation. They are real people, and whether the injury was the result of negligence or not, they, not the physicians burdened with a lawsuit, are the real victims. When asked, "What was wrong with the care you or your child received?" or "What complaints do you have about physicians?" patients respond rather specifically (Table 24.1).[4] As underscored by these data, the attorney is often the last person who is contacted, not the first. Indeed, most often patients are directed to an attorney by a member of the medical community.

Indeed, many are amazed when looking at medical malpractice cases, by the cold-blooded attitude so many defendants have taken toward patients who have been seriously, and sometimes

Table 24.1: Malpractice induced activities

Modality	Percent
Testing	76.2
Monitoring	73.3
Documenting	72.2
Informed Consent	61.6
Consulting MDs	58.0
Patient Information	51.2
Referrals	47.2
Staff Presence	21.8
ACOG — 1990	

grotesquely, harmed. Inhumanity and indifference to the suffering of others is in itself another form of injury. When patients file suit, they are often made to feel as though they had done something wrong, as if seeking legal redress and compensation was in some sense an affront to the system, a personal assault on the physician. Many plaintiffs feel pressured by all the parties involved to agree to a settlement. In some instances, such advice may come from the plaintiff attorney or even the sitting judge. Indeed, on occasion extraordinary amounts of offered settlement are turned down, not because of the size of the award, but because all the details of their case would then come out publicly—they would have their day in court.

Physicians believe themselves to be operating in an environment of zero tolerance for error. It is embedded in their oath and dedication to "do no harm", in their professed desires help others, and magnified by a historic paternalistic tendency to extend unrealistic expectations to their patients.[8] The physician who has erred is wounded, and suffers the consequences of guilt, fear of reprisal (from the patient, hospital and regulatory agencies), embarrassment (peer), and sorrow for having harmed someone (Levinson).[5,9] Because medicine, for centuries, has been loathe to identify negligent care (even in closed, protected settings) this system of justice has enfranchised the plaintiff's attorney, not especially trained for the purpose, to determine the medical and the legal merits of the case (they are not the same!). Under the contingency-fee relationship prevalent in the United States, the attorney takes a percentage of the award as a fee (often around 35%) to compensate for the costs, expenses and time absorbed in pursuing the case irrespective of the outcome; they take nothing if the defendant prevails. These expenses are not trivial; bringing a "bad baby" case to court, for example, may easily cost $100,000 of up front expenses. It is not undertaken lightly.[8]

But before the attorney can proceed, one of his first expenses will involve consultation with a medical expert (a physician) to determine whether the potential case satisfies two most critical criteria of the 4Ds: Was there a Deviation from a reasonable standard of care and was there a Direct causal relationship between that failure and the adverse outcome? Damages and Duty, generally, are self-evident. Traditionally, the "standard of care" is defined as the quality of care (customs and behavior) that would be expected of a reasonable practitioner in similar circumstances. These standards are drawn from members of the profession itself as well as documents that reflect a consensus on appropriate standards (plural) of care.

It should be emphasized that there is no single standard of care. Satisfying the need to do something "*reasonable under the circumstances*", indeed, may permit mutually exclusive choices to be within the standard of care. Because the law holds the arcane nature of medicine "a learned profession" to be beyond the grasp of common citizens, it requires the testimony of experts in the same field as the defendant.[9,10] Neither the courts nor the legislatures can reasonably establish detailed conduct for professional practice without "practicing medicine".[11]

Ideally, medical witnesses will be readily available and forthright, and medical standards will be determinable from readily available medical records that are well documented, readable and responsive to questions of whether or not the medical conduct met a reasonable standard of care. The medical consultant/potential expert witness will possess both current knowledge and experience with the issues at hand, but, at any time in the review process, is honor bound to use all available relevant information and to apply broadly understood, minimal, standards of care—not their own personal standards. An expert witness must elaborate the standard for medical care at the time of the plaintiff's injury and give an opinion on whether the defendant's conduct met this standard. The standard is not unique to the expert, but rather must reflect general principles applicable to all practitioners, at the same time specific to the individual patient's circumstances. Ideally, it should be supported by scholarly literature. While it need not prescribe a single course of action, it must either (for the plaintiff) proscribe the defendant's conduct or (for the defense) endorse the defendant's conduct as an acceptable alternative. Therein lies the conflict.

While the courts expect that medicine, as a learned, science-based discipline, will have articulated standards for practice in most circumstances they also recognize that not all standards are formalized or even well-defined, not all clinical circumstances can be circumscribed in some obvious standard of care, and that there is "art" to the practice of medicine. To overcome these hurdles, the courts using their own *legal* (not medical) standards of witness acceptability, allow appropriately qualified expert witnesses to express expert opinions. Indeed, the expert witness is the only party in the lawsuit who may express opinions; everyone else is only entitled to the "facts" of the case. Ideally, the expert will not be an advocate, except perhaps of his own opinion, and will honestly present his or her understanding of the applicable standards without tailoring his responses to serve the single-minded ends of the lawyer engaging the expert.

Obtaining expert testimony has always been the most difficult part of medical malpractice litigation. Historically, experts were readily available to testify against competing medical disciplines including homeopathic physicians and chiropractors, although they were expected to remain silent about the misconduct of members of their own profession (omerta). To abolish these vituperative, economic rivalries, the courts established the doctrines of "school of practice" and "locality rule" as bases for qualifying expert witnesses.

The school of practice rule permits the differentiation of physicians into self-designated specialties depending upon whether the case concerns procedures and expertise that are intrinsic to the specialty or general medical knowledge and techniques that are common to all physicians. Thus, obstetrical cases may involve family practitioners, midwives, obstetrician/gynecologist as well as members in training; the potentially significant differences in their individual standards may indeed require expert witnesses from each of these specialties.

Before the standardization of medical training and certification that prevails today, there was a tremendous gulf between the skills and abilities of university-trained physicians and the graduates of "less reputable" schools issuing diplomas. Thus, in many parts of the country, a physician's ability to serve as an expert would be determined by comparison with the other physicians in the community, or at least in similar neighboring communities. For obvious reasons, this rule essentially precluded injured patients from finding supportive expert testimony—effectively preventing most medical malpractice litigation. Reasonably, there is no longer a justification for any rule that impedes evaluation of what have become national standards of care on the sole basis that it is the norm for a given community. While most states have explicitly abolished the locality rule, it is being reinvigorated in some states as a tort reform measure (and omerta) to deal with the problems of access to care and facilities in rural areas.

A national standard of care implies that the rural and urban physicians will have the same training and exercise the same level of judgment and diligence. The rule does not require that the rural physician have the same medical facilities, consultants or other resources available. If the community does not have facilities for an emergency cesarean section, for example, the physician cannot be found negligent for failing to do this surgery within the 15 minutes that might be the standard in a well-equipped urban hospital. However, to comply with the standard of care, the physician must inform the patient of the limitations of the available facilities and recommend prompt transfer, if indicated. He must also make reasonable efforts to deal with the inevitability of requiring an emergency section—even in a rural community. Proper informed consent allows patients to balance the convenience of local care against the risks of inadequate facilities.

At trial, judges and jurors (the triers of fact) have no alternative but to judge the testimony of witnesses whether expert or percipient (fact) on the personal credibility of the witness. For the experts and the defendants, positive factors such as academic degrees, specialty board certification and publications influence credibility. So do factors such as physical appearance, race, gender, command of English and personality. For each of these, the objective is to be believed. The defendant also has to be believed, but his role is much more focused; he has but one chore: to convince *anyone* who will listen (judge, juror, attorney, stenographer, bailiff, passerby) that he/she is a thoughtful, caring, concerned human being who did what was reasonable under the circumstances. The defendant has no other job. Performing research, providing expert opinion or combating the opinions of the opposing expert are all some else's function. As mentioned above, his demeanor in deposition or trail (as well as with his patients) has a great deal to do both with the likelihood of lawsuit and its resolution. For the expert witness, the foremost requirements are effective presentation and teaching ability. The expert must educate the judge and jury in the technical matters at hand.

Until 1993, Federal courts had used the "general acceptance" test, set forth in Frye vs. United States, to assess the admissibility of expert scientific testimony.[12] In 1993, the United States Supreme Court modified the standard for determining the admissibility of expert scientific testimony in federal trials. In Daubert, the court stated that Frye test did not comport with the Federal Rules of Evidence and that "a rigid 'general acceptance' requirement would be at odds with the 'liberal thrust' of the Federal Rules and their general approach to relaxing the traditional barriers to opinion testimony".[12] Accordingly, the court emphasized that a trial judge must screen the proposed scientific testimony to ensure that the testimony is relevant and reliable before allowing the testimony to be presented at trial. Rule 702 reflects the need for screening.[12-14]

If scientific, technical or other specialized knowledge will assist the trier of fact to understand the evidence or to determine a fact in issue, a witness qualified as an expert by knowledge, skill, experience, training or education may testify thereto in the form of an opinion or otherwise. It is a judicial decision, not a medical one.[14,15]

The court set forth four factors that may be used to assist the trial judge in determining "whether the expert is proposing to testify to scientific knowledge that will assist the trier of fact to understand or determine a fact in issue". The factors that may be considered when determining the validity of a scientific theory or technique are:

1. Whether the theory or technique can be tested.
2. Whether the theory has been subject to peer review and publication.
3. The rate of error, and the acceptance of the theory of technique within the community. The court cautioned that "the focus ... must be solely on principles and methodology, not on the conclusions that they generate". The court emphasized that these factors are not exclusive.

Thus, under Daubert, a defendant doctor may be considered negligent for treatment and diagnosis even though he presents evidence from a number of medical experts genuinely of the opinion that the defendant's care followed customary medical practice. The court must determine for itself the appropriateness and the logic of the professional opinion and find reassurance that the body of opinion relied upon was not created for defensive purposes (see below). It is a curiosity that an expert's position may fail a Daubert challenge in one case, but may continue to be offered in other cases! It seems counterintuitive that a lay judge is qualified to be asked to determine the qualifications and credibility of an expert. Some believe that the selection of medical experts should be the purview of medically trained peers. Indeed, there is an argument to be made that the specialty societies develop a list of "true" experts that are available to either side or the judge himself.

At least in Federal Court the expert's legal activities over the last 5 years must be listed with the court prior to his appearance. Federal rules also give a judge the authority to

- Limit cumulative evidence, i.e. more than one expert testifying to the same issues unrelated to qualifications.
- Retain experts to assist the court.
- With mutual consent appoint a single expert witness.

Despite these available options, especially in "bad baby cases", there is an increasing tendency to line up a broad array of qualified experts on both sides including an obstetrician, perinatologist, placental pathologist, neonatologist, neurologist, nurse, economist, neuroradiologist, etc. There is at least some evidence that this proliferation of experts (and costs), more likely driven by the defense, is counterproductive. Bors-Koffelt, et al. found that the use of multiple defense expert witnesses decreased the chances of a successful defense.[16]

Many jurisdictions have attempted to insinuate the expert witness into the proceedings prior to the case being filed. In several states a report or affidavit of merit from the expert is required to launch the suit, in others only the testimony by the lawyer that he has contacted an expert is required. By and large there is no standard format for expert reports, and they are normally quite minimal and nonspecific. There is also no requirement that the "expert" who gave an affirmative opinion to the attorney, whether he signed the letter of merit or not, will subsequently be involved in the case, a deplorable circumstance as will be discussed below. Even if he/she were later involved, there are no mechanisms short of deposition or interrogatory to amplify on the experts' allegations. In some states, the expert cannot be deposed before trial and indeed his identity is unknown to the opposing side until he is called to the stand—widely referred to as "trial by ambush".

While the expert's opinion is normally protected by the doctrine of witness immunity, this does not protect the witness from fraud or from professional malpractice liability[17] or from other forms of harassment. "The goal to insuring that the path to truth is unobstructed and the judicial process is protected, by fostering an atmosphere where the expert witness will be forthright and candid in stating his or her opinion, is not advanced by immunizing the expert witness from…negligence in forming the opinion".[17] In one instance, a consulting expert was sued for failing to testify on behalf of the plaintiff in trial. The expert believed that causation could not be satisfactorily proven.

It is perhaps instructive here to deal with the terms, "meritorious" and "frivolous" as applied to malpractice cases. As a short-hand, whether the case is meritorious or not is a function not of the result, but of whether there is a substantive question about the standard of care and its relationship to the outcome. In a frivolous case, there is no substantive question, the 4 Ds cannot be shown or linked, or any question of negligence is readily answered in the negative simply with the most cursory examination of the evidence. Often, the complaints that prompt the visit to the attorney derive from actual or perceived slights by the physician related to a poor "bedside manner", a disputed bill, a lack of timely response, etc. In this respect, it is important to understand how, given the unrequited emotional needs associated with adverse outcomes, malpractice litigation serves the purpose of emotional vindication.[18,19] Such complaints are usually dismissed out of hand by the attorney in the first interview with the patient or secondarily on the basis of the review by the consulting expert. It is not widely appreciated but the vast majority of patients that approach lawyers with complaints about their physicians are turned down (probably in excess of 90%). Some patients are actually grateful to know that they did not receive substandard care, and equally important, that they themselves did not contribute to the adverse outcome. Despite any anger or frustration, they may have with the conduct or deportment of the physician they often harbor notions of their own complicity in an adverse outcome, especially when there has been a brain-damaged baby—if they had only not skipped an appointment, not used the hot tub, not gained so much weight, etc. Being turned down in a request to sue a physician may have positive benefits of closure. It may, indeed help them to forgive themselves. While it is quite uncommon to pursue a lawsuit based solely on an emotional misdemeanor by the physician, it becomes a powerful incentive to bring a lawsuit if the care has also been negligent. As will be seen in the statistics below, many negligent physicians are exculpated or avoid lawsuits entirely not because of the facts of the case, but by becoming a demeanor to the patient or to the jury. Other physicians have been found negligent, not because of their care, but by their indifference toward the patient. It is this author's experience that the minute the jury perceives that the physician does not care vindication of his medical conduct is not possible.

Thus, to label as "frivolous", as many physicians have, all cases that plaintiffs lose, or are settled "for economic reasons" or are dismissed, trivializes the tort system, the lawyers, the patients, the opposing expert witness, and in its way, impedes the solution of the malpractice problem and foments more error. This posture reveals an inadequate understanding of the dynamics of expert allegations, settlements, jury verdicts and even the process of peer review.

Given the affirmative report by his expert, the attorney is legally *obligated* to pursue discovery—the accession of all the relevant clinical data from the medical records or other sources. To flesh out the records and to understand something of the personality of the defendants, depositions are taken of the relevant treating or factual witness—sometimes including the custodian of records, etc. and the various medical experts.

The defense against the allegation of failing to meet the standard of care of a malpractice case centers around issues of customary practice, clinical practice guidelines, informed consent and differentiating error from complication. In judging the conduct of the physician in a court of law the court is guided by a notion called "reasonable conduct". Indeed, it is sufficiently vague as to require the participation of an expert witness to state what is and what is not "reasonable" conduct. At least theoretically, the creation of clinical practice guidelines would simplify and implement broadly understood practices subscribing to a quality care that could be objectively measured. At the same time, the quality of care would be improved and iatrogenic injury diminished.

There has been a broad implementation of "clinical practice guidelines" from various hospitals, professional organizations and the government itself. A clinical practice guideline is any guide to the clinical management of a patient. These guidelines vary widely according to the purpose for which they are written and who has been selected to write them. They may be driven by medicolegal issues, by the cost of care, or by the quality of care. While great emphasis has now been placed on the process of writing guidelines, many providers have become concerned with the basic precepts of guidelines, including the possible emergence of "cookbook" medicine, the effect of patient variability, and the need to keep guidelines flexible, current and credible.[20, 21]

Clearly, one impetus for the creation of clinical practice guidelines for specific medical conditions and their treatment was the notion that they would help avoid or defend malpractice claims. Indeed, someday they might replace the "reasonable conduct" standards and their dependence upon expert testimony in medical cases and thereby discourage both defensive medical practices and spurious claims—after all it is the medical profession and not the juries that establishes the standard of care; the jury just attempts to find out what were the standards that the medical profession had set for itself in any given situation and then to determine whether those guidelines were appropriately and reasonably followed. There are several problems with the use of "guidelines". First, they may not be usable (admissible in evidence) at all. Because of the wide range of reasons for creating guidelines (care, costs, medicolegal protection) in many states such guidelines constitute "hearsay" in great measure because their author is not in court to be cross-examined. Finally, having followed the guidelines may not mean malpractice was not committed. Scrupulous adherence to the relevant guidelines for an amputation, for example, avails nothing if the wrong leg has been amputated. Thus, it is that the notion that compliance with guidelines renders the clinician immune from lawsuit has not been upheld. Consensus, after all, is not necessarily wisdom, or applicable in all cases!

When the opinions of the opposing experts conflict irreconcilably over this issue the jury comes face to face with the logical conundrum. Is the disagreement related to lack of awareness of the standards or is one of the experts lying? The jury assesses the credentials and the credibility and various other sources of information to help them decide which expert is more credible in relating the individual patient's care to the prevailing standards.

One of the most widely quoted and misunderstood guidelines require that institutions should be capable of instituting an emergency cesarean section within 30 minutes of decision.[22] Some institutions cannot meet these guidelines reliably while others maintain a standard that can result in an emergency cesarean section in 10 minutes or less. While several studies have attempted to determine the reasonableness of "the 30 minute rule", neither the "studies" nor the "guidelines" take into account certain realities or certain remedies.[22] The "30 minute rule" is shorthand designation for a more encompassing principle that, under certain conditions performance of a cesarean section should be carried out as quickly as possible consistent with concern for the health and well-being of the mother and fetus, preferably within 30 minutes. But what is the standard if there is already one cesarean section in progress or two? Under these circumstances, a delay becomes "reasonable under the circumstances", notwithstanding the fact that standard of care required earlier cesarean section. However, if a physician is late in realizing the need for cesarean section or is ready to operate within 20 minutes but fritters away 10 minutes beforehand, his conduct cannot possibly comport with a reasonable standard of care, even if the patient is delivered within 30 minutes. Further, it stands to reason, that institutions normally unable to consistently meet the 30-minute rule must modify their practices and exhibit a willingness to prepare for cesarean sections early (even if it proves unnecessary) in anticipation of problems and make special arrangements for unique situations such as vaginal birth after cesarean (VBAC). Thus, the failure to meet the 30-minute rule is rarely by itself a telling a plaintiff's allegation. Much more frequently, the plaintiff's allegation is that the failure to properly interpret the fetal monitoring tracing or to properly estimate the feasibility of safe vaginal delivery hopelessly delayed the decision in the first place, irrespective of the "decision to incision" interval.

There is frequent debate over whether "official" pronouncements such as the "30-minute rule" are to be construed as monolithic "standards of care". More reasonably, it seems, that irrespective of whether these writings are entitled practice parameters, guidelines, standards, apocrypha, hints, clues, etc. the imprimatur of an official body, gives any statement about care the force of a "standard". Indeed during litigation, both sides are opt to offer these professional publications as standards to support their case irrespective of the disclaimer that these recommendations are guidelines rather than standards of care. Thus, guidelines, whatever their provenance, are never "medicolegally binding" and can be directly and reasonably contravened by a thoughtful, alternative choice of care—that is annotated!

INFORMED CONSENT

Similarly, the patient has rights, no matter how appropriately they may be exercised, to influence decisions about her care. In dealing with matters of informed consent, most courts in the United States look to what a reasonable patient would want to know, not what a "reasonable physician" would have said. The courts have on several occasions been asked to intervene in circumstances involving the refusal of treatment by a pregnant woman, refusal which nominally threatens the life and well-being of her fetus and herself. While the courts' responses have been varied there is general consensus amongst the specialties that these ethical (not legal) issues should not be resolved in court and that considerable ethical weight should be given to the mother's decision as long as the consent has been proper and there been no coercion. Lawsuits based entirely on informed consent are quite uncommon, but most such cases in obstetrics seem to involve VBAC the use of operative delivery and the decision to induce labor with a previous history of shoulder dystocia. If the "informed consent" document in such cases is to truly represent "informed consent" it must reveal the patient's understanding that she may either undergo an elective repeat Cesarean section or, if she is a suitable candidate, attempt a VBAC. She must understand that not all patients are candidates for VBAC and that not all VBAC attempts will result in successful vaginal delivery. She must be aware that some of the determinable clinical factors that affect the success of VBAC become apparent only in labor. The patient must also understand that all pregnancies carry a small risk to both mother and fetus, whether or not the mother has had a previous cesarean section. In patients with a previous cesarean section, the risk of uterine rupture during a VBAC is approximately 1% and this occasionally may result in serious, potentially life-threatening complications for the mother or the baby. If the patient initially agrees to attempt VBAC, she needs to understand that she is entitled to an updating of the likelihood of success and to change her mind at any reasonable time and to obtain a cesarean section, even during labor. Finally, the patient should understand that no decision, however thoughtfully made, or how reasonably pursued, guarantees a normal outcome for the mother or the infant.

The reader may now compare this approach with the deliberations in an "informed consent" case that was decided by the Wisconsin Supreme Court and that stretched the limits to which some physicians would go to reduce their cesarean delivery rate. In this case (Schreiber), a patient presented with a history of two previous cesarean sections, the first undertaken for arrest of labor after 17 hours (the second was elective); she had agreed prior to labor to attempt VBAC.[23] During labor, in the face of slow progress and severe abdominal pain, she changed her mind and repeatedly requested a cesarean section. Just as often, the obstetrician maintained that it was unnecessary. The obstetrician commented, "if I performed cesarean section on every woman who wanted one then all deliveries would be by cesarean section". Intimidated, the patient no longer requested cesarean section. Ultimately, the uterus ruptured and the child was hopelessly injured despite delivery within 30 minutes. The physician defended his conduct on the ground that the original informed consent should prevail throughout the labor and that the standard of care had been met by the "timely" delivery within 30 minutes. He noted that the patient had reaffirmed upon admission her earlier willingness to undergo a trial of labor and he maintained that labor continued "without objection".

The court (inviting the implication that the patient had been coerced) rejected the defense position that the patient's resignation implied acceptance of a continued trial of labor.[23] The court did not comment on the change in the medical situation (dysfunctional labor, unexplained abdominal pain) that required medical reconsideration of the case and updating of the informed consent. The court did, however, conclude that the legal situation had changed. "Where two or more medically acceptable options for treatment are present", the court held, "the competent patient has the absolute right to select from among those treatment options after being informed of the relative risks and benefits of each approach. But consent, once given, is not categorically immutable and the patient was entitled to withdraw her consent to VBAC. That indisputable withdrawal placed the patient and her physician in their original position—a blank slate on which the parties must again diagram their plan which in this case would have resulted in cesarean section." It was foreseeable that as a backlash to the alarm generated by this verdict along with other reports and settlements, many hospitals no longer permit VBAC deliveries and an increasing number of malpractice insurers are limiting their indemnification of physicians performing VBAC deliveries! (ob-gyn news, vol 40 no.3 Feb, 1, 2003).

COMPLICATION OR ERROR?

The "recognized risk defense", asserts that the undesirable outcome or injury in question is nothing more than an unavoidable complication—an understandable and acceptable risk of a properly considered and provided treatment. Accordingly, so long as the patient is reasonably apprised of the more serious and the commonplace risks and participates in the decision then in theory there can be no issue of negligence. A typical example is subgaleal or intracranial hemorrhage in the newborn following vacuum assisted delivery. Indeed, every obstetrical text devotes significant space to such complications but only rarely do they include a full discussion about preventability or even the distinction between complication and negligence. Is intracranial/subgaleal hemorrhage following vacuum extraction, for example, an unavoidable risk or, in some instances, the result of negligence and how would that be determined?[24] Similarly, is brachial plexus injury after shoulder dystocia a foreseeable event related to excessive lateral traction on the fetal neck, anticipated by multiple risk factors, or is it a totally unpredictable, unpreventable injury *always* unrelated to the care of the physician during delivery. In the courtroom, the plaintiff's attorney will use the statistics on complications as follows: A "recognized complication" does not preclude that the "complication" was caused by negligence. Indeed, none, all, or only a part of such complications may represent negligence. For example, if 2% of all drivers run red lights, running red lights is a known complication of driving, but it is also negligent. The most likely situation is that some of the injury is potentially avoidable.

Thus, that a given adverse outcome is a known complication of a procedure, tells an attorney nothing. The attorney wants to know why the complication occurs and, more importantly, why it occurred in this particular case.

PURSUING THE CASE

If the case is pursued, it may be settled by an agreement of the parties or go to trial. While the physician believes himself disadvantaged in this system of finding fault, in reality the law gives health care providers considerable advantage. They are advantaged by the presumption of nonnegligence. They do not have to be right in their care, just reasonable. The law denies the jury the right to decide medical issues and even requires "expert witnesses" from the profession itself. After an agreement to settle the case or after an adjudication that finds the defendant negligent, his insurance company bears the costs of both economic losses (lost earnings and medical bills) and the noneconomic losses, so-called "pain and suffering". The system is maintained in balance by the provision of insurance for both hospitals and physicians based on a pooling of risk, historically through separate lines of insurance.[11,25] This minimizes the risk of bankruptcy by a single large pay out and that resources are available to compensate patients. The cost of insurance coverage for hospitals is typically linked to the history of claims from year to year, an arrangement known as "experience rating". Physicians, on the other hand, unless their experience is extreme, are generally not risk rated, a potentially contrived actuarial practice.[26]

In practice, this theoretically balanced system falls short of its objectives as illustrated in the "ire and angst" of contemporary malpractice litigation.[11] This chapter, therefore, being written at the end of 2004, will attempt to review some of the competing, nay dueling, agendas that are being brought to bear in the medical, legal and political arenas. The enterprise redounds with myth and divisive and often contradictory data—sometimes of dubious provenance. The dust of the latest in these, increasingly disagreeable, epochal skirmishes for the malpractice "high road" has not yet settled and is unlikely to be settled to everyone's satisfaction in the near future. In the authors' view, this situation prevails because each side, for its particular, reasons, is unwilling to make the tort system work as it was designed to. Indeed some of the issues raised are ethical in nature, beyond the purview of the courts and the legislature.

MALPRACTICE MYTHOLOGY—THE FAILURE OF MEDICOLEGAL EDUCATION

An enduring feature of the malpractice upheaval in the United States (and almost nowhere else) is the ignorance of malpractice doctrine in the medical community and beyond. Not only is there widespread fear of being sued, but there is a great misperception about the requirements for proof of malpractice, the outcomes of lawsuits and the reasons patients sue. There is little appetite to deal with the major litogen (a factor promoting lawsuit)—physician behavior.

Some current mythology includes: "Malpractice relates to the incompetence of a few bad physicians." "Anyone can sue, everyone wins." "Every case resulting in CP will come to lawsuit." "The system is unfair and favors the plaintiff." "Patients who sue are greedy, ingrates." "Judges and juries cannot understand medicine." "Losing a lawsuit raises premiums and besmirches the physician's name in the community." "The plaintiff's attorney and the expert are the enemy, along with the judge, jury and insurance company". "Malpractice does not make care better." "The majority of suits in medicine are frivolous whether they are settled, dropped, go to jury trial or lose." "We are living in a time when people have a higher expectation from physicians—that until proven otherwise, it is the doctor's fault". "The system is overrun with runaway juries and jackpot justice, with sinister lawyers and opportunistic plaintiffs preying on virtuous corporations, hospitals and doctors in search of that big pay out from the lawsuit lottery".[27]

There is almost universal belief that the injured child's appearance in the courtroom elicits sufficient sympathy from the jury for the plaintiff to win the case. Physicians, however, win about 80% of lawsuits that do go to court. It is naïve to believe that these were the cases in which the plaintiff's attorney forgot to bring the affected child into the courtroom. More reasonably, it is the thoughtful, compassionate physician who manifests his sympathy and compassion that most easily obtains the jury's favor and a favorable verdict.

The defendant is often unaware of the statistics that about 40% of cases are dropped, about 50% settle, sometimes as befitting the merits of the case and sometimes as a calculated strategy that limits exposure of assets. The physician who is terrified by an *ad damnum* clause (demand for damages) that greatly exceeds his insurance policy limits is rarely in our experience reassured by his own attorney that the risk to a physician's assets is essentially nil. The author is unaware of any malpractice suit involving an obstetrician who was covered by a reasonable policy and who, despite a verdict that exceeded the policy limits, had to pay any money out of his own pocket. Despite counseling, the frightened obstetrician does "not want to be the first one". To some extent the defense attorney may be excused for failing to understand how impoverished the physician's medicolegal education is. As one physician put it: "I fought in the battle of the bulge in World War II. We were trained, we were fighting a good cause and we were armed. I felt safer than I do in a malpractice suit".

Education is the antidote to disabling myth. Medical and legal organizations have long recognized the importance of legal medicine and have repeatedly recommended its study by physicians in training—with minimal success. In 1952 the AMA advised that "No medical student should be permitted to receive his medical degree without instruction in legal duties". Four decades later, less than 50% of medical schools had medicolegal courses, considering the subject too unimportant to teach. Even fewer schools have any formal instruction on communication and dispute management skills. Many medical schools feel that the intense curriculum leaves no room for such instruction, and that the ability to communicate and deal with conflict is part of the student selection process, that is to be refined following their didactic medical school training, during their apprentice/mentor training of internship and residency.

Kollas in 1997 studied the medicolegal knowledge base of senior residents in internal medicine. Only 28% felt they had been adequately trained in the subject. Only 26% could list the requirements for proof of malpractice, i.e. the 4 Ds.[28,29]

A national survey of physicians in 1999 revealed that 58% had faced malpractice charges and that more than 20% had been sued at least three times. Almost 70% expected to be sued during their career. Despite the fact that physicians win the vast majority of cases that go to court, more than 75% of physicians polled felt that lay juries were not capable of deciding malpractice cases! While ready to admit that everyone makes mistakes and that they had made mistakes in other cases, virtually all physicians believe that the cases filed against them have no merit. Something (read tort reform) must be done, physicians cry, to stem the tide, to eliminate the reign of terror by the plaintiff's attorneys. Plaintiff's attorneys and some consumer groups also want to stem the tide as they see it —the tide of medical error, the tide of unsympathetic, unapologetic and ill-informed physicians.

When all of these myths are wiped away, the most devastating myth or fiction about malpractice, the one that resides deepest beneath the surface, is that the allegation of malpractice represents the allegation of incompetence or misanthropy or malice. In fact, it simply represents an allegation of fallibility—being human and being capable of error. Imagine the response of the physician who believes that he or she is being accused of malice—the intention to do harm. The allegation of malice is precluded by the precepts of tort law and is rendered improper by the Hippocratic Oath in which the physician swears to, "First, do no harm," and by implication, to "intend no harm, i.e. malice". Judges and jurors understand that the physician, like the speeding driver, did not intend harm. But the physician's good intentions are not the test of reasonable performance and the profession will be unlikely to regulate itself without first understanding that the rules of negligence exclude malice. Indeed Institute of Medicine's (IOM), "To Err is Human", and Chaudry's, uncovered an alarming incidence of medical errors within institutions, which was associated with a high resistance, among physicians, to report errors (IOM, Chaudry). The "culture of secrecy" may in fact represent a "culture of fear."

I will attempt, in passing, to deal with these notions, but perhaps the following experiences will assist the reader to focus on the issue of patients' expectations of a perfect outcome. I delivered my first baby as a medical student in about 1963. After the delivery, the first words out of the mother's mouth were, "Is my baby alright?" I would deliver my last baby about 40 years later and the first question this mother asked me was exactly the same as the question asked by the mother 40 years earlier. In the intervening 40 years the ultrasounds, computers and monitors of every description have allowed us to visualize the fetus, characterize its genetic composition, and determine its behavior, its growth and its tolerance to hypoxia. As a result there has been a dramatic reduction in the risk of fetal anomaly or death, especially during labor. Labor rooms have become intensive care suites with remote surveillance capabilities. Indeed, it has never in history been safer to deliver a baby, or perversely, to be sued for negligent care. Everyone, patients and physicians included, understand that there are no guarantees with pregnancy and under the best of circumstances, considering the stakes, not all outcomes are perfect. As with all medical care, there is always an element of uncertainty—about care, and about outcome. Are lawsuits generated by those patients who fail to understand this principle, or by the physician who confronted with a bad outcome fails not only to educate such a patient but also fails to respond compassionately?

With regard to the notion that the presentation of the handicapped child in the courtroom dooms the defense case because of sympathy for the child, the author has witnessed the following situation in the courtroom in the case of a neurologically handicapped infant. After their deliberations, the jury returned to the courtroom to announce their verdict before the judge and the various parties. When the judge asked for the decision of the jury, the foreman arose and asked the judge if he could first make a preliminary statement on behalf of each of the jury. With tears in his eyes, the foreman acknowledged that over the course of the trial the members of the jury felt that they had come to know and care for the parents and the afflicted child. He further stated that he wanted to extend from each member of the jury both their best wishes for the future and their considerable concerns about the future support of the child. They did not find the physician negligent.

In medicine today there is considerable enthusiasm for "evidence-based medicine", epidemiologically-driven decisions, and structured reimbursement. There seems much less appetite for "evidence-based law". The initiatives derived from "evidence-based medicine" seem to be driven as much by motives of cost control as by the hope for better health care services. Similarly, the avoidance of error such as the use of automated medication ordering and dispensing, and the efforts of risk management (safeguarding assets) while contributory may not directly enhance the quality of care. The extraordinary response to the IOM study has led to a nationwide movement to find ways to reduce error and increase patient safety. The foundation of these efforts is based on increasing the ease and confidentiality for error reporting, as well as the facilitation of root cause analysis systems, team approach techniques, and improved communication and dispute management techniques, all with the goal of improving patient care. Legislative bills such as HR663 are aimed at such lofty goals, but to date no proposed legislation has answered all the needs, and the ones that have been endorsed by medical associations only given tepid support.

In this way, the avoidance of error and the efforts of risk management (safeguarding assets) have become as important, if not more important than assuring the quality of care. The breadth of malpractice mythology and the detestation and fear of the malpractice system by the physicians and organized medicine has distracted our attention from the public's concern about the ineffectual efforts to improve outcome whether by the adoption of higher standards, improved educational processes or the meaningful activities of peer review committees and professional societies.

Peer Review

In 1973, the United States Congress enacted legislation requiring physicians to initiate Peer Review Organizations to monitor the utilization and the quality of hospital and physician services in the federally funded Medicare program. Now more than 30 years later, we must acknowledge the lack of a gold-standard, medical or legal, for reviewing allegations of negligence and dealing meaningfully with medical error. Peer reviews produce inconsistent agreement and operate without formal rules or guideline for review.[38] They are left to the local hospital;[30] although the ACOG has attempted to provide outside review to individual hospitals, there is no analysis of such efforts.[31] The majority of "true" peer review exercises are driven by adverse outcomes and do not represent systemic reviews of the numerous latent processes promoting adverse outcome. These are left to the occasional review of a "sentinel event". With peer review the rules for reviewing records and for obtaining agreement about either the severity of any departure or impact on the offending physician are inconstantly applied and haphazardly administered. Peer review requires the presence of the physician, an overt acknowledgment of the fact that medical records are often silent about important questions whose understanding is necessary to determine the standard of care. Despite the physician's presence, the deliberations of the peer review committee are not backed up by systemic reviews of the physician's conduct with similar cases. The system is not designed to promote either patient education or an apology.

Peer review in obstetrics is especially problematic. The medical records of the infant may not be present, nor may there be anyone (neonatologists/pediatrician) present to discuss the infant's course and the impact of the obstetrical care on that course. The patient, moreover, is rarely, if ever, questioned about her perceptions of the care! Invariably, there is no long-term follow-up, especially if the infant is transferred to another hospital. Imagine, therefore, a discussion at a Peer Review Meeting of the medical conduct in a case of shoulder dystocia and brachial plexus injury. The medical record is silent about the use of fundal pressure—as it should be —fundal pressure should not be used to relieve shoulder dystocia. As a result the physician who had carefully documented a normal sequence of maneuvers was exonerated. During the malpractice case, however, incontrovertible evidence was produced that the 263 pound anesthesiologist was exerting sufficient force on the top of the patient's abdomen to produce considerable pain and broad ecchymoses. The case settled in behalf of the plaintiff!

Other complaints of lack of due process and poor reproducibility plague discussions of the peer review process. There is evidence that the knowledge of an adverse outcome (hindsight bias) may cause the peer review committee, like the expert in a malpractice case, to criticize retrospectively the decisions of the treating doctor.[32,33] While it might be better to withhold outcome information in both circumstances, this seems neither practical nor enforceable.

Peer reviews are conducted by people from the same department of the hospital and in many states are safeguarded from legal scrutiny under the common law privilege of self-critical analysis, a privilege that protects and encourages quality assessment, but that secrecy, in the final analysis, may be counterproductive for the ultimate objective of improved patient care and better transparency of medicines self-governance.[34,35] At its most collegial, colleagues of the physician being reviewed are likely to minimize error on the notion that when my turn comes, similar cordiality and extenuation will prevail.

Sometimes, however, peer review meetings may not be cordial and the meeting may be the appropriate venue for criticism, removal of privileges or dismissal. Sometimes, the purpose is not strictly medical, political, economic and administrative, described under such appellations as "economic credentialing" or "sham peer review". At these times, generally, hostility will prevail, the physician will hire a lawyer and the battle will be joined. It is the law not medicine, that will safeguard due process. If it can be shown that peer review was being used for purposes other than medical care, the deliberations of the committee may no longer be protected.

In either circumstance, it is an expensive, unsatisfying, experience for which physicians have little appetite—whatever the outcome.

A study by Cheney, et al. about agreement among anesthesiologists assessing twelve actual malpractice cases whose verdict was known has implications both for malpractice and peer review.[36] They showed a high intra-observer agreement amongst observers (>80%). Of the eight cases with complete or virtually complete agreement between respondent anesthesiologists, three (37.5%) disagreed with the verdict rendered by the actual juries. In addition, anesthesiologists showed significant disagreement (>30%) among themselves in four of the case scenarios, indicating there may not be agreement regarding the standard of care in these clinical circumstances. Finally, anesthesiologists predicted jury verdicts poorly, with success rates of 50% or less in seven of the twelve case scenarios. One wonders what the results would be if this study were performed in cases of peer review. Finally, peer review is a parochial matter; only rarely does it obtain information from the patient or review from bonafide experts in the field. These potential sources of enlightenment are available in the courtroom.

Gawande, in an article in The New Yorker, describes a surgical peer review exercise and the limitations of this process. He admits that he made a serious medical error, but he was not obligated to face the peer review committee directly, and the committee did not deal directly with the error itself in any remedial way.[37] Under the heading of "the banality of injury", Gawande acknowledges that medial error is ubiquitous and makes the point that medical error is NOT the province of a selective few culprits as common wisdom suggests. There are no "incompetent, unethical, negligent few", no basket of "bad apples" that conspire to taint all of medicine.

While there are correlations between risk of lawsuit and medical school prestige, physician intuition, gender and even the apparently perverse inverse relationship between current medical knowledge and the likelihood of being sued, the fact is that most obstetricians are sued at least once in their professional life.[38] Repeat offenders may sometimes occur, but are not a common problem. As Gawande poignantly asks, "How do we keep good physicians from harming patients?" We may also ask, what is the value of either peer review or even malpractice suits in improving care?[37]

A study (generally known as the Harvard study) commissioned by New York State in 1986, and released in 1990, showed that actual malpractice is relatively rare, it is nevertheless underreported. If anything, they believed that there were too few lawsuits.[39-41] Further, they wrote, that "Physicians tended to equate a finding of negligence with a judgment of incompetence. Thus, although willing to admit that 'all doctors make mistakes', physicians were often unwilling to label substandard care as negligent and were opposed to compensation for iatrogenic injury". Given the medicine's delayed response to the problem of medical error, including the limitations of peer review, the public's only alternative, therefore was for individual patients to try to hold individual practitioners, one at a time, to whatever medical standards could be upheld by lawyers and expert witnesses (Mohr, 2000). It may be true that to "address the problem of iatrogenic injuries seriously, we must reform the system of malpractice litigation." What seems equally true is that the problems of iatrogenic injury and physician conduct cannot be contingent on changing the tort system alone.

The Role of the Physician

These complaints about the system also serve to camouflage the physician's role in the genesis of malpractice suits. It has been estimated that, the risk of lawsuit "seems not to be predicted by patient characteristics, illness complexity, or even physicians' technical skills". Instead, risk appears related to patients' dissatisfaction with their physicians' ability to establish *rapport*, develop trust, provide access, administer care and treatment consistent with reasonable *expectations*, deal effectively with conflict, and *communicate* effectively".[4] In an article by Hickson, et al. patients who saw physicians with the highest number of lawsuits were more likely to complain that their physicians *would not listen or return telephone calls, were rude, and did not show respect.*[2] Such complaints, furthermore, were similar to those documented in interviews with families who sued their physicians. Patients are less likely to sue (about 50%), even for moderate and severe mistakes, if the physician informs them of the mistake (basically, apologizes).

For reasons mentioned above, physicians are untrained in the art of apology. It may seem counterintuitive for many physicians that one can accept responsibility for an outcome, without admitting blameworthiness.[42,43]

In an analysis of 500 claims in obstetrics and gynecology B-Lynch, et al. show that 46% were misguided allegations about, half were due to incompetent care, an error of judgment, lack of expertise, poor supervision or inadequate staffing. The other half were due to poor communication and "misguided allegations" for which they recommend alternative course of dispute resolution combined with improved communication.[44] Parenthetically, the more time the physician spends with a patient the greater is the satisfaction of both patient and physician (Woods). In a survey reported by the ACOG, physicians reported wholesale changes in their practices and their fees as a result of malpractice —including greater consultation with the patient.

In 1997, a highly publicized article recommended that when doctors make a mistake that harms a patient, they should tell the patient what happened, apologize and do whatever it takes to repair the damage.[45] Basic professional ethics aver that patients have a right to know what happened to them. It seems like the right thing to do as part of the physician's responsibility to his patient and it may be therapeutic for the physician who may feel guilt and distress. Telling the truth may also strengthen patient's faith in the doctor while a cover-up that fails, as many do, may anger patient and make them more inclined to sue. Cover-ups also antagonize juries. Medicine is a human enterprise and error (i.e. fallibility) is part of being human. "We are programmed for error".

Understandably, the notion of admitting error has drawn skeptical review from the medical community, the insurance companies and the defense bar.[46] They fear that admitting mistakes will "open the floodgates" to lawsuits and hurt their reputations and careers. They also fear that without tort reform to decrease the number of malpractice suits and large settlements, and to reduce the punitive implications of existing reporting, few doctors could risk owning up to errors. The notion that telling the truth, apologizing and reaching out to a family in grief can defuse some anger and polarization that characterize a typical lawsuit becomes hostage to the notion that every word you uttered in consolation or contrition is an admission that can be used against you in a court of law. On top of that, defense lawyers then order doctors to say nothing until all the facts are in, and then to say nothing. It seems obvious to state that until legislative protections maintaining such admissions are enacted, it is very likely that lawyers will continue to order doctors to say nothing until all the facts have been ascertained through discovery, and then to say nothing. But is this a medicolegal problem, or is it an ethical problem?[45,47,48] Baldwin suggests that increased levels of moral reasoning may diminish the risk of malpractice suit.[49] making legislative protection unnecessary.

The Joint Commission on Hospital Accreditation (JACHO) standards require the disclosure of sentinel events and other unanticipated outcomes of care to patients and to their family members when appropriate. Hospital administrators, fearing medical liability suits, are reluctant to comply with this standard.[50] If disclosure is taken a step further to the offer of an apology, hospitals and physicians are even more likely to gravitate to traditional "defend and deny" behaviors. Apology as it turns out is yet one more control that physicians exert over the risk of lawsuit. Thus, a prompt explanation of what is understood about what happened and its probable effects; assurance that an analysis will take place to understand what went wrong; follow-up based on the analysis to make it unlikely that such an event will happen again; and an apology will likely reduce the risk of lawsuit and heal, rather than harm, the physician-patient relationship.[51] In fact, a growing number of hospitals, doctors and insurers have come to accept that genuine disclosure and apology may reduce error-related payouts and the frequency of litigation.[52-55] Further, a growing number of states are passing ("I am sorry") laws that protect an apology from being used against a doctor in court.[52] Despite the ethical imperatives underlying such disclosure, it seems likely that more such fundamental protections will be needed before these practices become commonplace.

Common Areas of Litigation during Labor

General problems relating to litigation in medicine include documentation, communication, to institute chain of command, or internal systems conflicts, when there is unresolved disagreements between individuals, departments, and all levels of healthcare providers, such as between physicians and nurses or physicians and administrators. Most concerning are the attitudinal problems involving the interaction of nurses and physicians which receive too little emphasis and are particularly difficult to change. Their potential serious impact on the ability of an obstetrical unit to provide "high reliability care" has been discussed at length by Simpson and Knox.[25] Of the many specific types of cases only several will be briefly discussed here: the failure to properly interpret fetal monitoring tracings, poor conduct of operative vaginal delivery, management of the large infant and shoulder dystocia resulting in either brain damage with death or subsequent CP or the infant with brachial plexus injury (sometimes both).

Along with the measures taken by physicians in response to the threat of malpractice, the profession, especially obstetrics, has embarked upon a series of defensive "scientific" initiatives to *modify* its vocabulary and its accountability. Defensive medicine is a practice designed not for the purpose of answering clinical questions or directing therapy, but for the purpose of preventing lawsuits or counteracting plaintiff testimony in court. The ACOG, for example, has recommended the elimination of such universally applied terms of art as "fetal distress", "perinatal asphyxia" and "stat cesarean section" and have modified the definitions of "low" and "mid forceps".[57-59] Further articles have created definitive, unyielding requirements for the diagnosis of birth-related injury and suggest that labor related injury is rare and perhaps irreducible.[60]

Irrespective of motivation, these publications have not been accompanied by any decrease in lawsuits, any improvement in outcome or any less defensive posture on the part of the obstetrical community. These efforts to make our specialty "fair of speech" and litigation proof, discount important mechanisms of injury, diminish notions of medical judgment, inhibit scientific inquiry into the timing and mechanism of fetal injury and delay the testing of new paradigms for dealing with adverse outcome. These articles attempt to influence the defense in these cases in several ways: an inexperienced lawyer may turn down a meritorious case because, as the guideline states, "It is not possible to ascertain retrospectively whether earlier obstetric intervention could have prevented injury or cerebral damage in any individual case where no detectable sentinel hypoxic event occurred", or because the umbilical artery pH was >7.0 despite obvious injury during labor or delivery. In addition, by insisting that extreme derangements in pH values are required to begin to make the correlation between labor events and subsequent neonatal injury, these criteria modify the level of proof normally required in malpractice suits. The burden of proof in these suits requires that the level of confidence in the relationship between the events and the outcome be more probable than not. It is well to compare these pronouncements with a widely respected authority of neonatal brain injury. "Brain injury in the intrapartum (period) does occur, (it) effects a large absolute number of infants worldwide... and represents a large source of potentially preventable neurological morbidity. Among the many adverse consequences of the explosion in obstetrical litigation there has been a tendency in the medical profession to deny the importance or even existence of intrapartum brain injury (Volpe, Neurology of the Newborn (3rd ed.) 1995). These issues have also been discussed at some length for the brain-damaged infant[61,62] and for brachial plexus injury.[63]

Fetal Cardiotocography

In part because of the pivotal role they play in malpractice cases, there have been attacks on fetal monitoring that have come both from within the profession and from without. In an article in the Stanford University Law Review, Margaret Lent, a young defense lawyer, argues that the widespread use of EFM is both medically and legally unsound.[64] Ms. Lent points to selected clinical trials to demonstrate that EFM does not reduce fetal mortality, morbidity or cerebral palsy rates. She argues that because EFM has a very high false positive rate and its usage correlates strongly with a rise in cesarean section rates so it offers no medical advantage over auscultation. Similarly, she argues, EFM provides no protection in the courtroom. Though obstetricians believe that they should use EFM because its status as the standard of care will protect them from liability, Ms Lent argues that given its failings it may in fact expose them to liability. She further argues that auscultation, at least as safe and effective as EFM is also more likely to protect physicians from liability. Ms Lent concludes that obstetricians have an obligation to their patients and to themselves to adopt auscultation as the new standard of care. She finds "no excuses left to defend the continued use of EFM". The medical literature, can be used to justify any position on monitoring, including those of Ms Lent. Thus, it may be shown that CTG increases the risk of CP and that "substandard care" protects against subsequent CP.

While failure on the part of the health care provider to recognize clear FHR abnormalities is frequently alleged in malpractice cases, to isolate the CTG tracing under these circumstances frequently oversteps its permissive role in obstetrical care. A normal CTG pattern permits ongoing labor only as long as the safe vaginal delivery is a reasonable option. If the pattern turns abnormal (rising baseline, decreasing variability along with variable/late decelerations) especially in the second stage then the questions are several. Can the pattern be ameliorated (by reducing the oxytocin, moderating the pushing efforts)? If the pattern cannot be ameliorated what is the feasibility of safe vaginal delivery given the estimated fetal weight, previous obstetrical history, position, presentation of the fetal head and progress in labor to this point? Experience suggests that the vast majority of cases hinge far more on the reasonableness of conduct of the obstetrical care (especially the second stage) than on the interpretation of the fetal monitor. Irrespective, reviewers of malpractice cases consistently find that the CTG tracing has been frequently misinterpreted in allegations of negligence.[65]

THE LEGAL CLIMATE

Most changes in both the medical and legal professions are evolutionary and it is often difficult to define any sea change. *The last three decades, however*, have witnessed a number of remarkable and epochal changes in the medicolegal climate in the United States, with doubtless more to come. Many of the changes derive from periodic surges in malpractice premiums, reduced availability of insurance coverage and the exodus of major insurers from the market first in the early 1970s, again in the mid-1980s, a lesser event in the 1990s and more recently in the new millennium. In each epoch, affected providers clamored for policy changes to inhibit litigation.[66] In the 1970s legislatures established joint underwriting associations to serve as insurers of last resort,[67] special state patient-compensation funds were introduced to absolve commercial insurers of responsibility for specified dollar portions of malpractice payments, and public reinsurance mechanisms were established to fill gaps in the underwriting market. By the late 1970s, the malpractice crisis had abated—only to recur less than a decade later. In Washington State between 1984 and 1986, for example, malpractice premiums for obstetrics jumped approximately 100%. As a consequence, obstetricians marched on legislatures or joined many family physicians and midwives in an exodus from obstetric practice. Those remaining in practice became more reluctant to care for high-risk obstetric patients and less willing to accept indigent patients and reduced fees, irrespective of the fact that indigent patients, in fact, appear less likely to sue.[68]

In many rural locales across the US obstetric care became virtually unobtainable. Periodically, these circumstances galvanize legislative activity in virtually every state and lead to further far-reaching reforms of existing tort and insurance law[69,70] with some stabilization of premiums—at least initially. After almost a decade of essentially flat premiums are rising exponentially; it is said to be due to an increasing size of awards and by insurers leaving the medical malpractice business because of diminishing returns on investment. This has been aggravated by rising health care costs ($1.6 trillion in 2002 and increasing yearly), and efforts to control physician income. The average annual increase in health care costs from 2000–2004 was 12–16% with predictions (Towers Perrin) that, whether or not derived from negligent care, will rise by a further 8% in 2005 and with likely little containment beyond that

It is important to emphasize that premium levels are responsive to a variety of factors besides litigation dynamics, including previous losses, past and expected investment returns, business strategies, and the degree of state regulation of rate changes.[71] A January 2004 study found that nationwide, average premiums for all physicians between 2000 and 2002 rose by 15%—a rate of rise almost twice as fast as per capita total health care spending. Certain specialties had even greater increases including: obstetricians/gynecologists (22%) and internists and general surgeons (33%)[72] Neurosurgeons, obstetricans, orthopedists and ER physicians are particularly likely to have premium rate increases. The rates for obstetricians/gynecologists vary nationally, but according to ACOG, between 2002 and 2003 about half of obstetricians/gynecologists were experiencing increases of 10–49% in their insurance premiums.

Premiums may influence physicians' decisions to join and leave the labor force, their choice of a medical specialty, and their decision of where to locate, creating the potential for underserved patient populations in certain specialties or geographic areas. Rising malpractice premiums may also encourage physicians to practice "defensive medicine", performing more tests and procedures than necessary in order to reduce exposure to lawsuits. Parenthetically, however, "defensive medicine" (ordering a test not for the purpose of furthering patient care, but for the legal protection of the physician) is indefensible in court. Imagine the physician-defendant responding to a question about the indication for a certain test with the answer: "I didn't want to get sued". Both rising malpractice premiums and defensive medicine practices may contribute to the rising health care costs and thus to an increase in health insurance premiums.

The choices for the obstetricians—short of some windfall protection scheme—is 1) leave practice, move to a "more compliant" state, give up obstetrics, obtain employment where malpractice insurance is provided, raise fees, discontinue seeing patients with restrictive payment structures, or go bare, i.e. not obtain any malpractice insurance. For many, there is not a good option and their future will hinge on the least inimical choice. Beyond physicians, these rapidly rising medical malpractice premiums have again become an issue of increasing concern about the health care system for policy makers and the general public.

Underwriter Data Claims Payments

The insurance industry also has its problems. In 2003 insurers were paying out in claims and expenses, 1.38 dollars for every medical malpractice premium dollar collected (National Underwriter Data Services). Results have deteriorated steadily from 1998 when the rate of return was 7.6. Medical malpractice insurers' return on net worth was a negative 7.4% in 2002, down from a negative 4.7% in 2001 (National Association of Insurance Commissioners). Results in 2002 were worst in the following states: Arkansas, Nevada, Montana, Mississippi, Illinois and Missouri, with return on net worth ranging from minus 33.7% in Arkansas to minus 24.4% in Missouri. In reality, even in good years, premiums rarely cover payouts. The system works in part because premiums are invested and with at least a modest return permit the insurance company to make a profit. This is abetted by the fact that malpractice suits, especially, take a long time to resolve—about 4 years on average.

The average claim payment rose almost 8% per annum from $95,000 in 1986 to $320,000 in 2002 despite the fact that the frequency of claims per 100 doctors has remained more or less constant. Only about 30% of claims result in insurance payouts, but expenses for cases, especially obstetrical (brain injured baby cases) where there is no payout are considerable. Concurrently, insurance companies, along with the population at large, faced reduced income from investments to help offset underwriting losses.

Another study in 2004 found that hospital professional liability and physician liability claims costs have increased at a steady 9.7% since 2000 and are likely to rise at the same rate in 2004. Frequency, or the number of claims, is growing at 3% a year; claim severity (the dollar amount) is increasing 6.5% annually. Hospital liability claim costs for 2004 are expected to reach almost $150,000 per claim, compared with $79,000 per claim in 1996. The average claim against a physician is expected to reach $178,000, compared with $120,000 in 1996 (AON Risk Services).

Jury Awards and Settlements

In early 2005 a Towers Perrin study found that over the 28 years since 1975, when they were first identified separately, medical malpractice cost increases have outpaced other tort areas, rising at an average of 11.8% a year, compared with 9.2% for all other tort costs. In 2003 medical malpractice, at almost $27 billion, cost each American an average $91 a year. This compares with $5 a year in 1975 (January 2005, Towers Perrin - U.S. Tort Costs: 2004 Update). Recent data suggests that jury awards are stabilizing, but the range of awards is moving upward. Median medical malpractice jury awards have held steady at about $1 million over the 3 years from 2000 to 2002 (From Jury Verdict Research). However, awards ranged from a low of $11,000, almost double the amount the previous year, to a high of $95 million. The average award in 2002 hit $6.25 million, up from $3.91 million in 2001. However, only a small fraction of cases go to trial and very large awards are frequently reduced after the fact and after the publicity.

The costs of perinatal injury are quite high, related not only to the costs of settlement and defense, but also in terms of personal and professional upheaval for all concerned. As Simpson and Knox have pointed out[56] from the perspective of human and system factors reveals themes, context and conditions common to accidental injury in other high risk domains. According to the Jury Verdict Research Series (JVRI 2001), in 2000 the median jury award for neonatal neurological injury had increased to .$5 million compared to $725,000 in 1994 with 76% of the jury awards valued at greater than $1 million (compared to 40% in 1994). Higher awards were more likely to occur when the hospital was the sole defendant compared to when both were defendants.

Conventional wisdom holds several contributing factors to account for the increased incidence of malpractice claims:

1. People are more litigious; it is part of our culture and extends everywhere from lawyers themselves to city governments.

2. Given the media coverage and watchdog groups there has been an increasing understanding of public of the fallibility of physicians. The Public Citizen Health Research Group, and more recently formed groups emphasizing both medical error

and the need to improve care as part of tort reform have also helped fuel the public's demand for change.[35]

3. The diminishing intimacy of the patient-doctor relationship fomented in part by larger changes in the way health care is distributed (HMOs), by increasing overhead and by deteriorating reimbursement schedules.

4. The increasing availability of medical experts to testify in malpractice cases (the breakdown of OMERTA).

5. The increasing assertiveness of the courts and the increasing sophistication of the plaintiff's bar with more careful selection of meritorious suits.

6. The need to assistance with financing medical bills. Indeed, there is seeming growth in the frequency of lawsuits for the "bad baby", in part because of the large verdicts sometimes realized but also because of the increasing incidence of CP related to increasing survival of low birthweight infants and the costs thereof.

Several clinical practices and media attention would seem also to be impacting on the frequency and type of lawsuit. As an example, the United States Food and Drug Administration (FDA) issued a national advisory on the risks of vacuum extractors.[73] This was rapidly followed by a nationwide television program emphasizing some of the disastrous results with vacuums. In turn, there has been a dramatic increase both in the reporting of adverse events associated with vacuum deliveries to the FDA and lawsuits alleging negligent care in the use of vacuums. Similarly, the methods undertaken to lower the cesarean section rate in the US have perhaps been achieved at the expense of an increased risk of ruptured uterus, shoulder dystocia and lawsuit.[74] While all authorities would agree that any woman with one previous cesarean section and no other adverse features may be eligible for an attempt at—if she chooses to do so after being carefully explained the options. Some health maintenance organizations (HMO) refused to accede to the mother's choice and have required that every patient with a previous cesarean be given a trial of labor—a horrific, medically indefensible recommendation. One institution in California that adopted this policy was assessed almost $25 million as a result of 48 women who suffered adverse outcome as a result of this policy.

Prevalence of Medical Malpractice

A study (generally known as the Harvard study) commissioned by New York State in 1986, and released in 1990, showed that actual malpractice is relatively rare, it is nevertheless underreported. If anything, they believed that there were too few lawsuits. When hospital medical records from New York State were examined, the incidence of adverse events or injuries resulting from medical "interventions" or treatment, was 3.7%. The percentage of adverse events due to what the physician team characterized as "negligence" (not necessarily a legal definition) was 1%. However, only one in eight who suffered from an adverse event due to negligence filed a medical malpractice claim, and only one in 15 received compensation. Most adverse events resulted in only minimal and transient disability and most of the patients' medical care expenses were paid for by health insurance. This helps to explain why only a small percentage of patients who are injured as a result of negligence file medical malpractice claims. However, a significant portion (22%) of patients who did not file medical malpractice claims suffered moderate or greater incapacity. In a second phase of the study, researchers confirmed that some of the tort claims filed provided little or no evidence of medical malpractice or even an adverse event, suggesting that the tort system is "very error-prone", at least in its initial stages (related to the expert) This inefficiency in both the medical and legal systems, not withstanding, the study noted that, "if anything, there are too few lawsuits". The inference here is that more patients with adverse outcomes related to negligence should be suing.[39,40,75,76]

There are several studies of closed claims in obstetrics and their relationship to negligence or the adherence to guidelines. Julian, et al. reviewed the files of 220 obstetric closed-claim cases to identify common factors predisposing to claims and to suggest preventative measures. Identification of common obstetric risks and correct management of these risks was poor in these cases. Only 54% of the risks were recognized; of these, only 32% were correctly managed. A high percentage of risks were thought to be directly related to the obstetric outcome leading to the claim (66%). The authors feel obstetric closed claims can be studied and suggestions made to aid obstetricians in providing care. They concluded that obstetric malpractice closed claims are amenable to study; physicians and their patients would benefit from better data collection systems to identify risks in individual pregnancies, along with available resources to aid their management of patients. They felt that suits can be avoided through modification of physician behavior.[77]

In 1990, Rosenblatt and Hurst reviewed all closed obstetric claims in the records of a major physician-sponsored malpractice insurer from 1982 to 1989. Of the 54 files closed during the 6.5-year period covered by this study, 21 (39%) involved physician reports of bad outcomes that did not lead to a formal claim. Of the 33 formal claims, 14 (42%) were dismissed, either by the plaintiff's attorney or by the courts. Eighteen of the remaining 19 claims were settled before trial, with an average payment to the plaintiff of $185,000. The one suit that went to trial resulted in a defense verdict. A review of the case histories demonstrated that in the majority of cases when a payment was made, probable medical negligence had taken place. Nonmeritorious claims were not compensated. For those cases in which a payment was made, the size of the settlement was commensurate with the seriousness of the injury, which almost always involved damage to the infant. Poor physician judgment was the most common source of error.[78]

The surviving, handicapped infant, continues to represent the highest payout/case. There are numerous representative reviews of closed cases (Table 24.2). An analysis of 353 closed claims involving obstetrician-gynecologists revealed that the 40 highest-paid claims (11.3%) accounted for 88.7% of the total dollars spent. The majority of these 23 (57.5%) were obstetrical including the five highest claims and 17 of the first 20 highest-paid awards.

Obstetrical negligence represented over $5 million (76.5%) of the total expense. Of the 40 cases, 23 (60%) were resolved with a compromise settlement, 9 claims (22.5%) resolved with indemnity payment on the basis of verdict or pretrial compromise, 7 (17.5%) had no indemnity payment because of a jury verdict or voluntary dismissal. These seven were in the highest-paid claims group only because of expenses.[73,78]

Of the 40 case, none were considered frivolous; 28 (70%) were judged to be meritorious; and 12 (30%) were judged to be non-meritorious. Seven of the latter settled without indemnity

Table 24.2: Why patients sue (Hickson et al.[4])

Cited deficiencies of care	
Recognizing fetal distress	53%
Managing fetal distress	57%
Timely cesarean section	35%
Physician unavailable	29%
Birth injury (forceps)	28%
Consultation or transfer	10%
What prompted lawsuit?	
Person outside family	33%
Medical personnel	23/41 (56%)
Lawyer	8/41 (20%)
Money for long-term care	24%
Physician deception	24%
Child would have no future	20%
Find out what happened	20%
Deter malpractice/Revenge	19%
Complaints about physicians	
Not informed about injury potential	70%
Misled patient	48%
Would not talk or answer questions	32%
Would not listen	13%

costs, including four that went to trial with a defense verdict and three that were dismissed, leaving five others in this group with proper treatment and indemnity costs. Expenses to defend all 12 cases of proper treatment totaled over $500,000. Irrespective of the absence of strict negligence, each of these "nonmeritorious claims" illustrated substantial deficits with the medical record or system failures—inviting the allegation of negligence and lawsuit (making the case appear meritorious). These analyses clearly reveal that bad outcomes may not be the fault of the physician, but that physician behavior in the conduct of the case and the conduct of the medical record contribute heavily to successful allegations of malpractice.

Ogburn, et al. reviewed 153 closed claims involving perinatal injury or death filed from 1980 through 1982 with the St. Paul Fire and Marine Insurance Company. The claims included were those in which an indemnity was paid or $1,000 or more was expended on the legal defense. Cases were classified as to the presence or absence of medical negligence. Most of the complications leading to claims arose during labor and delivery. Many claims resulted from the failure to evaluate or treat in a manner consistent with accepted standards of care. Many lacked documentation of the physician's recognition of the risk factors involved. In the opinion of the reviewers, medical negligence occurred in 47% of the cases. Indemnity payment occurred with most (but not all!) of the claims judged to be associated with medical negligence. Payment to the claimant was also made in a number of cases in which the reviewer thought no malpractice had occurred. The authors concluded that these results suggest that improvements are needed in prenatal and perinatal health care as well as in the legal system used to address the problem of perinatal medical negligence.[79]

In a study published in 2003, Ransom et al. tried to estimate whether guideline compliance affected medicolegal risk in obstetrics and whether malpractice claims data can provide useful information about compliance.[80] From the claims experience of a large health system delivering approximately 12,000 infants annually, they retrospectively identified 290 delivery-related (diagnosis-related groups 370–374) malpractice claims and 262 control deliveries between 1988 and 1998. Clinical pathways for vaginal delivery and cesarean section, implemented in 1998, were used as a "standard of care". They compared rates of noncompliance with the pathways in the claims and control groups. They found that noncompliance with the clinical pathways was significantly more common among claims than controls (43.2% versus 11.7%, P <.001; odds ratio = 5.76, 95% CI 3.59, 9.2). In 81 (79.4%) of the claims involving noncompliance with the pathway, the main allegation in the claim related directly to the departure from the pathway. The excess malpractice risk attributable to noncompliance explained approximately one-third (104 of 290) of the claims filed (attributable risk = 82.6%). They concluded that malpractice data is a useful resource in understanding breakdowns in processes of care and that adherence to clinical pathways might:

- Reduce clinical variation.
- Improve the quality of care.
- Might protect clinicians and institutions against malpractice litigation.

A study by Greenwood, et al. from the National Perinatal Epidemiology Unit, Oxford, UK compared the prevalence of criteria suggesting acute intrapartum hypoxia in children with cerebral palsy according to whether a lawsuit was brought alleging obstetrical negligence. The subjects were singleton children with cerebral palsy born between 1984 and 1993, excluding cases with a recognized postnatal cause for cerebral palsy. Only one-fifth (27/138) of all singleton CP children were the subject of a lawsuit. The greater the number of criteria suggesting intrapartum insult the more likely was a legal claim (P < 0.01), but 36% (4/11) of those satisfying all required criteria did not make a claim. Of the 27 claims, 12 were discontinued, 8 were settled and in 7 the legal process is still pending at the time of the article. Furthermore, the presence of the three essential criteria for acute intrapartum hypoxia did not increase the likelihood of a legal claim being settled.[81]

Other studies have focused on the costs and outcomes of litigation but not on culpability.[16] Closed claims provide valuable data, but because, on average, a medical liability case takes 3–5 years to come to closure, (GAO 7) Opportunities for timely intervention in unsafe practices are lost. The research value is further compromised when the details of cases that reach settlement are suffocated by "gag clauses" that mandate silence not only about the amount of award, the allegations and the admission or even acknowledgment of wrong-doing, thereby removing an obvious incentive to make care better. Hatlie has suggested that gag orders are counterproductive.[35]

Medical Records

Unfortunately, the opinions that serve to launch medical or medicolegal proceedings are most often based on a review of medical records that are frequently silent on the intentions of the provider or their exercise of "medical judgment". They may be silent, as well, on fundamental details of the obstetrical care. As a result, medical records, which represent both a medical document and a legal document, often promote or perpetuate cases and confound their defense. A cost analysis of 3,205 multispecialty claims showed an average cost per claim of $22,584.[82] Deficits in the medical record, e.g. inadequate instructions, delayed entries, inadequate notes, and consent-form issues, more than doubles the average cost. System failures nearly tripled the average cost. Thus, while an erroneous decision may be defensible if the reasons leading to it are recorded in the chart, the changed record and the contradictory record are almost impossible to defend. Until medical records objectively communicate the findings, the attention paid, the comprehension that was achieved and offer a reasonable plan followed by appropriate and consistent action, their appearance in court will continue to be an uphill battle for the physician and he/she will get little credit for the thought process or use to his/her advantage the testimony of "a witness whose memory never dies".

As an aside, the reader is invited to compare the two enclosed notes regarding a midforceps procedure (Table 24.3). In the first example, the note invites lawsuit if there is an adverse outcome. The note provides no indication for, or detail about, the procedure. It is more a personal memorandum than a responsible medical description relevant for decisions about care in future pregnancies, for example. The second note, on the other hand, would seem to protect against lawsuit in several ways. The note:

- Clearly bespeaks thoughtfulness.
- It bespeaks understanding of the medical issues and alternatives.
- It underscores the physician's efforts to provide forthright explanation to the patient and her husband—all powerful disincentives to lawsuit. Naked may be the best disguise!

One can readily blame the plaintiff attorney for the bringing to suit apparently a frivolous case, but who is to blame (i.e. what has been learned?) for the negligent care and adverse outcome in situations where no suit is brought despite negligent care or where no award is made despite a suit and the physician's care is vindicated? Should the plaintiff attorney be blamed for pursuing a case that his expert has told him, based on a review of the medical records only, is negligent care? Each of the articles that evaluated closed cases found appreciable amounts of agreed upon negligent care. Each emphasizes:

- The need for better data,
- The inculpating role of physician behavior and
- importance of the review of malpractice claims to identify problem-prone clinical processes and suggest interventions that may improve outcome and reduce negligence.[83]

It must be readily apparent from even these limited studies that not all meritorious suits succeed and not all nonmeritorious (not the same as frivolous) lose. These articles leave open to speculation why patients victimized by obvious medical negligence do not sue or why they are not compensated by the system in the face of agreed upon negligence. Clearly, patients without demonstrable evidence of negligence bring suit and sometimes they are rewarded in the system. It does not work perfectly, but these studies from various specialties and perspectives strongly suggest that it is not a lottery. Given the nonmedical issues that incite or color a case, physicians squander much of the advantage they have in the system! Thus, it is with some justification that critics of malpractice litigation point out that it is unrealistic to expect that increased levels of

Table 24.3: Operative delivery notes

Operative Delivery Note (A)	Translation
Operative delivery note: MF, OP >> OA, Mid epis, no lac Apgar 8,9 P and M intact EBL 400, M and B left DR in good condition Signature	Operative Delivery Note: Midforceps, occiput posterior (OP) to occiput anterior (OA), Midline episiotomy, no lacerations Apgar scores 8,9 at 1,5 minutes. Placenta and membranes expressed intact Estimated blood loss 400 mL Mother and infant left the delivery room in good condition.
Operative Delivery Note (B) Procedures: Findings:	Trial of forceps, midforceps rotation, episiotomy repaired. Gyneocoid pelvis, normal active phase, +3 station, minimal molding, direct OP, epidural anesthesia, second stage = 2.5 hours, pushing inadequate, patient tired.
	EFW = 3000 Prev. baby = 2800
Indications: Informed consent:	Persistent occiput posterior, prolonged second stage, secondary arrest of descent, tired patient. Discussed options with patient and husband who agree and understand that if any difficulty is encountered, the forceps will be abandoned and cesarean section undertaken. The operating room has been alerted.
Methods:	Midline episiotomy Kielland forceps—Direct application to OP without difficulty. Gentle rotation: ROT to OA. Kiellands removed, Simpson forceps applied. Gentle traction—Delivered as OA
Fetal Outcome: Resuscitation: Maternal Outcome:	3,200 gm male infant APGAR 8, 9 (see individual features in chart). Oxygen only, no evidence of trauma to skull forceps marks reveal appropriate placement. Perineum intact, episiotomy repaired, no lacerations. Placenta and membranes intact. Estimated blood loss: 300 cc. Mother left delivery room in good condition.

litigation will make compensation for injuries more "just" or health care better. *A reductio ad absurdum* argument suggests that immunity from lawsuit, perhaps the true goal behind physicians' notion of tort reform, will, by eliminating lawsuits achieve these goals. Some conventional tort reforms appear to be effective in reducing litigation costs and stabilizing insurance markets, they are not, however, designed to remedy the fundamental failings of the malpractice system—making care better and making the physician patient relationship better. Fulfillment of these objectives may not require more sweeping tort reform, perhaps more sweeping "thought reform", or alternatively, trying to make the system work as it was supposed to. These reforms may only come from the medical community.

Legal Vulnerability

The last several decades have also witnessed the development of new bases for lawsuit in reproductive matters including wrongful birth and wrongful life. In the former the parents with an injured child may bring suit alleging that negligent treatment or advice deprived them of the opportunity to avoid conception or terminate a pregnancy. The latter, brought on behalf of the child born with birth defects, alleges that the child would not have been born but for negligent advice to, or negligent treatment of, the parents. It should be emphasized that such allegations are actionable in some states but not in others. While not strictly related to malpractice, a mother who pleaded with her hopelessly premature infant's caretakers to discontinue resuscitation was not heeded, resulting in the survival of a severely handicapped child and a provisional $42 million verdict for the plaintiff.

TORT REFORM MEASURES

Most Liability Reform Acts have four major components:

1. Reforms directly addressing the size of awards—Under the heading of caps on damages.

2. Reforms intended to modify liability rules, to control the number of claims and size of payouts by eliminating joint and several liability for cases in which a plaintiff found to be partially at fault becomes responsible for a disproportionate share of the damages.

3. Reforms limiting access to the courts, through shortening statutes of limitation. A reduction in the length of time during which lawsuit can be brought.

4. Periodic payments—The latitude to pay future economic damages overtime. Other initiatives have legislated review panels to pass on the merit of a case prior to the institution of suit, while others attempted to remove the infant who is brain damaged during birth from the medicolegal arena by the institution of no-fault insurance. Still other initiatives have attempted to increase the percentage of any award that goes to the patient by limiting the attorney's fees.

The most popular of these, caps on premiums, have had the benefit of moderating the increases in insurance payments. A publication from the Rand Corporation has cast doubt on the likely benefit of caps on the high award cases where economic damages are large and "pain and suffering" may be much smaller. It seems axiomatic that caps should not apply to frivolous suits where the cap should be zero.

In the 1970s 22 states legislated some form of prelitigation processes, including screening panels and mandatory binding and nonbinding arbitration: only two remain active and neither has been effective. The costs of constitutional battles over due process rights for binding processes and the failed reduction of litigated cases in non-binding processes, led to further soaring legal costs, rather than reductions. The only lasting "tort reform", although as discussed later, questionable material impact on malpractice frequency and awards, has been "Caps" on noneconomic damages, with the "gold standard" being that of California's Medical Injury Compensation Reform Act of 1975 (MICRA).

Tort reform, the mantra of both the ACOG and the Bush administration to deal with high medical malpractice costs, makes sense only from the political aspect. (New York Times Editorial–Malpractice Mythology 1/9/2005). Capping awards on malpractice suits may offend trial lawyers, but it helps or holds harmless special interests in the insurance, drug and health care industries. It provides no assistance to patients who suffer grievous harm as a result of negligent care nor does it improve the delivery of medical care. To many, a $250,000 cap (the cap placed on noneconomic damages in California) is poor acknowledgment indeed for the physical and emotional damage done to people who have suffered total paralysis, permanent blindness or severe brain injury because of medical errors. Indeed, many states burdened with high premiums have already set their own caps, but generally at more reasonable levels. It would seem more useful to consider making it harder for insurance companies to gain rate increases.

Guidelines for judges and juries might be enacted to help determine what compensation is reasonable in a given circumstance. Similar guidelines could help ensure that punitive damages, sometimes masquerading as noneconomic damages are high enough to deter bad conduct; $250,000 would hardly amount to a wrist slap.

The problem with frivolous lawsuits is best addressed by raising the hurdles for filing a malpractice suit, for example, requiring an expert judgment on the merits of a case before it can proceed through the courts. As mentioned above, there seems to be no place for the expert witness to certify a case as meritorious if that same expert will not appear on the record for (public) report, deposition and trial, if necessary.

The notion that the crisis of escalating malpractice insurance premiums is forcing doctors out of business remains murky. Insurance companies have substantially raised premiums for malpractice coverage for doctors in high-risk specialties like obstetrics and neurosurgery in some states, leading at least some doctors to curtail their services, retire or move. But when the Government Accountability Office visited five of the hardest hit states in 2003, it found only scattered problems and was unable to document wide-scale lack of access to medical care.[71]

None of the tort reform proposals deal with the underlying need to diminish malpractice and to identify harmed patients and provide them with fair, prompt compensation or provide tools for healthcare providers to properly prepare patients and to deal effectively with unanticipated outcomes. Although, they do solve the health care industry and the insurance companies' desire for fewer big court awards, they do not materially impact the frequency of suit. But they do act as a roll back of the legal rights of patients who are injured.

The Center for Justice and Democracy, a consumer advocacy group, recently commented that, "It may be hard to understand why 'tort reform' is even on the national agenda at a time when insurance industry profits are booming, tort filings are declining, only 2% of injured people sue for compensation, punitive damages are rarely awarded, liability insurance costs for businesses are minuscule, medical malpractice insurance and claims are both less than 1% of all health care costs in America, and premium-gouging underwriting practices of the insurance industry have been widely exposed".

Despite claims by the insurance industry, there is no evidence that soaring malpractice premiums are the result of sharp increases in the amounts of money paid out for malpractice claims. And, tellingly, industry executives have carefully acknowledged that tort reforms will not result in substantial premium reductions—only an improvement in care can do that (Bob Herbert, Malpractice Myths NYT 6/21/04 Editorial NYT – Feb 2005).

Caps do not limit lawsuits. More reasonably, caps are intended to increase the hurdles to a lawsuit by diminishing the economic value of a suit. In cases where there is little economic loss (irrespective of negligence) victims may not be able to find lawyers to take their cases (www.saynotocaps.org/newsarticles/ WSJEffect of Caps.html) because malpractice cases can cost plaintiff's lawyers hundreds of thousands of dollars out of pocket to prosecute, with no guarantee of recouping those expenses. As pointed out by the Rand Corporation study, caps have little impact on lawsuits where there are substantial economic losses, e.g. brain damaged infant, maternal death, etc. A one-size-fits-all cap cannot encompass the unique facts in any case, and, in fact, more reasonably creates a system of "one size fits none". It unfairly discriminates against victims with no economic losses, such as children, stay-at-home moms, the elderly, the poor and the mentally handicapped. The media unflinchingly promulgates numerous cases tragic, ineffable medical error where such arbitrary limits (originally set in 1979) seem inadequate, if not inadequate, arbitrary.

Caps will not lower doctors' malpractice insurance premiums (www.saynotocaps.org/reports/ Premium Deceit.pdf: The Failure of Tort 'Reform' To Cut Insurance Rates"). Average premiums are actually 16% higher in states with caps. In states that have recently adopted caps, most notably Texas and Florida, insurance rates are continuing to increase. Indeed the only thing keeping rates down in California—a state often cited as a model for caps—is insurance industry regulation provided by Proposition 103.

The amount of money awarded on pain and suffering is unknown. In the majority of awards, those reached by settlement out of court, there was no distinction between economic and non-economic damages. In jury trials economic and noneconomic damages are awarded separately, but there appears to be no calculation of either the amount or the propriety. Nor has there been any compilation of those extreme awards that are reduced, sometimes drastically, by judicial review. In three cases where the jury awarded over $220 million, the total cumulative amount received was $14 million (6 cents on the dollar!). There was no publication of the reduction! (www.saynotocaps.org/reports/Public Citizen.pdf). When adjusted for the skyrocketing rate of health care inflation, total payouts in malpractice cases remained flat up until 2001. (www.say-notocaps.org/reports/Stable Losses Unstable Rates.pdf). In the 3 years since, total payouts have declined each year (www.saynotocaps.org/newsarticle/Lower-Payouts.htm). Furthermore, data released in March 2004 by the Pennsylvania Supreme Court show malpractice case filings have decreased by nearly 30% statewide since 2000.

Many states have enacted legal reforms which have effectively eliminated any lawsuits that could be construed as "frivolous" by requiring a "certificate of merit" from a physician certified in the same medical specialty as the doctor being sued. There have also been laws enacted to prevent "venue shopping" for a more favorable jury has been eliminated. Indeed a Republican state Senator from Pennsylvania declared that "There is no such thing as a frivolous lawsuit anymore" in Pennsylvania. In addition, again in Pennsylvania, one of the "red alert states", there has been a significant increase in the number of physicians over the past several years prompting one state legislator to call such claims of a doctor exodus as "scare tactics".

It is far from clear that malpractice costs are driving up the costs of health care. Malpractice costs account for less than 2% of the US health care budget. The Congressional Budget Office, in a report released in January 2004, found that legislation to cap damages in medical malpractice lawsuits would "do little to hold down health care spending" or eliminate the practice of "defensive medicine". There is little evidence that the threat of malpractice lawsuits contributes to the practice of "defensive medicine". Rather, it has been suggested that doctors order additional tests because it is good medical practice; doctors make money from additional testing; and managed care discourages unnecessary testing, or "bad" defensive medicine.[71]

Faulty underwriting and misfeasance by malpractice underwriters are additional factors contributing to the rise in premiums. In Pennsylvania in the late 1990s half dozen major malpractice insurers became insolvent because of risky premium underpricing, poor investment strategies and Enron-style malfeasance, leaving doctors to pay for their mismanagement (*www.saynotocaps.org/reports/ InsolvencySummary.pdf.*).

There is no basis for the notion that insurance companies routinely settle lawsuits just to make them go away. This seems more like a strategy for self-destruction and is contradicted by the closed-claims data presented above (*www.saynotocaps.org/factsandfigures/fibsysfacts.html#settle*).

There can be little doubt that there is an immediate question of affordability which must be dealt with acutely. Indeed several states have contributed significant amounts of public money to subsidize insurance premiums. Physician remain the highest-paid professionals in the state, according to US. Census data, indeed the incomes of obstetricians the physicians most affected by higher premiums—are rising. For many, on average, doctors spend 1–5% of their gross revenues on medical malpractice insurance. It seems obvious also that many doctors supplement their incomes with fees from attorneys for providing "independent medical evaluations" in malpractice cases.

Alternative System Reforms

Experts have suggested a number of approaches, including special health courts with judges trained to deal with malpractice issues, required mediation, mandatory reporting of errors by doctors and prompt offers of compensation. Some of these will be reviewed briefly here (JCAHO). Not strictly part of tort reform, alternative dispute resolution has much to recommend it.[44]

Strict Liability (No-Fault) Administrative System supports creation of a just patient safety culture and encourages reporting (and prevention) of adverse events. It has the advantages of dispensing with trial and supports open disclosure to the patient (not the public) as the deliberations are administrative. In this system the provider is accountable for all avoidable medically related losses and the matter can be resolved promptly. It eliminates the requirement of proving negligence, but the patient must establish that their injury was actually caused by the treatment. As a generalization, eligibility is based on avoidability rather than providers being strictly responsible for medically related losses. There is, unfortunately, the common perception that "no-fault" means "no accountability". Examples include NICA in Florida and Virginia.

Although, the system of No-Fault is modeled after that of Workers Compensation and Automobile No-Fault claims, the complexity of determining causal and avoidable medical injury claims is very different. Although it removes negligence as a basis for claim, it does not replace the regulatory system of reporting and resultant physician fear, nor does it address the inbred philosophy of the "do no harm", "zero tolerance." Since premiums in any no-fault system are based on injury rates, this creates an incentive to conceal injuries and reduce the admission of high-risk specialists to medical staffs.

It may also discriminate against patients at high-risk for injury. It is uncertain how the establishment of a no-fault system will impact cost. Some test programs have demonstrated that costs of a general no-fault system would exceed that of the present tort system. Finally, the introduction and administration of a no-fault medical injury system, whether public or private, will be complicated and likely politically encumbered.

Preventable Events (ACES) represents consensus on what constitutes an avoidable event (Rosenblatt, 1999).[66] These are predetermined events that should not occur in quality health care delivery. They encourage prevention of avoidable events that can trigger eligibility for early compensation offer. ACE's make "avoidability" and therefore, eligibility for compensation, transparent to providers and patients alike. They standardize eligibility for compensation and provide quicker identification of eligible cases. There is, however, no comprehensive ACE list currently available, and concern exists as to who is to develop the categories of avoidable events. Brain damaged infants, for example, would not be covered. Development of the list will, of course, require an array of expert consensus (selected by whom?). The use of ACE's provides a basis to determine eligibility for alternative and conventional compensation systems. It can also be paired with a standardized compensation fee schedule.

MEDIATION

Mediation represents a highly efficient option for nonadversarial resolution of healthcare conflicts. It is a process in which the parties to the conflict, themselves, not lawyers, craft their own unique resolution to a conflict. Mediation is essentially facilitated communication and negotiation using a neutral third party. The process itself is nonbinding and does not prevent the patient from moving forward to litigation. However, if a resolution is reached, it becomes binding under contract law and may even be brought as an order of the court. Mediation is highly cost efficient, time sparing in that it makes response to adverse events and their resolution more timely and boasts a greater than 90% resolution rate. It is widely excepted and highly successful in many "industries" such as real estate and education but has met with much resistance in the healthcare "industry", especially in medical malpractice. It intensifies pressure on patients to settle thus reducing or avoiding litigation. Because confidentiality has been stripped from the mediation process in medical malpractice disputes by medical regulatory boards and reporting agencies, and therefore has crippled the successful application of the mediation process in physician/patient conflicts. Although, confidentiality in error reporting is a foundation for most of the proposed legislation, it has not been extended to the resolution of conflicts arising from alleged medical errors. The statutory obligation physicians have to report settlements of disputes involving quality of care issues creates a perverse incentive for physicians to move forward in litigation, especially when one considers the high attrition rate of malpractice claims and the likelihood of a physician prevailing in those cases that persist. It is likely that even in the face of tort reform, mediation will remain an infrequently used medium for physician/patient dispute resolution.

Arbitration

As with mediation, arbitration provides economical and prompt adjudication of adverse events. Like mediation, it provides prompt, private settlement and compensation, yet is also subject to reporting requirements and regulatory oversight. The processes differ, however, in a few major factors: with arbitration the decision maker is a third party, the arbitrator(s), and the process is highly formalistic and adversarial. There are two forms of arbitration, binding and nonbinding. The later is similar to mediation in that if either party disagrees with the arbitrator's decision, they may move on to litigation. The former, however, is a binding decision, which cannot be appealed. Binding arbitration for malpractice claims has met with considerable legal opposition and nonbinding arbitration has met with low utilization and increased litigation costs. Such systems intensifies pressure on patients to settle thus reducing or avoiding litigation. It may be used with current tort system—as well as with no fault and ACEs. Kaiser Permanente, for example, "requires enrollees to sign a 'willingness to arbitrate' agreement". With this approach, the health plan undertakes to resolve disputes through arbitration then go through the courts. This of course is not the same as a waiver of liability.

Specialized Medical Malpractice Courts

There are three types of specialized courts under consideration: the Health Court, the Medical Board Administrative Adjudication System and Tripartite Panel.

Health Court involves the creation of an alternative court system within the federal court system. This proposal will, as touted by the consumer advocate group, Common Good, presumably make judgments more reliable and provide clearer lessons for deterrence of adverse outcome. In theory they can provide more timely access, provide faster resolution of claims along with more reliable and standardized compensation. It requires appointment of special expert courts to hear medical cases or administer compensation based on avoidable events. Health courts also make the system more transparent by providing public access to settlement and adjudication findings. It will require judges who have special knowledge or training in medicine. Although proponents believe that this form of adjudication will offer more consistent and informed decisions than the traditional trier of fact, a lay jury, many studies find that in comparison with expert's reviews, the present jury system is quite consistent.

Health courts may be paired with ACEs and standardized compensation schedule and may even add a trial option to an administrative system. There are precedents for these types of courts in certain tax and patent infringement and worker's compensation laws.

Medical Board Administrative Adjudication System—In 1988 the AMA, 31 medical specialty associations, the Physician Insurer's Association of America (PIAA), and the Counsel of Medical Specialty Societies created the Medical Liability Project to develop an equitable and efficient method to handle malpractice claims. They proposed a claims adjudication process based on fault and suggested that the states' medical boards act as the trier of fact in addition to their regulatory and disciplinary roles. This system would initially screen cases, offer free legal counsel for cases passing review and offer limited judicial review. In a parallel development, the AMA considers that the provision of expert testimony constitutes "the practice of medicine"? and that it should be subject to peer review by state medical boards. The AMA encourages the state medical associations to work with the licensing boards to develop effective disciplinary measures for fraudulent testimony.

Tripartite Panel—Also in 1988 PIAA proposed an administrative system similar to that used in Workers' Compensation in the hope that patients would elect this more speedy system through the offer of incentives. The panel would consist of a judge, a physician, and a lay person and function much like the few state screening panels that remain active. In cases where malpractice was found, all medical expenses would be paid under a specific method of computation, all noneconomic awards would be based on a fixed schedule of benefits, and their would be a limit on attorney's fees.

Pretrial Screening Panels

This is a system that is modeled after state programs that are presently functioning, with those of Maine and Vermont most recognized. To enlist the Panel, the patient provides written notice to physician and with the Superior court to be acted upon within 90 days. The Superior Court selects a Panel Chair from a pool of retired judges and/or mediators with judicial or legal experience. The chair selects from a Court issued list, one attorney and one physician panelist, of the same or relevant specialty. The parties may challenge the selection for cause.

There is Prehearing discovery then a Pretrial screening hearing that follows the format of an arbitration. Depositions are admissible, but expert testimony unusual. The panel has prior access to written briefs, complete medical records and deposition transcripts. The panel then acts as both the trier of fact and law, under the standard used by lay juries, "preponderance of the evidence". It evaluates the case on the basis of the Four Ds of negligence. Unanimous decisions by the panel on negligence and causation are admissible in court, both in favor of patient or provider. The decision of the panel, like in nonbinding arbitration does not bind either party from pursuing litigation and trial. Some systems allow recovery of costs by the losing party, but as stated previously, if it is the plaintiff, actual recovery is unlikely.

Enterprise Liability

Enterprise liability provides incentive for prioritization of enterprise-wide safety. It shifts liability from individual provider to a provider organization such as an integrated medical staff, IPO, large group practice or hospital capable of influencing care across the systems. Enterprise liability essentially makes these organizations "strictly liable" in both a legal and economic sense by their responsibility for liability premiums for all staff involved in the organization, which could potentially impact the present punitive reporting system and allow for a freer flow of error reporting. Such a system would promote institutional safety and potentially stabilize liability insurance fees. Legal provisions (Stark laws) may prohibit liability insurance coverage of nonemployee physicians. It works equally well with alternatives as well as the current tort system. "The Department of Health and Human Services" Office of Inspector

General (OIG) historically has concerned that a hospital's subsidy of malpractice insurance premiums for potential referral sources, including hospital medical staff, may implicate the antikickback statute, because the payments may be used to influence referrals. There is a particular concern where subsidies are offered in a conditional or selective manner that reflects current or anticipated referrals from the subsidized practitioners. Hospitals may be able to subsidize the malpractice insurance of local obstetricians without triggering antikickback sanctions, according to an advisory opinion issued by the OIG. In the opinion, OIG outlines a specific case in which it would not impose antikickback sanctions against a medical center that provides subsidies to four community-based obstetricians who hold staff privileges at the medical center but are not employees of the facility (OB-GYN NEWS October 15, 2004, p. 25).

Tort reform in many of its guises, however, has historically not been universally "friendly" to the physician. In 1988, the US Congress established a National Practitioner Data Bank authorizing the collection of data about physicians and dentists from malpractice settlements, awards and disciplinary actions; these data were to be supplied by insurers, hospitals and HMOs.[4] Queries of the Data Bank might be made by hospitals and physicians, but there is to be no access by the public or actual or prospective litigants including patients and attorneys although expanded access to this information is the subject of much debate. This tracking by the Data Base has probably decreased the willingness of physicians to settle cases, but has probably not decreased the frequency of malpractice. The NPDB reporting system is primarily based on the reporting of any formal written claim of malpractice that results in even one penny changing hands, regardless of admission of blame or severity of injury. Such reports carry great weight in considerations for staff privileges, provider contracts and malpractice premium rates. Hatlie has argued that the NPDB should be abandoned.[35]

Even more recently has come the increasing attention of the amount of medical error that has heretofore gone unnoticed and undocumented. The AMA has created a Patient Safety Initiative and the Federal Government is considering legislation that will likely reorient the approach to error. Indeed, since the publication of the prestigious Institute of Medicine's "To Err is Human" which claims that between 44,000 and 98,000 hospitalized patients die per year as a result of medical error, and subsequent studies such as that of Sarwat Chaudry, et al., patient safety has become the mantra of the Joint Commission on Accreditation which has now embellished the requirements for disclosure of error (JACHO). Programs for the evaluation of route cause analyses of reported errors and resulting error reducing actions have become, as they should, a national priority.

Also potentially threatening to the physician, are those tort reforms that are linked (politically) to the establishment of enhanced physician review panels, the creation of "3 strikes and you are out rules", etc. In Texas, for example, along with a stringent tort reform bill passed in 2003, the Texas legislature gave the Texas State Board of Medical Examiners new authority to regulate medical practice through the passage of SB 104. This bill gave the board increased funding for expert consultants and staff. These resources were used to assess the approximately 6,000 complaints the board receives each year. As a result, Board enforcements have increased dramatically. Before the augmentation, cases were filed against physicians immediately and immediately affected their records. The new system provides more due process, but is more

far ranging. Opponents of this feature of Texas Health litigation argue that standard of care issues should be left to local community medical societies or hospital peer review and credentialing societies. But when the shoe is on the other foot, these organizations engage in sham peer review or economic credentialing physicians complain about their unfair practices (see below). Physician groups complaining about SB 104 want the presumption of innocence, the right to access details of the complaints against them, the right of discovery, the right to present witnesses and cross-examine witnesses and the right to appeal. How seductive is the illusion of a new idea—all of these features are present in current malpractice law—the beneficiary of 200 years of accumulated jurisprudence. Public Citizens's Health Research Group ranked Texas 23 out of the 50 states.

Reviews of the impact tort reform on premiums suggest that while premiums do respond to increases in payments, they do not increase dollar for dollar (http://www.nber.org/papers/w10709). This suggests that other factors may also be important in explaining the recent jump in malpractice premiums, such as a less competitive insurance industry or a decline in insurers' investment income. There is little evidence that changes in malpractice premiums are linked to changes in either the total number of physicians or the number of physicians working in obstetrics/gynecology, surgery or internal medicine. Weak evidence suggests that the entry decisions of young physicians and the exit decisions of older physicians may be affected by malpractice premiums. Stronger evidence suggests that rural physicians are more sensitive to change in premiums—a 10 percent increase in premiums results in a 1% decrease in rural physicians per capita and a 2% decrease in older rural MDs (http://www.nber.org/papers/w10709).

Although there is no change in the frequency of most treatments, some data suggests that physicians may increase the use of screening procedures in response to higher premiums. Such practices, however, have had little effect on total Medicare expenditures, suggesting that the costs associated with defensive medicine practices may be small, at least for this age group. Thus, it is far from clear that state tort reforms will avert local physician shortages or lead to greater efficiencies in care. The stabilization of premiums, the initial response to most rounds of tort reform, may not indeed be the result of the tort reform legislation. Normally, it takes years before legislative tort reform has a direct impact on malpractice premiums and several, but not all state courts have invalidated the cap on damages, the component of the law with the greatest potential to reduce premiums (Zuckerman, et al. 1989). Malpractice premiums are affected by a constellation of additional factors, including the general investment climate, interest rate cycles and insurance regulations [Department of Health and Human Services. Report of the Task Force on Medical Liability and Malpractice, August 1987 (Washington, DC: United States Government Printing Office, 519–216/63040, 1988)].

Whether driven by legislation or not, it seems reasonable that stable malpractice insurance premiums offered by experienced, reputable companies are important reasons for maintaining physician availability and equilibrium.

There is no evidence that tort reform has resulted in better care or more realistic confrontation of error. Tort reform simply "tinkers with certain aspects of the system in a piecemeal fashion without having to grapple with fundamental reform of either the health care delivery system, the reimbursement system or physician behavior".

Tort Reform and Finances—Litigation and Risk Management

There is universal agreement that the medical needs of those with adverse outcome need more attention, whether it is related to negligence or not. There is also universal agreement that the present functioning of the medicolegal system is an anachronism neither efficient nor error-free in reaching settlement or that the distribution of money is equitable. In the United States, only about 28 cents of every premium dollar goes to injured patients after an average delay of 4.9 years to dispose of a case.

Is no fault insurance better? To determine whether Florida's implementation of a no-fault system for birth-related neurological injuries reduced lawsuits and total spending associated with such injuries, and whether no-fault was more efficient than customary tort procedures in distributing compensation, Sloan, et al. compared claims and payments before and after implementation of a no-fault system in 1989.[6] They found that the number of tort claims for permanent labor-delivery injury and death indeed fell by about 16–32%. However, when no-fault claims were added to tort claims, the total claims frequency rose by 11–38%. Further, of the estimated 479 children suffered birth-related injuries annually, only 13 were compensated under no-fault. Total combined payments to patients and all lawyers did not decrease, but under no-fault, a much larger portion of the total went to patients. Thus, less than 3% of total payments went to lawyers under no-fault versus 39% under tort—a new equilibrium. Some claimants with birth-related injuries were winners, taking home a larger percentage of their awards than their tort counterparts. Lawyers clearly lost under no-fault, but so did many children with birth-related neurologic injuries who did not qualify for coverage because of the narrow statutory definition.

SOLVING THE MALPRACTICE PROBLEM

While the focus of clinical risk management intuitively rests on the analysis of adverse events, it seems clear that this is a most inefficient way of reducing or eliminating harm to the patient. In the current climate risk management tends to deal more with avoidance of blame and litigation than in the avoidance of harm to patients.

One of health care's principal patient safety success stories is anesthesiology. In the 1980s, in the midst of a separate medical liability crisis, the rate of anesthesia-related deaths was one in 10,000; 6,000 people per year who had undergone anesthesia died or suffered brain damage, and anesthesiologists' liability insurance premiums had sharply escalated.[68] Following a national news magazine broadcast which pilloried the field for these outcomes, the American Society of Anesthesiologists (ASA) decided to seize the opportunity presented by the crisis to improve anesthesiology safety.

It started with the hiring of a systems engineer. Through close scientific examination of 359 anesthesia errors, every aspect of anesthesia care—equipment, practices, and caregivers—was analyzed. Eventually, with the commitment of leadership and resources toward the task, the many system failures revealed by the study were re-engineered, and anesthesia-related death rates fell to one in more than 200,000 cases.[69]

The ASA uses case analysis to identify liability risk areas, monitor trends in patient injury and design strategies for prevention. Today, the ASA Closed Claims Project—created in 1985—contains 6,448 closed insurance claims. Analyses of these claims have, for example, revealed patterns in patient injury in the use of regional anesthesia, in the placement of central venous catheters and in chronic pain management. Results of these analyses are published in the professional literature to aid practitioner learning and promote changes in practices that improve safety and reduce liability exposure.

Closed claims data analysis is the one way in which the current medical liability system helps to inform improvements in care delivery. However, reliance on closed claims for information related to error and injury is cumbersome at best. It may take years for an insurance or malpractice claim to close. These are years in which potentially vital information on substandard practices remains unknown. Providing patient safety researchers with access to open claims, now protected from external examination, could vastly improve efforts aimed at identifying worrisome patterns in care and designing appropriate safety interventions.

In addition to anesthesiology's early work in identifying the human factors and system failures that cause error, anesthesiology has also promoted reliance on standards and guidelines to support optimal anesthesiology care. Anesthesiology has also been at the forefront in the use of patient simulation for research, training and performance assessment. With simulation, no patients are at risk for exposure to novice caregivers or unproven technologies.[70]

Anesthesiology is still far from perfect. But, its "institutionalization of safety",[71] continues to serve the field well as it tackles the continuing threats to patient safety that are endemic to modern medicine.

Medicine is different from industry in that the medical system has not adjusted to the realities of human fallibility. The circumstances of contemporary malpractice situation continue to compromise both the provision and safety of health care as well as our notions of justice of access to the law and to health care. This state of affairs benefits neither the patient, nor in the long run, the physician. While in some instances the fear of lawsuit has increased the amount of surveillance and may have even had a salutary effect on outcome, there is little argument that the present format for dealing with allegations of negligence provides any incentive to the profession to practice better medicine, to provide better peer review or in the occasional instance, restrict the future practice of the physician whatever his conduct. True reform will require a systemic approach to error in medicine as elsewhere and some refinement of our ethics and an appreciation of the paradoxes of contemporary malpractice. To lower the risk of malpractice we must continue to attempt to raise the standards of care. We need this more than we need the identification of the "bad apples" of our specialty. We must increase communication with the patient and remain their advocate. We must address the formal teaching of communication skills, conflict management, and team development techniques throughout medical school and residency. We must construct effective error reporting and systems analyses programs that promote error reduction, while protecting physicians from being punished by arbitrary and ineffective reporting systems. We must not squander our greatest asset, the medical record, and stop acting the role of victim. Often the ultimate failure is often not the individual provider but the latent, systemic errors, errors for which our systems are programmed, but which are functionally immune from lawsuit. A law suit cannot make "the system" a defendant. Finally, we must be willing to participate in the process of uncovering error and make the patients our allies in these efforts.

REFERENCES

1. Keeton WP, Keeton RE, Owens DG. Prosser and Keeton on the law of torts, 5th edition St. Paul, Minn: West Publishing; 1984.
2. Hickson GB, Clayton EW, Entman SS, et al. Obstetricians' prior malpractice experience and patients' satisfaction with care. JAMA. 1994;272(20):1583-7.
3. Hickson GB, Federspiel CF, Pichert JW, et al. Patient complaints and malpractice risk. JAMA. 2002;287(22):2951-7.
4. Hickson GB, Clayton EW, Githens PB, et al. Factors that prompted families to file medical malpractice claims following perinatal injuries. JAMA. 1992;267(10):1359-63.
5. Ambady N, Laplante D, Nguyen T, et al. Surgeons' tone of voice: A clue to malpractice history. Surgery. 2002;132(1):5-9.
6. Sloan FA, Whetten-Goldstein K, Hickson GB. The influence of obstetric no-fault compensation on obstetricians' practice patterns. Am J Obstet Gynecol. 1998;179(3 Pt 1):671-6.
7. Gibson S. Wall of Silence.
8. Kritzer H. The Justice Broker: Lawyers and Ordinary Litigation. New York: Oxford University Press; 1990.
9. Hyams AL, Shapiro DW, Brennan TA. Medical practice guidelines in malpractice litigation: an early retrospective. J Health Polit Policy Law. 1996;21(2):289-313.
10. Peters K. The role of the jury in modern malpractice law. Iowa Law Rev. 2002:909-69.
11. Studdert DM, Mello MM, Brennan TA. Medical malpractice. N Engl J Med. 2004;350(3):283-92.
12. Fry v. United States F. In.
13. Shea vs. Esensten F, 3d 625m 629 (8th Cir.). In; 1997.
14. Daubert v. Merrell Dow Pharmaceuticals I, 509 US 579. In; 1993.
15. Kumho Tire Co. LVC, 119 S. Ct. 1167. In; 1999.
16. Bors-Koefoed R, Zylstra S, Resseguie LJ, et al. Statistical models of outcome in malpractice lawsuits involving death or neurologically impaired infants. J Matern Fetal Med. 1998;7(3):124-31.
17. LLMD of Michigan IvJ-C, Co. In; 1999.
18. Ross BK. ASA closed claims in obstetrics: Lessons learned. Anesthesiol Clin North America. 2003;21(1):183-97.
19. Meyers AR. 'Lumping it': The hidden denominator of the medical malpractice crisis. Am J Public Health. 1987;77(12):1544-8.
20. Meeker CI. A consensus-based approach to practice parameters. Obstet Gynecol. 1992;79(5 (Pt 1)):790-3.
21. Meeker WC. The future impact of clinical practice guidelines. J Manipulative Physiol Ther. 1995;18(9):606-10.
22. Lavery JP, Janssen J, Hutchinson L. Is the obstetric guideline of 30 minutes from decision to incision for cesarean delivery clinically significant? J Healthc Risk Manag. 1999;19(1):11-20.
23. Schreiber v. Physicians Insurance Company of Wisconsin 223 Wis. 2d 417. In; 1996.
24. Plauche WC. Subgaleal hematoma. A complication of instrumental delivery. Jama. 1980;244(14):1597-8.
25. Calbresi G. The cost of accidents: A legal and economic analysis. New Haven, Conn: Yale University Press; 1970.
26. Schwartz W, Mendelson D. Physicians who have lost their malpractice insurance: Their demographic characteristics and the surplus-lines companies that insure them. JAMA. 1989;262:1335-41.
27. Brooks R. Editorial - Malpractice Mythology. New York Times, 2005.
28. Kollas CD. Medicolegal program for resident physicians. Pa Med. 1997;100(9):28-9.
29. Kollas CD, Frey CM. A medicolegal curriculum for internal medicine residents. J Gen Intern Med. 1999;14(7):441-3.
30. Spaeth RG, Pickering KC, Webb SM. Quality assurance and hospital structure: How the physician-hospital relationship affects quality measures. Ann Health Law. 2003;12(2):235-47.
31. Gluck PA, Scarrow PK. Peer review in obstetrics and gynecology by a national medical specialty society. Jt Comm J Qual Saf. 2003;29(2):77-84.
32. Hugh TB, Tracy GD. Hindsight bias in medicolegal expert reports. Med J Aust. 2002;176(6):277-8.
33. Meadow W, Lantos JD. Expert testimony, legal reasoning, and justice. The case for adopting a data-based standard of care in allegations of medical negligence in the NICU. Clin Perinatol. 1996;23(3):583-95.
34. Donohue SK. Health care quality information liability & privilege. Ann Health Law. 2002;11:147-58.
35. Hatlie MJ, Sheridan SE. The medical liability crisis of 2003: Must we squander the chance to put patients first? Health Aff (Millwood). 2003;22(4):37-40.
36. Cheney FW, Posner K, Caplan RA, et al. Standard of care and anesthesia liability. JAMA. 1989;261(11):1599-603.
37. Gawande AA. Ubiqity of error. New Yorker. 2003.
38. Reding R. The role of intuition in medical malpractice. Zentralbl Chir. 1999;124 (Suppl 3):50-2.
39. Brennan TA, Hebert LE, Laird NM, et al. Hospital characteristics associated with adverse events and substandard care. JAMA. 1991;265(24):3265-9.
40. Brennan TA, Leape LL. Adverse events, negligence in hospitalized patients: Results from the Harvard Medical Practice Study. Perspect Healthc Risk Manage. 1991;11(2):2-8.
41. Localio AR, Lawthers AG, Brennan TA, et al. Relation between malpractice claims and adverse events due to negligence. Results of the Harvard Medical Practice Study III. N Engl J Med. 1991;325(4):245-51.
42. Hobgood C, Peck CR, Gilbert B, et al. Medical errors-what and when: What do patients want to know? Acad Emerg Med. 2002;9(11):1156-61.
43. Witman AB, Park DM, Hardin SB. How do patients want physicians to handle mistakes? A survey of internal medicine patients in an academic setting. Arch Intern Med. 1996;156(22):2565-9.
44. B-Lynch C, Coker A, Dua JA. A clinical analysis of 500 medico-legal claims evaluating the causes and assessing the potential benefit of alternative dispute resolution. Br J Obstet Gynaecol. 1996;103(12):1236-42.
45. Finkelstein D, Wu AW, Holtzman NA, et al. When a physician harms a patient by a medical error: Ethical, legal, and risk-management considerations. J Clin Ethics. 1997;8(4):330-5.
46. Grady D. Doctors Urged to Admit Mistakes. New York Times. 12/9/1997.
47. Hebert PC, Levin AV, Robertson G. Bioethics for clinicians: 23. Disclosure of medical error. Cmaj. 2001;164(4):509-13.
48. Nowicki M, Chaku M. Do healthcare managers have an ethical duty to admit mistakes? Healthc Financ Manage. 1998;52(10):62-4.
49. Baldwin DC Jr., Adamson TE, Self DJ, et al. Moral reasoning and malpractice. A pilot study of orthopedic surgeons. Am J Orthop. 1996;25(7):481-4.
50. Lamb RM, Studdert DM, Bohmer RM, et al. Hospital disclosure practices: Results of a national survey. Health Aff (Millwood). 2003;22(2):73-83.
51. Physician Apology. Wall Street Journal 2004 May 18, 2004.
52. Zimmerman R. Doctors' new tool to fight lawsuits: saying 'I'm sorry,. Malpractice insurers find owning up to errors soothes patient anger. 'The risks are extraordinary'. J Okla State Med Assoc. 2004;97(6):245-7.

53. Mazor KM, Simon SR, Yood RA, et al. Health plan members' views about disclosure of medical errors. Ann Intern Med. 2004;140(6):409-18.

54. Gallagher TH, Waterman AD, Ebers AG, et al. Patients' and physicians' attitudes regarding the disclosure of medical errors. JAMA. 2003;289(8):1001-7.

55. Michael S, Woods MD. "Healing Words: The Power of Apology in Medicine." (info@doctorsintouch.com.); 2004.

56. Simpson KR, Knox GE. Common areas of litigation related to care during labor and birth: Recommendations to promote patient safety and decrease risk exposure. J Perinat Neonatal Nurs. 2003;17(2):110-25; quiz 26-7.

57. ACOG. Technical Bulletin, No. 196, Operative Vaginal Delivery. 1994.

58. ACOG. Committee Opinion No. 197—Inappropriate Use of the Terms Fetal Distress and Birth Asphyxia). 1998.

59. Schifrin BS. Polemics in perinatology: Disengaging forceps. J Perinatol. 1988;8(3):242-5.

60. ACOG. Technical Bulletin, No. 163, Fetal and Neonatal Neurologic Injury. 1992.

61. Schifrin BS. The CTG and the timing and mechanism of fetal neurological injuries. Best Pract Res Clin Obstet Gynaecol. 2004;18(3):437-56.

62. Dear P, Newell S. Establishing probable cause in cerebral palsy. How much certainty is enough? BMJ. 2000;320(7241):1075-6.

63. O'Leary JA. Shoulder Dystocia and Birth Injury: Prevention and Treatment. New York: Mcgraw-Hill; 1992.

64. Margaret Lent. The Medical and Legal Risks of the Electronic Fetal Monitor. In: 51 Stan L Rev 807 April, 1999: 51 Stan. L. Rev. 807 April, 1999; 1999.

65. Ennis M. Obstetric accidents: A review of 64 cases BMJ.; 300(6736):1365-7. BMJ 1990;300(6736):1365-7.

66. Rosenblatt RA, Bovbjerg RR, Whelan A, et al. Tort reform and the obstetric access crisis. The case of the WAMI states. West J Med. 1991;154(6):693-9.

67. Weiler P. Medical malpractice on trial. Cambridge, Mass: Harvard University Press; 1991.

68. Burstin HR, Johnson WG, Lipsitz SR, et al. Do the poor sue more? A case-control study of malpractice claims and socioeconomic status. JAMA. 1993;270(14):1697-701.

69. Sloan FA, Whetten-Goldstein K, Githens PB, et al. Effects of the threat of medical malpractice litigation and other factors on birth outcomes. Med Care. 1995;33(7):700-14.

70. The effects of medical professional liability on the delivery of obstetrical care. Washington, DC: Institute of Medicine, National Academy Press; 1989.

71. Medical malpractice insurance: Multiple factors have contributed to increased premium rates. In: General Accounting Office W, DC, ed.: US Government; 2003.

72. Limiting Tort Liability for Medical Malpractice. In: Office CB, ed.: US Government, Washington, DC; 2004.

73. FDA. Advisory: Food and Drug Administration; 1998.

74. Sachs BP, Kobelin C, Castro MA, et al. The risks of lowering the cesarean-delivery rate. N Engl J Med. 1999;340(1):54-7.

75. Brennan TA, Leape LL, Laird NM, et al. Incidence of adverse events and negligence in hospitalized patients: Results of the Harvard Medical Practice Study I. 1991. Qual Saf Health Care. 2004;13(2):145-51; discussion 51-2.

76. Brennan TA, Localio AR, Leape LL, et al. Identification of adverse events occurring during hospitalization. A cross-sectional study of litigation, quality assurance, and medical records at two teaching hospitals. Ann Intern Med. 1990;112(3):221-6.

77. Julian TM, Brooker DC, Butler JC Jr, et al. Investigation of obstetric malpractice closed claims: Profile of event. Am J Perinatol. 1985;2(4):320-4.

78. Rosenblatt RA, Hurst A. An analysis of closed obstetric malpractice claims. Obstet Gynecol. 1989;74(5):710-4.

79. Ogburn PL Jr, Julian TM, Brooker DC, et al. Perinatal medical negligence closed claims from the St. Paul Company, 1980-1982. J Reprod Med. 1988;33(7):608-11.

80. Ransom SB, Studdert DM, Dombrowski MP, et al. Reduced medicolegal risk by compliance with obstetric clinical pathways: a case control study. Obstet Gynecol. 2003;101(4):751-5.

81. Greenwood C, Newman S, Impey L, et al. Cerebral palsy and clinical negligence litigation: A cohort study. BJOG. 2003;110(1):6-11.

82. Richards BC, Thomasson G. Closed liability claims analysis and the medical record. Obstet Gynecol. 1992;80(2):313-36.

83. Kravitz RL, Rolph JE, McGuigan K. Malpractice claims data as a quality improvement tool. I. Epidemiology of error in four specialties. JAMA. 1991;266 (15):2087-92.

SECTION 3

Evidence-based Medicine and Epidemiology

Z Alfirevic, L Cabero-Roura

25 Epidemiology in Perinatal Medicine

LS Bakketeig

DEFINITIONS

For a long time, it has been recognized that events during pregnancy and childbirth influence the health and development of the newborn. This recognition has led to the establishment of perinatology as a medical specialty, which bridges the gap between the obstetrician's concern for the pregnant woman and the pediatrician's care of the newborn.

Population-based studies of these phenomena are labeled "perinatal epidemiology", which has evolved into a major subspecialty of epidemiology, representing an important contribution to perinatal medicine. Traditionally, perinatal epidemiologists have focused on exposures and outcomes occurring in the perinatal period, which most commonly covers the time from conception through to birth and the first part of life (1 week, 1 month or the first year of life). In recent years, though, it has been realized that events or exposures that take place in utero, or shortly after birth, can also affect development and health even into adult life. We also have come to realize that even events occurring long before pregnancy, sometimes intergenerationally, can affect our reproduction.

An Austrian pediatrician suggested nearly 75 years ago that stillbirths and deaths during the first week of life should be treated as one statistical entity in the analysis of causes of death.[1] The term "perinatal mortality" was increasingly used from the 1940s onward.[2-4] The increasing attention being paid to perinatal mortality was caused by the observation that the fall in infant mortality (death during the first year of life) in the first half of the 20th century derived mainly from the reduction in mortality of infants surviving beyond the first week of life.[5] It appeared that the progress made was mostly a result of the success in combating deaths due to infectious diseases in early infancy. Mortality among infants shortly after birth, as well as fetal mortality, had decreased far less.[5]

Perinatal mortality is the most commonly used death rate as an indicator of perinatal health. The other death rates used in perinatal epidemiology are stillbirth, neonatal, postneonatal and infant death rates, illustrated. The death rates are defined as the number of deaths per 1,000 births, or per 1,000 livebirths for the latter three rates.

PERINATAL SURVEILLANCE

Perinatal surveillance can be based on the perinatal and infant death rates, but also on other health indicators such as the frequency of different congenital anomalies or the frequency of preterm births or low-birthweight births. Some countries, for example, the Scandinavian countries, have established medical birth registries where all births in the country are monitored. Thus, the occurrence of different adverse outcomes can be monitored and changes in frequencies can be detected and further investigated. The thalidomide disaster in the early 1960s was the main reason why

such a medical registration system was established in Norway in 1967. This was the first national population-based registration of births ever established.[6] Later, similar registration systems were established in Denmark, Sweden and Finland.

The medical registration of births contains information of the parents (a few items on civic and medical information), the course of pregnancy and delivery and, finally, some information about the newborn baby. Therefore, the medical birth registration information can be used for perinatal audit purposes beyond the surveillance of congenital anomalies. Perinatal audit represents a current assessment of the quality of perinatal care, based on the structure of care, the process of care and the outcome of care. The information collected through the medical birth registration represents a valuable basis for assessing at least the process and the outcome of care, while data on the structure of care will have to be collected separately.

The medical birth registration forms the basis of the Medical Birth Registries in the Nordic countries. The child and its parents are identified by unique identification numbers. This facilitates the linkage of the information with other data sources, like the death registry, the census data and the education registry. Also, the identification number makes it possible to link the medical birth registries with other morbidity registries, such as the cancer registries, which represent high-quality data sources in the Nordic countries.

RISK FACTORS

Perinatal epidemiology focuses on different risk factors associated with pregnancy and childbirth. Births with an adverse outcome are compared with controls and whether one group has more often been exposed to the risk factor under study than the controls (case-control study). An outstanding example of such a study is the discovery of the strong association between the use of diethylstilbestrol in pregnancy to prevent miscarriages and the risk of vaginal cancer in the female offspring of these women when they reach their early reproductive years.[7]

The other approach in studying associations between exposures and adverse outcomes is the use of cohort studies, where two groups of women are selected, one being and one not being exposed to the suspected risk factor, and then comparing the outcomes in the groups. In Table 25.1, an example is shown of such a cohort study which focuses on the risk of small-for-gestational-age (SGA) births for groups of women with established risk factors at the start of their pregnancies, and evaluates the additional risk associated with cigarette smoking. The data shown in the table are based on a longitudinal study of fetal growth.[8] For women with no known risk factors at the beginning of the pregnancy, 6.5% will have a SGA birth. If the women smoke cigarettes, the

Table 25.1: The frequency of small-for-gestational-age (SGA) births in cohorts of women with different risk factors, including cigarette smoking, at start of pregnancy

Risk factor	Women (n)	SGA births		Relative risk	95% Confidence interval
		n	%		
None*					
Nonsmoker	3,190	208	6.5	1.0	
Smoker	1,515	179	11.8	1.8	(1.5, 2.2)
Previous low-birthweight birth					
Nonsmoker	286	44	15.4	2.4	(1.7, 3.3)
Smoker	238	84	35.3	5.4	(4.2, 7.0)
Low prepregnancy weight (< 50 kg)					
Nonsmoker	164	20	12.2	1.9	(1.2, 3.0)
Smoker	175	45	25.7	3.9	(2.9, 5.4)

*Defined as the absence of the following risk factors: previous low birthweight birth, low prepregnancy weight, previous perinatal death or chronic maternal diseases (essential hypertension, heart disease or renal disease)

Table 25.2: Prediction of low birthweight (LBW), preterm and small-for-gestational-age (SGA) second births based on birth weight and gestational age of first birth (76,398 mothers with first two births 1967–73). From reference 10

First birth	Risk of second birth					
	LBW		Preterm		SGA	
	%	Relative risk	%	Relative risk	%	Relative risk
LBW	15.2	5.6	15.4	3.7	20.5	4.1
Preterm	11.8	4.1	16.4	4.0	11.5	1.5
SGA	7.7	2.8	6.6	1.4	22.1	3.9

risk increases to 11.8% [relative risk (RR) = 1.8]. If the women have had a previous low birthweight (LBW) birth (birthweight below 2,500 g), then the risk of a SGA birth is more than doubled (RR = 2.4), and if they smoke cigarettes, there is a further doubling of the risk (RR = 5.4).

Case control and cohort studies are both observational studies. Furthermore, within perinatal epidemiology as well as other areas of epidemiology, observational studies are the dominant tools in addition to more descriptive and even hypotheses generating studies. The more powerful experimental approaches are obviously less suitable. However, in evaluating perinatal care, one can use randomized controlled trials, applying either individual or cluster randomization. This approach can also be applied in the evaluation of preventive programs. Here, the cluster randomization approach ought to be used more often. For example, in evaluating a new program for antenatal care, instead of randomizing individuals, one could randomize areas, counties, municipalities or clinics to alternative programs and then compare the results.[9]

RECURRENCE RISKS

The feasibility of linking parents and child in the medical birth registries makes it possible to study the recurrence of pregnancy and childbirth events within sibships. This has been done extensively, based on the Norwegian Medical Birth Registry data over the last 20 years, starting with a paper in 1977 which demonstrated the strong tendency to repeat preterm, low birthweight and SGA births in successive pregnancies in the same woman.[10]

As it turned out, as shown in Table 25.2, low birthweight (LBW) was the best predictor of subsequent LBW, preterm birth was the best predictor of later preterm birth, and SGA birth was the best predictor of subsequent SGA births. These and later analyses have indicated that women are 'programmed' to have births of a similar size in subsequent pregnancies.

The first births included in the Norwegian Medical Birth Registry from 1967 onward have now since long started to reproduce themselves, which facilitates the study of intergenerational effects. As it turns out, birthweight correlates across generations, but gestational age correlates to a lesser extent.[11] A recent analysis is based on 105.104 mother/child pairs recruited from females in the Norwegian Medical Birth Registry born since 1967 and reproducing through 1995. Based on 101.579 single mother/child units, the recurrence risks across generations are shown in Table 25.3. The recurrence risk for low birthweight is of the same magnitude as the recurrence within sibships.[10] However, for gestational age, the recurrence risk across generations is much weaker compared to the recurrence within sibships. This could indicate that genetic factors affect fetal growth more than the duration of pregnancy and that gestational age might be more affected by environmental factors. Further studies of paternal effects and the association among paternal and maternal half-siblings might help to clarify these relationships.

Table 25.3: Recurrence risks across generations

	Relative risk
Preterm birth (<37 weeks)	1.18
LBW birth (<2500 g)	2.25
SGA birth (sex and parity specific)	2.57

FUTURE PERSPECTIVES OF PERINATAL EPIDEMIOLOGY

The idea that health in adult life may reflect circumstances in childhood, or even earlier in life, dates back many years.[12] The notion that at least some adult diseases may originate in utero has recently captured attention across a wide range of biomedical sciences. Editorial comments have ranged from being enthusiastic, claiming a "paradigm shift"[13] to being more critical and septical.[14]

Barker has introduced a series of hypotheses of relationships between perinatal events and later health.[15] For example, Barker and colleagues have examined the association between blood pressure and measures of size and shape at birth, indicating that the ratio of birthweight to placental weight is an important predictor of subsequent blood pressure, where men who were light at birth, but with a relatively heavy placenta, had the highest blood pressure.[16]

Most of these associations will require more sophisticated studies before the issues can be resolved. In the Nordic countries we have some advantages in approaching some of these challenges, particularly since we have relatively homogeneous populations where the individuals can be traced over time due to our identification number system, which thus facilitates longitudinal studies with follow-up over a long time.[17]

Epidemiology certainly has an extremely important role to play in perinatal medicine, and genetic and molecular epidemiology are likely to introduce new and more effective analytical methods, which will provide the basis for improved prevention of adverse outcomes of perinatal events, regardless of when these outcomes occur.

ACKNOWLEDGMENT

I wish to thank Liv Knurvik for skillful technical assistance in preparing this manuscript.

REFERENCES

1. Peller S. Proper delineation of the neonatal period in perinatal mortality. Am J Public Health. 1965;55:1005-11.
2. Wallgren A. The neonatal mortality in Sweden, from a pediatric point. Acta Paediatr Scand. 1942;29:372-86.
3. Baird D, Thomson AM, Duncan, EH. The causes and prevention of stillbirths and first week deaths. J Obstet Gynaecol Br Emp. 1953;60:17-30.
4. World Health Organization. Epidemiological and Vital Statistics. Report 57. 1957. pp. 506-11.
5. Taylor W. The changing pattern of mortality in England and Wales. I. Infant mortality. Br J Prev Soc Med. 1954;8:1-9.
6. Bjerkedal T, Bakketeig LS. Surveillance of congenital malformations and other conditions of the newborn. Int J Epidemiol. 1975;4:31-6.
7. Schlesselman JI. Case-Control Studies. New York: Oxford University Press; 1982.
8. Bakketeig LS, Jacobsen G, Hoffman HJ, et al. Pre-pregnancy risk factors of small-for-gestational age births among parous women in Scandinavia. Acta Obstet Gynaecol Scand. 1993;72:273-9.
9. Bakketeig LS. Methodological problems and possible endpoints in the evaluation of antenatal care. Int J Technol Assess Health Care. 1992;8(Suppl 1):33-9.
10. Bakketeig LS. The risk of repeated preterm or low-birth-weight delivery. In: Reed DM, Stantey FJ (Eds). The Epidemiology of Prematurity. Baltimore-Munich: Urban and Schwarzenberg; 1977.
11. Magnus P, Bakketeig LS, Skjærven R. Correlations of birth weight and gestational age across generations. Ann Hum Biol. 1993;20:231-8.
12. Kuh D, Davey Smith G. When is mortality risk determined? Historical insights into a current debate. Soc Hist Med. 1993;6:101-23.
13. Robinson RJ. Is the child father of the man? (editorial). Br Med J. 1992;304:789-90.
14. Paneth N, Susser M. Early origin of coronary heart disease ("the Barker hypothesis") (editorial). Br Med. J 1995;310:411-2.
15. Barker DJ. Fetal and infant origins of adult disease. Br Med J. 1992.
16. Barker DJ, Bull AR, Osmond C, et al. Fetal and placental size and risk of hypertension in adult life. Br Med J. 1990;301:259-62.
17. Bakketeig LS. Perinatal epidemiology—A Nordic challenge. Scand J Soc Med. 1991;19:145-7.

26 Structure of Perinatal Care Systems

GA Little

Pregnancy outcomes are clearly dependent upon the availability and effective delivery of reproductive care. Advances in knowledge and technology have resulted in improvement in national perinatal statistics such as survival of low birthweight infants, but the degree of improvement is dependent upon the care environment. Structure, the systematic organization of perinatal care, is a primary determinent of the degree of success in meeting the needs of a population.

Constant improvement of pregnancy outcomes is a logical objective. The optimal state of health involves functioning at full individual potential, without disease or abnormality. The ultimate positive expression of reproductive health would be pregnancies without adverse medical outcomes occurring as intended events within a healthy emotional and social environment. A zero adverse outcome rate may not seem attainable at this time, but there is no reason to believe that there is an irreducible minimum of poor outcome that cannot eventually be overcome.

This chapter discusses organization of perinatal care in the effort to improve outcomes of pregnancy. While each geopolitical entity—population, region or country—must be analyzed and subject to individualized planning and intervention, there are common concepts that apply.

THE PROBLEMS

Throughout the world, disease associated with reproduction represents a dominant portion of medical need and is a major contributor to mortality and long-term morbidity. Even if that portion of reproductive system pathology not necessarily associated with pregnancy, such as infertility and sexually transmitted diseases, is removed, the human and economic cost of pregnancy-related disease remains very high in both developed and less fortunate countries.

The disparity between developed and developing regions is especially dramatic in the area of reproductive health. Thirty-nine of 50 million yearly deaths worldwide (approximately four-fifths) occur in the developing countries where maternal, perinatal and communicable causes are said to be responsible for 40% of deaths as compared to 5% in developed countries. Pregnancy-related conditions are estimated to be responsible for 18% of the burden of disease in women between 15 years and 44 years of age, and in children under 5 years of age about 19% of loss of healthy life is said to be due to perinatal complications.[1] Of five essential groups of clinical interventions for developing countries identified in a world development report—prenatal and delivery care, family planning services, management of the sick child, treatment of tuberculosis and case-management of sexually transmitted diseases—three involve perinatal and reproductive health.[2,3]

Within developed countries there have been remarkable advances in outcomes over recent decades but persistent differences between countries. Furthermore, expenditure of greater resources per capita and availability of proportionately more providers does not necessarily result in better outcomes. The United States despite greater application of resources to neonatal intensive care does not appear to have better birthweight specific mortality than some other countries.[4]

INDICATORS

Perinatal systems of care have traditionally used vital statistics indicators to quantify relative magnitude of outcomes. The following are illustrative of indicators that are based upon events that are relatively easy to define and record such as death, birth weight and gestational age.

Maternal mortality, usually defined as death of a woman during or within 42 days of pregnancy of any cause other than accidental or incidental, remains a problem in the industrialized world where deaths approximate 10–20 per 100,000 live births. This indicator is said to document the widest disparity of human reproductive outcomes yet reported, with some sections of the world, notably Sub-Saharan Africa and South Asia, apparently experiencing an incidence as much as 200 times higher than the safest areas.[5]

Fetal, neonatal or infant mortality serve as valuable indicators by themselves or when included in various rates and ratios. Perinatal mortality, including all newborns, live and stillborn, of 1,000 g and greater and up to 168 hours or 7 days (early neonatal), is used frequently. Neonatal mortality, deaths up to 28 days, is part of infant mortality (deaths in the first year) and the two, independently or when analyzed together, give valuable insights into the health of a population and availability of care. For example, it has become evident that improvement in infant mortality in some countries such as Egypt has exceeded the rate of improvement in neonatal mortality, suggesting that advances in perinatal care for the fetus and neonate may lag behind advances in care for conditions of infancy, as programs such as oral rehydration for diarrheal diseases make an impact.[6]

The low birthweight rate and *birthweight-specific mortality* provide information about the general health of a population and relative success of intervention, especially for the population of prematurely born babies (< 37 weeks of gestation). Within the United States, for example, the low birthweight rate varies by a factor of 3 or 4 times for various subpopulations and has not responded favorably to interventions, while birthweight-specific mortality has improved considerably, probably due to neonatal intensive care and regional programs. The result is a situation where individual low birthweight babies do relatively well and birthweight-specific mortality is perhaps the best in the world, but the number of low birthweight babies per thousand births remains higher than in many other countries.

Figure 26.1 serves to illustrate the breadth of possible perinatal outcome indicators. Identified values can be used to derive indicators. Traditional outcomes based on vital statistics address a small portion of the value and outcome spectrum. The clinical value compass model can be applied to all aspects of a care delivery process including parent perspective of the neonatal intensive care experience.[7] Perinatal care systems in all stages of development will rely on vital statistics based indicators. Those in complex environments that are complex and market-driven with a strong interest in consumer or family-centered care may also employ a variety of indicators.

RISK ASSESSMENT, NEED IDENTIFICATION AND RESOURCE ALLOCATION

Risk assessment is a key concept in perinatal care systems. The process of evaluating the possibility that a patient has or will have a specific problem is an integral part of all medical practice including perinatal medicine. *Needs* are identified and quantified for both individual patients and populations. *Resources* can then be allocated to meet identified or anticipated needs.

Risk assessment has furthered care and improved outcomes through identification of populations and individuals at increased risk for specific conditions. It also can result in false positives and negatives. Furthermore, there is legitimate concern that the concept of risk has meant to some that pregnancy is never normal except retrospectively. These shortcomings must be managed.

A method entitled the *risk approach* has been developed to improve availability and use of existing health care resources and systems especially in resource poor areas. Health problems, including their associated risk factors and populations, are identified, the status of function of the existing health-delivery system is assessed, interventions to deal with risk and performance are put in place, and these are followed by monitoring and evaluation.[8] This process has been applied to construct programmatic approaches to population-based maternal and child health care. Shortcomings have been discussed, including inability in some situations to recognize or evaluate all forms of risk, inadequate preparation or training of personnel, lack of complete understanding of determinants of risk including cultural factors, and inability to achieve balance between preventive and curative services.[9,10]

PATIENT CARE AND THE NEED FOR STRUCTURE

The individual perinatal patient has benefited greatly from advances in care. For example, if access to preventive and acute care is available then timely, all of the five main causes of maternal mortality hemorrhage, unsafe abortions, hypertensive disorders, sepsis and obstructed labor can be managed successfully. Most of the common causes of fetal and neonatal mortality and morbidity, such as peripartum asphyxia, prematurity and infections, respond to assessment of fetal well-being, obstetric intervention, neonatal resuscitation and intensive care. Although there are many diagnostic and therapeutic challenges that remain such as prevention of prematurity, the simple fact is that most of the world's perinatal pathology can be detected and treated successfully with available knowledge and structured care.

Because it is not possible to meet all needs in all places a structured system that allows for efficient use of resources and maximizes outcomes is a logical objective.

HEALTH CARE PYRAMID

The World Health Organization (WHO) has presented an ideal health care pyramid with three levels: family/community, health center and district hospital.[3] With slight modification (Fig. 26.2), this model can serve as a conceptual framework for the structure of perinatal health care in countries and societies at all stages of development. The basic importance of the family/community sector is emphasized; it is here that the need for clinical intervention arises and moves to health center and hospital when necessary (See referral arrow in Fig. 26.2). The arrow on the right pointing down suggests a family/community objective for supervision in the WHO model; the guidance and management terms were added to this illustration to suggest proactive clinical and educational interventions that originate in health care institutions.

A problem associated with improving pregnancy outcomes is the need for both comprehensive preventive and acute care for an entire population. One without the other will not be successful. As the health care pyramid suggests, an effective and efficient framework or structure of component activities is necessary.

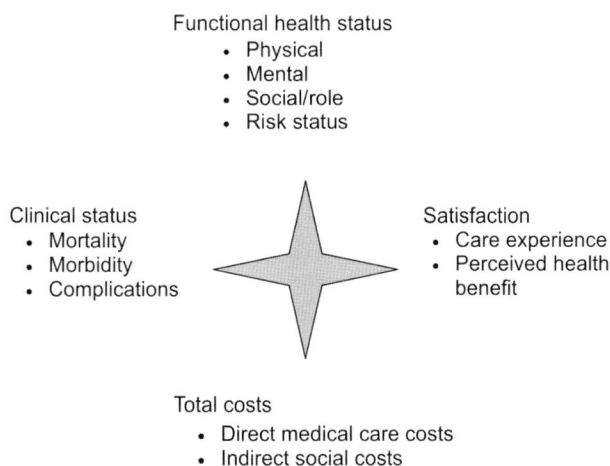

Fig. 26.1: The clinical value compass model has been used to derive the four parental neonatal intensive care outcome groupings. A wide range of outcome indicators can be developed for each of these groupings[7]

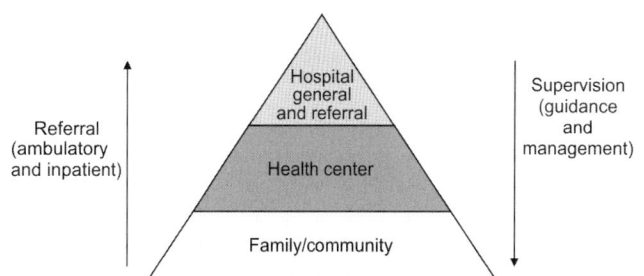

Fig. 26.2: The World Health Organization health care pyramid. Modified from World Health Organization[3]

PERINATAL SYSTEMS

Systems consist of components functioning together for common goals and objectives. Understanding of the complexity and breadth of activities associated with perinatal care is essential if systems are to be effective.

Perinatal System Activities

Table 26.1 provides an overview of the basic activities associated with systematic efforts to improve pregnancy outcomes of a population. Patient care is essential and must be facilitated by administration and management. If standards of care and outcomes are to be maintained and improved, ongoing data collection, evaluation and research must take place to provide the substrate for quality improvement. Training and education of personnel must be available either from within the system itself or available from a co-operating resource.

System Development

Much of the effort of system development in technically-advanced nations has focused on hospital inpatient services. The hospital is usually the community institution where knowledge and technology are concentrated, with individual members of the community coming to that location. In developing and less fortunate environments, a single regional institution such as a district hospital receives designated governmental support, while in more affluent areas there may be multiple hospital alternatives that, in fact, may compete.

Perinatal systems and their patients originate from communities and families. The focus on hospitals as an identified community resource and site of a many if not most births leads to a challenge for systems to adequately address needs in the ambulatory and education sectors. Preconception and prenatal care tends to be less well addressed in many systems as inpatient services.

In the ideal situation, need assessment followed by resource allocation to guide initial development of a basic perinatal system for a defined population is a relatively uncomplicated exercise. As previously discussed, vital statistics and perinatal indicators can help to quantify the magnitude of the need and support solutions that direct resources toward systems and comprehensive program activities. The reality of perinatal systems development is complex, with each situation involving different medical, economic, social and political determinants.

Perinatal Regionalization in the United States: Evolution of a Systems Approach

During the 1960s and early 1970s, significant advances in perinatal care, especially in hospital-based services, were occurring in the United States, Canada and many countries in Europe and elsewhere. Neonatal intensive care in particular was emerging, as was the concept of interhospital transfer, including care instituted prior to and during movement to established centers. Perinatal providers and their organizations, including the American Academy of Pediatrics (AAP) and the American College of Obstetricians and Gynecologists (ACOG), became convinced that a systems or programmatic approach to perinatal care could improve outcomes. With the assistance of a private foundation, The National Foundation-March of Dimes, the AAP and ACOG, joined by the American Medical Association and American Academy of Family Physicians, formed an ad hoc Committee on Perinatal Health.

Toward improving the outcome of pregnancy: Recommendations for the regional development of maternal and perinatal health services was formally released in 1976.[11] The first sentence states that to make optimal care available for each person, "a systems approach is essential".

The publication, now known as TIOP I, while directed broadly at maternal and perinatal services, focused heavily on the third trimester and neonatal period and on the hospital or inpatient

Table 26.1: Perinatal system activities

Patient Care	Date Acquisition, Evaluation and Research	Administration	Education

Primary (basic)
  pregnancy planning
  preconception
  prenatal
  peripartum
  postpartum
  maternal
  infant
	Vital statistics
	Pregnancy outcomes
	  maternal
	  neonatal/infant
	Technology assessment
	Professional/provider
	Medical and social
	  science
		Clinical services
		System development and
		  maintenance
		Institutions
		  clinics
		  hospitals
		Quality assessment and
		  improvement
			Public
			Patient
			  prevention
			  preparation
			  training and
			  continuing
			System (outreach)

Specialty (consultative, referral)
  genetics
  high-risk obstetrics
  (maternal-fetal)
Neonatal (medical and surgical)
  psychological and social
  ancillary services
  radiology/imaging
  anesthesia
  laboratory
Transportation
  (interhospital care)
  maternal-fetal
  neonatal
		Fiscal	

sectors primarily. Central to the recommendations and subsequent influence of TIOP I was a three-level categorization of perinatal services. The level framework was promoted to introduce co-operative interaction and organization into a system having as its only objective the improvement of pregnancy outcome (Fig. 26.3).[11,12]

By the mid-1980s, perinatal regionalization, including the level concept of organization, had been implemented throughout the United States with most authorities agreeing that it had been responsible for improvement in outcomes.[13] The degree of governmental involvement in the form of leadership and regulation varied widely across the 50 states. The three-level categorization was broadly accepted, although some argued for a four-level system with a few perinatal centers, usually academic, to provide the most technologically demanding care as another level. Others argued for a two-level system involving primary, routine or specialty care and a referral level for subspecialty care. Some felt that the level system inappropriately centralized care, although the TIOP documents clearly state that that is not intended. Recently the AAP released, after considerable collection of practice data and debate, a new categorization of levels of newborn care that maintained a basic three-level framework with subcategorization based upon functional capabilities.[14] The rationale utilized, while applied to neonatal care, is seemingly also applicable to obstetric units. As perinatal services in hospitals and within systems are interrelated, assigning level of perinatal service is an important aspect of structure.

By the late 1980s, a great deal of concern was being expressed by US professionals and health planners that so-called "deregionalization" was occurring and that outcomes might be worsening or at best the rate of improvement was inadequate. Some argued that the levels categorization had outlived its usefulness. It is important to place this concern into a context of a nationwide deliberation about the entire system of care and health care reform. A movement to review and revise TIOP I emerged.

TIOP II, *Toward Improving the Outcome of Pregnancy, The 90s and Beyond* was released in 1993 by a reconstituted and expanded Committee on Perinatal Health.[15] Included is a review of past development of US prenatal services, consideration of indicators of outcome, and recommendations for improvement that are broad and strongly state that successful interventions such as intensive obstetrical and neonatal hospital-based interventions must be maintained, while a newly energized focus on ambulatory care, especially in the preconception, prenatal and postpartum intervals should be instituted. The level categorization is supported but with a recommendation that review and revision on a local or state basis should be undertaken as part of an emphasis on the need for regional systems to be community focused. Also stressed are health awareness and promotion, universal access to care, and a recognition that social and fiscal, as well as medical factors must be addressed. TIOP II is also not a laissez-faire document; it recommends that community resources as well as professionals should play a role in a system that includes a forum, usually government led, for addressing accountability, access and progress.[16]

Thus, in the United States, the need for structure in delivery of perinatal care that includes risk identification, patient referral and possible transport to a site of available service, and categorization of levels of care has been debated and largely accepted. Agreement on specifics of system implementation and management is not as universal. In some states, structure has evolved informally, while in others, considerable structure has been mandated. The care-related activities presented in Table 26.1 are largely in place, while some, such as continuous quality improvement involving an entire geopolitical unit such as a state, are not. The current movement toward managed care and competition on one hand supports the development of systems of care that are internally structured and largely self-contained, while on the other hand urging freedom to compete and limited external structure and review. In many areas, there are regionalized perinatal networks that function in parallel, with limited interaction including assessment.

In this millennium the US perinatal system continues to evolve while there is ongoing questioning of resource allocation. The dominance of hospital based services including obstetric high-risk and neonatal intensive care is being debated from the perspective of whether it improves outcomes.[17] Availability of neonatal intensive

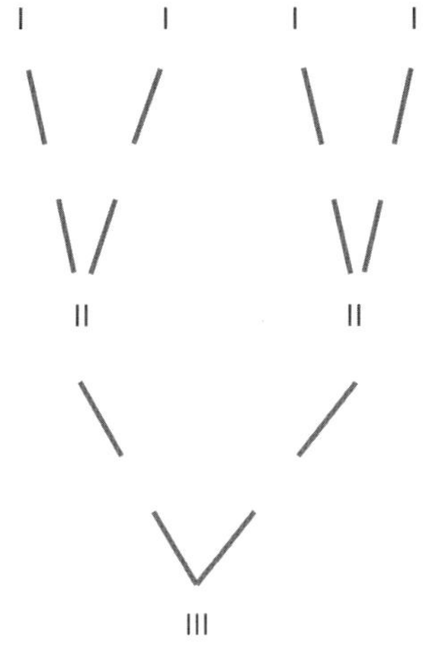

Activity	Location
Usual level of patient entry Risk assessment Uncomplicated care Stabilization of unexpected problems Data collection Sponsor of local education	Community or district clinics and hospitals
Level I activities plus: diagnosis and treatment of selected high-risk pregnancies and neonatal problems education for part of network	Large community hospitals with many support services
Level I and II activities plus: diagnosis and treatment of most perinatal problems regional transport research and outcome surveillance regional education regional administration	Large medical centers with comprehensive, often academic programs

Fig. 26.3: Level of hospital perinatal services originally recommended in the United States in 1976[12]

care capacity is thought to be responsible for a significant portion of improvement in outcomes such as low birthweight survival with obstetric care contributing a smaller but definite portion.[18] There is research that supports a concern that neonatal intensive care capacity may be excessive and not able to contribute further to improved pregnancy outcomes.[19]

A cross-national study of reproductive care involving the US, Australia, Canada and the United Kingdom determined that the US has more neonatal intensive care capacity with 6.1 neonatologists per 10,000 live births compared with 3.7, 3.3 and 2.7 for the others respectively. Neonatal bed capacity was also greater in the US. Birthweight specific mortality outcomes were not the best in the US where proportionately less resources are allocated to such efforts as preconception, prenatal, and other maternal and child health services.[4] This study questions the effectiveness of current distribution of reproductive care resources, as did TIOP II,[15] and should serve as resource for other perinatal systems in development and evolution.

PRESENT AND FUTURE CHALLENGES

Access to Clinical Care

Implementation and improvement of perinatal systems remains challenging across the spectrum of economic development and political structure. In the less developed situations, certain key system components, such as the first referral level for emergency obstetric care and the ability to perform operative interventions like cesarean sections, are yet to be made universally available. In others access may be less than optimal due to organizational or economic factors. System structure may have to be modified or individualized to meet prioritized acute care needs. In situations where care is readily available and perhaps even oversubscribed, such as neonatal care, there are challenges related to relative priority of technologies and services. Dissemination of evidence-based innovations has been pointed to as a challenge in all industries including health care.[20]

Data Acquisition and Analysis

The ability now is available to perinatal system management to use existing computer technology to provide data about events and outcomes in a practical and real-time fashion. Individual providers, centers or hospitals and systems can record data economically, and through analysis derive information to effect improvement and change. Efforts such as the Oxford Database for Perinatal Trials,

the emergence of measures of acuity[21,22] and the growing worldwide presence of collaborative networks such as the Vermont-Oxford Neonatal Network[23] with its international cumulative database of 400–1,500-g-birthweight babies from over 400 units provide opportunity for evidence based collaborative research.[24] These tools need to be supported, developed further and used by perinatal systems.

Quality Improvement

The concept of continuous quality improvement employed with success in business and in health care is not foreign to perinatal care. In fact, an emphasis on measurement and improvement of outcomes has always been a fundamental part of perinatal care, as evidenced by the Apgar Score and neonatal follow-up efforts. Perinatal systems can benefit from advances in quality management being championed in other sectors, including competitive business. Data acquisition and analysis is essential in this effort and the productive linkage of data with quality improvement is a systems function.[25]

Expectations and Accountability

Perinatal systems, their institutions and personnel are formally and informally considered to be accountable for their actions and outcomes. Accountability is well-defined in some areas such as procedures on patients in hospitals and less evident in other concerns such as who is responsible for patients who receive inadequate prenatal care. Problems such as maternal mortality in developing countries and infant mortality in subpopulations of some advanced countries may become part of a political process that asks for identification of responsible party and improvement. In such situations the media may become involved by publicizing issues and asking for accountability and change.

Families and communities in this era of patient or consumer involvement in health care have expectations . They can profoundly influence care. For example, perinatal parents have successfully advocated for change leading to presence of fathers at operative delivery and increased involvement in decision-making in the neonatal intensive care unit.[26]

A basic principle of public health is to involve the entire population in analysis and efforts for improvement. Many perinatal systems across the economic and political spectrum of countries study portions of the total population. Accountability or responsibility for less than the total cohort is inadequate. If more than one perinatal network, program or system exists within a population, then responsibility must rest somewhere, often with the government, for total cohort accountability.

REFERENCES

1. Murray CJ, Lopez AD. Global Comparative Assessments in the Health Sector: Disease Burden, Health Expenditures and Intervention Packages. World Health Organization, Geneva; 1994.
2. The World Bank. World Development Report 1993: Investing in Health. New York: Oxford University Press; 1993.
3. World Health Organization. Care of Mother and Baby at the Health Centre: A Practical Guide. Report of a Technical Working Group, WH0/FHE/MSM/94.2. World Health Organization, Geneva; 1994.
4. Thompson LA, Goodman DC, Little GA. Is more neonatal intensive care always better? Insights from a cross-national comparison of reproductive care. Pediatrics. 2002;109(6):1036-43.
5. Tinker A, Koblinsky MA. Making Motherhood Safe. The World Bank, Washington; 1992.
6. Little GA, El Kassas M, Eissa AN. The Egyptian National Neonatal Care Program: A practical strategy to improve neonatal outcomes. Int Child Health. 1996;VII:31-8.

7. Conner JM, Nelson EC. Neonatal intensive care: satisfaction measured from a parent's perspective. Pediatrics 1999;103 (Suppl 1): 336-49.

8. World Health Organization. The Risk Approach in Maternal and Child Health. (WHO Offset Publication No. 39). World Health Organization, Geneva; 1978.

9. McCarthy BJ, Kowal D. The risk approach in maternal and child health. In Wallace HM, Giri K, Serrano CV (Eds). Health Care of Women and Children in Developing Countries, 2nd edition. Oakland: Third World Publishing; 1995.

10. Backett EM, Davies AM, Petros-Barvazian A. The Risk Approach in Health Care, Public Health Papers, No 76. World Health Organization, Geneva; 1983.

11. Committee on Perinatal Health. Toward Improving the Outcome of Pregnancy (TIOP #1): Recommendations for the Regional Development of Maternal and Perinatal Health Services. White Plains, NY: National Foundation-March of Dimes; 1976.

12. Frigoletto FD, Little GA, (Eds). Guidelines for Perinatal Care, 2nd edition. Elk Grove, Washington: American Academy of Pediatrics, American College of Obstetricians and Gynecologists; 1988.

13. Phibbs CS, Bronstein JM, Boxton E, et al. The effects of patient volume and level of care at the hospital of birth on neonatal mortality. J Am Med Assoc. 1996;276:1054-9.

14. American Academy of Pediatrics, Committee on Fetus and Newborn, Policy Statement, Levels of Neonatal Care, Pediatrics. 2004;114(5):1341-7.

15. Committee on Perinatal Health. Toward Improving the Outcome of Pregnancy, The 90's and Beyond (TIOP #2). White Plains, NY: National Foundation-March of Dimes; 1993.

16. Little GA, Merenstein GB. Toward improving the outcome of pregnancy, 1993: Perinatal regionalization revisited (commentary). Pediatrics. 1993;92(4):611-2.

17. Grumbach K. Specialists, technology, and newborns – Too much of a good thing. New Eng J of Med. 2002;346:1574-5.

18. Richardson DK, Gray JE, Gortmaker SL, et al. Declining Severity Adjusted Mortality: Evidence of Improving Neonatal Intensive Care. Pediatrics. 1998;102(4):893-9.

19. Goodman DC, Fisher ES, Little GA, et al. The Relation Between the Availability of Neonatal Intensive Care and Neonatal Mortality, New Eng J of Med. 2002;346:1538-42.

20. Berwick DM, Disseminating Innovations in Health Care, JAMA. 2003;15:1069-975.

21. International Neonatal Network. The CRIB (clinical risk index for babies) score: A tool for assessing initial neonatal risk and comparing information of neonatal intensive care units. Lancet 1993;342:193-8.

22. Richardson DK, Gray JE, McCormick MC, et al. Score for neonatal acute physiology: A physiology severity index for neonatal intensive care. Pediatrics 1993;91(3):617-23.

23. Horbar JD. The Vermont Oxford Neonatal Network: Integrating research and clinical practice to improve the quality of medical care. Semin Perinatol 1995;19:124-31.

24. Lucey JF, Rowan CA, Shiono P, et al. Fetal Infants: The Fate of 4172 Infants with Birth Weights of 401-500 Grams – The Vermont-Oxford Network Experience (1996-2000) Pediatrics 2004;113(6):1559-66.

25. Horbar JD, Rogowski JD, Plsek P, et al. Collaborative Quality Improvement in Neonatal Intensive Care. Pediatrics 2001;107(1): 14-22.

26. Harrison H. The Principles for family-centered neonatal care. Pediatrics 1993; 92(5):643-50.

27 Perinatal Quality Indicators and Perinatal Audit

G Lindmark, J Langhoff-Roos

INTRODUCTION

Health care services should be evaluated not only in quantitative terms, which is still often the case, but also with respect to the quality. The qualitative dimensions of health care are fundamental for its impact on health. Clients, not least in maternal health care, increasingly demand to be considered as individuals and not only as objectives of the health care activities. Resources are restricted even in the most affluent parts of the world and do not allow unlimited use of health care interventions. Critical scrutiny and assessment of the quality of health care is therefore mandatory.[1]

In maternal and perinatal health care, survival of mother and baby without short- or long-term morbidity are the first and fundamental needs. However, in childbearing there are other needs related to social, cultural and existential dimensions, which also have to be considered in the care of mothers and infants. One obvious reason to acknowledge these dimensions is their importance for acceptance of and compliance with care.

To maintain and improve quality in health care, it is necessary to clearly define goals and objectives related to patient's needs and assess available resources.[2] For such a process to be possible, good communication and collaboration must be present. It is also essential that health workers at all levels feel themselves as subjects and part of the process, and not as objects of scrutiny or criticism.

To define quality as the extent to which the care is meeting the expectations and needs of the patient is attractive, and implies that also other outcomes than the strict medical ones must be considered. However, the expectations on the health care do not come only from the patient but also from society and from the agencies that cover the cost of the care. Therefore, not only individual but also public health outcomes must be considered, and the effective use of available resources will therefore be a quality aspect of great interest. When comparisons of quality of perinatal care are performed, it is common to relate only to indicators of outcome or process, and not mention indicators of structural input. Also, single process or outcome indicators—like rates of cesarean section and perinatal mortality—have been used to measure quality without considering the relation with other important aspects of care.

It will be increasingly important to define quality also as cost-effectiveness, in any case, if the ambition is to offer universal high-quality care to all mothers and newborns.

INDICATORS OF QUALITY

A weighted sum of all essential indicators, including fetal and maternal, short-term and long-term outcomes, as well as maternal satisfaction and the impact on future pregnancies and deliveries, would be the ideal measure of quality. This will imply that an unrealistic high amount of resources are spent to collect quantitative as well as qualitative data, at least in the same population. The most important source for quality improvement activities is the routinely collected indicators at the local and regional level. However, we still need to supplement with results from other and larger regions. Published descriptive-analytical clinical research will also in the future constitute one of the backbones of regional quality assessment activities.

Decisions on the best indicators must consider not only the relevance for assessment of the objectives of the care, but also their feasibility. For an indicator to be useful, it must be constructed from data that is possible to collect within the available resources, and both these variables and the indicator itself must be clearly defined. The usefulness of quality indicators for comparisons over time or between regions is depending on agreement on these definitions and continuous data collection by all the participating health facilities.

Quality assessment of the *structure* of care includes organization, resources, qualifications of staff, and availability of structured and adequate programs of care. The *process* or utilization of resources in the provision of health care can be assessed so that each activity for screening, prevention, diagnosis or therapy is correctly applied, and used for the intended or appropriate purpose. Assessment of process quality should ascertain that the care is carried out according to evidence-based guidelines or recommendations.

In perinatal care the *result* of the health care process in terms of mortality and morbidity traditionally has been discussed most often. Nowadays, patient satisfaction and provision of relevant and reliable information are products of care generally appreciated as important not just in cases with perinatal complications but also in the majority of cases in which everything is normal from a strictly medical perspective.

These quality indicators are useful for constructive discussions about the content and quality of perinatal health care. The variations in outcome are not related to physical resources in a simplified way, but must be discussed in the wider context of attitudes, practices and training of health staff at all levels. Assessment of results of care should not be limited to intermediate variables such as results of tests or examinations, but focus on essential patient-related indicators. In perinatal care, it is common that a screening procedure or an intervention during pregnancy is validated by parameters that are indirectly related to actual health outcome of mother or infant or even to the result of another test or examination. Variables that are indirectly related to health outcome, such as low birthweight and preterm birth and to some extent low Apgar score, may be useful, however, if there is a direct relationship with short- and long-term morbidity.

DATA COLLECTION

Since quality assessment includes both the general level of care in all cases as well as serious adverse events, variables and indicators must include both information about all mothers and newborns, and special information in selected cases of special interest. The data collection system must therefore include both routine registration of basic information and more detailed information on complicated events—usually to be retrieved from the medical record.

Existing routinely collected data, for example from medical birth registers, should be used whenever possible in order to limit resources needed.[3] Studies show that the quality of routine data in maternity services can be adequate for quality control.[4]

In some countries, routine data may be retrieved from clinical information systems in hospitals or primary care, or civil registers of births and deaths. In the Scandinavian countries, national medical birth registers provide important information. In some countries, routine surveys of reproductive health outcomes are performed at regular intervals and data from routine child health care may be used for quality assessment purposes. However, register data and standard data collected without a specific purpose or unrelated to specific quality improvement activities may be of questionable validity. Registers may also be unreliable regarding causes of death, diagnoses of complications or autopsy data. Terms such as hypoxia, placental dysfunction or preeclampsia are frequently used without clear and uniform definitions of the variables.

For comparisons—not only of trends over time in one specific region, but also, between regions or using the data compiled for international comparisons—it is essential that all variables are defined according to international standards.

Definitions of basic concepts such as perinatal mortality, gestational age, and diagnoses describing maternal and infant condition must be uniform. It is particularly important that all extremely preterm deliveries and infants with the lowest birthweight are included, because of their high risk of mortality and morbidity.

The patient record is an important quality instrument if it is standardized, and contains specified and well defined data. It is nowadays often in a computer format and can be used directly to produce data for special purposes. However, there must be specified definitions for registration to make a variable useful for quality assessment. All data that are the result of a subjective interpretation are also less reliable than absolute values of test results.

Specific surveys and interviews, as well as observations of the process of care, are valuable instruments for assessment of quality, but cannot usually be routinely used since they are more resource demanding and also require training and skills of the data collectors. Thus, these methods will be limited to specific, short-period projects.

Validity of Data

The most common problem in the initial discussions about choice of indicators is that people underestimate the difficulties to perform continuous data collection in routine care over long periods of time.

The validity of the data registration must therefore be given attention before the data registration begins as well as regularly over time. Also it is important that definitions and indications are not changed too often. A change should not be considered unless a significant improvement is foreseen to follow, considering both the

initial rather poor validity of data during the first phase and the loss of longitudinal aspects of data collection.

In order to secure valid registration of indicators, it is important that health personnel is provided with regular and immediate feedback based on registered data and that regular proper validation based on internal registry analyses and external studies based on case notes are performed.

Validation of reported indicators depend on whether the data are aggregated, anonymous case-based or case-based linked to a personal ID. At an aggregated level validation may be achieved by logic checks for outliers, at a case-based anonymous level by logic checks for relations between indicators (such as compatibility cesarean section versus sphincter rupture), whereas at a case-based level where case notes are traceable a proper external validation may be carried out.

Sets of Indicators for Quality Assessment

Many quality assurance projects have used process indicators in the health care, often recorded as proportions of cases subject to various interventions. Several national and international agencies and scientific societies have developed lists of essential quality indicators for maternal and perinatal care.[5] An example of a set of clinical quality indicators for monitoring results have been developed by the American College of Obstetricians and Gynecologists[2] (Table 27.1). Other sets reflect a more public health oriented perspective. Usually they are a mix of input from clinicians (obstetricians or midwives) and public health professionals. Clinicians usually focus more on indicators of specific areas to be improved by clinical interventions (process-outcome indicators), indicators such as cesarean section, sphincter rupture, and asphyxia at delivery. Public health professionals focus more on areas that are public health issues (structure-outcome indicators) such as maternal age, marital status, congenital malformations, length of hospital stay for childbirth, etc.

By comparison, these sets of indicators are quite heterogeneous and show a considerable amount of diversity, reflecting differences in interest, but also characterized by a number of common indicators that were found to be essential such as maternal, perinatal and infant death.

A recent European collaborative effort, PERISTAT—a part of the European Commission's Health Monitoring Program—has developed indicators of perinatal health for health professionals, policy makers, researchers and health service users who wish to monitor and evaluate perinatal health. The aim of this project, which included 13 countries, was to facilitate monitoring and comparison by harmonizing indicator definitions and encouraging the collection of comparable data based on the following priorities:

- Assess maternal and infant mortality and morbidity associated with events in the perinatal period

- Describe the evolution of risk factors for perinatal health outcomes in the population of childbearing women including demographic, socioeconomic and behavioral characteristics

- Monitor the use and consequences of medical technology in the care of women and infants during pregnancy, delivery and the postpartum period.

In 2003, a list of recommended indicators (Table 27.2) was published on the internet together with the figures for year 2000 from most of the participating countries.[6]

Table 27.1: Obstetric clinical indicators developed by the American College of Obstetricians and Gynecologists

Maternal indicators

- Maternal mortality
- Unplanned readmission within 14 days
- Cardiopulmonary arrest
- In-hospital initiation of antibiotics 24 hours or more after term vaginal delivery
- Unplanned removal, injury or repair of organ during operative procedure
- In-hospital maternal red blood cell transfusion or hematocrit < 22 vol% or hemoglobin of <7.0 g or decrease in hematocrit of 11 vol% or hemoglobin of 3.5 g or more
- Maternal length-of-stay more than 5 days after vaginal delivery or more than 7 days after cesarean delivery
- Eclampsia
- Delivery unattended by the "responsible" physician*
- Postpartum return to delivery room or operating room for management
- Induction of labor for an indication other than diabetes, premature rupture of membranes, pregnancy-induced hypertension, postterm gestation, intrauterine growth retardation, cardiac disease isoimmunization, fetal demise or chorioamnionitis
- Cesarean delivery required
- Primary cesarean delivery for fetal distress
- Primary cesarean delivery for failure to progress
- Delivery of an infant with a birthweight <2,500 g or respiratory distress syndrome following induction of labor.

Neonatal indicators

- Perinatal mortality of a fetus or infant surviving less than 28 days and weighing 500 g or more at delivery
- Intrapartum death, in hospital, of a fetus or infant weighing 500 g or more
- Neonatal mortality of an inborn infant with a birthweight of 750–999 g in an institution with a neonatal intensive care unit**
- Delivery of an infant weighing <1,800 g in an institution without a neonatal intensive care unit
- Transfer of a neonate to a neonatal intensive care unit in another institution
- Term infant admitted to a neonatal intensive care unit
- Apgar score of 4 or less at 5 minutes
- Birth trauma (#767 in ICD-9 directory) such as shoulder dystocia, cephalohematoma, Erb palsy and clavicular fracture but not caput
- Diagnosis of fetal "massive aspiration syndrome (#770.1 in ICD-9-CM")
- Inborn term infant with clinically apparent seizures recorded before discharge

* To be defined by each institution
** An inborn infant is one born in this hospital rather than transferred from another institution.

ANALYSIS OF INDICATORS

Differences in quality indicators are usually interpreted as mainly related to the care itself, but it is also important to consider differences in the population. Even when comparing area-based populations, differences in maternal characteristics such as parity, multiple pregnancy, preterm birth rate, etc. influence the rates of interventions and outcome. Differences in social and economic conditions may be important for outcomes, but are difficult to assess in reliable way.

Analyses also depend on the level at which data are reported. Aggregated data merely provide a basis for frequencies and predefined tables, whereas case-based data allow ad hoc analyses involving all variables or indicators recorded. When cases have an ID-number with a link to the newborns personal ID, longitudinal follow-up of maternal and infant morbidity and mortality, and even intergenerational studies are possible.

When data are reported at a case-based level, regional differences may be adjusted by multivariate analyses. This is often used in epidemiological analyses for a scientific purpose. Multivariate analyses have the advantages that adjustment may be made in a model that considers several variables/risk factors and ends up in a single Odds ratio with confidence intervals. The disadvantages are that the analysis only considers very simple mathematical relations, that the procedure is not easy to explain, and that the analysis often is perceived as something happening in a black box.

STANDARD POPULATIONS OR RISK STRATIFICATION

Another way to adjust for differences in maternal characteristics is to apply "standard populations". One of the first standard populations used in perinatal quality assessment is the "standard primipara".[7] The standard primipara is a 20–35 year old parturient without pregnancy complications, admitted in spontaneous labor at term with vertex presentation. This "standard primipara" is only one of several possible standard populations that adjust for clinically relevant preconditions, and, not least, reflect a risk of interventions and complications that occur in a specific group of mothers. Thus, the results from these analyses are relevant for that specific group of women when informed to choose mode of delivery.

It is possible to construct a structure of mutually exclusive standard populations that constitute the whole population.[8] In this way, the variables primi/ multiparity, preterm/term, vertex/breech-transverse, singleton/multiple pregnancy and elective delivery

Table 27.2: PERISTAT[6] working list of indicators

Category	Core	Recommended	Future development
Neonatal health	Fetal mortality rate Neonatal mortality rate Infant mortality rate Distribution of birthweight Distribution of gestational age	Prevalence of congenital anomalies Distribution of APGAR score at 5 minutes	Causes of perinatal death Prevalence of cerebral palsy Prevalence of hypoxic-ischemic encephalopathy
Maternal health	Maternal mortality ratio	Maternal mortality by cause of death Severe maternal morbidity Prevalence of trauma to the perineum	Prevalence of fecal incontinence
Population characteristics or risk factors	Multiple birth rate by number of fetuses Distribution of maternal age Distribution of parity	Percent of women who smoke during pregnancy Distribution of mothers' education	Distribution of mothers' country of origin
Heath care services	Distribution of births by mode of delivery	Percent of all pregnancies following fertility treatment Distribution of timing of first prenatal visit Distribution of births by mode of onset of labor Distribution of place of birth Percent of infants breastfeeding at birth Percent of very preterm births delivered in units without a NICU	Indicator of support to women Indicator of maternal satisfaction

(induction of labor/cesarean section) have been used to define standard populations.

National birth statistics stratified by place of birth and standard population may be useful for clients choosing place of birth and midwives and obstetricians as a basis for discussions on quality improvement issues.[9]

To compare regional differences of cesarean section rates in a population with an average rate of 23%, a specific low risk standard population was defined and used for comparison.[10] The low-risk standard population, which constituted 49% of the population, consisted of women of all parities without previous cesarean section, spontaneous labor at term, vertex presentation and without specific pregnancy complications or fetal malformations. The average rate in this standard population was 5.8%. Places of birth were categorized by a higher, lower or average rate of cesarean section in the low risk group. With this method it could be demonstrated that neonatal morbidity was increased in centers where the cesarean section rates were either higher or lower than average.

AUDIT OF PERINATAL DEATHS

Perinatal audit can be performed at different levels: local, regional and national. The levels are of importance when discussing the methodology and outcome of an audit.

Audit at *local level* is often performed on materials that cannot be compared in a quantitative way because of the small sample sizes. However, they are very useful for improvement in structure and process. Depending on whether the audit is performed by a selected group (leaders) or by all involved in the care (all midwives, all obstetricians, a keen pathologist, all neonatologists), the audit process will be perceived as a superior control or as constructive discussion how to improve within the team. It is very important that audit meetings of the latter type are supervised in a permissive way to underline the fact that by discussing our mishaps openly we share with each other experience that probably will reduce the risk of repetition. This can also reduce the guilt that may carry subsequent to a more or less preventable adverse outcome.

For practical reasons, audit at a *regional level* will not take place very close to the obstetrical or neonatal department where the event took place. Regional audits, however, can work as a forum for discussion of guidelines and attitudes. Also, since the distance from the auditors to the local department where implementation should take place is not very far, often at least one participant in the activity will represent the local department or hospital. Quantitative analyses of common events will sometimes be possible at a regional level, and comparisons between regions are often valuable for initiating quality improvement activities. The results of qualitative activities, such as auditing in different regions, however, may be difficult to compare unless audit procedures are identical and the auditors are well matched. In addition, historical comparisons in the same region imply that criteria are explicit and identical, and that auditors do not change their sense of judgment over time.

At a *national level*, epidemiological analyses of clinical indicators and well-defined categories can be used for surveillance and provision of subgroups for audit, in order to identify health care structures or processes that should be changed to improve perinatal health care on a national level.

The premise for a valuable international audit is that indicators and categories are similarly defined. The major advantage of the higher level is the larger sample sizes that in many cases reach a magnitude suitable for statistical analyses with confidence intervals that allow differences to be detected and addressed.

Classification of Perinatal Deaths

One of the main objects of perinatal care is to avoid serious adverse outcomes. Most perinatal audit activities have focused on perinatal deaths, which is the most important fetal adverse outcome to be avoided. However, perinatal deaths are heterogeneous, and chains of events and causes of death differ widely. Clearly, some deaths are potentially more avoidable than others. A perinatal death classification, which stratifies the perinatal deaths in appropriate groups aiming for quality improvement, including qualitative analyses by audit, and comparison between regions may be helpful as a basic tool. It should rely on simple, routinely recorded variables for allocation into mutually exclusive groups, which should be associated with specific areas for health care interventions.

In an investigation that analyzed the differences in perinatal mortality rate between Denmark and Sweden, a new perinatal death classification was proposed in order to categorize the perinatal deaths in relevant groups for further qualitative audit. This classification was discussed and evaluated at a Nordic Baltic collaborative workshop with obstetricians, pediatricians and perinatal epidemiologists. The final classification system was named the Nordic-Baltic Perinatal Death Classification[11] (Table 27.3). Perinatal deaths with fetal malformations were placed in a separate category, and subsequently the rest were categorized by time of death (before, during or after delivery), gestational age, Apgar score, plurality and birthweight (considering intrauterine growth restriction, IUGR) in mutually exclusive groups.

This classification can be applied both to medical records data and, because of the simple structure, to register data.

Table 27.3: The Nordic-Baltic perinatal death classification[11]

Thirteen mutually exclusive groups
I Fetal malformation
II Antenatal death. Single growth restricted fetus ≥28 weeks of gestation
III Antenatal death. Single fetus ≥28 weeks of gestation
IV Antenatal death. Before 28 weeks of gestation
V Antenatal death. Multiple pregnancy
VI Intrapartum death. After admission. ≥28 weeks of gestation
VII Intrapartum death. After admission. Before 28 weeks of gestation
VIII Neonatal death. 28–33 weeks of gestation. Apgar score >6 after 5 minutes
IX Neonatal death. 28–33 weeks of gestation. Apgar score <7 after 5 minutes
X Neonatal death. >33 weeks of gestation. Apgar score >6 after 5 minutes
XI Neonatal death. >33 weeks of gestation. Apgar score <7 after 5 minutes
XII Neonatal death. Before 28 weeks of gestation
XIII Unclassified

Qualitative Audit

It is possible to continue the analysis of cases in subgroups in a qualitative way. Applying the Nordic-Baltic perinatal death classification, a panel from Denmark and Sweden found that there were significantly more intrapartum deaths of nonmalformed infants in Denmark than in Sweden. By subsequent qualitative audit on case notes blinded by nationality, a panel of Nordic obstetricians concluded that there was more insufficient care and a higher rate of potentially avoidable deaths among the Danish cases. It was proposed that a cardiotocographic (CTG) recording should be done on admission, and that more swift intervention during delivery should be implemented in Denmark.[12]

Register-based Subanalysis

When comparing Lithuania with the Nordic countries, the higher perinatal mortality in Lithuania was mainly explained by a doubled rate of malformed infants, a threefold increase in intrapartum, and two-to-fivefold increase in neonatal deaths of nonmalformed infants.[13] Since qualitative audit by case notes was not feasible, a register based subanalysis of the type of malformation was performed. The higher rate of malformed perinatal deaths was explained by a four times higher mortality from neural tube defects.

Perinatal Deaths in Europe

In the Euronatal Study, a research project contracted by the European Union for the period from 1996 to 2000, factors related to differences in populations and health care were studied to explain the differences in perinatal death rates. To determine whether suboptimal factors were present in the cases of perinatal deaths, a regional case-based audit was performed in 10 European regions,[14] using the Nordic-Baltic perinatal death classification. The groups in which care and treatment were most likely to have a significant impact on the outcome were audited: singleton fetal deaths and intrapartum deaths of 28 weeks of gestation or more, and neonatal deaths in children born after 34 weeks of gestation or more.

Suboptimal factors were mostly identified in the antenatal care period, often related to professional care delivery, with failure to detect severe intrauterine growth retardation as the most prominent factor. Maternal smoking was also a significant suboptimal factor among potentially avoidable deaths.

Perinatal Quality Assessment and Audit in Low-income Countries

In low-income countries, regions are not always clearly defined and referral systems are often not working even if there is a structure proposed. The most common situation is that the regional center with its better resources is overloaded with fairly normal deliveries whereas the complicated cases may not even reach the first level of care. The denominator for any area-based assessment of outcome is therefore very uncertain and also the process-related indicators will reflect only what happens to a minor part of the obstetric population. Still, there is an agreement that especially in settings with limited resources and large health problems, quality assessment of care is even more important than in affluent regions. It is essential that quality assessment activities in low-income countries are focused and their results implemented to improve quality of care.

The baseline registration of data in low-income countries is usually limited to a delivery book in which all mothers who are coming for delivery are noted. This registration is done on admission, and the information about complications and interventions that occur later is usually not complete. Usually, the outcome of the baby is not registered beyond a notation of stillbirth. In uncomplicated cases, the neonatal observation time is very short and can be a few hours. If the newborn baby needs special care, it is separated from the mother and the information is not available in her file.

Therefore, routine registration needs to be improved at several levels before it is valid for regional quality assessment activities. Until then local and focused quality improvement activities are needed to motivate staff for relevant routine registrations.

Perinatal audit is such an activity, which is suitable for all levels irrespective of the standard of care and has been found to increase motivation in staff and quality of care. The introduction of this process, however, needs good leadership and careful introduction to overcome initial suspicion and cultural barriers.

REFERENCES

1. Meeker CI. Quality improvement: then and now. Clin Obstet Gynecol. 1994;37:115-21.
2. Loegering L, Reiter RC, Gambone JC. Measuring the quality of health care. Clin Obstet Gynecol. 1994;37:122-36.
3. Hall M. Audit of antenatal care. Fetal Maternal Med Rev. 1993;5: 19-27.
4. Cleary R, Beard RW, Coles J, et al. The quality of routinely collected maternity data. Br J Obstet Gynaecol. 1994;101:1042-7.
5. Zeitlin J, Wildman K, Breart G, et al. Selecting an indicator set for monitoring and evaluating perinatal health in Europe: Criteria, methods and results from the PERISTAT project. Eur J Obstet Gynecol Reprod Biol. 2003;111(Suppl 1):S5-14.
6. PERISTAT Monitoring and evaluating perinatal health in Europe. Available from http://europeristat.aphp.fr.
7. Cleary R, Beard RW, Chapple J, Coles J. The standard primipara as a basis for inter-unit comparisons of maternity care. Br J Obstet Gynaecol. 1996;103:223-9.
8. Robson MS. Can we reduce the caesarean section rate? Best Pract Res Clin Obstet Gynaecol. 2001;15:179-94.
9. Danish Medical Birth Statistics. Available from http://www.dsog.dk.
10. Gould JB, Danielsen B, Korst LM, et al. Cesarean delivery rates and neonatal morbidity in a low-risk population. Obstet Gynecol. 2004;104:11-9.
11. Langhoff-Roos J, Borch-Christensen H, Larsen S, et al. Potentially avoidable perinatal deaths in Denmark and Sweden 1991. Acta Obstet Gynecol Scand. 1996;75:820-5.
12. Westergaard HB, Langhoff-Roos J, Larsen S, et al. Intrapartum death of nonmalformed fetuses in Denmark and Sweden in 1991. A perinatal audit. Acta Obstet Gynecol Scand. 1997;76:959-63.
13. Langhoff-Roos J, Larsen S, Basys V, et al. Potentially avoidable perinatal deaths in Denmark, Sweden and Lithuania as classified by the Nordic-Baltic classification. Br J Obstet Gynaecol. 1998; 105:1189-94.
14. Richardus JH, Graafmans WC, Verloove-Vanhorick SP, et al. Differences in perinatal mortality and suboptimal care between 10 European regions: Results of an international audit. Br J Obstet Gynecol. 2003;110:97-105.

28 Audit in Perinatal Medicine

JM Thomas, S Paranjothy

DEFINITION

Research is concerned with discovering the right thing to do; audit is concerned with ensuring that the right thing is done.[1] Clinical audit aims to improve patient care and outcome by reviewing the care provided to patients against explicit quality criteria and implementating change to improve the quality of care as a result. The structure, processes and outcomes of care can be selected and systematically evaluated against explicit criteria. Where indicated, changes are implemented at an individual, team or service level, and further monitoring is used to confirm improvement in health care delivery.[2]

IS AUDIT EFFECTIVE AT IMPROVING

A review of the evidence by NICE concluded that audit is an effective method for improving the quality of care. The same review also described the audit methods associated with successful audit projects.[2] These findings are drawn upon in this document to give practical advice for undertaking audit.

WHAT CAN BE AUDITED?

Audit may evaluate the structure (organization or provision) of services, the process of care or the outcome of care against an agreed standard.

Measure of Structure or Service Provision

Audit can provide an overview of service provision. For example, research evidence shows that the outcome for patients with ovarian cancer is better if they are operated on by an appropriately trained gynecologist and managed within the framework of a multidisciplinary team.[3–9] An audit of the referral and management of patients with ovarian cancer can provide an overview of service provision in this area. Good quality health care services need to be patient-centered and acceptable to those who use them. Measuring the views of those who use services enables health care providers to assess the service delivered from the patient's perspective.

Process Measure

Process measures are clinical practices that have been evaluated in research and shown to have an influence on outcome. For example, research evidence shows that the use of antenatal steroids has improved perinatal outcome. Evaluation of this process of care would entail measuring the proportion of appropriate women who received antenatal steroids. Process measures may be used to assess the quality of care and have some advantages over outcome measures:

- They provide a more direct measure of the quality of care provided
- They occur more frequently, so smaller samples are needed
- The findings are easier to interpret
- As smaller audits are needed, they cost less to achieve.

Outcome Measure

Outcome measure is the physical or behavioral response to an intervention for example, the health status (dead or alive), cure following surgery for stress incontinence, level of knowledge or satisfaction (e.g. users' views on the care they have received). Outcomes can be desirable, for example, improvement in the patient's condition or quality of life, or undesirable, e.g. adverse effects of a treatment. The assessment of outcomes such as cancer survival rates is fundamental to measuring quality of care but the use of outcomes alone in assessing quality of care has limitations:

1. Outcomes are not a direct measure of the care provided, ascribing causal factors too
2. Variation in care may be problematic, e.g. social and health inequalities may contribute to variation in mortality rates
3. Not all patients who experience substandard care will have a poor outcome
4. Many factors contribute to eventual outcome (e.g. disease severity, health status, and social and health inequalities); therefore, mechanisms to account for these differences are required (e.g. case-mix adjustment for comorbidity)
5. Outcomes may be delayed
6. Research evidence about the impact of some care processes on outcome is limited
7. Adverse outcomes occur less frequently so larger samples will be needed.

Despite all the difficulties associated with the interpretation of outcome measures, mortality and morbidity measures are important and this is a major justification for regular monitoring. "Critical incident" or "adverse event" reporting involves the identification of patients where an adverse event has occurred, such as the Confidential Enquiries into Maternal Deaths (CEMD), the Confidential Enquiry into Stillbirths and Deaths in Infancy (CESDI) and the National Confidential Enquiry into Perioperative Deaths (NCEPOD). These are examples[6] of outcome reporting. However, only adverse events are reported.

AUDIT CYCLE

Audit can be considered to have five principal steps, commonly referred to as the audit cycle:

1. Selection of a topic.
2. Identification of an appropriate standard.

3. Data collection to assess performance against the prespecified standard.

4. Implementation of changes to improve care, if necessary.

5. Data collection for a second, or subsequent, time to determine whether care has improved.

Audit projects require a multidisciplinary approach with the involvement of stakeholders (including consumers or users of the service provided) and the local audit department at the planning stage. Good planning and resources are also necessary to ensure its success.

Selecting a Topic for Audit

It is essential to establish clear aims and objectives at this stage, so that the audit is focused and addresses specific issues within the selected topic. A key consideration is "how will we use the results of this audit to change or improve practice?"

In selecting a topic for audit, priority should be given to common health concerns, areas associated with high rates of mortality, morbidity or disability, and those where good research evidence is available to inform practice or aspects of care that use considerable resources. It is important to involve those who will be implementing change at this stage of the audit process.

Identifying an Appropriate Audit Standard

Review Criteria

These are defined as "systematically developed statements that can be used to assess specific health care decisions, services and outcomes". In audit, review criteria are generally used for assessing care; this approach is sometimes referred to as criterion-based audit. The criterion is the reference point against which current practice is measured (Table 28.1). High-quality evidence-based guidelines can be used as the starting point for developing criteria. Where this is not possible, criteria should be agreed by a multidisciplinary group including those involved in providing care and those who use the service. Where criteria are based on the views of professionals or other groups, formal consensus methods are preferable. Review criteria should be explicit rather than implicit and need to:[2]

- Lead to valid judgments about the quality of care, and therefore should be based on research evidence about the importance of those aspects of care

Table 28.1: Examples of audit and review criteria

Audit Topic	Review Criteria
Induced abortion	Screening for lower genital tract organisms and treatment of positive cases among women undergoing induced abortion should be carried out to reduce postabortion infective morbidity
Cesarean section	A thromboprophylaxis strategy should be part of the management of women delivered by cesarean section
Hysterectomy	Transcervical resection of the endometrium or endometrial ablation should be available and offered to women with dysfunctional uterine bleeding as an alternative to hysterectomy

- Relate to aspects of care that are important either to patients or in terms of clinical outcome
- Be measurable.

Standard and Target Level of Performance

This is defined as "the percentage of events that should comply with the criterion" (e.g. the proportion of women undergoing induced abortion who were screened for lower genital tract organisms, the proportion of women delivered by cesarean section who received thromboprophylaxis, the proportion of women with dysfunctional uterine bleeding who were offered transcervical resection of the endometrium or endometrial ablation). Information about the levels of performance that can be achieved may be helpful when making plans for improvement. Target levels of performance should be examined periodically. The most common approach for setting target levels of performance is informal agreement among the group leading the audit or among health professionals. In some settings, external standards can be useful. However, in many audits no explicit targets are set and the aim is to improve upon current performance.

Target levels of performance have been most used in screening programs. For example, in screening for cervical cancer there are quality criteria to be met, such as the proportion of cervical smears that have endocervical cells.

The term "standard" has been used to refer to different concepts, sometimes as an alternative word for "clinical guidelines" and "review criteria", either with or without a stated target level of performance and, somewhat confusingly, also refer to the observed or desired level of performance. However, it has been defined as "the percentage of events that should comply with the criterion" in the interests of clarity.

Benchmarking

This is the "process of defining a level of care set as a goal to be attained". There is insufficient evidence to determine whether it is necessary to set target levels of performance in audit. However, in some audits, benchmarking techniques could help participants in audit to avoid setting unnecessarily low or unrealistically high target levels of performance. Reference to the levels achieved in audits undertaken by other professionals is useful. National audits may provide data for benchmarking. For example, the National Sentinel Cesarean Section Audit Report[7] gives regional and national data for comparison on topics such as the use of regional anesthesia in women having cesarean section.

Data Collection to Assess Performance Against the Prespecified Standard

Data collection in criterion-based audit is generally undertaken to determine the proportion of cases where care is in accordance with the criteria. In practice, the following points need to be considered.

What Data Items to Collect?

Consideration needs to be given to which data items are needed in order to answer the audit question. For example, if undertaking an audit on cesarean section rates, collecting information on the number of cesarean sections alone will not give sufficient information to measure the cesarean section rate. Data on the number of other births that took place is also required. In general, for audit projects with clear aims, objectives and well-defined review criteria, it is easier to identify those data items that require collection. Definitions need to be clear so that there is no confusion about what is being collected. The definitions will depend upon the review criterion that is being assessed. For example, if collecting data on rupture of membranes, it may need to be specified whether this is spontaneous or artificial. Data collectors should always be aware of their legal responsibilities regarding confidentiality and having electronic patient data such as under the Data Protection Act in the UK and the Caldicott Principles.[8] Under the Data Protection Act 1998, it is an offence to collect personal details of patients such as name, address or other items that are potentially identifiable for the individual without consent. It is rarely necessary or acceptable to use patient identifiers, such as names and addresses, but some form of pseudoanonymized identifiers may be used. Clinical audit may be considered part of direct patient care and therefore consent to use of data for audit can be implied through consent to treatment, provided that information is given to patients that their data may be used in this way. Audit project protocols should be submitted to the local research and development committee and ethics committees to seek approval if necessary. Guidance on how to do this can be obtained from the respective bodies.

Data Collection

Sources of data include:

- Routinely collected data if available (e.g. birth registers); this enables repeated data collections with the minimum of extra effort
- Clinical records
- Data collection through direct observation or from questionnaire surveys of staff or patients.

Routinely collected data can be used if all the data items required are available. It will be necessary to check the definitions for data items that are used within the routine database to ensure its usefulness for the aims of the audit. Also, the completeness and coverage of the routine source needs to be known.

Where the data source is clinical records, training of data abstractors and use of a standard proforma can improve accuracy and reliability of data collection. The use of multiple sources of data may also be helpful. However, this can also be problematic, as it will require linking of data from different sources with common unique identifiers.

Questionnaire surveys of staff or patients are often used for data collection. There are several validated questionnaires on a wide range of topics that may be adapted to a specific audit project. There is also literature on developing these.

Developing a Questionnaire

There is a large amount of literature on how to develop questionnaires.[11,12] Some of the general principles involved are presented here. Questionnaires are often used as a tool for data collection. Questions may be open or closed. Generally, questionnaire design using open questions, e.g. "What was the indication for cesarean section?" (followed by space for free text response) is easier. However, analysis of these data is difficult, as there will be a range of responses and interpretation can be problematic. Open questions may be more difficult and time-consuming to answer and can lead to nonresponse, which results in loss of data.

Questionnaires can be composed entirely of closed questions (i.e. with all possible answers predetermined). More time is needed to develop this type of questionnaire but the analysis is generally easier. An example of this type of questionnaire is:

Which of the following statements most accurately describes the urgency of this cesarean section?

A. Immediate threat to life of the fetus and the mother.

B. Maternal or fetal compromise that is not immediately life-threatening.

C. No maternal or fetal compromise but needs early delivery.

D. Delivery timed to suit the woman and staff.

Closed questions assume that all possible answers to the question are known but not the distribution of responses. Time and consideration needs to be given to the options available for response as, if a desired response is not available, the question may just be missed out and it may put people off completing the rest of the questionnaire. For some questions, the "other" category can be used with the option "please specify", which gives an opportunity for the respondent to write in a response. However, if this is used, thought must be given a priori as to how these free text responses will be coded and analyzed. In some situations, not having a category of "other" may lead to the question not being answered at all, which means that data will be lost.

If questionnaires are developed for a specific project, they need to be piloted and refined to ensure their validity and reliability before use as a tool for data collection. While those who developed the questionnaire understand the questions being asked, the aim of piloting is to check that those who have to fill in the questionnaire are able to understand and respond with ease. Questionnaires that are not user friendly are associated with lower response rates, the quality of data collected will be poor and hence results will be of little value.

Data Management

Thought needs to be given to who will collect the data, as well as the time and resources that will be involved. In small audit projects it may be feasible for the principal investigators to go through clinical notes for data abstraction. However, for larger projects, e.g. a prospective audit on induction of labor practices within a maternity unit, it may be more appropriate for those involved in the care of the woman giving birth (e.g. midwives or obstetricians) to fill in standard data collection sheets. Where available, audit support staff should be involved.

Data that are collected on paper forms are usually entered on to electronic databases or spreadsheets such as Microsoft Access®, Epi Info® or Microsoft Excel® for cleaning and analysis. Data entry may be done by optical character recognition (OCR) software, optical mark readers (OMR) or manually. OCR is most accurate for questionnaire data using tick boxes but less accurate for free text responses. The method of data entry needs to be taken into account when designing the questionnaire or data collection sheet. For manual data entry, accuracy is improved if double data entry is used. However, this can be a time-consuming exercise. If the facilities and resources are available, electronic collection of data can be considered. In this case, data are entered immediately, at source, into a computer and saved to disk. While this is quick and requires minimal storage space, it can be difficult to handle unexpected responses. As information is entered directly into a computer it cannot be verified or double-entered.[9]

Consideration also needs to be given to the coding of responses on the database. For ease of analysis of closed questions it is generally better to have numeric codes for responses. For example, yes/no responses can be coded to take the value 0 for no and 1 for yes. Missing data will also need to be coded; for example, with the number 9. The code assigned for missing data should be distinguished from those where the response is "not known" (if this was an option on the questionnaire).

It is advisable to incorporate consistency checks as data are being entered, in order to minimize errors. For example, if there are two questions:

a. How many previous pregnancies of at least 24 weeks of gestation has this woman had?

b. How many previous cesarean sections has she had?

A consistency check will highlight entries with responses other than 0 to question (b) if the response to question (a) is 0.

Data Analysis

Simple statistics are often all that is required. Statistical methods are used to summarize data for presentation in the form of summary statistics (means, medians or percentages) and graphs.[10]

Statistical tests are used to find out the likelihood that the data obtained has arisen by chance and how likely it is that a real difference exists between two groups. Before data collection has started it is essential to know what data items will be collected, whether comparisons will be made and the statistical methods that will be used to make these comparisons.

Data items that have categorical responses (e.g. yes/no or A/B/C/D) can be expressed as percentages. Some data items are collected as continuous variables, for example, mother's age, height and weight. These can either be categorized into relevant categories and then expressed as percentages, or if they are normally distributed, the mean and standard deviations can be reported. These summary statistics (percentages and means) are useful for describing the process, outcome or service provision that was measured.

Comparisons of percentages between different groups can be made using a chi-square test; tests can be used to compare means between two groups, assuming that these are normally distributed. Nonparametric statistical methods can be used for data that are not normally distributed. These comparisons are useful in order to determine whether there are any real differences in the observed findings, for example, when comparing audit results obtained at different time points or in different settings. In some situations a sample-size calculation may be necessary to ensure that the audit is large enough to detect a clinically significant difference between groups, if one exists. In this situation, it is important to consult a statistician during the planning stages of the audit project.

These simple statistics can be easily done using Microsoft Excel spreadsheets and Microsoft Access databases. Other useful statistical software packages include Epi Info, SAS, SPSS, STATA and Minitab.

Implementation of Changes to Improve Care if Necessary

Data analysis and interpretation will lead to the identification of clinical areas that should be addressed. There are many methods by which this can be done. The feedback of audit findings is most commonly used, for example, presentation at regular audit meetings will stimulate discussions and solutions may be agreed. The NICE review[2] identified several audits in which change in care had occurred. Simple methods were occasionally effective, for example:

- Feedback of data collected
- Provision of clear data, perhaps using modern information systems, supported by active teamwork
- Support from the organization for teamwork
- Use of several methods together within the context of an implementation plan

Change does not always occur in audit and consideration of the reasons for failure may take place after the second data collection. Resistance to change among local professionals or in the organizational environment or team should be considered. Patients themselves may have preferences for care that make change difficult.

The significance of teamwork, culture and resistance to change has led several authors to propose frameworks for planning implementation. These usually include analysis of the barriers to change and use of theories of individual, team or organizational behavior to select strategies to address the barriers. For some topics, such as adverse incidents, systems for continuous data collection may be justified.

ORGANIZATION OF AUDIT

The NICE review[2] found that some methods of organizing audit programs were better than others. The following features are associated with successful audit:

- Structured programs with realistic aims and objectives
- Leadership and attitude of senior management
- Nondirective, hands-on approach
- Support of staff, strategy groups and regular discussions
- Emphasis on teamworking and support
- Environment conducive to conducting audit.

Common Reasons Why Audits Fail

- Failure to participate and attitudes to audit: Involving all stakeholders (including service users) in the project can encourage participation. It is important to recognize the attitudes of those whose behavior is being audited, and to modify the audit process to accommodate these views.

Failure to continue and complete the audit cycle: This makes it impossible to determine whether the audit has led to any improvements in care.

- Failure to provide a supportive environment for audit: Perceived lack of support at all stages, together with a range of structural and organizational problems, is associated with poor progress in conducting audit. Research has pointed to a theory-practice gap for clinicians carrying out audit, one solution being to change the organizational culture to one in which clinical audit is supported and actively encouraged.

- Lack of resources, especially time: This includes lack of protected time to investigate the audit topic, collect and analyze data, and the time to complete an audit cycle. It follows that audit should be recognized as an important part of clinical practice and those directly involved in audit need to be allocated protected time.

- Lack of training in audit methodology and evidence-based skills: Health professionals and audit support staff require adequate knowledge and skills for undertaking audit, and they should be keen to learn. Barriers identified in the literature include a lack of training in evidence-based audit skills and the failure to apply what has already been established.

- Cost: It must be recognized that audit requires appropriate funding and that improvements in care resulting from clinical audit can increase costs.

REFERENCES

1. Smith R. Audit and research. [see comments]. BMJ. 1992;305:905.
2. NHS, National Institute for Clinical Excellence, Commission for Health Improvement, Royal College of Nursing, University of Leicester. Principles for Best Practice in Clinical Audit. Oxford: Radcliffe Medical Press; 2002. Available from www.nelh.nhs.uk/BestPracticeClinicalAudit.pdf [Accessed September 2003].
3. Junor EJ, Hole DJ, Gillis CR. Management of ovarian cancer: referral to a multidisciplinary team matters. Br J Cancer. 1994;70:363-70.
4. Woodman C, Baghdady A, Collins S, et al. What changes in the organisation of cancer services will improve the outcome for women with ovarian cancer? Br J Obstet Gynaecol. 1997;104:135-9.
5. Department of Health. The NHS Cancer Plan. London: Department of Health; 2000.
6. Penney GC. Audit. In: O'Brien PM, Broughton Pipkin F, (Eds). Introduction to Research Methodology for Specialists and Trainees. London: RCOG Press; 1999. pp. 95-106.
7. Royal College of Obstetricians and Gynaecologists, Clinical Effectiveness Support Unit. The National Sentinel Caesarean Section Audit Report. London: RCOG Press; 2001.
8. Department of Health. Data Protection Act 1998. Protection and Use of Patient Information. London: Department of Health. 1998.
9. McKenzie-McHarg K, Ayres S. Data management. In: O'Brien PM, Broughton Pipkin F, (Eds). Introduction to Research Methodology for Specialists and Trainees. London: RCOG Press; 1999. pp. 140-6.
10. Brocklehurst P, Gates S. Statistics. In: O'Brien PM, Broughton Pipkin F, (Eds). Introduction to Research Methodology for Specialists and Trainees. London: RCOG Press; 1999. pp. 147-60.
11. Gillham B. Developing a Questionnaire. London: Continuum; 2000.
12. McColl E, Jacoby A, Thomas L, et al. Design and use of questionnaires: A review of best practice applicable to surveys of health service staff and patients. Health Technol Assess. 2001;5(31):1-256.

29 Systematic Reviews in Perinatal Medicine

Z Alfirevic

INTRODUCTION

The principles of evidence-based medicine are not disputed. What constitutes the evidence, however, is hotly debated. Traditionally, medical textbooks and review articles written by experts and opinion leaders have been the main sources of evidence. Recommendation on diagnostic and therapeutic interventions in such material was predominantly based on personal clinical experience and easily accessible literature. Although there has always been some concern about possible biases inherent in this traditional approach to teaching and information sharing, a more formal criticism gathered momentum in the early nineties. For example, Antman, et al. published in JAMA a comparison between treatment recommendations for myocardial infarction extracted from review articles and textbook chapters on one hand and randomized clinical trials on the other.[1] The evidence that thrombolytic therapy saves lives had been available in early 1970 when a combined reduction in deaths from 10 clinical trials with around 2,500 enrolled patients reached statistical significance. Unfortunately, there were no attempts to analyze the results from the different studies together and further clinical trials continued well into 1990s with tens of thousands of patients exposed unnecessarily to placebo and many more to no treatment at all. Even more worryingly, it took more than 15 years for this evidence to start appearing in medical textbooks and authoritative review articles. In perinatal medicine, the evidence that antenatal corticosteroids cannot only reduce neonatal respiratory distress syndrome, but also reduce the risk of neonatal intracranial hemorrhage and perinatal death was available from early 1970s. Even if early studies could have been seen as hypothesis generating, the reluctance to consider the totality of evidence on this topic in the late eighties was inexcusable.

Systematic reviews have emerged as one of the most effective ways of bridging the gap between already available evidence and clinical recommendations. The main differences between traditional and systematic reviews are summarized in the Table 29.1. Numbers of published systematic reviews have risen quite considerably in the last decade (Fig. 29.1) and such reviews are now considered not only an integral part of clinical guidelines, but also a prerequisite for any planned research on diagnostic and therapeutic interventions.

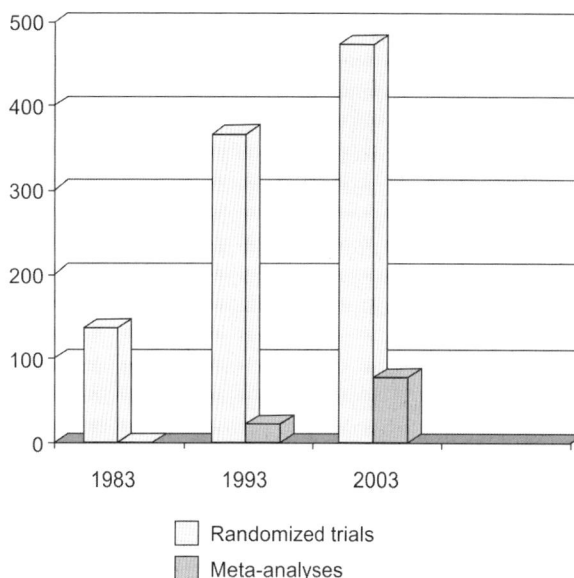

Fig. 29.1: Progressive increase in the number of randomized trials and meta-analyses related to pregnancy included in the PubMed (number of hits for three separate 12-month periods using keywords: pregnan* or labor or labour)

The term meta-analysis is often used as a synonym for a systematic review in this context because of the misconception that systematic review must always include a quantitative synthesis of the data to yield a summary statistics (meta-analysis). This is clearly not the case, as systematic reviews may fail to identify studies suitable for statistical pooling.

COCHRANE REVIEWS

Major advances in the scientific rigor and availability of systematic reviews in perinatal medicine have come from the Cochrane Collaboration—an international, not for profit organization established in 1993.[2] The aim of the Cochrane Collaboration is to facilitate the preparation, maintenance and dissemination of up-to-date systematic reviews of the effects of healthcare interventions.

Table 29.1: The main differences between traditional and systematic reviews

	Narrative reviews	Systematic reviews
Defined clinical questions	Rarely	Common
Reproducible, clearly defined literature search	No	Mandatory
Defined exclusion criteria for potentially eligible studies	Rarely	Common
Prespecified comparisons and outcomes of interest	No	Common
Statistical pooling of the results (meta-analysis)	No	Common
Peer review before publication	Rarely	Common

The Cochrane Collaboration Pregnancy and Childbirth Group (CCPC) was the first registered review group within the Cochrane Collaboration and was subsequently joined by around 50 other topic-based groups, each of them working under the guidance of an international editorial team. The CCPC remains the largest and most productive Cochrane Review Group with more than 400 registered reviewers from 27 countries.

The distinguishing features of the Cochrane Reviews published quarterly in the electronic publication *The Cochrane Library* are transparent peer-reviewed protocols published in anticipation of each new review, significant input from consumers and consumer advocates throughout the reviewing process[3] and a commitment to keep Cochrane Reviews regularly updated. The main criticism of Cochrane Reviews is a limitation of any evidence-based solely on randomized trials.

The criticism that systematic reviews of randomized trials ignore the wealth of knowledge generated by observational studies and basic science is valid. However, the restriction of Cochrane Reviews to randomized trials is primarily pragmatic. The methodology for systematic searches of observational studies is nowhere near as sophisticated as searches restricted to randomized trials. The current register of randomized trials compiled by the Cochrane Pregnancy and Childbirth Group contains more than 10,000 trial reports the majority of which are yet to be included in the Cochrane Reviews. It is anticipated that any similar register of all literature relevant to the evaluation of health interventions related to pregnancy could contain more than million records.

OTHER TYPES OF SYSTEMATIC REVIEWS

Two other types of systematic reviews have gathered momentum recently as a welcome addition to the already established analyses of aggregate data from randomized trials—systematic reviews of diagnostic and screening tests and individual patient data analysis.

Systematic reviews of diagnostic tests differ from standard reviews in the assessment of study quality and statistical methods used to combine results (pooled sensitivities, specificities, likelihood ratios and summary receiver operating curves).[4] Most published systematic reviews of diagnostic tests are hindered by the poor quality of the included studies. It is also important to note that the evaluation of diagnostic accuracy of a test is only one aspect of clinical usefulness; the most accurate test can still be clinically useless or, even worse, harmful.

Methods of undertaking a meta-analysis of several studies may involve collecting either aggregate data or data on each patient individually. The advantages of the latter approach, described as the "yardstick"[5] include a more complete analysis of "time of event" outcomes and a more powerful analysis of whether treatment is more or less effective in particular subgroups. The drawbacks can include the increased use of time, staff and financial resources and the lack of availability of the original data for some trials.

CONCLUSION

Systematic reviews in perinatal medicine have made an important contribution to perinatal medicine by reinforcing the evidence about effective therapies like antenatal corticosteroids in threatened preterm labor and highlighting ineffective interventions like thyrotropin-releasing hormone in the same clinical scenario. Equally important has been the role of systematic reviews in identifying gaps in our knowledge. The challenge for the future is to provide regularly updated unbiased summaries of observational, randomized and qualitative data in a format that is understandable to both patients and health professionals. We have nothing to fear. The time currently spent on information gathering and the haphazard critical appraisal of incomplete evidence will be much better spent talking with our patients and helping them to achieve perinatal care and outcomes that truly suit their needs.

REFERENCES

1. Antman EM, Lau J, Kupelnick B, et al. A comparison of results of meta-analyses of randomized control trials and recommendations of clinical experts. Treatments for myocardial infarctions. JAMA. 1992;268:240-8.
2. Sakala C, Gyte G, Henderson S, et al. Consumer-professional partnership to improve research: The experience of the Cochrane Collaboration's Pregnancy and Childbirth Group. Birth. 2001;133-7.
3. Chalmers I. The Cochrane Collaboration: Preparing, maintaining and disseminating systematic reviews of the effects of health care. Annals of the New York Academy of Science. 1993;703:156-65.
4. Deeks JJ. Systematic reviews of evaluations of diagnostic and screening tests. BMJ. 2001;323:157-62.
5. Stewart LA, Parmar MK. Meta-analysis of the literature or of individual patient data: Is there a difference? Lancet. 1993;341:418-22.

30 Cost-benefit in Perinatal Medicine

Z Stembera

INTRODUCTION

Greatly increased advances in medicine lead on one hand to a high quality of care expected and demanded by both the health-care professionals and the patients, but on the other hand the resources available for responding to the expectations and demands are becoming increasingly stretched. Even in the high-income countries, the available resources are scarce in relation to these demands.

Because of this, more and more has appeared in the expert medical literature of these countries in the last two decades trying to solve the disproportion between the increasing investments in health care and the principal factors that have led to basic improvements in health by means of methods of economic evaluation.

The key question on how best to choose between the different and competing ways of using the resources that are available has considerable importance in perinatal medicine, whose share in the costs of health care is quite high. This has three reasons: first is that the number of users pregnant and childbearing women and their infants is quite high. Second is that, the number of preventive screening examinations and preventive hospitalizations in the course of pregnancy is increased. Third is that, the number of special, sometimes very expensive, examinations using technological advances in medicine increases.

The approach to preparation of these studies and to their exploitation exhibits considerable variations. It is different in the professionals within the perinatal field who wish to make optimal use of the budgets and resources that are available to them, than in the planners who must decide on the appropriate level of funding for the maternity care. There are also differences between the views of the patient, of the hospital, as well as of the government or a community at large.

METHODS OF ECONOMIC EVALUATION

When discussing the already classical studies of Drummond and colleagues[1] and Mugford and Drummond,[2] it is necessary first to quote some basic considerations related to the role of economics in the evaluation of care:

1. The first consideration must be that the care for which the resources are used is likely to do more good than harm. Only afterward comes the consideration of both the most cost-effective or efficient use of the resources available for perinatal care, and the extent to which the society's resources should be allocated to perinatal care.
2. Economic evaluation requires a contrast between alternative courses of action, in term of both costs and consequences.

3. There are three main stages of economic evaluation: first, the likely costs and benefits must be enumerated; second, they must be measured; and third, they must be expressed in comparable units.
4. To the most important methods of economic evaluation of perinatal care programs belong the cost-minimalization, or marginal, cost-effectiveness, cost-utility and cost-benefit analyses.

The nature and scale of any economic evaluation will vary according to the question that is being asked. While all approaches involve to some extent deriving a balance sheet of the costs and benefits of the different strategies compared, some approaches are more complex than others.

COST-MINIMALIZATION ANALYSIS

This probably most simple analysis comes from the presumption that benefits of treatments that are compared are equal, which makes it possible to compare the resource costs without any need to measure benefits. A different length of hospitalization of a woman subsequent to a spontaneous delivery and physiological pregnancy, who delivered a healthy, term newborn, whose adaptation to extrauterine life was normal in the first hours of life, could serve as an example. This is the problem that is being solved at present in the Czech Republic. Before the transformation of health care to the conditions of market mechanism, that is, before 1990, hospitalization after delivery in the given case lasted for 5–6 days, whereas in the majority of high-income countries with advanced perinatal care, such hospitalization lasts for half that time on average without adversely influencing the health condition of the woman or her child.

From the given example concerning the calculation of decreased costs with the same benefit, it explicitly emerges that it is possible to save the costs of hospitalization for 2–3 days. On the other hand, however, new costs arise for visits of every mother and infant at home when women are discharged earlier from hospital after delivery. This has to last at least until the time of separation of the umbilical stump in the child, and healing of the perineal wound in the woman. Even if, in comparison with the more expensive hospital care, the cheaper home care clearly decreases the costs of postnatal care, this change opens new concerns:

1. A deteriorated satisfaction of Czech women (predominantly primiparae) in consequence of the shorter spell of rest after delivery and the early care of the newborn at home.[3]
2. A choice of the optimal method for cord care associated with a reduction of the number of home visits by midwives.[4] However, these types of studies fall within other methods of economic evaluation.

MARGINAL ANALYSIS

Such analysis would be particularly useful in the case of routine and repeated testing that is so common in the care of women during pregnancy and childbirth. But the key question is: how many of them should we use? There may be a general agreement that certain screening tests should be applied to high-risk pregnancies. But should they be applied routinely to all pregnant women and possibly also repeatedly? When analyzing the majority of screening tests performed in the course of pregnancy, it should be first taken into account that there exist complex factors affecting the mother's health. It is consequently extremely difficult to evaluate the effectiveness of the analyzed test, because many other variables that influence maternal and fetal health are interacting at the same time and confound the findings. These variables are considerably different in developing and industrial countries, where the most important ones influencing the outcome of pregnancy include socioeconomic factors, level of education, desire for pregnancy and maternal age. Taking into account the above background information and limitations, we shall try to ascertain the effectiveness of these screening tests and subsequent measures from the following two aspects:

1. Biological: Each intervention is considered in terms of what it intended to achieve.

2. Programmatic: Do the maternal health programs successfully deliver the biologically effective intervention to the intended target population?

The widely used practice of ultrasound imaging of the fetus during pregnancy can be employed as a typical example. From the biological point of view this method is routinely performed up to the 20th week of pregnancy since it:

1. defines more precisely the expected date of confinement, hence reducing the induction rate in pregnancies mistakenly diagnosed as post-term;

2. allows an earlier diagnosis of twin pregnancies, leading to a reduced premature labor connected with an increased mortality and morbidity of these newborns; and

3. improves the detection of malformed fetuses, which is followed by termination of pregnancy if the pregnant woman agrees, thereby reducing the number of impaired babies.

Repeated routine ultrasound examinations at the beginning of the third trimester improve a timely diagnosis of fetal growth retardation and placenta previa leading to reduced mortality and morbidity in newborns.

In a series of studies, the routinely and repeatedly performed ultrasound examinations in the course of pregnancy were compared with only selective examinations for predicting the expected date of delivery and for assessing subsequent measures upon the occurrence of adverse outcomes. From the programmatic point of view, the health resources implications of such screening programs between the two strategies of care can be considered on the basis of costs which include equipment, trained staff and clinic accommodation. These then vary with the number of cases treated and differ between the two types of care offered. Of the mentioned studies concerning the effectivity of ultrasound screening programs, only a few refer explicitly to health resource implications.[5] However, since several of the above-mentioned pregnancy complications are studied at the same time in the course of one ultrasound examination, it is very difficult, if not impossible, to earmark out of the total cost of this examination, the partial cost of diagnosing only one of these conditions. For instance, in the Czech Republic, it was possible to successively eliminate anencephaly out of the population of newborns by means of routine ultrasound screening, which is performed in 94% of all pregnant women before the 20th week of pregnancy.[6]

In an effort to limit some relatively expensive and, in the majority of cases, invasive tests connected with a certain, albeit very small, physical risk, but enabling a reliable and timely diagnosis of a serious pathological condition, the procedure was divided from the programmatic point of view into two levels. The timely diagnosis of some chromosomal or genetic disorders in the fetus can be taken as an example. By means of a routine screening program using relatively cheap and noninvasive tests, a high-risk group is selected from the total population of women on the first level. Only in the small group of women selected in this way are reliable diagnostic methods allowing a timely identification of the disease used. Here belong, for example, chorionic villus sampling or examination of fetal cells after obtaining a sample of amniotic fluid by amniocentesis. Over the past few years in the Czech Republic, such a programmed procedure has decreased the incidence of neural tube defects and Down Syndrome to a half, similar to the majority of high-income countries.[7]

COST-EFFECTIVENESS ANALYSIS

Cost-effectiveness analysis of any intervention requires calculation of the change in costs divided by the change in outcome of the intervention; the outcomes are measured in units of health (for example, survival rates or life-years saved).

Change in Cost

The best economic analysis will consider all costs, regardless of who has to pay: the health insurance company, the hospital, the patient, the family or the community at large. A distinction has to be made between charges and costs. Only in some cases will the charge for a service equal the cost, and only under such circumstances can charge be substituted for costs.

Change in Survival Rates

A differentiated approach to the change in survival rate can be demonstrated with the example of care for newborns of a very low birthweight. When evaluating the effectivity of the care for these newborns in the sense of their survival, the following considerations are taken into account:

1. Birthweight of the newborn: The lower the birthweight, the longer the time of hospitalization in the neonatal intensive care unit (NICU) and the higher the costs of the treatment, because the two factors are combined.

2. Whether the evaluation concerns a country-wide or regional program, all livebirths or only neonatal intensive care in the hospital.

3. Whether the newborn was delivered in a perinatologic center where there is a NICU, or whether the newborn was transported to the NICU only after delivery, because out-born newborns have a different prognosis.

4. Whether all liveborns are evaluated, or whether certain newborns are excluded, for example, those with lethal malformations, whose death is not influenced by the quality of intensive perinatal care.

The results of this deliberation determine which newborns must be accounted for in the denominator of any calculation of survival rate.

An internationally recommended objective criterion for the intensive care for newborns of a very low birthweight differentiated in this way is the birthweight-specific neonatal death rate (potentially after exclusion of lethal malformations), which can be further differentiated into death during the first 7 days after delivery (early neonatal death) or during the subsequent 3 weeks (late neonatal death).[8,9]

COST-UTILITY ANALYSIS

In cost-utility analysis, the social value of the outcome is determined. The analysis requires calculation of the change of costs, which is the same as for cost-effectiveness analysis, divided by the change in outcome adjusted for the quality-adjusted life saved, or quality-adjusted life-years saved. From the point of view of utility, the outcome is also the satisfaction gained from consumption of a service.

Change in Quality-adjusted Life-years or Survival Rate

The major difficulty is the inability to define what constitutes a normal quality of life, and what is the possibility of measuring the health status and health-related quality of life. The broad definition of health as formulated by the World Health Organization (WHO) is: "a state of complete physical, mental and social well-being and not merely the absence of disease or infirmity". WHO has also developed a classification of impairment, disability and handicap.[10] Conventionally, an outcome with normal health and quality of life is allotted a utility of 1, and death is allotted a utility of 0.[11] Any outcome of less than normal health or quality of life has a value of less than 1. But many handicapped children lead productive lives, and their health-related quality of life might be fairly good. In this respect, measurement of health-related quality of life adds a different, additional and important dimension to the standard description of cognitive and motor functioning in outcome studies. It is therefore clear that the available adult measures cannot be applied directly to children, whose life experiences and daily activities differ substantially from those of adults. Therefore, the six-component multi-attributable system known as the health utilities index (HUI) was worked out to describe the quality of life of children, and this includes sensory and communication ability, happiness, self-ability, freedom from moderate to severe pain, learning and school difficulty, and physical ability.[12] In spite of this, there still remains series of factors that may influence the measurement of the health-related quality of life of these children, for example:

1. Children of different ages have varying capabilities, and with increasing age they develop new and more advanced skills and challenges. Therefore, the dimensions of any measure of health-related quality of life have to take these changes into consideration.[13]

2. Health status measured by health professionals, self-assessment and parental score might not be consistent.[14]

3. Children with the same disability might view their quality of life very differently.

A particular problem represents the justification of estimating the health status at the time of a striking decline in neonatal monitoring of very immature newborns, although improvements in morbidity of these children have not been significant. Offering intensive care to all newborns of borderline viability without having the possibility to predict reliably the quality of life gained in every individual case is being questioned by both parents and health care providers. It is well-recognized that parents, health professionals and members of society may have different views on both the dimensions of importance and the values placed on different health states.[15] The fundamental question, however, is whose values are important for consideration of allocation of health care resources and for decision making.

Another criterion for analogous decision making, for example, between neonatal intensive care versus other programs, is the probability of the length of life gained by means of intensive care. Most surviving adults admitted to intensive care will be dead within a shorter time than the neonates admitted to the NICU, out of whom the surviving ones may live well for 70 years or more.

However, cost-utility is also used from the point of view of utility to women. For example, pregnant women may be anxious about their genetic history, or because of their age that they may be carrying a fetus with one or more abnormalities. It is precisely the above-mentioned two-level screening performed in these women that will affect an unnecessary prolongation of their anxiety up to the time of assessment of the correct diagnosis on the second level, since there exists a certain percentage of false-positive results on the first level. The anxiety of the women will be also prolonged if the correct final diagnosis is made by amniocentesis, which can only be performed in the second trimester. On the other hand, the examination by means of chorionic villus sampling can be performed earlier, in the first trimester.

However, routine ultrasound screening also has a psychosocial benefit in some cases. A mother's attitude to her pregnancy can be positively affected by the observation of first fetal movements on the screen of the ultrasound apparatus, even more than by their perception.[16] It is, in this way, possible to create a relationship with the child before it is born.

Another example of utility to women represents the lower satisfaction of women in connection with the shortened time of hospitalization after delivery that is mentioned in the section "Cost-minimalization analysis".

COST-BENEFIT ANALYSIS

This method of economic analysis in perinatal care, the last one to be mentioned, similarly allows the outcome to be converted into monetary terms. The cost-benefit analysis of perinatal intensive care requires the subtraction of additional costs per livebirth from additional earnings per livebirth; the results can be expressed in units of currency and would be termed the net economic benefit or net economic loss, if negative.

The data used for the change in cost are the same ones as mentioned in the section "Cost-effectiveness analysis". The major difficulty is to estimate the lifetime earnings of a survivor, when such imponderables as life expectancy, career choice (including the possibility of unemployment) and inflation have to be predicted so far into the future. Affected children may have different skills and capacities than unaffected children, different health care, education and other needs throughout their lives.

Another important point of view when taking into account the timing of costs and benefits is a generational view, when, for example, the favorable result of treatment of a pregnant woman 40 years ago may have an adverse effect on the fertility of her offspring, as happened in the case of diethylstilbestrol.[17]

The already classical randomized trial of MacDonald and associates[18] concerning the economic evaluation of electronic fetal heart monitoring versus intermittent auscultation achieved the same outcome of care. Since, however, the whole course of labor in every individual woman was always followed by one midwife, and if, rather than her salary bill, the time necessary for such a follow-up should be measured, we would find that hardly any workplace would have sufficiently numerous staff for such a procedure.

Costs and benefits arise from changes in uses not only of a community's, but also of a family's, resources. Returning back to the example of early postnatal discharge from hospital, it is likely that more family resources will be needed for informal home care and support for a mother who comes back home very soon after delivery.

INTERNATIONAL COMPARATIVE STUDIES

The cost-effective analysis for better health outcome is also solved in the form of international comparative studies. To some above-mentioned problems, for example, that the costs have to be standardized if different areas are compared, further sources of confusion arise when comparing different countries due to the fluctuations in the respective currency rates over time.

Out of these studies, the World Bank data[19] on infant mortality and life expectancy in 21 high-income and 27 low-income countries are meaningful. For each country, the differences between actual and predicted values were calculated for health expenditure per capita on the basis of per capita gross national product and health. From the results of this comparison, it emerged that for high-income countries, the marginal return of health expenditure per capita as measured by mortality is negligible. This means that improvement in health and reduction in mortality can be expected to arise not from further increases in costs, but from greater efficiency in the use

of resources, more reliance on preventive measures, and advances in lifestyle, behavior and medical technology.[20]

It was the preventive measures to which a comparative epidemiological study was devoted, concerning the effect of bed rest during pregnancy upon two internationally accepted indicators of maternal morbidity: rate of eclampsia and neonatal rate of low birthweight.[21] Incidence of these indicators in the Czech Republic was compared with the incidence in Hessen (one of the federal states of the Federal Republic of Germany), where there is a lower rate of prenatal hospital admissions, while the system of perinatal care and the perinatal mortality rate is similar. From the economic point of view, it was calculated under the conditions of the Czech Republic that:

1. The increase of expenses for hospitalization of women is higher by 7% in the Czech Republic (predominantly because of hospitalization for different lengths of time for preventive reasons) (Table 30.1).

2. There is a decrease of expenses for specialized care in the NICU due to a 0.5% lower incidence of low birthweight infants in the population (further differentiated into four groups according to birthweight) (Table 30.2).

The two fold lower sum spared from the NICU costs against the sum paid for the higher percentage of preventively hospitalized women does not include the benefit attained in the second analyzed indicator, that is, the decreased incidence of eclampsia (one case per 2,556 deliveries/year in the Czech Republic compared with a more than two fold incidence in Hessen, that is, one case per 1,328 deliveries/year). However, it is not possible to express this benefit in monetary terms.

CONCLUSION

In the economy at large, the costs and benefits of activities are made visible through the market system. However, the market mechanism in general either does not apply, or works imperfectly in the health care field. This is also true of use of the terms "cost" and "benefit" during economic evaluation of perinatal care. Economists thus have to use other approaches in estimating the benefits of health care programs. The most promising approach appears to be the evaluation of health improvements not in monetary terms. Also, the monetary cost is often an inadequate measure of the true economic cost. From this point of view, the main methods that economists consider in evaluation of health care alternatives and in comparison of health care programs were described. These methods of economic evaluation should also ensure wise spending during allocation of resources.

Table 30.1: Increase of costs for hospitalization of pregnant women. The data are based on a comparison of two groups of pregnant women: Czech Republic (n = 106,680) and Hessen (58,430) in 1994. The costs are calculated in accordance with the rate table of the Czech Health Insurance Company in Czech crowns

| | Hospitalizations of Pregnant Women in Population | | | Cost increase | |
Length of hospitalization (days)	Czech Republic (%)	Hessen (%)	Difference (%)	Czech crown (millions)	
1–7	10.9	10.1	0.7	0.8	
8–21	9.8	7.6	2.2	10.4	
> 21	6.6	3.1	3.5	47.8	
Total	27.3	20.8	6.4	59.0	

Table 30.2: Decrease of costs for the care of low birthweight newborns in consequence of their decreased incidence in the population. The data are based on a comparison of two groups of newborns: Czech Republic (n = 107,721) and Hessen (n = 59,198) in 1994. The costs are calculated in accordance with the rate table of the Czech Health Insurance Company in Czech crowns

	Incidence of low birthweight newborns		Cost increase	
Birth weight (g)	Czech Republic (%)	Hessen (%)	Difference (%)	Czech crown (millions)
< 1,000	0.30	0.37	0.07	69.9
1,000–1,499	0.55	0.62	0.07	34.1
1,500–1,999	1.07	1.23	0.16	18.6
1,500–1,999	3.55	3.82	0.27	7.3
Total	5.47	6.04	0.57	129.9

The application of the methods of economic evaluation in perinatal care cannot overcome the moral dilemmas that arise in the choice of different screening or therapeutic methods or allocation of resources. It does, however, provide a framework within which such factors become less easily avoided and more readily discussed from the point of view of both the care givers and the care receivers.

REFERENCES

1. Drummond MF, Stoddart GL, Torrance GW. Methods for the Economic Evaluation of Health Care Programmes. Oxford: Oxford University Press; 1986.
2. Mugford M, Drummond MF. The role of economics in the evaluation of care. In Chalmers I, Enkin M, Keirse MJ, (Eds). Effective Care in Pregnancy and Childbirth. Oxford: Oxford University Press; 1991. pp. 86-96.
3. Goldberg H, Velebil P, Stembera Z, et al. Czech Republic Reproductive Health Survey 1993. Atlanta, USA: Centers for Disease Control and Prevention; 1995.
4. Mugford M, Somchaiwong M, Waterhouse I. Treatment of umbilical cords. Report of a randomized controlled trial. Midwifery. 1986;2:177-86.
5. Bakketeig LS, Eik-Nes SH, Jacobsen G, et al. Randomized controlled trial of ultrasonographic screening in pregnancy. Lancet. 1984;2:207-9.
6. Sípek A, Gregor V, Chudobová M. Incidence of birth defects and effectivity of prenatal diagnosis in the Czech republic 1993 (in Czech). Cs Pediatrie. 1996;2:114-23.
7. International Clearinghouse for Birth Defects Monitoring System. ICBDMS, Annual report 1994. Rome: ISSN 0743-5703. 1996. pp. 52-123.
8. Dunn PM, McIlwaine G. Perinatal audit. Prenat Neonat Med. 1996;1:160-94.
9. World Health Organization. International Statistical Classification of Diseases, 10th revision. Statistical presentation. Geneva: World Health Organization. 1993;2:124-38.
10. World Health Organization. International Classification of Impairments. Disabilities and Handicaps. Geneva: World Health Organization 1980.
11. Bennett KJ, Torrance GW. Measuring health state preference and utilities rating scale time trade-off, and standard gamble techniques.

In: Spilker B, (Ed). Quality of Life and Pharmacoeconomics in Clinical Trials. Philadelphia: Lippincott-Raven; 1996. pp. 253-65.
12. Torrance GW, Furlong W, Feeny D, et al. Multiattribute preference functions: Health Utilities Index. Pharmacoeconomics 1995;7: 503-20.
13. Saigal S, Szatmari P, Rosenbaum P, et al. Cognitive abilities and school performance of extremely low- birth-weight children and matched term control children at age 8 years: A regional study. J Pediatr. 1991;118:751-60.
14. Saigal S, Feeny D, Rosenbaum P, et al. Self-perceived health status and health-related quality of life of extremely low-birth-weight teenagers: comparison with term controls. J Am Med Assoc. 1996;276:453-9.
15. Saigal S, Rosenbaum PL, Feeny DH, et al. Comparison of preferences of health professionals and parents for health outcomes of neonatal intensive care (abstr). Pediatr Res. 1996;39:no. 1654.
16. Reading AD, Campbell S, Cox DN, et al. Health beliefs and health care behaviour in pregnancy. Psychosom Med. 1982;12:379-83.
17. Herbst AL, Ulfelder H, Postkanzer DC. Adenocarcinoma of the vagina: association of maternal stilbestrol therapy with tumor appearance in young women. N Engl J Med. 1971;284:878-81.
18. MacDonald D, Grant A, Sheridan-Pereira M, et al. The Dublin randomised trial of intrapartum fetal heart monitoring. Am J Obstet Gynecol. 1985;152:524-39.
19. The World Bank. World Development Report 1993: Investing in Health. New York: Oxford University Press; 1993.
20. Shmueli A. Cost-effective outlays for better health outcomes. World Health Forum. 1995;16:287-92.
21. Stembera Z, Holub J. Hospitalization during pregnancy: professional versus economic aspect (in Czech). Ces Gynek. 1996;61:332-7.

SECTION 4

Ultrasound

A Kurjak, Y Ville

31 3D-4D Ultrasound Evaluation of the Embryo and the Early Fetus

F Bonilla-Musoles, LE Machado, F Raga

INTRODUCTION

Following the USA Food and Drug Administration (FDA) approval of 3D in November 1997, interest in the technique has soared to the extent that reports on 3D in Obstetrics and Gynecology are now in the thousands. Moreover, any international or national Ultrasound Congress or Meeting of our specialty contains main lectures, courses or workshops dedicated to this issue.

Today, 3D is an integrated part of US not only in Obstetrics and Gynecology but also in other medical steams.

Most important, the FDA with its strict guidelines has highlighted the importance of this technology for the future of medicine.

Because of the most recent advances in informatics, several important innovations have appeared recently.

The first 3D instruments that appeared in 1991 took 25 seconds to store an image and minutes to hours to reconstruct the 3D rendering. Then the defocused instruments[87,88] formed 3D images in real time. Current software have improved to the extent that images are stored in tenths of second and being able to reconstruct spatial images immediately, in 1 second. In this way, images are obtained in quasi-real time showing embryonic or fetal movements, the so-called 4D.

The newest instruments limit the field of vision (a disadvantage similar to 2D) and eliminate distorted echoes. They also store transparency systems allowing immediate visualization an avoiding loss of time. The smaller and easier to handle transducers and the better proportionate image quality are also definitive improvements.

But not only 3D has changed and improved in the past only 2 years, in our opinion two amazing improvements have been introduced:

1. The combination in "quasi-real time" at the same time and in the same frame of the 2D and 3D images. This advantage allows a rapid and better orientation and, for those with scarce experience, to an easier identification of structures and planes
2. The integration of successive images in only 1 second allowing the visualization of embryonic or fetal movements.

But these are not the final consequences of the new computer's technology:

Recently, we used Japanese new prototypes of 3D machines which were able to produce six images per second, with a store capacity of minutes (the nowadays existing store only 10 seconds) and with an incredible image quality.

Today more than 11 commercial houses dispose 3D, but not all are good. Many use insufficient "work stations" which obligate to spend time (and money) after the exam. These are not real 3D machines and, do not forget, that what the patient, and the sonographer, wants is to visualize here baby on the frame.

In our opinion and until very recently no one of the "work stations" were good enough. Recently, a new one has been approved by the FDA (but not yet approved in the European community) with important advantages:

- The software program is cheap (15,000)
- Adaptable to all ultrasound machines (also the small ones) and transducer images
- Excellent image quality
- Immediate free-hand 3D rendering image of an excellent quality
- No store space limitation, as it occurs with all existing 3D transducers
- Very rapid 3D rendering allowing the study of the heart motion
- Adaptable to old stored clinical cases, and not only in ultrasound machines but also in videos, PC, DVD, etc. some problems remain to be solved:
  - There is a shortage of learning centers where interested professionals can learn about new techniques, learn how to use the new instruments, and become acquainted with the variety of equipment that is constantly appearing on the market
  - Health care professionals must be aware that not only all commercial instruments are equipped with all of the latest technological advantages

    They also must know that every month new machines are being offered with new and better technology
  - The three first and more important statistics on fetal malformations (Merz, Pretorius, Bonilla-Musoles) need to be reproduced by other investigators. All the recently appeared articles show isolated cases, superficial malformations or works with few cases.

As a summary, we would recommend to start working with 3D, IT IS THE FUTURE.

HISTORY OF 3D

The 3D reports started 10 years ago. The first descriptions were dedicated to emphatice the diagnostic possibilities in OB/GYN[1,3,13,14,17,19,47,54,55,58,63,76,77,88,89,111,127,128,132,139,140,149,150,152,155,166,170,178-205,209,211,213,215,217,230,246,250,262,263,266]

Sporadic reports of normal[3,8,13,14,17-19,23,24,26,27,46,54,55,63,70,77,81,82,85,88,89,103-105,144,147,155,251] and malformed fetuses[9,23,24,26,43,53,74,88,98,99,100,104,105,112,113 116,117,120-133,136,144,157,187,198,203,220,254] followed.

Soon after, descriptive images of specific organs and areas were available:

- Craneum and fontanelles[138,151]
- Central nervous system[221,224,257,265,269,275]

- Head[49,139,279]
- Face[49,56,58,100,110,114,131,140,153,188]
- Lips[154,157]
- Forehead[176]
- Eyes [175]
- Thorax and vertebral column[76,110,138,143,162,163,166,173,183,186,271]
- Heart[44,106,137,142,176,177,214,215,210,222,252-254,256]
- Fingers[36-38,70,104,146,170,173]
- Genitalia, normal or ambiguous.[7,68,69,135,248,258]

Comparative 2D/3D biometric studies of fetal weight[33,34,207,223,233,242,247,270,274] and organ volumes[35,58,141,171,207,223] showed that 3D provides more accurate results.

Specific organ studies allowed to have available nomograms regarding:

- Anatomic structures (e.g. long bones)
- Volumetry of organs (e.g. the gestational sac, lung)[48,51,96,101,147,207,223]
- Functions (e.g. the heart)[42-44,106,137,142,176,177,214,215]
- Vascularization[206,218,219,236,237,244,245,247,272,280]
- Estimation of the fetal weight or fat content through the calculation of the muscle circumference.[52]

Extensive casuistics have shown that 3D improves the diagnostic accuracy of 2D in more than 70% of malformations.[23,24,27,120-132,227,228] Also the more recent specific reports on selected malformations, such as facial,[100,204] lips,[154] head, neck and spine,[23,138] abdominal wall,[118,213] limbs,[99,146] have confirmed these findings.

Regarding to the first trimester fetus, many either abdominal or transvaginal descriptions have been published.[10,14,17,18,20,23,24,26-29,31,32,54,57,65-67,79,93,108,115,134,136,151,201,212,225] The most outstanding are those related to studies from the cerebral cavities.[10,13,18,19,20-27,257,265,275] Also uterine introduced 10 MHz transducers were used[65] without success.

Gestational sac and secundines have been volumetrically studied.[59,91,181,184]

A new field of publications concerning the early diagnosis of malformations has appeared. They show the ability to study important markers of chromosomal anomalies such as the nucal translucency,[23,27,93] ectopia cordis[108] trisomy 18 affected fetuses[212] or conjoined twins.[24,28,74,115]

Outside of the prenatal diagnosis same important articles have been published related with assisted reproduction,[205,212,216,231,238,249,261,264,267,268,273,281] the cervix in pregnancy,[208] urogynecology,[214,276,277] gynecological and breast cancer.[234,235,239-241,243,260,279]

This chapter deals with the appearance chronology of embryonic and fetal structures up to week 16 based on our own previous published investigations.[13,14,17-20, 23,24,26,27]

ABDOMINAL ULTRASOUND

When using 2D, the transvaginal approach is much superior to the transabdominal for 3D in the first trimester. Abdominal 3D should not be recommended.

Nevertheless, in this chapter, we are showing the 3D schedule images of the abdominal US, because all machines are equipped with abdominal transducers but not all dispose of transvaginal transducers. These are an acquired option.

In our book "Atlas de ecografia obstetrica" of 1988, the schedule of apparition of embryonic and fetal structures according to the gestational week was established.

This embryologic-echographic schedule is totally adaptable still today to the first trimester abdominal 3D (Graphics 31.1 and 31.2).

Because of its low interest and the difficulty in obtaining good 3D first trimester abdominal images, there is a scarcity of publications. However, with a careful examination exceptional quality 3D images can be obtained:

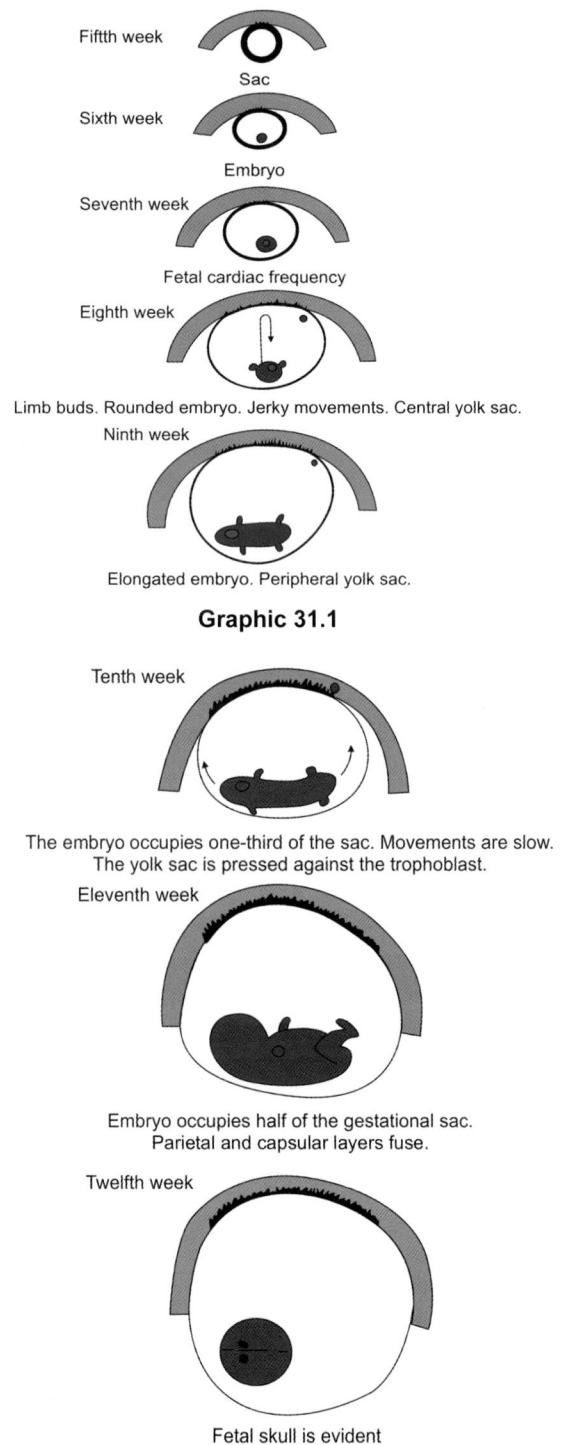

Fiftth week — Sac

Sixth week — Embryo

Seventh week — Fetal cardiac frequency

Eighth week
Limb buds. Rounded embryo. Jerky movements. Central yolk sac.

Ninth week
Elongated embryo. Peripheral yolk sac.

Graphic 31.1

Tenth week
The embryo occupies one-third of the sac. Movements are slow. The yolk sac is pressed against the trophoblast.

Eleventh week
Embryo occupies half of the gestational sac. Parietal and capsular layers fuse.

Twelfth week
Fetal skull is evident

Graphic 31.2

Fifth Week

The gestational sac can be observed with the following characteristics:

- Oval or round shaped with limpid boundaries
- Homogeneous trophoblastic rim greater than 5 mm
- No internal contour irregularities
- Progressive growth (1 mm per day).

The abdominal 3D gestational sac vision at this age does not result easy, and there is no improvement when compared with 2D. At the present only the transvaginal route is useful.

The sac's shape is round between the fifth and sixth week and becomes oval later on. Irregular forms such as enlarged, comma-like shaped, should not be considered abnormal if not accompanied by other anomaly/ies, such as:

- Irregular growth: no growth, to slow, to rapid
- Decidual refringency changes
- Contour irregularities
- Embryo not visible (vanishing), etc.

Abnormal sac forms in normal evolution pregnancies are common in cases of myomas, ovarian cysts, distended bladder or sigmoid, etc.

The gestational sac wall thickness decreases as the gestation progresses due to the progressive atrophy of the deciduas capsularis and parietalis.

Following the visualization of the embryo, the crown-rump length should be measured. This measurement should be made from the cephalic pole to the rump taking care to measure the embryonic curvature. The crown-rump length should be measured across the dorsal curvature.

Sixth Week

The most important finding is the embryonic visualization. It appears as an echorefringent round structure located in the inferior pole because of its specific gravity greater than that of the amniotic fluid. Its length is of approximately 10 mm.

The gestational sac grows approximately 1.15 mm per day, so that at the end of the sixth week it measures 20 mm, up from 10 mm at the beginning of this week.

The embryonic growth is of 1 mm per day, reaching 15–17 mm at the end of the sixth week.

Seventh Week

Along with the increasing size of the embryo and sac, the most important feature is the visualization of the cardiac activity. The embryo remains round.

Eighth Week

The limb buds appear in an embryo that is still rounded in shape. So-called jerky embryonic movements are detectable. We say so-called, because the embryo in fact moves up and down repeatedly within the sac.

The yolk sac can be observed in a location near the gestational sac.

Ninth Week

For the first time, the embryo appears elongated with definite cranial and caudal poles. The limbs are fully developed, although the fingers are not yet visible. The yolk sac is in a more peripheral location.

From this week on, 3D visualization is superior to 2D due to the amount of the existing amniotic fluid (Fig. 31.1)

Tenth Week

So-called slow and lazy movements appear. They are characterized by fetal rotations around its longitudinal axis, balancing and movement of the extremities.

The fetus occupies more than a third of the space in the gestational sac; it can be well defined with 3D along with the yolk sac (Figs 31.2 to 31.4).

Eleventh Week

There is fusion of the parietal and capsular decidual layers, eliminating in this way what is considered a gestational sac.

The fetus occupies now half of the amniotic cavity. Structures in the head, abdomen and limbs are clearly visible.

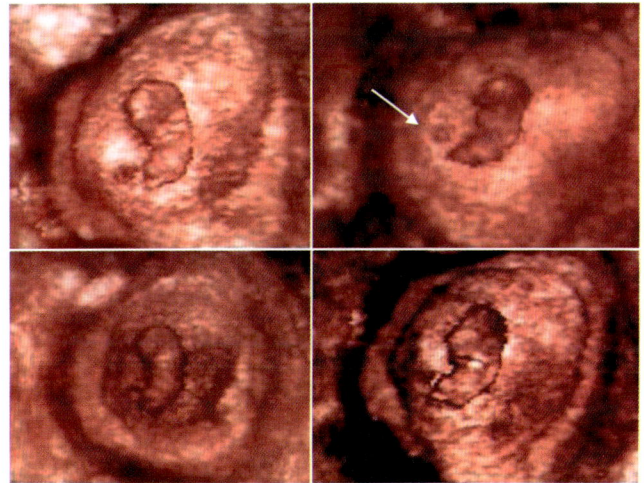

Fig. 31.1: Abdominal 3D US in 9+6 weeks. Observe the profile of the embryo lying over the placenta, showing well defined cranial and caudal poles. The yolk sac can be seen in the upper pictures (arrow). The remaining pictures show the lower limbs

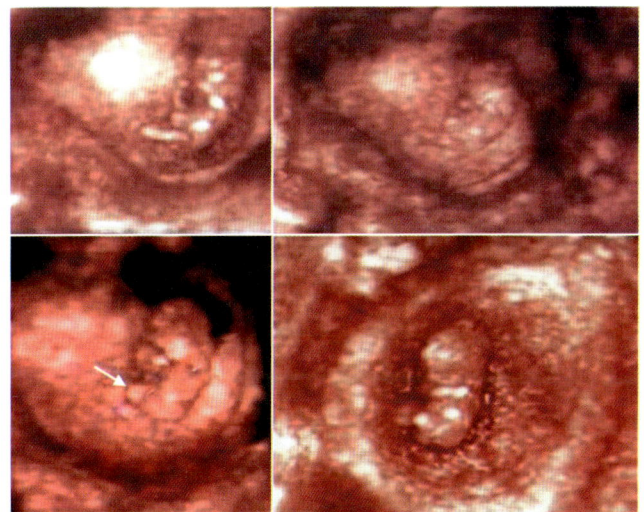

Fig. 31.2: Abdominal 3D US first trimester. 10+1 weeks. The fetal head, abdomen and extremities are clearly defined. The ossification nuclei of the jaw and the face profile along with the four limbs are visible. The physiological herniation is depicted in the two lower pictures

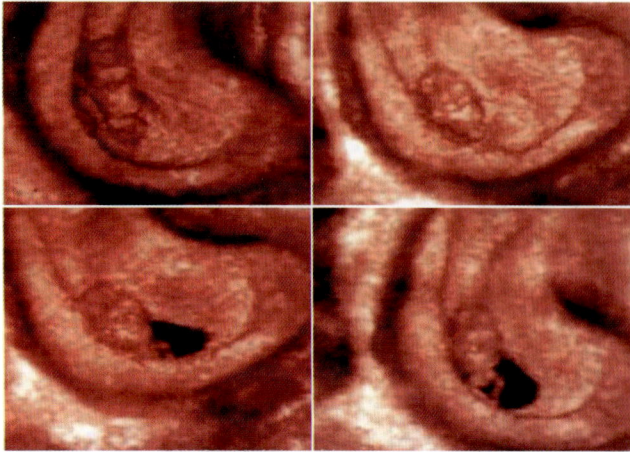

Fig. 31.3: 3D abdominal US. 10+3 weeks. Frontal view of the fetus showing semi-extended legs. The fetus is resting on the placenta (left upper and lower pictures), seen in a frontal view where the face can be observed (bottom right) and the feet already formed (bottom pictures)

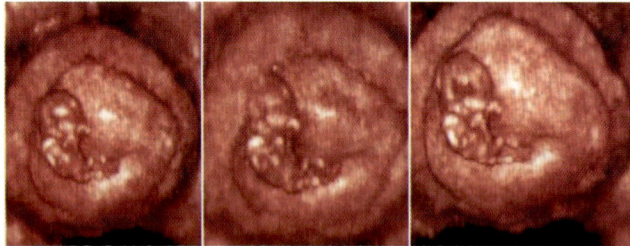

Fig. 31.4: Abdominal 3D US 10+4 weeks. The extremities are complete. The fetus lies over the placenta. Fully developed fetus with well-formed arms and legs lying over the placenta

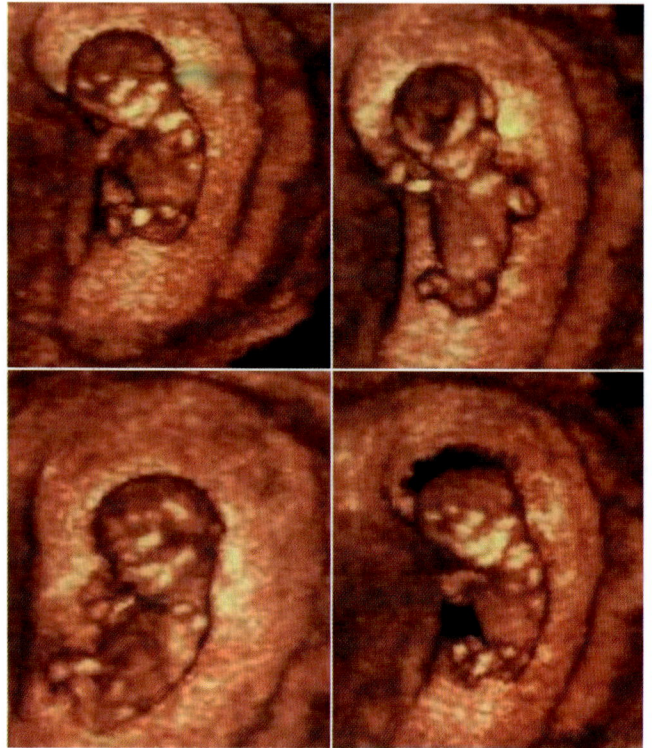

Fig. 31.5: Abdominal 3D US in first trimester. 13 weeks. In this fully developed fetus the physiological herniation has disappeared. The orbits, nose, mouth, and limbs with hands and feet can be seen

Twelfth till Sixteenth Week

In week twelve, the skull is fully formed (Figs 31.5 and 31.6). Facial and abdominal structures can be observed. Hands and feet are fully developed. Finger and toes are identified.

From week thirteenth on the normal fetal development can be followed (Figs 31.7 to 31.12).

Twin Pregnancy

Twin pregnancy can be diagnosed after week 6, when two gestational sacs are clearly visible, each one with its own embryo.

It is not acceptable to miss a diagnosis of twins by transabdominal ultrasound examination after the 8 weeks of pregnancy (Fig. 31.11).

The gestational sac appears round or oval in shape, perfectly delimited by an echogenic zone greater than 3 mm: the trophoblastic rim. At this time, the gestational sac size is of 2–3 mm (Graphic 31.3).

One day after, the yolk sac appears. It is round, central, well delimited and measuring 3–4 mm in diameter (day 32 ± 1 day). He is linked through the omphalomesenteric duct to the embryo.

On day 33 (± 1 day) the embryo can be seen, laminar, small, wide, refringent and 2 mm in length. The yolk sac is always visible facing the ventral surface of the embryo.

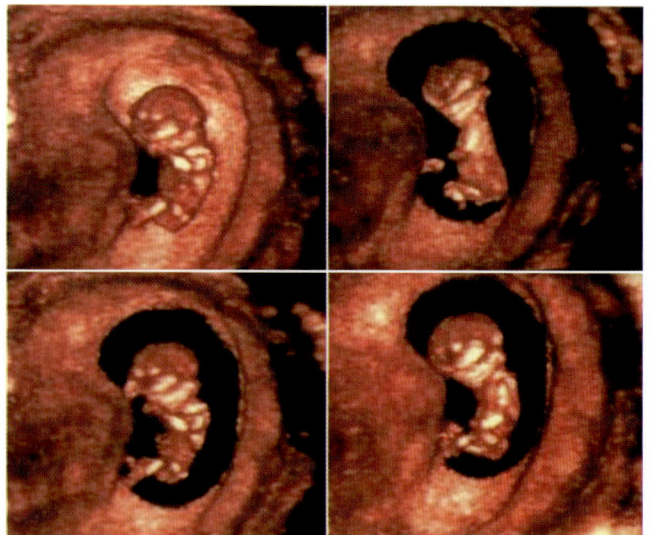

Fig. 31.6: Thirteen weeks days. This image shows hands and feet with fingers and toes

TRANSVAGINAL 3D ULTRASOUND

Fourth Week (from 4+0 to 4+6 days)

The first structures observed with 3D as with transvaginal 2D are obtainable between weeks 4 and 5.

The first suspicious image of a pregnancy is the persistence proximal to the menstrual days of a decidual transformed endometrium accompanied by a vascular active corpus luteum (Fig 31.13).

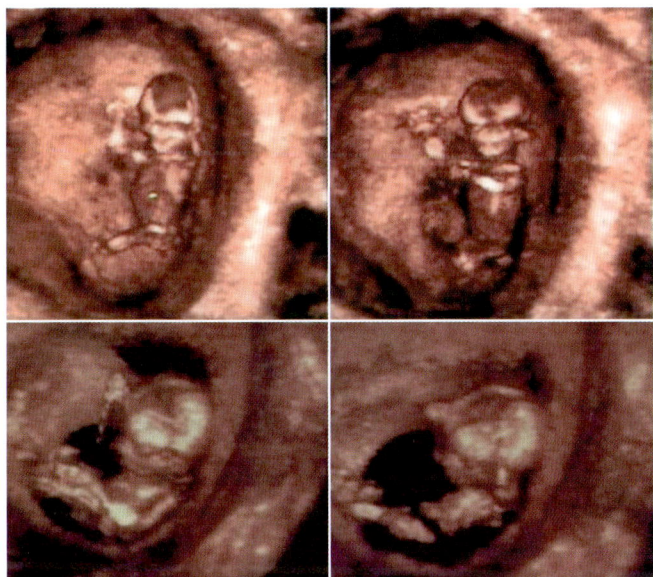

Fig. 31.7: Fourteen weeks and one day gestation (above). Observe the frontal view of the fetus with uplifted arms, the superciliary arches, the nose, ears and hands. Bottom: Fourteen weeks and four days gestation. Fetal profile, superciliary arches, eyes, sutures and fontanelles

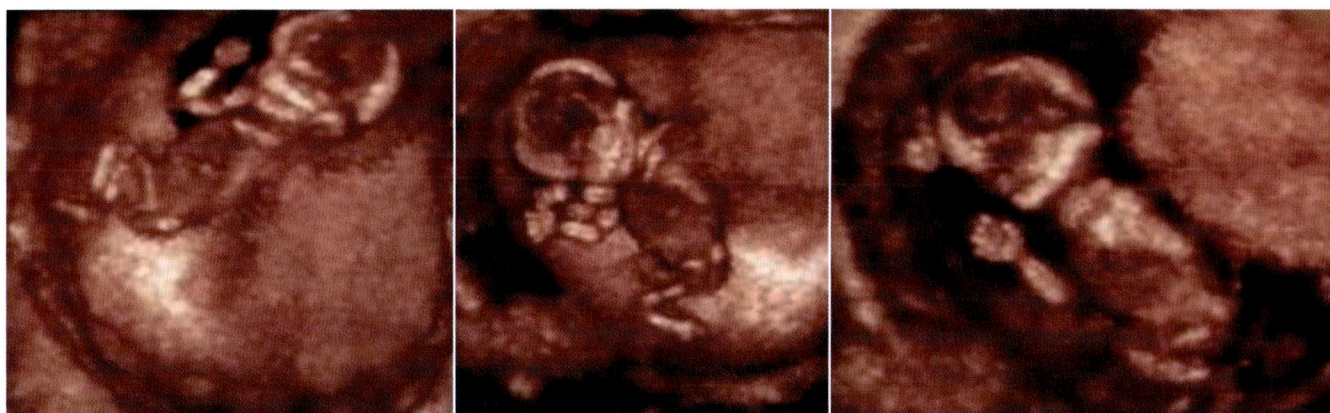

Fig. 31.8: Fourteen weeks and five days pregnancy. This lying fetus reveals arms and hands with clearly defined fingers. The mouth can be seen on the profile view of the face (left)

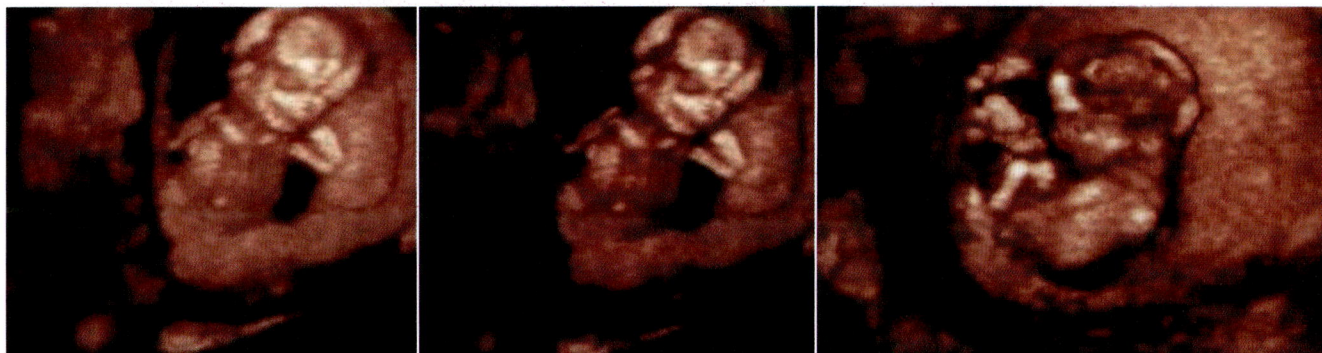

Fig. 31.9: Fifteen weeks plus one day pregnancy. Frontal view of a fetus. Skull bones along with sutures, fontanelles, orbital sockets, mouth and lower limb bones. The right figure shows the profile, forehead, eyes, nose and mouth

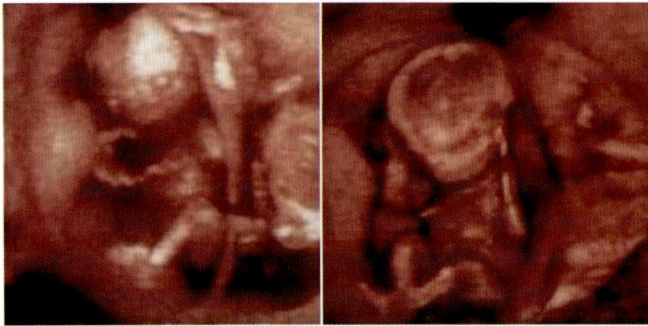

Fig. 31.10: Gestations of fourteen plus four and plus five days. At the left, the fetus shows open eyes. At the right, the eyes are closed

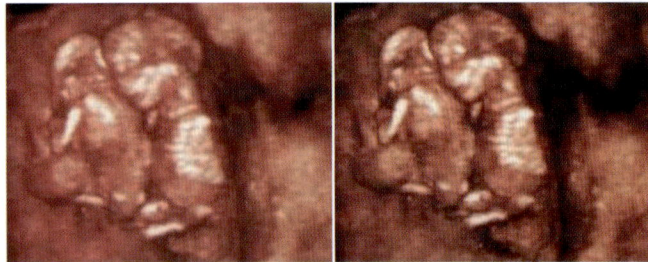

Fig. 31.11: Monochorionic twin gestation at 13 weeks and 3 days. Discordant fetuses are already evident. The fetus on the left side is already evident. The fetus on the left side is already smaller

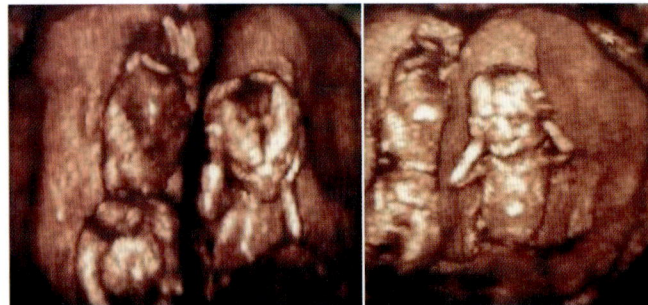

Fig. 31.12: Dichorionic diamnionic twin pregnancy at 14 weeks and 5 days. Both fetuses are aligned longitudinally, one in cephalic and the other in breech position. The face, sutures, and fontanelles of one of them can be observed

What is first observed is the gestational sac (day 31 ± 1), and the visualization threshold is nowadays established when the ß-hCG values have surpassed the 1000 mUI.

Being able to observe in the three orthogonal planes and with 3D rendering allows observation of the exact site of implantation in the endometrium (Figs 31.14 to 31.21).

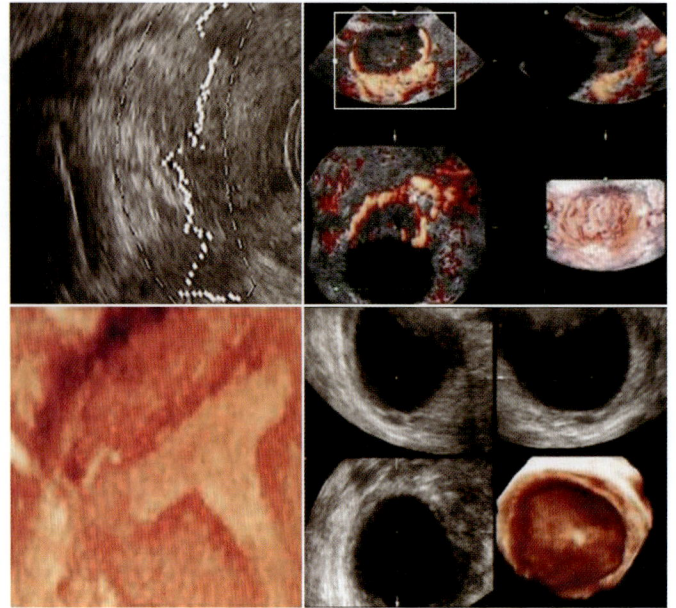

Fig. 31.13: Left images 2D and 3D of the decidua. To the right, the corpus luteum with its vascularization. The gestation is not yet defined

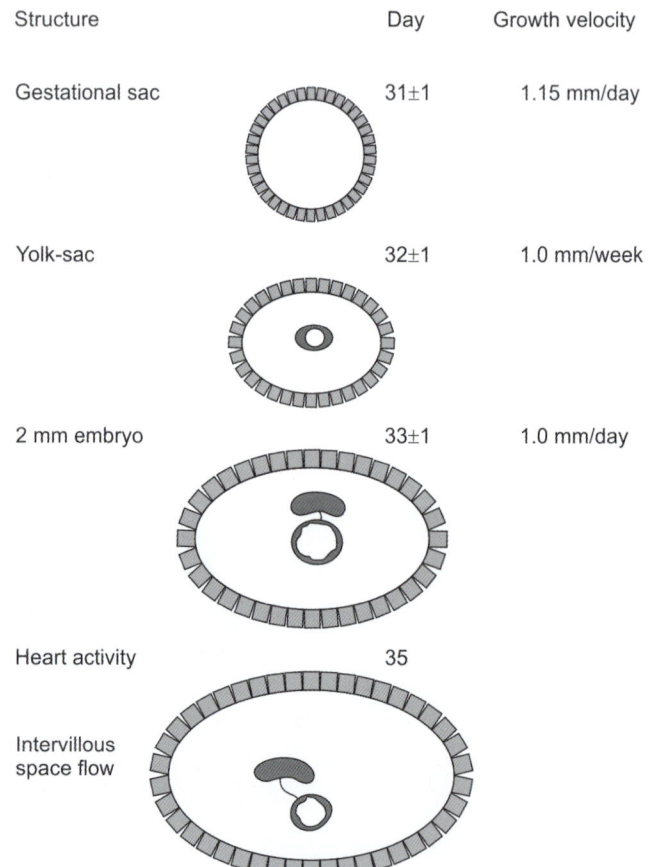

Structure	Day	Growth velocity
Gestational sac	31±1	1.15 mm/day
Yolk-sac	32±1	1.0 mm/week
2 mm embryo	33±1	1.0 mm/day
Heart activity	35	
Intervillous space flow		

Graphic 31.3

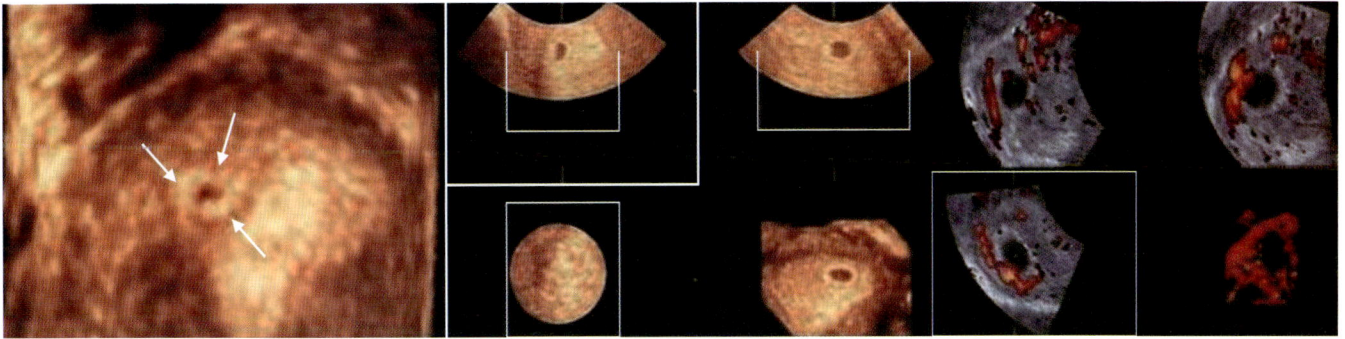

Fig. 31.14: Beginning of pregnancy. Weeks 4 to 5. Round or oval implanted gestational sac and its vascularization

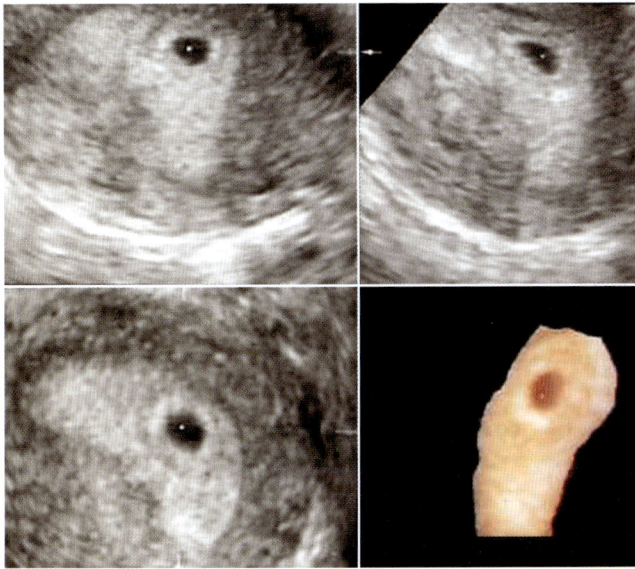

Fig. 31.15: Four weeks and three days pregnancy. The decidua and the gestational sac are showed. Observe the rim

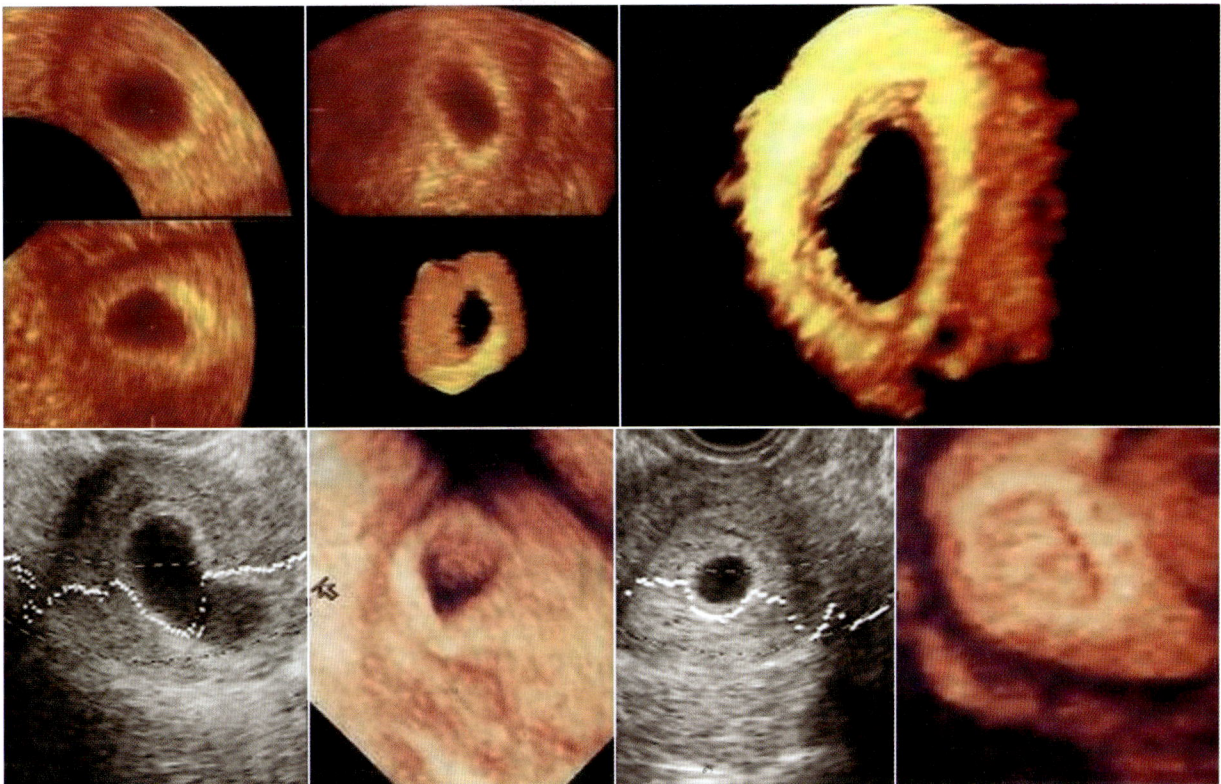

Fig. 31.16: 3D normal gestational sacs. The trophoblastic rim is clearly depicted and can be measured. Its thickness has to be bigger than 5 mm

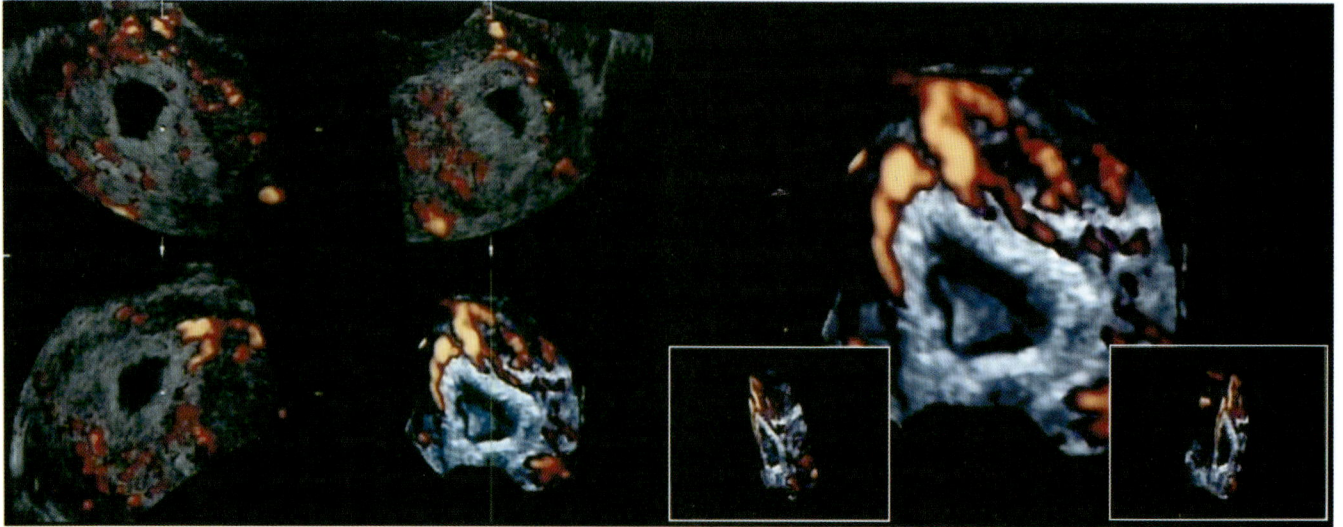

Fig. 31.17: 4D color Doppler of a normal gestational sac vascularization. Observe the trophoblastic rim

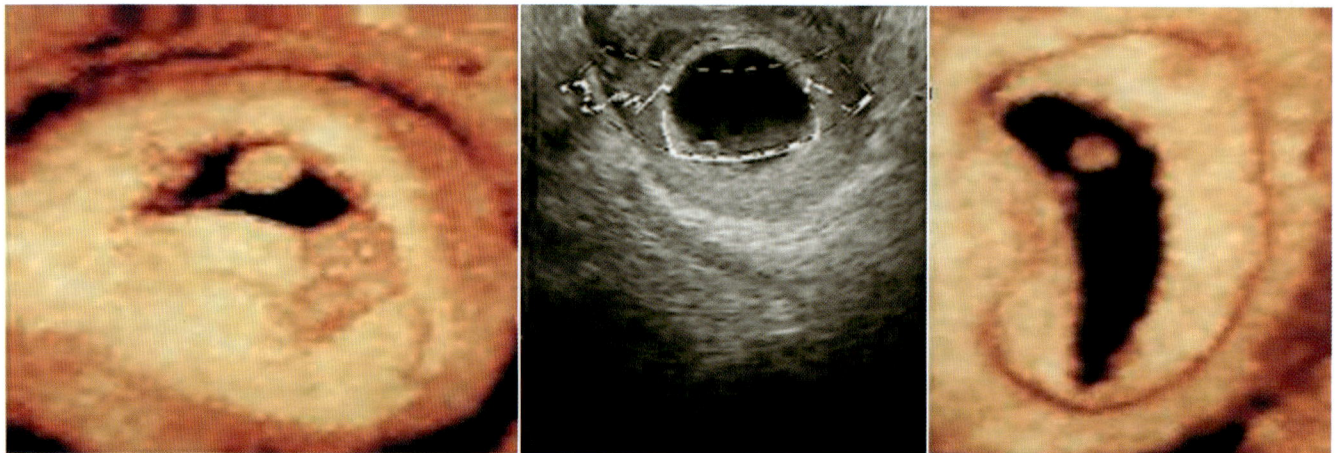

Fig. 31.18: Day 32. The yolk sac appears. A small segment of the omphalomesenteric duct can be observed in the left image

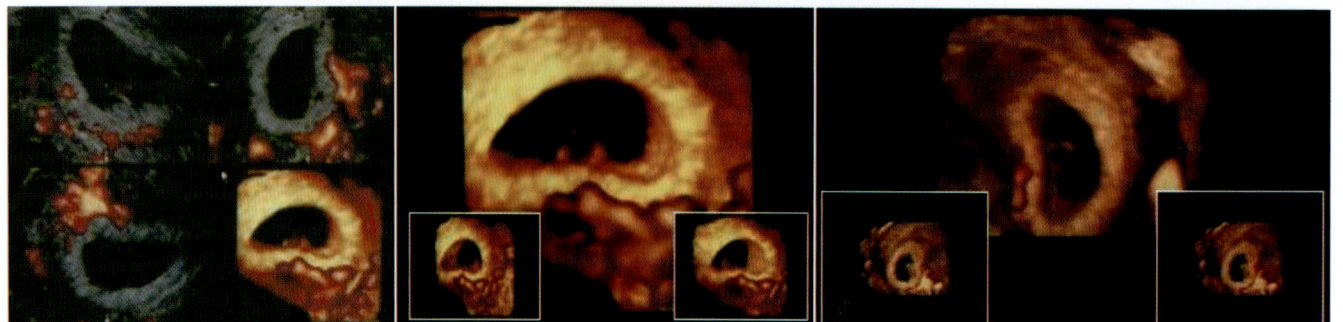

Fig. 31.19: 4D pictures of normal yolk sacs, gestational sacs trophoblast and vascularization

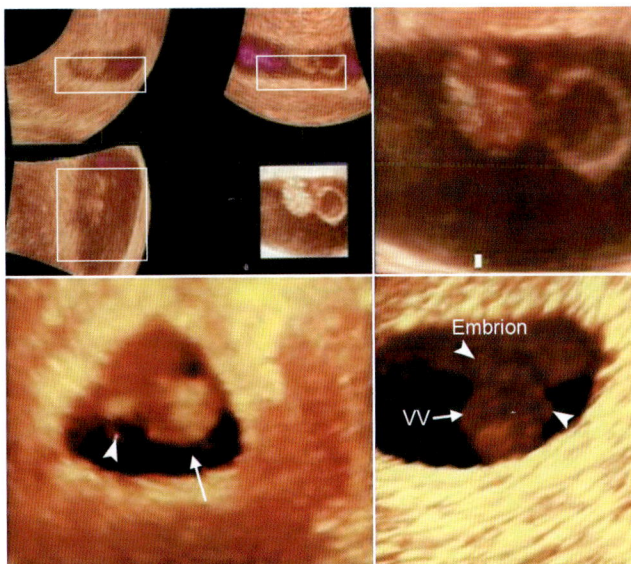

Fig. 31.20: Day 33 the embryo is visible measuring 2 to 3 mm. The yolk sac is faced to the abdominal embryonic wall. The embryo growths very rapid, and only days after is bigger than the yolk sac

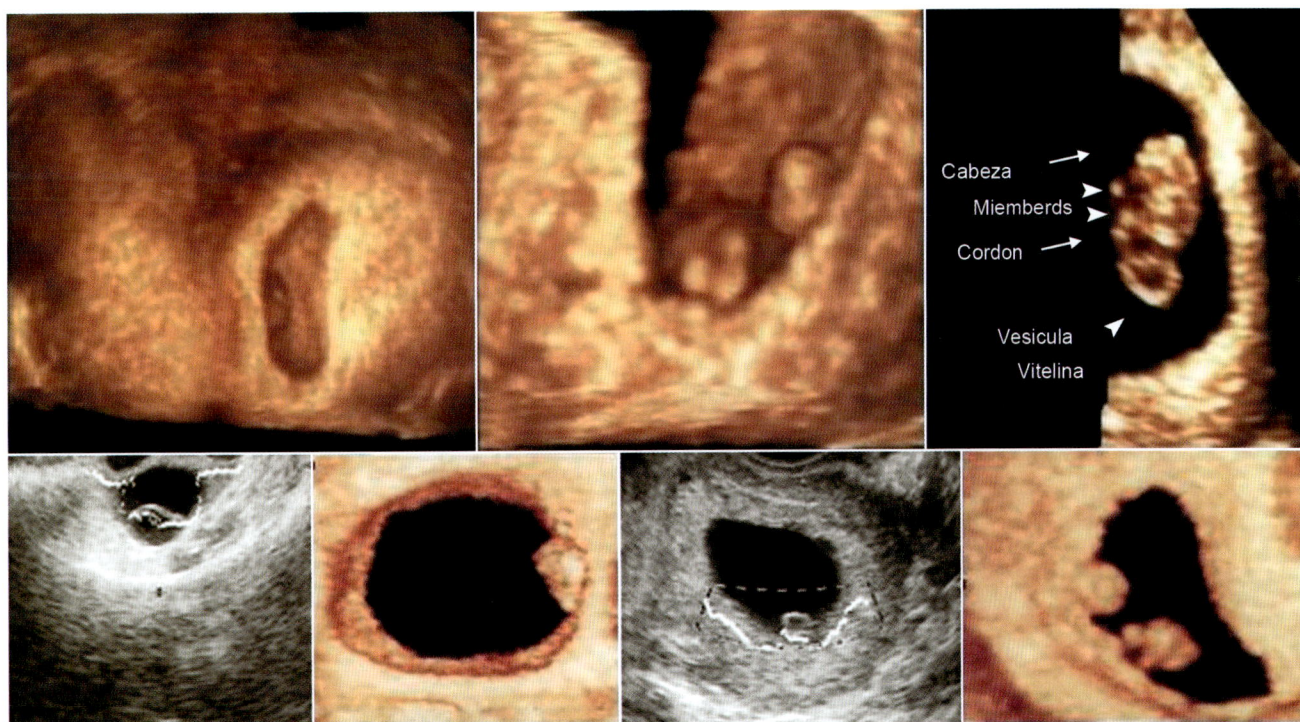

Fig. 31.21: Visualization of the embryo. Days 33–35. The embryo takes a laminar form. Two poles are depicted

In cases of multiple pregnancies, monochorial or bichorial, sacs and embryos can be observed. (Figs 31.22 to 31.26). Two sacs and two embryos in bichorionic or two embryos in one sac in cases of monoamnionic twin gestation.

Fifth Week

By the end of week 5, all these structures are evident; the embryo enlarges and is connected to the yolk sac by a long and slender duct (Figs 31.27 to 31.29).

From week fifth on, different organs and structures will appear and will be visible according to the schedule showed in (Graphics 31.4 and 31.5).

Sixth Week

In only on week, the embryo enlarges, allowing the observation of two well differentiated poles: the cranial and the caudal. Also the limb buds can be visualized, especially the superior, which appear earlier. This finding occurs earlier than what we have seen in transvaginal 2D US.

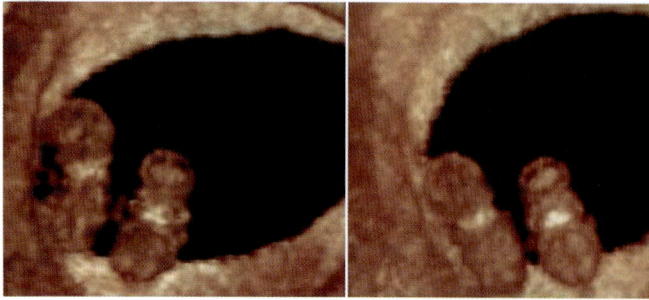

Fig. 31.22: Seventh week monochorionic monoamniotic twin pregnancy

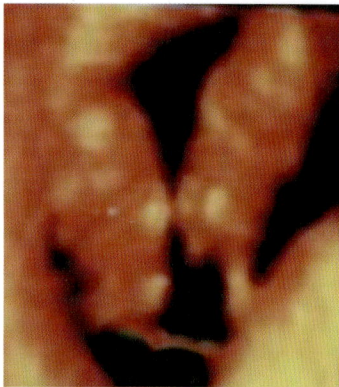

Fig. 31.23: Eight weeks monochorionic twin

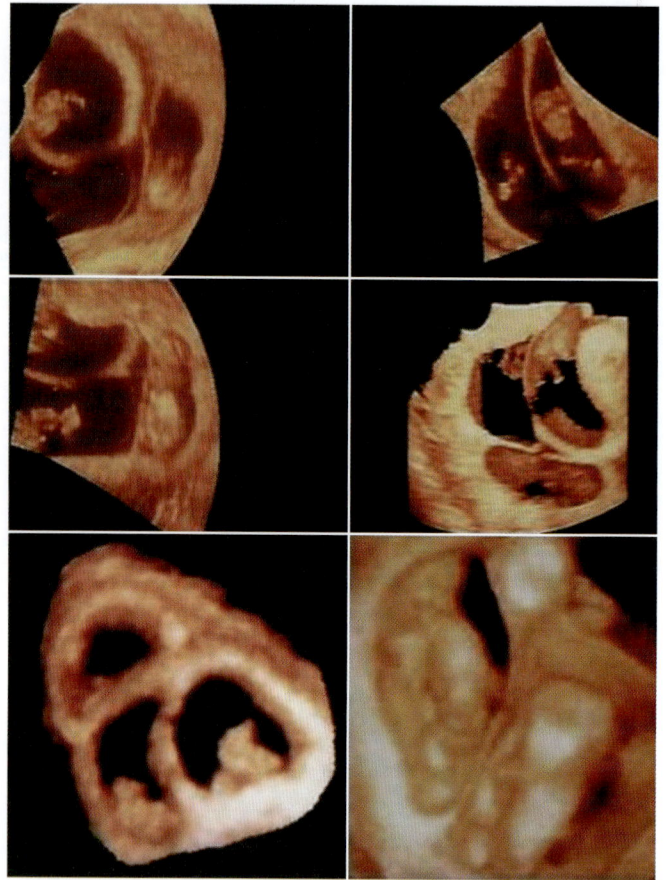

Fig. 31.24: Comparison between bichorial biamniotic with lambda sign twin (left) with a monochorial monoamniotic one (right)

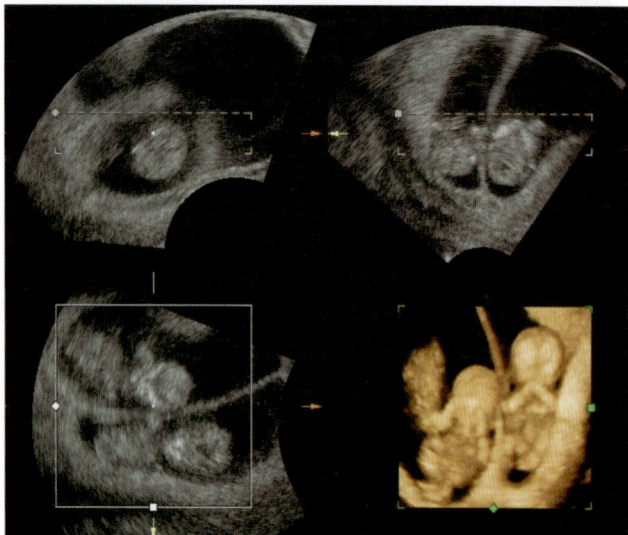

Fig. 31.25: Orthogonal planes and 3D rendering of a twelfth week twin pregnancy

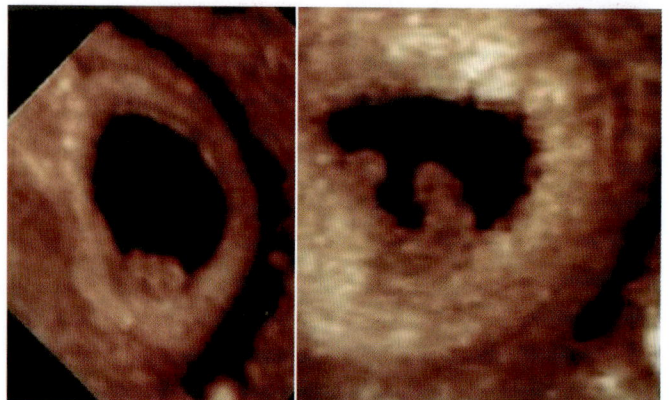

Fig. 31.26: Different cases of triplets. Above in week tenth and the bottom pictures in week sixth (left) and thirteenth (right)

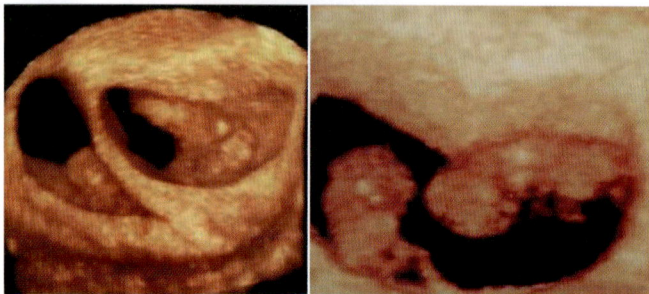

Fig. 31.27: Five weeks pregnancy. Elongated embryo with two poles. The yolk sac is visible on the left side of the right image

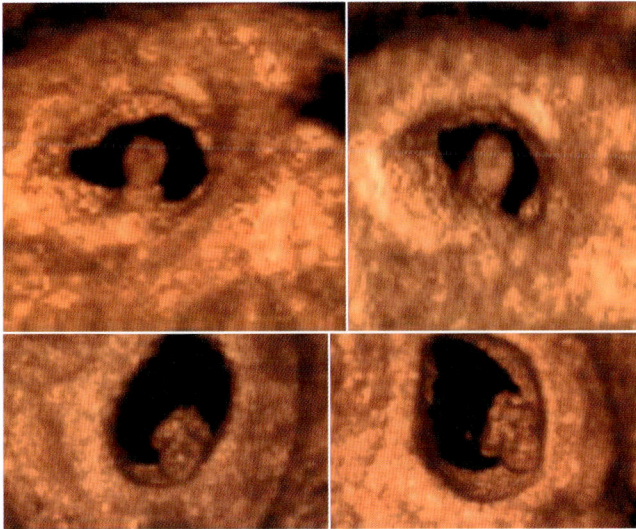

Fig. 31.28: Five weeks pregnancy. These four images show the embryo, still smaller and elongated, and the yolk sac round and faced to the embryo

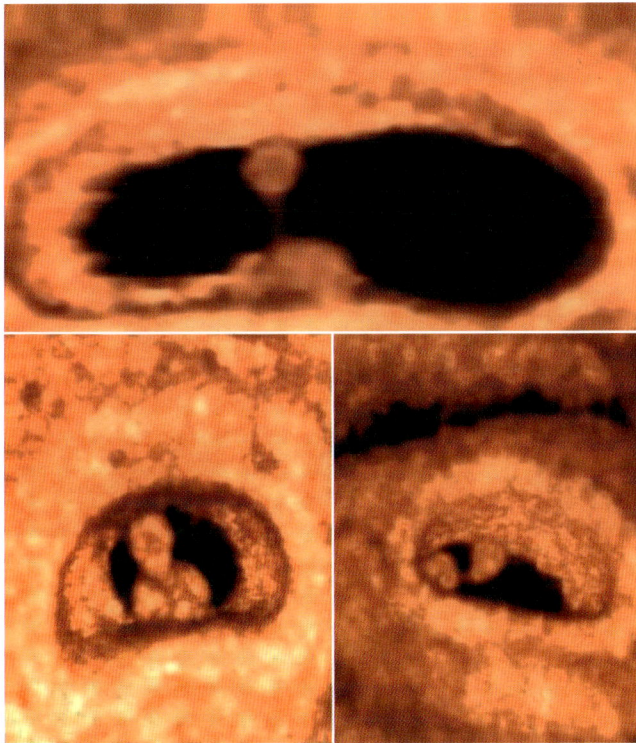

Fig. 31.29: The same case of Fig. 31.10. Five weeks pregnancy showing the embryo with a thin omphalomesenteric duct linking the yolk sac

Structure	Week
• Amnion • Two poles • Aortic flow • Cord flow	6 + 0 day
• Full amnion • Extraembryonic mesenchyme • Umbilical cord	6 + 6 day

Graphic 31.4

Structure	Week
• Extremities begining • Movements • Cerebral flows	7
• Extremities complete • Mesencephalon • Rombencephalon • Skeletal • Stomach	8
• Septum lucidum • Lateral ventricles • Choroid plexus	9

Graphic 31.5

Another interesting finding is that at this age in the distal portion of the caudal pole the cauda is visible. This structure is not observable with other ultrasound techniques.

In this week, it is especially remarkable to study the secundines:

The amnios appears as a very thin membrane in the surface of the dorsum of the embryo, just on the opposite side from where the yolk sac is visible. The amnion will soon surround the entire embryo, leaving out the extraembryonic mesenchyme and the yolk sac (Figs 31.30 to 31.33).

The yolk sac remains visible until weeks 13 to 14. It is always round and grows very slowly: 1 mm a week.

As the cord forms, its anchoring site narrows and thins out.

Seventh Week

The embryo clearly shows the limb buds. This detail is used to establish the gestational age (Figs 31.34 and 31.35).

The cephalic pole is flexed. It is very interesting that in the back of the embryo two parallel layers are observable which represent

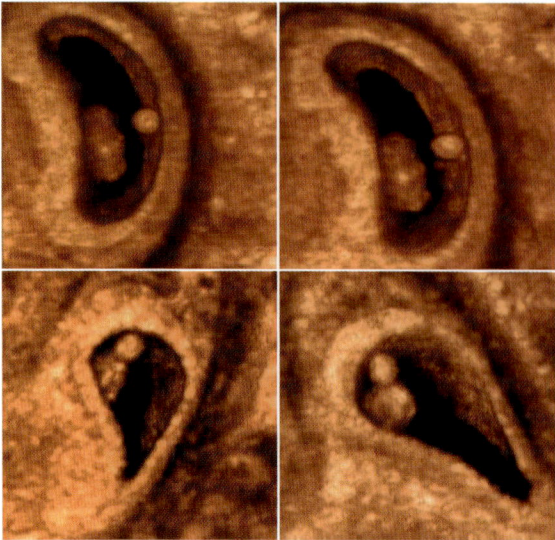

Fig. 31.30: Beginning of week 6. The embryo is much bigger than in week 5, shows clearly two poles, the craneal and the caudal, and the upper and lower buds of the extremities can be depicted. The cauda appears between the lower extremities buds

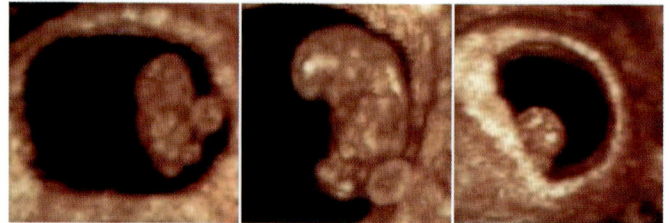

Fig. 31.31: End of week 6. The embryo shows a bigger size, the cephalic pole is slightly angulated, and the extremities buds are longer

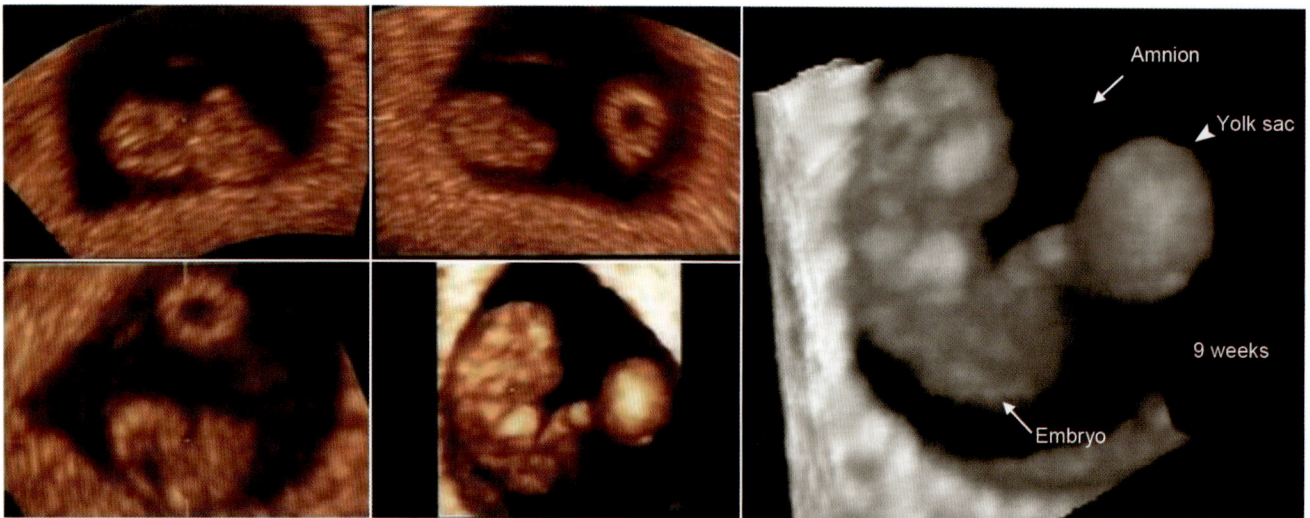

Fig. 31.32: These two figures show the 3D image of the whole omphalomesenteric duct and the yolk sac in week 6

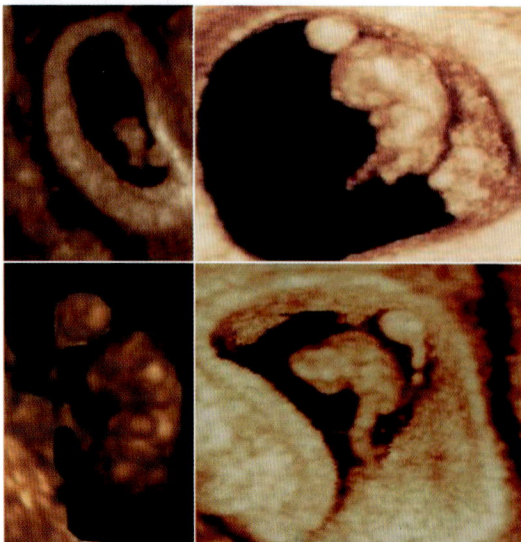

Fig. 31.33: End of week 6. The embryo shows in detail the curved cephalic pole and an elongated, sometimes thick sometimes thin but very long omphalomensenteric duct

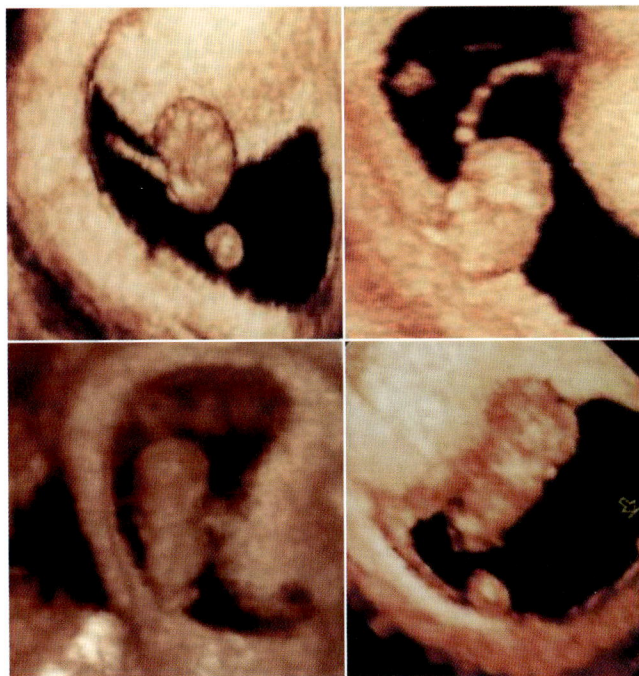

Fig. 31.34: Seventh week pregnancy. Observe the cephalic pole, the extremity buds, and a long coiled umbilical cord. The yolk sac lies away from the embryo

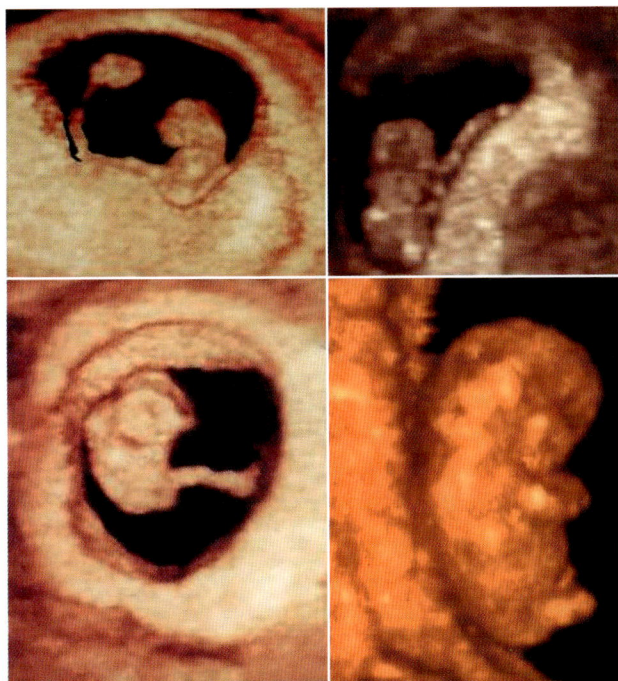

Graphic 31.6

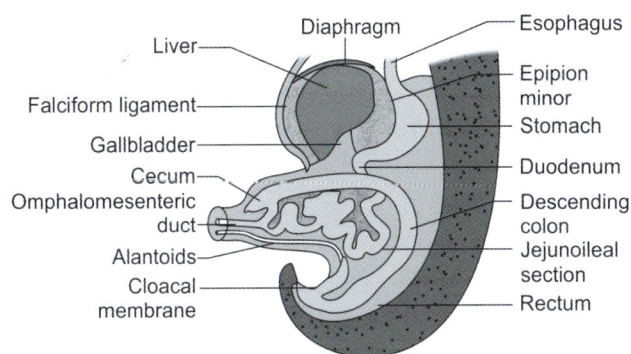

Fig. 31.35: Seventh week pregrancy, fetuses showing the cauda, the buds and a very long omphalomesenteric duct

the first vision of what will be the fetal spine. This finding is only visible with 2D TV ultrasound in the 8 weeks.

Eighth Week

The configuration of the embryo is completed. The cranial pole is large and voluminous. The profile, face, orbits, mouth, jaw and maxilla can be identified.

The caudal pole shows large limb buds with stubby ends that resemble hands and feet. Joints and articulations are visible.

The spine is completely formed, and appears as a white line in the dorsum. The superior portions (axis and atlas) still remain separate.

It is important to notice that at this week the physiologic herniation can be seen. It is a round and well defined structure, refringent, and linked to the abdominal wall at the site of the umbilical cord insertions (Graphic 31.6).

Its refringency is that of the abdominal wall, its size is small, less than 7 mm, and always disappears between the eleventh and twelfth week.

Although at this week the profile, forehead, nose and mouth are visible they will be clearly defined by the tenth week (Figs 31.36 to 31.39).

Ninth Week

At this week the head appears always flexed anteriorly and the finger and toes buds appear (Figs 31.40 to 31.42).

Tenth Week

The fetus is completely formed. Generally, the head is flexed over the thorax, but even so, we have been able to see the face with big orbits, lips mouth, etc. We can visualize prominent fontanelles and sutures on the forehead.

On the remainder of the fetal body, the arms are well developed with elbow and knee flexions as well as hands and feet visible (Figs 31.43 to 31.47).

The umbilical cord is very long and thick, proportionally larger and thicker than at the end of the pregnancy. By using the transparency system, we can observe for the first time, and identify, the femur, tibia, fibula, humors, radius and ulna. At the beginning of the eleventh week the superciliar arch, the orbits, eyes, forehead, nose, ears and jaw can be observed (Figs 31.44 and 31.45).

OTHER ORGANS AND STRUCTURES

The fingers and toes are clearly observed in the eleventh and twelfth weeks, and are better defined than what is seen with 2D TV US. (Figs 31.48 and 31.49).

It is of interest to note how these structures move independently. It is possible to notice that the thumb opposes the other fingers. The phalanges can be observed in fingers and toes.

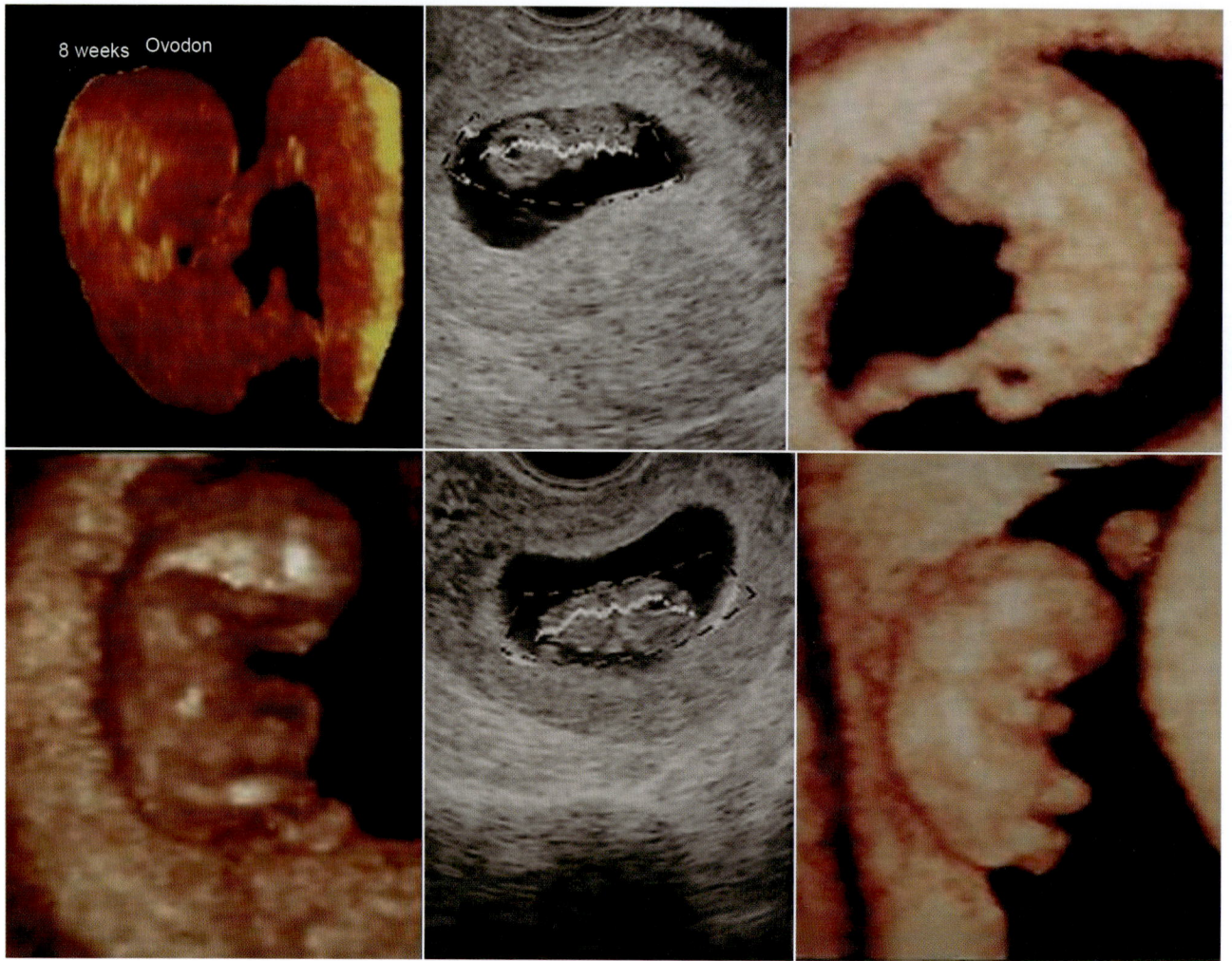

Fig. 31.36: Eight weeks pregnancy. The embryo shows full extremities. The profile can be identified. The umbilical cord is fully formed

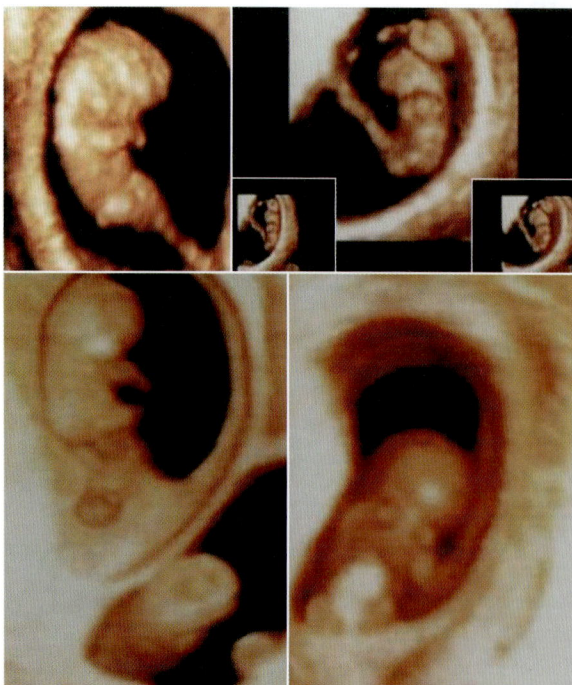

Fig. 31.37: Frontal and sagittal 4D view of an eighth week embryo

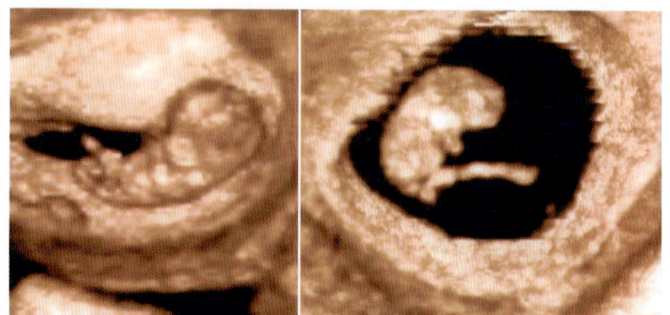

Fig. 31.38: This picture shows the ossification nuclei of jaw and maxilla. The mouth is visible as well as the complete extremities

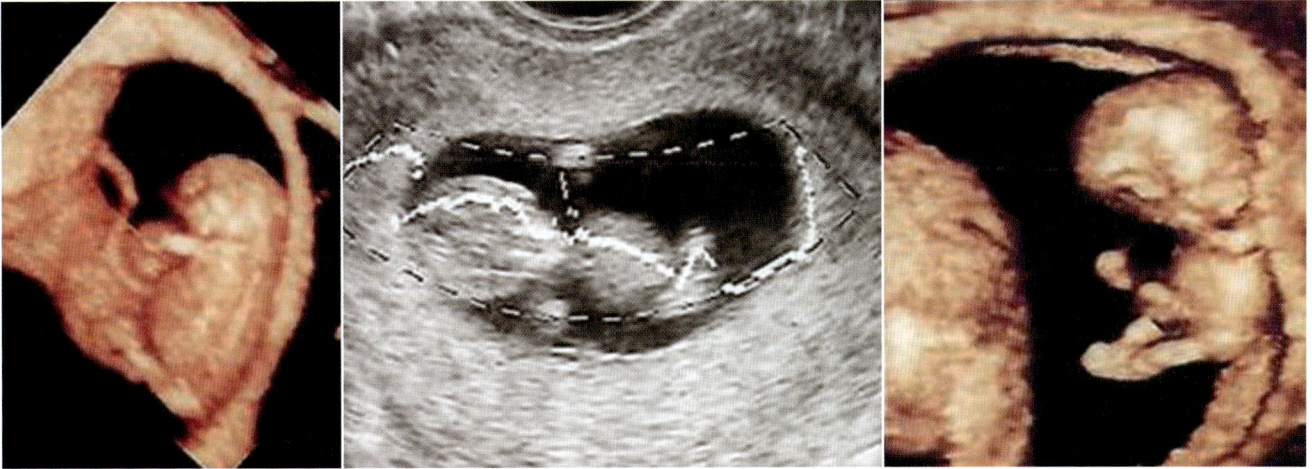

Fig. 31.39: Eigth weeks twin pregnancy showing the both fetuses the hand and feet

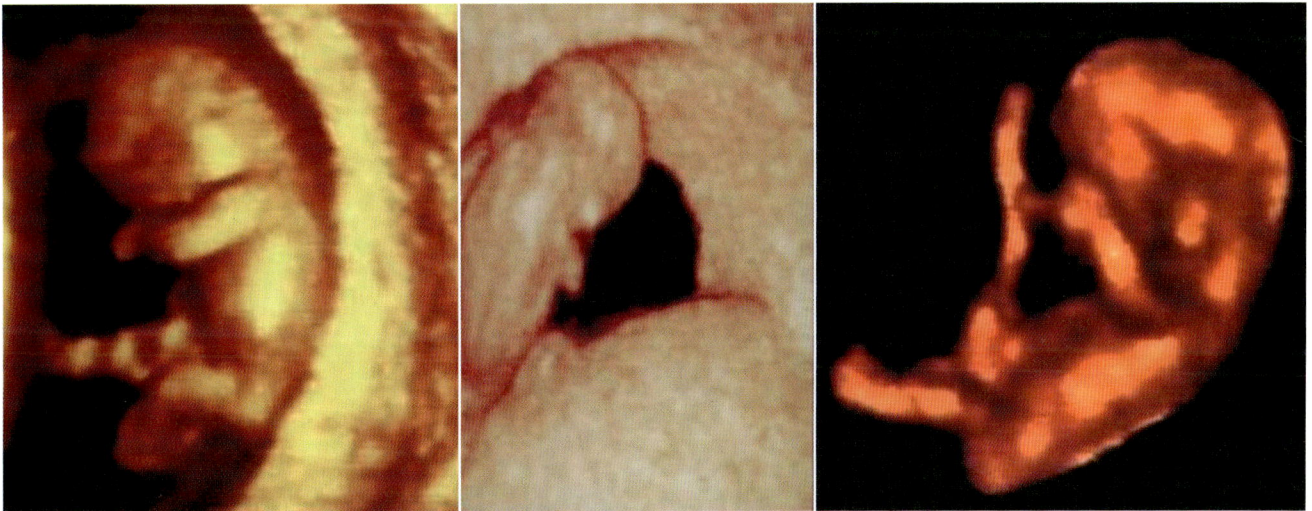

Fig. 31.40: Ninth week pregnancy showing the back with the medullary canal (center), a coiled (left) and a not coiled cord (right) and the physiological herniation (right)

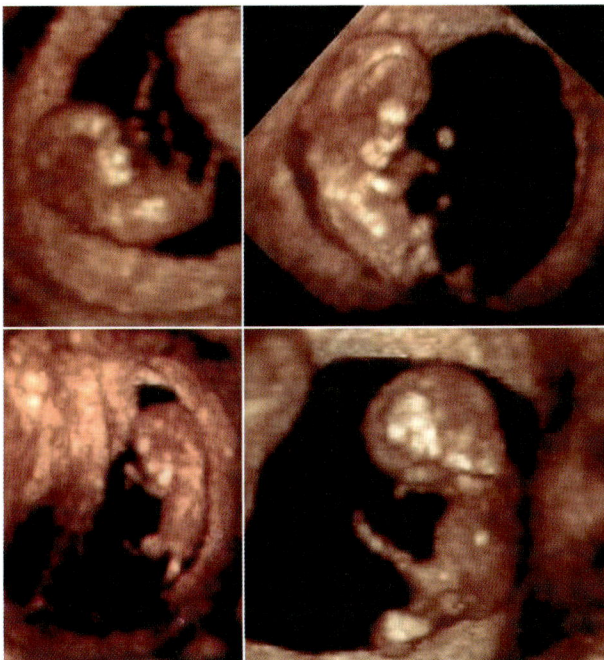

Fig. 31.41: These pictures showed different varieties of normal physiological herniations. Also the fetal profile is clearly depicted, showing the mouth, jaw and maxilla. See the feet

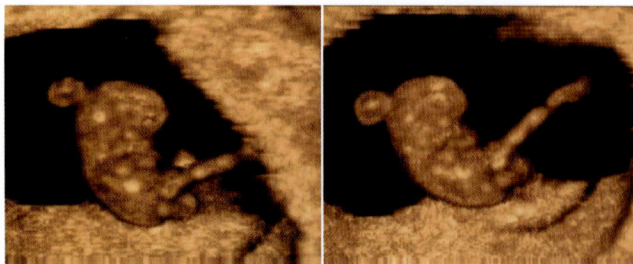

Fig. 31.42: Ninth week pregnancy. The fetus shows the yolk sac near the occipital bone. The profile, eyes, abdominal wall with the physiologic herniation, extremities and umbilical cord are clearly depicted

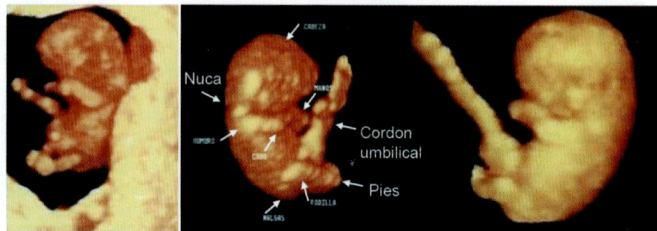

Fig. 31.43: Ten weeks fetuses showing a long umbilical cord with physiologic herniation. Hands and feet are visible

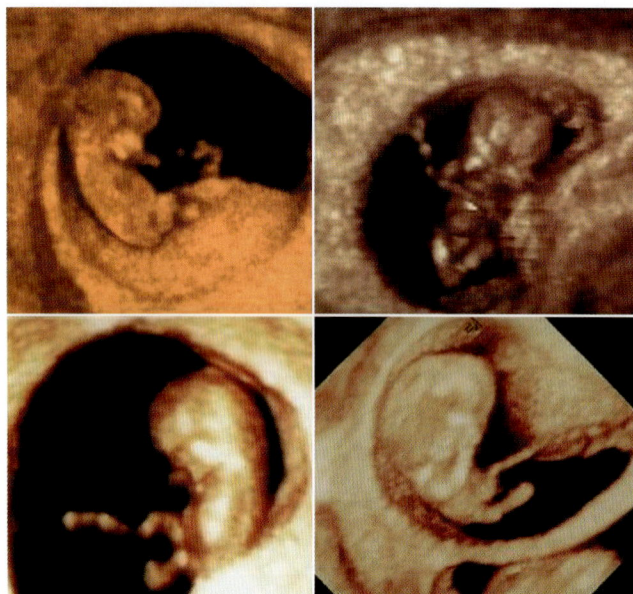

Fig. 31.44: Ten weeks fetuses. Frontal and sagittal view showing the mouth, nose, supercilliary arch, hands and feet. The umbilical cord is very long and coiled

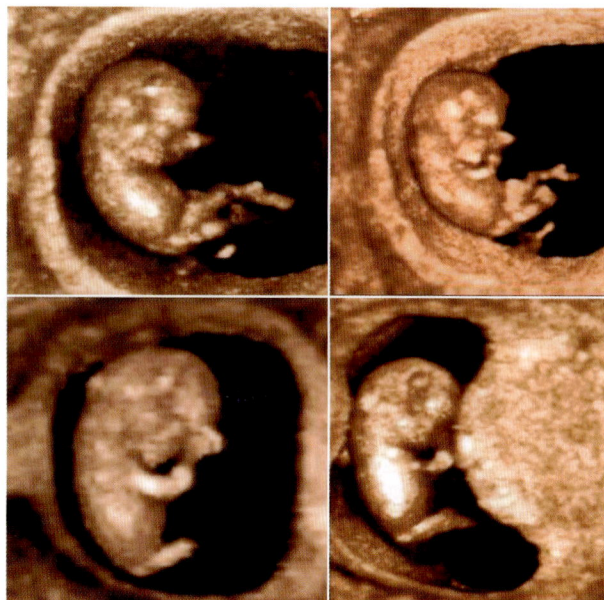

Fig. 31.45: Ten weeks fetuses. The hands are showing the finger boots. Eyes are also visible

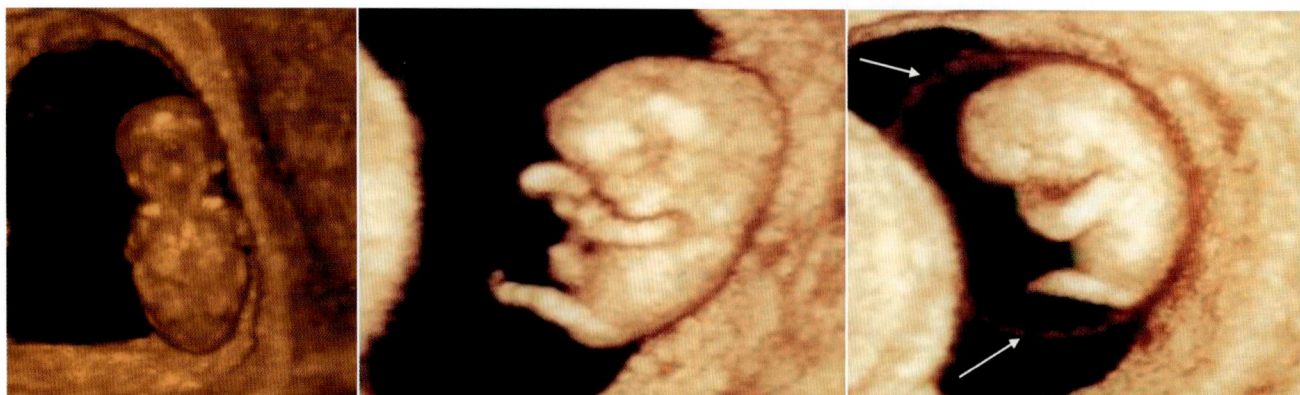

Fig. 31.46: Above, shoulder of a 10 weeks fetus looking at the sky. Observe the ears and the claviculae. Bottom, 10 weeks normal fetus surrounded by the amnion (arrows)

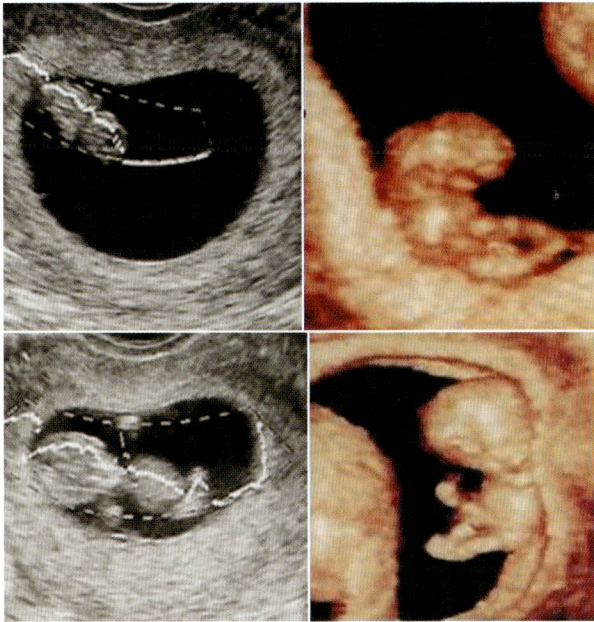

Fig. 31.47: Ten weeks of pregnancy. The fetus shows the profile and the eyes and it is involved by the amnion. Extremities, hands and feet are clearly depicted

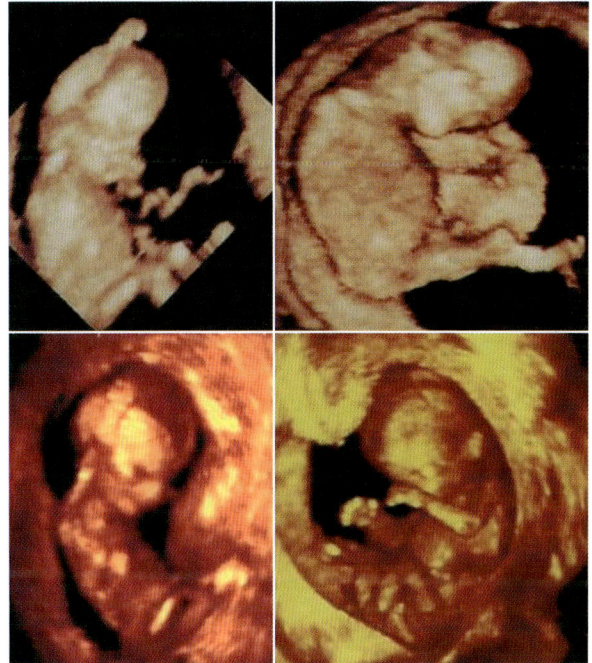

Fig. 31.48: Eleventh week fetuses. The herniation is getting smaller

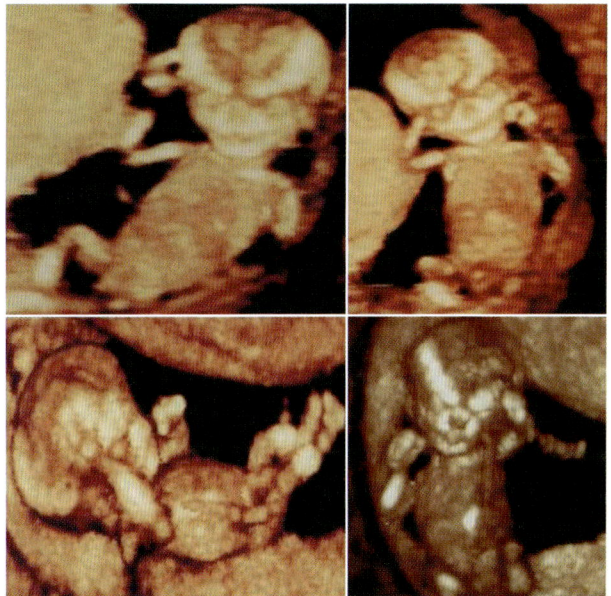

Fig. 31.49: Twelfth week fetuses. Visualization of the whole fetus, umbilical cord and placenta

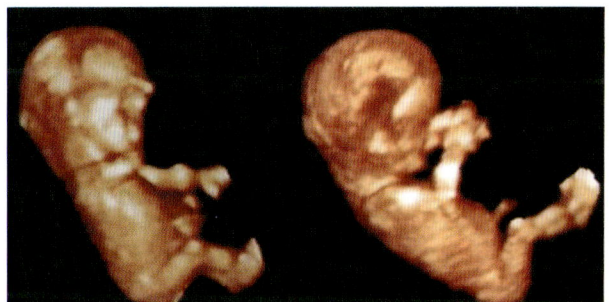

Fig. 31.50: Visualization of fetuses of thirteenth weeks, showing intense arm and leg movements

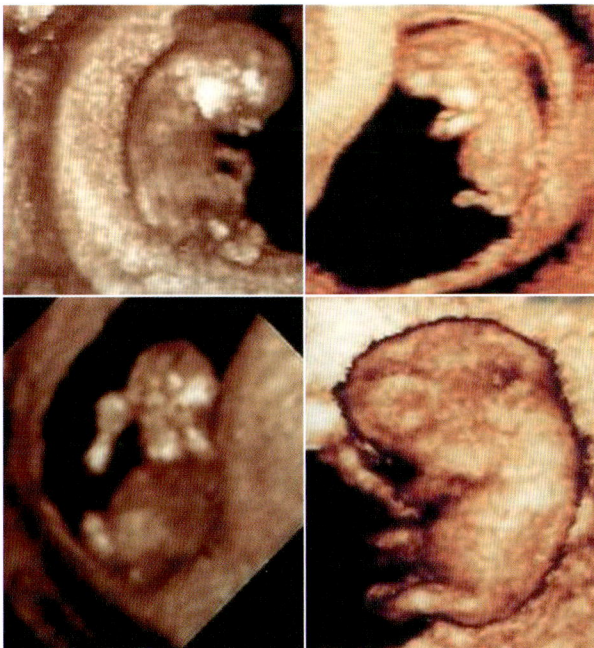

Fig. 33.51: Frontal view of thirteenth week fetuses showing the development of the face. Special details can be observed from the development of the nose, eyes and mouth

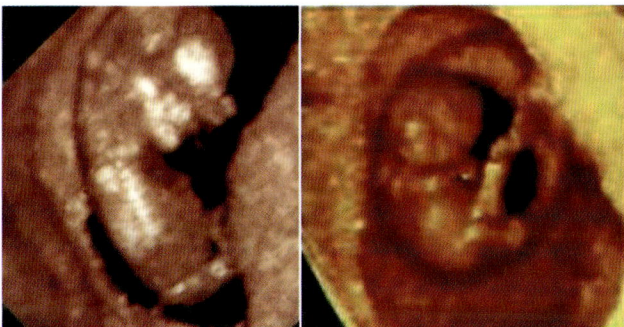

Fig. 31.52: 4D thirteenth week fetus showing complete developed arms and legs

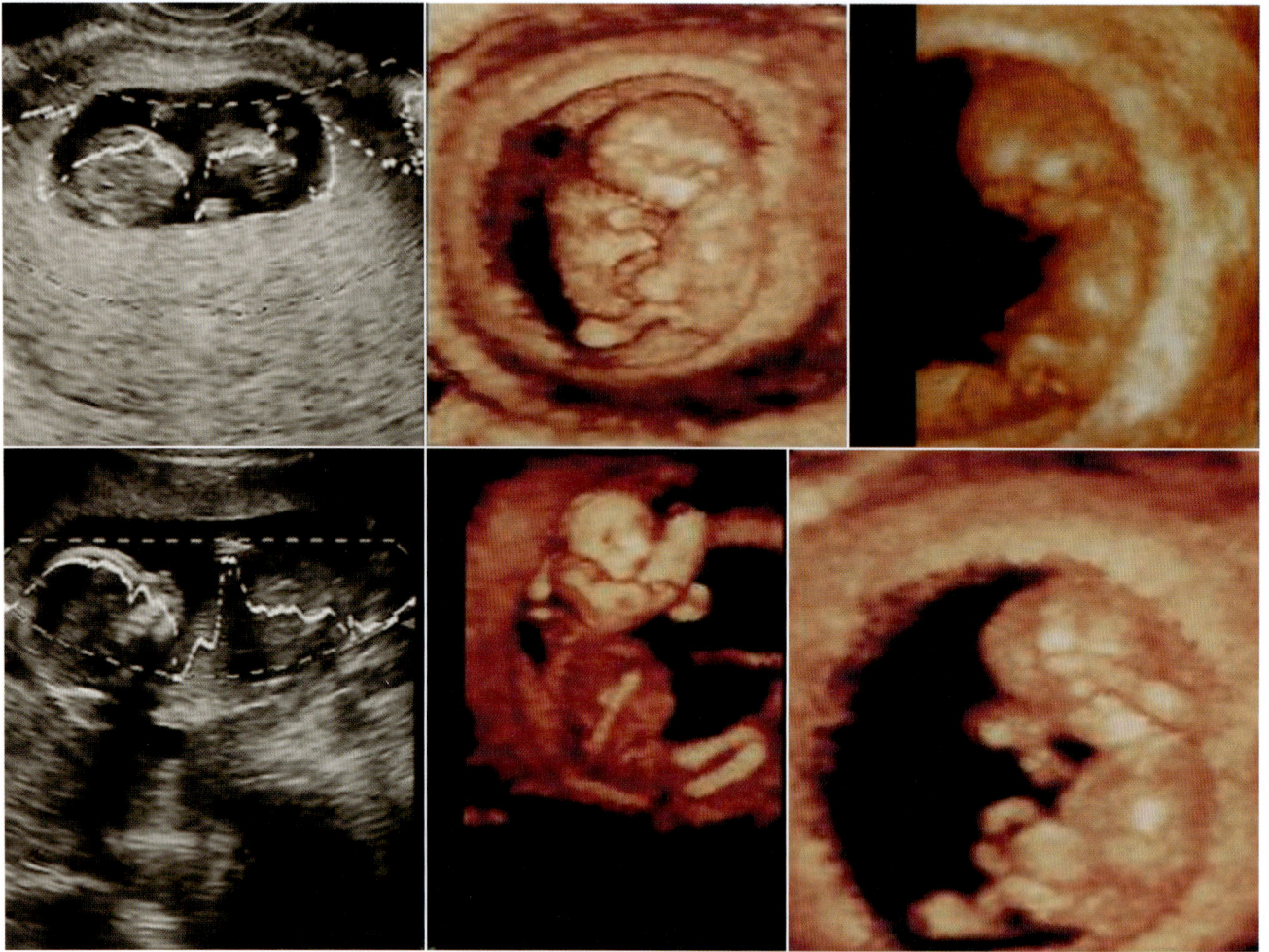

Fig. 31.53: 3D and 4D visualization of thirteenth week fetuses. The herniation has disappeared. The femur, tibia and ulna are visible

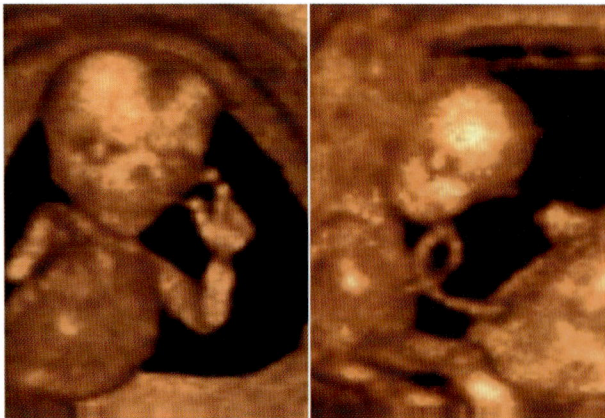

Fig. 31.54: Fourteenth week fetuses showing the face, the fingers and the palm, as well as the arm bones

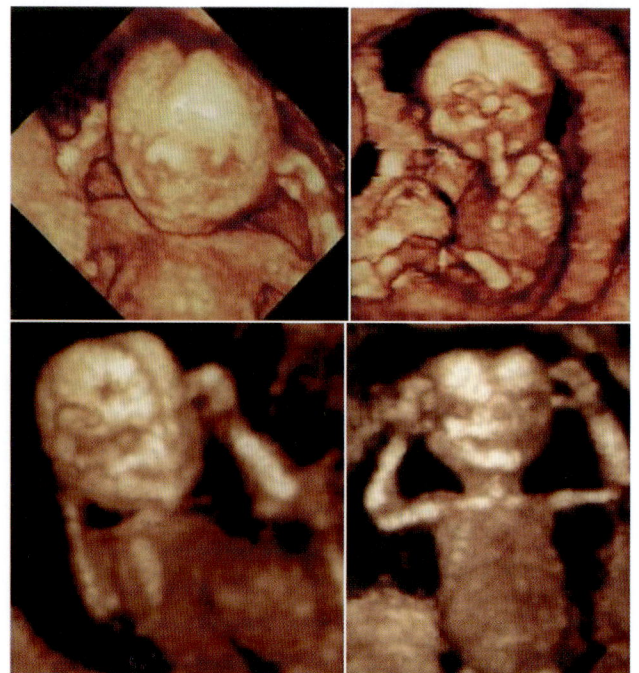

Fig. 31.55: Fourteenth week fetuses showing the whole face

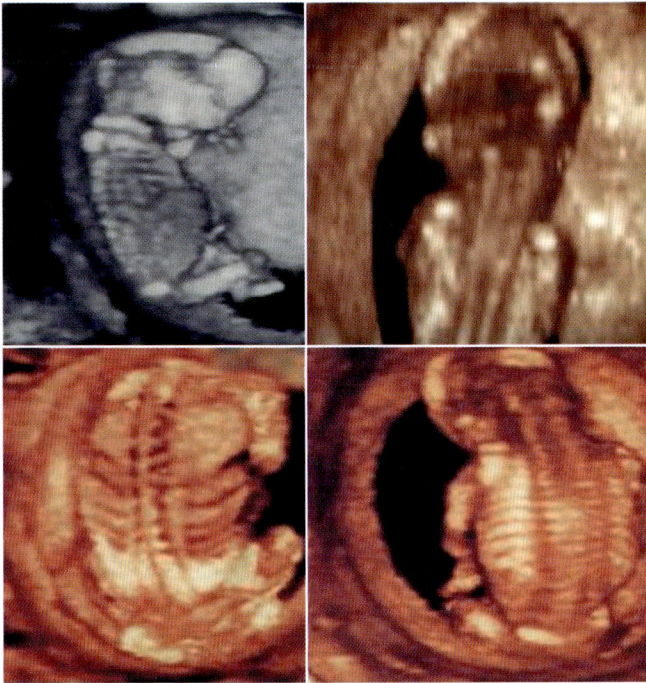

Fig. 31.56: Either the use of the transparence system or introducing the ROI into the thorax allows to study the thoracic cage, ribs, vertebrae and medullary canal

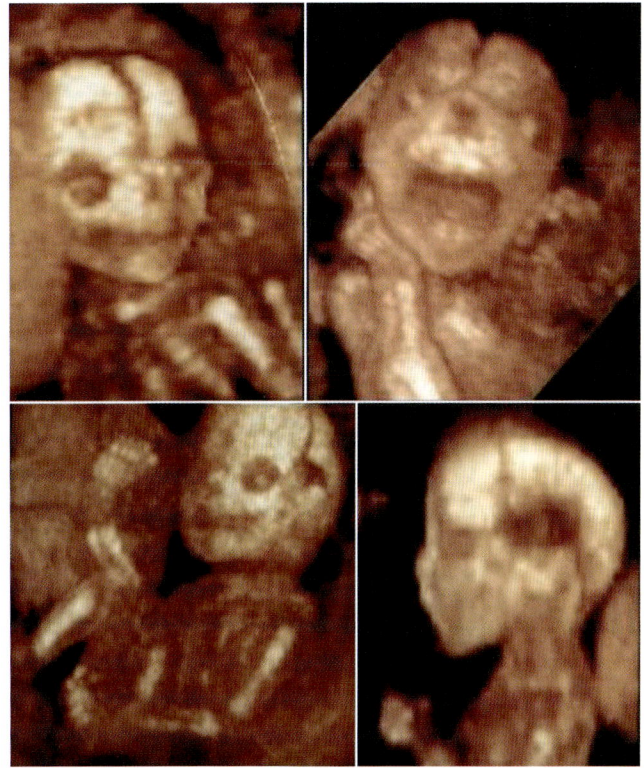

Fig. 31.58: Eighteenth weeks of pregnancy. The upper images are showing a fetus opening the mouth. The bottom images show the skull bones, fontanelles and sutures

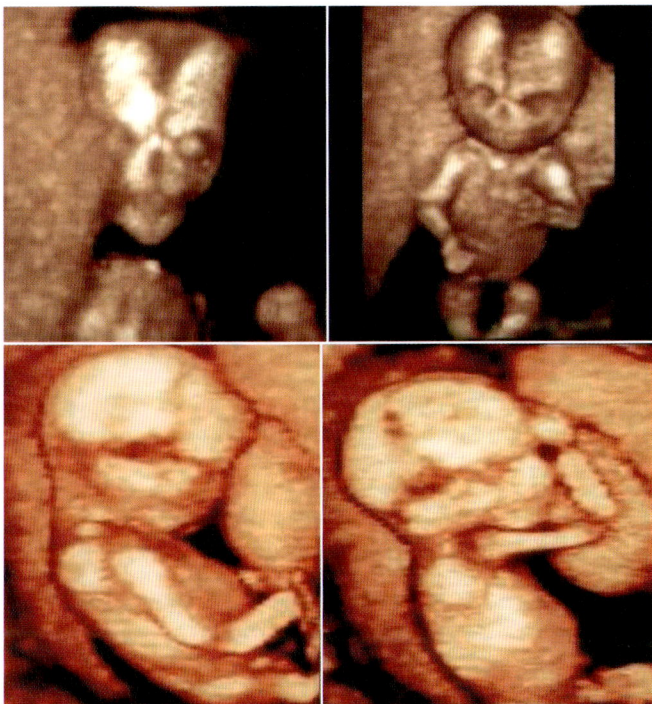

Fig. 31.57: Frontal and sagittal view of fetuses between week fourteenth and sixteenth showing the whole skull development. See the clear view of all bones and sutures

Although, we have observed movement since the seventh week, by the eighth week we can observe the fetus flexing its arms and legs across the abdomen. These movements, as well as others like opening and closing the mouth, etc. are better observed by using the 4D system available today (Fig. 31.50).

We consider the use of the transparency and X-ray systems essential for the study of the spine and pelvic bones after week twelve. In this way, the medullary canal, vertebrae, the ossification nuclei in the ribs can be visualized. It is important to remember that the high portion of the spine is not completely closed until the end of week 12 (axis and atlas). This is of great importance for cases of hygroma colli (see the corresponding chapter), and we think that this will also serve in the future for early diagnosis of neural tube defects. (Fig. 31.56).

At the same time the ribs can be seen, principal pelvic bones (ischium and ilium) and their ossification. All of this will be useful to measure the intervertebral spaces.

Normally, fetuses are flexed, and cover their faces with their hands. But after the tenth week they can deflex, showing in this manner their faces. The orbits and eyes are more visible and the lids are evident (Figs 31.51 to 31.58).

The nose is more protuberant and is completely formed between weeks 10 and 13. The mouth, lips and jaw are perfectly defined. The sutures and fontanelles will approximate progressively (Figs 31.51, 31.53 and 31.57).

Finally, in some cases we have observed the fetal sex clearly as early as the thirteenth week only in male fetuses. The labia of female fetuses can occasionally be distinguished clearly during the sixteenth week.

REFERENCES

1. Achiron R (Ed). The art of ultrasound in obstetrics: from abstraction to hyperrealism. Ultrasound Obstet Gynecol. 1995;6:1-3.
2. Ayida G, Kennedy S, Barlow D, et al. Contrast sonography for uterine cavity assessment: a comparison of conventional two-dimensional with three-dimensional transvaginal ultrasound. Fertil Steril. 1996;66:848-50.
3. Baba K, Okai T, Kozuma S. Real-time processable three-dimensional fetal ultrasound. Lancet. 1996;348:1307.
4. Baba K, Satoh K, Sakamoto S, et al. Development of an ultrasonic system for three-dimensional reconstruction of the foetus. J Perinat Med. 1989;17:19-24.
5. Balen FG, Allen CM, Gardener JE, et al. Three-dimensional reconstruction of ultrasound images of the uterine cavity. Brit J Radiol. 1993;66:588-91.
6. Benoit B. Early fetal gender determination. Ultrasound Obstet Gynecol. 1999;13:299-300.
7. Berardi JC, Mouilis M, Dlanete A, et al. Echographie en 3-dimensions (3D) en Obstetrique. Avantages et limites. J Gynec Obster Biol Rep. 1997;26:520-4.
8. Bernaschek G, Deutinger J. Vluvision fetaler Fehlbindungen. Ultraschall Klin Prax. 1993;8:154-7.
9. Blaas HG, Eik-Nes SH, Kiserud T, et al. Three-dimensional imaging of the brain cavities in human embryos. Ultrasound Obstet Gynecol. 1995;5:228-32.
10. Blaas HG, Eik-Nes SH, Berg S, et al. In-vivo three-dimensional ultrasound reconstructions of embryos and early fetuses. Lancet. 1998;ii:1182-6.
11. Blohmer JU, Bollmann R, Heinrich G, et al. Die dreidimensionale Ultraschalluntersuchung (3D-Sonographie) der weiblichen Brustdrüse. Geburtsh Frauenh. 1996;56:161-5.
12. Bonilla-musoles F, Raga F, Osborne N, et al. Ecografia tridimensional en Obstetricia y Ginecologia. Obstet Ginecol Espaň. 1994;3:233-50.
13. Bonilla-musoles F, Raga F, Blanes J, et al. Three-dimensional ultrasound in reproductive medicine: preliminary report. Human Reprod Update. Vol. 1,4 Item 21 CD Rom; 1995.
14. Bonilla-musoles F, Raga F, OS Borne N, et al. Control of inserted devices (IUD's) by using three-dimensional ultrasound (3D). It is the future? J Clin Ultrasound. 1996;24:263-7.
15. Bonilla-musoles F, Raga F, Osborne N. Three-dimensional ultrasound evaluation of ovarian masses. Gynecol Oncol. 1995;59:129-35.
16. Bonilla-musoles F, Pellicer A, Raga F, et al. Review: three-dimensional (3D) ultrasound in reproduction, obstetrics and gynecology. Ass Reprod Reviews. 1995;5:170-88.
17. Bonilla-musoles F, Raga F, Osborne N, et al. The use of three-dimensional (3D) ultrasound for the study of normal and pathologic morphology of the human embryo and fetus: preliminary report. J Ultrasound Med. 1995;14:757-65.
18. Bonilla-Musoles F, Raga F, Blanes J, et al. A tridimensao ecografica em Obstetricia e Ginecologia: futuro da nosa especialidade? Ginecol Obstet Attual (Brazil). 1995;7:29-45.
19. Bonilla-Musoles F. Three-dimensional visualization of the human embryo: a potential revolution in prenatal diagnosis. Ultrasound Obstet Gynecol. 1996;7:393-7.
20. Bonilla-musoles F, Raga F, Blanes J, et al. La tridimensión ecográfica en tumores ováricos. Obstet Ginecol Espaň. 1995;4:193-210.
21. Bonilla-musoles F, Raga F, Blanes J, et al. Three dimensional hysterosonographic evaluation of the normal endometrium: comparison with transvaginal sonography and three-dimensional ultrasound. J Gynecol Surg. 1997;13:101-7.
22. Bonilla-musoles F, Raga F, Osborne N, et al. Three-dimensional evaluation of embryonic and fetal malformations: comparison with two-dimensional ultrasound. In: Kurjak A (Ed). Perinatology. Lancs UK: Parthenon Publishing Group; 1998. pp. 228-35.
23. Bonilla-musoles F, Raga F, Osborne N, et al. La triple dimensión ecográfica en el estudio del embrión y del feto normales durante el primer trimestre del embarazo e inicio del segundo. In: Carrerajm Y, Kurjak A (Eds). Masson Barcelona: Medicina del embrión; 1997. pp. 163-88.
24. Bonilla-musoles F, Raga F, Osborne N, et al. Three-dimensional hysterosonography (3D-HSSG), for the study of endometrial tumors; comparison with conventional transvaginal sonography, hysterosalpingosonography and hysteroscopy. Gynecol Oncol. 1997;65:245-52.
25. Bonilla-musoles F, Raga F, Blanes J, et al. Avances en el diagnóstico prenatal: empleo de la angiografía digital Doppler y la tridimensión ecográfica. Rev Iberoamer Fertil. 1997;14:295-318.
26. Bonilla-musoles F, Raga F, Villalobos A, et al. First-trimester neck abnormalities: three-dimensional evaluation. J Ultrasound Med. 1998;17:419-26.
27. Bonilla-musoles F, Raga F, Bonilla FJ, et al. Early diagnosis of conjoined twins using two-dimensional color Doppler and three-dimensional ultrasound. J Nat Med Assoc. 1998;90:552-6.
28. Bonilla-musoles F, Machado l, Raga F, et al. Ecografia tridimensional interactiva Doppler color en el primer trimestre del embarazo. In: Kurjak A, Carreras JM (Eds). Barcelona: Medicina Perinatal Masson; 2000. pp. 213-30.
29. Bonilla-musoles F, Martinez Molina V, Blanes J, et al. Three-dimensional ultrasound investigation for identification and control of intrauterine devices. In: Merz E (Ed). 3-D Ultrasound in Obstetrics and Gynecology. Philadelphia: Lippincott Williams and Wilkins; 1999. pp. 31-6.
30. Bonilla-musoles F, Raga F, Villalobos A, et al. Demonstration of early pregnancy with three-dimensional ultrasound. In: Merz E (Ed). 3-D Ultrasound in Obstetrlcs and Gynecology. Philadelphia: Lippincott Williams and Wilkins; 1999. pp. 81-94.
31. Brlnkley JF, Mc Callum WD, Muramatsu SK. Fetal weight estimation from length and volumes found by three-dimensional ultrasonic measurements. J Ultrasound Med. 1984;3:162-9.
32. Brinkley LF, Mc Callum WD, Muramatsu SK. Fetal weight estimation from ultrasonic three-dimensional head and trunk reconstructions: evaluation in vitro. Am J Obstet Gynecol. 1982;144:715-20.
33. Brunner M, Obruca A, Bauer P. Feichtingerw: clinical application of volume estimation based on three-dimensional ultrasonography. Ultrasound Obstet Gynecol. 1995;6:358-61.
34. Budorick NE, Pretorius DH, Tartar MK, et al. Three-dimensional US of the fetal hands: normal and abnormal findings. Radiology. 1996;201(P):160.
35. Budorick NE, Pretorius DH, Johnson DO, et al. Three-dimensional ultrasound examination of the fetal hands: normal and abnormal. Ultrsound Obstet Gynecol. 1998;12:227-34.
36. Budorik NE, Pretorius OH, Johnson DO, et al. Three-dimensional ultrasonography of the fetal distal lowerextremity: normal and abnormal. J Ultrasound Med. 1998;17:649-60.
37. Carson PL, Moskalika P, Govil A, et al. The 3D and 2D colour flow display of breast masses. Ultrasound Med Biol. 1997;23:837-49.
38. Carson PL, Adler DO, Fowlkes LB, et al. Enhanced color flow imaging of breast cancer vasculature: continuous wave Doppler and three-dimensional ultrasound display. J Ultrasound Med. 1992;11:377-85.
39. Casanas-roux F, Nissole M, Marbaix E, et al. Morphometric, inmunohistological and three-dimensional evaluation of the endometrium of menopausal woman treated by oestrogen and crinone, a new slow-release vaginal progesterone. Human Reprod. 1996;11:357-63.
40. Chan L, Lin M, Uerpairojkit B, et al. Evaluation of adnexal masses using three-dimensional ultrasonographic technology: preliminary report. J Ultrasound Med. 1997;16:349-54.

41. Chang FM, Hsu KF, Ko HC, et al. Fetal heart volume assessment by three-dimensional ultrasound. Ultrasound Obstet Gynecol. 1997;9:42-8.

42. Cheng-yang Chou, Ken-fu Hsun, Shan-Tairwang, et al. Accuracy of three-dimensional ultrasonography in volume estimation of cervical carcinoma. Gynecol Oncol 1997;65:89-93.

43. Chevernak A, Kurjak A, Comstock CH. Ultrasound and the fetal brain. Progress in Obstetric and Gynecological Sonography Series. The Parthenon Publishing Group; 1995. pp. 221-36.

44. Chiba Y, Hayashi K, Yamazaki S, et al. New technique of ultrasound, thick slicing 3D imaging and the clinical aspects in the perinatal field. Ultrasound Obstet Gynecol. 1994;4:337.

45. D'arcy TJ, Hughes SW, Chiu WSC. Estimation of fetal lung volume using enhanced 3-dimensional ultrasound: a new method and first results. Brit J Obstet Gynecol. 1996;103:1015-20.

46. Devonald KJ, Ellwood D, Griffiths K, et al. Volume imaging: three-dimensional appreciation of the fetal head and face. J Ultrasound Med. 1995;14:919-26.

47. Dolz N, Osborne NG, Blanes J, et al. Polycystic ovarian syndrome: assessment with color Doppler angyography and three-dimensional ultrasound. J Ultrasound Med. 1999;18:303-13.

48. Duncan KR, Baker PN, Johnson IR. Estimation of fetal lung volume using enhanced 3-dimensional ultrasound: a new method and first results. Brit J Obstet Gynecol. 1997;86:971-2.

49. Favre R, Nisand K, Bettahar K, et al. Measurement of limb circumference with three-dimensional ultrasound for fetal weight estimation. Ultrasound Obste Gynecol. 1993;3:176-9.

50. Favre R. Echographie tridimensionelle dans ledespistage des malformations. J Med Foetale. 1994;19:22-9.

51. Feichtinger W. Transvaginal three-dimensional imaging. Ultrasound Obstet Gynecol. 1993;3:375-8.

52. Feichtinger W. Follicle aspiration with interactive three-dimensional digital imaging (Voluson*): a step toward real-time puncturing under three-dimensional ultrasound control. Fertil Steril. 1998;70:374-7.

53. Fujiwaki R, Hata T, Hata K, et al. Intrauterine sonographic assessments of embryonic development. Am J Obstet Gynecol. 1995;173:1770-4.

54. Gregg A, Steiner H, Staudach A, et al. Accuracy of 3D sonographic volume measurements. Am J Obstet Gynecol. 1993;168:348.

55. Gregg A, Steiner H, Bogner G, et al. The gestational sac and 3D volumetry. Am J Obstet Gynecol. 1993;168:348.

56. Gruboeck K, Jurkovic D, Lawton F, et al. The diagnostic value of endometrial thickness and volume measurements by three-dimensional ultrasound in patients with menopausal bleeding. Ultrasound Obstet Gynecol. 1996;8:272-6.

57. Hafner E, Philipp T, Schuchter K, et al. Second-trimester measurements of placental volume by three-dimensional ultrasound to predict small for gestational age infants. Ultrasound Obstet Gynecol. 1998;12:97-102.

58. Hamper UM, Trapanatto V, Sheth S, et al. Three-dimensional US: preliminary clinical experience. Radiology. 1994;191:397-401.

59. Harita G, Gabriel R, Carre-Pigeon F. Primary application of three-dimensional ultrasonography to early diagnosis of ectopic pregnancy. Eur J Obstet Gynecol. 1995;60:110-20.

60. Hata T, Manabe A, Makihara K, et al. Assessment of embryonic anatomy at 6-8 weeks of gestation by intrauterine and transvaginal sonography. Human Reprod. 1997;12:1873-6.

61. Hata T, Aoki S, Manabe A, et al. Three-dimensional ultrasonography in the first trimester of human pregnancy. Human Reprod. 1997;12:1800-4.

62. Hata T, Manabe A, Aoki S, et al. Three-dimensional intrauterine sonography in the early first trimester of human pregnancy: preliminary study. Human Reprod. 1998;13:740-3.

63. Hata T, Aoki S, Manabe A, et al. Visualization of fetal genitalia by three-dimensional ultrasonography in the second and third trimesters. J Ultrasound Med. 1998;17:137-9.

64. Hata T, Aoki S, Hata K, et al. Three-dimensional ultrasonographic assessment of fetal development. Obstet Gynecol. 1998;91:218-23.

65. Hata T, Aoki S, Akiyama M, et al. Three-dimensional ultrasonographic assessment of fetal hands and feet. Ultrasound Obstet Gynecol. 1998;12:235-9.

66. Hata T, Yanaglhara T, Hayashi K, et al. Three-dimensional ultrasonographic evaluation of ovarian tumours prelimlnary study. Human Reprod.1999;14:858-61.

67. Hosli JM, Tercanli S, Herman A, et al. In-vitro volume measurement by three-dimensional ultrasound: comparison of two different systems. Ultrasound Obstet Gynecol. 1998;11:17-22.

68. Johnson DD, Pretorius DH, Budorick N. Three-dimensional ultrasound of conjoined twins. Obstet Gynecol. 1997;90:701-2.

69. Johnson DD, Pretorius DH, Riccabona M, et al. Three-dimensional ultrasound of the fetal spine. Obstet Gynecol. 1997;89:434-8.

70. Jurkovic D, Jauniaux E, Campbell S. Three-dimensional ultrasound in obstetrics and gynecology. In: Kurjak A, Chervenak FA (Eds). The Fetus as a Patient. Carnforth, UK: Parthenon Publishing Group; 1995. pp. 135-40.

71. Jurkovic D, Geipel A, Gruboeck K, et al. Three-dimensional ultrasound for the assessment of uterine anatomy and detection of congenital anomalies: a comparison with hysterosalpingography and two-dimensional sonography. Ultrasound Obstet Gynecol. 1995;5:233-7.

72. Jurkovic D, Jauniau E. Ultrasound and early pregnancy. Progress in Obstetric and Gynecological Sonography Series. The Parthenon Publishing Group; 1996.

73. Kelly IMG, Gardener JE, Lees WR. Three-dimensional fetal ultrasound. Lancet. 1991;i(339):1062-4.

74. Kelly IMG, Gardener JE, Brett AD, et al. Three-dimensional US of the fetus. Work in progress. Radiology. 1994;192:253-9.

75. King DL, King DL Jr, Shao MY. Evaluation of in vitro measurements accuracy of a three-dimensional ultrasound scanner. J Ultrasound Med. 1991;10:77-82.

76. King DL, King DL Jr, Shao MY. Three-dimensional spatial registration and interactive display of position and orientation of real-time ultrasound images. J Ultrasound Med. 1990;9:625-32.

77. Kirbach D, Whittingham TA. 3D ultrasound. The Kretztechik voluson approach. Eur J Ultrasound. 1994;1:85-9.

78. Kossoff G, Griffiths A, Warren PS. Real-time quasi three-dimensional viewing in sonography, with conventional grey-scale volume imaging. Ultrasound Obstet Gynecol. 1994;4:211-6.

79. Kossoff G. Three-dimensional ultrasound. Technology push or market pull. Ultrasound Obstet Gynecol. 1995;5:217-8.

80. Kratochwil A. Versuch der 3-dimensionalen Darstellung in der Geburtshilfe. Ultraschall Med. 1992;13:183-6.

81. Kuo HC, Chang FM, Wu CH, et al. The primary application of three-dimensional ultrasonography in obstetrics. Am J Obstet Gynecol. 1992;166:880-6.

82. Kupesic S, Kurjak A. Septate uterus: detection and prediction of obstetrical complications by different forms of ultrasonography. J Ultrasound Med. 1998;17:631-6.

83. Kurjak A, Kupesic S, Breyer B, et al. The assessment of ovarian tumour angiogenesis: what does three-dimensional power Doppler add? Ultrasound Obstet Gynecol. 1998;12:136-46.

84. Kyei-Mensah A, Zaidi J, Pittrof R, et al. Transvaginal three-dimensional ultrasound: accuracy of follicular volume measurements. Fertil Steril. 1996;65:371-6.

85. Kyei-Mensah A, Maconochie N, Zaidi J, et al. Transvaginal three-dimensional ultrasound: reproducibility of ovarian and endometrial volume measurements. Fertil Steril. 1996;66:718-22.

86. Laudy JAM, Janssen MMM, Struyk PC, et al. Three-dimensional ultrasonography of normal fetal lung volume: a preliminary study. Ultrasound Obstet Gynecol. 1998;11:13-6.

87. Laudy JAM, Janssen MMM, Struyk PC, et al. Fetal liver volume measurements by three-dimensional ultrasonography: a preliminary study. Ultrasound Obstet Gynecol. 1998;12:93-6.

88. Lee A, Deutinger J, Bernaschek G. Voluvision: three-dimensional ultrasonography of the fetal malformations. Am J Obstet Gynecol. 1994;170:1312-4.

89. Lee A, Kratochwil A, Deutinger J, et al. Three-dimensional ultrasound in diagnosing phocomelia. Ultrasound Obstet Gynecol. 1995;5:238-40.

90. Lee A, Deutinger J, Bernaschek G. Three-dimensional ultrasound: abnormalities of the fetal face in surface and volume rendering mode. Brit J Obstet Gynecol. 1995;102:302-6.

91. Lee A, Kratochwil A, Stümpflen L, et al. Fetal lung volume determination by three-dimensional ultrasonography. Am J Obstet Gynecol. 1996;175:588-92.

92. Lee A, Eppel W, Sam C, et al. Intrauterine device localization by three-dimensional transvaginal sonography. Ultrasound Obstet Gynecol. 1997;10:289-93.

93. Lees WR, Gardener JE, Gilliams A. Three-dimensional US of the fetus. Radiology. 1991;181:131-2.

94. Levaillant JM, Rotten D, Billon C, et al. Three-dimensional ultrasound imaging of the female breast and human fetus in utero. Preliminary results. Ultrasound Imaging. 1989;11:149-50.

95. Levaillant JM, Benoit B, Bady J, et al. Echographie tridimensionelle apport technique etclinique en echographie osbtetricale. Reprod Humaine Hormone. 1995;3:341-7.

96. Leventhal M, Pretorius DH, Sklansky MS, et al. Three-dimensional ultrasound of the normal fetal heart. A comparison with two-dimensional imaging. J Ultrasound Med. 1998;17:341-8.

97. Lev-Toaff AS, Rawool NM, Kurtz AB, et al. Three-dimensional sonography and 3D-transvaginal US: a problem solving tool in complex gynecologic cases. Radiology. 1996;20(P):384.

98. Liang RI, Huang SE, Chang FM. Prenatal diagnosis of ectopia cordis at 10 weeks of gestation using two-dimensional and three-dimensional ultrasonography. Ultrasound Obstet Gynecol. 1997;10:137-9.

99. Lin MT, Chen GD, Lin LY, et al. Measurements of follicle size and the volume of follicular fluid by 3-dimensional ultrasound scanning compared with aspirated findings in IVF programs. J Obstet Gynecol Rep China. 1991;30:47-50.

100. Ludomirski A, Khandelwal M, Uerpairojkit B, et al. Three-dimensional ultrasound evaluation of fetal facial and spinal anatomy. Am J Obstet Gynecol. 1996;174(Supple):318.

101. Ludomirski A, Uerpairojkit B, Whiteman VE, et al. New technology in three-dimensional obstetrical ultrasonography: technique, advantages and limitations. Am J Obstet Gynecol. 1996;174(Supple):328.

102. Machado LE, Chamusca L, Chagas K, et al. Ecografia tridimensional (3D) en tiempo "quasi real" en la segundamitad del embarazo. Obstet Ginecol Españ. 1999;8:7-18.

103. Machado LE, Bonilla-Musoles F, Chamuscal, et al. Diagnóstico de toracópagos mediante el empleo deecografía tridimensional. Obstet Ginecol Españ. 1999;8:19-27.

104. Maymon R, Halperin R, Weinraub Z, et al. Three-dimensional transvaginal sonography of conjoined twins at 10 weeks: a case report. Ultrasound Obstet Gynecol. 1998;11:292-4.

105. Matsumi H, Kozuma S, Baba K, et al. Three-dimensional ultrasound is useful in diagnosing the fetus with abdominal wall defects. Ultrasound Obstet Gynecol. 1996;8:356-8.

106. Meinel K, Guntermann E. Transparente 3D-Sonographie bei fetalen Fehlbildungen. Ultraschall Med. 1998;19:120-5.

107. Meng-Hsing MO, Chao-Chin H, Yue-Shan L. Three-dimensional ultrasound and hysteroscopy in the evaluation of intrauterine retained fetal bones. J Clin Ultrasound. 1997;25:93-5.

108. Meng-Hsing MO, Chao-Chin H, Ko-En H. Detection of congenital Müllerian duct anomalies using three-dimensional ultrasound. J Clin Ultrasound. 1997;25:487-92.

109. Merz E, Macchiela O, Bahlmann F, et al. Fetale Fehlbildungsdiagnostik mit Hilfe der 3D-Sonographie. Ultraschall Klin Prax. 1991;6:147-52.

110. Merz E, Macchiella D, Bahlmann F, et al. Three-dimensional ultrasound for the diagnosis of fetal malformations. Ultrasound Obstet Gynecol. 1992;2:137-44.

111. Merz E, Bahlmann F, Weber G, et al. Volume 3D-scanning. A new dimension in the evaluation of fetal malformations. Ultrasound Obstet Gynecol. 1993;3:131-6.

112. Merz E, Weber G, Macchiella O, et al. 3D-Volumensonographie in der transvaginalen Diagnostik Ultraschall. Klin Prax. 1993;8:154-62.

113. Merz E, Bahlmann AF, Weber G. 3D-Volumensonographie in der transvaginalen Diagnostik. Med Bild. 1994;8:43-51.

114. Merz E. Volume (3D) scanning in the evaluation of fetal malformation. Ultrasound Obstet Gynecol. 1994;4(Is):339.

115. Merz E, Bahlmann AF, Weber G. Volume scanning in the evaluation of fetal malformations: a new dimension in prenatal diagnosis. Ultrasound Obstet Gynecol. 1995;5:222-7.

116. Merz E, Weber G, Bahlmann AF, et al. Transvaginale 3D-Sonographie in der Gynakologie. Der Gynäkologe. 1995;28:270-5.

117. Merz E, Bahlmann F, Weber G. Three-dimensional ultrasonography in prenatal diagnosis. J Perinat Med. 1995;23:213-22.

118. Merz E, Einsatz der. 3D-Ulltrschalltechnik in derpranatalen Diagnostik. Ulltraschall Med. 1995;16:154-61.

119. Merz E. Three-Dimensional ultrasound in the evaluation of fetal anatomy and malformations. In: Chervenak FA, Kurjak A (Eds). Current perspectives on the fetus as a patient. New York, London: Parthenon Publishing Group; 1996. pp. 75-87.

120. Merz E, Weber G, Bahlmann AF, et al. Application of transvaginal and abdominal three-dimensional ultrasound for the detection or exclusion of malformations of the fetal face. Ultrasound Obstet Gynecol. 1997;9:237-43.

121. Merz E. Aktuelle technische Möglichkeiten der 3D-Sonographie in der Gynakologie und Geburtshilfe. Ulltraschall Med. 1997;18:190-5.

122. Merz E. Three-dimensional ultrasound—a requirement for prenatal diagnosis? Ultrasound Obstet Gynecol. 1998;12:225-7.

123. Merz E, Bahlmann F, Welter C, et al. Transvaginale 3D-Sonographie in der Frühgraviditat Gynäkologe. 1999;32:213-9.

124. Merz E, Miric-Tesanic D, Bahlmann F, et al. Prenatal diagnosis of fetal ambiguous gender using three-dimensional sonographic. Ultrasound Obstet Gynecol. 1999;13:217-8.

125. Merz E. 3-D Ultrasound in Obstetrics and Gynecology. Philadelphia: Lippincott Williams and Wilkins; 1998.

126. Meyer-Wittkopf M, Cook A, Mclennan A, et al. Evaluation of three-dimensional ultrasonography and magnetic resonance imaging in assessment of congenital heart anomalies in fetal cardiac specimens. Ultrasound Obstet Gynecol. 1996;8:303-8.

127. Müller GM, Weiner CP, Yankowitz J. Three-dimensional ultrasound in the evaluation of fetal head and spine anomalies. Obstet Gynecol. 1996;88:372-8.

128. Nelson TR, Pretorius DH. Three-dimensional ultrasound of fetal surface features. Ultrasound Obstet Gynecol. 1992;2:166-74.

129. Nelson TR, Pretorius DH. 3D-ultrasound volume measurements (abstract). Med Physics. 1993;201:927.

130. Nelson TR, Pretorius DH, Skansky M, et al. Three-dimensional echocardiographic evaluation of fetal heart anatomy and function: acquisition, analysis and display. J Ultrasound Med. 1996;15:1-2.

131. Nelson TR, Pretorius DH. Visualization of the fetal thoracic skeleton with three-dimensional sonography: a preliminary report. Am J Roentgenol. 1995;164:1485-8.

132. Nelson TR, Downey DB, Pretorius DH, et al. Three-dimensional ultrasound. Philadelphia: Lippincott Williams and Wilkins; 1999.

133. Pellicer A, Villalobos A, Raga F, et al. Three-dimensional ultrasound in low responders. Fertil Steril. 1998;70:671-5.

134. Ploeckinger-Ulm B, Ulm MR, Lee A, et al. Antenatal depiction of fetal digits with three-dimensional ultrasonography. Am J Obstet Gynecol. 1996;175:571-4.

135. Pohls UG, Rempen A. Fetal lung volumetry by three-dimensional ultrasound. Ultrasound Obstet Gynecol. 1998;11:6-12.

136. Pretorius DH, Nelson TR, Jaffe JS. Three-dimensional US of the fetus. Radiology. 1990;177:194.

137. Pretorius DH, Nelson TR. Three-dimensional ultrasound imaging in patient diagnosis and management: the future (opinion). Ultrasound Obstet Gynecol. 1991;1:381-3.

138. Pretorius TH, Nelson TR, Jaffe JS. Three-dimensional sonographic analysis based on color flow Doppler and grey scale image data. A preliminary report. J Ultrasound Med. 1992;11:225-32.

139. Pretorius DH, Nelson TR. Prenatal visualization of cranial sutures and fontanelles with three-dimensional ultrasonography. J Ultrasound Med. 1994;13:871-6.

140. Pretorius DH, Nelson TR. Three-dimensional ultrasound. Ultrasound Obstet Gynecol. 1995;5:219-21.

141. Pretorius DH, Nelson TR. Fetal face visualization using three-dimensional ultraonography. J Ultrasound Med. 1995;4:349-56.

142. Pretorius DH, House M, Nelson TR, et al. Evaluation of normal and abnormallips in fetuses: comparison between three and two dimensional sonography. Amer J Roentgenol. 1995;165:1233-7.

143. Pretorius DH, Nelson TR. Three-dimensional US in obstetrics. In: Fleischer AC, Manning FA, Jeanty P, Romero R (Eds). Principles and Practice of Ultrasonography in Obstetrics and Gynecology, 5th edition. Norwalk: Appleton and Lange; 1995. pp. 119-26.

144. Pretorius DH, Nelson TR, Baergen R. 3-dimensional ultrasound and power Doppler imaging of placental vasculature (abstract). Academ Radiol. 1995;2:1154.

145. Retorius DH, Johnson DD, Budorick NE, et al. Three-dimensional ultrasound of the fetal lip and palate. Radiology. 1997;205(s):245.

146. Pretorius DH, Richards RD, Budorick NE. Three-dimensional ultrasound in the evaluation of fetal anomalies. Radiology. 1997;205(s):245.

147. Pretorius DH, Nelson TR. Three-dimensional ultrasound in gynecology and obstetrics. A review. Ultrasound Q. 1998;14:218-33.

148. Raga F, Bonilla-Musoles F, Blanes J, et al. Accuracy of three-dimensional ultrasound diagnosis in congenital Müllerian anomalies. Fertil Steril. 1996;65:523-8.

149. Raga F, Bonilla-Musoles F, Blanes J, et al. Uterine anomalies with three-dimensional ultrasound (Müllerian duct malformations) Ass Reprod Reviews. 1996;6:126-41.

150. Rempen A. The shape of the endometrium evaluated with three-dimensional ultrasound: an additional predictor of extrauterine pregnancy. Human Reprod. 1998;13:450-4.

151. Riccabona M, Nelson TR, Pretorius DH, et al. Distance and volume measurements using three-dimensional ultrasound. J Ultrasound Med. 1995;14:881-6.

152. Riccabona M, Johnson D, Pretorius DH, et al. Three-dimensional ultrasound: display modalities in the fetal spine and thorax. Eur J Radiol. 1995;22:141-5.

153. Riccabona M, Nelson TR, Pretorius DH, et al. In vivo three-dimensional sonographic measurement of organ volume: validation in the urinary bladder. J Ultrasound Med. 1996;15:637-42.

154. Riccabona M, Pretorius DH, Nelson TR, et al. Three-dimensional ultrasound: display modalities in obstetrics. J Clin Ultrasound. 1997;25:157-67.

155. Rotten D, Billon C, Rua P. Three-dimensional ultrasound imaging of the female breast and human fetus in utero. Preliminary results. Ultrasound Imaging. 1989;11:149-50.

156. Rotten D, Levaillant JM, Constancis E, et al. Three-dimensional imaging of solid breast tumours with ultrasound: preliminary data and analysis of its possible contribution to the understanding of the standard two-dimensional sonographic images. Ultrasound Obstet Gynecol. 1991;1:384-90.

157. Schwartz G. Three-dimensional volume measurement. Ultrasound Obstet Gynecol. 1998;11:4-5.

158. Schild RL, Fimmers R, Hansmann M. Kann die3 D-Volumetrie von fetalem Oberarm und Oberschenkel konventionelle 2D-Gewichtsschätzungen verbessern? Ultraschall Med. 1999;19:31-7.

159. Schild RL, Wallny T, Fimmer R, et al. Fetal Lumbar spine volumetry by three-dimensional ultrasound. Ultrasound Obstet Gynecol. 1999;13:335-9.

160. Shih JC, Shyu MK, Lee CN, et al. Antenatal depiction of the fetal ear with three-dimensional ultrasonography. Obstet Gynecol. 1998;91:500-5.

161. Sivan E, Chan L, Uerpairojkit B, et al. Growth of the fetal forehead and normative dimensions developed by three-dimensional ultrasonographic technology. J Ultrasound Med. 1997;16:401-6.

162. Sklansky MS, Nelson TR, Pretorius TH. Usefulness of gated three-dimensional fetal echocardiography to reconstruction and display structures not visualized with two-dimensional imaging. Am J Cardiol. 1997;80:665-8.

163. Sklansky MS, Nelson TR, Pretorius DH. Three-dimensional fetal echocardiography: gated versus nongated techniques. J Ultrasound Med. 1998;17:451-7.

164. Steiner H, Staudach A, Spitzer D, et al. Bietet die 3D-Sonographie neueperspektive in der Gynakologie and Geburtshilfe? Geburtsh Frauenheilk. 1993;53:779-82.

165. Steiner H, Spitzer D, Diem A, et al. Staudach Aa Outcome nach artifizielle Fruchtwasser-Instillation (AFI) bei früher Oligohydramnie. Geburtsh Frauenheilk. 1993;53:559-63.

166. Steiner H, Gregg AR, Bogner G, et al. First trimester 3-D ultrasound volumetry of the gestational sac. Ultrasound Obstet Gynecol. 1993;3(s):168.

167. Steiner H, Staudach A, Schaffer H. Dreidimensionale Ultraschalldiagnostik in der Geburshilfe und Gynakologie. Medizin im Bild. 1994;1:19-23.

168. Steiner H, Staudach A, Zajc M, et al. Verbesserte Diagnostik am fetalenSkelett mittels 3D-Sonographie. Ultraschall Klin Prax. 1994;8:154-7.

169. Steiner H, Gregg AR, Bogner G, et al. First trimester three-dimensional ultrasound volumetry of the gestational sac. Arch Gynecol Obstet. 1994;255:165-70.

170. Steiner H, Staudach A, Spitzer D, et al. Three-dimensional ultrasound in obstetrics and gynecology; technique, possibilities and limitations. Human Reprod. 1994;9:1773-8.

171. Steiner H, Spitzer D, Weiss-Wichert PH, et al. Three-dimensional ultrasound in prenatal diagnosis of skeletal dysplasia. Prenat Diagn. 1995;15:373-7.

172. Steiner H. Potential der dreidimensionalen (3D) Sonographie in del Fehlbildungsdiagnosrik. Gynäkologe. 1995;28:315-20.

173. Steiner H, Merz E, Staudach A. Three-dimensional fetal facing. Human Reprod Update. 1995;1.

174. Sohn C, Grotepass J, Swobodnik W. Moglichkeiten der 3-dimensionalen ultra-schalluntersuchung. Ultraschall Med. 1989;10:307-13.

175. Sohn CH, Grotepa SJ, Schneider W, et al. Dreidimensionale Darstellung in der Ultra-schalldiagnostik. Erste Ergebenisse. Dtsch Med Wschr. 1988;113:1743-7.

176. Sohn CH, Grotepa SJ, Schneider W, et al. Erste Untersuchungen zur Dreidimensionalen Darstellungmittels Ultraschall. Z Geburtsh Perinatol. 1988;192:241-8.

177. Sohn CH, Grotepa SJ, Menge KH, et al. Klinische Anwendung der dreidimensionalen Ultra-schall Dartellung. Dtsch Med Wsch. 1989;114:534-7.

178. Sohn CH, Rudofsky G. Die dreidimensionale Ultraschalldiagnostik. Ein neues Verfahren für die klinische Rourine? Ultraschall Klin Prax. 1989;4:219-24.

179. Sohn CH, Grotepass J. Die 3-dimensionale Organdatstellung mittels Ultraschall. Ultraschall Med. 1990;11:295-301.

180. Sohn C, Stolz W, Nuber B, et al. Die dreidimensionale Ultraschalldiagnostik in Gynäkologie und Geburtshilfe. Geburtsh Frauenheilk. 1991;51:335-40.

181. Sohn C, Bastert G. Dreidimensionale Ultraschalldatstellung. Deutsch Med Wschr. 1992;117:467-72.

182. Sohn CH, Stolz W, Kaufmann M, et al. Die dreidimensionale Ultraschalldarstellung benignerund maligner Brusttumoren. Erste klinische Erfahrungen. Geburtsh Frauenheilk. 1992;52:520-5.

183. Sohn C, Bastert G. Die 3D-Sonographie in derpränatalen Diagnostik. Z Geburtsh Perinatol. 1993;197:11-19.

184. Sohn C, Bastert G. Dreidimensionale Ultraschalldiagnostik. Springer Publsh Heidelber; 1994.

185. Sohn C, Bastert G. The technical requirements of stereoscopic three-dimensional ultrasound imaging. Sonoace Internacional. 1996;3:16-25.

186. Suren A, Osmers R, Kuhn W. 3D color power angioimaging. A new method to assess intracervical vascularization in benign and pathological conditions. Ultrasound Obstet Gynecol. 1998;11: 133-7.

187. Tan SL. Clinical applications of Doppler and three-dimensional ultrasound in assisted reproductive technology. Ultrasound Obstet Gynecol. 1999;13:153-6.

188. Tulandi T, Watkin K, Tan SL. Reproductive performance and three-dimensional ultrasound volume determination of polycystic ovaries following laparoscopic ovarian drilling. Int J Fertil Womens Med. 1997;42:436-40.

189. Ulm MR, Kratochwil A, Ulm B, et al. Three-dimensional ultrasound evaluation of fetal tooth germs. Ultrasound Obstet Gynecol. 1998;12:240-3.

190. Van Wymersch, Favre R. Interét de l'échographie tridimensionnelle en Obstétrique et Gynécologie. References en Gynecologie Obstetrique. 1995;3:82-7.

191. Watkin KL, Khalife S, Nuwayhid B, et al. Three-dimensional reconstruction of freehand abdominal and vaginal ultrasonic images. Ultrasound Obstet Gynecol. 1993;3(s):185.

192. Weber G, Merz E, Bahlmann F, et al. Sonographische Beurteilung von Ovarialtumoren-Vergleich zwischen transvaginaler 3D-Technik und konventioneller 2-dimensionaler Vaginosonographie. Ultraschall Med. 1997;18:26-30.

193. Weinraub Z, Maymon R, Shulman A, et al. Three-dimensional saline contrast hysterosonography and surface rendering of uterine cavity pathology. Ultrasound Obstet Gynecol. 1996;8:277-82.

194. Wisser J, Schar J, Kurmanavicius J, et al. Anwendung von 3D-Ultraschall als neuerWegzur Bestimmung von Geburtstraumen am Beckenboden. Ultraschall Med. 1999;19:15-8.

195. Wu MH, Hsu CC, Huang KE. Detection of congenital Müllerian duct anomalies using three-Dimensional ultrasound. J Clin Ultrasound. 1997;25:487-92.

196. Zarca D, Bady J, Levaillant JM, et al. Desimages et des nombres. Gynecol Int. 1996;5:6-10.

197. Zosmer N, Jurkovic K, Gruboeck K, et al. Three-dimensional fetal echocardiography: the identification of arterial connections on planar reformatted sections. Ultrasound Obstet Gynecol. 1994;4(s):359.

198. Zosmer N, Jurkovic D, Jauniaux E, et al. Selection and identification of standard cardiac views from three-dimensional volume scans of the fetal thorax. J Ultrasound Med. 1996;15:25-32.

199. Bonllla-Musoles F, Machado L. Ultrasonidosy Reproduction. Madrid: Panamericana Ed; 2000.

200. Bonilla-Musoles F. Ecografia Vaginal, Doppler y Tridimensional. Madrid: Panamericana Ed; 2000.

201. Andrist LA, Katz VI, Elijah R. Developing a plan for routine 3D surface rendering in Obstetrics. JDMS. 2001;17:16-21.

202. Andrist LA, Katz VI, Elijah R. Visualization of fetal anomalies with surface 3-dimensional ultrasound: a case study. JDMS. 2001;17: 88-93.

203. Axt-Flietner R, Hendrick HJ, Ertan K, et al. Course and outcome of a pregnancy with a giant fetal cervical teratoma diagnosed prenatally. Ultrasound Obstet Gynecol. 2001;18:543-6.

204. Baba K, Ishihara O, Hayashi N, et al. Three-dimensional ultrasound in embryotransfer. Ultrasound Obstet Gynecol. 2000;16:372-3.

205. Bahlmann F. Three-dimensional color power angiography of an aneurysm of the vein of Galen. Ultrasound Obstet Gynecol. 2000;15:341-1.

206. Bahmaei A, Hughes SW, Clark T, et al. Serial fetal lung volume measurement using three-dimensional ultrasound. Ultrasound Obstet Gynecol. 2000;16:154-8.

207. Bega G, Lev-Toaff A, Kuhlman K, et al. Three-dimensional multiplanar transvaginal ultrasound of the cervix in pregnancy. Ultrasound Obstet Gynecol. 2000;16:351-8.

208. Bega G, Lev-Toaff A, Kuhlman K, et al. Three-dimensional ultrasonographic imaging in obstetrics. J Ultasound Med. 2001;20:391-408.

209. Bega G, Kuhlman K, Lev-Toaff A, et al. Application of three-dimansional ultrasonography in the evaluation of the fetal heart. J Ultasound Med. 2001;20:307-13.

210. Blaas HG, Eik-Nes SH, Berg S. Three-dimensional fetal ultrasound. Baillieres Best Pract Res Clin Obstet Gynaecol. 2000;14:61-27.

211. Bonilla-Musoles F, Raga F, Blanes J, et al. Current status of three-dimensional ultrasound in reproductive medicine. Middle East Fertility Society Journal. 2000;5:169-77.

212. Bonilla-Musoles F, Machado L, Bailao LA, et al. Abdominal wall defects. Two-versus three-dimensional ultrasonographic diagnosis. J Ultraound Med. 2001;20:379-89.

213. Bonilla-Musoles F, Raga F, Blanes J, et al. Ecografía tridimensional enuroginecología. Progresos Obstet Ginecol. 2001;44:237-44.

214. Bonilla-Musoles F, Serra V, Machado LE, et al. Tridimension y diagnóstico prenatal. Cuadernos Med Reprod. 2001;7:123-38.

215. Bordes A, Bory AM, Benchaid M, et al. Reproducibility of transvaginal three-dimensional endometrial volume measurements with virtual organ computer-aided analysis (VOCAL) during ovarian stimulation. Ultrasound Obstet Gynecol. 2002;19:76-80.

216. Campbell S. 4D or not 4D: that is the question. Ultrasound Obstet Gynecol. 2002;19:1-5.

217. Chaoui R, Kalache KD, Hartung J. Application of three-dimensional power Doppler ultrasound in prenatal diagnosis. Ultrasound Obstet Gynecol. 2001;17:22-9.

218. Chaoui R, Kalache KD. Three-dimensional power Doppler ultrasound of the fetal great vessels. Ultraosund Obstet Gynecol. 2001;17:455-6.

219. Dyson RL, Pretorius DH, Budorick NE, et al. Three-dimensional ultrasound in the evaluation of fetal anomalies. Ultrasound Obstet Gynecol. 2000;16:321-8.

220. Endres LK, Cohen L. Reliability and validity of three-dimensional fetal brain volumes. J Ultrasound Med. 2001;20:1265-70.

221. Guerra FA, Isla AI, Aguilar RC, et al. Use of free-hand three-dimensional ultrasound software in the study of the fetal heart. Ultrasound Obstet Gynecol. 2000;16:329-34.

222. Hafner E, Schuchter K, Van Leeuwen M, et al. Three-dimensional sonographic volumetry of the placenta and the fetus between weeks 15 and 17 of gestation. Ultrasound Obstet Gynecol. 2001;18:116-20.

223. Hata T, Yanagihara T, Matsumoto M, et al. Three-dimensional sonographic features of fetal central nervous system anomaly. Acta Obstet Gynecol Scand. 2000;79:635-9.

224. Hull AD, James G, Salerno CC, et al. Three-dimensional ultrasonography and assessment of the first-trimester fetus. J Ultrasound Med. 2001;20:287-93.

225. Jackson DN, Aptekar I, Thompson KK, et al. Counselling impact of three-dimensional imaging in perinatal consultation. Ultrasound Rev Obstet Gynecol. 2001;1:216-47.

226. Jackson DN, Braun I, Keel-Thompson K. Comparison of rapid MRI (HASTE) procedure to volume mode planar imaging in the management of fetal abnormalities. J Med Ultrasonics. 2000;27: 1-3.

227. Jackson DN, Braun I, Keel-Thompson K. Volume mode planar imaging in patients with non-surface fetal abnormalities: techniques and efficacy. J Med Ultrasonics. 2000;27:14-9.

228. Jackson DN, Aptekar LH, Keel-Thompson K. Technique of 3D volume mode sectional planar imaging. Ultrasound Obstet Gynecol. 2000;16(s):26.

229. Jones D, Reyes M, Gallagher P, et al. Three-dimensional sonographic imaging of a highly develop fetus in fetu with spontaneous movement of the extremities. J Ultrasound Med. 2001;20:1357-64.

230. Kiyokawa K, Masuda H, Fuyuki T, et al. Three-dimensional hysterosalpingo-contrast sonography (3D-HyCoSy) as an outpatient procedure to assess infertile women: a pilot study ultrasound. Obstet Gynecol. 2000;16:648-54.

231. Kratochwil A, Lee A, Schoisswohl A. Networking of three-dimensional sonography volume data. Ultrasound Obstet Gynecol. 2000;16:335-40.

232. Kuno A, Akiyama M, Yamashiro C, et al. Three-dimensional sonographic assessment of fetal behavior in the early second trimester of pregnancy. J Ultrasound Med. 2001;20:1271-7.

233. Kupesic S, Kurjak A. Contrast-enhanced, three-dimensional power Doppler sonography for differenciation of adnexal of masses. Obstet Gynecol. 2000;96:452-8.

234. Kupesic S, Kurjak A, Ujevic B. B-mode, color Doppler and three-dimensional ultrasound in the assessment of endometrial lesions. Ultrasound Rev Osbtet Gynecol. 2001;1:50-71.

235. Kupesic S, Bekavac I, Bejelos D, et al. Assessment of endometrial receptivity by transvaginal color Doppler and three-dimensional power Doppler ultrasonography in patients undergoing in-vitro fertilization procedures. J Ultrasound Med. 2001;20:125-34.

236. Kupesic S. Clinical implications of sonographic detection of uterine anomalies for reproductive outcome Ultrasound. Obstet Gynecol. 2001;18:387-400.

237. Kupesic S. The present and future role of three-dimensional ultrasound in asisted reproduction. Ultrasound Obstet Gynecol. 2001;18:191-4.

228. Kurjak A, Kupesic S, Anic T, et al. Three-dimensional ultrasound and power Doppler improve the diagnosis of ovarian lesions. Gynecol Oncol. 2000;76:28-32.

239. Kurjak A, Kupesic S, Jacobs Y. Preoperative diagnosis of the primary Fallopian tube carcinoma by three-dimensional static and power Doppler sonography. Ultrasound Obstet Gynecol. 2000;15:246-50.

240. Kurjak A, Kupesic S, Sparac V, et al. Three-dimensional ultrasonographic and power Doppler characterization of ovarian lesions. Ultrasound Obstet Gynecol. 2000;16:365-71.

241. Kurjak A, Hafner T, Kos M. Three-dimensional sonography in prenatal diagnosis: a luxury or a necessity? J Perinat Med. 2000;28:194-209.

242. Kurjak A, Kupesic S. The use of echo-enhancing contrasts in gynecology. Ultrasound Rev Obstet Gynecol. 2001;1:85-95.

243. Lee TH, Shih JC, Peng SSF, et al. Prenatal depiction of the angioarchitecture of an aneurysm of the vein of Galen with three-dimensional color power angiography. Ultrasound Obstet Gynecol. 2000;15:345-5.

244. Lee W, Kirk JS, Comstock CH, et al. Vasaprevia: prenatal detection by three-dimensional ultrasonography. Ultrasound Obstet Gynecol. 2000;16:384-7.

245. Lee SL, Tan A. Lymphangiectasis with iniencephaly. Ultrasound Obstet Gynecol. 2001;18:552-3.

246. Lee W, Deter R, Ebersole J, et al. Birth weight prediction by three-dimensional ultrasonography: fractional limb volume. J Ultrasound Med. 2001;20:1283-92.

247. Lev-Toaff AS, Ozhan S, Pretorius D, et al. Three-dimensional multiplanar ultrasound for fetal gender assignment: value of the mid-sagittal plane. Ultrasound Obstet Gynecol. 2000;16:345-50.

248. Lever AS, Pinheiro LW, Bega G, et al. Three-dimensional multiplanar sonohysterography: comparison with conventional two-dimensional sonohysterography and X-ray hysterosalpyngoraphy. J Ultrasound Med. 2001;20:295-306.

249. Maymon R, Herman A, Ariely S, et al. Three-dimensional vaginal ultrasonography in obstetrics and gynecology. Hum Reprod Update. 2000;5:475-84.

250. Merz E, Miric-Tesanic D, Welter C. Value of the electronic scalpel (cut mode) in the evaluation of the fetal face. Ultrasound Obstet Gynecol. 2000;16:564-8.

251. Meyer-Wittkopf M, Rappe N, Sierra F, et al. Three-dimensional (3D) ultrasonography for obtaining the four and five chamber view: comparison with cross-sectional (2D) fetal sonographic screening. Ultrasound Obstet Gynecol. 2000;15:397-402.

252. Meyer-Wittkopf M, Cole A, Cooper SG, et al. Three-dimensional quantitative echocardiographic assessment of the ventricular volume in healthy human fetuses and in fetuses with congenital heart disease. J Ultrasound Med. 2001;20:317-27.

253. Meyer-Wittkopf M, Cooper SG, Vaughan J, et al. Three-dimensional echocardiographic (3D) analysis of congenital heart disease in the fetus: comparison with cross-sectional (2D) fetal echocardiography. Ultrasound Obstet Gynecol. 2001;6:485-492.

254. Michailidis GD, Simpson JM, Tulloh R, et al. Retrospective prenatal diagnosis of scitimar syndrome aided by three-dimensional power Doppler imaging. Ultrasound Obstet Gynecol. 2001;17:449-52.

255. Michailidis GD, Simpson JM, Karidas C, et al. Detailed three-dimensional fetal echocardiography facilitated by and internet link. Ultrasound Obstet Gynecol. 2001;18:325-8.

256. Monteagudo A, Timor-Tritsch IE, Mayberry P. Three-dimensional transvaginal neurosonography of the fetal brain: "navigating" in the volume scan. Ultrasound Obstet Gynecol. 2000;16:307-13.

257. Naylor C, Carlson D, Santulli T, et al. Use of three-dimensional ultrasonography for prenatal diagnosis of ambiguous genitalia. J Ultrasound Med. 2001;20:1365-9.

258. Nelson TR, Pretorius DH, Hull A, et al. Sources and impact of artefacts on clinical three-dimensional ultrasound imaging. Ultrasound Obstet Gynecol. 2000;16:374-83.

259. Orden MR, Gudmundsson S, Kirkinrn P. Contrast-enhanced sonography in the examination of benign and malignant adnexal masses. J Ultrasound Med. 2000;19:783-9.

260. Pal A, Babinski A, Vajda G, et al. Diagnosis of Asherman's syndrome with three-dimensional ultrasound. Ultrasound Obstet Gynecol. 2000;15:341.

261. Pedersen MH, Larsen T. Three-dimensional ultrasonography in obstetrics and gynecology. Ugeskr Laeger. 2001;163:594-9.

262. Platt LD. Three-dimensional ultrasound. Ultrasound Obstet Gynecol. 2000;16:295-8.

263. Poehl M, Hohlagschwandtner R, Doerner V, et al. Cumulus assessment by three-dimensional ultrasound for In-Vitro Fertilization. Ultrasound Obstet Gynecol. 2000;16:251-3.

264. Pooh RK, Pooh K. Transvaginal 3D and Doppler ultrasonography of the fetal brain. Semin Perinatol. 2001;25:38-43.

265. Pretorius DH, Nelson TR. Fetal three-dimensional ultrasonography. today or tomorrow? J Ultrasound Med. 2001;20:283-6.

266. Raine-Fenning N, Campbell B, Collier J, et al. The reproductibility of endometrial volume acquisition and measurements with the VOCAL imaging program. Ultrasound Obstet Gynecol. 2002;19: 69-75.

267. Sabbagha R. The endometrium and the role of three-dimensional sonohysterography. Ultrasound Rev Obstet Gynecol. 2001;1:72-84.

268. Salerno CC, Pretorius H, Hilton SW, et al. Three-dimensional ultrasonographic imaging of the neonatal brain in high-risk neonates; preliminary study. J Ultrasound Med. 2000;19:549-56.

269. Schild RL, Fimmers R, Hansmman M. Fetal weight estimation by three-dimensional ultrasound. Ultrasound Obstet Gynecol. 2000;16:445-52.

270. Schild RL, Wallny T, Fimmers R, Hansmman M. The size of the fetal thoracolumbar spine: a three-dimensional ultrasound study. Ultrasound Obstet Gynecol. 2000;16:468-72.

271. Schild RL, Holdhaus S, D'Alquen J. Quantitative assessment of subendometrial blood flow by three-dimensional ultrasound is an important predictive factor of implantation in an in-vitro fertilization programme. Human Reprod. 2000;15:89-94.

272. Sladkevicius P, Ojha K, Campbell S, et al. Three-dimensional power Doppler imaging in the assessment of fallopian tube patency. Ultrasound Obstet Gynecol. 2000;16:644-7.

273. Song TB, Moore TR, Lee JY, et al. Fetal weight prediction by thigh volume measurement with three-dimensional ultrasonography. Obstet Gynecol. 2000;96:157-61.

274. Timor-Tritsch IE, Monteagudo A, Mayberry P. Three-dimensional ultrasound evaluation of the fetal brain: the three horn view. Ultrasound Obstet Gynecol. 2000;16:302-6.

275. Toots-Hobson P, Kuhllar V, Cardozo L. Three-dimensional ultrasound: a novel technique for investigating the urethral sphincter in the third trimester of pregnancy. Ultrasound Obstet Gynecol. 2001;17:421-4.

276. Umek WH, Obermair A, Stutterecker D, et al. Three-dimensional ultrasound of the female urethra: comparing transvaginal and transrectal scanning. Ultrasound Obstet Gynecol. 2001;17:425-30.

277. Wang P. Obstetrical three-dimensional ultrasound in the visualization of the intracranial midline and corpuscallosum of fetuses with cephalic position (Letter). Prenat Diagn. 2000;20:518-20.

278. Weisman CF, Forstner R, Prokop E, et al. Three-dimensional targeting: a new three-dimensional ultrasound technique to evaluate needle position during breast biopsy. Ultrasound Obstet Gynecol. 2000;16:359-64.

279. Welsh AW, Taylor MJO, Cosgrove D, et al. Free hand three-dimensional Doppler demonstration of monochorionic vascular anastomoses in vivo: a preliminary report. Ultrasound Obstet Gynecol. 2001;18:317-24.

280. Woelfer B, Salim R, Banerjee S, et al. Reproductive outcomes in women with congenital uterine anomalies detected by three-dimensional ultrasound screening. Obstet Gynecol. 2001;98:1099-103.

281. Bonilla-Musoles F, Machado LE, Raga A. Three- and four-dimensional images of fetal malformations. In: Kurjak A, Jackson D (Eds). An Atlas of Three-and-Four-Dimensional Sonography in Obstetrics and Gynecology. London: Taylor & Francis Ed; 2004. pp. 67-127.

282. Bonilla-Musoles F, Machado LE. 3D-4D in Obstetrics. Madrid: Panamericana Ed; 2004.

32 Malformations of the Gastrointestinal System

V D'Addario, L Di Cagno

INTRODUCTION

A correct ultrasonic examination of the fetal gastrointestinal tract includes the visualization of the following structures:

- The stomach (Fig. 32.1)
- The small and large bowels (Fig. 32.2)
- The liver with its main vessels and the gallbladder (Fig. 32.1)
- The abdominal wall and the insertion of the umbilical cord (Fig. 32.3)
- The diaphragm (Fig. 32.4).

The systematic evaluation of the above mentioned structures allows the recognition of several congenital anomalies of the gastrointestinal system. The reported sensitivity of ultrasound in diagnosing gastrointestinal malformations varies from 24% to to 86%, according to different Authors' results. This wide variation is due to the different study designs (mainly the numbers of scans performed during pregnancy), inclusion criteria, levels of examination. Since many gastrointestinal malformations appear late in pregnancy, the best results are obtained when the screening design includes a scan also in the third trimester.

The malformations of gastrointestinal tract and abdominal wall can be divided in four groups:

1. Anterior abdominal wall defects
2. Diaphragmatic defects
3. Bowel disorders
4. Non-bowel cystic masses.

ANTERIOR ABDOMINAL WALL DEFECTS

The congenital abdominal wall defects include gastroschisis, omphalocele and body stalk anommaly.[1]

The ultrasonic prenatal diagnosis of these defects is relatively simple and possible in the first half of pregnancy. However, it must be remembered that there is a physiological herniation of the small intestine outside the abdominal cavity between the fifth and the eleventh weeks of gestation (Fig. 32.5) and therefore a prenatal diagnosis of abdominal wall defect cannot be made in the earliest stage of pregnancy.[2]

Gastroschisis

This malformation consists in a paraumbilical full thickness defect of the anterior abdominal wall which is usually located to the right side of the umbilical cord insertion, associated with evisceration of abdominal organs.

The incidence ranges from 1:10,000 to 1:15,000 live births.

Gastroschisis is considered a sporadic event with a multifactorial etiology, but cases of familial occurrence have been reported. Young maternal age, maternal cigarette use and vasoactive drugs consumption during first trimester are considered as possible etiological factors.

The malformation results from vascular compromise of either the umbilical vein or the omphalomesenteric artery. The abdominal wall defect is generally small but the amount of bowel protruding from the defect and floating freely in the amniotic fluid may be

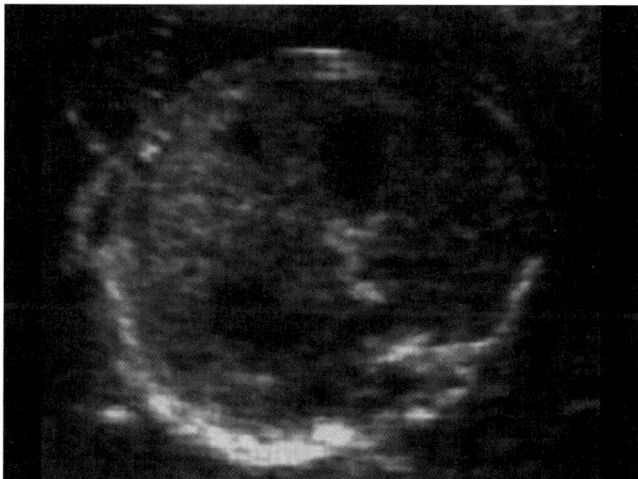

Fig. 32.1: Transverse scan of the fetal abdomen showing the stomach, the liver, the intrahepatic tract of the umbilical vein and the gallbladder

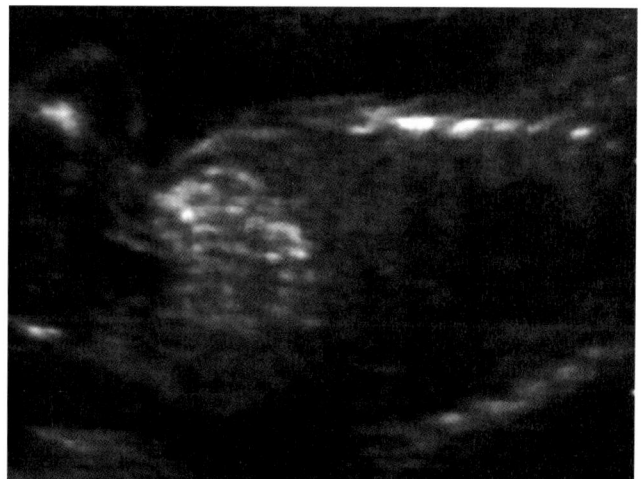

Fig. 32.2: The echogenic bowel is seen below the liver

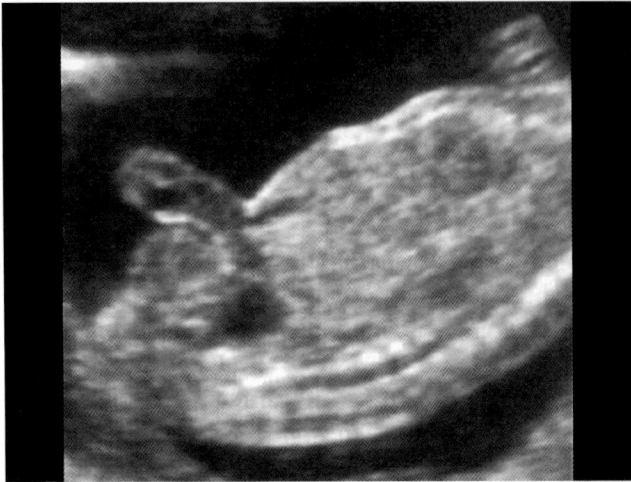

Fig. 32.3: Insertion of the umbilical cord into the abdominal wall

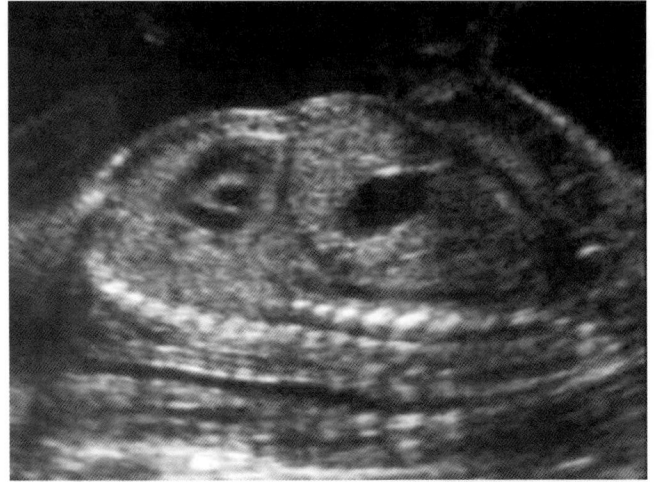

Fig. 32.4: Longitudinal scan on the fetal chest and abdomen showing the diaphragm between the lung and the liver

disproportionately large. The herniated organs include mainly bowel loops that are not protected by a membrane but usually covered by an inflammatory exudate, possibly resulting from chemical irritation by exposure to amniotic fluid.

The ultrasonographic diagnosis of gastroschisis is suggested by the finding of a partly solid, partly cystic mass adjacent to the anterior abdominal wall and freely mobile in the amniotic fluid (Fig. 32.6) which has a cauliflower-like appearance. The differential diagnosis from omphalocele is based on the presence of a normal insertion of the umbilical cord, the lateral location of the mass and the absence of a membrane covering the herniated mass.

In contrast to omphalocele, gastroschisis is rarely associated with other malformations and chromosomal anomalies, but additional gastrointestinal abnormalities (malrotation, atresia, volvulus, infarction) may occur in 20–40% of the cases.[3,4] A high percentage of fetuses with gastroschisis (77%) presents intrauterine growth retardation and preterm labor occurs in one-third of cases. The extent of bowel damage is variable and strictly affects the prognosis. Most of the bowel damage is caused by constriction at the site of the abdominal wall defect: the sonographic evidence of small bowel dilatation and mural thickening correlates with severe intestinal damage and poor clinical outcome.

The mode of delivery of fetuses affected by gastroschisis is still controversial although there is no striking evidence for cesarean section over vaginal delivery. Maternal transfer before delivery to a tertiary care center is recommended. The mortality rate ranges from about 8% to 28%.

Omphalocele

Omphalocele is a ventral wall defect characterized by an incomplete development of abdominal muscles, fascia and skin and the herniation of intra-abdominal organs (bowel loops, stomach, liver) into the base of umbilical cord, with a covering amnioperitoneal membrane. The defect is thought to be caused by an abnormality in the process of body infolding. The classic omphalocele is a mid-abdominal defect although there is also a high or epigastric omphalocele (typical of the pentalogy of Cantrell) and a low or hypogastric omphalocele (as seen in bladder or cloacal exstrophy),

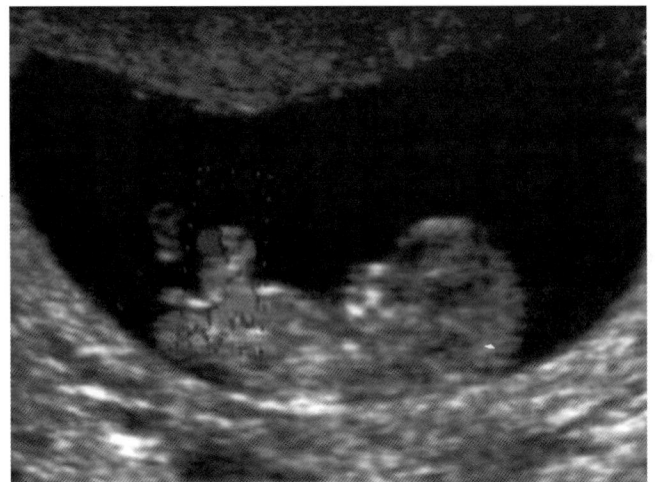

Fig. 32.5: Physiological herniation of the midgut at 10 weeks of gestation

due respectively to cephalic and caudal folding defects. The incidence of omphalocele ranges from 1:4,000 to 1:7,000 live births. It is more frequent in older women; most cases are sporadic, although a familial occurrence with a sex-linked or autosomal pattern of inheritance has been reported.

The ultrasonographic appearance of omphalocele varies according to the type of defect, the presence of ascites and the organs herniated. The principal diagnostic features are: the umbilical cord insertion into the membrane covering the abdominal wall defect, the presence of the intrahepatic portion of the umbilical vein coursing through the central portion of the defect, and the presence of a limiting membrane that can occasionally rupture (Fig. 32.7).

There are different syndromes that include omphalocele, such as pentalogy of Cantrell (midline supraumbilical abdominal defect, lower sternum defect, deficiency of diaphragmatic pericardium, anterior diaphragm defect, cardiac abnormality) and Beckwith-Wiedemann syndrome (macroglossia, visceromegaly, omphalocele). Although most cases of omphalocele are sporadic, a familial occurrence of this anomaly with a sex-linked or autosomal pattern of inheritance has been reported.

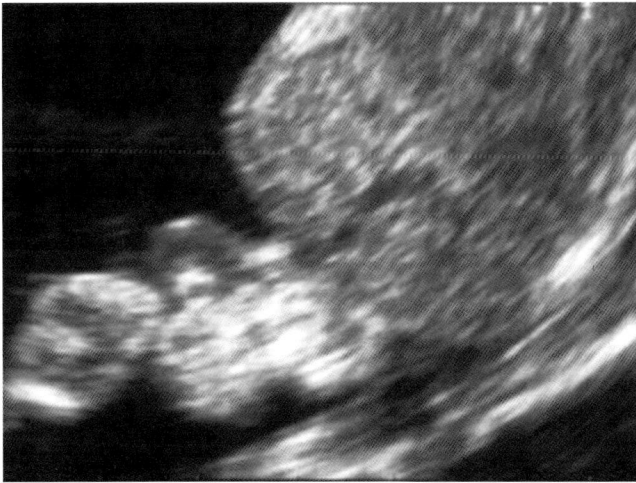

Fig. 32.6: Gastroschisis: a cauliflower-like mass protrudes from the abdominal cavity into the amniotic fluid

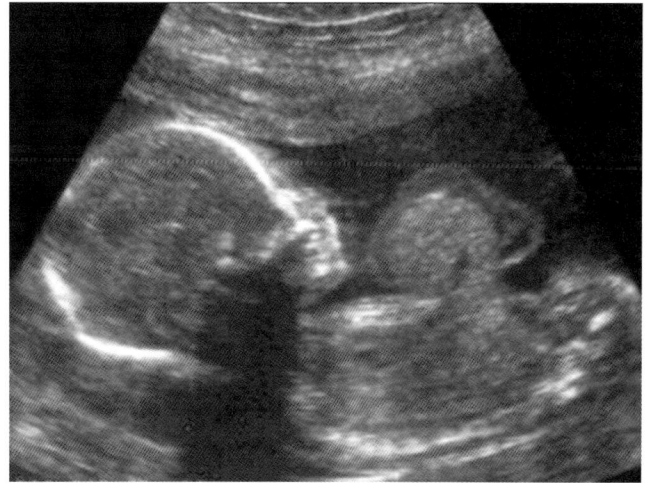

Fig. 32.7: Omphalocele: a round solid mass, covered by a thin membrane, protrudes from the anterior abdominal wall

The most important prognostic variable is the presence of associated malformations (50–70% of cases) or chromosomal abnormalities (30% of cases).[5] Some authors have demonstrated that small defects containing only bowel are associated with an increased risk of chromosomal abnormalities, as opposed to large defects that have exposed liver. The main associated malformations are cardiac anomalies (up to 47% of cases), genitourinary abnormalities (40% of cases) and neural tube defects (39% of cases). Fetal mortality highly depends on associated malformations but also respiratory complications account for a significant percentage of morbidity and mortality.

The mode of delivery of fetuses with omphalocele has been debated in literature. The goal in the management is to deliver the fetus as close to term as possible in tertiary care centers. Cesarean section may be necessary to avoid dystocia or sac rupture in large omphaloceles. In the case of small defects vaginal delivery is recommended.

Body Stalk Anomaly

The body stalk anomaly is a severe abdominal wall defect caused by the failure of formation of the body stalk; it is characterized by the absence of umbilical cord and umbilicus and the fusion of the placenta to the herniated viscera. The incidence is 1:14,000 births. This malformation is caused by a developmental failure of the cephalic, caudal and lateral embryonic folds.

The ultrasonographic diagnosis is suggested by the finding of a large anterior wall defect attaching the fetus to the placenta or uterine wall, the absence of umbilical cord, and the visualization of abdominal organs in a sac outside the abdominal cavity (Fig. 32.8).[6,7] The position of the fetus may lead to scoliosis and kyphosis. Multiple malformations such as neural tube defects, gastrointestinal and genitourinary anomalies, may be associated. The body stalk anomaly is a uniformly fatal condition.

DIAPHRAGMATIC DEFECTS

The classification of these malformations is based on the location of the diaphragmatic defect:

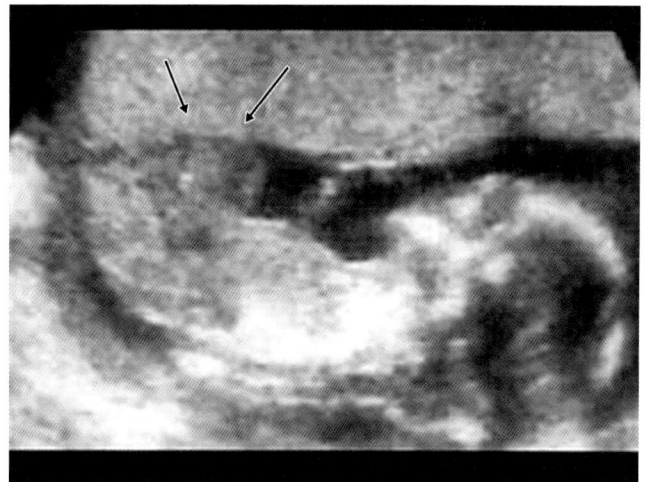

Fig. 32.8: Body stalk anomaly: a large anterior abdominal wall defect attaches the fetus directly to the placenta

1. Diaphragmatic hernia (Bochdalek and Morgagni types)
2. Septum transversum defects (defect of the central tendon)
3. Hiatal hernia (congenital large esophageal orifice)
4. Eventration of the diaphragm
5. Agenesis of the diaphragm.

A diaphragmatic hernia is a defect in the diaphragm, due to failure of the pleuroperitoneal canal to close between 9 and 10 weeks of gestation thus determining the protrusion of the abdominal organs into the thoracic cavity.

The incidence of congenital diaphragmatic hernia is 1:3,000–1:5,000 live births. This entity can be either sporadic or a familiar disorder but its etiology is quite unknown. The most common type of diaphragmatic hernia is the Bochdalek type which is a posterolateral defect mostly located on the left side (80% of cases), less frequently on the right side (15%) on bilateral (5%). Stomach, spleen and colon are the most frequently herniated organs. When the hernia is on the right side, the main organs involved are the liver and the gallbladder.

The Morgagni type is usually a very small hernia which occurs in 1–2% of cases. It is a parasternal defect located in the anterior portion of the diaphragm; it contains liver, which may limit the degree of herniation. In the case of eventration of diaphragm, this structure appears to be weak so that the abdominal contents are displaced in the thoracic cavity.

Eventration of the diaphragm consists of an upward displacement of abdominal organs into the thoracic cavity secondary to a congenitally weak diaphragm which has the aspect of an aponeurotic sheet. It occurs in 5% of diaphragmatic defects and it is more common on the right side.

Diaphragmatic hernia can be either a sporadic or a familiar disorder and although the etiology is unknown this abnormality has been described in association with maternal ingestion of drugs such as thalidomide, quinine and anticonvulsivants. There are two hypotheses to explain the mechanism responsible for the origin of a diaphragmatic defect:

1. Delayed fusion of the diaphragm and
2. A primary diaphragmatic defect.

In addition to this classification, another one has been proposed concerning a late onset of this anomaly:

i. Herniation occurring early during bronchial branching causing a severe bilateral pulmonary hypoplasia and lately death.

ii. Herniation at the stage of distal bronchial branching leading to unilateral hypoplasia, with survival depending on a balance between pulmonary vascular and ductal resistances.

iii. Late herniation in pregnancy which causes a compression of otherwise normal lung and a good prognosis.

iv. Postnatal herniation without pulmonary pathology and with good chances of viability.

The prenatal sonographic diagnosis of diaphragmatic hernia is mainly based on the visualization of abdominal organs at the same level of the four chamber view of the heart in the transverse section of the fetal chest. The heart is usually shifted on the right side of the chest (Fig. 32.9).

The visualization of the fluid-filled bowel or the stomach bubble in the thoracic cavity is highly diagnostic. The presence of peristalsis of bowel loops may help making the differential diagnosis with other conditions such as cystic adenomatoid malformation of the lung, bronchogenic cysts and mediastinal cysts. Polyhydramnios is common and is secondary to the bowel obstruction.

The rate of associated anomalies is 25–75% increasing to 95% in stillborns. Such anomalies include central nervous system, cardiac and chromosomal abnormalities, omphalocele and oral cleft.

The prognosis for this malformation is still very poor and becomes poorer if other malformations are associated. The poor prognosis mainly depends on the severity of pulmonary hypoplasia induced by the prolonged compression of the lungs by the herniated viscera. For this reason experimental prenatal surgery has been suggested to prevent the lung damage. The different outcome is related to variation in the timing of entry of abdominal organs into the chest (the earlier is the entrance, the worse is the prognosis). Due to the complexity of this malformation and the different diagnosis

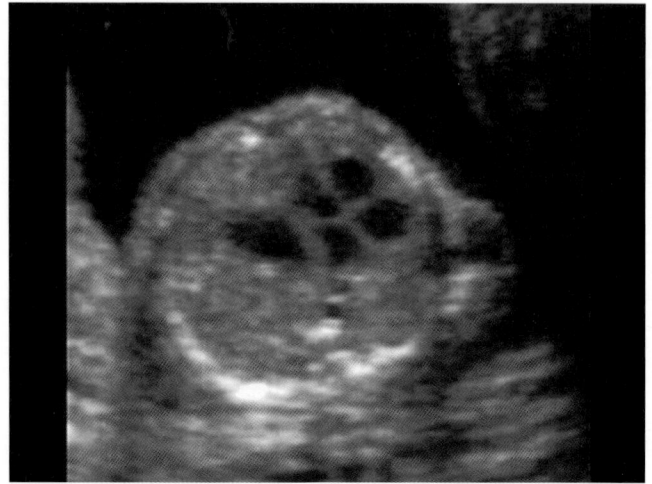

Fig. 32.9: Transverse section of the fetal chest in a case of diaphragmatic hernia: the heart is displaced to the right side by the presence of the stomach and bowel loops in the thoracic cavity

and treatment, the ultrasound examination is very essential. Management relies on protecting the contralateral lung hoping that it is normally formed, which depends on the gestational age at diagnosis. If the fetus is less than 24 weeks of gestation, parents may choose to terminate the pregnancy, to continue the pregnancy with postnatal care or even to consider repair of the defect in utero. Between 24 and 32 weeks, parents may choose between conventional postnatal therapy and fetal surgery. Anytime a diaphragmatic defect is diagnosed, prenatal karyotyping and detailed ultrasound examination to detect associated anomalies are recommended. There are no indications for preterm delivery or for cesarean section. The delivery should be planned in a tertiary care center.

BOWEL DISORDERS

Prenatal ultrasound examination allows the detection of the majority of gastrointestinal malformations because they are often associated with a dilated bowel, cystic masses or intra-abdominal calcifications, although the prenatal diagnosis generally does not influence the mode or the timing of delivery (except in the cases with polyhydramnios that can cause premature labor or delivery). Moreover, it allows maternal referral to a center with appropriate perinatal, neonatal and surgical expertise which, in some cases, may improve the outcome.

Esophageal Atresia

This anomaly consists in the absence of a segment of the esophagus and is often associated with a tracheoesophageal fistula (86–90% of cases). Five types of esophageal atresia may be distinguished:

1. Isolated (type I);
2. Associated with a fistula connecting only the proximal part of the esophagus and the trachea (type II);
3. Associated with a fistula connecting the lower part of the esophagus and the trachea (type III);
4. Associated with proximal and distal fistulas (type IV) and
5. Tracheoesophageal fistula without esophageal atresia (type V).

Among different types, the most common is the esophageal atresia associated with a fistula connecting the proximal part of the esophagus and the trachea (80% of the cases). The incidence varies between 1:800 and 1:5,000 live births and the etiology is unknown.

The prenatal diagnosis is possible in only 10% of the cases and should be suspected in the presence of polyhydramnios with absent stomach bubble in several and repeated ultrasound examinations or visualizing a dilated proximal tract of the esophagus with absent stomach (Fig. 32.10); however, this malformation can occur even in presence of a normal or small stomach, due to the frequently associated tracheoesophageal fistula.[8]

Associated anomalies are present in 50–70% of the cases, including cardiac, genitourinary, chromosomal (trisomy 21), additional gastrointestinal and muscaloskeletal anomalies. A characteristic association is the "VACTERL" (Vertebral, Anorectal anomalies, Cardiac anomalies, Tracheoesophageal fistula, Esophageal atresia, Renal anomalies, Limb anomalies). Fetal karyotyping is suggested. The prognosis depends on the associated malformations and on the severity of polyhydramnios, which can facilitate preterm delivery.

Duodenal Atresia or Stenosis

The incidence of this malformation is 1:10,000 live births and its genesis goes back to the eleventh week of gestation due to a failure of canalization of the primitive bowel. In most cases the etiology is unknown. Atresia is more common than stenosis (70% of cases) and could be associated with chromosomal abnormalities (trisomy 21), skeletal defects and other anomalies.[9]

The most typical sonographic finding is the characteristic "double bubble" sign caused by the simultaneous dilatation of the stomach and the proximal duodenum (Fig. 32.11). The diagnosis is usually made in the late second trimester.[10] Up to half of duodenal atresia cases are complicated by polyhydramnios and this can contribute to preterm labor, but the main cause of death are the associated anomalies. This malformation can present late complications (motility disorders, megaduodenum, gastroesophageal and duodenal-gastric reflux, gastritis, blind loop syndrome) and late death even months or years after management.

Bowel Obstruction

The incidence of bowel stenosis and atresia is 2–3:10,000 births and the most common locations are distal ileum (36%) and proximal jejunum (31%). There are four types of intestinal atresias:

1. Type I: Presence of a transverse diaphragm of mucosa or sub-mucosa (20%);
2. Type II: Presence of blind ends of bowel loops connected by a fibrous band (32%);
3. Type III: Complete separation of blind ends with a corresponding mesenteric defect (48%) and
4. Type IV: Absence of a large tract of small bowel with the typical "apple peel" deformity, resulting from loss of the superior mesenteric artery.

These defects are usually sporadic, although familial cases have been described.

According to the site of the obstruction the defects are divided in: (1) jejunoileal atresia and stenosis, (2) colonic atresia and (3) imperforate anus.

The sonographic prenatal appearance varies according to the level of the defect. In the case of jejunoileal atresia multiple dilated bowel loops in the fetal abdomen may be seen in association with polyhydramnios (Fig. 32.12).[11,12] In colon atresia (that usually occurs proximal to the splenic flexure with a significant segment of absent colon with distal microcolon) the sonographic finding is similar to distal ileal occlusion and the differential diagnosis may not be possible. In the imperforate anus dilated intestinal loops with increased peristalsis may be seen as well as intraluminal hyperechogenic small areas referring to meconium (Fig. 32.13).[13]

The diagnosis of bowel obstruction is usually made in the third trimester: the lower is the obstruction the latter is the appearance of the sonographic signs.

The prognosis of these malformations mainly depends on the level of obstruction (the lower the obstruction, the better the outcome), the length of remaining intestine and birth weight. Other important prognostic factors are the presence of associated malformations (especially gastrointestinal anomalies including

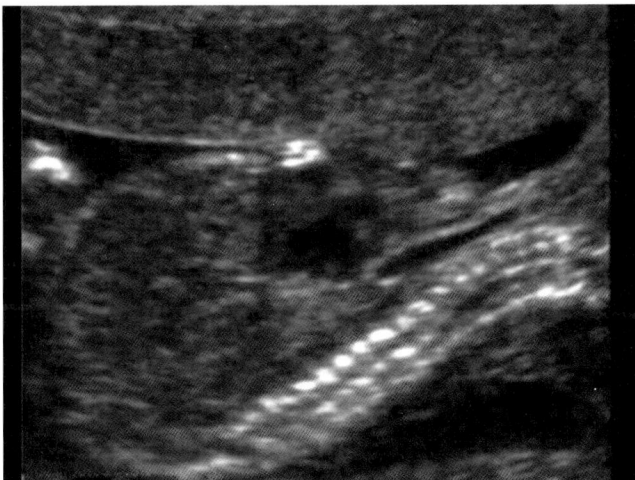

Fig. 32.10: Esophageal atresia: the diagnosis is suspected by the association of absent stomach and dilatation of the proximal tract of the esophagus

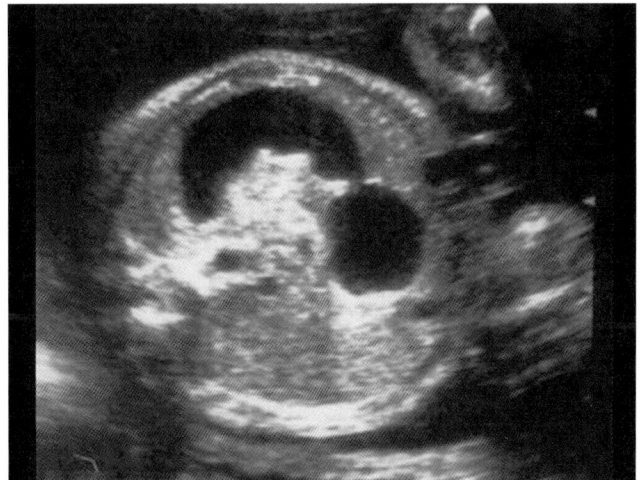

Fig. 32.11: Duodenal atresia: the dilated stomach and proximal duodenum are clearly recognized

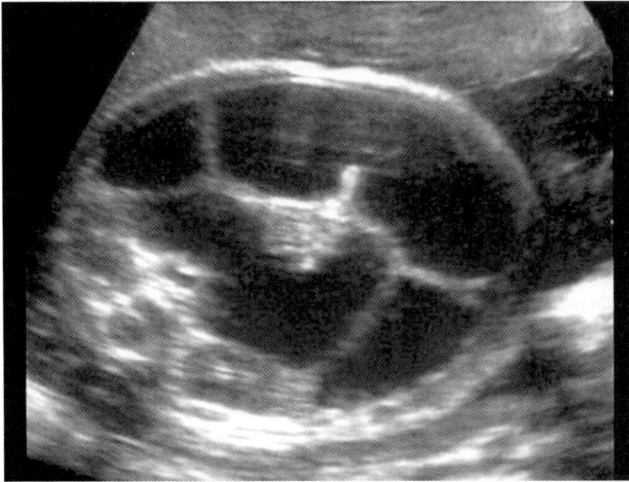

Fig. 32.12: Jejunal atresia: multiple dilated bowel loops are present in the fetal abdomen

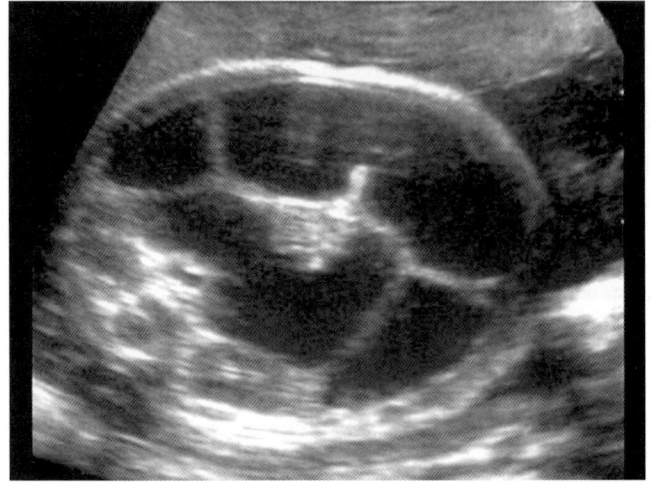

Fig. 32.13: Imperforate anus in a third trimester fetus

bowel malrotation, esophageal atresia, microcolon and intestinal duplication), meconium peritonitis and intrauterine growth restriction.

Meconium Peritonitis

This condition is the consequence of in utero perforation of the bowel with spread of meconium into the peritoneal cavity leading to a local sterile chemical peritonitis. The peritonitis may be localized, with the development of a dense calcified mass or fibrous tissue, or diffuse, with a fibrous reaction leading to bowel adhesions and pseudocyst formation. Inflammatory reaction leads to an exudative process and ascites. Its incidence is 1:35,000 live births. Bowel perforation involves the proximal tract, with some form of obstruction such as intestinal atresia (65% of cases), meconium ileus, volvulus, gastroschisis or Meckel's diverticulum.

The prenatal sonographic appearance of meconium peritonitis varies according to the underlying anatomical finding: main signs are intrabdominal calcifications (85% of cases), polyhydramnios, fetal ascites caused by exudate and bowel dilatation.

Postnatal management depends on the etiology of meconium peritonitis; up to one-third of all cases have cystic fibrosis.

Echogenic Bowel

Sonographically, "echogenic bowel" is defined as echogenicity of the bowel loops equal to or greater than the density of the iliac wing (Fig. 32.14). 1:200 mid-trimester fetuses present this feature which might depend on a slow or delayed transit of the meconium along the bowel. This finding has been considered as a "soft marker" of chromosomal abnormalities but actually the increased risk of chromosomopathy in the presence of such an isolated marker is extremely low.[14] The risk increases when further sonographic markers are present. The "echogenic bowel" may also be the first sign of cystic fibrosis or can be seen in cases of intra-amniotic bleeding.[15] However, it is important to stress that the recognition of hyperechogenic meconium does not always represent a pathological condition but might be a normal variant and an isolated finding.[16]

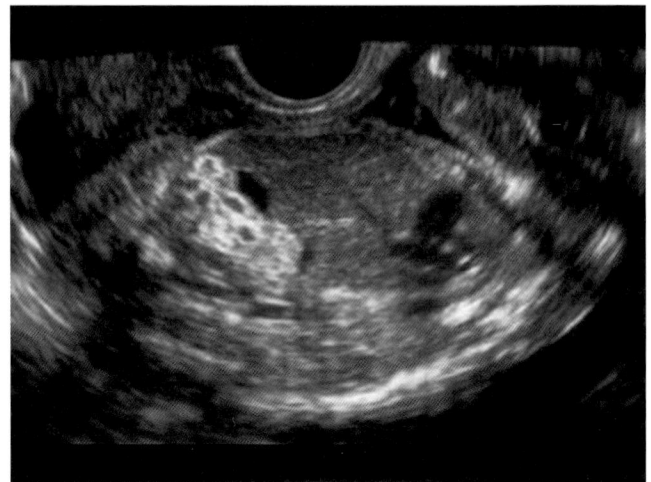

Fig. 32.14: Echogenic bowel

NON-BOWEL CYSTIC MASSES

Choledochal Cysts

Choledochal cyst is a rare congenital cystic dilatation of the common bile duct. The incidence is about 1:2,000. The cysts can be single or, in rare cases, multiple involving the intrahepatic or extrahepatic portion of the biliary tree. Choledochal cysts are classified into four types: (1) Fusiform dilatation of the common bile duct, (2) Diverticular dilatation of the common bile duct, (3) Intramural dilatation of the common bile duct and (4) Intrahepatic biliary duct dilatation. Its sonographic appearance is that of a cystic structure located in the upper right abdomen with dilated proximal ducts. Differential diagnosis includes duodenal atresia, hepatic cyst, dilated gallbladder, ovarian cyst and biliary atresia. The cystic size and the association with biliary obstruction affect the prognosis.[17]

Mesenteric and Omental Cyst

These benign malformations consist in cystic structures located in the small or large bowel mesentery or in the omentum filled with serous or chilous fluid. Its sonographic appearance is that of a thin-walled, unilocular or multilocular cystic mass. It is difficult to make a differential diagnosis with other intra-abdominal cystic conditions such as choledocal, ovarian and hepatic cysts.

Hepatic Masses

Hepatic masses might origin from an obstruction of the hepatic biliary system or might have a tumoral origin (hemangioma, amartoma, etc.).

Their sonographic appearance changes depending on the origin: mesenchymal hamartomas usually appear as irregular hyperechoic areas (Fig. 32.15), while hemangioma appears hypoechoic, hyperechoic or mixed depending on the degree of fibrosis and stage of involution.[18] Hepatoblastomas and adenomas have a solid appearance. Polyhydramnios may be associated; many cases of reduction in volume or even disappearance in utero have been described.

The management is expectant in terms of monitoring the size and evolution of the tumor; for large tumors the cesarean section is indicated.[19]

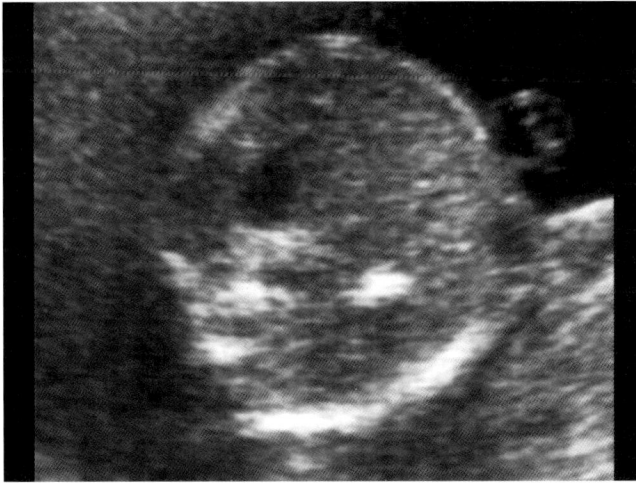

Fig. 32.15: Hepatic hamartoma appearing as an isolated intrahepatic area

REFERENCES

1. Martin RW. Screening for fetal abdominal wall defects. Obstet Gynecol Clin North Am. 1998;25(3):517-26.
2. Kurkchubasche AG. The fetus with an abdominal wall defect. Med Health RI. 2001;84(5):159-61.
3. Oguniemy D. Gastroschisis complicated by midgut atresia, absorption of bowel, and closure of the abdominal wall defect. Fetal Diagn Ther. 2001;16(4):227-30.
4. Morris-Stiff G, al-Wafi A, Lari J. Gastroschisis and total intestinal atresia. Eur J Pediatr Surg. 1998;8(2):105-6.
5. Boyd PA, Bhattacharjee A, Gould S, et al. Outcome of prenatally diagnosed anterior abdominal wall defects. Arch Dis Child Fetal Neonatal Ed. 1998;78(3):F209-13.
6. Cadkin A, Strom C. Prenatal diagnosis of body stalk anomaly in the first trimester of pregnancy. Ultrasound Obstet Gynecol. 1997;10(6):419-21.
7. Takeuchi K, Fujita I, Nakajima K, et al. Body stalk anomaly: prenatal diagnosis. Int J Gynaecol Obstet. 1995;51(1):49-52.
8. Shulman A, Mazkereth R, Zalel Y, et al. Prenatal identification of esophageal atresia: the role of ultrasonography for evaluation of functional anatomy. Prenat Diagn. 2002;22(8):669-74.
9. Sugimoto T, Yamagiwa I, Obata K, et al. Choledochal cyst and duodenal atresia: a rare combination. Pediatr Surg Int. 2002;18(4):281-3.
10. Lawrence MJ, Ford WD, Furness ME, et al. Congenital duodenal obstruction: early antenatal ultrasound diagnosis. Pediatr Surg Int. 2000;16(5-6):342-5.
11. Uerpairojkit B, Charoenvidhya D, Tanawattanacharoen S, et al. Fetal intestinal volvulus: a clinico-sonographic finding. Ultrasound Obstet Gynecol. 2001;18(2):186-7.
12. Ogunyemi D. Prenatal ultrasonographic diagnosis of ileal atresia and volvulus in a twin pregnancy. J Ultrasound Med. 2000;19(10):723-6.
13. Has R, Gunay S. 'Whirlpool' sign in the prenatal diagnosis of intestinal volvulus. Ultrasound Obstet Gynecol. 2002;20(3):307-8.
14. Al-Kouatly HB, Chasen ST, Streltzoff J, et al. The clinical significance of fetal echogenic bowel. Am J Obstet Gynecol. 2001;185(5):1035-8.
15. Berlin BM, Norton ME, Sugarman EA, et al. Cystic fibrosis and chromosome abnormalities associated with echogenic fetal bowel. Obstet Gynecol. 1999;94(1):135-8.
16. Slotnik RN, Abuhamad AZ. Study of fetal echogenic bowel (FEB) and its implications. J Ultrasound Med. 1999;18(1):88.
17. Chen CP, Cheng SJ, Chang TY. Prenatal diagnosis of choledochal cyst using ultrasound and magnetic resonance imaging. Ultrasound Obstet Gynecol. 2004;23(1):93-4.
18. Macken MB, Wright JR Jr, Lau H, et al. Prenatal sonographic detection of congenital hepatic cyst in third trimester after normal second-trimester sonographic examination. J Clin Ultrasound. 2000;28(6):307-10.
19. Tsao K, Hirose S, Sydorak R, et al. Fetal therapy for giant hepatic cysts. J Pediatr Surg. 2002;37(10):E31.

33 Ultrasound Diagnosis of Urinary Tract Anomalies

P Prats, N Maiz, A Rodriguez

EMBRYOLOGY AND ANATOMY OF THE NEPHROUROLOGIC SYSTEM

The nephrourologic system has the functions of production and conduction of the urine toward the exterior by means of two independent nephrourologic tracts, but with the same functions that converge toward a reservoir that is the bladder, where the urine produced by the kidneys is stored, and it is excreted to the exterior through the urethra.

Embryology

The nephrourologic system has its embryonic origin in the intermediate mesoderm, located on both sides of the dorsal wall of the body. As the embryonic development advances it suffers transformations and specifications that will be translated into different anatomical parts of the urinary tract.

It would be possible to say that the embryonic development of the nephrourologic system occurs in two areas but in a synchronous way.

The superior nephrourologic system consists of kidneys (nephrons), collecting tubules, papillary ducts, calyces, renal pelvis and ureters.

Toward the fifth week of gestation, the paraspinal mesoderm differentiates into pronephros and mesonephros, which present some structural changes to become the metanephric blastema (that would be undifferentiated mesenchyma from the nephrogenic crest, which will give place to the future kidneys).

At the sacral level, there are also some paraspinal structures of mesodermic origin named ureteral gemmae from where some canals arise in caudocephalad direction address denominated mesonephric ducts or Wolffian ducts that in their ascent penetrate inside the metanephric blastemas and ramify in their interior until a total of 15 generations.

In the seventh week of gestation, the functional units of the kidney, the nephrons, begin to differ due to the inductive influence of the ureteral gemma.

In the twentieth week of gestation, the collecting system has already been formed are: collecting tubules, papillary ducts, calyces, renal pelvis and ureters and 30% of the total population of nephrons starting from this week and until the thirty-sixth week of gestation, an exponential increment in the total number of nephrons will take place.

The lower nephrourologic system consists of bladder and urethra. Both structures are unique and they take charge of transporting the urine produced in the superior nephrourologic system toward the exterior.

They arise from the mesoderm and the paramesonephric ducts (that also participate in the formation of the genital system) that will give place at the pelvic level to an embryonic structure called cloaca.

The cloaca, among the fourth and sixth weeks of gestation, presents a tabication by means of the urorectal septum that divides the cloaca into two parts: a posterior one that will be the rectum and another anterior one that will be the primitive urogenital sinus whose superior portion together with the allantois will give place to the bladder that will receive posterolaterally the ureters from the ureteral gemmae.

The inferior portion of the primitive urogenital sinus will give place to the membranous urethra and vaginal introitus in females, and to the membranous and prostatic urethra in males.

Normal Anatomy and Variants

With the transvaginal ultrasonography, the kidneys and the bladder can be detected in the fetus from the ninth week of gestation. From the twelfth week, the kidneys look like bilateral echogenic structures in the paraspinal region (Fig. 33.1). The renal pelvis can be identified central to the medial hypoechogenic. The bladder is in the pelvis and looks like a round anechoic structure that is well defined. Its position can be confirmed with the Doppler technique to identify the two umbilical arteries that surround it.

From 18 weeks to 20 weeks of gestation, the kidneys can be defined clearly as oval masses lateral to the psoas muscles and below the suprarenal glands using coronal or sagittal sections. These look like hypoechoic triangular that delimit the superior pole of the kidneys. In the traverse plane, the kidneys look like round paravertebral structures and the renal pelvis looks like anechoic areas medial to the kidneys (Figs 33.2 and 33.3). The renal pelvis is measured better in the anteroposterior projection, whether the fetus' column is up or down. The normal limit is 4 mm until thirty-third weeks of gestation and 7 mm from this date until the term. The normal values of the renal dimensions have been published, including the renal longitude, the anteroposterior diameter and the renal circumference.

With high-resolution devices, the renal pyramids can be seen as hypoechoic areas in the renal cortex, which should not be confused with renal cysts.

The ureters are not usually seen, and if they are identified they are suspected for a renal obstruction or vesicoureteral reflux.

In the first trimester, the bladder looks like a round anechoic structure with the rectum behind. It is often possible to differentiate it from the intestine that surrounds it. However, it is better to measure the wall thickness at the umbilical artery level when this surrounds the bladder. The normal limit for the bladder wall thickness is 2 mm.

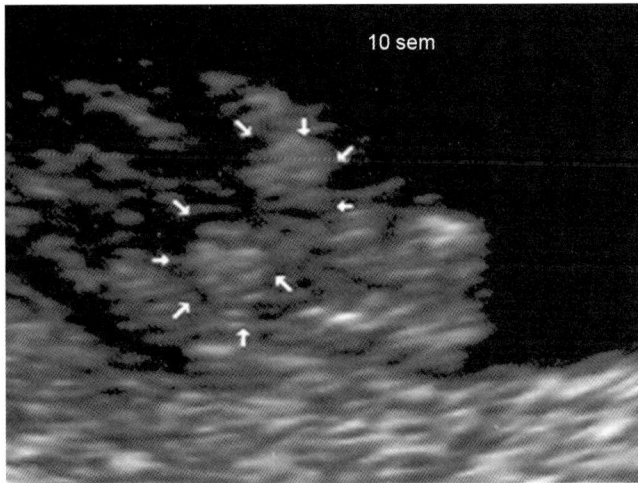

Fig. 33.1: Kidneys at tenth weeks of gestation. Bilateral echogenic structures in the paraspinal region

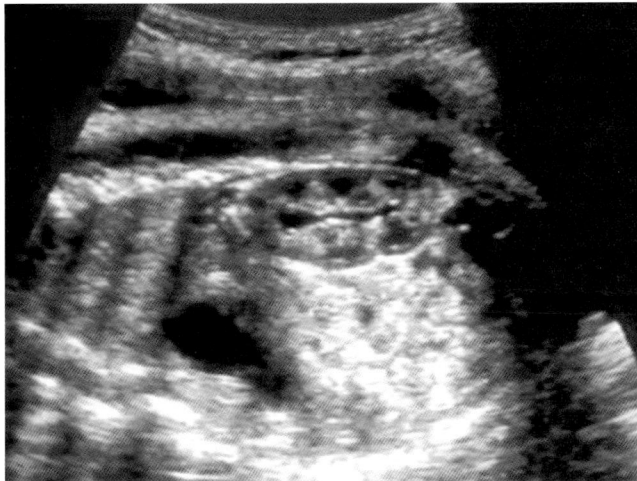

Fig. 33.2: Sagittal scan of the kidney

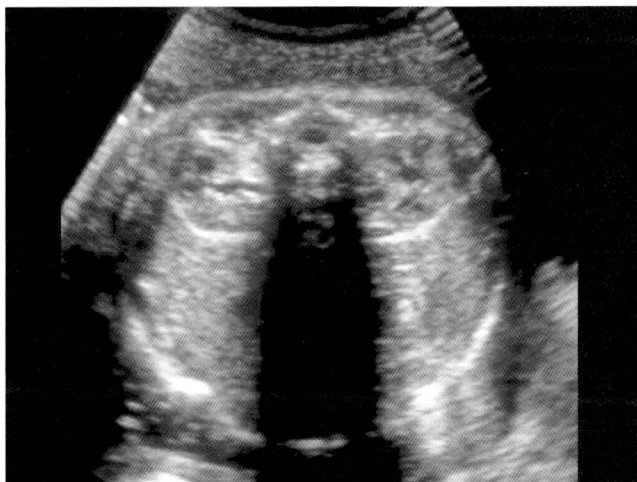

Fig. 33.3: Coronal scan of the kidney

Ultrasonographic Study

The ultrasonographic study of the fetal urinary system involves the evaluation of the kidneys, the bladder and the volume of amniotic fluid. It is also necessary to eliminate the associated anomalies.

Fetal Kidneys

First, it is imperative to confirm if two kidneys are present. If a kidney is not present, it is necessary to look for it in ectopic positions like the pelvis. If it is not found, it is necessary to consider the possibility of unilateral renal agenesis. The bilateral renal agenesis usually associates to a severe oligoamnios, mainly starting from 17 weeks of gestation. When a renal anomaly is detected, it is fundamental to explore the contralateral kidney to confirm or to exclude a bilateral renal illness.

The size and echogenicity of both the kidneys should be valued. The hyperechoic kidneys can be normal, but it is also necessary to think about the possibility of a cystic renal disease, particularly when they are big.

The presence of macroscopic cysts usually indicates a multicystic kidney, but it is necessary to make sure that the cysts do not spread, because there are cases of multicystic kidneys with a great central cyst and smaller outlying cysts that can be mistaken for hydronephrosis. If there is only one cyst, it can be considered a simple cyst.

The collector system of both kidneys should be evaluated not only with respect to the size but also the number. If two collector systems are seen, it is necessary to discard a double kidney and to explore the bladder to rule out an ureterocele.

The dilatation of the collector system forces us to consider the possibility of a renal obstruction. The grade of dilatation of renal pelvis, ureter and bladder usually suggests the level of obstruction. When there is a dilatation of the collector system, it is necessary to value the renal cortex echogenicity and the presence or absence of renal cysts to rule out secondary renal dysplasia.

Bladder

Bladder exploration includes size evaluation and, when it is large, the visualization of the posterior urethra, because if this is dilated it is necessary to think of an obstruction of the vesical exit. The thickness of the vesical wall can be measured at the level of the umbilical artery. It is necessary to rule out the existence of the ureterocele, particularly when there is a renal duplicity. In a period of 30–40 minutes, it is usually possible to demonstrate vesical filling and drainage.

Volume of Amniotic Fluid

This volume can be evaluated in different ways. Most echographers carry out a subjective evaluation first and then they adopt more objective approaches if they find that there is too much or too little. It seems that the best technique is the calculation of the index of amniotic fluid from the measures in the four uterine quadrants and its half-value. Severe oligoamnios of the second trimester usually has a bad prognosis and if it excludes premature rupture of membranes (PROM) and a severe intrauterine growth restriction (IUGR), it usually indicates the presence of a severe bilateral renal illness.[1-4]

URINARY TRACT MALFORMATIONS

Renal Agenesis

Renal agenesis is the absence of one or two of the kidneys. The incidence of unilateral renal agenesis is 1 per 1000 births, and bilateral is 1 per 4000 births.[5] The etiology is ignored. Some cases of unilateral agenesis could be secondary to an intrauterine regression of a dysplastic multicystic kidney.[6] The embryological origin of the renal agenesis is the lack of union or penetration of the ureteral sprouting in the metanephric blastema, so that the primitive collecting tubules do not induce nephron formation starting from metanephric mesoderm.[7]

Diagnosis

Bilateral agenesis: Echographic diagnosis is carried out for:

- The absence of kidneys in renal fossae that is difficult to evaluate because of the oligohydramnios in many cases
- Severe oligoamnios
- No bladder visualization[8]
- The absence of renal arteries by means of the color Doppler study[9,10] (Fig. 33.4)
- The "lying down adrenal sign" where the renal fossae is not occupied by the suprarenal glands[11] (Fig. 33.5)
- Fetuses in podalic presentation where transvaginal ultrasound will help to improve the image[12,13]
- The infusion of intra-amniotic and intraperitoneal physiologic salt solution to improve the image quality.[14,15]

Unilateral agenesis: For diagnosis, a meticulous evaluation of both renal fossae must be carried out. Ultrasound findings will be:

- Absence of kidney in the renal fossa
- Absence of ipsilateral renal artery by means of color Doppler (Fig. 33.6)
- Absence of pelvic kidney or renal ectopy, for this the renal pelvis and contralateral kidney needs to be evaluated.

The contralateral kidney can be increased in size because of compensatory hypertrophy[16] (Fig. 33.7).

Differential Diagnosis

Differential diagnosis will be mainly carried out for other causes of severe oligoamnios:

- Renal pathology
- Bilateral multicystic kidneys: The kidneys are usually evident for their cysts
- Infantile polycystic kidney disease (PKD): The kidneys are usually big and echogenic
- Uretral obstruction: The bladder is usually much evident

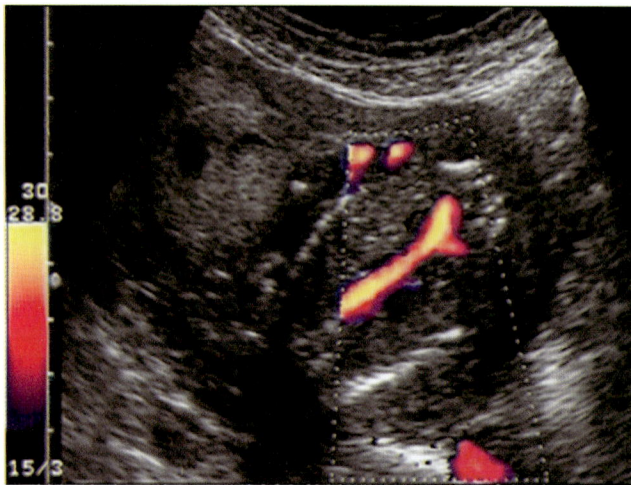

Fig. 33.4: Bilateral renal agenesis. Absence of the renal arteries

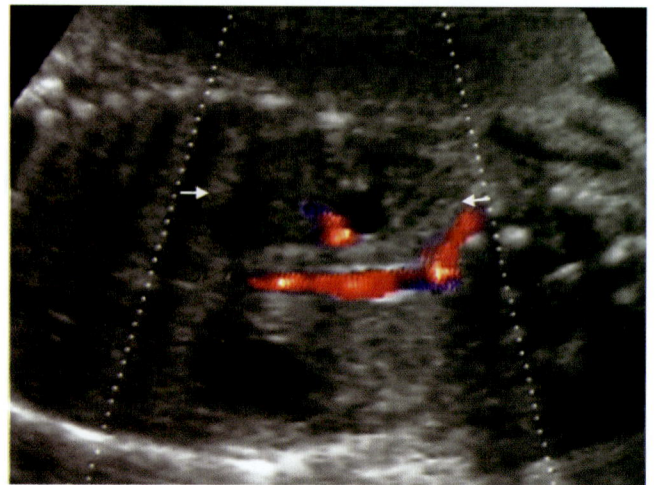

Fig. 33.6: Unilateral renal agenesis. Renal artery in Doppler color. Notice the absence of the renal artery

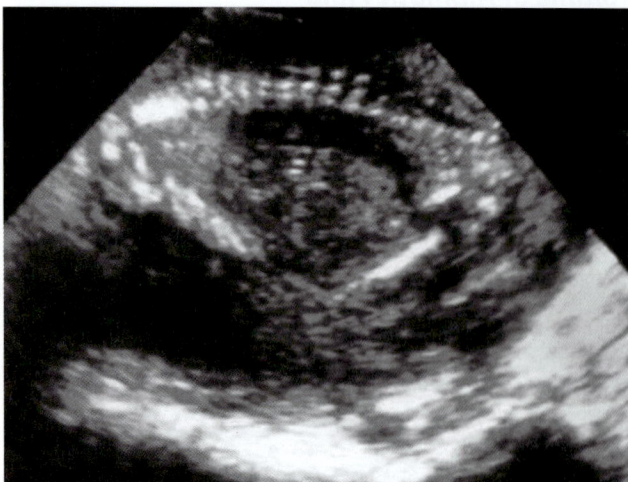

Fig. 33.5: Bilateral renal agenesis. Note the enlarged adrenal gland

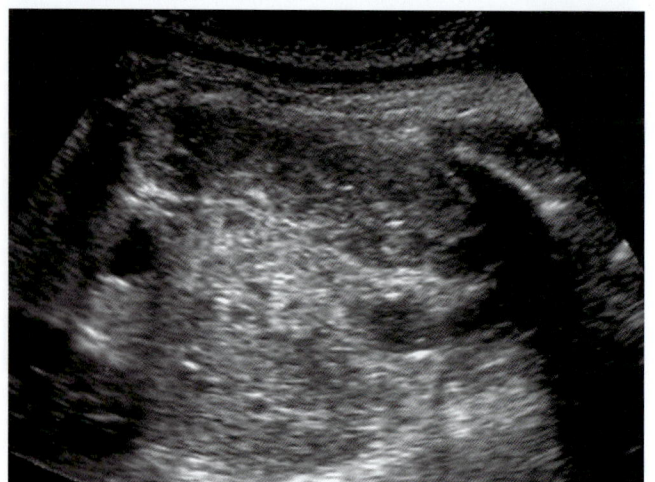

Fig. 33.7: Unilateral renal agenesis. Note the large kidney

- IUGR. The kidneys and the bladder are present. It is usually accompanied by an alteration in the flow wave speed of the umbilical artery
- PROM: It usually has an antecedent of loss of vaginal liquid. The kidneys and the bladder are present.

Associated Anomalies

Bilateral agenesis

- The Potter sequence (wide and plane nose, ears of low implantation, hypertelorism, receding chin, deformities of extremities) appears as a consequence of the severe oligoamnios.
- Fifty percent present other associated anomalies
- Cardiovascular
- VATER (vertebral defects, anal atresia, tracheoesophageal, radial and renal anomalies)
- Gastrointestinal (anal and duodenal atresia, omphalocele)
- Phrenic hernia
- Musculoskeletal: Sirenomelus, digital anomalies
- Central nervous system (CNS): Neural tube defects.

Associate Syndromes

- Fraser syndrome
- Cerebro-oculo-facio-skeletal syndrome
- Acrorenal mandibular syndrome
- Branchiootorenal syndrome.

Unilateral agenesis

- Anomalies of the contralateral kidney in 48% of the cases
  - Vesicoureteral reflux
  - Obstruction of vesicoureteral junction
  - Obstruction of ureteropelvic junction.

Prognosis

- *Bilateral agenesis:* The prognosis is very poor. All newborns die in the first few hours or days similar to the consequence of lung hypoplasia.
- *Unilateral agenesis:* In general, the prognosis of these newborns is very good, although it will much depend on any anomalies associated with the contralateral kidney.

Management

- *Bilateral agenesis:* A pregnancy interruption may be offered due to the lethal prognosis. If the mother decides to continue with the pregnancy, it will be opted by a conservative behavior, a vaginal delivery will always be attempted, and reanimation maneuvers will not be made in the neonate.
- *Unilateral agenesis:* During the pregnancy, normal controls are followed as much during the pregnancy as in the newborn. The appearance of anomalies will be watched over in the contralateral kidney.

The recurrence risk of the bilateral renal agenesis is approximately 4%.[17] About 9% of first grade relatives of the fetuses or newborns with renal impotence will have asymptomatic renal malformations. If the renal agenesis is part of a syndrome, the recurrence risk will depend on the inheritance type.

Renal Ectopy

Ectopic kidney is that which is located outside the renal fossa. The most frequent locations are the pelvis (pelvic kidney) and the crusader of the other side (ectopia renal crusade); other less frequent ones are lumbar or thoracic. The incidence is approximately 1/1200 and 1/1900 respectively.[18,19]

Pelvic Kidney

The lack of ascent of the kidneys originates the pelvic kidneys and other ectopic forms.

Diagnosis: The echographic signs that will be found are:

- Absence of the kidney in the renal fossa: In these cases, it is very important to make an exploration of the fetal pelvis and the contralateral side in search of a possible ectopic kidney.
- Localization of the kidney adjacent to the bladder or the wing of the ileum:[18] In some cases, it may be difficult for its echogenicity to be similar to the adjacent intestine (Figs 33.8 and 33.9)

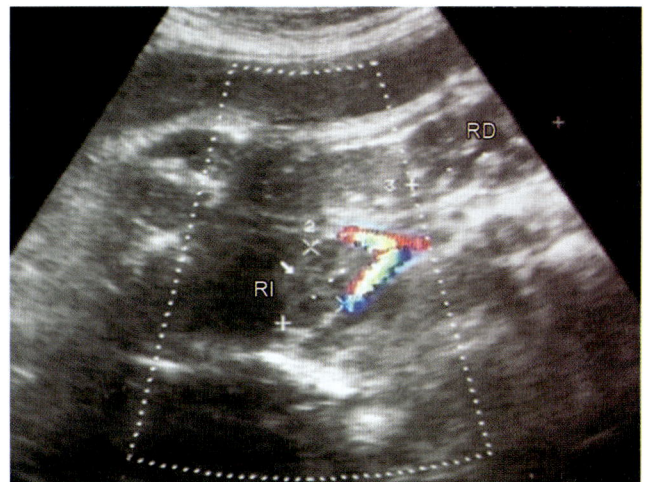

Fig. 33.8: Ectopic pelvic kidney. Between iliac arteries

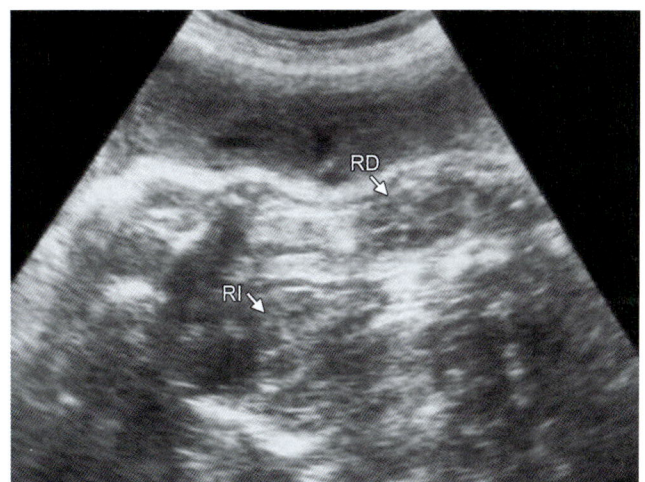

Fig. 33.9: Ectopic pelvic kidney. Between iliac arteries

Differential diagnosis
- Unilateral renal agenesis.

Associated anomalies: Other anomalies have been described as:
- Gynecological anomalies
- Gastrointestinal, cardiovascular anomalies and skeletal defects[18]
- Unique umbilical artery
- Contralateral kidney anomalies, as vesicoureteral reflux.

Prognosis: The prognosis is very good, although it will depend on the associated anomalies of the contralateral kidney.

Crossed Ectopic Kidney

During the renal ascent, a kidney crosses to the other side, resulting in crossed renal ectopy.

Diagnosis
- Absence of kidney in the renal fossa
- Big contralateral kidney and bilobate[20]

Differential diagnosis
- Unilateral renal agenesis with compensatory hypertrophy: In these cases, the kidney is not bilobed and it does not present a second collector system.
- Renal tumor: The contralateral kidney is present. A collector system is not identified in the tumor.

Associated anomalies
- Vertebral anomalies (myelomeningocele, sacral agenesis)
- Anal atresia
- Urinary anomalies like ureterovesical reflux, hydronephrosis, urinary infections, etc.

Prognosis: If it is presented in an isolated way, the prognosis is good.

Horseshoe Kidney

Horseshoe kidney is the union of the lower, or occasionally, the upper extremities of the two kidneys by a band of tissue extending across the vertebral column. The incidence is 1 per 400–600 births.[21,22] Because of their proximity, the kidneys fuse before completing their ascent, so that the root of the inferior mesenteric artery will avoid completing their ascent.

Diagnosis

Because of subtle findings, it is underdiagnosed. The echographic diagnosis is based on the demonstration of the presence of a renal tissue bridge that connects both the kidneys. Generally, in the inferior poles, it can be identified both in the transverse and coronal sections.

Associated Anomalies

- Urogenital anomalies: Hydronephrosis, vesicoureteral reflux, hypospadias and cryptorchidism
- Extraurological anomalies: Anomalies of CNS (neural tube defects)[23], cardiovascular, gastrointestinal anomalies and musculoskeletal defects[24]

- Chromosomal anomalies: Turner's syndrome,[25] Trisomy 18[26,27]
- Renal tumors: In children, it has been associated to the Wilms' tumor,[28] and in adults, it has been associated to a higher incidence of adenocarcinoma[29] and transitional cells tumor.[30]

Prognosis

The prognosis is excellent. A higher incidence of vesicoureteral reflux, renal stone, infection and hydronephrosis must be kept in mind.

Obstructive Uropathies

The fetal kidney responds in different ways to an obstruction depending on the gestational age in which it occurs. Very precocious obstructions, in the first trimester or beginning of the second, will give place to polycystic dysplastic kidneys. Later obstructions (after the twenty-second week) can produce hydronephrosis.

A particular difficulty in the diagnosis of renal obstruction is the high proportion of false-positive estimates in 36–81%. This is due to the mild hydronephrosis that is solved at the end of the pregnancy or in the neonatal stage. In order to avoid these false positives, limiting values of the anteroposterior diameter of the renal pelvis have been defined, for which the obstruction should be suspected. Unfortunately, these cut-off points vary from 4 mm to 10 mm in the second trimester and from 7 mm to 10 mm in the third trimester.

For some authors, the best echographic approach to predict postnatal uropathies is an anteroposterior diameter of the renal pelvis greater than or equal to 7 mm in the third trimester with a 69% positive predictive value.[31,32] Other authors have calculated echographic false negatives below 10%[33] and negative predictive values of 98%.[34]

Diameters of the renal pelvis above 15 mm have a high predictive value of renal pathology that needs postnatal surgery.[35]

The group that has more problems is those that have pelvic diameters from 4 mm to 10 mm in the twentieth week because 10–30% of children will present a vesicoureteral reflux that could damage the renal function without follow-up.[31]

These cases should be re-evaluated toward the twenty-eighth week of gestation and in the neonatal period to rule out a possible progression of the pyelectasis.

A sign of serious concern of the hydronephrosis is the presence of caliectasis, because it bends the necessity of surgery with regard to when the hydronephrosis is only present.[36]

Another aspect is the association between the dilatation of the urinary tract and chromosomal anomalies. In most of the cases, they are part of a multisystemic alteration secondary to a genetic alteration.[37] In the case of isolated mild hydronephrosis, the association with chromosomopathies is less clear; according to Nicolaides, it would be a 3% in isolated hydronephrosis.[38]

Obstruction at the Pyeloureteral Junction Level

Obstruction at the pyeloureteral junction level is the most common cause of obstruction at renal level with an unknown real incidence; some authors have calculated it in 1/2000 born alive.[39] It is more common in males, and in 30%, it is bilateral; when it is unilateral, it is more frequently on the left side. It is produced by a stenosis at the pyeloureteral junction level. The obstruction is, in most of the cases, functional, so it would result in a urine propulsion failure.

Histologically, the ureter frequently shows signs of chronic inflammation with disruption and disorganization of the collagen and muscular fibers in its wall. In 69% of the cases, a muscular anomaly exists so that there is an absence of the longitudinal fibers.[40]

With less frequency, there are anatomical causes of obstruction like fibrous adhesions, bands, anomalous ureteral insertion and obstruction for double kidneys.

Diagnosis: In the sonographic scan, a dilated renal pelvis will be seen with or without dilation of the renal calyces and without ureteral or vesical dilation (Figs 33.10 to 33.13).

In cases of severe obstructions, dilation of the renal chalices takes place with weight loss of the renal cortex (Fig. 33.14). In rare cases, an abdominal cyst will be present, or it will rupture with consequent perirenal urinoma (Fig. 33.15).

The volume of the amniotic fluid is usually normal; however, it can cause polyhydramnios for increase of urine production. The appearance of oligoamnios is not normal.

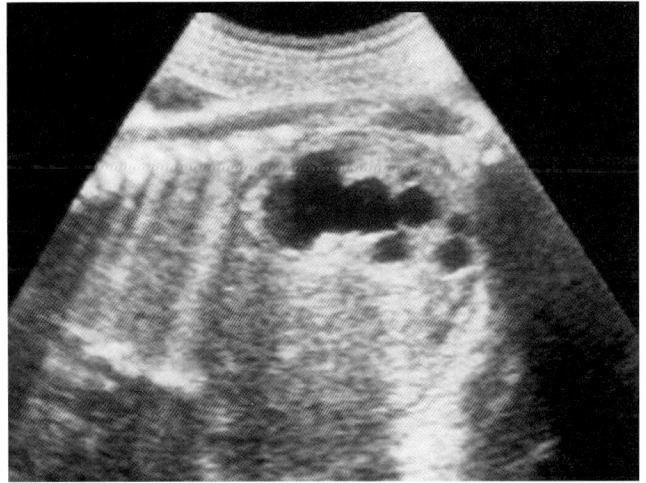

Fig. 33.12: Moderate dilatation of the collecting system and the renal pelvis

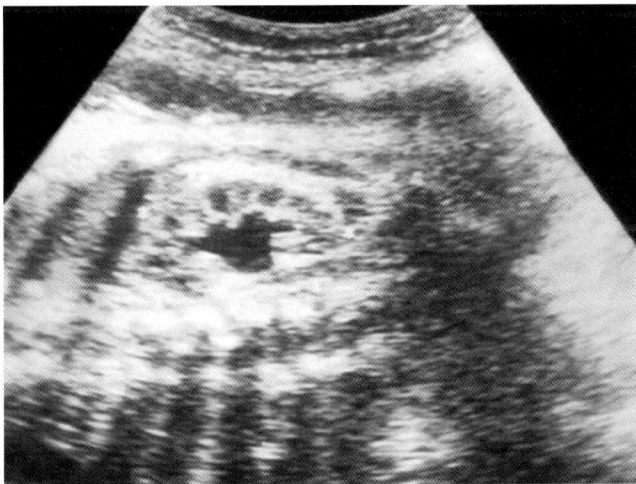

Fig. 33.10: Mild dilatation of the renal pelvis

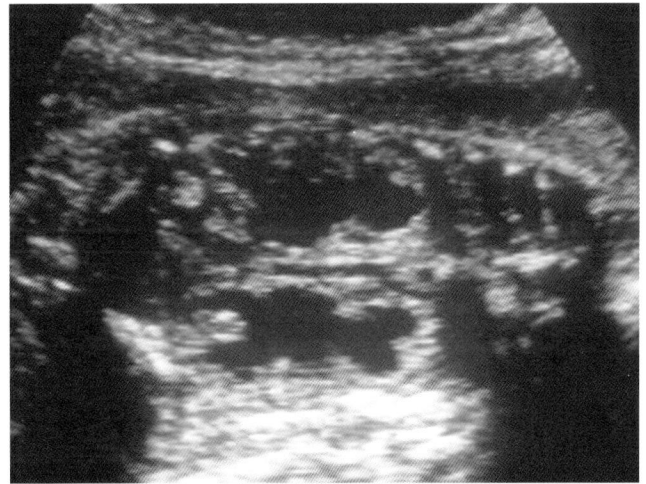

Fig. 33.13: Moderate dilatation of the collecting system and the renal pelvis

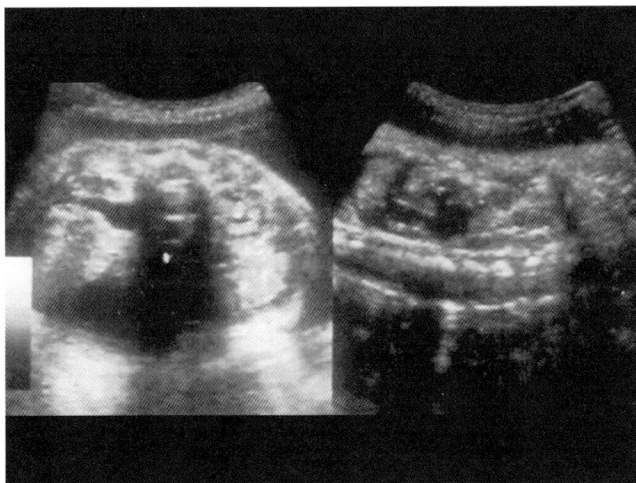

Fig. 33.11: Mild dilatation of the renal pelvis

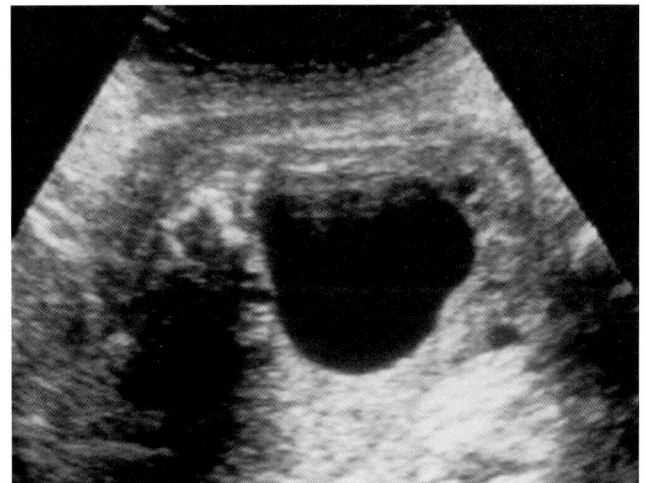

Fig. 33.14: Hydronephrosis. Severe dilatation of the renal pelvis and calyces. Enlarged kidney

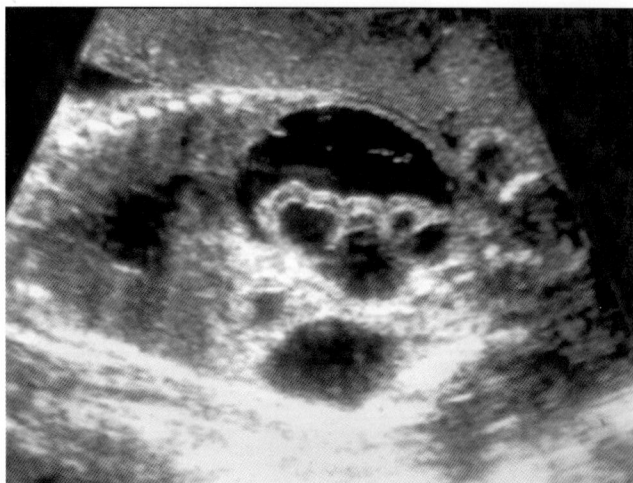

Fig. 33.15: Urinoma. Note the thinning of the cortex

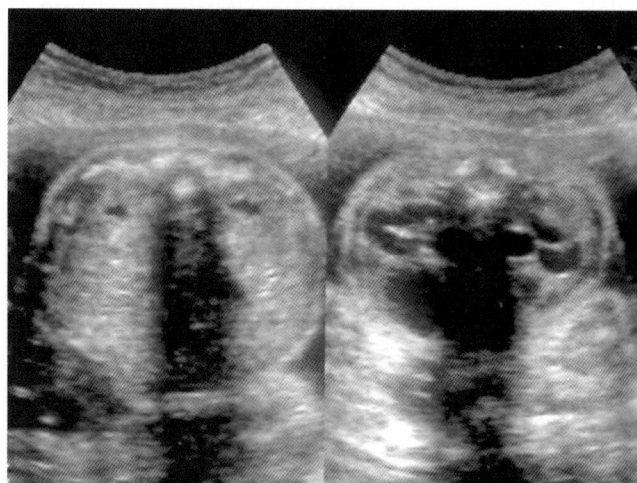

Fig. 33.16: Dilatation of the ureters

Differential diagnosis: It is necessary to consider other causes of lower renal obstruction where the ureters appear usually dilated like those of the vesicoureteral junction, vesical exit and the bilateral vesicoureteral reflux. It will also be necessary to consider polycystic kidneys, simple renal cysts or urinomas.

Associated anomalies: In the cases of pyeloureteral obstruction, we should study both kidneys in detail in search of possible associated anomalies (25–27%) as agenesis, multicystic dysplasia, vesicoureteral reflux, as well as possible extrarenal anomalies (12–19%) like cardiovascular anomalies, neural tube or digestive anomalies, and chromosomal anomalies.[41]

Prognosis: The postnatal prognosis is usually good and the hydronephrosis grade is usually correlated with the renal function.[35]

Prenatal management is usually conservative with the echographic follow-up in the third trimester. In the newborn, antibiotic prophylaxis is prescribed and a complete evaluation is carried out with echography, isotopic renogram and cystourethrography. The examinations are delayed for about 10 days except in the cases that present severe bilateral affectation.[42]

In most cases, postnatal management is conservative except when an increment of the hydronephrosis or decrease of the differential renal function exists, where pyeloplasty is the surgery of choice.[43]

Though most of the cases are sporadic, family forms of dominant inheritance have been described.[44]

Obstruction of the Ureterovesical Junction

This is the second cause of hydronephrosis, affecting 1/6500 newborns.[39] It is more common in males (ratio 2:1). It can be bilateral in 25% of the cases.

The obstruction is generally due to a regional malfunction or stenosis at the ureteral end, without evidence of vesicoureteral reflux or obstruction of the vesical exit. This is also called primary megaureter or megaureter without reflux.

Diagnosis: The affected kidney is shown with pyelectasis and a tortuous ureteral course (Figs 33.16 and 33.17).

The intravesical urine volume and amniotic fluid volume are usually normal, although they can be diminished in some cases of severe bilateral obstructions.

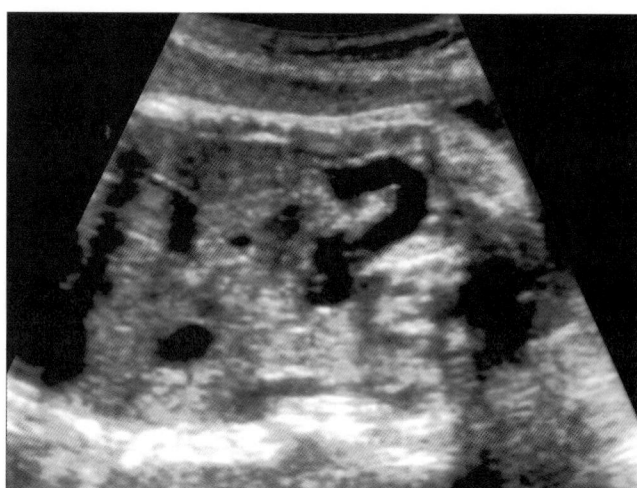

Fig. 33.17: Dilatation of the ureters

Differential diagnosis: The dilated ureter can be easily differentiated from intestine because the urine is anechoic while the intestinal content transmits low echogenicity.

A differential diagnosis with the vesicoureteral reflux should be carried out, which can have the same prenatal echographic appearance and not to be able to exclude until the realization of a cystourethrography in the neonatal period. It will also be necessary to carry out the differential diagnosis with strange cases of obstructions in the exit of the bladder that produce a massive ureteral reflux, and in the cases of double kidneys, where the ureteral dilatation is produced by an ureterocele, in this situation it is usual that the superior pole is hydronephrotic and that the ureterocele is visualized inside the bladder.

Associated anomalies: The contralateral kidney will present anomalies in 16% of the cases, including pyeloureteral obstruction, multicystic renal dysplasia, pelvic kidney, renal agenesis and vesicoureteral reflux.[45]

Prognosis: It is generally good so that up to 40% is resolves postnatally in a spontaneous way. Ureters with diameters of less than 6 mm are associated with low surgery incidence, while those that have a diameter above 10 mm have a higher incidence of surgical corrections.[46,47]

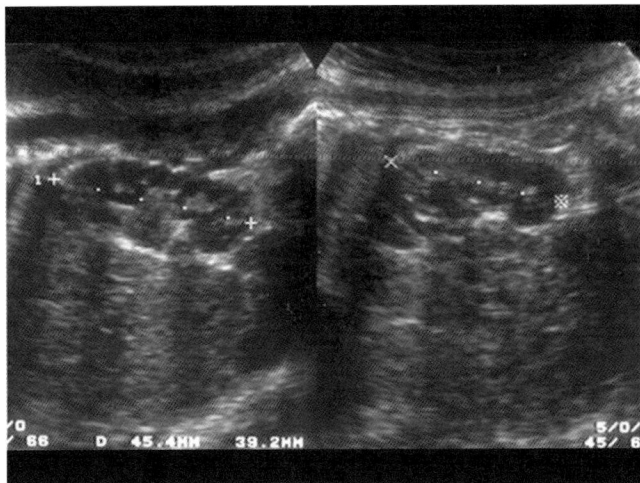

Fig. 33.18: Duplex kidney. A sagittal scan through a duplex kidney shows two collecting systems

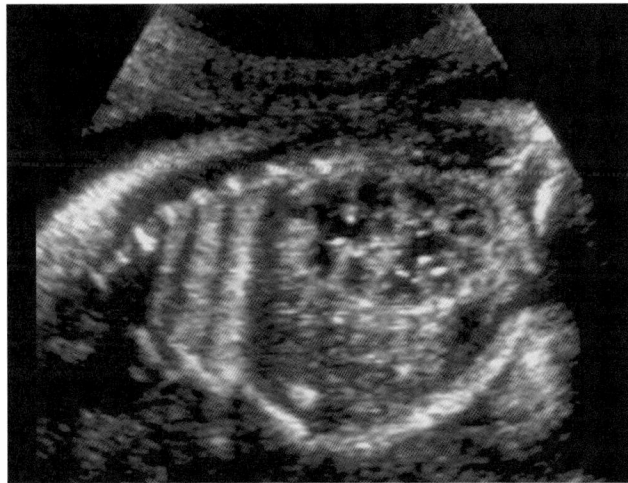

Fig. 33.19: Duplex kidney. A sagittal scan through a duplex kidney shows two collecting systems

A neonatal follow-up should be carried out with cystourethrography and a renogram to evaluate the renal function. Those that present a poor renal function will be candidates for surgery with ureteral reimplantation.

It is sporadic with a low recurrence risk.

Secondary Obstruction to Ureterocele and Ectopic Ureter

The ureterocele is a cystic dilation of the distal ureter in its intravesical portion. An ectopic ureter is that which is not inserted near the posterolateral angle of the trigone.

An ectopic ureter can end in the urethra, in the neck of urinary bladder or in the trigone, in an inferomedial localization regarding the normality. In girls, it can also be inserted in the vestibule of the vagina, vagina or uterus and in males in the seminal vesicle, ductus deferens or ejaculatory ducts.

The incidence is difficult to determine. There are studies that estimate it in 1/9000 newborns.[39]

The ureteroceles frequently associates in girls (up to 80%) with double renal systems being located in these cases the ureterocele in the superior system.[48]

However, in 40% of children the ureteroceles drain to a unique collector system. The ureteroceles and the ectopic ureters are bilateral in 10–15% of the cases. The double systems occur for the development of two ureteral gemmae starting from the mesonephric duct. In the double systems, the place where it drains is reversed, so the ureter of the superior pole drains into a more inferior and more medial place, and the inferior pole drains into a superior and lateral place. The presence of ureterocele will produce hydronephrosis in the superior pole, which can produce dysplasia and deterioration of the renal function. In the inferior pole, it can also have hydronephrosis, but it is usually due to vesicoureteral reflux.

Diagnosis: In the absence of hydronephrosis, it may be difficult to diagnose prenatally a double system. In these cases, a meticulous echographic study would demonstrate a kidney of increased size with two collector systems. The prenatal diagnosis of the double system is usually carried out during the second half of the pregnancy with the presence of two or more of the following signs: limited hydronephrosis to a kidney pole, double renal pelvis not communicated, ipsilateral megaureter and ureterocele[49] (Figs 33.18 and 33.19).

When hydronephrosis exists, the superior pole is usually affected and the ureterocele can be demonstrated if the bladder is full. The ureterocele cannot be seen for different reasons: dysplasia of the superior pole that makes little urine excretion, empty bladder, large ureterocele that confuses with the own bladder. An ectopic ureter will be suspected when hydronephrosis exists in the superior system of a double system, and this dilated ureter seems to end below the base of the bladder without ureterocele. The utility of the magnetic resonance has been described in doubtful cases[50] (Figs 33.20 and 33.21).

The ureteroceles can be large enough to produce obstruction of the exit of the urine from the bladder. They can be bilateral in 15% of the cases[51] (Figs 33.22 to 33.24). The amniotic fluid is usually normal in unilateral cases.

Differential diagnosis: With the reflux and the vesicoureteral obstruction. Also with posterior urethral valves in cases of ureteroceles that occlude the urethra, the posterior urethral valves occur only in males.

Associated anomalies: The vesicoureteral reflux is presented in the inferior pole in 50% of the fetuses with ureterocele in the superior pole.[52] Higher association with other anomalies does not exist.

Prognosis: It is better when a prenatal diagnosis is carried out. The necessity to carry out second surgery is reduced when it has been diagnosed prenatally.[53] The renal function will depend on the grade of dysplasia of the superior pole that is usually higher in ectopic ureters than in ureteroceles. In cases of severe reflux in the inferior pole, dysplasia and worsening of the renal function can also exist.

Prenatal follow-up ultrasound will be carried out to evaluate the progression of the hydronephrosis.

In the postnatal period, it will be re-evaluated with echography, renogram and cystourethrography. In cases with good renal function, the ureterocele can be punctured through the urethra by

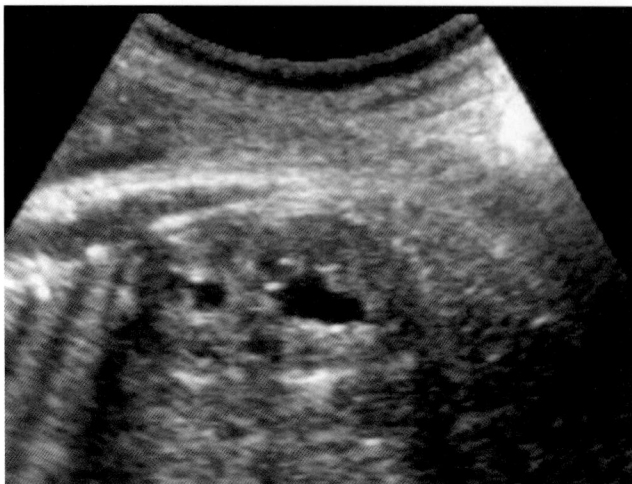

Fig. 33.20: Duplex kidney. A sagittal scan through a duplex kidney shows two collecting systems

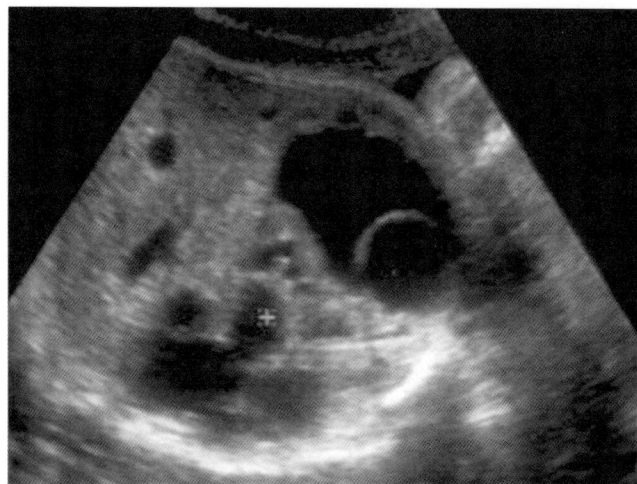

Fig. 33.23: Ectopic ureterocele in the bladder

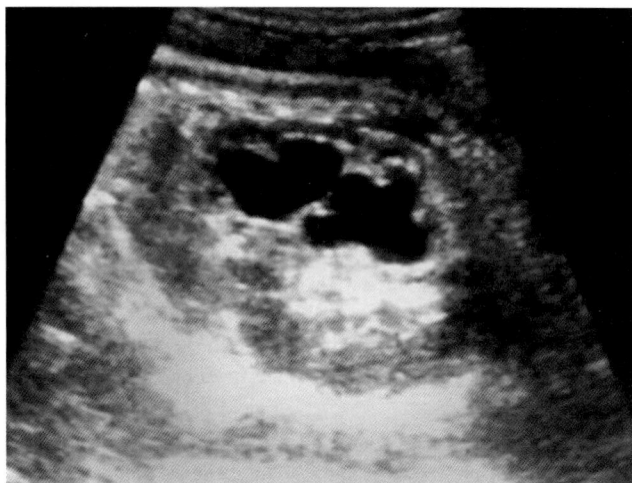

Fig. 33.21: Duplex kidney. A sagittal scan through a duplex kidney shows two collecting systems

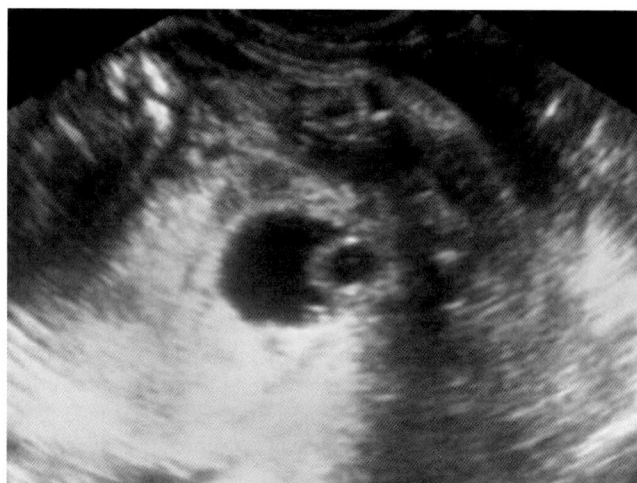

Fig. 33.24: Ectopic ureterocele in the bladder

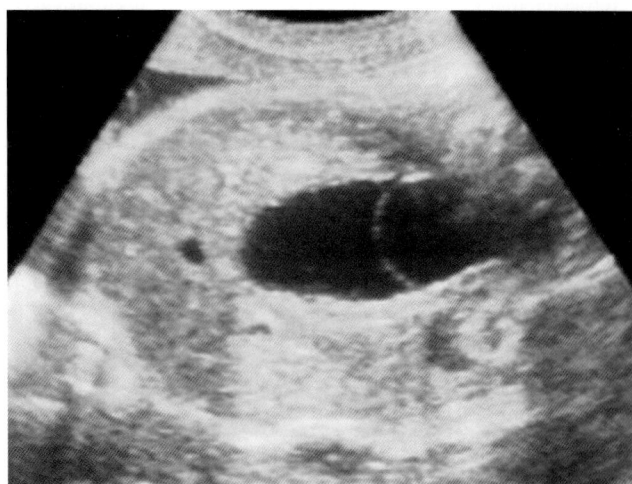

Fig. 33.22: Ectopic ureterocele in the bladder

cystoscopy, which although has a risk of increasing the reflux in 30% does not seem to increase the necessity of second surgeries.[54] The non-functional superior poles are usually resected.[55–58] It is sporadic with a low risk of recurrence.

Posterior Urethral Valves

This is the most frequent cause of severe obstructive uropathy in children, constituting 9% of the cases of fetal urinary obstruction.[55] The approximate incidence is 1 in each 5000–8000 children. It only affects males.

It is produced by folds of membranous tissue with a fibrous stroma that go from the prostatic urethra to the external urinary sphincter producing a more or less severe difficulty of the urine exit from the bladder.[59] The etiology is unknown; one of the theories is an anomalous insert of the mesonephric conduit into the cloaca.[60]

Diagnosis: It is usually diagnosed in the second and third trimester. The characteristic echographic findings will be bladder dilatation

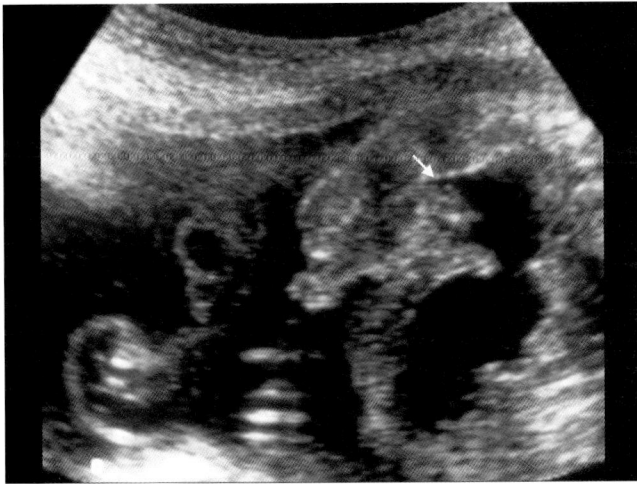

Fig. 33.25: Dilated bladder and a "keyhole" deformity of the posterior urethra

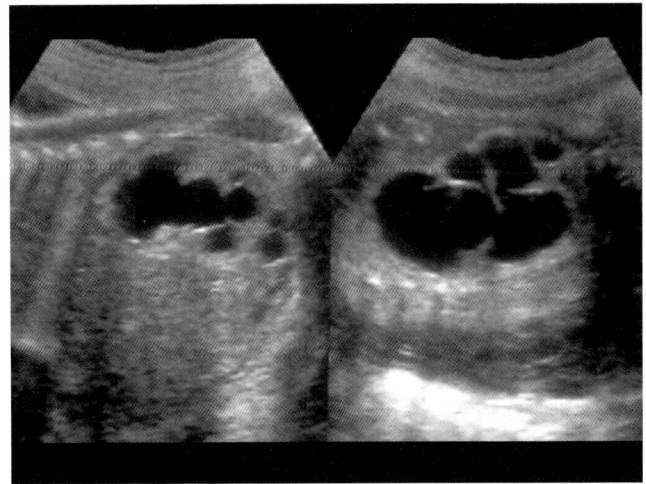

Fig. 33.26: Kidney showing moderate dilatation

with wall thickening (due to a detrusor thickening) and dilatation of the posterior urethra. It can exist in secondary way renal dysplasia recognized echographically for echogenic kidneys whether or not accompanied by cortical cysts (Fig. 33.25).[61]

It is usually associated with a variable grade of bilateral ureterohydronephrosis (Fig. 33.26).[60] The vesical distension can give place to its rupture causing urinary ascites, this ascites is considered a sign of good prognosis, since it liberates the kidneys from pressure due to obstruction and therefore diminishes the risk of dysplasia.[55–62,63]

They can also break the renal chalices giving place to perirenal urinomas, which is a sign of bad prognosis since it is associated with renal dysplasia.[64]

It can exist as an asymmetric hydronephrosis by a massive reflux to a kidney that is practically destroyed; this can be a protection mechanism for the contralateral kidney.[65] The amniotic fluid can be diminished, which is a sign of poor prognosis.

Differential diagnosis: It is mainly with severe bilateral vesicoureteral reflux. Sometimes diagnosis is not easy. It may be useful to observe that in the reflux the bladder wall is usually thin, the dilatation of the posterior urethra also will not be seen.

We will also carry out the differential diagnosis with the ureteral atresia in which a marked vesical distension usually exists of precocious detection in the first trimester or second initial trimester usually accompanied by oligoamnios.

We will also consider other rare causes of obstruction of the exit of the bladder like the congenital megalourethra, where a distal obstruction in the penile urethra exists and cystic images among the fetal legs can be observed in the ultrasound,[66] the cloacal persistence and hydrometrocolpos associated with a urogenital sinus that only takes place in girls,[67] and the megacystis-microcolon syndrome where bilateral hydronephrosis and vesical dilatation can exist, but it can be polyhydramnios and stomach distention. It affects the females more, and it is of recessive autosomal inheritance.[68,69]

Associated anomalies: They will be associated with a sequence of anomalies in variable grade secondary to the obstruction: megacystis, megaloureter, hydronephrosis, paraurethral diverticula

and dilatation of the proximal urethra. Other associated urinary anomalies are: megalourethra,[70] cryptorchidism, hypospadias and urethral duplications. Anomalies in other organs are also very frequently found (up to 43% of the fetuses)[71] such as tracheal hypoplasia, persistent ductus arteriosus, skeletal anomalies, imperforate anus, VACTERL syndrome[72,73] and frequent association of chromosomal anomalies.

When a precocious oligoamnios exists, lung hypoplasia will occur and the typical findings of the Potter's syndrome (low ear implantation, micrognathia, hypertelorism, limbs contracture) will be observed.

It can be the cause of the prune belly syndrome (thickening of the abdominal wall muscles, urinary tract alterations and undescended testes) due to the abdominal distension secondary to the vesical distension.

Prognosis: The prognosis is variable depending on the graveness of the obstruction that in turn will be translated in the ultrasound findings, so that the most serious cases diagnosed before the twenty-fourth week will have a perinatal mortality or chronic renal failure in 53%, while those diagnosed later will have a bad evolution risk of 7%.

The precocious oligoamnios, signs of renal dysplasia as the echogenic kidneys, cortical cysts, the perirenal urinoma and the association with other anomalies are the signs of a poor prognosis.

A determination of urine electrolytes is used to evaluate the renal function, with serial determinations to avoid the stagnated urine (Table 33.1). According to the result, it will also be able to classify as good or bad prognosis.

Table 33.1: Poor prognostic values in fetal urine

Sodium	100 mEq/L
Chlorine	90 mEq/L
Osmolarity	280 mOsm/L
Calcium	2 mmol/L
Phosphate	2 mmol/L
β_2 microglobulin	2 mmol/L

It will also be convenient to carry out a fetal karyotype.

In the fetuses diagnosed before 32 weeks without signs of renal dysplasia but with oligoamnios, the decompression of the urinary tract should be evaluated by means of the realization of a vesico amniotic bypass.[74] After the thirty-second week, it will be necessary to evaluate the finalization of the gestation for the decompression of the urinary tract in the proximate neonatal period. Nowadays, an option of intrauterine fetal therapy exists, which can be carried out by means of valvular resection with endoscopy. The criteria for this intrauterine surgery will be the absence of echographic dysplasia findings, normal karyotype and some appropriate values of electrolytes in the vesicocentesis.[75,76] It is sporadic with a low recurrence risk.

Atresia Urethral

The real incidence is ignored. It affects males more. Etiology is ignored. It is characterized by the complete obstruction from the urethra secondary to the obliteration of the membranous urethra.

Diagnosis: It can be seen as a much dilated bladder with oligoamnios in the echograph. Detection can be carried out very early, on occasion starting from the tenth week. Frequently, an anhydramnios exists with such a loosened bladder that it is difficult to explore the fetal anatomy (Figs 33.27 to 33.29).

In some occasions, a vesicocutaneous fistula is developed being able to be the amniotic liquid normal.[77]

Differential diagnosis: With other causes of vesical exit obstruction: posterior urethral valves, megalourethra, megacystis-microcolon syndrome, persistent cloaca and severe vesicoureteral reflux.[78]

Associated anomalies: They are very frequent (more than 50%) but difficult to diagnose because of the oligoamnios. Among them are: heart anomalies, diaphragmatic hernia, polydactyly, VACTERL syndrome and chromosomal anomalies. It is one of the causes of the prune belly syndrome.[79]

Prognosis: It is always poor and almost always lethal. Due to the oligoamnios or anhydramnios they develop a lung hypoplasia. The development of a vesicocutaneous fistula can improve the neonatal survival; however, they usually develop a renal failure that makes a renal transplantation necessary with a bigger surgical reconstruction or hemodialysis.[77]

Due to the possibility of an early diagnosis an appropriate option is the interruption of the pregnancy. If the gestation is continued the possibility of the realization of a vesicoamniotic shunt will be evaluated.[80] It is sporadic with a low recurrence risk.

Vesicoureteral reflux

This is the backward flow of urine from bladder into ureter and the pyeloureteral system. This reflux occurs in around 1% of all the children. Fetal vesicoureteral reflux presents a masculine prevalence of up to 80% and a high frequency (20%) of high grade reflux (III–IV).[81,82] Around 60% is bilateral. It represents 11% of the prenatal hydronephrosis cases.[83]

The etiology seems to be multifactorial. The neonatal reflux seems to have its origin in a distortion of the vesicoureteral junction in utero, secondary to the high casting pressures that some fetuses present.[81]

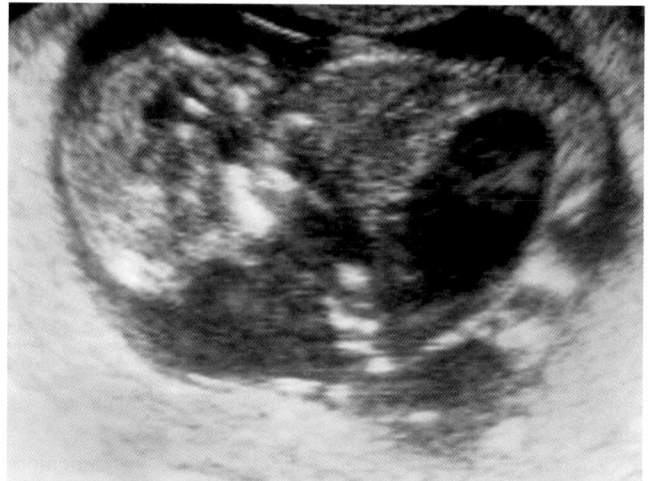

Fig. 33.28: Axial plane through the fetal abdomen demonstrating fetal megacystis

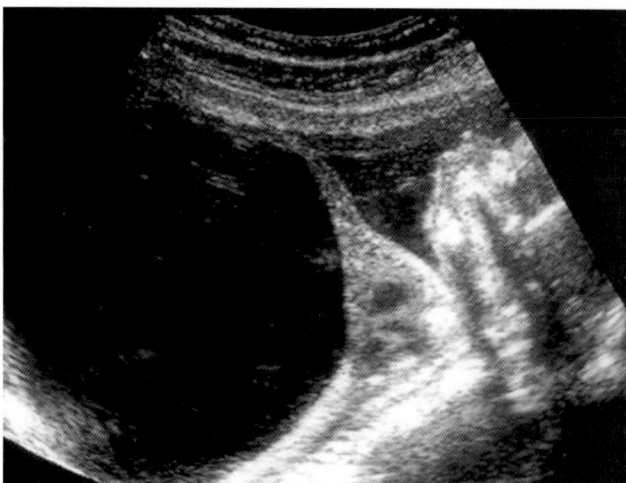

Fig. 33.27: Axial plane through the fetal abdomen demonstrating fetal megacystis

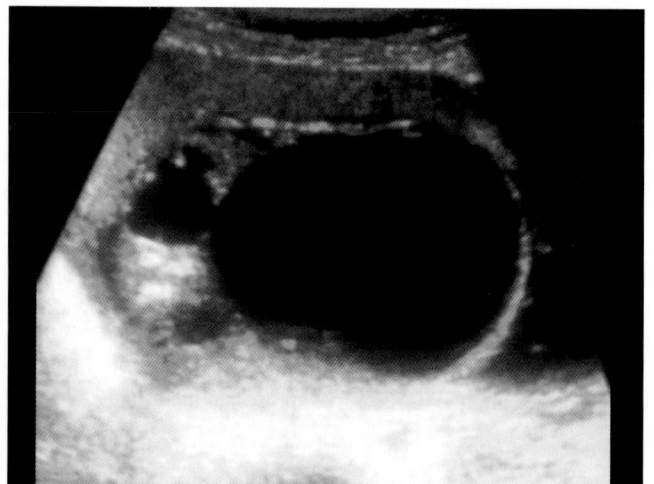

Fig. 33.29: Kidney showing moderate dilatation

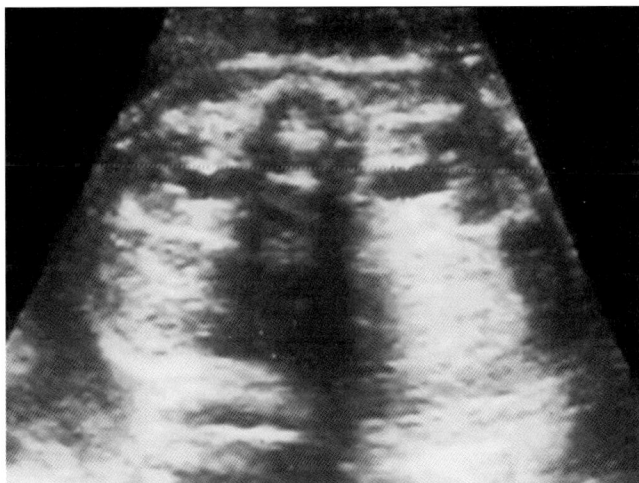

Fig. 33.30: Moderate pyelectasis with vesicoureteral reflux

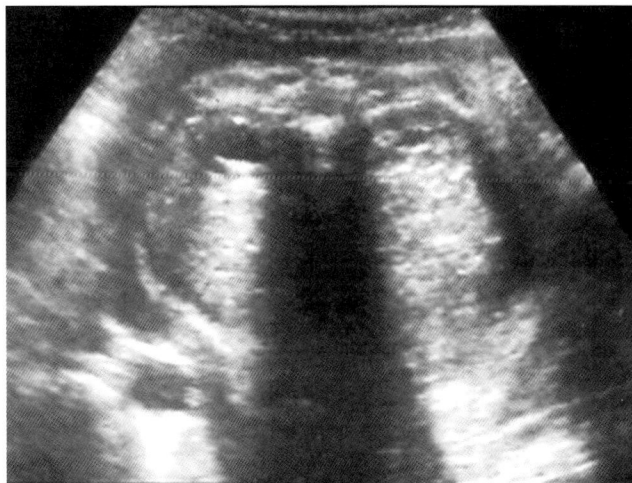

Fig. 33.31: Moderate pyelectasis with vesicoureteral reflux

Pathology

- Urinary tract infection, which is more frequent in this group, is typically associated to parenchymatous affectation.
- Up to 50% of the infants with sterile vesicoureteral reflux can present parenchymatous renal anomalies, which suggests a congenital etiopathology of renal lesion independent of the urinary infection[84,85]

Diagnosis

- *Hydronephrosis:* It is the main echographic finding. It can be unilateral or bilateral (Figs 33.30 and 33.31)
- *Hydroureter and a dilated bladder with a thinner wall:* These are findings that we could find in the most severe cases. It may be confused with some posterior ureteral valves
- The amniotic fluid volume is normal
- The moderate pyelectasis (4–10 mm) can also be associated to vesicoureteral reflux.

Differential Diagnosis

Other hydronephrosis causes should be considered

- *Unilateral:* Obstruction of pyeloureteral or vesicoureteral junction
- Bilateral: Posterior urethral valves.

Associated Anomalies

These are mainly anomalies of the contralateral kidney.

- Obstruction of the pyeloureteral junction
- Multicystic kidney
- Renal agenesis
- Renal or ureteral duplicity.

Prognosis

- Many resolve completely spontaneously. A total of 60% grade III, 50% grade IV and 28% grade V were resolved in 14 months.[83]

- Thirty percent of these fetuses present renal scars, and two-thirds of them present widespread renal lesions.
- The reflux is the cause of 25% of the renal failure in children and 15% in adults.

Management

- If there is a hydronephrosis:
  - Prenatal control: In utero, we must make an echographic follow-up of the hydronephrosis and of the volume of amniotic fluid.
  - Postnatal control:
    - Echography starting from 48 hours of life
    - Antibiotic prophylaxis
    - Serial cystourethrography
- If there is a moderate pyelectasis:
  - Postnatal echography
  - Echography up to 3 months
  - Urologic follow-up.

Treatment will be surgical in those cases that present new renal scars, a high reflux grade, a progressive reflux, or persistent urinary infections.

The recurrence risk in brothers of the affected cases is 34%[86] and in children of the affected cases is 66%.[87]

Renal Cystic Diseases

Renal cystic disease compromises a mixed group of heritable, developmental and acquired disorders. Because of their diverse etiology, histology and clinical presentation, no single scheme of classification has gained acceptance.[88]

The Potter classification (Potter 1972),[89] does cover the most important conditions seen prenatally (Table 33.2).

Many of the terms used to describe kidney malformations, such as the Potter classification, are confusing since they are based on histology and do not take account of recent advances in molecular biology and genetics. A more straightforward approach is to divide the abnormalities into groups based on the underlying cell biology, such as aberrant early development or defects in "terminal" maturation.[90]

Table 33.2: Potter classification of cystic renal disease

Type I	Autosomal recessive (infantile) polycystic renal disease
Type II	Multicystic renal dysplasia
Type III	Autosomal dominant (adult) polycystic renal disease
Type IV	Obstructive cystic dysplasia

The aberrant early development group includes dysplastic kidney:[90]

- Large multicystic dysplastic (Potter type IIa).
- Small organs with a combination of hypoplasia/dysplasia (Potter type IIb).
- Severely obstructed kidneys (Potter type IV). Kidney malformations associated with syndromes are also included within this category.[90]

Defects in terminal maturation are observed in PKD. Initial nephron and collecting duct formation is unremarkable in these kidneys, but there is a later cystic dilatation of these structures causing secondary loss of adjacent normal structures. The most common types are autosomal dominant and autosomal recessive PKD. Both may present prenatally.[90]

Polycystic Kidney Diseases

Two forms of PKD will be discussed in this chapter:

1. Autosomal recessive polycystic kidney disease (infantile) (ARPKD).
2. Autosomal dominant polycystic kidney disease (adult) (ADPKD).

Both diseases may present prenatally or during infancy. Cysts only arise from collecting ducts in ARPKD, whereas they arise from all area of the nephron or collecting duct in ADPKD. In addition, there are usually numerous small cysts in ARPKD whereas there are fewer, larger cysts in the dominant disease. Associated abnormalities in other organ systems are quite different in both conditions.[90]

Autosomal recessive polycystic kidney disease (Potter I): The condition is characterized by symmetric enlargement of both kidneys secondary to renal collecting tube dilatation. This is associated with varying degrees of hepatic fibrosis and biliary ectasia.[91]

It is an autosomal recessive condition with an incidence of 1/40,000–50,000 live births.[92]

There is likely to be a defect in the collecting ducts resulting in the formation of cystic dilatations of the collecting tubules.[93] The hepatic fibrosis could be due to overgrowth of the biliary epithelium. The gene for ARPKD is located on chromosome 6p.[103]

Pathology: The kidneys are symmetrically enlarged, and this is produced by cystic dilatations of the collecting tubules, which are arranged radially throughout the renal parenchyma.[93] The earlier-forming distal collecting tubules are more severely affected than the proximal collecting tubules. There is no proliferation of the connective tissue. Clinically the disease has been classified into four subtypes[94] (Table 33.3).

Diagnosis: The typical appearance is of enlarged kidneys showing increased echogenicity associated with small or absent bladder and oligohydramnios[95,96] (Fig. 33.32).

Table 33.3: Manifestations of ARPKD according to the subclassification of Blyth and Ockenden

Type	Proportion of dilated renal tubules (%)	Extent of portal fibrosist	Lifespan
Perinatal	90	Minimal	Hours
Neonatal	60	Mild	Months
Infantile	20	Moderate	10 years
Juvenile	< 10	Gross	50 years

These sonographic features may not be present until the third trimester; however, and it is well documented that fetuses with their condition may look absolutely normal at the 20-week scan. Thus, this condition cannot be excluded until well into the third trimester.[97–99]

A few cases diagnosed by transvaginal scanning at 12–14 weeks of gestation have been reported.[100] Careful measurements of both kidneys are important to the diagnosis because affected kidneys have a faster growth profile than normal kidneys.[101]

Molecular genetics studies provide a useful adjunct to ultrasound for diagnosing ARPKD, and these should be discussed with high-risk families. It is possible to make a prenatal diagnosis at 11–12 weeks of gestation from chorionic villus sampling.

Magnetic resonance imaging (MRI) has also been used to diagnose ARPKD in utero, but this technique is not in regular use in most centers.[102]

Associated anomalies: The main association is hepatic fibrosis.

Differential diagnosis: The differential diagnosis for ARPKD is quite large. However, one important consideration is ADPKD, which can look identical except that liquor volume is usually normal. The other main diagnoses are outlined in Table 33.4.

Prognosis: The outcome is predicted from the severity of the renal disease with the poorest outlook for the perinatal type. Infants usually die from respiratory failure rather than renal problems, although

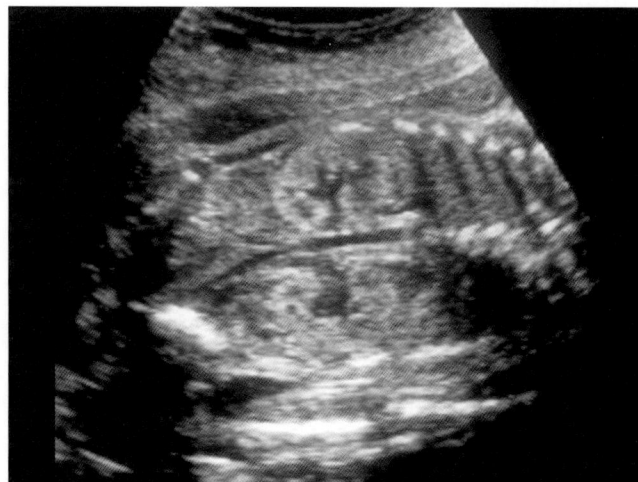

Fig. 33.32: Autosomal recessive polycystic kidney disease. The images show enlarged kidneys with echogenic parenchyma and oligohydramnios. The bladder is not visible

Table 33.4: Echogenic kidneys: Antenatal ultrasound appearances and clinical findings

Condition	Renal size	Cysts present?	Hydronephrosis	AF	Cysts in parents' kidneys	Family history	Associated findings
ARPKD	Large	No	No	→	No	Yes, in sibling	Hepatic fibrosis
ADPKD	Large	Sometimes	No	Normal	Yes >20 years	Yes, in loss parent	Occasionally cysts in parents' liver, spleen
Obstructive cystic dysplasia	Small	Often	No	Depends on degree of renal obstruction	No	No	Hydronephrosis usually urethral obstruction
Finnish type nephrotic syndrome	Large	No	No	Normal	No	Yes, in sibling	Raised serum alpha-fetoprotein
Beckwith–Wiedemann syndrome	Large	No	No	Normal ↑	No	Occasionally	Macrosomia, large liver, macroglossia, omphalocele
Perlman syndrome	Large	No	Sometimes	Normal ↑	No	Yes, in sibling	Macrosomia, hepatosplenomegaly ascites, micrognathia, depressed nasal bridge
Meckel–Gruber syndrome	Large	Sometimes	No	→	No	Yes, in sibling	Polydactyly, encephalocele
Trisomy 13	Large	Sometimes	No	Normal	No	No	Facial clefting, holoprosencephaly, cardiac defects, polydactyly
CMV infection	Large	No	No	Normal	No	No	Microcephaly, hydrocephaly, intracranial calcification, large liver and spleen, hydrops
Renal vein thrombosis	Large, usually unilateral	No	No	Normal	No	No	Maternal diabetes, maternal pyelonephritis
Normal	Normal	No	No	Normal	No	No	

aggressive ventilatory support and emergency nephrectomy may improve the outcome. The outcome is progressively better with later presentation and decreasing severity of renal involvement.

Long-term complications include severe systemic hypertension, urinary tract infection and hepatic fibrosis with portal hypertension leading to hypersplenism and gastroesophageal varices.[104]

Management: When scanning demonstrates bilaterally enlarged echogenic kidneys with oligohydramnios and there is family history of autosomal recessive polycystic renal disease, the outlook is likely to be very poor. In such a setting a termination of the pregnancy could be offered to the mother before viability.

When there is no family history and the amniotic fluid is normal, other conditions that have better prognosis should be considered. In such cases, conservative management is more appropriate.

The presence of associated abnormalities recommends karyotype. Follow-up scans are of value to assess liquor volume in pregnancy. There is a 25% risk of recurrence.

Autosomal dominant polycystic renal disease (Potter III): This condition is much more common than ARPKD. However, it is much less common or ADPKD to present prenatally or in early childhood. The ADPKD classically present bilaterally with cystic dilatation of the nephrons. It is the most common of the hereditary renal cystic disease, with an incidence of 1/1000 live births.[105]

The condition is caused by a mutation near the telomere of chromosome 16 in 90% cases.[106] Five percent of cases are caused by abnormality of chromosome 4.[107] Ninety percent of cases are linked to the PKD1 gene on the short arm of chromosome 16[106] and 5% are linked to the PKD2 gene on chromosome 4.[107] Prenatal diagnosis is possible by gene probes from chorion sampling.[104]

Pathology: It is a systemic disorder characterized by cysts formation in ductal organs, particularly the kidneys and liver. Cysts may also be present within the pancreas, spleen and CNS.[88] In the kidneys, only 5% of nephrons are cystic in the early part of the disease.

Diagnosis: In adults, almost all patients present one cyst, at least, at age of 30 years.[108,109] The sonographic appearance is well known: enlarged hyperechogenic kidneys, with a mixture of small and large cysts (Fig. 33.33).[110]

Some cases diagnosed prenatally have been reported. The most common sonographic finding is large kidneys.[111-113] The sonographic appearance is similar to the ARPKD: symmetrically enlarged and hyperechogenic kidneys. The bladder is generally present and the amniotic fluid is normal. The corticomedullary junction may appear accentuated or may be indistinct.[114] Some reports have described the presence of macroscopic cysts within the echogenic kidneys.[90]

Brun et al.[27] determined a new specific echographic pattern: moderately enlarged kidneys (1–2 SD > mean) with, in the majority of cases, a hyperechogenic cortex and relatively hypoechogenic medulla that occurs in the third trimester. This hyperechogenic cortex is probably related to the presence of multiple microcysts within renal cortex.

Sonographic diagnosis is usually made in the third trimester with a mean of 28 weeks.[114] Some cases of earlier sonographic diagnosis have been reported but mostly in cases with known family history.[115,116]

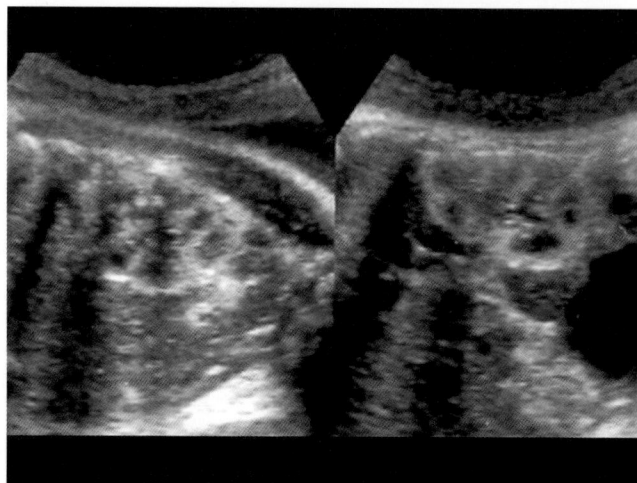

Fig. 33.33: Adult polycystic kidney disease. Brightly echogenic kidneys with accentuation of the corticomedullary junction and a small bladder with decreased fluid

Follow-up scans are essential because in the second trimester the kidneys can look normal. Very rarely, the condition can be unilateral.[117,118]

Differential diagnosis: Several conditions may exhibit enlarged hyperechogenic kidneys. This echographic feature may correspond to different renal diseases with different outlooks and perinatal outcomes: obstructive dysplasia, multicystic renal dysplasia, autosomal recessive polycystic renal disease, genetical syndromes (Perlman syndrome, Beckwith–Wiedemann syndrome, Bardet–Biedl syndrome, Meckel syndrome), nefroblastomatosis, renal vein thrombosis, toxic injured, infections (cytomegalovirus), ischemia, aneuploidy and, sometimes, normality.

In ADPKD few cases are diagnosed prenatally. The diagnosis is based on family history, amniotic fluid, associated abnormalities and genetic analysis.

Associated anomalies: The most important associated anomalies are cysts in the liver, spleen and pancreas. Noncystic anomalies include cardiac disease, skeletal anomalies, pyloric stenosis and intracranial aneurysms.[88] Tract urinary malformations associated with this condition have also been described.[114]

Prognosis: The condition is often asymptomatic and usually presents in the fifth decade with hypertension and end-stage renal failure.[105]

The outlook for those cases diagnosed in utero is difficult to determine because to date only 83 cases of adult-type polycystic renal disease presenting prenatally or in the first few months of life have been reported. MacDermot et al.[104] reported that in prenatal cases, 43% of babies die within the first year of life and 67% of survivors develop hypertension. The best indicators for outcome are the presence of oligohydramnios and the perinatal outcome from a previously affected sibling.

Management: Management of the pregnancy depends in large part on the parents' knowledge of this condition. The diagnosis of this condition requires very careful counseling with regards to both the short-term and long-term outlooks. Follow-up scans in the third trimester are of value to assess liquor volume. There is a 50% risk of recurrence.

Dysplastic Kidneys: Multicystic Renal Dysplasia (Potter II)

The diagnosis is inferred from the 'bright' echogenic appearance caused by the lack of normal renal parenchyma and structurally abnormal kidneys.

Dysplastic kidneys can be of any size, ranging from massive distended with multiple large cysts up to 9 cm in diameter, which are commonly termed "multicystic dysplastic kidneys" (MCDK), to normal or small kidneys with or without cysts. Dysplasia can be unilateral or bilateral. MCKD is one of the most common causes of abdominal masses in the newborn.[90]

It is the most common form of renal cystic disease in childhood. It has an incidence of 1/3000 live births and is more common in boys.[119,120] The majority is unilateral, but it can be bilateral up to 23% of cases.[119]

Multicystic dysplastic kidney are attached to atresia of the ureter and renal pelvis. This may be related to incomplete, but severe obstruction to the kidney early in nephrogenesis.[121]

Pathology: The kidney is replaced by multiple smooth-walled cysts of varying size.[88] Between the cysts is a dense stroma, but usually no normal renal tissue.[122,123] Typically, the renal artery is either absent or very small.

Diagnosis: The prenatal diagnosis for the unilateral condition is variable and depends on its severity. It is usually straightforward in the midtrimester scan. The classical presentation of MCDK is a multiloculated abdominal mass consisting of multiple thin-walled cysts, which do not appear to be connected. The kidneys are usually enlarged with an irregular outline and no renal pelvis can be demonstrated (Figs 33.34 and 33.35). Circumferential cysts may occasionally be detected in kidneys of more normal size, particularly in association with lower tract obstruction. Parenchymal tissue between the cysts is often hyperechogenic[90] (Figs 33.36 and 33.37). Bladder and amniotic fluid are usually normal in the unilateral condition.[120,121]

The bilateral form is usually diagnosed earlier because oligohydramnios is present and bladder is not seen. MCDK usually

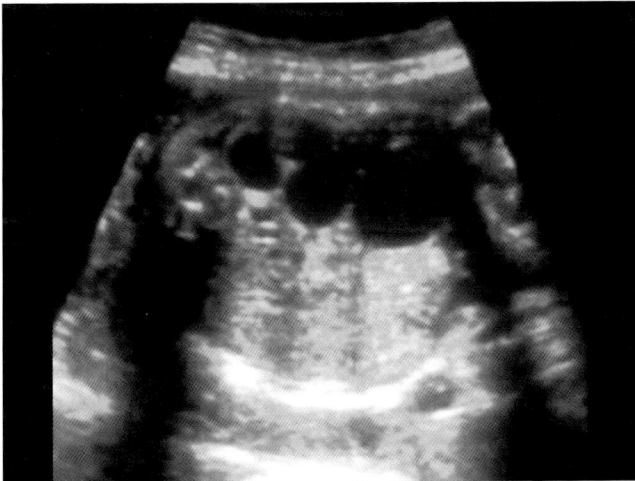

Fig. 33.34: Multicystic dysplastic kidney disease. The kidney appears enlarged with multiple cysts. The contralateral kidney is normal

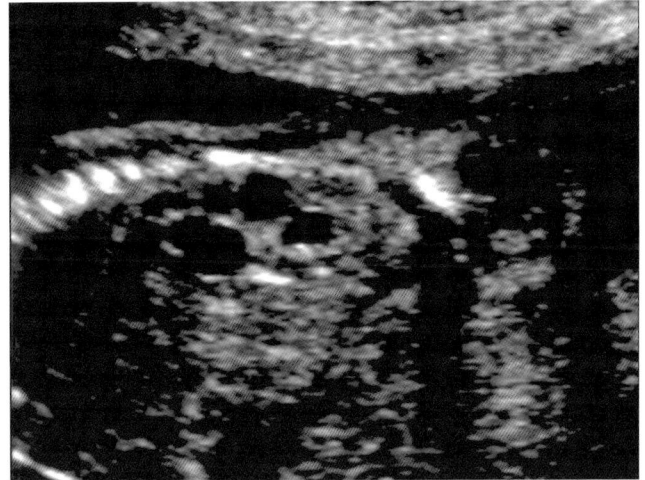

Fig. 33.36: Multicystic dysplastic kidney disease. Parenchymal tissue between the cysts is often hyperechogenic

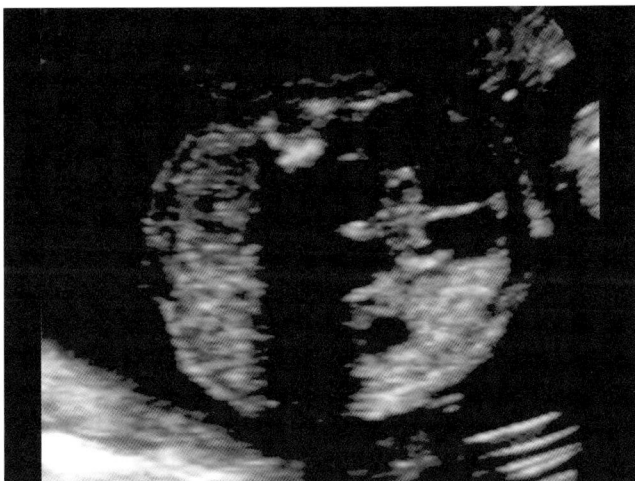

Fig. 33.35: Multicystic dysplastic kidney disease. The kidney appears enlarged with multiple cysts. The contralateral kidney is normal

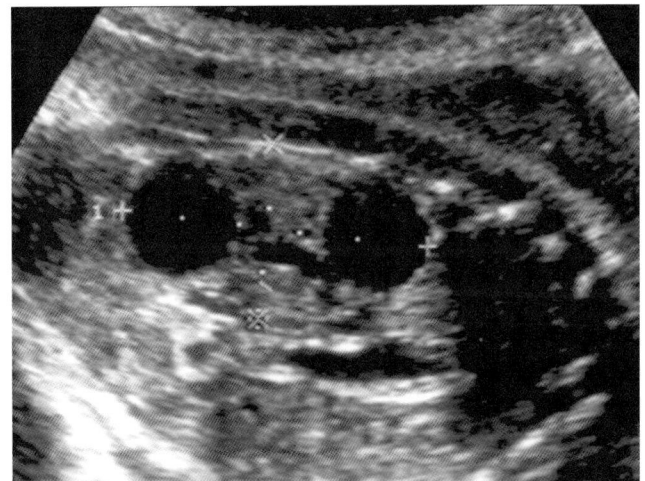

Fig. 33.37: Multicystic dysplastic kidney disease. Parenchymal tissue between the cysts is often hyperechogenic

affects the whole kidney; however, occasionally, only part of the kidney is involved, usually the upper pole of a duplex kidney.[124]

Careful attention should be paid to assessment of the contralateral kidney because the incidence of contralateral renal anomalies is high (39%). A search should be made for nonrenal anomalies.[110]

There is a high association between dysplasia and obstruction: dysplastic kidneys are classically attached to atresic ureter; renal dysplasia is associated with lower urinary tract malformations.[90]

Color Doppler assessment may be useful in determining the diagnosis since the renal artery is always small or absent in MCKD, and the Doppler waveform, when present, is markedly abnormal with reduced systolic peak and absent diastolic flow (Fig. 33.38). Differential diagnosis includes upper urinary tract dilatations and other cystic abdominal masses.

Associated anomalies: Associated anomalies are seen in the contralateral kidney in 30–50% of cases: vesicoureteric reflux is the most common, followed by renal agenesis, renal hypoplasia and pelviureteric junction obstruction.[125,126]

Detection of dysplastic kidneys should stimulate a detailed examination of the fetus for other structural abnormalities, including heart, spine, gastrointestinal, CNS, cleft palate, limb anomalies and umbilical cord as up to 35% may have extrarenal anomalies. These are more likely to occur in fetuses with bilateral than unilateral MCDKD.[127] Chromosome analysis should also be discussed with the parents, particularly when structural abnormalities are detected or dysplasia is bilateral. Risks of chromosomal defects are low if there is isolated renal dysplasia.

Lazebnik et al.[127] reported 102 prenatally detected cases. In their experience, the condition is unilateral in 76% of cases, 10% have normal karyotype, but in all cases they found associated nonrenal anomalies.

Prognosis: Unilateral multicystic dysplastic kidney has a good outcome provided the contralateral kidney is normal. If an associated renal anomaly is present, the prognosis depends on the severity of the associated abnormality. The presence of multiple anomalies confers a poorer prognosis.

Bilateral multicystic kidneys have a very poor prognosis, and all babies succumb, in the early neonatal period, to pulmonary hypoplasia.

Management: Unilateral multicystic kidney can be managed conservatively with follow-up scans in the third trimester to assess both the multicystic and contralateral kidney. Bilateral multicystic kidney has a very poor prognosis, and a termination of pregnancy is an appropriate management strategy. The risk of recurrence is small, about 2–3%, but it can be higher if it is associated with a genetic syndrome.

Obstructive Cystic Dysplasia (Potter IV)

It occurs secondary to obstruction in the first or early second trimester of pregnancy.[128]

The incidence of this condition is difficult to determine because only a small proportion of obstructed kidneys progress to renal dysplasia. There is an approximate incidence of 1 in 8000 live births, with 40% being bilateral dysplasia.[92,129] This condition is caused by early renal obstruction. Unilateral disease can be caused by a pelviureteric or vesicoureteric junction obstruction. Bilateral obstructive dysplasia is caused by severe bladder outlet obstruction (urethral atresia or posterior urethral valves).

Pathology: The kidney is usually small with disorganized epithelial structures surrounded by fibrous tissue. Cortical cysts are often present.[129]

Diagnosis: The sonographic appearance is small echogenic kidneys with peripheral cysts. In the bilateral condition, bilateral hydronephrosis may be present, bladder with thick walls and usually collapsed and severe oligohydramnios may be seen.

The renal cortex assessment is very important. The presence of cortical cysts and hydronephrosis is suggestive of dysplasia.[129] Although increased echogenicity is a good sign of renal dysplasia, normal renal echogenicity does not exclude this condition[128] (Figs 33.39 and 33.40).

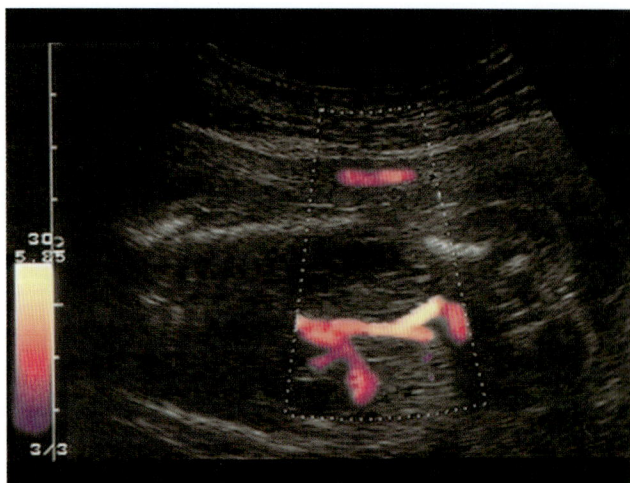

Fig. 33.38: Multicystic dysplastic kidney disease. Color Doppler shows that the renal artery is always small or absent

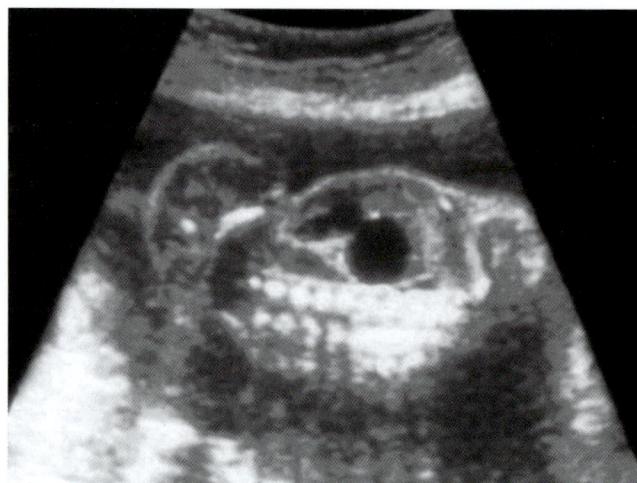

Fig. 33.39: Obstructive cystic dysplasia. Peripheral cortical cysts and echogenic parenchyma

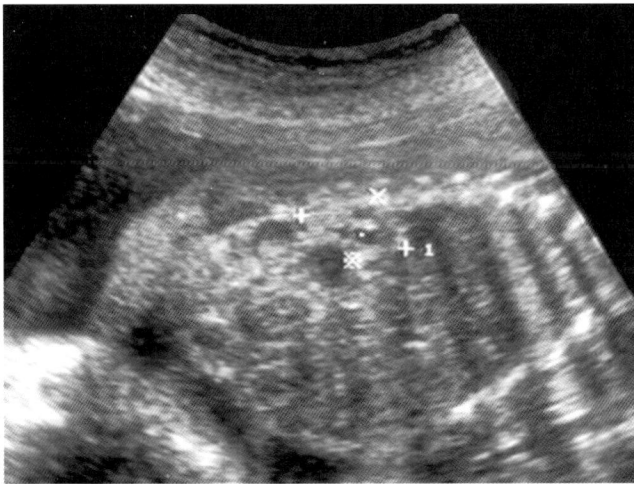

Fig. 33.40: Obstructive cystic dysplasia. Peripheral cortical cysts and echogenic parenchyma

Occasionally, the obstructive dysplasia can affect part of a kidney.[130]

Differential diagnosis: The differential diagnosis is established between multiple conditions, as shown in Tables 33.4 and 33.5.

Associated anomalies: The main anomalies seen are cardiac and the VACTERL association (vertebral anomalies, anorectal atresia, cardiac anomalies, tracheo-esophageal fistula, renal anomalies and limb abnormalities). Other less common associations are hydrocephalus, cloacal malformation, malrotation and ambiguous genitalia.[131]

Prognosis: The prognosis depends on whether the condition is bilateral or unilateral. Bilateral disease has a poor prognosis, and most of newborn succumb in neonatal period to pulmonary hypoplasia. In unilateral disease, the outcome depends on the presence of renal anomalies affecting to the contralateral kidney and the presence or absence of associated abnormalities.

Management: Due to the very poor outcome of the bilateral condition, interruption of pregnancy can be offered to the parents.

Unilateral condition can be managed conservatively in the absence of contralateral kidney disease and associated abnormalities. The condition is sporadic.

Echogenic Large Kidneys or "Bright" Kidneys

Large "bright", or hyperechogenic kidneys are occasionally seen at the time of a routine ultrasound scan or indeed later in pregnancy when a woman is scanned for another clinical indication.[132]

Table 33.5: Syndromes associated with renal cystic disease

Syndrome	Clinical features
Meckel–Gruber	Large echogenic kidneys, polydactyly, encephalocele
Patau	Hyperechogenic large kidneys, polydactyly, holoprosencephaly, facial clefting
Jeune	Echogenic kidneys, dwarfism, small thorax
Beckwith–Wiedemann	Large echogenic kidneys, macrosomia, hepatosplenomegaly, macroglossia, omphalocele
Short rib-polydactyly (Majewski type)	Large echogenic kidneys, dwarfism, polydactyly, small thorax
Laurence–Moon (Bardet–Biedl)	Renal cysts, retinal dystrophy, polydactyly, mental deficiency, hypogonadism
Zellweger	Cystic kidneys, hypotonicity, limb contractures, congenital cataracts, hypoplastic corpus callosum, heterotopia
Perlman	Macrosomia, hepatosplenomegaly, ascites, micrognathia, depressed nasal bridge
Tuberous sclerosis	Epilepsy, mental retardation, cutaneous lesions, cardiac rhabdomyomas (in utero)

Table 33.6 Conditions associated with large, "bright" kidneys

	AF	Renal cysts	Renal pelvis dilatation	Macrosomy	Other abnormalities	Heart abnormalities	Inheritance	Alternative prenatal diagnosis
Dysplasia	N/Oligo	+/–	+/–	–	+/–	–	10% (AD)	–
Obstruction	N/Oligo	+/–	+	–	+/–	–	Sporadic	
ARPKD	N/Oligo	–	–	–	–	–	AR	DNA
ADPKD	N/Oligo	+	–	–	–	–	AD	DNA
Beckwith–Wiedemann	N/Oligo	–	+/–	+	+	–	AD or Disomy	Cyto/DNA
Perlman	N/Oligo	–	+/–	+	+	–	AR	–
Simpson–Golabi–Behmel	?	?	?	+	+	+/–	X-linked	DNA
Trisomy 13	N/Oligo	–	+/–	–	+	+/–	Sporadic	Cyto
Meckel-Gruber	N/Oligo	–	–	–	+	+/–	AR	DNA
Nephrocalcinosis	N	–	–	–	–	–	Sporadic	–

Abbreviations: AD, autosomal dominant; AR, autosomal recessive; ADPKD, autosomal dominant polycystic kidney disease; ARPKD, autosomal recessive polycystic kidney disease

They represent a difficult diagnostic dilemma, particularly in the presence of a normal liquor volume, since their underlying etiologies are relatively diverse. A list of the more common underlying pathologies is shown in Table 33.6.[90] Only a few of these conditions can be identified prenatally, usually on the basis of associated abnormalities, liquor volume and targeted invasive test. In many instances, however, definitive diagnosis is dependent upon postnatal investigations.

Sonographic detection of large, "bright" kidneys should stimulate a detailed examination of the rest of the fetus paying particular attention to the rest of the renal tract and other measurements. If the bladder is enlarged, with or without dilated ureters, then the findings reflect an obstructive uropathy. If the kidneys and all measurements lie above the 95th percentile, then an overgrowth syndrome (Beckwith–Wiedemann, Perlman, Simpson–Golabi–Behmel syndromes, etc.) could be considered (Figs 33.41 and 33.42). Karyotyping should be discussed, particularly when other malformations are detected.

If the fetus has isolated hyperechogenic kidneys and a normal karyotype with no evidence of renal tract obstruction, then the etiology lies between renal dysplasia, autosomal recessive polycystic kidney dysplasia, autosomal recessive polycystic dysplasia, nephrocalcinosis or a variant of normal.

Accurate prediction of the prognosis can be difficult, although liquor volume is a key indicator since reduced volume or its absence indicates that the outcome is likely to be poor and the pregnancy will frequently end in a neonatal death subsequent to pulmonary hypoplasia, as well as renal failure. In these circumstances, termination of pregnancy is a reasonable option.

In the presence of normal amniotic fluid, serial scanning should be undertaken to monitor the size of the kidneys and renal function as indicated by liquor volume.

Simple Renal Cysts

The incidence of simple renal cysts varies with gestational age. Scanning at 14–16 weeks of gestation is 1/1100[132] and at 20 weeks is 1/2400.[133]

The etiology is unclear, but there are two main theories:[134,135]
1. They are retention cysts resulting from the obstruction of renal tubules secondary to local vascular damage or inflammation.
2. The second to fourth generations of uriniferous tubules fail to degenerate or unite with later generations of collecting tubules, persisting as cystic collections.

The cysts are usually solitary and unilocular with no communication with the renal pelvis. The rest of the kidney is normal.[133]

Diagnosis: The cysts appear as a unilocular round or oval anechoic structure with well-defined borders, usually near the periphery of the kidney. Cysts vary in size (2–4 mm).[133]

The differential diagnosis is established between:
- Hydronephrosis of the upper pole moiety of a duplex kidney.
- Perinephric urinoma.
- Cysts arising from structures close to the kidneys (duplication or mesenteric cysts).

Associated anomalies: Most simple cysts are asymptomatic and rarely associated with structural or other abnormalities. Occasionally they are associated with.[133,136,137]
- Pelviureteric junction obstruction
- Posterior urethral valves
- Turner's syndrome
- Trisomy 13
- Trisomy 18
- Trisomy 21 (5% are associated with simple renal cysts).

Prognosis: The outcome is good for fetuses with simple cysts.[133] When cysts do become symptomatic, simple aspiration under ultrasound control is the treatment of choice.[138]

Management: Simple cysts seen in the first half of pregnancy can be followed up with scans during the third trimester. The majority resolves, and those that persist do not need any postnatal investigations.

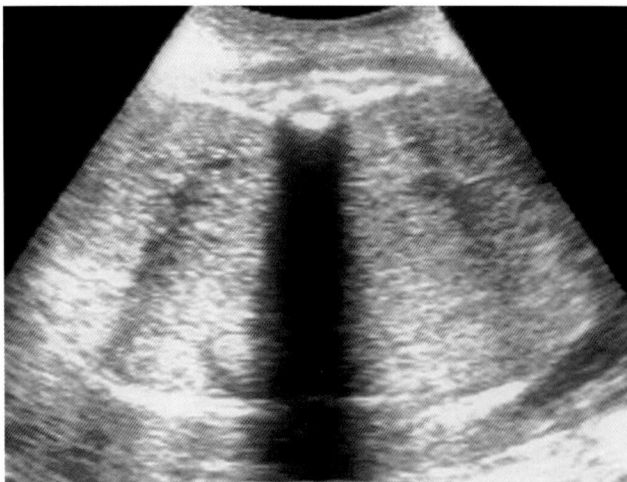

Fig. 33.41: Meckel–Gruber syndrome. Distended abdomen due to the cystic renal dysplasia

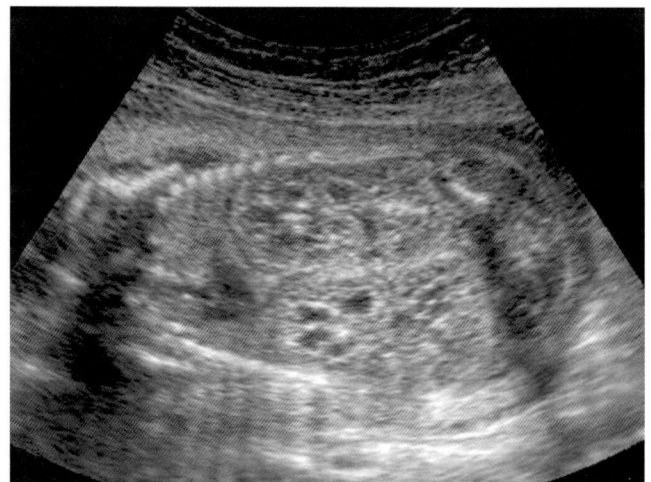

Fig. 33.42: Large and bright kidneys with oligohydramnios

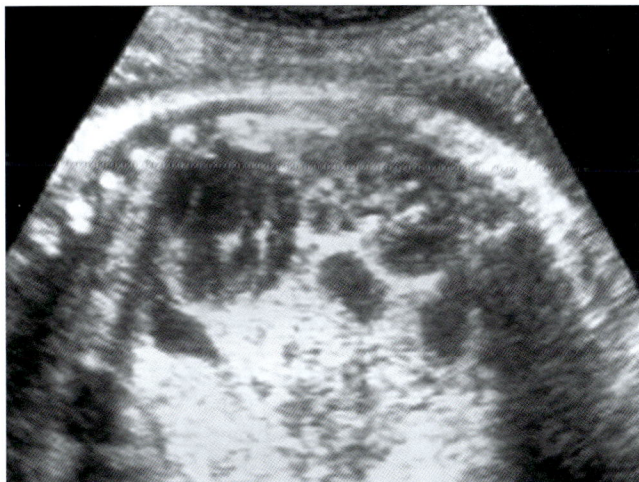

Fig. 33.43: Neuroblastoma. Solid tumor and heterogenous

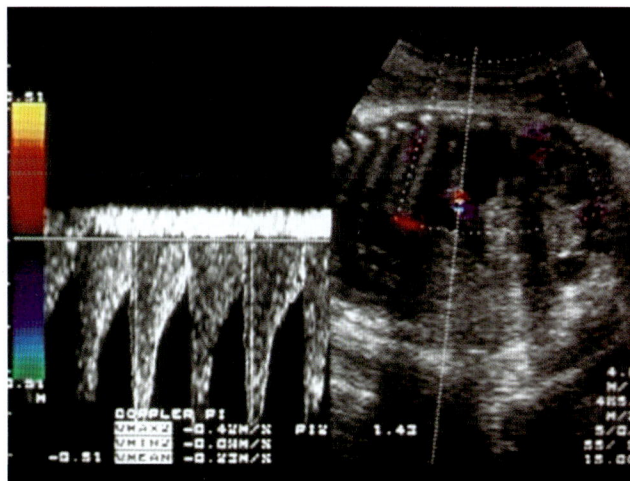

Fig. 33.44: Neuroblastoma. Solid tumor and heterogenous color Doppler shows artery blood flow

Renal tumors

Congenital renal tumors are rare. The incidence is 1 per 125,000 newborns.[139] The most frequent tumor is the mesoblastic nephroma. It is a benign tumor that presents continuity with the normal nephrons. Wilms' tumor is rare in the fetus. The etiology is unknown.

Diagnosis

The diagnosis will generally be made before the presence of a polyhydramnios and an abdominal mass at level of renal fossa in third trimester[140] (Figs 33.43 and 33.44).

- The mesoblastic nephroma is unilateral and on ultrasonography appears as a solid mass. Occasionally, cysts can be identified, many of them are located near the renal hilus, and almost all affect the renal parenchyma. On occasions, the tumor can be adjacent to the kidney and compress it. The mesoblastic nephromas is usually well defined.
- It can have polyhydramnios in 70% of the cases, resulting from the polyuria secondary to the hypercalcemia.[141]
- The hydrops is uncommon, and it has a poor prognosis.[142]
- Wilms' tumor presents very similar echographic characteristics and an anatomopathological study should be carried out for its diagnosis.[143]

Differential Diagnosis

- *Neuroblastoma:* It usually displaces inferior to the kidney
- Suprarenal hemorrhage

- Retroperitoneal teratoma
- Extralobar subphrenic sequestrum.

Associated Anomalies

- The mesoblastic nephroma unusually associates to anomalies.
- Wilms' tumor associates to anomalies in 15% of the cases: aniridia, genitourinary anomalies and hemihypertrophy.[144]

Genetic Markers

The genes WT1 and WT2 located in chromosome 11 have been implicated in the development of the Wilms' tumor, as well as the gene WT3 of chromosome 16 in Beckwith–Wiedemann syndrome and Denys–Drash syndrome.[144]

Prognosis

Treatment is surgical and it is usually curative. The presence of hydrops involves a very bad prognosis.[142]

Management

- During the pregnancy it is necessary to control the polyhydramnios to avoid premature childbirth and the PROM.
- Childbirth should take place in a tertiary level hospital, where there are neonatology unit, pediatric surgery and pediatric oncology.

 This tumor appears sporadically.

REFERENCES

1. Twining P. Anomalías fetales. Diagnóstico ecográfico. 2002;13:270-8.
2. Larsen WJ. Human Embryology. London: Churchill Livingstone; 1993.
3. Wendell Smith CP, Williams PL, Treadgold S. Basic Human Embryology. London: Pitman Publishing; 1984.
4. Elder JS. Tratado de Pediatría Nelson, 16a edición. Transtornos urológicos Embriología. 2;1767-96.
5. Bronshtein M, Amil A, Achiron R, et al. The early prenatal diagnosis of renal agenesis: techniques and possible pitfalls. Prenat Diagn. 1994;14:291-7.

6. Mesrobian HG, Rushton HG, Bulas D. Unilateral renal agenesis may result from in utero regression of multicystic renal dysplasia. J Urol. 1993;150:793-4.

7. Moore KL, Persaud TVN. The Developing Human: Clinically Oriented Embryology. Philadelphia: WB Saunders; 1998.

8. Romero R, Cullen M, Grannum P, et al. Antenatal diagnosis of renal anomalies with ultrasound, III: Bilateral renal agenesis. Am J Obstet Gynecol. 1985;151:38-43.

9. Mackenzie FM, Kingston GO, Oppenheimer L. The early prenatal diagnosis of bilateral renal agenesis using transvaginal sonography and color Doppler ultrasonography. J Ultrasound Med. 1994;13:49-51.

10. Sepulveda W, Stagiannis KD, Flack NJ, et al. Accuracy of prenatal diagnosis of renal agenesis with color flow imaging in severe second-trimester oligohydramnios. Am J Obstet Gynecol. 1995;173:1788-92.

11. Hoffman CK, Filly RA, Callen PW. The "lying down" adrenal sign: a sonographic indicator of renal agenesis or ectopia in fetuses and neonates. J Ultrasound Med. 1992;11:533-6.

12. Benacerraf BR. Examination of the second trimester fetus with severe oligohydramnios using transvaginal scanning. Obstet Gynecol. 1990;175:491-3.

13. Hill LM, Rivello D. Role of transvaginal sonography in the diagnosis of bilateral renal agenesis. Am J Perinatol. 1991;8:395-7.

14. Gembruch U, Hansmann M. Artificial instillation of amniotic fluid as a new technique for the diagnostic evaluation of cases of oligohydramnios. Prenat Diagn. 1988;8:33-45.

15. Nicolini U, Santolaya J, Hubinont C, et al. Visualization of fetal intra-abdominal organs in secondtrimester severe oligohydramnios by intraperitoneal infusion. Prenat Diagn. 1989;9:191-4.

16. Glazebrook KN, McGrath FP, Steele BT. Prenatal compensatory renal growth: Documentation with US. Radiology. 1993;189:733-5.

17. Roodhooft AM, Birnholz JC, Holmes LB. Familiar nature of congenital absence and severe dysgenesis of both kidneys. N Engl J Med. 1984;310:1341-5.

18. Hill L, Peterson CS. Antenatal diagnosis of fetal pelvic kidneys. J Ultrasound Med. 1987;6:393-6.

19. Hill LM, Grzybek P, Mills A, et al. Antenatal diagnosis of fetal pelvic kidneys. Obstet Gynecol. 1994;83:333-6.

20. Greenblatt AM, Beretsky I, Lankin DH, et al. In utero diagnosis of crossed renal ectopia using high resolution real-time ultrasound. J Ultrasound Med. 1985;4:105-7.

21. Moore KL, Pesrsaud TVN. The urogenital system. In: Moore KL, Persaud TVN (Eds). The Developing Human: Clinically Oriented Embryology, 6th edition. Philadelphia: WB Saunders; 1998. p II:330.

22. Weizer AZ, Silverstein AD, Auge BK, et al. Determining the incidence of horseshoe kidney from radiographic data at a single institution. J Urol. 2003;170:1722-6.

23. Hunt GM, Whitaker RH. The pattern of congenital renal anomalies associated with neural-tube defects. Dev Med Child Neurol. 1987;29:91-5.

24. Boatman DL, Kolln CP, Flocks RH. Congenital anomalies associated with horseshoe kidney. J Urol. 1972;107:205-7.

25. Canki N, Warburton D, Byrne J. Morphological characteristics of monosomy X in spontaneous abortions. Ann Genet. 1988;31: 4-13.

26. Kravtzova GI, Lazjuk GI, Lurie IW. The malformations of the urinary system in autosomal disorders. Virchows Arch A Pathol Anat Histol. 1975;368(2):167-78.

27. Scott JE, Renwick M. Screening for fetal urological abnormalities: How effective? Br J Urol Int. 1999;84:693-700.

28. Huang EY, Mascarenhas L, Mahour GH. Wilms' tumor and horseshoe kidneys: a case report and review of the literature. J Pediatr Surg. 2004;39:207-12.

29. Rubio Briones J, Regalado Pareja R, Sanchez Martin F, et al. Incidence of tumoural pathology in horseshoe kidneys. Eur Urol 1998;33:175-9.

30. Smith-Behn J, Memo R. Malignancy in horseshoe kidney. South Med J. 1988;81:1451-2.

31. Ismaili K, Hall M, Donner C, et al. Results of systematic screening for minor degrees of fetal renal pelvis dilatation in an unselected population. Am J Obstet Gynecol. 2003;188:242-6.

32. Ismaili K, Hall M, Avni FE. Management of isolated fetal dilatations of the kidney pelvis. Rev Med Brux. 2003;24:29-34.

33. Eckoldt F, Heinick C, Wolke S, et al. Prenatal diagnosis of obstructive uropathies-positive predictive value and effect on postnatal therapy. Z Geburtshilfe Neonatol. 2003;207:220-4.

34. Moorthy I, Joshi N, Cook JV, et al. Antenatal hydronephrosis: negative predictive value of normal postnatal ultrasound a 5 year study. Clin Radiol. 2003;58:964-70.

35. Barrer AF, Cave MM, Thomas DFM, et al. Fetal pelvi-ureteric junction obstruction: predictions of outcome. Br J Urol. 1995;76:649-52.

36. Lepercq J, Beaudoin S, Bargy F. Outcome of 116 moderate renal pelvis dilatations at prenatal ultrasonography. Fetal Diagn Ther- 1998;13:79-81.

37. Benacerraf Br, Mandell J, Estroff JA, et al. Fetal pyelectasis: a possible association with Down syndrome. Obstet Gynecol. 1992;76:58-60.

38. Nicolaides KH, Cheng HH, Abbas A, et al. Fetal renal defects: associated malformations and chromosomal defets. Fetal Diagn Ther. 1992;7:1-11.

39. James CA, Watson AR, Twining P, et al. Antenatally detected urinary tract abnormalities: changing incidence and management. Eur J Pediatr. 1998;157:508-11.

40. Antonakoupoulos GN, Fuggle WJ, Newman J, et al. Idiopathic hydronephrosis. Arch Pathol Lab Med. 1985;109:1097-101.

41. Bosman G, Reuss A, Nijman JM, et al. Prenatal diagnosis, management and outcome of fetal uretero-pelvic junction obstruction. Ultrasound Med Biol. 1991;17:117-20.

42. Grapin C, Auber F, de Vries P, et al. Postnatal management of urinary tract anomalies after antenatal diagnosis. J Gynecol Obstet Biol Reprod (Paris). 2003;32:300-13.

43. McAleer IM, Kaplan GW. Renal function before and after pyeloplasty: Does it improve? J Urol. 1999;162:1041-4.

44. Buscemi M, Shanke A, Mallet E. Dominantly inherited ureteropelvic junction obstruction. Urology. 1985;24:568-71.

45. Rickwood AMK, Jee LD, Williams MPL, et al. Natural history of obstructed and pseudo-obstructed megaureters detected by prenatal ultrasonography. Br J Urol. 1992;70:322-5.

46. Manzoni C. Megaureter. Rays. 2002;27:83-5.

47. McLellan DL, Retik AB, Bauer SB, et al. Rate and predictors of spontaneous resolution of prenatally diagnosed primary nonrefluxing megaureter. J Urol. 2002;168:2177-80.

48. Sherer DM, Hulbert WC. Prenatal sonographic diagnosis and subsequent conservative surgical management of bilateral ureteroceles. Am J Perinatol. 1995;12:174-7.

49. Vergani P, Ceruti P, Locatelli A, et al. Accuracy of prenatal ultrasonographic diagnosis of duplex renal system. J Ultrasound Med. 1999;18:463-7.

50. Sozubir S, Lorenzo AJ, Twickler DM, et al. Prenatal diagnosis of a prolapsed ureterocele with magnetic resonance imaging. Urology. 2003;62:144.

51. Kang AH, Bruner JP. Antenatal ultrasonographic development of ureteroceles. Implications for management. Fetal Diagn Ther. 1998;13:157-9.

52. Winters WD, Lebowitz RL. Importance of prenatal detection of hydronephrosis of the upper pole. Am J Radiol .1990;155:125-9.

53. Upadhyay J, Bolduc S, Braga L, et al. Impact of prenatal diagnosis on the morbidity associated with ureterocele management. J Urol. 2002;167:2560-5.

54. Castagnetti M, Cimador M, Sergio M, et al. Transurethral incision of duplex system ureteroceles in neonates: Does it increase the need for secondary surgery intravesical and ectopic cases? Br J Urol Int. 2004;93:1313-7.

55. Elder JS. Antenatal hydronephrosis fetal and neonatal management. Pediatr Clin North Am. 1997;44:1299-321.
56. Edkoldt F, Heling KS, Stover B, et al. Retrospective analysis of differential therapeutic measures in children with double kidney and ureter and hydronephrosis. Urologe A. 2003; 42:1087-91.
57. Arena F, Nicotina A, Cruccetti A, et al. Can histologic changes of the upper pole justify a conservative approach in neonatal duplex ectopic ureterocele? Pediatr Surg Int. 2002;18:681-4.
58. Cendron M, D'Alton ME, Crombleholme TM. Prenatal diagnosis and management of the fetus with hydroneprosis. Semin Perinatol. 1994;18:163-81.
59. Dinnen MD, Duffy PG. Posterior urethral valves. Br J Urol. 1996; 78:275-81.
60. Manzoni C, Valentini AL. Posterior urethral valves. Rays. 2002; 27:131-4.
61. McHugo J, Whittle M. Enlarged fetal bladders: aetiology, management and outcome. Prenat Diagn. 2001;21:958-63.
62. Silveri M, Adorisio O, Pane A, et al. Fetal monolateral urinoma and neonatal renal function outcome in posterior urethral valves obstruction: the pop-off mechanism. Pediatr Med Chir. 2002;24: 394-6.
63. De Vries SH, Klijn AJ, Lilien MR, et al. Development of renal function after neonatal urinary ascitis due to obstructive uropathy. J Urol. 2002;168:675-8.
64. Lee E, Thonell S. Posterior urethral valves causing urinomas: two case reports. Australas Radiol. 2002;46:101-5.
65. Peters CA. Lower urinary tract obstruction: clinical and experimental aspects. Br J Urol. 1998;81(Suppl 2):22-32.
66. Perrotin F, Ayeva-Derman M, Lardy H, et al. Prenatal diagnosis and postnatal outcome of congenital megalourethra. Report of two cases. Fetal Diagn Ther. 2001;16: 123-8.
67. Geifman-Hotzman O, Crane SS, Winderl L, et al. Persistent urogenital sinus: prenatal diagnosis and pregnancy complications. Am J Obstet Gynecol. 1997;176:709-11.
68. McNarama HM, Onwude JL, Thornton JG. Megacystismicrocolon-intestinal hypoperistalsis syndrome: a case report supporting autosomal recessive inheritance. Prenat Diagn. 1994;14:153-4.
69. Hsu CD, Craig C, Pavlik J, et al. Prenatal diagnosis of megacystis-microcolon-intestinal hypoperistalsis syndrome in one fetus of a twin pregnancy. Am J Perinatol. 2003;20:215-8.
70. Sharma AK, Kothari SK, Goel D, et al. Megalourethra with posterior urethral valves. Pediatr Surg Int. 1999;15:591-2.
71. Hayden SA, Russ PD, Pretorius DH, et al. Posterior urethral obstruction. Prenatal sonographic findings and clinical outcome in fourteen cases. J Ultrasound Med. 1988;7:371-5.
72. Krapp M, Geipel A, Germer U, et al. First-trimester sonographic diagnosis of distal urethral atresia with megalourethra in VACTERL association. Prenat Diagn. 2002; 22:422-4.
73. Hutton KAR, Thomas PFM, Arthur RJ, et al. Prenatally detected posterior urethra valves: Is gestational age at detection a predictor of outcome? J Urol. 1994;152:698-701.
74. Holmes N, Harrison MR, Baskin LS. Fetal surgery for posterior urethral valves: Long-term postnatal outcomes. Pediatrics. 2001; 108:E7.
75. Quintero RA, Johnson M, Muñoz H. In utero endoscopic treatment of posterior urethral valves. Prenat Neonat Med. 1998;3:208-16.
76. Quintero RA, Morales WJ, Allen MA, et al. Fetal hydrolaparoscopy and endoscopic cystotomy in complicated cases of lower urinary tract obstruction. Am J Obstet Gynecol. 2000;183:324-33.
77. González R, De Filippo R, Jednak R, et al. Urethral atresia: Long-term outcome in 6 children who survived the neonatal period. J Urol. 2001;165:2241-4.
78. Reinberg Y, Chelimsky G, González R. Urethral atresia and the prune-belly syndrome. Report of 6 cases. Br J Urol. 1993;72: 112-4.
79. Jennings RW. Prune belly syndrome. Semin Pediatr Surg. 2000;9: 115-20.
80. Leeners B, Sauer I, Schefels J, et al. Prune belly syndrome: therapeutic options including in utero placement of a vesicoamniotic shunt. J Clin Ultrasound. 2000;28:500-7.
81. Elder JS. Commentary: Importance of antenatal diagnosis of vesicoureteral reflux. J Urol. 1992;148:1750-4.
82. Scott JE, Renwick M. Screening for fetal urological abnormalities: How effective? Br J Urol Int. 1999;84:693-700.
83. Farhat W, McLorie G, Geary D, et al. The natural history of neonatal vesicoureteral reflux associated with antenatal hydronephrosis. J Urol. 2000;164(3, Pt2):1057-60.
84. Orsola A, Fraga Rodriguez GM, Parra Roca J, et al. Congenital renal abnormalities in neonates with fetal vesicoureteral reflux. Detection by 99m-technetium(m)- dimercaptosuccinic acid renal scintigraphy (in Spanish). An Pediatr (Barc). 2003;59(4):345-51.
85. Nguyen HT, Bauer SB, Peters CA, et al. 99m Technetium dimercapto-succinic acid renal scintigraphy abnormalities in infants with sterile high grade vesicoureteral reflux. J Urol. 2000;164:1674-8.
86. Noe HN. The long-term results of prospective sibling reflux screening. J Urol. 1992;148:1739-42.
87. Noe HN, Wyatt RJ, Peeden JN Jr, Rivas ML. The transmission of vesicoureteral reflux from parent to child. J Urol. 1992;148(6): 1869-71.
88. Thomsen MS, Levine E, Meilstrup JW, et al. Renal cystic diseases. Eur Radiol. 1997;7:1267-75.
89. Potter EL. Normal and Abnormal Development of the Kidney. Chicago, IL: Year Book Medical Publishers Inc; 1972.
90. Winyard P, Chitty L. Dysplastic and polycystic kidneys: Diagnosis, associations and management. Prenat Diagn. 2001;21:924-35.
91. Zerres K. Autosomal recessive polycystic disease. Clin Invest. 1992;70:794-801.
92. Tsuda H, Matsumota M, Imanaka M, et al. Measurement of fetal urine production in mild infantile polycystic kidney disease – a case report. Prenat diagn. 1994;14:1083-5.
93. Osathanondh V, Potter EL. Pathogenesis of polycystic kidneys. Type I due to hypoplasia of intersticial portions of collecting tubules. Arch Pathol. 1964;77:466-73.
94. Blyth H, Ockenden BG. Polycystic disease of kidneys and liver presenting in childhood. J Med Genet. 1971;8:257-84.
95. Romero R, Cullen R, Janty P, et al. The diagnosis of congenital renal anomalies with ultrasound II. Infantile polycysytic kidney disease. Am J Obstet Gynecol. 1984;150:259-62.
96. Wissser J, Hebisch G, Froster U, et al. Prenatal sonographic diagnosis of autosomal recessive polycystic kidney disease during the early second trimester. Prenat Diagn. 1995;15:868-71.
97. Mahony B, Cullen PW, Filly R, et al. Progression of infantile polycystic kidney disease in early pregnancy. J Ultrasound Med. 1984;3:277-9.
98. Barth R, Gillot A, Capeless E, et al. Prenatal diagnosis of autosomal recessive polycystic kidney disease: Variable outcome in one family. Am J Obstet Gynecol. 1992;166:560-7.
99. Zerres K, Hansmann M, Mallmann R, et al. Autosomal recessive polycystic kidney disease. Problems of prenatal diagnosis. Prenat Diagn. 1988;8:215-29.
100. Bronshtein M, Bar-Hava I, Blumenfeld Z. Clues and pitfalls in the early prenatal diagnosis of "late onset" infantile polycystic kidney. Prenat Diagn. 1992;12:293-8.
101. Kogutt MS, Robichaux W, Boineau F, et al. Asymmetric renal size in autosomal recessive polycystic kidney disease: a unique presentation. Am J Radiol. 1993;160:835-6.
102. Cassart M, Massez A, Metens T, et al. Complementary role of MRI after sonography in assessing bilateral urinary tract anomalies in the fetus. AJR Am J Roentgenol. 2004;182:689-95.
103. Guay-Woodford LM, Meucher G, Hopkins SD, et al. The severe form of autosomal recessive polycystic kidney disease maps to chromosome 6p21.1-p12: Implications for genetic counseling. Am J Hum Genet. 1995;56:1101-7.

104. MacDermot KD, Saggar-Malik AK, Economides SJ. Prenatal diagnosis of autosomal dominant polycystic kidney disease (PKD1) presenting in utero and prognosis for very early onset disease. J Med Genet. 1998;35:13-6.

105. Parfrey PS, Bear JC, Morgan J, et al. The diagnosis and prognosis of autosomal dominant polycystic kidney disease. N Engl J Med. 1990;323:1085-90.

106. Reeders ST, Breuning MH, Davies KE, et al. A highly polymorphic DNA marker linked to adult type polycystic kidney disease on chromosome 16. Nature. 1985;317:542-4.

107. Kimberling WJ, Kimar S, Gabow P. Autosomal dominant polycystic kidney disease: localization of the second gene to chromosome 4p13-q23. Genomics. 1995;18:467-72.

108. Demetriou K, Tziakouri C, Anninou K, et al. Autosomal dominant polycystic kidney disease-type 2. Ultrasound, genetic and clinical correlations. Nephrol Dial Transplant. 2000;15:205-11.

109. Nicolau C, Torra R, Bianchi L, et al. Autosomal dominant polycystic kidney disease types 1 and 2: Assessment of US sensitivity for diagnosis. Radiology. 1999;213:273-6.

110. Aubertin G, Cripps S, Coleman G, et al. Prenatal diagnosis of apparently isolated unilateral multicystic kidney: Implications for counseling and management. Prenat Diagn. 2002;22:388-94.

111. Journel H, Guyor C, Barc RM, et al. Unexpected ultrasonographic prenatal diagnosis of autosomal dominant polycystic kidney disease. Prenat Diagn. 1989;9:663-71.

112. Michaud J, Russo P, Girgnon A, et al. Autosomal dominant polycystic kidney disease in the fetus. Am J Med Genet. 1994;51:240-6.

113. Friedmann W, Vogel M, Dimer JS, et al. Perinatal differential diagnosis of cystic kidney disease and urinary tract obstruction: anatomic pathologic, ultrasonographic and genetic findings. Eur J Obstet Gynecol Reprod Biol. 2000;89:127-33.

114. Brun M, Maugey-Laulomk B, Eurin D, et al. Prenatal sonographic patterns in autosomal dominant polycystic kidney disease: a multicenter study. Ultrasound Obstet Gynecol. 2004; 24:55-61.

115. Tsatsaris V, Gagnadoux MF, Aubry MC, et al. Prenatal diagnosis of bilateral isolated fetal hyperechogenic kidneys. Is it possible to predict long-term outcome? BJOG Br J Obstet Gynaecol. 2002;109:1388-93.

116. Ceccherini I, Lituania M, Cordone MS, et al. Autosomal dominant polycystic kidney disease: prenatal diagnosis by DNA analysis and sonographic at 14 weeks. Prenat Diagn. 1989;9:751-8.

117. Hartmann SS. Unilateral adult polycystic kidney. J Ultrasound Med. 1982;1:371-4.

118. Middlebrook PF, Nizalik E, Schillinger JF. Unilateral renal cystic disease: a case presentation. J Urol. 1992;148:1221-23.

119. Gough DCS, Postlethwaite RJ, Lewis MA, et al. Multicystic renal dysplasia diagnosed in the antenatal period: a note of caution. Br J urol. 1995;76:244-8.

120. Rickwood AMK, Anderson PAM, Williams MPL. Multicystic renal dysplasia detected by prenatal ultrasonography. Natural history and results of conservative management. Br J Urol. 1992;69:538-40.

121. Van Eijk L, Cohen-Overbeek TE, Den Hollander NS, et al. Unilateral multicystic dysplasia kidney: a combined pre- and postnatal assessment. Ultrasound Obstet Gynecol. 2002;19:180-3.

122. D'Alton M, Romero R, Grannum P, et al. Antenatal diagnosis of renal anomalies with ultrasound IV: bilateral multicystic kidney disease. Am J Obstet Gynecol. 1986;54:532-7.

123. Hashimoto B, Filly R, Callen P. Multicystic dysplastic kidney in utero: changing appearance in ultrasound. Radiology. 1986;159:107-9.

124. Diard F, le Dosseur P, Cadier L, et al. Multicystic dysplasia in the upper component of the complete duplex kidney. Pediatr Radiol. 1984;14:310-3.

125. De Klerk DF, Marshall FF, Jeffs RD. Multicystic dysplastic kidney. J Urol. 1977;118:306-8.

126. Karmazyn B, Zerin J. Lower urinary tract abnormalities in children with multicystic dysplastic kidney. Radiology. 1997;203:223-6.

127. Lazebkik N, Bellinger MF, Fergurson JE, et al. Insights into the pathogensis and antural history of nfetuses with multicystic dysplastic kidney disease. Prenat Diagn. 1999;19:418-23.

128. Saunders RC, Nussbaum AR, Solez K. Renal dysplasia: sonographic findings. Radiology. 1988;167:623-6.

129. Mahony BS, Filly R, Callen PW, et al. Fetal renal dysplasia: sonographic evaluation. Radiology. 1984;152:143-6.

130. Newman LB, McAlister WH, Kissane J. Segmental renal dysplasia associated with ectopic ureteroceles in childhood. Urology. 1974;3:23-6.

131. Blane CE, Barr M, Dipietro MA, et al. Renal obstructive dysplasia: ultrasound diagnosis and therapeutic implications. Pediatr Radiol. 1991;21:274-7.

132. Braithwaite JM, Armstrong MA, Economides DL. Assessment of fetal anatomy at 12 to 13 weeks of gestation by transabdominal and transvaginal sonography. Br J Obstet Gynaecol. 1996;103:82-5.

133. Blazer S, Zimmer E, Bumenfeld Z, et al. Natural history of fetal simple renal cysts detected in early pregnancy. J Urol. 1999;162:812-4.

134. Paduano L, Giglio L, Bembi B, et al. Clinical outcome of fetal uropathy. I. Predictive value of prenatal echography positive for obstructive uropathy. J Urol. 1992;146:1094-6.

135. Siegel MJ, McAlister WH. Simple cysts of the kidney in children. J Urol. 1980;123:75-8.

136. Herman TE, Siegel MJ. Renal cysts associated with Turner' syndrome. Pediatr Radiol. 1994;24:139-40.

137. Ariel I, Wells TR, Landing BH, et al. The urinary system in Down syndrome: a study of 124 autopsy cases. Pediatr Pathol. 1991;11:879-88.

138. Steinhardt GF, Slovis TL, Perlmutter AD. Simple renal cysts in infants. Radiology. 1985;155:349-50.

139. Apuzzio JJ, Unwin W, Adhate A, et al. Prenatal diagnosis of fetal renal mesoblastic nephroma. Am J Obstet Gynecol. 1986;154: 636-7.

140. Goldstein I, Shoshani G, Ben-Harus E, et al. Prenatal diagnosis of congenital mesoblastic nephroma. Ultrasound Obstet Gynecol. 2002;19:209-11.

141. Fung TY, Fung YM, Ng PC, et al. Polyhydramnios and hypercalcemia associated with congenital mesoblastic nephroma: Case report and a new appraisal. Obstet Gynecol. 1995;85(5, Pt 2):815-7.

142. Liu YC, Mai YL, Chang CC, et al. The presence of hydrops fetalis in a fetus with congenital mesoblastic nephroma. Prenat Diagn. 1996;16:363-5.

143. Applegate KE, Ghei M, Perez-Atayde AR. Prenatal detection of a Wilms' tumor. Pediatr Radiol. 1999;29(1):65-7.

144. Vadeyar S, Ramsay M, James D, et al. Prenatal diagnosis of congenital Wilms' tumor (nephroblastoma) presenting as fetal hydrops. Ultrasound Obstet Gynecol. 2000;16:80-3.

CHAPTER
34
Fetal Echocardiography

C Mortera, JM Carrera

INTRODUCTION

Prenatal diagnosis of fetal cardiovascular malformations is generally based on the use of ultrasound and echocardiography techniques during pregnancy.[1,2]

Anatomical cardiac anomalies[3,4] are identifiable throughout the use of two-dimensional (2D) echocardiography, providing fetal anatomical cardiac structures.[2,4] Current use to 3D echocardiography provides images that may improve anatomical structural relationship.[5,6] However, Doppler echocardiography studies allow for additional dynamic information to the cardiologist[7] and interested obstetrician[8,9] in prenatal diagnosis. Consequently, the application of such methods in normal and abnormal fetal cardiac structures and function leads to an accurate congenital heart disease diagnosis inside the uterus.[10,11]

In order to successfully diagnose cardiac malformations throughout the use of fetal echocardiography, a number of integrated conceptual areas need to be thoroughly understood to achieve a complete cardiovascular diagnosis. First it is required a profound knowledge of cardiovascular fetal physiology[12] and anatomy as well as fetal cardiovascular pathology and cardiac rhythm disturbances and second to understand the causes and concepts of heart failure to identify the signs and causes of fetal heart failure.[13]

However, the goal of prenatal echocardiography is to make a prediction of the pregnancy outcome, offering medical[14] and surgical cardiac prognosis about the short- and long-term surgical management.[15]

FETAL CARDIOVASCULAR ANATOMY

The fetal cardiovascular system is developed during the first 9 weeks of gestation. Extraordinarily, the heart is the only organ in the fetus capable of functioning while it is being developed. The "foramen ovale" and "ductus arteriosus" become the only different features in a developed fetal heart[16] when compared to an adult heart. The right atrium is presented as a slightly larger cavity than the left atrium. The superior and inferior vena cava are identifiable as they meet with the right atrium. Pulmonary veins tend to be smaller in size due to the reduced pulmonary blood flow; however, they become apparent in mature fetuses.

The tricuspid and mitral valves present similar features under echocardiographic analysis (Fig. 34.1). Two papillary muscles constitute the subvalvular apparatus of the mitral valve, when only one is observed in the tricuspid valve. The tricuspid septal leaflet is distinctively apparent because it attaches to the septum at a closer location than the mitral valve from the apex of the heart. This separation in valve positioning allows for effective visual recognition if the ventricles are pathologically inverted.

To ensure normal ventriculoarterial connections[8,17] a "crossing" by the pulmonary and aortic outflows tracts and arteries must be identified when examine with echo (Fig. 34.2). A parallel position of both great vessels at their origin from the heart would suppose a "transposition of the great arteries".[8]

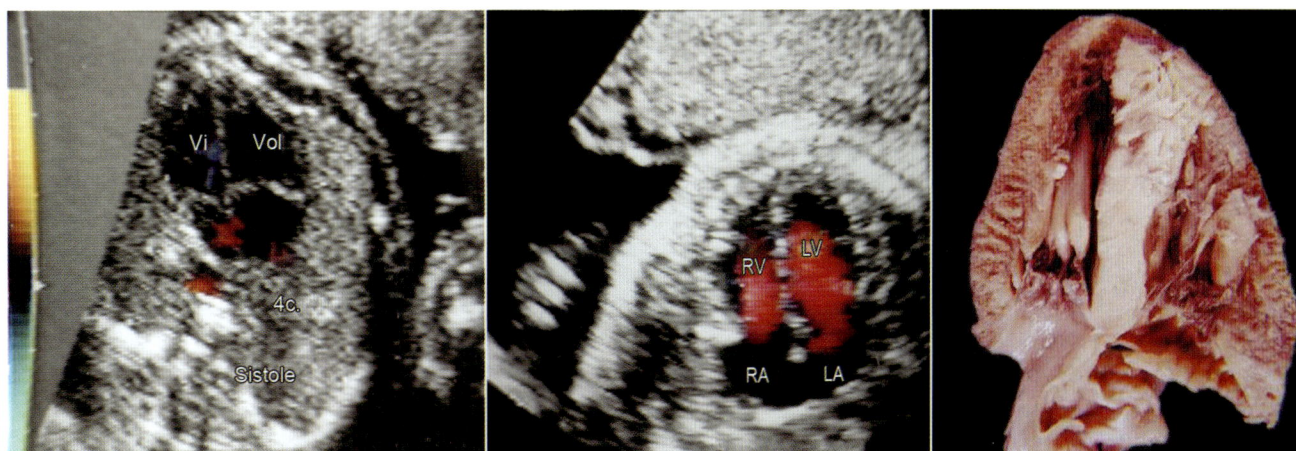

Fig. 34.1: Normal four chamber view. Systolic and diastolic color flow Doppler phases at the A-V valves. Anatomic correlation with the heart specimen

In order to differentiate the "aortic arch from the ductal arch", (Fig. 34.3) three supra-aortic vessels must be attached to the curve of the aortic arch before it extends into the descending aorta. Positioned beneath the ductal arch is recognizable by its continuity from the pulmonary artery into the ductus arteriosus and the descending thoracic aorta.

FETAL CARDIOVASCULAR PHYSIOLOGY

The normal fetal heart structure and blood circulation differ physiologically[12] from that of the adult. The placenta and the fetoplacental circulation become the major source of oxygen in the uterus during fetal life as opposed to the adult lung autonomous respiratory system.

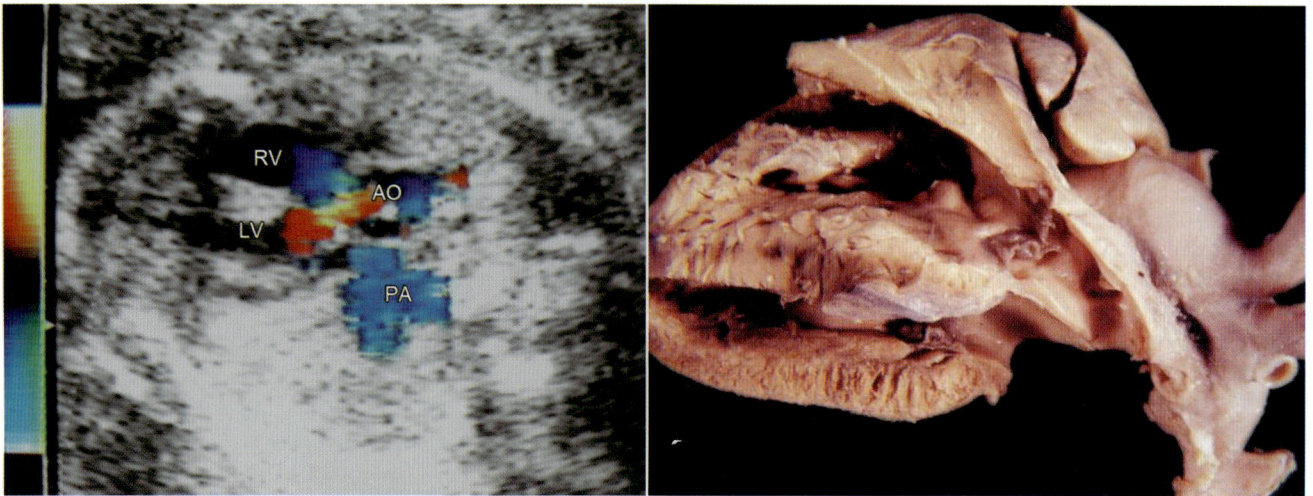

Fig. 34.2: Normal longitudinal color flow Doppler cuts at lateral dorsum. Crossing of the outflow tracts and arteries and anatomic correlation

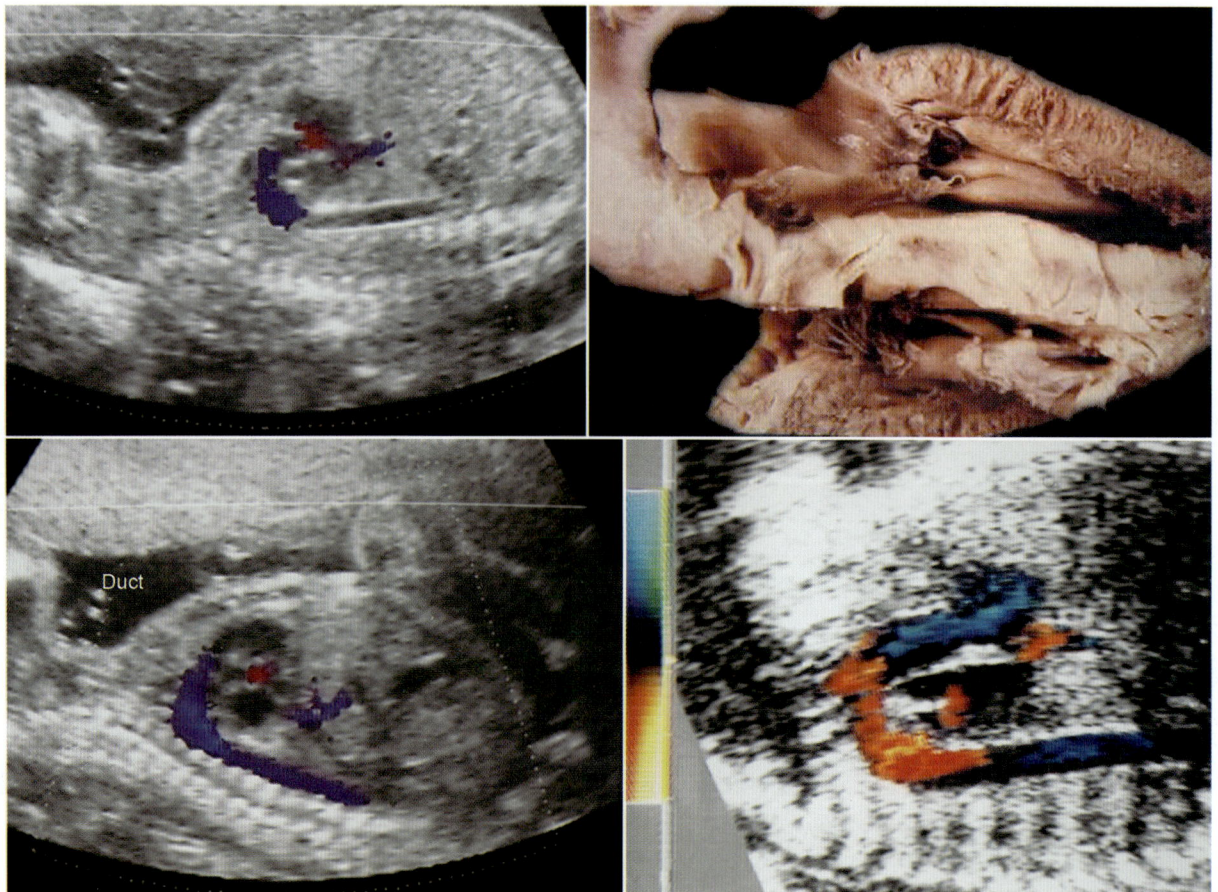

Fig. 34.3: Normal aortic arch at posterior/anterior dorsum. Normal ductus arteriosus arch at posterior dorsum

Two major fetal intracardiac shunts appear, one at the foramen ovale level and other at the ductus arteriosus. These allow for a *right to left* direction of the almost total fetal cardiac output. Approximately half of this circulatory blood volume will be sent to the placenta to be oxygenated, returning subsequently to the fetus, resulting in two major circulations: the Fetal circulation and the fetoplacental circulation.[16]

Fetoplacental venous circulation is characterized by the entry of the umbilical vein through the fetal liver. Oxygenated blood travels from the placenta entering the fetus through the "ductus venosus" which is an extension of intrahepatic umbilical vein. It has been found that the flow dynamics of the circulatory system in this specific area are crucial for the fetal oxygenation process. The diameter of the ductus venosus is reduced as it meets with the inferior vena cava. This reduction in diameter accelerates the oxygenated blood creating a directional jet toward the foramen ovale and left atrium. The entry of this oxygenated blood stream is cyclically regulated by the fetal heart rate. The change in volume in right atrial cavity imposes the cardiac filling pattern. This allows the oxygenated blood to be propelled through the left atrium and left ventricle toward the coronary arteries and fetal brain fetal brain. Less oxygenated blood returning from the peripheral fetal body, coming from "superior vena cava and inferior vena cava", enters the right atrium, right ventricle and the pulmonary artery. At this last point, most of the blood is diverted through the "ductus arteriosus" toward the descending aorta, leaving the pulmonary circulation at minimum flow.

The lower part of the fetal body has low oxygen requirements. This area is supplied by part of less oxygenated blood coming from the descending aorta. The rest of the blood at this level is directed toward the placenta through the umbilical arteries and umbilical cord. The blood oxygenation process takes place at the placenta, which is then returned to the fetus, closing the fetoplacental circulation.

Thus, two main circulatory systems are them developed during fetal life: fetal and fetoplacental circulation. Both circulatory systems are maintained by the fetal heart. Consequently, high fetal cardiac output is required to keep both circulations functioning. This is translated in elevated heart rates (130–160 bpm) rates which are also partially imposed by the limited ventricular compliance of the fetal heart.

Another representative feature only present in the fetal circulatory system is the similar systolic pressure levels between the right ventricle/pulmonary artery and the left ventricle/aorta at a systemic level. Therefore right to left intracardiac shunts are dependable on systemic vascular resistance as well as changes in cardiac and vascular blood volume adjustment.

ASSESSING THE FETAL HEART

Instrumentation and Technique

The study of the fetal heart requires the combination of several dynamic ultrasounds techniques and sequential cardiac analysis.[18]

The equipment to perform intracardiac fetal echocardiographic studies requires a range-gated 2D and pulsed Doppler to perform selective interrogation of blood flow, across the AV valves, ventricles and great arteries, ductus arteriosus, descending aorta as well as the aortic arch. The scanning should also include the hepatic duct and veins, the inferior vena cava, atrial flows, foramen ovale and when possible the pulmonary veins. The equipment should also include CW Doppler to sample high velocity jets.

Color flow mapping increases the diagnostic accuracy and understanding of fetal cardiovascular circulation.[8,9] Color flow displayed must be performed with the instrumentation settings at a high pulse repetition frequency in order to avoid aliasing. Intracardiac blood velocities are higher than in the periphery, therefore color Doppler settings must be set up at high frame rates, reduced angle and high filter to obtain good color resolution. However, diagnostic misinterpretation of color intracardiac Doppler may occur in complex congenital heart disease if previous analysis of 2D cardiac malformed anatomy has not been properly done.

1. Two-dimensional echocardiography identifies anatomical structures, spatial relationship, position of the heart, myocardial thickness and myocardial function. The superimposition of color Doppler technique allows to perform selective cardiovascular flow dynamics in each heart structure.

2. "Pulsed Doppler" is used for selective flow studies in each cavity or vessel and the instrument setting have to be adjusted according to the sampling site. "Continuous Doppler" is necessary to identify high velocity blood signals as well as to quantify intracardiac and intravascular pressure gradients. "Color Doppler" opacification of the blood flow in cardiac cavities and vessels allows to detect abnormal turbulent accelerated flows produced by valve regurgitation and stenosis or other cardiac defects.

3. "M-mode color Doppler flow" is used to measure accurately the cavity size and vessels as well as to evaluate cardiac rhythm disturbances and cardiac function.

4. Fetal position within the uterus must be understood to evaluate the spatial orientation of the different heart structures in order to trace the best Doppler signal and map the color flow Doppler displayed in anatomical position.

"Anterior dorsum" and "Posterior dorsum" are usually the best fetal position to study the color flow displayed in the aortic arch and the aorta as well as the ductus arteriosus arch.

"Posterior dorsum" is the most favorable position to obtain the four chamber view to evaluate the ventricular filling pattern across the AV valves, obtaining information about atrial and ventricular size and anatomy, integrity of the atrioventricular septum and inlet septum, the AV valves and atrioventricular connections.

"Lateral dorsum" identifies best the opacification of the right and left outflow tracts and outlet septum, as well as ventriculoarterial connections.

Transabdominal cardiac Doppler studies can be performed with adequate level of cardiac definition from the 17 weeks of gestation onward, using a 3.5 MHz transducer. Cardiac scanning should include at least three anatomical and functional cuts to demonstrate structural and functional normal assessment.

Normal Anatomical and Functional Fetal Echocardiographic Features

A number of normal features should be identified in the echocardiographic evaluation of the fetus:

1. The normal position of the heart within the thorax is of levocardia (the heart is usually to the left, opposite to the liver and superior to the stomach). In four chamber view, the

thoracic aorta should be in the left in close relationship with the left atrium. The fetal heart lies in a more horizontal position due to the large liver.

2. Septal integrity should be present although weakening of inlet/outlet septum may give the impression of a ventricular septal defect in the early stages of pregnancy; no posterior confirmation have been possible, probably due to a transitional echo view which cuts part of the left outflow tract and the interventricular septum.

3. The patent foramen ovale should be a visible atrial communication of approximately the same size as the ascending aorta but no larger than 6 mm along pregnancy and with detectable moving membrane.

4. Normal separation between the septal leaflet implantation of the mitral and tricuspid valves should identify right and left AV valves (Figs 34.4A to D).

5. Myocardial contractility presents an out of systolic phase, paradoxical septal movement; however, movement of the anterior and posterior heart walls should be identified to evaluate ventricular myocardial movement and function.

6. A pericardial space translucency may be visualized in the absence of pericardial effusion.

7. The heart rate should be between 120 and 180 bpm.

8. Normal ventriculoarterial connections should be established when normal crossing of both ventricular outflow tracts and arteries are seen (Fig. 34.2).[8]

9. Normal vessel relationship is seen by the transverse three vessel view from left to right the pulmonary artery, the Ao and the SCV are seen in the same transverse plane.[19]

10. The aortic arch should give origin to the three supra-aortic arteries.

11. The ductus arteriosus arch should be identified as a vascular structure in continuity with the descending aorta, in a right angle curvature when it meets the aorta.

12. Superior and inferior vena cava should be visualized in continuity entering the right atrium.

13. The pulmonary veins should be seen entering the left atrium.

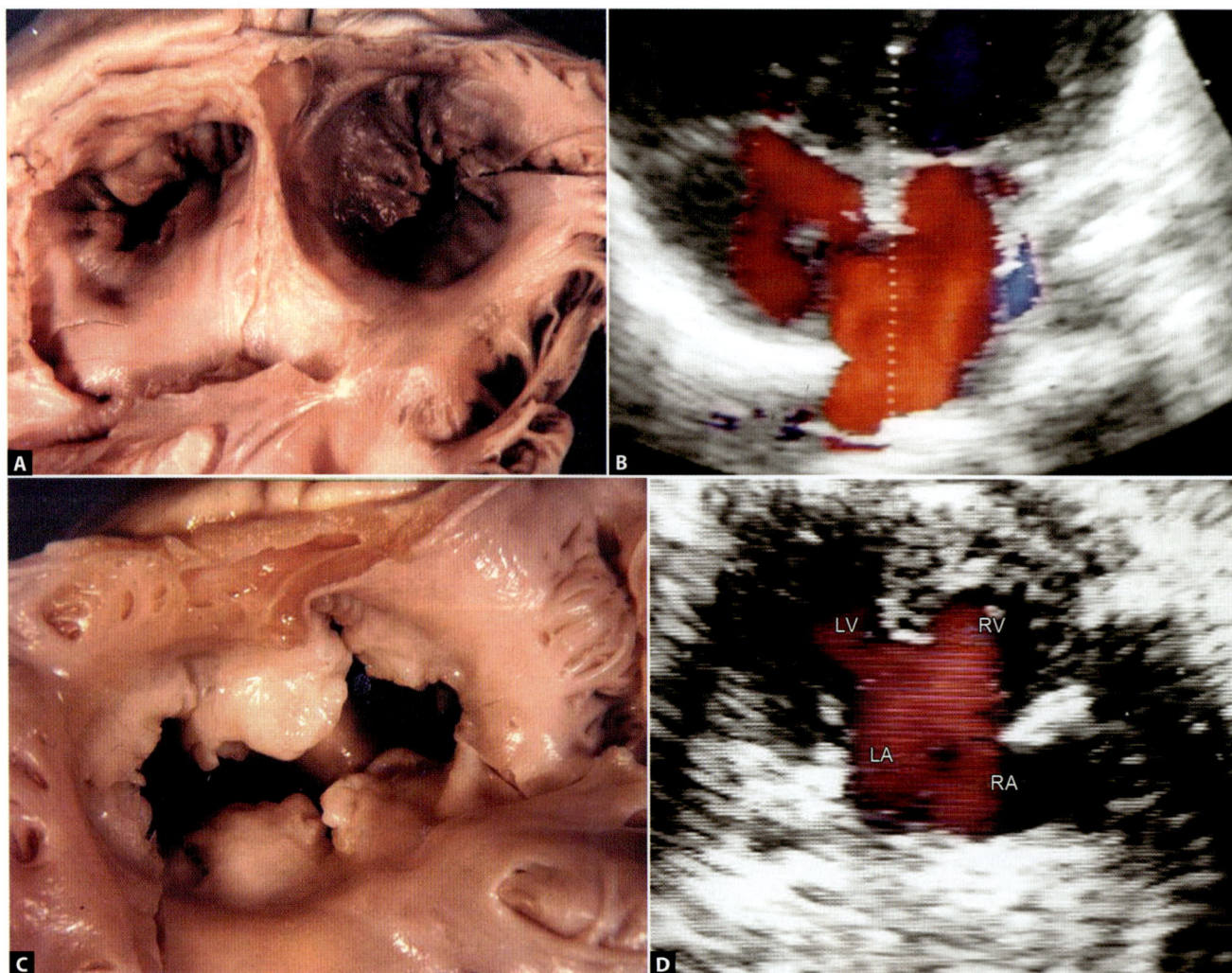

Figs 34.4A to D: Inflow of the heart with two normal AV valves. Color Doppler also identifies the PFO. Inflow of a heart specimen with one common AV valve in atrioventricular septal defect (Echo/Anatomy correlation)

Normal Doppler Fetal Hemodynamics

Peripheral Venous Return of the Umbilical Vein and Ductus Venosus

Doppler sample at the umbilical vein level shows a low velocity no pulsatile waveform slightly influenced by diaphragmatic respiratory movements. The intrahepatic umbilical vein continuous with the ductus venosus as it meets the inferior vena cava (IVC). The diameter of the ductus venosus is reduced as it meets with the inferior vena cava. This reduction in diameter accelerates the blood flow converting the non-pulsatile Doppler venous wave of the umbilical vein into a high velocity triphasic wave form directly influenced by the cycling cardiac filling pattern. The first peak (S) represents the systolic cardiac phase; the second peak (D) represents the diastolic phase, which is followed by the atrial contraction inflection (A).

Right/Left Atrium and Foramen Ovale

Doppler interrogation of the foramen ovale demonstrates a right-left shunting. Premature closure of the foramen ovale has been described.[20] Doppler tracing in the pulmonary veins is also triphasic as in the systemic veins; the lowest-velocity deflection occurs during atrial contraction. Timing of the phases in the venous flow of the pulmonary veins may be useful to diagnose "premature atrial contractions".

Increase in right atrial or ventricular filling pressure may lead to right heart failure. This increase in resistance to umbilical venous flow accentuates the atrial contraction and the corresponding Doppler inflection wave at the "ductus venosus", creating a negative deflection wave that may exceed the zero line at the venous return, this Doppler form should be recognized as a sign of heart failure.

The less oxygenated blood returning from the peripheral fetal body, coming from "superior vena cava and inferior vena cava" as the blood enters the right atrium, presents a Doppler venous flow with triphasic wave form related to the same cardiac filling cycle; this wave form exhibits more pronounced atrial inflection but less flow velocity that the waves obtained in "ductus venosus".

Inflow Heart and Atrioventricular Valves

Doppler interrogation of the inlet heart examines the diastolic filling function. Doppler wave forms through the tricuspid and mitral valve are similar, representing the ventricular filling pattern, the first peak E is followed by the A wave due to atrial contraction an increase in "A" happens in early phases of pregnancy and may represent a transient restricted compliance of the ventricles; normal velocity across the AV valves increases along pregnancy. High heart rate may produce single wave changes in morphology. AV valve stenosis or volume overload alter the morphology and increases velocity across the valves.

Regurgitation of an AV valve is detected within the atrial cavity. Although quantification of a regurgitant flow by Doppler is difficult, detection of a significant regurgitant jet in fetal life represents a considerable hemodynamic dysfunction.[13]

The integrity of the atrioventricular septum in continuity with the inlet septum should be seen as color Doppler fills the ventricles. Weakening of the inlet septum may give the impression of a ventricular septal defect in early stages of pregnancy; but no posterior confirmation has been possible, being probably due to a transitional echo cut. However, an AV septal defect has to be excluded (Figs 34.5A to C).

Outflow Heart, Semilunar Valves and Arteries

Color Doppler has become an extremely effective tool in identifying crossing flow patterns versus parallel flows at arterial level. The different color opacification of each artery indicates opposing flow directions that represent normal crossing of the pulmonary and the aortic outflow tracts and arteries[8] and normal ventriculoarterial connection (Fig. 34.2). A single color representation in both arteries identifies parallel relationship of the great arteries, being the most frequent anatomical arterial relationship seen in transposition of the great arteries (Figs 34.6A and B). However, careful attention should be paid to fetal spatial orientation in the uterus in lateral dorsum to evaluate arterial crossing relationship by color Doppler.[24]

Color Doppler also gives information about the integrity of the outlet septum when both outflow tracts are identified. Subarterial and Infundibular VSD will be seen during this examination.

Semilunar valve systolic flow examination by Doppler allows to measure time intervals to assess systolic function, but may give also information about the presence of valve stenosis and/or regurgitation. Blood velocity across a semilunar should not exceed 130 cm/sec, therefore an increase above this velocity could be due to valvular stenosis or increase blood volume. A turbulent high Doppler flow is usually produced by valve stenosis; the degree of obstruction is the key for measuring the severity of this lesion. In fetal life, each semilunar valve allows the passage of approximately

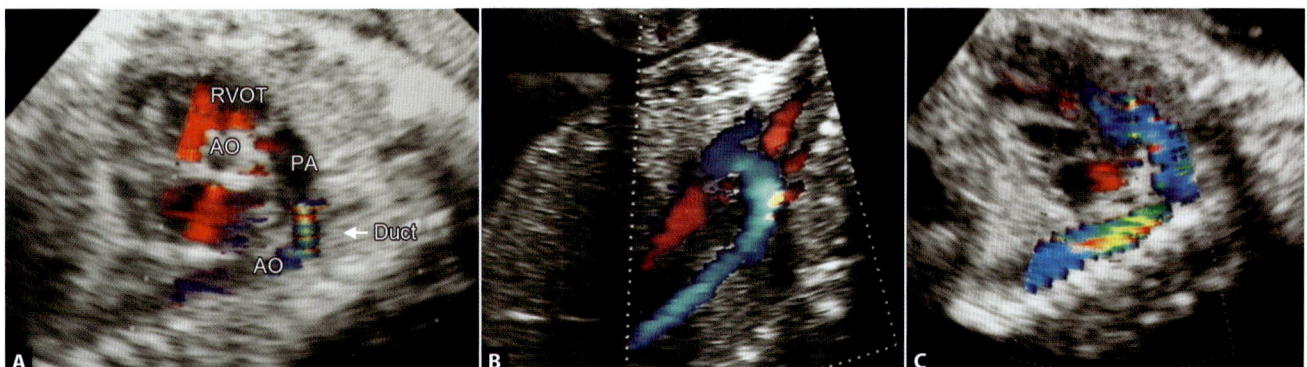

Figs 34.5A to C: (A) Ductus arteriosus constriction under indomethacin therapy. Color flow Doppler shows a turbulent ductal flow. (B) Normal aortic arch. (C) Coarctation of the aorta. Color flow detects a turbulent flow at the descending aorta

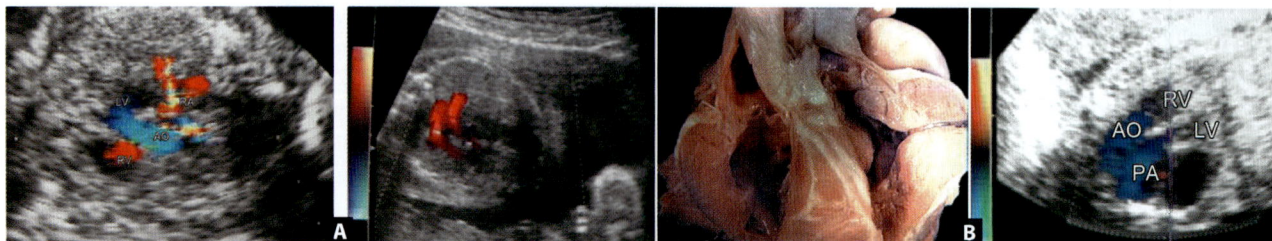

Figs 34.6A and B: (A) Normal outflow right and left ventricular tracts and arteries. The opposite code opacification shows the normal crossing relationship. (B) Heart specimen from a transposition of the great arteries. Color flow Doppler shows parallel opacification of both arteries

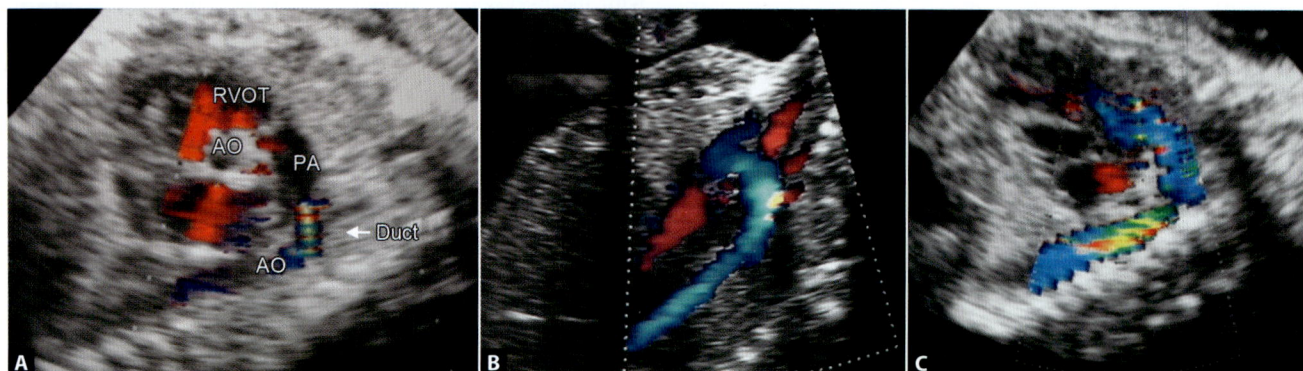

Figs 34.7A to C: (A) Ductus arteriosus constriction under indomethacin therapy. Color flow Doppler shows a turbulent ductal flow. (B) Normal aortic arch. (C) Coarctation of the aorta. Color flow detects a turbulent flow at the descending aorta

half of the blood volume that will transverse the valve after birth; this reduced blood volume will cause an underestimation of the obstruction and of the valve pressure gradient, making the fetal assessment difficult. Valvular regurgitation produces a backward flow into the left or right ventricular outflow tract that in the fetus with normal heart rate (>130 bpm) represents structural valvular dysfunction.

Ductus Arteriosus and Descending Aorta

The pulmonary artery receives approximately have of the total blood flow ejected by the right fetal heart. At this point most of the blood is diverted through the "ductus arteriosus" toward the descending aorta, leaving the pulmonary circulation at minimum flow. The ductus arteriosus is a vascular structure in continuity with the descending aorta, forming almost a right angle curvature when it meets the aorta; the ductus at this level may impose a degree of flow restriction however this is compensated with the active systolic contraction of the right ventricle; Doppler wave form shows a slight increase systolic velocity as the ductus meets the Aorta. However, an abnormal increase in systolic and diastolic velocity above 130 cm/seg is produced during ductal constriction with marked elevation of systolic and diastolic velocity. Patients in indomethacin treatment should be Doppler control to detect signs of ductal constriction (Figs 34.7A to C) and medication should be stop. Sudden increase of duct constriction leads to increase in afterload with tricuspid regurgitation.[25,26]

Systolic arterial Doppler wave in the abdominal aorta is followed by continuous diastolic flow as blood entering the intra-abdominal umbilical arteries go in the umbilical cord toward the placenta.

Abnormal Anatomical and Functional Echocardiographic Fetal Features

Abnormal features of echocardiography include:

1. Malposition of the heart is established when atrial and visceral (liver/stomach) are seen in a wrong position: the usual place for these structures is termed as "Situs solitus". "Situs inversus" involves reversal of the normal atrial and ventricular positions. "Situs ambiguous" describes an undefined medial visceral position. Dextrocardia, mesocardia, levocardia are terms which define the location of cardiac apex.
2. Comparative disproportion between atrial and ventricular cavities, as well as arterial size; may lead to demonstrate pathological dilatation or reduced diameter of these heart structures (Figs 34.8 and 34.9).
3. A single ventricular cavity.
4. A single atrium.
5. A single atrioventricular valve (Fig. 34.4).
6. Specific valvular anomalies. Ebstein's anomaly.
7. Parallel ventricular outflow tracts and arteries (Fig. 34.6).
8. A single arterial trunk (truncus).
9. A septal defect.
10. Ventricular inversion.
11. Regurgitant valvular jets (by Doppler).
12. Cardiomegaly.
13. Signs of heart failure: pericardial effusion, ascitis, hydrops.
14. Arteriovenous fistula.
15. Arrhythmias; tachyarrhythmia, bradycardia.

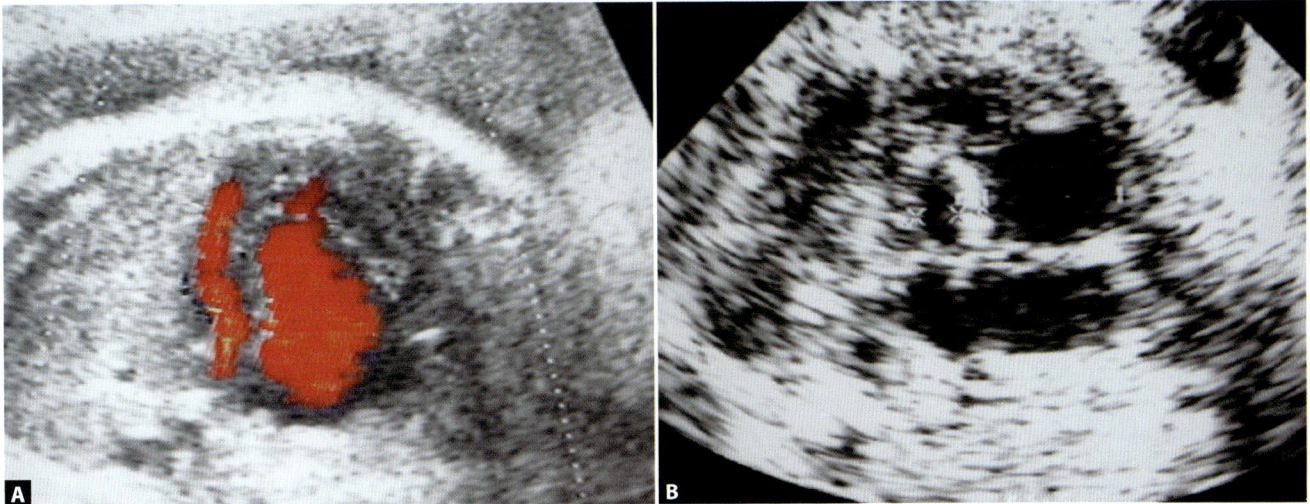

Figs 34.8A and B: Four chamber cut in left heart asymmetry due to hypoplastic left heart

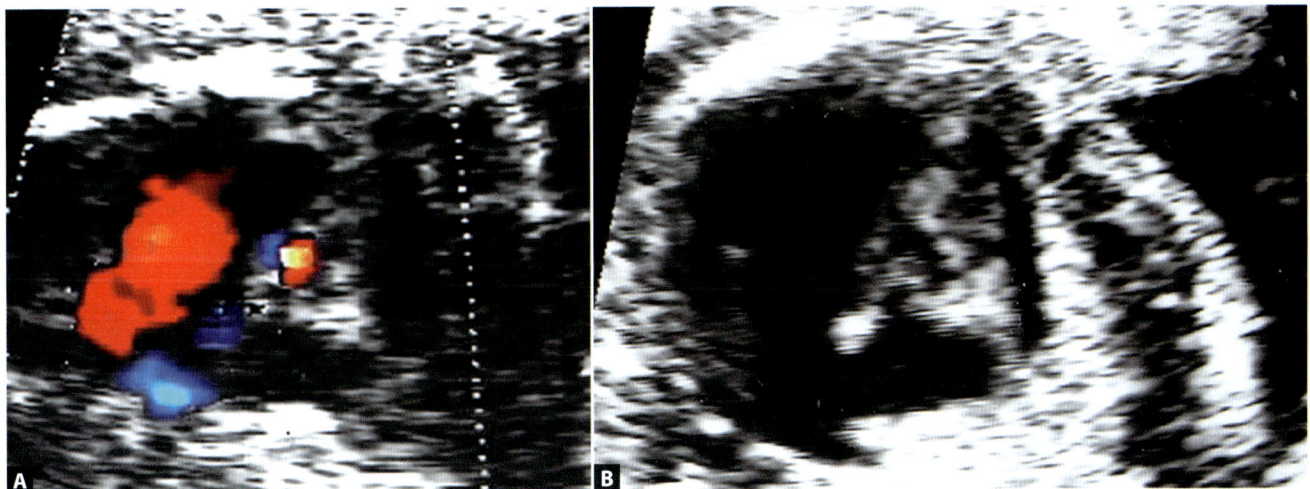

Figs 34.9A and B: Tricuspid atresia and hypoplastic right heart. The color Doppler helps to identify small right ventricular cavity

Fetal Cardiovascular Pathology

Identification by two-diamensional echocardiography and Color Doppler.

Congenital heart disease (CHD) appears as a result of "structural malformations" developed during fetal early phases of fetal life.[2,3] The severity of each malformation marks the future prognosis of the newborn with a perinatal death as high as 50% mortality,[4] when congenital heart disease has been diagnosed in fetal life.[21] Chromosomal abnormalities may be found as high as 42% of the fetal cases referred because of CHD.[22] However, "functional cardiac anomalies" may occur as transitory disturbance during fetal intrauterine growth and usually present a good prognostic outlook at term.

In an attempt to simplify congenital heart disease complexity, cardiac malformations may occur at two basic levels following a segmental approach:[7]

1. The inflow level, including malformations at systemic and pulmonary veins, atriums, atrial septum, inlet valves, inlet/trabecular septum and ventricular cavities.

2. The outflow level, which includes ventricles, outlet septum, outflow tracts, semilunar valves and arteries.

Inflow Level

The veins are identified by using the four chamber view as they meet with the right atrium and left atrium. Anomalous connections of the systemic veins as well as pulmonary veins may be visually identified.[23] The relative sizes of the right and left atrium should be compared. Usually the right atrium is larger than the left atrium. Early closure or reduction of the foramen ovale[20] (atrial septal aneurysm) may be identified as well as a distended foramen. The ventricles should be of similar size although right ventricular dominance may be normally present.

Congenital cardiac malformations and conditions at inflow level include:

1. Anomalous venous connections of the systemic venous return or the pulmonary veins.

2. Atrial septal defects: ostium primum, ostium secundum, and sinus venosus defects and patent foramen ovale with septal aneurismatic membranous septum.

3. Atrioventricular valve anomalies: mitral/tricuspid atresia, mitral/tricuspid stenosis/hypoplasia (Figs 34.9 and 34.10). Atrioventricular valve regurgitation. Single common valve, Ebstein's anomaly.

4. Ventricular development: hypoplastic left heart, hypoplastic right heart, single ventricle (univentricular heart), single inlet, double inlet, atrioventricular canal complete and partial, and ventricular inversion (atrioventricular discordance) corrected transposition.

5. Ventricular septal defect: inlet portion (perimembranous), trabecular (muscular) and apical.

6. Pericardium (effusion).

7. Myocardium: ventricular anatomy (right ventricle heavily trabeculated containing the tricuspid valve with a confluent papillary muscle/left ventricle smooth endocardial walls with the mitral valve and two well-defined papillary muscles. Left ventricular myocardial contractility, function and hypertrophy.

8. Cardiomyopathies: hypertrophic (diabetes, etc.) dilated (endocardial fibroelastosis, etc.).

9. Cardiac tumors.

Outflow Level

Color Doppler has become an extremely effective tool in identifying "crossing flow patterns" versus "parallel flows".[8] The different color code opacification of each artery indicates opposing blood flow directions that represent normal ventriculoarterial connections (Fig. 34.6).[24] Although the key to the diagnosis is to demonstrate the origin of the pulmonary artery arising from the left ventricle and the aorta from the right ventricle.

Single color code opacification in both arteries identifies parallel arterial relationship which represents a discordance ventricular-arterial connection, so-called transposition of the great arteries (Fig. 34.6). Single opacification of one single arterial trunk, truncus.

Congenital cardiac malformation and conditions at the outflow level include:

1. Aortic valve/pulmonary valve: atresia, stenosis and regurgitation.

2. Hypoplastic aortic arch/pulmonary trunk.

3. Coarctation of the aorta (Fig. 34.7)/aortic arch interruption.

4. Coronary arteries anomalies.

5. Absent pulmonary valve syndrome.

6. Single arterial trunk (truncus arteriosus).

7. Tetralogy of Fallot (Figs 34.11A to C)/Pulmonary atresia + VSD.

8. Double outlet right ventricle (Figs 34.12A and B).

9. Double outlet right ventricle and transposition of the great arteries. (Figs 34.12A and B).

10. Ventricular septal defect: infundibular, perimembranous, subarterial and trabecular.

11. Aortopulmonary window.

12. Anomalies of the aortic arch.

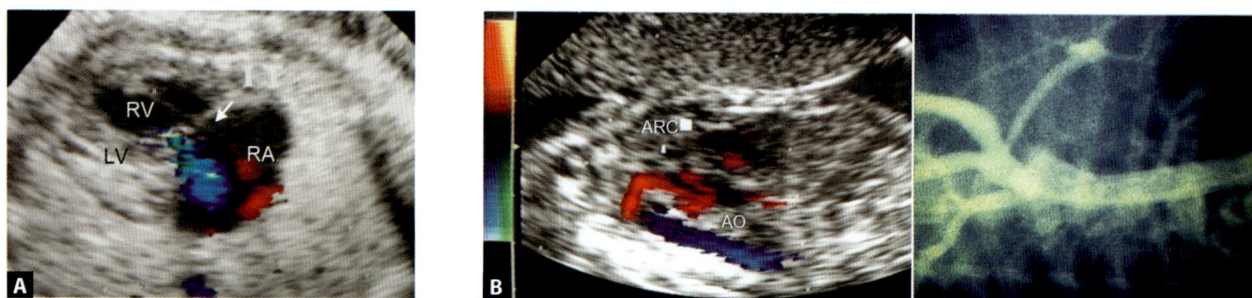

Figs 34.10A and B: Hypoplastic left heart syndrome with mitral atresia and aortic atresia. (A) Single ventricular cavity corresponding to the right ventricular. Tricuspid regurgitation is seen. (B) Eco/Angiogram shows the retrograde aortic arch opacification as no blood is ejected through the aortic valve

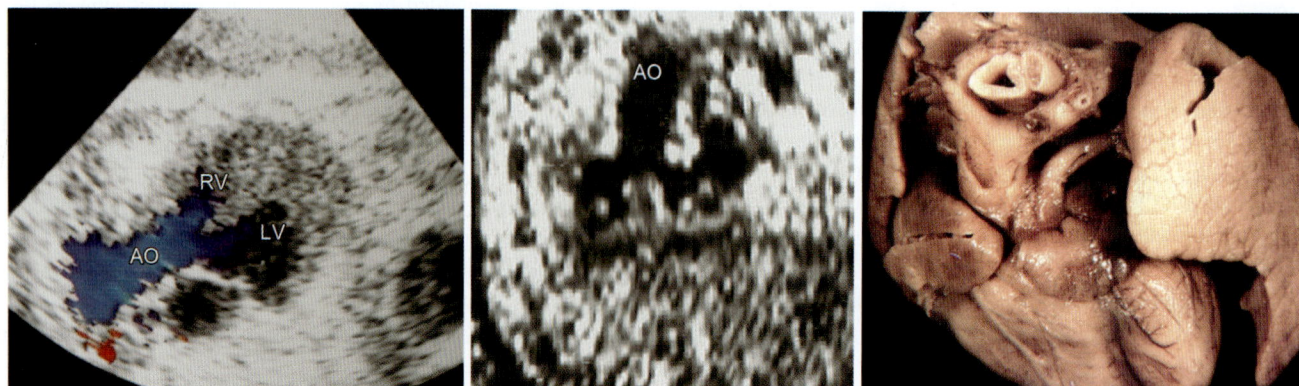

Figs 34.11A to C: Tetralogy of Fallot. The heart specimen shows reduced pulmonary artery compared to the ascending aorta. A double aortic arch was present as well. Aortic-septal overriding can be seen by Eco demonstrates the Subarterial VSD

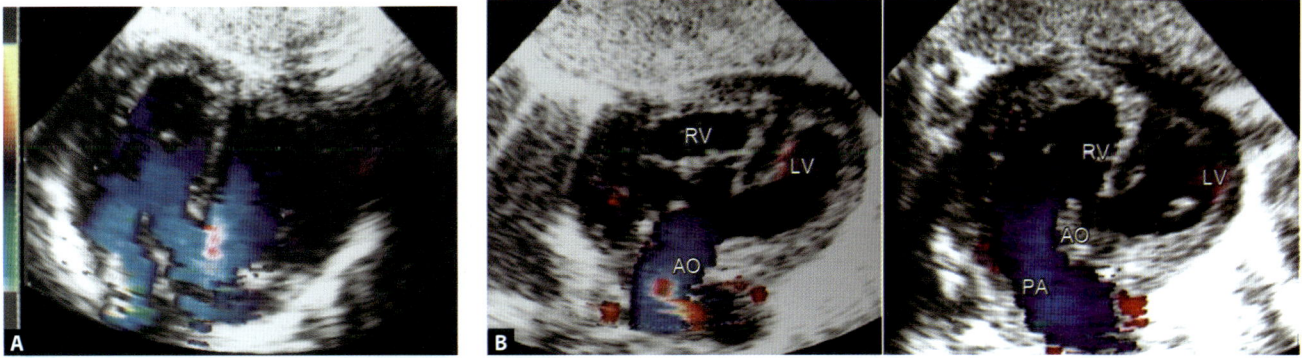

Figs 34.12A and B: Double outlet right ventricle: (A) two parallel outflow tracts and arteries are seen coming of the right ventricle with subpulmonary VSD. In double outlet right ventricle with TGA. (B) Double outlet right ventricle with normally related arteries with subaortic VSD

13. Hypoplastic aortic arch and coarctation of the aorta (Fig. 34.7) versus interrupted aortic arch.

The diagnosis of structural and functional heart disease is possible during fetal life although not always can be made with the amount of precision required. There are a number of congenital heart malformations in which it is extremely difficult to establish the before birth, as the fetal heart is not yet fully adapted to the future adult circulation that will take place after birth.

In the newborn with congenital heart disease, as the pulmonary circulation and lung oxygenation process begins, cardiac malformations will further developed. The intracardiac fetal shunts will close down as pulmonary artery pressure is reduced to one-quarter of the systemic pressure.

During pregnancy some fetal heart defects such as ostium secundum atrial defect, anomalous pulmonary venous return and some small ventricular septal defects will be impossible to evaluate. Also in some cases of Fallot's tetralogy in which fetal pulmonary blood obstruction is not yet well established during prenatal period, it may be difficult to identify the obstruction as the main functional/anatomical feature of this malformation. During fetal life, malformations and vascular anomalies such as persistent ductus arteriosus, aortopulmonary window, coarctation of the aorta and interruption of the aortic arch are extremely difficult to diagnose because no dysfunctional changes take place before birth although indirect cardiac signs as enlargement of right heart cavities have been described.

Coronary artery anomalies are also difficult to suspect. The diagnosis of atrioventricular or semilunar valve stenosis is similarly difficult; the degree of obstruction to blood flow is the key to measuring severity in these lesions. In fetal life, each cardiac valve allows the passage of only half of the blood volume that will transverse the valve after birth because fetal intracardiac circulation pattern; this reduced blood volume will cause an underestimate of the obstruction and valve pressure gradient making the diagnosis by Doppler difficult.

Diagnosis and Prognosis of Fetal Heart Failure

The echocardiographic examination of the cardiovascular system provides much information about the well-being of the fetus. Heart failure is established when low cardiac output produces inadequate tissue perfusion. This results in series of complex hormonal reflexes and vascular adaptations to improve direct flow to vital organs. Peripheral vasoconstriction increases the fetal systemic resistances in response to cardiovascular stress with excess production of catecholamines and natriuretic factor together with other complex humeral agents to maintain arterial redistribution of fetal cardiac output for the survival of the fetus.

The diagnosis of fetal heart failure is established through the analysis of a number of cardiovascular features.

1. The cardiothoracic size. Cardiomegaly is the universal sign of heart failure. This is measured using the CT cardiac/chest circumference ratio (normal = 0.5).
2. Myocardial function. Assessment of cardiac function by global myocardium fiber shortening fraction is calculated by using the difference between the diastolic and systolic dimensions divided by the diastolic diameter (normal, >0.30).
3. Increased atrial reversal contraction at the venous Doppler triphasic pattern in the hepatic duct and IVC. This may be a sign of increased end diastolic ventricular pressure. Increase A:S ratio peak atrial reversal divided by peak ventricular systole (Figs 34.13A to F). Normal values should be less than 7%. In the fetus with CHD the venous filling patterns should be normal with exception of tricuspid/pulmonary atresia with intact septum of restrictive filling compliance lesions.
4. Analysis of Doppler detection of valve leak at the heart.

Fetal Cardiac Arrhythmias

Fetal cardiac dysrhythmias[27,28] are rhythm disturbances caused by irregular cardiac beats "extrasystoles" or by regular accelerated tachycardias produced by ectopic heart beats superior to 180 bpm. On the contrary, bradycardias are slow regular heart rhythms, below 80 bpm.

Cardiac dysrhythmias count for 1–2% of rhythm alterations during pregnancy. Fetal arrhythmias are also associated with a higher incidence of congenital heart disease. However, irregular cardiac rhythms caused by extrasystoles count for 80–85% of benign rhythm disturbances in normal fetus with no need for specific treatment. Management of these dysrhythmias during pregnancy only requires maternal rest and withdraw of stimulants.

Taquy-bradycardias[29] are frequent cause of heart failure and hydrops. They usually require in utero treatment via maternal

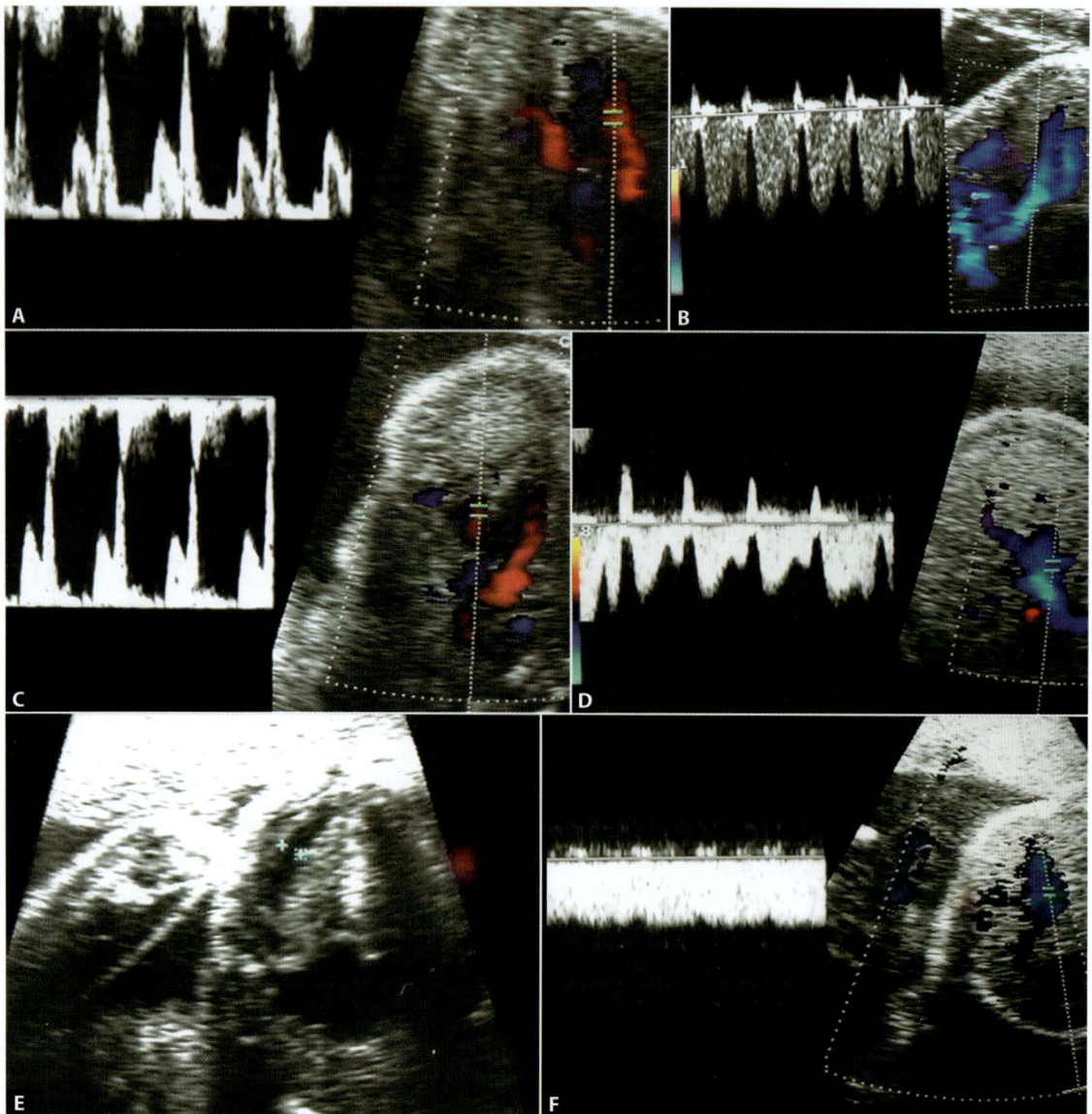

Figs 34.13A to F: A number of Doppler signs can predict fetal heart failure. Increase "a" in AV flow. Deep diastolic phase at ductus venosus flow prominent and negative "a" wave at the IVC small pericardial effusion pulsatile deflection at the umbilical flow

administration of antiarrhythmic agents, premature delivery and cardiac pacing of the newborn as in the case of congenital heart block.

Classification of Cardiac Arrhythmias

Irregular Heart Beats (Figs 34.14A to C)

Extrasystoles: Extrasystoles constitute the most frequent arrhythmia in the fetus and in the newborn; no treatment is required, only observation.

It has been associated to high fetal catecholamines, maternal hyperthyroidism and stimulants.

Sinus Arrhythmia: In this disorder, there is variability between the sinus atrial contractions. It is recognized by the variable space between Doppler pulsed waves.

Premature Atrial Contraction: Premature atrial contraction is the most frequent ectopic arrhythmia often causing extrasystoles. It may be the origin of supraventricular tachycardia.

Premature Ventricular Contraction: Premature ventricular contractions are ventricular ectopic beats; they are rare in the fetus.

Regular Fast Heart Rate

Sinus Tachycardia: This is a persistent cardiac rhythm above 160 bpm, but below 200 bpm, that may be related to fetal response to catecholamines, anemia, etc.

Pathological Tachycardias: They are regular fast heart rhythms above 200 bpm, divided in two main groups: supraventricular and ventricular tachycardia.

1. Supraventricular tachycardia (Figs 34.15A to C) include:
   a. "Atrial tachycardia", produced by an ectopic atrial beat.
   b. "Atrial flutter" a rapid atrial contraction of 300–400 bpm. The atrial activity is blocked at the atrioventricular (AV) node with ventricular response of 220 bpm. The p wave can

be identified at the movement of the atrial wall by m-mode echo.

c. "Intranodal Tachycardia", the most common fetal and newborn tachycardia, presents with a ventricular response between 220–280 bpm and a 2/1 atrioventricular block.

d. "Atrioventricular tachycardia with accessory pathway" with conduction via the Kent or Mahian intranodal and extranodal pathway conduction. In the Wolf-Parkinson-White syndrome, tachycardias are produced by a circular re-entry mechanism; atrial activity is not visualized by echo, therefore no specific diagnosis of this syndrome can be reliably made in utero.

2. Ventricular tachycardia is rare in the fetus, and newborn usually associated to myocardial dysfunction or intramyocardial tumor.

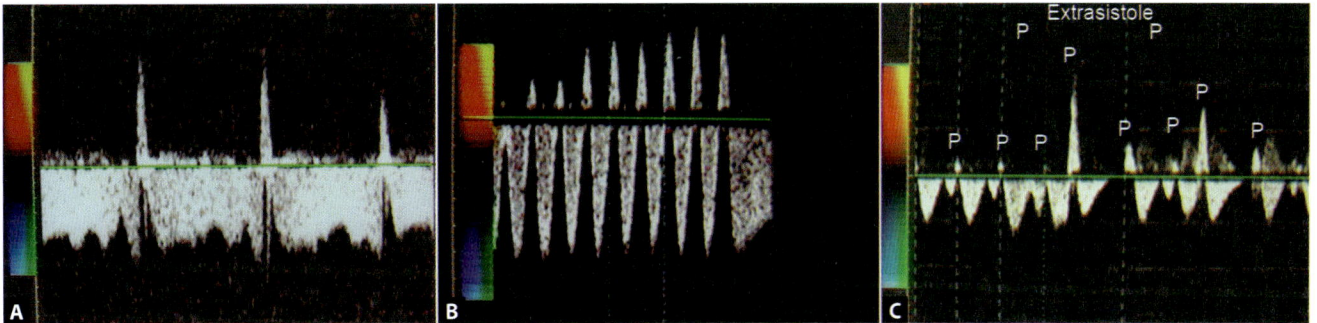

Figs 34.14A to C: Supraventricular ectopic beats seen at ductus venosus flow and IVC (negative deflections)—Run of supraventricular tachycardia

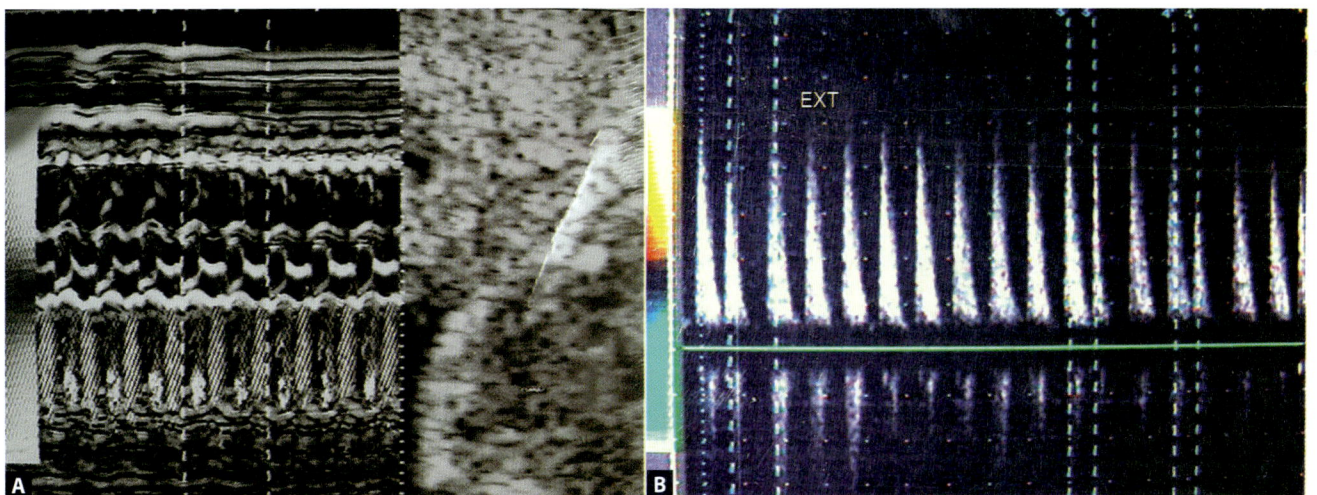

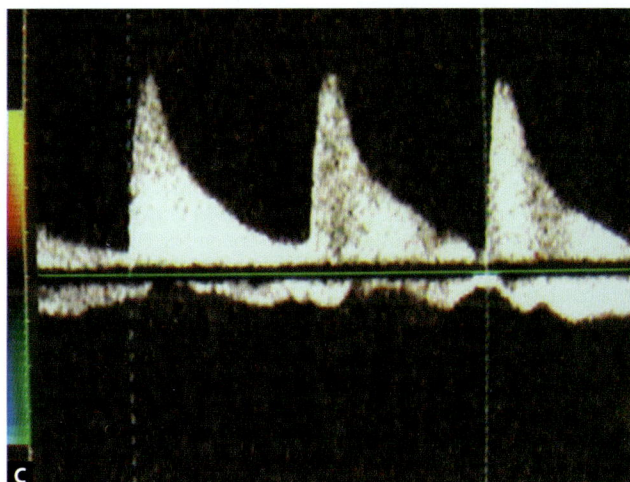

Figs 34.15A to C: (A) Supraventricular tachycardia using m-mode echo to establish a 2/1 atrioventricular rate comparing the atrial wall movements and the aortic valve opening. (B) Ventricular bradycardia in a congenital complete AV block

The ventricular heart rate is not as fast as in the supraventricular tachycardia and is in the range of 180 bpm. This dysrhythmia may present runs of tachycardia with irregular heart beats and no relationship can be established between atrial and ventricular contractions.

Regular Slow Heart Rate

Bradycardias: Bradycardia is a slow cardiac rhythm with heart rates below 80 bpm. The bradycardia include:

a. "Transient sinus bradycardia" which can occur during ultrasound examination. In this situation vagal stimulation over the head of the fetus may produce transient bradycardia with spontaneous recovery. Persistent bradycardia may be the consequence of fetal hypoxia or congenital heart block with or without structural congenital heart disease.

b. "Congenital heart block" is the result of a delay or a block in the transmission of atrial electrical impulse along the atrioventricular conduction system. Three degrees may be present.

- "First degree block" is produced by a delay in AV conduction system and is not recognized by echo.
- "Second degree heart block" occurs when an incomplete AV conduction delay results in an isolated atrial impulse, which is not conducted through the AV node, resulting in a missed ventricular contraction.

- "Third degree heart block" produces an atrioventricular dissociation. The atrial contraction is independent from the ventricles, it follows the sinus beats at atrial rate of 150 bpm. Atrioventricular conduction is blocked and ventricular contraction is established at an autonomous ventricular rate of 50–60 bpm (Figs 34.15A to C). Atrioventricular dissociation is the usual presentation of congenital heart block.

c. Congenital heart block and persistent fetal bradycardia are associated either with congenital heart disease or with a structurally normal heart. However, a normal fetal heart and congenital heart block can be related to autoimmune maternal disease as lupus erythematosus,[30] Sjögren's syndrome and rheumatoid arthritis not always diagnosed before pregnancy. Anti-Ro and anti-LA antibodies are most likely to be detectable in maternal blood.[31]

d. Congenital heart block with heart rates above 60 bpm seems to have a reasonable outcome. Pacemaker therapy in the newborn should be implanted when ventricular heart rate is below 70 bpm. Fetal hydrops and heart failure are related to slow ventricular heart rate below 50 bpm. Fetal management should include maternal administration of terbutaline or sympathomimetics agents, as well as premature delivery and pacemaker implantation in the newborn.[32]

REFERENCES

1. Allan LD, Tynan MJ, Campbell S, et al. Doppler echocardiography and anatomical correlates in the fetus. B Heart J. 1987;57:528-33.
2. Allan LD. A practical approach to fetal heart scanning. Sem Perinatol. 2000;24:324-30.
3. Cohen MS. Fetal diagnosis and management of congenital heart disease. Clin Perinatol. 2001;28:11-29.
4. Mortera C, Salvador JM, Torrens M, et al. Diagnostico prenatal de las Cardiopatias Congenitas mediante Ecocardiografia Doppler. In: Masson-salnot (Ed). Doppler en Obstetricia. Hemodinamica Perinatal. 1992.
5. Chaoui R, Hoffmann J, Heling KS. Three-dimensional (3D) and (4D) color Doppler fetal echocardiography using spatio-temporal image correlation. Ultrasound Obstet Gynecol. 2004;23(6):535-45.
6. Maulik D, Nanada NC, Singh V, et al. Live three-dimensional echocardiography of human fetus. Echocardiography. 2003;20(8):715-21.
7. Mortera C. Diagnostico prenatal de las cardiopatias congenitas: valor de la ecocardiografia. Doctoral thesis. Universidad de Barcelona; 1989.
8. Mortera C, Carrera JM, Torrents M. Doppler pulsado codificado en color: mapa Doppler color de la circulacion fetal. In: Masson-Salvat (Eds). Doppler en Obstetricia. Hemodinamica Perinatal. 1992.
9. Copel JA, Morotti R, Hobbins JC, et al. The antenatal diagnosis of congenital heart disease using fetal echocardiography: is color flow mapping necessary. Obstet Gynecol. 1991;78(1):1-8.
10. Chiba Y, Kanzaki T, Kobayashi H, et al. Evaluation of fetal structural heart disease using color flow mapping. Ultrasound Med Biol. 1990;16(2):221-9.
11. Kovalchin JP, Silverman NH. The impact of fetal echocardiography. Pediatr Cardiol. 2004;25:299-306.
12. Rychick J. Fetal cardiovascular physiology. Pediatr Cardiol. 2004;25:201-9.
13. Huhta JC. Guidelines for the evaluation of heart failure in the fetus with or without hydrops. Pediatr Cardiol. 2004;25:274-86.
14. Small M, Copel JA. Indications for fetal echocardiography. Pediatr Cardiol. 2004;(25):250-52.
15. Mortera C. Fetal ultrasound in the preliminary diagnosis of cardiac anomalies for management of the new born with interventional cardiac catheterization. The perinatal medicine of the new millennium. The 5th World Congress of Perinatal Medicine. 2001. pp. 177-80.
16. Rudolph AM. Congenital Heart Disease. Chicago: Year Book Medical. 1974. pp. 17-28.
17. DeVore GR. The aortic and the pulmonary outflow tract screening examination in the human fetus. J Ultrasound Med. 1992;11:345-8.
18. Allan L. Technique of fetal echocardiography. Pediatr Cardiol. 2004;25:223-33.
19. Yoo SJ, Lee YH, Kim ES, et al. Three-vessel view of the fetal upper mediastinum: an easy means of detecting abnormalities of the ventricular outflow tracts and great arteries during obstetric screening. Ultrasound Obstet Gynecol. 1997;9:173-82.
20. Eyck J, Stewart PA, Wladimiroff JW. Human fetal foramen ovale flow velocity waveforms relative to fetal breathing movements in normal term pregnancies. Ultrasound Obstet Gynecol. 1991;1:5-7.
21. Cohen MS. Fetal diagnosis and management of congenital heart disease. Clin Perinatol. 2001;28:11-29.
22. Allan LD, Sharland GK, Chita SK, et al. Chromosomal anomalies in fetal congenital heart disease. Ultrasound Obst Gynecol. 1991;1:8.
23. Wessels MW, Frohn-Mulder IM, Cromme-Dijkhuis AH, et al. In utero-diagnosis of infradiaphragmatic total anomalous pulmonary venous return. Ultrasound Obstet Gynecol. 1996;8:206-9.
24. Mortera C, Maroto C, Maroto. Echocardiografia Doppler de la circulacion fetal. In principios y practica del Doppler Cardiaco. New York: McGraw-Hill; 1995. pp. 365-89.

25. Achiron R, Lipitz S, Kidrons D, et al. In utero congestive heart failure due to maternal indomethacin treatment for polyhydramnios and premature labour in a fetus with antenatal closure of the foramen ovale. Prenatal Diagnosis. 1996;16:652-6.

26. Kim HS, Sohn S, Park MY, et al. Coexistence of ductal constriction and closure of the foramen in utero. Pedatr Cardiol. 2003;24(6):588-90.

27. McCurdy CM, Reed KL. Fetal arrhythmias. Doppler en Obstetrics and Gynecology. New York: Raven Press; 1995. pp. 253-70.

28. Kleiman CS, Copel JA. Electrophysiological principles and fetal antiarrhythmic therapy. Ultrasound Obstet Gynecol. 1991;1:284-97.

29. Lynn LS, Marx G. Diagnosis and treatment of structural fetal cardiac abnormality and dysrhthmia. Seminar in Perinatology. 1994;18(3):215-27.

30. Silverman E, Mamula M, Hardin JA, et al. Importance of the immune response to Ro/La particle in the development of congenital heart block and neonatal lupus erythematosus. J Rheumatol. 1991;18:120-4.

31. Schmidt KG, Ulmer HE, Silverman NH, et al. Perinatal outcome of fetal complete atrioventricular block. Bloqueo Auriculoventricular Completo Congénito A multicenter experience. J Am Cardiol. 1991;91:1360-6.

32. Comas C, Mortera C, Figueras J, et al. Diagnóstico Prenatal y Manejo Perinatal. Rev Esp Cardiol. 1997;50(7):498-506.

CHAPTER 35

Three-dimensional Ultrasound in Prenatal Medicine

E Merz

INTRODUCTION

During the past two decades, three-dimensional (3D) ultrasound has evolved from a relatively tedious laboratory technique to a highly sophisticated technique for daily routine examinations, particularly in prenatal diagnosis.

In 1989 the first commercially available ultrasound scanner (Combison 330) with special 3D probes for transabdominal and transrectal scanning was launched by Kretztechnik AG, Austria.[1] This system allowed fully automated volume acquisition and multiplanar reconstruction of the 3D data set in three orthogonal planes. Due to rapid developments in computer and transducer technology, image quality and processing speed improved tremendously in the following years. With the latest 4D technology of Voluson® 730 Expert (GE Medical Systems Kretz Ultrasound), volume acquisition and volume display can be accelerated in such a way that the fetus can be visualized three-dimensionally in real-time. This gives the examiner a direct impression of the fetal surface and movements.

Additional 3D/4D techniques have been developed within the past 2–3 years: glass body rendering, volume contrast imaging (VCI-A and VCI-C) and spatio-temporal image correlation (STIC).

TECHNICAL ASPECTS

All 3D/4D ultrasound examinations consist of four main steps[2,3]: (1) data acquisition, (2) 3D/4D visualization, (3) volume analysis/image processing, and (4) storage of volumes, rendered images or image sequences (cine clips) (Table 35.1).

Table 35.1: Steps required in transvaginal and transabdominal 3D ultrasound (after Merz[3])

(1) Data acquisition
- Orientation in the 2D image
- Definition of the region of interest (ROI)
- Volume acquisition

(2) 3D visualization
- Multiplanar display
- Surface-rendered image (surface mode, light mode)
- Transparent image (maximum mode, X-ray mode)
- Vascular image (combination of surface or transparent rendering and color Doppler)
- Animated image (rendering of image sequences)

(3) Volume/image processing
- Electronic scalpel
- Filtering
- Contrast and brightness control
- Color image

(4) Storage of volumes, rendered images and image sequences

3D Data Acquisition

For volume acquisition, the ultrasound beam has to be moved over the object of interest. This procedure can be performed manually with external acquisition systems or automatically with internal acquisition systems.

External Acquisition Systems

These freehand systems do not require a specially designed transducer. The scans are performed using a freehand technique with a conventional 2D probe, whose position and movement in space are tracked by an add-on system.[4-6] However, the freehand systems are not able to achieve 4D ultrasound.[3]

Internal Acquisition Systems

These systems use specific probes with a fully automated scanning technique.[1,3,7] The automated scanning movement can be achieved by using mechanical gears and/or electronic scanning techniques such as steered phased arrays and/or curved/linear arrays in which different groups of elements are excited.[1] These probes can be used for 3D and 4D ultrasound as well.

3D DISPLAY

In contrast to conventional 2D ultrasound which provides only one imaging mode to demonstrate the fetus, present 3D technology offers the ability to review the fetus in several different display modes:

Triplanar (or Multiplanar) Mode

The triplanar mode allows re-slicing of acquired volumes in any direction.[3,8,9] Thus any arbitrary plane can be shown, even image planes that are not accessible with conventional 2D ultrasound. The simultaneous display of all three perpendicular sectional planes, provides an ideal basis for a detailed tomographic survey of the fetus and allows the demonstration of a specific plane to be precisely controlled (Figs 35.1 and 35.2).

Surface Mode

The surface mode can provide 3D images of the outer and inner fetal surfaces (Figs 35.3 to 35.5).[2,3,10,11] For this purpose, the region of interest has to be framed with a volume box. For many years, this volume box was only variable in size, but nowadays it is variable in size and shape. Various rendering algorithms (surface mode, soft surface mode, light mode, soft light mode) can be used in surface rendering, either individually or in different combinations.[3]

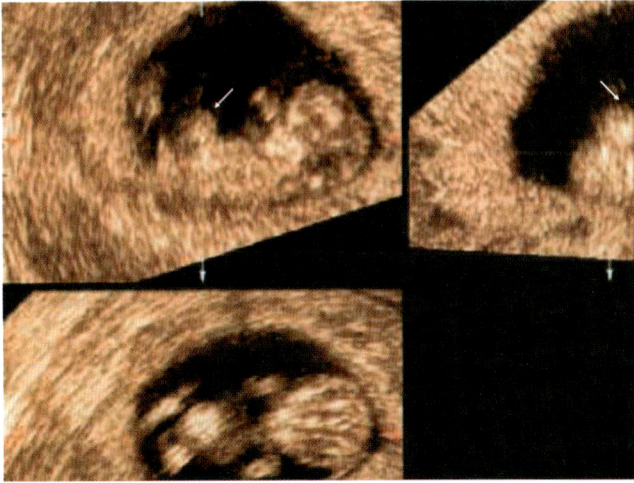

Fig. 35.1: Fetus with physiologic umbilical hernia (←) (9 weeks) in the multiplanar display. Upper left: midsagittal scan. Upper right: transverse scan. Lower left: coronal scan

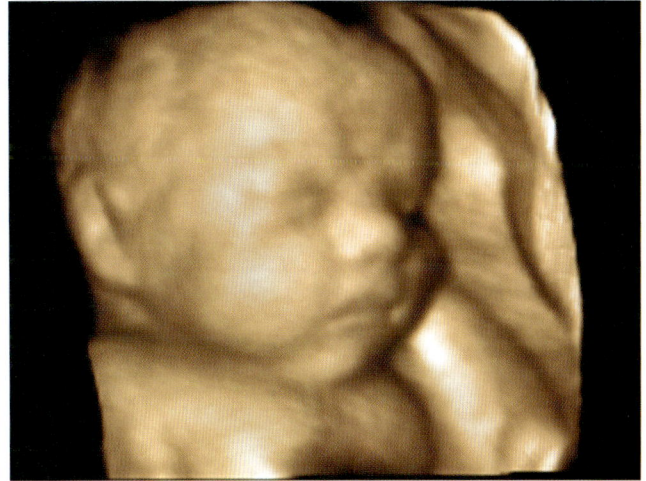

Fig. 35.4: Surface view of a fetal face at 32 weeks of gestation

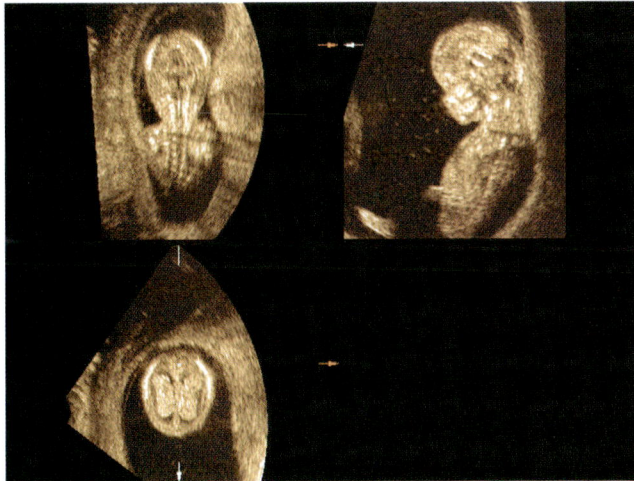

Fig. 35.2: Multiplanar display of a fetus at 13 weeks of gestation. Upper left: coronal scan. Upper right: midsagittal scan. Lower left: transverse scan of the head

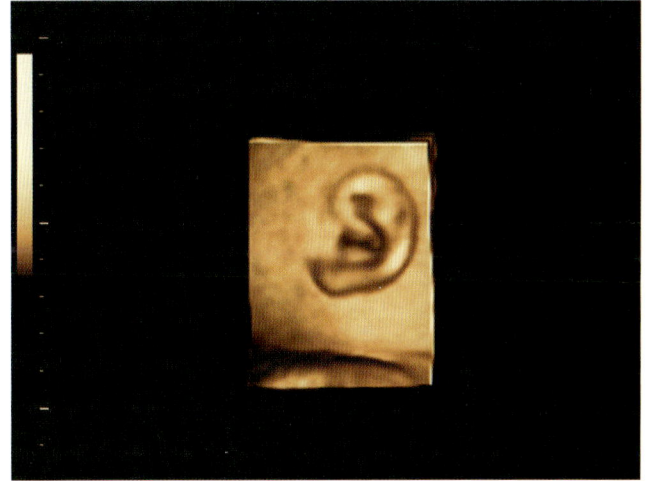

Fig. 35.5: Surface view of a fetal ear at 38 weeks of gestation

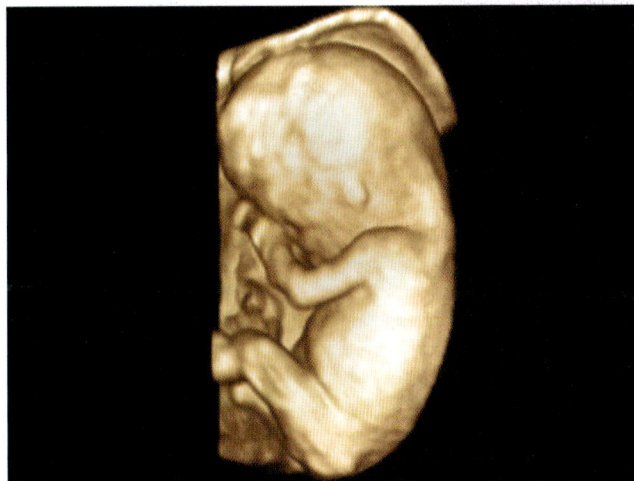

Fig. 35.3: Surface view of a fetus at 12 weeks of gestation

A basic requirement for all 3D surface rendering is the presence of an adequate fluid pocket in front of the structure being imaged. Overlying or adjacent structures such as the placenta, fetal limbs, and loops of the umbilical cord tend to obscure the structure of interest and must be removed with the electronic scalpel.[12]

Transparent Mode

The transparent mode provides a complete survey of the fetal skeleton (Fig. 35.6).[13-14] Two different rendering algorithms (maximum mode and X-ray mode) can be used, either individually or in combinations with the smooth surface mode or the gradient light mode.

Glass Body Rendering

The combination of 3D color Doppler or power Doppler and gray-scale 3D images enables the physician to analyze the fetal vascular system (Figs 35.7A and B).

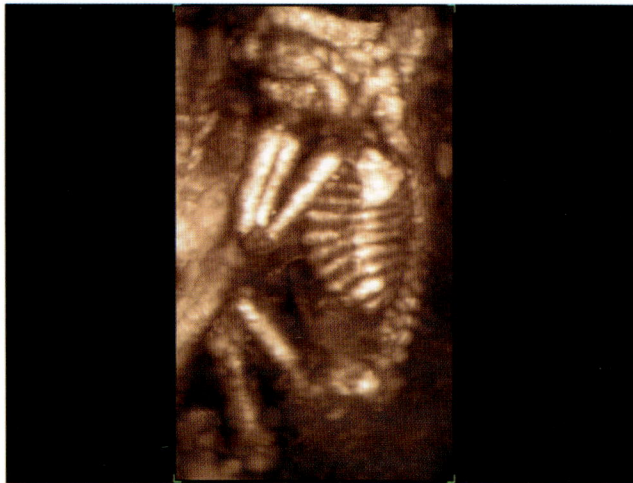

Fig. 35.6: Transparent view (maximum mode) of a normal fetal skeleton at 20 weeks of gestation

3D Cine Mode

In order to obtain an overall 3D impression of the object of interest, a certain number of rendered views are displayed in a fast sequence. In this way the observer can see the object of interest rotating on the screen. The 3D cine mode can be used with the surface mode, the transparent mode and the glass body rendering.

4D DISPLAY

4D Ultrasound

With the acquisition of up to 25 volumes per second, both the surface and movements of the fetus can be demonstrated on the screen. This enables the parents to observe the movements of the fetus and allows the examiner to study the behavior of the fetus. The 4D cine loop allows the examiner to scroll back through volumes to achieve the best surface demonstration of the region of interest (Fig. 35.8). For 4D volume rendering, two rendering modes are always applied simultaneously.

4D Cine Sequence

A 4D image cine sequence can be created with a Voluson® 730 series machine in the real-time 4D mode. After storage as an AVI file, such a sequence can be shown with a movie program in any personal computer.

DiagnoSTIC™ (Spatio-temporal Image Correlation)

DiagnoSTIC or STIC is a new technique for assessment of the fetal heart, based on the automatic acquisition technology. It allows off-line multiplanar analysis of the fetal heart. For DiagnoSTIC™, a slow-motion (7.5 sec, 10 sec or 12.5 sec) volume scan of the fetal heart is performed. The data is then rearranged and stuck together by correlation of its temporal and spatial domains. An EGC trigger is not necessary. The result is a 4D real-time data set presenting one heart cycle in motion. This data set can also be rotated and analyzed in the triplanar view while the heart is beating at any stage of the cycle.

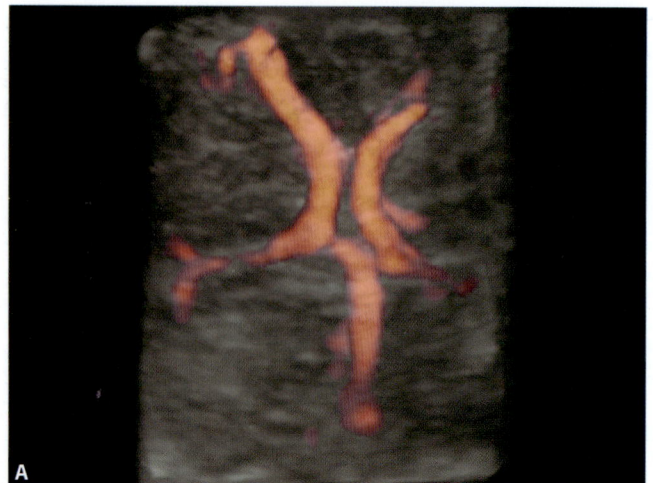

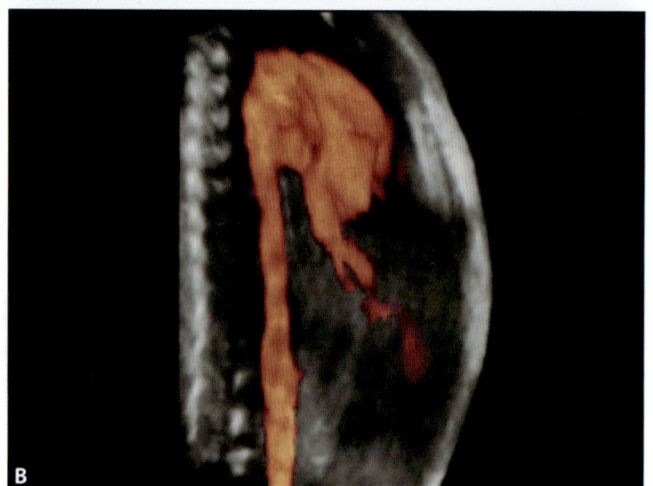

Figs 35.7A and B: Glass body rendering: The combination of transparent mode and power Doppler displays the vascular system of the fetus. (A) Circle of Willis (35 weeks). (B) Fetal heart and aorta (30 weeks)

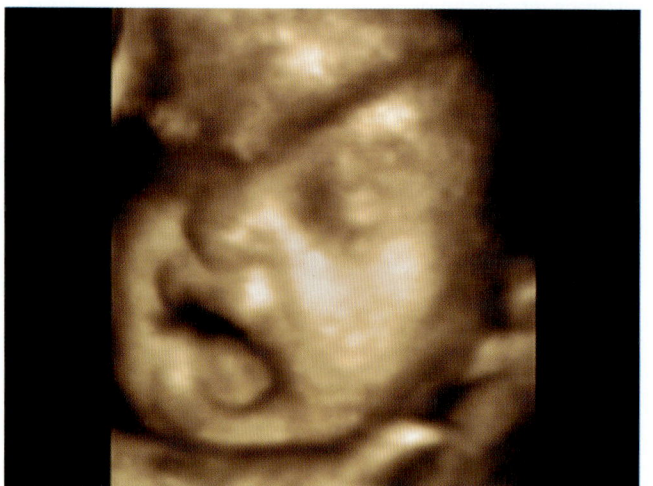

Fig. 35.8: Surface-rendered view of fetal yawing at 32 weeks. The 4D cine loop allows scrolling back to the most interesting movement

STIC-Color (Spatio-Temporal Image Correlation with Color Doppler)

In this technique, the STIC technique is combined with color Doppler information. This facilitates the recognition and confirmation or exclusion of congenital heart defects (septal defects, transposition of the great vessels, etc.) (Fig. 35.9).[3,15-18]

Volume Contrast Imaging

In VCI the probe is applied in the same way as in conventional 2D ultrasound and so is an easy approach to 4D, even for the novice. This volume rendering process is based on thick slice tissue data[3] and it is possible to select a slice thickness between 3 mm and 20 mm. Displayed as a thick slice, the VCI technique allows a 4D volumetric data acquisition.

The development of this tool has facilitated a marked improvement in tissue contrast resolution in real-time and therefore enables inhomogeneous areas or subtle lesions to be detected. It provides additional information simultaneously with conventional 2D imaging, without the processing time of off-line 3D reconstruction. In VCI technology, a mixture of surface mode and transparent maximum mode rendering is employed.

VCI-A

Volume contrast imaging in the A-plane provides the examiner with an easy 4D approach. It reveals the same anatomical region as in the 2D ultrasound image, but the tissue contrast is better with VCI-A (Fig. 35.10).

VCI-C

Volume contrast imaging in the C-plane allows an easy 4D real time approach in the coronal plane of the region of interest (Fig. 35.11). VCI-C offers great potential in prenatal diagnosis because it scans planes which are not accessible with conventional B-mode scanning. This is particularly important when the fetus is in an unfavorable position.

VOLUME/IMAGE PROCESSING

In many cases, the acquired data sets require post-processing. In order to obtain a high quality surface image, adjacent or overlapping structures which are obscuring the fetus have to be removed with an electronic scalpel. Low-level echoes in the amniotic fluid may be filtered out by increasing the threshold value. In color Doppler the angio threshold removes small motion artifacts and color noise.

Image brightness and contrast can be set to any desired value in all 3D/4D display modes just as in 2D ultrasound. In glass body rendering, the color and gray-scale areas can be adjusted independently of one another. All changes are immediately visible on the monitor. These interactive control features make it easy to display any object with optimal brightness and contrast.[3,19]

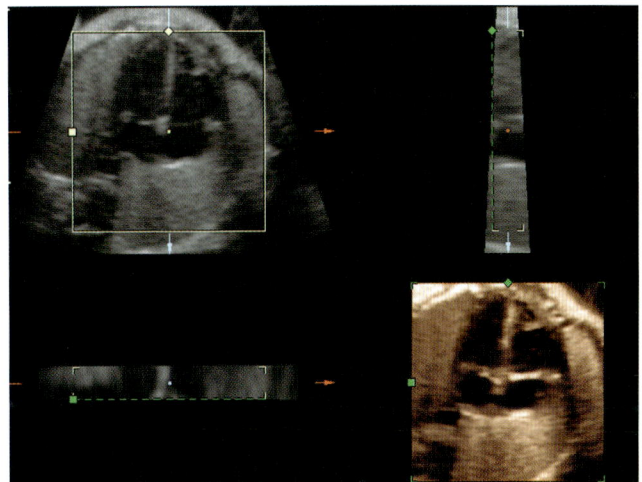

Fig. 35.10: VCI-A (volume contrast imaging in the A-plane) of the fetal heart (29 weeks). This technique shows the same anatomical region as in the 2D ultrasound (upper left), but the contrast is better in VCI-A (lower right)

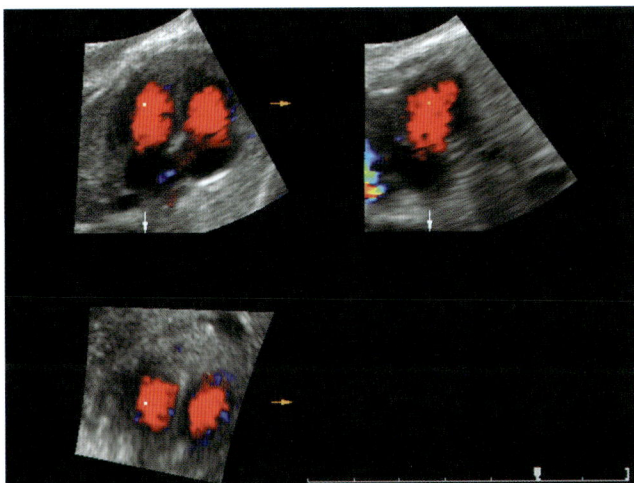

Fig. 35.9: Fetal heart at 36 weeks. The STIC (spatio-temporal image correlation) technique combined with color Doppler displays blood flow in all three orthogonal planes at the same time

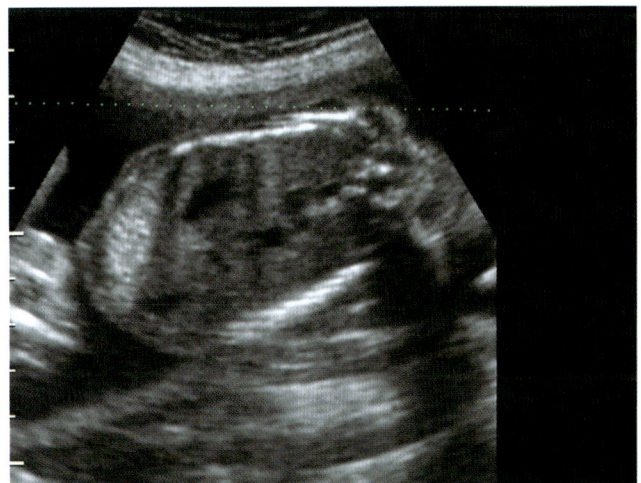

Fig. 35.11: VCI-C (volume contrast imaging in the C-plane). This simple technique yields detailed morphologic information of the plane perpendicular to the marked green line in the conventional 2D plane. Here 3D information of the fetal chest in the coronal view (20 weeks)

STORAGE OF VOLUMES, RENDERED IMAGES AND IMAGE SEQUENCES

Long-Term Storage

Three-dimensional/four-dimensional ultrasound gives us the capability to store volumes, rendered images, 3D and 4D cine sequences digitally. Today, various media are available for the long-term storage of these volumes, such as removable hard disks, magneto-optical disks (MOD) and DVD.

When findings of interest are stored digitally on non-degrading media, the examiner can retrieve the volumes at any time and navigate through them in the absence of the patient.[7] This is of particular value in the diagnosis of fetal anomalies, as it enables the examiner to take the time to fully scrutinize equivocal findings without upsetting the patient by lingering at a particular site with the probe, which is often a problem in conventional 2D examinations.[3]

Clinical Applications

For the examination in the first trimester, the transvaginal 3D/4D probe is usually applied, and for the second and third trimester examinations, the abdominal 3D/4D probe is used. If the fetus is in a cephalic presentation, the transvaginal 3D/4D probe can also be used in the second or third trimester to assess the fetal brain in a higher resolution.[9,20]

The advantage of all the different 3D/4D rendering modes is that it is possible to visualize the normal embryonic and fetal development at all stages.[21-23] The first view of the fetal face has an important psychological effect on the parents to whom the detailed images are much better recognizable than the 2D pictures. With the use of glass body rendering (3D and power Doppler) even the vascular system can be observed by the parents.

For the sonographer, however, the detection of a fetal malformation is of more importance.[24-33] Despite the fact that, with conventional 2D ultrasound examinations, most of the fetal abnormalities can be detected by the experienced examiner, 3D/4D ultrasound provides additional information, particularly for the experienced examiner.[7] 3D ultrasonography can depict many image planes that are inaccessible with conventional 2D ultrasound. In the first trimester the tri-planar demonstration is particularly helpful in the verification of a true mid-sagittal section which is necessary for an exact nuchal translucency (NT) measurement (Fig. 35.12).[34-36] In NT demonstration and measurement, the examination time can be dramatically reduced, especially in case of an unfavorable fetal position and the quality of the requested image can be improved.[36]

In the second and third trimesters, the photorealistic surface view of the fetus offers interesting opportunities for the detection of abnormalities, especially in subtle defects (Figs 35.13 and 35.14).[24-33] In some cases, it is also possible to find defects which were not revealed with conventional 2D ultrasound.[7] In other cases, the surface mode can also provide impressive 3D images of the inner fetal surfaces (Fig. 35.15).

Four-dimensional ultrasound provides an excellent real-time 3D view of the fetus. With the STIC technique even 4D fetal echocardiography has become reality. The triplanar demonstration of the beating heart enables a comprehensive assessment of the fetal heart morphology including the great vessels. Due to the fact that the volume can be rotated and re-sliced in all three dimensions even complex anomalies of the fetal heart can be demonstrated

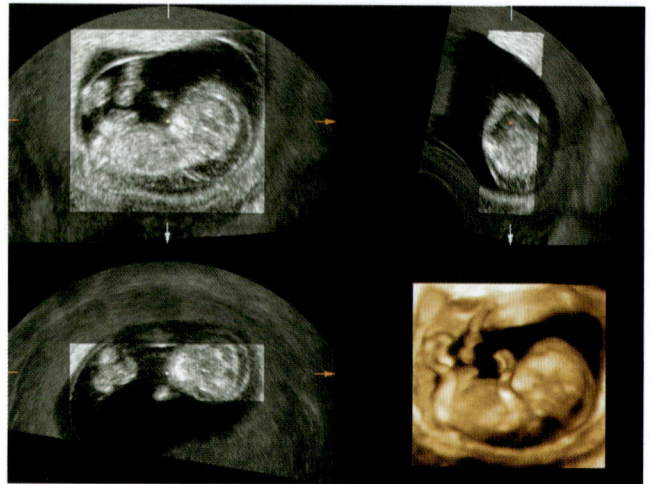

Fig. 35.12: Multiplanar demonstration of a fetus with increased nuchal translucency thickness of 6.2 mm (11+4 weeks). Karyotype: Trisomy 18. Upper left: precise midsagittal scan. Upper right: Transverse scan at neck level. Lower left: Coronal scan. Lower right: Surface view

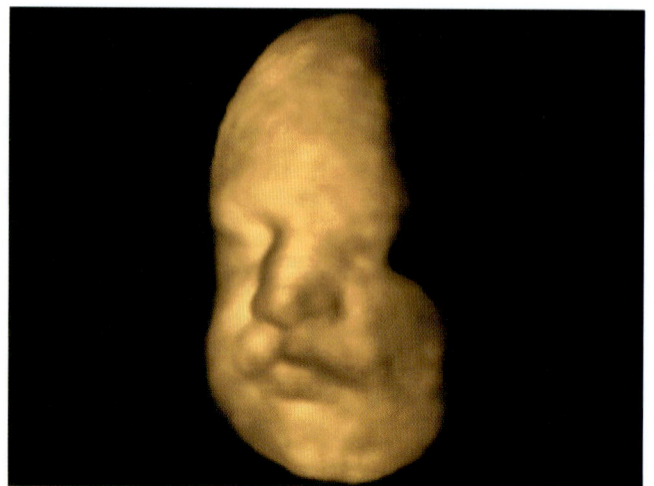

Fig. 35.13: Surface-rendered view of a small cleft lip at the right side (38 weeks)

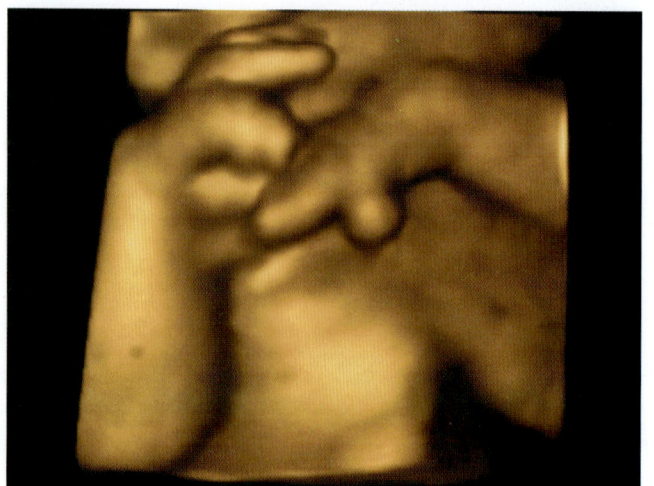

Fig. 35.14: Surface-rendered view of the left hand with postaxial hexadactyly (31 weeks)

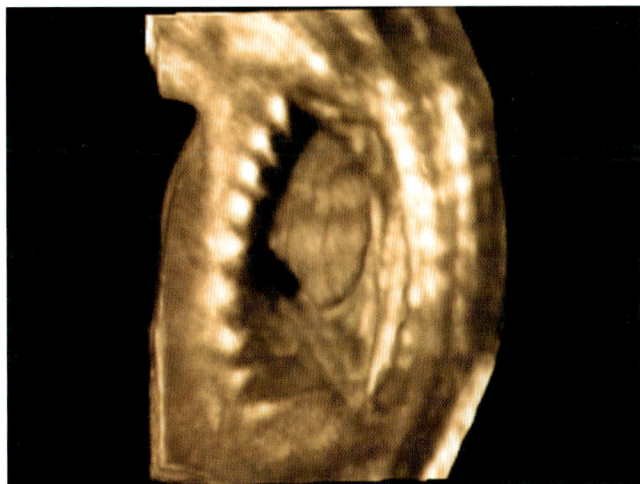

Fig. 35.15: Surface-rendered view of a fetus with left-sided hydrothorax at 30 weeks of gestation. The fetal chest has been partly "removed" with the electronic scalpel, displaying the surface of the small left lung

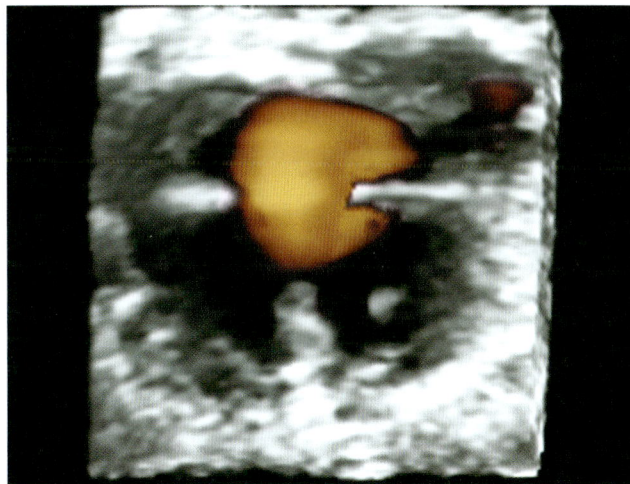

Fig. 35.16: Glass body rendering (surface-rendered image) of an AV canal (23 weeks). The combination of transparent mode and power Doppler displays the defect in the valvular plane

precisely. The combination of STIC and color Doppler allows an exact control of the cardiac blood flow while the heart in motion (Fig. 35.16).

The interactive display in 3D/4D ultrasound is particularly useful for the detection of specific abnormalities, making it possible to identify fetal surface abnormalities and define the extent of a defect in all dimensions. The same applies to the targeted exclusion of fetal anomalies. Particularly in cases with an increased recurrence risk, the various display options of 3D/4D ultrasound provide a selective exclusion of a fetal defect and parents can see for themselves that the 3D surface image demonstrates a normal fetus.

REFERENCES

1. Wiesauer F. Methodology of three-dimensional uktrasound. In: Kurjak A, Kupesic S (Eds). Clinical application of 3D sonography. London: Parthenon Publishing Group; 2000. pp 1-6.
2. Merz E. 3D ultrasound in prenatal diagnosis. Curr Obstet Gynaecol. 1999;9:93-100.
3. Merz E. 3D Ultrasound in prenatal diagnosis. In: Merz E (Ed). Ultrasound in Obstetrics. Stuttgart: Thieme. 2004.
4. Sakas G, Schreyer L, Grimm M. Preprocessing, segmenting and volume rendering 3D ultrasonic data. In: IEEE Computer Graphics and Applications. 1995;15:47-54
5. Guerra FA, Isla AI, Aguilar RC, et al. Use of free-hand three-dimensional ultrasound software in the study of the fetal heart. Ultrasound Obstet Gynecol. 2000;16:329-34.
6. Prager R, Gee A, Treece G, et al. Freehand 3D ultrasound without voxels: Volume measurement and visualisation using the Stradx system. Ultrasonics. 2002;40(1-8):109-15.
7. Merz E, Bahlmann F, Weber G, et al. 3D ultrasonography in prenatal diagnosis. J Perinatal Med. 1995;23:213-22.
8. Kratochwil A. Importance and possibilities of multiplanar examination in three-dimensional sonography. In: Merz E (Ed). 3D ultrasound in Obstetrics and Gynecology. Philadelphia: Lippincott Williams and Wilkins; 1998. pp 105-8.
9. Timor-Tritsch IE, Monteagudo A, Mayberry P. Three-dimensional ultrasound evaluation of the fetal brain: the three horn view. Ultrasound Obstet Gynecol. 2000;16:302-6.
10. Benoit B. Three-dimensional surface mode for demonstration of normal fetal anatomy in the second and third trimesters. In: Merz E (Ed). 3D Ultrasound in Obstetrics and Gynecology. Philadelphia: Lippincott Williams and Wilkins; 1998. pp 95-100.
11. Pretorius DH, House M, Nelson TR. Fetal face visualization using three-dimensional ultrasonography. J Ultrasound Med. 1995;14:349-56.
12. Merz E, Miric-Tesanic D, Welter C. Value of the electronic scalpel (cut mode) in the evaluation of the fetal face. Ultrasound Obstet Gynecol. 2000;16:364-8.
13. Yanagihara T, Hata T. Three-dimensional sonographic visualization of fetal skeleton in the second trimester of pregnancy. Gynecol Obstet Invest. 2000;49:12-6.
14. Benoit B. The value of three-dimensional ultrasonography in the screening of the fetal skeleton. Childs Nerv Syst. 2003;19: 403-9.
15. DeVore GR, Falkensammer P, Sklansky MS, et al. Spatio-temporal image correlation (STIC): new technology for evaluation of the fetal heart. Ultrasound Obstet Gynecol. 2003;22:380-7.
16. Goncalves LF, Lee W, Chaiworapongsa T, et al. Four-dimensional ultrasonography of the fetal heart with spatiotemporal image cor-relation. Am J Obstet Gynecol. 2003;189:1792-802.
17. Chaoui R, Hoffmann J, Heling KS. Three-dimensional (3D) and 4D color Doppler fetal echocardiography using spatio-temporal image correlation (STIC). Ultrasound Obstet Gynecol. 2004;23:535-45.
18. Vinals F, Poblete P, Giuliano A. Spatio-temporal image correlation (STIC): A new tool for the prenatal screening of congenital heart defects. Ultrasound Obstet Gynecol. 2003; 22:388-94.
19. Nelson TR, Pretorius DH. Interactive acquisition, analysis and visualization of sonographic volume data. Int J Imag Systems Technol. 1997;8:26-37.
20. Pooh RK, Pooh KH. The assessment of fetal brain morphology and circulation by transvaginal 3D sonography and power Doppler. J Perinat Med. 2002;30:48-56.

21. Bonilla-Musoles F. Three-dimensional visualization of the human embryo: a potential revolution in prenatal diagnosis. Ultrasound Obstet Gynecol. 1996;7:393-7.

22. Benoit B, Hafner T, Kurjak A, et al. Three-dimensional sonoembryology. J Perinat Med. 2002;30: 63-73.

23. Rotten D, Levaillant JM. Two- and three-dimensional sonographic assessment of the fetal face. 1. A systematic analysis of the normal face. Ultrasound Obstet Gynecol. 2004;23:224-31.

24. Merz E, Bahlmann F, Weber G. Volume (3D) scanning in the evaluation of fetal malformations—a new dimension in prenatal diagnosis. Ultrasound Obstet Gynecol. 1995;5:222-7.

25. Pretorius DH, House M, Nelson TR, et al. Evaluation of normal and abnormal lips in fetuses: Comparison between three- and two-dimensional sonography. AJR. 1995;165:1233-7.

26. Lee A, Deutinger J, Bernaschek G. Three-dimensional ultrasound: abnormalities of the fetal face in surface and volume rendering mode. Br J Obstet Gynaecol. 1995;102:302-6.

27. Mueller GM, Weiner CP, Yankowitz J. Three-dimensional ultrasound in the evaluation of fetal head and spine anomalies. Obstet Gynecol. 1996;88:372-8.

28. Merz E, Weber G, Bahlmann, et al. Application of transvaginal and abdominal three-dimensional ultrasound for the detection or exclusion of malformations of the fetal face. Ultrasound Obstet Gynecol. 1997;9:237-43.

29. Lee W, Kirk JS, Shaheen KW, et al. Fetal cleft lip and palate detection by three-dimensional ultrasonography. Ultrasound Obstet Gynecol. 2000;16:314-20.

30. Dyson RL, Pretorius DH, Budorick NE, et al. Three-dimensional ultrasound in the evaluation of fetal anomalies. Ultrasound Obstet Gynecol. 2000;16:321-28

31. Kos M, Hafner T, Funduk-Kurjak B, et al. Limb deformities and three-dimensional ultrasound. J Perinat Med. 2002;30:40-7.

32. Xu HX, Zhang QP, Lu MD, et al. Comparison of two-dimensional and three-dimensional sonography in evaluating fetal malformations. J Clin Ultrasound. 2002;30:515-25.

33. Krakow D, Williams J III, Poehl M, et al. Use of three-dimensional ultrasound imaging in the diagnosis of prenatal-onset skeletal dysplasias. Ultrasound Obstet Gynecol. 2003;21:467-72.

34. Chung, BL, Kim HJ, Lee KH. The application of three-dimensional ultrasound to nuchal translucency measurement in early pregnancy (10-14 weeks): a preliminary study. Ultrasound Obstet Gynecol. 2000;15:122-5.

35. Eppel W, Worda C, Frigo P, et al. Three- versus two-dimensional ultrasound for nuchal translucency thickness measurements: comparison of feasibility and levels of agreement. Prenat Diagn. 2001;21:596-601.

36. Welter C, Merz E. Nuchal translucency-screening using 2D and 3D ultrasound. Ultrasound Obstet Gynecol. 2003;22(Suppl 1):13.

36 Ultrasound-guided Fetal Invasive Procedures: Current Status

JM Troyano, M Alvarez de la Rosa, I Martinez-Wallin

INTRODUCTION

Since the early eighties a varied amount of experiences and trials of fetal puncture (fine needle aspiration) have been carried out with diagnostic aims.[1-5] At the beginning, the only possible way to enter the fetal environment was with the support of a fetoscope but the spectacular development of the already well known ultrasonography has permitted the invasion of the intrauterine environment with tools that are more and more harmless in the use, especially in the gradually tighter sections and the evolution of certain characteristics of the new needles that are now being incorporated into the new biopsy techniques.[3,6,7] Fetal puncture with diagnostic aims is technically possible, provided it is done by adequately trained hands, but the essential problem lies in establishing the correct indications which are not yet quite defined.[8]

TECHNIQUE GENERALIZATION

Whatever, the location of the fetal puncture may be a certain number of requirements are imperative.

1. The operator must have sufficient working experience in invasive echography.

2. The room should have surgical consideration or rank, it is necessary to have an aseptic room for echographic intervention. A sterile wrap is recommended for the ultrasound probe. We use a surgical glove for an airtight seal.

3. The characteristics of the surgical equipment or the obtaining of the sample.

   As the tendency is to obtain samples with the maximum diagnostic guarantee and a minimal risk to the integrity of the pregnancy, it is of capital importance, with few exceptions, to use sectio needles no smaller than 18 G.

   It is clear that depending on the tissue sample we are aiming to obtain, it is not always possible to use innocuous tools. Clear examples are the devices used to date for skin biopsies to diagnose some types of *genodermatosis*, which consist on clipper forceps measuring 2.5 mm.

   These methods in many cases require the use of an anesthetic, including in some, general anesthesia, previous to the incision in the maternal abdomen, with a scalpel, and the introduction of a trocar sheath equivalent section to needle that serves as a guide vehicle for the mentioned system or method.

The complications derived from the use of 2.5 mm section needles and the transabdomen forceps method are closer to those of the fetoscope, added to the fact that the great flexibility in many cases of the method itself, having the availability of a great variety of needles of relatively small caliber (18 G standard), obtaining very good biopsies, including in skin samples and visceral solid areas (Fig. 36.1).[2,7]

Within the organs that are intrauterinally reachable. With worthy guarantees, the one that follows in difficulties after the skin sampling, is the kidney, fundamentally due to its histological parenchymal stratum constitution.[9]

We can only consider satisfactory the samples or cylinders that include corticomedullar stratum. The fetal availability in respect of its intrauterine position, the distance and the interposed tissue to the kidney (skin, muscle) as well as perirenal fat and the very capsule, are the elements that obstruct the obtaining of valid samples.

The use in these cases of a catheter of 14–16 G caliber with isometric aspiration techniques with constant vacuum, allow to obtain valid samples, between 69% and 80%, while the use of 18–20 G caliber catheter obtains the very best specimens between 25% and 30%. This means that isometric (fine needle) puncture-aspiration techniques do not always offer the results hoped for on solid organs, fundamentally the kidney, unless

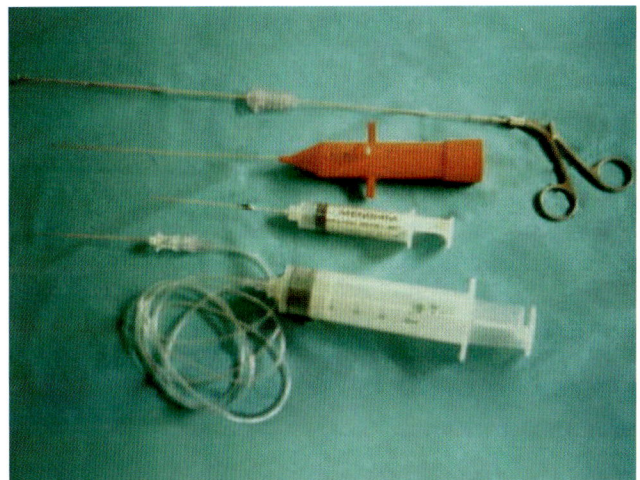

Fig. 36.1: Different types of needles and system for fetal biopsy

wider catheters are used, that are far from the "harmless philosophy" that should prevail in these processes.

For these cases and others that are similar that could present themselves, depending on the tissue characteristics, the use of methods such as the *Aspiration Biopsy Set* that includes an 18 G bisided trocar syringe in all its circumference, acting as a circular blade, and a conical sheath with vacuum suction embolus contriving through its interior which allows to obtain cylinders of 2–5 mm in maximum length, with optimal safety conditions and histological quality, similar to those of the *Tru-Cut* method.

Of all the viscus solid organs within reach, the one that offers the least problem is the liver, its spongy tissue constitution and its great size and volume in the fetal abdomen allows optimal accessibility and consequently offers samples in practically 100% of all cases, using a conventional fine needle of 18–20 G.

The obtention of muscle tissue samples offers one of the main difficulties due to the topographic and anatomical characteristics of the skeleton, also the important motorous innervation. For this reason, it is necessary to correctly select the spot and the muscular area least susceptible to provoke indelible functional lesions.

The most accessible topographic areas are the external face of either thigh, but it is technically more attainable the vastus externus muscle (Fig. 36.2); it is a zone covered by the subtrochanteric fascia lata in an orbicular direction descending towards the fetal femur. The use of the *Sure Cut* systems 18 G with incorporated vacuum aspiration allows a successes rate over 75%. Conventional spinal needles with complementary aspiration by 50 cc syringe vacuum allow to obtain sample with great difficulties.

When the puncture area has liquid characteristics, the echographic view is wide ranged, allowing a large field of action.

4. In general, technically it is precise to choose the most direct route, avoiding any interpositioning obstacles, being also of interest to avoid the placenta if at all possible.

5. Once the crucial point to puncture has been determined, the needle should be introduced within the field of view of the probe, frame by frame until reaching the fetus.

6. It is recommended to approximate the puncture point without making direct contact with it in the first instance, until quite certain of the needles angle to the chosen spot, being of capital importance to enter with only one *sudden jab* to avoid sudden fetal jolts or movements.

7. It is advisable in all *free-hand* fetal punctures carried out, that the operator should take into account the dynamic variations of fetal positions.

8. For better manipulation, an assistant should be in charge of carrying out the isometric aspiration process at a prudential distance, approximately a meter away from the surgical table, interplacing a serum of the same length between the needle and the syringe.

9. Except in exceptional circumstances such as pericardiac and pleural overflow that need an operating time of about 15–30 minutes, it is absolutely feasible to carry out without any anesthetic procedures.

Aspiration in cystic disorders will fundamentally orientate the diagnosis. Aspiration on ovarian cysts is only indicated in complex cases derived from its dynamic volume or due to rare structural types with therapeutic aims more than to diagnostic ones.

We collect suspicious chylous collections, where the presence of high lymphocyte concentrations practically give a sure diagnosis also the fact that it allows a genetic study in very few days, justifies this type of procedures (Fig. 36.3).

The puncture of pericardiac discharges has also the same diagnostic aims as well as being therapeutic.

Concerning brain punctures, the most representative, the *ventriculocentesis*, also allows us to accomplish serological marker studies in RCL, independent to any derived therapeutic attitude, although in this last case the efficiency of the derivative procedures in hydrocephalic is uncertain (Fig. 36.4).

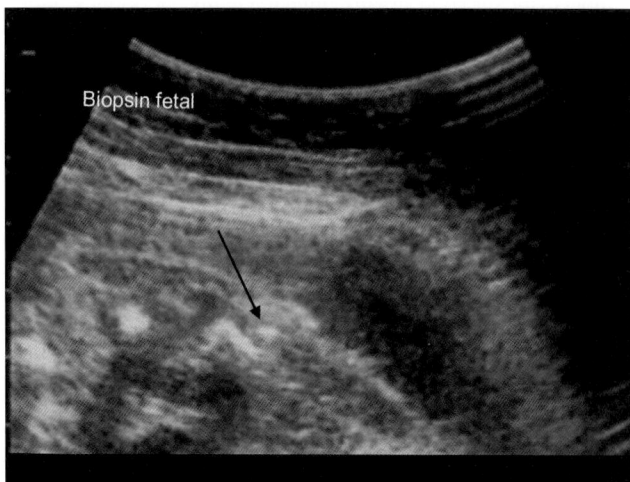

Fig. 36.2: Subtrochanteric muscle biopsy: Echographic monitoring. The arrow indicates the puncture position obliquely to the fetal femur

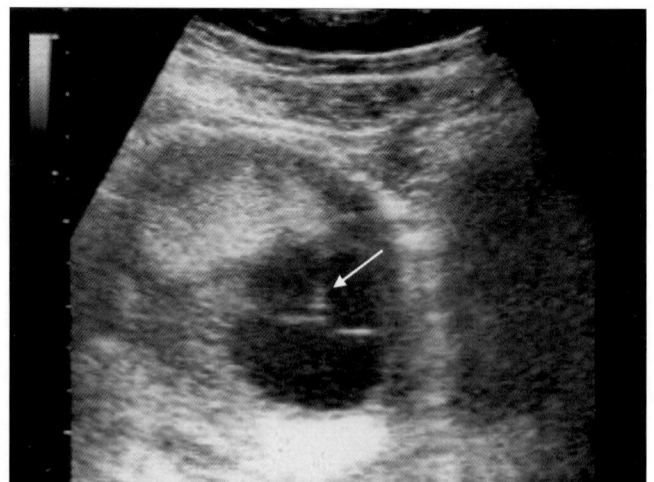

Fig. 36.3: Cystic lymphangioma: Percutaneous puncture determines qualitative and genetic characteristics (lymphocytes)

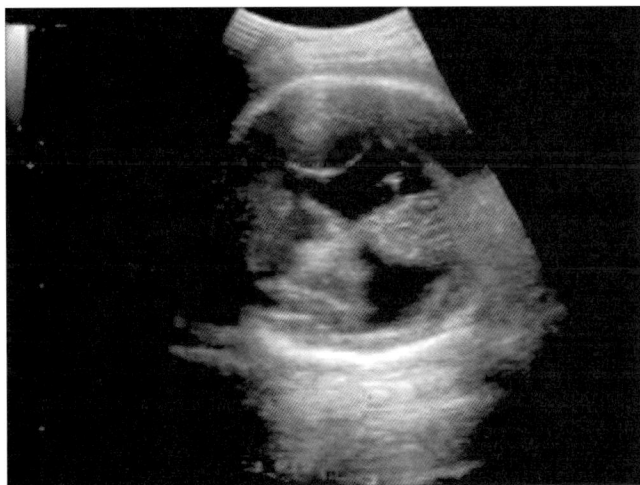

Fig. 36.4: Ventriculocentesis: Obtaining cephalo raguideos liquid determines the presence of viral bodies by polymerase chain reaction

Of all the structurally cystic processes, the obtention of fetal urine in dilated urological pathology represents the greatest and highest interest for diagnosis value. The biochemical analysis of the fetal urine allows us to detect irreversible tubular lesions from those which have a normal renal function.

There is no doubt that the incorporation of biological molecular techniques and deoxyribonucleic acid (DNA) studies allow to establish in many of the cases, the alterations of any determined genetic locus.[10-13]

Occasionally, we may find that we do not have enough material due to the lack of family records of deceased relations, in these cases, the absence of this previous information constitutes a serious inconvenience in order to establish a prenatal diagnosis, as this is based only on a small chorionic villi, funicular or amniotic sample.[11,14]

This situation is where sampling directly from the fetal tissue is of special relevance for the diagnose of one or the other, or in order to rule out any pathological suspicion of family inheritance that are being submitted to any particular study.

The taking of fetal samples by biopsy techniques is justified only in cases when the prenatal diagnosis of any specific pathological illness is not possible, or is frankly difficult, using any of the existing conventional techniques.

LIVER BIOPSY

Technique

Fetal transabdominal aspiration-puncture using 18 G needles with conic catheter or spinal needles of the same sectio with isometric vacuum aspiration using a 50 cc syringe and serum system. Once introduced into the fetal kidney, soft brief *inward outward* movements should be made in the same direction as the puncture.

Firstly, the aspiration system should be extracted and last of all the needle, to avoid contaminating any other tissue. The spot to be punctured should be situated between the belly bottom and the border of the rib. This fate is helped by the physiological hepatomegalia, introducing the needle approximately 1 cm under strict echographic monitoring. Preferably the external third of the right lobe, should

be chosen, as it offers a minor principal vascularization, if not, the suprahepatic vessels should be avoided (Fig. 36.5).

If the diagnosis being sought for is histological, the cylinder should be conserved in formaldehyde if on the contrary it is enzymatic, it should then be airtight sealed in carbonic snow.

The gestational age recommended should be around 20 weeks, provided that the hepatic metabolism and main enzymatic processes are well or practically established.

Indications

Prenatal diagnosis, fundamentally of enzymatic alterations and of lethal metabolic characteristics.[15,16]

Ornitil Transcarbamylase (OTC) Deficiencies

This mitochondrial enzyme of the urea cycle is synthesized in the liver or the intestines. Sex-linked disorders tied to the sex, are shown on the screening data of mothers who have urine excretion of orotic acid.

Primary Hyperoxaluria

This is severe, charted renal insufficiency of rapid evolution, that is characterized by the presence of calcic oxalate deposits in the renal tubule, microlithiasis and interstitial fibrosis. The hepatic level is accompanied by a total absence of alanine, inactivity of the catalytic gliosilate aminotransferase and immunoreactive proteins. This is incompatible with life.

For diagnosis, it is fundamental to have the previous family clinical history available.

Carbamoyl Phosphate Synthetase Deficiency

This is an enzymatic defect of the urea cycle with recessive autosomic inheritance. Other autosomic recessive disorders may be detected by means of hepatic biopsy, including:

- Non-ketotic hyperglycinemia
- Prenatal diagnosis of infantile neuronal ceroid-lipofuscinosis
- Biliar atresia (type I cysts)
- Long-chain 3-hydroxyacyl-CoA dehydrogenase.[17-20]

Complications

The prenatal liver biopsy has few risks on a tissular level, due to its own visceral characteristics. Those risks are derived from the main vascular tears which will have great bleeding resulting in fetal death. In our experience (seven prenatal punctures), we have observed no complications (Table 36.1).

FETAL PUNCTURE IN THE EVALUATION OF RENAL STATUS

The correction of a theoretic renal obstruction problem is possible, in spite of the difficulties and risks that it holds, even if in the majority of cases, it is not necessary. We should start by stating that an ultrasound echography diagnosis of the obstructed renal pathology does not necessarily imply an irreversible function alteration. In this sense, the amniotic volume can be used as an indirect marker of the actual renal function, but this does have the inconvenience that it includes the possible measuring of the intrinsic clearance function.

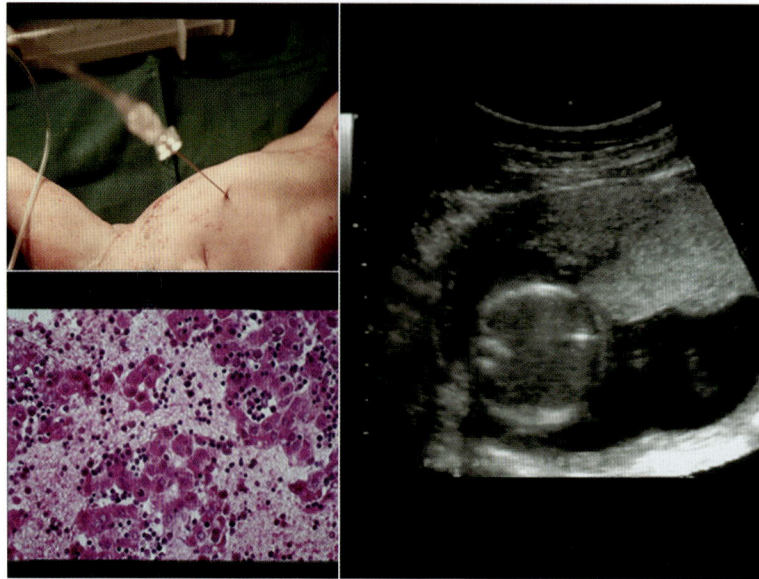

Fig. 36.5: Liver biopsy: Echographic monitoring and histological samples of fetal liver (19 weeks). Extramedullar hematopoietic foci can be detected

Table 36.1: Experience with seven prenatal punctures for liver biopsy

Reasons for biopsy	Number of cases
OTC diseases in the same family	4
Previous affected brother	1
Mitochondrial respiratory deficit	1
Non-ketotic hyperglycinemia	1
Results	
Prenatally confirmed diagnosis of OTC deficiency	2
Prenatally non-confirmed diagnosis with neonatal exitus by hyperammonemia	1
Prenatally confirmed as non-affected fetuses	4

Abbreviation: OTC, Ornitil Transcarbamylase Deficiency

Table 36.2: Fetal nephrouropathy: Echographic prediction

Tissue marker	Sensibility	Specificity
Corticomedullar cysts	70%	100%
Hyperechogenity	60%	90%
Hydronephrosis	75%	70%
Hydronephrosis + cysts	90%	100%

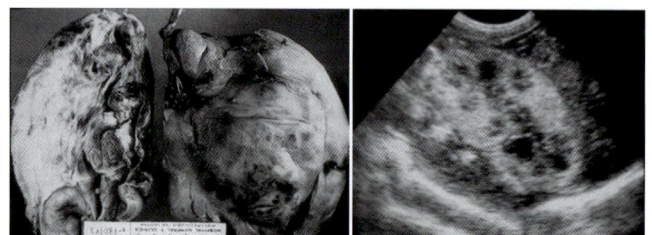

Fig. 36.6: Fibro-cortical dysplasia associated with corticomedullar cyst and renomegalia

When taking into account the possibility of practicing an intrauterine derived therapy, this can only be justifiable in those fetuses in whose kidneys there has been no irreversible damage. However, this makes it essential to establish a precise evaluation of the renal function, in order to adequately select those fetuses that will benefit from prenatal therapy.

The most conflictive situation is the renal dysplasia. In the latter coexist tissular phenomena that are characterized by fibrosis, dysplasia, cartilagenosis, frequently associated to corticomedullar cysts, although not always so (Fig. 36.6).

Approximately 90% of all kidney dysplasia is associated to dilated or obstructive disorders. In these cases, it can be remarked that any derived therapeutic action is unnecessary.

The high resolution echography has turned into the unquestionable kidney evaluation processes; however, it does have a few diagnostic limitations (Table 36.2).

In our experience, the obstruction of a kidney without objectable cysts or hyperechos does not, however, exclude dysplasia. This quite alarming fact occurs approximately in 25–30% of all cases.[8-21]

From this, we can deduce that the echography on its own does not diagnose all renal dysplasias, and for this reason fetuses with pelvic dilation are subsidiary of derived drainage.

A biochemical study of fetal urine is capital data in the managing of these fetuses. The composition of the fetal urine stays constant, practically throughout the pregnancy and with hypotonic characteristics. This fact has automatically demonstrated an optimal and reliable renal function and on the contrary and iso or hypertonic urine, a deficiency in renal function with an infastous prediction.

The biochemical markers that have close relation with a renal function are defined by the Na^+, Cl^- and osmotic urine.

Another determining factor in the normal renal clearance function derived from the near high reabsorptive tubular activity,

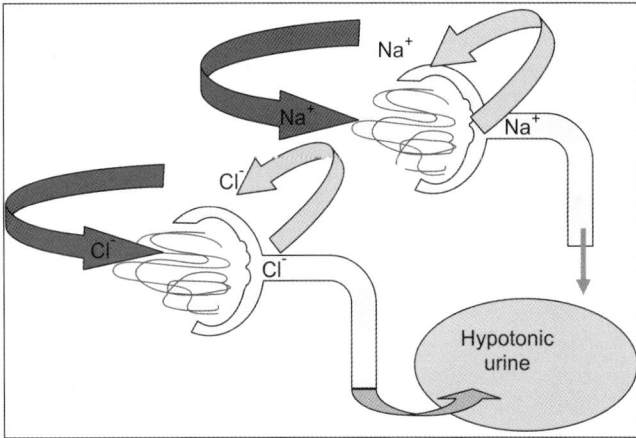

Fig. 36.7: Biochemical markers that have close relation with a renal function are defined by the Na$^+$, Cl$^-$ and osmotic urine derived from the near high reabsorptive tubular activity. Fetal urine stays constant, practically through the pregnancy and with hypotonic characteristics

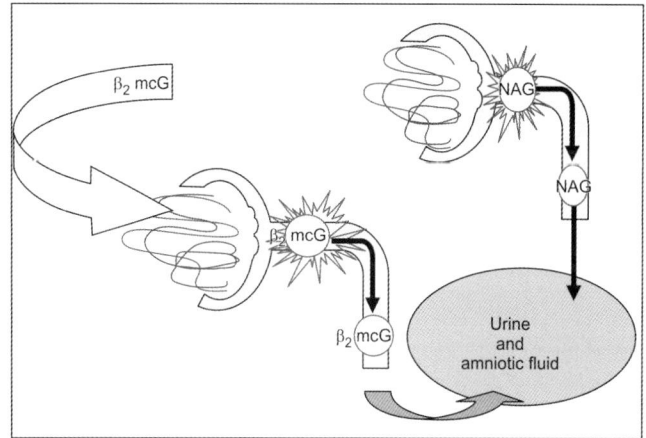

Fig. 36.8: Another determining factors in the normal renal clearance function correspond to lysosomal proteins exclusive of the proximal tubular structure [N-Acetyl-D-glucosamine (NAG)], if it is present in fetal urine and in the amniotic fluid in large quantities, it is indicative of tubular tissue destruction, β-2 microglobulin would be considered in the same manner

is the establishing of specific proximal tubular lesion selective markers.

These markers correspond to lysosomial proteins exclusive of the proximate tubular structure and become expressed by NAG (N-Acetyl-D-glucosamine). Low molecular weight proteins filtered by the glomerular system and reabsorbed practically in their totality by the proximal tube, if it is present in fetal urine and in the amniotic fluid in large quantities (higher than 8 U/L), it is indicative of tubular tissue destruction.

The detection of β-2 microglobulin would be considered in the same manner. (Figs 36.7 and 36.8). We found that the levels of biochemical markers are sensibly low in the physiological urine in comparison with the cases affected with irreversible renal disorder. The same outcome occurs with the tissue markers, NAG and β2 microglobuline (Table 36.3).

When we compare the relationship between the ionic concentrations and the osmolarity (Na$^+$ and Cl$^-$) of the fetal urine, and those of the amniotic liquid, we do not find significant differences between fetuses with conserving and fetuses with pathological functionalities. But comparing the levels of NAG and β2 microglobulin, a significantly greater concentration of the two markers in the amniotic liquid of the affected fetuses have been observed (Tables 36.4 and 36.5).

The increase in concentration of NAG and β-2 microglobulin increase possibly due to the cumulative effect of the amniotic clearance mechanism.

This opens the field of study of nephrouropathies through the determination of these and other parameters in the amniotic liquid, without the need for invasive study of the fetal urine.[21]

The K$^+$ and creatinine concentrations are different in their predictive evaluation as there exists a great clearance effect in the placenta and great variability in its ionic charge, that makes the potassium filtration very dispersed, in the other hand 90% of the K$^+$ concentration are intracellular.[8,21]

Summarizing, we can venture a prediction of renal viability in relation to those parameters expressed. In the Table 36.6 taking into account that these values are applicable to any gestational age.

Table 36.3: Fetal urinary aspiration: Pathological biochemical markers and their values

	18–20 Weeks	20–30 Weeks	>32 Weeks
Na$^+$ (mEq/mL)	120.0	126.44 ± 11.50	139.60
Cl$^-$ (mEq/mL)	119.0	132.50 ± 7.18	141.00
OsM (mOsm)	240	261.50 ± 24.20	281.00
NAG (U/L)	18.0	25.83 ± 0.85	25.73
β-2 Microglobin (mL/L)	26.0	38.97 ± 1.30	38.72
K$^+$ (mEq/mL)	3.1	3.41 ± 0.66	3.90
Creatinine (mL/L)	1.2	2.54 ± 0.83	3.70

Abbreviation: NAG, N-Acetyl-D-glucosamine

Table 36.4: Physiological values: Urine versus amniotic liquid

Urine/amniotic liquid	18–20 Weeks	20–30 Weeks	>32 Weeks
Na$^+$ (mEq/mL)	42/137	42/140	47/140
Cl$^-$ (mEq/mL)	23/109	47/109	41/108
OsM (mOsm)	98/267	102/273	102/271
NAG (U/L)	2.0/3.6	2.7/3.62	2.0/4.69
β-2 Microglobulin (mL/L)	4.7/4.5	5.1/5.0	5.3/5.8
K$^+$ (mEq/mL)		41/140	
Creatinine (ml/L)		1.9/.6	

Abbreviation: NAG, N-Acetyl-D-glucosamine

Table 36.5: Pathological values: Urine versus amniotic liquid

Urine/amniotic liquid	18–20 Weeks	20–30 Weeks	>32 Weeks
Na$^+$ (mEq/mL)	120/132	126.4/140	139.6/140
Cl$^-$ (mEq/mL)	119/107	132.5/149	141/158
OsM (mOsm)	240/267	261.5/273	281/296
NAG (U/L)	18/16.9	25.83/20.34	25.73/20.8
β-2 Microglobulin (mL/L)	26/22.3	38.9/28.74	38.72/30.0
K$^+$ (mEq/mL)	3.1/138	3.4/140.6	3.9/148
Creatinine (mL/L)	1.2/0.7	2.54/0.82	3.7/0.9

Abbreviation: NAG, N-Acetyl-D-glucosamine

Table 36.6: Fetal urine: Biochemical markers applicable to any gestational age, echographic image and amniotic liquid volume to determine a renal function status

Prediction	Bad	Good
Echographic image	Hyperechogenity + cyst	Normal echography
Amniotic liquid	Oligoamnios	Normal
Fetal Urine		
Na+	> 100 mEq/mL	< 100 mEq/mL
Cl-	> 90 mEq/mL	< 90 mEq/mL
Osmolarity	> 210	< 210
NAG	> 8 U/L	< 8 U/L
β-2 microglobulin	> 4 mg/L	< 4 mg/L
K+	Indifferent	Indifferent
Creatinine	Indifferent	Indifferent

Abbreviation: NAG, N-Acetyl-D-glucosamine

The intrauterine determination of the characteristics of fetal urine offers absolute diagnostic possibilities about the normal renal clearance function.

Urine aspiration puncture with diagnostic aims is technically feasible, using conventional spinal needles of 18 G having an aspiration system connected to a 20 cc syringe. The way to this approach depends on the fetal position available.

If at the posterior back position we would not find any great inconveniences in puncturing the bladder whilst for a lateral or anterior back where a nephrostomic aspiration is chosen (Fig. 36.9).

In neither one nor the other, can any noticeable complications be found, at least in our experience.[8,21]

The nephrostomy aspiration allows us firstly to re-evaluate the echostructural characteristics of the expanded kidney parenchyma, and secondly, as long as we use the 16 G *sure cut* aspiration system, to carry out at the same time a renal biopsy without any technical difficulties.

For this, once the nephrostomy urine aspiration has been done, without taking the needle out move it towards the renal parenchyma and carry out the aspiration with a *swing* movement over the corticomedullar area.

The obtaining of samples of 2 mm in length is enough for the detection of the histological characteristics that define a kidney dysplasia.[8,9,21-23]

But the use of 16 G catheters *Aspiration Biopsy Set* (Fig. 36.3), once the technical problems of involving tissues have been solved, allows to obtain samples in the 65% of the cases. If conventional 18 G catheters are used but inocuous, only 30% of the cases are obtained. (J Troyano, Ian Donald, School Interuniversity of Medical Ultrasound, Dubrovnik, August 1996, unpublished observations).

SKIN BIOPSY

As already stated in the general section about fetal biopsies, the skin biopsy entails the most serious difficulties in the obtaining of adequate or sufficient samples that would allow correct histopathological diagnosis or prediction.

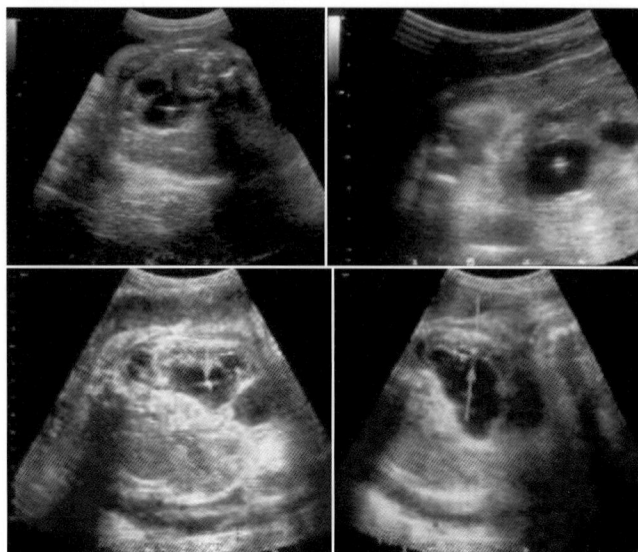

Fig. 36.9: Aspirative nephrostomy: Echographic monitoring

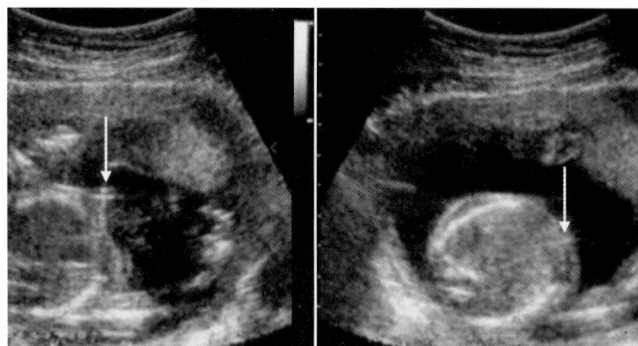

Fig. 36.10: Left: Skin biopsy in fetal abdomen, side longly scratching. Right: Mature histological cutaneous samples where keratohyalin and hemidesmosomes are detected

The most important aspect is the obtention of valid samples, for this we need at least 1 mm strips of skin and no smaller in surface area and that also include a thickness of the epithelial stratum, and comprising of conjunctive areas and basal membrane. Only by this an acceptable reading can be obtained.[24]

The second aspect to be taken into account is the surgical biopsy material. We have already exposed previously that the use of section 2.5 mm clipping tongs (forceps/clippers) introduced into the amniotic environment by trocar, will allow the obtention of skin samples in 100% of all cases, and it is true that the residual skin lesions and any pregnancy complications there maybe, will not render any noticeable benefits in relation to the diagnostic data.

The use of conventional needles and isometric aspiration practicing the *slice* technique, that consists in inserting the needle side longly over the skin and make *scratching* or *scraping* movements, as this will allow us to obtain skin strips of optimum quality with minimum damage to the integrity of the pregnancy (Fig. 36.10).[25-28]

The third aspect to consider is the place selected to proceed for the taking of the sample, as depending on the disorder that we aim to diagnose prenatally, the biopsy area would be different. Not always the same area of the fetal skin wrap will be valid, or will suit the purpose of the biopsy.

Technique

Skin samples should, if possible, be taken from different areas of the fetus.

The pregnancy stage recommended for this is around 20 weeks, as after this time, the pilose follicles and keratinization mechanisms begin to develop. The study of the elements involved in the keratinization (keratohyalin and tonofibers), initially give suspicions of the disorder.

On the other hand, at this stage in the pregnancy, the dermoepidermical junction has definitively been established, and the gradual rise of intercellular desmosomes is a great help for the diagnosis of different forms of epidermolysis.

The sequence should follow the following steps:

- Echographic monitoring
- If it is possible, the placenta must be avoided
- Take into consideration the fetal position as on some occasions it will be necessary to obtain samples from different skin areas
- Rigorous sterilization
- Optional local anesthesia, depending on the surgical timing
- Oblique needle incidence in the thickness and surface of the skin, making a scraping or scratching movement without pulling back
- Try to obtain at least 1 mm strips. The use of the vacuum needles allow the collection of various fragments from the interior without the need of withdrawing the needle
- Immediately proceed to swim the samples in saline serum for their histological staining and fixing process or for electronic microscopy analysis.

Indications

They are most frequently based on the diagnosis of some type of genodermatosis or congenital dermoepidermic disorders of dominating autosomic transmission as well as recessive types, the majority being lethal in short or medium terms.

These disorders can be classified as follows:

- Bullous epidermolysis: Fetuses with large scale blistered areas that once the blisters break, set off intensive erosive zones with a fast loss of electrolytes are affected.[6,10,29,30]
- Anhidrotic ectodermic dysplasias: Recessive disorder linked to the sex. The fetuses are born without pilose follicles, without any hair or sudoriparous glands. They develop hyperthermic affectation by disregulation and general dryness syndromes.[31]
- Keratinization disorders: Also called *Collodion baby syndrome*, characterized by the appearance of *reptile skin* due to epidermic membranes that are of quick *shedding*. Severe and lethal dehydrating disorders.[32,33]
- Pigmentary atopies: Ocular syndromes with severe intolerance to light and early or premature development of skin cancers.[31,34,35]

The diagnostic problems faced with these dermatosis are due to the development of the lesion has different topographic origins, so the need to select the puncture spot has to be in accordance to the illness that one is trying to detect.

The diagnostic possibilities of skin biopsies are summarized as shown in Table 36.7.

It is fundamental to have objective family history in order to determine the biopsy spot.[34,36,37]

Complementary Requirements

The study of the samples will be based on the ultrastructural features stated beforehand. A great deal of experience in fetal dermatology using electronic microscopy is required to make the diagnosis.

It is fundamental to have objective family history knowledge in order to determine the prenatal dermoepidermic structural markers.

It is recommended to have kept previous samples in order to be used as a *study bank*.

Complications

Now the tendency is to propose minimally invasive techniques by the use of conventional needles.[38]

The use of conventional needles does not withhold more risks than the amniocentesis. On the other hand, the trocar techniques and the 2.5 mm sectio biopsy provoke around 5% of miscarriages due to iatrogenic amniorexis, although similarly some indelible fetal skin lesions have been described (Fig. 36.14). This does not occur in cases where the *scalp* technique is carried out with the use of conventional needles.

Table 36.7: Diagnoses possible from fetal skin biopsies

- Keratinization disorders:
  Harlequin fetus
  Colodion baby
  Sjögren-Larsson syndrome
  Congenital ichthyosis
  The puncture spot is in trunks and buttocks (Fig. 36.11)

- Ampollous diseases:
  Herlitz ampollous junctional disease
  Hallopeau-Siemens ampollous dermolytic disease
  Inverse dystrophic ampollous disease
  Cockayne-Touraine dystrophic ampollous disease
  The puncture spot is in waist, skin folds, abdomen and buttocks (Fig. 36.12)

- Pigmentary disorders:
  Negative tyirosinase oculocutaneous albinism
  Chediak-Higashi disease
  Anhidrotic ectodermic disease
  The puncture spot in the skin-head (scalp) (Fig. 36.13)

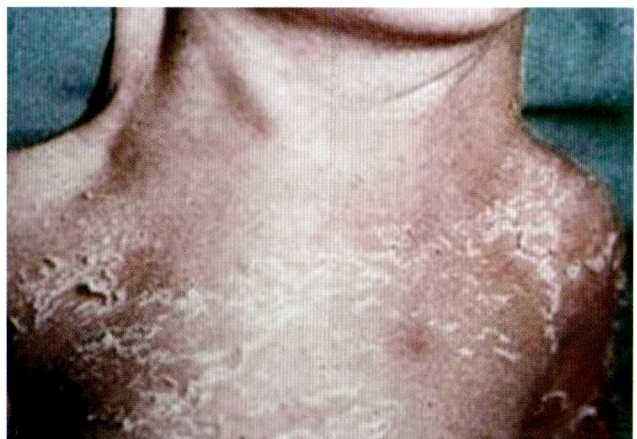

Fig. 36.11: Keratinization disorder

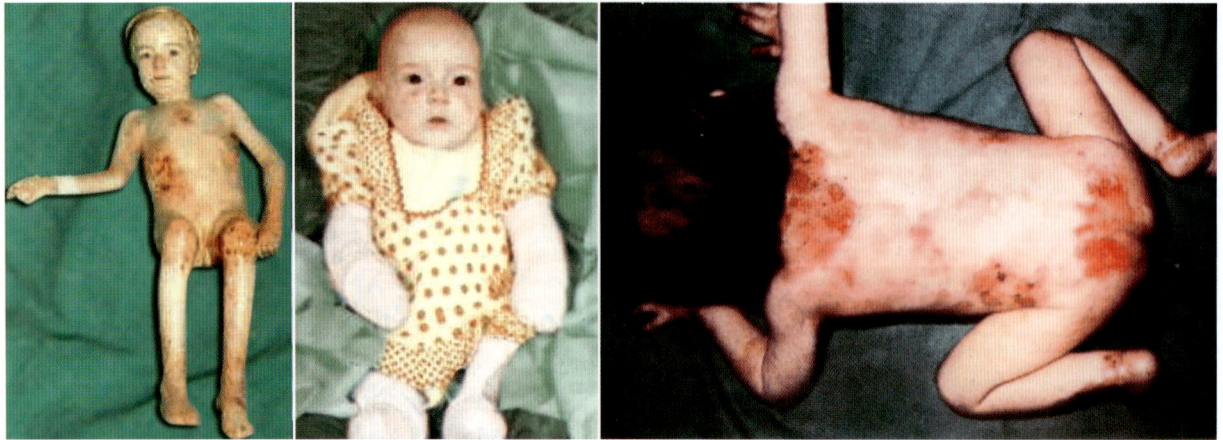

Fig. 36.12: Ampollous diseases

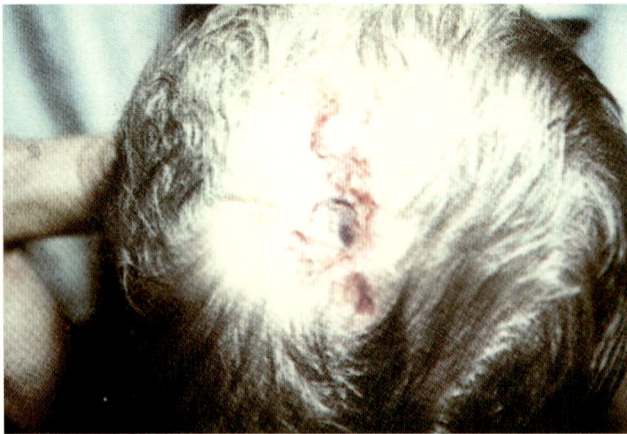

Fig 36.13: Pigmentary disorder (scalp lesions)

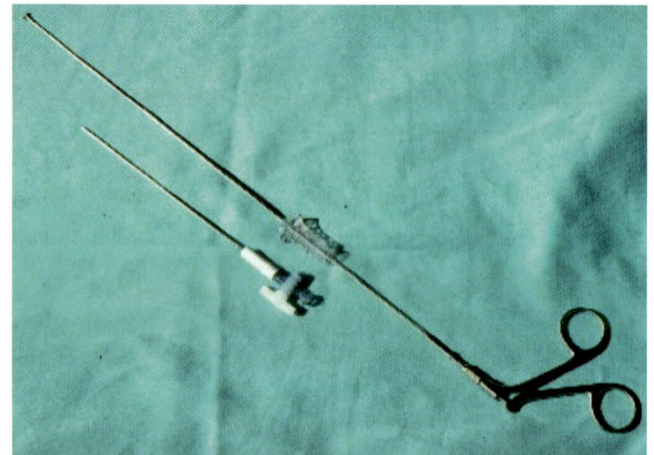

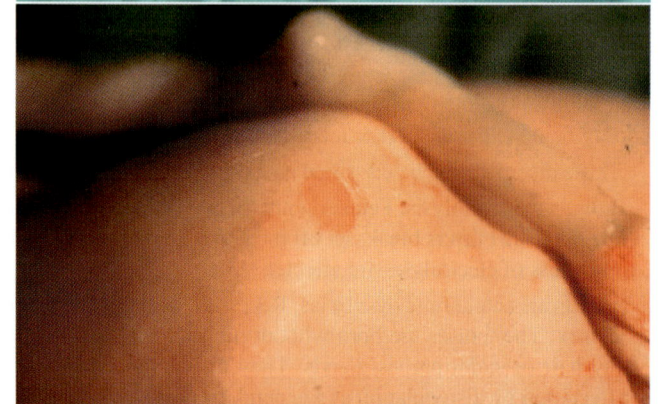

Fig. 36.14: Residual cutaneous lesion after biopsy with clipper system

MUSCLE BIOPSY

This is carried out preferably for the prenatal diagnosis of Duchenne's muscular dystrophy (DMD), although it is also possible to detect other hereditary myopathies as long as there is some clinical family history of these disorders.[11,38,39]

For the diagnosis of DMD, it is usual for the DNA analysis to be used. When the recombinations within the DMD gene or the DNA analysis are not sufficiently informative, or if from the family history it is not clear if there are possible carriers, so the direct examination of the muscle and its analysis is the only way to give the basis of an objective prenatal diagnosis.

The marker used is the dystrophin, its determination by means of immunofluorescence allows to differentiate the features of affected muscles from those of the healthy ones. The absence of this protein from the skeletal muscles is practically pathognomonic of DMD (Fig. 36.15).[11,14,39,40]

Some other times, the prenatal diagnosis of DMD may be impossible when there is only one previously affected male in the family, and there is no identifiable detection.

The absence of dystrophin in a skeleton muscle, is worth in itself the determination of the screening of the DMD. Nevertheless, this diagnosis can be reinforced by detecting a rise in phosphocreatine kinase of more than 10 times its normal value in fetal blood.

Within the possibilities that can reinforce a prenatal DMD diagnosis or prediction we have:

- Sex linked
- High values of phosphocreatine kinase
- Absence of dystrophin
- Degenerated muscle
- Fat infiltration
- Connective infiltration
- Nuclear and cellular morphological alterations (Fig. 36.16).

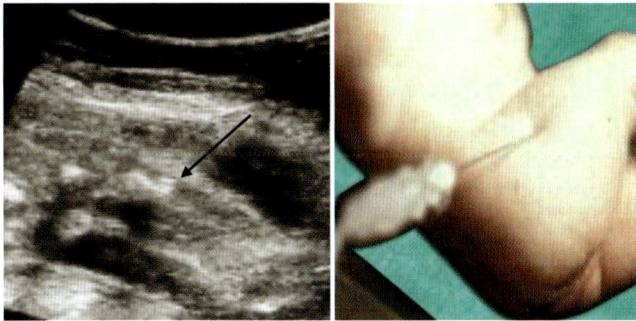

Fig. 36.15: Subtrochanteric muscle biopsy; the detection of dystrophine by immunofluorescence determines healthy muscle

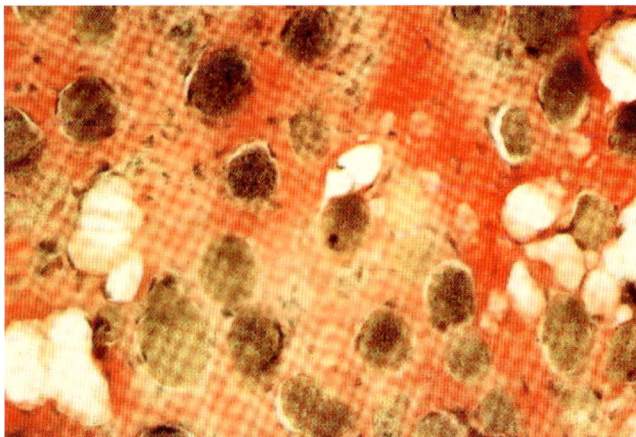

Fig. 36.16: Duchenne's muscular dystrophy; degenerated muscle as an associated sign: Fat and connective infiltration, and morphological cellular alterations and leukocytes infiltration

Technique

Any muscular skeleton area is good, preferably of the external face of any of the thighs or knuckle areas, avoiding topographic places with innervation or vital vascularization, in this manner indelible functional lesions will not be provoked. Preferably using 18 G conventional needles or even better, the *sure cut* method that have already been described (Fig. 36.2).[8,38,41-43]

Carrying out subtrochanteric punctures in a descending obliquest manner as possible, orientated towards the fetal femur (Fig. 36.2).

The puncture success rate is of 75%.

It is essential to determine muscle dystrophy by immunofluorescence, being advisable but not determining the detection of phosphocreatine kinase and the study of the muscular structure at a morphological muscular level, fat and connective infiltration.

No complications are described.

The fetus is susceptible to being studied by invasive techniques. These techniques are only justified by the seriousness of a possible inherited illness, or by any other disorder detected during pregnancy; in the latter the need for biopsy diagnosis is exceptional, as the thoracocentesis, pericardiocentesis and punctures of other thoracoabdominal, primary seek a therapeutic attitude, using the extracted material for studying its analytical components.

Other punctures on fetal tumor formations (sacrococcygeal teratomas, solid cervical teratomas, etc.), or liquid collections, such as pericardiocentesis, do not have an acceptable justification from a therapeutic or diagnostic point of view, as the echographic evaluation and the present application of biophysical methods (color Doppler amongst them) give an acceptable identification of their vascularization and origin, including those of suspicious neoplasm.[44,45] (A Kurjak, Ian Donald. University School of Medical Ultrasound 16th Course, Granada, Spain, June 14th–16th 1993, Unpublished).

In agreement with our philosophy, we would like to express this thought:

The fetus has been endowed by nature to confront several inconveniences provided by the 40 weeks of development. It is a real "Titan" that can face any adversity, and its adaptability is exceptional.

Let us not disturb it!

Let us not invade its privacy aggressively!

Let us observe it minutely. When it needs us, which generally happens in few occasions, it will advise us; then let us help it.

JM Troyano-Luque (1993)

REFERENCES

1. Bahado-Singh RO, Morotti R, Pirhoren J, et al. Invasive techniques for prenatal diagnosis: current concepts. J Assoc Acad Minor-Phys. 1995;6:28-33.
2. Cadrin C, Golbus MS. Fetal tissue sampling indications, techniques, complications and experience with sampling of fetal skin, liver and muscle. West J Med. 1993;159:269-72.
3. Golbus MS, Sagebield RW, Filly RA, et al. Prenatal diagnosis of congenital icthyosiform erythroderma (epidermolytic hyperkeratosis) by fetal skin biopsy. N Engl J Med. 1980;302:93.
4. Kouseff BG, Matsouca LY, Stenn RS, et al. Prenatal diagnosis of Sjögren-Larsson syndrome. J Pediatr. 1082;101:998.
5. Robjn AJ, David B, Gardner A, et al. Prenatal diagnosis of oculocutaneous albinism by electron microscopy of fetal skin. J Invest Dermatol. 1983;80:210-12.
6. Dolan CR, Smith LT, Syber UP. Prenatal detection of epidermolysis bullosa fetalis with pyloric atresia in a fetus by abnormal ultrasound and elevated alphafetoprotein. Am J Genet. 1993;47:395-400.
7. Rodeck CH. Fetoscopy guided by real-time ultrasound for pure fetal samples, fetal skin samples and examination of the fetus in utero. Br J Obstet Gynaecol. 1980;87:449-56.
8. Troyano JM, Padron E, Clavijo M. Fetal biopsy and puncture. Actual status. Balkan Ohrid's School of Ultrasound. Advanced Ultrasound II. Ohrid, Macedonia: Dobri S. Filipche. 1996;9:51-61.
9. Campbell WA, Yamase HT, Salafia CA, et al. Fetal renal biopsy: technique development. Fetal Diagn Ther. 1993;8:135- 43.
10. Dunnill MG, Rodeck CH, Richards AJ, et al. Use of type VII collagen gene (COL7A1) markers in prenatal diagnosis of recessive dystrophic epidermolysis bullosa. J Med Genet. 1995;32:749-50.

11. Evans MI, Farrell SA, Greb A, et al. In utero fetal muscle biopsy for the diagnosis of Duchenne musular dystrophy in a female fetus "suddenly at risk". Am J Med Genet. 1993;46:309-12.

12. Fox J, Hack AM, Fenton WA, et al. Prenatal diagnosis of ornithine transcarbamylase deficiency with the use of DNA polymorphisms. N Engl J Med. 1986;315:1205.

13. Matilla I, Corral J, Miranda M, et al. Prenatal diagnosis of Werdnig-Woffmann disease: DNA analysis of a mummified umbilical cord using closely linked microsatellite markers. Prenat Diagn. 1994;14:219-22.

14. Kuller JA, Hoffman EP, Fries MH, et al. Prenatal diagnosis of Duchenne muscular dystrophy by fetal muscle biopsy. Hum Genet. 1992;90:34-40.

15. Illum N, Lavard L, Danpure ZJ, et al. Primary hyperoxaluria type 1: clinical manifestation in infancy and prenatal diagnosis. Child Nephrol Urol. 1992;12:225-7.

16. Rodeck CH, Patrick AD, Pembrey ME, et al. Fetal liver biopsy for prenatal diagnosis of ornithine carbamyl transferase deficiency. Lancet. 1982;1:297-9.

17. Goebel HH, Vesa J, Reiter B, et al. Prenatal diagnosis of infantile neuronal ceroidlipofuscinosis: A combined electron microscopic and molecular genetic approach. Brain Dey. 1995;17:83-8.

18. Murotsuki J, Vehara S, Okamura K, et al. Fetal liver biopsy for prenatal diagnosis of carbamoyl phosphate synthetase deficiency. Am J Perinatol. 1994;11:160-2.

19. Tsushida Y, Kawarasaki H, Iwanaka T, et al. Antenatal diagnosis of biliary atresia (type 1 cyst) at 19 weeks of gestation: differential diagnosis and etiologic implications. J Pediatr Surg. 1995;30:607-9.

20. Von Dobeln V, Venizelos N, Westgren M, et al. Long chain 3-hydroxyacyl-CoA dehydrogenase in chorionic villi, fetal liver, and fibroblasts and prenatal diagnosis of 3-hydroxyacyl-CoA dehydrogenase. J Inherit Metab Dis. 1994;17:185-8.

21. Troyano JM, de la Fuente P. Prenatal features of fetal kidney physiopathology and their intra and extrauterine treatment. A multidisciplinary problem. Santa Cruz de Tenerife: University Hospital of the Canary Islands; 1993:35-9.

22. Greco P, Loverro G, Carusso G, et al. Diagnostic potential of fetal renal biopsy. Prenat Diagn. 1994;14:415.

23. Gubler MC, Levy M. Prenatal diagnosis of Nail-Patella syndrome by intrauterine kidney biopsy. Am J Med Genet. 1993;47:122-4.

24. Elias S, Emerson DS, Simpson JL, et al. Ultrasound-guided fetal skin sampling for prenatal diagnosis of genodermatoses. Obstet Gynecol. 1994;83:337-41.

25. Bakharev VA, Aivazyan AA, Karetnikova NA, et al. Fetal skin biopsy in prenatal diagnosis of some genodermatoses. Prenat Diagn. 1990;10:1-12.

26. Buckshee K, Parveen S, Mittal S, et al. Percutaneous ultrasound-guided fetal skin biopsy: A new approach. Int J Gynaecol Obstet. 1991;34:267-70.

27. Holbrook KA, Wapner R, Jackson L, et al. Diagnosis and prenatal diagnosis of epidermolysis bullosa herpetiformis (Dowling-Meara). In a mother, two affected children and an affected fetus. Prenat Diagn. 1992;12:725-39.

28. Suzumori K, Kanzak I. Prenatal diagnosis of Harlequin ichthyosis by fetal skin biopsy: report of two cases. Prenat Diagn. 1991;11:451-7.

29. McGrath JA, McMillan JR, Dunnill MG, et al. Genetic bases of lethal junctional epidermolysis bullosa in an affected fetus: implications for prenatal diagnosis in one family. Prenat Diagn. 1995;15:647-54.

30. Shirnizu H, Onodera Y, Ikeda S, Ogawa H, et al. Prenatal diagnosis of epidermolysis bullosa: first successful trial in Asia. Dermatology. 1994;188:46-9.

31. Shimizu H, Ishko A, Kikushi A, et al. Prenatal diagnosis of tyrosinase negative oculocutaneous albinism by an electron microscopic dopa-reaction test of fetal skin. Prenat Diagn. 1994;14: 442-50.

32. Akiyama M, Kim DK, Main DM, et al. Characteristic morphologic abnormality of Harlequin ichthyosis detected in amniotic fluid cells. J Invest Dermatol. 1994;102:210-3.

33. Rizzo WB. Sjögren-Larsson syndrome. Semin Dermatol. 1993;12:210-8.

34. Akeo K, Shirai S, Okisaka S, et al. Histology of fetal ages with oculocutaneous albinism. Arch Ophthalmol. 1996;114:613-6.

35. Shimizu H, Niizeki H, Suzurnori K, et al. Prenatal diagnosis of oculocutaneous albinism by analysis of the fetal tyrosinase gene. J Invest Dermatol. 1994;103:104-6

36. Holbrook KA, Smith LI, Elias S. Prenatal diagnosis of genetic skin disease using fetal skin biopsy samples. Arch Dermatol. 1993;129:1437-54.

37. Normand J, Karasek MA. A method for the isolation and serial propagation of keratinocytes, endothelial cells and fibroblasts from a single punch biopsy of human skin. In vitro Cell Dey Biol Anim. 1995;31:447-55.

38. Evans MI, Krivchenia EL, Johnson MP, et al. In utero fetal muscle biopsy alters diagnosis and carrier risks in Duchenne and Becket muscular dystrophy. Fetal Diagn Ther. 1995;10:71-5.

39. Fanin M, Pegoraro E, Angelini C. Absence of dystrophin and spectrin in regenerating muscle fibers from Becket dystrophy patients. J Neurol Sci. 1994;123:88-94.

40. Lindahl M, Backman E, Henriksson KG, et al. Phospholipase A2 activity in dystrophinopathies. Neuromusc Disord. 1995;5:193-9.

41. Benzie RJ, Ray P, Thompson D, et al. Prenatal exclusion of Duchenne muscular dystrophy and fetal muscle biopsy. Prenat Diagn. 1994;14:235-8.

42. Evans MI, Hoffman EP, Cadrin C, et al. Fetal muscle biopsy: Collaborative experience with varied indications. Obstet Gynecol. 1994;84:913-7.

43. Evans MI, Quintero RA, King M, et al. Endoscopically assisted, ultrasound-guided fetal muscle biopsy. Fetal Diagn Ther. 1995;10:167-72.

44. Troyano JM, Clavijo MT, Clemente I, et al. Kidney and urinary tract diseases: Ultrasound and biochemical markers. Ultrasound Rev Obstet Gynecol. 2002;2(2):92-109.

45. Bebatar A, Vaughan J, Nicolini U, et al. Prenatal pericariocentesis: its role in the management of intrapericardial teratoma. Obstet Gynecol. 1992;79(5):859.

37

The Role of Ultrasound Examination of the Cervix in Pregnancy

P Rozenberg, Y Ville

INTRODUCTION

Preterm delivery is the main cause of perinatal mortality and morbidity.[1] Its prevalence has been stable for the last 20 years accounting for 5.9% and 11% of all deliveries in France and in the USA respectively.[2-4] This is mainly due to poor therapeutic results and the inadequacy of the diagnostic criteria for preterm labor. Risk scoring for preterm birth have both low sensitivity and positive predictive value (PPV).[5-8] Only 15% of women with a previous history of preterm delivery will do so in a subsequent pregnancy.[8] Routine digital cervical examinations during pregnancy increases the risk for admission in hospital without decreasing the incidence of prematurity.[9] In threatened preterm labor as defined by painful contractions, cervical changes on digital examination and frequency of contractions both remain poor predictors of preterm delivery.[10-13]

Different strategies have been developed to refine the risk of preterm delivery, including the use of transvaginal sonography (TVS) to measure and examine the length and shape of the cervix. TVS has been studied in three different populations: (1) symptomatic women with threatened preterm labor, i.e. regular and painful contractions together with changes on digital examination of the cervix; (2) asymptomatic women at high risk of delivering prematurely, as defined by a history of preterm delivery, late miscarriage, conization, maternal exposure to diethylstilbestrol (DES) during her fetal life, uterine malformation or a current multiple pregnancy; (3) asymptomatic women without any relevant history.

THREATENED PRETERM LABOR

The Risk of Preterm Delivery is Significantly Associated with two Ultrasound Features—Shortening of the Cervical Length and Cervical Wedging: Cervical length measured by transvaginal ultrasonography less than 20 mm, less than 25 mm, or less than 30 mm on admission had positive and negative predictive values (NPVs) of 100% and 72%, 70% and 82%, and 65% and 100%, on preterm delivery respectively. These patients delivered preterm despite tocolytic therapy during hospitalization.[14] Thus, the risk of preterm delivery is especially high in women whose cervical length on admission is less than 20 mm, whereas a cervical length greater than or equal to 30 mm is reassuring. Preterm delivery is also significantly associated with the presence of cervical wedging together with a short cervical length. This led to sensitivity, specificity, positive and NPV of 100%, 74.5%, 59.4%, and 100% respectively.[15]

Ultrasound Examination is more Accurate than Digital Examination of the Cervix in Preterm Labor: In preterm labor with intact membranes, Gomez et al.[10] showed that despite cervical dilatation of less than 3 cm, cervical length and cervical wedging (P < 0.005) were highly predictive of preterm delivery, but digital examination of the cervix (dilatation and effacement) failed to do so. Survival analysis demonstrated a shorter admission-to-delivery interval for patients with an abnormal cervical length (P less than 0.005). In preterm labor following completion of a course of IV tocolysis, cervical sonography performed better than digital examination to predict delivery before 36 weeks and even 34 weeks, with a best cutoff of 30 mm on receiver operating characteristic (ROC) curve analyses.[11,16] The PPV and NPV were of 15% and 36%, and 97% and 100% in singleton and twin pregnancies respectively, when assessed at between 23 weeks and 33 weeks' of gestation. When analyzed for delivery before 37 weeks this held true for singletons but not for twins.

The comparison of cervical fetal fibronectin (fFN) assay and TVS of the cervix to predict preterm delivery remains a controversial issue: We found that prediction performances of vaginal fFN assay greater than or equal to 50 ng/mL and of a cervical length of lesser than or equal to 26 mm in threatened preterm labor between 24 weeks and 34 weeks were similar with a high NPV 86.6% and 89.1% respectively.[17] The combination of both tests performed better with a NPV of 94.4% but the PPV remained at around 50% although the odds ratio (OR) for delivering before 34 weeks was high (13.9,95% CI;3.7–52.2).

Rizzo et al.[18] reported that cervical fFN greater than or equal to 60 ng/mL performed better than the association of cervical length and the presence of funneling on ultrasound. Furthermore, in patients with cervical fFN greater than or equal to 60 ng/mL a shorter admission-to-delivery interval was found in the presence of an abnormal cervical index.

More recently, multiple logistic regression analysis found that only positive fibronectin testing (OR 11.25, P = 0.005) and functional cervical length lesser than or equal to 20 mm (OR 8.18, P = 0.027) were independently associated with preterm delivery.[19] In the group with cervical length of 20–31 mm positive fFN was found in 71.4% of patients delivered within 28 days and in 7.4% delivered after 28 days (P = 0.001). Fibronectin testing could therefore be performed only in patients with a short cervix to discriminate further those at true high risk of prematurity. With specificity, PPV and NPV predictive values of 86%, 90%, 63%, and 97% respectively, in predicting delivery within 28 days.

ASYMPTOMATIC WOMEN AT HIGH RISK OF PRETERM DELIVERY

There are four types of clinical studies addressing this issue: (1) observational studies examining the natural course, (2) observational studies examining the course of those treated with cervical cerclage, (3) non-randomized interventional studies, and (4) randomized interventional trials.

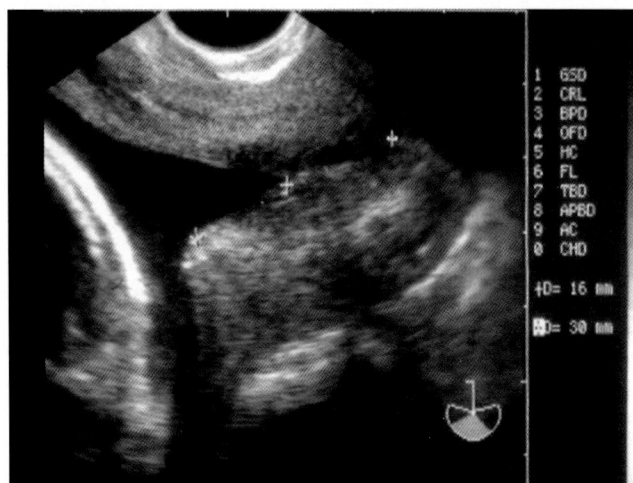

Fig. 37.1: Dilatation of the internal os

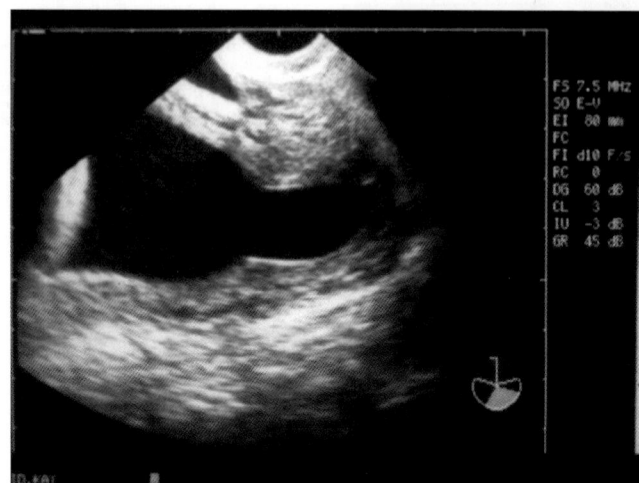

Fig. 37.2: Sacculation of the membranes into the cervix

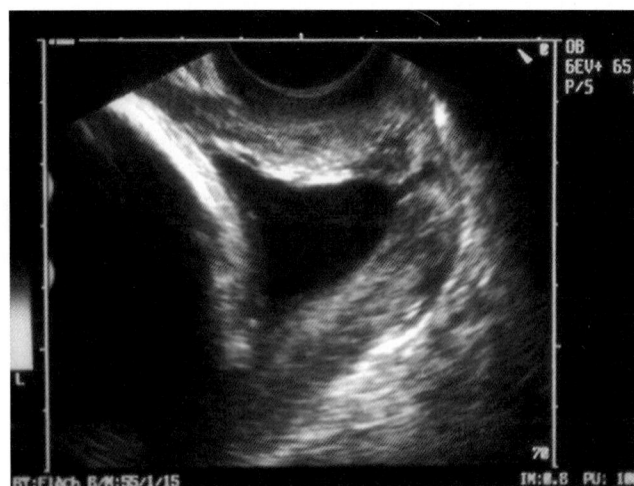

Fig. 37.3: Funneling with shortening of the functional cervical length

Observational Studies of Ultrasound Features Suggestive of Cervical Incompetence: Three ultrasound features are suggestive of cervical incompetence.

Dilatation of the internal os (Fig. 37.1) was the first ultrasound feature suggesting cervical incompetence and thus increased risk of preterm delivery. Dilatation of the internal os more than 5 mm before 30 weeks of gestation is associated with preterm delivery in 33.3% versus 3.5% when the internal os remained closed (P less than 0.01). Digital cervical examination noted dilatation of the internal os in only 10 of the 26 (38.5%) patients in whom ultrasound showed cervical dilatation.[20]

Sacculation or prolapse of the membranes into a shortening cervix (Fig. 37.2), either spontaneously or induced by transfundal pressure, can be seen even when digital cervical examination shows a long and closed cervix.[21]

Another study, in which ultrasound examinations were performed at between 15 and 24 weeks, compared three methods to detect cervical incompetence: transfundal pressure, coughing and standing.[22] The transfundal pressure was the most predictive (sensitivity specificity, PPV and NPV of 83.3%; 97.2%; 88.2%; and 95.8% respectively).

Shortening of the cervix in the absence of uterine contractions is also suggestive of cervical incompetence. A cervical length less than 10th percentile (22 mm) and funneling at the internal os (Fig. 37.3) at between 16 weeks and 30 weeks were associated with delivery within 2 transfundal pressure 4 weeks and before 35 weeks [33% vs 0 ($P = 0.01$); 67% vs 0%, ($P < 0.001$); and 100% vs 19%, $P < 0.001$ respectively].[23] Within this high-risk group, women with medical or obstetrical complications (including multiple gestation and ruptured membranes), symptoms of preterm labor and history of incompetent cervix that required cerclage were excluded. A short cervix or funneling beyond 20 weeks of gestation were also associated with an increased risk of preterm delivery before 35 weeks but not with an increased risk of delivering within 2–4 weeks following TVS.

Prospective longitudinal evaluation of a large cohort of 469 high-risk pregnancies by TVS and transfundal pressure on 1,265 occasions at between 15 weeks and 24 weeks[24] compared various sonographic cervical parameters to predict spontaneous preterm birth. ROC curve analysis showed that cervical length lesser than or equal to 25 mm alone performed as well as a combination of risk factors, CL, funneling and transfundal pressure. The sensitivity for delivery at less than 28, less than 30, less than 32 and less than 34 weeks of gestation was 94%, 91%, 83% and 76% respectively, while the NPV was 99%, 99%, 98% and 96% respectively. Shortening of cervical length, at weekly assessment helps in differentiating cervical competence from cervical incompetence in high-risk women (-0.3 vs -4.1 mm/week; $P < 0.001$).[25] Ultrasound diagnosis of cervical incompetence was defined as progressive shortening of the endocervical canal to 20 mm or less before 24 weeks of gestation.

In this high-risk group, cervical length less than 25 mm by TVS of the cervix performs better than cervical length less than 16 mm by digital cervical examination in assessing the risk of delivery before 35 weeks with relative risks of 4.8 and 2.0 respectively.[26]

In multiple pregnancies at between 24 weeks and 28 weeks, a cervical length lesser than or equal to 25 mm by TVS was the best predictor of preterm delivery before 32 weeks, before 35 weeks and before 37 weeks.[27] There is a continuous increase of 5% to 17% and 80% for this risk with cervical length shortening down to 40 mm and 20 mm and 8 mm respectively.[28] Cervical length of lesser than or equal to 20 mm seems to perform as well as any combination of clinical and ultrasound features at predicting preterm birth,[29] whereas cervical length more than 35 mm before 26 weeks seems to accurately identify a sub-group of twin pregnancies at low-risk to deliver prematurely (3% to 4%). [30,31]

Although series are smaller, the predictive value of TVS of the cervix seems to hold true in triplets.[32,33] Cervical length of lesser than or equal to 25 mm between 21 weeks and 24 weeks of gestation was the best cutoff for the prediction of spontaneous preterm birth less than 28 weeks of gestation (86%, 79%, 40%, 97% for sensitivity, specificity, positive predictive PPV, and NPV, respectively).[34]

Follow-up Studies in Cervical Incompetence Diagnosed by TVS and Treated by Cerclage:
It has been established that cervical cerclage is followed by a measurable increase in cervical length. This applies to both rescue cerclage[35,36] and elective procedures.[35,37,38] However, the relation of this increase with outcome is controversial and the longer the pre-cerclage cervical length the more likely a delivery near term.[39] The value of cervical length shortening following cerclage is also controversial. A decrease of at least 10 mm is significant to predict delivery before 36 weeks.[36,37,40] However, this may not be significant when 34 weeks is considered as a cutoff. [38]

The value of Non-randomized Interventional Studies based Upon Ultrasound Diagnosis of Cervical Incompetence is Controversial:
TVS together with transfundal pressure can be used in high-risk women to define cervical incompetence at between 16 weeks and 24 weeks whenever this causes dilatation of the internal os or membranes protrusion.[41]

Serial TVS suggests that evidence for cervical incompetence can be established by 24 weeks.[42] In a retrospective analysis, Kurup[43] compared the outcome in three categories of cerclage—elective cerclage indicated by the patient's history, ultrasound-indicated cerclage performed in asymptomatic patients with cervical changes by ultrasound, and rescue procedure performed in symptomatic patients. This shows that the performance of ultrasound-indicated cerclage in terms of preterm delivery rate and gestational age at delivery performed better than emergency procedures. The benefit of cerclage in this group is however uncertain when compared to elective cerclage on the basis of a relevant history.[44,45] This therefore suggests that a new indication for cerclage can be defined as cervical changes on serial TVS in a high-risk group.

Randomized Trials Assessing Ultrasound-based Indications for Cerclage in High-risk Women:
There are two such randomized trials published and their results are apparently contradictory. Althuisius et al. studied patients with a history of delivery before 34 weeks with suspected cervical incompetence or preterm rupture of membranes at less than 32 weeks without preceding contractions.[46] In subsequent singleton pregnancies, they were randomized into two groups, with a ½ ratio, for either prophylactic cerclage ($N = 23$) or a follow-up cervical TVS ($N = 44$). In the follow-up group, a cervical length less than 25 mm before 27 weeks led to a second randomization for either therapeutic cerclage or expectant management. The obstetrical characteristics of the prophylactic cerclage and observational groups were similar. There was no significant difference in the rate of delivery before 34 weeks (13.0% vs 13.6%) in

these 2 groups. A cervical length less than 25 mm before 27 weeks was found in 18 (41%) patients in the observational group with a mean cervical length of 18.2 ± 5.9 mm at a mean gestation of 19.1 ± 2.9 weeks. The incidence of deliveries less than 34 weeks was significantly lower in the therapeutic cerclage group when compared (1/10 vs 5/8) with the bed rest group ($P = 0.04$).

There might therefore be a double benefit in performing cerclage for ultrasound indication only among asymptomatic patients at high risk:

- First, this would allow a significant reduction in the number of prophylactic cerclage. Indeed, in this study, cerclage was performed in only 40% of the cases.

- Second, therapeutic cerclage before 27 weeks may reduce the incidence of premature delivery before 34 weeks among patients with a cervical length less than 25 mm.

More recently, Althuisius et al.[47] published the Final results of their trial on 35 women with definite risk factors of cervical incompetence and shortening of the cervix down to less than 25 mm at before 27 weeks, 19 were allocated randomly to the cerclage group and 16 to the bed rest group. Both groups were comparable for mean cervical length and mean gestational age at time of randomization. Preterm delivery before 34 weeks was significantly more frequent in the bed rest group than in the cerclage group (7 of 16 vs none, respectively; $P = 0.002$). The compound neonatal morbidity, defined as admission to the neonatal intensive care unit or neonatal death, was significantly higher in the bed rest group than in the cerclage group (8 of 16 vs 1 of 19 respectively; $P = 0.005$).

The other randomized trial by Rust et al.[48] led to different conclusions but addressed a different population. Screening in the general population and detecting cervical funneling more than 25% or cervical length less than 25 mm at between 16 weeks and 24 weeks for Rust et al. were randomized into cerclage group or expectant management. Except for the cerclage, all patients were treated identically before and after randomization. Cerclage did not affect the perinatal outcome in any of the two trials.

Several differences between these studies[47,48] may explain these contradictory results. Low-risk patients were screened for a short cervical length to be included in Rust trial. In Althuisius, all but one patients had risk factors for cervical incompetence.

The main difference is therefore the initial selection of potential candidates. In Rust trial, measurement of the cervical length was performed in patients who had risk factors for preterm birth. In Althuisius trial, they were performed in patients who had risk factors for cervical incompetence.

All three trials included patients with short cervical length, which implies high risk of preterm delivery but not necessarily high risk of cervical incompetence. Rust et al. hypothesized that these ultrasonographic findings of the cervix during the second trimester demonstrate a potential final common pathway of multiple pathophysiological processes, such as infection, immunologically mediated inflammatory stimuli, and subclinical abruptio placentae. This hypothesis is supported by a 14.8% incidence of abruptio placentae in their study. Abruptio placentae was not found in any of the women in Althuisius study. This difference in prevalence of abruptio placentae confirms that the study populations in both trials are basically different.

TVS OF THE CERVIX IN CLINICAL TRIALS IN THE GENERAL POPULATION

There is a relation between the risk of preterm delivery and the functional length of the cervix in the general population. In a prospective multicenter observational study, Iams et al.[49] performed TVS of the cervix in women with a singleton pregnancy at 24 weeks ($N = 2,915$) and 28 weeks ($N = 2,531$) of gestation. Delivery before 35 weeks occurred in 126 (4.3%) of the 2915 patients examined at 24 weeks. Cervical length was normally distributed at 24 weeks (35.2 ± 8.3 mm) and at 28 weeks (33.7 ± 8.5 mm). The risk of preterm delivery was inversely correlated with the length of the cervix.

Heath et al.[50] measured cervical length by TVS at 23 weeks in 2,567 singleton pregnancies in women attending routine antenatal care. The risk for delivery at lesser than or equal to 32 weeks decreased from 78% at a cervical length of 5 mm to 4% at 15 mm and 0.5% at 50 mm.

To et al.[51] measured the cervical length in 6819 singleton pregnancies at 22–24 weeks and looked for the presence of funneling to evaluate possible additional risk. Funneling of the internal os was present in about 4% of pregnancies and the prevalence decreased from 98% when the cervical length was less than or equal to 15 mm to less than 1% at lengths of more than 30 mm. The rate of preterm delivery was 6.9% in those with funneling compared to 0.7% in those without funneling (P less than 0.0001). However, logistic regression analysis demonstrated that funneling did not provide a significant additional contribution to cervical length in the prediction of spontaneous delivery before 33 weeks.

Taipale et al. and Hassan et al.[52,53] confirmed the relation between the risk of preterm delivery and the functional length of the cervix but showed the limitations of this screening method in the general population. Indeed routine TVS of the cervix performed between 18 weeks and 22 weeks helped to identify patients at risk of preterm delivery; nonetheless, the low prevalence of preterm births in these populations (2–3%) at low obstetrical risk is a limitation to the development of such method of screening which would bring either a high false positive rate if the cutoff is 29 mm (3.6%), or a low sensitivity if the cutoff is 15 mm (8.2%).[52,53]

Non-randomized interventional studies among patients in whom ultrasound images are suggestive of a shortened cervix reported encouraging results.[54] Cervical length was 15 mm in 1.6% of the cases at 23 weeks in an unselected population of singleton pregnancies.[54] The attending physician decided upon performing a cerclage or expectant management. The two groups did not differ for ethnic or obstetrical characteristics. The median cervical length was 10 mm in both groups. In the cerclage group, the prevalence of preterm delivery before 32 weeks was 5%, whereas it was 52% in the expectant management group.

There is one randomized trials among patients with ultrasound images suggestive of cervical incompetence, that was initiated following the results of Heath' study. To et al.[50] chose a cutoff cervical length of less than 15 mm at 23 weeks for To et al. in the general population, with an overall low incidence of preterm deliveries. In To et al. cervical length was measured indication. Randomization into cerclage or expectant management did not lead to any difference in the mean maternal age nor in neonatal morbidity.

CONCLUSION

Transvaginal ultrasound of the cervix is an objective evaluation. Cervical biometry as well as anatomical survey looking for funneling and protrusion of the membranes through the cervix. Dynamic functional examination of the cervix evaluates the changes in the internal os in response to uterine contractions or transfundal pressure. It has the advantage of screening for dilatation of the internal os even when the external os is unchanged. Similarly it enables early detection of shortening of the supravaginal portion of the cervix, which is not amenable to clinical examination. We can hope that this early diagnosis will improve the efficacy of tocolytics.

Transvaginal ultrasound is a more discriminant approach than digital examination of the cervix both in terms of PPV and NPV. Among high-risk symptomatic patients (threatened preterm delivery), the data in the literature are sufficient to justify the systematic use of TVS for a more accurate evaluation of the risk of preterm delivery before any decision of hospital admission.

Cervical ultrasound might also be useful at selecting patients with complete or partial cervical incompetence among asymptomatic women at high risk (history of preterm delivery, late miscarriage, conization, maternal DES treatment, uterine malformation or a current multiple pregnancy). Among asymptomatic patients at high risk, progressive cervical incompetence may be a primary uterine condition which could trigger premature labor. Searching for funneling or protrusion of the membranes into the cervix is therefore extremely useful. In their absence, cervical incompetence should be sought by transfundal pressure. Compared with a single cervical measurement at 16–18 weeks and 6 days gestation, serial measurements up to 23 weeks 6 days significantly improved the prediction of spontaneous preterm birth.[21,25,55] A shortened cervix, although non-specific and rarely observed in the absence of uterine contractions, could also be the only warning of cervical incompetence. On the basis of Guzman's studies, ultrasound surveillance of such patients should begin by the fifteenth week.

In the general population, TVS of the cervix should be a useful complement to ultrasound examination performed at 22–24 weeks of gestation and help clinicians to better identify patients at low risk of preterm delivery (NPV = 96.7% and PPV = 47.6%).[53] High-risk patients as defined by short cervical length or the presence of cervical funneling could benefit from weekly cervical ultrasound assessment in order to define further intervention including cerclage, tocolytics, steroids injection for lung maturation.

REFERENCES

1. Hall MH, Danielian P, Lamont RF. The importance of preterm birth. In: Elder MG, Lamont RF, Romero R (Eds). Preterm Labor. New York: Churchill Livingstone; 1997. pp 1-28.
2. Blondel B, Du Mauzaubrun C, Bréart G. Enquête nationale périnatale 1995. Rapport de fin d'étude. Paris: INSERM, Feburary. 1996.
3. Ventura SJ, Martin JA, Curtin SC, et al. Final data for 1997: National Vital Statistics Reports (Vol 47, No. 18). Hyattsville (MD): National Center for Health Statistics; 1998.
4. Ventura SJ, Martin JA, Curtin SC, et al. Report of final natality statistics, 1996: Monthly Vital Statistics Report (Vol 46, No. 11; Suppl). Hyattsville (MD): National Center for Health Statistics; 1998.

5. McLean M, Walters WA, Smith R. Prediction and early diagnosis of preterm labor: A critical review. Obstet Gynecol Surv. 1993;48:209-25.

6. Keirse MJ. An evaluation of formal risk scoring for preterm birth. Am J Perinatol. 1989;6:226-33.

7. Shiono PH, Klebanoff MA. A review of risk scoring for preterm birth. Clin Perinatol. 1993; 20:107-25.

8. Creasy RK, Merkatz IR. Prevention of preterm birth: clinical opinion. Obstet Gynecol. 1990;76(Suppl 1): 2S-4S.

9. Buekens P, Alexander S, Boutsen M, et al. Randomised controlled trial of routine cervical examinations in pregnancy. European Community Collaborative Study Group on Prenatal Screening. Lancet. 1994;344:841-4.

10. Gomez R, Galasso M, Romero R, et al. Ultrasonographic examination of the uterine cervix is better than cervical digital examination as a predictor of the likelihood of premature delivery in patients with preterm labor and intact membranes. Am J Obstet Gynecol. 1994;171:956-64.

11. Iams JD, Paraskos J, Landon MB, et al. Cervical sonography in preterm labor. Obstet Gynecol. 1994;84:40-6.

12. Berghella V, Tolosa JE, Kuhlman K, et al. Cervical ultrasonography compared with manual examination as a predictor of preterm delivery. Am J Obstet Gynecol. 1997;177:723-30.

13. Iams JD, Newman RB, Thom EA, et al. The National Institute of Child Health and Human Development Network of Maternal-Fetal Medicine Units. Frequency of uterine contractions and the risk of spontaneous preterm delivery. N Engl J Med. 2002;346:250-5.

14. Murakawa H, Utumi T, Hasegawa I, et al. Evaluation of threatened preterm delivery by transvaginal ultrasonographic measurement of cervical length. Obstet Gynecol. 1993;82:829-32.

15. Timor-Tritsch IE, Boozarjomehri F, Masakowski Y, et al. Can a "snap-shot" sagittal view of the cervix by transvaginal ultrasonography predict active preterm labor? Am J Obstet Gynecol. 1996;174:990-5.

16. Crane JM, Van den Hof M, Armson BA, et al. Transvaginal ultrasound in the prediction of preterm delivery: singleton and twin gestations. Obstet Gynecol. 1997;90:357-63.

17. Rozenberg P, Goffinet F, Malagrida L, et al. Evaluating the risk of preterm delivery: A comparison of fetal fibronectin and transvaginal ultrasonographic measurement of cervical length. Am J Obstet Gynecol. 1997;176:196-9.

18. Rizzo G, Capponi A, Arduini D, et al. The value of fetal fibronectin in cervical and vaginal secretions and of ultrasonographic examination of the uterine cervix in predicting premature delivery for patients with preterm labor and intact membranes. Am J Obstet Gynecol. 1996;175:1146-51.

19. Hincz P, Wilczynski J, Kozarzewski M, et al. Two-step test: the combined use of fetal fibronectin and sonographic examination of the uterine cervix for prediction of preterm delivery in symptomatic patients. Acta Obstet Gynecol Scand. 2002;81:58-63.

20. Okitsu O, Mimura T, Nakayama T, et al. Early prediction of preterm delivery by transvaginal ultrasonography. Ultrasond Obstet Gynecol. 1992;2:402-9.

21. Guzman ER, Vintzileos AM, McLean DA, et al. The natural history of a positive response to transfundal pressure in women at risk for cervical incompetence. Am J Obstet Gynecol. 1997;176:634-8.

22. Guzman ER, Pisatowski DM, Vintzileos AM, et al. A comparison of ultrasonographically detected cervical changes in response to transfudal pressure, coughing, and standing in predicting cervical incompetence. Am J Obstet Gynecol. 1997;177:660-5.

23. Andrews WW, Copper R, Hauth JC, et al. Second trimester cervical ultrasound: Association with increased risk for recurrent early spontaneous delivery. Obstet Gynecol. 2000;95:222-6.

24. Guzman ER, Walters C, Ananth CV, et al. A comparison of sonographic cervical parameters in predicting spontaneous preterm birth in high-risk singleton gestations. Ultrasound Obstet Gynecol. 2001;18:204-10.

25. Guzman ER, Mellon C, Vintzileos AM, et al. Longitudinal assessment of endocervical canal length between 15 and 24 weeks of gestation in women at risk for pregnancy loss or preterm birth. transfudal pressure, coughing, and standing in predicting cervical incompetence. Obstet Gynecol. 1998;92:31-7.

26. Berghella V, Tolosa JE, Kuhlman K, et al. Cervical ultrasonography compared with manual examination as a predictor of preterm delivery. Am J Obstet Gynecol. 1997;177:723-30.

27. Goldenberg RL, Iams JD, Miodovnik M, et al. The preterm prediction study: Risk factors in twin gestations. Am J Obstet Gynecol. 1996;175:1047-53.

28. Skentou C, Souka AP, To MS, et al. Prediction of preterm delivery in twins by cervical assessment at 23 weeks. Ultrasound Obstet Gynecol. 2001;17: 7-10.

29. Guzman ER, Walters C, O'Reilly-Green C, et al. Use of cervical ultrasonography in prediction of spontaneous preterm birth in twin gestations. Am J Obstet Gynecol. 2000;183:1103-7.

30. Imseis HM, Albert TA, Iams JD. Identifying twin gestations at low risk for preterm birth with a transvaginal ultrasonic cervical measurement at 24 to 26 weeks of gestation. Am J Obstet Gynecol. 1997;177:1149-55.

31. Yang JH, Kuhlman K, Daly S, et al. Prediction of preterm birth by second trimester cervical sonography in twin pregnancies. Ultrasound Obstet Gynecol. 2000;15:288-91.

32. Ramin KD, Ogburn PL, Mulholland TA, et al. Ultrasonographic assessment of cervical length in triplet pregnancies. Am J Obstet Gynecol. 1999;180:1442-5.

33. To MS, Skentou C, Cicero S, et al. Cervical length at 23 weeks in triplets: prediction of spontaneous preterm delivery. Ultrasound Obstet Gynecol. 2000;16:515-8.

34. Guzman ER, Walters C, O'Reilly-Green C, et al. Use of cervical ultrasonography in prediction of spontaneous preterm birth in triplet gestations. Am J Obstet Gynecol. 2000;183:1108-13.

35. Funai EF, Paidas MJ, Rebarber A, et al. Change in cervical length after prophylactic cerclage. Obstet Gynecol. 1999;94:117-9.

36. Guzman ER, Houlihan C, Vintzileos A, et al. The significance of transvaginal ultrasonographic evaluation of the cervix in women treated with emergency cerclage. Am J Obstet Gynecol. 1996;175:471-6.

37. Althuisius SM, Dekker GA, van Geijn HP, et al. The effect of therapeutic McDonald cerclage on cervical length as assessed by transvaginal ultrasonography. Am J Obstet Gynecol. 1999;180:366-9.

38. El-Azeem SA, Samuels P, Fullana M, et al. Perioperative transvaginal sonography as an adjunct to cervical cerclage. Am J Obstet Gynecol. 2000;182(1):117.

39. Dijkstra K, Funai EF, O'Neill L, et al. Change in cervical length after cerclage as a predictor of preterm delivery. Obstet Gynecol. 2000;96:346-50.

40. Andersen HF, Karimi A, Sakala EP, et al. Prediction of cervical cerclage outcome by endovaginal ultrasonography. Am J Obstet Gynecol. 1994;171:1102-6.

41. Guzman ER, Rosenberg JC, Houlihan C, et al. A new method using vaginal ultrasound and transfundal pressure to evaluate the asymptomatic incompetent cervix. Obstet Gynecol. 1994;83: 248-52.

42. Macdonald R, Smith P, Vyas S. Cervical incompetence: the use of transvaginal sonography to provide an objective diagnosis. Ultrasound Obstet Gynecol. 2001;18:211-6.

43. Kurup M, Goldkrand JW. Cervical incompetence: elective, emergent, or urgent cerclage. Am J Obstet Gynecol. 1999;181:240-6.

44. Guzman ER, Forster JK, Vintzileos AM, et al. Pregnancy outcomes in women treated with elective versus ultrasound-indicated cervical cerclage. Ultrasound Obstet Gynecol. 1998;12:323-7.

45. Berghella V, Daly SF, Tolosa JE, et al. Prediction of preterm delivery with transvaginal ultrasonography of the cervix in patients with high-risk pregnancies: does cerclage prevent prematurity ? Am J Obstet Gynecol. 1999;181:809-15.

46. Althuisius SM, Dekker GA, van Geijn HP, et al. Cervical incompetence prevention randomized cerclage trial (CIPRACT): study design and preliminary results. Am J Obstet Gynecol. 2000;183: 823-9.

47. Althuisius SM, Dekker GA, Hummel P, et al. Final results of the cervical incompetence prevention randomized cerclage trial (CIPRACT): therapeutic cerclage with bed rest versus bed rest alone. Am J Obstet Gynecol. 2001;185:1106-12.

48. Rust OA, Atlas RO, Reed J, et al. Revisiting the short cervix detected by transvaginal ultrasound in the second trimester: why cerclage therapy may not help. Am J Obstet Gynecol. 2001;185:1098-1105.

49. Iams JD, Goldenberg RL, Meis PJ, et al. The National Institute of Child Health and Human Development Maternal Fetal Medicine Unit Network. The length of the cervix and the risk of spontaneous premature delivery. N Engl J Med. 1996;334:567-72.

50. Heath VC, Southall TR, Souka AP, et al. Cervical length at 23 weeks of gestation: prediction of spontaneous preterm delivery. Ultrasound Obstet Gynecol. 1998;12:312-7.

51. To MS, Skentou C, Liao AW, et al. Cervical length and funneling at 23 weeks of gestation in the prediction of spontaneous early preterm delivery. Ultrasound Obstet Gynecol. 2001;18:200-3.

52. Taipale P, Hiilesmaa V. Sonographic measurement of uterine cervix at 18-22 weeks of gestation and the risk of preterm delivery. Obstet Gynecol. 1998;92:902-7.

53. Hassan SS, Romero R, Berry SM, et al. Patients with an ultrasonographic cervical length = 15 mm have nearly a 50% risk of early spontaneous preterm delivery. Am J Obstet Gynecol. 2000;182:1458-67.

54. Heath VCF, Souka AP, Erasmus I, et al. Cervical length at 23 weeks of gestation: the value of Shirodkar suture for the short cervix. Ultrasound Obstet Gynecol. 1998;12:318-22.

55. To MS, Skentou C, Liao AW, Cacho A, Nicolaides KH. Lancet, 2004.

38 Labor and Puerperium

A Mulic-Lutvica, O Axelsson

LABOR

There is no doubt that labor is a dangerous period of our life and may result in birth-related disorders. Preterm and post-date deliveries, multiple gestations, preterm rupture of the membranes, intrauterine growth disturbances, breech presentations and intrapartum bleeding are associated with a considerable perinatal morbidity and mortality. Healthy newborns with expected good quality of life are the main goal of modern obstetrics. Numerous different methods have been developed to achieve this goal. One of the most widely used is without doubt ultrasound. Although the value of ultrasound in antenatal care is well established, it is surprising that the clinical knowledge of its advantages during the intrapartum or postpartum period is sparse. Nowadays, however, it is becoming increasingly common for obstetricians to use bedside ultrasound and to have ultrasound equipment permanently available in labor and delivery suites. By means of an ultrasound admission test a selection of high-risk patients should be made. The uterus with its contents, including the fetus, placenta, umbilical cord and amniotic fluid, as well as the cervix, can be assessed in detail by ultrasound. Even the maternal pelvis has become the subject of growing interest from sonographers. Ultrasound can also assist during the performance of some obstetrical procedures including external version of a breech fetus, intrapartum twin management, or manual or instrumental placental evacuation, as well as for confirmation of an empty uterus after the completed procedure. Intrapartum ultrasound imaging is difficult due to discomfort in women caused by pain, supine hypotension, and loss of the "acoustic window" after rupture of the membranes, low station of the presenting part, and lack of appropriate ultrasound equipment in the labor and delivery suite as well as inadequately trained examiners.[1-3]

Ultrasound Admission Test

Laboring women with inadequate or no prenatal care should be carefully examined with ultrasound when arriving at the labor and delivery unit.

Diagnosis of Fetal Life or Death

Ultrasound diagnosis of fetal life or death is simple, prompt and accurate. The fetal heart should be identified and the absence of fetal heart motion by real-time ultrasound and/or color Doppler implies fetal death. A completely quiescent fetus without body or breathing movements is an additional sign of fetal death. If the fetus has been dead for several days, the ultrasound signs of fetal death are oligohydramnios, overlapping skull bones, hyperflexion of the spine and the presence of hydrops.

Fetal Number

The presence of two separate heads, two spines and two heart motions is enough to identify a twin pregnancy. However, it is rare but not impossible to miss a multiple gestation even by ultrasound in a busy labor and delivery room, and especially if one of the fetuses is dead. Moreover, as the number of fetuses increases, the accuracy of intrapartum ultrasound diagnosis decreases. One of the possible explanations may be crowding and shadowing of one fetus by another, which creates a very confusing ultrasound image. Therefore, a thorough systematic approach should be adopted. All quadrants of the uterus must be explored in order to avoid missing a multiple gestation. Furthermore, ultrasound can be used to estimate the amount of amniotic fluid, and to give information on fetal presentation, growth discordance, signs of hydrops and fetal malformations. A correct intrapartum diagnosis and painstaking management of delivery with the assistance of ultrasound are essential for an optimal outcome in cases with multiple gestations.

Fetal Presentation

The presenting part of the fetus, be it head, breech, shoulder or compound presentation, can be simply and accurately diagnosed by ultrasound. It should always be done before labor induction, cesarean sections, preterm deliveries, deliveries of multiple gestations and in cases of planned vaginal deliveries after previous cesarean sections.

Placenta Location

Intrapartum vaginal bleeding and transverse lie are diagnosis in which ultrasound can be of assistance to confirm or rule out placenta previa, or low-lying placenta. Prior to cesarean delivery, ultrasound can be an aid to locate the placenta and help to decide the type of uterine incision.

Intrapartum Assessment of Amniotic Fluid

Ultrasound has made it possible to assess the amount of amniotic fluid. Several semiquantitative methods for evaluation of amniotic fluid volume, such as the largest vertical pocket and amniotic fluid index (AFI) have been published. A single largest vertical pocket of less than 2 cm was labeled as oligohydramnios and a pocket of more than 8 as hydramnios. Phelan and co-workers[4] described a four-quadrant method to measure the amount of amniotic fluid. A value of AFI less than 5 cm was designated as oligohydramnios and a value of AFI more than 24 cm as polyhydramnios. The umbilical cord and fetal limbs should be excluded from the measurement.[4-6]

Since its introduction in clinical praxis, AFI has been widely accepted as an accurate method to estimate amniotic fluid volume. In antepartum surveillance, an AFI less than 5 cm was considered to be associated with an increased risk for adverse pregnancy outcome and cesarean section for fetal distress.[7-9] Likewise an intrapartum AFI less than 5 cm was considered to be associated with neonatal metabolic acidosis.[5,10] Premature rupture of membranes, growth deficiency, postdate pregnancy and fetal renal anomalies are related to reduced amount of amniotic fluid. A marked reduction in amniotic fluid increases the risk for cord compression and fetal death during labor, especially in post-date pregnancies.[6] Oligohydramnios in early labor should alert the obstetrician, and it is recommended that careful intrapartum surveillance be used. However, in the past several years AFI has been questioned as the appropriate method of defining oligohydramnios. Results from randomized trials showed that the use of AFI compared with the largest vertical pocket was associated with significantly higher rate of suspected oligohydramnios.[11] The use of the test may increase interventions without improving neonatal outcome.[11,12] A meta-analysis of 42 reports found only one study that correlated intrapartum AFI with the rate of umbilical arterial pH less than 7.00.[13]

Moreover, Moses[14] showed in a randomized study of 499 pregnancies that neither the AFI nor the single pocket technique that was undertaken as a fetal admission test intrapartum identified a pregnancy that was at risk for an adverse outcome. As regards amnioinfusion for umbilical cord compression, in a systematic review of 12 studies it appears to reduce the occurrence of variable decelerations, lower the use of cesarean section for suspected fetal distress and it is associated with a reduction in puerperal infection.[15-17] Amnioinfusion can also reduce the incidence of meconium aspiration.[17,18] Hofmeyr[18] performed a systematic review of two studies of 285 women related to prophylactic versus therapeutic amnioinfusion for oligohydramnios in labor. There is no advantage of prophylactic amnioinfusion over therapeutic amnioinfusion carried out only when fetal heart rate (FHR) decelerations or thick meconium staining of the liquor occurred.[18] Likewise, in one study of 66 women serial amnioinfusion for preterm rupture of membranes did not detect significant differences concerning cesarean section rate, low Apgar score or neonatal death rate. Author does recommend the use of serial amnioinfusion for preterm rupture of membranes.[19]

Fetal Malformations

|Preterm labor, breech presentations and multiple gestations imply an increased risk of fetal malformations. Ultrasound can be used to look for fetal malformations in these clinical situations. The detection of an unsuspected fetal malformation may change the obstetrical management.[20] Anencephaly or infantile polycystic kidneys have a dismal prognosis, and cesarean section should be avoided on fetal indications. The vaginal probe and a diagnostic amnioinfusion may permit a definitive diagnosis of bilateral renal agenesis or Potter syndrome with severe oligohydramnios. That diagnosis is not possible with the poorer resolution of the transabdominal approach.[21] In addition, Color Doppler ultrasonography is useful to demonstrate the presence or absence of renal arteries. Diaphragmatic hernia as well as some structural or functional abnormalities of the fetal heart may require prompt surgical or medical treatment after delivery, so an accurate diagnosis before delivery is a prerequisite for appropriate neonatal management. Conjoined twins or sacrococcygeal teratoma may cause soft tissue dystocia, and cesarean section should be advised. In addition, ultrasound detection of a severe fetal malformation in preterm labor can exclude the need for tocolytic therapy.

Estimation of Fetal Weight

Accurate knowledge of fetal weight in early labor is important. Many clinical situations in an acute care setting require quick decision-making, often based on estimated birth weight. Intrauterine growth retardation, preterm labor, post-term gestations, suspicion of macrosomia, and twin and breech presentations are some of the clinical situations in which prediction of fetal weight may influence the management decision. Clinical estimation of fetal weight by abdominal palpation may be highly inaccurate, especially in the extremes of fetal size.[22,23] Since the introduction of ultrasound in obstetrics, a variety of equations using biparietal diameter (BPD), head circumference (HC), abdominal diameter (AD), abdominal circumference (AC) and femur length (FL) have been evaluated in order to find the most accurate way to predict fetal weight. It is now generally accepted that ultrasound estimation of fetal weight is more reliable than clinical estimation. Ultrasound has contributed to an improvement in estimation of birth weight,[22-26,29-31] although a few reports have questioned its accuracy.[27-28] The accuracy of ultrasound estimation of fetal weight is ± 10–15%. To avoid errors caused by a low station of the fetal head and molding or dolichocephaly in breech presentations, formulas based on FL and AC or adjusting BPD using cephalic index or HC should be used intrapartum.[24-25,29-32] In spite of inherent difficulties, the accuracy of intrapartum estimations of fetal weights performed by the house staff in a busy labor and delivery unit is comparable to that reported by more experienced examiners.[24,25] Furthermore, Pattersson[24] found that amniotic fluid volume, cervical dilatation or station of the fetal head did not influence the accuracy of intrapartum estimation of fetal weight.

Fetal Well-being during Labor
The Biophysical Profile

Several methods for assessing the fetal well-being and for identifying a fetus at risk for intrauterine death or injury have been evaluated. Manning,[33,34] originally described the biophysical profile. The ability to see the fetus, its activities and environment yielded the concept of the "fetus as a patient". The four components included in the biophysical profile based on ultrasound parameters are fetal breathing movements, fetal body movements, fetal tone and amniotic fluid index. A reassuring biophysical profile score of more than 8 confers a high probability of perinatal survival, and it accurately predicts antepartum umbilical venous pH.[34,35] FHR and fetal body movements are the most sensitive indicators for impending asphyxia antepartum. Oligohydramnios is associated with chronic fetal stress, and the absence of fetal body movements is predictive of impending fetal demise.[34] As labor progresses, a decrease in the fetal motor activity is a normal finding.[36,37] Fetal apnea is also a normal phenomenon during labor and has no adverse prognostic significance.[37] Sasson et al.[38] did not find correlation between the intrapartum biophysical profile and umbilical pH. Chua et al.[39] tried to select the best screening test to identify fetal compromise during labor. They concluded that women in early labor with an equivocal admission test should be assessed by an additional test like amniotic fluid index, umbilical artery Doppler or vibroacoustic stimulation, which might be of some help to detect a fetus with an increased risk of adverse outcome. Although observational studies[33-35,40] found that biophysical profile score gives the best prediction of both acute and chronic fetal compromise, a systematic review of randomized controlled trials (RCTs) (four studies of 2,849 patients) do not support the use of the biophysical profile as a test of fetal well-being in high risk pregnancies.[41] However, the power of these studies is not strong enough to prove that biophysical profile score is without value.[42] Kim et al.[40] has recently found that cessation of any ultrasound component of biophysical profile intrapartum significantly increased the risk of cesarean delivery and admission to the neonatal intensive care unit (NICU).

Intrapartum Doppler

Antepartum Doppler studies have shown an association between Doppler velocimetry and fetal well-being,[43] and the use of Doppler for antepartum surveillance in high-risk pregnancies can significantly reduce perinatal mortality in these cases.[43-46] The first intrapartum Doppler studies were performed with continuous and pulsed wave Doppler. Later, color Doppler and the transvaginal approach came into use. The most commonly examined vessels are the umbilical artery, uterine artery, fetal middle cerebral artery and aorta. There are three semiquantitative parameters that evaluate velocity waveform—pulsatility index (PI), resistance index (RI), and systolic/diastolic ratio (S/D). Uterine contractions, fetal breathing movements and frequent alterations in maternal position during painful contractions, as well as engagement of the fetal head in the bony pelvis, may make it difficult to get intrapartum Doppler signals.[47] Fairlie et al.[48] have, however, shown that the reproducibility of umbilical artery Doppler recordings during labor was comparable to the corresponding reproducibility from antepartum recordings. There is no significant change in the umbilical artery resistance during normal labor.[47-50] Neither amniotomy nor oxytocin infusion changes the umbilical artery resistence.[48] Likewise, epidural block with enough replacement has no negative effect on the S/D ratio.[51] Although Feinkind et al.[52] found that intrapartum screening with Doppler was sensitive enough to identify the fetus at risk for poor perinatal outcome, its use as a labor admission test is uncertain. At least two studies observed that intrapartum umbilical artery Doppler velocimetry is not good predictor of fetal distress among unselected patients.[53, 54]

Only in a high-risk population has a correlation been observed between the umbilical S/D ratio and umbilical cord pH.[48,52] The intrapartum umbilical artery S/D ratio might be of help in differentiating between variable decelerations caused by hypoxia or by mechanical occlusion.[55] It can also distinguish between true- and false-positive intrapartum late decelerations.[56] In the uterine arteries and their branches, a markedly reduced blood flow during normal labor has been noticed by several investigators.[47-49, 51] Apart from intrauterine growth retardation and preeclampsia, preterm labor is also associated with a significantly higher uterine artery S/D ratio, probably due to decidual vascular abnormalities.[51] The few studies on fetal aortal blood flow have shown decreased flow during labor if intrapartum analgesia with pethidine and with a paracervical block were used.[47, 57] In cases with no analgesia or with epidural blocks, an increased intrapartum fetal aortic blood flow was noticed.[57] Doppler studies of fetal cerebral blood flow in labor may help to explain the pathophysiology of intrapartum asphyxia. Published data are, however, considerably controversial.[58-62] The aims of future investigations should be to elucidate the possible factors influencing the waveform pattern and possible reasons for discrepancy in current reports.

Term and Preterm Premature Rupture of the Membranes

In cases of premature rupture of the membranes, ultrasound assessment may be of diagnostic help in the labor and delivery unit. The amniotic fluid volume assessment, biophysical profile and cervix status are ultrasound parameters of importance for evaluation of fetal well-being as well as for estimation of the conditions for induction of labor. In order to look for evidence of subclinical infection, a diagnostic amniocentesis may be performed. In patients with premature rupture of the membranes, it has been shown that the overall biophysical profile of the healthy fetus is not altered.[63,64] The most important parameters to evaluate fetal well-being are the amount of amniotic fluid and fetal breathing movements. Thus, premature rupture of the membranes with severe oligohydramnios is accompanied by variable decelerations due to cord compression, an increased risk of metabolic acidosis, chorioamnionitis, and a higher rate of cesarean section.[9, 63-65] It seems that FHR alone and biophysical profile are poor predictors of intrauterine infection. In a prospective study of 225 pregnancies complicated by preterm premature rupture of the membranes (PPROM) with delivery between 24 weeks and 32 weeks of gestation, AFI less than 5 cm was the only significant risk factor independently associated with early-onset neonatal sepsis and chorioamnionitis.[66] Nowak also concluded that oligohydramnios might be associated with increased risk of chorioamnionitis.[67] While Vintzileos[68] recommended frequent estimation of the biophysical profile as a simple test to predict the fetus at risk for developing sepsis, and questioned amniocentesis as a method to detect the fetus at risk for infection, Yoon[69] found amniotic fluid white blood cell count to be the best predictor of positive amniotic fluid culture, histological and clinical chorioamnionitis and neonatal morbidity. In a review of 12 studies Hofmeyr found that amnioinfusion to prevent infection in women with membranes ruptured for more than 6 hours was associated with a reduction in puerperal infection.[17] Amnioinfusion for umbilical cord compression in labor reduced FHR decelerations, cesarean section for suspected fetal distress, neonatal hospital stay more than 3 days, and maternal hospital stay more than 3 days.[15] The assessment of fetal age, weight and presentation is important when determining optimal management. Tsoi et al.[70] studied 101 women presented with preterm prelabor amniorrhexis. He measured cervix length by transvaginal ultrasound and concluded that prediction of delivery within 7 days is provided by cervical length, gestation and presence of contractions at presentations.

Threatened Preterm Labor

More than 70% of women presenting with threatened preterm labor do not progress to active labor and delivery. When confronted with a potential of preterm labor, ultrasound evaluation can provide important information such as gestational age, fetal weight, presentation, biophysical profile and the status of the cervix. Doppler velocimetry can detect cases associated with uteroplacental impairment. Severe fetal malformations and placental abruption should be excluded prior to institution of tocolytic therapy. Gestational age and birth weight are the most important predictors of neonatal survival. None of the various formulas for estimation of fetal weight seems to have superiority when applied to preterm labor.[71] In very low-birth-weight fetuses, ultrasound estimation of fetal weight is very accurate and correlates with neonatal survival.[72] Fetal presentation can drastically change the delivery management. The value of the biophysical profile to predict impending preterm delivery has been studied.[73] The individual biophysical parameters, especially fetal tone rather than the total score, demonstrate a strong relationship with the time interval to delivery.[74] It has been shown that the presence or absence of fetal breathing movements might be helpful in differentiating between true and false preterm labor.[73] Rising fetal prostaglandin levels during either term or preterm labor affect the fetal respiratory center, and provide a possible explanation of the cessation of fetal breathing movements during labor.[75, 76] Recently published systematic review regarding the accuracy of absence of fetal breathing movements in predicting preterm birth confirmed that the absence of fetal breathing has the potential to be useful test in predicting preterm birth both within 7 days and within 48 hours of testing.[77] Future researches are needed.

Cervical sonography allows determination of cervical length, funneling, the cervical index (funnel length +1/endocervical length), originally described by Andersen and colleagues,[78] and dynamic changes in cervical anatomy.[79] With the transvaginal approach, errors due to a low presenting part, maternal obesity or an overdistended bladder can be avoided.[80] The transperineal or translabial approach is a good alternative for departments where vaginal probes are not available in the labor and delivery suite. Prolapse of the amniotic sac through a dilated internal cervical os can also be observed and has been described as the "hourglass membranes."[81]

Although ultrasound assessment of the cervix seemed to be better than digital examination to predict preterm delivery,[78-83] qualitative analysis of nine studies using a cervical length cut-off 18–30 mm, showed that transvaginal ultrasound assessment of cervical dilatation or length has poor predictive value.[84] The sensitivity for predicting preterm birth varied from 68% to 100% and the specificity ranged from 54% to 90%. The most recently published studies of women with threatened preterm labor, cervical length cutoff less than 5 mm seemed to have higher probability to predict preterm delivery within 7 days.[85,86] Thus sonographic measurement of cervical length helps to distinguish between true and false labor and to avoid overdiagnosis of preterm labor.[85,86]

Intrapartum Vaginal Bleeding

Two major clinical causes of vaginal intrapartum bleeding, which may require ultrasound expertise, are placenta previa and placental abruption. The transabdominal approach may result in high false positive (2–7%) and false negative (2–8%) rates for placenta previa, depending on the time of scanning.[87,88] An overdistended bladder, maternal obesity, a posterior location of the placenta, the presence of fresh blood clots and an acoustic shadowing from the fetal head are factors that make the diagnosis of placenta previa difficult. Considerable improvement has been achieved by transvaginal ultrasound where false-positive rate of 1% and a false-negative rate of 2% have been observed.[87] The focal zone of the vaginal probe is 2–8 cm, which provides optimal imaging of the internal os. It is enough to insert the probe to a distance of 2 cm remote from the external os to avoid severe bleeding.

Tan et al.[89] studied the role of transvaginal sonography in the diagnosis of placenta previa and performed transvaginal sonography in 70 women diagnosed to have placenta previa by transabdominal sonography. The diagnostic accuracy of the transvaginal approach

was 92.8%, compared with 75.7% for the transabdominal route. They concluded that transvaginal sonographic localization of the placenta is superior to the transabdominal approach for type 1 and 2 placenta previa but no better for type 3 and 4. Transvaginal color Doppler seems promising in the diagnosis of placenta previa accreta.[90] The ultrasound appearance of placental abruption can vary. A high false-negative rate is a problem. The normal anechoic retroplacental area with signs of venous flow identified by pulsed Doppler should not be interpreted as a placental abruption.[91] Nyberg et al.[92] reported results of 57 cases of placental abruption, retrospectively reviewed. The location of the hemorrhage was subchorionic in 81%, retroplacental in 16% and preplacental in 4% of the cases. The fetal mortality rate was 20% with a placental abruption including 20% of the placenta. The ultrasound findings varied with the size and location of the hematoma, as well as with the time of the sonogram. Furthermore, the risk of fetal demise was greater in retroplacental and preplacental cases than in cases with subchorionic hematoma. In most of the cases with clinically suspected abruption, ultrasound findings are negative.[93] It is likely that the free passage of blood through the cervical os prevented the formation of a hematoma large enough to be visualized.[94] An acute hemorrhage is usually hyperechoic to isoechoic, and then gradually becomes anechoic during the following 1–2 weeks.[94-95] Rivera et al.[96] suggest that the use of ultrasound and nonstress testing in the expectant management of placental abruption could result in a decrease in maternal and perinatal mortality and morbidity. It must, however, be remembered that a negative ultrasound finding should not postpone essential treatment when there is a clinical suspicion of placental abruption.

Dystocia in Early and Late Labor

Dystocia—"poor progress of labor" is one of the leading indications for operative delivery, and it has previously been shown that mechanical problems in labor are responsible for a great number of all cesarean sections.[97] Cephalopelvic disproportion should be suspected in cases with an unengaged fetal head during labor, or in women with previous cesarean section due to dystocia. Efforts have been made to establish ultrasound diagnostic criteria to estimate cephalopelvic disproportion during early labor, based on results from ultrasound determination of the true conjugate and the transverse diameter of the pelvic inlet before labor.[98, 99] This requires, however, special equipment and considerable expertise. Dystocia in late labor can be caused by persistent occiput position. Clinical evaluation of the position of the fetal head by digital palpation is sometimes uncertain and inaccurate due to scalp edema, which causes difficulties in recognition of the sutures and the fontanelles. Akmal et al.[100] studied the accuracy of intrapartum routine digital examination in defining the position of the fetal head and found that digital examination during labor failed to identify the correct fetal position in the majority of 496 cases. Likewise, he found among 64 women that digital examination during instrumental delivery failed to identify the correct fetal head position in 26.6% of cases.[101] Ultrasound diagnosis of persistent occiput posterior position is simple, by visualization of the facial bones and orbits anteriorly and the spine posteriorly. By contrast, persistent occiput anterior position is confirmed when the facial bones and orbits are placed posteriorly and the spine anteriorly. The risk of cesarean section can be estimated during the early stage of active labor by the sonographically determined occiput position.[102] Rayburn et al.[103] studied 86 patients with arrested labor and showed that intrapartum ultrasound significantly improved the diagnosis of persistent occiput position, and could be of help in the management of delivery. Chou[104] confirmed this recently. If midpelvic forceps or vacuum extraction is to be performed, precise knowledge of the position of the fetal head is mandatory; a more proper forceps application and proper axis of traction may then be applied. Persistent occiput anterior position associated with labor dystocia is indicative of fetal macrosomia, and shoulder dystocia can be expected.[103] A new method to assess the descent of the fetal head in labor with transperineal ultrasound has been presented.[105] Head deflection may cause either a brow or a face presentation and then an abnormally broad diameter makes the passage through the maternal pelvis difficult. Such head deflection can be detected by ultrasound. Clinically, face presentation can be mistaken for breech presentation, especially if there is facial edema. Ultrasound examination can accurately exclude such an unpleasant surprise in the delivery unit. Knowledge of the position of the mentum anterior and occiput posterior are mandatory for allowing vaginal delivery in cases with face presentation, and this can be confirmed by ultrasound. With a brow presentation, engagement of the fetal head and delivery usually cannot take place if it persists. The brow presentation can, however, be converted to either a vertex or face presentation to allow vaginal delivery.[106] With a transverse lie during early labor, the position of the head and back as well as the location of the placenta should be identified before an external version or a cesarean section is undertaken. When the back is anterior, the risk of cord prolapse is greater. Information obtained from ultrasound can facilitate the performance of the cesarean section.

Breech Presentation

Recently published review of RCTs concerning preferred method of delivery for breech at term, showed that cesarean delivery occurred in 550/227(45%) of those women allocated to a vaginal delivery protocol.[107] Perinatal mortality and morbidity was greatly reduced in planned cesarean section group [relative risk (RR) = 0.31, 95% confidence interval (CT) 0.19–0.52]. Reviewers concluded that planned cesarean section for breech at term should be preferred method of delivery. Result of this review has considerably influenced obstetrical praxis regarding delivery mode for breech at term.

Nowadays there is enough evidence that external cephalic version reduces not only breech presentation at delivery, but, caesarean section rate.[108] Ultrasound may be of help during an external version of a breech fetus at term. Ferguson et al.[109] performed successful external version in 11 of 15 women at term who presented in active labor. In contrast, review of three RCTs of 889 women shows that external cephalic version (ECV) is not useful in preterm breech presentations.[110] However if ECV fails and vaginal breech delivery is woman's preference or if a breech presentation is diagnosed during early labor, a thorough and targeted ultrasound evaluation should be performed. Valuable information that can be obtained by ultrasound includes:

1. Type of breech (frank, complete or footling)
2. Estimated birth weight
3. Amniotic fluid volume assessment
4. Placental location (rule out placenta previa)
5. Rule out malformations (anencephaly, infantile polycystic kidneys).

Additional information that substantially influences the decision-making can also be obtained by ultrasound, i.e:

1. Fetal head position (hyperextension)
2. Nuchal or extended arm
3. Nuchal cord
4. Cord presentation
5. Cephalopelvic disproportion.

The gold standard for evaluation of the maternal pelvis has long been X-ray pelvimetry. This technique can expose both fetus and mother to possible long-term radiation hazards.[106] Rojansky et al.[98] proposed a simple ultrasound method for diagnosis of hyperextension of the fetal head by measurement of the cranio-spinal angle, and a method to measure the obstetrical conjugate by transabdominal ultrasound. He studied 72 laboring women with breech presentations and performed both traditional X-ray and ultrasound evaluation of the head position, type of breech and pelvic adequacy. A highly significant correlation between the two methods was demonstrated. He suggests that the ultrasound approach is reliable and may replace the X-ray method in management of breech presentation in labor. Although similar suggestions had been proposed previously[99,111,112] sonographic pelvimetry has not yet become a routine praxis.

Ultrasound indications for Cesarean sections, according to Rojansky, are a cranio-spinal angle of 150°, an obstetrical conjugate of less than 10 cm, and certain non-frank breech presentations. Ballas et al.[113] suggest that hyperextension of the fetal head (angle >90°) that was present on radiographic assessment, should be a contraindication to labor. Among twenty babies reported to have an angle more than 90°, 8 of 11 delivered vaginally, sustained cervical cord lesions. The nine babies delivered by cesarean section had no cervical damage. Sherer[114] suggests an additional indication for abdominal delivery, namely "nuchal arm" (extension of an arm behind the fetal head). This condition can be diagnosed by ultrasound. He pointed out that nuchal arm is a cause of severe birth trauma, and can result in persistent Erb's palsy, torticollis and convulsions. Ultrasound can identify a nuchal cord with single or multiple coils, although its clinical value is still controversial.[115] Lange et al.[116] defined cord presentation as the finding on ultrasound of loops of the umbilical cord below the fetal body and occupying the lower segment. Estimation of birth weight should be performed in patients with breech presentations who prefer vaginal delivery; weights between 2000 g and 4000 g are reasonable limits within which a trial of labor can be permitted.[117,118] When fetal weight is estimated in breech presentations, dolichocephaly should be identified by the cephalic index, and corrections made for this. For the purpose of avoiding errors due to dolichocephaly, formulas based on femur length, abdominal diameter or abdominal circumference should be used.[31, 32]

Intrapartum Management of Multiple Gestations

Ultrasound is an indispensable diagnostic tool for intrapartum management of multiple gestations. Presentations and estimated weights are most important when deciding on the mode and route of delivery. Estimation of fetal weight in twin gestations during labor seems to be reliable regardless of presentation, gestational age or the presence of discordant twins.[119,120] There is a general aim for vaginal delivery unless presenting twin nonlongitudinal lie. A retrospective study comparing neonatal morbidity in term twins delivered by cesarean section with vaginal delivery found that neonatal respiratory disorders were significantly more common in the first group.[121] In vertex/vertex twins, vaginal deliveries are most often planned. It has to be remembered, however, that in about 20%, the second twin will change position once the first is delivered.[122] Therefore, ultrasound assessment should always be performed after delivery of the presenting twin, so that a transverse lie can be turned into a longitudinal lie.[122-125] Moreover, ultrasound should be used to assess the FHR of the second twin, and may be of help if a suddenly compromised second twin needs a swift delivery by internal version and extraction. The same maneuver should be done if external version of the second twin to longitudinal lie fails. If there is a vertex/nonvertex presentation, the ultrasonic estimated birth weight will be of vital importance when deciding upon the route of delivery. Estimated birth weights between 2000 g and 4000 g can be allowed for breech deliveries,[123] provided there is a pelvic adequacy, no substantial growth discordance, no cord presentations, nuchal cord, extended arm or head deflection. Retrospective study of 408 twin deliveries showed that external cephalic version of the second twin and subsequent vaginal delivery in vertex/nonvertex was successful in 75% of cases. Internal podalic version and assisted breech delivery was performed in 20 cases and the remaining two were delivered by cesarean section. Apgar scores were not significantly different among the various groups and no complications arouse from external cephalic version performed on second nonvertex twin.[126]

Induction of Labor

Preeclampsia, intrauterine growth retardation, postdate pregnancies and diabetic pregnancies are common causes of labor induction. In post-date pregnancies, the presence of severe oligohydramnios, fetal macrosomia and unfavorable cervix can be revealed by ultrasound. Bishop[127] originally described evaluation of the cervix before induction of labor by digital vaginal examination. Results of numerous studies concerning the evaluation of the cervix by ultrasound are contradicting.[128-135] An unfavorable cervix results in failed induction in 3–5%. A careful evaluation of the cervix before induction of labor may help to avoid complications such as failed inductions leading to cesarean section. Since the introduction of transvaginal ultrasound cervicometry, it has been possible to assess the cervical status more objectively, and our ability to predict the course of labor seemed to be improved.[128] A sagittal section of the cervix can be seen between the anterior anechogenic bladder and echogenic rectum. Although the cervical length and dilatation can be objectively measured by ultrasound, the consistency of the cervix can be assessed only by digital vaginal examination. Therefore, a combination of digital examination and vaginal ultrasound assessment was recommended. The Bishop score would seem to be the best and most cost-effective method to assess the cervix and predict the likelihood of success of labor induction and the duration of such an induction. It seems that transvaginal ultrasound does not predict successful labor induction in post term pregnancy as well as digital cervical examination.[129] Reis et al.[130] obtained similar results concerning induction at term. They found ultrasound measurement of the cervix and fibronectin test failed predicts accurately the outcome of induced labor. Digital examination and obstetric history were the only variables independently associated with labor duration and predicted accurately vaginal delivery within 24 hours. Roman et al.[136] showed that neither the Bishop

score nor cervical length by ultrasound was good predictor for the outcome of labor induction in an unfavorable cervix. In contrast recently published studies as regard the value of ultrasound in the prediction of successful induction of labor found sonographic parameters (cervical length, occipital position posterior, cervical angle) being superior to the Bishop score.[131, 132] The same authors studied induction of labor for prolonged pregnancy and found cervical length and parity to be significant independent prediction of the likelihood of cesarean section, prediction of induction to delivery interval and the likelihood of vaginal delivery within 24 hours of induction.[133, 134] In postdate pregnancies or diabetic pregnancies, fetal macrosomia should be ruled out since large-for-date infants have an increased risk of traumatic birth injury.[135-137] Formulas based on femur length and abdominal circumference has the best correlation with actual birth weight in macrosomia.[138] Great efforts have been made to diminish the numbers of shoulder dystocia, which is a nightmare for the obstetrician.[139-142] A cutoff value of 1.4 cm for the difference between the chest diameter and biparietal diameter[142] or 26 cm for the difference between abdominal diameter and biparietal diameter[143] can be helpful in estimating the risk of shoulder dystocia, and can thus be helpful in deciding the appropriate route of delivery. The fetal subcutaneous tissue/femur length ratio is an additional gestational age-independent parameter for the intrapartum identification of a macrosomic fetus.[144] Vaginal birth after cesarean section has been advocated as a safe method to reduce the increasing cesarean section rate.[145] Prior to a trial of labor, the myometrial thickness in the area of the prior cesarean scar can be examined by ultrasound. It has been shown that defects in the lower uterine segment or abnormal uterine thickness can be visualized by ultrasound.[147]

Third Stage of Labor

Herman et al.[148] investigated the third stage of labor by dynamic ultrasound. They showed that, immediately after delivery of the fetus, the placenta-free uterine wall became thick and the uterine wall at the site of the placenta remained thin. As soon as the contraction phase began, the wall behind the placenta contracted gradually and only when it attained its final thickness did the placenta detach. No hematoma was observed between the placenta and the uterine wall. Ultrasound during the third stage of labor can help to clarify whether the placenta has already detached or still is adherent to the uterine wall. Directly after the delivery of the placenta, the uterine cavity is visualized as a thin bright central line. Krapp et al.[149] has shown that the disappearance of blood flow between the basal part of the placenta and the myometrium is the hallmark of normal placental separation—persistent blood flow due to abnormal vascular connections is suggestive of placenta accreta. Although this method can be helpful in making an early diagnosis and thus preventing heavily postpartum hemorrhage by early manual removal of placenta, the clinical application is of limiting value due to lack of appropriate ultrasound equipment at delivery suites.

Intrapartum Uterine Rupture

The actual site of uterine rupture is usually difficult to visualize by ultrasound.[150] Indirect ultrasound signs of uterine rupture are retroperitoneal hematoma and free peritoneal blood, most often localized in the cul-de-sac, the paracolic gutters, or the subdiaphragmatic areas.[151,152] Sometimes an extruded fetus or placenta can be seen. Although the clinical signs and symptoms of uterine rupture are most important, the use of ultrasound may be of additional aid in diagnosing this dangerous complication.

PUERPERIUM

Normal Ultrasound Appearance of the Postpartum Uterus

The puerperium is defined as the period of 6–8 weeks after birth during which the reproductive tract anatomically and physiologically returns to the nonpregnant state. When faced with puerperal abnormalities, it is useful to know the normal ultrasound appearance, and the dynamic changes of the uterus during the puerperium, in order to better distinguish pathological from normal conditions. The involution changes concerning the size, shape and position of the uterus, as well as the appearance of the uterine cavity, can be evaluated by ultrasound.[153-160] In the early puerperium, transabdominal ultrasound examinations are to be recommended. The woman should have a moderately filled urinary bladder. Gentle compression with the probe should be used and measurements should be made between uterine contractions to avoid uterine distortion. During the middle or late puerperal period, the transvaginal approach is preferable. Color Doppler[161–163] and transvaginal duplex Doppler[164] with high resolution have made it possible to study the vascular changes of the uterine involution non-invasively, and these methods have improved our ability to recognize puerperal abnormalities. The puerperal uterus should be assessed in sagittal, coronal and transverse sections (Figs 38.1 and 38.2). The coronal section is preferable for investigation of uterine malformations. Some ultrasound pictures are typical for the puerperium.[165] The involution of the uterus is a dynamic process that has no parallel in normal adult life. The uterine dimensions and the uterine cavity diminish progressively and substantially during the puerperium. There are two physiological lifesaving processes occurring soon after placenta delivery—thrombotamponade (enhanced blood clotting activity) and myotamponade (compression of the vessels by myometrial contraction). The appearance of ultrasound finding during early puerperium reflects these physiological changes. The normal shape of the uterus in the sagittal plane during the first postpartum days has been described as a "hockey stick",[166] or a "crescent".[156] This form of the uterus is typical only in the early puerperium and it is artificial. An extremely great degree of uterine deformability is caused by a heavy uterine corpus, a hypotonic lower uterine segment and supine position of the examined woman. In the 2nd postpartum week, the shape changes and becomes more globular. The position of the uterus also changes. In the early period the uterus arches over the sacral promontory in a retroverted position. Wachsberg et al.[166] pointed

out the importance of this uterine angulation and its effect on the measurements of uterine length.

The uterus rotates along its internal cervical os and in majority of women it achieves an anteverted position in the beginning of the second postpartum week. This position is then retained. In only a few women does the uterus return to a retroverted position at the end of puerperium.[165] Concomitantly with the changes in dimension, shape and position of the uterus, the uterine cavity goes through a marked process of involution. During the first 3 postpartum days lifesaving uterine contraction approaches anterior and posterior uterine walls and just virtual cavity appears. It is empty and decidua appears as a thin white line from the fundus to the level of the internal cervical os. Sometimes this line can be irregular and thicker which probably depends on the amount of retained decidua. The separation of the placenta and membranes generally occurs in the spongy layer, however the level varies. Already in the 1931, Williams wrote concerning the line of separation of the placenta and membrane. "*While separation generally occurs in the spongy layer, the line is very irregular so that in places a thick layer of decidua is retained, in others only a few layers of cells remain, while in still others the muscularis is practically bare.*"[167] The variation in sonographic appearance of the cavity could be seen as a demonstration of these physiological variations in retained decidua. The thin white line seen on ultrasound might possibly represent cases in which only the basal decidual layer is retained or if the muscularis is practically bare. Whereas the thicker and more irregular lines might represent cases with retention of more spongy decidual layer and perhaps fragments of membranes. It is unusual to find a collection of fluid or any echogenic masses in the upper part of the cavity at that time. In the lower uterine segment, however, a collection of fluid with mixed echo patterns is almost always present. It comprises blood clots and probably small fragments of retained membranes.[165, 166,168,169] This finding has no clinical significance and the mass is usually expelled spontaneously. Small echogenic or echolucent dots in the cavity are harmless physiological findings.[168] In contrast Sokol et al.[170] found in 16 of 40 women echogenic material in the uterine cavity within 48 hours after normal vaginal delivery. On the posterior wall of the uterus the prominent uterine vascular channels are regularly seen.[160] From days 7 to 14, endometrial fluid can be seen in the whole cavity, not only in the lower segment (Figs 38.2B and C). Moreover, echogenic and nonechogenic areas are seen in the whole uterine cavity, probably comprising a mixture of blood, blood clots and offcasts of necrotic decidua. The diameter of the cavity in the upper part of the uterus may then be quite wide, which reflects a normal healing process of the placental site inside uterine cavity, necrotic changes of retained decidua and an abundant shedding of lochia. In contrast Edwards et al.[171] found an echogenic mass in a great proportion of normal puerperal women. At 4 weeks postpartum, the uterus is again empty and the uterine cavity is seen as a thin central line. Sometimes a small amount of fluid can be seen. By 8 weeks postpartum the involution process is complete, and the uterus has non-pregnant dimensions. It lies in an anteverted position in 88% of cases.[165] In 12% of cases the uterus has a retroverted position corresponding well to normal prevalence of retroversion of the uterus in general population. Decidua and necrotic vessel ends are exfoliated, the placental site is recovered and a new endometrium is regenerated from the basal layer of the decidua adjacent to the myometrium. In 1953 Sharman performed endometrium biopsies and identified fully restored endometrium from the 16th postpartum day.[172] Ultrasonically the cavity appears

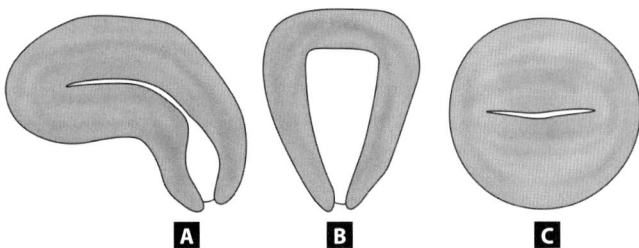

Figs 38.1A to C: Three standard sections of the puerperal uterus: (A) A longitudinal; (B) A coronal; and (C) A transverse

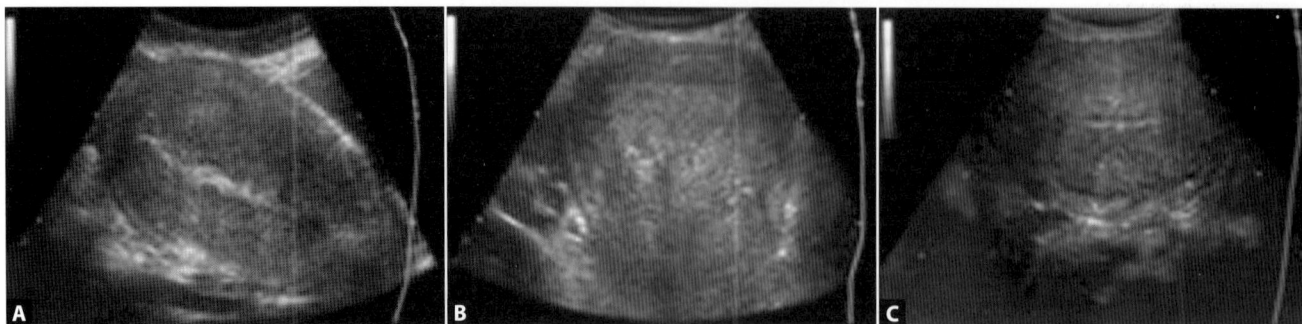

Figs 38.2A to C: Transabdominal ultrasound scans of a normal puerperal uterus on day 1: (A) Longitudinal scan; (B) A coronal scan, and (C) A transverse scan

as a thin white line. This corresponds to an inactive endometrium and reflects the hypoestrogenic state of the puerperium (the physiologic menopause). It is not common to find fluid or echogenic masses in the uterine cavity at that time. There are conflicting data about the presence of gas in the uterine cavity during the normal puerperium. Previous studies have suggested a correlation between gas and endometritis caused by *E. coli* or *C. perfringens*.[159,178] These conditions are, however, nowadays very rare. Wachsberg and Kurtz[173] detected gas in the uterine cavity in 21% of the normal population, and suggested that gas in the uterine cavity did not necessarily indicate endometritis but could be considered as a normal finding. Other investigators have not been able to confirm this.[165,168,169] Whether or not a small amount of gas is seen in the uterine cavity has, however, no clinical significance. Lavery and Shaw[160] described the prominent uterine vascular channels in the normal early postpartum period. With color Doppler a venous blood flow could be demonstrated, which usually disappears during the 2nd and 3rd postpartum weeks. Besides conventional ultrasound, Doppler technology is used to study hemodynamic events occurring during the puerperium.[161-164, 181-182] Normal pregnancy requires the growth of many new vessels. Consequently during puerperium dramatically regressive changes occur. The physiological destruction of the uterus involves not only muscle cells and decidua but also the arteries. Tekay[161] and Kirkiinen[162] assessed the peripheral vascular resistance of the uterine arteries in the postpartum period and found that the PI value started to increase in the early puerperium, remained unchanged during the next 6 weeks and finally increased to reach the non-pregnant values about 3 months after delivery. The prediastolic notch is also detected in the early puerperium and these hemodynamic changes can be partly explained by the immediate contraction of the uterus[161,162] Fluid collections in the fossa of Douglas are not a common finding during the puerperium.[165, 169]

Retained Placental Tissue

Retained placental tissue in the uterine cavity postpartum is associated with a high risk of excessive bleeding, either immediate or delayed. Immediate postpartum bleeding requires urgent management; manual evacuation of the uterine cavity is warranted. Ultrasound can be a valuable aid to confirm an empty uterine cavity after the evacuation by demonstrating the easily visible bright echogenic linear echo in the middle part of the uterus. Delayed postpartum hemorrhage occurs in about 1-2% of cases. It is most often the result of abnormal involution of the placenta site in the

uterine cavity and endometritis, but it may be caused by retention of placental tissue. In developed countries, half of postpartum women who are admitted to hospital with this condition undergo uterine surgical evacuation. In developing countries it is a major contributor to maternal death.[174] Two etiological factors were identified as risk factors, namely primary postpartum hemorrhage and a history of manual removal of a retained placenta. Uterus curettage was performed in 63% of cases. Histological confirmation of residual placental tissue was obtained in 37% following ultrasound diagnosis and in 33% without previous ultrasound examination. The decision whether to perform uterine evacuation for retained placental tissue depends on both, clinical finding and the ability to visualize retained placenta by ultrasound. Although prompt curettage seems to be necessary in many cases it usually does not remove identifiable placental tissue.[175] Moreover it is more likely to traumatize the implantation site and incite more bleeding. Consequently the complications rate is high. Hoveyda et al.[176] reported in his review regarding secondary postpartum hemorrhage that the frequency of perforation of the uterus was 3% and hysterectomy about 1%. Alexander et al.[174] identified 45 papers about the management of women with secondary postpartum hemorrhage and they concluded that no information was available from randomized trials to inform the management of women with this condition. Since curettage in the postpartum period can be dangerous, it is of great value to have a tool that can diagnose retained placental tissue. Many conflicting data exist about the ultrasound appearance of retained placenta tissue. The first studies were performed with old static ultrasound equipment.[154,177,178] They described various ultrasound images of retained placental tissue, and the rate of false-positive diagnosis was high. Despite the markedly improved imaging possibilities in the 1990s, confirmation or exclusion of retained placental tissue is still difficult.[163,164,168,169,176-180] We cannot expect the same ultrasound picture during early (Fig. 38.3) and late period of the puerperium. The ultrasound appearance of retained placental tissue may vary depending on the presence of different kinds of intrauterine contents. Necrotic decidua, blood, blood clots and inflammatory necrotic changes may essentially influence the ultrasound image. Nevertheless the most common finding associated with retained placental tissue is an echogenic mass.[164,168, 169, 177-179] In contrast, Edwards et al.[171] found in his study an echogenic mass on day 7 in 51% of normal cases, in 21% on day 14 and in 6% on day 21. He questioned ultrasound finding of an echogenic mass in uterine cavity as a sign of retained placental tissue. The definition of an echogenic mass was not specified. Even Sokol et al.[170] found "echogenic material" in 40% of cases during 48 hour after normal

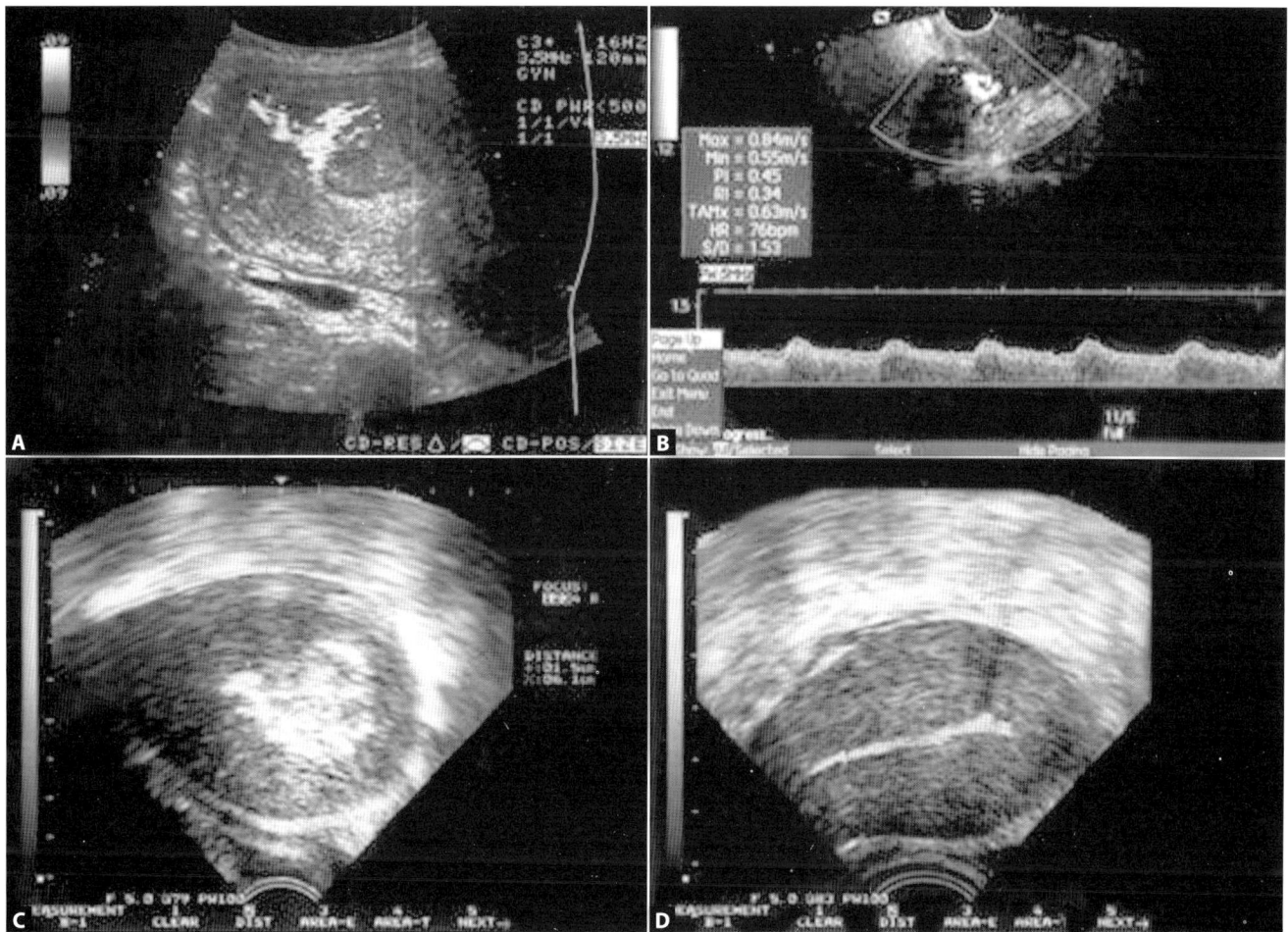

Figs 38.3A to D: Puerperal abnormalities as seen by the transvaginal (A, B) or transabdominal (C, D) approach. (A) Retained placental tissue is seen as an echogenic mass surrounded by a distinct halo and easy detectable flow on the side of the mass; (B) Retained placental tissue which has persisted for a long time postpartum and is seen as "a stippled pattern"; (C) After cesarean section gas is observed in the uterine cavity with clean and dirty shadowing well visualized; (D) A necrotic myoma which caused dysfunctional puerperal bleeding is seen in the uterine cavity

delivery. However, echogenic material was localized in lower uterine segment in 14 of 16 women. On the other side ultrasound appears as a valuable tool to confirm an empty cavity. Lee and Mandrazzo[178] found empty cavity in 20 of 27 patients with late puerperal bleeding. In only one case retained placental tissue was confirmed. The same authors reported that histological confirmation was obtained in eight of nine patients with ultrasound suspected retained placenta tissue. If ultrasound finding shows an empty uterus with a thin white decidua/endometrium, pure endometrial fluid or only small echolucent or hyperechogenic dots, a clinically significant amount of retained placental tissue is unlikely.[164, 165,168,169] Patients with persistent dysfunctional postpartum bleeding are highly suspected of having retained placental tissue, and they often show a typical ultrasound image with a "stippled pattern" of scattered hyperechogenic foci.[168] Later on, retained placental tissue becomes increasingly echogenic and the scattered appearance disappears.[168] A heterogeneous pattern may cause confusion since retained placental tissue and necrotic decidua with organized blood clots can give similar images during the 1st or 2nd postpartum week. Neil et al.[180] compared ultrasound with clinical assessment for the diagnosis of retained placental tissue related to secondary postpartum hemorrhage. They concluded that both,

clinical assessment and ultrasound scan have limited diagnostic accuracy. Transabdominal two-dimensional imaging alone is not specific enough. Transvaginal ultrasound has been advocated[164] with the use of a high frequency (6.5 MHz) transvaginal probe to better differentiate between retained placental tissue and blood clots mixed with necrotic decidua. Transvaginal pulsed and color Doppler is promising non-invasive methods to improve the diagnostic accuracy of ultrasound concerning retained placental tissue.[161-163] Achiron et al.[164] looked at the myometrial arterial blood flow around intracavitary contents and found that patients with a RI below 0.35 had residual tissue. These patients are suitable for invasive treatment. A resistance index above 0.45 should exclude diagnosis. Values between 0.35 and 0.45 were designated as a "gray zone". These patients could be treated conservatively with repeated ultrasound examinations, and curettage should be performed only if conservative treatment failed. Alcazar et al.[181] found a RI value less than 0.45 to be suggestive of retained placental tissue. We observed easily detectable flow, always on the side of the circumscript echogenic mass, that was histological proven to be retained placental tissue. It may be speculated that this highly vascularized area is responsible for the blood supply to retained placental tissue. Kelly et al.[198] described a rare cause of severe secondary postpartum hemorrhage—arteriovenous malformation of the uterus. By color Doppler ultrasound, a localized area of increased vascularity within the myometrium may be detected. Pulsed Doppler usually reveals a low resistance turbulent flow. Thus uterine artery embolization may be performed and unnecessary curettage should be avoided. In contrast Van Schobroeck[182] found enhanced myometrial vascularity (EMV) to be a common transient ultrasound finding if asymptomatic and it does not require treatment. On the other side, if in symptomatic patients residual placental tissue is suspected on ultrasound, EMV is an additional ultrasonic finding which can help guiding the appropriate management. It has recently been evaluated the accuracy of transvaginal sonohysterography and compared it with transvaginal ultrasound.[163,183] It seems to be this new method more effective for evaluation of residual trophoblastic tissue. Power Doppler and three-dimensional ultrasound seems to be new unexplored modalities that could improve our abilities to diagnose clinically significant retained placental tissue. All of these new modalities need further evaluation before their usefulness can be recommended.

Postpartum Endometritis

Whenever the obstetrician is faced with postpartum bleeding accompanied by signs of endometritis, the most important question is whether there is retained placental tissue in the cavity or not. Previously, it has been considered that ultrasound finding of retained placental tissue and endometritis overlap. Recent studies have, however, contradicted this view.[169] Only if endometritis is the result of retained placental tissue can a similar ultrasound appearance be observed. An isolated endometritis without retained placental tissue has no pathognomonic ultrasound finding. Confusion can sometimes arise in the presence of large retained and organized blood clots in the uterine cavity, that may mimic retained placental tissue. Clinical improvement following conservative treatment with antibiotics and uterotonic medications speaks against the presence of retained placental tissue. Uterine involution could be delayed in cases of endometritis, particularly if endomyometritis is present.[184] The detection of gas in the uterine cavity has been considered as a sign of endometritis. Madrazo[159] found endometrial gas in 15% of patients with proven puerperal endometritis. Wachsberg and Kurtz,[166] however, observed gas in 21% of women postpartum; none of these women developed endometritis. Whenever gas is present in the uterine cavity a follow-up ultrasound should be performed to confirm its disappearance. It usually resolves during the first 2 postpartum weeks. If ultrasound is performed after intrauterine manipulations or cesarean sections, it should kept in mind that highly echogenic foci caused by air are normal findings that must not be misinterpreted as retained placental tissue or endometritis. Kirkiinen found that blood flow to the infected uterus could be different from normal.[162] Deutchman and Hartman[184] have described an uncommon result of endometritis postpartum pyometra. A lucent area within the uterus with no echogenic components is suggestive of pus. Ultrasound can assist in the proper diagnosis and be of help in guiding a drainage procedure.

Septic pelvic thrombophlebitis, well known as an "enigmatic puerperal fever" is another uncommon complication of the puerperium. It most commonly presents in early postpartum period and antibiotic treatment is usually unsuccessful. Rudoff et al.[192] suggest ultrasound examination in case of clinical suspicion of pelvic thrombophlebitis. Although ultrasound diagnosis of ovarian vein thrombophlebitis is well described,[193-195] the diagnosis is still difficult and an ultrasound expertise is needed. Asymmetric dilatation of the ovarian or other pelvic vein may sometimes be observed.[193] Furthermore a complex or hypoechoic mass near the lower pole of the kidney particularly in clinical setting of an "enigmatic puerperal fever" should suggest thrombophlebitis. An echogenic intracaval mass is considered diagnostic and anticoagulation treatment should be added.[195]

Cesarean Section

Nowadays when cesarean section rates are continuously rising, higher incidence of all puerperal complications should be expected. The ultrasound appearance of the uterus after cesarean section usually shows three distinctive patterns: (1) gas in the cavity (2) a small rounded area at the incision site that reflects tissue reaction due to localized edema[185-187] and (3) some echogenic dots at the incision site, which is related to the type of closure and the suture material used.[187] All these characteristics are normal findings and no correlation with pathological conditions is found. The ultrasound appearance of endometrial gas is an intensively hyperechogenic focus equivalent in echogenic to bowel gas with clean or dirty shadowing or reverberation artifacts.[173,188] Fat and calcium have a similar ultrasound appearance. The gas usually disappears during the first 2 weeks after surgery. The involution rate of the uterus following cesarean section is not different from the involution rate after vaginal delivery. Nakai et al.[197] studied uterine blood flow resistance after cesarean section and concluded that the resistance index for the uterine artery did not show any change during the early postpartum period. The significant infectious morbidity is associated with cesarean section. Ultrasound may be useful in postpartum women with clinical suspicion of a postoperative complication like phlegmona,[186] abscess, pyometra, hematometra, wound infection, subfascial hematoma. If surgical drainage is chosen as therapy, ultrasound guidance can be helpful. Ultrasound can also confirm the suspicion of an intraabdominal postoperative hemorrhage by visualization of free fluid in the abdomen. Baker et al.[185] described bladder flap hematoma after a low uterine transverse cesarean section. A solid or complex mass between the posterior bladder wall and the anterior uterine wall may be observed by ultrasound. An abscess appears as a cystic structure with internal debris surrounded by thicker irregular walls. An infected hematoma initially has similar ultrasound appearance. During the resolution process, it may change and appears more solid. However, the physician must be aware that ultrasound diagnosis is just a complement and clinical condition of the patient should guide the therapeutic approach.

Uterine Myoma

Myoma may obstruct the birth canal and thus be a cause for cesarean section. Intracavitary myoma may cause problems such as placental detachment with subsequent postpartum bleeding. Ultrasound is the best tool to make a correct diagnosis. A myoma is characterized by hypoechogenicity. Due to degenerative processes, a myoma may appear as a bizarre heterogeneous pattern of solid and fluid areas, and thus, be misinterpreted as retained placental tissue. Pinpoint tenderness on palpation may direct the ultrasound examination and reveal the presence of a necrotic myoma.

Developmental Abnormalities of the Uterus

The prevalence of the congenital uterine malformations in general population is unknown. Failed fusion of the two Müllerian ducts to form the genital organs may cause reproductive, fetal and maternal hazards. In addition to an increased risk of premature labor and abnormal fetal presentations, retained placental tissue with postpartum hemorrhage may be a consequence of this uterine abnormality. It is well known that uterine anomalies may remain undiscovered except when they are associated with reproductive or obstetric problems. Already in 1976, Bennett suggested puerperal ultrasonic hysterography as a screening procedure prior to radiological examination in women whose reproductive performance suggests a diagnosis of congenital malformation of the uterus.[189] Since that a few studies concerning the issue were published.[190,191] Szoke and Kiss[190] examined in 1977 patients where manual examination revealed a uterus differing in shape from normal, the patient had a breech presentation in her previous or present pregnancy and the involution of the uterus was slow. The ultrasound echo technique was applied and uterine anomalies were found in five cases postpartum. In 1984, Land et al.[191] performed ultrasonic hysterography in 104 patients between the 2nd and 5th postpartum day. An unexpectedly high number of women (16%) showed an abnormal uterine configuration. The coronal section seems to be the most appropriate section in order to reveal uterine cavity anatomy. It is difficult to obtain the coronal section by abdominal examination in non-pregnant patients. However, the puerperium when the uterus is extremely large makes an exception. The ultrasound examination should perform in the early puerperium because a large uterus lies in near proximity to the ultrasound probe and highly echogenic decidua outlines well the shape of the cavity. Puerperal ultrasound can detect such an abnormality, providing an explanation for complications in labor and the puerperium.

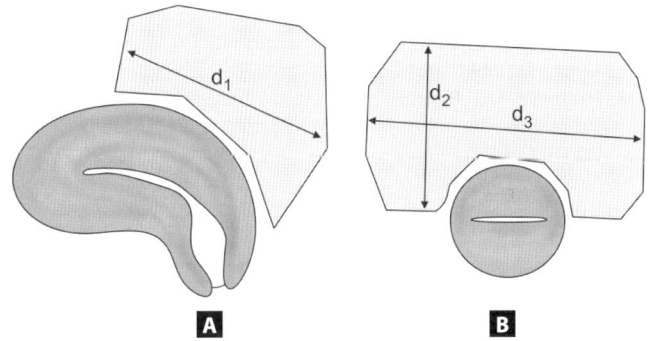

Fig. 38.4: Residual urine volume measurement

Postpartum Urinary Retention

Postpartum urinary retention is a relatively common condition and incidence ranges between 1% and 18%.[196] According to the International Continence Society, 100 mL is considered as the upper limit of residual urine. Ultrasound is the method of choice when assessing urinary bladder and residual urine postpartum. Invasive catheterization with the discomfort and the risk of infection can be avoided. Conventional bladder scanner is not to be recommended during the puerperium. Large uterus may content fluid and thus, a misinterpretation may be done. Many different techniques for bladder volume measurement are used and the accuracy of the method varies widely.

We prefer a method where the longest distance of the maternal bladder (d_1) is measured in a longitudinal section, and then two perpendicular diameters (d_2 and d_3) are measured in the transverse section (Fig. 38.4). The estimated amount of residual urine can be calculated using the formula for approximation of the ellipsoid:

$$\text{Volume (mL)} = (d_1 \times d_2 \times d_3)/2 \text{ (Fig. 38.4)}.$$

REFERENCES

1. Treacy B, Smith C, Rayburn W. Ultrasound in labor and delivery. Obstet Gynecol Surv. 1990;45:213-9.
2. Deutchman ME, Sakornbut EL. Diagnostic ultrasound in labor and delivery. Am Fam Physicians. 1995;51:145-54.
3. Benito CW, Guzman ER, Vintzileos AM. The use of ultrasonography in the labor and delivery suite. Clin Perinatol. 1996;23:117-39.
4. Phelan JP, Ahn MO, Smith CV. Amniotic fluid index measurements during pregnancy. J Reprod Med. 1987; 32:601.
5. Chauhan SP, Rutherford SE, Sharp TW, et al. Intrapartum amniotic fluid index and neonatal acidosis, a pilot study to determine the correlation. J Reprod Med. 1992;37:868-70.
6. Phelan JP. The role of ultrasound assessment of amniotic fluid volume in the management of the post-date pregnancy. Am J Obstet Gynecol. 1985;151:304.
7. Robson SC, Crawford RA, Spencer JA. Intrapartum amniotic fluid index and its relationship to fetal distress. Am J Obstet Gynecol. 1992;166:78.
8. Gonik B, Bottoms SF, Cotton DB. Amniotic fluid volume as a risk factor in preterm premature rupture of the membranes. Obstet Gynecol. 1985;65:456.
9. Romero R, Gomez R, Galasso M. Is oligohydramnios a risk factor in term premature rupture of the membranes? Ultrasound Obstet Gynecol. 1994;4:95.
10. Sarno AP, Ahn MO, Harbinder SB. Intrapartum Doppler velocimetry, amniotic fluid volume, and fetal heart rate as predictors of subsequent fetal distress. Am J Obstet Gynecol. 1989;161:1508.
11. Chauhan SP, Doherty DA, Magann EF. Amniotic fluid index versus single deepest pocket technique during modified biophysical profile: a randomised clinical trial. Am J Obstet Gynecol. 2004;19(2): 661-7.
12. Alfirevic Z, Luckas M, Walkinshow SA, et al. A randomized comparison between amniotic fluid index and maximum pool depth in the monitoring of pos-term pregnancy. BJOG. 1997;104:207-11.
13. Chauhan SP, Sanderson M, Hendrix NW, et al. Perinatal outcome and amniotic fluid index in the antepartum and intrapartum periods: a meta analysis. Am J Obstet Gynecol. 1999;181:1473-8.
14. Moses J, Doherty DA, Magann EF, et al. A randomized clinical trial of the intrapartum assessment of amniotic fluid volume: amniotic fluid index versus the single deepest pocket technique. Am J Obstet Gynecol. 2004;190(6):1564-9.
15. Hofmeyr GJ. Amnioinfusion for umbilical cord compression in labour. Cochrane Database of Syst Rev. 2012;1:CD000013.
16. Moen MD, Besinger RE, Tomich PG, et al. Effect of amnioinfusion on the incidence of postpartum endometritis in patients undergoing cesarean delivery. J Reprod Med. 1995;40:383-6.

17. Sadovsky Y, Amon E, Bade ME. Prophylactic amnioinfusion during labor complicated by meconium: a preliminary report. Am J Obstet Gynecol. 1989;161:613.

18. Hofmeyr GJ. Prophylactic versus therapeutic amnioinfusion for oligohydramnios in labour. Cochrane Database Syst Rev. 2000;2:CD000176.

19. Hofmeyr GJ. Amnioinfusion for preterm rupture of membranes. Cochrane Database Syst Rev. 2000;2: CD000942.

20. Vintzileos AM, Campbell WA, Nochimson DJ. Antenatal evaluation and management of ultrasonically detected fetal anomalies. Obstet Gynecol. 1987;69:640.

21. Benacerraf BR. Examination of the second-trimester fetus with severe oligohydramnios using transvaginal scanning. Obstet Gynecol. 1990;75:491-3.

22. Hadlock FP, Harrist DB, Carpenter RJ. Sonographic estimation of fetal weight. Radiology. 1984;150:535.

23. Hadlock FP, Harrist RB, Sharman RS, et al. Estimation of fetal weight with the use of head, body and femur measurements–a prospective study. Am J Obstet Gynecol. 1984;151:333-7.

24. Pattersson RM. Estimation of fetal weight during labor. Obstet Gynecol. 1985;65:330-2.

25. Platek DN, Divon MY, Anyaegbunam A, et al. Intrapartum ultrasonographic estimates of fetal weight by the house staff. Am J Obstet Gynecol. 1991;165:842-5.

26. Yarkoni S, Reace EA, Wan M. Intrapartum fetal weight estimation: a comparison of three formulae. J Ultrasound Med. 1986;5:707-10.

27. Chauhan SP, Lutton TC, Bailey KJ, et al. Intrapartum prediction of birth weight: clinical versus sonographic estimation based on femur length alone. Obstet Gynecol. 1993;81:695-7.

28. Chauhan SP, Lutton PN, Bailey KJ, et al. Intrapartum clinical sonographic and parous patients' estimates of newborn birth weight. Obstet Gynecol. 1992; 79:956-8.

29. Shanley KT, Landon MB. Accuracy and modifying factors for ultrasonic determination of fetal weight at term. Obstet Gynecol. 1994;84:926.

30. Shepard MJ, Richard VA, Berkowitz RL, et al. An evaluation of two equations for predicting fetal weight by ultrasound. Am J Obstet Gynecol. 1982;142:47-54.

31. Doubilet PM, Greenes RA. Improved prediction of gestational age from fetal head measurements. Am J Roentgenol. 1982;142:47.

32. Kasby CB, Poll V. The breech head and its ultrasound significance. Br J Obstet Gynaecol. 1982;89:106.

33. Manning FA, Morrison I, Lange IR. Fetal assessment based on fetal biophysical profile scoring. Am J Obstet Gynecol. 1985;151:343.

34. Manning FA. Dynamic ultrasound based fetal assessment: The fetal biophysical profile score. Clin Obstet Gynecol. 1995;38:26-44.

35. Manning FA, Morrison I, Harman CR, et al. Fetal assessment based on fetal biophysical profile scoring in the management of the growth restricted fetus. Ultrasound Obstet Gyncol. 1987;16: 399-40.

36. Whitman BK, Davison BM, Lyons E. Real-time ultrasound observation of fetal activity in labor. Br J Obstet Gynaecol. 1979;86: 278.

37. Boylan P, Lewis PJ. Fetal breathing in labor. Obstet Gynecol. 1980;56:35

38. Sasson DA, Castro LC, Davis JL. The biophysical profile in labor. Obstet Gynecol. 1990;76:360.

39. Chua S, Arulkumaran S, Kurup A, et al. Search for the most predictive test of fetal well being in early labor. J Perinat Med. 1996;24:199-206.

40. Kim SY, Khandelwal M, Gaughan JP, et al. Is the intrapartum biophysical profile useful? Obstet Gynecol. 2003; 102(3):471-6.

41. Alfirevic Z, Neilson JP. Biophysical profile for fetal assessment in high-risk pregnancies. Cochrane Database Syst Rev. 2000;(2): CD000038.

42. David KJ, Mahomed K, Stone P, et al. Evidence Based Obstetrics. Philadelphia: Saunders, Elsevier Science;2003.

43. Jouppila P, Kiirkiinen P. Umbilical vein blood flow as an indicator of fetal hypoxia. Br J Obstet Gynecol. 1984; 91:107.

44. Farmakides G, Weiner Z, Mammapolos M, et al. Doppler velocimetry. Clin Perinatol. 1994;21:849-61.

45. Almström H, Axelsson O, Gnattingius S. Comparison of umbilical artery velocimetry and cardiotocography for surveillance of small for gestational age fetuses. A multicenter randomised controlled trial, abstr. J Matern Fetal Invest. 1991;1:127.

46. Alfirevic Z, Neilson JP. Doppler ultrasonography in high-risk pregnancies: systematic review with metaanalysis. Am J Obstet Gynecol. 1995;172:1379-87.

47. Kurjak A, Dudenhausen J, Kos M, et al. Doppler information pertaining to the intrapartum period. J Perinat Med. 1996;24: 271-6.

48. Fairlie FM, Lang GD, Sheldon CD. Umbilical artery flow velocity waveforms in labour. Br J Obstet Gynaecol. 1989;96:151.

49. Fleischer A, Anyaegbunam A, Shulman H, et al. Uterine and umbilical artery velocimetry during normal labor. Am J Obstet Gynecol. 1987;157:40.

50. Brar HS, Platt LD, De Vore GR, et al. Qualitative assessment of maternal uterine and fetal umbilical artery blood flow and resistance in labouring patients by Doppler velocimetry. Am J Obstet Gynecol. 1988;158:952.

51. Strigini FA, Lencioni G, De Luca G, et al. Uterine artery velocimetry and spontaneous preterm delivery. Obstet Gynecol. 1995;85: 374-7.

52. Feinkind L, Abulafia O, Delke I, et al. Screening with Doppler velocimetry in labor. Am J Obstet Gynecol. 1989;161:765-70.

53. Malcus P, Gudmundsson S, Marsal K, et al. Umbilical artery Doppler velocimetry as a labor admission test. Obstet Gynecol. 1991;77:106.

54. Sarno AP, Ahn MO, Brar HS, et al. Intrapartum Doppler velocimetry, amniotic fluid volume, and fetal heart rate as predictors of subsequent fetal distress an initial report. Am J Obstet Gynecol. 1989;161:1508-4.

55. Weis E, Hitschold T, Berle P. Umbilical artery blood flow velocity waveforms during variable decelerations of the fetal heart rate. Am J Obstet Gynecol. 1991;164:534-9.

56. Brar HS, Platt LD, Paul RH. Fetal umbilical blood flow velocity waveforms using Doppler ultrasonography in patients with late decelerations. Obstet Gynecol. 1989;73:363-6.

57. Lindblad A, Bernow J, Marshal K. Obstetric analgesia and fetal aortic blood flow during labor. Br J Obstet Gynaecol. 1987;94-306.

58. Ueno N. Studies on fetal middle cerebral artery blood flow velocity waveform in the intrapartum period. Nippon Sanka Fujinka Gakkai Zasshi. 1992;44:97.

59. Vyas S, Campbell S, Bower S, et al. Maternal abdominal pressure alters fetal cerebral blood flow. Br J Obstet Gynaecol. 1990;97:140.

60. Mirrro R, Gonzales A. Perinatal anterior cerebral artery Doppler flow indexes: methods and preliminary results. Am J Obstet Gynecol. 1987;156:1227.

61. Maesel A, Lingman G, Marsal K. Cerebral blood flow during labor in human fetus. Acta Obstet Gynecol Scand. 1990;69:493.

62. Yagel S, Anteby E, Lavy Y, et al. Fetal middle cerebral artery blood flow during normal active labour and in labour with variable decelerations. Br J Obstet Gynaecol. 1992;99:483.

63. Vintzileos AM, Campbell WA, Nochimson DJ. The use of fetal biophysical profile improves pregnancy outcome in premature rupture of the membranes. Am J Obstet Gynecol. 1987;157:236.

64. Vintzileos AM. Antepartum surveillance on preterm rupture of membranes. J Perinat Med. 1996;24:319.

65. Goldstein I, Romero R, Merill S. Fetal body and breathing movements as predictors of intra-amniotic infection in preterm premature rupture of membranes. Am J Obstet Gynecol. 1988;159:363.

66. Vermillion ST, Kooba AM, Soper DE, et al. Amniotic fluid index values after preterm premature rupture of the membranes

and subsequent perinatal infection. Am J Obstet Gynecol. 2000;183:271-6.

67. Nowak M, Oszukowski P, Szpakowski M, et al. Intrauterine infections. I. The role of C-reactive protein, white blood cell count and erythrocyte sedimentation rate in pregnant women in the detection of intrauterine infection after preliminary rupture of the membranes. Ginekol Pol. 1998;69:615-22.

68. Vintzileos AM, Campbell WA, Nochimson DJ. Fetal biophysical profile versus amniocentesis in predicting infection in premature rupture of the membranes. Obstet Gynecol. 1986;68:488.

69. Yoon BH, Jun JK, Park KH, et al. Serum C-reactive protein, white blood cell count, and amniotic fluid blood cell count in women with preterm premature rupture of membranes. Obstet Gynecol. 1996;88:1034-40.

70. Tsoi E, Fuchs I, Henrich W, et al. Sonographic measurement of cervical length in preterm prelabor amniorrhexis. Ultrasound Obstet Gynecol. 2004; 24(5):550-3.

71. Main DM, Hadley CB. The role of ultrasound in the management of preterm labor. Clin Obstet Gynecol. 1988;31:53.

72. Weinberger E, Cyr DR, Hirsh JH. Estimating fetal weights less than 2000 g. An accurate and simple method. Am J Roentgenol. 1984;141:973.

73. Besinger RE, Compton AA, Hayashi RH. The presence or absence of fetal breathing movements as a predictor of outcome in preterm labor. Am J Obstet Gynecol. 1987;157:753-7.

74. McFarlin BL, Baumann P, Sampson MB, et al. The biophysical profile as a tool for prediction of preterm delivery. Obstet Gynecol. 1995;50:413-14.

75. Weitz CM, Ghodaonkar RB, Dubin NH. Prostaglandin F metabolite concentration as a prognostic factor in preterm labor. Obstet Gynecol. 1986;67:496.

76. MacKenzie IZ. Induction of labor–a review of the use of prostaglandins. J Obstet Gynecol. 1988;8:s7.

77. Honest H, Bachmann LM Sengupta R, et al. Accuracy of absence of fetal breathing movements in predicting preterm birth a systematic review. Ultrasound Obstet Gynecol. 2004;24:194-100.

78. Andersen HF, Nugent CE, Wanty SD, et al. Prediction of risk for preterm delivery by ultrasonographic measurement of cervical length. Am J Obstet Gynecol. 1990;163:859.

79. Van Dessel HJ, Friijns JH, Kok FT, et al. Ultrasound assessment of cervical dynamics during the first stage of labour. Eur J Obstet Gynecol Reprod Biol. 1994;53:123-7.

80. Gomez R, Galasso M, Romero R, et al. Ultrasonographic examination of the uterine cervix is better than cervical digital examination as a predictor of the likelihood of premature delivery in patients with preterm labor and intact membranes. Am J Obstet Gynecol. 1994;171:956-64.

81. McGahan JP, Phillips HE, Bowen MS. Prolapse of the amniotic sac "hourglass membranes": ultrasound appearance. Radiology. 1981;140:463-6.

82. Romero R. The uterine cervix and preterm delivery. Presented at the VI World Congress of Ultrasound in Obstetrics and Gynecology, Rotterdam. 1996;257.

83. Iams JD, Paraskos J, Landon MB, et al. Cervical sonography in preterm delivery. Obstet Gynecol. 1994; 84:40-6.

84. Vendittelli F, Volumenie J. Transvaginal ultrasonography examination of the uterine cervix in hospitalized women undergoing preterm labour. Eur J Obstet Gynecol Reprod Biol. 2000;90:3-11.

85. Tsoi E, Akmal S, Rane S, et al. Ultrasound assessment of cervical length in threatened preterm labor. Ultrasound Obstet Gynecol. 2003;6:552-5.

86. Fuchs IB, Henrich W, Osthues K, et at. Sonographic cervical length in singleton pregnancies with intact membranes presenting with threatened preterm labor. Ultrasound Obstet Gynecol. 2004;5:554-7.

87. Laing FC. Placenta previa: avoiding false-negative diagnosis. J Clin Ultrasound. 1981;9:109.

88. Timor-Trish IE, Rottem S. Transvaginal sonography. New York: Elsevier; 1987.pp.:1-13.

89. Tan NH, Abuy M, Woo JL. The role of transvaginal sonography in the diagnosis of placenta previa. Aust N Z J Obstet Gynecology. 1995; 35: 42-5.

90. Patel F, Bornet C, Moodley J. The use of transvaginal color Doppler ultrasound in the diagnosis of placenta previa accreta. Ultrasound Obstet Gynecol. 1996;8(1):78.

91. McGahan JP, Phillips HE, Reid MH. The anechoic retroplacental area. Radiology. 1980;134:47.

92. Nyberg DA, Cyr DR, Mack LA, et al. Sonographic spectrum of placental abruption. Am J Roentgenol. 1987; 148:161-4.

93. Hurd WW, Miodovnik M, Hertzberg V. Selective management of abruptio placentae: a prospective study. Obstet Gynecol. 1983;61:467-72.

94. McGahan JP, Phillips HE, Reid MH. Sonographic spectrum of retroplacental hemorrhage. Radiology. 1982;142:481.

95. Spirt BA, Kagan EH, Rozanski RM. Abruptio placenta: sonographic and pathologic correlation. Am J Roentgenol. 1979;133:877-81.

96. Rivera Alsima ME, Saldana LR, Maklad N. The use of ultrasound in the expectant management of abruptio placentae. Am J Obstet Gynecol. 1983;146:924-7.

97. Macara LM, Murphy KW. The contribution of dystoci to the cesarean section rate. Am J Obstet Gynecol. 1994;171:71-7.

98. Rojansky N, Tanos V, Lewin A, et al. Sonographic evaluation of fetal head extension and maternal pelvis in cases of breech presentation. Acta Obstet Gynecol Scand. 1994;73:607-10.

99. Deutinger J, Bernaschek G. Vaginosonographical determination of the true conjugate and the transverse diameter of the pelvic inlet. Arch Gynecol. 1987;240: 24-16.

100. Akmal S, Tsoi E, Kametas N, et al. Intrapartum sonography to determine fetal head position. J Matern Fetal Neonatal Med. 2002;12(3):172-7.

101. Akmal S, Tsoi E, Kametas N, et al. Comparison of transvaginal digital examination with intrapartum sonography to determine fetal head position before instrumental delivery. Ultrasound Obstet Gynecol. 2003;21(5):437-40.

102. Akmal S, Tsoi E, Nicolaides KH. Intrapartum sonography to determine fetal occipital position: Interobserver agreement. Ultrasound Obstet Gynecol. 2004;24(4): 421-4.

103. Rayburn WR, Siemers KH, Legino LJ. Dystoci in late labor: determining fetal position by clinical and ultrasonic techniques. Am J Perinatol. 1989;6:161-89.

104. Chou MR, Kreiser D, Taslimi MM, et al. Vaginal versus ultrasound examination of fetal occiput position during the second stage of labor. Am J Obstet Gynecol. 2004;191(2):521-4.

105. Barbera A, Pombar X, Perugino G, et al. A new method to assess fetal head descent in labor with transperineal, ultrasound. Ultrasound Obstet Gynecol. 1996;8(1): 95.

106. Pritchard JA, MacDonald PC, Gant NF. Williams Obstetrics, 17th edition. Norwalk: Appleton-Century-Crofts; 1985.pp.660.

107. Hofmeyr GJ, Hannah ME. Planned cesarean section for term breech delivery. Cochrane Database Syst Rev. 2001;(1):CD000166.

108. Hofmeyr GJ, Kulier R. External cephalic version for breech presentation at term. Cochrane Database Syst Rev. 2000;(2): CD000083.

109. Ferguson JE, Dyson DC. Intrapartum external cephalic version. Am J Obstet Gynecol. 1985;152:297.

110. Hofmeyr GJ. External cephalic version for breech presentation before term. Cochrane Database Syst Rev. 2006;(1):CD000084.

111. Kratochwil A, Zeibekis N. Ultrasonic pelvimetry. Acta Obstet Gynecol Scand. 1972;240:241-6.

112. Schlensker KH. Ultrasonographic examinations of the true conjugate. Geburshilfe Frauenheilkd. 1979;37:333-7.

113. Ballas S, Toaff R. Hyperextension of the fetal head in breech presentation radiological evaluation and significance. Br J Obstet Gynecol. 1976;83:201-4.
114. Sherer DM. Sonographic detection of a nuchal arm in the intrapartum assessment of the breech-presenting fetus (letter). J Ultrasound Med. 1993;12:524.
115. Giacomello F. Ultrasound determination of nuchal cord in breech presentation (letter). Am J Obstet Gynecol. 1988;159: 531.
116. Lange IR, Masning FA, Morrison, et al. Cord prolapse: is antenatal diagnosis possible? Am J Obstet Gynecol. 1985;151:1083.
117. Gimovsky ML, Paul R. Singleton breech presentation in labor. Experiences in 1980. Am J Obstet Gynecol. 1982;143:733.
118. Scorza WE. Intrapartum management of breech presentation. Clin Perinatol. 1996;23:31-49.
119. Chauhan S, Washburne J, Martin J. Intrapartum assessment by house staff of birth weight among twins. Obstet Gynecol. 1993;82:523.
120. Lukacs HA, MacLennan AH, Verco PW. Ultrasonic fetal weight estimation in multiple and singleton pregnancy. Aust Pediatr J. 1984;20:59-61.
121. Chasen ST, Madden A, Chervenak FA. Cesarean delivery of twins and neonatal respiratory disorders. Am J Obstet Gynecol. 1999;181:1052-6.
122. Houlihan C, Knuppel RA. Intrapartum management of multiple gestations. Clin Perinatol. 1996;23:91.
123. Chervenak F, Johnson R, Youcha S. Intrapartum management of twin gestation. Obstet Gynecol. 1985; 65:119.
124. Chervenak F, Johnson RE, Berkowitz RL, Hobbins JC. Intrapartum external version of the second twin. Obstet Gynecol. 1983;62:160.
125. Hays PM, Smeltzer JS. Multiple gestations. Clin Obstet Gynecol. 1986;29:264.
126. Kaplan B, Peled Y, Rabinerson D, et al. Successful external version of B twin after the birth of A twin for vertex non vertex twins. Eur J Obstet Gynecol Reprod Biol. 1995;58:157-60.
127. Bishop EH. Pelvic scoring for elective induction. Obstet Gynecol. 1964;24:266.
128. Boozarjomehri F, Timor-Trisch I, Chao C. Transvaginal sonography– an objective evaluation of the cervix in labor: presence of cervical wedging is associated with shorter duration of labor for induction. Am J Obstet Gynecol. 1994; 170:374.
129. Sujata Chandra S, Crane JMG, Hutchens DRN, et al. Transvaginal ultrasound and digital examination in predicting successful labor induction. Obstet Gynecol. 2001;98(1):2-6.
130. Reis FM, Gervasi MT, Florio P, et al. Prediction of successful induction of labor at term, role of clinical history, digital examination, ultrasound assessment of the cervix, and the fetal fibronectin assay. Am J Obstet Gynecol. 2003;189:1361-7.
131. Rane SM, Guirgis RR, Higgins B, et al. The value of ultrasound in the prediction of successful induction of labor. Ultrasound Obstet Gynecol. 2004;24 (5):538-49.
132. Yang SH, Roh CR, Kim JH. Transvaginal ultrasonography for cervical assessment before induction of labor. J Ultrasound Med. 2004; 23;375-82.
133. Rane SM, Guirgis RR, Higgins B, et al. Pre induction sonographic measurement of cervical length in prolonged pregnancy the effect of parity in the prediction of the need for Cesarean section. Ultrasound Obstet Gynecol. 2003;22(1):45-8.
134. Rane SM, Pandis GK, Guirgis RR, et al. Pre induction sonographic measurement of cervical length in prolonged pregnancy the effect of parity in the prediction of induction to delivery interval. Ultrasound Obstet Gynecol. 2003;22(1):40-4.
135. Mastrogiannis DS, Knuppel RA. Critical management of the very low birth weight infant and macrosomic fetus. Clin Perinatol. 1996;23:51-89.
136. Roman H, Verspyck E, Vercoustre L, et al. Does ultrasound examination when the cervix is unfavourable improve the prediction of failed labor induction? Ultrasound Obstet Gynecol. 2004;23(4): 357-62.
137. Wikström I, Bergström AR, Meirik O. Traumatic injury in large for dates infants. Obstet Gynecol Surv. 1989; 44:616-7.
138. Hirata GI, Medearis AI, Horenstein J. Ultrasonographic estimation of fetal weight in the clinically macrosomic fetus. Am J Obstet Gynecol. 1990;162:238.
139. Wiznitzer A. Obstructed labor and shoulder delivery. Curr Opin Obstet Gynecol. 1995;7:486-914.
140. Pearson JF. Shoulder dystocia. Curr Obstet Gynecol. 1996;6:30-4.
141. Smith RB, Lane C, Pearson JF. Shoulder dystocia: what happens at the next delivery? Br J Obstet Gynecol. 1994;101:713-5.
142. Eliot JP, Garite TJ, Freeman RK, et al. Ultrasonic prediction of fetal macrosomia in diabetic patients. Obstet Gynecol. 1982;60:159-62.
143. Cohen B, Penning S, Major C, et al. Sonographic prediction of shoulder dystocia in infants of diabetic mothers. Obstet Gynecol. 1996;88:10-3.
144. Santolaya-Forgas TJ, Meyer WJ, Gauthier DW, et al. Intrapartum fetal subcutaneous tissue/femur length ratio: An ultrasonographic clue to fetal macrosomia. IS J Obstet Gynecol. 1994;171:1072.
145. Martins ME. Vaginal birth after cesarean section. Clin Perinatol. 1996;23:141-53.
146. Rayburn W, Haraman M, Legino L, et al. Routine preoperative ultrasonography and cesarean section. Am J Perinatol. 1988;5:297-9.
147. Michaels WH, Thompson HO, Boutt A, et al. Ultrasound diagnosis of defects in the scarred lower uterine segment during pregnancy. Obstet Gynecol. 1988;71:112.
148. Herman A, Weinraub Z, Bukovsky I, et al. Dynamic ultrasonographic imaging of the third stage of labor: New perspectives into third-stage mechanisms. Am J Obstet Gynecol. 1993;168:1496-9.
149. Krapp M, Baschat AA, Hankeln M, et al. Gray scale and color Doppler sonography in the third stage of labor for early detection of failed placental separation. Ultrasound Obstet Gynecol. 2000;15:138-142.
150. Bedi DG, Salmon A, Wisett MZ et al. Ruptured uterus: sonographic diagnosis. J Clin Ultrasound. 1986;14:529-33.
151. Schiotz HA. Rupture of the uterus in labour. An unusual case followed with sonography. Arch Gynecol Obstet. 1991;249:43-5.
152. Suonio S, Saarikoski S, Kääriäinen J, et al. Intrapartum rupture of uterus diagnosed by ultrasound: a case report. Int J Gynecol Obstet. 1984;22:411-3.
153. Robinson HP. Sonar in the puerperium. Scott Med J. 1972;17:364-6.
154. Szoke B, Kiss D. The use of the ultrasonic echo technique in examining the normal and pathological involution in the puerperium. Int J Gynecol Obstet. 1976;14:513-6.
155. Rodeck CH, Newton JR. Study of the uterine cavity by ultrasound in the early puerperium. Br J Obstet Gynaecol. 1976;83:795-801.
156. Defoort P, Benijts G, Martens G, et al. Ultrasound assessment of puerperal uterine involution. Eur J Obstet Gynecol Reprod Biol. 1978;8:95-7.
157. Van Rees D, Bernstine R, Crawford W. Involution of the postpartum uterus: an ultrasonic study. J Clin Ultrasound. 1981;9:55-7.
158. Seeds JW, Chescheir NC, Wade RV. Postpartum ultrasound. Practical Sonography in Obstetrics and Gynecology, 2nd edition. Philadelphia, New York: Lippincott-Raven; 1986. pp. 347-8.
159. Madrazo BL. Postpartum Sonography. In the principle and Practice of Ultrasonography in Obstetrics and Gynecology, 3rd edn. East Norwalk: Appleton-Century-Crofts; 1985. pp. 449-56.
160. Lavery JP, Shaw LA. Sonography of the puerperal uterus. J Ultrasound Med. 1989;8:481-6.
161. Tekay A, Jouppila P. A longitudinal Doppler ultrasonographic assessment of the alterations in peripheral vascular resistance of uterine arteries and ultrasonographic findings of the involuting uterus during the puerperium. Am J Obstet Gynecol. 1993;168: 190-8.

162. Kirkinen P, Dudenhausen J, Baumann H, et al. Postpartum blood flow velocity waveforms of the uterine arteries. J Reprod Med. 1988;33:745-74.

163. Zalel Y, Gamzu R, Lidor A, et al. Color Doppler imaging in the sonohysterographic diagnosis of residual trophoblastic tissue. J Clin Ultrasound. 2002;30:222-5.

164. Achiron R, Goldenberg M, Lipitz S, et al. Transvaginal duplex Doppler ultrasonography in bleeding patients suspected of having residual trophoblastic tissue. Obstet Gynecol. 1993;81:507-11.

165. Mulic-Lutvica A, Bekuretzion M, Axelsson O, et al. Ultrasonic evaluation of the uterus and uterine cavity after normal, vaginal delivery. Ultrasound Obstet Gynecol. 2001;18:491-8.

166. Wachsberg RH, Kurtz AB, Levine CD, et al. Real-time ultrasonographic analysis of the normal postpartum uterus: technique, variability and measurements. J Ultrasound Med. 1994;13:215-21.

167. Williams JW. Regeneration of the uterine mucosa after delivery with special reference to the placental site. Am J Obstet Gynecol. 1931;22:664.

168. Hertzberg BS, Bowie JD. Ultrasound of the postpartum uterus, prediction of retained placental tissue. J Ultrasound Med. 1991;10:451-6.

169. Sakki A, Kirkiinen P. Ultrasonography of the uterus at early puerperium. Eur J Ultrasound. 1996;4:99-105.

170. Sokol ER, Casele H, Haney EI. Ultrasound examination of the postpartum uterus what is normal? J Maternal Fetal Neonat Med. 2004;15:95-9.

171. Edwards A, Ellwood DA. Ultrasonographic evaluation of the postpartum uterus. Ultrasound Obstet Gynecol. 2000;16:640-3.

172. Sharman A. Reproductive Physiology of the Post-Partum Period. Edinburgh: Livingston;1966.

173. Wachsberg RH, Kurtz AB. Gas within the endometrial cavity at postpartum US. A normal finding after spontaneous vaginal delivery. Radiology. 1992;183:431-3.

174. Alexander J, Thomas P, Sanhghera J. Treatments for secondary postpartum haemorrhage. Cochrane Database Syst Rev. 2002;(1):CD002867.

175. Dewhurst C. Secondary postpartum hemorrhage. J Obstet Gynaecol Br Commonwealth. 1966;73:53-8.

176. Hoveyda F, MacKenzie IZ. Secondary postpartum haemorrhage: incidence, morbidity and current management. Br J Obstet Gynaecol. 2001;108:927-30.

177. Malvern J, Campbell S, May P. Ultrasonic scanning of the puerperal uterus following secondary postpartum hemorrhage. J Obstet Gynecol Br Commonw. 1973;80:320-4.

178. Lee CY, Madrazo B, Drukker BH. Ultrasonic evaluation of the postpartum uterus in the management of postpartum bleeding. Obstet Gynaecol. 1981;58:227-32.

179. Carlan SJ, Scott WT, Pollack R, et al. Appearance of the uterus by ultrasound immediately after placental delivery with pathologic correlation. J Clin Ultrasound. 1997; 25(6):301-8.

180. Neill AMC, Nixon RM, Thornton S. A comparison of clinical assessment with ultrasound in the management of secondary postpartum hemorrhage. Eur J Obst Gynecol Reprod Biol. 2002;104:113-5.

181. Alcazar JL, Lopez-Garcia G, Zornoza A. A role of color velocity imaging and pulsed Doppler sonography to detect retained trophoblastic tissue. Ultrasound Obstet Gynecol. 1996;8(1):41.

182. Van Schoubroeck D, Van den Bosch T, Scharpe K, et al. Prospective evaluation of blood flow in the myometrium and uterine arteries in the puerperium. Ultrasound Obstet Gynecol. 2004;23:378-81.

183. Wolman I, Hartoov J, Amster R, et al. Transvaginal sonohysterography for the early detection of residual trophoblastic tissue. Ultrasound Obstet Gynecol. 1996; 8(1):37.

184. Deutchman ME, Hartmann KJ. Postpartum pyometra: a case report. J Fam Pract. 1993;36:449-52.

185. Baker ME, Bowie JD, Killam AP. Sonography of post cesarean-section bladder-flap hematoma. Am J Roentgenol. 1984;144:757-9.

186. Lavery JP, Howell RS, Shaw L. Ultrasonic demonstration of a phlegmona following Caesarean section – case report. J Clin Ultrasound. 1985;13:134-6.

187. Burger NF, Dararas B, Boes EGM. An echogenic evaluation during the early puerperium of the uterine wound after caesarean section. J Ultrasound Med. 1983;2:18.

188. Carson PL. Clean and dirty shadowing at US a reappraisal. Radiology. 1991;181:231-6.

189. Bennett MJ. Puerperal ultrasonic hysterography in the diagnosis of congenital uterine malformations. Br J Obstet Gynaecol. 1976;83(5):389-92.

190. Szoke B, Kiss D. The use of ultrasonic echo technique in the diagnosis of developmental anomalies of the uterus. Ann Chir Gynaecol. 1977;66(1):59-61.

191. Land JA, Stoot JE, Evers JL. Puerperal ultrasonic hysterography. Gynecol Obstet Invest. 1984;18(3):165-8.

192. Rudoff JM, Astranskas LJ, Rudoff JC, et al. Ultrasonographic diagnosis of septic pelvic thrombophlebitis. J Ultrasound Med. 1988;7:287-291.

193. Warhit JM, Fagelman D, Goldman MA, et al. Ovarian vein thrombophlebitis: diagnosis by ultrasound and CT. J Clin Ultrasound. 1984;12:301.

194. Wilson PC, Lerner RM. Diagnosis of ovarian vein thrombophlebitis by ultrasonography. J Ultrasound Med. 1983;2:187.

195. Sherer DM, Fern S, Mester J, et al. Postpartum ultrasonographic diagnosis of inferior vena cava thrombus associated with ovarian vein thrombosis. Am J Obstet Gynecol. 1997;177(2):474-5.

196. Weissman A, Grisarn D, Shenhav M, et al. Postpartum Surveillance of urinary retention by ultrasonography: the effect of epidural analgesia. Ultrasound Obstet Gynecol. 1995;6:130-4.

197. Nakai Y, Imanaka M, Nishio J, et al. Uterine blood flow velocity waveforms during early postpartum course following caesarean section. Eur J Obstet Gynecol Reprod Biol. 1997;74(2):121-4.

198. Kelly SM, Belli AM, Campbell S. Arteriovenous malformation of the uterus associated with secondary postpartum hemorrhage. Ultrasound Obstet Gynecol. 2003;21:602-5.

39 Safety of Diagnostic Ultrasound in Obstetrics

B Breyer, A Kurjak, K Maeda

INTRODUCTION

Diagnostic ultrasound has become an integral component of perinatal care. Even after widespread use for almost four decades there has not been a single known instance of identifiable adverse effects caused by the diagnostic intensity of ultrasound. Nevertheless, the need for continuing vigilance for biosafety is well recognized. It has long been recognized that, given certain circumstances, ultrasound exposure can influence biological systems. Diagnostic medical insonation, however, is generally assumed to be safe.

This chapter addresses some complex issues about safety, and presents a review of available data from literature as well as from personal experience of the authors.

PHYSICAL BACKGROUND

Ultrasound Waves

Ultrasound waves convey mechanical energy through matter by passing energy from particle to particle. Longitudinal waves induce pressure variations along their way. In soft tissues, these waves are the most common type. Other modes, like transverse or shear waves, can spread an appreciable distance, only in solids. When transmitted into bodily liquids, such waves are absorbed within a very small distance. Waves that spread only very short distances are not really of interest from a diagnostic point of view, but when considering safety, such absorption within a short distance is exactly the type of phenomenon that may be of concern. All waves attenuate very strongly in bone.

Describing Ultrasound Waves

Ultrasound waves and pulses can be described using the following parameters:

- *Propagation speed.* The average speed for longitudinal waves in human soft tissue is 1540 m/s. In calcified bones, the speed is about twice that in soft tissues. In gasses, it is about 330 m/s. Shear waves travel more slowly.

- *Wavelength* (λ) is inversely proportional to frequency. It greatly influences the resolution of diagnostic machines. The higher the frequency, the shorter the wavelength. For example, the wavelength in the body at 3 MHz is approximately 0.5 mm.

- The *pulse length* for Doppler measurements is often longer than for B-mode imaging. These pulses are transmitted at a repetition frequency typically of the order of a few kilohertz (kHz).

- The *attenuation* of ultrasound is proportional to frequency. Absorption causes heating of tissues.

- *Ultrasound pressure amplitude* is the maximum pressure induced by the compressional wave at a point in the tissue. If we operate with continuous wave [as in fetal cardiotocographic (CTG) monitoring] the wave is continuous. If, however, we use pulses (such as in imaging), ultrasound is transmitted in the form of short pulses and the maximum positive (compressional), maximum negative (rarefaction) and average pressure during the pulse or during the total time must be taken into account.

Energy is measured in watt seconds or joules; *power* is measured in watts and *intensity* is measured in watts per square meter or centimeter. The *attenuation* property is measured in decibels per centimeter per megahertz.

In diagnostic applications, ultrasound waves are mainly used in the form of beams and are usually transmitted in the form of pulses. In pulse applications, the energy flow exists in time only during the pulse. Considering an example when the pulse duration is one-thousandth of the repetition period, then the intensity during the pulse is about 1,000 times higher than the overall time average intensity.

Ultrasound beams can be focused in various ways, but the important feature from the safety standpoint is that focusing concentrates ultrasound energy and thus, potentially, increases the hazard. For safety consideration, only transmission focusing is relevant. In scanning applications the beam moves, while in Doppler spectrometry and M-mode imaging one tends to keep the beam in one position for a prolonged time.

The ultrasound pulse consists of a few pressure oscillations around the static atmospheric pressure. When considering safety, the positive peak pressure p_c and the negative peak pressure p_r play a role. At p_c high intensities the positive peak pressure may become a few times higher than the negative peak pressure. These effects are much more expressed in liquids in which there is little attenuation compared to human tissues in which attenuation is much greater.

Acoustic Parameters used to Describe Ultrasound Exposure

In order to concisely and exactly describe ultrasound waves in regard to their potential hazard a multitude of parameters are used. Intensity was the first such parameter. Later, it was recognized that this was not enough and, therefore, additional parameters were introduced:

- *Acoustic power* output is the total acoustic power that exits from a transmitting transducer. In commercial B-mode instruments the power ranges between 0.3 mW and 280 mW; in color Doppler mapping between 15 mW and 400 mW; in pulsed Doppler spectrometry between 10 mW and 450 mW.[1–3]

- *Spatial peak temporal average intensity* (I_{SPTA}) is the intensity averaged over time, but measured in the position of the spatial peal (focus). When considering the potential hazard of heating, we take this I_{SPTA} into account. In commercial B-mode instruments this ranges between 0.3 mW/cm^2 and 990 mW/cm^2; in color Doppler mapping between 20 mW/cm^2 and 2000 mW/cm^2; and in pulse Doppler spectrometers between 170 mW/cm^2 and 9000 mW/cm^2.

- The intensity at the point of maximum pressure in a pulse is the *pulse peak intensity*. This is the temporal peal intensity.
- When considering the potential hazard of cavitation, *spatial peak pulse average* (I_{SPPA}) is among the significant parameters. In commercial pulsed Doppler instruments this ranges between 1 W/cm^2 and 770 W/cm^2.
- *Peak negative pressure* is also among the parameters for evaluation of the cavitation probability. It is easier to measure than the peak positive pressure, which may be greatly distorted in shape. The peak pressure varies in all types of modern equipment between 0.4 MPa and 5 MPa.[1–3]

The above parameters play a role in the body, but are far easier to measure in water. In addition, it is much easier to standardize them in water. Two approaches are used: the measurement of all parameters in water or the immediate calculation of the in situ values taking into account conventional standard attenuation values, e.g. 0.3 dB/cm MHz. The bone is considered to be very attenuating, so that nearly all the energy is absorbed within a short path. Various organ or situation models have been conceived to represent specific situations, e.g. full bladder and uterus with an embryo.

Instrument Properties and Acoustic Output

In purely practical terms, it is necessary to know what properties of the scanners are important for their safe use, both when acquiring a new machine and when using existing ones. Some properties are inherent to the instrument while others depend on the application and the way in which the instrument is used.

Heating of tissues is proportional to I_{SPTA} in situ. The general trend for an increase in the output of diagnostic ultrasound instruments.[1] Since 1980s, there have been instruments in the market with I_{SPTA} above 1 W/cm^2 in pulsed Doppler operation regimens.[2] The actual intensity greatly depends on the mode of operation and settings (ALARA principle[4,5] should be obeyed). The lowest intensity is used in fetal heart monitors [continuous wave (CW) Doppler systems with the intensity below 100 W/cm^2], and then in order of increasing intensities: B-mode imaging scanners, 2D Doppler machines and pulsed Doppler instruments. In many instruments, it is possible to operate in various regimens. High-end scanners normally have the possibility of quasi-parallel operation in various regimens, e.g. gray scale, 2D flow mapping and Doppler spectrometry "at the same time". In fact, the scanner switches quickly between the various modes.

The actual acoustic power and pressures in the pulses greatly depends on the mode of operation, depth and length of examination also influence the exposure. The frequency influences the penetration ability and thus may influence the acoustic power used. For example, the use of higher frequency intracavitary probes implies two opposite effects, i.e. the scanning distance (range) is reduced, but the frequency is increased and therefore, the attenuation per centimeter is reduced. Thus, the acoustic energy traversing the region of interest is about the same.

In the current commercially available instrumentation, I_{SPTA} varies with the mode: in B-mode imaging the median in 35 mW/cm^2; in M-mode the median is about 100 mW/cm^2; in 2D velocity mapping (color Doppler) the median is about 290 mW/cm^2 and in pulsed Doppler the median is 1200 mW/cm.^{2} The factor of increase of intensity between the various modes is about three from mode to mode.[1–3]

Another source of heat may be heating of the transducer because of internal dissipation. When intracavitary probes are used this may be a factor for serious consideration. The extent of heating depends on the probe design and materials used.

Cavitation is less likely with short pulses. In B-mode imaging, the pulse length is usually less than 0.5 μs, but in pulsed Doppler applications it can be up to 20 μs. It is possible to control this length by varying the "sample volume". Shorter "sample volumes" generally yield smaller I_{SPTA}.

ULTRASOUND THERAPY

In order to have a feeling of what these intensities may mean it is worth mentioning that the ultrasound machines used in physical therapy operates at intensities between 0.5 mW/cm^2 and 3 mW/cm^2. Therapy using these machines is based on tissue heating, particularly heating of boundaries between soft and connective tissue and bones. There exists an extensive body of data[1–3] on ultrasound machine outputs.

There is the ever-developing ultrasound-treatment field that includes lithotripsy, physiotherapy and "ultrasound knives" of various types, particularly of brain and liver surgery. Therefore, it is sensible to consider how these applications, where the biological effect is the essence of the application, compare to diagnostic applications where, in ideal cases, information is gathered without causing any biological effect.

Physiotherapy devices use continuous waves or very long pulses of intensity between 0.5 W/cm^2 and 3 W/cm^2. The mechanism used is heating. The therapist must continuously move the probe in order not to overheat some structure in the patient.

Lithotripsy is done with short pulses that "bang" on the stones. Their average intensity is fairly low compared to the effects on the stones. However, their acoustic pressures are very high, reaching nearly 10 Mpa. The range of pressures overlaps with the diagnostic equipment.

The important difference between these therapy applications and the diagnostic applications is the frequency, normally 10–50 times lower in therapy.

The application of ultrasound for treatment of disease in the mother may inadvertently lead to damage to the fetus if serious precautions are not taken.

SAFETY OF DIAGNOSTIC ULTRASOUND IN OBSTETRICS

Obstetrics is a particularly sensitive field. A general rule is that fast growing and developing tissues are more sensitive to outside influences. This applies to embryonic and fetal tissues in particular. The potential hazard varies in extent and nature during the intrauterine development.

Before implantation, physical stress can cause abortion. After implantation, various tissues and organs become susceptible to damage at different times. Between 5 weeks and 10 weeks of gestation, the neural tube is prone to damage; the forebrain development is particularly important until the 20th week of gestation. The development of the right and left side of the brain is not symmetrical in time, and nor is the end result. Thus, it is important to be aware of possible neurological effects and that such effects may show as some sort of sidedness.

Heating and its Effects

The human body is a thermodynamic system. Chemical reactions depend on the temperature. The sensitivity of the reactions dictates the very narrow temperature span in which the human body operates well.

A very long temperature increase of 1.5°C above 37°C does not present a health hazard for humans.[6–10] It has been shown that exposure of mouse embryos for 5 minutes to a temperature increase of 4°C is hazardous for their development. The temperature range between the two extremes both in temperature and duration is the present "gray zone" of knowledge. Consensus is that exposure of adult proliferative tissue to heat at 42°C for up to 2 hours[11] can cause only reparable damage. The effects are proportional to I_{SPTA} and absorption coefficient. The absorption coefficient is proportional to frequency. Absorption also depends on the tissue type. In the case of longitudinal waves, absorption is at least an order of magnitude greater in bone than in soft tissues. Bodily fluids absorb very little, so that they are unlikely to heat up due to the traversing of ultrasound. Tissues with high connective tissue content absorb more. However, they allow little attenuated ultrasound to reach structures positioned beyond them. On the other hand, the absorption of shear waves is very high in soft tissues and thus, if any shear wave is induced in a bone it will be absorbed within a millimeter in the adjacent soft tissue. This may then significantly increase the temperature on such a boundary. Blood vessels and perfusion in the target area act as a cooling system and take the heat away. If the perfusion is poor the heat may accumulate. Fatty tissue and bones are structures with relatively poor perfusion and little consequent cooling. The heating may have multiple maxima, i.e. near the transducer at the focus and at specific media interfaces. The main problem may be the heating of nervous tissue caused by absorption within itself, by heating at the adjacent bone/soft tissue boundaries (skull vertebrae). The same applies to bone marrow.[12] While it is known that hyperthermia can be teratogenic in animals, there is no confirmed study in large mammals confirming that diagnostic ultrasound-induced hyperthermia causes such effects. It should be borne in mind that a higher body temperature, e.g. due to fever, may increase the damaging ultrasound energy.

Non-thermal Effects

Effects other than thermal are conceivable. In 1972, Hill considered the possibility of mechanical effects.[13] Either cavitation, or other forces induced by altering compression, and rarefaction forces may damage the molecules of which the body is composed. Transient cavitation is known to have damaging potential, since collapsing bubbles generate shock waves that disrupt nearby structures. The temperature at the point of implosion is extremely high (a few thousand degrees). In addition, relatively stable, oscillating bubbles induce microstreaming of liquids around them, possibly causing changes in metabolism or mechanical damage to cell membranes. If cavitation is a possible cause of hazard then the mechanical index (MI)[14,15] accepted by the Food and Drug Administration[16] might yield some means of comparing various scanners and modes of operation.

In order to measure the pressure in situ, it is necessary to take into account the attenuation in the intervening tissue. Using this convention, the attenuation is taken to be 0.3 dB/cm MHz. It is a good idea to have this index displayed on the screen in order to choose the operation regimen that yields the required data while maintaining the MI as low as possible.

Streaming[17,18] of absorbing and attenuating liquids due to ultrasound passage is due to the variation of energy concentration along the path (actually it is the change of the impulse). It depends on the attenuation coefficient of the liquid and its viscosity. Particles in the liquid can contribute to streaming. A particular type of streaming is microstreaming around an oscillating gas bubble.

The basic biological effect that would cause concern in the case of collapsing bubbles is the generation of free radicals. This could lead to alteration of chromosomes. If the free radicals are formed outside the membrane, the time needed for transport of such radicals to the nucleus is longer than their half-life. However, there is no confirmed evidence of chromosomal effects, particularly in living mammals.

Another possible non-thermal mechanism may be due to direct mechanical vibration of cell membranes. This might cause changes in ion (calcium in particular) permeability.[4]

The soft-tissue to gas boundary may present a particularly favorable situation for mechanical effects since the gas side presents very low resistance. Rarefaction pressures may present a potential hazard when using high-energy Doppler with the beam hitting the lung.[19] However, the fetal lung is not at such risk since it is not filled with air. The reports of change in neurological development such as speech and handed-ness[20–22] have not been confirmed by independent studies.

Clinical Aspects

The whole body of knowledge concerning the biological effects of ultrasound is relevant only if it helps in the estimation of whether diagnostic ultrasound as used today is hazardous for the patients and, if so, to what extent. It should be noted that even a significant change in rare conditions (for example those that appear once in 10,000) may not be detectable because the statistics require to a great number of controlled cases. In such investigations, we must concentrate on the type of damage that is most likely to occur, based on the understanding of the underlying mechanisms. Due to the bone/soft tissue interface the central nervous system is the most likely candidate for thermal damage. Damage of a small area in the brain may not yield easily detectable consequences unless it affects a sensory mechanism (vision, hearing, etc.). Other organs, once they consist of a large number of cells, can repair partial mechanical damage. If the damage happens early, destruction of a small number of cells may have very serious late consequences in the form of defective development.

While there is no independently confirmed experimental proof of such damage, the indications are that any effects are obtained only when the temperature rises by more than 2°C for a few minutes. Using scanned beams and modern equipment, it is very improbable that such a long time would be spent at one spot.

The application of echo/contrasts ought to be restricted to adult scanning for the time being since the existence of microbubbles may increase the probability of non-thermal effects.

In vitro experiments yield a variety of demonstrated effects.[13,23,24] Such experiments can help indicate the direction of investigation in whole organisms, but they lack the important property of living tissues, namely that the individual cells are interconnected in a tissue unlike cells suspended in a culture. Under such conditions, the probability of non-thermal mechanisms occurring is much higher than in whole tissues.

All the experimental indications of damage caused by diagnostic ultrasound, although independently confirmed, indicate that the probability is low. This means that in practice caution is advised, but no absolute recommendation against the use of diagnostic ultrasound measurements is advised.

Standards and Labeling Recommendations

There are no easy methods for measuring the temperature increase in a patient in vivo. Thus, it is necessary to resort to estimates based on experimental work. Present solutions to this problem are certainly approximate and partial, but the pressure of the reality warrants such approaches. The National Council on Radiation Protection and Measurements (NCRP) and the American Institute of Ultrasound in Medicine/National Electrical Manufacturers Association (AIUM/NEMA)[14] have developed models. The latter body has devised an index for estimating the heating likelihood that is not expected to be exceeded under normal circumstances. This so-called thermal index (TI) may be displayed on the screen to give the operator real-time relative guidance on the potential heating of the tissues scanned. The value applies to the situation in situ. There exists no internationally accepted standard for any of the proposed indicators of thermal hazard. The AIUM/NEMA TI provides an estimate of temperature increase. By convention, TI is the ratio of total acoustic power to the acoustic power required to raise tissue temperature by 1°C. Although, its basis is an approximate calculation of the actual temperature increase for a "standard" tissue at a distance, it may not be interpreted literally. It is a relative indication of the possible temperature increase. The subvariants of the TI are meant for specific situations, i.e. TIS for homogeneous soft tissue, TIC for temperature increase of bone near the surface (e.g. skull) and TIB for temperature increase at the bone boundary in the beam focus area. Using this labeling standard, if the scanner is not capable of producing a TI of more than 1, it does not have to be displayed. Other national and international bodies have conceived other estimation means. The capability of an ultrasound system to cause heating may be described by the ratio of acoustic power to the maximum temperature rise. The idea is to perform an actual worst-case calculation and to define the conditions (and instrument settings) that yield the maximum temperature increase, so that all else is less hazardous. This is still in development as a consensus about the tissue and beam properties has not been achieved.[11] Various sources give differing data[9,25–28] on ultrasound absorption in tissues and its action upon them. Nevertheless, the ultimate aim should be a consensus in recommendations given by various bodies and organizations. This should be based on realistic estimates of the possibility of ultrasound-induced heating. This is, among other things, an important guideline for the industry to discontinue the increase in ultrasound energy outputs in new apparatus models.

This leads to guideline conclusions by expert groups, e.g. European Federation of Societies of Ultrasound in Medicine and Biology (EFSUMB) Watchdogs or the AIUM bioeffects committee that came to the consensus that when using the I_{SPTA} of 720 mW/cm², the maximum temperature rise in situ would not exceed 2°C, thus will be safe to use. The present FDA regulation gives I_{SPTA} values of

720, 430, 94, 17 mW/cm² for peripheral vessel, cardiac, fetal and ophthalmic (i.e. eye lens) applications, respectively. The regulation is not limited to I_{SPTA} but includes a MI. Measurements in humans would be difficult or unduly aggressive and thus are impossible. Experiments on excised tissue or experimental animals can not be directly extrapolated to humans but give important guidelines as to where to look for danger. The time-limited soft-tissue experiments with ultrasound pulses equivalent to pulsed Doppler mode have shown heating below 2.5°C in various experiments. However, higher temperature increases have been measured in animals at skull bone/brain boundaries.[11]

THE SAFETY OF DOPPLER ULTRASOUND

In general, it is emphasized that ultrasonic examination should be performed only for medical indications, and diagnostic ultrasound users should recognize the sensitivity of young biological tissues of developing embryos and fetuses exposed to intense ultrasound.[10] The users also should know ultrasonic intensity of their devices, the mechanisms of ultrasound bio-effect, and the prudent use of the devices, because they are responsible for the ultrasound safety. An important ultrasound bioeffect is thermal effect due to temperature rise induced by ultrasound absorption, because malformations were reported in the exposure of animal embryos and fetuses to high temperature in biological experiments. No hazardous thermal effect is expected when the temperature rise of exposed tissue is less than 1.5°C, and local temperature is lower than 38.5°C.[32] Five minutes exposure to 41°C temperature can be hazardous to the tissue. Inertial cavitation and other mechanical effects are concerned in the non-thermal bioeffects of ultrasound.

The Intensity of Doppler Ultrasound

No hazardous thermal effect is expected in common B-mode imaging device because of minimum heat production due to low ultrasound intensity, i.e. World Federation of Ultrasound in Medicine and Biology (WFUMB)[32] concluded that the use of simple imaging equipment is not contraindicated on thermal grounds. The real-time B-mode, simple three-dimensional (3D) and four-dimensional (4D) imaging devices, ultrasonic fetal heart beat detector and fetal monitor are included in the category. Diagnostic ultrasound safety was established in Japan, after the Japanese Industrial Standard regulated the output power of diagnostic ultrasound devices below 10 mW/cm² in 1980, which was 1/100 of hazardous CW ultrasound[38-40] intensity at 1 w/cm². However, ultrasound safety has been discussed again after the introduction of Doppler flow velocity measurement, because pulsed Doppler method required definitely higher power than B-mode ultrasound.

Maximum intensity of commercial Doppler ultrasound is 1–3 W/cm². It is definitely higher than that of B-mode imaging, and it is the level of ultrasound physiotherapy for the tissue heating. Ultrasound safety is warned even in the physiotherapy, e.g. therapeutic transducer should be always moved on the bone, young bone and pregnant woman is contraindicated to the physiotherapy. The difference between therapeutic ultrasound and pulsed Doppler is exposure duration, i.e. it is short in Doppler flow measurement and long in therapeutic ultrasound. Therefore, thermal effect is big concern in Doppler ultrasound bioeffect. Temperature rises not only at the sample volume, but also in all tissues passed by the ultrasound beam. The International Society of Ultrasound in Obstetrics and gynecology (ISUOG) also discussed the safe use of

Doppler ultrasound.[37] Ultrasound intensity is less in color/power Doppler flow mapping than pulsed Doppler due to the scanning procedure than stable irradiation of pulsed Doppler. Also temporal averaging intensity of common color Doppler ultrasound is less than 720 mW/cm[2], which is lower than pulsed Doppler devices, and lower than FDA regulation.[16] Thermal effect is discussed in the first place, due to possible teratogenicity of heating. Exposure duration is important for the safety of Doppler velocimetry.

The Effect of Heating on Mammal Fetuses

A teratogenic effect was reported by the biologists after the exposure of animal embryos and fetuses to high temperature, namely, malformations were found in various species by experimental heating. The temperature was 39° to 50°C. Teratogenic effect on mammals are summarized in the report of National Council for Radiation Protection and Measurement (NCRP).[33] A discrimination line is found between the hazardous and no hazardous areas in the NCRP report. There is no malformation, if the fetus is heated in the area under the discrimination line which is determined by connecting the points of high temperature/short exposure and low temperature/long exposure. Non-hazardous exposure is as short as 1 minute in 43°C, and infinite in physiological body temperature. In case of ultrasound irradiation, TI indicates the temperature rise, therefore, absolute temperature is obtained by summing 37°C and the temperature rise derived from TI.

Non-Hazardous Exposure Time of the Fetus to the Heating

The guideline on the safety of mammals against the heat can be found in the revised safety statement of American Institute of Ultrasound in Medicine (AIUM)[35] published in 1998, which is based on the NCRP report in 1992, where inverse relation was found between hazardous temperature level and exposure time.

AIUM[35] stated that the fetus tolerates 50 hours at 2°C rise (absolute temperature is 39°C), and 1 minute at 6°C rise (43°C). They also showed the relation of the temperature rise (T) above 37°C and non-hazardous exposure time *(t* min) by the equation 1, and non-hazardous time *(t* min) is known with the equation 2, which is revised from equation 1:

$$T\ (°C) = 6 - \{(\log_{10} t)/0.6\} \tag{1}$$
$$t = 10^{(3.6-0.6T)} \tag{2}$$

The relation of non-hazardous exposure time and the temperature rise as well as absolute temperature is known by the equation 2 (Table 39.1 and Fig. 39.1). The safety regarding

Table 39.1: Non-hazardous exposure time (*t* min) to the temperature rise above 37°C and absolute temperature is calculated by the equation 2 which is obtained from the results of experimental heating of animal fetus[33]

Temperature rise (°C)	Absolute temperature (°C)	Non-hazardous exposure time; *t* (*t* min)	Log *t*
1	38	1000.0	3.00
2	39	251.8	2.40
3	40	63.10	1.80
4	41	15.85	1.20
5	42	3.98	0.60
6	43	1.0	0

the thermal effect of ultrasound can be discussed by the relation of exposure time and the temperature, when the heat production of Doppler ultrasound is estimated from TI, which indicates the temperature rise above 37°C in the worst-case of temperature rise in ultrasound exposure to standardized tissue model, i.e. maximum temperature rise is known by TI.

Keeping the Safety of Doppler Sonography

General Safety of Diagnostic Ultrasound Device

Electrical and mechanical safety is proved in ultrasound devices by the manufacturer under international and domestic guidelines. In a Doppler scanner, TI, MI, transducer temperature and other related indices are displayed on the monitor screen[34] making the users to keep the safety of ultrasound diagnosis by themselves. Obstetric setting should be confirmed before Doppler flow velocity measurements during pregnancy. Ultrasonic examinations should be done under medical indications. Although ISUOG safety statement [37] reported that there is no reason to withhold the use of scanners that have received current FDA clearance in the absence of gas bodies, AIUM[35] stated that for the current FDA[16] regulatory limit of 720 mW/cm[2], the best available estimate of the maximum temperature increase can exceed 2°C. Pulsed ultrasound intensity threshold to suppress cultured cell-growth curve was 240 mW/cm[2] in our studies.[40] The FDA regulation may be still controversial from the opinions and reports.

Thermal Effect of Doppler Scanner

The TI is a useful index of temperature rise induced by ultrasound exposure. Standard tissue models are exposed to ultrasound and TI is determined in the worst-case, i.e. the highest temperature rise is the base of TI.[34] One TI stands for one degree C temperature elevation, and in the same manner, temperature rises for 3°C above 37°C, and absolute temperature is 40°C, if TI is 3. Local temperature rise is estimated only by TI at present, therefore, TI is the index to estimate tissue temperature in ultrasound examination, to study ultrasonic thermal effect, and to avoid possible thermal hazard of intense ultrasound. TI is small and temperature rise is low in the soft tissue exposure, and TI is large and temperature rise is high in the bone exposure. Soft tissue TI (TIS) is, therefore, used in

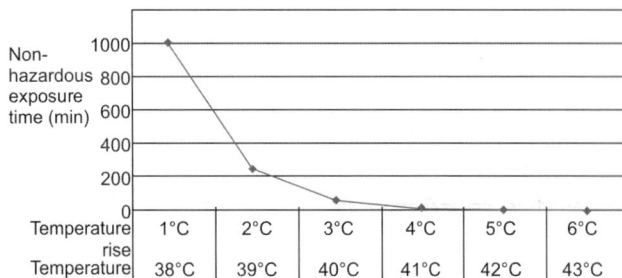

Fig. 39.1: Non-hazardous exposure time to the temperature rise between 1°C and 6°C above 37°C (38° – 43°C of absolute temperature) in experimental heating of animal fetuses[33] (graphed by the equation 2)

case of embryo which has no bone before 10 weeks of pregnancy, and bone TI (TIB) is applied in the fetus with bone after 10 weeks. Cranial TI (TIC) is the index for the intracranial flow examination.

No hazardous thermal effect is expected when the temperature rise of exposed tissue is less than 1.5°C, and local temperature is lower than 38.5°C, while 5 minutes duration of 41°C can be hazardous to the tissue. Its temperature rise is 4°C above 37°C, and TI can be 4. Ultrasound examination is totally safe in the exposure with the TI less than one. In common daily practice, therefore, TI should be less than one, particularly in long fetal examination, screening of pregnancy, or the research study of no limit. The output power is reduced, if the TI is higher than one on the monitor, then TI decreases to the level lower than one.[34] Clear flow velocity wave form is recorded even output power is reduced to 60% in the author's experiment on the small hand artery.

Revised safety statement of American Institute of Ultrasound in Medicine (AIUM)[35] stated that equal or less than 2°C temperature rise above 37°C showed no adverse effects with exposure duration up to 50 hours, and that the upper limit of safe exposure duration was 16 minutes at 4°C rise and 1 minutes at 6°C rise above normal, respectively. The AIUM opinion on the effect of high temperature is similar to the report of NCRP,[33] and the safety statement is acceptable, if the temperature rise is accurately determined by the TI, because TI indicates the worst tissue temperature elevation due to ultrasound exposure in clinical study.

Although revised safety statement is useful in a retrospective safety confirmation after ultrasound exposure of known exposure time and TI, fetal exposure to the temperature rise for 4–6°C may be controversial, where absolute temperature is 41–43°C. Non-hazardous exposure time at such temperature higher than 40°C is critically short in the NCRP report[33] and AIUM statement,[35] where safe margin remains very narrow, excess heating may not be completely avoided, and it may be imperfect to precisely keep strict exposure time in the highest temperature. The aim of this report is, therefore, to propose practically applicable safe exposure time in the prospective situation before a Doppler ultrasound diagnosis.

Two Modes in the Exposure Time to Diagnostic Ultrasound

Two modes can be classified in the use of Doppler ultrasound. The TI lower than one (AIUM), or the temperature rise below 1.5°C (WFUMB) after temperature equilibrium can be adopted for the infinite exposure. Therefore, the mode is suitable for research work, where exposure duration is hardly expected before studying. TI may also be lower than one in the screening of fetus during pregnancy and in the fetal heart rate monitoring.

A pulsed Doppler study is another situation, where the user requires improved Doppler flow wave by using higher TI than one. In some ultrasound lectures, speakers used to tell us higher TI than one in the Doppler studies, where they proved the safety by shortened exposure. The technique is the same as the NCRP report[33] which proved non-hazardous short exposure to high temperature. Therefore, the Doppler examination with the TI higher than one can be also non-hazardous by the short exposure.

The relation among non-hazardous exposure to high temperature, high temperature rise, and large TI is achieved by the application of the author's equation 2 (Table 39.1 and Fig. 39.1). Exposure time is as long as 250 minutes, about 4 hour, when TI is 2

and temperature is 39°C, 1 hour if TI is 3 and temperature 40°C, and 15 minutes even if TI is 4, where the temperature is 41°C according to the reports of NCRP[33] and AIUM.[35] These criteria is extremely useful in the retrospective confirmation of Doppler ultrasound safety of past examination. However, the prospective exposure time setting before examination should be further discussed.

Prospective Exposure Time Setting before Doppler Examination

Exposure time is preset before the Doppler examination, where the TI is voluntarily increased to be higher than one with the intension to improve Doppler flow. NCRP report is the base of decision, where non-hazardous exposure time is determined by the temperature rise estimated by TI (Tables 39.1 and 39.2, Fig. 39.1). It is unique in the present proposal that obtained non-hazardous exposure time is divided by the "safety factor" of 3 – 100, and actual exposure time is obtained. The procedure was the same as the past regulation of simple ultrasound devices in Japan, where hazardous threshold intensity of CW ultrasound in our experimental study was divided by the safety factor of 100 and output intensity was regulated to be lower than 10 mW/cm^2. There was no problem in the safety of diagnostic ultrasound before the introduction of Doppler flow studies. Although, the factor is voluntarily changed by the user, appropriate value will be discussed in this paper. As ultrasound intensity may increase for about 3 times in case of standing wave, 3 is the lowest safety factor. The intensity increases due to the distortion of ultrasound wave, and possible estimation error of TI[11] or others are further added the safety factor.

For example, non-hazardous exposure time is 252 minutes at 39°C (Table 39.1), where the temperature rises for 2°C and corresponding TI is 2. If the safety factor is 50, 252 minutes is divided by 50, and the exposure time is 5 minutes. By the same procedure, 1 minutes' exposure time is preset when TI is 3 (Table 39.2). The safety factor of 100 may be too conservative, although the factor can be selected by the user. Mildly longer exposure than preset value may be included in the safety factor in most cases. Possibly 50 is appropriate safety factor in the actual Doppler examination. The exposure time setting is coincidentally close to the safety statement of British Medical Ultrasound Society (BMUS),[41] where the exposure time is 4 minutes when the TI is 2 and 1 minutes if TI is 2.5.

The users can voluntarily change the safety factor and prolong the exposure time, because they are responsible to the ultrasound safety. However, they may also be responsible at the same time for the increased risk factor caused by the reduction of safety factor.

Other Thermal Issues

Ultrasound thermal effect has been discussed mainly in the relation to teratogenicity in the first trimester, whereas animal fetal skull or the brain surface was heated and the temperature elevation was more than 4°C by the exposure to intense ultrasound.[36] Thermal damage of the brain can not be denied in the case. Therefore, the use of maximum intensity level of Doppler ultrasound is inadvisable in the flow study even in late pregnancy.

Caution should be paid regarding the temperature of the tissue exposed to Doppler ultrasound in febrile patients, where the basic temperature is higher than 37°C. For example, if TI is 2 in 38°C febrile patient, the temperature rise above physiologic

Table 39.2: Thermal index (TI), tissue temperature, non-hazardous exposure time in the NCRP report 2, the safety factors and exposure time to ultrasound are listed. Although the user can voluntarily set the safety factor and exposure time, the author recommends to choose the safety factor at 50 and exposure time at 5 minutes when TI is 2

TI	Absolute temperature (°C)	Non-hazardous exposure time of NCRP report 2 (min)	Exposure time (min) obtained by dividing non-hazardous exposure time of NCRP report 2 by various safety factors			
				Safety factor		
			3	10	50	100
6	43	1	0.3	0.1	.02	0.01 (no use)
4	41	16	5	0.2	.03	0.02 (no use)
3	40	64	21	6	1	0.6
2	39	256	85	25	5	2.5

condition is 3°C, the situation is the same as TI 3 in non-febrile normal temperature case, and therefore, 1 minute of exposure time is allowed if the safety factor is 50.

Exposure duration should be recorded by the user in every study of voluntarily increased exposure time, while TI which appeared on the monitor screen are recorded on the photograph or computer memory. The safety indices including TI and MI are recommended to be described in the "Methods" of the reports of Doppler ultrasound study on human subjects.

Transducer Temperature in Transvaginal Scan

Transvaginal scan user should be careful on the direct heating of the attached tissue due to high surface temperature of the transducer, which directly attach vaginal wall, and the subjects are closer to the transducer than to abdominal ultrasound. The transducer temperature, which is displayed on the monitor screen, should be lower than 41°C. Every intracavitary scan user should also be careful on the transducer temperature.

Mechanical Effects of Diagnostic Ultrasound

Mechanical index is used for the estimation of mechanical bioeffect. It is rarefactional sound pressure expressed in Mega-Pascal (MPa), divided by square root of ultrasound frequency (MHz). The MI indicates non-thermal bioeffect of ultrasound particularly in the collapse of gas bubbles in various liquids. Although gynecologic examination by contrast medium is still infrequent, its common use in adult circulation should be carefully studied in the mechanical bioeffect. Although common B-mode imaging devices are low in the thermal effect, its mechanical effect is similar to the Doppler devices because instantaneous intensity of its ultrasound pulse is not much different from Doppler machines, and therefore, even simple imaging devices should be carefully handled in the relation to mechanical effect. It is rare to use contrast medium in obstetrical tissue, free radicals formed in the liquid due to inertial cavitation hardly reaches floating cells because of their short life, and no

cavitation may occur within the cell due to the high viscosity of cell plasma. However, biological effects of acoustic streaming, capillary blood cell stasis by the standing wave, or the direct ultrasonic pressure require further basic studies. As hemorrhage is found in the lung of neonatal animals after the exposure to intense ultrasound, lower MI than one is recommended particularly in neonatal lung examination. International Electrotechnical Commission (IEC) is working on the classification of diagnostic ultrasound devices by the MI.

CONCLUSION

Diagnostic ultrasound safety has been mainly discussed on the thermal effect. Simple real-time B-mode, 3D and 4D imaging devices, fetal heart detector and fetal monitor, are not contraindicated due to thermal effect, because of their very low ultrasound intensity. Doppler flow machines are mainly discussed with thermal effect, because of their definitely high ultrasound intensity. Safe fetal exposure time to ultrasound determined by the NCRP criteria on the exposure to high temperature estimated by TI is useful in the retrospective evaluation of past ultrasound examination. In prospective estimation of ultrasound safety in daily practice, the principle of safe diagnostic ultrasound is the reduction of ultrasonic intensity and exposure time when displayed TI is above one. The research work and pregnancy screening follow the principle. Moderately higher TI is allowed in clinical study when the users require more improved Doppler flow wave by increased intensity, where a limited short exposure time is prescribed and the users adhere the preset time by their own responsibility. The author recommends to use non-hazardous exposure time of NCRP report after dividing it by the safety factor of 50, where exposure time is 5 minutes if TI is 2, and 1 minutes if TI is 3. Higher TI or longer exposure may be applied by reducing safety factor under the users' responsibility. Attention should be paid to the decreased safety in febrile patient. Transvaginal transducer should be used under 41°C. The mechanical effect may be similar in simple B-mode to Doppler devices. MI is recommended to be less than one in ultrasound examination, particularly in the studies on air containing neonatal lung.

REFERENCES

1. Starrit HC, Duck FA. A comparison of ultrasound exposure in therapy and pulsed Doppler fields. Br J Radiol. 1992;65:557-63.
2. American Institute of Ultrasound in Medicine (AIUM). Acoustical Data for Diagnostic Ultrasound Equipment. AIUM. 1993.
3. Henderson J, Willson K, Jago JR, et al. A survey of acoustic outputs of diagnostic ultrasound equipment in current clinical use. Ultrasound Med Biol. 1995;21:699-705.
4. International Commission on Radiation Protection. Recommendation for Radiation Protection, ICRP Publication 26. New York: Pergamon. 1977.
5. International Commission on Radiation Protection. Recommendation for Radiation Protection, ICRP Publication 60. New York: Pergamon. 1991.
6. MacDonald W, Newham J, Gurrin L, et al. Effect of frequent prenatal ultrasound on birthweight: follow-up at one year of age. Lancet. 1996;348:482.
7. Lyons EA, Dyke C, Toms M, et al. In utero exposure to diagnostic ultrasound: a 6 year follow-up. Radiology. 1988;166:687-90.
8. Smith CB. Birthweights of fetuses exposed to diagnostic ultrasound. J Ultrasound Med. 1984;3:395-6.
9. Saari Kemppainen A, Karjalainen O, Ylostalo P, et al. Ultrasound screening and perinatal mortality: controlled trial of systemic one-stage screening in pregnancy. The Helsinki Ultrasound Trial. Lancet. 1990;336:387-91.
10. Barnett SB, Ter Haar G, Ziskin MC, et al. Current status of research on biophysical effects of ultrasound. Ultrasound Med Biol. 1994;20:205-18.
11. Barnett SB, Kossoff G, et al. Issues and Recommendations Regarding Thermal Mechanisms for Biological Effects of Ultrasound--WFUMB Symposium on Safety and Standardization in Medical Ultrasound and Chapter 3 therein--Reasonable Worst Case Tissue Models, by Kossoff G, Carson P, Carstensen E and Preston R, pp 759-768, Ultras. in Med. & Biol., Special Issue, 18:9, 731-814, 1992.
12. Barnett SB, Edwards MJ, Martin P. Pulsed ultrasound induces temperature elevation and nuclear abnormalities in bone marrow cells of guinea pig femurs. Presented at the 6th World Congress of Ultrasound in Medicine, Copenhagen, Denmark. 1991;3405.
13. Hill CR. Ultrasonic exposure thresholds for changes in cells and tissues. J Acoust Soc Am. 1972;52:667-72.
14. American Institute of Ultrasound in Medicine. AIUM/NEMA Standard for Real-time Display of Thermal and Mechanical Acousitc Output Indices on Diagnostic Ultrasound Equipment. AIUM Publications. 1992.
15. Food and Drug Administration. Guide for Measuring and Reporting Acoustic Output of Diagnostic Ultrasound. Rockville, MD: Food and Drug Administration, Devices and Radiological Health. 1992.
16. Food and Drug Administration. Revised 510(k) diagnostic ultrasound guidance for 1993. Rockville, MD: Food and Drug Administration. 1993.
17. Nyborg WL. Acoustic streaming due to attenuated plan waves. J Acoust Soc Am. 1953;25:68-5.
18. Starrit HC, Duck FA, Humphrey VF. An experimental investigation of streaming in pulsed diagnostic ultrasound beams. Ultrasound Med Biol. 1989;15:363-73.
19. Tarantal AF, Canfield DR. Ultrasound induced lung hemorrhage in the monkey. Ultrasound Med Biol. 1994;20:65-72.
20. Salvesen KA, Vatten LJ, Eik-Nes S, et al. Routine ultrasonography in utero and subsequent handedness and neurological development. Br Med J. 1993;307:159-64.
21. Campbell JD, Elford RW, Brant RF. Case control study of prenatal ultrasonography exposure in children with delayed speech. Can Med Assoc J. 1993;149:1435-40.
22. Salvesen KA, Vatten LJ, Bakketig LS, et al. Routine ultrasonography in utero and speech development. Ultrasound Obstet Gynecol. 1994;4:101-3.
23. Holland CK, Zheng X, Apfel RE, et al. Direct evidence of cavitation in vivo from diagnostic ultrasound. Ultrasound Med Biol. 1996;22:917-25.
24. Hefer-Lauc M, Latin V, Breyer B, et al. Glycoprotein and ganglioside changes in human trophoblasts after exposure to pulsed Doppler ultrasound. Ultrasound Med Biol. 1995;21:579-84.
25. Duck FA. Acoustic streaming and radiation pressure in diagnostic applications: what are the implications? In Barnett SB, Kossoff G (Eds). Safety of Diagnostic Ultrasound. Carnforth, UK: Parthenon Publishing, 1998;87-98.
26. American Institute of Ultrasound in Medicine. Medical Ultrasound Safety. AIUM Publications. 1994.
27. International Electrotechnical Commission. IEC International Standard, IEC/CEI 1157. Geneva: Bureau Central de la Commission Electrotechnique Internationale. 1992.
28. Dyson M. The susceptibility of tissues to ultrasound. In Docker FM, Duck FA, eds. The Safe use of Diagnostic Ultrasound. BIR. 1991;24.
29. Eropean Committee for Ultrasound Radiation Safety tutorial paper: thermal and medical indices. Eur J Ultrasound. 1996;4:145.
30. ter Haar G. Commentary: Safety of diagnostic ultrasound. Br J Radiol. 1996;69:1083-5.
31. EFSUMB. European Committee for Ultrasound Radiation Safety–the Watchdogs, clinical safety statement. Eur J Ultrasound. 1996;3:283.
32. Barnett SB, Kossoff G. WFUMB symposium on safety and standardisation in medical ultrasound: Issues and recommendations regarding thermal mechanisms for biological effects of ultrasound. Hornbick, 1991, Ultrasound in Med & Biol. 1992; 18:v-xix,731-814.
33. National Council on Radiation Protection and Measurements; Exposure Criteria for Medical Diagnostic Ultrasound: I. Criteria Based on Thermal Mechanisms. NCRP Report No. 113. 1992.
34. American Institute of Ultrasound in Medicine/National Electrical Manufacturers Association; Standard for Real Time Display of Thermal and Mechanical Acoustic Output Indices on Diagnostic Ultrasound Equipment. 1992.
35. AIUM Official Statement Changes: Revised statements; Clinical safety, AIUM Reporter. 1998;154(1):6-7.
36. Barnett SB, Rott HD, Ter Haar GR, et al. The sensitivity of biological tissue to ultrasound. Ultrasound in Med & Biol. 1997;23:805-12.
37. ISUOG Bioeffects and Safety Committee; Safety statement, 2000 (reconfirmed 2002). Ultrasound Obstet Gynecol. 2002; 19:105.
38. Ide M. Japanese policy and status of standardisation. Ultrasound in Med & Biol. 1986;12:705-8.
39. Maeda K, Ide M. The limitation of the ultrasound intensity for diagnostic devices in the Japanese Industrial standards. IEEE Trans Ultrasonics, Ferroelectrics and Frequency Control. 1986; UFFC-33: 241-4.
40. Maeda K, Murao F, Yoshiga T, et al. Experimental studies on the suppression of cultured cell growth curves after irradiation with CW and pulsed ultrasound. IEEE Trans Ultrasonics, Ferroelectrics and Frequency Control. 1986; UFFC-33: 186-93.
41. The Safety Group of the British Medical Ultrasound Society. Guidelines for the safe use of diagnostic ultrasound equipment. BMUS Bulletin. 2000;3:29-33.

40 Behavioral Perinatology Assessed by Four-dimensional Sonography

A Kurjak, U Honemeyer, P Antsaklis

INTRODUCTION

Three-dimensional (3D) ultrasound has been available for more than 10 years. However, the 3D image freezes the object and therefore does not provide information on movements or any information about the dynamic changes of the object of interest. A technique was needed that would enable 3D imaging to be performed in a real-time mode. This technique has been recently introduced and has been called four-dimensional (4D) sonography, because time becomes a parameter within the 3D imaging sequence.

Four-dimensional ultrasound provides a new tool for observation of the fetal face. Simultaneous imaging of complex facial movements was not possible using real-time two-dimensional (2D) ulrasound. 4D ultrasound integrates the advantage of the spatial imaging of the fetal face with the addition of time. This new technology, therefore, allows the appearance and duration of each facial movement and expression to be determined and measured.

In a relatively short period of time, 4D sonography has stimulated many multicentric studies on fetal behavior and even fetal awareness with more convincing imaging and data than those obtained by conventional ultrasonic and non-ultrasonic methods. The purpose of this chapter is to review and illustrate presently available data on 4D ultrasound fetal behavior imaging in all three trimesters of pregnancy.

NEUROPHYSIOLOGY OF FETAL BEHAVIOR

For centuries, maternal registration of fetal movements and obstetrical auscultation of fetal heartbeats were the only methods of the follow-up of fetal well-being in utero. However, during the past few decades, development of ultrasonic techniques has enabled the direct visualization of fetus in utero, as well as the real-time assessment of fetal activity. Ultrasonic studies have revealed the fascinating diversity of fetal intrauterine activities. It has been shown that fetal activity occurs as early as the late embryonic period, which is far earlier than a mother can sense it. Furthermore, qualitative and quantitative aspects of behavioral patterns expand rapidly as the pregnancy progresses, and the random movements of the fetal body, which are the earliest sign of fetal activity, change into the well-organized behavioral patterns observed late in gestation. Analysis of the dynamics of fetal behavior has led to the conclusion that fetal behavioral patterns directly reflect developmental and maturational processes of the fetal central nervous system. Nevertheless, the ultrasound findings and their relevance in the assessment of the development of the central nervous system can be interpreted only in comparison with the structural developmental events in the particular period of gestation. Therefore, understanding the relation between fetal behavior and developmental processes in different periods of gestation may make possible the distinction between normal and abnormal brain development, as well as the early diagnosis of various structural or functional abnormalities.

Structural Development of Human Central Nervous System

All the neurons and glial cell originate from embryonic ectoderm, precisely a structure called the neural plate. During the fourth postconceptional week, the neural plate bends into a neural tube, whose further growth reshaping and histological characteristics directly reflect complicated histogenetic processes. The results of those processes are specific transitional embryonic zones, which cannot be observed in an adult brain. Three embryonic zones, ventricular, intermediary and marginal zone (seen from ventricular to pial surface), are present in all parts of neural tube, whereas telencephalon contains additional two zones, subventricular and subplate zone.[1]

Histogenetic processes are proliferation, migration and differentiation of neurons and glial cells, as well as the synaptogenesis and development of chemical specificity of neurons. The dynamics of the main histogenetic processes is shown in Table 40.1.

It is important to point out that proliferation of neurons and glial cells occurs only in the ventricular zone and in the subventricular zone of telencephalon. All the future neurons and glia originate from these zones, form other transitional zones during their migration toward the pial surface and finally reach their permanent position and form the permanent synapses. Early appearance of interneuronal connections, shown on Table 40.1, implicates a possibility of an early functional development. However, these first synapses exist only temporarily and disappear due to the normal developmental processes. Namely, simultaneously with

Table 40.1: Dynamics of the most important progressive processes in the development of the human brain

	Beginning	The most intensive period	Ending
Proliferation	3–4 weeks of gestation	8–12 weeks of gestation	Approximately 20 weeks of gestation
Migration	Simultaneously with proliferation	18–24 weeks of gestation	38 weeks of gestation
Synaptogenesis	8 weeks of gestation	13–16 weeks of gestation, after 24 weeks of gestation, 8th month to 2 year of postnatal life	Puberty

these progressive processes, so-called reorganization processes occur. Some embryonic zones, types of neurons and glia and synapses that play the crucial role in certain periods of fetal brain development eventually disappear, significantly changing structure and function of the brain. Reorganization processes include apoptosis, disappearance of redundant synapses, axonal retreat and transposition, and transformation of the neurotransmitters' phenotype. The temporal overlapping of the major histogenetic processes during the fetal brain development can be seen only in primates.

Obviously, development of human brain is not completed at the time of delivery. In an infant born at term, characteristic cellular layers can be observed in motor, somatosensory, visual and auditory cortical areas. Although proliferation and migration are completed in a term infant, synaptogenesis and neuronal differentiation continue very intensively.[2] Brainstem demonstrates high level of maturity, whereas all histogenetic processes actively persist in cerebellum.[3] Therefore, only subcortical formations and the primary cortical areas are developed completely in a newborn. Associative cortex, barely visible in a newborn, is scantily developed in a 6-month old infant. Postnatal formation of synapses in associative cortical areas, which intensifies between 8th month and 2nd year of life, precedes the onset of first cognitive functions, such as speech. Following the 2nd year of age, many redundant synapses are eliminated. The elimination of synapses begins very rapidly, and continues slowly until the puberty, when the same number of synapses as seen in adults is reached.[3]

Functional Development of Fetal Nervous System

The functional development of the human fetus cannot be studied directly, but ultrasonic studies have made possible the visualization of the fetal motor activity in utero. The ultrasonic studies of fetal spontaneous motor activity and motor responses to stimulation, in comparison with morphological studies and experiments on animal models have given us insight into the complex dynamics of fetal development. The overview of the functional development of fetal nervous system, which will be discussed further in the text, is given in Table 40.2.

Fetal Motor Development

First synapses in the human nervous system appear approximately simultaneously with the formation of the cortical plate, i.e. around 8th postconceptional week.[4,5] It is the period when earliest electrical activity and transmission of information[6] occurs. First spontaneous fetal movements were observed at 7.5th postconceptional week. These movements, consisting of slow flexion and extension of the fetal trunk accompanied by the passive displacement of arms and legs[7] and appearing in irregular sequences, were described as "vermicular".[8] In a little while, they are replaced by various general movements, that include head, trunk and limb, such as "rippling" seen at 8th week, "twitching" and "strong twitching" at 9th and 9.5th week respectively, and "floating" "swimming" and

Table 40.2: Chronology of the functional development of fetal nervous system (detailed description is given in the text)

Weeks of gestation	Motor system	Sensor system	Circadian rhythm
6	Earliest spontaneous movements, gross body movements	Development of taste buds; development of nociceptors	
7		Generalized movements after cutaneous stimulation	
8	Movements of extremities, head and trunk, isolated limb movements	Localized movements after cutaneous stimulation	
9			
10	Sporadic breathing movements; spontaneous movements observed over 15% of 24 hour time	Peripheral afferents from nociceptors to spinal cord begin to form—reflexive reactions to pain; cutaneous reflexes seen in hands	
11			
12			
13			Spontaneous movements and breathing movements associated with heart rate acceleration
14	Facial movements—swallowing, yawning, grimacing, very intensive motor activity, 15 different types of body movements can be observed; sporadic eye movements	Legs sensitive to cuntaneous stimulation–reflexes	
15		Secretion of leptin and VIP-possible regulators of appetite	
16			

Contd…

Contd…

Weeks of gestation	Motor system	Sensor system	Circadian rhythm
17			
18		Alterations in cerebral blood flow in response to painful stimuli	
19			
20		Nociceptors present all over the body	
21			
22			
23		Elevation of cortisol and beta endorphin levels in response to painful stimuli	
24	Breathing movements observed over 14% of 24 hours period		Consolidation of eye movements—alternation of eye movement (EM) and non-eye movement (NEM) periods
25		Cochlear function established (22–25 week) response to vibroacoustic stimulation without lag time	
26			
27			
28			
29			
30	Number of breathing movements change in response to alteration in CO_2 concentration in maternal blood	Fetus responds to purely acoustic stimulation	
31			
32	The number of spontaneous movements begins to decrease		
33			Rapid eye movement (REM) periods and slow eye movement (SEM) periods can be distinguished
34	Breathing movements sensitive to the maternal plasmatic glucose concentration		
35			
36			
37			
38			Constant duration of EM and NEM periods, integration of eye movements with other parameters of fetal activity (heart rate, movements)
39			
40			

"jumping" at 10th week.[9] Isolated limb movements appear almost simultaneously with the generalized movements.

Simultaneously with the onset of spontaneous movements, earliest cutaneous reflex activity can be observed, allowing the assumption of the existence of first afferent-efferent circuits (Table 40.2). The first reflex movements are massive and indicate a very limited number of synapses in a cutaneous reflex pathway.[10] At that time, head tilting after perioral stimulation was noted. During the 8th week of gestation these massive reflex movements are replaced with local movements, probably due to an increase in the number of axodendritic synapses. Hands become sensitive at 10.5 weeks and lower limbs begin to participate in these reflexes approximately at 14th week.[10–14] From 10th week onward, the number and frequency of movements increase. By 14–19 weeks, fetuses are very active with the longest period of inactivity lasting only 5–6 minutes. In the 15th week 15 different movements can be observed. Besides the general body movements and isolated limb movements, retroflection, anteflexion and rotation of the head can easily be seen. Moreover, face movements, such as mouthing, yawning, hiccups, suckling, and swallowing, can be added to a wide repertoire of fetal motor activity in this period (Table 40.2).[15] However, in such an early gestation, dynamic pattern of neuronal production and migration, as well as the limited cerebral circuits are considered too immature for the cortical involvement in the motor behavior (for review see Reference 16). Only at the end of this period a quantifiable number of synapses appear in the structures preceding the cerebral cortex, probably forming a substrate for the first cortical electric activity, noted at the 19th week.[16] Studies of anencephalic fetuses have also provided apparent evidences that around 17th–20th gestational week motor behavior becomes influenced by the supraspinal structures. Namely, in these fetuses, the incidence of movements was normal or even increased, but the complexity of movement patterns changed dramatically and movements were stereotyped and simplified.[17,18]

The number of spontaneous movements tends to increase until a peak around 32 weeks whereupon it decreases again.[19–21] By term, average number of generalized movements per hour was found to be approximately 31 with the longest period between movements ranging from 50–75 minutes.[22] This decrease is considered rather as a result of cerebral maturation processes, than as consequence of reduced amniotic fluid volume. Simultaneously with the decrease in the number of generalized movements, an increase in facial movements, including opening/closing of the jaw, swallowing and chewing, can be observed. These movements can be seen mostly during absence of generalized movements, and this pattern is considered to reflect a normal neurological development of the fetus.[19] However, not only the changes in the number of movements, but also in their complexity are shown to be the result of maturational processes. Recent 4D ultrasound studies, which will be described later in the text, have shown even a wider repertoire of fetal face and hand movements in the third trimester of gestation, than it has been previously described.[23] Obviously, the story of fetal intrauterine activity is far from being completed and the development of new recording techniques could enrich our perspective of the intrauterine life. It has been demonstrated that the fetal movement patterns in the second half of pregnancy are almost identical to those observed after birth,[24,25] although the repertoire of movements in newborns includes some patterns that cannot be observed in the fetus, such as the Moro reflex,[26] which may be related to the transition from intrauterine micro-gravity to full gravity postpartum. The detailed description of fetal movement patterns at different gestational age, studied by conventional as well as 4D ultrasound will be given later in the text.

Many factors, such as cigarette smoking[27] or injection of corticosteroids for fetal lung maturation,[28] were proved to decrease the number of spontaneous fetal movements. Furthermore, fetal activity is increased in mothers suffering some kind of emotional stress.[29] The quality of fetal movement patterns is altered in fetuses suffering intrauterine growth restriction. The movements become slower, monotonous, resembling cramps, and their variability in the strength and amplitude is reduced. These changes could indicate the existence of brain lesions in growth restricted and possibly hypoxic fetuses. Namely, despite earlier assumptions, the alterations in the amplitude and complexity of movements in these fetuses do not appear due to the oligohydramnios. In cases of premature rupture of fetal membranes and a subsequently reduced volume of amniotic fluid, movements occur less frequently, but their complexity resembles that of movements performed in a normal volume of amniotic fluid (for review see Reference 30). Obviously,

the qualitative as well as quantitative analysis of fetal movements reveal the integrity of the fetal nervous system, and can be used for the detection of various cerebral dysfunctions, and probably neuromuscular diseases.[29,30]

Development of Specialized Movements

Studies on animals, especially various species of mammals, as well as their comparisons with the ultrasonic recordings of human fetuses, have revealed that some specialized movement patterns, crucial for the survival of newborns, such as swallowing or rhythmic respiratory movements, develop and mature during gestation. Although these patterns somewhat differ from adult patterns, in the near term fetuses they are developed sufficiently to enable the survival of the fetus.

In human fetuses, breathing movements occur around 10th week of gestation.[31] Early in gestation, they are present almost continually and are associated with activity of postural muscles of neck and limbs. However, the frequency and complexity of the breathing pattern changes as pregnancy progresses. Total breathing time in a 24-hour interval extends, as well as the duration of individual breathing and non-breathing intervals.[32,33] Changes in breathing patterns are considered to be a result of the maturation of fetal lungs and respiratory and sleep centers in the fetal central nervous system. In 38th and 39th week of gestation, the frequency of breathing movements decreases to 41 breaths per minute and the movements become as regular as in the postnatal period.[34] Approximately at the 30th week of gestation, the regulation of fetal breathing movements by the plasmatic level of carbon dioxide is established and the number of breaths increases following an excess of carbon dioxide in maternal blood.[35,36] This sensitivity to the alterations in the plasmatic carbon dioxide level is connected to the maturation of fetal respiratory neural centers, which is thought to occur during the last 10 weeks of pregnancy (Table 40.2).[37] The process of maturation of fetal breathing movements is accelerated in some conditions such as premature rupture of membranes. For instance, decrease in fetal breathing has been observed following premature rupture of membranes[38,39] and during the 3 days prior to the initiation of labor.[37,40] Kisilevsky et al. compared body movements and breathing patterns in normal fetuses at 24–33 weeks of gestation and fetuses threatening to deliver prematurely. High-risk fetuses had a reduced level of body movements and an earlier onset of extended periods of breathing, which occurred at 30 weeks in contrast to 33 weeks in the control group.[41] However, in this study accelerated maturation of breathing was not observed in the presence of ruptured membranes. Fetuses delivered prematurely had less breathing than those delivered at term. Maternal consumption of alcohol or methadone, and according to some authors, even cigarette smoking, is known to decrease incidence of breathing movements.[42–44] On the other hand, aminophylline, used for the treatment of bronchial asthma, as well as conjugated estrogens and betamethasone increase the frequency of breathing.[45,46] Increased number of fetal movements following the elevation of the glucose concentration in maternal blood has been noted at 34th week of gestation.[47,48]

Another indispensable prerequisite for the survival of the newborn is the ability to feed, i.e. to ingest food. In the human fetus, swallowing was noted as early as 11 weeks of gestation,[49] with daily swallowing rates near term of 200–500 mL.[50,51] Swallowing of amniotic fluid proteins and growth factors contributes to the growth and maturation of fetal gastrointestinal tract, and possibly to the fetal somatic growth.[52] Namely, amniotic fluid provides 10–14% of the nitrogen requirements in the normal fetus, and esophageal atresia is often associated with lower birth weight.[53] Many authors agree that swallowing patterns develop in utero in all species in which there is significant fetal fluid excretion (urine and lung liquid) into the amniotic cavity. Thus, fetal swallowing contributes to the regulation of amniotic fluid volume.[52] In some, although not all cases with fetal esophageal atresia, the volume of amniotic fluid is increased. The normal volume of amniotic fluid in some of these cases could be explained by the coexistence of a tracheoesophageal fistula which could allow the intake of liquid during respiratory movements (for review see Reference 54). Furthermore, polyhydramnios sometimes, though not always, develops in anencephalic fetuses. However, some of these fetuses have an intact swallowing reflex, whereas the cases with normal amniotic fluid volume and decreased fetal swallowing have been described (for review see Reference 54). Spontaneous fetal swallowing is, like most motor patterns, correlated with neurobehavior. The development of dypsogenic mechanisms and their influence on fetal swallowing will be described later in the text. Here we have to emphasize that fetal swallowing patterns differ significantly from those seen in the adult and that the fetus daily swallows 5–10 times more fluid per body mass unit.[55]

Development of Fetal Sensory System

The combination of ultrasonic studies, pathoanatomical examinations and the studies of premature infants have provided a wide spectrum of evidence that the ability to register vibrations, acoustic stimuli, and even light is acquired during intrauterine life. It is well known that the fetus can sense pain and respond to the painful stimulus with a variety of responses, such as movements, circulatory and hormonal responses, although the question of the emotional response to pain or memorization of the unpleasant events in utero still remains unresolved. The fetus can also sense the taste of amniotic fluid and even functions such as appetite, satiety and thirst seem to be developed during intrauterine life (Table 40.2).

Fetal Vestibular and Auditory System

It is generally accepted that reflexes of the brainstem, which includes vestibulary, olfactory and auditory reflexes, develop early in gestation.[56] Vestibular ganglionic cells mature earlier than the neurons of lateral and inferior vestibular nuclei, which are functional from the 9 gestational weeks onward.[57] Vestibular stimulation is thought to contribute to the development of fetal movements. Namely, the gravity-free environment in utero appears to promote the development of vestibulary reflexes.[58] According to electrophysiological examinations of the evoked potentials in prematurely delivered healthy infants, cochlear function develops between 22 and 25 weeks of gestation, whereas its maturation continues during the first 6 months upon delivery.[59-61] Maternal heartbeats and motility of the gastrointestinal tract during digestion appear to generate a 90 decibel noise[62] level in utero. However, fluid in the fetal ear, as well as the immaturity of cochlea, complicate the sound transmission, so that only strong acoustic stimuli can produce fetal reflex movements, such as startle motion of the trunk and/or flexion of the extremities, accompanied by changes in the heart rate. These are seen during or soon after vibroacoustic stimulation.[61] Applying acoustic stimulation with wide spectrum of frequencies directly on the maternal abdomen, Shahidullah

et al. have registered reflex movements with a short lag time in 20 week old fetuses, and movements without the lag time in 25 week old fetuses.[63] However, these movements were explained as a reflex response to vibroacoustic stimulation or proprioceptor stimulation. Kisilevsky et al. reported an increase of number of fetal movements and heart rate during acoustic stimulation performed with the sound transmitter placed 10 cm above the maternal abdomen, in 30 week old fetuses.[64]

Fetal Vision

Intrauterine environment is not completely deprived of light. Moreover, some experimental results indicate that the development of visual and auditory organs could not be possible without any light or acoustic stimulation.[62] Although structural development of sensor pathways is a prerequisite for functional development, final organization of brain circuitries relies predominantly on guidance from external input. In cortical area 17 synaptogenesis perisits between 24 weeks and 8 months after delivery,[65] whereas myelinization of the optical tract begins at 32 weeks of gestation[66] and cones of the central foveola reach the adult proportions late in childhood.[67]

Fetal Pain

During the past decade, fetal perception of pain has been not only an object of interest for scientists, but also an important issue in public debates, in relation to late abortion and an increasing number of intrauterine operations. The pain consists of two components; perception of stimulus and an emotional reaction or unpleasant feeling of the noxious stimulus. These occur in two anatomically and physiologically distinct systems in the brain. The response to painful stimulation can be regarded at three different levels; somatosensory response, pain-induced autonomic and endocrinological reflexes, and pain related behavior (for review see Reference 68). In the human fetus, the first nociceptors appear at the 7th week of gestation and by the 20th week these are present all over the body. Peripheral afferents begin to make synapses to the spinal cord, approximately during weeks 10–30.[69] The myelination of these pathways[70] and the development of functional spinal reflex circuitry develop almost simultaneously.[70,71] Higher parts of pain pathways include the spinothalamic tract, established at the 20th week and myelinized by 29 weeks of gestation[72] and thalamocortical connections which begin to grow into the cortex at 24–26 weeks.[66] Finally, at the 29th week, evoked potentials can be registered from the cortex, indicating that the functional connection between periphery and cortex operates from that time onward.[71,73]

Earliest reactions to painful stimuli are motor reflexes, resembling withdrawal reflexes. These reactions are completely reflexive and are guided by the spinal cord. Higher perception or processing of painful sensation does not exist at this stage.[10] However, some investigators indicate that facial reflexes in response to somatic stimulation, which could indicate the emotional reaction to pain, develop rather early in gestation.[13] These reflexes are thought to be coordinated by subcortical systems and probably reflect development of these lower brain circuitries.[74] As for the autonomic responses to pain, an elevation of cortisol and beta-endorphin levels in plasma in response to needle pricking of the innervated hepatic vein was registered in a 23-week old fetus, whereas the stimulation of the uninnervated umbilical cord had no effect.[75,76] Alterations in cerebral blood flow, i.e. blood flow redistribution during invasive procedures, were noted in an 18-week old fetus.[77] These results indicate that painful stimuli trigger wide spectra of reactions in the central nervous system, such as activation of the hypothalamic pituitary axis or autonomic reflexes, even without reaching the cortex. Furthermore, we have to emphasize that these hormonal, autonomic and metabolic responses can be neutralized by analgesics such as fentanyl.[77,78] The reduction of fetal responses to pain is extremely important because many studies have shown the influence of the early pain experiences on the later behavioral variables or on the later developmental outcomes.[79] One of the most important effects of painful experience is a prolonged stress response.[80] It includes fluctuations in blood pressure and cerebral blood flow, and hypoxemia, which may predispose to intracranial hemorrhage.[77] Experiments on animals have revealed that elevated cortisol levels, equivalent to those secreted during the stress response in humans, were associated with degenerative changes in fetal hypothalamus.[81] Finally, long-term follow-up studies of fetuses treated in the intensive care units (ICU) and exposed to pain and/or stress have demonstrated the correlations between the stay in ICU and altered pain thresholds and abnormal pain-related behavior later in life.[80,82] All these findings underline the importance of a stress-free environment for normal physiological and psychological development.

Fetal Taste, Appetite and Satiety

It is generally believed that appetite and satiety functions develop during the intrauterine period in all precocial species. In the human fetus, taste buds are developed from the 7th week of gestation onward.[83] Sucrose increases swallowing in the human fetus, whereas the incidence of swallowing movements decreases following the injection of lipiodol, a bitter extract of poppy seeds, into the amniotic fluid.[83] The main endocrine regulators of appetite, leptin and neuropeptide Y (NPY) are secreted as early as 15 and 18 weeks, respectively, in the human fetus, but the ontogeny and functions of their regulatory pathways have not been delineated in the human fetal brain.[84-86] However, experiments on animals have shown the increase of swallowing upon injection of NPY.[87] Swallowing was increased following the injection of leptin, which is in contradiction with leptin function in adults.[88] Therefore, some authors postulated that the presence of NPY pathways and the immaturity of leptin pathways may potentiate feeding and facilitate weight gain in newborns, despite high body fat levels.[52]

Development of Dipsogenic Mechanisms

Experiments on animal models, especially fetal lambs, have shown that dipsogenic mechanisms begin to modulate fetal swallowing during intrauterine life. For instance, in fetal lambs swallowing and arginine vasopressin secretion increase following the central administration of hypertonic saline and angiotensin II.[89,90] Ross et al. have identified the hypertonicity-activated neurons in dipsogenic hypothalami nuclei, such as the parvocellular and magnocellular division of periventricular nucleus and supraoptic nucleus in near-term ovine fetus.[91-93] These authors also suggested that exaggerated fetal swallowing under physiologic conditions (5–10 times more liquid in proportion to the adult) might be the result of tonic activation of angiotensin II receptors and production of nitric oxide.[94,95] Nevertheless, the fetus appears to have reduced sensitivity to osmotic stimuli.[96-98] when compared to the adult,

despite the intact dipsogenic nuclei. Reduced swallowing during systemic hypotension despite the elevated renin plasma levels, together with the increased amount of liquid swallowed under normal conditions, indicates that fetal dipsogenic response might differ from the adult.[99]

Cyclic Behavior and Development of Circadian Rhythms

Fetal life in utero is organized in cyclical patterns. Periods of activity alternate with periods of rest. The observation of human infants resulted in the hypothesis that the alternations of activity and inactivity periods reflect the elementary ultradian rhythm of the fetal central nervous system, uninfluenced by external input.

For instance, eye movements, which become observable at 16–18 weeks of gestation, begin to consolidate at 24–26 weeks of gestation, and the periods of eye movements begin to alternate with non-eye movement periods. During the last 10 weeks of gestation, both switching and maintaining mechanisms responsible for this ultradian rhythms mature, and constant mean values of duration of eye movement (EM) and non-eye movement (NEM) periods are achieved by 37–38 weeks. At that time, EM and NEM last 27–29 and 23–24 minutes respectively, which is similar to the values in neonate.[100] In the adult human, rapid eye movements (REM) are present during the active sleep, alternate with the slow eye movements (SEM), or deep sleep and are accompanied by changes in electrocortical activity.[101] In the fetus, REM and SEM movements can be registered at 33 weeks of gestation. At 36–38 weeks of gestation, they become integrated with other parameters of fetal activity, such as heart rate and fetal movements, into organized and coherent behavioral states.[102]

In animal fetuses, simultaneous measurements of fetal electrocortical activity, eye and body movements have shown that deep sleep, characterized by high voltage waves and decreased fetal activity, occurred during 54% of the total time each day. The total length of REM sleep period, characterized by low voltage waves and rapid eye movements lasted 40% of the total time each day. Wakeful state (6% of a day) is characterized by low voltage waves.[103] In human premature newborns, born 4 weeks prior to the term, 60–65% of the total sleep period is REM sleeping, whereas in a term newborn, the REM sleep period includes 50% of total 16 hours of sleep.[104] Intensive activity of neuronal circuits during the REM sleep is thought to contribute to the development of central nervous system.[104]

Circadian system is a kind of biological clock that receives information from the environment and sends efferent outputs that orchestrate circadian rhythms.[105] In mammals, the major role in orchestration of these rhythms is played by the suprachiasmatic nucleus (SCN) of the hypothalamus that oscillates with a period of close to 24 hours. Biological oscillations of SCN are entrained by the light/darkness cycle, which is registered by retinal receptors and transmitted by the retinohypothalamic tract. Efferent pathways from SCN include projections into the various nuclei of the hypothalamus, and possibly, endocrine SCN secretion. In the human fetus, as well as other mammal species, SCN is developed by mid-gestation, but its maturation continues after birth, as shown by an increase in the number of neurons containing adrenaline-vasopressin (AVP) and vasoactive intestinal polypeptide (VIP) during the 1st year of postnatal life (for review see Reference 105). Circadian rhythms in behavior, cardiovascular function and hormones are present in human fetuses, as well as in fetal sheep and monkey, and are entrained to the light/darkness cycle. However, the question whether that rhythm is generated by the fetus itself or influenced by maternal rhythms, remains to be resolved, although some animal experiments indicate the importance of the maternal SCN. In this case, the transmission of the signal to the fetus would necessarily require an endocrine mediator, but no such a molecule has been identified yet. Latest results suggest the role of maternal pineal hormone melatonin. This hormone is present in humans, as well as in other mammals, and its plasma concentrations exhibit daily variations, with the peak during the night. Therefore, its role in sleep induction has been suggested (for review see Reference 105). Seasonal alterations in melatonin concentrations have also been reported. Daily oscillations of melatonin concentrations in plasma are present throughout gestation,[105] and various human tissues including the central nervous system express some types of melatonin receptors.[106,107] However, its role in the orchestration of fetal circadian rhythms remains to be confirmed.

BASIC TECHNOLOGY OF 4D SONOGRAPHY

The rapid development of digital ultrasound systems allows 3D image reconstructions and lately 4D real time inspection of anatomical regions and pathological changes. However, 3D images are static and do not provide information of movements and dynamic changes of the object of interest.[23] Moreover, fetal movements are the source of significant artifacts and volume scanning should be performed during the fetal inactive phase, i.e. whenever the fetus is active, a 3D image of good quality is unobtainable. This fact limits the usage of classic 3D ultrasound. 4D ultrasound overcomes above mentioned disadvantages, making it possible to obtain a good quality 3D image, regardless of fetal movements. The only limiting factor for 4D sonography is the quantity of adjacent amniotic fluid.

The acquisition of volume datasets is performed by using special transducers (linear, convex, transvaginal) designed for 2D scans, 3D and real time 4D volumes.[108] The real time 4D mode is obtained from simultaneous volume acquisition and computing of 3D images, which is in fact multi-dimensional ultrasound.[109] The movement of the ultrasound beam over the region of interest (ROI) is automatic. Such design enables simplified 3D and 4D acquisition. Ultrasound probes include a scanning mechanism moved a built-in electromotor. The processing speed allows continuous acquisition and processing of 4D volumes.

The volume acquisition begins with a 2D image and superimposed volume box. The initial 2D image is the central 2D image of the volume. According to the dimensions of the volume box, the volume scan sweeps between the margins of the volume box. The volume box is set to frame the ROI. The following steps are important for producing reliable 4D images:

1. Orientation in real time 2D mode.
2. Selection of ROI.
3. Starting the volume scan. Volume data is shown in a multiplane display on the monitor (transverse, sagittal and coronal).

During the 3D and 4D acquisition, sweep time depends on the volume box size, scan quality and adjusted scan parameters, such as depth, number of focuses and other parameters which affect the B-mode image frame rate.

4D Rendering

The pixel is the smallest element of 2D images while the voxel is the smallest information unit in 3D and 4D imaging. Volume rendering provides visualization of animated voxel-based images on a 2D screen. Because of recent computer technology development and fast data transmition, volume acquisition and data processing are accelerated to enable 3D rendering in real time (4D). Fast volume data processing enables calculation of 5–30 volumes per second depending on the system hardware and size of the render box. As 4D imaging is almost in "real time", since there is always some delay as a result of time needed to reconstruct 3D image from 2D scans. It is always desirable to achieve as many volumes per second (volume rate) as possible. Number of volumes per second is some kind of trade-of between image quality and frame rate. 3D and 4D image quality mostly depends on 2D image quality. Prior to volume acquisition, it is important to achieve the best 2D image quality by carefully adjusting depth, focus position and number of focuses, frequency and gain. All 2D image artifacts will be also present on 3D and 4D image reconstruction. Good 4D image acquisition depends on the following important points: ROI size and volume box size, ROI position or direction of view and accessibility to the object. The render box determines the contents that will be rendered. Structures that are not selected by the volume box will be cut from 3D reconstruction.

The ROI can be sized, moved and rotated in all directions arbitrarily by operator. Volume data can be acquired from different 2D modes: grayscale-, color Doppler-, and power Doppler imaging. There are different rendering modes available: Surface, transparent (maximum, minimum, X-ray) and Light, some of them can be active simultaneously in real time.

Volume rendering is a process of visualization of 3D structures on an animated 2D screen and render modes determine how the 3D image will be presented on screen.

Surface Rendering or Gray Scale Rendering

In the surface-rendering mode, only signals from the surface of ROI are extracted and displayed in the plastic appearance. Surface rendering examination of the fetus focuses the sonographer's attention exclusively on fetal external anatomy (Figs 40.1A to C).

This mode is capable of clear visualization of fetal normal surface anatomy or surface anomalies such as myelomeningocele, omphalocele, cleft lip/palate, macroglossia and limb defects (Figs 40.2 to 40.6). Furthermore, visualization of the spatial relationship between surface structures enables accurate diagnosis of subtle malformations and anomalies such as micrognathia, overlapping fingers, hexadactilia and auricular malposition or malformation.

The surface image can be displayed in "textural" mode. The gray values can be colored by different color maps, but the most successful map for 4D images is the "body heat" map. The texture mode can also be "smoothed", showing smooth surfaces on 4D reconstructions. Texture and smooth surface displays are suitable for use in applications such as fetal face, abdominal wall, genitals, umbilical cord (Fig. 40.7), and the surfaces of urinary bladder.[110-112]

The surface can be displayed in "light" mode. Closer structures are brighter while distant structures are displayed darker. Variation of the light mode is "gradient light mode" showing virtual illumination from a spotlight source.[113]

Transparent Mode

In the transparent mode, contrary to surface mode, only the signals from the inner layers of ROI are extracted providing spatial reconstruction of internal structure of ROI. According to the echogenicity of the extracted signals, there are two sub-

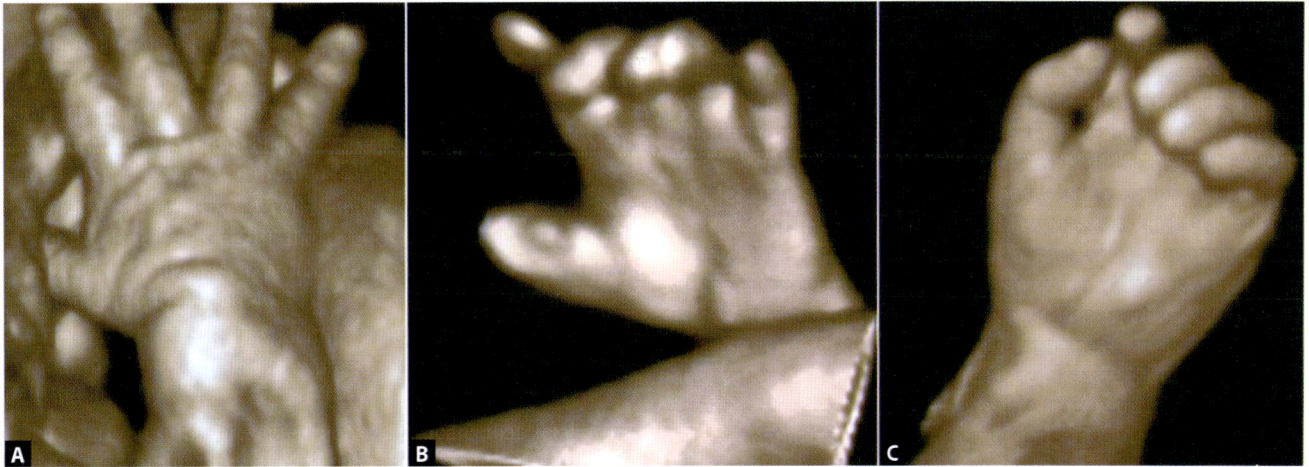

Figs 40.1A to C: (A to C) 3D surface rendering of the normal hand movement. Note the alteration of the palm position

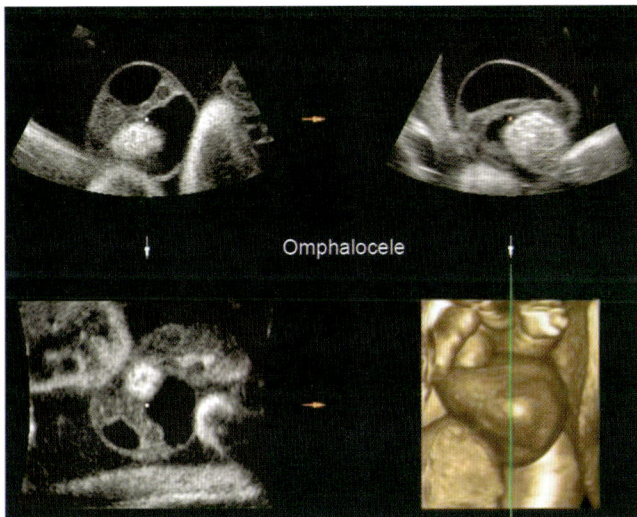

Fig. 40.2: 3D surface rendering of omphalocele

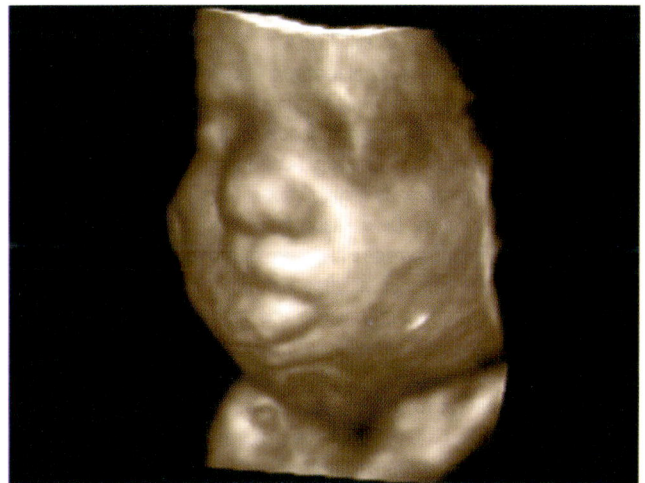

Fig. 40.3: 3D surface rendering of macroglossia

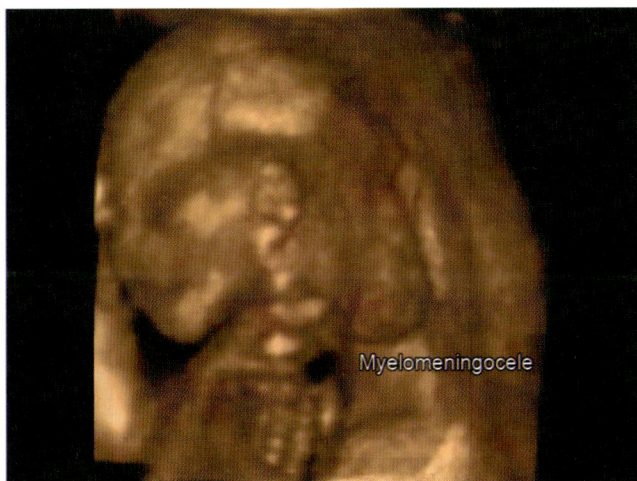

Fig. 40.4: 3D surface rendering of myelomeningocele

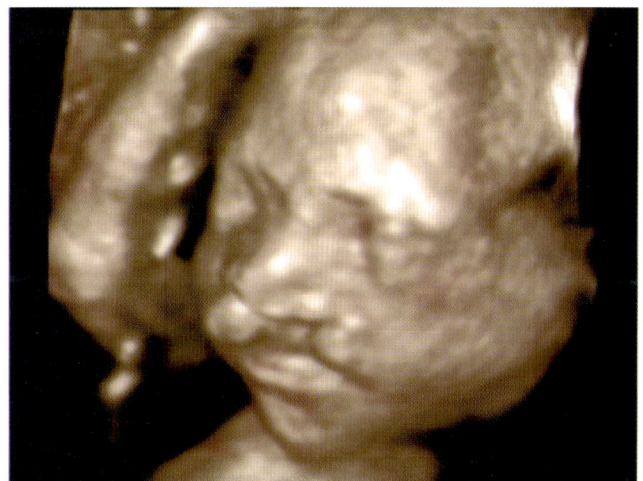

Fig. 40.5: 3D surface rendering of bilateral cleft lips

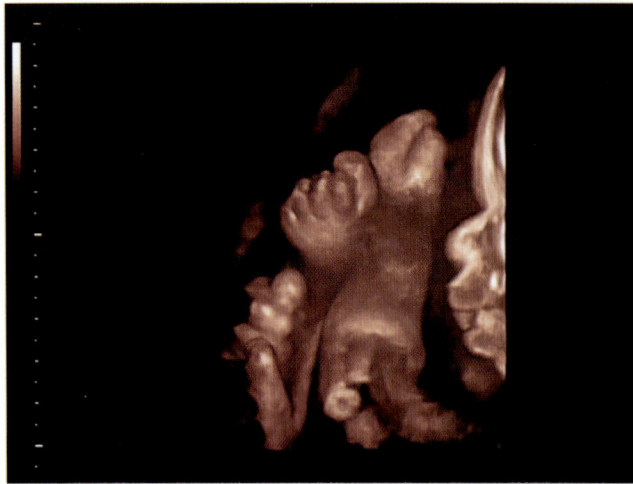

Fig. 40.6: 3D surface rendering of arthrogryposis of the fingers showing rigid and fixed posture. Surface rendering gives the best result when ROI structures are surrounded by fluid or hypoechoic tissue. Any change of the threshold parameter influences the quality of the surface rendered image: by selecting the threshold level, voxels with gray values below the selected level are not shown on the reconstructed image

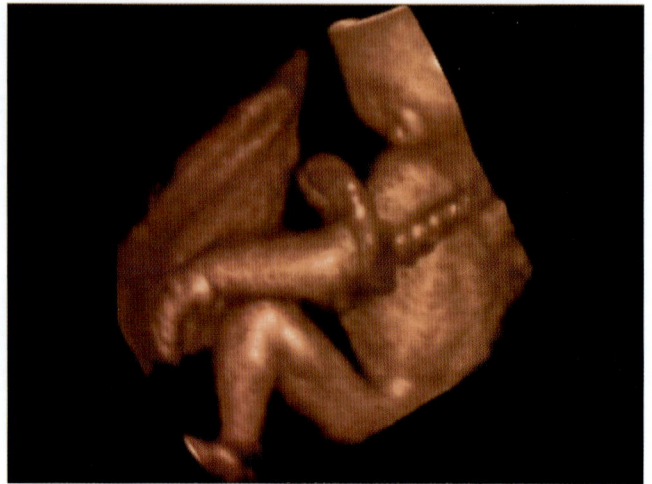

Fig. 40.7: 3D surface rendering of umbilical cord around the arm

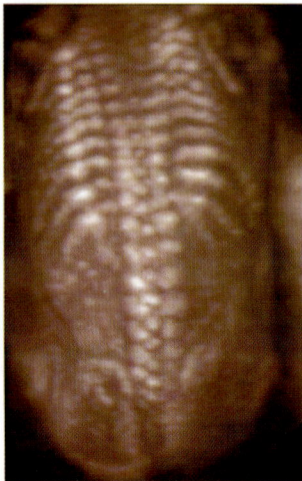

Fig. 40.8: 3D Maximum mode showing the vertebral column

modalities: maximum and minimum mode. In the maximum mode only the signals of highest echogenecity are selected, whereas in the minimum mode only the signals of lowest echogenicity are extracted from the entire volume. In the transparent mode only maximum gray values are displayed. This mode is suitable for visualization of fetal bones, endometrium and breast.

Minimum Mode

Minimum gray values are displayed for visualization of vessels, cystic structures and parenchyma of different organs.[114]

Maximum Mode

Maximum gray values are displayed. It is suitable for visualization of fetal bone structures and is the method of choice for imaging of the spatial relationships between bones.[115] Moreover, this modality

offers an option of complete visualization of curved bones such as ribs or clavicle on single image.

Evaluation of the complete skeleton, particularly the thoracic skeleton in the developing fetuses often is difficult with 2D US because of curvature of the bones. Ribs can be completely observed using the 3D US transparency mode. This modality reduces the echogenicity of soft tissues, leaving behind echogenic structures namely the bones. The curvature and relationship of the rib ends to the vertebral bodies and the anterior chest wall can be demonstrated as well as the entire length.

The vertebral column is originally curved anteroposteriorly. If it is pathologically curved laterally, it is impossible to display the whole vertebral column in a single sectional image by 2D US. The advantage of 3D ultrasound (Fig. 40.8) is the ability to visualize both curvatures at the same time. Anomalies such as scoliosis, kyphosis, lordosis and spina bifida may be overlooked by 2D ultrasound, but are easy to recognize by using the 3D maximum mode. Congenital malformations of the fetal spine can be identified easier using 3D surface and transparent mode reconstruction together. Specific vertebral body levels may be accurately identified by simultaneous evaluating of axial planes of the spine within the volume rendered image. It is difficult to acquire the entire spine in a single volume and thus multiple volumes are often necessary to evaluate the spine completely.

Volume Contrast Imaging (VCI)

Using 4D, it is possible to make high contrast 2D images. The rendered algorithm is a combination of surface texture mode and minimum transparency 4D mode. It is possible to display a volume slice with a thickness of only a few millimeters, showing very good contrast between different tissues. The operator can define the thickness of the slice that is scanned, by using 4D image rendering. The reconstructed image shows improved tissue contrast. VCI is used for better visualization of nodular or diffuse lesions in parenchyma of organs such as liver and spleen.

Spatio-Temporal Image Correlation in Fetal Echocardiography

Spatio-temporal image correlation (STIC) is a new method for clinical investigation of the fetal heart. The reconstructed volume scan offers a user friendly technique to acquire data from the fetal heart for visualization in a 4D sequence. The volume acquisition occurs in two ways: First, data acquisition is performed by a single, automatic volume sweep. In the second step, the system examines the data in proportion to their spatial and temporal domain and processes a 4D sequence. This sequence presents the heart beating in real-time in a multi-planar display. After the volume acquisition, the heart can be assessed off-line, without being dependent on the patient.[116,117]

Removing Overlaying Structures

This option is called "magic cut" or "electronic scalpel". During 3D and 4D scanning in most cases, there are structures that are interfering or are superimposed to the reconstructed image. Magic-cut tool enables successful removal of overlaying structures using 3D imaging. Unwanted structures can be cut off from the image in all three directions along the x, y, and z axes. There is also a possibility of using this tool to remove some structures from real time 4D volumes. The cutting tool enables the operator to have improved visibility to the object from all directions.[118]

Data Review and Networking

Volume data sequences can be stored on the hard disk of the ultrasound unit or by means of different media (CD-R, MO-Disc) in various formats: 2D image, 2D cine (selected sequence of 2D images), 3D volume (sequence of 3D rotating images) and 4D volume. Since the complete volume data set is saved, it is possible to review saved examinations without any loss of image quality. Stored data can be interactively processed with additional 3D reconstruction possibility.

The 3D and 4D imaging provides additional dimensions to conventional 2D sonography. The main advantage of ultrasound in general is dynamic imaging of the human body. 4D imaging is following this tradition permitting visualization of dynamic changes inside body and organs. Using 4D ultrasound in obstetrics, it is possible for the first time to monitor quality and quantity of fetal movements on 3D real time reconstructed images.

ASSESSMENT OF FETAL BEHAVIOR

Prenatal motility is considered to reflect the developing nervous system but also involves functional and maturational properties of fetal hemodynamics and the muscular system. Despite medical reports from 100 years ago and 25 years of systematic research initiated by Prechtl and associates, the study of prenatal behavior is in its infancy.

Fetal behavior can be defined as fetal activities observed or recorded with ultrasonographic equipment. As it is not yet possible to assess functional development of the CNS directly, investigators started to analyze fetal behavior as a measure of neurological maturation.[119]

A turning point in the assessment of fetal behavior was the introduction of real-time ultrasound. This technique allowed the investigation of spontaneous fetal motor activity in utero.[18,120] For the first time, studies of spontaneous prenatal movements and behavior in utero were performed and published. Since fetal body movements give important information about the condition of the fetus, their quantitative as well as qualitative aspects were analyzed. De Vries and colleagues described the developmental pathway of fetal movements in a longitudinal study of 12 healthy nulliparous women.[15] They reported not only how to describe a particular movement, but also how these movements were performed in terms of speed and amplitude.[15]

Assessment of Fetal Movements

Using ultrasound imaging, de Vries and colleagues focused on the first half of pregnancy while Roodenburg and coworkers investigated the second half of pregnancy.[24,121] In the classic paper de Vries and her team classified at least up to 13 different movement patterns.[24]

Classification of Movement Patterns

1. Just discernible movements (between 7 and 8.5 weeks)
2. Startle
3. General movements (Figs 40.9A to F)
4. Hiccup
5. Breathing

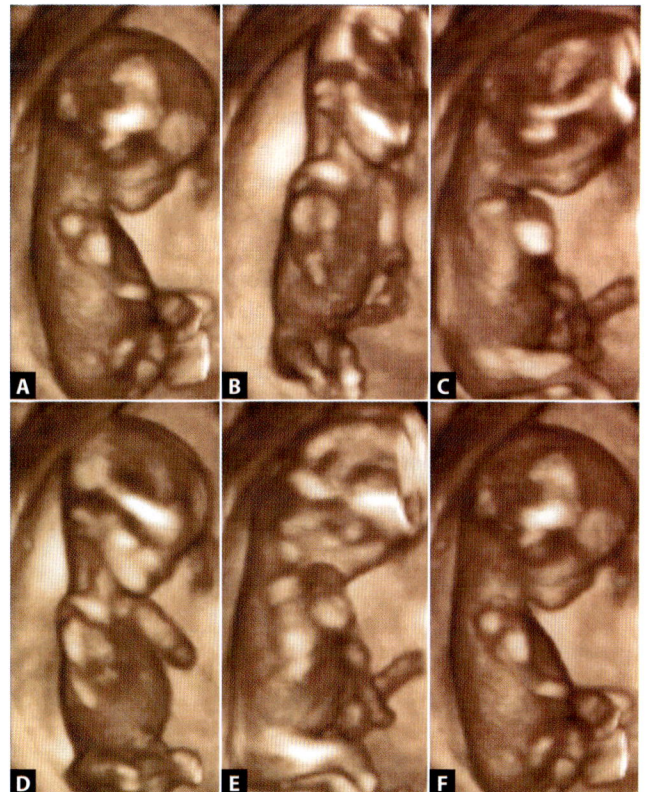

Figs 40.9A to F: Four-dimensional ultrasound sequence of the fetus at 12 weeks of gestation showing general movements. The complex movements of the limb, trunk and head are clearly visible and cause a shift in fetal position. In the first sequence, the right limb is bent in elbow joint. In the next sequence, the fetus has dropped the hand and has begun to deflect the elbow joint. In the last sequence, further elevation of hand is seen

6. Isolated arm or leg movement
7. Isolated retroflexion of the head
8. Isolated rotation of the head
9. Isolated anteflexion of the head
10. Jaw movements
11. Hand-face-contact: In this pattern of movement, the hand slowly touches the face, the fingers frequently extend and flex (Figs 40.10 to 40.15)
12. Stretch
13. Rotation of the fetus.

However, the lack of definition specificity and long-term follow-up and the reliability of descriptions have limited the usefulness of some of these studies. In only two studies, fetal motor behavior has been described. The descriptor of "general movements" has been applied to the movement of preterm newborns.

Relying on the observations of apparently typical spontaneous human fetal movements, de Vries and coworkers recorded variations in "general movements" that they believed suggested abnormalities of the CNS.[122] Following their lead, other researchers have selected, as a dependent variable, general movements or "gross movements" involving the whole body.[123] Fetal motor behavior has been described.[124,125] The descriptor of "general movements" has been applied to the movement of preterm newborns.[126] Unfortunately, the lack of definition specificity, long-term follow-ups and the reliability of descriptions have limited the usefulness of some of these studies. Nevertheless, careful observation and analysis of fetal movements

could be useful in the assessment of the integrity of fetal central nervous system, as will be described later in the text.

The Zagreb group has evaluated the advantages of 4D over 2D real-time sonography in the assessment of early fetal behavior.[118] With 4D transvaginal sonography these authors found body movements at 7 weeks of pregnancy (Table 40.3).[118] The observed body movements consisted of the changing position of the head toward the body. Therefore, this technology enables the visualization of the moving phenomenon 1 week earlier than 2D ultrasound. At 7 weeks of gestation, the dominant embryonic feature is the head, which is strongly flexed anteriorly. Upper and lower limb buds are visible on the lateral aspects of the embryo. However, embryonic movements are not frequent and consist mainly of moving of the head toward the rest of the body. At 8–9 weeks, the head is less flexed and the changes of the position of the head toward the body are clearly visible.

General movements are the first complex fetal movement patterns observable by 2D ultrasound.[15] They can be recognized from 8–9 weeks of pregnancy and continue to be present until 16–20 weeks after birth.[127] According to Prechtl, these are gross movements, involving the whole body.[128] Movements of the limbs, trunk and head are of variable speed, but smooth in appearance. They wax and wane in intensity, force and speed, and they have a gradual beginning and end.[128] The qualitative characteristics of general movements can be altered in some pathological conditions, such as in fetuses of women with type 1 diabetes mellitus or fetuses with anencephaly.[17,129] The range of the movements varies

Table 40.3: The incidence of spontaneous embryonic/fetal movement according to gestational age

Gestational age (weeks)	CRL (mm)	No movements	Gross body movements	Limb movements	Complex limb movements
7–8	0–15	31	12	0	0
9–10	16–30	26	11	7	0
11–12	31–50	19	16	12	8

CRL; crown-rump length (*Source:* Adapted from Reference 118)

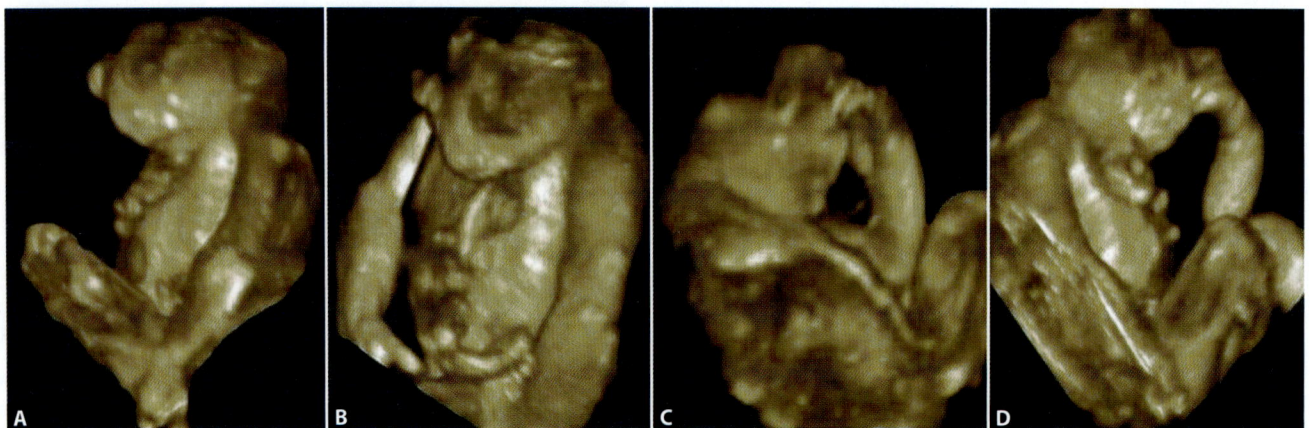

Figs 40.10A to D: (A to D) 4D sequence of anencephalic fetus at 19 weeks of pregnancy, only hand to head movement in one direction of the left arm could be seen, their onset was abrupt and jerky. Body movements in anencephalic fetus showed lack of positional changes with waxing and waning in intensity. Using this technique, the function of lower level CNS responsible for these forceful, monotonous changes is evaluated

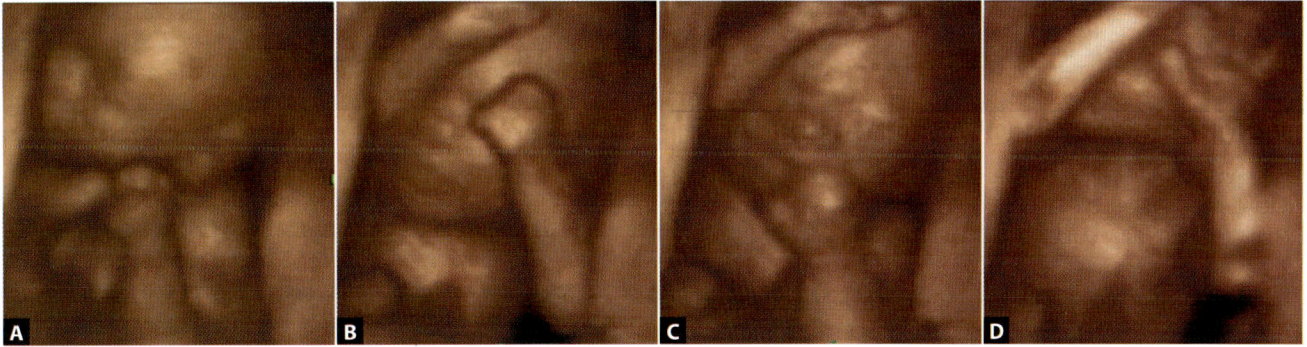

Figs 40.11A to D: (A to D) 4D 4D sequence of a normal fetus at the same age as Figure 40.10, hand movement could be observed in any direction. We can see head movement (retroflexion and rotation) followed by palm opening. Qualitative alteration of movements can be used as a marker of the severity of associated neurological disability

from forceful and jerky in character and of large amplitude in anencephalic fetuses (Figs 40.10A to D), to the monotonous and rigid or chaotic in diabetic pregnancies. Qualitative alterations of general movements (Figs 40.11A to D) seem to be useful in the assessment of the severity of associated neurological disability. The complex sequences of extension and flexion of the legs and arms (Figs 40.9A to F), may be better assessed with 4D ultrasound. Furthermore, 4D sonography seems to be the method of choice for detecting subtle changes such as superimposed rotations and changes in direction of the movements. The application of this new technique could improve the analysis of fetal movements and could allow the definition of precise criteria for the assessment of the integrity of fetal nervous system.

In the literature, there is a range between 8 and 12 weeks concerning the first appearance of limb movements.[15,129] De Vries found isolated arm and leg movements at 8 weeks of pregnancy.[15] With 4D ultrasound, the limb movements were detected at 8–9 weeks of gestation (Table 40.3).[118] In this interval, limbs are elongated and their segments are discernible. Isolated arm and leg movements were clearly visible and consisted of changes in position of the extremities toward the body without observable flexion or extension in joints.

Limb movements become more complex with advancing gestational age. Specific movements can be recognized at 14 weeks by 2D ultrasound. The organization of the movement pattern occurs as their frequency increases.[130] It seems that fetal arms explore the surrounding environment and cross the midline, while the palmar surface is oriented toward the uterine wall. The fetal legs are extended to the uterine wall. This phenomenon can be seen 2 weeks earlier using 4D ultrasound.[118] Despite its presence, these movement patterns are less organized in comparison with those observed at 14 weeks by 2D ultrasound. Complex limb movement consists of changes in position of the limb segments toward each other, seen by 4D ultrasound. More limb joints are active and move simultaneously, for example, as extension or flexion in arm and elbow or hip and knee. The elevation of the hand, extension of the elbow joint, with a slight change in direction and rotation, can be seen simultaneously.

Sparling and Wilhelm also described spontaneous movements in fetuses from 12 to 35 weeks of gestation (Table 40.4) and recorded the characteristics of hand movement.[130] Many movements appeared to be directed to a body part or the uterine wall. The hands of the fetuses moved with a variety of frequencies and apparent force. Joint ranges of motion changed throughout movements rather than remaining the same, as in floating. These movements suggested

Table 40.4: Developmental motor characteristics cord

Gestational Age (weeks)	description
8	Trunk flexion and extension
12	Isolated random-appearing movement of extremities
14	All movement patterns present; an increased frequency of movement that is more "organized" in appearance compared with movement at 12 weeks; arms appear to "explore" while legs extend against uterine wall; arm crosses midline, extending palmar surface to opposite uterine wall
16	Decreased frequency of movements from 14 weeks, with pincr grasps, thumb in mouth
20	More bilateral movement (e.g. legs extend together against uterine wall, arms flex, and hands are often held together near the face)
26–32	Independent movement of extremities to all parts of the uterus and specific body parts; no cephalocaudal development; but apparent distal-proximal development in extremities
37–38	Decreased frequency of movements; hand often molded to occiput, or dorsum of hand rests against uterine wall

Source: Adapted from Reference 126

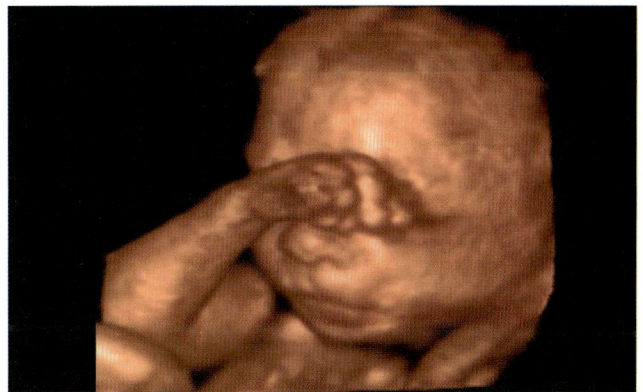

Fig. 40.12: This picture shows the hand-to-face contact

primary and secondary circular reactions in which a movement is repeated, presumably because it has functional importance to the organism.[131,132] During later gestational periods, the fetuses' hands were directed to and manipulated body parts and features of the environment, such as the umbilical cord.

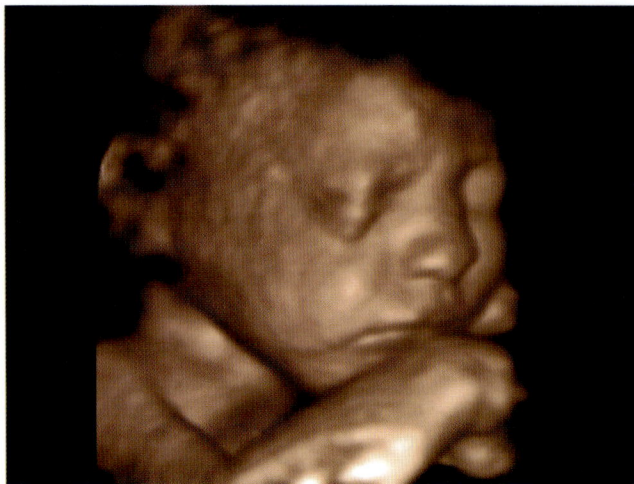

Fig. 40.13: The hand movement into direct contact to the mouth

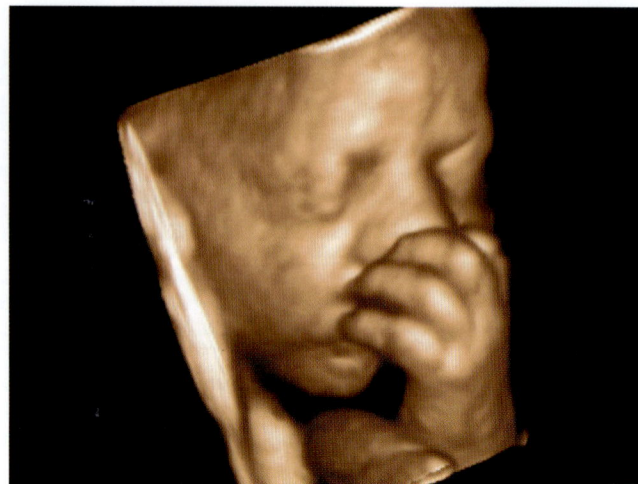

Fig. 40.14: 3D image showing the direction of hand movement to the nose

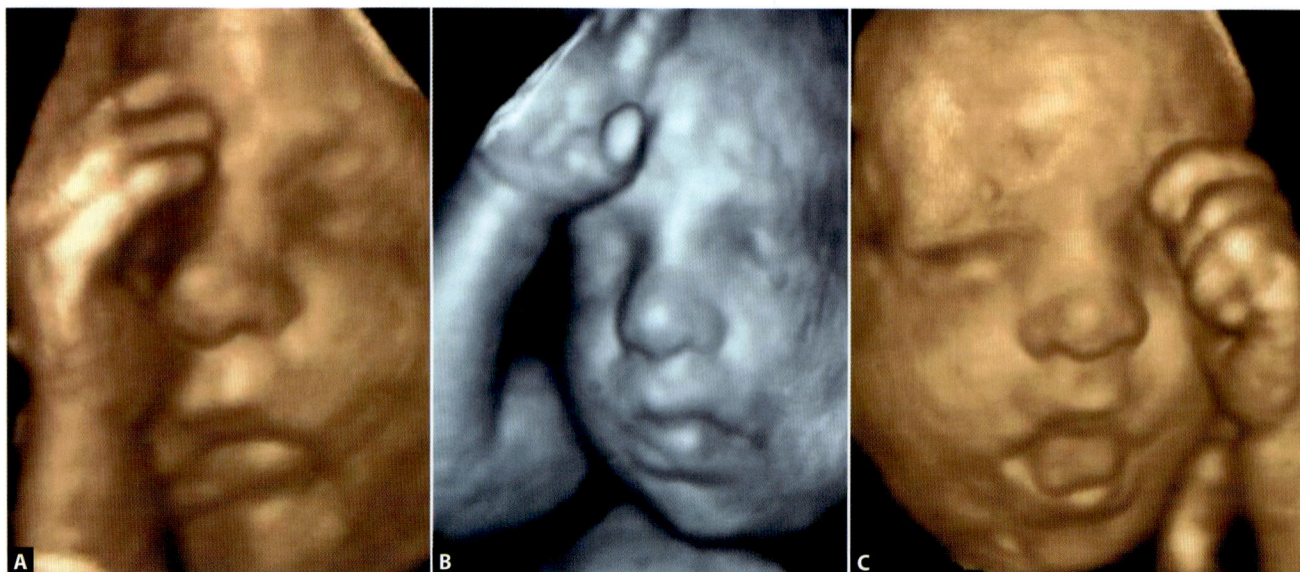

Figs 40.15A to C: Several 3D images of hand direction (A) to the face, (B) to the head, (C) to the eye

Our recent study, performed by 4D sonography, has shown that the amount of isolated arm movements decreases gradually from 13 through 16 weeks (Table 40.5A). All recordings have been made during 15-minutes intervals. The incidence varied between 50 and 120 with a median value of 60 at 13 weeks, 17 and 27 with a median value of 23 at 14 weeks, 0 and 6 with a median value of 2 at 15 weeks, 18 and 28 with a median value of 25 at 16 weeks. The highest range was registered at 13 weeks of gestation. Data from Table 40.5B demonstrate the incidence of hand-to-head movements (Fig. 40.15). There is notable decrease in their incidence, followed by a plateau at 14 weeks of gestation. The incidence varied from 4 to 29 at 13 weeks and from 0 to 7 at 16 weeks of gestation. Table 40.5C shows the incidence of hand-to-mouth movements (Fig. 40.13). The incidence varied between 0 and 4 with a median value of 2 at 13 weeks, and between 0 and 2 with a median value of 2 at 16 weeks.

The highest range was found at 15 weeks of gestation. At 13 weeks, a plateau was observed and was present until 16 weeks.

Although this plateau was evident, mild fluctuations occurred. In contrast to most other movement patterns, hand near mouth movements (Table 40.5D) decreased gradually from 13 weeks onward with a single fluctuation in 14th week (it varied between 0 and 3 with a median value of 1). The incidence of hand-to-face movement (Figs 40.12 and 40.15) is characterized by a decrease at 14 weeks followed by a plateau (Table 40.5E and Fig. 40.14). From 13 weeks onward, the hand-near-face movement pattern was visible in all 15 fetuses with an incidence of 2 to 9 and a median value of 8. At 16 weeks, the range was from 1 to 7 with a median value of 3. Although the plateau was observed, mild fluctuation was evident, especially at 15 weeks. From Table 40.5F, we can recognize that the incidence of hand-near-face movement is stable between 13 and 16 weeks of gestation with slight increase at 14 and 15 weeks. At 13 weeks, the range was the widest (from 0 to 12), with the median value of 3. The incidence of hand to ear movements decreased between 13 and 16 weeks (Table 40.5G). It varied between 4 and 12 with a median value of 8 at 13 weeks, and 0 and 3 with a median

Table 40.5: The incidence of several characteristics of hand movements from 13 to 16 gestational weeks showed by 4D sonography. (A) Isolated hand movement; (B) Hand to head movements; (C) Hand to mouth movements; (D) Hand near mouth movements; (E) Hand to face movements; (F) Hand near face movements (G) Hand to ear movements; (H) Hand to eye movements

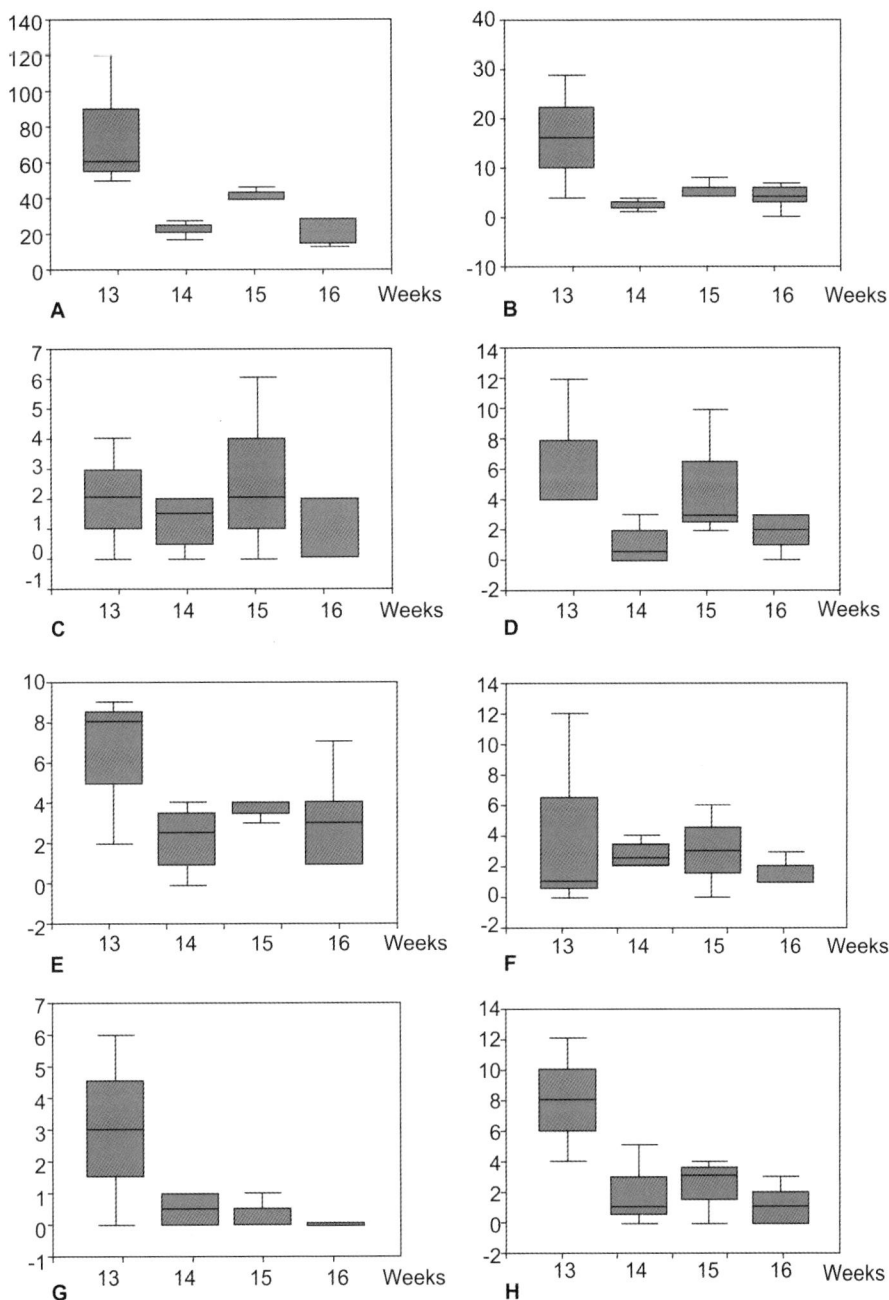

Source: Adapted from Reference 23

value of 0 at 16 weeks. The incidence of the hand-to-eye movement (Fig. 40.15) pattern showed the same developmental trend as hand-to-head and hand-to-face movement patterns (Table 40.5H). At 13 weeks, the incidence was between 4 and 12 occurrences per 15 minutes observation time with a median value of 8. At 16 weeks, the range was from 0 to 3 with a median value of 1.[23]

Other developmental tendencies in hand movement have been noted.[133] Movements such as thumb-in-mouth and bilateral leg extension against the uterine wall were considered as functionally important. The frequently observed leg extension against the uterine wall was believed by the authors to be a possible precursor to later participation in the birthing process. Early movements of

the arms appeared to assist the fetus in identifying components of its environment. Attributing function to any of these early movements, however, does not imply that the assigned function is preliminary to or necessary for the appearance of a spontaneous behavior.[25,133-137]

Assessment of Fetal Facial Expressions by 4D Ultrasound

Recent studies have demonstrated that during the second and third trimester, it is possible to study total fetal facial activities. In addition to yawning, sucking and swallowing described by 2D real-time imaging, it is now possible to study a full range of facial expressions including smiling, crying, and eyelid movements.[23,134]

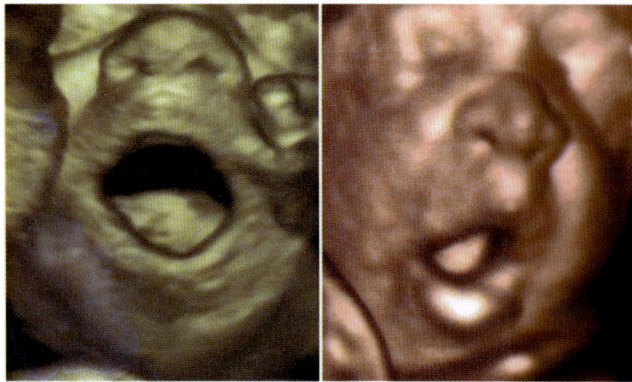

Fig. 40.16: Yawning expression of the fetus. An involuntary wide opening of the mouth, with maximal widening of the jaw, followed by quick closure often with retroflexion of the head and sometimes elevation of the arms

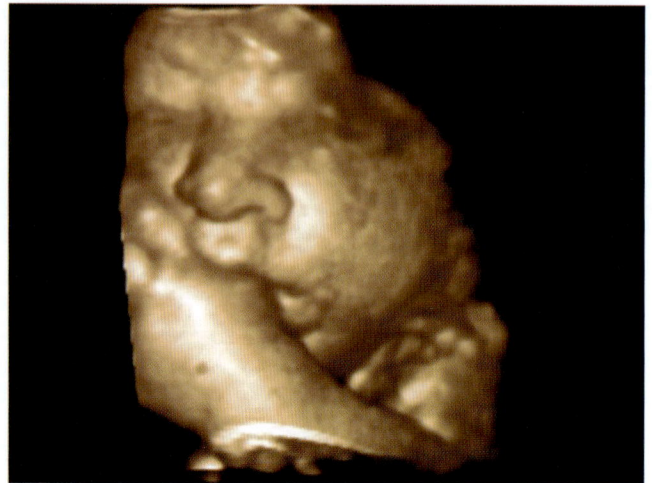

Fig. 40.17: Shows sucking expression of the fetus. The fetus is placing the thumb into the mouth, probably on the roof of the mouth and sucking with lips closed

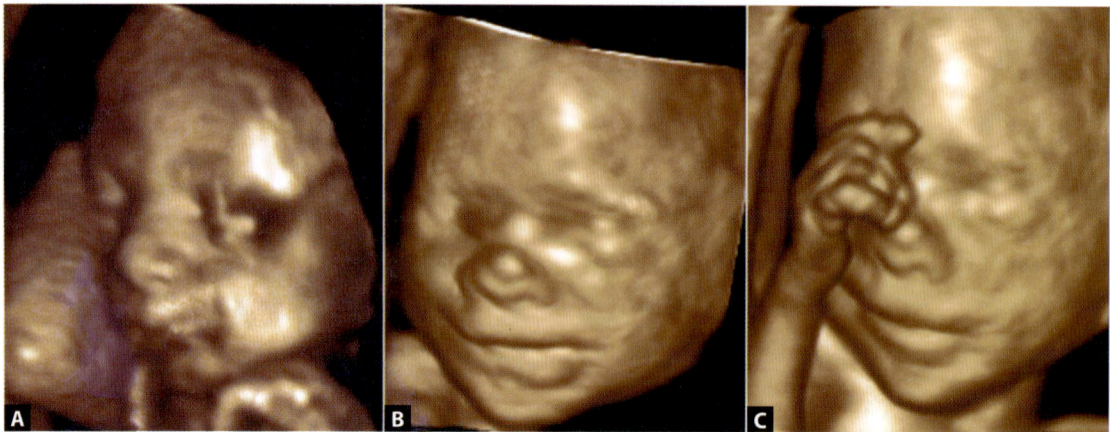

Figs 40.18A to C: (A to C) Several facial expressions characterized by turning up the corners of the mouth shows the smiling fetus

The fetal behavioral patterns have been evaluated in 10 gravidas in the third trimester between 30–33 weeks of gestation.[23] The incidence of eyelid movements ranged between 4 and 20 with a median value of 17, mouthing movements ranged between 2 and 19 with a median value of 12, mouth and eyelid movements ranged between 0 and 13 with a median value of 5. The incidence of pure mouth movements such as the mouth opening ranged between 4 and 13 with a median of 5, tongue expulsion ranged between 0 and 2 with a median of 2, yawning ranged between 0 and 2 with a median of 1 and pouting ranged between 0 and 9 with a median of 3. The incidence of facial expressions such as smiling ranged between 2 and 7 with a median of 2 and scowling between 2 and 4 with a median of 2. It is evident that eyelid and mouthing movements dominate at this gestational age. The continuity between fetal and neonatal behavior has also been suggested.[133] These findings may stimulate multicentric studies of the fetal behavior and responsiveness as a sign of neurological maturation. In the long-term, fetal behavioral studies may become a means of assessing fetal well-being.[23]

The Zagreb group has attempted to evaluate 4D sonography in the assessment of fetal facial expression. They have classified eight different facial expressions.

Classification of Facial Movement Patterns

1. *Yawning:* This movement is similar to the yawn observed after birth. An involuntary wide opening of the mouth, with maximal widening of the jaws followed by quick closure often with retroflexion of the head and sometimes elevation of the arms. This movement pattern is non-repetitive (Fig. 40.16).

2. *Swallowing:* Indicating that the fetus is drinking amniotic fluid. Swallowing consists of displacements of tongue and/or larynx. Swallowing activity develops earlier than sucking in the course of fetal development.

3. *Sucking:* Rhythmical bursts of regular jaw opening, and closing at a rate of about one per second. Placing the finger or thumb on the roof of the mouth behind the teeth and sucking with lips closed. Thumb sucking is a very frequent fetal behavioral pattern (Fig. 40.17).

4. *Smiling:* A facial expression characterized by turning up the corners of the mouth (Fig. 40.18).

5. *Tongue expulsion:* A facial expression characterized by expulsion of the tongue (Fig. 40.19).

6. *Grimacing:* The wrinkling of the brows or face in frowning for expression of displeasure (Fig. 40.20).
7. *Mouthing:* A facial expression characterized by mouth manipulation to investigate an object. Mouthing is most common in the fetus and it may develop into a persistent, stereotyped behavior pattern (Figs 40.21A to I).
8. *Isolated eye blinking:* A reflex that closes and opens the eyes rapidly. Brief closing of the eyelids by involuntary normal periodic closing, as a protective measure, or by voluntary action (Figs 40.18 and 40.22).

They have also tried to identify emotional expressions as the combinations of several facial expressions mentioned above (Figs 40.20 and 40.22).

The early results, presented above, indicate that fetal facial grimaces, resembling the emotional expressions in adults are present during the third trimester of gestation. However, the precise criteria for a distinction of theses expressions in the fetus remain to be established. The option to study fetal facial expressions allows dealing with new research questions and indicates a great potential for 4D sonographic studies in the psychological and fetal behavioral sciences. Facial expressions are an important channel of nonverbal communication. The characteristics of facial expressions can provide a different mode to the expert for understanding the hidden side of the fetus in utero, a side that may not be accessible in the form of any verbalizations. However, the clear evidences that fetal emotional processing exists in the third trimester of gestation or that it is related to facial expressions are still lacking and extensive multicentric studies should be conducted in order to clarify this area. We believe that the fetal facial expressions and fetal behaviors related to emotions could reveal a part of the emotional aspect of the intrauterine life. If this assumption becomes confirmed, it is possible to imagine that we could construct a system, which relates the discrete emotions, like happiness, anger, sadness, etc. and various intensities of the fetal facial expressions in utero to the external events. It might be possible to construct a system where componential and general internal states like pleasure control each parameter unit and establish a pleasure score of the fetus that can be used evaluate facial expressions.

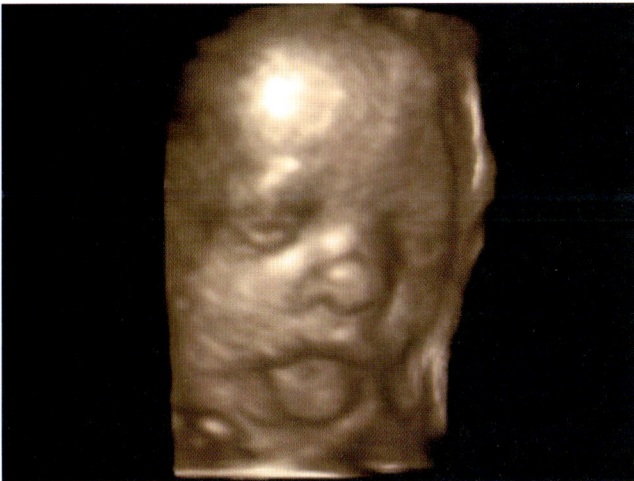

Fig. 40.19: Facial expression characterized by tongue expulsion

WHAT IS KANET?

The KANET system for assessment of fetal and neonatal behavior was developed mainly as a diagnostic tool for the early detection of brain dysfunction.[138] KANET is a new scoring system for the assessment of fetal neurobehavior that has been recently introduced and is based on prenatal evaluation of the fetus by 3D/4D ultrasound.[139] This scoring system is a combination of some parameters consisting of fetal general movements (GMs) and of postnatal Amiel-Tison neurological assessment at term (ATNAT) signs, which can be easily visualized prenatally by using 4D ultrasound.[140-142] Several papers have shown that there is a continuity of behavior from prenatal to postnatal life and it has been observed that all movements that are present in neonates are also present in fetal life, with the exception of Moro's reflex, which cannot be demonstrated in fetuses.[143] This is probably due to the different environment to which fetus and neonate are exposed. The fetus lives in an environment of microgravity, while the newborn is exposed to full gravity, which creates certain obstacles for neurodevelopment in the 1st month of life.[144] The parameters were chosen based on developmental approach to the neurological assessment and on the theory of central pattern generators of GMs emergence, and were the product of multicentric studies conducted for several years.[140,145]

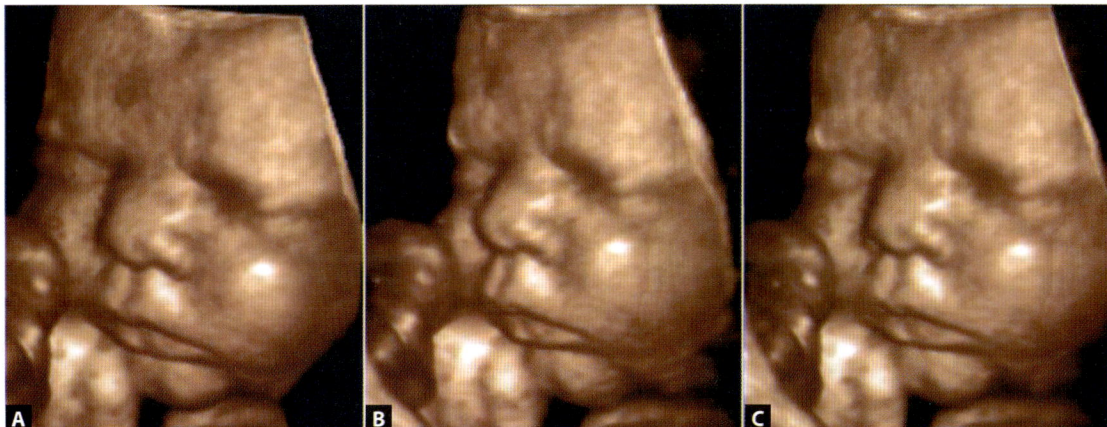

Figs 40.20A to C: (A to C) In these pictures, the fetus shows wrinkling of the brows or face in frowning, may be to express displeasure or anger. The frontalis muscle can also be responsible for the appearance of grimacing. However, the main actor responsible for the appearance of scowling is the corrugator muscle

KANET is a combination of assessments of fetal behavior, GMs and three out of four signs which have been postnatally considered as symptoms of possible neurodevelopmental impairment (neurological thumb, overlapping sutures and small head circum-ference).[146] KANET test was standardized in Osaka, Japan, on the 24th of October 2010, to improve reproducibility and applicability for fetal medicine specialists.[146] According to the Osaka consensus statement the KANET should be performed in the third-trimester of pregnancy, between 28 and 38 weeks. The duration of the examination should be between 15 and 20 minutes, and fetuses should be examined while they are awake. If the fetus is in the sleeping period, the assessment should be postponed for 30 minutes or for the following day, at a minimum period of 14–16 hours. In cases of grossly abnormal or of borderline score, the test should be repeated every 2 weeks until delivery. Special attention should be paid to the facial movements and to eye blinking, which are prenatally very informative and important ("the face is the mirror of the brain"). The frequency of facial and mouth movements should be 0–5 and more than 5. Overall number of movements should be defined in very active or inactive fetuses and compared with normal values of previous studies.[140,145] All the examiners should have extensive hands-on education for the application of KANET test, both in low and in high-risk pregnancies. Intraobserver and intraobserver variability should be available. It is advisable to use 4D ultrasound machines, with a frame rate of minimum 24 volumes/ second. The Osaka consensus statement concluded that the KANET should use eight parameters rather than ten, for the assessment of the fetus (Table 40.6). A score range of 0–5 is characterized as abnormal, a score calculated from 6 to 9 is considered borderline and a score range of 10–16 is normal (Table 40.7). After delivery, neonates should be followed up for neurological development for a 2-year period.

Advantages of KANET

The test evaluates quantitative as well as qualitative aspects of fetal motor behavioral patterns. This technique supplies more convincing images/video sequences than conventional ultrasonic and nonultrasonic methods, enabling to observe fetal movements in their full repertoire and variability (Figs 40.23A to F).

The parameters examined by this test are partly based on observation of GMs. A second group of parameters is adopted from ATNAT.[147,148] The criterion of quality and quantity of spontaneous GMs is believed to have excellent reliability in evaluating the integrity of fetal CNS.[119,149]

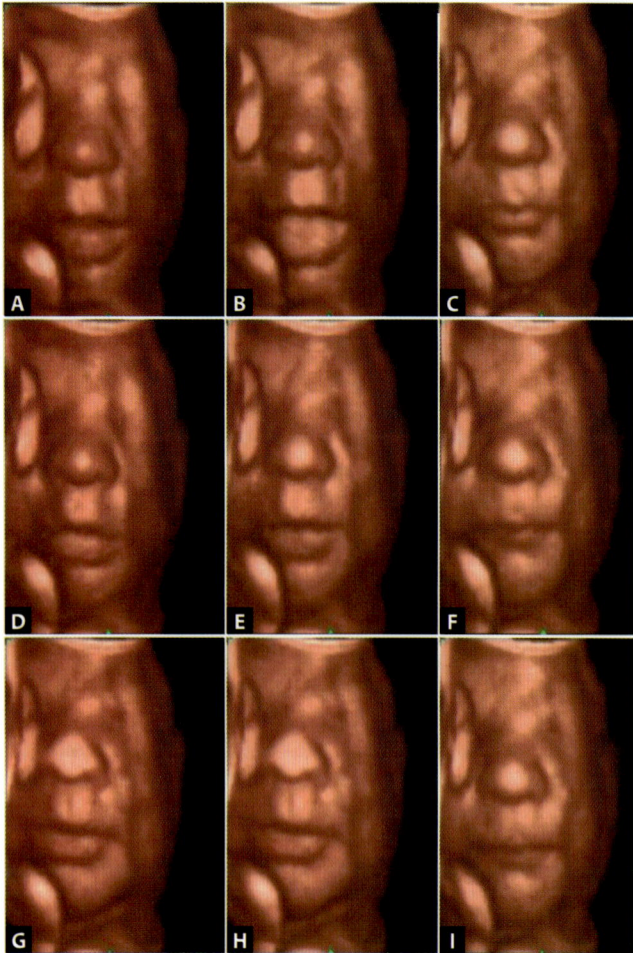

Figs 40.21A to I: (A to I) On this image sequence, mouthing could be observed as a facial expression pattern. We can see a series of rhythmic movements involving the mandible and tongue, characterized by constant frequency and duration until disappearance

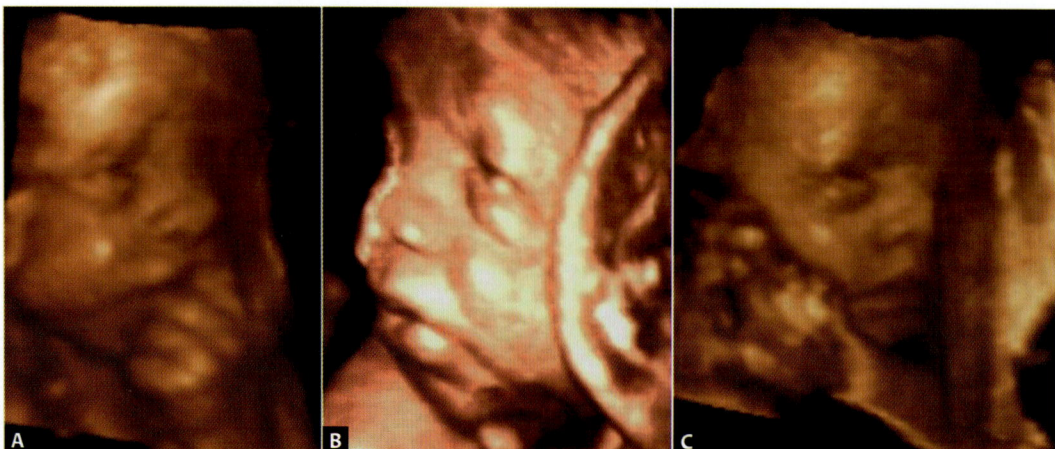

Figs 40.22A to C: (A to C) Fear expressions of the fetus. We can see the hand to the mouth movement together with eyelid opening. We assumed that this complex expression could be related to the imminent possibility of fetal danger, a nearby threat, a displeasure position, or of bodily harm

Table 40.6: The KANET scoring system

Sign	Score			Sign Score
	0	1	2	
Isolated head anteflexion	About	Small range (0–3 times of movement)	Variable in full range, many alternation (>3 times of movements)	
Cranial sutures and head circumference	Overlapping of cranial sutures	Normal cranial sutures with measurement of HC below or above the normal limit (–2 SD) according to GA	Normal cranial sutures with normal measurement of HC according to GA	
Isolated eye blinking	Not present	Not fluent (1–5 times of blinking)	Fluency (>5 times of blinking)	
Facial alteration (grimace or tongue expulsion) or Mouth opening (yawning or mouthing)	Not present	Not fluent (1–5 times of alteration)	Fluency (>5 times of alteration)	
Isolated leg movements	Cramped	Poor repertoire or Small in range (0–5 times of movement)	Variable in full range, many alternation (>5 times of movements)	
Isolated hand movements or Hand to face movements	Cramped of abrupt	Poor repertoire or Small in range (0–5 times of movement)	Variable in full range, many alternation (>5 times of movements)	
Fingers movements	Unilateral or bilateral clenched fist, (neurological thumb)	Cramped invariable finger movements	Smooth and complex, variable finger movements	
Gestalt perception of GMs	Definitely abnormal	Borderline	Normal **Total score**	

Source: Stanojevic et al. Osaka Consensus Statement. DSJUOG. 2011;5(4):317-29.

Table 40.7: Interpretation of test scores

Total score	Interpretation
0–5	Abnormal
6–9	Borderline
10–16	Normal

Source: Stanojevic et al. "Osaka Consensus Statement. DSJUOG. 2011;5(4):317-29.

Furthermore, a continuity of behavioral patterns from prenatal to the postnatal period has been proven.[133,150,151] This continuity suggests to use the same parameters in ultrasonography which are used for neurologic evaluation of the newborn. Both these facts justify the choice of the parameters used in this test, making KANET theoretically appropriate for the assessment of fetal behavior. According to previous reports,[152-157] KANET easily recognizes serious functional impairment associated with structural

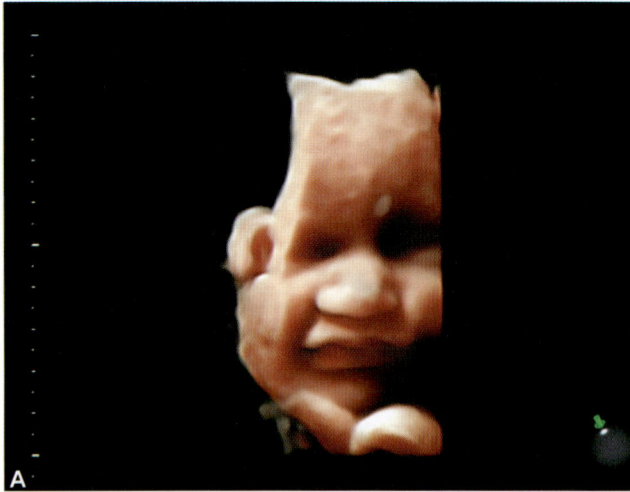

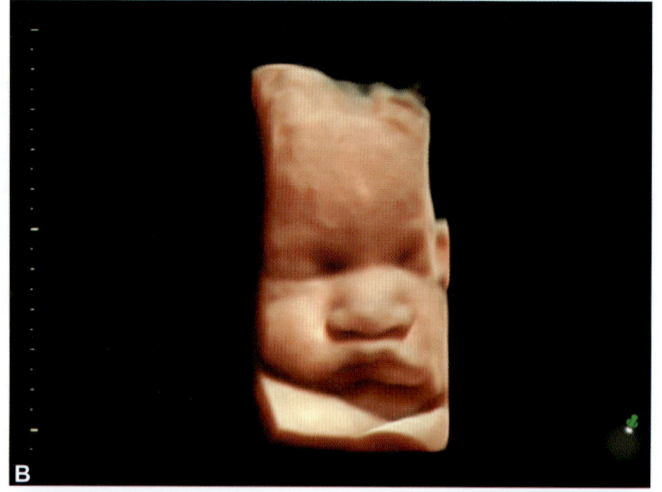

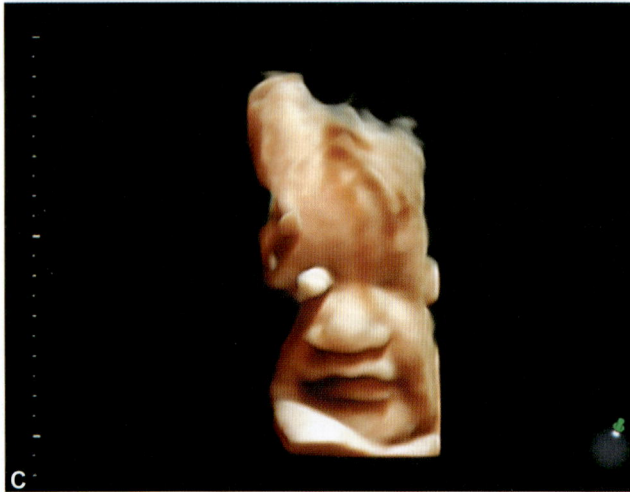

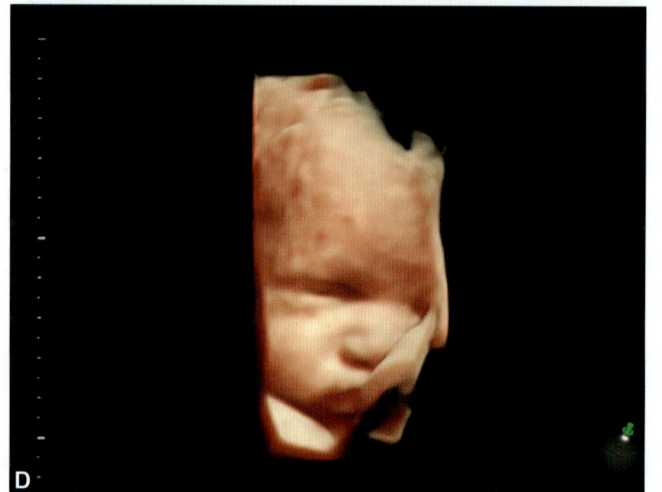

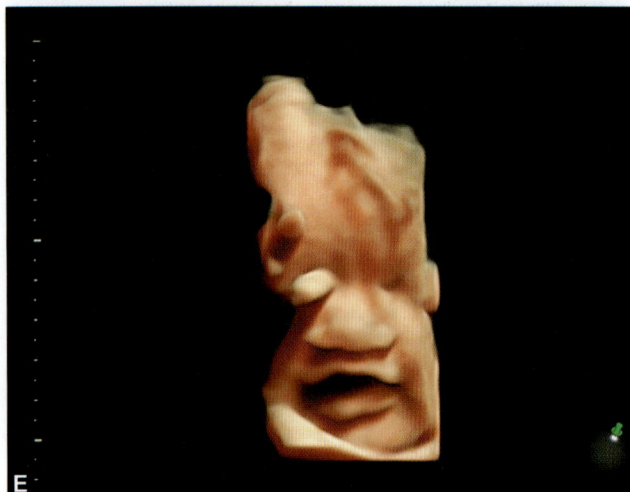

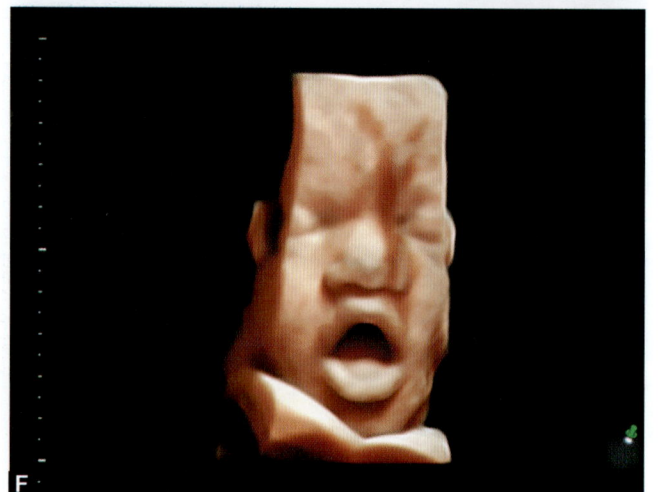

Figs 40.23A to F: Facial expressions

abnormalities. Recent studies have shown that the application of KANET in both low- and high-risk populations has given very promising results about the outcome of the fetuses. Especially in high risk populations, the result of KANET may provide extremely useful information and guidelines for the counseling of the neurological outcome of these fetuses.[138]

The KANET is the first test which is based on 4D ultrasound, with an original scoring system and has been standardized, so it can be implemented in everyday practice, overcoming the practical difficulties and covering the gaps of methods that were used in the past for the evaluation of fetal behavior.[159-162] More recent studies show evidence that KANET is easily applicable to the majority of pregnancies, that the learning curve is short for physicians who already have training in obstetrical ultrasound, and that the actual time of the KANET is very reasonable, ranging from 15 to 20 minutes. These characteristics support a wide implementation of KANET as a tool for fetal neurological assessment.[152] As a conclusion, the results of recent, large multicenter studies show that KANET is an easily applied, standardized test, which utilizes the advantages of 4D ultrasound, such as better analysis of facial expressions and quality (variability and complexity) of fetal movements, in order to distinguish between normal and abnormal behavioral patterns of the fetus, with the aim of early recognition of fetal brain impairment.[146]

Exploration of the environment: palm of the hand to uterine wall (Figs 40.24A to D).

FETAL BEHAVIOR AND RISK ASSESSMENT

Several studies have proven that presence or absence of fetal movements has significance for fetal wellbeing.[163-167] Different types of high-risk pregnancies have been found to go along with reduced fetal movements (RFM).

Altered fetal behavior may be functional expression of anomalies of the Central Nervous System (CNS) (Figs 40.25A to G).[168-170]

Decreased fetal movements (DFM) may represent a fetal behavioral response, to compensate stages of moderate hypoxemia, and can be compared to fetal adaptation to chronic hypoxemia by redistribution of oxygenized blood to essential organs, i.e. heart, brain, and adrenal glands.

Persistent DFM can indicate impending decompensation of fetal adaptive strategies, and—when hypoxemia becomes more severe and prolonged—even imminent IUFD.[171-176]

Absence or diminution of a given fetal biophysical variable like movements does not necessarily signal pathology. Normal intrinsic fetal rhythms, such as the deep stage of quiet sleep, may reduce the

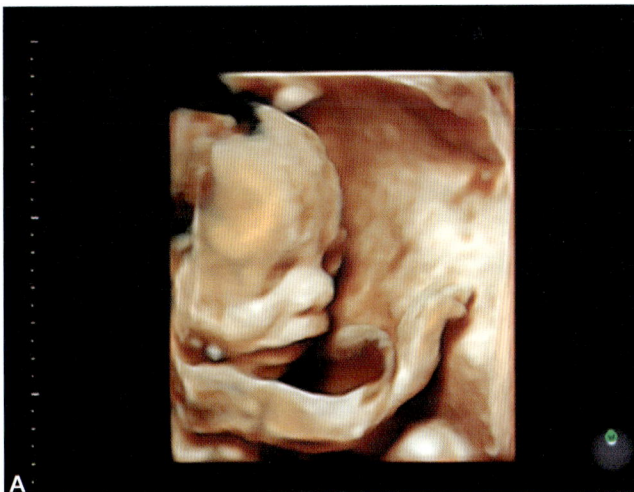

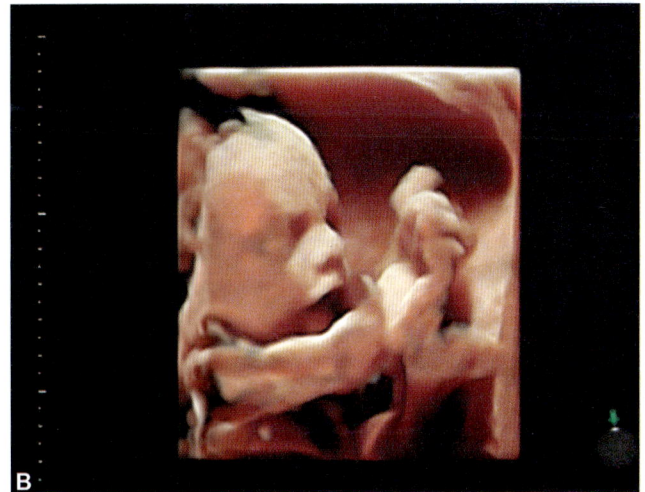

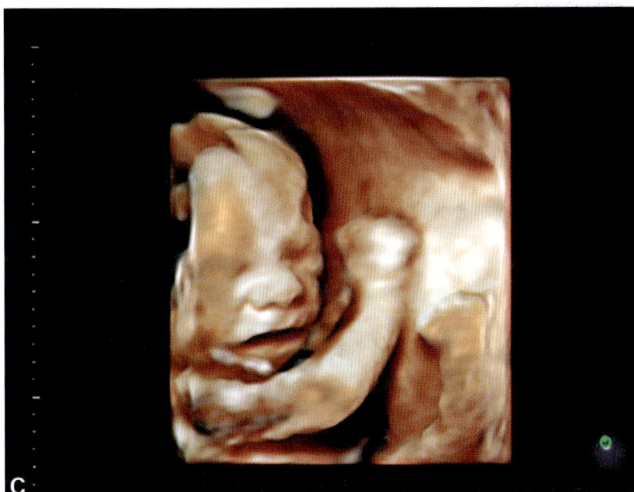

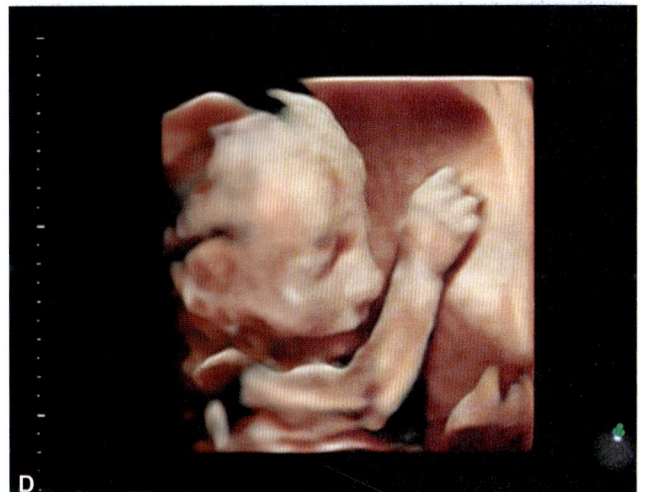

Figs 40.24A to D: (A to D) Hand to uterine wall

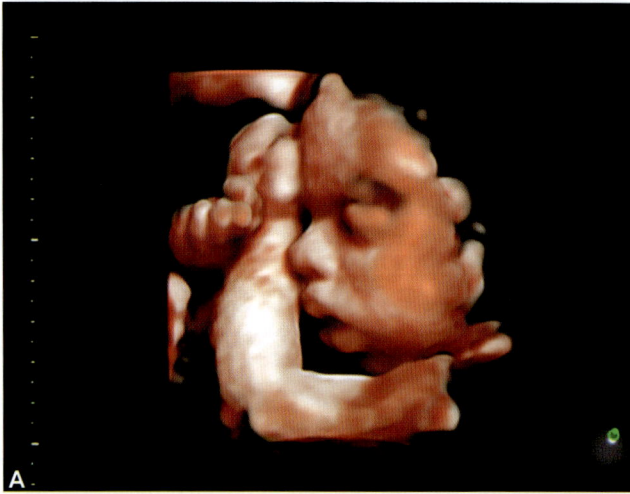

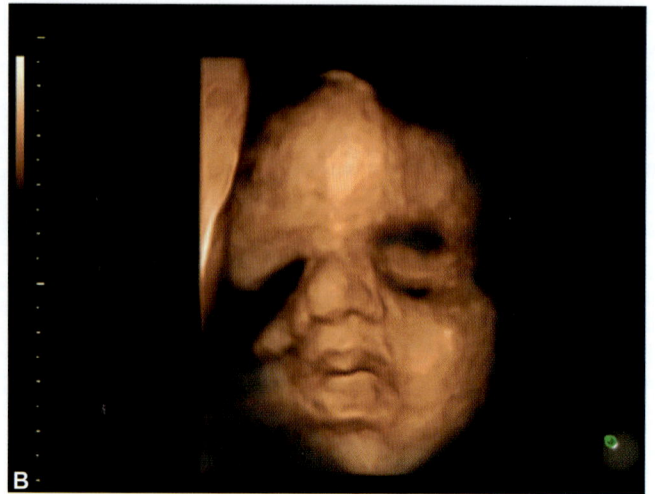

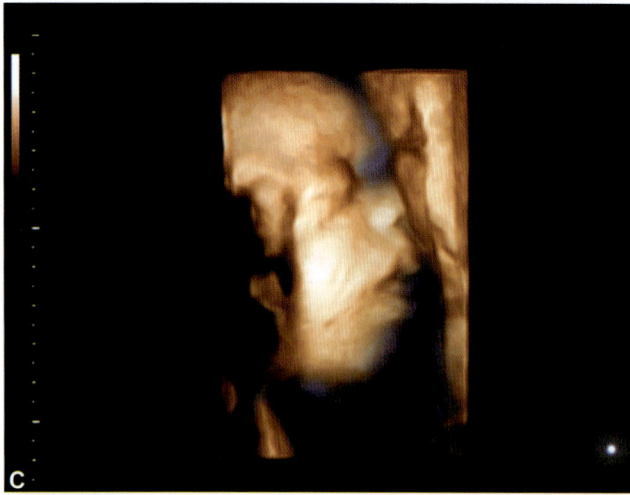

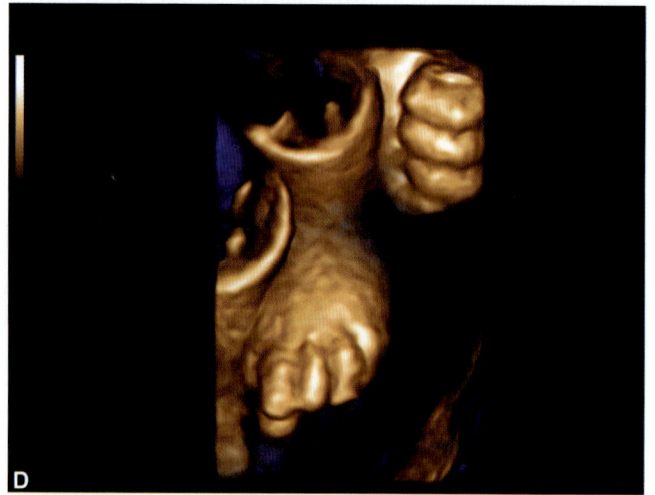

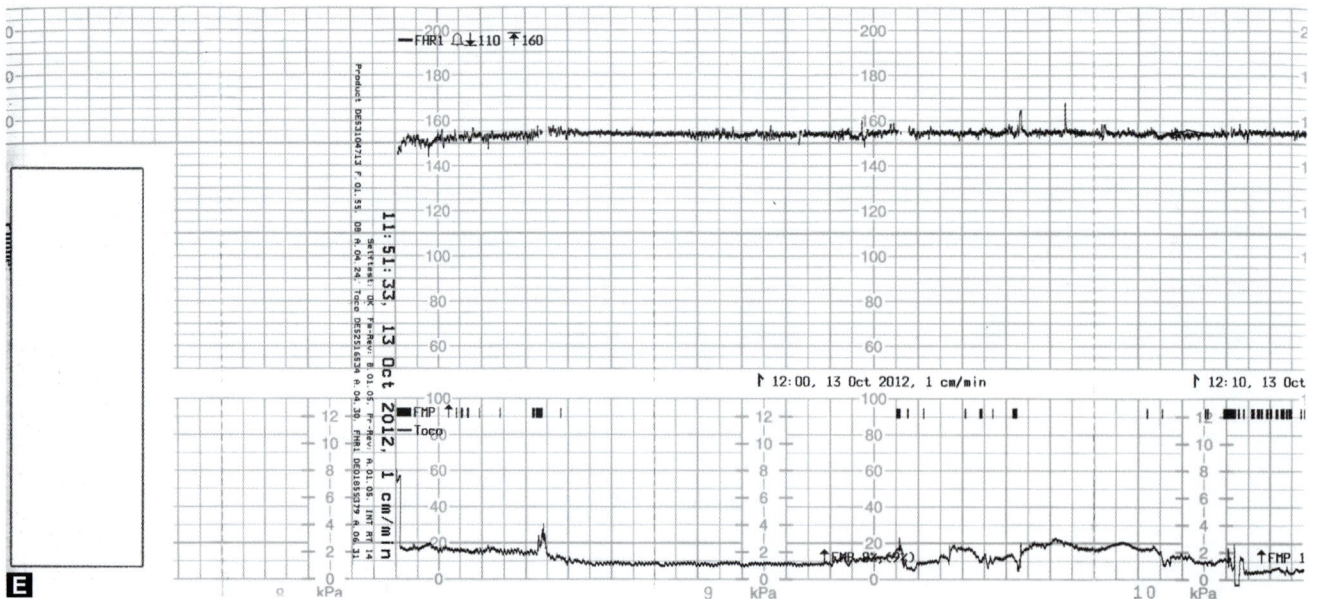

Contd…

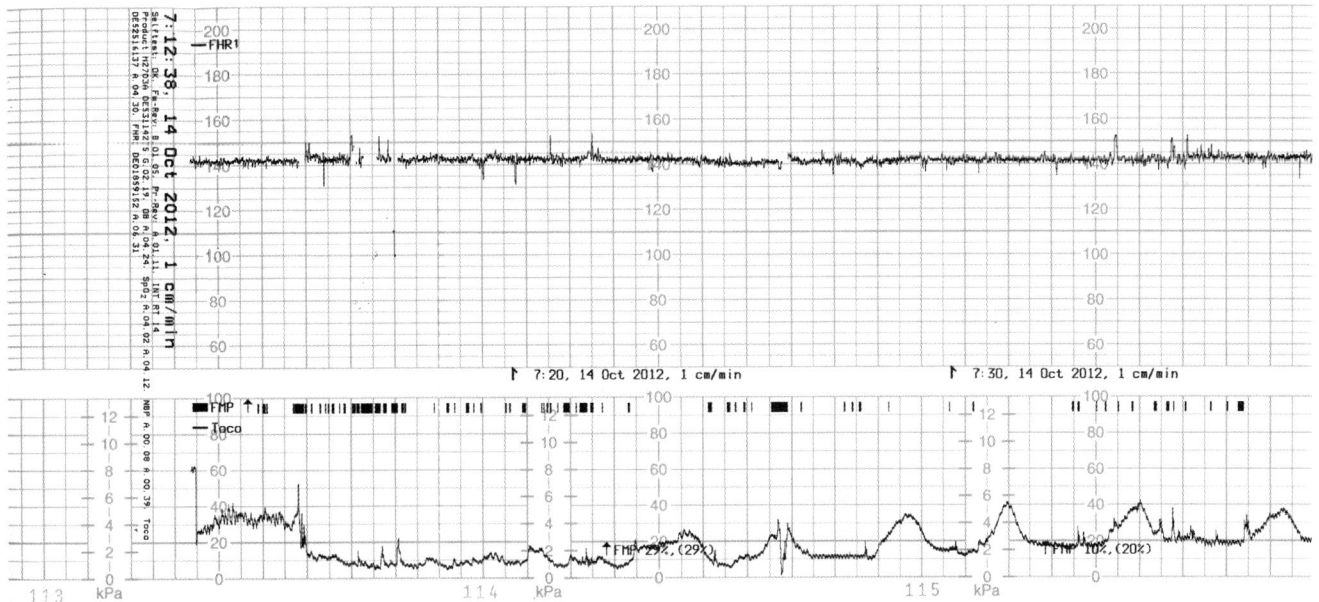

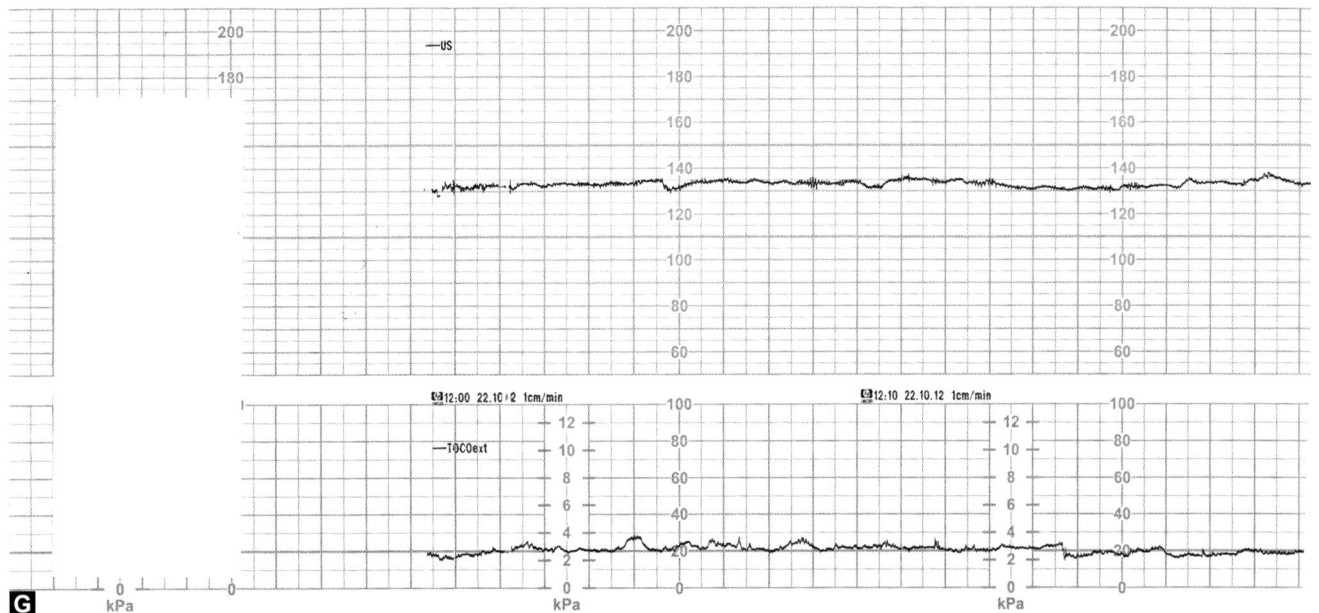

Figs 40.25A to G: In this case of Akinesia-Deformation Sequence at 30 weeks, with normal karyotype, normal fetal Doppler and only mild IUGR, with (still) normal neurosonoanatomy, it was repeated abnormal KANET to reveal the true extent of fetal compromise, initiate further diagnostic measures, and appropriate counseling and mental preparation of the parents for an unfavorable pregnancy outcome. (A) Note bilateral clenched fists; (B) Note open mouth with slightly protruding tongue; (C) Lateral aspect of B; (D) Note clenched fist with adducted thumb and fixed position of first digit of the right foot; (E to G) Note fixed heart rate with loss of variability on all three CTGs within an interval of 9 days (decerebration pattern) (for further review see Reference 177)

activity of regulatory centers in the fetal CNS and suspend fetal motoric activity.

Behavioral state in the fetus, with periods of activity and inactivity, is—as stated above—a result of maturation of the central nervous system.[159,178]

It is obvious that any method assessing fetal wellbeing, which is based on fetal behavior, may be affected by fetal ultradian rhythm, i.e. fetal quiet sleep. This may be reason for misinterpretation of fetal behavior. Fetal and maternal daily

rhythms run with a reverse phase: the fetus between 36–40 weeks develops a sleep-like "quiet" state from 4 am to 9 am and from 2 pm to 7 pm, with "active" periods from 9 am to 2 pm and evening-night 7 pm to 4 am.[179,180]

According to the occurrence rate of state 1F = Quiet Sleep of 15% at 36 and 30% at 38 weeks (31), it would be expected to find low KANET scores in 15–30% at 36–38 weeks.[159,181]

How often and when should KANET be performed during pregnancy? Prenatal screening for neurological disability should come early enough and should be repeated to detect conversion from normal to abnormal behavior, because timely neuroprotective fetal therapy could be helpful in certain cases.[187,188]

About one-third of cases of Cerebral Palsy are estimated to be caused by prenatal impacts. These events seem to take place as a sequence of interdependant adverse events.[189,190]

There are a growing number of studies providing evidence that certain risk pregnancies go along with quantitative and qualitative deviation of fetal behavior assessed by KANET[139,152-155,158,182-186,191-198] (Table 40.8).

CONCLUSIONS

One of the greatest challenges of obstetrical ultrasonography is the better understanding of fetal neurological function.[199,200]

Neurological problems such as CP, which has for many years been a huge scientific and medicolegal problem for obstetricians, is poorly understood and often is falsely attributed to intrapartum events, while for the majority of CP cases this is not true.[201-203]

So the question of how could we define normal and abnormal fetal neurological function in utero, both for low-risk fetuses and for

Table 40.8: List of studies that have applied Kurjak's antenatal neurodevelopmental test to different populations[192]

Author	Year	Study	Study Design	Study Population	Indication	No	GA (weeks)	Time (mins)	Result	Summary
Kurjak et al.[139]	2008	Cohort	Retrospective	High-risk	Multiple	220	20–36	30	Positive	A new scoring system for the assessment of neurological status of fetuses, for antenatal application was proposed, based on retrospective observations
Kurjak et al.[154]	2010	Multicenter	Prospective	High-Risk	Multiple	288	20–38	30	Positive	KANET showed potential for antenatal detection of serious neurological fetal problems. KANET appeared to be able to identify serious structural abnormalities associated with brain impairment
Miskovic et al.[152]	2010	Cohort	Prospective	High-risk	Multiple	226	20–36	30	Positive	Statistically significant moderate correlation of KANET and ATNAT tests was found. KANET confirmed the differences of fetal behavior between the high-risk and normal pregnancies
Talic et al.[153]	2011	Multicenter Cohort	Prospective	High-risk	Multiple	620	26–38	15–20	Positive	KANET test showed a potential of detection and discriminate normal from border line and abnormal fetal behavior in normal and in high risk fetuses. Low KANET scores were predictable of either intrauterine or postnatal death.
Talic et al.[182]	2011	Multicenter Cohort	Prospective	High-risk	Ventriculomegaly	240	32–36	10–15	Positive	KANET in normal pregnancies and pregnancies with ventriculomegaly showed statistically significant differences. Abnormal KANET scores and most of the borderline-scores were found among the fetuses with severe ventriculomegaly associated with additional abnormalities
Honemeyer et al.[183]	2011	Cohort	Prospective	Unselected	Unselected	100	28–38	N/A	Positive	Normal prenatal KANET scores were significantly predictive for normal postnatal neurological assessment of newborns
Lebit et al.[184]	2011	Cohort	Prospective	Low-risk	Normal 2D examination	144	7–38	15–20	Positive	A pattern of fetal behavior for each trimester of pregnancy was identified

Contd...

Contd…

Author	Year	Study	Study Design	Study Population	Indication	No	GA (weeks)	Time (mins)	Result	Summary
Abo-Yaqoub et al.[155]	2012	Cohort	Prospective	High-risk	Multiple	80	20–38	15–20	Positive	The difference in KANET score was significant. All cases with abnormal KANET proved to be abnormal postnatally
Vladareanu et al.[185]	2012	Cohort	Prospective	High-risk	Multiple	196	24–38	N/A	Positive	Most fetuses with normal KANET were low-risk, those with borderline were IUGR fetuses with increased MCA RI and most fetuses with abnormal KANET were threatened PTD with PPROM. There was statistical significant difference fetal movements in the two groups.
										In normal pregnancies, most fetuses (93.4%) achieved a normal KANET score compared to 78.5% of the fetuses from high risk pregnancies.
Honemeyer et al.[186]	2012	Cohort	Prospective	High and Low Risk	Multiple	56	28–38	30 max	Positive	Introduction of the average KANET score, which derived from the mean value of total KANET score during pregnancy. Showed connection of fetal diurnal rhythm with pregnancy risk.

Abbreviations: KANET, Kurjak's antenatal neurological test; No, number of patients; IUGR, intrauterine growth restriction; MCA, middle cerebral artery; PTD, preterm delivery; PPROM, preterm premature rupture of membranes.

fetuses at risk for neurological problems, irrespective of intrapartum management, has been one of the great obstetrical problems and has remained unanswered for many years.[202-204]

Normal axis of lower arm and hand, normal finger position (Figs 40.26A and B) abnormal lower arm-hand axix, abnormal finger position at 28w4d (Fig. 40.26C).

Indeed, assessment of the integrity of the fetal nervous system is a major task in modern perinatal medicine.[154]

It is well-established that fetal behavioral patterns are directly reflecting developmental and maturational processes of fetal CNS.[202-204] It has been suggested that the assessment of fetal behavior and developmental processes in different periods of gestation may make possible the distinction between normal and abnormal brain development, as well as early diagnosis of various structural or functional abnormalities.[205] The innovation in fetal imaging, which enabled the study of fetal activity in explicit detail, was made by the introduction of high-quality 3D and 4D ultrasound, which allowed the performance of real-time observation of the fetus, with sufficient dynamics and good image resolution, allowing the evaluation of even the face and small anatomic parts of the fetus, and especially the movements of the mouth, eyes (facial expressions) and fingers.[134,206-208]

The first test that succeeded to combine all these parameters and form a scoring system that would assess the fetus in a comprehensive and systematic approach, in the same way that neonatologists perform a neurological assessment in newborns, in order to determine their neurological status during the 1st days of their life, is the KANET test.[209] KANET has already been shown

to be useful in standardization of neurobehavioral assessment with the potential for antenatal detection of fetuses with severe neurobehavioral impairment.[133,156,210]

KANET has also succeeded to verify the good neurological outcomes of fetuses that had normal KANET scores, showing a great positive predictive value and offering reassurance for the neurological outcome of these pregnancies.[159,183]

The first results prove that the prenatal neurological findings as estimated by KANET test are in concordance with their postnatal outcome.[154]

Of course, more studies are required to draw safe conclusions. Of great importance for this issue was the standardization of the test to make it reproducible and more easily applied, according to the Osaka Consensus Statement, during the International Symposium on Fetal Neurology of the International Academy of Perinatal Medicine (24th of October 2010).[146]

The importance of postnatal follow-up was also emphasized, especially in infants with abnormal or borderline KANET. Following the suggestions of the Osaka consensus statement on the standardization of the method, the KANET can be introduced in everyday clinical practice as a reproducible and sensitive prenatal screening neurological test, on which future studies can be designed. The results of these ongoing studies will investigate sensitivity, specificity, negative and positive predictive values, intraobserver and interobserver variability and reproducibility of the KANET, and these outcomes will form the base for the guidelines of fetal neurosonography and neurobehavior assessment.[194]

KANET appears to be a promising diagnostic tool for obstetricians, in detecting fetal brain and neurodevelopmental alterations,

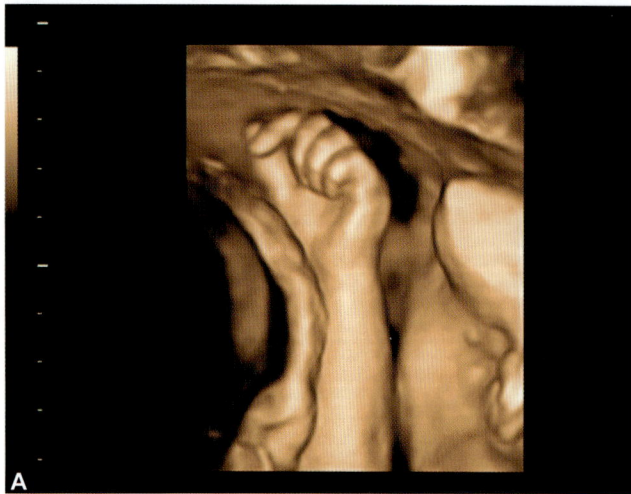

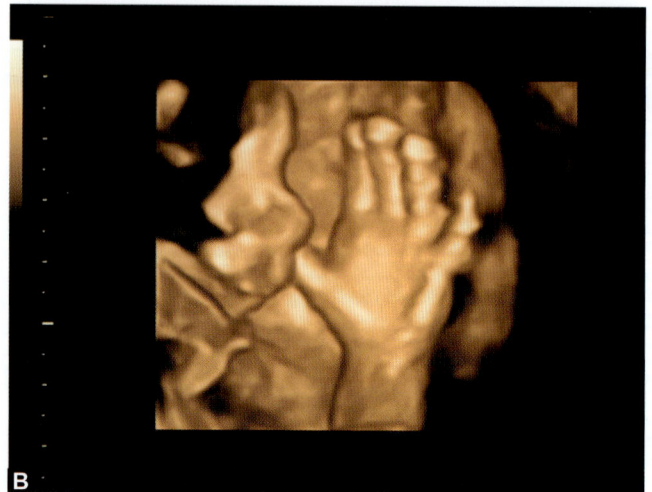

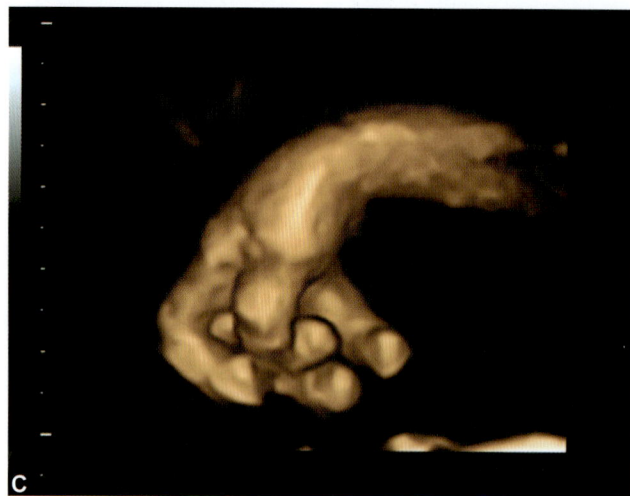

Figs 40.26A to C: Normal and abnormal arm-hand axis

due to in utero brain impairment, that is inaccessible by any other method.[140]

Representative evaluation of fetal behavior requires repeated assessment over appropriate pregnancy interval. The revised KANET score appears to correlate sufficiently with pregnancy risk status, fetal outcome and postnatal follow-up. Correlation appears even better when average KANET is applied. Fetal sleep pattern seems to have an impact on KANET scores in late third trimester.

Additional studies in large populations are needed before recommending the test in routine clinical practice. The results from the first studies on KANET are very optimistic and new results from bigger, ongoing multicenter studies are on their way.

REFERENCES

1. Judaš M, Kostović I. Temelji Neuroznanosti, 1st edition. MD Zagreb; 1997. pp. 24-31, 622-42, 353-60.
2. Schacher S. Determination and differentiation in the development of the nervous system. In: Kandel ER, Schwartz JH (Eds). Principles of Neural Science, 2nd edition. New Elsevier Science Publishing; 1985. pp. 730-2.
3. Kostović I. Prenatal development of nucleus basalis complex and related fibre system in man: a histochemical study. Neuroscience. 1986;17:1047-77.
4. Molliver ME, Kostovic I, Van der Loos H. The development of synapses in cerebral cortex of the human fetus. Brain Res. 1973;50:403-7.
5. Kostovic I. Zentralnervensystem. In: Hinrichsen KV (Ed). Humanembryologie. Berlin: Springer-Verlag; 1990. pp. 381-448.
6. Kurjak A (Ed). Očekujući Novorođenče. Zagreb: Mladost; 1984. pp. 18, 30.
7. Ultrasound studies of human fetal behaviour. Early Hum Dev. 1985;12(2):91-8.
8. Ianniruberto A, Tajani E. Ultrasonographic study of fetal movements. Semin Perinatol. 1981;4:175-81.
9. Goto S, Kato TK. Early movements are useful for estimating the gestational weeks in the first trimester of pregnancy. In: Levski RA, Morley P (Eds). Ultrasound. New York: Pergamon Press; 1983. pp. 577-82.

10. Okado N. Onset of synapse formation in the human spinal cord. J Comp Neurol. 1981;201(2):211-9.
11. Okado N. Development of the human cervical spinal cord with reference to synapse formation in the motor nucleus. J Comp Neurol. 1980;191(3):495-513.
12. Fitzgerald M. An Update on Current Scientific Knowledge. London: Department of Health; 1995.
13. Humphrey T. Some correlations between the appearance of human fetal reflexes and the development of the nervous system. Prog Brain Res. 1964;4:93-135.
14. De Vries JIP, Visser GHA, Prechtl HFR. Fetal motility in the first half of the pregnancy. In: Prechtl HFR (Ed). Continuity of Neural Functions from Prenatal to Postnatal Life. Philadelphia, PA: Lippincott; 1984. pp. 44-64.
15. De Vries JIP, Visser GHA, Prechtl HFR. The emergence of fetal behavior I. Qualitative aspects. Early Human Dev. 1982;7:301-22.
16. Kostovic I, Judas M, Petanjek Z, et al. Ontogenesis of goal-directed behavior: anatomo-functional considerations. Int J Psychophysiol. 1995;19(2):85-102.
17. Visser GHA, Laurini RN, Vries JIP, et al. Abnormal motor behaviour in anencephalic fetuses. Early Human Dev. 1985;12:173-83.
18. Visser GHA, Prechtl HFR. Perinatal neurological development. Proceedings of the Third International Conference on Fetal and Neonatal Physiological Measurements III. 1989. pp. 335-46.
19. D'Elia A, Pighetti M, Moccia G, et al. Spontaneous motor activity in normal fetus. Early Human Dev. 2001;65(2):139-44.
20. Natale R, Nasello-Paterson C, Turlink R. Longitudinal measurements of fetal breathing, body movements, and heart rate accelerations, and decelerations at 24 and 32 weeks of gestation. Am J Obstet Gynecol. 1985;151:256-63.
21. Eller DP, Stramm SL, Newman RB. The effect of maternal intravenous glucose administration on fetal activity. Am J Obstet Gynecol. 1992;167:1071-4.
22. Patrick J, Campbell K, Carmicheal L, et al. Patterns of gross fetal body movements over 24-hour observation intervals during the last 10 weeks of pregnancy. Am J Obstet Gynecol. 1982;142:363-71.
23. Kurjak A, Azumendi G, Vecek N, et al. Fetal hand movements and facial expression in normal pregnancy studied by four-dimensional sonography. J Perinat Med. 2003;31(6):496-508.
24. De Vries JIP, Visser GHA, Prechtl HFR. The emergence of fetal behavior. II Quantitative aspects. Early Hum Dev. 1985;12:99-120.
25. De Vries JIP, Visser GHA, Prechtl HFR. The emergence of fetal behavior. III. Individual differences and consistencies. Early Hum Dev. 1988;16:85-103.
26. Prechtl HF. Fetal behaviour. Eur J Obstet Gynecol Reprod Biol. 1989;32(1):32.
27. Graca LM, Cardoso CG, Clode N, et al. Acute effects of maternal cigarette smoking on fetal heart rate and fetal movements felt the mother. J Perinat Med. 1991;19:385-90.
28. Katz M, Meizner I, Holcberg G, et al. Reduction or cessation of fetal movements after administration of steroids for enhancement of lung maturation. Israel J Med Science. 1988;24:5-9.
29. Kurjak A. Kada ivot počinje. OKO. 1981;232:14.
30. Prechtl HFR, Einspieler C. Is neurological assessment of the fetus possible? Eur J Obstet Gynecol Reprod Biol. 1997;75:81-4.
31. Patrick J, Gagnon R. Fetal breathing and body movement. In: Creasy RK, Resnik R (Eds). Maternal-Fetal Medicine: Principles and Practice, 2nd edition. Philadelphia: WB Saunders Company; 1989. pp. 268-84.
32. Natale R, Nasello-Paterson C, Connors G. Patterns of fetal breathing activity in the human fetus at 24 to 28 weeks of gestation. Am J Obstet Gynecol. 1988;158:317-21.
33. Patrick J, Campbell K, Carmichael L, et al. Patterns of human fetal breathing during the last 10 weeks of pregnancy. Obstet Gynecol. 1980;56:24-30.
34. Patrick J, Campbell K, Carmichael L, et al. A definition of human fetal apnea and the distribution of fetal apneic intervals during the last 10 weeks of pregnancy. Am J Obstet Gynecol. 1978;136:371-7.
35. Ritchie K. The response to changes in the composition of maternal inspired air in human pregnancy. Seminars Perinatol. 1980;4:295-9.
36. Richardson B, Campbell K, Campbell L, et al. Effects of external physical stimulation on fetuses near term. Am J Obstet Gynecol. 1981;139:344-52.
37. Richardson B, Natale R, Patrick J. Human fetal breathing activity during induced labour at term. Am J Obstet Gynecol. 1979;133:247-55.
38. Roberts AB, Goldstein I, Romero R, et al. Fetal breathing movements after preterm rupture of membranes. Am J Obstet Gynecol. 1991;164:821-5.
39. Kivikoski A, Amon E, Vaalamo PO, et al. Effect of third-trimester premature rupture of membranes on fetal breathing movements: a prospective case-control study. Am J Obstet Gynecol. 1988;159:1474-7.
40. Besinger RE, Compton AA, Hayashi RH. The presence or absence of fetal breathing movements as a predictor of outcome in preterm labor. Am J Obstet Gynecol. 1987;157:753-7.
41. Kisilevsky BS, Hains SMJ, Low JA. Maturation of body and breathing movements in 24-33 week old fetuses threatening to deliver prematurely. Early Hum Dev. 1999;55(1):25-38.
42. Fox HE, Steinbrecher M, Pessel D, et al. Maternal ethanol ingestion and occurrence of human breathing movements. Am J Obstet Gynecol. 1978;132:354-61.
43. Richardson B, O'Grady JP, Olsen GD. Fetal breathing movements in response to carbon dioxide in patients on methadone maintenance. Am J Obstet Gynecol. 1984;150:400-4.
44. Manning FA, Wym Pugh E, Boddy K. Effect of cigarette smoking on fetal breathing movements in normal pregnancy. Br Med J. 1975;1:552-8.
45. Ishigava M, Yoneyama Y, Power GG, et al. Maternal teophylline administration and breathing movements in late gestation human fetus. Obstet Gynecol. 1996;88(6):973-8.
46. Cosmi EV, Cosmi E, La Torre R. The effect of fetal breathing movements on the utero-placental circulation. Early Pregnancy. 2001;5(1):51-2.
47. Natale R, Patrick J, Richardson B. Effects of maternal venous plasma glucose concentrations on fetal breathing movements. Am J Obstet Gynecol. 1978;132-41.
48. Patrick J, Natale R, Richardson B. Patterns of human fetal breathing activity at 34 to 35 weeks gestational age. Am J Obstet Gynecol. 1978;132(5):507-13.
49. Diamant NE. Development of esophageal function. Am Rev Respir Dis. 1985;131:S29-32.
50. Pritchard JA. Fetal swallowing and amniotic fluid volume. Obstet Gynecol. 1966;28:606-16.
51. Abramovich DR, Garden A, Jandial L, et al. Fetal swallowing and voiding in relation to hydramnios. Obstet Gynecol. 1979;54(1):15-20.
52. Abramovich DR. Fetal factor influencing the volume and composition of liquor amnii. J Obstet Gynecol Br Commonw. 1970;77(10):865-77.
53. Pitkin RM, Reynolds WA. Fetal ingestion and metabolism of amniotic fluid protein. Am J Obstet Gynecol. 1975;123:356-63.
54. Ross MG, Nijland JM. Development of ingestive behavior. Am J Physiol. 1998;274(4, Pt 2):R879-93.
55. Ross MG, El Haddad M, DeSai M. Unopposed orexic pathways in the developing fetus. Physiol Behav. 2003;79(1):79-88.
56. Humphrey T. The embryologic differentiation of the vestibular nuclei in man correlated with functional development. International symposium on vestibular and occular problems. Tokyo: Society of vestibular research. University of Tokyo; 1965. pp. 51-6.

57. Hooker D. Fetal reflexes and instinctual processes. Psychosom Med. 1942;4:199-20.
58. Starr A, Amlie RN, Martin WH, et al. Development of auditory function in newborn infants revealed by auditory brainstem potentials. Pediatrics. 1991;60:831-8.
59. Morlet T, Collet L, Solle B, et al. Functional maturation of cochlear active mechanisms and of the medial olivocochlear system in humans. Acta Otolaringol (Stockholm). 1993;113(3):271-7.
60. Morlet T, Collet L, Duclaux R, et al. Spontaneous and evoked otoacustical emissions in preterm and full term neonates: is there a clinical application? Int J Pediatr Otorhinolaryngol. 1995;33:207-11.
61. Leader LR, Baille P, Martin B, et al. The assessment and significance of habituation to a repeated stimulus by human fetus. Early Human Dev. 1982;7:211-8.
62. Liley AW. Fetus as a person. Speech held at the 8th meeting of the psychiatric societies of Australia and New Zealand. Fetal Therapy. 1986;1:8-17.
63. Schahidullah S, Hepper P. The developmental origins of fetal responsiveness to an acoustic stimulus. J Reprod Infant Psychol. 1994;12:143-54.
64. Kisilevsky BS, Pang LH, Hains SMJ. Maturation of human fetal responses to airborne sound in low- and high-risk fetuses. Early Human Dev. 2000;58:179-95.
65. Huttenlocher PR, deCourten CH. The development of synapses in striate cortex of man. Human Neurobiol. 1987;6:1-9.
66. Magoon EH, Robb RM. Development of myelin in human optic nerve tract. A light and electron microscopic study. Arch Ophtalmol. 1981;99:655-9.
67. Hendrickson AE, Youdelis C. The morphological development of the human foveola. Ophtalmol. 1981;91:603-12.
68. Vanhatalo S, van Nieuvenhuizen O. Fetal pain? Brain Dev. 2000;22(3):145-50.
69. Fitzgerald M. Development of pain mechanisms. Br Med Bul. 1991;47:667-75.
70. Okado N, Kojim T. Ontogeny of central nervous system: neurogenesis, fibre connections, synaptogenesis and myelination in the spinal cord. In: Prechtl HFR (Ed). Continuity of Neural Functions from Prenatal to Postnatal Life. Philadelphia PA: Lippincott; 1984. pp. 31-45.
71. Anand KJS, Hickey PR. Pain and its effects in the human neonate and fetus. N Engl J Med. 1987;317:1321-9.
72. Anand KJS, Phil D, Carr DB. The neuroanatomy, neurophysiology, and neurochemistry of pain, stress and analgesia in the newborns and children. Ped Clin North Am. 1989;36:795-822.
73. Fitzgerald M. Fetal pain: an update of current scientific knowledge. London: Department of Health; 1995.
74. Holstege G. Descending motor pathways and the spinal motor system: limbic and non-limbic components. Prog Brain Res. 1991;87:307-421.
75. Giannakoulopoulos X, Sepulveda W, Kourtis P, et al. Fetal plasma cortisol and beta endorphin response to intrauterine needling. Lancet. 1994;344:77-81.
76. Giannakoulopolous X, Teixeira J, Fisk N, et al. Human fetal and maternal noradrenaline responses to invasive procedures. Pediatr Res. 1999;45:494-9.
77. Smith RP, Gitau R, Glover V, et al. Pain and stress in the human fetus. Eur J Obstet Gynecol Reprod Biol. 2000;92:161-5.
78. Anand KJS, Sippell WG, Aynsley-Green A. Randomized trial of fentanyl anesthesia in preterm babies undergoing surgery: effects of the stress response. Lancet. 1987;1:62-6.
79. Guinsburg R, Kopelman BI, Anand KJS, et al. Physiological, hormonal and behavioural responses to a single fentanyl dose in intubated and ventilated preterm neonates. J Pediatr. 1998;132:954-9.
80. Anand KJS. Clinical importance of pain and stress in preterm neonates. Biol Neonate. 1998;73:319-24.
81. Uno H, Lohmiller L, Thieme C, et al. Brain damage induced by prenatal exposure to dexamethasone in fetal rhesus macaques. I. Hippocampus. Brain Res Dev. 1990;53:157-67.
82. Grunau RVE, Whitfield MF, Petrie JH, et al. Early pain experience, child and family factors, as precursors of somatization: a prospective study of extremely premature infants and fullterm children. Pain. 1994;56:353-9.
83. Bradley RM, Mistretta CM. The developing sense of taste. U: Olfaction and Taste VDA. Denton and JP Coghlan, New York: Academic; 1975. pp. 91-8.
84. Kawamura K, Takebayashi S. The development of noradrenaline-, acetylcholinesterase-, neuropeptide Y- and vasoactive intestinal polypeptide-containing nerves in human cerebral arteries. Neurosci Lett. 1994;175:1-4.
85. Cetin I, Morpurgo PS, Radaelli T, et al. Fetal plasma leptin concentrations: relationship with different intrauterine growth patterns from 19 weeks to term. Pediatr Res. 2000;48:646-51.
86. Jaquet D, Leger J, Levy-Marchal C, et al. Ontogeny of leptin in human fetuses and newborns: effect of intrauterine growth retardation on serum leptin concentrations. J Clin Endocrinol Metab. 1998;83:1243-6.
87. Roberts TJ, Caston-Balderrama A, Nijland MJ, et al. Central neuropeptide Y stimulates ingestive behavior and increases urine output in the ovine fetus. Am J Physiol Endocrinol Metab. 2000;279(3):E494-500.
88. Roberts TJ, Nijland MJ, Caston-Balderrama A, et al. Central leptin stimulates ingestive behavior and urine flow in the near term ovine fetus. Horm Metab Res. 2001;33:144-50.
89. Ross MG, Kullama LK, Ogundipe OA, et al. Ovine fetal swallowing response to intracerebroventricular hypertonic saline. J Appl Physiol. 1995;78:2267-71.
90. Ross MG, Kullama LK, Ogundipe OA, et al. Central angiotensin II stimulation of ovine fetal swallowing. J Appl Physiol. 1994;76(3):1340-5.
91. McDonald TJ, Li C, Nijland MJM, et al. Fos response of the fetal sheep anterior circumventricular organs to an osmotic challenge in late gestation. Am J Physiol. 1997;275(2 Pt 2):H609-14.
92. Xu Z, Nijland MJ, Ross MG. Plasma osmolality dypsogenic thresholds and c-fos expression in the near-term ovine fetus. Pediatr Res. 2001;49(5):678-5.
93. Caston Balderrama A, Nijland MJM, McDonald TJ, et al. Central Fos expression in fetal and adult sheep following intraperitoneal hypertonic saline. Am J Physiol. 1999;276:H725-35.
94. El Haddad MA, Chao CR, MA SX, et al. Neuronal NO modulates spontaneous ANG II-stimulated fetal swallowing behavior in the near-term ovine fetus. Am J Physiol Regul Integr Comp Physiol. 2002;282:R1521-7.
95. El Haddad MA, Chao CR, Sayed AA, et al. Effects of central angiotensin II receptor antagonism on fetal swallowing and cardiovascular activity. Am J Obstet Gynecol. 2001;185:828-33.
96. Davison JM, Gilmore EA, Durr J. Altered osmotic thresholds for vasopressin secretion and thirst in human pregnancy. Am J Physiol. 1984;246:F105-9.
97. Ross MG, Sherman DJ, Schreyer P, et al. Fetal rehydration via amniotic fluid: contribution of fetal swallowing. Pediat Res. 1991;29:214-7.
98. Nijland MJM, Kullama LK, Ross MG. Maternal plasma hypo-osmolality: effects on spontaneous and stimulated ovine fetal swallowing. J Mater-Fetal Med. 1998;7:165-71.
99. Ross MG, Sherman DJ, Ervin MG, et al. Fetal swallowing: response to systemic hypotension. Am J Physiol. 1990;257:R130-4.
100. Inoue M, Koyanagi T, Nakahara H. Functional development of human eye-movement in utero assessed quantitatively with real-time ultrasound. Am J Obst Gynec. 1986;155:170-4.
101. Aserinski E, Kleitman N. Two types of ocular motility occurring in sleep. Journal of Applied Physiology. 1955;8:1-10.

102. Parmelee AH, Stern E. Development of states in infants. In: Clemente CD, Purpura DP, Mayer FE (Eds). Sleep and the maturing central nervous system. New York: Academic Press; 1972. pp. 100-215.

103. Ruckenbush Y, Gaujoux M, Eghbali B. Sleep cycles and kinesis in the fetal lamb. Electroenceph Clin Neurophysiol. 1977;42:226-33.

104. Kelly DD. Sleep and dreaming. In: Kandell ER, Schwartz JH (Eds). Principles of Neural Science, 2nd edition. New York-Amsterdam-Oxford: Elsevier Science Publishing; 1985. p. 651.

105. Seron Ferre M, Torres C, Parraguez VH, et al. Perinatal neuroendocrine regulation. Development of the circadian time-keeping system. Mol Cell Endocrinol. 2002;186:169-73.

106. Vanecek J. Cellular mechanisms of melatonin action. Physiol Rev. 1998;78:687-721.

107. Yie SM, Niles LP, Younglavi EV. Melatonin receptors on human granulosa cell membranes. J Clin Endocrinol Metab. 1995;80:1747-9.

108. Hu W, Wu MT, Liu CP, et al. Left ventricular 4D echocardiogram motion and shape analysis. Ultrasonics. 2002;40:949-54.

109. Kossoff G. Basic physics and imaging characteristics of ultrasound. World J Surg. 2000;24:134-42.

110. Timor-Tritsch IE, Platt LD. Three-dimensional ultrasound experience in obstetrics. Curr Opin Obstet Gynecol. 2002;14:569-75.

111. Lee W. 3D fetal ultrasonography. Clin Obstet Gynecol. 2003;46:850-67.

112. Arzt W, Tulzer G, Aigner M. Real time 3D sonography of the normal fetal heart-clinical evaluation. Ultraschall Med. 2002;23:388-91.

113. Yanagihara T, Hata T. Three-dimensional sonographic visualization of fetal skeleton in the second trimester of pregnancy. Gynecol Obstet Invest. 2000;49:12-6.

114. Mangione R, Lacombe D, Carles D, et al. Craniofacial dysmorphology and three-dimensional ultrasound: a prospective study on practicability for prenatal diagnosis. Prenat Diagn. 2003;23:810-8.

115. Kurjak A, Hafner T, Kos M, et al. Three-dimensional sonography in prenatal diagnosis: a luxury or a necessity? J Peranatal Med. 2000;28:194-209.

116. De Vore GR, Falkensammer P, Sklansky MS, et al. Spatio-temporal image correlation (STIC): new technology for evaluation of the fetal heart. Ultrasound Obstet Gynecol. 2003;22:380-7.

117. Vinals F, Poblete P, Giuliano A. Spatio-temporal image correlation (STIC): a new tool for the prenatal screening of congenital heart defects. Ultrasound Obstet Gynecol. 2003;22:388-94.

118. Kurjak A, Vecek N, Hafner T, et al. Prenatal diagnosis: what does four-dimensional ultrasound add? J Perinat Med. 2002;30:57-62.

119. Nijhuis JG, (Ed). Fetal Behaviour: Developmental and Perinatal Aspects. Oxford: Oxford University Press; 1992.

120. Azumendi G, Kurjak A. Three-dimensional and four-dimensional sonography in the study of the fetal face. Ultrasound Rev Obstet Gynecol. 2003;3:1-10.

121. Roodenburg PJ, Wladimiroff JW, van Es A, et al. Classification and quantitative aspects of fetal movements during the second half of normal pregnancy. Early Hum Dev. 1991;25:19-35.

122. De Vries JIP, Laurini RN, Visser CHA. Abnormal motor behaviour and developmental postmortem findings in a fetus with Fanconi anemia. Early Hum Dev. 1994;36:137-42.

123. Prechtl HFR. Qualitative changes of spontaneous movements in fetus and preterm infant are a marker of neurological dysfunction. Early Hum Dev. 1990;23:151-8.

124. Ververs IAP, De Vries JIP, Van Geijn HP, et al. Prenatal head position from 12–38 weeks, I: developmental aspects. Early Hum Dev. 1994;39:83-91.

125. Hepper PG, Shahidullah S, White R. Handedness in the human fetus. Neuropsychologia. 1991;29:1107-11.

126. Geerdink JJ, Hopkins B. Effects of birthweight status and gestational age on the quality of general movements in preterm newborns. Neonate. 1993;63:215-24.

127. Hopkins B, Prechtl HFR. A qualitative approach to the development of movements during early infancy. In: Prechtl HFR (Ed). Continuity of Neural Functions from Perinatal to Postnatal Life. Oxford: Blackwell Scientific Publications; 1984. pp. 179-97.

128. Prechtl HFR. Qualitative changes of spontaneous movements in fetus and preterm infant are a marker of neurological dysfunction. Early Hum Dev. 1990;23:151-8.

129. Kainer F, Prechtl HF, Engele H, et al. Assessment of the quality of general movements in fetuses and infants of women with type-I diabetes mellitus. Early Hum Dev. 1997;50(1):13-25.

130. Sparling JW, Wilhelm IJ. Quantitative measurement of fetal movement: fetal-posture and movement assessment (F-PAM). Phys Occup Ther Pediatr. 1993;12:97-114.

131. Piaget J. The Origins of Intelligence in Children. New York: International Universities Press; 1952.

132. Butterworth G, Hopkins B. Hand-mouth coordination in the new-born baby. Br J Dev Psychol. 1988;6:303-14.

133. Kurjak A, Stanojevic M, Andonotopo W, et al. Behavioral pattern continuity from prenatal to postnatal life—a study by four-dimensional (4D) ultrasonography. J Perinat Med. 2004;32:346-53.

134. Kozuma S, Baba K, Okai T, et al. Dynamic observation of the fetal face by three-dimensional ultrasound. Ultrasound Obstet Gynecol. 1999;13:283-4.

135. Arabin B. Two-dimensional real-time ultrasound in the assessment of fetal activity in single and multiple pregnancy. Ultrasound Rev Obstet Gynecology. 2004;4(2).

136. Arabin B, Van Straaten I, Van Eyck J. Fetal hearing. In: Kurjak A (Ed). Textbook of Perinatal Medicine. London: Parthenon Publishing; 1998. pp. 756-75.

137. Arabin B, Bos R, Rijlaarsdam R, et al. The onset of inter-human contacts: longitudinal ultrasound observations in early twin pregnancies. Ultrasound Obstet Gynecol. 1996;8(3):166-73.

138. Yigiter AB, Kavak ZN. Normal standards of fetal behavior assessed by four-dimensional sonography. J Matern Fetal Neonatal Med. 2006;19(11):707-21.

139. Kurjak A, Miskovic B, Stanojevic M, et al. New scoring system for fetal neurobehavior assessed by three- and four-dimensional sonography. J Perinat Med. 2008;36(1):73-81.

140. Kurjak A, Stanojevic M, Andonotopo W, et al. Fetal behavior assessed in all three trimesters of normal pregnancy by four-dimensional ultrasonography. Croat Med J. 2005;46(5):772-80.

141. Antsaklis P, Antsaklis A. The assessment of fetal neurobehaviour with four-dimensional ultrasound: the Kurjak antenatal neurodevelopmental test. DSJUOG. 2012;6(4):362-75.

142. Gosselin J, Gahagan S, Amiel-Tison C. The Amiel-Tison neurological assessment at term: conceptual and methodological continuity in the course of follow-up. Ment Retard Dev Disabil Res Rev. 2005;11(1):34-51.

143. Stanojevic M, Kurjak A, Salihagic-Kadic A, et al. Neurobehavioral continuity from fetus to neonate. J Perinat Med. 2011;39:171-7.

144. Haak P, Lenski M, Hidecker MJ, et al. Cerebral palsy and aging. Dev Med Child Neurol. 2009;51(Suppl 4):16-23.

145. Kurjak A, Andonotopo W, Hafner T, et al. Normal standards for fetal neurobehavioral developments—longitudinal quantification by four-dimensional sonography. J Perinat Med. 2006;34(1):56-65.

146. Stanojevic M, Talic A, Miskovic B, et al. An attempt to standardize Kurjak's antenatal neurodevelopmental test: Osaka consensus statement. Donald School J Ultrasound Obstet Gynecol. 2011;5:317-29.

147. Pooh RK, Pooh K, Fetal VM. Donald School J Ultrasound Obstet Gynecol. 2007;1(4):40-6.

148. Kurjak A, Ahmed B, Abo-Yaquab S, et al. An attempt to introduce neurological test for fetus based on 3D and 4D sonography. Donald School J Ultrasound Obstet Gynecol. 2008;2:29-44.

149. Kuno A, Akiyama M, Yamashiro C, et al. Three-dimensional sonographic assessment of fetal behavior in the early second trimester of pregnancy. J Ultrasound Med. 2001;20(12):1271-5.

150. Koyanagi T, Horimoto N, Maeda H, et al. Abnormal behavioral patterns in the human fetus at term: correlation with lesion sites in the central nervous system after birth. J Child Neurol. 1993;8(1):19-26.

151. Stanojevic M, Kurjak A. Continuity between fetal and neonatal neurobehavior. Donald School J Ultrasound Obstet Gynecol. 2008;2:64-75.

152. Miskovic B, Vasilij O, Stanojevic M, et al. The comparison of fetal behavior in high risk and normal pregnancies assessed by four-dimensional ultrasound. J Matern Fetal Neonatal Med. 2010;23:1461-7.

153. Talic A, Kurjak A, Ahmed B, et al. The potential of 4D sonography in the assessment of fetal behavior in high risk pregnancies. J Matern Fetal Neonatal Med. 2011;24(7):948-54.

154. Kurjak A, Abo-Yaqoub S, Stanojevic M, et al. The potential of 4D sonography in the assessment of fetal neurobehavior—multicentric study in high-risk pregnancies. J Perinat Med. 2010;38:77-82.

155. Abo-Yaqoub S, Kurjak A, Mohammed AB, et al. The role of 4D ultrasonography in prenatal assessment of fetal neurobehaviour and prediction of neurological outcome. J Matern Fetal Neonatal Med. 2012;25(3):231-6.

156. Andonotopo W, Kurjak A, Kosuta MI. Behavior of an anencephalic fetus studied by 4D sonography. J Matern Fetal Neonatal Med. 2005;17(2):165-8.

157. Andonotopo W, Kurjak A. The assessment of fetal behavior of growth restricted fetuses by 4D sonography. J Perinat Med. 2006;34(6):471-8.

158. Talic A, Kurjak A, Stanojevic M, et al. The assessment of fetal brain function in fetuses with ventrikulomegaly: the role of the KANET test. J Matern Fetal Neonatal Med. 2012;25(8):1267-72.

159. Nijhuis JG, Prechtl HF, Martin CB Jr, et al. Are there behavioural states in the human fetus? Dev Psychobiol. 1982;34(4):257-68.

160. Horimoto N, Koyanagi T, Maeda H, et al. Can brain impairment be detected by in utero behavioural patterns? Arch Dis Child. 1993;69(1 Spec No):3-8.

161. Morokuma S, Fukushima K, Yumoto Y, et al. Simplified ultrasound screening for fetal brain function based on behavioral pattern. Early Hum Dev. 2007;83(3):177-81.

162. Prechtl HF, Einspieler C. Is neurological assessment of the fetus possible? Eur J Obstet Gynecol Reprod Biol. 1997;75(1):81-4.

163. Ferrari F, Prechtl HF, Cioni G, et al. Posture, spontaneous movements, and behavioural state organisation in infants affected by brain malformations. Early Hum Dev. 1997;50(1):87-113.

164. Frøen JF. A kick from within—fetal movement counting and the cancelled progress in antenatal care. J Perinat Med. 2004;32:13-24.

165. Habek D, Kovačević M. Adverse pregnancy outcomes and long-term morbidity after early fetal hypokinesia in maternal smoking pregnancies. Arch Gynecol Obstet. 2011;283(3):491-5.

166. Hata T, Dai SY, Marumo G. Ultrasound for evaluation of fetal neurobehavioural development: from 2-D to 4-D Ultrasound Inf. Child Dev. 2010;19:99-118.

167. Hata T, Kanenishi K, Sasaki M. Four-dimensional sonographic assessment of fetal movement in the late first trimester. Int J Gynaecol Obstet. 2010;109(3):190-3.

168. Iwasaki S, Morokuma S, Yumoto Y, et al. Acute onset antenatal fetal neurological injury suspected prenatally based on abnormalities in antenatal testing: a case report. J Matern Fetal Neonatal Med. 2009;22(12):1207-10.

169. Chen YT, Hsu ST, Tseng JJ, et al. Cardiotocographic and Doppler ultrasonographic findings in a fetus with brain death syndrome. J Obstet Gynecol. 2006;45(3):279-82.

170. Zimmer EZ, Jakobi P, Goldstein I, et al. Cardiotocographic and sonographic findings in two cases of antenatally diagnosed intrauterine fetal brain death. Prenat Diagn. 1992;12(4):271-6.

171. Patrick J, Campbell K, Carmichael L, et al. Patterns of gross fetal body movements over 24-hour observation intervals during the last 10 weeks of pregnancy. Am J Obstet Gynecol. 1982;142(4):363-71.

172. Petrović O, Finderle A, Prodan M, et al. Combination of vibroacoustic stimulation and acute variables of mFBP as a simple assessment method of low-risk fetuses. J Matern Fetal Neonatal Med. 2009;22(2):152-6.

173. Prechtl HF. The behavioural states of the newborn infant (a review). Brain Res. 1974;76(2):185-212.

174. Prechtl HF. Qualitative changes of spontaneous movements in fetus and preterm infant are a marker of neurological dysfunction. Early Hum Dev. 1990;23:151-8.

175. Rotmensch S, Liberati M, Celentano C, et al. The effect of betamethasone on fetal biophysical activities and Doppler velocimetry of umbilical and middle cerebral arteries. Acta Obstet Gynecol Scand. 1999;78(9):768-73.

176. American College of Obstetricians and Gynecologists, American Academy of Pediatrics. Neonatal Encephalopathy and Cerebral Palsy: Defining the Pathogenesis and Pathophysiology. Washington, DC: American College of Obstetricians and Gynecologists; 2003. p. 768.

177. Honemeyer U, Kasirsky J, Pour-Mirza A, et al. Diagnosis of fetal akinesia deformation sequence at 30 weeks. Donald School J Obstet Gynecol. 2013;7(4):500-5.

178. Morokuma S, Fukushima K, Yumoto Y, et al. Simplified ultrasound screening for fetal brain function based on behavioral pattern. Early Hum Dev. 2007;83:177-81.

179. Natale R, Richardson B, Patrick J. The effect of maternal hyperglycemia on gross body movements in human fetuses at 32–34 week of gestation. Early Hum Dev. 1983;8(1):13-20.

180. Nijhuis JG. Fetal behavior. Neurobiol Aging. 2003;24:41-46.

181. Patrick J, Campbell K, Carmichael L, et al. Patterns of gross fetal body movements over 24-hour observation intervals during the last 10 weeks of pregnancy. Am J Obstet Gynecol. 1982;142:363-71.

182. Kurjak A, Talic A, Honemeyer U, et al. Comparison between antenatal neurodevelopmental test and fetal Doppler in the assessment of fetal well being. J Perinat Med. 2013;41(1):107-14.

183. Honemeyer U, Kurjak A. The use of KANET test to assess fetal CNS function. First 100 cases. 10th World Congress of Perinatal Medicine 8-11 November 2011. Uruguay. Poster Presentation 209.

184. Lebit DF, Vladareanu PD. The role of 4D ultrasound in the assessment of fetal behaviour. Maedica (Buchar). 2011;6(2):120-7.

185. Vladareanu R, Lebit D, Constantinescu S. Ultrasound assessment of fetal neurobehaviour in high-risk pregnancies. DSJUOG. 2012;6(2):Q132-47.

186. Honemeyer U, Talic A, Therwat A, et al. The clinical value of KANET in studying fetal neurobehavior in normal and at-risk pregnancies. J Perinat Med. 2013;41(2):187-97.

187. Stanojevic M, Kurjak A. Continuity from fetal to neonatal behavior: lessons learned and future challenges. DSJUOG. 2011;5(2):107-18.

188. Spittle AJ, Orton J, Doyle LW, et al. Early developmental intervention programs post hospital discharge to prevent motor and cognitive impairment in preterm infants. Cochran Database Syst Rev. 2007;(2):CD005495.

189. Himmelmann K, Hagberg G, Uvebrant P. The changing panorama of cerebral palsy in Sweden. Prevalence and origin in the birth-year period 1999-2002. Acta Paediatrica. 2010;99:1337-43.

190. Rees S, Harding R. Brain development during fetal life: influences of the intrauterine environment. Neursci Lett. 2004;361:111-14.

191. Talic A, Kurjak A, Honemeyer U. Effect of maternal fever on fetal behavior assessed by KANET test. DSJUOG. 2012;6(2):160-5.

192. Talic A, Kurjak A, Badreldeen A, et al. The potential of 4D sonography in the assessment of fetal behavior in high risk pregnancies. Metern Fetal Neonatal Med. 2011;24(5):764-7.

193. Kurjak A, Predojevic M, Stanojevic M, et al. The use of 4D imaging in the behavioral assessment of high risk fetuses. Imaging Med. 2011;3(5):557-69.

194. Kurjak A, Predojevic M, Salihagic Kadic A. Fetal brain function: lessons learned and future challenges of 4D sonography. Donald School Journal of Ultrasound in Obstetrics and Gynecology. 2011;5(2):85-92.

195. Kurjak A, Tikvica Luetic A, Stanojević M, Talić A, Zalud I, Al-Noobi M, et al. Further experience in the clinical assessment of fetal neurobehavior. Donald School Journal of Ultrasound in Obstetrics and Gynecology. 2010;4:59-71.

196. Kurjak A, Predojević M, Stanojević M, et al. Intrauterine growth restriction and cerebral palsy. Acta Medica Informatica. 2010;18: 64-83.

197. Kurjak A, Talic A, Stanojevic M, et al. The study of fetal behavior in twins in all three trimesters of pregnancy. Accepted for publication in J Matern Fet Neonat Med.

198. Honemeyer U, Kurjak A. Prenatal beginnings of temperament formation—myth or reality? Case Study of a Twin Pregnancy. DSJUOG. 2012;6(2):148-52.

199. Tomasovic S, Predojevic M. 4D Ultrasound—medical devices for recent advances on the etiology of cerebral palsy. Acta Inform Med. 2011;19(4):228-34.

200. Hepper PG. Fetal behavior: who so sceptical? Ultrasound Obstet Gynecol. 1996;8(3):145-8.

201. Greenwood C, Newman S, Impey L, et al. Cerebral palsy and clinical negligence litigation: a cohort study. BJOG. 2003;110(1):6-11.

202. Strijbis EM, Oudman I, van Essen P, et al. Cerebral palsy and the application of the international criteria for acute intrapartum hypoxia. Obstet Gynecol. 2006;107(6):1357-65.

203. de Vries JI, Fong BF. Changes in fetal motility as a result of congenital disorders: an overview. Ultrasound Obstet Gynecol. 2007;29(5):590-9.

204. de Vries JI, Fong BF. Normal fetal motility: an overview. Ultrasound Obstet Gynecol. 2006;27(6):701-11.

205. de Vries JI, Visser GH, Prechtl HF. The emergence of fetal behaviour. II. Quantitative aspects. Early Hum Dev. 1985;12(2):99-120.

206. Rosier-van Dunné FM, van Wezel-Meijler G, Bakker MP, et al. General movements in the perinatal period and its relation to echogenicity changes in the brain. Early Hum Dev. 2010;86(2):83-6.

207. Hata T, Kanenishi K, Akiyama M, et al. Real- time 3-D sonographic observation of fetal facial expression. J Obstet Gynaecol Res. 2005;31(4):337-40.

208. Kurjak A, Azumendi G, Andonotopo W, et al. Three- and four-dimensional ultrasonography for the structural and functional evaluation of the fetal face. Am J Obstet Gynecol. 2007;196(1):16-28.

209. Kurjak A, Tikvica A, Stanojevic M, et al. The assessment of fetal neurobehavior by three-dimensional and four-dimensional ultrasound. J Matern Fetal Neonatal Med. 2008;21(10):675-84.

210. Kurjak A, Pooh R, Tikvica A, et al. Assessment of fetal neurobehavior by 3D/4D ultrasound. Fetal Neurology. 2009. pp. 222-50.

41

Fetal Central Nervous System

RK Pooh, K Pooh

INTRODUCTION

Recent advances of prenatal imaging technologies such as transvaginal ultrasound, three-dimensional (3D) ultrasound, magnetic resonance imaging (MRI) have been remarkable and contributed prenatal evaluation of fetal abnormalities in utero. Owing to those technologies, fetal malformations have been reliably diagnosed with increasing accuracy and at earlier gestation. As for fetal central nervous system (CNS) assessment, a new field of "*neurosonography*"[1] has been established. Many of congenital CNS anomalies, which were disclosed in the late pregnancy or after birth, have been recently demonstrated by the use of high frequency transvaginal sonography before viability. More advances of technological development will clarify unknown neuropathological facts during fetal period.

Diagnostics of the fetal CNS is one of the most difficult fields in Perinatology. There are several reasons why the prenatal CNS evaluation is difficult; *lack of essential knowledge of CNS anatomy and pathology, rapid changes of normal CNS development during pregnancy, inexperience of CNS neuroimaging techniques.* When the beginners start prenatal CNS imaging, these three may be the most frequent reasons of toughness in prenatal assessment. However, after overcoming those problems, there still exist difficulties in assessment of fetal CNS diseases, because of difficulty in prediction of neurological prognosis and existence of gray zone between normality and abnormality.

CENTRAL NERVOUS SYSTEM DEVELOPMENT

The brain is a 3D structure and should be comprehended in the three orthogonal views of sagittal, coronal and axial section. During fetal period, the embryonal premature CNS structure develops to mature structure (Fig. 41.1). Within this rapid change of development, various developmental disorders and/or insults result in various phenotypes of fetal CNS abnormalities. For understanding of fetal CNS diseases, basic knowledge of the development of the nervous system is essential. The developmental stages and their major disorders are described in Table 41.1.

It is believed that the brain anatomy must be complicated and there must be lots of terms to remember. In this chapter, essential anatomical structures are selected for neuroimaging and comprehension of fetal CNS diseases. Figures 41.2 and 41.3 show the basic anatomy in the axial, sagittal and anterior coronal sections of the brain. For understanding of hydrocephalus, ventriculomegaly and/or other intracranial lesions, the ventricular system (Fig. 41.4) and cerebrospinal fluid (CSF) circulation (Fig. 41.5) should be understood.

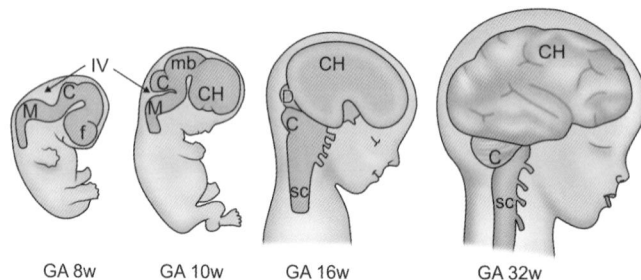

GA 8w   GA 10w   GA 16w   GA 32w

Fig. 41.1: Developing brain and spinal cord during pregnancy. Fetal central nervous system changes in size and appearance from early premature structure into late mature structure with gyral formation

Abbreviations: CH, cerebral hemisphere; C, cerebellum; D, diencephalon; M, medulla; SC, spinal cord; f, forebrain; mb: midbrain; IV: fourth ventricle

Table 41.1: Developmental stages and major disorders

Developmental stages	Disorders
Primary neurulation (3-4 week of gestation),	Spina bifida aperta, cranium bifidum
Caudal neural tube formation (secondary neurulation, from 4 week of gestation) Prosencephalic development (2-3 months' gestation)	Occult dysraphic states Holoprosencephaly Agenesis of the corpus callosum Agenesis of the septum pellucidum Septo-optic dysplasia
Neuronal proliferation (3–4 months' gestation) Neuronal migration (3–5 months' gestation)	Micrencephaly, macrencephaly Schizencephaly Lissencephaly, pachygyria
Organization (5 months' gestation – years postnatal) Myelination (birth – years postnatal)	Idiopathic mental retardation Cerebral white matter hypoplasia

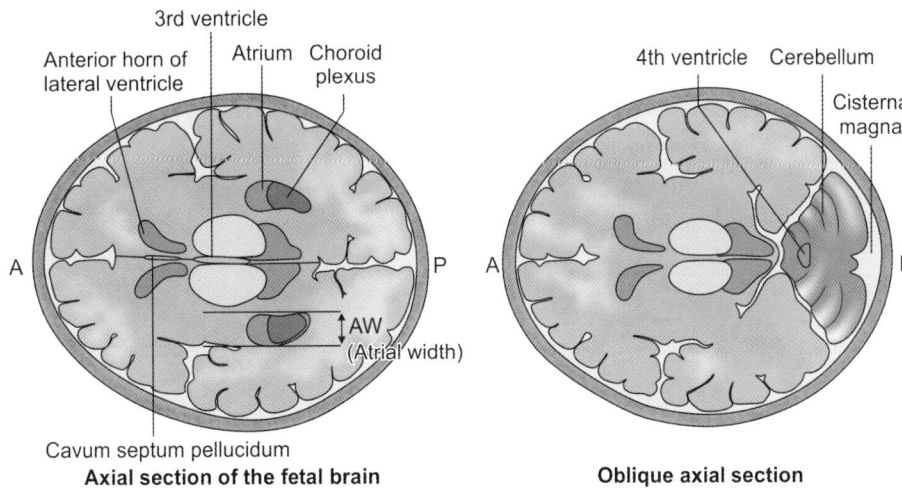

Fig. 41.2: Basic anatomical knowledge

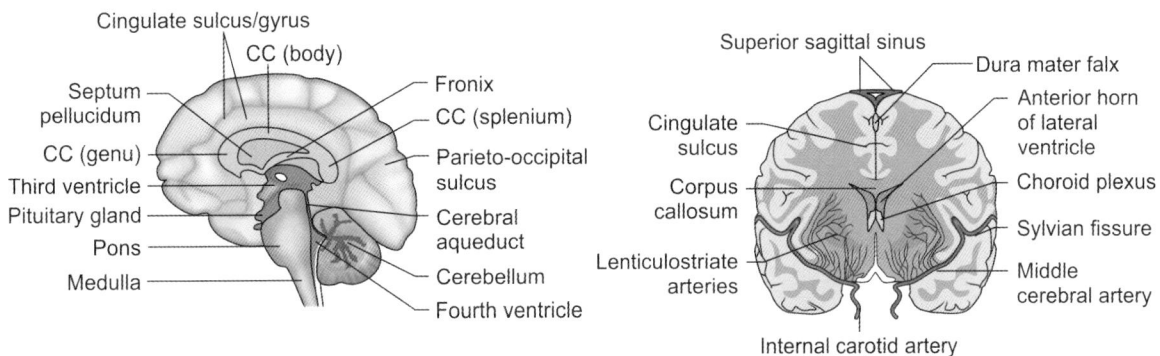

Fig. 41.3: Basic anatomical knowledge of sagittal (left) and anterior coronal cutting sections of the brain (CC, corpus callosum)

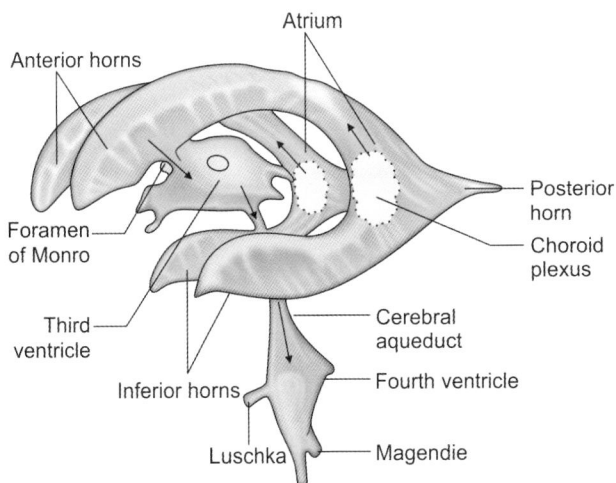

Fig. 41.4: Basic anatomical knowledge of ventricular system and cerebrospinal fluid (CSF) flow

TECHNOLOGY

Transabdominal sonographic technique, by which it is possible to observe the fetal internal organs through maternal abdominal wall and uterine wall, has been most widely used for fetal imaging diagnosis. By transabdominal approach, fetal brain structure mostly in the axial section and fetal back structure including the vertebrae and spinal cord in the sagittal section can be well demonstrated. However, in transabdominal approach to the fetal CNS, there are several obstacles such as maternal abdominal wall, placenta and fetal cranial bones.

Introduction of high-frequency transvaginal transducer has contributed to establishing "sonoembryology"[2] and recent general use of transvaginal sonography in early pregnancy enabled early diagnoses of major fetal anomalies.[3] In the middle and late pregnancy, fetal CNS is generally evaluated through maternal abdominal wall. The brain, however, is 3D structure, and should be assessed in basic three planes of sagittal, coronal and axial sections. Sonographic assessment of the fetal brain in the sagittal and coronal sections requires an approach from fetal parietal direction (Fig. 41.6). Transvaginal sonography of the fetal brain opened a new field in medicine, "neurosonography".[1] Transvaginal approach to the normal fetal brain during the second and third trimester was introduced in the beginning of 1990s. It was the first practical application of 3D CNS assessment by two-dimensional (2D) ultrasound.[4] Transvaginal observation of the fetal brain offers sagittal and coronal views of the brain from fetal parietal direction[5-8] through the fontanelles and/or the sagittal suture as ultrasound windows. Serial oblique sections[3] via the same ultrasound window reveal the intracranial morphology in detail. This method has contributed to the prenatal assessment of congenital CNS anomalies and acquired brain damage in utero.

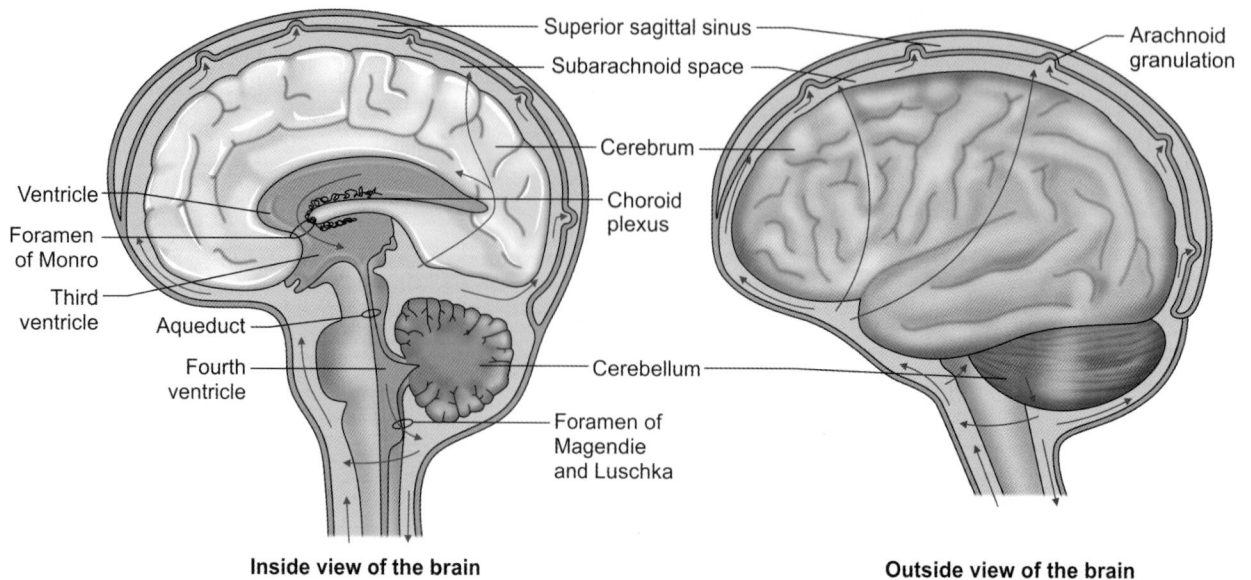

Fig. 41.5: Cerebrospinal fluid (CSF) circulation. Inside and outside views of the brain. CSF is produced from choroid plexus of ventricles. CSF runs through the third ventricle, aqueduct and fourth ventricle, goes to surface of the brain and spinal cord, and then absorbed by arachnoid granulation

Source: "Handbook on Hydrocephalus for Patients", Research Committee of "Intractable Hydrocephalus", Japanese Ministry of Health and Welfare, ©1993, with permission. (Schema by courtesy of chairman of the Committee, Professor Mori K)

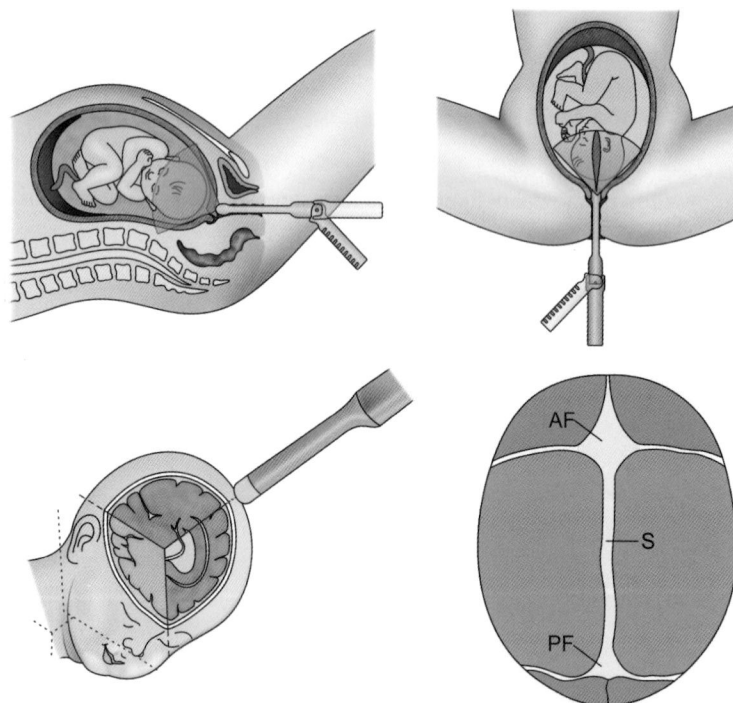

Fig. 41.6: Schema of transvaginal sonography. (Upper left) lateral view of vertex presenting fetus and transvaginal transducer. (Upper right) frontal view of transvaginal approach. Clear imaging is possible by rotating and angle-changing of the transducer. (Lower left) scheme of transfontanelle/trans-sutural approach of the fetal brain

Abbreviations: AF, anterior fontanelle; S, sagittal suture; PF, posterior fontanelle. Those spaces are used as ultrasound windows

Three-dimensional ultrasound is one of the most attractive modality in a field of fetal ultrasound imaging. There are two scanning methods of freehand scan and automatic scan. Automatic scan by dedicated 3D transducer produces motor driven automatic sweeping and is called as a fan scan. With this method, a shift and/or angle-change of the transducer is not required during scanning and scan duration needs only several seconds. After acquisition of the target organ, multiplanar imaging analysis is possible. Combination of both transvaginal sonography and 3D ultrasound[9-12] may be a great diagnostic tool for evaluation of 3D structure of fetal CNS. There are several useful functions in 3D ultrasound as follows:

- Surface imaging of the fetal head

- Bony structural imaging of the calvaria and vertebrae
- Multiplanar imaging of the intracranial structure
- 3D sonoangiography of the brain circulation
- Volume calculation of target organs, such as intracranial cavity, ventricle, choroid plexus and intracranial lesions
- Simultaneous volume contrast imaging by four-dimensional (4D) ultrasound.

In multiplanar imaging of the brain structure, it is possible to demonstrate not only the sagittal and coronal sections but also the axial section of the brain, which cannot be demonstrated from parietal direction by a conventional 2D transvaginal sonography. Parallel slicing provides a tomographic visualization of internal morphology similar to MR imaging. Volume extracted image and volume calculation of the fetal brain in early pregnancy was reported in 1990s.[13,14] We used Voluson 730 expert (GE Medical Systems, Milwaukee, USA) with transvaginal 3D transducer and 3D view version 3.2 software (Kretztechnik AG, Zipf, Austria) for volume extraction and volume estimation of the brain structure. Furthermore, with application of 4D ultrasound, real-time images with increased contrast resolution can be obtained in not only the same plane as 2D cutting section but also vertical plane to 2D image.[15] Fetal neuroimaging with advanced 3D/4D technology is easy, non-invasive, and reproducible methods. It produces not only comprehensible images but also objective imaging data which can be graphed in volume calculation.

Easy storage/extraction of raw volume data set enables offline analysis and consultation to neurologists and neurosurgeons.[16,17]

Fast MR imaging is being used increasingly as a correlative imaging modality because it uses non ionizing radiation, provides excellent soft tissue contrast, has multiple planes for reconstruction, and a large field of view.[18] Recent advances in fast MR imaging technology, such as half-Fourier and the 0.5-signal-acquired single-shot fast spin-echo (SE), half-Fourier rapid acquisition with relaxation enhancement (RARE) sequences, has remarkably improved the T2-weighted image resolution despite a short acquisition time, and minimized fetal and/or maternal respiratory motion artifacts without needs of fetal sedation.[19] MR imaging has a great potential especially in the evaluation of CNS and several reports have published on normal and abnormal CNS anatomy by using fast MR imaging techniques.[20-23]

NORMAL FETAL CENTRAL NERVOUS SYSTEM IMAGING

The calvaria and its major sutures develop between 12 weeks and 16 weeks of fetal life, with dura as guiding tissue in the morphogenesis of the skull.[24] The cranial bones are detectable by sonography from 10 weeks of gestation. At 12 weeks, premature cranial bones and sutures are detectable (Fig. 41.7). The sagittal suture, lambdoid sutures and posterior fontanelles are recognizable from 13 weeks. As the fetal parietal portion has the anterior/posterior fontanelles and sagittal suture which is the widest suture among the fetal cranial sutures,[25] transvaginal approach to the fetal brain using those spaces as ultrasound windows, demonstrates the detailed brain structure without obstacles of the cranial bone, and is the most reasonable way for brain assessment. Recent advanced 3D ultrasound has been able to depict vertebral body, intervertebral disk space and vertebral lamina (Figs 41.8 and 41.9).

From 8 weeks of gestation, premature sonolucent ventricular system is detectable (Fig. 41.10). Before 16 weeks of gestation, lateral ventricles are occupied by the choroid plexus (Fig. 41.11). Basic knowledge of images in several cutting sections obtained by transvaginal scanning is shown in Figure 41.12. Three orthogonal views by 3D ultrasound are useful for obtaining easy orientation. Multiplanar image analysis is possible (Fig. 41.13). By 3D ultrasound, the brain structure can be observed in parallel cutting slices of any sections (Fig. 41.14). 3D transvaginal power Doppler demonstrates clear anatomical vascular formation (Fig. 41.15). Vertebrae and spine should be observed carefully for detection of back abnormalities such as spina bifida or scoliosis. Fetal sagittal sectional screening is preferable (Fig. 41.16).

Volume analysis by 3D ultrasound provides exceedingly informative imaging data.[15] Volume analysis of the structure of interest provides an intelligible evaluation of the brain structure in total, and longitudinal and objective assessment of enlarged ventricles and intracranial occupying lesions. Any intracranial organ can be chosen as a target for volumetry, no matter how distorted its shape and appearance may be (Fig. 41.17).

HYDROCEPHALUS AND VENTRICULOMEGALY IN UTERO

Both "hydrocephalus" and "ventriculomegaly" are the terms, used to describe dilatation of the lateral ventricles. However, those two should be distinguished from each other. Hydrocephalus signifies

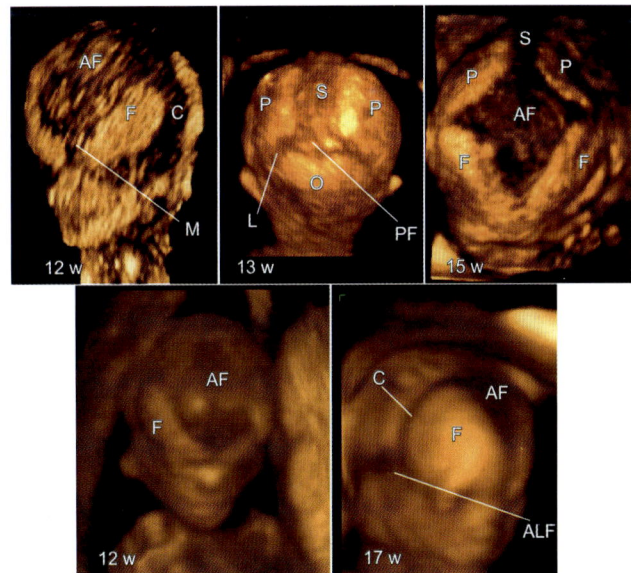

Fig. 41.7: Fetal cranial structure in early gestation [three-dimensional ultrasonography (3D US) images]. (Upper left) 12 weeks, from the oblique front. (Upper middle) 13 weeks, from the back. (Upper right) 15 weeks, from the top of head. (Lower left) 12 weeks, from the front. (Lower right) 17 weeks. Oblique position. Premature shape of cranial bones, sutures, and fontanelles at 12–13 weeks change its appearance to the neonatal shape

Abbreviations: AF, anterior fontanelle; PF, posterior fontanelle; ALF, anterolateral fontanelle; F, frontal bone; P, parietal bone; O, occipital bone; C, coronal suture; M, metopic suture; S, sagittal suture; L, lambdoid suture

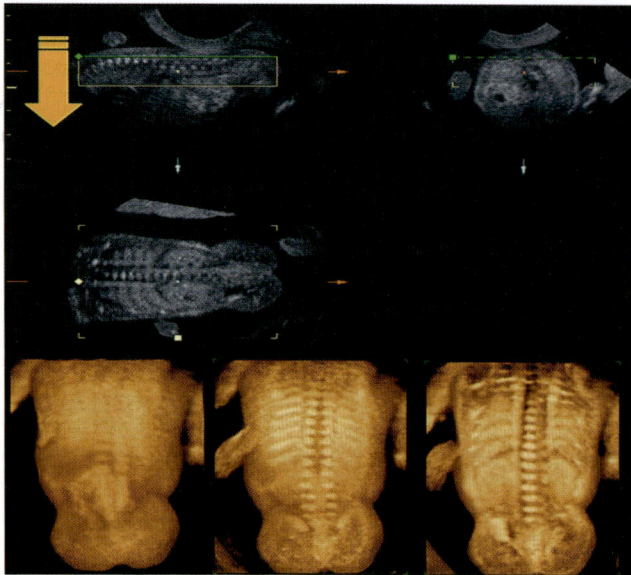

Fig. 41.8: Three orthogonal views and three-dimensional (3D) reconstructed image of normal fetus at 16 weeks of gestation. Movement of region of interest (arrow) provides 3D reconstruction image of the surface level (lower left), neural arch level (lower middle) and vertebral body level (lower right).

dilated lateral ventricles resulted from increased amount of CSF and intracranial pressure, while ventriculomegaly is a dilatation of lateral ventricles without increased intracranial pressure due to hypoplastic cerebrum or other intracerebral abnormalities such as agenesis of corpus callosum. Of course, ventriculomegaly can sometimes change into hydrocephalic state. In sonographic imaging, those two intracranial conditions can be differentiated by visualization of subarachnoid space and appearance of choroids plexus. In normal

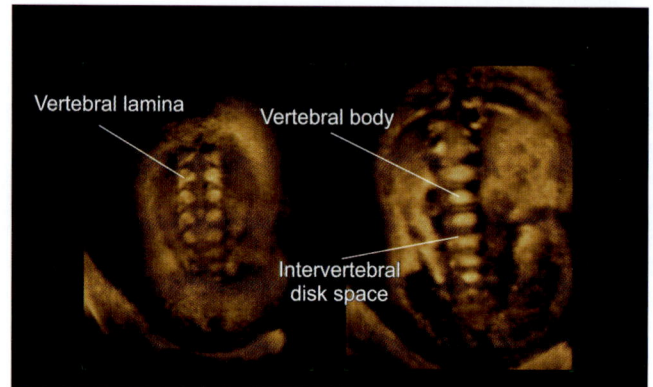

Fig. 41.9: Fetal vertebral structure by three-dimensional ultrasonography (3D US) at 21 weeks of gestation

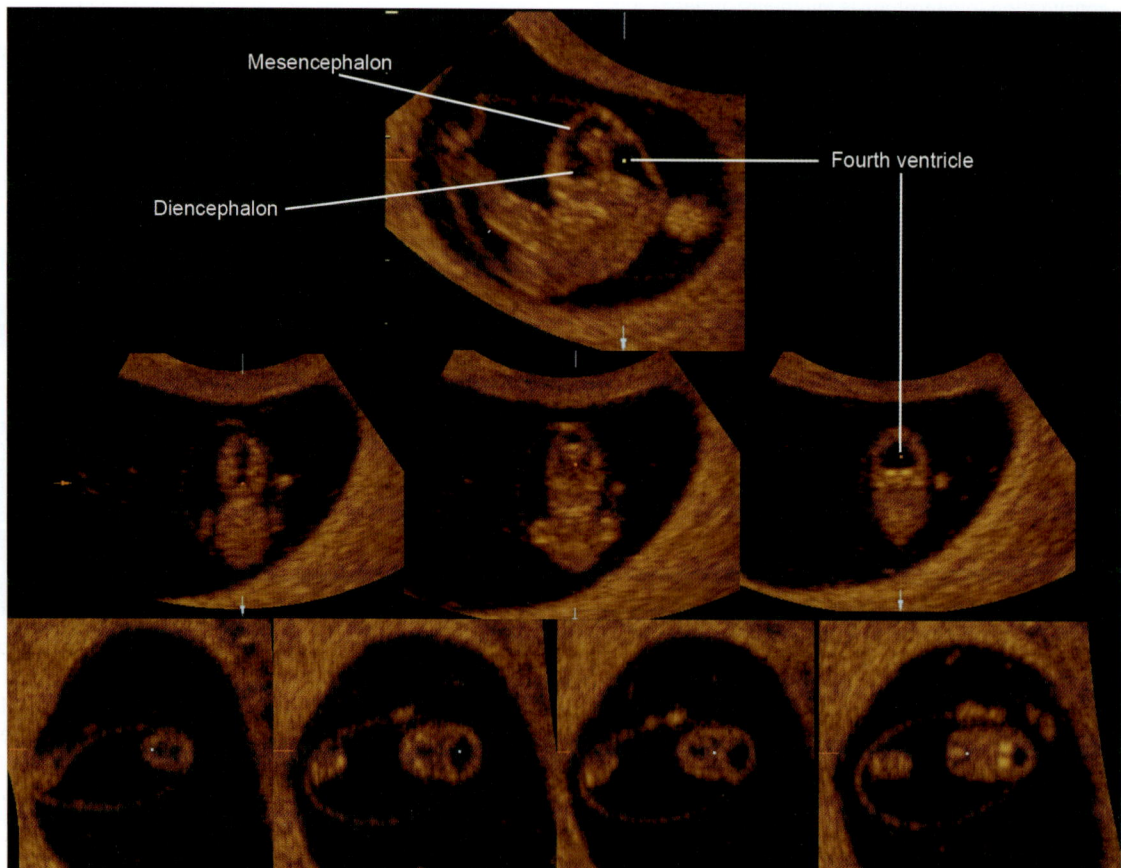

Fig. 41.10: Normal intracranial structure at 8 weeks of gestation in parallel cutting slices of three orthogonal views—sagittal, coronal, axial sections from above. Premature sonolucent ventricular system is visible

condition, subarachnoid space, visualized around the both cerebral hemispheres is preserved during pregnancy (Fig. 41.18). Choroid plexus, which secretes CSF within the ventricles, is a soft fissure and easily affected by pressure. Obliterated subarachnoid space

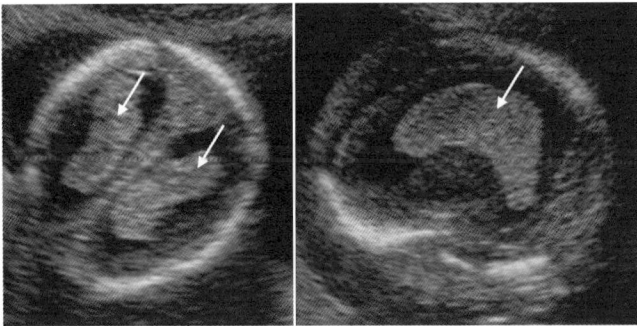

Fig. 41.11: Normal intracranial structure at 14 weeks of gestation. Axial view (left) and parasagittal view (right). Choroid plexus (arrows) occupies most of the lateral ventricle

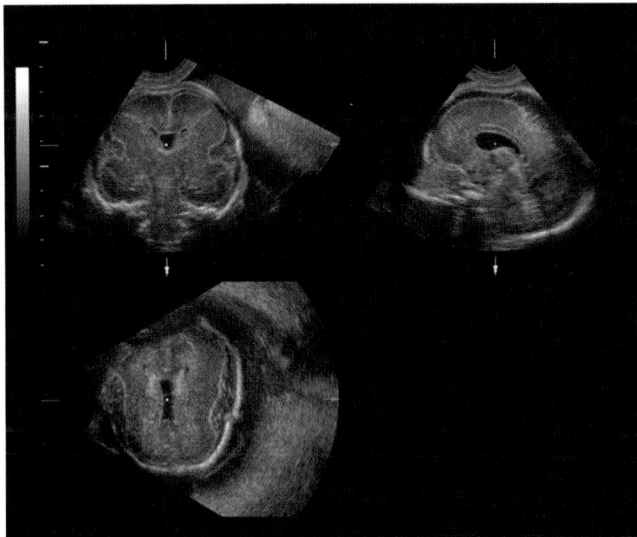

Fig. 41.13: Three-dimensional (3D) multiplanar image analysis (normal brain at 23 weeks of gestation). Three orthogonal view is useful to obtain orientation of the brain structure. Coronal (left upper), sagittal (right upper) and axial (left lower) images can be visualized on a single screen. Any rotation of the brain image around any (x, y, z) axis is possible

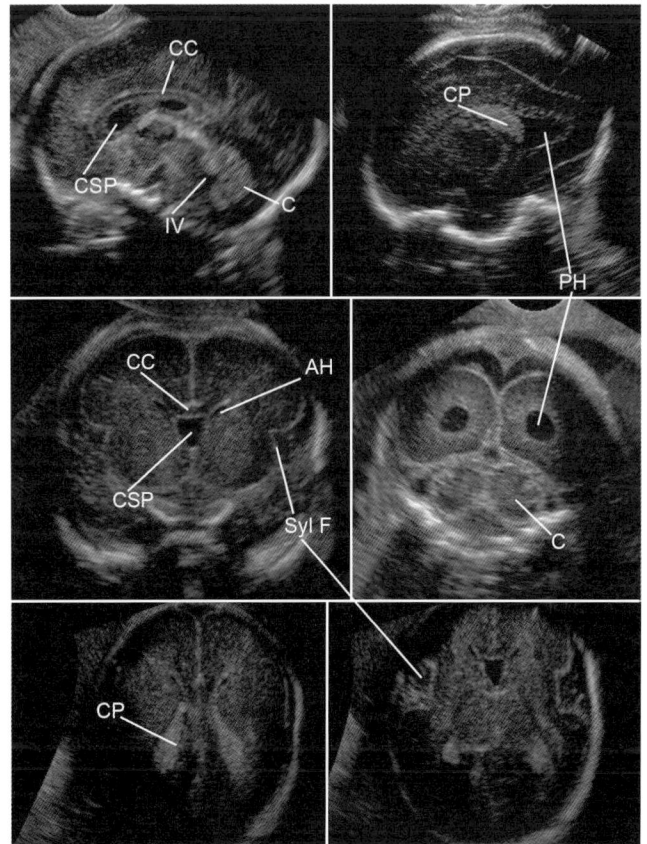

Fig. 41.12: Normal views of fetal brain at 26 weeks of gestation. Sagittal (upper), coronal (middle) and axial (lower) sections

Abbreviations: CC, corpus callosum; CSP, cavum septum pellucidum; C, cerebellum; IV, 4th ventricle; AH, anterior horn of the lateral ventricle; PH, posterior horn of the lateral ventricle; CP, choroid plexus; Syl F, Sylvian fissure

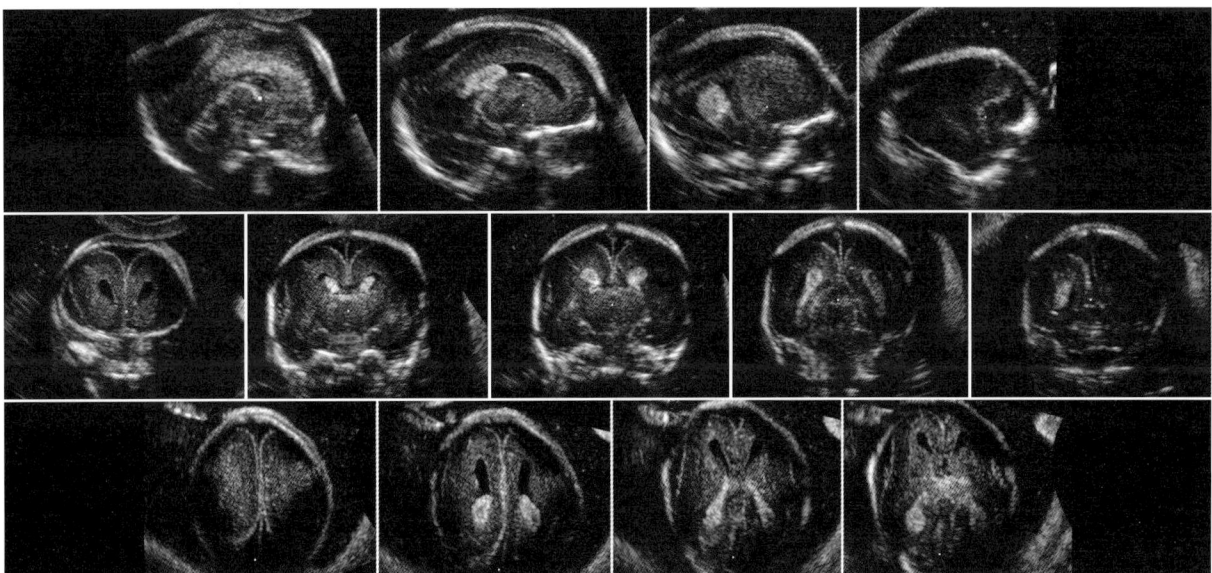

Fig. 41.14: Normal intracranial structure at 19 weeks of gestation in parallel cutting slices of three orthogonal view—sagittal, coronal, axial sections from above

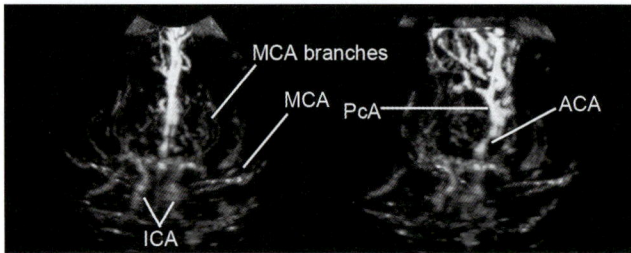

Fig. 41.15: Three-dimensional (3D) power Doppler image of fetal brain circulation. (Left) View from the front. Bilateral internal carotid arteries (ICA) and middle cerebral arteries (MCA) and branches of MCA are demonstrated. (Right) Oblique view. Anterior cerebral artery (ACA) and pericallosal artery (PcA) are demonstrated

and dangling choroid plexus in the case of hydrocephalus (Figs 41.19 and 41.20). In contrast, the subarachnoid space and choroid plexus are well preserved in cases of ventriculomegaly (Fig. 41.21). It is difficult to evaluate obliterated subarachnoid space in the transabdominal axial section and this method may not differentiate accurately hydrocephalus with increased intracranial pressure from ventriculomegaly without pressure. Therefore, it is suggested that the evaluation of fetuses with enlarged ventricles should be evaluated in the parasagittal and coronal views by transvaginal way or 3D multidimensional analysis. In some cases with hydrocephalus,

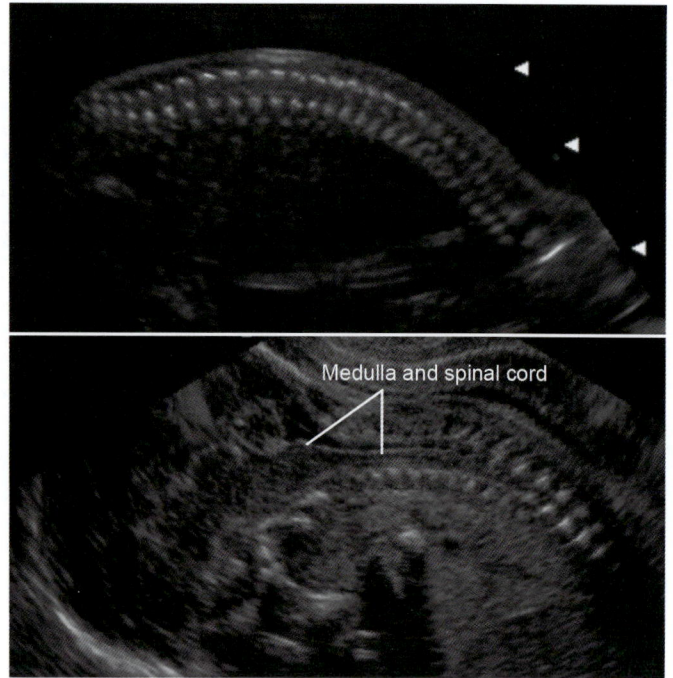

Fig. 41.16: Normal vertebral structure in the sagittal section at 19 weeks of gestation. Lower figure shows the medulla and spinal cord in the craniospinal region

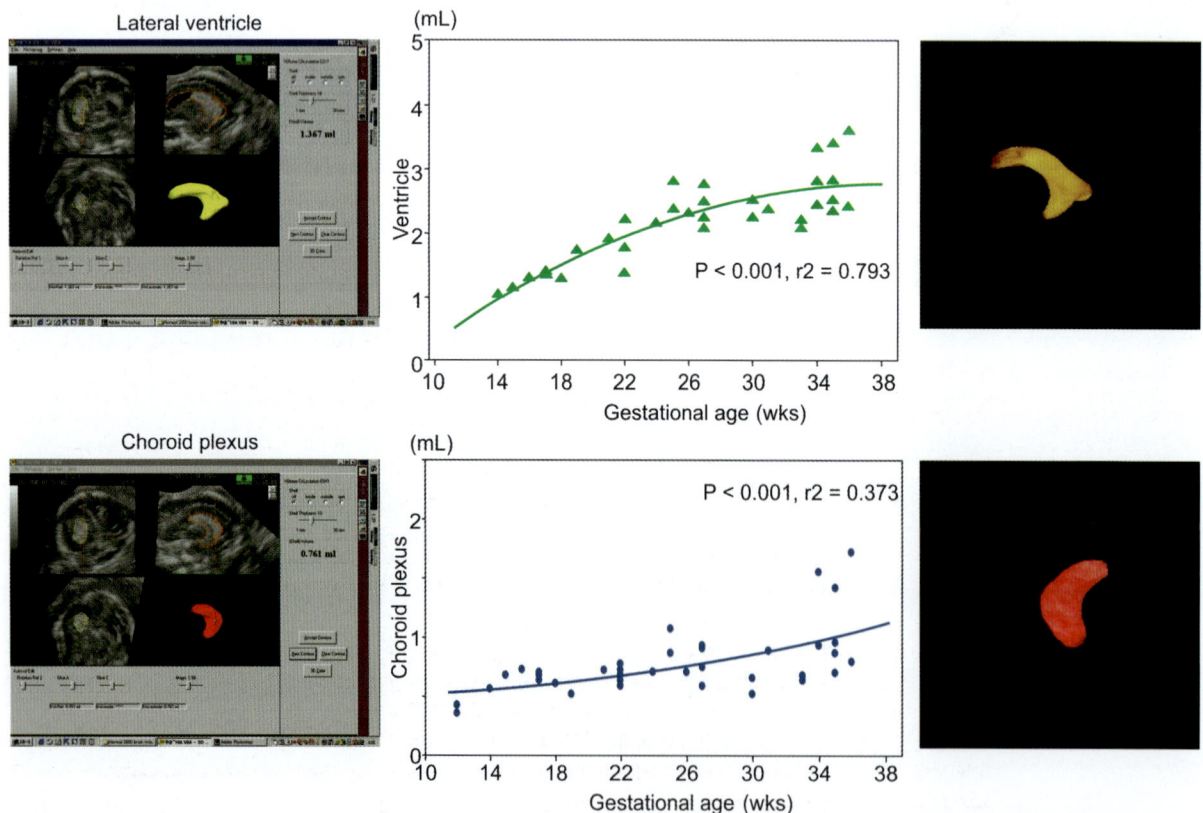

Fig. 41.17: Three-dimensional (3D) volume extraction and volumetric analysis of lateral ventricle and choroid plexus. On three orthogonal sections, the target organ can be traced automatically or manually with rotation of volume imaging data. After tracing, volume extracted image (right) is demonstrated and volume calculation data is shown. Middle graphs show normograms of ventricular size (upper) and choroid plexus size (lower) during pregnancy

the septum pellucidum is destroyed and both ventricles are fused with each other (Fig. 41.19). This condition should be differentiated from lobar type of holoprosencephaly. Furthermore, intracranial venous blood flow may be related to increased intracranial pressure. In normal fetuses, blood flow waveforms of dural sinuses, such as superior sagittal sinus, vein of Galen and straight sinus have pulsatile pattern[26] (Fig. 41.22). However, in cases with progressive hydrocephalus, normal pulsation disappears and blood flow waveforms become flat pattern[26] (Fig. 41.23). In cases with progressive hydrocephalus, there may be seven stages of progression (Fig. 41.24); (1) increased fluid collection of lateral ventricles, (2) increased intracranial pressure, (3) dangling choroids plexus, (4) disappearance of subarachnoid space, (5) excessive extension of the dura and superior sagittal sinus, (6) disappearance

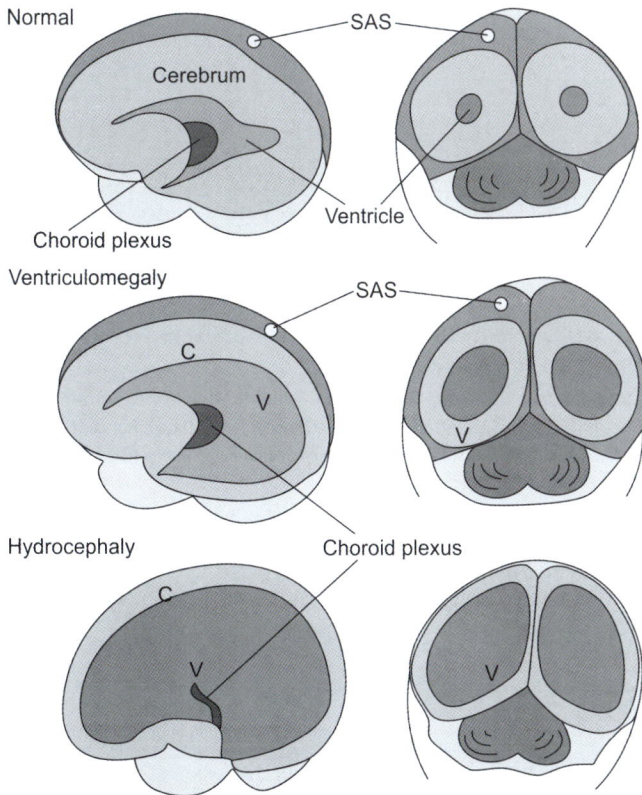

Fig. 41.18: Schema of ventriculomegaly and hydrocephaly. In cases of ventriculomegaly without increased intracranial pressure, subarachnoid space (SAS) and choroid plexus appearance are well preserved, while in cases of hydrocephaly with increased intracranial pressure, dangling choroid plexus and gradual disappearance of SAS are seen

Abbreviations: V, ventricle; C, cerebrum

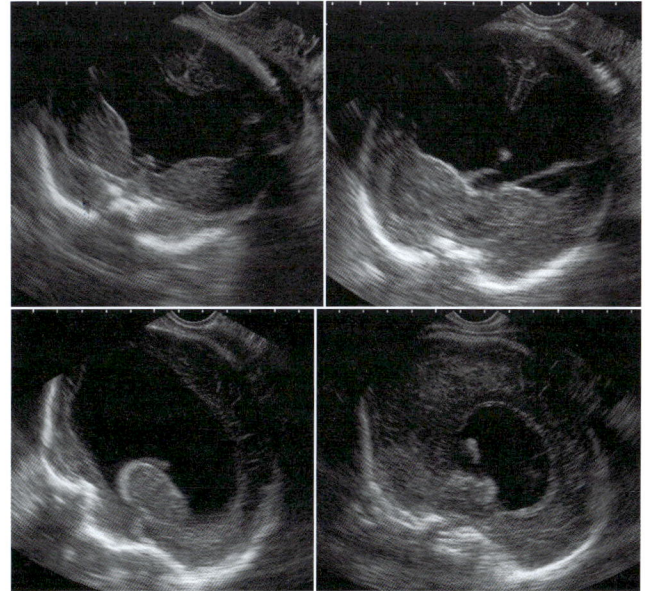

Fig. 41.19: Ultrasonography (US) images of hydrocephalus at 34 weeks of gestation. (Upper) Coronal images. Septum pellucidum was destroyed may be due to enlargement of bilateral ventricles and both ventricles were fused. Dangling choroid plexus is seen. (Lower) Parasagittal and sagittal images. Dangling choroid plexus and obliterated subarachnoid space are seen

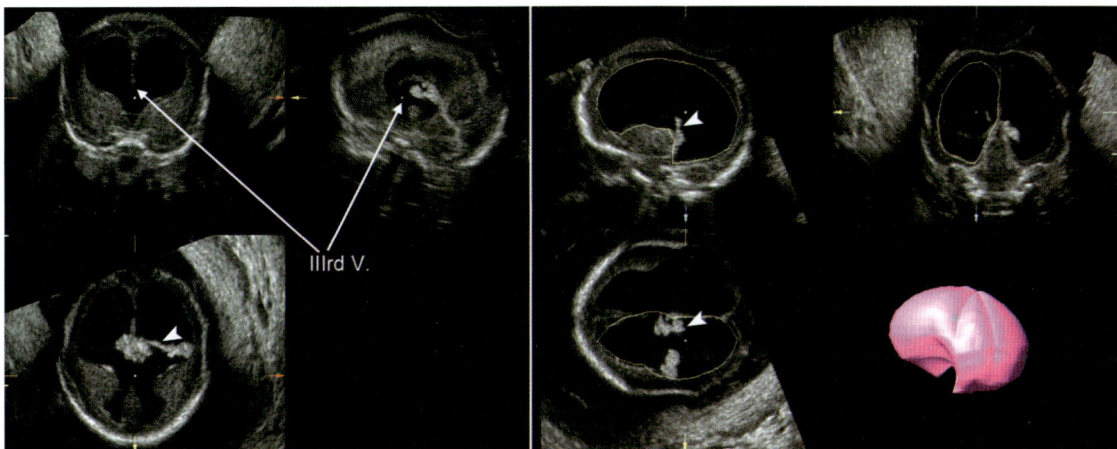

Fig. 41.20: Hydrocephalus due to aqueductal obstruction at 19 weeks of gestation
Left figure: Three orthogonal views with anterior coronal (upper left), median sagittal (upper right) and axial (lower left) slices. Bilateral ventriculomegaly and third ventriculomegaly (IIIrd V) are seen. No enlargement of forth ventricle indicates obstruction of the aqueduct. *Right figure*: Three orthogonal views with parasagittal (upper left) and posterior coronal (upper right) and axial (lower left) slices. Subarachnoid space is already obliterated and dangling choroid plexus (arrowheads) is seen. Lower right pink figure shows extracted 3D ventricular image by vocal mode. Ventricle in this case was ten-fold size of normal 19-week-ventricle

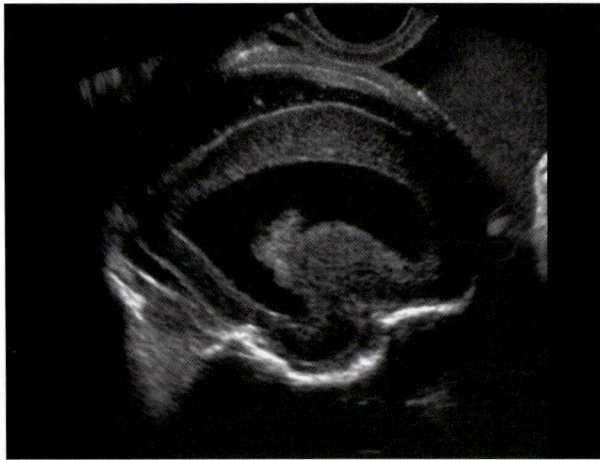

Fig. 41.21: Ultrasonography (US) image of ventriculomegaly at 29 weeks of gestation. Enlarged ventricle exists but subarachnoid space is well preserved and no dangling choroid plexus is seen. From those findings, non-increased intracranial pressure (ICP) is estimated. This condition should be differentiated from hydrocephalus with increased ICP

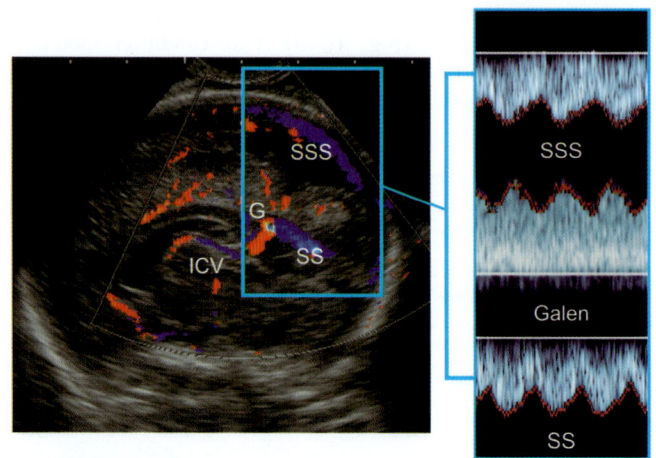

Fig. 41.22: Normal cerebral venous circulation. (Left) Sagittal image of color Doppler.

Abbreviations: SSS, superior sagittal sinus; ICV, internal cerebral vein; G, vein of Galen; SS, straight sinus; (right) Normal blood flow waveforms of dural sinuses. In normal fetuses, venous flow always has pulsations

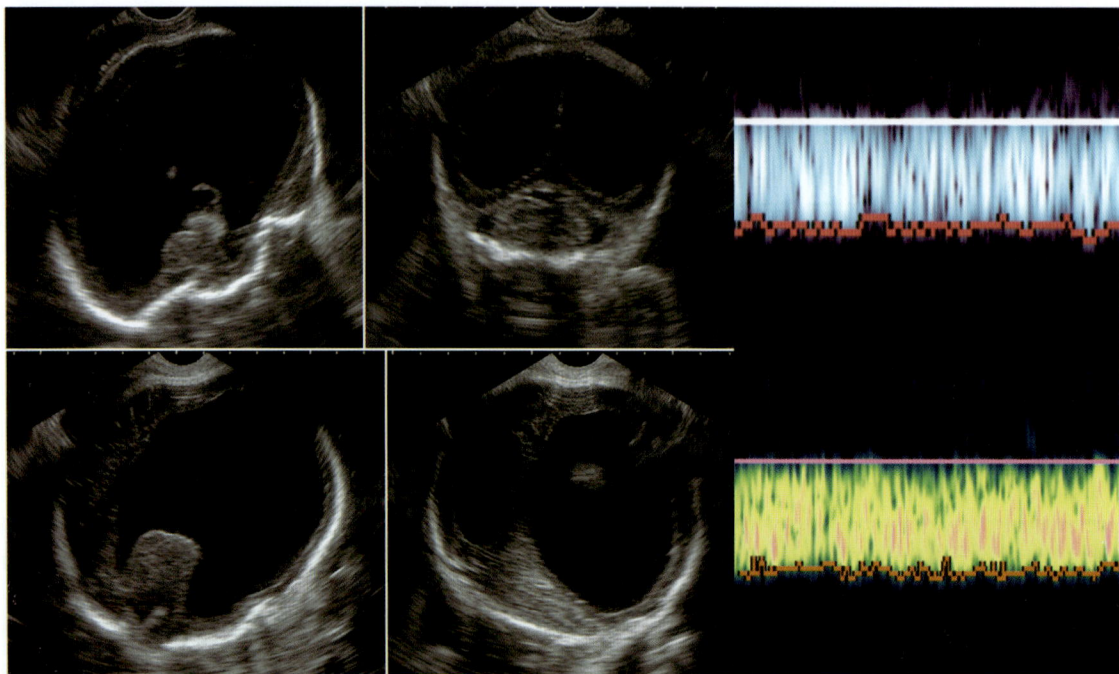

Fig. 41.23: Disappearance of venous pulsation in cases with hydrocephalus. Normal dural sinuses have pulsatile patterns of flow waveform (Fig. 41.22). In cases with progressive hydrocephalus, venous pulsation disappeared (right figures) may be because of excessive extension of the dura and dural sinuses

of venous pulsation, and finally, (7) enlarged skull. In general, both hydrocephalus and ventriculomegaly are still evaluated by the measurement of biparietal diameter (BPD) and atrial width (AW) in transabdominal axial section. As a screening examination, the measurement of AW is useful with a cut-off value of 10 mm.[27,28] As described above, however, hydrocephalus and ventriculomegaly should be differentiated from each other and hydrocephalic state should be assessed by changing appearance of intracranial structure. To evaluate enlarged ventricles, examiners should carefully observe the structure below and specify causes of hydrocephalus:

- Choroids plexus, dangling or not
- Subarachnoid space, obliterated or not
- Ventricles, symmetry or asymmetry
- Visibility of third ventricle
- Pulsation of dural sinuses
- Ventricular size (3D volume calculation if possible)
- Other abnormalities.

Genetic hydrocephalus is rare but important in counseling of couples on subsequent pregnancy. X-linked hydrocephalus (HSAS,

Increased fluid collection of lateral ventricles

↓

Increased ICP

↓

Dangling CP

↓

Disappearance of SAS

↓

Excessive extension of the dura and SSS

↓

Disappearance of venous pulsation

⬇

Enlarged skull

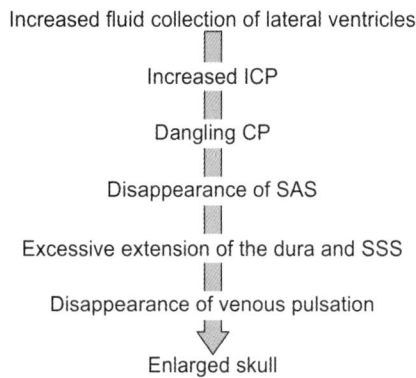

Fig. 41.24: Progressive stages of hydrocephalus

Abbreviations: ICP: intracranial pressure; CP: choroid plexus; SAS: subarachnoid space

hydrocephalus due to stenosis of the aqueduct of Sylvius), MASA (mental retardation-aphasia-shuffling gait-adducted thumbs) syndrome, X-linked complicated spastic paraparesis (SP1) and X-linked corpus callosum agenesis (ACC) are all due to mutations in the L1 gene.[29] The gene encoding L1 is located near the telomere of the long arm of the X chromosome in Xq28. Therefore, it was suggested to refer this clinical syndrome with the acronym CRASH, for corpus callosum hypoplasia, retardation, adducted thumbs, spastic paraplegia and hydrocephalus.[29] It has been reported that mutations which produce truncations in the extracellular domain of the L1 protein are more likely to produce severe hydrocephalus, grave mental retardation or early death than point mutations in the extracellular domain or mutations affecting only the cytoplasmic domain of the protein.[30] For the families, prenatal CNS diagnosis of male infants is important. Morphology-based approach becomes feasible between postmenstrual weeks 15 and 20. Prior to this gestational age, the diagnosis should rely on molecular biology tests.[31]

Borderline ventriculomegaly is defined as a width of the atrium of the lateral cerebral ventricles of 1,015 mm. The majority of prenatally detected isolated mild ventriculomegaly are developmentally normal.[32] Pilu et al.[33] reviewed 234 cases of borderline ventriculomegaly including an abnormal outcome in 22.8% and concluded that borderline ventriculomegaly carries an increased risk of cerebral maldevelopment, delayed neurological development and, possibly, chromosomal aberrations.

The treatment of hydrocephalus includes a miniature reserver,[34,35] shunt procedure and neuroendoscopy. Ventriculoperitoneal shunt is the most popular procedure. Effectiveness of shunt procedure for congenital hydrocephalus has been proven from earlier. However, it has been known that there are various complications of shunting, such as shunt infection, obstruction of the shunt tube, over drainage, under drainage, and slit ventricle syndrome. To reduce those complications, various types of shunt devices, such as antisiphon device or pressure programmable valve shunt device have been developed. Third ventriculostomy by neuroendoscopy has recently become performed in children with obstructive hydrocephalus, and the number of shunt-independent cases has been increased. It has been controversial, however, whether infants less than the age of one have a higher risk of treatment failure after neuroendoscopic procedures than older children. Some concludes that neuroendoscopy presents an effective alternative for the treatment of hydrocephalus in cases under the age of one.[36] However, third ventriculostomy still does not seem to be effective in neonates because of their prematurity of absorption ability in neonates and small infants.

CONGENITAL CENTRAL NERVOUS SYSTEM ANOMALIES

Cranium Bifidum

Prevalence: Anencephaly—0.29/1,000 births,[37] overall neural tube defect (NTD)—0.58–1.17/1000 births,[38–40] many reported remarkable reduction of prevalence of NTDs after using folic acid supplementation and fortification,[37–40] although some reported no decline of anencephaly rate.[41]

Definition: As in spina bifida, cranium bifidum is classified into four types of encephaloschisis (including anencephaly and exencephaly), meningocele, encephalomeningocele, encephalocystocele, and cranium bifidum occulutum. Encephalocele occurs in the occipital region in 70–80%. Acrania, exencephaly and anencephaly are not independent anomalies. It is considered that dysraphia (absent cranial vault, acrania) occurs in very early stage and disintegration of the exposed brain (exencephaly) during the fetal period results in anencephaly.[42]

Etiology: Multifactorial inheritance, single mutant genes, specific teratogens (valproic acid), maternal diabetes, environmental factors, predominant in females.

Pathogenesis: Failure of anterior neural tube closure or a restricted disorder of neurulation.

Associated anomalies: Open spina bifida (iniencephaly), Chiari type III malformation, bilateral renal cystic dysplasia and postaxial polydactyly with occipital cephalocele (Meckel-Gruber syndrome), hydrocephalus, polyhydramnios.

Prenatal diagnosis: Acrania in Figure 41.25, anencephaly in Figure 41.26 and early detection of iniencephaly in Figure 41.27.

Differential diagnosis: Amniotic band syndrome (ABS). In cases of ABS, cranial destruction occurs secondarily to an amniotic band, similar appearance is observed. However, ABS has completely different pathogenesis from acrania/exencephaly.

Prognosis: Anencephaly is a uniformly lethal anomaly. Other types of cranium bifidum, various neurological deficits may occur, depending on types and degrees.

Recurrence risk: Used to be high recurrence risk of 5–13%, however, recently declined by use of folic acid supplementation and fortification.

Obstetrical management: Termination of pregnancy can be offered in cases with anencephaly.

Neurosurgical management: For other cranium bifidum, surgical operation aims at transposition of cerebral tissue into the intracranial cavity. Ventriculoperitoneal shunt for hydrocephalus.

Spina Bifida

Prevalence: 0.22/1,000 births,[37] overall NTD; 0.58-1.17/1,000 births,[38-40] many reported remarkable reduction of prevalence of NTDs after using folic acid supplementation and fortification.[37-41]

Definition: Spina bifida aperta, manifest form of spina bifida is classified into four types: (1) meningocele, (2) myelomeningocele, (3) myelocystocele, and (4) myeloschisis. Spina bifida occulta is a generic term of spinal diseases covered with normal skin tissue, and does not indicate spinal diseases, which cannot be diagnosed

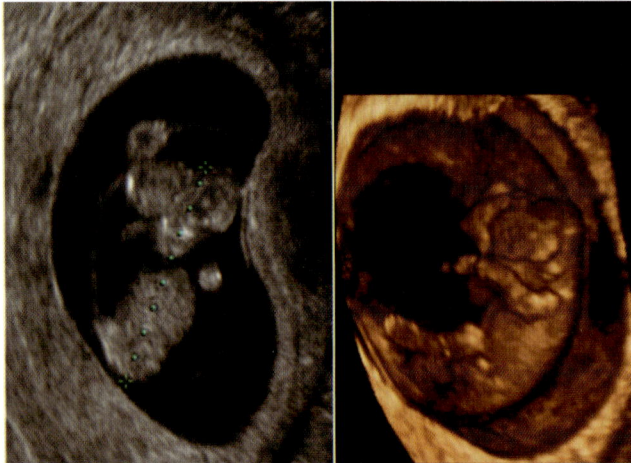

Fig. 41.25: A crania at 10 weeks of gestation. (Left) Ultrasonography (US) coronal image at 10 weeks. Note the normal appearance of amniotic membrane, which indicates this condition is not amniotic band syndrome. (Right) 3D US image of the same fetus as left image

by external appearance, cutaneous abnormalities near the spinal lesion are found; skin bulge (subcutaneous lipoma), dimple, hair tuft, pigmentation, skin appendage and hemangioma. In case with thickened film terminale, dermal sinus, or diastematomyelia (split cord malformation), abnormal tethering and fixation of the spinal cord occur.

Etiology: Multifactorial inheritance, single mutant genes, autosomal recessive, chromosomal abnormalities (trisomy 18, 13), specific teratogens (valproic acid), maternal diabetes, environmental factors, predominant in females.

Pathogenesis: Spina bifida aperta, an impairment of neural tube closure.

Spina bifida occulta: Caudal neural tube malformation by the processes of canalization and retrogressive differentiation.

Associated anomalies: Chiari type II malformation, hydrocephalus, scoliosis (above L2), polyhydramnios, additional non-CNS anomalies,

Prenatal diagnosis: Figures 41.28 to 41.31.

Differential diagnosis: Sacrococcygeal teratoma.

Prognosis: Disturbance of motor, sensory and sphincter function. Depends on lesion levels. Below S1; Enable to walk unaided, above L2; wheelchair dependent, variable at intermediate level.

Recurrence risk: Decreased, almost no recurrence rate[43] by use of folic acid supplementation and fortification.

Obstetrical management: In case with spina bifida aperta, especially with defect of skin, cesarean section is preferable to protect the spinal cord, nerves and prevent infection.

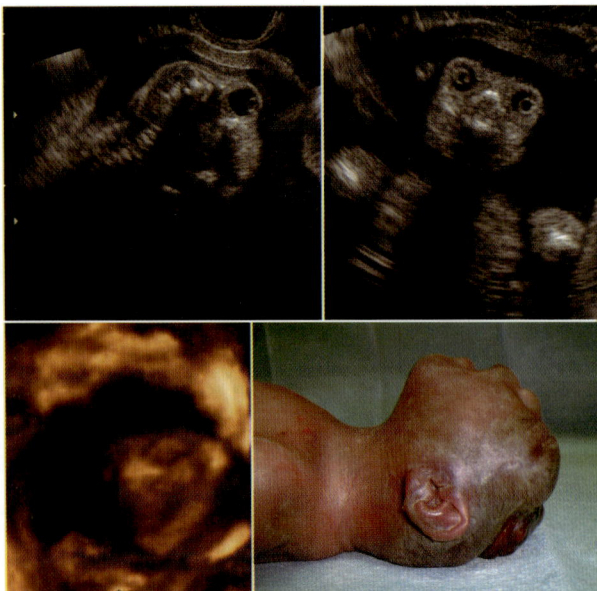

Fig. 41.26: Anencephaly in middle gestation. (Same case as Fig. 41.25). (Upper left) Ultrasonography (US) sagittal image at 23 weeks of gestation. (Upper right) US coronal image. (Lower left) 3D US image. (Lower right) External appearances of stillborn fetus at 25 weeks of gestation. It is clear that exenephalic brain tissue scattered in the amniotic space compared with this case at 10 weeks

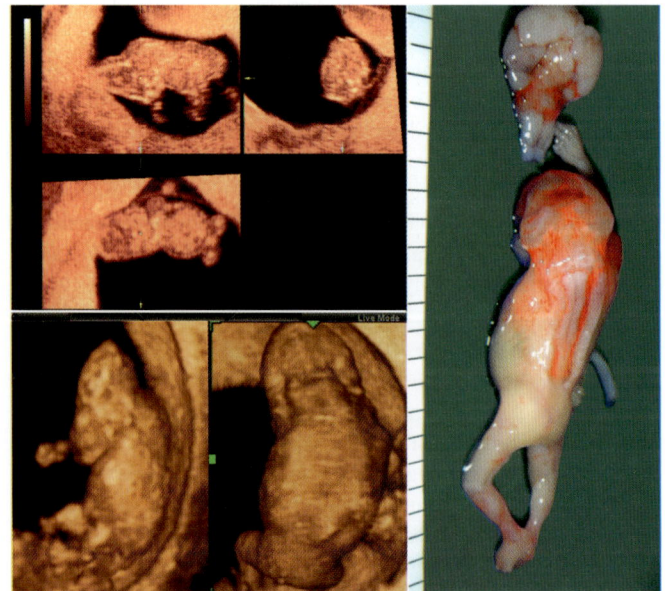

Fig. 41.27: Three-dimensional (3D) detection of a fetus with iniencephaly and acrania at 10 weeks of gestation. (Upper left) three orthogonal views of the fetus. Spina bifida (arrow) was demonstrated in the coronal section. (Lower left) 3D images show the fetal lateral and dorsal views. (Right) external appearance of aborted fetus at the end of 11 weeks of gestation. The brain and a part of spinal cord was detached at delivery

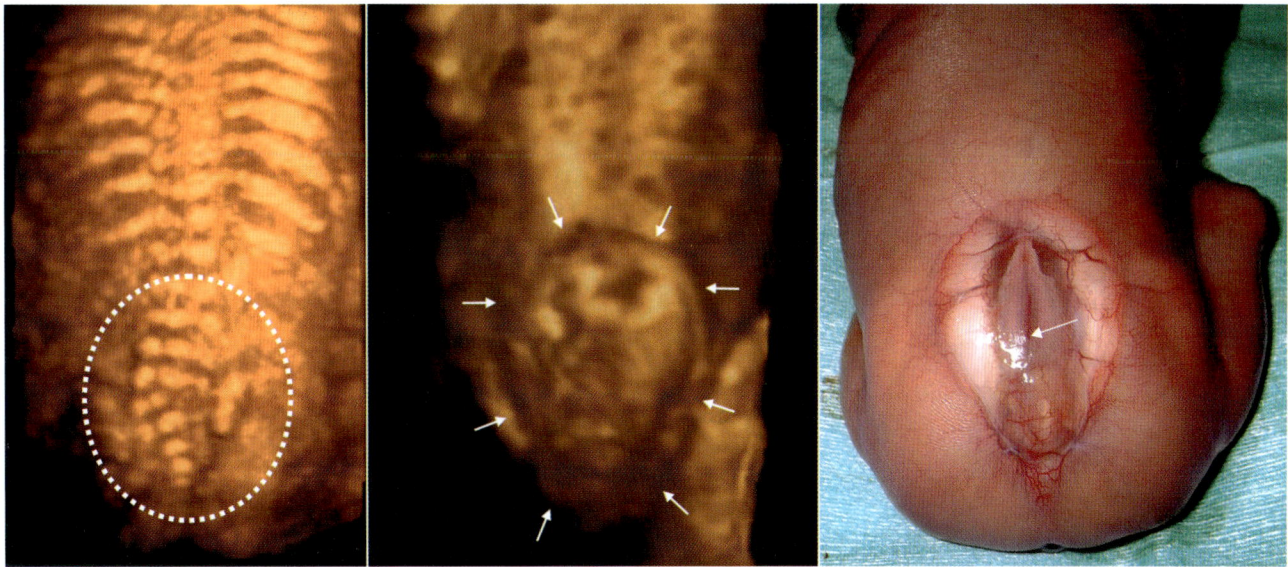

Fig. 41.28: Prenatal ultrasonography (US) image of myelomeningocele, spina bifida at 20 weeks of gestation. (Left) Three-dimensional (3D) bony demonstration of lumbar spina bifida. 3D ultrasound shows the exact level of spina bifida. (Middle) 3D surface reconstruction of large myelomeningocele (white arrows). (Right) external appearance of aborted fetus at 21 weeks of gestation. Note the central canal of the spinal cord (black arrow) in large myelomeningocele

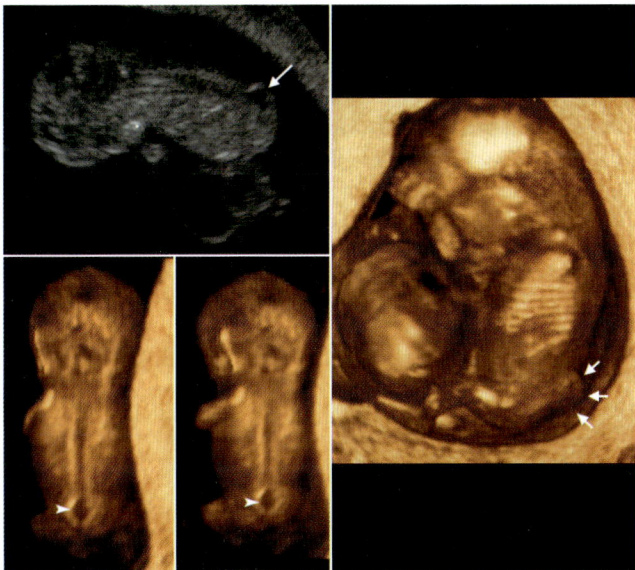

Fig. 41.29: Myelomeningocele in early pregnancy. 2D sagittal view at 9 weeks of gestation (upper left) shows the cystic lesion (arrow). Three dimensional dorsal views at 9 weeks (lower left) clearly demonstrate a neural tube defect at the lower lumber and sacral level (arrowheads). Right figure shows the same fetus at 12 weeks of gestation. Arrows indicate the lumbosacral myelomeningocele

Neurosurgical Management

1. Spina bifida aperta: In cases with defect of normal skin tissue, immediate closure of spina bifida after birth reduces spinal infection. Spinal cord reconstruction is the most important role of operation. Miniature Ommaya reservoir placement and subsequent ventriculoperitoneal shunt are required for hydrocephalus. For symptomatic Chiari malformation, posterior fossa decompressive craniectomy and/or tonsillectomy is performed.

2. Spina bifida occulta: The aim of surgical treatment for is decompression of the spinal cord and cutting off tethering to the spinal cord (Figs 41.32 and 41.33).

Chiari Malformation

Prevalence: Depends on prevalence of spina bifida (Chiari type II malformation). According to recent remarkable reduction of prevalence of NTDs after using folic acid supplementation and fortification, prevalence has declined. Other types are rare.

Definition: Chiari classified anomalies with cerebellar herniation in the spinal canal into three types by contents of herniated tissue; contents of type I is a lip of cerebellum, type II part of cerebellum, fourth ventricle and medulla oblongata, pons, and type III large herniation of the posterior fossa. Thereafter, type IV with just cerebellar hypogenesis was added. However, this classification occasionally leads to confusion in neuroimaging diagnosis. Therefore, at present, the classification as below is advocated.

i. Type I: Herniation of only cerebellar tonsil, not associated by myelomeningocele.

ii. Type II: Herniation of cerebellar tonsil and brainstem. Medullary kink, tentorial dysplasia, associated with myelomeningocele.

iii. Type III: Associated with cephalocele or craniocervical meningocele, in which cerebellum and brainstem herniated.

iv. Type IV: Associated with marked cerebellar hypogenesis and posterior fossa shrinking.

Synonyms: Arnold-Chiari malformation.

Etiology: Depends on the types.

Pathogenesis: Schematic picture and macroscopic findings, MRI images are in Figures 41.32 and 41.33. Chiari malformation occurs according to: (1) Inferior displacement of the medulla and the fourth ventricle into the upper cervical canal, (2) elongation and thinning of the upper medulla and lower pons and persistence of the embryonic flexure of these structures, (3) inferior displacement of

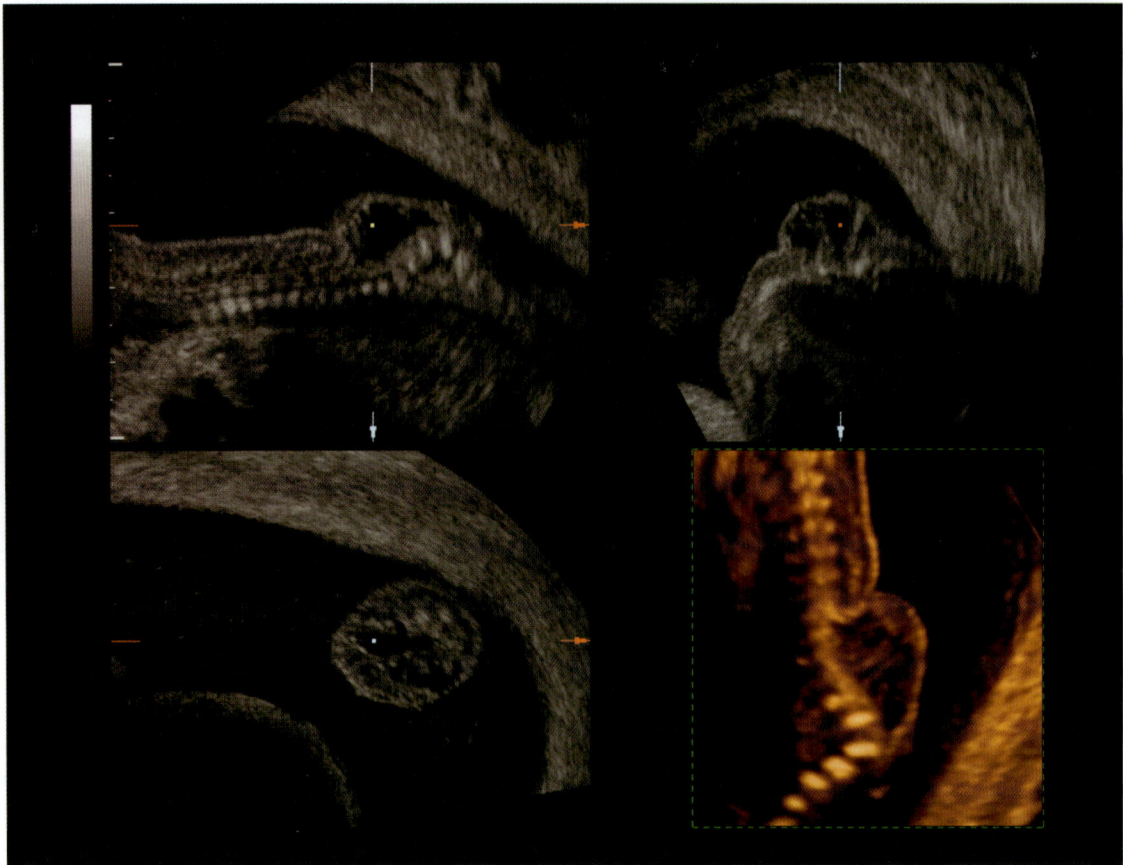

Fig. 41.30: Three-dimensional ultrasonography (3D US) image of myelomeningocele with kyphosis at 16 weeks of gestation. Three orthogonal views and surface reconstruction image. (Upper left) sagittal US image. Spinal cord completely protrude into the sac surface from spinal canal and severe kyphosis are seen (upper right) axial US view. (Lower left) coronal US view of myelomeningocele. Lower right figure demonstrates the sagittal vertebral bony structure by 3D thick slice

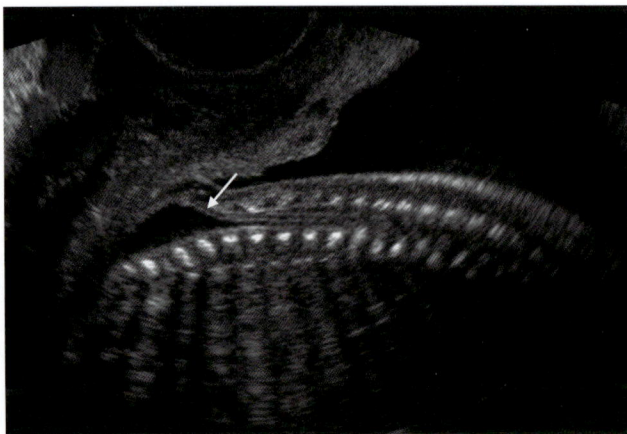

Fig. 41.31: Two-dimensional (2D) sagittal section of myelomeningocele at 19 weeks of gestation. The spinal cord (arrow) protrudes from spinal canal toward the sac surface of myelomeningocele

the lower cerebellum through the foramen magnum into the upper cervical region, and (4) a variety of bony defects of the foramen magnum, occiput, and upper cervical vertebrae.[44]

Associated anomalies: Hydrocephalus caused by obstruction of fourth ventricular outflow or associated aqueductal stenosis. Myelomeningocele or myeloschisis (type II), cephalocele or

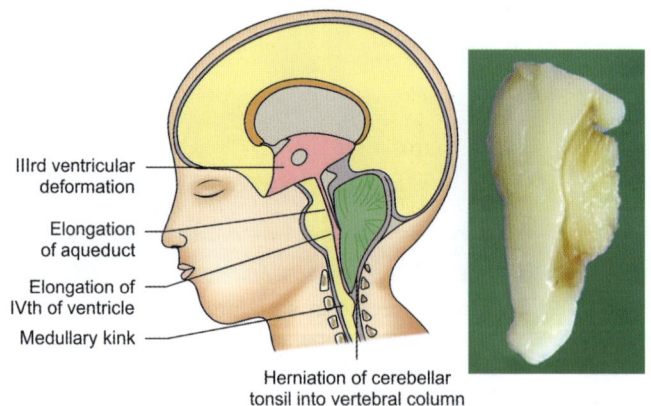

Fig 41.32: Schema and macroscopic finding of Chiari type II malformation. Chiari type II malformation is characterized by inferior displacement of the lower cerebellum through the foramen magnum with obliteration of the cisterna magna, inferior displacement of the medulla into the spinal canal, and elongation of the fourth ventricle and aqueduct. Right picture shows the macroscopic view of the elongated aqueduct, IVth ventricle and cerebellum from the specimen of an aborted fetus at 21 weeks of gestation

craniocervical meningocele (type III), cerebellar hypogenesis (type IV), and syringomyelia (type I).

Prenatal diagnosis: Prenatal ultrasonography diagnosis by features; lemon sign, which indicates deformity of the frontal bone, banana sign, which indicates abnormal shape of cerebellum without cisterna magna space (Figs 41.34A to C), medullary kink (Fig. 41.35), small clivus-supraocciput angle.[45]

Differential diagnosis: Craniosynostosis.

Prognosis: Nearly every case of myelomeningocele is accompanied morphological Chiari II malformation. Many cases with Chiari II are asymptomatic. However, clinical features due to Chiari malformation, such as feeding disturbances, laryngeal stridor or apneic episode, are found in approximately 9–30% of cases. In cases with these clinical features, vital prognosis is often poor.

Recurrence risk: Depends on types of Chiari malformation. Decreased according to decline of NTD recurrence rate by use of folic acid supplementation and fortification.

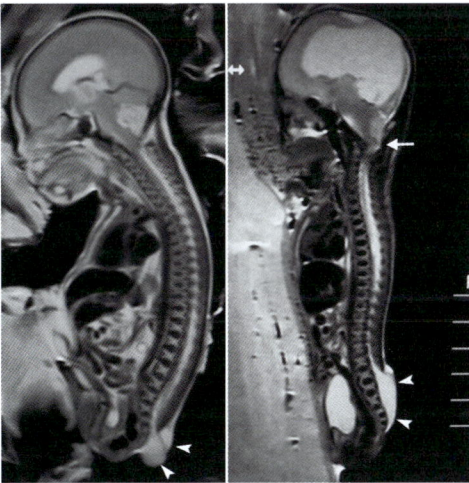

Fig. 41.33: Magnetic resonance (MR) images of aborted fetuses at 20–21 weeks of gestation. (Left) 20 weeks of gestation. Sacral myelomeningocele (arrowhead) and Chiari type II malformation are demonstrated. (Right) 21 weeks of gestation. Lumbosacral myelomeningocele with Chiari type II malformation is seen. This case, Myelomeningocele is complicated with holoprosencephaly. Normal karyotype. Severe medullary kink (arrow) is seen

Neurosurgical management: Neurosurgical decompression of foramen magnum (FMD) for any types of Chiari malformation. Syringo-subarachnoid shunt for Chiari type I.

Holoprosencephaly

Incidence: 1 in 15,000–20,000 live births, however, initial incidence may be more than sixty fold greater in aborted human embryos.[45-47]

Classification:[44] Holoprosencephalies are classified into three varieties:

1. Alobar type: A single-sphered cerebral structure with a single common ventricle, posterior large cyst of third ventricle (dorsal sac), absence of olfactory bulbs and tracts and a single optic nerve.
2. Semilobar type: With formation of a posterior portion of the interhemispheric fissure.
3. Lobar type: With formation of the interhemispheric fissure anteriorly and posteriorly but not in the midhemispheric region. The fusion of the fornices is seen.[48]

Etiology: 75% of holoprosencephaly has normal karyotype, but chromosomes 2, 3, 7, 13, 18 and 21 have been implicated in holoprosencephaly.[44] Particularly, trisomy 13 has most commonly been observed. Autosomal dominant (AD) transmission is rare.

Pathogenesis: Failure of cleavage of the prosencephalon and diencephalon during early first trimester (5–6 weeks) results in holoprosencephaly.

Associated anomalies: Facial abnormalities such as cyclopia, ethmocephaly, cebocephaly, flat nose, cleft lip and palate are invariably associated with horoprosencephaly. Extracerebral abnormalities are also invariably associated, such as renal cysts/ dysplasia, omphalocele, cardiac disease and or myelomeningocele.

Prenatal diagnosis: Alobar type in Figure 41.36 and semilobar type in Figure 41.37. Figure 41.38 shows facial appearance in cases of holoprosencephaly.

Differential diagnosis: Hydrocephalus, hydranencephaly.

Prognosis: Extremely poor in alobar holoprosencephaly. Uncertain in lobar type. Various but poor in semilobar type.

Recurrence risk: 6%,[49] but much lower in sporadic or trisomy cases, much higher in genetic cases.

Management: Chromosomal evaluation is offered.

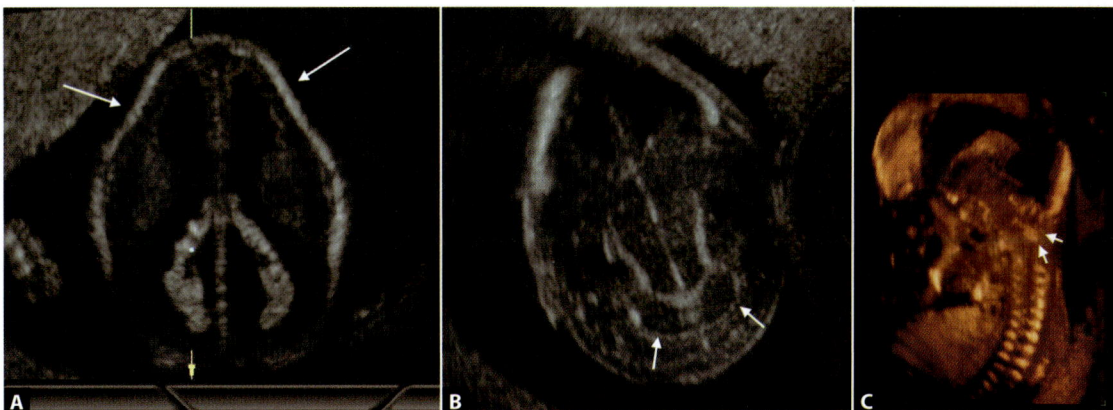

Figs 41.34A to C: Chiari type II malformation at 16 weeks of gestation. Chiari type II malformation is observed in most cases with myelomeningocele and myeloschisis. (A) typical lemon sign (arrows). (B) typical banana sign (arrows). (C) Three-dimensional (3D) reconstruction internal image of Chiari type II malformation (arrows)

Agenesis of the Corpus Callosum

Prevalence: Uncertain, but 3–7:1,000 in the general population is estimated.

Definition: Absence of the corpus callosum, which may be divided into (complete) agenesis, partial agenesis or hypogenesis of the corpus callosum.

Complete agenesis: Complete absence of the corpus callosum.

Partial agenesis (hypogenesis): Absence of splenium or posterior portion in various degrees.

Etiology: Chromosomal aberration in 20% of affected cases, such as trisomy 18, 8 and 13. Autosomal dominant, autosomal recessive, X-linked recessive, part of Mendelian syndromes such as Walker-Warburg syndrome, and X-linked dominant such as Aicardi syndrome.

Pathogenesis: Uncertain, but callosal formation may be associated with migration disorder.

Associated anomalies: Colpocephaly (ventriculomegaly with disproportionate enlargement of trigones, occipital horns and temporal horns, not hydrocephalus), superior elongation of the third ventricle, interhemispheric cyst, lipoma of the corpus callosum.

Prenatal diagnosis: Median sonographic images in Figures 41.39 and 41.40 and fetal MRI in Figure 41.41. Colpocephaly is shown in Figure 41.42.

Diagnosis: As the corpus callosum is depicted after 17 or 18 weeks of gestation by ultrasound, it is impossible to diagnose agenesis of the corpus callosum prior to this age.[50]

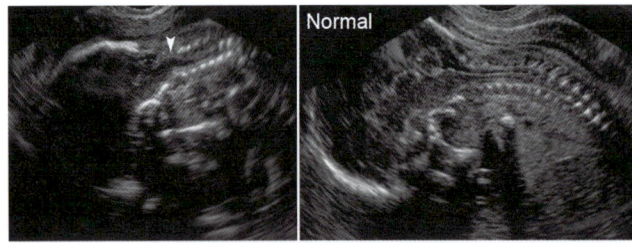

Fig. 41.35: Medullary kink in a case of Chiari II malformation at 19 weeks of gestation. (Left) medullary kink (arrowhead) associated obliterated cisterna magna is demonstrated. (Right) comparative normal image in the same cutting section at the same gestation. The cisterna magna, cerebellum and medullospinal portion are clearly demonstrated

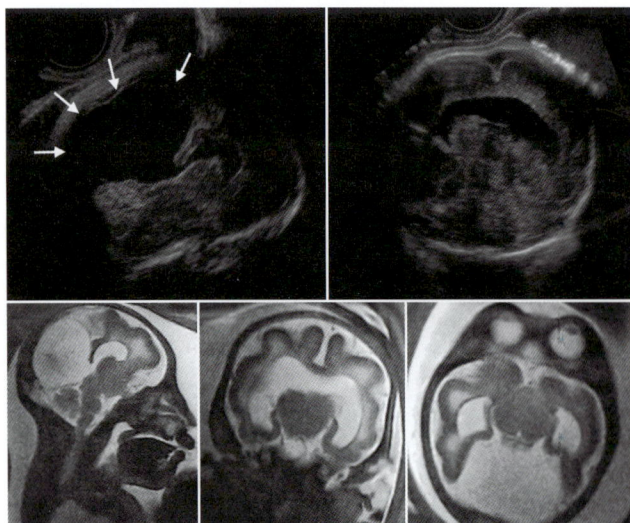

Fig. 41.36: Alobar holoprosencephaly at 15 weeks of gestation. Three orthogonal images of intracranial structure show a complete single ventricle within a single-sphered cerebral structure

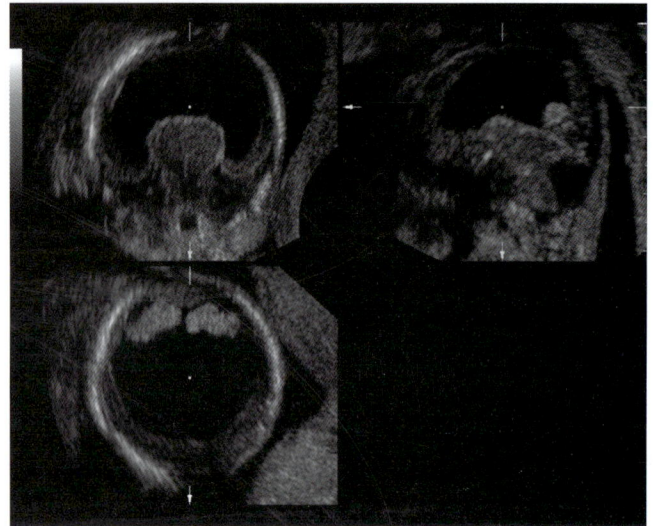

Fig. 41.37: Semilobar holoprosencephaly at 33 weeks of gestation. Upper left shows dorsal sac (arrows) in the median section. Upper right demonstrates the fused ventricle. Lower figures are fetal magnetic resonance (MR) images. Sagittal (left), coronal (middle) and axial (right) sections A blind end of nasal cavity and hypotelorism are seen in the sagittal and axial MR images respectively

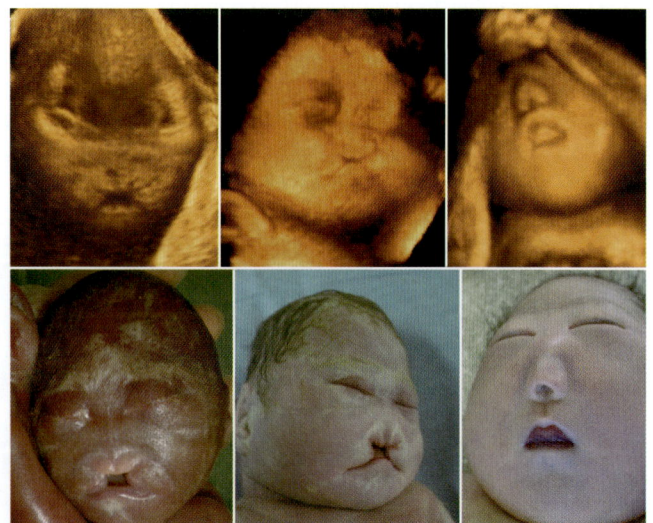

Fig. 41.38: Facial abnormalities in cases of holoprosencephaly. Upper figures are prenatal 3D facial images and lower figures show postpartum face appearance of each baby. Left; alobar holoprosencephaly at 20 weeks, Middle and right; semilobsr type in late pregnancy. Hypotelorism, and exophthalmos are common. Left and middle cases had cleft lip and palate and obstruction of the nasal cavity. Right case had a single and obstructed nasal cavity

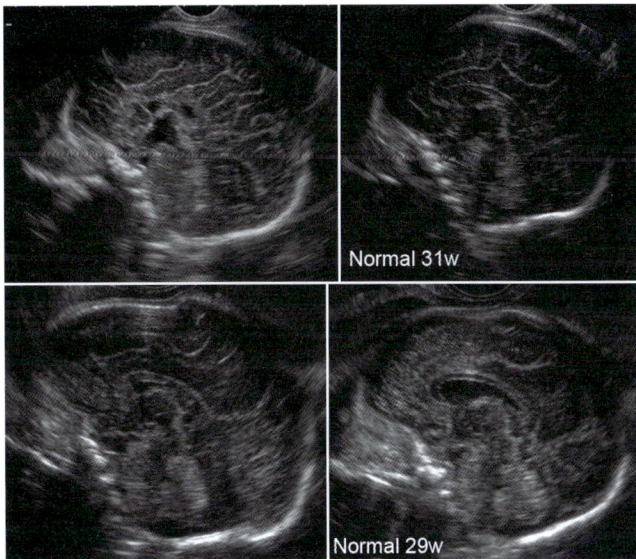

Fig. 41.39: Complete agenesis (upper) and hypogenesis (lower) of the corpus callosum. All images are transvaginal median (midsagittal) images. Right images are normal images of the corpus callosum at the same gestational age as each left image

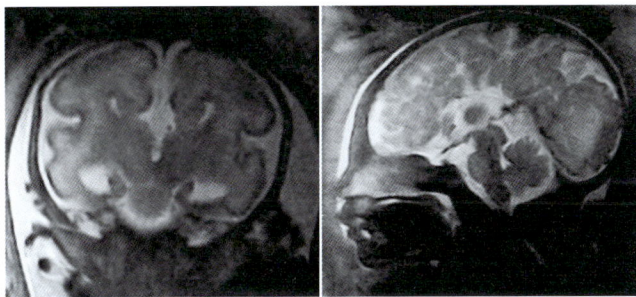

Fig. 41.41: Fetal magnetic resonance (MR) images of complete agenesis of the corpus callosum at 33 weeks of gestation. Anterior coronal section (left) and median section (right). No communicated bridge is seen. Note the bull's horn like appearance of the anterior horns of lateral ventricle in the coronal image

Prognosis: Various, depends on associated anomalies and most cases with isolated agenesis of the corpus callosum without other abnormalities are asymptomatic and prognosis is good. Complete agenesis has a worse prognosis than partial agenesis.[51] Epilepsy, intellectual impairment or psychiatric disorder[52] may occur later on.

Recurrence risk: Depends on etiology. Chromosomal: 1%, autosomal recessive: 25%, X-linked recessive male: 50%.

Management: Standard obstetrical care. Chromosomal evaluation is offered. In cases with interhemispheric cyst, postnatal fenestration or shunt procedure may be performed.

Absent Septum Pellucidum, Septo-Optic Dysplasia

Incidence: Unknown, rare.

Definition:

i. *Absent septum pellucidum*: Absence of the septum pellucidum with or without associated anomalies. The septum pellucidum can be destroyed by concomitant hydrocephalus or by contiguous ischemic lesions such as porencephaly. An isolated absent septum pellucidum[53] exists but rare.

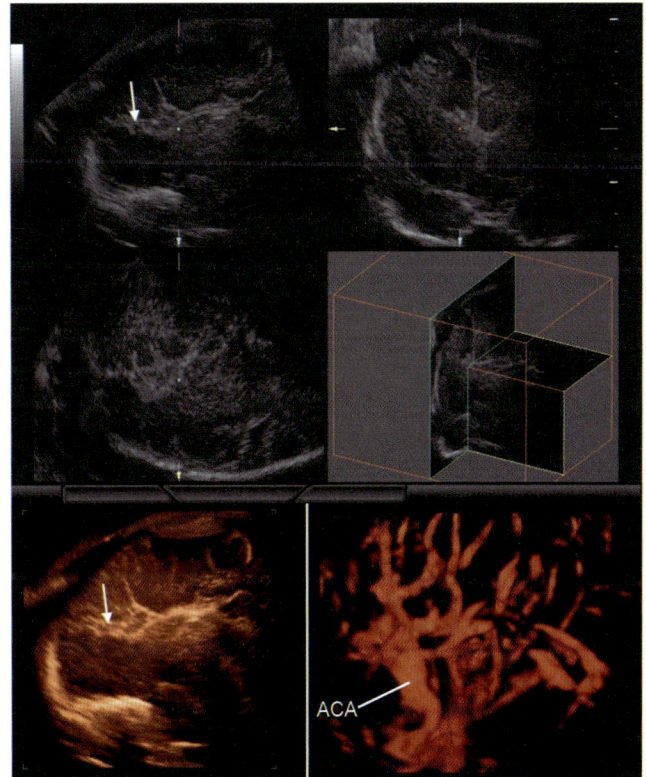

Fig. 41.40: Agenesis of the corpus callosum with abnormal gyration at 36 weeks of gestation. Upper figure shows the three orthogonal view of the brain with agenesis of the corpus callosum with an abnormal gyrus (arrow). Lower left figure is a thick slice of the sagittal section. Abnormal gyration (arrow) is more clearly demonstrated. Lower right shows the intracranial angiostructure by 3D power Doppler. Normal pericallosal artery does not exist and radial formation of the branches of anterior cerebral arteries (ACA) is seen

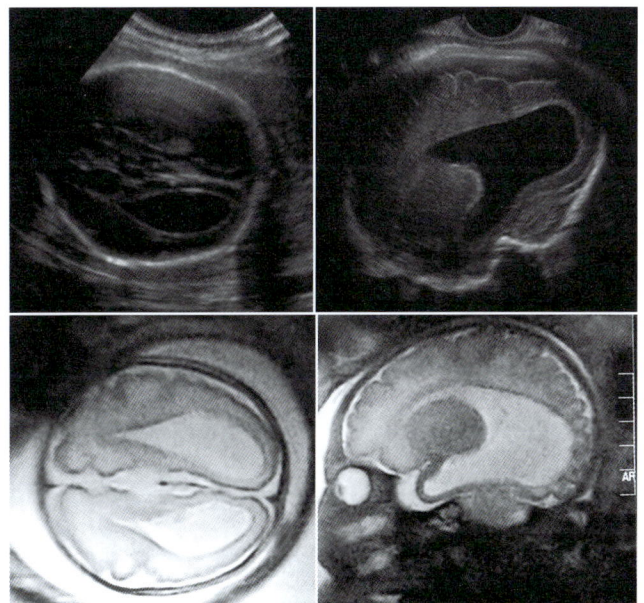

Fig. 41.42: Fetal ultrasonography (US) and magnetic resonance (MR) images of characteristic ventricular shape in a case with agenesis of the corpus callosum. Upper left: US axial image, upper right: US parasagittal image. Lower left: MR axial image, lower right: MR parasagittal image. Note the teardrop appearance of the lateral ventricles in the axial section. Ventricular appearance in the parasagittal section is called as "colpocephaly"

ii. *Septo-optic dysplasia*: Absence of the septum pellucidum and unilateral or bilateral hypoplasia of the optic nerve.

Synonyms: de Morsier syndrome (septo-optic dysplasia).

Etiology: Maternal drug (multidrug, valproic acid,[54] cocaine[55]), autosomal recessive, HESX1 homeodomain gene mutation.[56]

Pathogenesis: May occur as a vascular disruption sequence, with other prosencephalic or neuronal migration disorders.

Associated anomalies: Schizencephaly, gyral abnormalities, heterotopias, hypotelorism, ventriculomegaly, communicating lateral ventricles, bilateral cleft lip and palate, hypopituitarism.

Differential diagnosis: Dysgenesis of the corpus callosum, lobar holoprosencephaly.

Prognosis: Depends on associated anomalies. Variable degree of mental deficit, multiple endocrine dysfunction. In cases with isolated absent of septum pellucidum, prognosis may be good.

Recurrence risk: Unknown.

Management: Confirmation of diagnosis after birth is important for genetic counseling. Endocrine dysfunction should be searched and corrected. Shunt procedure in cases with progressive ventriculomegaly.

Lissencephaly

Incidence: Unknown, rare.

Definition: Characterized by a lack of gyral development and divided into two types:

1. *Lissencephaly type I*: A smooth surface of the brain. Cerebral wall is similar to that of an approximately 12-week-old fetus.[56] Isolated lissencephaly Miller-Dieker syndrome with additional craniofacial abnormalities, cardiac anomalies, genital anomalies, sacral dimple, creases, and/or clinodactyly.

2. *Lissencephaly type II*: Cobblestone appearance. Walker-Warburg syndrome with macrocephaly, congenital muscular dystrophy, cerebellar malformation, retinal malformation, Fukuyama congenital muscular dystrophy with microcephaly and congenital muscular dystrophy.

Synonyms: Agyria, Pachygyria, Walker-Warburg syndrome was known as HARD ±E syndrome (hydrocephalus, agyria, retinal dysplasia, with or without encephalocele).

Etiology: Isolated lissencephaly is link to chromosome 17p13.3 and chromosome Xq24-q24. Miller-Dieker syndrome is also link to chromosome 17p13.3. Walker-Warburg syndrome is autosomal recessive inheritance. Fukuyama congenital muscular dystrophy is link to chromosome 9q31, fukutin.[58]

Pathogenesis: Defective neuronal migration with four, rather than six layers in the cortex.

Associated anomalies: Polyhydramnios, less fetal movement, colpocephaly, agenesis of the corpus callosum, Dandy-Walker malformation, in Miller-Dieker syndrome, micrognathia, flat nose, high forehead, low-set ears, cardiac anomalies, genital anomalies in male are often observed in Walker-Warburg syndrome.

Prenatal diagnosis: Prenatal diagnosis[59-61] of lissencephaly without previous history of an affected child probably cannot be reliably made until 26–28 weeks of gestation.[42]

Prognosis: Type I—Hypotonia, paucity of movements, feeding disturbance, seizures. The prognosis is poor, and death occurs. Type II—Severe seizures, mental disorders, severe muscle disease with hypotonia. Death in the first year is common.

Recurrence risk: Depends on etiology.

Management: Karyotyping is recommended to detect the chromosomal defect. Standard obstetrical care.

Schizencephaly

Incidence: Rare.

Definition: A disorder characterized by congenital clefts in the cerebral mantle, lined by pia-ependyma, with communication between the subarachnoid space laterally and the ventricular system medially. 63% is unilateral and 37% bilateral. Frontal region in 44% and frontoparietal 30%.[57]

Etiology: Uncertain.

In certain familial case, a point mutation in the homeobox gene, EMX2 was found.[62,63] Cytomegalovirus infection was also related in some cases.[64]

Pathogenesis: Neuronal migration disorder.

Associated anomalies: Ventriculomegaly, microcephaly, polymicrogyria, gray matter heterotopias, dysgenesis of the corpus callosum, absence of the septum pellucidum, and optic nerve hypoplasia.

Differential diagnosis: Porencephaly, arachnoid cyst or other intracranial cystic masses. MR imaging is useful in diagnosis of schizencephaly.[65]

Prognosis: Variable.

Generally suffer, from mental retardation, seizures, developmental delay and motor disturbances.

Recurrence risk: unknown.

Management: Ventriculoperitoneal shunt for progressive hydrocephalus.

Dandy-Walker Malformation, Dandy-Walker Variant, Megacisterna Magna

Incidence: Dandy-Walker malformation has an estimated prevalence of about 1:30,000 births, and is found in 4–12% of all cases of infantile hydrocephalus.[66] Incidence of Dandy-Walker variant and megacisterna magna is unknown.

Definition: At present, the term Dandy-Walker complex[67] is used to indicate a spectrum of anomalies of the posterior fossa that are classified by axial computed tomography (CT) scans as it follows. Dandy-Walker malformation, Dandy-Walker variant, and megacisterna magna seem to represent a continuum of developmental anomalies of the posterior fossa.[67] Figure 41.43 shows the differential diagnosis of hypoechoic lesion of the posterior fossa.

i. *(Classic) Dandy-Walker malformation*: Cystic dilatation of fourth ventricle, enlarged posterior fossa, elevated tentorium and complete or partial agenesis of the cerebellar vermis.

ii. *Dandy-Walker variant*: Variable hypoplasia of the cerebellar vermis with or without enlargement of the posterior fossa.

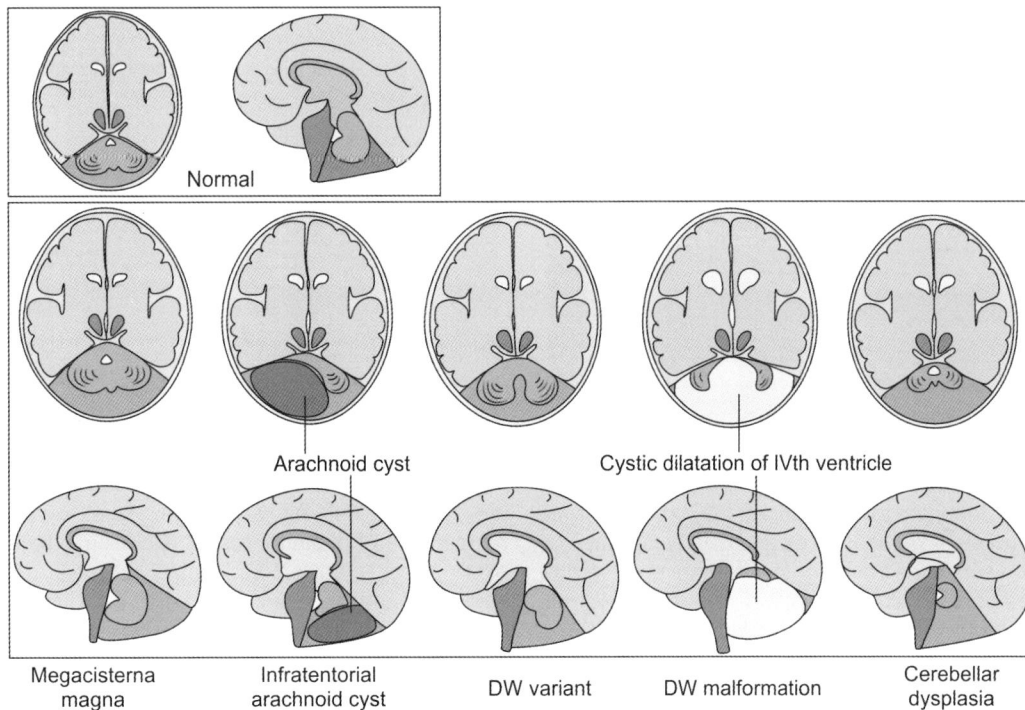

Fig. 41.43: Differential diagnosis of " hypoechoic lesion" of the posterior fossa

iii. *Megacisterna magna*: Enlarged cisterna magna with integrity of both cerebellar vermis and fourth ventricle.

Etiology: Mendelian disorders such as Warburg, chromosomal aberration such as 45, X, partial monosomy/trisomy, viral infections and diabetes.

Pathogenesis: During development of the fourth ventricular roof, a delay or total failure of the foramen of Magendie to open occurs, allowing a buildup of CSF and development of the cystic dilation of the fourth ventricle. Despite, the subsequent opening of the foramina of Luschka (usually patient in Dandy-Walker malformation), cystic dilatation of the fourth ventricle persists and CSF flow is impaired.

Associated anomalies of Dandy-Walker malformation: Hydrocephalus. Other midline anomalies, such as agenesis of the corpus callosum and holoprosencephaly and occipital encephalocele. Extracranial abnormalities, such as congenital heart disease, NTDs and cleft lip/palate. A frequency of additional anomalies ranging between 50 to 70%.

Prenatal diagnosis: Dandy-Walker malformation in Figures 41.44 and 41.45, Dandy-Walker variant in Figure 41.46. To observe the agenesis of the cerebellar vermis, axial cutting section is preferable. To observe the elevated tentorium, sagittal section is preferable.

Differential diagnosis: Infratentorial arachnoid cyst, other intracranial cystic tumor, hydrocephalus, cerebellar dysplasia (Fig. 41.47).

Prognosis: Progressive hydrocephalus, not observed in neonates but often progressive during the first one month. Cases diagnosed in utero or neonatal period, outcome is generally unfavorable. Nearly 40% die, and 75% of survivors exhibit cognitive deficits. Prognosis of Dandy-Walker variant is good. Clinical significance of megacisterna magna is uncertain.

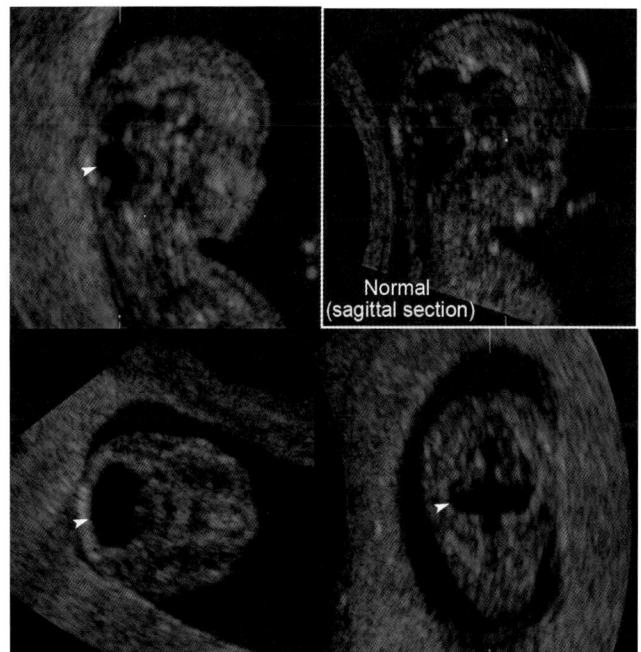

Fig. 41.44: Early stage of Dandy-Walker malformation at 11 weeks of gestation. Abnormal dilatation of the posterior fossa (arrowheads). Upper right figure is a sagittal image at the same gestational age in a normal case. Amniocentesis revealed trisomy 9 mosaicism and the fetus died in utero at 19 weeks

Recurrence risk: Depends on etiology. Generally 1-5% (Dandy-Walker malformation).

Management: Cystoperitoneal shunt, cysto ventriculoperitoneal shunt.

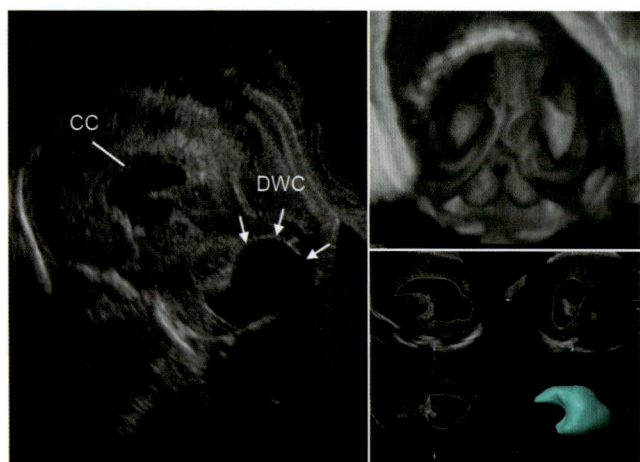

Fig. 41.45: Dandy-Walker malformation at 28 weeks of gestation. Left figure shows the median section of the brain. Corpus callosum (CC) is normally demonstrated and Dandy-Walker cyst (DWC, arrows) is seen in the posterior fossa. Right upper figure is a 3D view in the posterior coronal section. Hypoplastic vermis of the cerebellum (arrowhead) is seen. Right lower figures, three orthogonal views and an extracted ventricular appearance, demonstrate moderate ventriculomegaly in this case

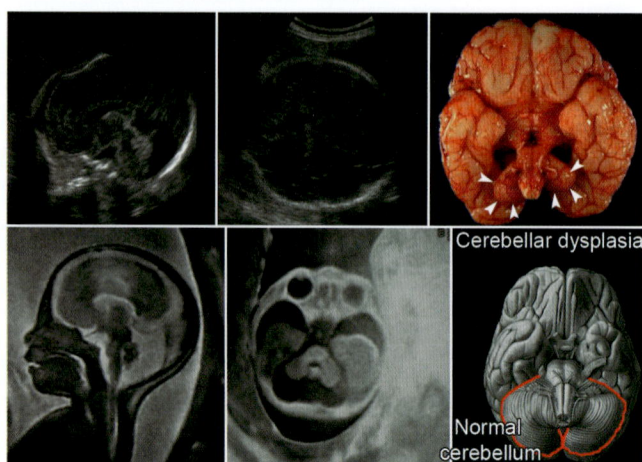

Fig. 41.47: Cerebellar dysplasia in a case of trisomy 18. (Upper left) transvaginal median image. Small cerebellum within a normal size of posterior fossa. (Upper middle) transabdominal axial image. (Lower left) fetal magnetic resonance (MR) sagittal image. (Lower middle) MR axial image. (Upper right) macroscopic photograph of cerebellar dysplasia in another case of trisomy 18. Compared with normal cerebellum shown in a right lower figure, hypo-plastic cerebellum is easily identified

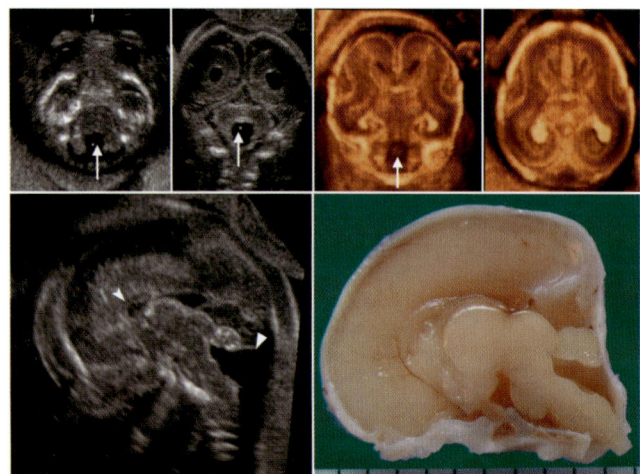

Fig. 41.46: Dandy-Walker variant at 20 weeks of gestation. Upper figures show the 2D axial, 2D posterior coronal, 3D thick slices of oblique coronal and axial sections from the left. Hypoplasia of the vermis (arrows) is demonstrated and no marked ventriculomegaly was seen. Lower left figure shows the median section. Partial agenesis of the corpus callosum (arrowhead), floated celebellum (triangle arrowhead) and cystic formation of the posterior fossa are seen. Lower right figure shows the median cutting section of the specimen of an aborted fetus at 21 weeks of gestation. This case had other complicated anomalies and the karyotype was partial trisomy of chromosome 10

Arachnoid Cyst

Prevalence: 1% of intracranial masses in newborns.

Definition: Congenital or acquired cyst, lined by arachnoid membranes, and filled with fluid collection, which is the same character as the cerebrospinal fluid. The number of cysts is mostly single, but two or more cysts can be occasionally observed. Location of arachnoid cyst is various; approximately 50% of cysts occurs from the Sylvian fissure (middle fossa), 20% from the posterior fossa, and 10–20% each from the convexity, suprasellar, interhemisphere, and quadrigeminal cistern. Interhemispheric cysts are often associated with agenesis or hypogenesis of the corpus callosum.

Etiology: Unknown.

Pathogenesis: Congenital arachnoid cyst is formed by maldevelopment of the arachnoid membrane. CSF accumulation in the subarachnoid space or intra-arachnoid layers from a choroid plexus-like tissue within the cyst wall, leads to a progressive distension of the lesion.

Associated anomalies: Unilateral or bilateral hydrocephalus, macrocrania.

Prenatal diagnosis: Figures 41.48 to 41.50. Detection in the first trimester was reported.[68]

Differential diagnosis: Porencephaly, schizencephaly, third ventriculomegaly, intracranial cystic type tumor, vein of Galen aneurysm, Dandy-Walker malformation, large cisterna magna, external hydrocephalus.

Prognosis: Generally good. Postnatally, many are asymptomatic and remain quiescent for years, although, others expand and cause neurological symptoms by compressing adjacent brain, ventriculomegaly, and/or expanding the overlying skull.

Recurrence risk: Unknown.

Obstetrical management: Arachnoid cysts may increase or decrease its size. Therefore, expectant management of antenatally diagnosed cases is suggested.[69] In cases with accompanied hydrocephalus, mode and timing of delivery may be modified.

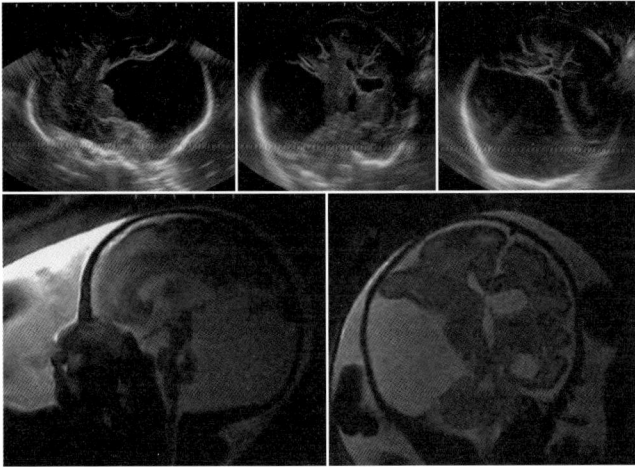

Fig. 41.48: Fetal arachnoid cyst at 31 weeks of gestation. (Upper) transvaginal ultrasonography (US) image. Sagittal (left) and coronal (middle, right) sections. (Lower left) fetal magnetic resonance (MR) sagittal image. The cyst occupies supra- to infratentorial space. Not only cerebrum but also cerebellum is compressed by the cyst. (Lower right) fetal MR coronal image. Midline is conspicuously arcuated. Unilateral scalp and skull bone are extended due to the existence of the huge cyst. Note the difference between right and left head size

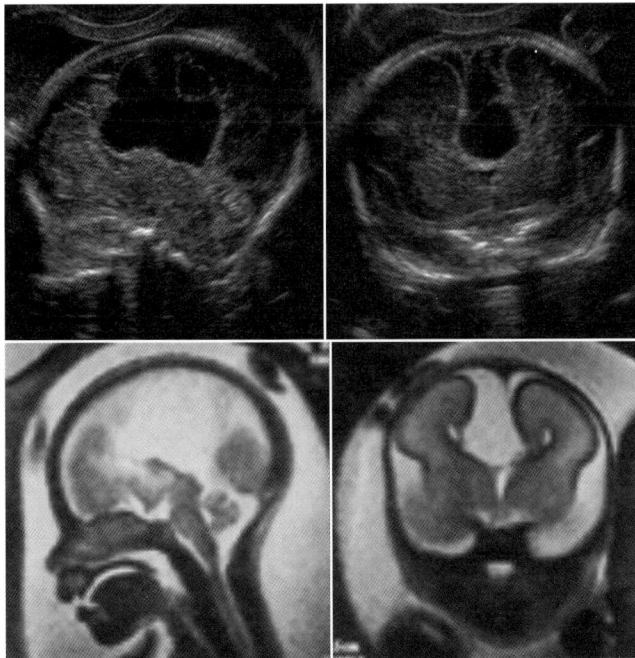

Fig. 41.49: Transvaginal ultrasonography (US) images of middle fossa arachnoid cyst at 29 weeks of gestation. (Upper) serial coronal sections. (Lower) serial sagittal sections. Compressed adjacent cerebrum is demonstrated

Craniotomy, shunting or neuroendoscopic method has been still controversial.[70,71]

Craniosynostosis

Incidence: unknown.

Definition: Premature closure of cranial suture, which may affect one or more cranial sutures. Simple sagittal synostosis is most common. Various cranial shapes depend on affected suture(s).

Sagittal suture	Scaphocephaly or dolichocephaly.
Bilateral coronal suture	Brachycephaly
Unilateral coronal suture	Anterior plagiocephaly
Metopic suture	Trigonocephaly
Lambdoid suture	Acrocephaly
Unilateral lambdoid suture	Posterior plagiocephaly
Coronal/lambdoid/metopic or squamous/sagittal suture	Cloverleaf skull
Total cranial sutures	Oxycephaly

Syndromes

i. *Crouzon syndrome*: Acrocephaly, synostosis of coronal, sagittal and lambdoid sutures with ocular proptosis, maxillary hypoplasia.

ii. *Apert syndrome*: Brachycephaly, irregular synostosis, especially coronal suture. With midfacial hypoplasia, syndactyly, broad distal phalanx of thumb and big toe.

iii. *Pfeiffer syndrome*: Brachycephaly, synostosis of coronal and/or sagittal sutures. With hypertelorism, broad thumbs and toes, partial syndactyly.

iv. *Antley-Bixler syndrome*: Brachycephaly, multiple synostosis, especially of coronal suture.

With maxillary hypoplasia, radiohymeral synostosis, choanal atresia, arthrogryposis.

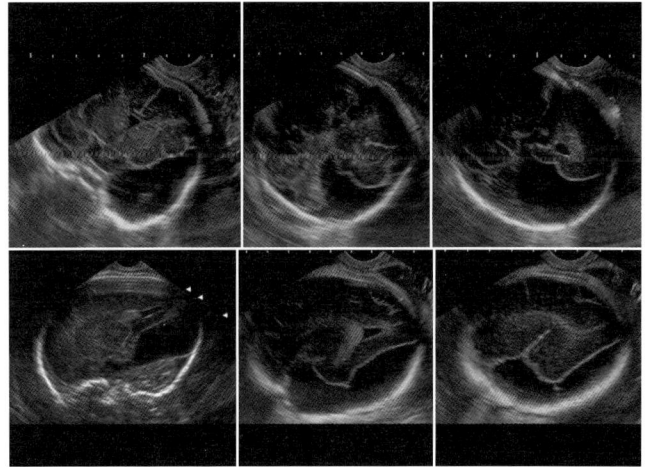

Fig. 41.50: Ultrasonography (US) and magnetic resonance (MR) images of interhemispheric cyst at 24 weeks of gestation. Upper left: US median section, upper right: US anterior coronal section, lower left: MR median section, lower right: MR anterior coronal section. Cystic lesion exists between hemispheres. Intracystic cyst is visible on US images

Postnatal management: In cases with those symptoms or with prospects of neurological symptoms, treatment should be considered. Operation methods include:

- Cyst fenestration by craniotomy
- Cyst fenestration by neuroendoscopy
- Cyst-peritoneal shunt.

Etiology: Crouzon (AD, variable), apert (AD, usually new mutation), Pfeiffer (AD), Antley-Bixler (AR). In five AD craniosynostosis syndromes (Apert, Crouzon, Pfeiffer, Jackson-Weiss and Crouzon syndrome with acanthosis nigricans) result from mutations in FGFR genes.[72]

Pathogenesis:[73] (1) Cranial vault bones with decreased growth potential, (2) asymmetrical bone deposition at perimeter sutures, (3) sutures adjacent to the prematurely fused suture compensate in growth more than those sutures not contiguous with the closed suture; (4) enhanced symmetrical bone deposition occurs along both sides of a non-perimeter suture continuing prematurely closed suture.

Associated anomalies: Hypertelorism, syndactyly, polydactyly, exophthalmos

Prenatal diagnosis: Figure 41.51 shows prenatal appearance in Apert syndrome and postnatal findings are shown in Figure 41.52. Abnormal craniofacial appearance can be detected by 2D/3D ultrasound.[74,75]

Prognosis: Various.

In some of trigonocephaly and syndromic types, prognosis is poor.

Recurrence risk: Depends on etiology.

Management: Operative aim of cranioplasty is improvement of intracranial pressure and cosmetic changes.

Vein of Galen Aneurysm

Incidence: Rare.

Definition: Direct arteriovenous fistulas between choroidal and/or quadrigeminal arteries and an overlying single median venous sac.

Synonyms: Vein of Galen malformation.

Etiology: Unknown.

Pathogenesis: Venous sac most probably represents persistence of the embryonic median prosencephalic vein of Markowski, not the vein of Galen, per se.[76]

Associated anomalies: Cardiomegaly, high cardiac output, secondary hydrocephalus, macrocrania, cerebral ischemia (intracranial steal phenomenon), subarachnoid/cerebral/intraventricular hemorrhages.

Prenatal diagnosis: 2D and 3D color/power Doppler detection is possible.

Differential diagnosis: Arachnoid cyst, porencephalic cyst, intracranial teratoma. Color/power Doppler is helpful for differential diagnosis.

Prognosis: According to earlier review, outcome did not differ between treated and non-treated group and over 80% of cases died.[77] However, recent advances in treatment have improved outcome, such that 60–100% survive and over 60% have a good neurological outcome.[78,79]

Recurrence risk: Unknown.

Management: Evaluation of the fetal high-output cardiac state for the proper obstetrical management. Percutaneous embolization by microcoils is recent main postnatal treatment and remarkably improved outcome.

Choroid Plexus Cysts

Incidence: 0.95-2.8% of all fetuses scanned.[80-82]

Definition: Cysts with fluid collection within the choroids plexus, which may exist unilaterally or bilaterally. They are depicted in the second trimester and usually resolve by the 24th week.

Etiology: Normal variant, chromosomal aberration such as trisomy 18 and others.

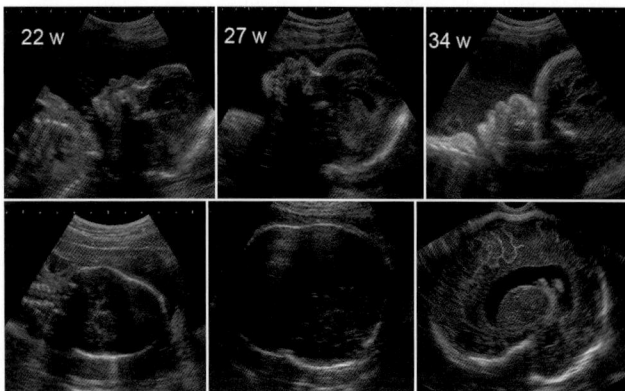

Fig. 41.51: Prenatal craniofacial appearance of Apert syndrome. (Upper) longitudinal changing appearance of frontal bossing and low nasal bridge at 22, 27 and 34 weeks of gestation in a case of Apert syndrome. (Lower left) irregular cranial shape at 20 weeks. (Lower middle) cranial shape at 34 weeks. Note the bilateral indentation. (Lower right) intracranial sagittal ultrasonography (US) image at 34 weeks. Mild ventriculomegaly is seen

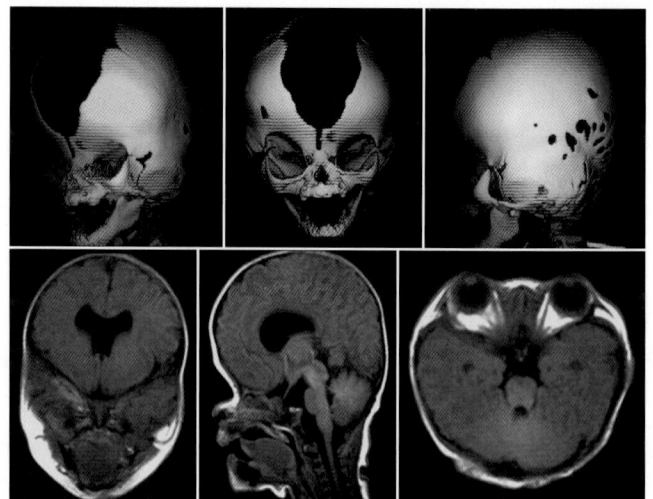

Fig. 41.52: Three-dimensional (3D) reconstruction of computed tomography (CT) scan and magnetic resonance (MR) images of Apert syndrome (the same case as Fig. 41.51). (Upper) 3D reconstruction of CT Scan. Fusion of bilateral coronal suture and squamous suture, defect of frontoparietal cranial structure and craniofacial bony dysplasia are recognizable. (Lower) postnatal MR images. Marked shortening of anterior cranial fossa is seen. Mild ventriculomegaly and absent septum pellucidum are seen

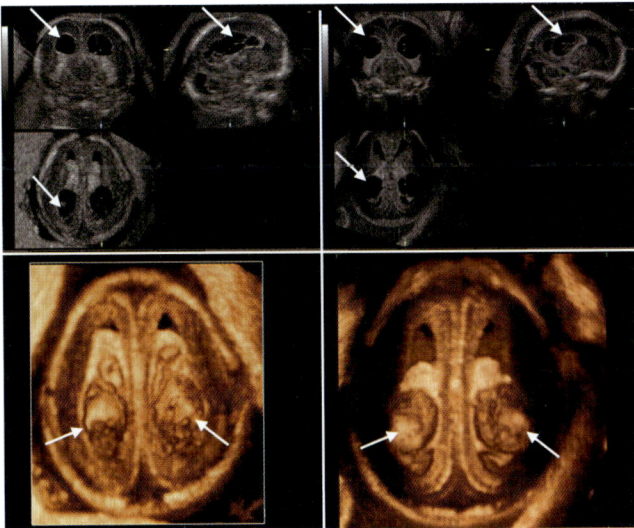

Fig. 41.53: Choroid plexus cysts (CPC) in cases of trisomy 18 (left) and normal karyotype (right). Left figure; three orthogonal views and inside 3D view of CPC in a case of trisomy 18 at 17 weeks of gestation. Various additional anomalies were detected. Right figure; three orthogonal views and inside 3D view of CPC in a case with normal karyotype at 16 weeks. No additional abnormalities. Normal postnatal course. Impossible to distinguish normal from abnormal karyotypes only by location and appearance of choroid plexus cyst. Detection of additional anomalies is important for differential diagnosis

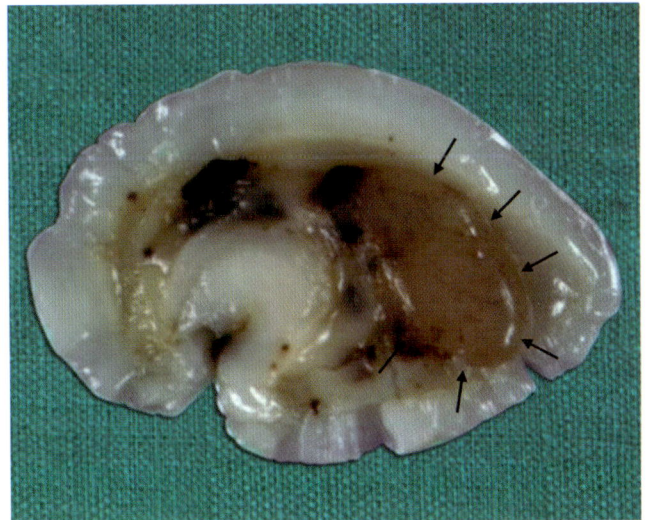

Fig. 41.54: Macroscopic appearance of choroid plexus cyst. Arrows indicate the choroid plexus cyst. The specimen was from an aborted fetus of trisomy 18 at 20 weeks of gestation

Pathogenesis: Choroid plexus is located within the ventricular system and produces CSF. Within the choroidal villi, choroid plexus cysts exists, surrounded by the loose stroma of the choroid plexus.[83]

Associated anomalies: In cases of trisomy 18, associated anomalies include growth retardation, congenital heart diseases such as ventricular septum defect and double outlet right ventricle, overlapping finger, facial anomaly, cerebellar dysplasia and others.

Prenatal diagnosis: (Fig. 41.53) Macroscopic photo is shown in Figure 41.54. It is impossible to distinguish normal from abnormal karyotypes only by location and appearance of choroid plexus cyst. Detection of additional anomalies is important for differential diagnosis.

Differential diagnosis: Intraventricular hemorrhage.

Prognosis: Choroid plexus cysts, per se, are usually asymptomatic and benign, but rarely, symptomatic and disturbs CSF flow.[84,85] Isolated choroids plexus cysts may be normal variation.

Recurrence risk: Unknown.

Management: Fetal karyotyping examination should be offered if additional abnormalities are found.

ACQUIRED BRAIN ABNORMALITIES IN UTERO

In terms of encephalopathy or cerebral palsy, "timing of brain insult, antepartum, intrapartum or postpartum" is one of the serious controversial issues including medico-socio-legal-ethical problems.[86] Although brain insults may relate to antepartum events in a substantial number of term infants with hypoxic-ischemic encephalopathy, the timing of insult cannot always be clarified. It is a hard task to give antepartum evidences of brain injury predictive of cerebral palsy. Fetal heart rate monitoring cannot reveal the presence of encephalopathy, and neuroimaging by ultrasound and MR imaging is the most reliable modality for disclosure of silent encephalopathy. In many cases with cerebral palsy with acquired brain insults, especially, term-delivered infants with reactive fetal heart rate tracing and good Apgar score at delivery, are not suspected having encephalopathy and often overlooked for months or years. Recent imaging technology has revealed brain insult in utero.

Brain Tumors

Incidence: Extremely rare.

Definition: Tumors located in the intracranial cavity.

Histological types: Brain tumors are divided into teratoma, most commonly reported and nonteratomatous tumor. Nonteratomatous tumors includes neuroepithelial tumor, such as medulloblastoma, astrocytoma, choroids plexus papilloma, choroids plexus carcinoma, ependymoma, ependymoblastoma, and mesenchymal tumor such as craniopharyngioma, sarcoma, fibroma, hemangioblastoma, hemangioma and meningioma, and others of lipoma of the corpus callosum, subependymal giant-cell astrocytoma associated with tuberous sclerosis (often accompanied by cardiac rhabdomyoma).[87,88]

Location of tumor: Supratentorial predominance in neonatal tumor. Infratentorial predominance in medulloblastoma. Choroid plexus papilloma is located within the lateral ventricles.

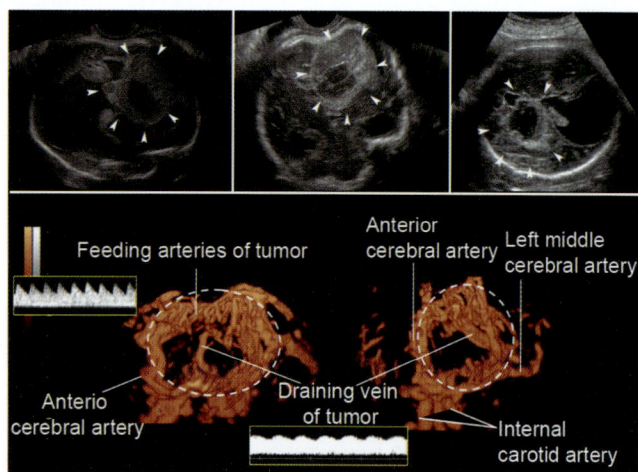

Fig. 41.55: Ultrasound images and tumoral vascular visualization by three-dimensional (3D) power Doppler in a fetus of intracranial tumor with interventricular hemorrhage (35 weeks and 5 days of gestation). (Upper) sagittal, coronal and axial ultrasonography (US) images. Huge tumor (arrowheads) with hemorrhage within the tumor in the frontoparietal lobe. Complicated with unilateral hydrocephalus with intraventricular hemorrhage (arrow). (Left lower) oblique sagittal view from fetal left side. (Right lower) oblique coronal view from fetal frontal side. Tumor is fed by numerous feeding arteries from anterior cerebral artery. Feeder arteries have low resistant flow waveform. One large vein, which drains blood from tumor is visible. The draining vein has pulsatile flow

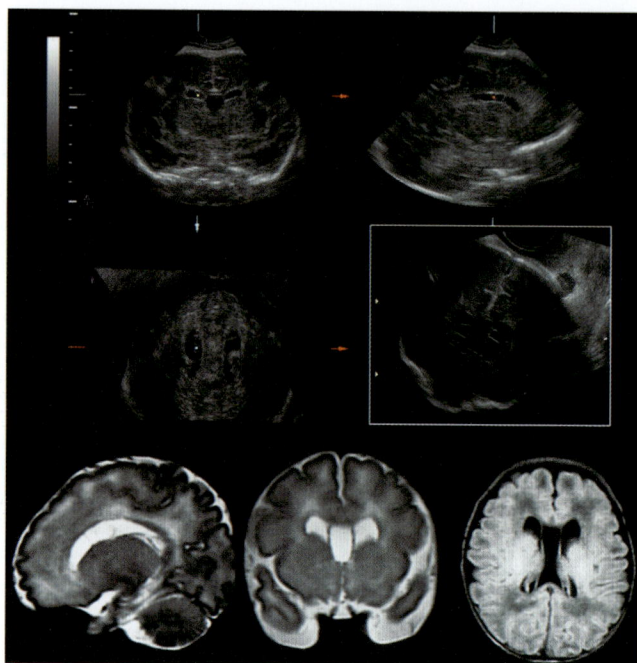

Fig. 41.56: Subependymal cysts [Fetal ultrasonography (US) images and neonatal magnetic resonance (MR) images]. (Upper) coronal and sagittal images. (Middle left) axial image. (Middle right) anterior coronal section. Note bilateral beads-like cystic formation. (Lower) MR sagittal, coronal and axial images at 3 days after birth. No neurological symptoms at the age of 1 year

Associated abnormalities: Macrocrania or local skull swelling, epignathus, secondary hydrocephalus, intracranial hemorrhage, intraventricular hemorrhage, polyhydroamnios, heart failure by high-cardiac output,[89] hydrops.

Diagnosis: Intracranial masses with solid, cystic or mixture pattern with or without visualization of hypervascularity by ultrasound and fetal MRI. Brain tumor should be considered in cases within explained intracranial hemorrhage.

Prenatal diagnosis: Prenatal diagnosis of intracranial tumor and its vascularization by 3D power Doppler is shown in Figure 41.55.

Differential diagnosis: Arachnoid cyst, vein of Galen aneurysm, porencephaly, schizencephaly, periventricular leukomalacia, subdural hemorrhage.

Prognosis: Fetal demise, stillborn may occur.

Prognosis in neonates is generally poor, but depends on timing of diagnosis and the histological type of tumor. Choroid plexus papilloma has minimal mortality rate and high likelihood of neonatal outcome. Mortality rate of teratomas is over 90%, medulloblastoma over 80%. Other tumors have various prognosis.

Recurrence risk: Unknown.

Management: Cesarean section may be considered. Neurosurgical tumor resection including subtotal hemispherectomy by craniotomy and chemotherapy are possible treatments for neonatal tumors. Radiation therapy is usually not indicated in neonates.

Subependymal Pseudocysts

Prevalence: 2.6-5% of all neonates, 1% of premature newborns, unknown in fetuses.

Definition: Cystic formation, which is located in the caudothalamic groove or in the caudate nucleus, lateral to the wall of the anterior horns of lateral ventricles.

Synonyms: Periventricular pseudocysts.[90,91]

Etiology: Infection (cytomegalovirus, rubella), subependymal hemorrhage, metabolic diseases, chromosomal deletions (del q6, delp4) cocaine exposure and others.

Pathogenesis: Cystic cavity is lined by a pseudocapsule, consisting of aggregates of germinal cells and glial tissue, but no epithelium can be found. Origin of pseudocysts is uncertain. Maybe cystic matrix regression or germinolysis.

Associated anomalies: Congenital infection such as cytomegalo virus, congenital heart diseases and associated CNS abnormalities.

Prenatal diagnosis: Shown in Figure 41.56.

Differential diagnosis: Periventricular leukomalacia.

Prognosis: Good in cases with isolated subependymal pseudocysts. In cases with accompanied abnormalities, such as cardiac disease, cytomegalovirus infection, other intracranial abnormalities, or cases with atypical pseudocysts, prognosis may be poor.[90-92]

Recurrence risk: Unknown.

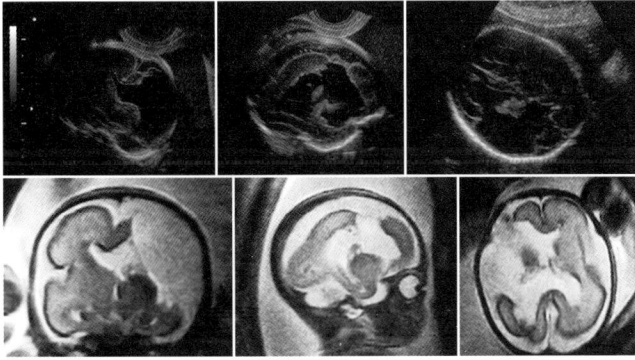

Fig. 41.57: Fetal ultrasonography (US) and magnetic resonance (MR) images of porencephaly at 25 weeks of gestation. (Upper left) transvaginal US coronal image. Defect of parietolateral part of the unilateral cerebrum. This case has also absent septum pellucidum. (Upper middle) parasagittal US image. Porencephalic part is fused with the unilateral ventricle. Echogenesity of inside ventricular wall indicates intraventricular hemorrhage. (upper right) Transabdominal US axial image. (Lower) fetal MR images at the same day. Coronal, parasagittal and axial sections from the left side

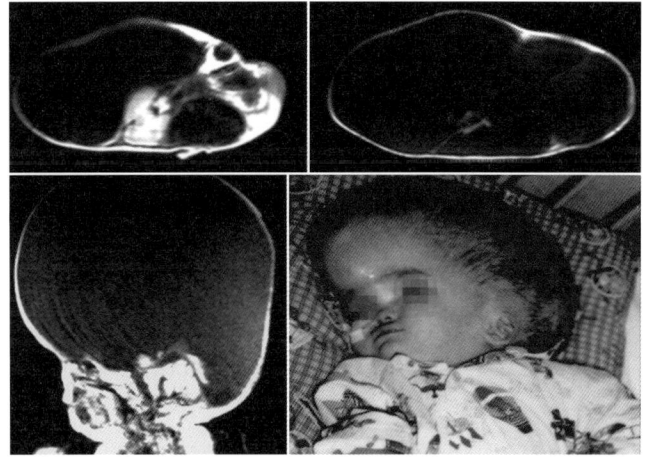

Fig. 41.58: Hydranencephaly. It is characterized by absence of the cerebral hemispheres with an incomplete or absent falx and a sac-like structure containing cerebral spinal fluid surrounding the brainstem and basal ganglia. In this case, tentorium and falx cerebri are recognized. Cerebral cortex is depicted in only a little part of occipital lobe. Brainstem and cerebellum are preserved to be normal. Cause of hydranencephaly may be obstruction of the bilateral internal carotid arteries. Note the remarkable increase of head circumference

Management: In many cases, cysts regress in several months afterbirth. Normal obstetrical/neonatal care.

Porencephaly

Incidence: Unknown.

Definition: Fluid-filled spaces replacing normal brain parenchyma and may or may not communicate with the lateral ventricles or subarachnoid space.

Synonyms: Porencephalic cyst.

Etiology: Ischemic episode, trauma[93] demise of one twin, intercerebral hemorrhage, infection.

Pathogenesis: Easy to occur when immature cerebrum has some factors with propensity of dissolution and cavitation, (high content of water, myelinated fiber bundles, deficient astroglial response). Timing of ischemic injury (maybe as early as second trimester) is strongly related to porencephaly, hydranencephaly.[94]

Associated anomalies: Intercerebral hemorrhage, interventricular hemorrhage, hydrocephalus.

Prenatal diagnosis (Fig. 41.57): Some cases in utero have been reported.[95,96]

Differential diagnosis: Schizencephaly, arachnoid cyst, intracranial cystic tumor, other cysts. Porencephalic cyst never causes a mass effect, which is observed in cases with arachnoid cyst or other cystic mass lesions.

This condition is acquired brain insult and differentiated from schizencephaly of migration disorder.

Prognosis: Various, depends on timing and size of lesion. Seizures, neurological deficits, cerebral palsy often occur.[97]

Recurrence risk: Unknown.

Management: Ventriculoperitoneal shunt if hydrocephalus progresses.

Hydranencephaly

Incidence: 1–2.5:10,000 births.

Definition: Absence of the cerebral hemispheres and a sac-like structure containing cerebral spinal fluid surrounding the brainstem and basal ganglia.

Etiology: Ischemic episode, trauma, demise of one twin, intercerebral hemorrhage, infection. There are several theories but bilateral occlusion of the supraclinoid segment of the internal carotid arteries[98] or of the middle cerebral arteries is one of the causes of subtotal defects of cerebral hemisphere.

Pathogenesis: Easy to occur when immature cerebrum has some factors with propensity of dissolution and cavitation, (high content of water, myelinated fiber bundles, deficient astroglial response). Timing of ischemic injury (maybe as early as second trimester) is strongly related to porencephaly and hydranencephaly.

Prenatal diagnosis: Recently hydranencephaly from 11 weeks of gestation has been reported.[99]

Associated anomalies: Large head (Fig. 41.58).

Differential diagnosis: Massive hydrocephalus, alober holoprosencephaly, porencephaly.

Prognosis: Extremely poor.

Recurrence risk: Unknown.

Management: No active treatment. Shunt procedure for progressive increase of infant's head.

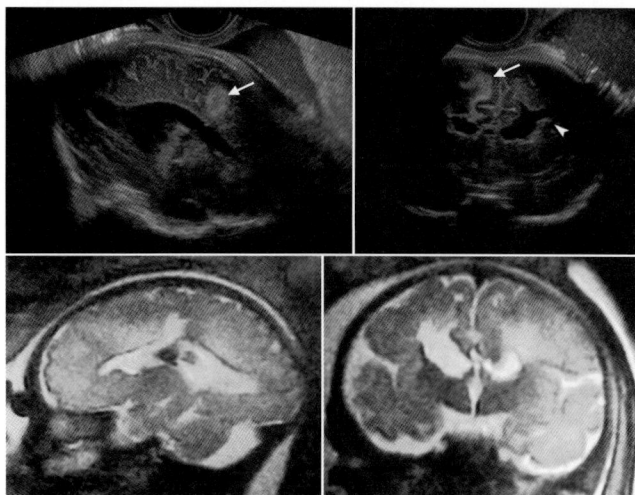

Fig. 41.59: Ultrasonography (US) and magnetic resonance (MR) images in a fetus with cerebral hemorrhage and mild ventriculomegaly at 35 weeks of gestation. Ultrasound parasagittal (upper left) and anterior coronal (upper right) images of the brain. Arrows indicate intracerebral hemorrhage. Arrowhead shows a porencephalic part fused with the lateral ventricle. Lower figures are MR images showing the same cutting sections as upper US images

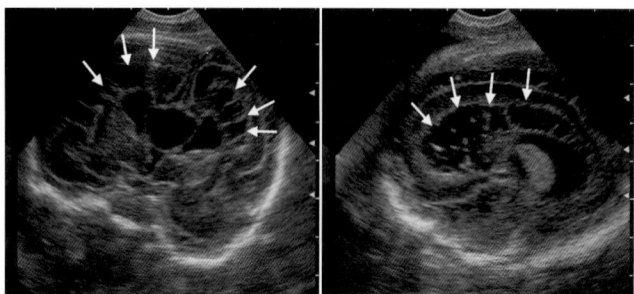

Fig. 41.60: Fetal periventricular leukomalacia (PVL) at 29 weeks of gestation. Bilateral wide-spread type PVL(arrows) was seen. No particular maternal episode existed before and during pregnancy

Intracranial Hemorrhage

Incidence: Unknown, rare in utero.

Definition: Hemorrhage, bleeding inside of the cranium. Intracranial hemorrhage includes subdural hemorrhage, primary subarachnoid hemorrhage, intracerebellar hemorrhage, intraventricular hemorrhage and intraparenchymal hemorrhage other than cerebellar.[100]

Etiology: Trauma, alloimmune and idiopathic thrombocytopenia, von Willebrand's disease, specific medications (warfarin) or illicit drug (cocaine) abuse, seizure, fetal conditions including congenital factor-X and factor-V deficiencies, intracranial tumor, twin-to-twin transfusion, demise of a co-twin, vascular diseases, or fetomaternal hemorrhage, extracorporeal membrane oxygenation (ECMO).[101,102]

Associated anomalies: Hydrocephalus, hydranencephaly, porencephaly, or microcephaly.

Prenatal diagnosis: Shown in Figure 41.59.

Differential diagnosis: Intracranial tumor.

Prognosis: Poor in premature infants. Apnea, seizures, and other neurological symptoms.

Recurrence risk: Depends on etiology.

Management: Ventriculoperitoneal shunt if hydrocephalus progresses.

FETAL PERIVENTRICULAR LEUKOMALACIA

Incidence: 25–75% of premature infants at autopsy are complicated with periventricular white matter injury. However, clinically, incidence may be much lower. 5–10% of infants less than 1500 g birth weight. In at term infants, fetal periventricular leukomalacia (PVL) is very rare.

Definition: Multifocal areas of necrosis found deep in the cortical white matter, which are often symmetrical and occur adjacent to the lateral ventricles. PVL represents a major precursor for neurological and intellectual impairment, and cerebral palsy in later life.

Etiology: Birth trauma, asphyxia and respiratory failure, cardiopulmonary defects, premature birth/low birthweight, associated immature cerebrovascular development and lack of appropriate autoregulation of cerebral blood flow in response to hypoxic-ischemic insults.[102]

Pathogenesis: Distinctive and consist primarily of both focal periventricular necrosis and more diffuse cerebral white matter injury. Two most common sites are at the level of the cerebral white matter near the trigone of the lateral ventricles and around the foramen of Monro. Volpe[94] describes three factors, such as (1) periventricular vascular anatomical and physiological factors, (2) cerebral ischemia, (3) intrinsic vulnerability of cerebral white matter of premature newborn, are strongly related to PVL.

Prenatal diagnosis: Shown in Figure 41.60.

Differential diagnosis: Subarachnoid (periventricular) pseudocysts, porencephaly, other intracranial cystic formation.

Prognosis: Neurological features of PVL in neonatal period is probable lower limb weakness and as features of long-term sequelae, spastic diplegia, intellectual deficits and visual deficits are observed.[94]

Recurrence risk: Unknown.

Management: Early rehabilitation.

REFERENCES

1. Timor-Tritsch IE, Monteagudo A. Transvaginal fetal neuro-sonography: standardization of the planes and sections by anatomic landmarks. Ultrasound Obstet Gynecol. 1996;8:42-7.
2. Timor-Tritsch IE, Peisner, DB, Raju S. Sonoembryology: an organ-oriented approach using a high-frequency vaginal probe. J Clin Ultrasound. 1990;18:286-98.
3. Pooh RK. B-mode and Doppler studies of the abnormal fetus in the first trimester. In: Chervenak FA, Kurjak A (Eds). Fetal medicine. Carnforth: Parthenon Publishing. 1999. pp. 46-51.
4. Monteagudo A, Reuss ML, Timor-Tritsch IE. Imaging the fetal brain in the second and third trimesters using transvaginal sonography. Obstet Gynecol. 1991;77:27-32.
5. Monteagudo A, Timor-Tritsch IE, Moomjy M. In utero detection of ventriculomegaly during the second and third trimesters by transvaginal sonography. Ultrasound Obstet Gynecol. 1994;4: 193-8.
6. Monteagudo A, Timor-Tritsch IE. Development of fetal gyri, sulci and fissures: a transvaginal sonographic study. Ultrasound Obstet Gynecol. 1997;9:222-8.
7. Pooh RK, Nakagawa Y, Nagamachi N, et al. Transvaginal sonography of the fetal brain: detection of abnormal morphology and circulation. Croat Med J. 1998;39:147-57.
8. Pooh RK, Maeda K, Pooh KH, et al. Sonographic assessment of the fetal brain morphology. Prenat Neonat Med. 1999;4:18-38.
9. Pooh RK. Three-dimensional ultrasound of the fetal brain. In Kurjak A (Ed). Clinical application of 3D ultrasonography. Carnfoth: Parthenon Publishing. 2000;176-80.
10. Pooh RK, Pooh KH, Nakagawa Y, et al. Clinical application of three-dimensional ultrasound in fetal brain assessment. Croat Med J. 2000;41:245-51.
11. Timor-Tritsch IE, Monteagudo A, Mayberry P. Three-dimensional ultrasound evaluation of the fetal brain: the three horn view. Ultrasound Obstet Gynecol. 2000;16:302-6.
12. Monteagudo A, Timor-Tritsch IE, Mayberry P. Three-dimensional transvaginal neurosonography of the fetal brain: 'navigating' in the volume scan. Ultrasound Obstet Gynecol. 2000;16:307-13.
13. Blaas HG, Eik-Nes SH, Kiserud T, et al. Three-dimensional imaging of the brain cavities in human embryos. Ultrasound Obstet Gynecol. 995;5:228-32.
14. Blaas HG, Eik-Nes SH, Berg S, et al. In-vivo three-dimensional ultrasound reconstructions of embryos and early fetuses. Lancet. 1998;352:1182-6.
15. Pooh RK, Pooh KH. Fetal neuroimaging with new technology. Ultrasound Rev Obstet Gynecol. 2002;2:178-81.
16. Pooh RK, Pooh KH. Transvaginal 3D and Doppler ultrasonography of the fetal brain. Semin Perinatol. 2001;25:38-43.
17. Pooh RK, Pooh KH. The assessment of fetal brain morphology and circulation by transvaginal 3D sonography and power Doppler. J Perinat Med. 2002;30:48-56.
18. Levine D. Magnetic resonance imaging in prenatal diagnosis. Curr Opin Pediatr. 2001;13:572-8.
19. Huisman TA, Wisser J, Martin E, et al. Fetal magnetic resonance imaging of the central nervous system: a pictorial essay. Eur Radiol. 2002;12:952-61.
20. Ertl-Wagner B, Lienemann A, Strauss A, et al. Fetal magnetic resonance imaging: indications, technique, anatomical considerations and a review of fetal abnormalities. Eur Radiol. 2002;12:1931-40.
21. Kubik-Huch RA, Huisman TA, Wisser J, et al. Ultrafast MR imaging of the fetus. AJR. 2000;174:1599-606.
22. Levine D, Barnes PD. Cortical maturation in normal and abnormal fetuses as assessed with prenatal MR imaging. radiology. 1999;210:751-8.
23. Huppert BJ, Brandt KR, Ramin KD, et al. Single-shot fast spin-echo MR imaging of the fetus: a pictorial essay. Radiographics. 1999;19:S215-27.
24. Smith DW, Tondury G. Origin of the calvaria and its sutures. Am J Dis Child. 1978;132:662-6.
25. Pooh RK. Fetal cranial bone formation: sonographic assessment. Margulies M, Voto LS, Eik-Nes S (Eds). 9th world congress of ultrasound in obstetrics and gynecology. Bologna, Italy: Monduzzi Editore. 1999. pp. 407-10.
26. Pooh RK, Pooh KH, Nakagawa Y, et al. Transvaginal Doppler assessment of fetal intracranial venous flow. Obstet Gynecol. 1999;93:697-701.
27. Alagappan R, Browning PD, Laorr A, et al. Distal lateral ventricular atrium: reevaluation of normal range. Radiology. 1994;193:405-8.
28. Almog B, Gamzu R, Achiron R, et al. Fetal lateral ventricular width: what should be its upper limit. A prospective cohort study and reanalysis of the current and previous data. J Ultrasound Med. 2003;22:39-43.
29. Fransen E, Lemmon V, Van Camp G, et al. CRASH syndrome: clinical spectrum of corpus callosum hypoplasia, retardation, adducted thumbs, spastic paraparesis and hydrocephalus due to mutations in one single gene, L1. Eur J Hum Genet. 1995;3:273-84.
30. Yamasaki M, Thompson P, Lemmon V. CRASH syndrome: mutations in L1CAM correlate with severity of the disease. Neuropediatrics. 1997;28:175-8.
31. Timor-Tritsch IE, Monteagudo A, Haratz-Rubinstein N, et al. Transvaginal sonographic detection of adducted thumbs, hydrocephalus, and agenesis of the corpus callosum at 22 postmenstrual weeks: the masa spectrum or L1 spectrum. A case report and review of the literature. Prenat Diagn. 1996;16:543-8.
32. Patel MD, Filly AL, Hersh DR, et al. Isolated mild fetal cerebral ventriculomegaly: clinical course and outcome. Radiology. 1994;192:759-64.
33. Pilu G, Falco P, Gabrielli S, et al. The clinical significance of fetal isolated cerebral borderline ventriculomegaly: report of 31 cases and review of the literature. Ultrasound Obstet Gynecol. 1999;14:320-6.
34. Wakayama A, Morimoto K, Kitajima H, et al. Extremely low birth weight infant with hydrocephalus; management of hydrocephalus using a miniature Ommaya's reservoir. No Shinkei Geka. 1991;19:795-800.
35. Morimoto K, Hayakawa T, Yoshimine T, et al. Two-step procedure for early neonatal surgery of fetal hydrocephalus. Neurol Med Chir. 1993;33:158-65.
36. Fritsch MJ, Mehdorn M. Endoscopic intraventricular surgery for treatment of hydrocephalus and loculated CSF space in children less than one year of age. Pediatr Neurosurg. 2002;36:183-8.
37. Perez JZ, Vazquez PA, Herrera RH, et al. Decline of neural tube defects cases after a folic acid campaign in Nuevo Leon, Mexico. Teratology. 2002;66:249-56.
38. Ray JG, Meier C, Vermeulen MJ, et al. Association of neural tube defects and folic acid food fortification in Canada. Lancet. 2002;360:2047-8.
39. Persad VL, Van den Hof MC, Dube JM, et al. Incidence of open neural tube defects in Nova Scotia after folic acid fortification. CMAJ. 2002;167:241-5.
40. Mathews TJ, Honein MA, Erickson JD. Spina bifida and anencephaly prevalence—United States, 1991-2001. MMWR Recomm Rep. 2002;51:9-11.

41. Green NS. Folic acid supplementation and prevention of birth defects. J Nutr. 2002;132:2356S-60S.

42. Monteagudo A, Timor-Tritsch IE. Fetal Neurosonography of congenital brain anomalies. In Timor-Tritsch IE, Monteagudo A, Cohen HL (Eds). Ultrasonography of the prenatal and neonatal brain. 2nd edition. New York: McGraw-Hill; 2001. pp. 151-258.

43. Stevenson RE, Allen WP, Pai GS, et al. Decline in prevalence of neural tube defects in a high-risk region of the United States. Pediatrics. 2000;106:677-83.

44. Volpe JJ. Neural tube formation and prosencephalic development. Neurology of the Neuborn, 4th edition. Philadelphia: WB Saunders; 2001. pp. 3-44.

45. D'Addario V, Pinto V, Del Bianco A, et al. The clivus-supraocciput angle: a useful measurement to evaluate the shape and size of the fetal posterior fossa and to diagnose Chiari II malformation. Ultrasound Obstet Gynecol. 2001;18:14-69.

46. Matsunaga E, Shiota K. Holoprosencephaly in hyman embryos: epidemiologic studies of 150 caswes. Teratology. 1977;16:261-72.

47. Cohen MM Jr. Perspectives on holoprosencephaly. I. Epidemiology, genetics and symdromology. Teratology. 1989;40:211-35.

48. Pilu G, Ambrosetto P, Sandri F, et al. Intraentricular fused fornices: A specific sign of fetal lobar holoprosencephaly. Ultrasound Obstet Gynecol. 1994;34:259-62.

49. Cohen MM. An update on the holoprosencephalic disorders. J Pediatr. 1982;101:865-9.

50. Pilu G, Porelo A, Falco P, et al. Median anomalies of the brain. In Timor-Tritsch IE, Monteagudo A, Cohen HL (Eds). Ultrasonography of the prenatal and neonatal brain, 2nd edition. New York: McGraw-Hill; 2001. pp. 259-76.

51. Goodyear PW, Bannister CM, Russell S, et al. Outcome in prenatally diagnosed fetal agenesis of the corpus callosum. Fetal Diagn Ther. 2001;16:139-45.

52. Taylor M, David AS. Agenesis of the corpus callosum: a United Kingdom series of 56 cases. J Neurol Neurosurg Psychiatry. 1998;64:131-4.

53. Schmidt-Riese U, Zieger M. Ultrasound diagnosis of isolated aplasia of the septum pellucidum. Ultraschall Med. 1994;15:286-92.

54. McMahon CL, Braddock SR. Septo-optic dysplasia as a manifestation of valproic acid embryopathy. Teratology. 2001;64:83-6.

55. Dominguez R, Aguirre Vila-Coro A, Slopis JM, et al. Brain and ocular abnormalities in infants with in utero exposure to cocaine and other street drugs. Am J Dis Child. 1991;145:688-95.

56. Dattani MT, Martinez-Barbera JP, Thomas PQ, et al. Mutations in the homeobox gene HESX1/Hesx1 associated with septo-optic dysplasia in human and mouse. Nat Genet. 1998;19:125-33.

57. Volpe JJ. Neuronal proliferation, migration, organization and myelination. Neurology of the newborn, 4th edition. USA: WB Saunders; 2001. pp. 45-99.

58. Kobayashi K, Nakahori Y, Miyake M, et al. An ancient retrotransposal insertion causes Fukuyama-type congenital muscular dystrophy. Nature. 1998;23;394(6691):388-92.

59. McGahan JP, Grix A, Gerscovich EO. Prenatal diagnosis of lissencephaly: Miller-Dieker syndrome. J Clin Ultrasound. 1994;22:560-3.

60. Greco P, Resta M, Vimercati A, et al. Antenatal diagnosis of isolated lissencephaly by ultrasound and magnetic resonance imaging. Ultrasound Obstet Gynecol. 1998;12:276-9.

61. Kojima K, Suzuki Y, Seki K, et al. Prenatal diagnosis of lissencephaly (type II) by ultrasound and fast magnetic resonance imaging. Fetal Diagn Ther. 2002;17:34-6.

62. Granata T, Farina L, Faiella A, et al. Familial schizencephaly associated with EMX2 mutation. Neurology. 1997;48:1403-6.

63. Brunelli S, Faiella A, Capra V, et al. Germline mutations in the homeobox gene EMX2 in patients with severe schizencephaly. Nat Genet. 1996;12:94-6.

64. Iannetti P, Nigro G, Spalice A, et al. Cytomegalovirus infection and schizencephaly: case reports. Ann Neurol. 1998;43:123-7.

65. Denis D, Maugey-Laulom B, Carles D, et al. Prenatal diagnosis of schizencephaly by fetal magnetic resonance imaging. Fetal Diagn Ther. 2001;16:354-9.

66. Osenbach RK, Menezes AH. Diagnosis and management of the Dandy-Walker malformation: 30 years of experience. Pediatr Neurosurg. 1991;18:179-85.

67. Barkovich AJ, Kjos BO, Normal D, et al. Revised classification of the posterior fossa cysts and cystlike malformations based on the results of multiplanar MR imaging. AJNR. 1989;10:977-88.

68. Bretelle F, Senat MV, Bernard JP, et al. First-trimester diagnosis of fetal arachnoid cyst: prenatal implication. Ultrasound Obstet Gynecol. 2002;20:400-2.

69. Elbers SE, Furness ME. Resolution of presumed arachnoid cyst in utero. Ultrasound Obstet Gynecol. 1999;14:353-5.

70. Ciricillo SF, Cogen PH, Harsh GR, et al. Intracranial arachnoid cysts in children. A comparison of the effects of fenestration and shunting. J Neurosurg. 1991;74: 230-5.

71. Nakamura Y, Mizukawa K, Yamamoto K, et al. Endoscopic treatment for a huge neonatal prepontinesuprasellar arachnoid cyst: a case report. Pediatr Neurosurg. 2001;35:220-4.

72. Hollway GE, Suthers GK, Haan EA, et al. Mutation detection in FGFR2 craniosynostosis syndromes. Hum Genet. 1997;99:251-5.

73. Delashaw JB, Persing JA, Broaddus WC, et al. Cranial vault growth in craniosynostosis. J Neurosurg. 1989;70:159-65.

74. Benacerraf BR, Spiro R, Mitchell AG. Using three-dimensional ultrasound to detect craniosynostosis in a fetus with Pfeiffer syndrome. Ultrasound Obstet Gynecol. 2000;16:391-4.

75. Pooh RK, Nakagawa Y, Pooh KH, et al. Fetal craniofacial structure and intracranial morphology in a case of Apert syndrome. Ultrasound Obstet Gynecol. 1999;13:274-80.

76. Raybaud CA, Strother CM, Hald JK. Aneurysms of the vein of Galen: embryonic considerations and anatomical features relating to the pathogenesis of the malformation. Neuroradiology. 1989;31:109-28.

77. Hoffman HJ, Chuang S, Hendrick EB, et al. Aneurysms of the vein of Galen. Experience at The Hospital for Sick Children, Toronto. J Neurosurg. 1982;57(3):316-22.

78. Campi A, Rodesch G, Scotti G, et al. Aneurysmal malformation of the vein of Galen in three patients: clinical and radiological follow-up. Neuroradiology. 1998;40(12):816-21.

79. Friedman DM, Verma R, Madrid M, et al. Recent improvement in outcome using transcatheter embolization techniques for neonatal aneurysmal malformations of the vein of Galen. Pediatrics. 1993;91(3):583-6.

80. Sullivan A, Giudice T, Vavelidis F, et al. Choroid plexus cysts: Is biochemical testing a valuable adjunct to targeted ultrasonography? Am J Obstet Gynecol. 1999;181:260-5.

81. Reinsch RC. Choroid plexus cysts—association with trisomy: prospective review of 16,059 patients. Am J Obstet Gynecol. 1997;176:1381-3.

82. Morcos CL, Platt LD, Carlson DE, et al. The isolated choroid plexus cyst. Obstet Gynecol. 1998;92:232-6.

83. Farhood AI, Morris JH, Bieber FR. Transient cysts of the fetal choroid plexus: morphology and histogenesis. Am J Med Genet. 1987;27:977-82.

84. Lam AH, Villanueva AC. Symptomatic third ventricular choroid plexus cysts. Pediatr Radiol. 1992;22:413-6.

85. Parizek J, Jakubec J, Hobza V, et al. Choroid plexus cyst of the left lateral ventricle with intermittent blockage of the foramen of Monro, and initial invagination into the III ventricle in a child. Childs Nerv Syst. 1998;14:700-8.

86. Pooh RK, Maeda K, Pooh KH. An atlas of fetal central nervous system disease. Diagnosis and Management. Parthenon CRC Press; 2003.

87. Wakai S, Arai T, Nagai M. Congenital brain tumors. Surg Neurol. 1984;21:597-609.
88. Volpe JJ. Brain tumors and vein of Galen malformation. Neurology of the Neuborn, 4th edition. Philadelphia; WB Saunders; 2001. pp. 841-56.
89. Sherer DM, Abramowicz JS, Eggers PC, et al. Prenatal ultrasonographic diagnosis of intracranial teratoma and massive craniomegaly with associated high-output cardiac failure. Am J Obstet Gynecol. 1993;168:97-9.
90. Lu JH, Emons D, Kowalewski S. Connatal periventricular pseudocysts in the neonate. Pediatr Radiol. 1992;22(1):55-8.
91. Malinger G, Lev D, Ben Sira L, et al. Congenital periventricular pseudocysts: prenatal sonographic appearance and clinical implications. Ultrasound Obstet Gynecol. 2002;20(5):447-51.
92. Bats AS, Molho M, Senat MV, et al. Subependymal pseudocysts in the fetal brain: Prenatal diagnosis of two cases and review of the literature. Ultrasound Obstet Gynecol. 2002;20(5):502-5.
93. Eller KM, Kuller JA. Porencephaly secondary to fetal trauma during amniocentesis. Obstet Gynecol. 1995;85:865-7.
94. Volpe JJ. Hypoxic-Ischemic Encephalopathy: Neuropathology and pathogenesis. Neurology of the Neuborn, 4th edition. Philadelphia; WB Saunders; 2001. pp. 296-330.
95. Meizner I, Elchalal U. Prenatal sonographic diagnosis of anterior fossa porencephaly. J Clin Ultrasound. 1996;24:96-9.
96. De Laveaucoupet J, Audibert F, Guis F, et al. Fetal magnetic resonance imaging (MRI) of ischemic brain injury. Prenat Diagn. 2001;21:729-36.
97. Scher MS, Belfar H, Martin J, et al. Destructive brain lesions of presumed fetal onset: Antepartum causes of cerebral palsy. Pediatrics. 1991;88:898-906.
98. Stevenson DA, Hart BL, Clericuzio CL. Hydranencephaly in an infant with vascular malformations. Am J Med Genet. 2001:15;104:295-8.
99. Lam YH, Tang MH. Serial sonographic features of a fetus with hydranencephaly from 11 weeks to term. Ultrasound Obstet Gynecol. 2000;16:77-9.
100. Sherer DM, Anyaegbunam A, Onyeije C. Antepartum fetal intracranial hemorrhage, predisposing factors and prenatal sonography: a review. Am J Perinatol. 1998;15:431-41.
101. Hardart GE, Fackler JC. Predictors of intracranial hemorrhage during neonatal extracorporeal membrane oxygenation. J Pediatr. 1999;134:156-9.
102. Rezaie P, Dean A. Periventricular leukomalacia, inflammation and white matter lesions within the developing nervous system. Neuropathology. 2002;22:106-32.

C H A P T E R

42

Ultrasound of the Fetal Thorax

A Khurana

INTRODUCTION

Technological advances in transducer and software technology have in recent years remarkably improved visualization of structures in the fetal thorax (Figs 42.1 to 42.4) way beyond the minimum requirement recommended by the American Institute of Ultrasound in Medicine[1] over the last few decades. Additionally, novel methods of in utero treatment, the evolution of neonatal surgical techniques and anesthesia, the newer understanding of the natural course of several malformations and the pressing social and legal need for informed parental counseling have placed a new responsibility on the shoulders of the practicing ultrasonologist.

There is now a pressing demand for an accurate diagnosis, the formulation of a prognosis and the institution of appropriate management whether it be expectant observation, in utero therapy or a referral to a tertiary care center.

This presentation reviews current concepts in the evaluation of the fetal thorax (excluding cardiac conditions).

EMBRYOLOGY

A knowledge of the embryology of the thoracic viscera is imperative to understand the outcome of congenital thoracic malformations and their direct bearing on fetal lung developments and ultimate fetal and neonatal outcomes.

Development of the lung begins at 5 weeks.[2] The epithelium of the respiratory system develops from endoderm. The connective tissue, cartilage and muscle develop from splanchnic mesoderm and neural crest cells.

At 26 days, the foregut evaginates to form a laryngotracheal diverticulum. This then gets separated from the foregut by longitudinal folds, which progress to form the tracheoesophageal septum. The lungs develop in four stages. From 5 weeks to 17 weeks all elements are developed except those involved in gas exchange. This is also called the pseudoglandular period. From 16 weeks to 25 weeks (canalicular period), the lumen of bronchi and bronchioles become larger, and respiratory bronchioles and alveolar ducts develop. Some terminal sacs develop and the tissue becomes more vascular. From 25 weeks to birth, many more terminal sacs

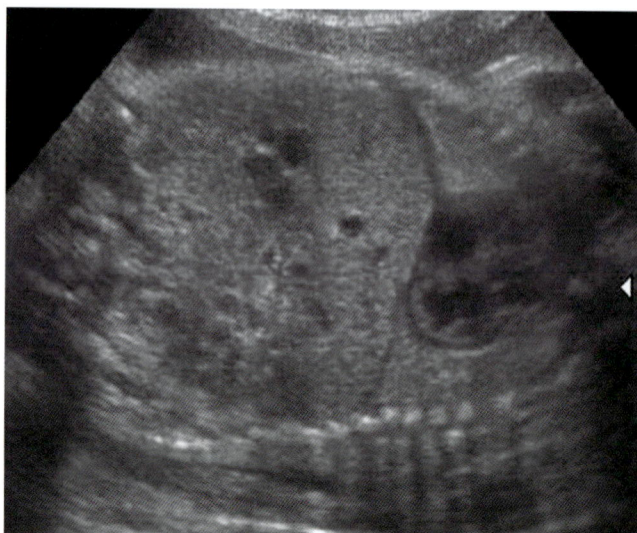

Fig. 42.2

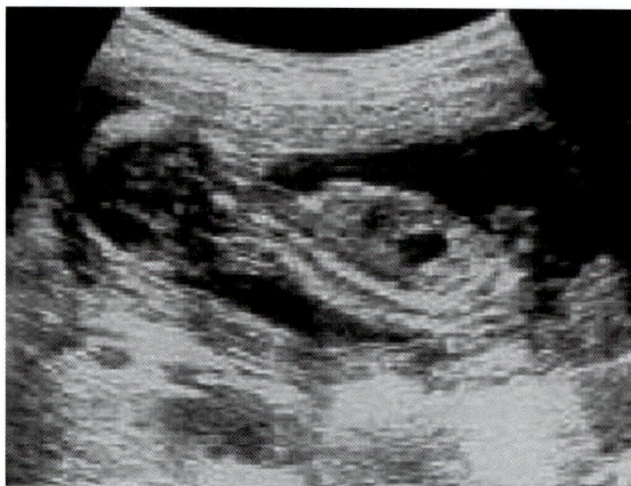

Fig. 42.1

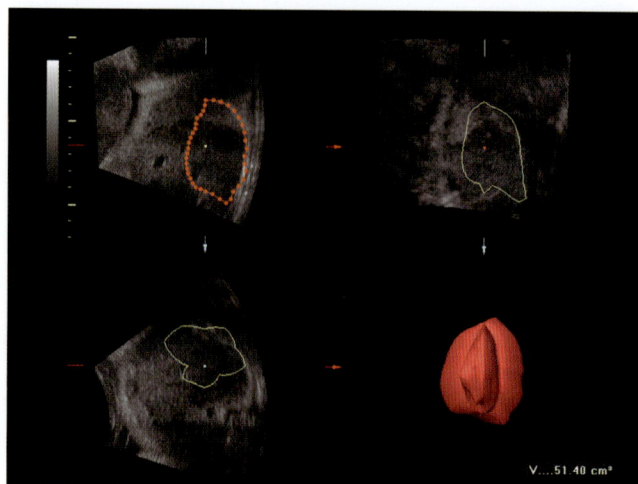

Fig. 42.3

develop, the epithelium becomes very thick, capillaries bunch into alveoli, Type I alveolar cells develop, and Type II alveolar cells begin producing surfactant. From late fetalhood and upto childhood, squamous epithelium forms and alveoli continue to form after birth.[3]

SONOANATOMY OF THE FETAL THORAX

The fetal thorax extends from the clavicles to the fetal diaphragm. The diaphragm is continuous, thin and hypoechoic (Fig. 42.5) and moves with respiratory movements in the third trimester of pregnancy. The thorax is bounded by the sternum anteriorly, the spine posteriorly and the ribs circumferentially. The heart is the most prominent structure in the thorax. The lungs are seen to surround it. The left lung is limited in its extent by the heart (Fig. 42.6). The lungs are homogeneously echogenic and largely isoechoic with other mediastinal structures. The heart occupies one-third to one-half of the thorax and its location and axis are important to identify and evaluate non-cardiac conditions as well. Cardiac and mediastinal shifts have a tremendous bearing on the prognosis of a chest lesion. No fluid is seen in normal pleural spaces. The pleural and pericardial space should be evaluated to assess for

hydrops, which again, is a prognostic factor in the assessment of a chest mass. With some effort and resort to color flow mapping (Fig. 42.7) and power Doppler studies, the aortic arch, pulmonary artery, ductus arteriosus, pulmonary veins, the trachea, esophagus and the thymus can be adequately evaluated.[4-6]

PULMONARY HYPOPLASIA

Adequate lung development is central to fetal viability.[7,8] Hypoplastic lungs show a low lung to body weight ratio and histologically demonstrate a reduced number of alveoli.[9] Pulmonary hypoplasia (PH) is rarely primary and unilateral.[10,11] It is usually secondary and consequent to any prolonged severe oligoamnios,[12-15] in skeletal dysplasias with a small bony thorax, in sizable intrathoracic masses,[16,17] consequent to neuromuscular dysfunction as in the Pena-Shokeir Syndrome,[18] in Trisomy 12, 18 and 21 and in conditions with decreased pulmonary artery perfusion.[19]

Thoracic perimeter measurements[20-23] (Fig. 42.8) are made at the level of the four-chamber view and should exclude the soft tissue areas beyond the ribs. The thoracic perimeter/abdominal perimeter ratio[24-26] is steady through the late second trimester and more than 0.80 in the third trimester: Lung lengths[27] although well

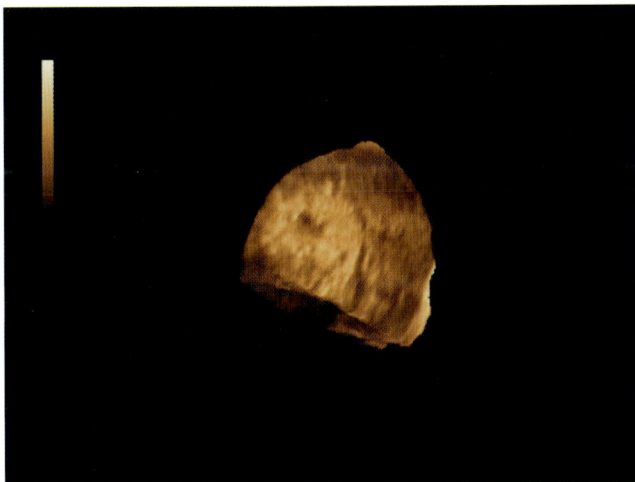

Fig. 42.4

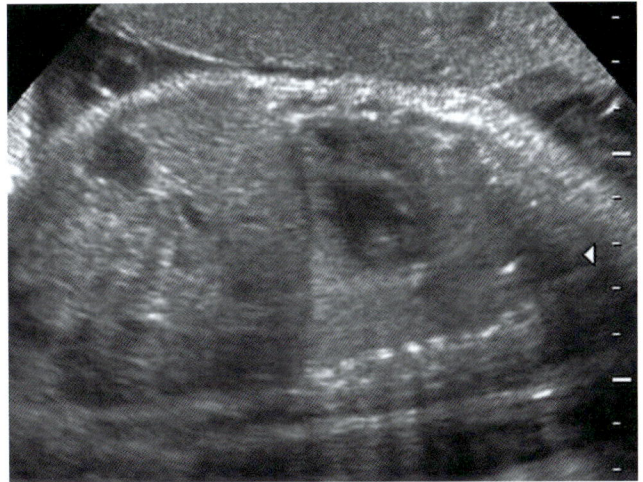

Fig. 42.5

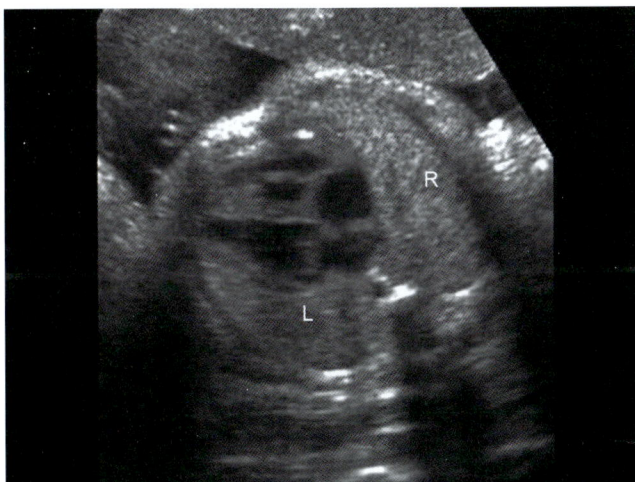

Fig. 42.6

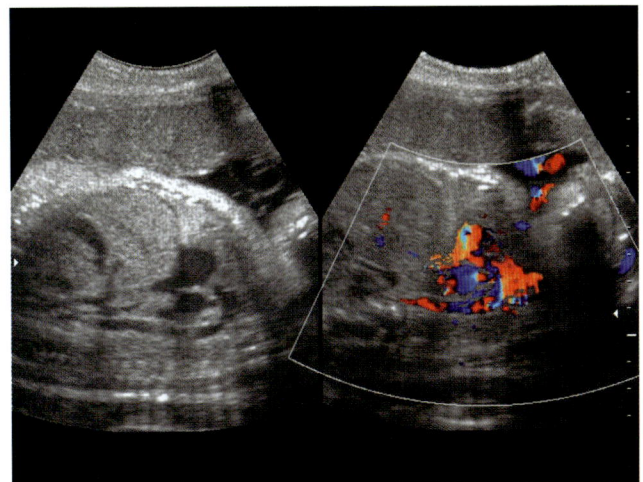

Fig. 42.7

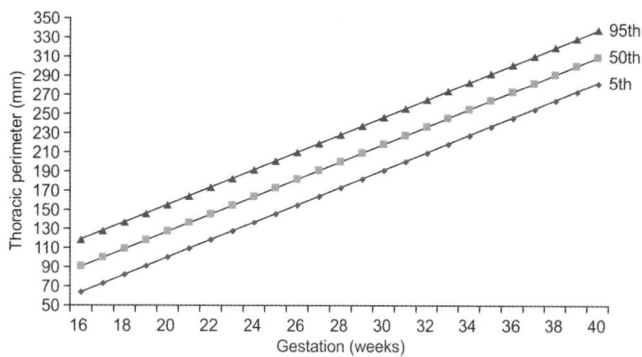

Fig. 42.8

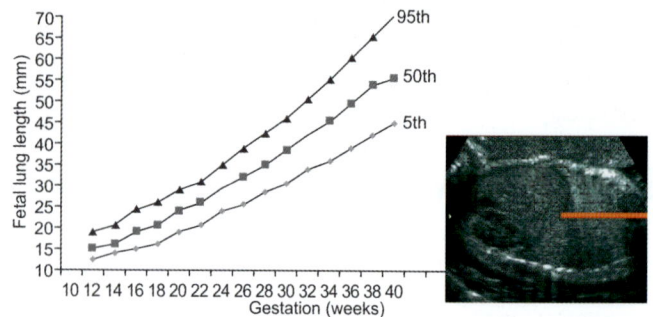

Fig. 42.9

studied (Fig. 42.9) are not easily reproducible. Fetal lung volumes by 3D reconstruction techniques (Fig. 42.10) are reliable and reproducible.[28,29]

The pathogenesis of PH commences with either inadequate thoracic space for growth, inadequate breathing movements of whatever cause, inadequate fluid within the lung and suboptimal quantities of amniotic fluid.[30] Lung echogenicity does not correlate with lung maturity.

General Features of Chest Masses

Not all lung masses can be delineated in the 18–20 weeks anomalies scan although embryologically they do exist.[31,32] Depending on their size and growth they result in unilateral or bilateral hypoplasia of the lungs. Prognosis depends on the size of the lesion, heart and mediastinal displacements, presence of hydrops, associated structural anomalies, underlying chromosomal abnormalities and the bearing of associated polyhydramnios on preterm premature rupture of membranes and prematurity.[33-35]

Common chest masses include congenital diaphragmatic hernia (CDH) and congenital cystic adenomatoid malformations (CCAM). Other lung masses include bronchogenic cysts, neurenteric cysts, congenital lobar emphysema (CLE), bronchial atresia, pulmonary gigantism, bronchopulmonary sequestration (BPS) and mediastinal masses. The mediastinal lesions include teratomas,[36] thymomas,[37] goiter, cardiac lesions such as rhabdomyoma, myxoma and fibroma,[38-40] esophageal duplication cysts,[41] enteric cysts[41] and neurenteric cysts,[42-44] and thoracic neuroblastoma. Mediastinal lesions are rare but important in the perspective of a differential diagnosis of a mass adjacent to the mediastinum but arising from the adjacent lung or from the abdomen.

CONGENITAL DIAPHRAGMATIC HERNIA

Congenital diaphragmatic hernia (CDH) has an incidence of 1–4.5/10,000 live births.[45] The incidence is higher in the fetus and a fair number are lost in utero or in the neonatal period prior to clinical identification. CDH is more common on the left side but not infrequently right sided or bilateral. The diaphragm forms between the 6th week and 14th week of pregnancy by fusion of the septum transversum, pleuroperitoneal membranes, mesentery of the esophagus and the body wall. Failure of fusion especially of the pleuroperitoneal membranes results in a herniation of abdominal contents into the thorax when the gut returns to the abdomen. The disorder is progressive and the organs that herniate

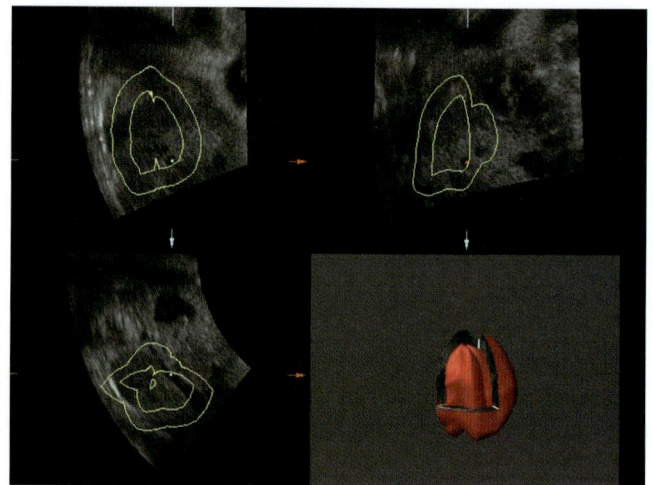

Fig. 42.10

include the stomach, liver, spleen, small bowel and colon. Left sided CDH usually involves the stomach. Right-sided CDH usually involves herniation of the liver. The herniation may be small, isoechoic and intermittent[46] and therefore go unrecognized except when the problem is specifically are looked for. Over four of five fetuses died in the neonatal period usually because of PH and pulmonary hypertension. Pulmonary hypertension is consequent to poorly understood but well documented medial wall muscular hypertrophy of the small pulmonary arteries extending up to the preacinar vessels. Newborns have a high incidence of feeding problems, gastroesophageal reflux, chronic lung disease and neurodevelopmental delays.[45,47] Sonographic signs[48] include a low abdominal perimeter, failure to visualize the fetal stomach in the fetal abdomen (Fig. 42.11), visualization of the herniated viscera in the thorax (Figs 42.12 and 42.13), cardiomediastinal shift, pleural effusions and hydrops. There may also be failure to delineate the diaphragm in its entire extent. Right-sided hernias are difficult to identify because of isoechoic lung and these should be evaluated by color Doppler to confirm the portal vein location in the thorax (Figs 42.14 and 42.15). Although identification of the liver is not critical for a diagnosis of CDH, it has a major bearing on the prognosis.[49,50] This is so because after surgical repair the ductus venosus and umbilical vein often get kinked or compromised thereby contributing to morbidity and often mortality. When bowel segments are not fluid-filled as is common in the second trimester, they may appear as a non specific chest mass (Fig. 42.16). Careful real time scanning would reveal peristalsis in the third trimester.

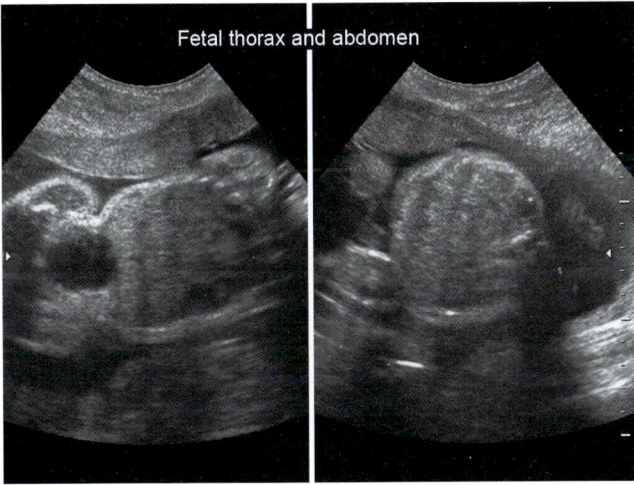

Fig. 42.11

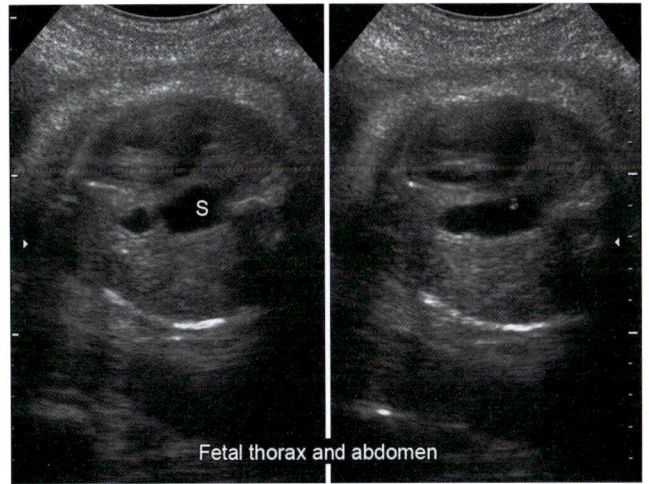

Fig. 42.12

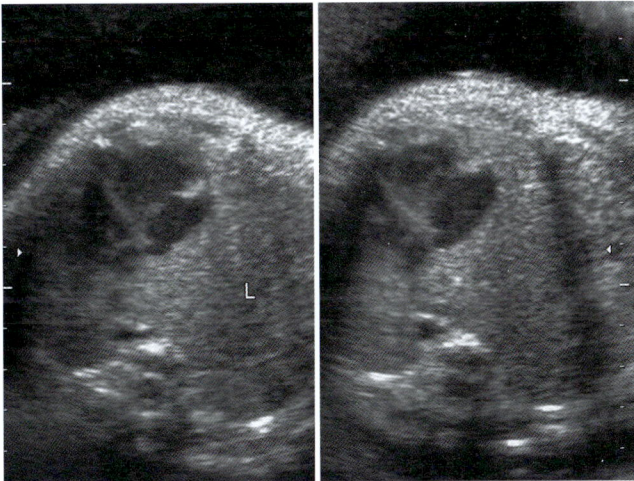

Fig. 42.13

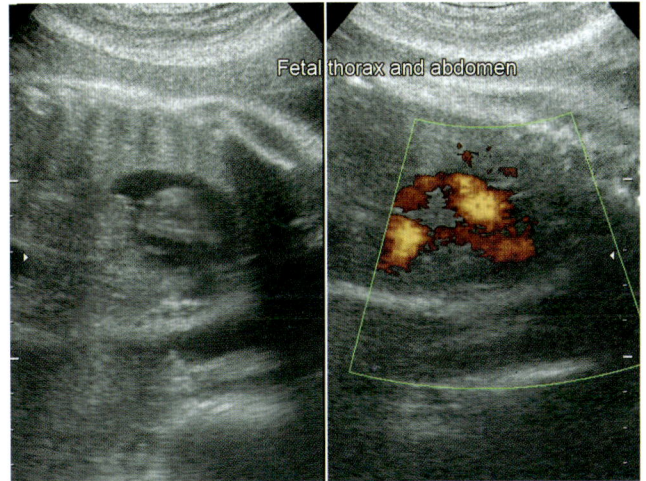

Fig. 42.14

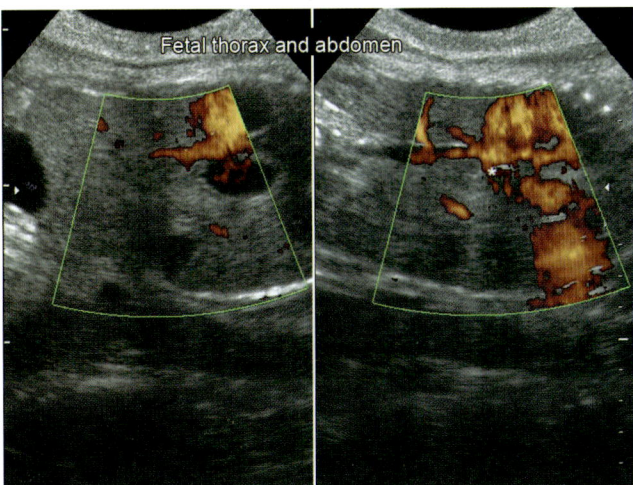

Fig. 42.15

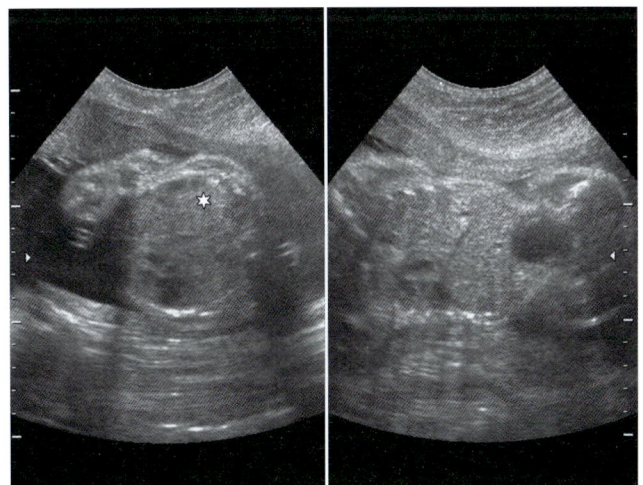

Fig. 42.16

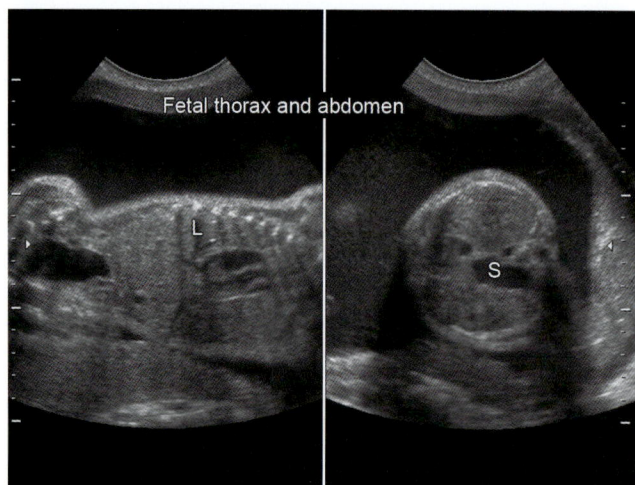

Fig. 42.17

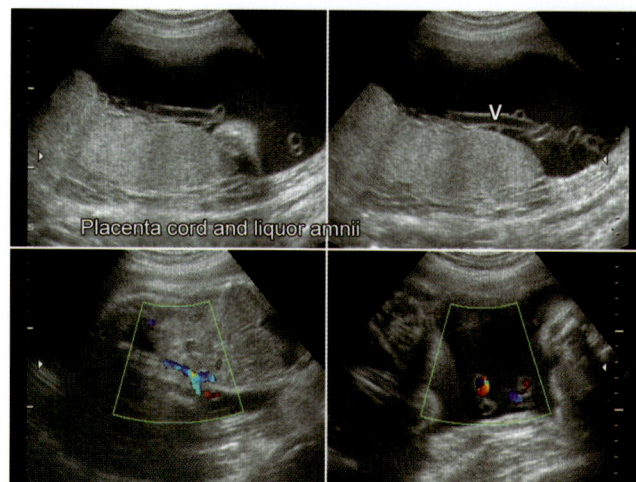

Fig. 42.18

Occasionally, a gall bladder may be seen in the CDH. Bilateral hernias may be difficult to detect because of no cardiomediastinal shift. Ascites within a herniation may be mistaken for a pleural effusion.

Not all fetuses with a CDH have a poor prognosis.[51-54] Prognosis depends on gestational age at diagnosis, particularly, if 24 weeks or earlier, large size, dilated stomach, presence of the liver, even its left lobe in left sided lesions, small contralateral lung, bilateral herniation (Fig. 42.17) and the presence of associated anomalies (Fig. 42.18). Because of the higher incidence of CDH in certain syndromes, a facial and cardiac survey merit special attention. These syndromes include Trisomy 18, Fryn's, Lethal pterygium, Beckwith-Wiedemann, Cornelia De Lange, Apert's, and Goldenhahr.[55,56]

Fetal therapy has found a reasonable place in the treatment of CDH.[57] The aim of surgery is to prevent lung hypoplasia. Although, to fetal therapy initially involved in reduction of the hernia by open repair in utero, current practice involves clipping of the trachea. Currently, videofetoscopic techniques are under evaluation. Tracheal occlusion results in increased lung volume and accelerated lung maturity similar to the pathophysiology seen in laryngeal and tracheal atresia.[58]

CONGENITAL CYSTIC ADENOMATOID MALFORMATIONS

Congenital cystic adenomatoid malformations occur consequent to failure of induction of mesenchyme by bronchiolar epithelium. Lack of normal cellular development is considered to be consequent to focal bronchial atresia. The lesion is hamartomatous and characterized by focal abnormal proliferation of bronchiolar like air spaces and absence of alveoli.[59] It is usually unilateral. Some may be associated with sequestration in the same lung. Diagnosis depends on the demonstration of a mass in the thorax.[60] This may be macrocystic (cysts 2–10 mm) (Fig. 42.19), microcystic (cysts 0.3-0.5 mm) (Fig. 42.20), or mixed (Fig. 42.21).[31,32] These may cause a cardiomediastinal shift, ipsilateral and contralateral lung compression, PH and hydrops. The lesion may regress spontaneously.[61]

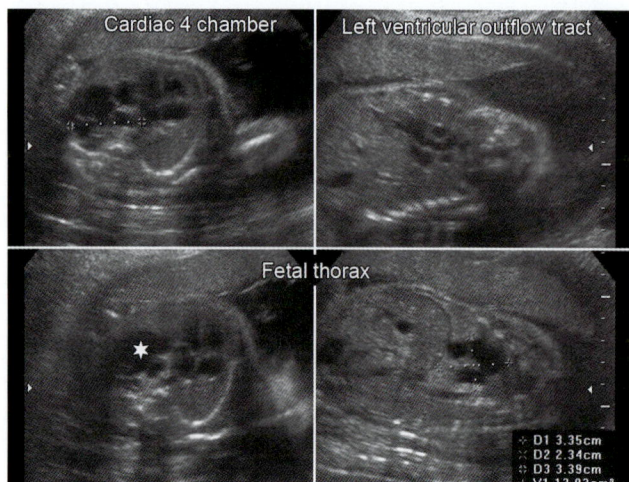

Fig. 42.19

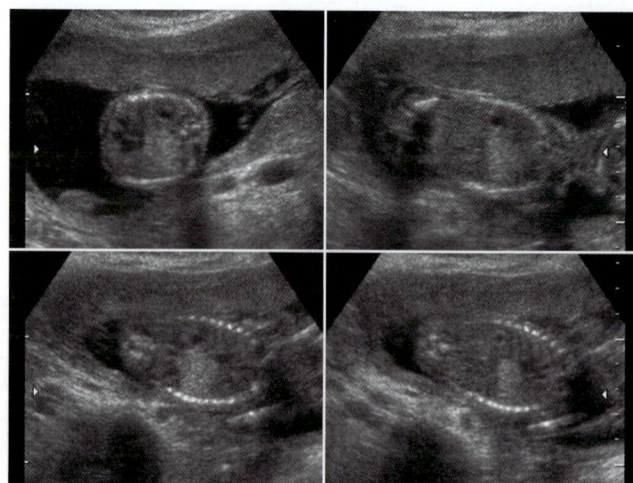

Fig. 42.20

Prognosis depends on associated PH pulmonary hypertension, hydrops, associated anomalies, polyhydramnios and prematurity (Fig. 42.22). Microcystic lesions are more likely to cause PH and hydrops. The arterial supply is via a pulmonary artery and drainage into a pulmonary vein. Treatment of the lesion consists of expectant management, monitoring for hydrops or premature/term delivery followed by lobectomy if necessary.[33] Referral to a tertiary care center is important because emergency thoracic surgery is often needed. Recurrence is rare in later pregnancies. Since, Klinefelter's syndrome and Trisomy 18 are known for an association with CCAMs, it is appropriate to obtain a karyotype when the condition is diagnosed.

In utero aspiration of a larger cyst, thoracoamniotic shunting of a larger cyst and in utero resections have been attempted and are methods of gaining time to achieve viability. In utero resection has been tried only in fetuses with the poorest prognosis, since the procedure itself carries a high morbidity and mortality.

Bronchopulmonary Sequestration

Also known as pulmonary sequestration and accessory lung, bronchopulmonary sequestration (BPS) is a congenital malformation consisting of lung parenchyma, which is separated from normal lung. It receives arterial supply of systemic origin and does not communicate with the normal tracheobronchial tree. Sequestrations arise from a supernumerary anomalous outpouching of the foregut. If these arise prior to closure of the pleura they have no separate pleural envelope and are called intralobar sequestrations. If these originate after closure of the pleura they are called extralobar sequestrations (ELS) and have their own pleura. Intralobar sequestrations drain into pulmonary veins

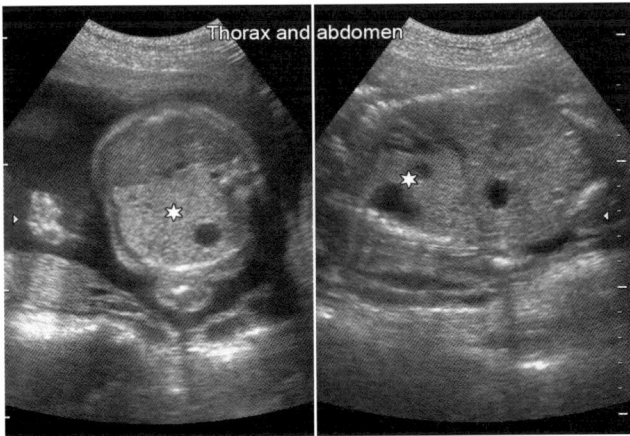

Fig. 42.21

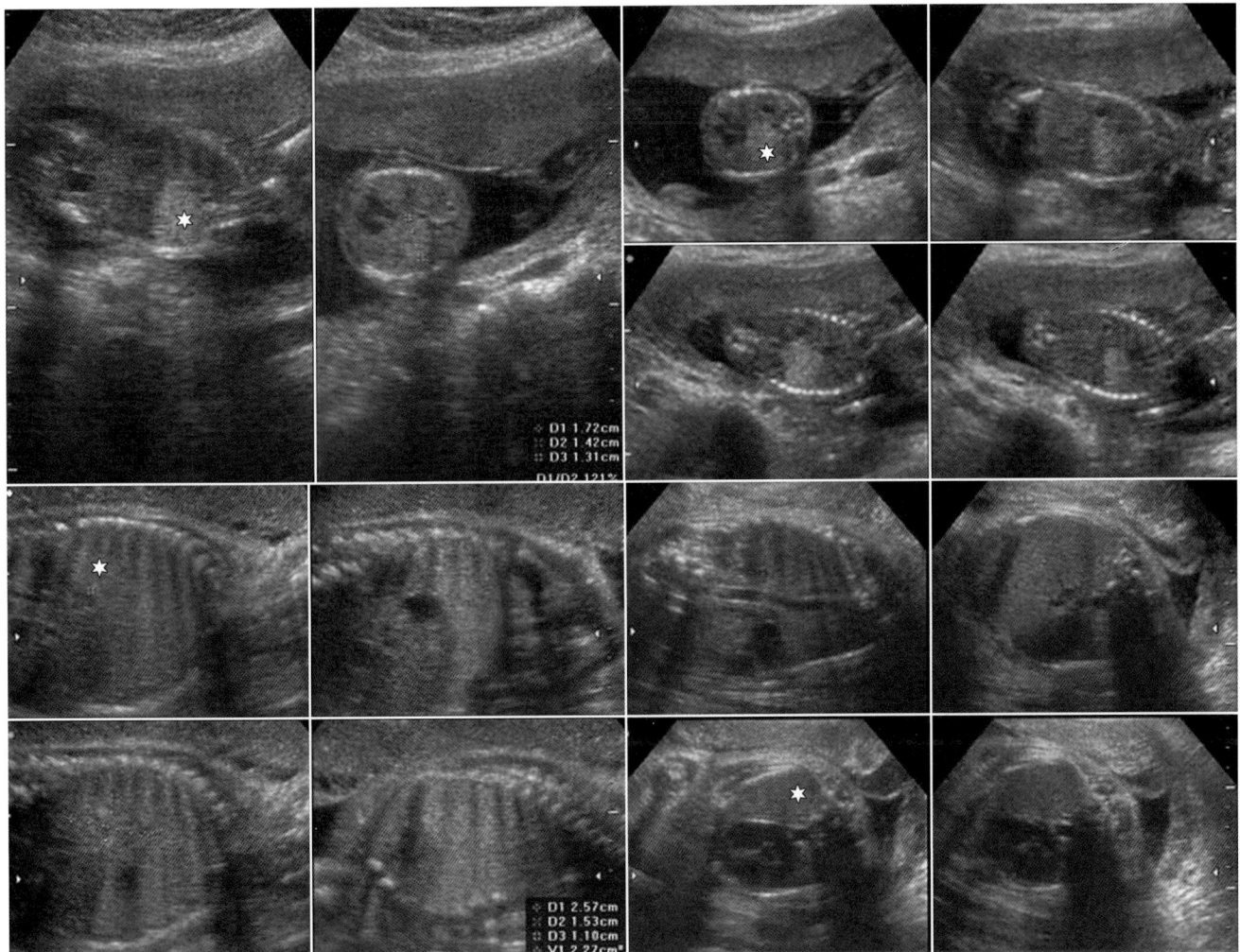

Fig. 42.22

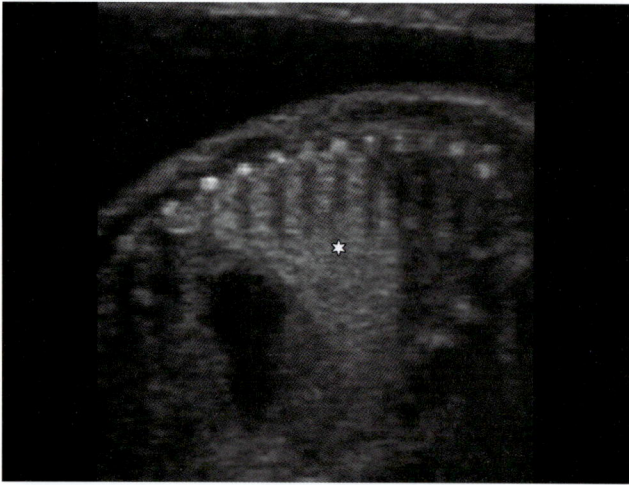

Fig. 42.23

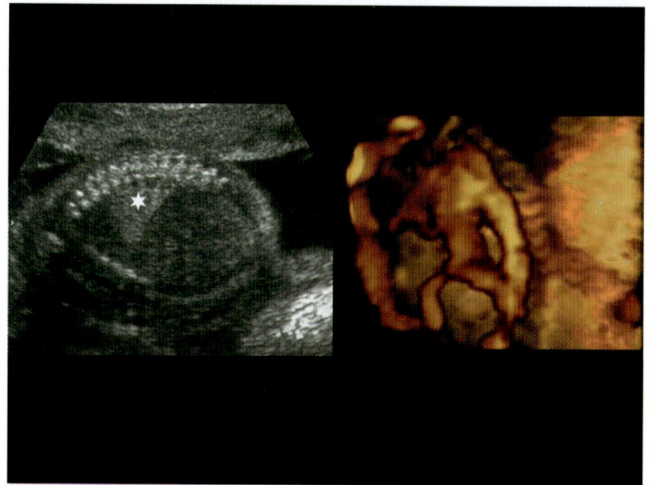

Fig. 42.24

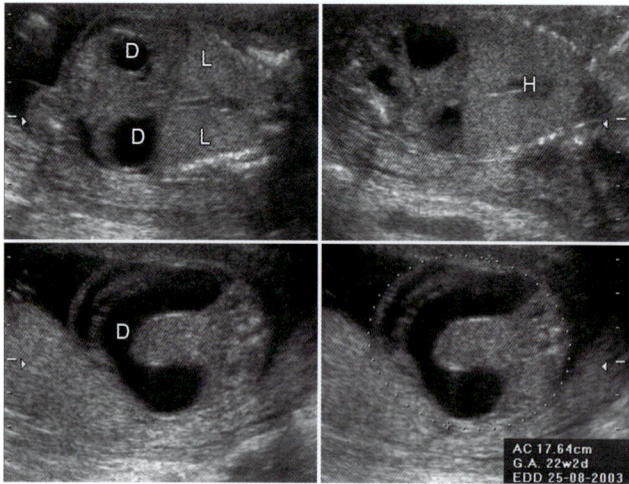

Fig. 42.25

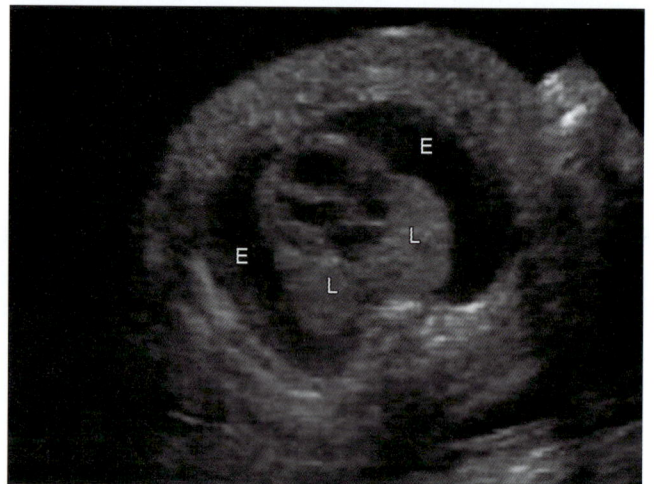

Fig. 42.26

and ELS usually drain into a systemic vein, usually the azygos, hemiazygos or inferior vena cava. Extralobar sequestrations may be thoracic or extrathoracic and may even communicate with the esophagus.[62] They are occasionally associated with other thoracic and foregut anomalies such as CDH, CCAMs, bronchogenic cysts and neurenteric cysts. A wide variety of extrapulmonary anomalies including congenital heart disease, renal anomalies and hydrocephalus have been reported to coexist with sequestrations. Many sequestrations show extensive subpleural lymphatics which account for ipsilateral pleural effusions. Typical sonographic appearances[63] include a lobar or triangular echogenic lesion in the lung base, usually left basal (Fig. 42.23). Color Doppler studies reveal a systemic arterial supply (Fig. 42.24).[64] There is a variable mediastinal shift and hydrops. Several sequestrations regress spontaneously.[65] No specific features indicate which sequestrations are likely to resolve. Persistent sequestrations may stabilize or may need surgical resection (postnatal).

Laryngeal and Tracheal Atresia

These are rare congenital anomalies, which are associated with demise soon after birth, unless treated antenatally. These arise consequently to either subglottic laryngeal atresia, tracheal stenosis or atresia, or tracheal webs or cysts and are also known as congenital high airways obstruction (CHAOS). Embryologically, persistent fusion of the sixth branchial arches is apparently involved. Pathologically, failure of efflux of fluid from the fetal lung results in exaggerated lung development. Ultrasound features[66,67] include symmetric enlargement of both lungs (Fig. 42.25) with anterior displacement of the heart. The lungs are homogeneously echogenic, often similar to autosomal recessive infantile polycystic kidneys, since the underlying lesion consists of numerous fluid-filled spaces. The diaphragm is flat or inverted and cutaneous edema is common as in hydrops. Polyhydramnios is seen consequent to esophageal compression. The distal trachea and bronchii may be identified as tubular bulging fluid laden structures in the mediastinum. Over half the fetuses with this abnormality have renal agenesis, facial anomalies and central nervous system malformations. To salvage a fetus with this anomaly it is necessary to establish a functional airway before the fetus is removed from placental support.[68]

Congenital Lobar Emphysema

Although, this condition has clinical manifestations in the pediatric age group, it can be seen in the fetus as a solid lung mass akin to a microcystic CCAM or an ELS. It is usually located in the upper lobe

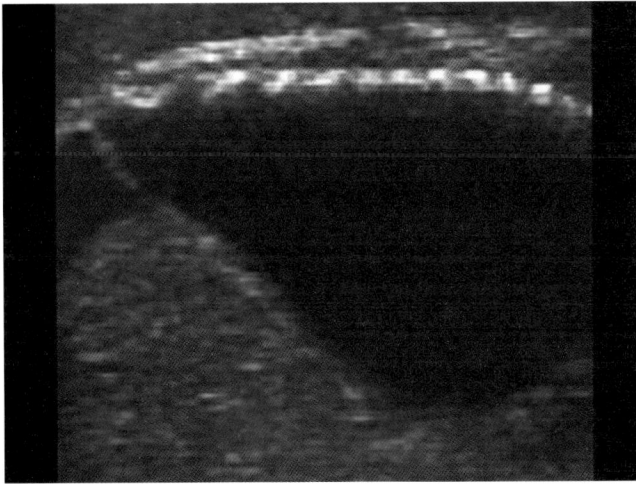

Fig. 42.27

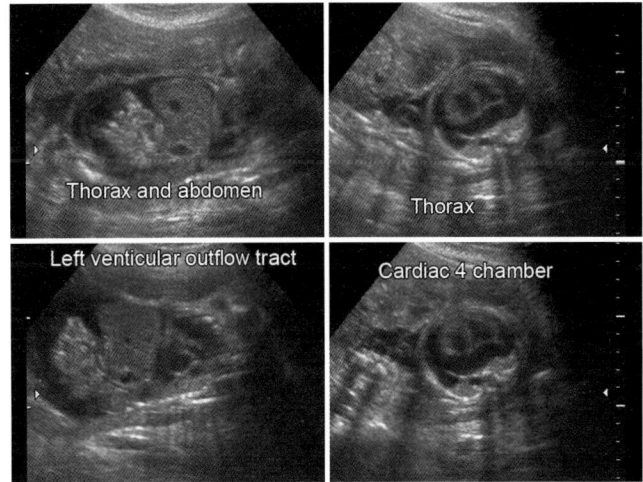

Fig. 42.28

unlike ELS. There is one case report of a spontaneous regression after indomethacin treatment.[69]

Pleural Effusion

Unlike a small amount of pericardial fluid, which may be physiological, a fetal pleural fluid collection is always abnormal.

Primary pleural effusions are accumulations of pleural fluid which may be idiopathic (Figs 42.26 and 42.27) or consequent to thoracic duct malformations.[70] They are unilateral, or if bilateral then markedly asymmetric. Mediastinal shifts are common and there are no associated findings except hydrops, which is an ominous finding. Pulmonary hypoplasia is common in large chronic effusions. The condition may resolve spontaneously and does very well after thoracentesis or thoracoamniotic shunting.[71,72]

Secondary pleural effusions are consequent to other fetal anomalies and are often the earliest sign of immune or non-immune hydrops fetalis (NIHF).[73] The causes, therefore, include anemia, infection, cardiac anomalies, anomalies with large arteriovenous shunts, chromosomal abnormalities, skeletal dysplasias and thoracic malformations. Secondary effusions are usually bilateral and often associated with early onset of other signs of hydrops (Fig. 42.28). Prior to instituting any treatment procedure it is wise to exclude an abnormal fetal karyotype and assess fetal anemia.

CONCLUSION

The current approach to a thoracic lesion involves the knowledge of sonographic features in order to make an accurate diagnosis. This should be followed by a careful evaluation for associated dysmorphic anomalies and identification of hydrops. An appropriate work-up for fetal anemia and fetal karyotype should be considered next. The prognosis then needs to be formulated in the perspective of prevention of PH, the possibility of spontaneous regression and referral to a tertiary care center. Ultrasound guided interventions in such a fetus would include amniocentesis or cordocentesis for a complete diagnosis, and from a therapeutic viewpoint, cyst aspiration, thoracentesis or a thoracoamniotic shunt.

REFERENCES

1. American Institute of Ultrasound in Medicine: guidelines for the performance of the antepartum obstetrical ultrasound examination. J Ultrasound Med. 1996;15:185.
2. Moore KL, Persaud TVN. The respiratory system: development of bronchi and lungs. Before we are born: essentials of embryology and birth defects, 5th edition. Philadelphia: WB Saunders; 1998. p. 246.
3. Hislop AA, Wigglesworth JS, Desai R. Alveolar development in the human fetus and infant. Early Hum Dev. 1986;13:1.
4. Felker RE, Cartier MS, Emerson DS, et al. Ultrasound of the fetal thymus. J Ultrasound Med. 1989;8:669.
5. Jeanty P, Romero R, Hobbins JC. Fetal pericardial fluid: a normal finding of the second half of gestation. Am J Obstet Gynecol. 1984;149:529.
6. Cooper C, Mahony BS, Bowie JD, et al. Ultrasound evaluation of the normal fetal upper airway and esophagus. J Ultrasound Med. 1985;4:343.
7. Kilbride HW, Yeast J, Thibeault DW. Defining limits of survival: lethal pulmonary hypoplasia after midtrimester premature rupture of membranes. Am J Obstet Gynecol. 1985;175:675.
8. Vergani P, Ghidini A, Locatelli A, et al. Risk factors for pulmonary hypoplasia in second trimester premature rupture of membranes. Am J Obstet Gynecol. 1994;170:1359.
9. Askenazi SS, Perlman M. Pulmonary hypoplasia: Lung weight and radial alveolar count as criteria of diagnosis. Arch Dis Child. 1979;54:614.
10. Bromley B, Benacerraf BR. Unilateral lung hypoplasia: Report of three cases. J Ultrasound Med. 1997;16:599.
11. Yancey MK, Richards DS. Antenatal sonographic findings associated with unilateral pulmonary agenesis. Obstet Gynecol. 1993;81:847.
12. McNamara MF, McCurdy CM, Reed KL, et al. The relation between pulmonary hypoplasia and amniotic fluid volume: lessons learned from discordant urinary tract anomalies in monoamniotic twins. Obstet Gynecol. 1995;85:867.
13. Nicolini U, Fisk NM, Rodeck CH, et al. Low amniotic pressure in oligohydramnios—is this the cause of pulmonary hypoplasia? Am J Obstet Gynecol. 1989;161:1098.
14. Alcorn D, Adamson TM, Lambert TF, et al. Morphological effects of chronic tracheal ligation and drainage in the fetal lamb lung. J Anat. 1977;123:649.

15. Hislop A, Hey E, Reid L. The lungs in congenital bilateral renal agenesis and dysplasia. Arch Dis Child. 1979;54:32.
16. Fewell JE, Lee CC, Kitterman JA. Effects of phrenic nerve section on the respiratory system of fetal lambs. J Appl Physiol. 1981;51:293.
17. Harrison MR, Bressack MA, Churg AM, et al. Correction of congenital diaphragmatic hernia in utero: II. Simulated correction permits fetal lung growth with survival at birth. Surgery. 1980;88:260.
18. Ohlsson A, Fong KW, Rose TH, et al. Prenatal sonographic diagnosis of Pena-Shokeir syndrome type I, or fetal akinesia deformation sequence. Am J Med Genet. 1988;29:59.
19. Mitchell JM, Roberts AM, Lee A. Doppler waveforms from the pulmonary arterial system in normal fetuses and those with pulmonary hypoplasia. Ultrasound Obstet Gynecol. 1998;11:167.
20. Nimrod C, Davies D, Iwanicki S, et al. Ultrasound prediction of pulmonary hypoplasia. Obstet Gynecol. 1986;68:495.
21. DeVore GR, Horenstein J, Platt LD. Fetal echocardiography: VI. Assessment of cardiothoracic disproportion – a new technique for the diagnosis of thoracic hypoplasia. Am J Obstet Gynecol. 1986;155:1066.
22. Songster GS, Gray DL, Crane JP. Prenatal prediction of lethal pulmonary hypoplasia using ultrasonic fetal chest circumference. Obstet Gynecol. 1989;73:261.
23. Chitkara U, Rosenberg J, Chervenak FA, et al. Prenatal sonographic assessment of the fetal thorax: normal values. Am J Obstet Gynecol. 1987;156:1069.
24. Vintzileos AM, Campbell WA, Rodis JF, et al. Comparison of six different ultrasonographic methods for predicting lethal fetal pulmonary hypoplasia. Am J Obstet Gynecol. 1989;161:606.
25. D'Alton M, Mercer B, Riddick E, et al. Serial thoracic versus abdominal circumference ratios for the prediction of pulmonary hypoplasia in premature rupture of the membranes remote from term. Am J Obstet Gynecol. 1992;166:658.
26. Yoshimura S, Masuzaki H, Gotoh H, et al. Ultrasonographic prediction of lethal pulmonary hypoplasia: comparison of eight different ultrasonographic parameters. Am J Obstet Gynecol. 1996;175:477.
27. Roberts AB, Mitchell JM. Direct ultrasonographic measurement of fetal lung length in normal pregnancies and pregnancies complicated by prolonged rupture of membranes. Am J Obstet Gynecol. 1990;163:1560.
28. D'Arcy TJ, Hughes SW, Chiu WS, et al. Estimation of fetal lung volume using enhanced 3-dimensional ultrasound. A new method and first result. Br J Obstet Gynecol. 1996;103:1015.
29. Lee A, Kratochwil A, Stumpflen I, et al. Fetal lung volume determination by three-dimensional ultrasonography. Am J Obstet Gynecol. 1996;175:588.
30. Rizzo G. Use ultrasound to predict preterm delivery: do not lose the opportunity [Editorial]. Ultrasound Obstet Gynecol. 1996;8:289.
31. Adzick NS, Harrison MR, Crombleholme TM, et al. Fetal lung lesions: management and outcome. Am J Obstet Gynecol. 1998;179:884.
32. Bromley B, Parad R, Estroff JA, et al. Fetal lung masses: prenatal course and outcome. J Ultrasound Med. 1995;14:927.
33. Thorpe-Beeston JG, Nicolaides KH. Cystic adenomatoid malformation of the lung: prenatal diagnosis and outcome. Prenat Diagn. 1994;14:677.
34. Rice HE, Estes JM, Hedrick MH, et al. Congenital cystic adenomatoid malformation. A sheep model of fetal hydrops. J Pediatr Surg. 1994;29:692.
35. Dommergues M, Louis-Sylvestre C, Mandelbrot L, et al. Congenital adenomatoid malformation of the lung: when is active fetal therapy indicated? Am J Obstet Gynecol. 1997;177:953.
36. Todros T, Gaglioti P, Presbitero P. Management of a fetus with intrapericardial teratoma diagnosed in utero. J Ultrasound Med. 1991;10:287.
37. de Miguel Campos E, Casanova A, Urbano J, et al. Congenital thymic cyst: prenatal sonographic and postnatal magnetic resonance findings. J Ultrasound Med. 1997;16:365.
38. Gushiken BJ, Callen PW, Silverman NH. Prenatal diagnosis of tuberous sclerosis in monozygotic twins with cardiac masses. J Ultrasound Med. 1999;18:165.
39. Green KW, Bors-Koefoed R, Pollack P, et al. Antepartum diagnosis and management of multiple fetal cardiac tumors. J Ultrasound Med. 1991;10:697.
40. Schmaltz AA, Apitz J. Primary heart tumors in infancy and childhood. Report of four cases and review of literature. Cardiology. 1981;67:12.
41. Reed JC, Sobonya RE. Morphologic analysis of foregut cysts in the thorax. AJR Am J Roentgenol. 1974;120:851.
42. Fernandes ET, Custer MD, Burton EM, et al. Neurenteric cyst: surgery and diagnostic imaging. J Pediatr Surg. 1991;26:108.
43. Macualay KE, Winter TC III, Shields LE. Neurenteric cyst shown by prenatal sonography. AJR Am J Roentgenol. 1997;169:563.
44. Wilkinson CC, Albanese CT, Jennings RW, et al. Fetal neurenteric cyst causing hydrops: case report and review of the literature. Prenat Diagn. 1999;19:118.
45. Katz AI, Wiswell TE, Baumgart S. Contemporaries controversies in the management of congenital diaphragmatic hernia. Clin Perinatol. 1998;25:219.
46. Lewis DA, Reickert C, Bowerman R, et al. Prenatal ultrasonography frequently fails to diagnose congenital diaphragmatic hernia. J Pediatr Surg. 1997;32:352.
47. Bernbaum J, Schwartz IP, Gerdes M, et al. Survivors of extracorporeal membrane oxygenation at 1 year of age. The relationship of primary diagnosis with health and neurodevelopmental sequelae. Pediatrics. 1995;96:907.
48. Guibaud L, Filiatrault D, Garel L, et al. Fetal congenital diaphragmatic hernia: accuracy of sonography in the diagnosis and prediction of the outcome after birth. AJR Am J Roentgenol. 1996;166:1195.
49. Albanese CT, Lopoo J, Goldstein RB, et al. Fetal liver position and perinatal outcome for congenital diaphragmatic hernia. Prenat Diagn. 1998;18:1138.
50. Bootstaylor BS, Filly RA, Harrison MR, et al. Prenatal sonographic predictors of liver herniation in congenital diaphragmatic hernia. J Ultrasound Med. 1995;14:515.
51. Dommergues M, Louis-Sylvestre C, Mandelbrot L, et al. Congenital diaphragmatic hernia. Can prenatal ultrasonography predict outcome? Am J Obstet Gynecol. 1996;174:1377.
52. Geary MP, Chitty LS, Morrison JJ, et al. Prenatal outcome and prognostic factors in prenatally diagnosed congenital diaphragmatic hernia. Ultrasound Obstet Gynecol. 1998;12:107.
53. Sharland GK, Lockhart SM, Heward AJ, et al. Prognosis in fetal diaphragmatic hernia. Am J Obstet Gynecol. 1992;166:9.
54. Losty PD, Vanamo K, Rintala RJ, et al. Congenital diaphragmatic hernia – does the size of the defect influence the incidence of associated malformations? J Pediatr Surg. 1998;33:507.
55. Sheffield JS, Twickler DM, Timmons C, et al. Fryns syndrome: prenatal diagnosis and pathologic correlation. J Ultrasound Med. 1998;17:585.
56. Harrison MR, Adzick NS, Estes JM, et al. A prospective study of the outcome for fetuses with diaphragmatic hernia. JAMA. 1994;271:382.
57. Geary M. Management of congenital diaphragmatic hernia diagnosed prenatally. An update. Prenat Diagn. 1998;18:1155.
58. Silver MM, Thurston WA, Patrick JE. Perinatal pulmonary hyperplasia due to laryngeal atresia. Hum Pathol. 1988;19:110.
59. Moerman P, Fryns JP, Vandenberghte K, et al. Pathogenesis of congenital cystic adenomatoid malformation of the lung. Histopathology. 1992;21:315.
60. Mayden KL, Tortora M, Chervenak FA, et al. The antenatal sonographic detection of lung masses. Am J Obstet Gynecol. 1984;148:349.

61. Budorick NE, Pretorius DH, Leopold GR, et al. Spontaneous improvement of intrathoracic masses diagnosed in utero. J Ultrasound Med. 1992;11:653.

62. Gerle RD, Jaretzki AD, Ashley CA, et al. Congenital bronchopulmonary-foregut malformation. Pulmonary sequestration communicating with the gastrointestinal tract. N Engl J Med. 1968;278:1413.

63. Lopoo JB, Albanese CT, Goldstein RB, et al. Fetal pulmonary sequestration. A favorable cystic lung lesion. Obstet Gynecol. 1999;94:567.

64. Hernanz-Schulman M, Stein SM, Neblett WW, et al. Pulmonary sequestration. Diagnosis with color Doppler sonography and a new theory of associated hydrothorax. Radiology. 1991;180:817.

65. Langer B, Donato L, Riethmuller C, et al. Spontaneous regression of fetal pulmonary sequestration. Ultrasound Obstet Gynecol. 1995;6:33.

66. Scott JN, Trevenen CL, Wiseman DA, et al. Tracheal atresia: ultrasonographic and pathologic correlation. J Ultrasound Med. 1999;18:375.

67. Choong KKL, Trudinger B, Chow C, et al. Fetal laryngeal obstruction: sonographic detection. Ultrasound Obstet Gynecol. 1992;2:357.

68. DeCou JM, Jones DC, Jacobs HD, et al. Successful ex utero intrapartum treatment (EXIT) procedure for congenital high airway obstruction syndrome (CHAOS) owing to laryngeal atresia. J Pediatric Surg. 1998;33:1563.

69. Richards DS, Langham MR Jr, Mahaffey SM. The prenatal ultrasonograhic diagnosis of cloacal exstrophy. J Ultrasound Med. 1992;11:507.

70. Longaker MT, Laberge JM, Dansereau J, et al. Primary fetal hydrothorax: natural history and management. J Pediatr Surg. 1989;24:573.

71. Benaceraff BR, Frigoletto FD Jr. Mid-trimester fetal thoracentesis. J Clin Ultrasound. 1985;13:202.

72. Wilkins Haug LE, Doubilet P. Successful thoracoamniotic shunting and review of the literature in unilateral pleural effusion with hydrops. J Ultrasound Med. 1997;16:153.

73. Weber AM, Philipson EH. Fetal pleural effusion: a review and meta-analysis for prognostic indicators. Obstet Gynecol. 1992;79:281.

43

Three-dimensional Ultrasound of Blood Flow in the Fetal Cardiovascular System

R Chaoui

INTRODUCTION

In the recent 5 years three-dimensional (3D) ultrasound moved from a toy of advertisement with the highlight of baby facing to a new powerful diagnostic tool in prenatal medicine. This was mainly achieved by the development of fast processors enabling rapid 3D-image acquisition and the advent of new software allowing new 3D image display.

The use of color and power Doppler ultrasound in the 1990s improved the prenatal diagnosis of malformations involving the cardiac and vascular system.[1-3] Malformations of the cardiovascular system are often complex and difficult to understand when only gray-scale imaging is used. Two-dimensional (2D) color or power Doppler ultrasound can help in a better assessment of fetal abnormalities, but they generally enable the visualization of only those vessels with a straight course or lying in a 2D plane.[4-6] In most cases the examiner is reconstructing mentally a spatial image of the examined vessels.[5]

In the recent years few cases reports and studies demonstrated that the 3D power Doppler ultrasound (3D-PDU) helps in the reconstruction of the vessels of interest and thus improves the understanding of the spatial appearance of the vascular tree.[4,7,8] Images produced were very similar to results known from radiology acquired either by X-ray[9-11] or magnetic resonance (MR) angiography. This chapter aims to present the actual possibilities of 3D ultrasound of the cardiovascular system in normal and abnormal pregnancies, looking for possible future applications of this method in prenatal diagnosis.

TECHNICAL BACKGROUND

The main aspects that have to be considered when evaluating a 3D imaging system are (1) the volume data acquisition, (2) the image rendering display.

Volume Data Acquisition

The acquisition of a volume with information of the fetal heart or the fetal vessels can be achieved either in 3D static mode, that means a volume consisting of a series of still images or in four-dimensional (4D) mode, which reflects the beating character of the heart. The latter can be acquired either in live real-time 3D or as offline 4D, which was possible recently by the advent of the new software of spatial and temporal image correlation (STIC).[12,13] In these acquisitions heart and vessels can be visualized either on gray scale mode, or in combination with color Doppler,[14] power Doppler or B-flow. The acquisition of a volume with gray scale information is reduced to the demonstration of the lumen of the heart or the vessels, whereas in Doppler or B-flow techniques blood flow is visualized. To acquire a volume with a potentially good 3D/4D image the examiner should spend time in optimizing the presetting of the color and power Doppler or B-flow or to increase the contrast on the gray scale.

Image Rendering

It is the process of creating a 3D visual representation of the parameters of interest. Generally, the principle used is the "planar geometric projection" of the 3D-image, i.e. a 2D-image, representing the 3-D data. For the 4D image it will be a 2D projection with cine-loop. The impression of the third dimension is generally given by the on-line rotation of the image on the screen and by different shadowing of anterior and posterior structures. Color maps can be used as well as different postprocessing means of increasing the brightness and transparency of color. The examiner can decide whether to visualize only the vessels of interest or in combination with gray scale information in the so called "glass body" rendering (Fig. 43.1). Interestingly, the system allows also a gradual increase of the transparency allowing at the beginning of the visualization of the surface in gray scale but with progression of transparency, the visualization of the vessels inside the structure of interest (Fig. 43.1).[7] For information using no Doppler assistance but only the gray scale information, there are two volume rendering features, permitting a 3D/4D appearance: The transparent minimum mode and the transparent inversion mode.

Most experience shared in this chapter was acquired with a Voluson 730 Expert system (GE Kretztechnik, Zipf, Austria) using mechanical transducers for acquisition and the 4D view software for 3D/4D volume reconstruction. The 4D of the fetal heart was achieved either with live 3D or by using the integrated STIC software as described elsewhere. Only the latter permitted a 4D of color or power Doppler information of the heart. It is expected that in near future other companies will provide new software with new possibilities of 3D/4D acquisition and rendering, but the fields of interest will probably remain unchanged.

CLINICAL APPLICATION

The clinical application of 3D/4D in prenatal visualization of the fetal cardiovascular system is closely related to the regions of interest known from the application of color and power Doppler ultrasound. We refer to reviews on the benefit of using color Doppler in fetal diseases.[2,3] Some years ago we examined in a study the application of 3D-PDU in prenatal diagnosis on 45 normal and 87 abnormal pregnancies including mainly vascular abnormalities.[4] In this study, we used a prototype system and satisfactory image information was collected in only 56 out of the 87 abnormal cases examined (64%). Following eight regions were found to be interesting: Vessels of the placenta, umbilical cord, abdomen, kidneys, lung, brain and fetal tumors as well as the heart and great vessels. In the following findings, some of the main regions of interest with the possible anomalies involving the vascular system were demonstrable on 3D ultrasound. The fetal heart will be separately discussed in the second part of this section.

Peripheral Vascular System in 3D
Umbilical Cord and Placenta

From our experience it seems to be the structure most easily accessible to 3D throughout pregnancy. Intraplacental vessel network architecture can be visualized with this method.[15] The umbilical cord can be rendered at different places from its insertion on the placental side (Figs 43.2 and 43.3) to its attachment on the fetal abdominal wall.[4] Abnormalities like placenta praevia, vasa praevia[16] or velamentous insertion (Fig. 43.3) can be demonstrated as well as single umbilical artery or less important conditions as the connecting vessels in twin pregnancies, nuchal cord or true and false knot (Fig. 43.4) or the free course of the umbilical cord (Fig. 43.5).

Intra-abdominal Vessels

The vessels of interest are the umbilical vein, the ductus venosus, the portal vein system, the hepatic veins, splenic vessels, inferior vena cava and abdominal aorta (Fig. 43.6). The visualization of the lower abdomen gives a good orientation in visualizing the umbilical arteries around the urinary bladder in normal conditions. Since, the application of color Doppler and the intensive study of the ductus venosus, abnormalities of intrahepatic venous system were detected to be more common as expected. Conditions to study by 3D power Doppler could involve the abnormal cord insertion on the abdomen (omphalocele, gastroschisis) (Fig. 43.7), abnormal umbilical vein size (varix or ectasia) but the main field of interest seems to be the absence of ductus venosus (Fig. 43.8) with the different possibilities of connection of umbilical vein. In these conditions 3D power Doppler demonstrates the spatial course of the aberrant vessel. Another interesting condition is the abnormal course of vessels in isomerism, i.e. interruption of inferior vena cava with azygous continuity (Fig. 43.9).

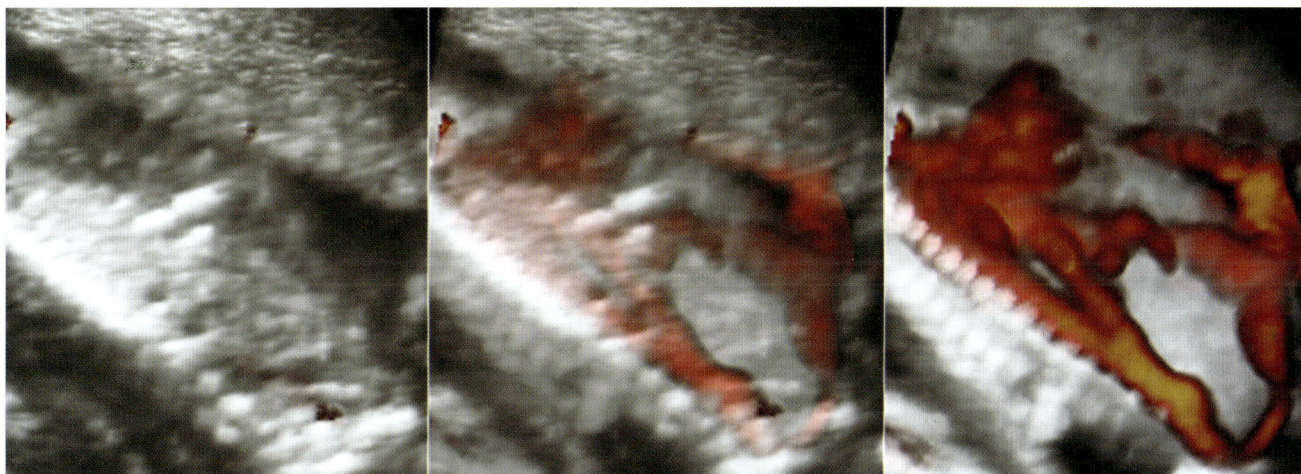

Fig. 43.1: A longitudinal view of the abdomen seen from the right side in glass body mode. From left to right, the transparency is gradually increased allowing a progressive visualization of power Doppler information

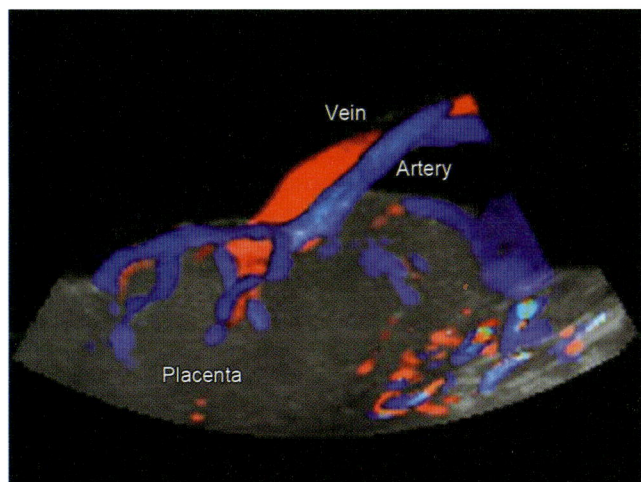

Fig. 43.2: Three-dimensional (3D) color Doppler ultrasound showing a posterior placenta with central insertion of the umbilical cord. There is a single umbilical artery

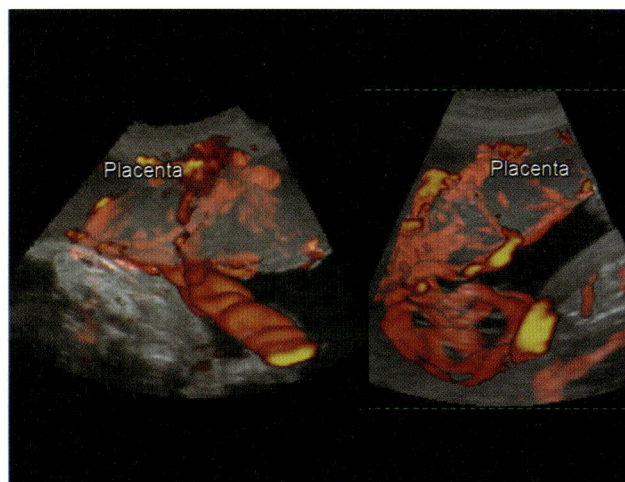

Fig. 43.3: Three-dimensional (3D) power Doppler ultrasound showing a central insertion of the umbilical cord (left) and a velamentous insertion (right)

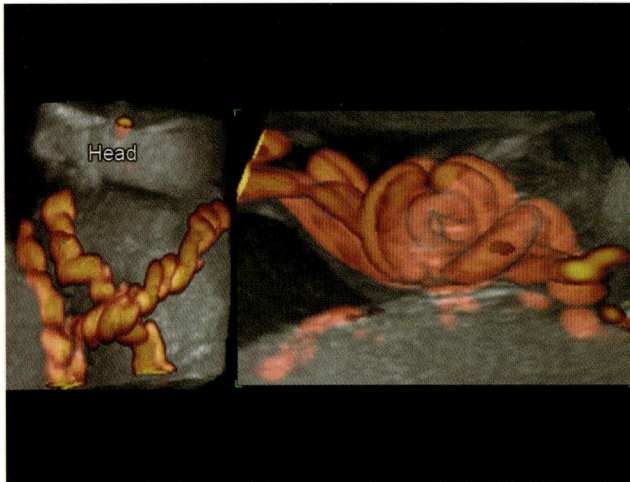

Fig. 43.4: Fetus seen from behind with the umbilical cord around the neck (left). False knot of the umbilical cord

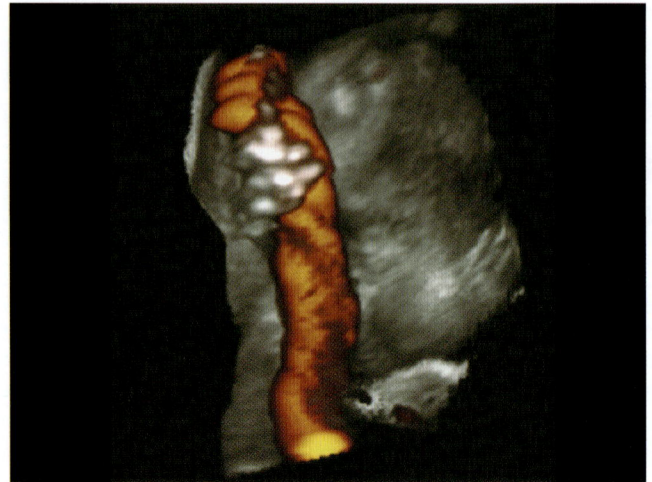

Fig. 43.5: Fetus holding the umbilical cord with the hand in front of its face

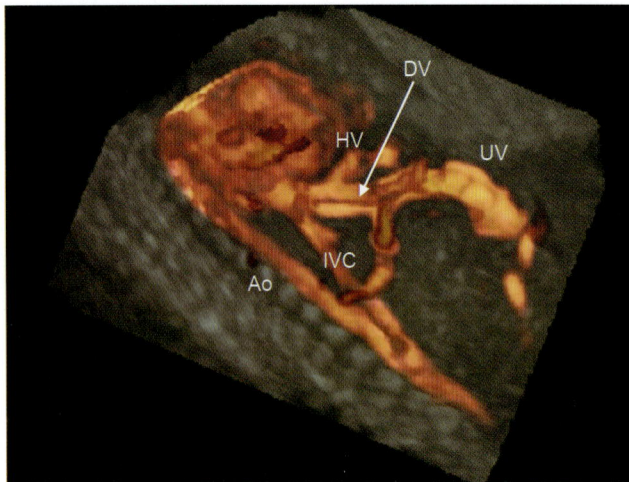

Fig. 43.6: Longitudinal view of the abdomen from the right side showing the descending aorta (AO), the inferior vena cava (IVC), the umbilical vein (UV) with ductus venosus (DV) as well as hepatic veins

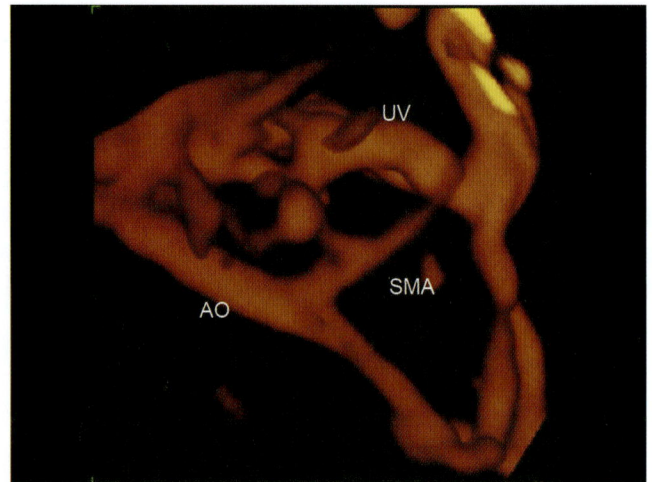

Fig. 43.7: Longitudinal view from the right side in a fetus with gastroschisis, showing in comparison to figure 43.6 the distortion in the course of the umbilical vein (UV), and the descending aorta (AO). The superior mesenteric artery is stretched and arises in direction of the abdominal wall

Renal vessels: The visualization of renal vessels is known to increase the accuracy of diagnosis of kidneys malformations in the fetus. The renal vascular tree is well visualized in a coronal plane with the descending aorta showing a horizontal course. Conditions with possible benefit of 3D-PDU application are agenesis of one or both kidneys, arteries in duplex kidney, horseshoe or pelvic kidney (Fig. 43.10), but the 3D rendering adds only few information to 2D color and was probably overestimated in our fewer investigations.

Intracerebral vessels: The anatomy of intracranial vessel architecture became more important in the recent years and is closely related to the structural anatomy of the brain. A transversal insonation allows easily the reconstruction of the circulus of Willis (Fig. 43.11), whereas a more sagittal approach enables the visualization of the pericallosal artery with its ramifications.[17] Choosing a lower velocity scale flow in the cerebral veins and sagittal sinus can be imaged as well. Main fields of interest are the abnormal anterior cerebral artery in agenesis of corpus callosum,

the aneurysm of the vein of Galen (Fig. 43.12) and disturbed vascular anatomy in cerebral malformations [holoprosencephaly (Fig. 43.13), hydrocephaly, encephalocele, etc.]. Improved image information can be reached by using transvaginal ultrasound of the fetal brain in fetuses with vertex position (Fig. 43.13).

Lung vessels: Proximal and peripheral lung arteries and veins can be seen from their origin into peripheral pulmonary segments (Fig. 43.14). Fields of interest are the analysis of the 3D vessel architecture in cystic lung malformation, congenital diaphragmatic hernia and in bronchopulmonary sequestration (Fig. 43.15).

The role of color or power Doppler in predicting pulmonary hypoplasia failed and it is not expected that the 3D demonstration of the vessels could be in this field of great interest in the near future.

Fetal tumors or aberrant vessels: Aberrant vessels can be visualized in the presence of several malformations like lung sequestration,

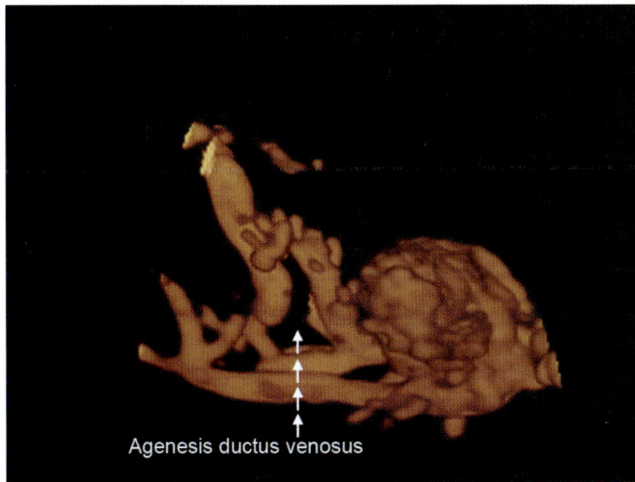

Fig. 43.8: Longitudinal view of the intra-abdominal vascular tree in a 22 weeks fetus with agenesis of ductus venosus and connection of the umbilical vein into the hepatic vein system

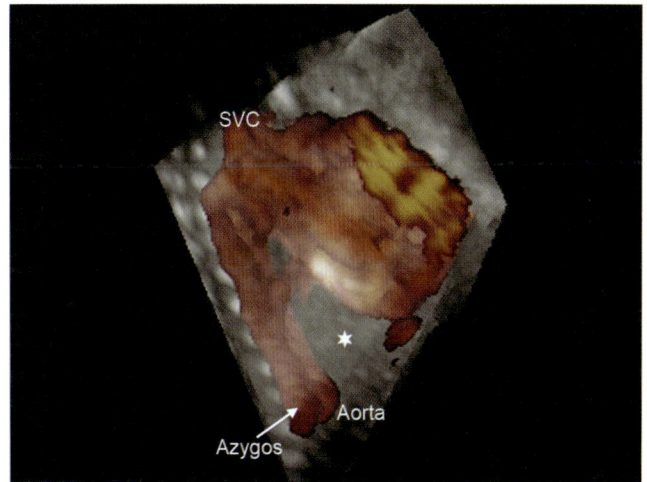

Fig. 43.9: Fetus with left isomerism (polysplenia) with an interruption of the inferior vena cava (*), which is absent on three-dimensional power Doppler ultrasound (3D-PDU). Venous blood from the inferior part of the body returns via the azygos vein, which is dilated and seen side by side near the aorta

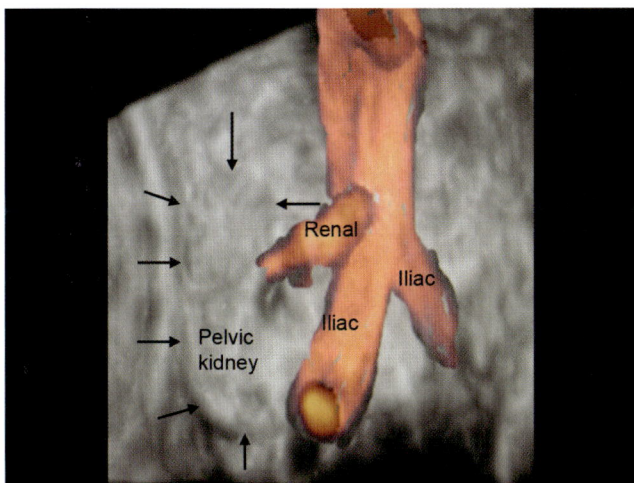

Fig. 43.10: Pelvic kidney showing the abnormal renal artery arising in the region of the bifurcation of the iliac arteries

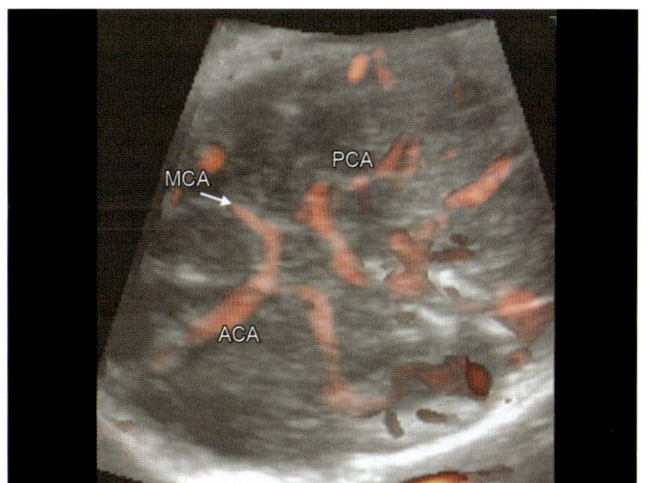

Fig. 43.11: Circulus of Willis as demonstrated with three-dimensional power Doppler ultrasound (3D-PDU), with the anterior cerebral artery (ACA), middle cerebral artery (MCA) and posterior cerebral artery (PCA)

chorangioma, lymphangioma or in (sacrococcygeal) teratoma, acardiac twin, etc. Fetal tumors can be of interest to be visualized not only for their risk of cardiac failure due to the presence of arteriovenous fistulae, but also to assess compression of shifting of neighboring organs (Fig. 43.16A and B). Some fields of interest are chorangioma, teratoma, lung sequestration, acrania [twin reversed arterial perfusion (TRAP)], hemangioma, renal tumors, and cardiac rhabdomyomas, etc.

The Fetal Heart in 3D and 4D

An extended fetal echocardiographic examination is achieved by acquiring and documenting different cross-sectional planes.[1,18] An examiner acquiring these cardiac cross sectional planes during different cycles is automatically reconstructing mentally the heart in the third and fourth dimension (3D+time). In the last decade

3D and 4D fetal echocardiography was investigated intensively in laboratories using external work stations, static volume sweep, matrix transducers and recently a new ultrasound equipment with integrated software (STIC™) was introduced allowing a reliable 3D and 4D fetal echocardiography.[12,14]

Surface rendering can be applied to the fetal heart by using the interface between the cavities and the cardiac walls. The views are however either the known views from 2D ultrasound (four-chamber and five chambers) or could be new views as well, which still to be defined.[19] Such views could focus on demonstrating the atrioventricular-valves or the interventricular or interatrial septum. The future will show, which views are appropriate for clinical application. This part will not be covered in this chapter mainly focusing on the 3D appearance of blood flow. First steps were acquired by combining power Doppler mode with 3D to get the image of the four-cavities (Fig. 43.17)[4] or the spatial arrangement

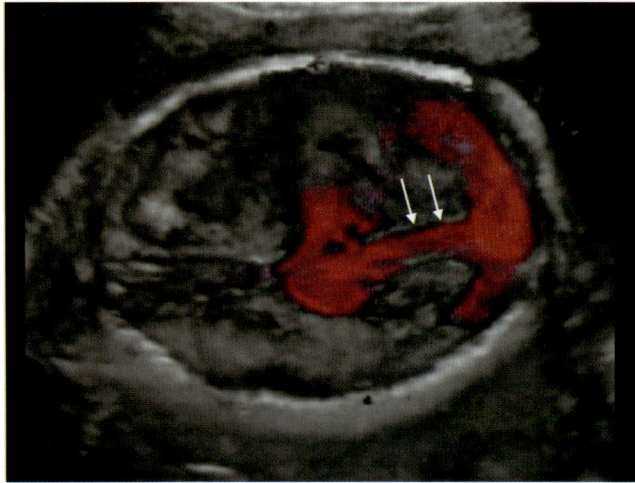

Fig. 43.12: Three-dimensional power Doppler ultrasound (3D-PDU) of a vein of Galen aneurysm at 22 weeks gestation with the dilated vessel between the hemispheres and in the posterior fossa

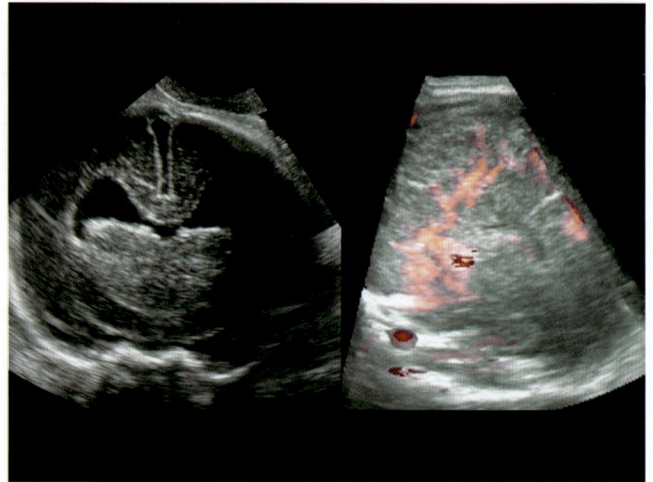

Fig. 43.13: Fetus with trisomy 13 and lobar holoprosencephaly as seen by transvaginal ultrasound (left). 3D power Doppler shows the aberrant bizarre course of the anterior cerebral artery

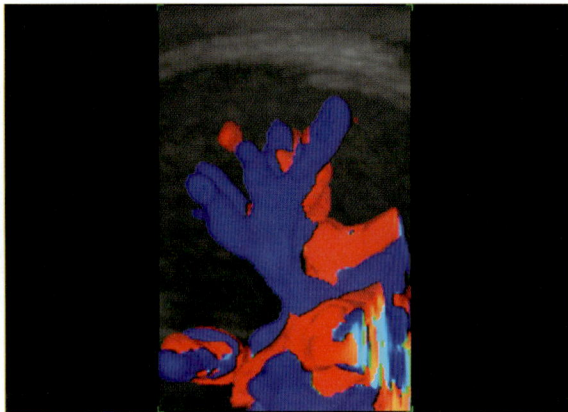

Fig. 43.14: Pulmonary veins and arteries are demonstrated with 3D color Doppler ultrasound

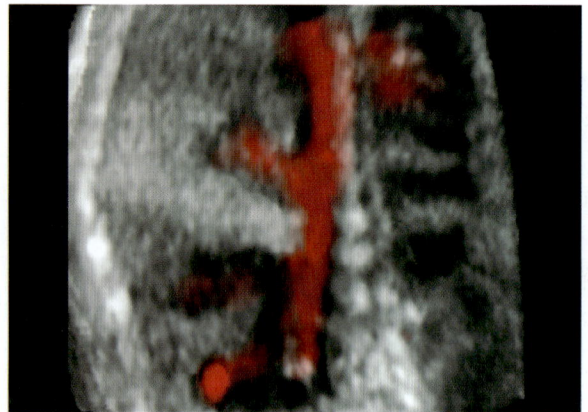

Fig. 45.15. In this fetus with an echogenic lung segment the diagnosis of bronchopulmonary sequestration is supported by the demonstration of an aberrant vessel arising from the descending aorta

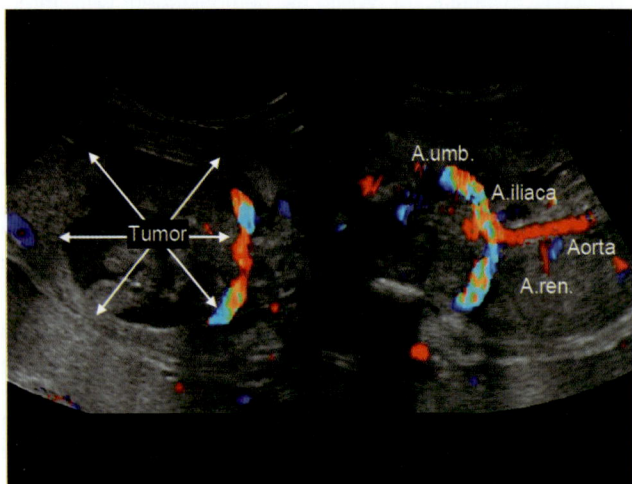

Fig. 43.16A: In this fetus at 27 weeks with sacrococcygeal teratoma there was an intra-abdominal masses as well (arrows). In different planes one recognizes the descending aorta, one renal artery and the bifurcation of iliac arteries with the arising of umbilical arteries (A.umb.), (A. iliaco, iliaco arteries; A. ren, renal arteries)

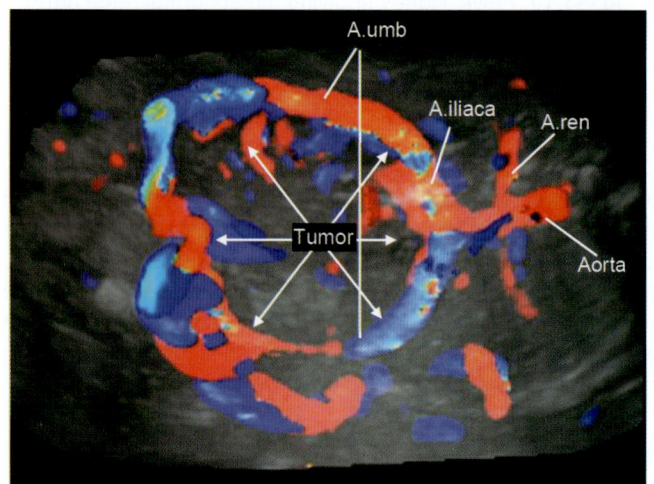

Fig. 43.16B: The 3D rendering gives the complete aspect of the tumor and the surrounding vessels, (A. iliaco, iliaco arteries; A ren, renal arteries)

of the great vessels.[11] These views could help in the demonstration of interventricular communications as a ventricular septal defect (Fig. 43.18). Their main potential could be the demonstration of the crossing of the great vessels and the aortic arch under normal conditions (Fig. 43.19) versus a transposition of the great arteries (Fig. 43.20).[4] The application of STIC with color Doppler and "glass body mode" allows a more precise and dynamic appearance of the relationship of the vessels to one each other (Fig. 43.21).[14]

An interesting rendering mode is the "transparent minimal mode" rendering (Figs 43.22 and 43.23 left), in which blood vessels can be seen as hypoechoic structures in a projection. Especially in a longitudinal view, the aortic and ductus arch can be seen properly. The use of the new software of "inversion mode" permits the demonstration of a negative image of the projection in minimum mode, but the image gets more plasticity and appears more three-dimensional than the minimal mode (Figs 43.23 right and 43.24).

2 years ago, the breakthrough was achieved by the software allowing the acquisition of the STIC volume combined with color Doppler or power Doppler information. We presented extensively this technique elsewhere.[14] Using this technique, the examiner is able to assess the hemodynamic spatial changes throughout the cardiac cycle. The 3D/4D volume rendering of color or power Doppler STIC provides images similar to an angiography, when the feature glass body is chosen.

Potential of 3D is that it facilitates not only the understanding of the spatial arrangement of the chambers showing their size and shape, but the course of the great vessels can be better understood. Crossing of vessels versus parallel course, abnormal course as seen in double aortic arch, right arch with a sling,[20] or simply tortuous hypoplastic aorta or pulmonary artery in different anomalies may be fields for future research.[21]

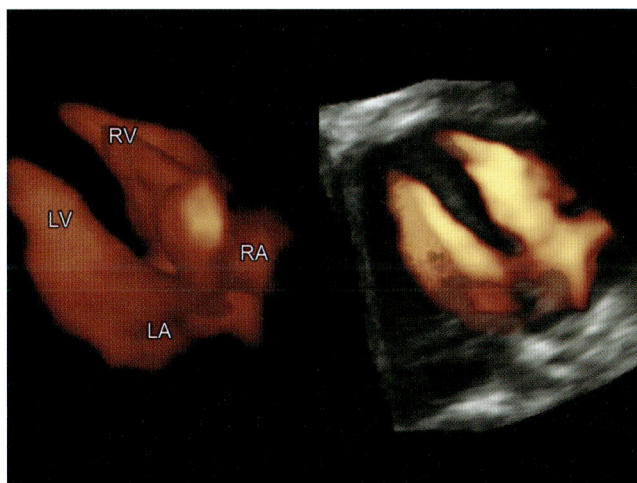

Fig. 43.17: Three-dimensional power Doppler ultrasound (3D-PDU) of a normal four-chamber-view (left) with right atrium (RA), left atrium (LA), right ventricle (RV) and left ventricle (LV) in 3D power mode (left) and glass body mode

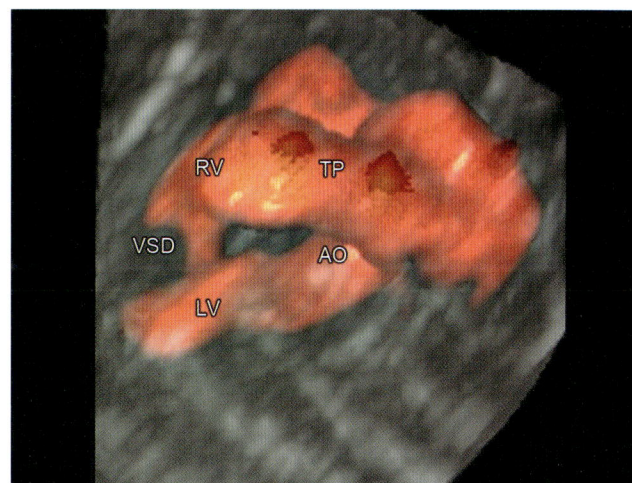

Fig. 43.18: A muscular ventricular septal defect (VSD) connecting both right and left ventricles, whereas the vessels show a regular crossing, right ventricle (RV), left ventricle (LV), pulmonary trunk (TP), aorta (AO)

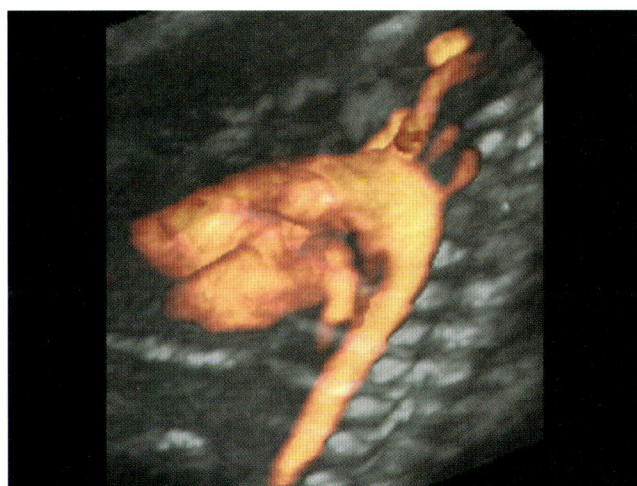

Fig. 43.19: Aortic arch with the origin of the cephalic vessels. Behind the brachiocephalic artery the superior vena cava is seen

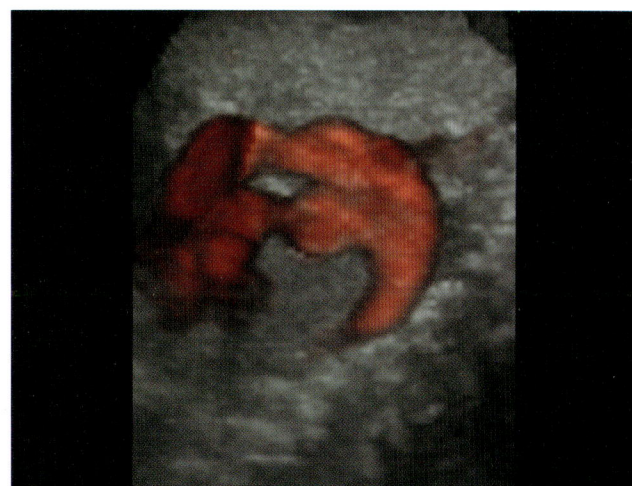

Fig. 43.20: Parallel course of the great vessels in transposition of the great vessels

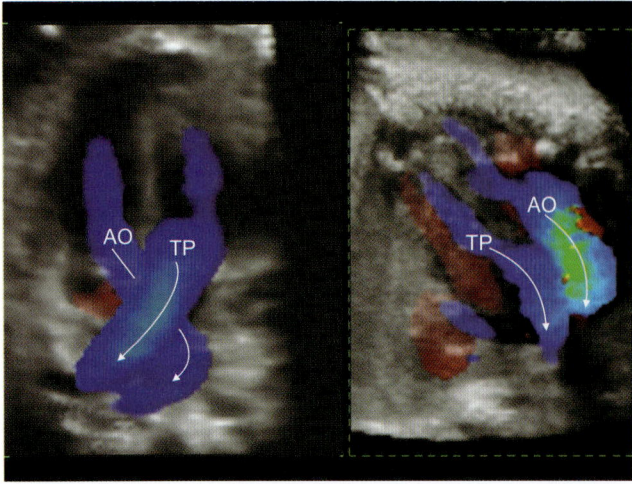

Fig. 43.21: 3D and 4D volume rendering with transparent gray scale and surface color Doppler of two fetuses: On the left a normal finding with the regular crossing of the great vessels. On the right a fetus with transposition of the great arteries with parallel course of both vessels, (TP, pulmonary trunk; AO, aorta)

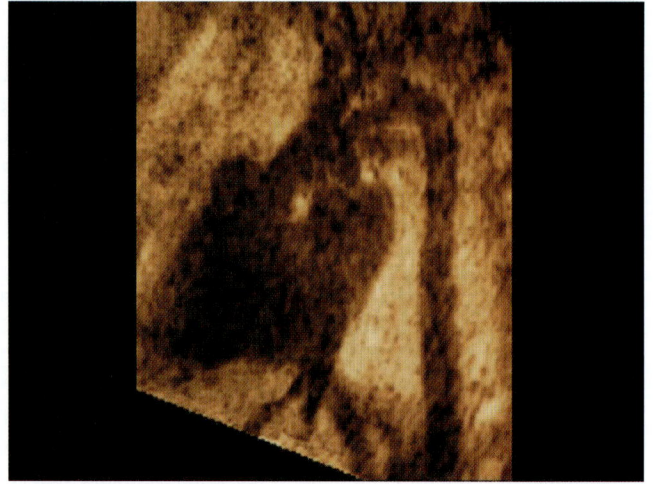

Fig. 43.22: Longitudinal view of the heart, the aortic arch and the hepatic vessels in transparent minimum mode

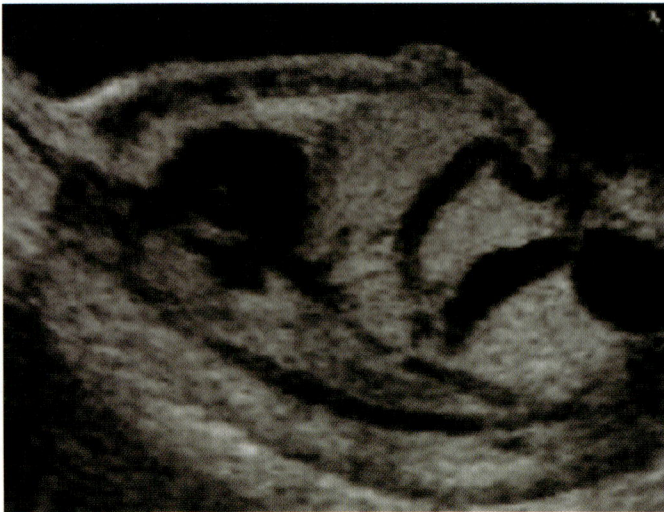

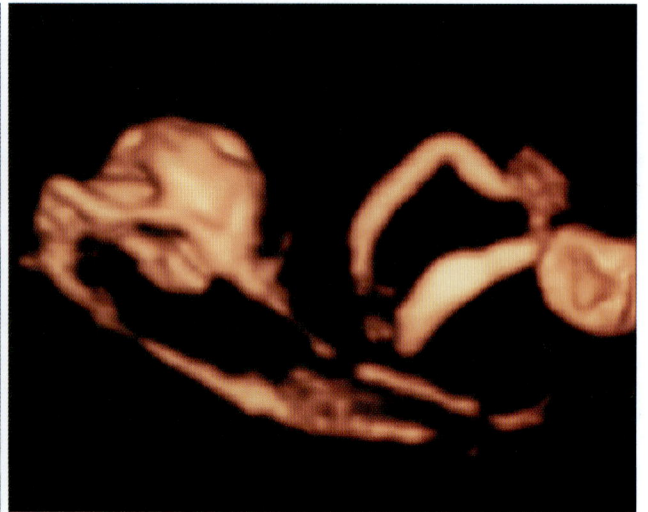

Fig. 43.23: A longitudinal view of a fetal abdomen in minimum mode (left) and inversion mode (right). No blood flow is visualized but hypoechoic structures as gallbladder and urinary bladder in addition to the usual vessels

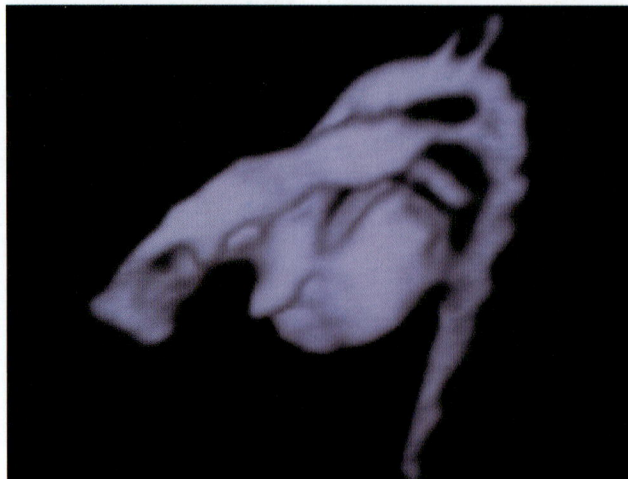

Fig. 43.24: Crossing of the great vessels as demonstrated with the inversion mode

REFERENCES

1. Chaoui R, McEwing R. Three cross-sectional planes for fetal color Doppler echocardiography. Ultrasound Obstet Gynecol. 2003;21(1):81-93.
2. Chaoui R. Color Doppler sonography in the assessment of the fetal heart. In: Nicolaides KH, Rizzo G, Hecher (Eds). Placental and fetal Doppler. London: Parthenon Publishing; 2003. pp. 171-86.
3. Chaoui R. Color Doppler sonography in the diagnosis of fetal abnormalitites. In: Nicolaides KH, Rizzo G, Hecher (Eds). Placental and fetal Doppler. London: Parthenon Publishing; 2000. pp 187-203.
4. Chaoui R, Kalache KD, Hartung J. Application of three-dimensional power Doppler ultrasound in prenatal diagnosis. Ultrasound Obstet Gynecol. 2001;17(1):22-9.
5. Chaoui R, Kalache KD. Three-Dimensional Color Power Imaging: Principles and First Experience in Prenatal Diagnosis. In: Merz E (Ed). 3D Ultrasonography in Obstetrics and Gynecology. Philadelphia: Lippincot Williams and Wilkins; 1998. pp. 35-42.
6. Chaoui R, Kalache KD, Bollmann R. Three-Dimensional color power Doppler in the assessment of fetal vascular anatomy under normal and abnormal conditions. In: Kurjak A (Ed). Three-Dimensional Power Doppler in Obstetrics and Gynecology. New York-London: Parthenon Publishing Group; 2000. pp. 113-9.
7. Lee W, Kalache KD, Chaiworapongsa T, et al. Three-dimensional power Doppler ultrasonography during pregnancy. J Ultrasound Med. 2003;22(1):91-7.
8. Hartung J, Kalache KD, Chaoui R. [Three-dimensional power Doppler ultrasonography (3D-PDU) in fetal diagnosis]. Ultraschall Med. 2004;25(3):200-5.
9. Heling KS, Chaoui R, Bollmann R. Prenatal diagnosis of an aneurysm of the vein of Galen with three-dimensional color power angiography. Ultrasound Obstet Gynecol. 2000;15(4):333-6.
10. Gagel K, Heling KS, Kalache KD, et al. Prenatal diagnosis of an intracranial arteriovenous fistula in the posterior fossa on the basis of color and three-dimensional power Doppler ultrasonography. J Ultrasound Med. 2003;22(12):1399-403.
11. Chaoui R, Kalache KD. Three-dimensional power Doppler ultrasound of the fetal great vessels. Ultrasound Obstet Gynecol. 2001;17(5):455-6.
12. DeVore GR, Falkensammer P, Sklansky MS, et al. Spatio-temporal image correlation (STIC): new technology for evaluation of the fetal heart. Ultrasound Obstet Gynecol. 2003;22(4):380-7.
13. Vinals F, Poblete P, Giuliano A. Spatio-temporal image correlation (STIC): a new tool for the prenatal screening of congenital heart defects. Ultrasound Obstet Gynecol. 2003;22(4):388-94.
14. Chaoui R, Hoffmann J, Heling KS. Three-dimensional (3D) and 4D color Doppler fetal echocardiography using spatio-temporal image correlation (STIC). Ultrasound Obstet Gynecol. 2004;23(6):535-45.
15. Pretorius DH, Nelson TR, Baergen RN, et al. Imaging of placental vasculature using three-dimensional ultrasound and color power Doppler: a preliminary study. Ultrasound Obstet Gynecol. 1998;12(1):45-9.
16. Lee W, Kirk JS, Comstock CH, et al. Vasa previa: prenatal detection by three-dimensional ultrasonography. Ultrasound Obstet Gynecol 2000;16(4):384-7.
17. Pooh RK, Pooh KH. The assessment of fetal brain morphology and circulation by transvaginal 3D sonography and power Doppler. J Perinat Med. 2002;30(1):48-56.
18. Chaoui R. The examination of the normal fetal heart using two-dimensional echocardiography. In: Yagel S, Silvermann N, Gembruch U, (Eds). London New York: Martin Dunitz; 2003. pp. 141-9.
19. Chaoui R, Hoffmann J, Heling KS. Basal Cardiac View on 3D/4D fetal echocardiography for the assessment of AV-Valves and great vessels arrangement. Ultrasound Obstet Gynecol. 2004;22:228-Abstract.
20. Chaoui R, Schneider MBE, Kalache KD. Right aortic arch with vascular ring and aberrant left subclavian artery: prenatal diagnosis assisted by three-dimensional power Doppler ultrasound. Ultrasound Obstet Gynecol. 2003;22(6):661-3.
21. Chaoui R, Kalache KD, Heling KS, et al. 3D Power Doppler Echocardiography: usefulness in spatial visualization of fetal cardiac vessels. Ultrasound Obstet Gynecol. 2003;22:Abstract.

Specific Aspects of Ultrasound Examination in Twin Pregnancies

E Quarello, Y Ville

INTRODUCTION

Although, twins account for only 2% of all pregnancies they are responsible for 20% of perinatal morbidity, and the incidence of twining has increased by 50% over the last 20 years. Embryologically, two-thirds twins are dizygotic, resulting from fertilization of two ovocytes by two spermatozoids. One-third of twins are, therefore, monozygotic resulting from the splitting of one fertilized egg. Depending the time of splitting after fecondation, one-third of monochorionic twins will be dichorionic when this occurs within the first 4 days. The majority, however, will be monochorionic. It is only when splitting occurs after 8 days in 5% of these that the twins are monoamniotic. When splitting occurs after 12 days, the siamese twins will share some organs. Among twin pregnancies, the incidence of perinatal mortality and morbidity is 2–6 times higher in monochorionic pregnancies. Both specific and non-specific complications justify closer surveillance by ultrasound. Indeed, ultrasound examination in twins is subjected to technical difficulties related to the presence of two fetuses in the uterine cavity and this impacts both on biometry, and morphological and functional assessment. Specific features should also be surveyed during ultrasound examination of all twin pregnancies.

DETERMINATION OF CHORIONICITY AND AMNIONICITY (FIGS 44.1A TO H)

Gestational sacs count should not be performed before 6 weeks. Indeed before that, one sac could be left unnoticed. Embryos can be counted from 7 weeks onward and yolk sacs can be identified between 8 and 12 weeks. Amnionicity should not be confirmed before 9 weeks. Prior to 9 weeks of gestation, amnionicity cannot be assessed reliably, even with the use of high frequency vaginal ultrasound probes.[1] Determination of chorionicity is the main determinant of both specific and non-specific complications in twin pregnancies. This is, therefore, the main aim of ultrasound examination in twins. Eighty percent of twin pregnancies are dichorionic. Diagnosis of chorionicity should be made in the first trimester of pregnancy, ideally between 9 and 12 weeks; however, this is still reliable until 14 weeks but it becomes uncertain thereafter when the twins are of the same sex.

Chorionicity Can Be Established Based On

* Gestational sacs count
* Presence of the lambda sign before 14 weeks, as opposed to the T sign in monochorionic pregnancies

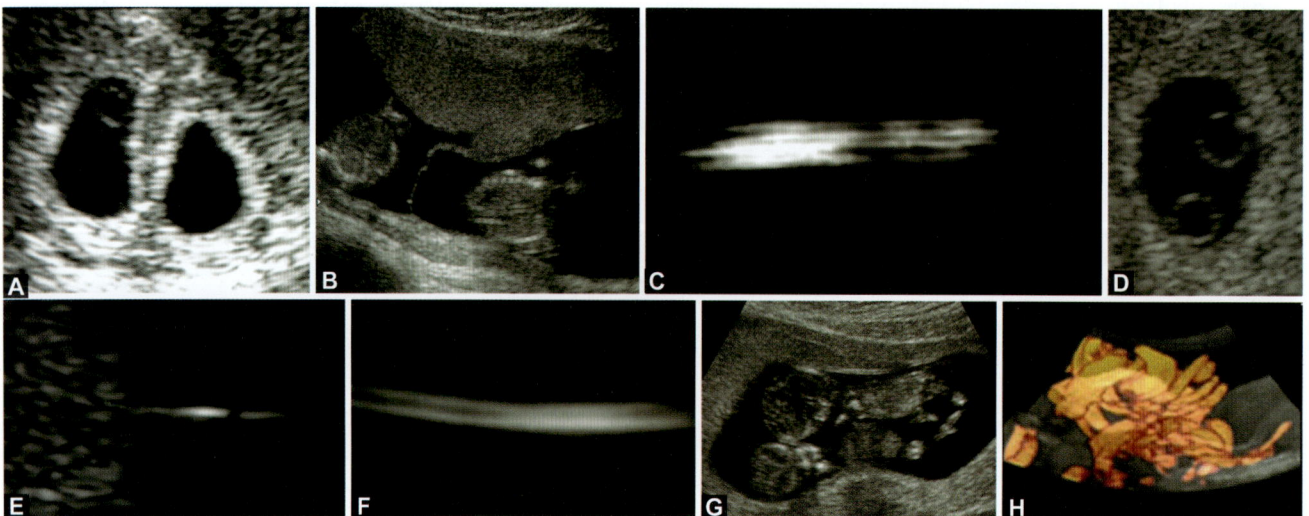

Figs 44.1A to H: Assessment of chorionicity and amnionicity. (A) Dichorionic pregnancy (DCP) before 9 weeks showing two gestational sacs; (B) DCP showing the lambda sign (λ) of the fused chorions; (C) Interamniotic membrane in a DCP at 22 weeks counting more than two layers; (D) Monochorionic pregnancy (MCP) before 9 weeks showing one gestational sac and two yolk sacs; (E) MCP at 12 weeks showing the T sign at the membrane attachment on the placenta without chorion interposition; (F) Interamniotic membrane in an MCP at 22 weeks counting only two layers; (G) Monoamniotic twins at 12 weeks; (H) Cord entanglement in a monoamniotic twin pregnancy at 17 weeks

- Presence of the twin peak
- Identification of two distinct placental masses
- Determination of different fetal genders
- Examination of the intertwin fetal membranes.

The "Lambda" sign[2] and the "twin peak"[3] are specific features of dichorionic pregnancies but have been described at two different gestational periods. They both appear as a thick hyperechoic or isoechoic triangular base of the intertwine membranes on a single placental mass. These feature the triangular projection of villous tissue at the union of two fused chorionic plates. In monochorionic placentae, a single chorionic layer cannot therefore project on the placenta; this features an abrupt junction on the placenta described as the T sign A lambda sign is the guarantee for a dichorionic pregnancy with a sensitivity close to 100%.[4] It can be found throughout the pregnancy but the significance of its absence is reliable only before 14 weeks. Non-visualization of the lambda sign with the presence of the T sign has a positive predictive value for monochorionicity close to 100%.

The presence of two placental masses is predictive of a dichorionic pregnancy; however, this may feature a placenta bipartita in up to 15% of these cases. Monochorionicity cannot be confirmed by the presence of a single placental mass since two separate placentae are frequently fused after 15 weeks. The presence of vascular anastomoses on the chorionic plate joining the two funicular circulations is a specific feature of monochorionicity but is time consuming and its reproducibility remains to be established.

Different fetal genders are specific of dichorionicity since it would confirm a dizygotic pregnancy. The reverse is not true.

Intertwin membrane is the result of the fusion of two amniotic and two chorionic layers in dichorionic pregnancies. This is made of only two amniotic layers in monochorionic-diamniotic pregnancies. In the late second and third trimester, ultrasound examination can assess the thickness of the intertwin membranes using cutoff measurements of 1.5 or 2 mm or better counting 2 or 4 layers in monochorionic and in dichorionic pregnancies respectively. Technically, this requires to use magnification and the lowest gain possible and an angle of insonation to the membranes close to 45°. A right angle, although theoretically more suitable is subjected to more artefactual images.

Amnionicity Can Be Determined Upon

- Visualization of the interamniotic membrane. However, non-visualization of the membrane in a diamniotic pregnancy can arise due to technical difficulties, mainly before 8 weeks of pregnancy or in obese patients.
- Visualization of the yolk sacs and extra-amniotic spaces. The number of yolk sacs and extra-amniotic spaces matches the number of amniotic sacs. Two yolk sacs are seen in monochorionic diamniotic pregnancies and only one in monoamniotic pregnancies.[5] They can be seen as non-contiguous in dichorionic pregnancies.
- Cords entanglement in monoamniotic twins can be best visualized using color Doppler. Doppler flow within the cord mass should also show a biphasic arterial flow.
- Conjoined twins can only be seen in monoamniotic pregnancies and can be suspected when visualizing close proximity of both twins which also show concomitant movements.

Examination before 15 Weeks

Examination before 15 weeks is critical and a well-documented picture should be kept in the notes in order to confirm chorionicity whenever clinically relevant later on in pregnancy.

NUCHAL TRANSLUCENCY MEASUREMENT IN TWIN PREGNANCIES

Nuchal translucency measurement can be used in twins to reliably screen for fetal aneuploidy. The false positive rate for each dichorionic twin is 5% and is, therefore, similar to that in singletons. However, in monochorionic twins, nuchal translucency is measured above the 95th centile for CRL in either twin in as much as 8.5% of the cases. Sebire et al. reported an 88% detection rate for a false positive rate per pregnancy of around 10% and 15% in dichorionic and in monochorionic pregnancies respectively.[6] Discordance of NT measurements between monochorionic twins is also predictive of the development of twin-to-twin transfusion syndrome (TTTS) with a sensitivity of 33% and a positive predictive value of 28%. The likelihood ratio of developing TTTS at 10–14 weeks of gestation is 4.2 (IC 95%, 3.0–6.0).[6]

SPECIFIC COMPLICATIONS OF MONOCHORIONIC TWINS

Twin-to-Twin Transfusion Syndrome (Figs 44.2A to G)

In all monochorionic pregnancies, a single placental mass implies that the two fetuses share some placental units with a shared vascularization of these cotyledons. An imbalance in placental sharing will arise in around 15% of monochorionic pregnancies.[6] Indeed the natural history of monochorionic twins as observed by serial ultrasound examination suggest that up to 28% of all monochorionic twins scanned at 12 weeks will show some discrepancy either in abdominal circumference or in amniotic fluid volume, with membrane folding at 16–18 weeks but only up to half of these (14% of the starting number) will develop twin-to-twin transfusion syndrome in the second or early third trimester;[6,7] Twin-to-twin transfusion syndrome results from an acute hemodynamic imbalance through the vascular placental anastomoses. The Donor twin becomes hypovolemic, oliguric and around two-thirds of these will also show some degree of growth restriction. Oligohydramnios develops in this sac. There is hypervolemia in the recipient twin who is therefore polyuric leading to polyhydramnios in its sac and is exposed to high output cardiac failure. Although a net transfer of blood is likely to initiate it, this is not the only mechanism involved in the syndrome. In order to maintain volemia, the fetal renin-angiotensin system is activated in the donor twin and suppressed in the recipient with preferential maternal-fetal transfer of fluid to the recipient.[8] A paradoxical effect of a transfer of renin toward the recipient twin through the placental anastomoses could also contribute to the development of hypertension and cardiomyopathy in this fetus. A velamentous insertion of the cord of either twin on the placenta is found in up to 30–50% of all monochorionic pregnancies and this is likely to play a significant role in creating hemodynamic imbalance between the two fetoplacental circulations.

The diagnosis of TTTS requires that the pregnancy is monochorionic and relies on the association of polyuria-related

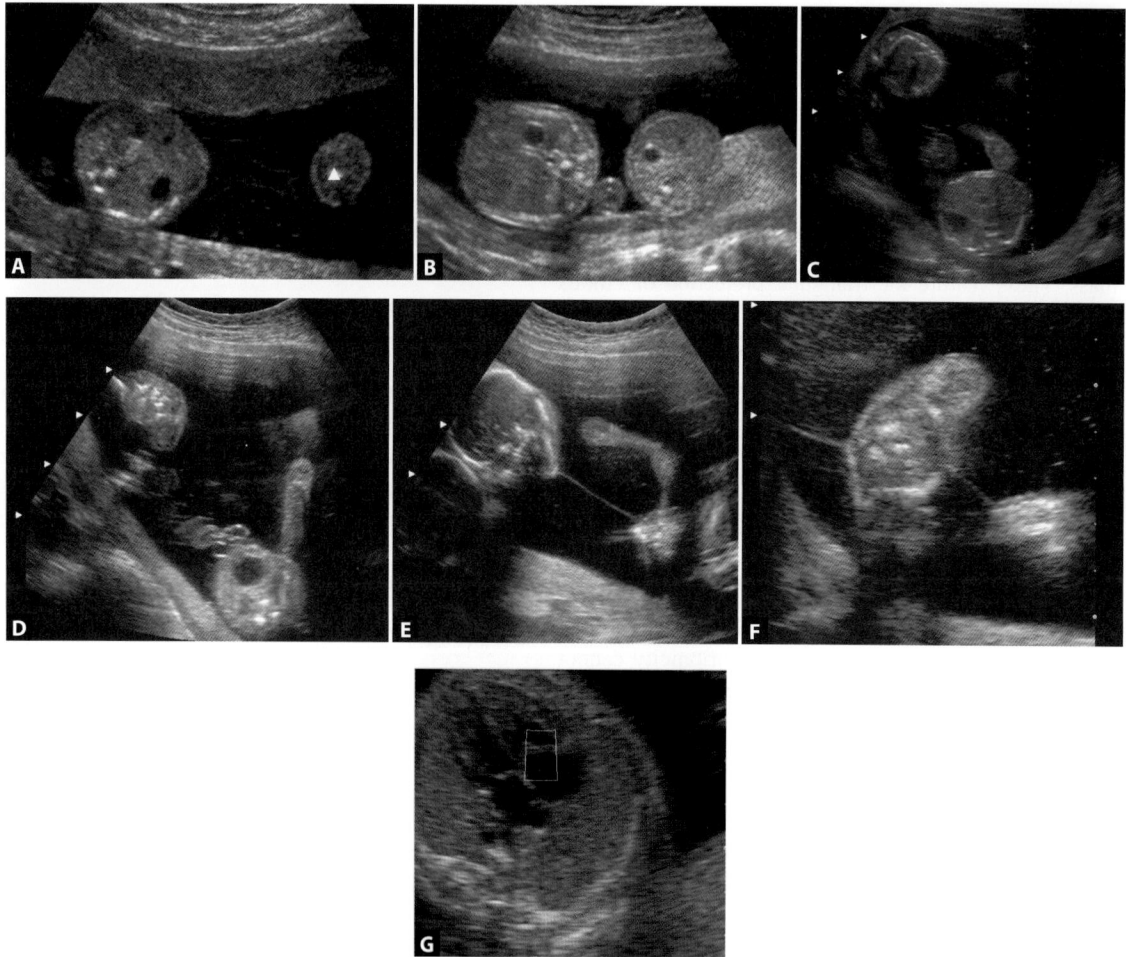

Figs 44.2A to G: (A) Folding of the membranes (arrowhead) in a monochorionic twin pregnancy at 17 weeks; (B) Cross section through the fetal abdomen of two monochorionic twins discordant for growth at 20 weeks; (C) Cross section through the fetal abdomen of the stuck donor twin in anhydramnios against the uterine wall and the recipient twin in polyhydramnios in twin-to-twin transfusion syndrome; (D) Cross section through the fetal pelvis of the stuck donor and of the recipient showing absent and distended bladder respectively; (E) The donor in anhydramnios is wrapped in its membranes as shown in a sagittal plane; F. and in a cross section through the pelvis showing an empty bladder. This "sling sign" could lead to the false impression that the amniotic fluid volume is normal on both sides of a floating intertwin membrane; (G) Examination of the recipient's 4-chamber view of the heart with color Doppler showing tricuspid regurgitation

polyhydramnios in the recipient-twin together with oliguria-related oligohydramnios in the donor twin. Polyhydramnios is defined by a vertical deepest pool of amniotic fluid of at least 8 cm before 20 weeks and 10 cm thereafter, and oligohydramnios is present when the deepest fluid is at least 2 cm. Up to 28% of all monochorionic twins seen at 12 weeks on ultrasound will develop some discrepancy in the volume of amniotic fluid and/or a discrepancy in size[6] by 16–18 weeks. This does not meet the criteria for TTTS and has led to a long-standing misunderstanding on the diagnosis and the prognosis of TTTS. It is only half of these, therefore 14% of the starting number which will develop the polyoligohydramnios sequence. The fetal size, although the recipient is usually appropriately grown and the donor is usually smaller is not an important criteria for the diagnosis of TTTS.

When oligohydramnios confines to anhydramnios, the intertwin membranes are difficult to visualize and the donor twin is "stuck" on the placenta or the uterine wall. This can lead to a false diagnosis of monoamniotic pregnancy or the suspicion of various malformations in the compressed donor twin. Pushing the abdominal wall in regard to the donor twin will demonstrate that this twin cannot move due to anhydramnios. Hypervolemia in the recipient often shows a cardiothoracic index of more than 0.55 with a thick myocardium and the presence of tricuspid regurgitation, which has no prognostic value when the recipient is not hydropic. The best first line treatment consists of fetoscopic surgery to coagulate the anastomotic chorionic plate vessels.[9]

Arterial and venous fetal Doppler can be normal or show absent or reverse end diastolic flow in the umbilical arteries. Absent or reverse flow in the A-wave of the ductus venosus usually corresponds to severe hypoxemia or cardiac overload in the donor or the recipient twin respectively. Peak-systolic velocities in the middle cerebral artery is sensitive to anemia and to polycythemia showing values above 1.5 MoM or below 0.7 MoM respectively.[10] However, a difference in hemoglobin is unusual in utero in most cases of TTTS.[11]

Quintero[12] has proposed a classification of TTTS in four stages, which has the advantage of homogenizing the diagnostic criteria. Stage 1 corresponds to the association of polyhydramnios in the recipient and oligohydramnios in the donor, which bladder is visible. Stage 2 is similar but the bladder cannot be visualized in the donor. In Stage 3, Doppler examination shows marked abnormalities with absent or reversed end diastolic flow or, absent or reversed a wave in the umbilical arteries or in the ductus venosus respectively. Stage 4 is characterized by the presence of hydrops in either twin. Stage 5 is when one or both twins have died in utero.

Twin-to-twin transfusion syndrome can also develop in monoamniotic pregnancies. Polyuric polyhydramnios is then seen together with a small or unseen bladder in its co-twin.

Acardiac Twin

The acardiac twin is defined by the presence of one monochorionic twins without a clearly anatomically defined heart; the co-twin is usually normal. Vascularization of the monochorionic placenta almost invariably shows the presence of two superficial anastomoses between the two cord insertions: one artery-to-artery and one vein-to-vein anastomoses flowing in opposite directions. There is usually a single umbilical artery in the cord of the acardiac twin and this sets the basis for an increased cardiac workload in the normal twin also named the pump-twin. The acardiac mass can grow and develop to various degrees, increasing the mass of tissue which the normal twin heart has to bear (Figs 44.3A to C). This can, therefore, lead to the development of high-cardiac output hydrops in up to 50% of pump-twins. The bigger the acardiac mass, the higher the likelihood for hemodynamic decompensation of the pump twin.[13] The acardiac twin usually bears several major malformations allowing for embryological classification,[13] the most frequent being the acardiac acephalus; however, rudimentary organs, especially limbs and spine, are often present. Early in the pregnancy, this is often mistaken for either an early embryonic demise or for a placental tumor. The key to the diagnosis is the use of color Doppler showing retrograde perfusion of the acardiac mass, and eventually demonstrating the placental anastomoses.

Monoamniotic Pregnancies

The fetuses will be seen in close proximity and both crossing of their limbs and cord entanglement as seen by color Doppler will establish the diagnosis.

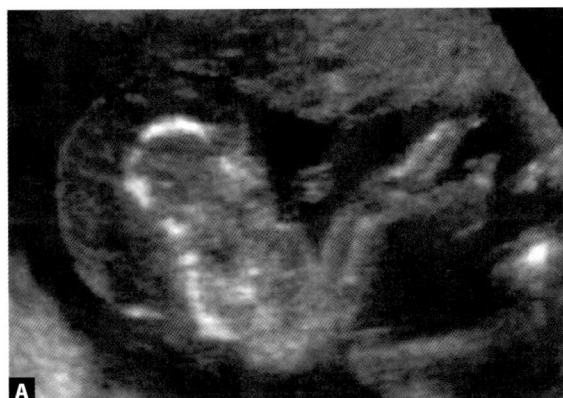

Conjoined Twins

These are 4–5% of all monochorionic-monoamniotic twins. The embryological classification refers to the part of their body through which they are attached; the most frequent type being thoracopagus.[14] Organ sharing can be symmetrical or asymmetrical. The extreme form of the latter constitutes the fetus-in-fetu where a rudimentary fetal mass can be found as a hyperechogenic tumoral mass into an otherwise usually normal fetus, child or even adult.

There is a clear benefit for an early diagnosis of a unique embryonic mass often characterized by the presence of two beating hearts. Embryonic/fetal movements are always simultaneous and a single umbilical cord with more than three vessels can be identified.

AMNIOTIC FLUID VOLUME IN TWIN PREGNANCIES

Oligohydramnios, Anahydramnios and the Stuck Twin Phenomenon

All causes of oligohydramnios in singleton can affect one or both twins and should be investigated in the same way. The stuck-twin phenomenon can, therefore, affect both monochorionic and dichorionic pregnancies to the same extent. However, when oligohydramnios affects only one twin, the twin with a normal amount of fluid is often unduly credited for having polyhydramnios and a wrong diagnosis of twin-to-twin transfusion syndrome is often suspected. It is therefore critical to use an objective measurement of the amniotic volume, mainly using the deepest pool measurement.[15] Another important pitfall is to consider that two layers of membranes tightly wrapped around the stuck-twin, featuring the "sling-sign"[16] could be mistaken as free-floating membranes separating two cavities with a normal amount of fluid in each sac. Etiologies that are more prone to affect twins include: low urinary tract obstruction, severe intrauterine growth retardation and preterm prelabor rupture of the membranes.

Polyhydramnios in Twins

All malformations seen in singletons such as anencephaly, bowel atresia are more frequent in twins.

Monochorionic twins, however, are the only one to see acute polyhydramnios developing polyhydramnios due to TTTS.

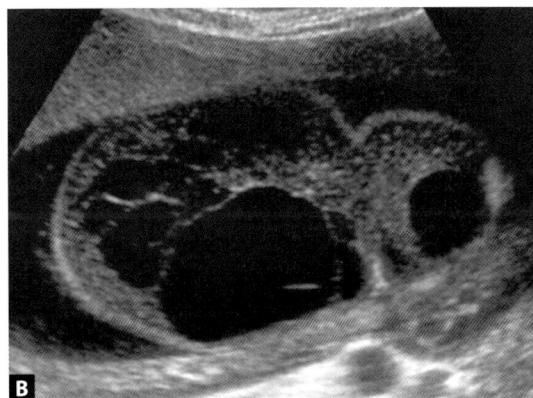

Figs 44.3 A and B: (A) Monochorionic twin pregnancy showing an acardiac twin at 13 weeks showing rudimentary head, spine and lower extremities; (B) Edematous acardiac mass at 25 weeks.

CERVICAL CHANGES IN TWIN PREGNANCIES

Although, twin pregnancies are 1% of all pregnancies and 2% of all deliveries, twins account for 15% of all maternal morbidity and mortality. This is mainly due to preterm delivery with 12% of all preterm neonates being twins.

The advantage of cervical ultrasound over digital examination has also clearly been shown in twins. Relative risk of preterm delivery within a week of cervical ultrasound examination has been reviewed by Ong et al.[17] as 4.1 (95% CI, 1.10–15.47) and 11.7. (95% CI, 4.23), respectively, for values lower than the thresholds of 25 mm and 20 mm.

GROWTH DISCORDANCE IN TWINS

This is the second most frequent complication in twins and the second contributor to neonatal mortality and morbidity. Conflict of interest may arise between twins as to define optimal timing for delivery. In the second and third trimesters of pregnancy, the cutoff value for EBW estimate is of at least 20%.

MALFORMATIONS IN TWINS

The presence of two embryos/fetuses increases the risk as compared to singletons. A recent series[18] has gathered data on 260,000 twin pregnancies among 12 millions births. Around 5,500 twin pregnancies carry at least one malformed twin outside specific risks associated with monochorionicity representing 2.14% vs 1.72% for singletons. Around 101 malformative sequences have been reported, 37 of which are more prevalent in twins. The prevalence of fetal malformations in twins is, therefore, of around 25% with relative risks of 8–60%. Dizygotic twins only carry non-specific malformations. Monochorionic twins will bear malformations both non-specific and specific to monochorionicity. Specific malformations include those arising from a delay in zygotic splitting or midline abnormalities as well as those resulting from a sequence of events following severe hemodynamic imbalance through placental anastomoses. Furthermore, only 5–20% of monozygotic pregnancies are concordant for fetal malformations.[19] These differences can also arise from post-zygotic genetic abnormalities, different susceptibility to their exposure to environmental factors.

INTRAUTERINE FETAL DEATH OF ONE TWIN

Perinatal mortality in twins is up to sevenfold higher than in singletons.[20] Intrauterine death of one twin can result from non-specific fetal complications such as these seen in singletons, including cord compression and severe growth restriction as well as from specific complications related to hemodynamic imbalance, including TTTS and collapse. In monochorionic twins, the death of one fetus will threaten its co-twin by causing an abrupt and profound drop in systemic blood pressure subsequent to the exsanguinations of the survivor in its dead co-twin and its placenta through the intertwin anastomoses. Peak-systolic velocities in the mid cerebral arteries of the survivor measured above 1.5 MoM within 24 hours of the co-twin's death will predict anemia/hypovolemia in this twin (sensitivity 90% for a 10% false positive rate).[10] Exsanguination will lead to fetal death or severe ischemic sequelae in the survivor in 25% and 25% of the cases respectively. Ischemia-related malformations include cerebral lesions such as periventricular leukomalacia, porencephaly, hydrocephalus and migrational anomalies; renal ischemia and mesenteric ischemia leading to bowel atresia. These lesions will only be amenable to prenatal diagnosis from 2–3 weeks following the acute event.

In dichorionic pregnancies, the co-twin will only be exposed to a persistent cause of death and to prematurity.[21,22]

REFERENCES

1. Monteagudo A, Timor-Tritsch IE, Sharma S. Early and simple determination of chorionic and amniotic type in multifetal gestations in the first fourteen weeks by high-frequency transvaginal ultrasonography. Am J Obstet Gynecol. 1994;170:824-9.
2. Bessis R, Papiernick E. Echographic imagery of amniotic membranes in twin pregnancies. In: Gedda L, Parisi P(Eds). Twin Research 3: Twin Biology and Multiple Pregnancy. New York: Alan R Liss; 1981. pp. 183-7.
3. Finberg HJ. The 'twin peak' sign: a reliable evidence of dichorionic twinning. J Ultrasound Med. 1992;11:571-7.
4. Sepulveda W, Sebire NJ, Hughes K, et al. The lambda sign at 10-14 weeks of gestation as a predictor of chorionicity in twin pregnancies. Ultrasound Obstet Gynecol. 1996;7:421-3.
5. Bromley B, Benacerraf B. Using the number of yolk sac to determine amnionicity in early first trimester monochorionic twins. J Ultrasound Med. 1995;14:415-9.
6. Sebire NJ, Souka A, Skentou H, et al. Early prediction of severe twin-to-twin transfusion syndrome. Human Reprod. 2000;15:2008-10.
7. Sebire NJ, d'Ercole C, Carvelho M, et al. Inter-twin membrane folding in monochorionic pregnancies. Ultrasound Obstet Gynecol. 1998;11:324-7.
8. Mahieu-Caputo D, Dommergues M, Delezoide AL, et al. Twin-twin transfusion syndrome. Role of the fetal renin-angiotensin system. Am J Pathol. 2000;156:629-6.
9. Senat MV, Deprest J, Boulvain M, et al. Endoscopic laser surgery versus serial amnioreduction for severe twin-to-twin transfusion syndrome. N Engl J Med. 2004;351(2):136-44.
10. Senat MV, Loizeau S, Couderc S, et al. The value of middle cerebral artery peak systolic velocity in the diagnosis of fetal anemia after intrauterine death of one monochorionic twin. Am J Obstet Gynecol. 2003;189:1320-4.

11. Denbow M, Fogliani R, Kyle P, et al. Haematological indices at fetal blood sampling in monochorionic pregnancies complicated by feto-fetal transfusion syndrome. Prenat Diagn. 1998;18:941-6.

12. Quintero R, Morales WJ, Allen MH. Staging of twin-to-twin transfusion syndrome. J Perinat. 1999;19:550-5.

13. Moore TR, Gale S , Benirschke K. Perinatal outcome of 49 pregnancies complicated by acardiac twining. Am J Obstet Gynecol. 1990;163:907-12.

14. Spencer R. Parasitic conjoined twins: external, internal, detached. Clin Anat. 2001;14:428-44.

15. Hill LM, Krohn M, Lazebnik N, et al. The amniotic fluid index in normal twin pregnancies. Am J Obstet Gynecol. 2000;182:950-4.

16. Al-Kouatly HB, Skupski DW. Intrauterine sling: a complication of the stuck twin syndrome. Ultrasound Obstet Gynecol. 1999;14:419-21.

17. Ong S, Smith A, Smith N, et al. Cervical length assessment in twin pregnancies using transvaginal ultrasound. Acta Obstet Gynecol Scand. 2000;79:851-3.

18. Mastroiacovo P, Castilla EE, Arpino C, et al. Congenital malformations in twins: an international study. Am J Med Gen. 1999;83:117-24.

19. Schinzel AAGL, Smith DW, Miller JR. Monozygotic twinning and structural defects. J Pediatr. 1979;95:921-30.

20. Benirschke K, Kim CK. Multiple pregnancy. N Engl J Med. 1973;14:1276-83.

21. Bajoria R, Wee LY, Anwar S, et al. Outcome of twin pregnancies complicated by single intrauterine death in relation to vascular anatomy of the monochorionic placenta. Human Reprod. 1999;14:2124-30.

22. Fusi L, Gordon H. Twin pregnancy complicated by single intrauterine death. Problems and outcome with conservative management. BJOG. 1990;97:511-6.

45 Echocardiography in Early Pregnancy: A New Challenge in Prenatal Diagnosis

C Comas, JM Martinez, A Galindo

INTRODUCTION

Prenatal detection of fetal congenital heart defects (CHD) remains the most problematic issue of prenatal diagnosis.[1] Major CHD are the most common severe congenital malformations, with an incidence of about 5 in a thousand live births, whenever complete ascertainment is done and minor lesions are excluded.[1,2] Congenital heart anomalies have a significant effect on affected children's life with up to 25–35% mortality rate during pregnancy and the postnatal period, and it is during the first year of life, when the 60% of this mortality occurs. Moreover, major CHD are responsible for nearly 50% of all neonatal and infant deaths due to congenital anomalies, and it is likely to be significantly higher if spontaneous abortions are considered. Although, CHD use to appear isolated, they are frequently associated with other defects, chromosomal anomalies and genetic syndromes. Their incidence is six times greater than chromosomal abnormalities and four times greater than neural tube defects.[1-3]

Most major CHD can be diagnosed prenatally by detailed transabdominal second trimester echocardiography at 20–22 weeks of gestation.[1,3-6] The identification of pregnancies at high-risk for CHD needing referral to specialist centers is of paramount importance in order to reduce the rate of overlooked defects.[6,7] However, the main problem in prenatal diagnosis of CHD is that the majority of cases take place in pregnancies with no identifiable risk factors. Therefore, there is wide agreement that cardiac ultrasound screening should be introduced as an integral part of the routine scan at 20–22 weeks. When applied to low-risk population, scrutiny of the four chamber view allows only the detection of 40% of the anomalies while additional visualization of the outflow tracts and the great arteries increase the rate up to 60–70%.[3-5]

Recently, the finding of an increased nuchal translucency[8,9] or an altered ductus venosus blood flow[10,11] at 10–14 weeks of gestation have been associated with a high-risk for CHD and their prevalence increase exponentially with the thickness of nuchal translucency[8] regardless the fetal karyotype. Since, earlier diagnosis of congenital malformations is increasingly demanded, the option of an early fetal echocardiography must be taken into account.[12-14] The use of high-frequency vaginal ultrasound probes along with substantial improvements in magnification and processing of the imaging, together with the introduction of color Doppler, have extensively contributed to the development of the technique, allowing better visualization of cardiac structures earlier in pregnancy.[12,15,16] Although, most of the groups perform early fetal echocardiography between 13 and 16 weeks of gestation, we can name it as so when performed before the 18th week of gestation. Despite several studies that stated that fetal heart examination could be incorporated in first or early second trimester examinations, its use is currently still limited to a few specialized centers.

TECHNICAL ISSUES

Regarding early fetal echocardiography, some institutions use predominantly the transvaginal (TV) approach[14,17-22] while others prefer the transabdominal one.[23-26] Most of the authors reporting early fetal echocardiography prefer the TV approach due to its increased resolution associated with higher frequency transducers and also because given that equivalent tranducers frequencies, the TV probes provide better quality images.[27] However, most importantly, authors with background training as pediatric cardiologists are more likely to use the transabdominal approach in contrast with most of obstetricians, who are well used to the TV route. The superiority of transvaginal sonography is usually well accepted before the 14th week. Between 15th and 18th week both transabdominal and transvaginal routes seem to offer similar advantages and disadvantages, and beyond the 18th week the transabdominal echocardiography seems to achieve better results.[1,5,16,27,28]

The combination of two-dimensional echocardiography with color Doppler flow imaging proved generally helpful, in particular by visualization of blood flow on both great arteries and of two divided ventricular inflows. The addition of color Doppler flow studies provides substantial improvement in the diagnostic accuracy of early echocardiography, as was also shown by DeVore for transabdominal sonography in the second half of pregnancy.[29]

When performing early fetal echocardiography, we firstly recommend to scan by the TV route, following the examination by the transabdominal probe when a complete study is not possible. The highest frequency must always be used, whatever the route is chosen. Obviously, a high-resolution real-time ultrasound has to be used. For color Doppler evaluation, the energy output levels have to be lower than 50 mW/cm^2 spatial peak-temporal average. Since color Doppler is dissipated over a wide area of interest, thermal effects resulting from Doppler insonation should not be a matter of concern, unlike pulse Doppler in which the whole energy of the beam is focused at a specific location. Besides, the embryonic developmental of the heart has been completed by the time the scan is performed.

ULTRASOUND ANATOMY OF THE NORMAL HEART

Embryonic heart beat can be detected as early as the fifth week of gestation, and normal development of its function shows an increasing heart rate from 80–90 beats per minute at 5 weeks of gestation to 170–180 beats per minute at the end of the 9–10th week. As pregnancy progresses, the control of the heart rate matures with increasing vagal dominance, and the baseline rate declines to 145–155 beats per minute with the appearance of beat to beat variation, most likely resulting from the functional adaptation to the development of the heart and autonomic nervous system maturation, and remains more or less constant during the rest of intrauterine life.[30,31]

The structural development of the heart begins on day 16 and it is finished by the 10th week. Early fetal echocardiography has the same goals that the standard one, and we advocate to perform it in a segmental approach. The first objective of the examination is to assess the normality of the four chamber view through a transverse section of the fetal chest: normal situs solitus; normal size and axis of the heart in relation to the chest; both atria equal in size, with the foramen ovale flapping within the left atrium; both ventricles equal in size and contractility; atrial and ventricular septa are of normal appearance; tricuspid and mitral valves are normally inserted, opening and closing together. Color and pulsed Doppler are particulary useful to confirm normal inflow to the ventricles and to detect turbulent flow or jets suggesting valve regurgitation. It is useful to assess the four-chambers in different views: apical, basal and long axis with the interventricular septum perpendicular to the ultrasound beam in order to visualize the better integrity of the septum. Then, the origin and double crossing of the great arteries must be correctly identified: the left ventricle outflow tract, with the continuity between the interventricular septum and the anterior wall of the ascending aorta; the right ventricle outflow tract, more superior, anterior, almost perpendicular to the axis of the ascending aorta and connecting to the descending aorta in the three vessels view. Color Doppler is also helpful to better visualize the outflow tracts, confirm anterograde flow through the semilunar valves and great arteries, and makes easier the examination of both aortic and ductal archs and their confluence. Pulsed Doppler may be used to assess blood flow through the aortic and pulmonic valves in order to confirm normal anterograde flow and to detect very high velocities suggesting valve stenosis. Finally, color and pulsed Doppler are also very useful to identify normal systemic and pulmonary venous return. Figures 45.1 to 45.10 illustrates images obtained at early fetal scan by 2D echocardiography and color Doppler in a structurally normal heart. In our experience, the average duration of the complete fetal cardiac scan is over 15 minutes. It essentially depends on the gestational age at the examination, and can be even shorter if there is a favorable fetal life. In our setting, a subsequent transabdominal echocardiography is scheduled for all our patients at 20–22 weeks of gestation.

Most of the authors agree that the best window of time to perform the early echocardiography is between the 13 weeks and 16 weeks of gestation, since a complete cardiac examination is rarely achieved before the 13th week of gestation.[14,17,18,20-22,26] Articles on early fetal echocardiography demonstrate an increase in visualization rates of the four-chamber view and the outflow tracts in the last decade, with visualization rates greater than 90% at 13 weeks of gestation.[28] To maximize the reduction of uninterpretable examinations, early fetal echocardiography should be preferably performed at 13 completed weeks of gestation. Using current technology, the four-chamber view and the outflow tracts are often demonstrated by two-dimensional echocardiography only, but color Doppler imaging enhances and makes the identification of the structures faster, increasing the success rate of the examination, and allows even earlier identification of the structures.

DIAGNOSIS OF CONGENITAL HEART DEFECTS

The first diagnosis of a CHD by early echocardiography was reported by Gembruch et al.[32] in 1990. A complete atrioventricular canal defect, with complete heart block and atrioventricular valve regurgitation was diagnosed at 11 weeks + 4 days' gestation using a 5-MHz transvaginal probe.

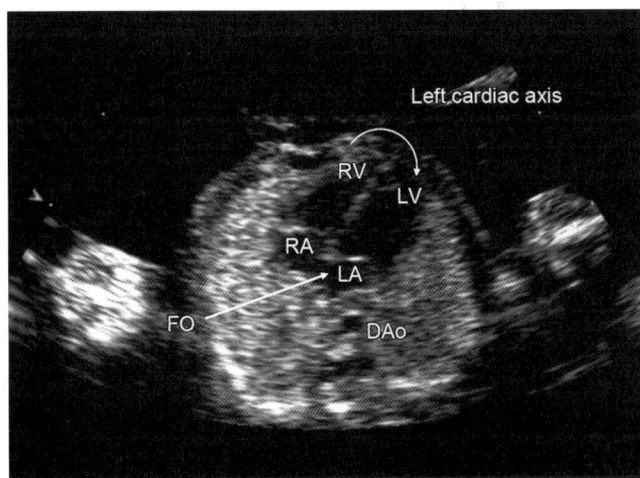

Fig. 45.1: Early fetal echocardiography by 2D in a structurally normal heart. The 4 chamber-view: normal situs solitus; normal size and axis of the heart in relation to the chest; both atria equal in size, with the foramen ovale flapping within the left atrium; both ventricles equal in size and contractility; atrial and ventricular septa are of normal appearance; tricuspid and mitral valves are normally inserted; RV, right ventricle; LV, left ventricle; RA, right atrium; LA, left atrium; FO, foramen ovale; DAo, descending aorta

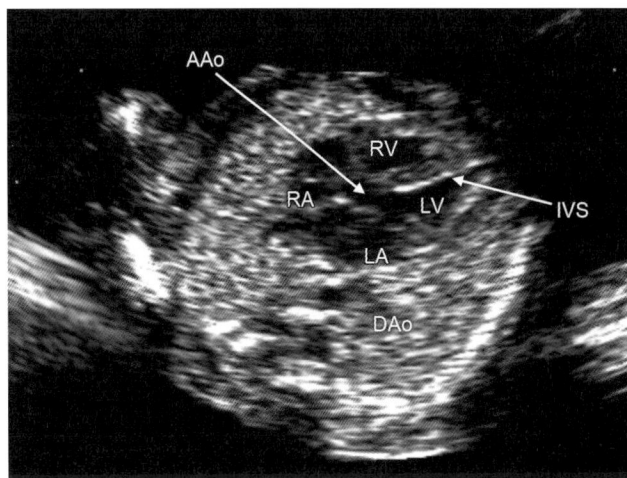

Fig. 45.2: Early fetal echocardiography by 2D in a structurally normal heart. The 5 chamber-view: left ventricle outflow tract in the long axis view showing the continuity between the interventricular septum and the anterior wall of the ascending aorta. RV, right ventricle; LV, left ventricle; RA, right atrium; LA, left atrium; AAo, ascending aorta; DAo, descending aorta; IVS, interventricular septum

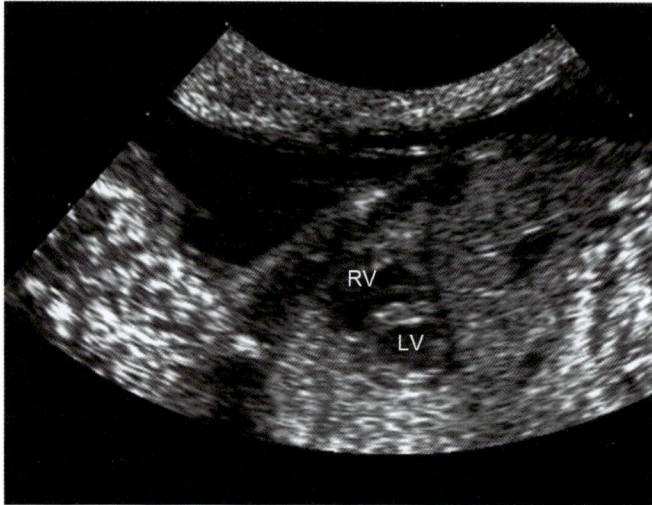

Fig. 45.3: Early fetal echocardiography by 2D in a structurally normal heart. The short axis view, showing an anterior right ventricle and a posterior left ventricle. RV, right ventricle; LV, left ventricle

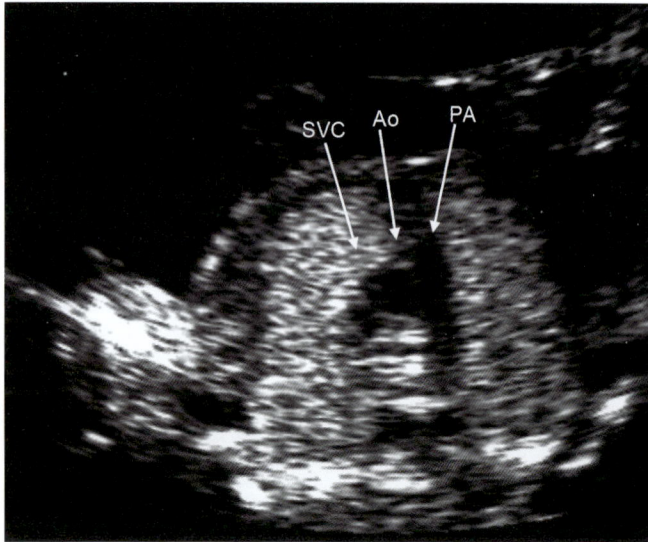

Fig. 45.4: Early fetal echocardiography by 2D in a structurally normal heart. The 3 vessel-view: Cross-sections of the pulmonary artery, ascending aorta and superior vena cava in a transverse view of upper mediastinum. In normal conditions, the structures in the 3 vessel-view are in descending order of size from left to the right. PA, pulmonary artery; Ao, aorta; SVC, superior vena cava

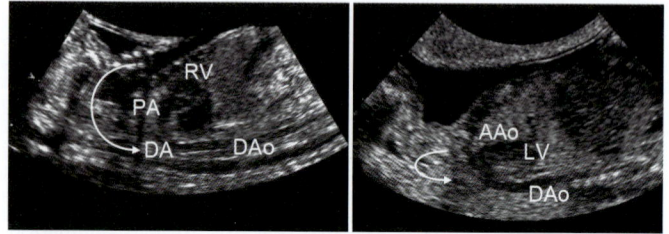

Fig. 45.5: Early fetal echocardiography by 2D in a structurally normal heart.The left sagital view of ductal and aortic archs. RV, right ventricle; LV, left ventricle; PA, pulmonary artery; DA, ductus arteriosus; DAo, descending aorta; AAo, ascending aorta

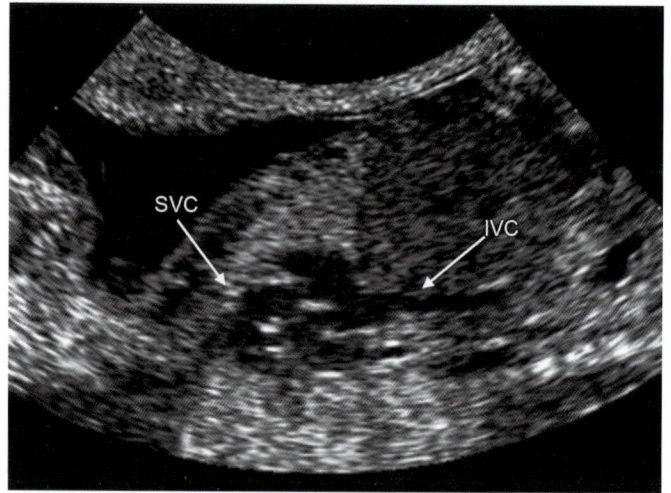

Fig. 45.6: Early fetal echocardiography by 2D in a structurally normal heart. Systemic venous return to the right atrium throw the superior and inferior vena cava. SVC, superior vena cava; IVC, inferior vena cava

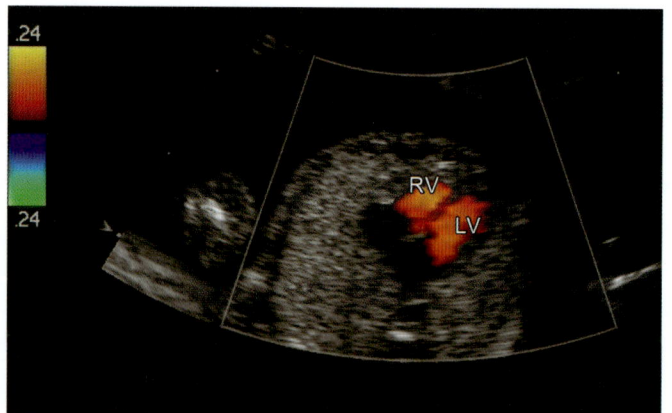

Fig. 45.7: Early fetal echocardiography by 2D and color Doppler in a structurally normal heart. Color Doppler in the 4 chamber view is particulary useful to confirm normal inflow to the ventricles and to detect turbulent flow or jets suggesting valve regurgitation. RV, right ventricle; LV, left ventricle

The same year, Bronshtein et al.[33] reported the diagnosis of a ventricular septal defect (VSD) with overriding aorta and a further case of an isolated VSD with pericardial effusion, both cases at 14 weeks of gestation. Since then, an increasing number of case reports and series on the early diagnosis of CHD have been reported, both in high-risk and low-risk population. Tables 45.1 and 45.2 summarizes some of the largest and most significant studies on the detection of CHD using early fetal echocardiography in high-risk and low-risk pregnancies.[14,17-22,24-26,34-39] Obviously, studies in unselected population report less encouraging results, with lower visualization rates and detection rates. The largest series so far is the one published by Bronshtein et al.[20] They report the diagnosis of 173 cases of CHD over 36,323 fetuses evaluated by transvaginal ultrasound at 11–17 weeks of gestation over a 14-year period of time, with 99%

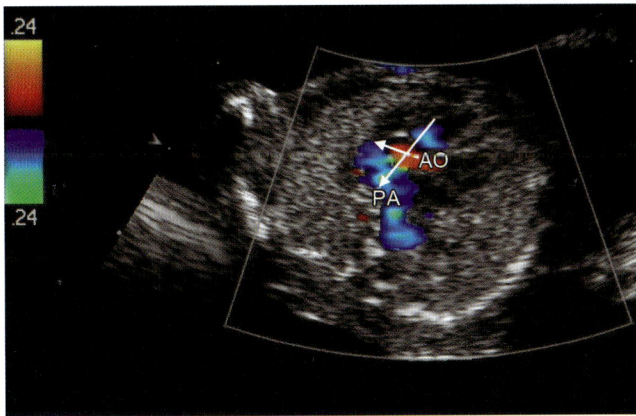

Fig. 45.8: Early fetal echocardiography by 2D and color Doppler in a structurally normal heart. Color Doppler is particulary useful to demonstrate the crossing of the great arteries. Ao, aorta; PA, pulmonary artery

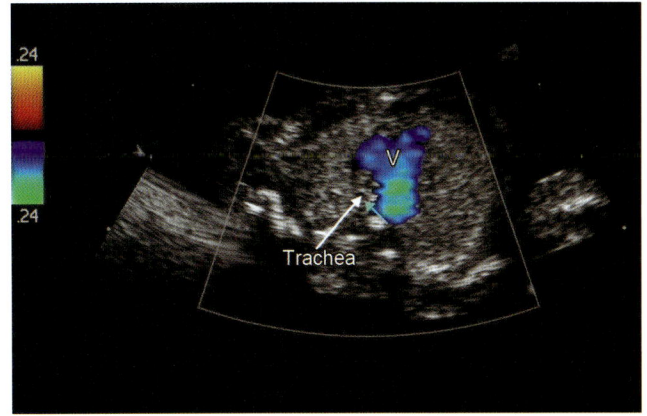

Fig. 45.9: Early fetal echocardiography by 2D and Color Doppler in a structurally normal heart. Color Doppler is particulary useful to demonstrate the normal V confluence of the ductal and aortic archs (V sign). Note that normally the trachea is located behind the aortic arch

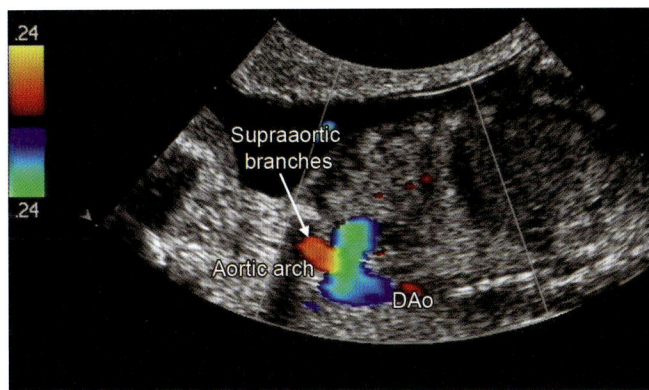

Fig. 45.10: Early fetal echocardiography by 2D and Color Doppler in a structurally normal heart. Color Doppler is particulary useful to demonstrate the aortic arch. DAo, descending aorta

Table 45.1: Results of early fetal echocardiography to diagnose cardiac defects in high-risk population (only series with at least 10 cardiac defects diagnosed)

Author, year	Route	GA	Success (%)	Risk	N	Cases	11-16 ws (%)	20-22 ws (%)
Gembruch,93[14]	TV	11–16	90.3	high	114	13	92	100
Zosmer, 99[24]	TA	13–17		high	323	27	89	96.3
Simpson, 00[25]	TA	12–15	98.7	high	229	17	76	94
Huggon, 02[26]	TA	10–14	86.8	high	478	68	94	
Haak, 02[22]	TV	10–13	95.5	high	45	13	54	
Bronshtein, 02[20]	TV	11–17	> 99	high	6175	46	>90	
Comas, 02[21]	TV	12–17	94.6	high	337	48	79	96
Lopes, 03[39]	TV	12–16	94,9	high	275	37	89	

Route:	main approach. TV: transvaginal, TA: transabdominal
GA:	range of gestational age at scan, in weeks
Success:	visualization success rate for the complete early fetal echocardiography
N:	total number of pregnancies scanned
Cases:	total number of cardiac defects (pre- and postnatally)
11-16 ws:	percentage of the cardiac defects identified at early echocardiography
20-22 ws:	percentage of the cardiac defects identified at mid-trimester echocardiography

Table 45.2: Detection rate of cardiac defects at early ultrasound to screen for congenital malformations in low-risk population

Author, year	GA	Success %	Risk	Normal	Cases	11-16 ws %	20-22 ws %
Achiron, 94[18]	13–15	98	low	660	6	50	50
Hernadi, 97[34]	12		low	3991	3	50	100
D'Ottavio, 97[35]	13–15		low	3490	8	25	80
Yagel, 97[17]	13–16	98	low	6924	66	64	81
Economides, 98[36]	12–13		low	1632	3	0	33
Whitlow, 99[37]	11–14		low	6443	10	40	60
Guariglia, 00[38]	10–16		low	3592	11	18	56
Rustico, 00[19]	13–15	<50	low	4785	41	10	32
Bronshtein, 02[20]	11–17	99	low	30148	127	97	99

GA: range of gestational age at scan, in weeks
Success: visualization success rate for the extended cardiac examination (4 chambers + outflow tracts)
Normal: total number of pregnancies screened
Cases: total number of cardiac defects (pre- and postnatally)
11-16 ws: percentage of the cardiac defects identified at early scan
20-22 ws: percentage of the cardiac defects identified at mid-trimester scan

Table 45.3: Fetal heart anomalies diagnosed at early echocardiography (true positive cases at early fetal echocardiography)

True +	A	B	C	D	E	F	G	H	I	J	K	L	M	N	O	P	Q	R	Overall
Gembruch, 93[14]				6		1	1			2			2						12
Zosmer, 99[24]			3	3	2	1	4	2	3	1			4				1		24
Rustico, 00[19]				2		1	1	1											5
Simpson, 00[25]			3	2			3	2					2	1					13
Huggon, 02[26]			5	29		12	9	1			3			1	1	1			60
Bronshtein,02[20]	4	1	4	13	2	9	25		31	22	5		18		17	3	2	13	169
Comas, 02[21]			4	8		10	4	1	3		2	2	1			3			38
Achiron, 94[18]				2					2		1				1	1	1		8
Hernadi, 97[34]						1													1
D'Ottavio, 97[35]							2										2		4
Whitlow, 99[37]				1			1									1			3
Rustico, 00[19]		1					2		1										4
Lopes, 03[39]			2	6		11	5	1	1	1	1	3	2						33
OVERALL	**4**	**2**	**21**	**71**	**5**	**46**	**54**	**9**	**43**	**24**	**12**	**5**	**29**	**2**	**19**	**9**	**6**	**13**	**374**

Note: A, abnormal venoatrial connections; B, atrial septal defects; C, tricuspid atresia or dysplasia; D, atrioventricular septal defect E, single ventricle; F, ventricular septal defects; G, aortic atresia, aortic stenosis, hypoplastic left heart H, pulmonary atresia or stenosis; I, tetralogy of Fallot; J, transposition of great arteries; K, truncus L, double outlet right ventricle; M, aortic arch anomalies; N, isomerism; O, miocardiopathy; P ectopia cordis Q, complex cardiac defect, others; R, vascular ring
* This series include cases with tetralogy of Fallot and double outlet right ventricle

of scans performed at 14–16 weeks of gestation and 86% of them in low-risk population. Recently, two institutions went further and reported their experience performing the echocardiography as early as between 10 weeks and 13 weeks of gestation.[22,26]

The most frequent fetal heart anomalies diagnosed at early echocardiography are summarized in Table 45.3 (true positive cases).[14,18-21,24-26,34,35,37-39] Note that only the main anomaly for each fetus is presented in the table, even though some fetuses had several cardiac anomalies. It should be noted that defects such as small isolated VSD or valvular stenoses are not reported in these studies.

Table 45. 4 summarizes the published cases of cardiac anomaly not detected in early pregnancy (false negative cases).[14,19-21,24-26,34-37,39]

The results of these studies support the use of early fetal echocardiography to detect the majority of major CHD in both low-risk and high-risk populations, during the first and early second trimester of pregnancy. The cardiac anomalies detected at this early stage of pregnancy are mainly defects involving the four-chamber view, such as large VSD, atrioventricular septal defects and malformations resulting in asymmetry of the ventricles, indicating that defects solely affecting the outflow tracts are

Table 45.4: Fetal heart anomalies not detected at early echocardiography (false negative cases at early fetal echocardiography)

False +	A	B	C	D	E	F	G	H	I	J	Overall
Gembruch, 93[14]					1						1
Hernadi, 97[34]	1			1							2
D'Ottavio 97[35]	1			3	2				1		7
Economides, 98[36]	1					1	1				3
Whitlow, 99[37]	2	1				2	1	1			7
Zosmer, 99[24]					1	1			1		3
Rustico, 00[19]	1				4	1	2		1		9
Simpson, 00[25]	3									1	4
Comas, 02[21]	4	1			3	1	1				10
Huggon, 02[26]	2		2			1			2		7
Bronshtein, 02[20]					1	1		1	1		4
Lopes, 03[39]	3							1			4
OVERALL	**18**	**2**	**2**	**1**	**13**	**10**	**5**	**3**	**6**	**1**	**61**

Note: A, ventricular septal defects; B, atrial septal defects; C, abnormal veno-atrial connections; D, tricuspid atresia or dysplasia; E, atrioventricular septal defect; F, aortic atresia, aortic stenosis, hypoplastic left heart; G, tetralogy of Fallot H, transposition of great arteries; I, aortic arch anomalies; J, miocardiopathy

difficult to diagnose in the first trimester of pregnancy. Heart defects diagnosed early in pregnancy tend to be more complex than those detected later, with a higher incidence of associated structural malformations, chromosomal abnormalities and spontaneous abortions. It is widely accepted that the spectrum of CHD diagnosed during prenatal life is different from that observed in postnatal series, with a higher incidence of associated extracardiac lesions and a significant relationship with chromosomal abnormalities in comparison with postnatal life.[3-5,17] Furthermore, when the cardiac defects are detected during the early pregnancy, they use to be even more complex, probably corresponding to the most severe spectrum of the disease[21,25,26] and use to cause more severe hemodynamic compromise in the developing fetus. A common finding is the presence of an hygroma or hydrops associated with CHD, whereas this is not so when the diagnosis is done later in pregnancy.[1,5,21] As a result, many of these fetuses are not going to survive long into the second trimester, but this does not argue against early diagnosis. Indeed, when the intrauterine demise of the fetus occurs days or weeks before the delivery, the pathological examination is certainly more difficult to perform. All these considerations should be taken into account when counseling the parents complex CHD.

This review presents our experience in the first multicenter trial in early fetal echocardiography performed in Spain.[21] In accordance with other studies, this experience stresses the usefulness of early echocardiography when performed by expert operators on fetus specifically at risk for cardiac defects. Our review of these additional 48 cases contributes to the expanding literature on the ability of TV ultrasonography to detect fetal heart defects in early pregnancy.

OUR EXPERIENCE IN EARLY PRENATAL DIAGNOSIS OF CONGENITAL HEART ANOMALIES

Methods

A multicenter study was made of 334 fetuses from 330 selected high-risk pregnant women, including four twin pregnancies. The women were attending the prenatal diagnosis units of either Institut Universitari Dexeus in Barcelona (Group I), Hospital 12 de Octubre in Madrid (Group II) or Institut Clínic d' Obstetrícia, Ginecologia i Neonatologia del Hospital Clínic in Barcelona (Group III) for ultrasound examination because of an increased a priori risk for heart anomalies. These are referral centers for prenatal diagnosis of CHD. Fetal echocardiography was performed combining transvaginal and transabdominal probes between 12 weeks and 17 weeks of gestation. When possible, we selected the 14th week of gestation as the optimal time for TV scan because the visualization of heart structures is better at this time. This is a prospective design study, performed from September 1999 to May 2001, where the overall group was reviewed focusing in the feasibility of diagnosing fetal CHD by early echocardiography. An informed consent was obtained from each patient and the study was approved by our ethics committees.

Epidemiological data are summarized in Table 45.5, for the overall group and according to the reference unit. Maternal age ranged from 17 years to 46 years (mean 33 years with 36% of women over 34 years). The median gestational age at scan was 14.2 weeks (range 12–17 weeks). The distribution of gestational ages was as follows: 23 cases at 12 weeks, 76 cases at 13 weeks, 101 cases at 14 weeks, 72 cases at 15 weeks, 54 cases at 16 weeks and 8 cases at 17 weeks.

Fetal echocardiography was performed in a population with an increased a priori high- risk for CHD. Criteria for inclusion were family history of CHD (n=37), ultrasound markers for chromosomal abnormalities (n=186), as increased nuchal translucency (NT) (NT >99th centile) or abnormal ductus venosus (DV) flow (pulsatility index for veins in the DV >95th centile), suspected cardiac or extracardiac anomalies at early second-trimester scan (n=43), maternal pregestational diabetes (n=33), pregnancy affected by a chromosomal abnormality (n=8), exposition to teratogens (n=3), genetic sonography (n=22) and as a screening test (n=2). These last two cases refer to two twin pregnancies in which the main indication for the echocardiography was an ultrasound marker for chromosomal abnormality in one fetus, but the echocardiographic examination was performed to both fetuses for practical reasons. For NT and DV assessment, measurements were made between 10

Table 45.5: Our experience:[21] Epidemiological DATA

	GROUP I	GROUP II	GROUP III	OVERALL (GROUP I+II+III)
n (pregnancies)	68 (4 twins)	130	132	330 (334 fetuses)
Study period	9/99 to 5/01			
GA (mean, range)	14.9 (12–17)	13.7 (12–16)	14.3 (13–16)	14.2 (12–17)
MA (mean, range)	33 (26–46) 30% > 34 years	33 (17–45) 37% > 34 years	32 (19–42) 38% > 34 years	33(17–46) 36% > 34 years
Ultrasound system	Toshiba SSH-140 5.0–7.5 MHz TV 3.0–6.5 MHz TA	Acuson 128 XP 5.0-7.0 MHz TV 3.5-5.0 MHz TA	Acuson 128 XP Aspen 5.0-7.0 MHz TV 3.5-5.0 MHz TA	–
Optimal visualization	65/72 (90.3%)	119/130 (91.5%)	132/132 (100%)	316/334 (94.6%)
Overall follow-up	44/72 (61.1%)	108/130 (83.1%)	129/132 (97.8%)	281/334 (84.1%)

Note: GA, gestational age (weeks); MA, maternal age (years); TV, transvaginal; TA, transabdominal

weeks and 16 weeks of gestation. NT was systematically assessed in all cases, while DV blood flow was only measured in Group I and II. We have used our own published nomograms to define increased NT or abnormal DV.[40] Genetic sonography was offered to high-risk population refusing invasive karyotyping test.

For each fetus, visualization of the 4-chamber view (with both atria, atrioventricular valves and ventricles), the origin and double-crossing of the great arteries, aortic and ductal archs and systemic venous return was attempted in a segmental approach. Two-dimensional mode and color/pulsed Doppler flow imaging were used in all cases, while M-mode was occasionally performed. The operators kept a record of optimal visualization (complete visualization of heart structures) or partial visualization (incomplete visualization of heart structures). In cases of partial visualization, only when an anomaly was suspected a second scan was arranged weeks later. Ultrasound examinations were performed using a multifrequency real-time vaginal probe (5.0–7.5 MHz) and convex abdominal probe (3.0-6.5 MHz) on a Toshiba ultrasound system (Toshiba SSH-140A, Toshiba Co., Tokyo, Japan), Acuson 128 XP or Aspen (Acuson Inc., Mountain View, CA), and General Electric Logic 400 or Logic 500 (GE Medical Systems, Milwaukee, Wisconsin). The ultrasound examination was mainly performed transvaginally, completed nearly always by the transabdominal route. For color Doppler evaluation, the energy output levels were lower than 50 mW/cm² spatial peak-temporal average. The duration of complete heart examination was less than 30 minutes. All the examinations were made by three experienced operators (CC, JMM and AG).

When indicated, fetal karyotyping by chorionic villus sampling or amniocentesis was offered. According to the policy of our institutions, invasive testing was recommended as a result of advanced maternal age (>35 years), family history of aneuploidy, biochemical screening for Down's syndrome higher than 1/270 or ultrasound anomalies (including malformations or NT more than 95th centile). Fluorescence in situ hibridization (FISH) studies to test for 22q11 deletion was also offered when a heart malformation affecting the great arteries was suspected. When possible, in those who continue their pregnancies, a follow-up detailed ultrasound scan was carried out at 20–22 weeks of gestation. When karyotyping

was not performed, chromosomal abnormalities were excluded at neonatal examination.

Reliability was assessed by conventional transabdominal echocardiography at 20–22 weeks, by postnatal follow-up in the first 3 months of life, and/or by autopsy in cases of termination of pregnancy (TOP). Minor cardiac anomalies described in the literature as difficult or impossible to diagnose early (atrial septal defects or patent ductus arteriosus) were not considered when calculating the validity of the early echocardiography.

Results

The rate of optimal visualization of the fetal heart was 94.6% (316/334). In 48 out of 334 (14.4%) fetuses, the final diagnosis was abnormal, including 48 cases of structural heart abnormalities (Table 45.6). In 38 out of 48 cases with heart defects the diagnosis was suspected at early echocardiography. These true positive cases were as follows: 13 cases of abnormal outflow tracts, 8 cases of atrioventricular defect, 4 cases of hypoplastic left heart (HLH), 5 cases of tricuspid atresia or dysplasia, 3 cases of isolated VSD, 3 cases of ectopia cordis, 1 case of aortic coartation and 1 severe complex heart defect. True positive diagnoses are summarized in Table 45. 7. Figures 45.11 to 45.15 illustrate some examples of detected CHD early in pregnancy.

There were ten false negative cases (2 cases of HLH, 3 cases of atrioventricular defect, 4 cases of VSD and 1 case of tetralogy of Fallot) (Table 45. 8). There were no false positive diagnoses. When considering the validity of the early echocardiography, we have excluded one case of isolated pericardial effusion, two cases of significant tricuspid regurgitation within a structurally normal heart, a child affected by an ostium secundum atrial septal defect, a structural normal heart in a Down's syndrome affected by a patent ductus arteriosus who had neonatal surgery.

Karyotyping was performed in 290 cases of our series (86.8%), including all cases with cardiac abnormalities. Among the whole series, 51 cases had an abnormal karyotype. These chromosomal abnormalities included trisomy 21 (n = 28), 45XO (n = 7), trisomy 18 (n = 6), trisomy 13 (n = 2), 22q11 microdeletion (n = 1), triploidy (n = 1), trisomy 7 (n

Table 45.6: Our experience:[21] congenital heart defects

	OVERALL (GROUP I + II + III)
Prevalence	48/334 (14.4%)
True positive	38/48 (79.2%)
False negative	10
False positive	0
Chromosomal abnormalities	27/48 (56.3%)
Extracardiac abnormalities	31/48 (64.6%)
Increased NT	21/48 (43.8%)
Abnormal DV	18/37 (48.6%)
Outcome	37 TOP 1 selective feticide 2 postnatal death 8 surviving
Follow-up	33/48 (68.8%)
Autopsy available	25/41 (61.0%)

Note: NT, nuchal translucency; DV, ductus venosus; TOP, termination of pregnancy

= 1), partial trisomy 15 (n = 1), rearrangement (n = 1) and others (n = 3). Among the heart defects, 27 cases (56.3%) had an abnormal karyotype (13 trisomy 21, 5 trisomy 18, 3 Turner' syndrome, 2 trisomy 13, 1 trisomy 7, 1 partial trisomy 15, 1 rearrangement and 1 case with a 22q11 microdeletion detected by FISH) and 31 cases (64.6%) showed additional sonographic extracardiac anomalies, including mainly cystic hygroma, congenital diaphragmatic hernia, abnormal situs visceralis, single umbilical artery, bilateral dysplastic kidneys, hydrops, limb-body wall complex, omphalocele, exencephaly, holoprosencephaly, pyelectasis, choroid plexus cysts, hemivertebra and pleural effusion.

In CHD group, increased NT at 10-16 weeks of gestation was noted in 21 fetuses (43.8%), while abnormal DV blood flow was found in 18 out of 37 fetuses with DV assessment (48.6%).

The outcome of fetuses with a CHD was poor. In 37 cases, a TOP was performed at parents request before 20 weeks of gestation and in one case, a selective feticide was offered in a twin pregnancy discordant for a CHD. The outcome of the surviving fetuses was poor, with two cases of neonatal death (1 VSD, 1 hypoplastic left heart) and 8 surviving children (1 VSD, 3 atrioventricular defects, 1 pulmonary stenosis, 1 VSD diagnosed of Noonan's

Table 45. 7: Our experience:[21] Fetal heart anomalies diagnosed at early echocardiography (true positive cases at early fetal echocardiography). Fetal data of true positives cases (congenital heart defects, gestational age at diagnosis, associated findings, karyotyping studies and follow-up)

Case	Case CHD	GA	Associated findings	Karyotype	Follow-up
1	AVSD	17	Increased NT	Trisomy 21	TOP, no autopsy
2*	Hypoplastic RV Tricuspid atresia Abnormal great arteries	16	Single UA	Normal	TA-echo confirmative Selective feticide
3	AVSD	14	Increased NT	Trisomy 21	TOP, no autopsy
4	AVSD	13	Cystic hygroma	Trisomy 21	TOP, no autopsy
5	VSD	17	Cystic hygroma	Normal	Surviving Follow-up confirmative Noonan syndrome
6	VSD Abnormal great arteries	15	Abnormal situs Single UA	22q11 deletion	TOP, autopsy: abnormal situs visceralis, VSD, hypoplastic RV, truncus
7	AVSD	12	Increased NT	Trisomy 21	TOP, no autopsy
8	Abnormal great arteries	14	Cystic hygroma	Normal	Surviving, postnatal echo: tetralogy of Fallot
9	HLH, DORV, Pulmonary atresia	16	Bilateral renal dysplasia	Normal	TOP, autopsy confirmative
10	VSD, DORV	16	Increased NT	Partial trisomy 15	TOP, autopsy confirmative
11	Truncus	15	Polimalformative fetus	Trisomy 13	TOP, autopsy confirmative
12	VSD, DORV, Pulmonary atresia	12	Exencephaly	Normal	TOP, no autopsy
13	VSD, DORV	16	Ventriculomegaly, single UA	Normal	TOP, no autopsy
14	Tetralogy of Fallot	16	Increased NT, bilateral renal dysplasia, omphalocele	Normal	TOP, no autopsy
15	Tetralogy of Fallot	13	Increased NT, bilateral renal dysplasia	Trisomy 7	TOP, no autopsy
16	AVSD	16	–	Normal	Surviving; Follow-up confirmative
17	AVSD	13	Increased NT Hydrops	Trisomy 21	TOP, autopsy confirmative

Contd...

Contd...

Case	Case CHD	GA	Associated findings	Karyotype	Follow-up
18	AVSD	13	Increased NT Omphalocele	Trisomy 21	TOP, autopsy confirmative
19	VSD	16	Holoprosencephaly	Trisomy 13	TOP, autopsy confirmative
20	VSD	13	Increased NT	Trisomy 21	TOP, autopsy confirmative
21	HLH	13	Exencephaly	Normal	TOP, no autopsy
22	HLH	12	Increased NT	45XO	TOP, no autopsy
23	HLH	12	Increased NT, hydrops	45XO	TOP, autopsy confirmative
24	Aortic coartation	16	Cystic hygroma, hydrops	45XO	TOP, no autopsy
25	Trisuspid atresia	16	Increased NT	Normal	TOP, autopsy confirmative
26	Tricuspid atresia	16	Increased NT	Normal	TOP, autopsy confirmative
27	Ectopia cordis	12	Limb-body wall complex	Normal	TOP, no autopsy
28	Ectopia cordis	14	Limb-body wall complex	Normal	TOP, autopsy confirmative
29	Ectopia cordis, Tricuspid atresia	14	Increased NT Limb-body wall complex	Trisomy 18	TOP, autopsy confirmative
30	Tricuspid dysplasia	13	Increased NT	Trisomy 21	TOP, no autopsy
31	VSD, overriding aorta	13	Increased NT Omphalocele	Trisomy 18	TOP, no autopsy
32	DORV+ mitral atresia	13	Increased NT	Trisomy 18	TOP, no autopsy
33	VSD, tricuspid atresia	14	Increased NT	Normal	TOP, autopsy confirmative
34	Pulmonary stenosis	15	–	Normal	Surviving Follow-up confirmative
35	Single ventricle, TGA	15	–	Normal	Surviving Follow-up confirmative[a]
36	VSD, pulmonary atresia	16	Increased NT	Rearrengement	TOP, autopsy confirmative
37	AVSD	16	Increased NT Abnormal situs	Trisomy 21	TOP, autopsy confirmative
38	HLH+ abnormal situs	16	Increased NT	Normal	TOP, autopsy confirmative

CHD, congenital heart defect; GA, gestational age (weeks); TOP, termination of pregnancy; TA-echo, transabdominal conventional second-trimester echocardiography; *twin pregnancy; AVSD, atrioventricular septal defect; VSD, ventricular septal defect; LV, left ventricle; RV, right ventricle; ASD, atrial septal defect; DO, double outlet; HLH, hypoplastic left heart; TGA, transposition of great arteries; UA, umbilical artery; CDH, congenital diaphragmatic hernia; NT, nuchal translucency
[a] death at 3 months of life after paliative surgery

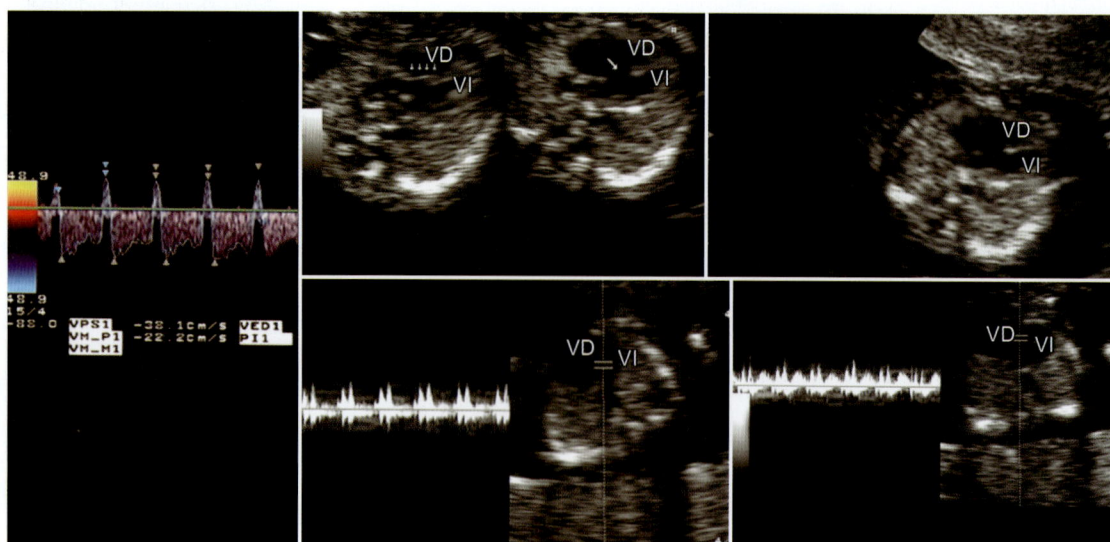

Fig. 45.11: Atrioventricular septal defect detected at 13 weeks of gestation in a fetus affected by cystic hygroma and trisomy 21. Note the abnormal reversed A wave in the ductus venosus

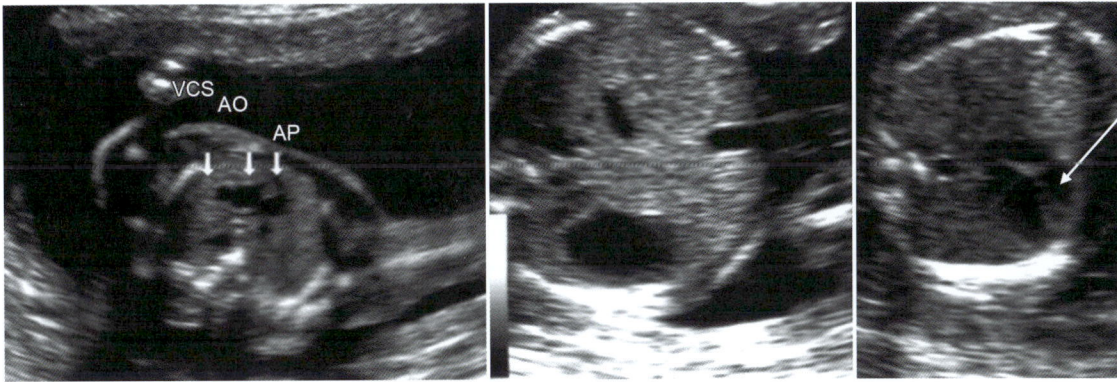

Fig. 45.12: Tetralogy of Fallot detected at 16 weeks of gestation in a fetus affected by cystic hygroma and normal karyotype. Note the left cardiac deviation and the dominance of the aorta compared with the small pulmonary artery at the 3 vessel view in the upper mediastinum; VCS, superior vena cava; AO, aorta; AP, pulmonary artery

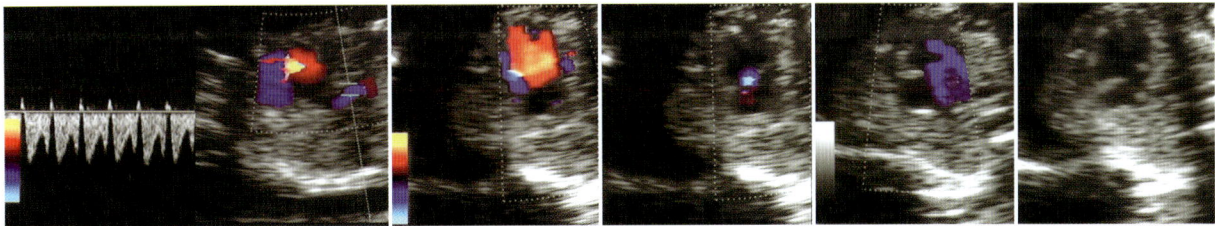

Fig. 45.13: Atrioventricular septal defect with unbalanced right ventricle dominance and double outlet: right ventricle at 15 weeks of gestation. Note the abnormal reversed A wave in the ductus venosus

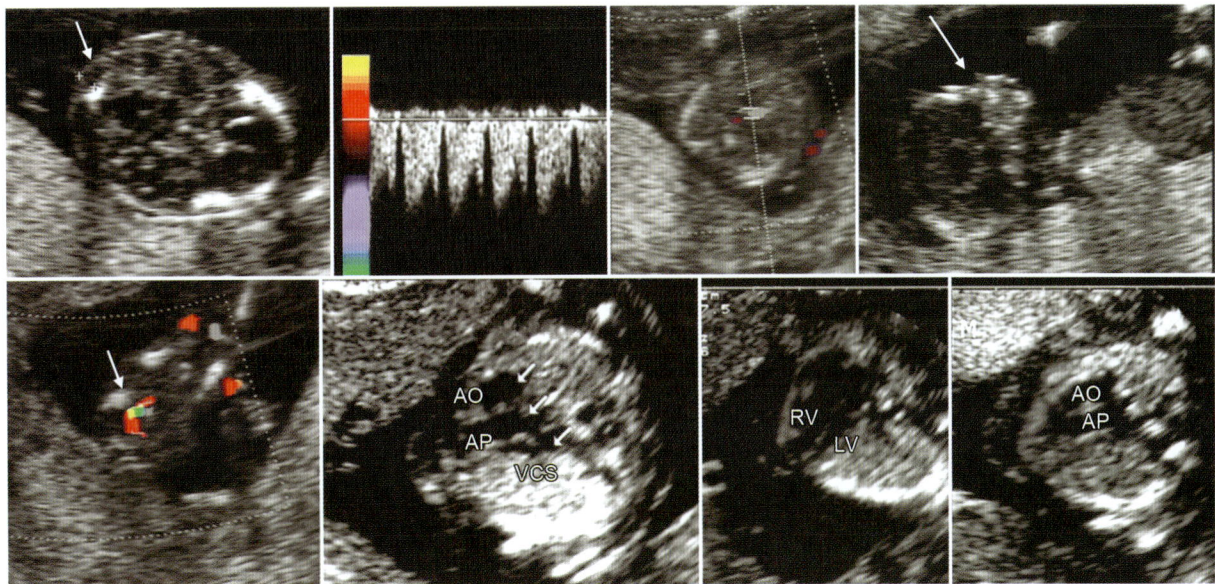

Fig. 45.14: Hypoplastic left heart and double outlet right ventricle at 15 weeks of gestation in a trisomy 18. Note the identification of multiple markers of chromosomal abnormality (increased nuchal translucency, abnormal ductus venosus flow, absent nasal bone, single umbilical artery)

syndrome, 1 case of tetralogy of Fallot, and 1 single ventricle with transposition of great arteries who died 3 months after palliative surgery). Pathological examination was performed in 25 cases. In 16 cases, the autopsy was not available, either because of the selective feticide in a twin pregnancy, or because the termination was performed in other hospital without fetal necropsy, or due to the unavailability of an adequate material for pathological exam (fragmentation), or because the parents declined the examination.

In our series of early echocardiography, a complete follow-up was possible in 281 cases (84.1%), 61.1% in group I, 83.1% in group II and 97.8% in group III . When a heart defect was detected, a complete follow-up was possible in 33 out of 48 cases (68.8%).

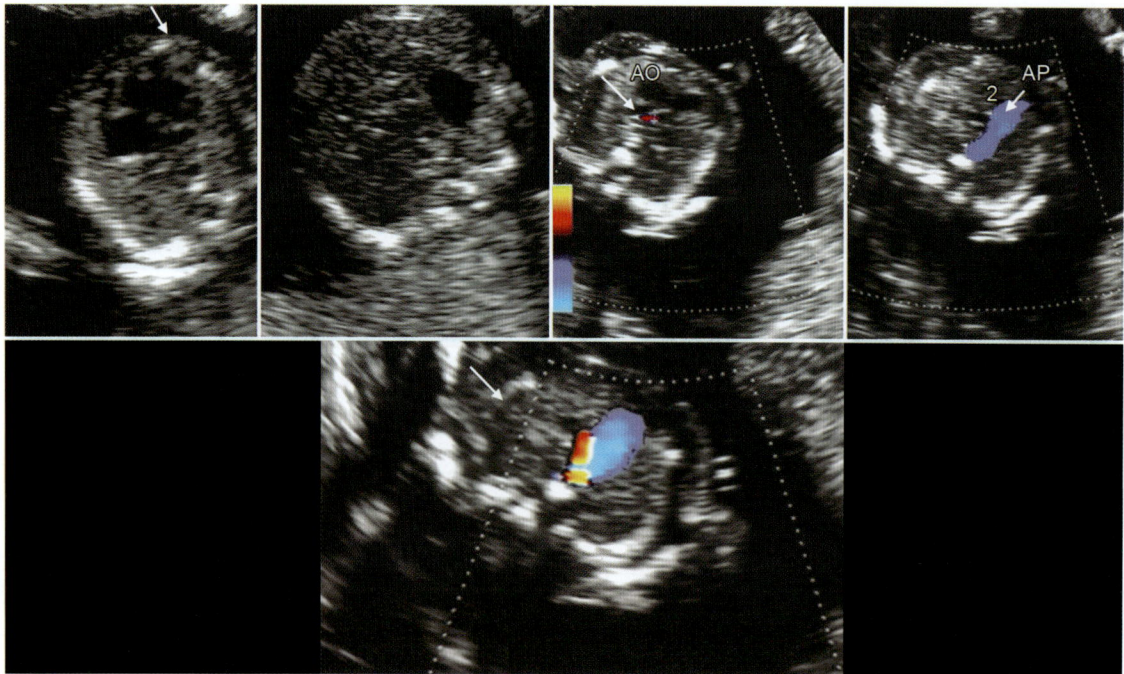

Fig. 45.15: Hypoplastic left heart and aortic stenosis at 17 weeks of gestation in a Turner syndrome. Note the left cardiac axis deviation, the opposite color flow in the V sign at the upper mediastinum level and the severe reduction of the aortic outflow tract compared to the main pulmonary artery

Table 45.8: Our experience:[21] Fetal heart anomalies not detected at early echocardiography (false negative cases at early fetal echocardiography). Fetal data of false negatives cases (congenital heart defects, gestational age at diagnosis, associated findings, karyotyping studies and outcome)

Case	CHD	GA1	GA2	Method diagnosis	Associated findings	Karyotype	Outcome
1*	HLH	14	20	TA-echo	Congenital Diaphragmatic hernia	Normal	Neonatal death after surgery
2	Ostium primum, ASD, HLH	14	20	Autopsy	Hydrops cystic higroma	Normal	TOP
3	AVSD	14	20	TA-echo	Single umbilical artery short femur	Trisomy 21	TOP
4	AVSD	16	33	TA-echo	Normal	Surviving	
5	AVSD	15	23	TA-echo	Echogenic foci pleural effusion	Trisomy 21	Surviving
6	VSD	12	14	Autopsy	Pyelectasis	Trisomy 21	TOP
7	VSD	15	28	TA-echo	Choroid plexus cysts Hemivertebra	Trisomy 18	Neonatal death
8	VSD	13	15	Autopsy	NTD48, XXY+18	TOP	
9	Tetralogy of Fallot	13	20	TA-echo	Pyelectasis	Trisomy 21	TOP
10	VSD	13	15	TA-echo	Normal	Surviving	

* twin pregnancy; CHD, congenital heart defect, GA[1] gestational age of the echocardiographic examination in early pregnancy (weeks); GA[2] gestational age at diagnosis (weeks); TOP, termination of pregnancy; HLH, hypoplastic left heart; TA-echo, transabdominal echocardiography; ASD, atrial septal defect; AVSD, atrioventricular septal defect; VSD, ventricular septal defect; NTD, neural tube defects

Fetal Heart Rate

The diagnosis of fetal arrhythmia early in pregnancy may rise the suspicion of a fetal chromosomal abnormality,[34-36] an increased risk for a later miscarriage[35,37,38,41] or the presence of a CHD.[42] The factors that control fetal heart rate in the first trimester are uncertain, so the underlying cause of the abnormal pattern in chromosomally abnormal fetuses remain obscure. A delay in maturation of sympathetic and parasympathetic systems as well as an abnormally developed and responsive myocardium have been proposed.[30,43] An alternative explanation could be that fetal arrhythmias are a reflection of an underlying structural heart disease, which are a common feature in trisomic fetuses.[35,42,44,45] Baschat et al.[46] reported four cases of severe CHD associated with bradycardia (likely to be atrioventricular block) during early echocardiography at 11–14 weeks of gestation. All cases had either increased NT or generalized edema and complex CHD. Most authors find a high correlation between abnormal heart rate and increased NT in chromosomally abnormal fetuses, thus supporting the hypothesis that cardiac defects may be involved in the physiologic basis of NT.[35,36,47]

Nuchal Translucency and Ductus Venosus

Nuchal translucency measurement at 10–14 weeks of gestation is a widely accepted method to screen for chromosomal abnormalities. Recent studies have suggested the potential role of an increased NT thickness[8,9,11,48-51] or an abnormal DV flow pattern[10,11,52,53] at early pregnancy as a screening tool for CHD, in addition to its role in screening for chromosomal defects. The risk of CHD after the finding of an increased NT seems to vary between 49%.[24,54] Recently, Galindo et al. have examined the prevalence, distribution and spectrum of cardiac defects in 353 chromosomally normal fetuses with increased NT, with a complete follow-up in 97% of the cases.[55] This multicenter spanish study present an overall prevalence of heart defects of 91%, increasing significantly from 53% in those with NT more than 95th centile to 24% when thickness more than 6 mm. Interestingly, most of the cardiac defects can be prenatally detected. A wide range of cardiac anomalies were observed in this series, with the most common being atrioventricular septal defects and tricuspid atresia. Hyett et al. reported that about 55% of major CHD were associated with a fetal NT thickness above 95th centile at 10–14 weeks of gestation.[8] However, others have failed to demonstrate such a strong association,[49,50,53,54,56-58] raising the matter that the routine assessment of the four chambers and great vessels at mid-second trimester remains as the most important screening tool for the detection of major CHD.[56,59] Theoretically, both types of screening used in combination should improve the overall sensitivity of prenatal diagnosis of major cardiac defects.

The physiopathogenic mechanism of this relationship is not easy to explain.[11,44,45,53,59-63] Pathological examination of fetuses with increased NT thickness at 10–14 weeks have demonstrated a high prevalence of cardiac defects and abnormalities of the great arteries and of subtle defects, such as widening of the aortic valve and ascending aorta, narrowing of the aortic isthmus and persistence of the left superior vena cava. Another proposed mechanism to explain the increased NT is an early cardiac function impairment suggested by an abnormal DV flow pattern. However, Matias et al.[10] reported that most of chromosomally normal fetuses with increased NT but normal DV flow did not have a CHD. This finding might contradict a cardiac involvement in the pathogenesis of the increased NT in most of the fetuses, and suggest that only fetuses with abnormal DV blood flow are those at high-risk of CHD. On the other hand, in cases with CHD and both enlarged NT and abnormal DV, because the type of cardiac defects cannot always explain the hemodynamic changes found in these fetuses, some other mechanisms seem to be envolved.[53]

Based on ultrasonographic and postmortem morphological studies, the findings in increased NT fetuses can be classified in three categories.[64] First, an association between increased NT and cardiac anomalies, combined with an abnormal ductus venosus flow pattern, has been described in some cases, leading to the theory that cardiac failure causes NT enlargement. Second, various types of abnormalities have been found in the extracellular matrix of the nuchal skin of fetuses with increased NT. Third, abnormal lymphatic development has been demonstrated in fetuses with increased NT. Many hypotheses on NT enlargement are based on associations and speculations. Therefore, wihin this context, it is not clear whether all these cardiovascular anomalies are the cause of the increased nuchal translucency or both events are the result of another pathophysiologic mechanism.

Chromosomal Abnormalities

The detection of a CHD may be the first clue to the diagnosis of a chromosomal abnormality or a genetic syndrome. The incidence of chromosomal defects in CHD diagnosed prenatally may be as high as 30–40%, and 15% when the CHD is presented isolated. These figures increase up to 40–60% when the CDH is diagnosed during the first trimester.[20-22,26] This is much higher than the incidence in liveborns. Also, the high rate of spontaneous abortion loss in early pregnancy suggest a higher rate of chromosomal abnormalities in first trimester fetuses with CHD. Therefore, whenever a CHD is diagnosed, karyotype evaluation is mandatory, including FISH test to rule out 22q11 deletion.[65-68]

Recently, the early finding of isolated tricuspid regurgitation or disproportion of the cardiac chambers and/or outflow tracts, has been regarded to be highly associated with fetal chromosomal abnormalities, even in the absence of structural heart disease, as it had been previously described during the second trimester.[26,69,70] The chromosomal defect most frequently found to be associated with tricuspid regurgitation was trisomy 21, but all types of karyotype anomalies were seen in association.[69] In view of these results, the authors propose to assess the four-chambers view and the outflow tracts for disproportion and to use color Doppler to rule out tricuspid regurgitation in each first or early second trimester ultrasound to screen for chromosomal anomalies.[26,27] Since, these unexpectedly good results were obtained in particularly high-risk fetuses, they remain to be confirmed in unselected population.

ADVANTAGES AND LIMITATIONS

The first benefit of performing early fetal echocardiography would be an early reassurance of normality in order to relieve anxiety and reduce emotional trauma to the parents at high-risk for CHD. Early prenatal diagnosis of CHD will allow us to optimize the genetic counseling to the parents by permitting further testing such as fetal karyotyping and in those cases with severe defects it may provide the parents with the option of an earlier and safer termination of pregnancy.[13,14,17] In selected cases, there is the possibility of pharmacological therapy. Furthermore, the correct timing and place for delivery may be planned and arranged well in advance.

However, there are certain disadvantages of the early scanning, which reduces its diagnostic accuracy compared with the conventional examination at 20–22 weeks of gestation.[1,5,13,14,17] The transvaginal technique requires a substantial amount of operator experience, yet it can not be learned from the second trimester examination as the early transabdominal scan. Unfavorable fetal position or limited angles of insonation due to the less mobile capacity of the transvaginal probe may not be overcome. Also, spatial orientation can be challenging by the transvaginal scan. In such cases, we recommend a transabdominal scan that will help us to quickly asses the situs and obtain a good spatial orientation. The small size of the fetal heart is an important limiting factor to obtain an optimal sonographic visualization, and also to obtain a successful pathological examination, particularly before the 13th week of gestation. At 13–14 weeks of gestation the transverse diameter of the heart at the four-chambers view ranges between 5 mm and 8 mm, and the great artery diameter at the level of the semilunar valves ranges between 0.8 mm[5] and 1.8 mm[5]. Moreover, this exploration is more time-consuming and requires a high level of training of the examiner. Finally, the biggest disadvantage of first-trimester echocardiography is the later manifestation of structural and functional changes in some CHD. Some cardiac lesions are progressive in nature, such as mild pulmonary and aortic stenosis or coarctation and even hypoplastic left heart syndrome. Some obstructive lesions, as a result of a reduced blood flow, may increase the severity of the lesions, resulting in a restricted growth in chambers or arteries. This may be the biggest disadvantage of performing the early scan. Progression usually is towards a more severe form of lesion that may be sometimes only discernible in the second or even in the third trimester, although, in some rare cases a regression to a less severe form may be observed. In this sense, the false negative cases published in literature are particularly instructive demonstrating these limitations (Table 45.4). Another disadvantage of early fetal echocardiography is the possible detection of defects that could resolve spontaneously in later pregnancy, such as muscular venticular septal defects, resulting in unnecessary anxiety in the parents.

Therefore, a normal early examination does not preclude a subsequent abnormal heart development at the second trimester ultrasound, or even in the third trimester or the postnatal period. After a normal early fetal echocardiography, a conventional transabdominal echocardiography at 20–22 weeks of gestation is strongly recommended.

PATHOLOGICAL CONFIRMATION

Pathological confirmation in the case of an early termination of pregnancy or perinatal death is particularly important in those areas where ultrasound diagnosis is most challenging. Only a complete diagnosis will make an individual genetic counseling possible and will validate the accuracy of early fetal echocardiography as a diagnostic technique. Therefore, we advocate that a precise pathological report have to be compulsory for an adequate assessment of the reliability of early fetal echocardiography. This is still a major drawback in most of the studies.[1,5,21,26]

Termination of pregnancy is an option only before 22 weeks of gestation in our country. Whenever a termination takes place, it is of vital importance to obtain permission for autopsy in order to confirm the diagnosis and to search for any other associated malformations. Ideally this should be performed by a pathologist who is familiar with the small size of the specimen and with special examination techniques such as dissection microscopy.[5,21,22,45] Current methods of terminating early pregnancies others than using prostaglandins are less recommended because do not usually allow the retrieval of suitable specimens for appropriate examination to correlate ultrasound and pathological findings.[45] This method allows a more gentle extraction of the embryo or fetus so that a pathological examination for verification of the prenatally diagnosed malformation can be performed. A pathological investigation after termination of pregnancy following the diagnosis of a CHD should be always

recommended, preferably in referral laboratories, being of paramount importance to validate early echocardiography. In particular, semilunar valve and aortic arch defects are usually underdiagnosed. We are aware of some cases in which Doppler findings, such turbulent flow and very high velocities, are more reliable to diagnose valve stenosis than pathological examination, even during the second trimester. Indeed, this is a problem and a major challenge not only for ultrasonographers but also for pathologists.

INDICATIONS OF EARLY FETAL ECHOCARDIOGRAPHY

Since, most CHD are detected in low-risk pregnancies, and knowing the high prevalence of heart defects in a non-selected population (incidence of CHD in low risk population 1/238),[20] some authors suggest that an early detailed cardiac examination should be performed in all pregnant women.[17,20] Indeed, very few cardiac defects have been identified in the pregnancies in which a family history was the main indication for the early fetal echocardiography, which is consistent with the recurrence rate of 2–3% for siblings. The main value of the early scan in such family-risk cases lies in the reassurance that it gives to the parents. As we have previously stated, in most of the studies, the early echocardiography is somewhat less reliable and may result in a higher false-negative and false-positive results in comparison with the 20–22 weeks transabdominal echocardiography. Besides, early echocardiography is most time-consuming and requires a high level of expertise of the examiner. Therefore, it is difficult to offer this scan as a screening test to the general population. In this context, the identification of a high-risk collective is of paramount importance.

Currently, the importance of the aforementioned limitations of early fetal cardiac examination justifies restriction of its use to fetuses at high risk of having cardiac anomalies.[5,10,14,18,21,22,26] The indications proposed for early fetal echocardiography are:

- Increased nuchal translucency (>95th or 99th centile) is the main indication of referral in all recently reported studies.
- Abnormal ductus venosus blood flow, regardless the measurement of the nuchal translucency.
- Fetuses affected by other structural malformations: hygroma, hydrops, omphalocele, situs inversus, arrythmia.
- Suspected cardiac anomalies at screening ultrasound.
- Pregestational diabetes of the mother.
- High-risk family, with a previously affected child, a first-degree relative affected by a congenital heart disease or a genetic disease in which CHD are common.
- Women at high risk of chromosomal abnormality declining invasive test for karyotyping.
- Pregnancies affected by a chromosomal abnormality.

Currently, as long as the sensitivity, specificity and predictive value of early echocardiography is still unclear, this examination should be generally reserved for patients at high-risk for CHD. However, only the accumulation of results from carefully collaborative studies as the present series will clearly define the role of early transvaginal echocardiography.

CONCLUSION

Fetal echocardiography performed by expert operators is reliable for an early reassurement of normal cardiac anatomy.

- Transvaginal sonography enables good visualization of fetal heart earlier in gestation. The four-chambers view and the extended examination to the great vessels can be imaged in almost 100% at 13–14 weeks of gestation. Less than 5% of patients will need a repeated scan because of inadequate visualization.
- The combination of transvaginal and transabdominal routes and the application of color Doppler enhances visualization.
- Most CHD are detected in low-risk population. As we can not perform a targeted fetal echocardiography as a screening test, we need to improve the identification of high-risk group pregnancies. Increased nuchal translucency at 10–14 weeks of scan and, maybe ductus venosus blood flow assesment seem to be the newest and most promising risk factors for fetal CHD, and may be particularly useful during the first trimester.
- Currently, early fetal echocardiography should be offered to high-risk pregnancies. Some authors advocate routine early extended cardiac examination in low-risk pregnancies. At present, as long as the sensitivity, specificity and predictive value of early echocardiography is still unclear, this examination should be generally reserved for patients at high-risk for CHD.

- Whenever a normal heart is diagnosed in the early scan, it has to be supplemented with the conventional transabdominal examination at 20–22 weeks of gestation.

Fetal echocardiography performed by expert operators is reliable to diagnose most major structural heart defects in the first and early second trimester of pregnancy:

- Cardiac defects diagnosed early in pregnancy tend to be more complex than those detected later on and use to cause more severe hemodynamic compromise in the developing fetus.
- Many CHD can be detected at the beginning of the second trimester.
- The incidence of associated structural malformations, chromosomal abnormalities and spontaneous abortions is significantly high.
- A complete work-up including pathological and karyotype evaluation should be warranted in order to provide parents with a proper genetic counseling, which is extremely difficult to obtain if spontaneous loss of the pregnancy occurs.
- The small size of specimens at this time of gestation renders pathological examination difficult and requires high expertise and careful inspection, irrespective of the technique used for termination.
- Clinical follow-up in the neonate and postmortem examination if termination of pregnancy is undertaken are essential to assess the actual role of early fetal ecocardiography.

REFERENCES

1. Campbell S. Isolated major congenital heart disease (Opinion). Ultrasound Obstet Gynecol. 2001;17:370-9.
2. Mitchell SC, Korones SB, Berendes HW. Congenital heart disease in 56,109 births. Incidence and natural history. Circulation. 1971;43:323-32.
3. Allan L, Sharland G, Milburn A, et al. Prospective diagnosis of 1006 consecutive cases of congenital heart disease in the fetus. J Am Coll Cardiol. 1994;23:1452-8.
4. Allan LD. Fetal cardiology. Curr Op Obstet Gynecol. 1996;8:142-7.
5. Gembruch U. Prenatal diagnosis of congenital heart disease. Prenat Diagn. 1997;17:1283-98.
6. Todros T. Prenatal diagnosis and management of fetal cardiovascular malformations. Curr Opin Obstet Gynecol. 2000;12:105-9.
7. Levi S, Schaaps JP, De Havay P, et al. End result of routine ultrasound screening for congenital anomalies. The Belgian Multicentric study 1984-92. Ultrasound Obstet Gynecol. 1995;5:366-1.
8. Hyett J, Perdu M, Sharland G, et al. Using nuchal translucency to screen for major cardiac defects at 10-14 weeks of gestation: population based cohort study. Br Med J. 1999;318:81-5.
9. Devine PC, Simpson LL. Nuchal translucency and its relationship to congenital heart disease. Semin Perinatol. 2000;24:343-51.
10. Matias A, Huggon I, Areias JC, et al. Cardiac defects in chromosomally normal fetuses with abnormal ductus venosus blood flow at 10–14 weeks. Ultrasound Obstet Gynecol. 1999;14:307-10.
11. Bilardo CM, Müller MA, Zikulnig L, et al. Ductus venosus studies in fetuses at high risk for chromosomal or heart abnormalities: relationship with nuchal translucency measurement and fetal outcome. Ultrasound Obstet Gynecol. 2001;17:288-94.
12. Johnson P, Sharland G, Maxwell D, et al. The role of transvaginal sonography in the early detection of congenital heart disease. Ultrasound Obstet Gynecol. 1992;2:248-51.
13. Bronshtein M, Zimmer EZ, Gerlis LM, et al. Early ultrasound diagnosis of congenital heart defects in high-risk and low-risk pregnancies. Obstet Gynecol. 1993;82:225-9.
14. Gembruch U, Knopfle G, Bald R, et al. Early diagnosis of fetal congenital heart disease by transvaginal echocardiography. Ultrasound Obstet Gynecol. 1993;3:310-17.
15. Achiron R, Tadmor O. Screening for fetal anomalies during the first trimester of pregnancy: transvaginal versus transabdominal sonography. Ultrasound Obstet Gynecol. 1991;1:186-91.
16. D'Amelio R, Giorlandino C, Masala L, et al. Fetal echocardiography using transvaginal and transabdominal probes during the first period of pregnancy: a comparative study. Prenat Diagn. 1991;11:69-75.
17. Yagel S, Weissman A, Rotstein Z, et al. Congenital heart defects: natural course and in utero development. Circulation. 1997;96:550-5.
18. Achiron R, Rotstein Z, Lipitz S, et al. First trimester diagnosis of congenital heart disease by transvaginal ultrasonography. Obstet Gynecol. 1994;84:69-72.
19. Rustico MA, Benettoni A, D' Ottavio G, et al. Early screening for fetal cardiac anomalies by transvaginal echocardiography in an unselected population: the role of operator experience. Ultrasound Obstet Gynecol. 2000;16:614-9.
20. Bronshtein M, Zimmer Z. The sonographic approach to the detection of fetal cardiac anomalies in early pregnancy. Ultrasound Obstet Gynecol. 2002;19:360-5.
21. Comas C, Galindo A, Martínez JM, et al. Early prenatal diagnosis of major cardiac anomalies in a high-risk population. Prenat Diagn. 2002;22:586-93.
22. Haak MC, Twisk JWR, Van Vigt JMG. How successful is fetal echocardiographic examination in the first trimester of pregnancy? Ultrasound Obstet Gynecol. 2002;20:9-13.

23. Carvalho JS, Moscoso G, Ville Y. First trimester transabdominal fetal echocardiography. Lancet. 1998;351:1023-7.

24. Zosmer N, Souter VL, Chan CS, et al. Early diagnosis of major cardiac defects in chromosomally normal fetuses with increased nuchal translucency. Br J Obstet Gynecol. 1999;106:829-33.

25. Simpson JM, Jones A, Callaghan N, et al. Accuracy and limitations of transabdominal fetal echocardiography at 12-15 weeks of gestation in a population at high risk for congenital heart disease. Br J Obstet Gynecol. 2000;107:1492-7.

26. Huggon IC, Ghi T, Cook AC, et al. Fetal cardiac abnormalities identified prior to 14 weeks of gestation. Ultrasound Obstet Gynecol. 2002;20:22-9.

27. De Vore GR. First trimester fetal echocardiographic: is the future now? Ultrasound Obstet Gynecol. 2002;20:68.

28. Haak MC, van Vugt JM. Echocardiography in early pregnancy: a review of the literature. J Ultrasound Med. 2003;22:271-80.

29. DeVore GR. Color Doppler examination of the outflow tracts of the fetal heart: a technique for identification of cardiovascular malformations. Ultrasound Obstet Gynecol. 1994;4:463-71.

30. Wladimiroff JW, Seelen JC. Doppler tachometry in early pregnancy. Development of fetal vagal function. Eur J Obstet Gynecol Reprod Biol. 1972;2:55-63.

31. Schats R, Jansen CAM, Wladimiroff JW. Embryonic heart activity: appearance and development in early human pregnancy. Br J Obstet Gynaecol. 1990;97:989-94.

32. Gembruch U, Knopfle G, Chatterjee M, et al. First-trimester diagnosis of fetal congenital heart disease by transvaginal two-dimensional and Doppler echocardiography. Obstet Gynecol. 1990;75:496-8.

33. Bronshtein M, Siegler E, Yoffe N, et al. Prenatal diagnosis of ventricular septal defect and overriding aorta at 14 weeks of gestation using transvaginal sonography. Prenat Diagn. 1990;10:697-705.

34. Hernadi L, Torocsik M. Screening for fetal anomalies in the 12th week of pregnancy by transvaginal sonography in an unselected population. Prenat Diagn. 1997;17:7539.

35. D'Ottavio G, Meir YJ, Rustico MA, et al. Screening for fetal anomalies by ultrasound at 14 and 21 weeks. Ultrasound Obstet Gynecol. 1997;10:375-80.

36. Economides DL, Braithwaite JM. First trimester ultrasonographic diagnosis of fetal structural abnormalities in a low risk population. Br J Obstet Gynaecol. 1998;105:53-7.

37. Whitlow BJ, Chatzipapas IK, Lazanakis ML, et al. The value of sonography in early pregnancy for the detection of fetal abnormalities in an unselected population. Br J Obstet Gynaecol. 1999;106:929-36.

38. Guariglia L, Rosati P. Transvaginal sonographic detection of embryonic-fetal abnormalities in early pregnancy. Obstet Gynecol. 2000;96:328-32.

39. Lopes LM, Brizot ML, Lopes MAB, et al. Structural and functional cardiac abnormalities identified prior to 16 weeks of gestation in fetuses with increased nuchal translucency. Ultrasound Obstet Gynecol. 2003;22:470-8.

40. Comas C, Antolín E, Torrents M, et al. Early screening for chromosomal abnormalities: new strategies combining biochemical, sonographic and Doppler parameters. Prenat Neonat Med. 2001;6:95-102.

41. Van Lith JMM, Visser GHA, Mantingh A, et al. Fetal heart rate in early pregnancy and chromosomal disorders. Br J Obstet Gynaecol. 1992;99:741-4.

42. Martinez JM, Comas C, Ojuel J, et al. Fetal heart rate patterns in pregnancies with chromosomal disorders or subsequent fetal loss. Obstet Gynecol. 1996;87:118-21.

43. Hyett JA, Noble PL, Snijders RJM, et al. Fetal heart rate in trisomy 21 and other chromosomal abnormalities at 10-14 weeks of gestation. Ultrasound Obstet Gynecol. 1996;7:239-44.

44. Achiron R, Tadmor O, Mahiach S. Heart rate as a predictor of first-trimester spontaneous abortion after ultrasound-proven viability. Obstet Gynecol. 1991;78:330-3.

45. Laboda LA, Estroff JA, Benacerraf BR. First trimester bradycardia: A sign ofimpending fetal loss. J Ultrasound Med. 1989;8:561-3.

46. Baschat AA, Gembruch U, Knopfle G, et al. First-trimester fetal heart block: a marker for cardiac anomaly. Ultrasound Obstet Gynecol. 1999;14:311-4.

47. Yagel S, Anteby E, Ron M, et al. The role of abnormal fetal heart rate in scheduling chorionic villus sampling. Br J Obstet Gynaecol. 1992;99:739-40.

48. Hyett JA, Moscoso G, Papapanagiotou G, et al. Abnormalities of the heart and grat arteries in chromosomally normal fetuses with increased nuchal translucency thickness at 11-13 weeks of gestation. Ultrasound Obstet Gynecol. 1996;7:245-50.

49. Moscoso G. Fetal nuchal translucency: A need to understand the physiological basis. Ultrasound Obstet Gynecol. 1995;5:6-8.

50. Mavrides E, Cobian-Sanchez F, Tekay A, et al. Limitations of using first-trimester nuchal translucency measurement in routine screening for major congenital heart defects. Ultrasound Obstet Gynecol. 2001;17:106-10.

51. Hyett JA, Perdu M, Sharland GK, et al. Increased nuchal translucency at 10-14 weeks of gestation as a marker for major cardiac defects. Ultrasound Obstet Gynecol. 1997;10:242-6.

52. Huisman TWA, Bilardo CM. Transient increase in nuchal translucency thickness and reversed end-diastolic ductus venosus flow in a fetus with trisomy 18. Ultrasound Obstet Gynecol. 1997:10:397-9.

53. Haak MC, Twisk JW, Bartelings MM, et al. Ductus venosus flow velocities in relation to the cardiac defects in first-trimester fetuses with enlarged nuchal translucency. Am J Obstet Gynecol. 2003;188:727-33.

54. Martinez JM, Echevarría M, Borrell A, et al. Fetal heart rate and nuchal translucency in detecting chromosomal abnormalities other than Down syndrome. Obstetrics and Gynecology. 1998;92: 68-71.

55. Galindo A, Comas C, Martínez JM, et al. Cardiac defects in chromosomally normal fetuses with increased nuchal translucency at 10-14 weeks of gestation. J Matern Fetal Neonatal Med. 2003;13:163-70.

56. Bilardo CM, Pajkrt E, De Graaf IM, et al. Outcome of fetuses with enlarged nuchal translucency and normal karyotype. Ultrasound Obstet Gynecol. 1998;11:401-6.

57. Maymon R, Jauniaux E, Cohen O, et al. Pregnancy outcome and infant follow-up of fetuses with abnormally increased first trimester nuchal translucency. Hum Reprod. 2000;15:2023-7.

58. Carvalho JS. Nuchal translucency, ductus venosus and congenital heart disease: an important association-a cautious analysis. Ultrasound Obstet Gynecol. 1999;14:302-6.

59. Snijders RJM, Noble P, Sebire N, et al. UK multicentre project on assessment of risk of trisomy 21 by maternal age and fetal nuchal transludcency thickness al 10-14 weeks of gestation. Lancet. 1998;351:343-6.

60. Brady AF, Pandya PP, Yuksel B, et al. Outcome of chromosomally normal livebirths with increased fetal nuchal translucency at 10-14 weeks of gestation. J Med Genet. 1998;35:222-4.

61. Schwärzler P, Carvalho JS, Senat MV, et al. Screening for fetal aneuploidies and fetal cardiac abnormalities by nuchal translucency thickness measurement at 10-14 weeks of gestation as part of routine antenatal care in an unselected population. Br J Obstet Gynaecol. 1999;106:1029-34.

62. Michailidis GD, Economides DL. Nuchal translucency measurement and pregnancy outcome in karyotypically normal fetuses. Ultrasound Obstet Gynecol. 2001;17:1025.

63. Hyett J, Moscoso G, Nicolaides K. Abnormalities of the heart and great arteries in first trimester chromosomally abnormal fetuses. Am J Med Genet. 1997;69:207-16.

64. Haak MC, van Vugt JM. Pathophysiology of increased nuchal translucency: a review of the literature. Hum Reprod Update. 2003;9:175 84.

65. Berg KA, Clark EB, Astemborski JA, et al. Prenatal detection of cardiovascular malformations by echocardiography: an indication for cytogenetic evaluation. Am J Obstet Gynecol. 1998;69:494-7.

66. Schwanitz G, Zerres K, Gembruch U, et al. Prenatal detection of heart defects as an indication for chromosome analysis. Ann Genet. 1990;33:79-83.

67. Gembruch U, Baschat AA, Knopfle G, et al. Results of chromosomal analysis in fetuses with cardiac anomalies as diagnosed by first- and early second-trimester echocardiography. Ultrasound Obstet Gynecol. 1997;10:391-6.

68. Lazanakis MS, Rodgers K, Economides DL. Increased nuchal translucency and CATCH 22. Prenat Diagn. 1998;18:507-10.

69. Huggon IC, DeFigueiredo DB, Allan LD. Tricuspid regurgitation in the diagnosis of chromosomal anomalies in the fetus at 11-14 weeks of gestation. Heart. 2003;89:1071-3.

70. Simpson JM, Sharland GK. Nuchal translucency and congenital heart defects: heart failure or not? Ultrasound Obstet Gynecol. 2000;16:30-6.

46 Prenatal Diagnosis of Fetal Cytomegalovirus Infection

Y Ville, O Picone, G Makridemas

INTRODUCTION

Congenital cytomegalovirus (CMV) infection is likely to have become the most prevalent infection-related cause of congenital neurological handicap since rubella vaccination has become universal in developed countries. However, prenatal diagnosis and screening policies have been rather incoherent for the last 25 years and obstetricians have showed great reluctance to tackle that issue.[2] Indeed, although, the infection is frequent with 1–2% of all neonates excreting CMV in their urine, 90% of these will remain asymptomatic.[3] However, among symptomatic neonates, half will be severely and one-third of these will die, while 60% will develop significant neurological and developmental sequelae. Among the moderately symptomatic neonates, 65–75% will develop normally whereas 25–35% will have some degree of handicap at long-term follow-up. Furthermore, between 5% and 15% of the asymptomatic cases will also develop long-term developmental abnormalities, mainly sensorineural hearing loss, which can be bilateral in up to 50% of the cases.[1,3,4] Epidemiological risk factors have been extensively reviewed elsewhere.[5] Maternal age below 25, low socioeconomic status and presence of children age 13 in the home are the more constantly quoted.. Preconceptional maternal immunity (RR 0.31; 95% IC 0.17–0.58) and maternal age of 25 years or older (RR 0.19;95% CI 0.07–0.49) are highly protective against congenital infection.[6]

The possibilities for prenatal diagnosis have emerged more rapidly than those for establishing the prognosis of an infected fetus and the possibilities of treatment are still experimental.[2] In this review, we will address the possibilities and limits of prenatal imaging and biology in assessing both the diagnosis and the prognosis of fetal CMV infection.

PRENATAL ULTRASOUND EXAMINATION

Overall, less than half of fetal infections are diagnosed by ultrasound[7-15] and multiple organ system involvement is present in more than 50% of the cases)[16] at the time of prenatal diagnosis, ranging from 15% to 100% (Table 46.1) and is very likely subjected to reporting bias.

Indeed, the review of the pediatric literature suggests that most symptomatic congenitally infected neonates obviously escaped ultrasound screening and one should be aware that ultrasound alone is not a sensitive test for fetal infection or affection.

Longitudinal observational surveys of intrauterine infection cases are lacking since the other half of prenatally diagnosed cases were recognized as a result of maternal screening. The majority of these cases reported to date were terminated on the basis of proven fetal infection without ultrasound findings or before they could eventually develop.[10,12] However, three small prospective series reported a 15–25% sensitivity for antenatal ultrasound.[12,14,15]

The predictive value of ultrasound, like that of any other diagnostic test, increases with the prevalence of the disease and, therefore, works better in a population preselected by screening for maternal seroconversion. However, even in such a high-risk population, at least 90% of infected fetuses are expected to be asymptomatic.[16] The ultrasound features of this progressive disease will also vary significantly with time and serial ultrasound follow-up is likely to perform better than routine cross-sectional examination at any fixed gestation.

The pathophysiology of fetal CMV infection allows to expect progressive and sometimes only subtle or transient findings on ultrasound in cases of fetal infection (Figs 46.1A and B). Indeed, irrespective of the mode of transmission to the mother, CMV is a viremic herpes virus with a prolonged latency within maternal monocytes, which will eventually reach the fetus via the umbilical circulation.

The placenta, where the virus replicates, will act both as a barrier against CMV but also as a reservoir, which may release the virus into the fetal circulation at any stage of the pregnancy, irrespective of the time of seroconversion.[17,18] Within 4–8 weeks following maternal viremia, an early but inconstant sign of vertical infection is, therefore, likely to be placentitis as defined by a thickness of 4 cm or more and a heterogeneous appearance typically with calcifications coexisting with hypoechoic areas (Figs 46.2A to F).[13]

Once the virus reaches the fetal circulation, the fetal kidney is hit early and preferentially, which may cause transient oligohydramnios and less often renal hyperechogenicity. This appears to be more frequent than polyhydramnios.[19] Viral enterocolitis often shows with transient or persistent appearance of at least grade-2 hyper-echogenic bowel as an early ultrasound finding, which may be accompanied by high human chorionic gonadotropin (hCG) and alpha fetoprotein (AFP) levels in maternal blood.[19-22] This usually represents meconial ileus or bowel perforation and meconial peritonitis.[23,24] Several weeks can elapse until other features of fetal infection, if any, show-up on antenatal ultrasound, and some of the formers may have disappeared by then.

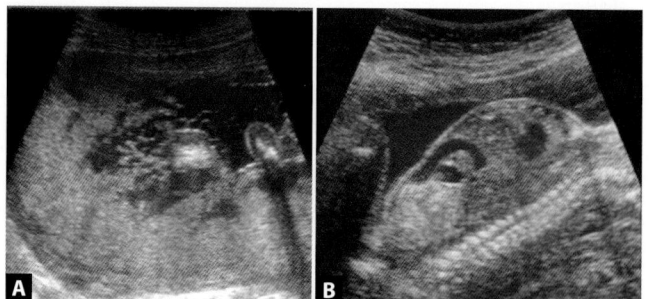

Figs 46.1A and B: Placentitis showing a thick and heterogeneous placenta (A). Hyperechogenic bowel and hepatomegaly (B) are not specific features of systemic fetal infection

Table 46.1: Fetal abnormalities diagnosed in utero in cases of congenital cytomegalovirus infection, except cerebral abnormalities (Table 46.2)

Series	Congenital CMV (n)	Fetuses with US findings (n)	Hyperechogenic bowel	Hepatomegaly	Splenomegaly	IUGR	Liver calcifications	Hydrops ascites	Cardiomegaly	Pericardial effusion	Placentomegaly	Pleural effusion	Oligohydramnios	Polyhydramnios	Skin edema
Enders et al. 2001[9]	189	41	12	15	4	3	2	2	2	3	1	2	2	4	1
Liesnard et al. 2000[10]	68	4	–	–	–	–	–	2	–	–	–	–	–	–	–
Lipitz et al. 1997[8]	51	11	6	1	2	–	1*	2 (1*)	–	–	–	–	–	–	–
Azam et al. 2001[11]	26	5	–	1*	–	–	–	1	–	1	–	–	1*	–	1
Lazzarotto et al. 2000[12]	25	3	1	–	–	–	–	–	1	2	1	–	–	–	–
Drose et al. 1991[13]	19	18	4 (1*)	4	–	1	3	–	1	–	3 (1*)	3 (1*)	5	6	7
Revello et al. 1999[14]	19	4	1*	2 (1*)	–	–	–	–	–	–	–	–	–	–	–
Preece et al. 1983[60]	9	–	–	–	–	–	–	–	–	–	–	–	–	–	–
Hohlfeld et al. 1991[46]	8	2	–	1*	1*	–	–	–	–	–	–	–	–	–	–
Malinger et al. 2003[30]	8	8	–	–	–	–	–	–	–	–	–	–	2	–	–
Lamy et al. 1992	7	2	–	–	–	–	–	–	–	–	–	–	–	–	–
Steinlin et al. 1996[61]	7	–	–	–	–	–	–	–	–	–	–	–	–	–	–
Lynch et al. 1991[52]	6	6	2 (1*)	1	1	–	–	1	–	–	–	–	–	3	–
Schneeberger et al. 1994[62]	4	1	1*	–	–	–	–	–	–	–	–	–	–	–	–
Grose et al. 1992[63]	3	2	1	–	–	1	–	–	–	–	–	–	–	1	–
Hogge et al. 1993[64]	3	2	–	1*	–	–	–	–	–	–	–	–	–	–	1
Tassin et al. 1990[65]	3	3	2	1	–	1	1	–	–	1	–	–	1	2	–
Agius et al. 1985[66]	2	–	–	–	–	–	–	–	–	–	–	–	–	–	–

Contd....

Contd…

Series	Congenital CMV (n)	Fetuses with US findings (n)												
		Hyperechogenic bowel	Hepatomegaly	Splenomegaly	Liver calcifications	Cardiomegaly	IUGR	Hydrops ascites	Placentomegaly	Pericardial effusion	Oligohydramnios	Pleural effusion	Polyhydramnios	Skin edema
Ahlfors et al. 1988[67]	2	–	–	–	–	–	–	–	–	–	–	–	–	–
Duvekot et al. 1990[68]	2	1*	–	–	–	–	–	–	–	–	–	–	–	–
Forouzan et al. 1992[20]	2	2	–	–	–	–	–	–	2	–	–	–	–	–
Gabrielli et al. 2003[69]	2	–	–	–	–	–	–	–	–	–	–	–	–	–
Inoue et al. 2001[70]	2	>	–	2	–	–	2	–	–	–	2	–	–	–
Morris et al. 1994[71]	2	–	–	–	–	–	–	–	–	–	–	–	–	–
Nigro et al. 1993[72]	2	–	–	–	–	–	–	–	–	–	–	–	–	–
Saigal et al. 1982[73]	2	–	–	–	–	–	–	–	–	–	–	–	–	–
Filloux et al. 1985[74]		–	–	tachycardia	–	–	–	–	–	–	–	–	–	–
Price et al. 1978[75]	1	1	–	1	–	–	–	–	–	–	–	1	–	1
Achiron et al. 1994[38]	1	1	–	–	–	–	–	–	–	–	–	–	–	–
Chaoui et al. 2002[25]	1	1	–	–	–	–	–	–	–	–	1	–	–	–
Heinrich et al. 2002[76]	1	1	–	1	1	–	–	–	–	–	–	–	–	–
Nigro et al. 1999[50]	1	1	–	–	–	1	–	–	–	–	–	–	–	–
Nigro et al. 1999[57]	1	1	–	–	–	–	–	–	–	–	–	1	–	–
Nigro et al. 1999[59]	1	1	–	–	–	–	–	–	1	–	–	–	1	1
Nigro et al. 2002[34]	1	1	–	–	–	–	–	–	–	–	–	–	–	1
Peters et al. 1995[22]	1	1	–	1	–	–	–	–	1	–	–	1	1	1

Contd…

Contd...

Series	Congenital CMV (n)	Fetuses with US findings (n)	Hyperechogenic bowel	Hepatomegaly	Splenomegaly	IUGR	Liver calcifications	Cardiomegaly	Hydrops ascites	Placentomegaly	Pericardial effusion	Pleural effusion	Oligohydramnios	Polyhydramnios	Skin edema
Pletcher et al. 1991[19]			1	–	–	–	–	–	1	–	–	–	–	–	–
Rousseau et al. 2000[77]			–	1	–	–	–	–	1	–	–	–	1	–	–
Seguin et al. 1988[78]			–	1	–	–	–	–	–	–	–	–	–	–	–
Soussotte et al. 2000[42]			–	1	–	–	–	–	–	–	–	–	–	–	–
Vogler et al. 1986[79]			1	–	–	–	–	–	–	–	–	–	–	–	–
Yamashita et al. 1989[80]			–	1	1	–	–	–	–	–	1	–	–	–	–
Watt-Morse et al. 1995[26]			–	1	1	–	–	–	–	–	–	1	–	–	–
TOTAL	490	130	37 (4*)	9 (1*)	32 (4*)	7	5 (1*)	6	13 (2*)	3	7 (1*)	5 (1*)	9 (1*)	17	8

IUGR: In utero growth restriction, US: Ultrasound, *Isolated abnormality

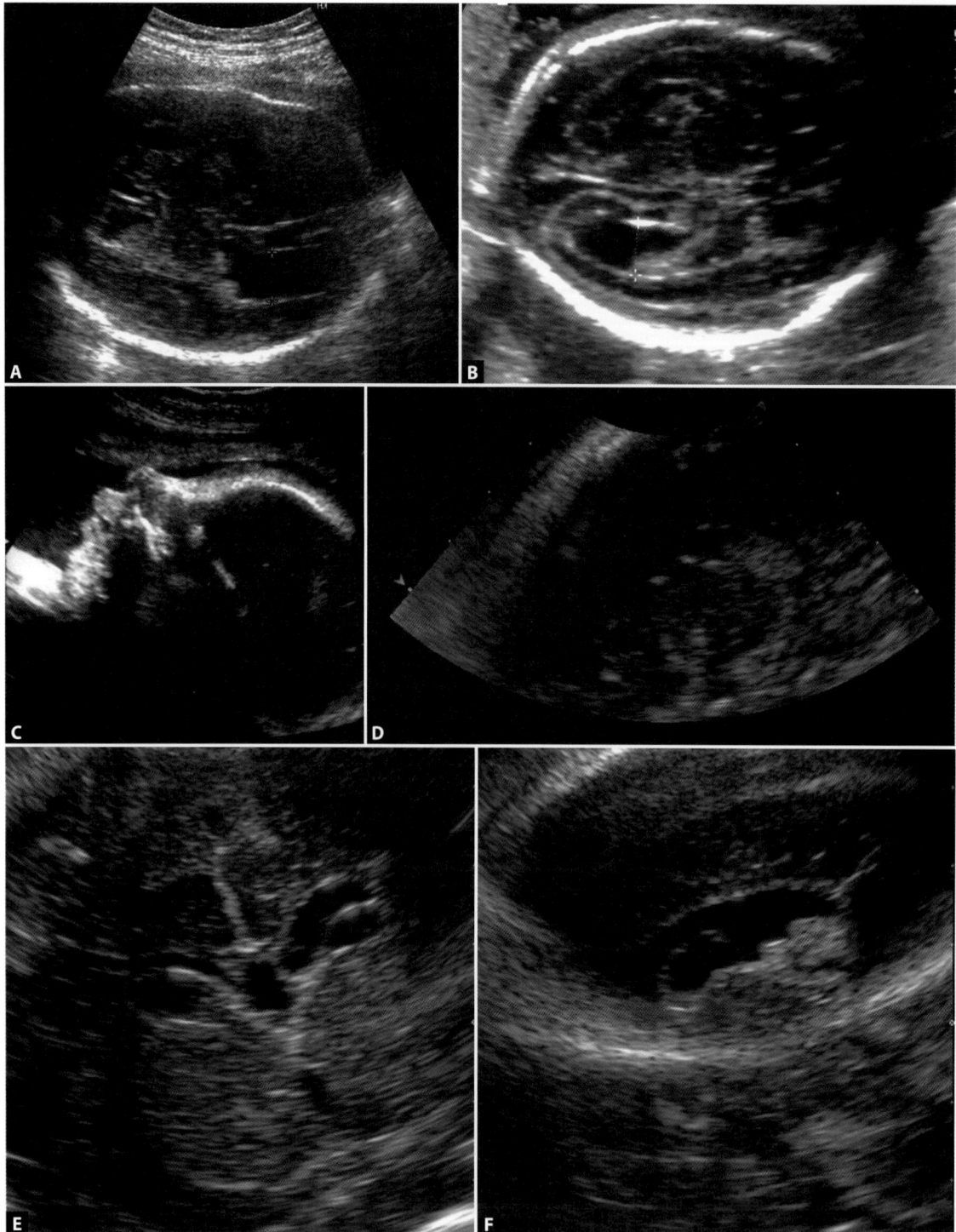

Figs 46.2A to F: (A) Cerebral features include ventriculomegaly (B) often preceding microencephaly (C) which in turn can precede microcephaly as illustrated by a sloping forehead on the profile view of the face. (D) More subtle features include parenchymal punctiform calcifications (E), subependymal cyst (F) and hyperechogenicity of the germinal matrix

Overt systemic disease will appear as hepatosplenomegaly and possibly ascites in the fetus as a result of cholestatic hepatitis and liver insufficiency).[25] Less often, generalized edema and ascites will suggest anemia-related hydrops due to the combined effect of liver failure and marrow infection. This spectacular presentation has also proven to eventually be transient with both ultrasound and biological normalization at follow-up.[26] Cardiomyopathy, expressed as cardiomegaly with a thick myocardium, which may

contain punctuate calcifications is a rare finding which could also participate to the development of fetal hydrops, eventually associated with tachyarrhythrnia.[13,25] Calcifications of the fetal liver, spleen, and even lungs could appear and remain as a result of a systemic disease.[27]

Intrauterine growth restriction (IUGR) may develop as a result of either fetal infection or placental infection or both. It can, therefore, be advised to screen for CMV as part of the assessment

Table 46.2: Fetal brain abnormalities diagnosed in utero in cases of congenital cytomegalovirus infection

Series	Congenital CMV (n)	Abnormal corpus callosum	Subependymal cysts	Ventriculomegaly	Reduced gyration	Hydrocephaly	Choroid plexus cyst	Microcephaly	Cystic structure in cerebellum	brain and periventricular calcifications	Lissencephaly	Agenesis or Hypoplastic or small Cerebellum
Enders et al. 2001[9]	189	7	7	12	3	2	–	2	2	2	–	–
Guerra et al. 2000[15]	68	4 (2*)	–	–	–	–	–	–	–	–	–	–
Boppana** et al. 1997[28]	56	4	–	–	3–	3	–	–	–	–	–	–
Liesnard et al. 2000[10]	55	1	2 (1*)	2	–	1	–	–	–	–	–	–
Lipitz et al. 1997[8]	51	3	–	–	1	–	1	–	–	–	–	–
Azam et al. 2001[11]	26	1	–	2 (1*)	–	–	–	–	–	–	–	–
Lazzarotto et al. 2000[12]	25	2 (1*)	–	–	1	1	–	–	–	–	–	–
Drose et al. 1991[13]	19	–	6 (1*)	2 (1*)	3	–	–	–	–	–	–	–
Barkovich** et al. 1994[41]	11	9	–	6	7	1	2	1	–	–	–	6
Malinger et al. 2003[30]	8	5	–	–	6	1	4	–	–	2 (1*)	–	3
Lamy et al. 1992	7	–	–	–	2*	–	–	–	–	–	–	–
Lynch et al. 1991[52]	6	3	–	1	1	–	–	–	–	–	–	–
Butt** et al. 1984[39]	4	4	–	–	4	–	–	–	–	–	–	2
Revello et al. 1999[14]	4	2	–	–	–	–	–	–	–	–	–	–
Hogge et al. 1993[64]	3	–	1	1	1	–	–	–	–	–	–	–
Tassin et al. 1990[65]	3	1	2	1	2	–	–	–	–	–	–	–
Inoue et al. 2001[70]	2	2	–	–	–	–	–	–	–	–	–	–
Nigro et al. 1999[57]	2	–	–	1	1	–	–	–	–	–	–	–
Ries** et al. 1990[81]	2	2	–	–	2	–	–	–	–	–	–	–
Seguin et al. 1988[66]	2	–	1	1	–	–	–	–	–	–	–	–
Twickler et al. 1993[35]	2	2	2	–	–	–	–	–	–	–	–	–
Achiron et al. 1994[38]	1	1	–	–	1	–	–	–	–	1	–	–
Chaoui et al. 2002[25]	1	1	–	–	–	1	–	–	–	–	–	–
Estroff et al. 1992[36]	1	1	–	1	1	–	–	–	–	–	–	–
Graham et al. 1982[82]	1	1	–	–	1	–	–	–	–	–	–	–
Mehta** et al. 2001[40]	1	1	–	–	1	1 (with Lipoma)	–	–	–	–	–	–
Mittelman-Handwerker et al. 1986[83]	1	1	1	–	1	–	–	–	1	–	1	–
Nigro et al. 1999[59]	1	–	–	–	–	–	1	–	–	–	–	1
Nigro et al. 2002[34]	1	1	–	–	–	–	–	–	–	–	–	–
Peters et al. 1995[22]	1	1	–	1	1	–	–	–	–	–	–	–
Pletcher et al. 1991[19]	1	1	–	–	1	–	–	–	–	–	–	–
Rousseau et al. 2000[65]	1	–	–	–	–	–	–	–	–	–	–	–
Soussotte et al. 2000[42]	1	–	–	1	1	–	1	–	–	–	–	1
Toma** et al. 1989[84]	1	–	1	1	1	–	–	–	–	–	–	–
Watt-Morse et al. 1995[26]	1	1	–	–	–	–	–	–	–	–	–	–
TOTAL	304	32 (3*)	13 (2*)	21 (2*)	21 (2*)	6	12	2	2	2	4 (1*)	14

of any IUGR fetus below the 5th centile. Indeed, this could be a completely isolated finding irrespective of placental or fetal Doppler values.[28,29]

Affection of the fetal brain shows mainly late and multiple suggestive and heterogeneous ultrasound features of fetal infection and of fetal affection (Table 46.2).[30] These can be present when the previously described features have resumed, therefore, weeks or months after the onset of maternal and even that of fetal infection.

Microcephaly is a major form of the disease, however this may prove to be a very difficult diagnosis to establish, especially in a growth retarded fetus.[31,32]

Ventriculomegaly, unilateral or bilateral, is a common entry to the diagnosis since around 5% of all ventriculomegaly diagnosed in utero are of infectious origin.[39] It can be of two types. Destructive ventriculomegaly is often moderate and will often precede microcephaly, showing even subtle enlargement of pericerebral spaces as an early sign of microencephaly. Obstructive ventriculomegaly can occur as a result of obstruction of the foramen of Monro and/or of Magendie and Lushka by ventriculitis-related edema or intraventricular hemorrhage.[34] The same mechanisms can lead to less common presentations such as mega cisterna magna, cerebellar hypoplasia or hemorrhage, pseudo-Dandy Walker malformations and schizencephaly.[30,35]

More subtle anomalies can be identified as associated findings with any of the features described above or as isolated findings, making the diagnosis more difficult. Non-specific vasculitis in the fetal thalami and basal ganglia[36] described as candle-stick images, punctuate echogenicity within the brain parenchyma or underlying the rim of the lateral ventricles together with strands across the lateral ventricles.[37,38] Germinolysis-related subependymal cysts can also be overlooked by routine fetal ultrasound examination when fetal infection is not known (Fig. 46.2A to 2F).[30,38,39] Rare cases of corpus callosum abnormalities have also been described in utero and postnatally.[30,40]

Abnormal myelinization and gyration of the fetal brain is another pitfall for fetal brain ultrasound examination and the development of fetal MRI is a recent and definite asset in the complete assessment of high-risk fetuses.[30,41,42] Lissencephaly could reflect injury before 16 or 18 weeks' whereas polymicrogyria could reflect injury at 18–24 weeks. Cases with normal gyral patterns have probably been injured during the third trimester showing diffuse heterogeneity in the white matter.[41] Both T1 and T2 sequences are therefore useful.

It is noteworthy that although the relationship between the ultrasound features described above and fetal CMV infection is well established, CMV is rarely reported in series of cases bearing these anomalies. This further emphasizes the poor performance of ultrasound to diagnose fetal CMV infection in the general population.

MATERNAL AND FETAL BIOLOGY

When the diagnosis of CMV infection is suspected on the basis of any of the ultrasound findings described above this can be excluded only if maternal serology shows negative IgG and negative IgM. Indeed, IgM, which can be present both in primary and non-primary infections are often negative at the time of a positive fetal ultrasound examination several weeks or months following maternal infection. At that time, both maternal viruria and viremia are also likely to be

negative although they have been found positive for 3–12 months following maternal infection.[43]

The diagnosis of fetal infection is made by recovery of the virus or by amplification of its genome in the amniotic fluid (AF) retrieved by amniocentesis.[5,44] Indeed, the AF is colonized once the virus has infected the fetal kidneys and replicates in the tubular epithelium to be passed in the urine. Viral DNA is therefore, accumulating in the AF as it does in the urine of infected individuals postnatally. This provides with clear guidelines for performing amniocentesis in CMV infection in pregnancy. Following seroconversion or reactivation, the process leading to CMV excretion in the fetal urine will take an average of 6–8 weeks and this interval should be recognized in order to avoid false negative prenatal diagnosis.[44] This should also be performed when fetal urination is well established and therefore not before 22 weeks.

Detection of infectious CMV in AF may be performed by the use of rapid virus isolation in cell cultures ("shell vial culture")[44,45] as well as CMV DNA detection by polymerase chain reaction (PCR) amplification. Sensitivity varies between 45% and 100% for both PCR and culture, the lowest figures being obtained when amniocentesis was performed before 21 weeks, and less than 6–8 weeks from maternal seroconversion.[8,46-51] However, the free interval can be even longer depending on the placental ability to contain infection.[52] The overall false negative rate of amniocentesis is around 12% (52/365) (0–25%)[9,10,12,43,49,51,52-57] Lipitz et al. 2002 have been reported to be much lower and even down to 0%, when the conditions of sampling were ideal.[45,56]

The variation in sensitivity may also account for the differences in PCR methods used. Each PCR method reported in the literature has its own protocol (e.g. single-round PCR, nested PCR, or commercial tests) and tested different volumes of fetal specimen, leading to variable sensitivities. Moreover, the CMV genome sequences amplified in these PCR tests varied with various fragments of the immediate early protein gene or of the glycoprotein B gene being most frequently used. Genetic diversity in those two genes is well recognize,[58] but the design of primers and probes did not always account for this.

False PCR positive results have also been reported when the neonate was not infected in 9/179 (5%) (030%) questioning the quality of the technique.[9,11,12,49,54,55,56,59] False positive diagnosis may be explained by contamination of the AF with the maternal blood during amniocentesis if the mother had a positive CMV DNAemia at the time of sampling. Indeed, Revello et al. showed that CMV DNA may be recovered in the blood of nearly 50% of immunocompetent patients up to 3 smonths after CMV primary infection.[43] Another explanation could be laboratory contamination occurring during PCR testing. Indeed, in some of these studies a nested CMV PCR was used, which is known to be a very sensitive technique but at high risk of contamination. Generalization of semiautomated real time PCR might help to overcome the risk of contamination and achieve absolute specificity for prenatal diagnosis of CMV infection. These results, however establish PCR as a reliable technique in reference laboratories. The question of performing a second amniocentesis when the result of the first examination is negative remains unanswered. However, to date, information available on 13 cases with a false negative result did not show any symptom at the age of up to 36 months although one neonate was growth-restricted.[9,52]

Another question without an answer today is that of the risk of fetal iatrogenic infection when maternal viremia is positive at the time of amniocentesis. However, the commonly understood pathophysiology of vertical transmission of CMV to the fetus makes this possibility unlikely.

PRENATAL DIAGNOSIS IN FETAL BLOOD

There are few data available on the prenatal diagnosis of CMV infection in fetal blood.

The sensitivity of IgM detection in fetal blood is around 50%.4,[10,4]. The sensitivity of CMV rapid or classic culture is even lower ranging from 0 to 40%[10,11,44] (Donner et al. 2000). This is probably due to the small volume retrieved by cordocentesis and PCR methods should be preferred. However, the sensitivity achieved by PCR in fetal blood varied greatly in three studies published, ranging from 40% to 92%.[9,10,44] Enders et al. reported a 100% sensitivity when combining amplification of CMV DNA in AF and in fetal blood.[9]

To date, CMV detection in fetal blood is, therefore, generally considered to be unsuitable for prenatal diagnosis. However, the value of viral quantification (DNA and IgM) in fetal blood to identify fetuses at risk of developing severe congenital infection is emerging and this issue will be developed in the second part of this review.[9,14,44]

CONCLUSION

Cytomegalovirus infection in pregnancy is not only when suggestive ultrasound features are diagnosed but also often questioned as a result of an individual or population-based screening result. Interpretation of maternal serology and indication for invasive and non-invasive testing requires some knowledge of the natural history of CMV transplacental infection.

Amniocentesis remains the gold standard invasive test to diagnose fetal infection and in the absence of ultrasound features, this should be performed after 22 weeks' and at least 6 weeks following maternal seroconversion.

REFERENCES

1. Stagno S, Pass RF, Gretchen Cloud MS, et al. Primary cytomegalovirus infection in pregnancy. J Am Med Assoc. 1986;256:1904-8.
2. Ville Y. The megalovirus. Ultrasound Obstet Gynecol. 1998;12:151-3.
3. Fowler KB, Stagno S, Pass RF et al. The outcome of congenital cytomegalovirus infection in relation to maternal antibody status. N Engl J Med. 1992;326:663-7.
4. Peckham C, Stark O, Dudgeon JA, et al. Congenital cytomegalovirus infection: A cause of sensorineural hearing loss. Arch Dis Child. 1987;62:1233-7.
5. Gaytant MA, Steegers E, Sommekrot BA, et al. Congenital cytomegalovirus infection: review of the epidemiology and outcome. Obst Gynecol Surv. 2002;57:245-56.
6. Fowler KB, Stagno S, Pass RF. Maternal immunity and prevention of congenital cytomegalovirus infection. J Am Med Ass. 2003;26:1008-11.
7. Hagay ZJ, Biran GB, Ornoy A, et al. Congenital cytomegalovirus infection: a long-standing problem still seeking a solution. Am J Obstet Gynecol. 1996;174:241-5.
8. Lipitz S, Yagel S, Shalev E, et al. Prenatal diagnosis of fetal primary cytomegalovirus infection. Obstet Gynecol. 1997;89:763-7.
9. Enders G, Bader U, Lindermann L, et al. Prenatal diagnosis of congenital cytomegalovirus infection in 189 pregnancies with known outcome. Prenat Diagn. 2001;21:362-77.
10. Liesnard C, Donner C, Brancart F, et al. Prenatal diagnosis of cytomegalovirus infection: prospective study of 237 pregnancies at risk. Obstet Gynecol. 2000;95:881-8.
11. Azam AZ, Vial Y, Fawer CL, et al. Prenatal diagnosis of congenital cytomegalovirus infection. Obstet Gynecol. 2001;97: 443-8.
12. Lazzarotto T, Varani S, Guerra B, et al. Prenatal indicators of congenital cytomegalovirus infection. J Pediatrics. 2000;137:90-5.
13. Drose JA, Dennis MA, Thickman D. Infection in utero: US findings in 19 cases. Radiology. 1991;178:369-74.
14. Revello MG, Zavattoni M, Sarasini A, et al. Prenatal diagnostic and prognostic value of human cytomegalovirus load and IgM antibody response in blood of congenitally infected fetuses. J Infect Dis. 1999;180:1320-3.
15. Guerra B, Lazzarotto T, Quarta S, et al. Prenatal diagnosis of symptomatic congenital cytomegalovirus infection. Obstet Gynecol. 2000;183:476-82.
16. Crino JP. Ultrasound and fetal diagnosis of perinatal infection. Clin Obstet Gynecol. 1999;42:71-80.
17. Goff E, Griffith BP, Booss J. Delayed amplification of cytomegalovirus infection in the placenta and maternal tissues during late gestation. Am J Obstet Gynecol. 1987;156:1265-70.
18. Kumazaki K, Ozono K, Yahara T, et al. Detection of cytomegalovirus DNA in human placenta. J Med Virol. 2002;68:363-9.
19. Pletcher BA, Williams MK, Mulivor RA, et al. Intrauterine cytomegalovirus infection presenting as fetal meconium peritonitis. Obstet Gynecol. 1991;78:903-5.
20. Forouzan I. Fetal abdominal echogenic mass: an early sign of intrauterine cytomegalovirus infection. Obstet Gynecol. 1992;80: 535-7.
21. McGregor SN, Tamura R, Sabbagha R, et al. Isolated hyperechoic fetal bowel: significance and implications for management. Am J Obstet Gynecol. 1995;173:1254-8.
22. Peters MT, Lowe TW, Carpenter A, et al. renatal diagnosis of congenital cytomegalovirus infection with abnormal triple-screen results and hyperechoic fetal bowel. Am J Obstet Gynecol. 1995;173:953-4.
23. Dechelotte PJ, Mulliez NM, Bouvier RJ, et al. Pseudo-meconium ileus due to cytomegalovirus infection: a report of three cases. Pediatr Pathol. 1992;12:73-82.
24. Huang YC, Lin TY, Huang CS, et al. Ileal perforation caused by congenital or perinatal cytomegalovirus infection. J Pediatr. 1997;129:931-4.
25. Chaoui R, Zodan Marin T, Wisser J. Marked splenomegaly in fetal cytomegalovirus infection: detection supported by 3-dimensional power Doppler ultrasound. Ultrasound Obstet Gynecol. 2002;20: 299-302.
26. Watt-Morse ML, Laifer, SA Hill LM. The natural history of fetal cytomegalovirus infection as assessed by serial ultrasound and fetal blood sampling: a case report. Prenat Diagn. 1995;15:567-70.
27. Stein B, Bromley B, Michlewitz H, et al. Fetal liver calcifications: sonographic appearance and post-natal outcome. Radiology. 1995;197:489-92.
28. Boppana SB, Fowler KB, Vaid Y, et al. Neuroradiographic findings in the newborn period and long term outcome in children with symptomatic congenital CMV infection. Pediatrics. 1997;99:409-14.

29. Conboy TJ, Pass RF, Stagno S, et al. Early clinical manifestations and intellectual outcome in children with symptomatic congenital cytomegalovirus infection. J Pediatr. 1987;111:343-8.

30. Malinger G, Lev D, Zahalka N, et al. Fetal cytomegalovirus infection of the brain: the spectrum of sonographic findings. Am J Neuroradiol. 2003;24:28-32.

31. Noyola DE, Demmler GJ, Williamson WD, et al. and the congenital CMV longitudinal study group. Cytomegalovirus urinary excretion and long term outcome in children with congenital cytomegalovirus excretion. Pediatr Infect Dis. 2000;19:505-10.

32. Ahlfors K, Ivarsson SA, Bjerre I. Microcephaly and congenital cytomegalovirus infection: A combined prospective and retrospective study of a swedish infant population. Pediatrics. 1986;78:1058-63.

33. Holzgreve W, Feil R, Louwen F, et al. Prenatal diagnosis and management of fetal hydrocephaly and lissencephaly. Child's Nerv Syst. 1993;9:51-4.

34. Nigro G, La Torre R, Sali E, et al. Intraventricular hemorrhage in a fetus with cerebral cytomegalovirus infection. Prenat Diagn. 2002;22:558-61.

35. Twickler DM, Perlman J, Maberry MC. Congenital cytomegalovirus infection presenting as cerebral ventriculomegaly on antenatal sonography. Am J Perinatol. 1993;10:404-6.

36. Estroff JA, Richard BP, Teele RL, et al. Echogenic vessels in the fetal thalami and basal ganglia associated with cytomegalovirus infection. J Ultrasound Med. 1992;11:686-8.

37. Fakhry J, Khoury A. Fetal intracranial calcifications; the importance of periventricular hyperechoic foci without shadowing. J Ultrasound Med. 1991;10:51-4.

38. Achiron R, Pinhas-Hamiel O, Lipitz S, et al. Prenatal ultrasonographic diagnosis of fetal cerebral ventriculitis associated with asymptomatic maternal cytomegalovirus infection. Prenat Diagn. 1994;14:523-6.

39. Butt W, Mackay RJ, De Crespigny L, et al. Intracranial lesions of congenital cytomegalovirus infection detected by ultrasound scanning. Pediatrics. 1984;73:611-4.

40. Mehta N, Hartnoll G. Congenital CMV with callosal lipoma and agenesis. Pediatr Neurol. 2001;24:222-4.

41. Barkovich AJ, Lindan CE. Congenital cytomegalovirus infection of the brain: imaging analysis and embryologic considerations. Am J Neuroradiol. 1994;15:703-15.

42. Soussotte C, Maugey-Laulom B, Carles D. Contribution of transvaginal ultrasonography and fetal cerebral MRI in a case of congenital cytomegalovirus infection. Fetal diagn Ther. 2000;15:219-33.

43. Revello MG, Zavattoni M, Sarasini A, et al. Human cytomegalovirus in blood of immunocompetent persons during primary infection: Prognostic implications for pregnancy. J Infect Dis. 1998;177: 1170-5.

44. Revello MG, Gerna G. Diagnosis and management of human cytomegalovirus infection in the mother, fetus and new born infant. Clin Microbiol Rev. 2002;15:680-713.

45. Gleaves CA, Smith TF, Shucter EA, et al. Rapid detection of cytomegalovirus in MRC-5 cells inoculated with urine specimens by using low-speed centrifugation and monoclonal antibody to an early antigen. J Clin Microbiol. 1984;19:917-9.

46. Hohlfeld P, Vial Y, Maillard-Brignon C, et al. Cytomegalovirus fetal infection: prenatal diagnosis. Obstet Gynecol. 1991;78:615-8.

47. Baldanti F, Sarasini FM, Zavattoni PE, et al. Polymerase chain reaction for prenatal diagnosis of congenital cytomegalovirus infection. J Med Virol. 1995;47:462-6.

48. Lamy H, Mulongo K, Gadissieux JF, et al. Prenatal diagnosis of fetal cytomegalovirus infection. Am J Obstet Gynecol. 2002;166:91-4.

49. Donner C, Liesnard C, Content J, et al. Prenatal diagnosis of 52 pregnancies at risk for congenital cytomegalovirus infection. Obst Gynecol. 1993;82:481-6.

50. Nigro G, La Torre R, Anceschi MM, et al. Hyperimmunoglobulin therapy for a twin fetus with cytomegalovirus infection and growth restriction. Am J Obstet Gynecol. 1999;180:1222-6.

51. Antsaklis A, Daskalakis G, Mesogitis S, et al. Prenatal diagnosis of fetal primary cytomegalovirus infection. Br J Obstet Gynaecol. 2000;107:84-8.

52. Lynch L, Daffos F, Emanuel D, et al. Prenatal diagnosis of fetal cytomegalovirus infection. Obstet Gynecol. 1991;165: 714-8.

53. Ruellan-Eugene G, Barjot P, Campet M, et al. Evaluation of virological procedures to detect fetal human cytomegalovirus infection: avidity of IgG antibodies, virus detection in amniotic fluid and maternal serum. J Med Virol. 1996;50: 9-15.

54. Bodeus M, Hubinont C, Bernard P, et al. Prenatal diagnosis of human cytomegalovirus by culture and polymerase chain reaction: 98 pregnancies leading to congenital infection. Prenat Diagn. 1999;19:314-7.

55. Gouarin S, Palmer P, Cointe D, et al. Congenital HCMV infection: a collaborative and comparative study of virus detection in amniotic fluid by culture and PCR. J Clin Virol. 2001;21: 47-55.

56. Revello MG, Zavattoni M, Furione M, et al. Quantification of human cytomegalovirus DNA in amniotic fluid of mothers of congenitally infected fetuses. J Clin Microbiol. 1999;37:3350-2.

57. Nigro G, La Torre R, Mazzocco M, et al. Multi system cytomegalovirus fetopathy by recurrent infection in a pregnant women with hepatitis B. Prenat Diagn. 1999;19:1070-2.

58. Chou S. Comparative analysis of sequence variation in gp116 and gp55 components of glycoprotein B of human cytomegalovirus. Virology. 1992;88:388-90.

59. Nigro G, Mazzocco M, Anceschi M, et al. Prenatal diagnosis of fetal cytomegalovirus infection after primary or recurrent maternal infection. Obstet Gynecol. 1999;94:909-14.

60. Preece PM, Blount JM, Glover J, et al. The consequence of primary cytomegalovirus infection in pregnancy. Arch Dis Child. 1983;58: 970-5.

61. Steinlin MI, Nadal D, Eich GF, et al. Late intrauterine cytomegalovirus infection: clinical and neuroimaging findings. Pediatr Neurol. 1996;15:249-53.

62. Schneeberger PM, Groendaal F, de Vries LS, et al. Variable outcome of a congenital cytomegalovirus infection in a quadruplet pregnancy after primary infection of the mother during pregnancy. Act Paediatr. 1994;83:986-9.

63. Grose C, Meehan T, Weiner CP. Prenatal diagnosis of congenital cytomegalovirus infection by virus isolation after amniocentesis. Pediatr Infect Dis. 1992;11:605-7.

64. Hogge WA, Buffone GJ, Hogge JS. Prenatal diagnosis of cytomegalovirus (CMV) infection: a preliminary report. Prenat Diagn. 1993;13:131-6.

65. Tassin GB, Maklad NF, Stewart RR, et al. Cytomegalic inclusion disease: intrauterine sonographic diagnosis using findings involving the brain. Am J Neuroradiol. 1991;12:117-22.

66. Agius G, Baillargeau E, Ranger S, et al. Infection congénitale à Cytomégalovirus chez des jumeaux dizygotes. Arch Fr Pediatr. 1985;42:63-4.

67. Ahlfors K, Ivarsson SA, Nilsson H. On the unpredictable development of congenital cytomegalovirus infection. A study in twins. Early Human Development. 1988;18:125-35.

68. Duvekot JJ, Theewes BA, Wesdrop JM, et al. Congenital cytomegalovirus infection in a twin pregnancy: a case report. Eur J Pediatr. 1990;149:261-2.

69. Gabrielli L, Lazzarotto T, Foschini MP, et al. Horizontal in utero acquisition of cytomegalovirus infection in a twin pregnancy. J Clin Microbiol. 2003;41:1329-1.

70. Inoue T, Matsumura N, Fukuoka M, et al. Severe congenital infection with fetal hydrops in a cytomegalovirus seropositive healthy women. Eur J Obstet Gynecol. 2001;95:184-6.

71. Morris DJ, Sims D, Chiswick M, et al. Symptomatic congenital CMV infection after maternal recurrent infection. Pediatr Inf Dis. 1994;13:61-4.

72. Nigro G, Clerico A, Mondaini C. Symptomatic congenital cytomegalovirus infection in two consecutive sisters. Arch Dis Child. 1993;69:527-8.

73. Saigal S, Lunyk O, Larke B, et al. The outcome of children with congenital cytomegalovirus infection. Am J Dis Child. 1982;136:986-01.

74. Fillioux F, Kelsey DK, Bose CL, et al. Hydrops fetalis with supraventricular tachycardia and cytomegalovirus infection. Clin Peadiatr. 1985;534-6.

75. Price JM, Fisch AE, Jacobson J. Ultrasonic findings in fetal cytomegalovirus infection. Journ Clin Ultras. 1978;6:215-94.

76. Henrich W, Meckies J, Dudenhausen JW, et al. Recurrent CMV infection during pregnancy: Ultrasound diagnosis and fetal outcome. Ultrasound Obstet Gynecol. 2002;19:608-11.

77. Rousseau T, Douvier S, Reynaud I, et al. Severe fetal cytomegalic inclusion disease after documented maternal reactivation of CMV during pregnancy. Prenat Diagn. 2000;20:333-6.

78. Seguin J, Cho CT. Congenital Cytomegalovirus Infection in one monozygotic twin. J Am Med Ass. 1988;260:22.

79. Vogler C, Kohl S, Rosenberg HS. Cytomegalovirus infection and fetal death in a twin. J. Reprod Med. 1986; 31:207-10.

80. Yamashita Y, Iwanaga R, Goto A, et al. Congenital cytomegalovirus infection associated with fetal ascites and intrahepatic calcifications. Acta Paediatr Scand. 1989;78:965-7.

81. Rics M, Deeg KH, Heininger U. Demonstration of perivascular echogenicities in congenital cytomegalovirus infection by colour Doppler imaging. Eur J Pediatr. 1990;150:34-6.

82. Graham D, Guidi SM, Sanders RC. Sonographic features of in utero periventricular calcification due to cytomegalovirus infection. J Ultrasound Med. 1982;1:171-2.

83. Mittelman-Handwerker S, Pardes JG, Post RC, et al. Fetal ventriculomegaly and brain atrophy in a woman with intrauterine cytomegalovirus infection. J Reprod Med. 1986;31;1061-4.

84. Toma P, Magnano GM, Mezzano, P, et al. Cerebral ultrasound images in prenatal cytomegalovirus infection. Neuroradiology. 1989;31:278-89.

47 Fetal Hydrops

T Marton, PM Cox

FETAL HYDROPS

Fetal hydrops is a combination of generalized soft tissue edema and fluid (effusion) in one or more body cavity.

Hydrops still has a high mortality causing fetal demise in more than 50% of the detected cases and postnatal mortality following live birth is also around 50%.[1] There may be many causes. According to the traditional classification, the hydrops can be divided into immune and non-immune types. A more clinically (fetal medicine) oriented approach could be to divide cases into those due to fetal anemia and non-anemia related hydrops. The practical reason for this categorization is that fetal anemia is still the most common cause of hydrops and in most cases fetal anemia is easily detectable in utero. It can often be treated with intrauterine transfusion and thus anemia related hydrops has a better prognosis than other forms.

In different parts of the world, there are different causes of hydrops. For example, in underdeveloped countries, Rhesus isoimmunization still remains a major cause; whereas in Southern China, fetal α-thalassemia is a main causative factor. In contrast, in the developed world structural and chromosomal anomalies and *Parvovirus* B19 infections are the most frequent causes of hydrops.

This chapter aims to be a comprehensive library of the various fetal conditions that play role in fetal hydrops and presents a few characteristic features.

ANEMIA-RELATED HYDROPS

It is well known that fetal anemia can be readily detected with the help of ultrasound/Doppler, measuring the middle cerebral artery velocity. For details see the relevant chapter of this book. The causes of fetal anemia should be subdivided, as they affect the prognosis for the pregnancy and fetus.

Immune Hydrops

Historically, immune hydrops (due to maternal anti-D iso-immunization) was the most common cause of fetal anemia and hydrops. Fortunately, these severe cases of anti-D isoimmunization are now very rarely seen, as a result of anti-D immunoglobulin prophylaxis for Rhesus negative mothers. In the absence of prophylaxis, the disease still occurs. Immune hydrops is the result of a maternal IgG-mediated hemolytic disease of the fetus, the severest form of which is erythroblastosis fetalis.

There are further antigens that can cause immune-mediated fetal hemolytic disease including: Rhesus anti-C, anti-c, anti-E, anti-e, anti-Kell, anti-MNS, anti-Duffy and anti-A or anti-B.

Isoimmunization due to the non-Rh groups such as Kell, MNS, and Kidd have assumed increasing importance as the incidence of Rh-D sensitization has decreased.

Anti-Kell disease has a particularly poor prognosis, probably because the anemia is partly hemolytic and partly the result of suppressed erythropoiesis.[2] A significantly higher incidence of polyhydramnios was found among fetuses with Kell isoimmunization and the maternal serum titer is much lower than in the RhD group.[3]

Genetically Determined Hemolytic Disease of the Fetus

There are a number of genetically determined hemolytic diseases of the fetus, which can rarely lead to fetal hydrops (Box 47.1).

> **Box 47.1:** Genetically determined hemolytic anemias causing fetal hydrops
>
> - Glucose phosphate isomerase deficiency (AD in adult cases, neonatal and fetal form most likely AR)[4] causes hemolytic crisis, very rarely fetal anemia and hydrops.
> - Dehydrogenase (G6PD) deficiency (X linked dominant) Hemolytic episodes.
> - Pyruvate kinase deficiency of erythrocyte (AR).[5]

Non-infectious Disorders of Erythrocyte Production

Alpha thalassemia (AD) is a common cause of fetal hydrops in Chinese population.[6] Thalassemias are a group of inherited abnormalities of the hemoglobin synthesis. Hemoglobin has an alpha and a beta chain. Homozygous alpha thalassemia (deletion of both α-chain alleles of the corresponding region of chromosome 16) is responsible for the fetal hydrops (Bart syndrome). Clinical classification, such as thalassemia major, intermedia and minor refer only to the clinical severity of the disease. It is also apparent that, at least in some cases, compound heterozygosity is responsible for the hydropic change of the fetus. Anemia in thalassemia is the result of short turnover time of erythrocytes with a reduced hemoglobin content.

Other inherited forms of dyserythropoiesis are listed in Box 47.2. These represent rarities.

Fetal Anemia as a Consequence of Fetal Blood Loss

Internal fetal hemorrhage may lead to severe anemia due to blood loss. The most common site of hemorrhage is the brain, but intrathoracic and intra-abdominal hemorrhages may also occur. Spontaneous fetal hemorrhage should always prompt a search for maternal antiplatelet antibodies to exclude alloimmune thrombocytopenia.[11,12]

> **Box 47.2:** Inherited dyserythropoietic conditions associated with fetal hydrops
>
> - Congenital dyserythropoietic anemia (AD)[7] is characterized by ineffective erythropoiesis and multinuclear erythroblasts.
> - Congenital erythropoietic porphyria (AR).[8]
> - Diamond-Blackfan syndrome (AD)[9] causes congenital hypoplastic anemia.
> - Leukemia (associated with Down syndrome).[10]

> **Box 47.3:** Obstruction of systemic venous return
>
> *Thorax:*
> - Congenital cystic adenomatoid malformation of the lung[25,26]
> - Pulmonary extralobar sequestration[27]
> - Large diaphragmatic hernia
> - Intrathoracic teratoma
> - Intrathoracic lymphangioma[28]
> - Cardiac or pericardial tumor[29]
> - Laryngeal atresia [Kalache, Chaoui, et al. 1997:174 /id].
>
> *Abdominal tumor or tumor-like lesion:*
> - Abdominal teratoma
> - Cystic kidneys
> - Obstructive uropathy
> - Hepatoblastoma
> - Ovarian cyst
> - Other tumor

Placental subchorial/intervillous hemorrhage can also originate from the fetus.

Fetomaternal hemorrhage (i.e. hemorrhage from the fetal into the maternal circulation) is common. Tiny hemorrhages are probably universal. Massive hemorrhage may be acutely fatal but smaller or recurrent bleeds may lead to an anemic, hydropic fetus. A maternal Kleihauer-Betke test is an essential part of the investigation of hydrops.[13] Hemorrhage can also occur into a necrotic congenital tumor.

Human Parvovirus B19 Infection

Parvovirus is one of the most important factors causing anemia and hydrops.

In pregnant women, it can cause miscarriage (6.5%),[14] hydrops and intrauterine death, although, most infected women give birth to healthy neonates without any intervention.[15] In a meta-analysis of 165 reported cases of antenatal HPV-B19 cases, there was a 10.2% excess risk of fetal death. Transplacental transmission was confirmed in 69 (24.1%) of 286 reported maternal infections. According to a separate meta-analysis HPV-B19 infection was present in 57 out of 299 (19.1%) non-malformed cases of non-immune hydrops fetalis.[16] *Parvovirus* affects not only the erythroid cell lines, inhibiting erythrocyte production, but also infects the cardiac myocytes. In most cases, the hydrops is a consequence of severe anemia, though at least in some chronic cases it appears that a direct effect on the heart cannot be excluded.

Infections, in which anemia plays a role in the hydrops are seen below.

NON-ANEMIA-RELATED HYDROPS

Infection-induced Fetal Hydrops[17]

The most common infections causing fetal hydrops are:

- *Parvovirus* B19 (see earlier section), *cytomegalovirus,[18] herpes simplex virus, Toxoplasma gondii, Treponema pallidum,* Coxsackievirus type B, Adenovirus. *Congenital Chagas'* disease is also reported to be associated with hydrops.[19]

- The mechanism, by which the different infections cause hydrops varies. For example, *Herpes simplex virus* causes liver damage, whilst coxsackievirus and adenovirus lead to myocarditis and fetal tachyarrhythmia.[20,21]

- Congenital syphilis results in generalized chronic infection,[22] with anemia, thrombocytopenia and later ascites. In congenital syphilis, the mother can be seronegative with an infected fetus,[23] and this may also be true for *Parvovirus* (personal observation).

> **Box 47.4:** Congenital heart conditions in fetal hydrops
>
> - Congenital heart disease[24,30]
> - Atresia of the aortic or pulmonary trunk
> - Various malformations of the great arteries
> - Atrioventricular septal defect
> - Right or left ventricular hypoplasia, divided right ventricle[31]
> - Cardiomyopathy[32]
> - *Fetal bradycardia:* Congenital heart block,[33] maternal SLE, Lupus anticoagulant
> - *Fetal tachycardia* with myocarditis, e.g. adenovirus, coxsackievirus, *parvovirus,* Chagas' disease or WPW syndrome[34,35]

Structural Anomalies

a. Tumors or tumor-like hamartomatous lesions within the body cavities may cause hydrops with compression or obstruction of the major vessels of the systemic venous return. The lesions that belong in this group are seen in Box 47.3. Fetal lung lesions associated with hydrops are almost always lethal.[24]

   Occlusions of the superior or inferior vena cava and ductus venosus are also reported to result in hydrops.

b. Cardiac disease, including developmental abnormalities, tachyarrhythmia and bradycardia may all cause fetal hydrops. A list of these conditions are in Box 47.4.

c. Vascular shunts result in high-output cardiac failure and subsequent hydrops.

   This occurs in fetal sacrococcygeal teratoma[36-38] and in arteriovenous malformations at various locations in the body. In the head, vein of Galen aneurysm, intracranial arteriovenous malformation and intracranial teratoma have been described.[39] Cervical, abdominal,[40] or cutaneous hemangiomas, AV malformations of the liver and lung, large placental chorangioma and angiomatosis of the fetus are also rare causes of hydrops.

   Hydrops can occur as a complication of *monocihorionic twinning,* often because of high output cardiac failure of one twin.[41] In twin-to-twin transfusion syndrome, volume overload in the recipient leads to failure and hydrops, whilst in TRAP sequence reversed perfusion of a large acardiac cotwin by the pump twin is the cause. There are also reported cases with myocardial infarct of the recipient in twin-to-twin transfusion syndrome[42] and transient hydrops of the donor after amniocentesis.[43]

Lysosomal storage disease:[48]
- Mucopolysaccharidosis type VII[49]
- Mucolipidoses I (Sialidosis III)[50]
- Mucolipidosis II (I-cell disease)
- Gaucher disease[51]
- Farber disease[52]
- GM1-gangliosidosis[53]
- Niemann-Pick disease[54]
- Morquio disease[55]

Glycogen storage disease:
- Type IIb (glycogen storage disease limited to the heart)[56]
- Type IV[57]

d. Other circulatory problems: It has been suggested that long, and/or over coiled umbilical cord with increased vascular resistance, may in some instances cause circulatory failure and consequent hydrops.[44]

Chromosome Abnormality (Including Turner Syndrome)

X monosomy (45, X0-Turner syndrome) is the most common chromosome aneuploidy related to hydrops. It appears that failure of the lymph vessel development causes the hydropic change.[45] It is also apparent that in 90% of the hydropic Turner syndrome fetuses, the heart weight is under the 2.5th centile and it has been suggested that this is a major cause of fetal demise in Turner syndrome fetuses.[46]

Trisomy 21: Hydrops or nuchal swelling was diagnosed in approximately 40% [cystic hygroma and increased nuchal fold thickness (30.5%), hydrops (9.6%)] according to a large series.[47]

Other karyotypic abnormalities associated with hydrops include: Trisomy 18, Trisomy 13, Trisomy 15 and Trisomy 10 mosaicism.

Metabolic and Storage Disease

Metabolic and storage disease represents less than 1% of all hydrops cases. These are individually rare, but important because of autosomal recessive inheritance and thus 25% recurrence risk. The relevant enzyme defects are listed in Box 47.5.

Further Genetic Causes

Box 47.6 contains the most frequent genetic syndromes that cause hydrops. Osteochondrodysplasias are important because of the inheritance and the number of recognized syndromes is growing.

MISCELLANEOUS

According to recent studies *fetal hemochromatosis* appears to be the result of fetal liver disease and in the late second trimester of pregnancy results in severe panhypoproteinemia with non-immune hydrops.[63,64]

Maternal indomethacin therapy mainly in the third trimester has been reported causing early closure of ductus arteriosus and consequent fetal hydrops.[65] One case of iatrogenic intrauterine hypothyroidism and subsequent fetal hydrops has also been published, which was caused by maternal propylthiouracil

Osteochondrodysplasias:
- Blomstrand type chondrodysplasia [(AR) short limbs, polyhydramnios, hydrops fetalis, facial anomalies, increased bone density, and a remarkable advanced skeletal maturation]
- Greenberg dysplasia [(AR) Radiological features: "motheaten" appearance of the markedly short long bones, bizarre ectopic ossification centers, and marked platyspondyly with unusual ossification centers][58]
- Conradi-Hunermann, chondrodysplasia punctata [(X linked - D), disorganization of the spine, premature echogenicity of femoral epipheses, and frontal bossing with depressed nasal bridge, polyhydramnios][59]
- Osteogenesis imperfecta congenita (AD)
- Achondrogenesis type IA [(AR) polyhydramnios, subgaleal edema, microcephaly, a narrow thorax, pericardial effusion, and a severe short-limbed dwarfism with unossified tubular bones and vertebral bodies][60]
- Achondrogenesis type IB [(AR) sulfate transporter gene mutation, severe rhizomelia, narrow chest, flat face, polyhydramnios, possible umbilical hernia]
- Achondrogenesis type II [(AD) marked micromelic dwarfism, barrel shaped, small chest, polyhydramnios]
- Short rib polydactyly syndrome Type II [(AR) short ribs, polydactyly (preaxial or postaxial), possible polycystic kidneys, median cleft lip][61]
- Short rib polydactyly syndrome Type IV (AR) markedly narrow ribs, micromelia, shortened limbs with postaxial heptasyndactyly polycystic renal dysplasia
- Fibrochondrogenesis (AR)
- Kniest like dysplasia (AR)
- Campomelic dysplasia (AR)

Other genetic syndromes associated with hydrops:
- Arthrogryposis multiplex
- Lethal multiple pterygium syndrome
- Fetal akinesia
- Beckwith-Wiedemann syndrome
- Simpson-Golabi-Behmel syndrome[62]
- Smith-Lemli-Opitz syndrome
- Tuberous sclerosis
- Congenital arterial calcification

medication for maternal Grave's disease.[66] In another case report fetal hyperthyreosis and hydrops, was caused by a hyperthyroid mother with Grave's disease by antithyroid antibodies.[67] Mother also had a history of three prior perinatal deaths between 26 and 28 weeks of gestation, all associated with fetal hydrops. After maternal therapy with propylthiouracil, resolution of non-immune hydrops was documented and a healthy neonate subsequently delivered to term.

INVESTIGATIONS IN HYDROPS[68,69]

Pathologic examination of fetuses with non-immune hydrops requires a multidisciplinary approach. The first and most important is the macroscopic description and identification of structural abnormalities. Developmental abnormalities may draw attention to the possibility of a chromosome abnormality thus cytogenetic studies are essential. (If cytogenetic culture fails, FISH studies should be performed to exclude common trisomies.) The pathologist has to be careful to save living cells for further biochemical studies in case of the suspicion of a metabolic disease. Osteochondrodysplasias cannot be diagnosed without proper X-ray documentation, and if necessary involvement of an experienced radiographer. Molecular biology and DNA investigation is also important. Microbiology with bacterial, viral cultures and if necessary PCR investigation may also be useful. Light microscopic examination is essential and in a significant proportion of the cases enough to make a diagnosis. Fortunately CMV, *Parvovirus* and Adenovirus antibodies are available to prove infection in paraffin embedded blocks of the fetal tissues. According to published figures a meticulous examination, including clinical studies, such as Kleihauer-Betke test and maternal auto-antibodies, leaves approximately 10–20% of cases unexplained.[68,69]

The proverb that a good clinical history is half the diagnosis is very true with regard to the pathologist's work while undertaking an autopsy of a hydropic fetus. Nowadays fetal hydrops is generally investigated prenatally. Clinical data can draw attention to subtle signs (which would otherwise be missed, especially in autolytic fetuses) and makes the pathologist widen the investigation in the relevant direction. Samples are taken that cannot be taken later, such as frozen tissue for metabolic studies or DNA, frozen sections for immunohistochemistry, especially fixed tissue for electron microscopy, instruction to the cytogenetic or histochemistry laboratory to save cells for biochemical studies, etc.

It is essential to seek for and document any prenatal finding, as it is an important feedback to the clinician and provides the parents with information.

In summary: Because of the wide spectrum of causes of hydrops, a multidisciplinary approach to diagnosis is recommended based on proper communication and exchange of information between the clinician and pathologist.

REFERENCES

1. Wy CA, Sajous CH, Loberiza F, et al. Outcome of infants with a diagnosis of hydrops fetalis in the 1990s. Am J Perinatol. 1999;16(10):561-7.
2. McKenna DS, Nagaraja HN, O'Shaughnessy R. Management of pregnancies complicated by anti-Kell isoimmunization. Obstet Gynecol. 1999;93(5Pt):667-73.
3. Babinszki A, Lapinski RH, Berkowitz RL. Prognostic factors and management in pregnancies complicated with severe kell alloimmunization: experiences of the last 13 years. Am J Perinatol. 1998;15(12):695-701.
4. Ravindranath Y, Paglia DE, Warrier I, et al. Glucose phosphate isomerase deficiency as a cause of hydrops fetalis. N Engl J Med. 1987;316(5):258-61.
5. Gilsanz F, Vega MA, Gomez-Castillo E, et al. Fetal anaemia due to pyruvate kinase deficiency. Arch Dis Child. 1993;69(5 Spec No): 523-4.
6. Chui DH, Waye JS. Hydrops fetalis caused by alpha-thalassemia: an emerging health care problem. Blood. 1998;91(7):2213-22.
7. Williams G, Lorimer S, Merry CC, et al. A variant congenital dyserythropoietic anaemia presenting as a fatal hydrops foetalis. Br J Haematol. 1989;72(2):289-90.
8. Pannier E, Viot G, Aubry MC, et al. Congenital erythropoietic porphyria (Gunther's disease): two cases with very early prenatal manifestation and cystic hygroma. Prenat Diagn. 2003;23(1):25-30.
9. McLennan AC, Chitty LS, Rissik J, et al. Prenatal diagnosis of Blackfan-Diamond syndrome: case report and review of the literature. Prenat Diagn. 1996;16(4):349-53.
10. Robertson M, De Jong G, Mansvelt E. Prenatal diagnosis of congenital leukemia in a fetus at 25 weeks of gestation with Down syndrome: case report and review of the literature. Ultrasound Obstet Gynecol. 2003;21(5):486-9.
11. Birchall JE, Murphy MF, Kaplan C, et al. European collaborative study of the antenatal management of fetomaternal alloimmune thrombocytopenia. Br J Haematol. 2003;122(2):275-88.
12. Khouzami AN, Kickler TS, Callan NA, et al. Devastating sequelae of alloimmune thrombocytopenia: an entity that deserves more attention. J Matern Fetal Med. 1996;5(3):137-41.
13. Biankin SA, Arbuckle SM, Graf NS. Autopsy findings in a series of five cases of fetomaternal haemorrhages. Pathology. 2004;35(4):319-24.
14. Levy R, Weissman A, Blomberg G, et al. Infection by Parvovirus B 19 during pregnancy: a review. Obstet Gynecol Surv. 1997;52(4):254-9.
15. Odibo AO, Campbell WA, Feldman D, et al. Resolution of human Parvovirus B 19-induced nonimmune hydrops after intrauterine transfusion. J Ultrasound Med. 1998;17(9):547-50.
16. Yaegashi N, Niinuma T, Chisaka H, et al. The incidence of, and factors leading to, Parvovirus B19-related hydrops fetalis following maternal infection; report of 10 cases and meta-analysis. J Infect. 1998;37(1):28-35.
17. Barron SD, Pass RF. Infectious causes of hydrops fetalis. Semin Perinatol. 1995;19(6):493-501.
18. Beksac MS, Saygan-Karamursel B, Ustacelebi S, et al. Prenatal diagnosis of intrauterine cytomegalovirus infection in a fetus with non-immune hydrops fetalis. Acta Obstet Gynecol Scand. 2001;80(8):762-5.
19. Okumura M, Aparecida dos-Santos V, Camargo ME, et al. Prenatal diagnosis of congenital Chagas' disease (American trypanosomiasis). Prenat Diagn. 2004;24(3):179-81.
20. Benirschke K, Swartz WH, Leopold G, et al. Hydrops due to myocarditis in a fetus. Am J Cardiovasc Pathol. 1987;1(1):131-3.
21. Oyer CE, Ongcapin EH, Ni J, et al. Fatal intrauterine adenoviral endomyocarditis with aortic and pulmonary valve stenosis: diagnosis by polymerase chain reaction. Hum Pathol. 2000;31(11):1433-5.
22. Hollier LM, Harstad TW, Sanchez PJ, et al. Fetal syphilis: clinical and laboratory characteristics. Obstet Gynecol. 2001;97(6):947-53.
23. Levine Z, Sherer DM, Jacobs A, et al. Nonimmune hydrops fetalis due to congenital syphilis associated with negative intrapartum maternal serology screening. Am J Perinatol. 1998;15(4):233-6.
24. Adzick NS, Kitano Y. Fetal surgery for lung lesions, congenital diaphragmatic hernia, and sacrococcygeal teratoma. Semin Pediatr Surg. 2003;12(3):154-67.
25. Laberge JM, Flageole H, Pugash D, et al. Outcome of the prenatally diagnosed congenital cystic adenomatoid lung malformation: a Canadian experience. Fetal Diagn Ther. 2001;16(3):178-86.
26. Diamond IR, Wales PW, Smith SD, et al. Survival after CCAM associated with ascites: a report of a case and review of the literature. J Pediatr Surg. 2003;38(9):E1-3.
27. Brus F, Nikkels PG, van Loon AJ, et al. Non-immune hydrops fetalis and bilateral pulmonary hypoplasia in a newborn infant with extralobar pulmonary sequestration. Acta Paediatr. 1993;82(4): 416-8.
28. Jung E, Won HS, Lee PR, et al. The progression of mediastinal lymphangioma in utero. Ultrasound Obstet Gynecol. 2000;16(7): 663-6.
29. Grebille AG, Mitanchez D, Benachi A, et al. Pericardial teratoma complicated by hydrops: successful fetal therapy by thoracoamniotic shunting. Prenat Diagn. 2003;23(9):735-9.
30. Knilans TK. Cardiac abnormalities associated with hydrops fetalis. Semin Perinatol. 1995;19(6):483-92.

31. Marton T, Hajdú J, Hruby E, et al. Intrauterine left chamber myocardial infarction of the heart and hydrops fetalis in the recipient fetus due to twin-to-twin transfusion syndrome. Prenat Diagn. 2002;22(3):241-3.

32. Pedra SR, Smallhorn JF, Ryan G, et al. Fetal cardiomyopathies: pathogenic mechanisms, hemodynamic findings, and clinical outcome. Circulation. 2002;106(5):585-91.

33. Eronen M, Heikkila P, Teramo K. Congenital complete heart block in the fetus: hemodynamic features, antenatal treatment, and outcome in six cases. Pediatr Cardiol. 2001;22(5):385-92.

34. Khositseth A, Ramin KD, O'Leary PW, et al. Role of amiodarone in the treatment of fetal supraventricular tachyarrhythmias and hydrops fetalis. Pediatr Cardiol. 2003;24(5):454-6.

35. Krapp M, Kohl T, Simpson JM, et al. Review of diagnosis, treatment, and outcome of fetal atrial flutter compared with supraventricular tachycardia. Heart. 2004;89(9):913-7.

36. Brace V, Grant SR, Brackley KJ, et al. Prenatal diagnosis and outcome in sacrococcygeal teratomas: a review of cases between 1992 and 1998. Prenat Diagn. 2000;20(1):51-5.

37. Neubert S, Trautmann K, Tanner B, et al. Sonographic prognostic factors in prenatal diagnosis of SCT. Fetal Diagn Ther. 2004;19(4):319-26.

38. Westerburg B, Feldstein VA, Sandberg PL, et al. Sonographic prognostic factors in fetuses with sacrococcygeal teratoma. J Pediatr Surg. 2000;35(2):322-5.

39. Bhattacharya B, Cochran E, Loew J. Pathologic quiz case: a 27-week female fetus with massive macrocephaly and generalized anasarca. Congenital immature intracranial teratoma with skull rupture and high output cardiac failure. Arch Pathol Lab Med. 2004;128(1):102-4.

40. Albano G, Pugliese A, Stabile M, et al. Hydrops foetalis caused by hepatic haemangioma. Acta Paediatr. 1998;87(12):1307-9.

41. Hayakawa M, Oshiro M, Mimura S, et al. Twin-to-twin transfusion syndrome with hydrops: a retrospective analysis of ten cases. Am J Perinatol. 1999;16(6):263-7.

42. Marton T, Hajdu J, Papp C, et al. Pulmonary stenosis and reactive right ventricular hypertrophy in the recipient fetus as a consequence of twin-to-twin transfusion. Prenat Diagn. 2001;21(6):452-6.

43. Morine M, Maeda K, Higashino K, et al. Transient hydrops fetalis of the donor fetus in twin-to-twin transfusion syndrome after therapeutic amnioreduction. Ultrasound Obstet Gynecol. 2003;22(2):182-5.

44. Machin GA, Ackerman J, Gilbert-Barness E. Abnormal umbilical cord coiling is associated with adverse perinatal outcomes. Pediatr Dev Pathol. 2000;3(5):462-71.

45. Chitayat D, Kalousek DK, Bamforth JS. Lymphatic abnormalities in fetuses with posterior cervical cystic hygroma. Am J Med Genet. 1989;33(3):352-6.

46. Barr MJ, Oman-Ganes L. Turner syndrome morphology and morphometrics: cardiac hypoplasia as a cause of midgestation death. Teratology. 2002;66(2):65-72.

47. Rotmensch S, Liberati M, Bronshtein M, et al. Prenatal sonographic findings in 187 fetuses with Down syndrome. Prenat Diagn. 1997;17(11):1001-9.

48. Stone DL, Sidransky E. Hydrops fetalis: lysosomal storage disorders in extremis. Adv Pediatr. 1999;46:409-40.

49. Cheng Y, Verp MS, Knutel T, et al. Mucopolysaccharidosis type VII as a cause of recurrent non-immune hydrops fetalis. J Perinat Med. 2003;31(6):535-7.

50. Godra A, Kim DU, D'Cruz C. Pathologic quiz case: a 5 day-old boy with hydrops fetalis. Mucolipidoses I (Sialidosis III). Arch Pathol Lab Med. 2003;127(8):1051-2.

51. Mignot C, Gelot A, Bessieres B, et al. Perinatal-lethal Gaucher disease. Am J Med Genet. 2003;120A(3):338-44.

52. van Lijnschoten G, Groener JE, Maas SM, et al. Intrauterine fetal death due to Farber disease: case report. Pediatr Dev Pathol. 2000;3(6):597-602.

53. Tasso MJ, Martinez-Gutierrez A, Carrascosa C, et al. GM1-gangliosidosis presenting as nonimmune hydrops fetalis: a case report. J Perinat Med. 1996;24(5):445-9.

54. Meizner I, Levy A, Carmi R, et al. Niemann-Pick disease associated with nonimmune hydrops fetalis. Am J Obstet Gynecol. 1990;193[1(Pt 1)]:128-9.

55. Applegarth DA, Toone JR, Wilson RD, et al. Morquio disease presenting as hydrops fetalis and enzyme analysis of chorionic villus tissue in a subsequent pregnancy. Pediatr Pathol. 1987;7(5-6):593-9.

56. Atkin J, Snow JWJr, Zellweger H, et al. Fatal infantile cardiac glycogenosis without acid maltase deficiency presenting as congenital hydrops. Eur J Pediatr. 1984;142(2):150.

57. Cox PM, Brueton LA, Murphy KW, et al. Early-onset fetal hydrops and muscle degeneration in siblings due to a novel variant of type IV glycogenosis. Am J Med Genet. 1999;86(2):187-93.

58. Greenberg CR, Rimoin DL, Gruber HE, et al. A new autosomal recessive lethal chondrodystrophy with congenital hydrops. Am J Med Genet. 1988;29(3):623-32.

59. Pryde PG, Bawle E, Brandt F, et al. Prenatal diagnosis of nonrhizomelic chondrodysplasia punctata (Conradi-Hunermann syndrome). Am J Med Genet. 1993;47(3):426-31.

60. Chen CP, Liu FF, Jan SW, et al. A case of achondrogenesis type IA with an occipital encephalocele. Genet Couns. 1996;7(3):193-9.

61. Montemarano H, Bulas DI, Chandra R, et al. Prenatal diagnosis of glomerulocystic kidney disease in short-rib polydactyly syndrome type II, Majewski type. Pediatr Radiol. 1995;25(6):469-71.

62. Terespolsky D, Farrell SA, Siegel-Bartelt J, et al. Infantile lethal variant of Simpson-Golabi-Behmel syndrome associated with hydrops fetalis. Am J Med Genet. 1995;59(3):329-33.

63. Moerman P, Pauwels P, Vandenberghe K, et al. Neonatal haemochromatosis. Histopathology. 1990;17(4):345-51.

64. Wisser J, Schreiner M, Diem H, et al. Neonatal hemochromatosis: a rare cause of nonimmune hydrops fetalis and fetal anemia. Fetal Diagn Ther. 1993;8(4):273-8.

65. Pratt L, Digiosia J, Swenson JN, et al. Reversible fetal hydrops associated with indomethacin use. Obstet Gynecol. 1997;90(4):676-8.

66. Yanai N, Shveiky D. Fetal hydrops, associated with maternal propylthiouracil exposure, reversed by intrauterine therapy. Ultrasound Obstet Gynecol. 2004;23(2):198-201.

67. Treadwell MC, Sherer DM, Sacks AJ, et al. Successful treatment of recurrent non-immune hydrops secondary to fetal hyperthyroidism. Obstet Gynecol. 1996;87[(5 Pt 2)]:838-40.

68. Lallemand AV, Doco-Fenzy M, Gaillard DA. Investigation of nonimmune hydrops fetalis: multidisciplinary studies are necessary for diagnosis—review of 94 cases. Pediatr Dev Pathol. 1999;2(5):432-9.

69. Rodriguez MM, Chaves F, Romaguera RL, et al. Value of autopsy in nonimmune hydrops fetalis: series of 51 stillborn fetuses. Pediatr Dev Pathol. 2002;5(4):365-74.

SECTION 5

Doppler Ultrasound

S Weiner, AK Ertan

48 3D/4D Color and Power Doppler in Obstetrics

G Bega, S Weiner

INTRODUCTION

Two-dimensional ultrasound (2DUS) derived color and power Doppler imaging is commonly used in fetal imaging. The information derived from 2DUS color and power Doppler images is displayed in a cross-sectional image plane. It is from these cross-sectional ultrasound planes that we develop a three-dimensional perception of the vascular anatomy. Nevertheless, the ability to visualize, fully understand and differentiate between normal and abnormal vascular anatomy with 2DUS is often limited. These limitations become especially important in complex anatomical abnormalities. Recent developments in digital signal processing and transducer design have made possible the acquisition of volume ultrasound data with color and power Doppler that can also be interactively manipulated through the volume. In three-dimensional ultrasound (3DUS) or volume ultrasound, a volume (rather than a slice) of ultrasonographic data is acquired and stored. The stored data can be analyzed and displayed in numerous ways, and new and more sophisticated tools are being introduced at a very fast rate. Although, these new and relatively complex applications are not widely known or understood in the field of ultrasound, there seems to be little doubt that these tools will become a routine part of our diagnostic imaging toolset. One of the most significant advantages of acquiring a volume ultrasound data is the ability to navigate through the saved volume and demonstrate any arbitrary plane and most importantly, even planes that are otherwise impossible to be obtained by the conventional 2DUS. In the multiplanar display, three perpendicular planes are displayed simultaneously. Correlation between these three planes is used to confirm a given desired plane, such as the mid-sagittal or mid-coronal plane. This process generally involves placing the planar center point at the point of interest in one of the planes and observing the location of the corresponding center points in the other two planes.[1,2]

In this manuscript, we intend to review the current and potential future applications of 3DUS and four-dimensional ultrasound (4DUS) color and power Doppler ultrasound in obstetrics. In the technical considerations section, the reader have been introduced to the basics of 3DUS volume acquisition, display, analysis, volume calculation and perfusion studies. The main clinical applications have been presented with a special section on techniques of 3D color and power Doppler in fetal echocardiography. The somewhat limited literature as related to 3D color and power ultrasound have been reviewed as well. Last but not least, networking capabilities have been discussed.

TECHNICAL ASPECTS OF ACQUISITION AND DISPLAY

Three-dimensional ultrasound acquires two-dimensional planar ultrasound data in a volume and as such represents an extension of the conventional 2DUS imaging. Considering this, 3DUS does not necessarily replace 2DUS but rather extends its capabilities in time and space. Being a 2DUS based technique makes 3DUS vulnerable to all drawbacks and limitations of 2DUS. As such, problems related to image resolution, penetration, depth, artifacts and body habitus are also present in 3DUS and are even made worse and compounded across a volume of data. Consequently, image and color, and power Doppler setting optimization plays a huge role in acquiring adequate information that could be used clinically. Using 3DUS color and power Doppler techniques generally requires an additional investment of time which in experienced hands, typically goes anywhere from 5 minutes to 20 minutes and at times, depending on the complexity of the case and the experience of the examiner, significantly more. This additional time is not so much related only to scanning and acquiring the data, which is only a portion of the learning curve, but to exploring the saved volume data afterwards in a meaningful way. Given the fact that this information can be digitally saved, either temporarily in the hard disk of the equipment or permanently in a removable disk such as CD-ROMs or DVD-ROMs, makes the exploration of the saved volume data after the patient is discharged a real possibility.

Important to understand is the concept of volume data and how they are acquired. The acquisition of one single volume of ultrasound data is called a 3DUS acquisition and the volume is commonly called a 3D volume. The introduction of dedicated transducers in the mid-nineties made possible the continuous acquisition of 3D volumes and on the fly display of either multiplanar or rendered views. This continuous acquisition displaying motion views of moving targets such as the fetus or the fetal heart was called the fourth dimension and the imaging technique, 4D. There are basically three methods of acquiring volumes of ultrasound data for 3DUS imaging. The first and the oldest one is the free-hand method, which utilizes a normal 2DUS transducer with a position sensing device mounted that can acquire multiple 2DUS images as the probe is manually swept through the region of interest. This method typically acquires one 3DUS volume and in principle cannot acquire 4D data, as that would require the operator to continuously move his/her hand at fast acquisition speeds, which is impossible in reality. The second one is the acquisition of volumes with a dedicated 3DUS transducer (Fig. 48.1). A mechanical device moves the transducer elements at a pre-selected speed and a preselected angle automatically in a fan shape through the region of interest.[3,4] While color and power Doppler ultrasound volumes can be reliably obtained with mechanically swept dedicated transducers, their acquisition time is typically slow as there simply is more information to acquire and process. There is a special fetal heart package that displays heart volumes with either color or power Doppler data in 4D, called spatio-temporal image correlation (STIC). This technique, which has been discussed in more detail the chapter Fetal Echo-

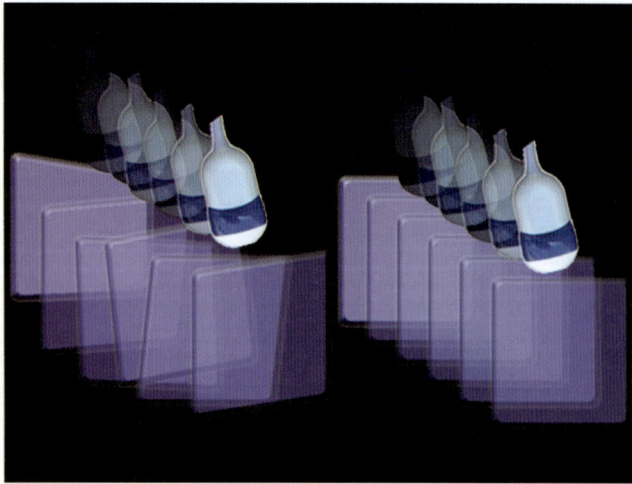

Fig. 48.1: This image illustrates the principle of image registration and the effect of a dedicated 3D volume transducer with a built-in position sensing device in it. The images in the right are represent a volume acquired with a free hand transducer and the images in the left represent a volume acquired with a dedicated volume transducer and appear well registered. The controlled acquisition and reliable registration are prerequisites for obtaining clinically useful ultrasound volumes with color or power Doppler

cardiography is an exception to the otherwise fact that currently mechanically swept transducers cannot display 4D color and power data. The third method is the volume acquisition through matrix array transducers. These newly introduced dedicated volume transducers have a very high number of transducer elements (typically as of this writing from 3000–4000 elements) and produce a thick ultrasound beam in all directions. All elements of the matrix array transducer transmit and receive. Interestingly, the first imaging and data processing take place in the transducer itself as it contains a built-in data processor. These transducers are electronically steered and have no need for mechanical sweeping. As such, they can produce very high acquisition speeds even with color or power Doppler.[5,6] These transducers are the future in volume imaging and will make a revolution in our capabilities of investigating fetal and/or placental vasculature with 3D/4D color and power Doppler. For the time being matrix array technologies are mainly being investigated in adult echocardiography but slowly studies are being conducted in obstetrics as well.[7] All of these methods rely on specialized three-dimensional software, which allows processing of the acquired volumes either on-line through a built-in computer or off-line on a workstation.

In this chapter, we have presented work with the dedicated mechanical volume transducers (the second method); as for the moment, this is the best and most commonly used technique of acquiring clinically useful data in obstetrics.

IMAGE OPTIMIZATION

One of the most common problems practitioners encounter in their learning curve of acquiring 3D color and power Doppler is optimization of the settings. While there is no fixed recipe for every occasion, there is a set of principles and techniques that if understood well should be helpful in obtaining adequate information. First we start with the 2D color or power Doppler information. Normal 2DUS principles of visualizing vessels with color and power

Doppler should be followed (and the following work better in a 3D volume acquisition as well), such as:

- Being as parallel to the vessel or vessels of interest as possible.
- Adjust the gain to avoid "bleeding" in the vessel wall by decreasing the gain at the minimally acceptable level, typically no more than 50–70%.
- Adjust the wall filter, usually the medium settings work better.
- Set the dynamic motion differentiation to avoid background noise signals.
- Sensitivity works better in medium scale.
- Priority set on high generally brings better signal.
- Pulse repetition frequency (PRF) should be adjusted according to the particular vessel size and blood flow, typically a higher PRF is needed for higher velocity vessels (i.e. intracardiac flow) and lower PRF is needed for small and/or branching vessels (i.e. brain) especially placental or retroplacental (venous) vessels.
- Start in 2D gray scale image with the highest frame rate as possible. That translates into a volume with the highest quality, as there will be more frames in a volume. Factors that affect the frame rate are the angle opening in the 2D beam (use the narrowest angle you can), the number of focal zones, and the amount of depth (the less the better). Harmonic imaging helps significantly in imaging in the near field but not much in the far field, but important to know is that it does slow down the frame rate.

The 2D power and color Doppler ultrasound principles above should be incorporated to adequate 3D volume acquisition principles, such as:

- Start with the slowest acquisition speed that is practically possible in order to leave time to the transducer to acquire the maximum amount of information. Typically, the slower the speed of acquisition the higher the quality of the obtained volume.
- Ask the mother to hold still for the expected time frame that the acquisition takes place. That is anywhere between 5 seconds and 15 seconds depending on the size of the volume box and the angle of acquisition.
- Try to acquire volumes at quiet fetal states to avoid motion artifacts.

Analyze the volume right after acquisition for possible acquisition related artifacts due to fetal breathing, respiration, or movement. Explore the B or the C window as those are the computer-generated views where the hidden artifacts can be depicted. Window A is the acquisition plane and as such may or may not show artifacts.

FLOW VOLUME AND PERFUSION STUDIES

For the first time 3DUS allows very accurate volume measurements. Multiple studies have shown that volume measurements are feasible and nomograms of several different organ systems in the fetus have been generated.[8-12] A very interesting aspect of obtaining power and color Doppler volumes is that this information can give an overall estimation of the blood supply of a given anatomical area. Many efforts have been made by the industry to further postprocess this information with the purpose of quantifying the amount of blood supply. One of the most useful programs is the so-called 3D-shell imaging method. In this method, a 3D volume is acquired with power Doppler; then a volume of interest (VOI) inside the initial acquired volume can be traced. Inside the VOI, the gray scale and color histograms can be evaluated together or separately and expressed as a mean value. The expected clinical value of these power and color Doppler volume quantification methods is better estimation of blood flow within the area of interest (i.e. tumor). For this purpose four indices have been proposed:

1. Average gray value of non-color voxels (MG).
2. Vascularization index (VI): Ratio of number of color voxels to total number of voxels inside VOI.
3. Flow index (FI): Ratio of sum of color intensities to number of color-voxels inside VOI.
4. Ratio of sum of color intensities to total number of voxels outside VOI (VFI).

Importantly, while these measurements provide a useful method in quantifying blood flow and vascularity in the acquired volumes, their information is based on digitized color voxel information. The accuracy of this information may change (i.e. improve) as software updates or better probes emerge that improve color or power Doppler sensitivity. Published nomograms for vascularity cannot be used for imaging with other types of machines or with different generations of the same probe because of variable color sensitivity. Nevertheless, the information obtained can provide important qualitative assessment of vascularization and blood flow changes in different normal and abnormal physiologic states. While a few studies have been conducted in gynecology, no studies have been reported in obstetrics yet.

CLINICAL APPLICATIONS

Color and power Doppler information in a volume have shown to be very useful in visualizing the fetal anatomy (Figs 48.2 to 48.10). Several authors have reported their positive experiences with the use of 3D Doppler.[13,14] Studies have shown that 3D color and power Doppler, as used with a free hand 3DUS system was useful in imaging tumors (chorioangioma, teratoma, hygroma, lung sequestration), the fetal brain (vein of Galen aneurism, corpus callosum agenesis, vascular malformations), kidneys (agenesis of the kidneys, renal arteries), fetal abdominal vessels, umbilical cord anomalies and placental disorders.[14] Lee, et al. demonstrated that 3D color and power Doppler, as acquired with an automated 3D probe, could visualize placental angiogenesis as early as 7.1 weeks of gestation, while cerebral and neck vessels as early as 12.9 weeks of gestation.[15] In an interesting study, Kalache described the use of 3D power Doppler ultrasound to identify vascular congenital anomalies of fetal portosystemic and umbilical venous system. He found 8 out of 310 fetuses with portosystemic venous malformations. When an umbilical vein or ductus venosus anomaly is suspected, the operator has to construct the 3D orientation of the vessels from cross-sectional 2D images. Power Doppler in 3D allows visualization of low velocity flow, blood flow is displayed independently of its velocity and the vessels a visualized throughout the volume ensuring spatial orientation[16] (Figs 48.11 and 48.12) and demonstrate how 3D color and power Doppler can have an important role in visualizing complex anatomical arrangements otherwise quite difficult with 2DUS.

Hull, et al. reported their experience in using 3D color and power Doppler in imaging the placenta.[17] They found that 3DUS with color Doppler imaging allowed a more accurate diagnosis of placenta percreta. They had seen several patients in whom the use of 3DUS with color flow and power Doppler imaging allowed refinement of the diagnosis of placental invasion, correctly predicting placenta percreta with bladder invasion. They feel that the multiplanar capability is the key to 3DUS utility. Other useful applications of 3D color and power Doppler reported by this group are placental cord insertion and vasa previa visualization.[17]

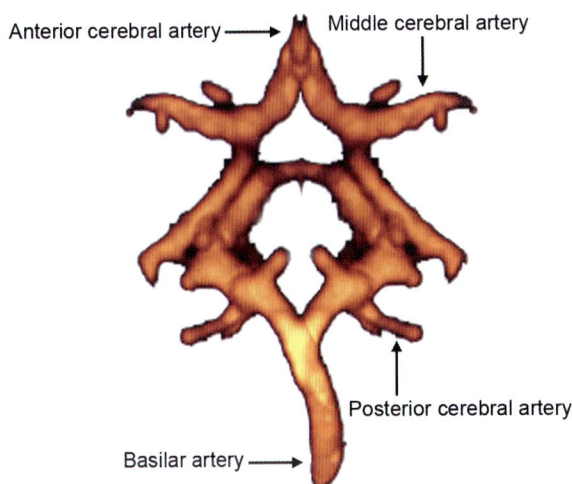

Fig. 48.2: This is a 3D power Doppler (without the gray scale) display of the circulus of Willis at 26 weeks of gestation. Note the anterior, middle and posterior cerebral arteries as well as the basilar artery

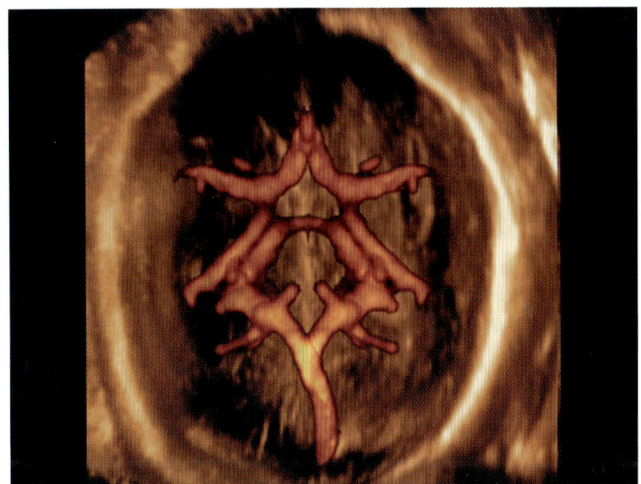

Fig. 48.3: The same case as Figure 48.2. A volume rendered in transparent mode in gray scale and 3D power Doppler information in the same display. This display is generally used to display the brain vasculature in power Doppler as well as the brain gray scale information simultaneously for better orientation and correlation. Typically, the color Doppler rendering can be combined with the gray scale at different percentages to the liking of the operator

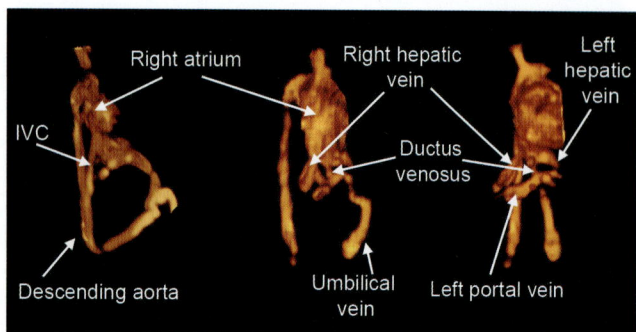

Fig. 48.4: This is a 3D power Doppler rendered volume of the fetal cardiovascular system of a normal 23 weeks of gestation fetus. This volume has been rendered only with the 3D power Doppler without the presence of any gray scale information. As this is volume data, it can be rotated to depict different views of the anatomy. Note the detailed visualization of descending aorta, inferior vena cava (IVC), right atrium, umbilical vein, right hepatic and left veins, left portal vein and ductus venosus

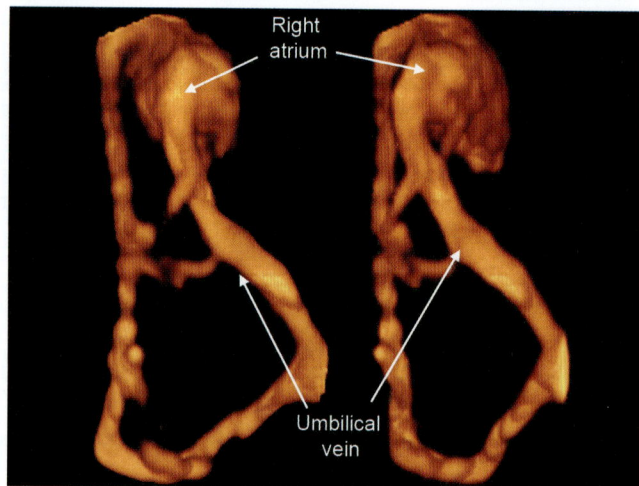

Fig. 48.5: Power Doppler rendered volume of a fetus at 20 weeks of gestation with Noonan syndrome. Note the absence of ductus venosus and the umbilical vein draining directly to the right atrium. Note the distorted angioarchitecture as compared to the normal fetus in Figure 48.4

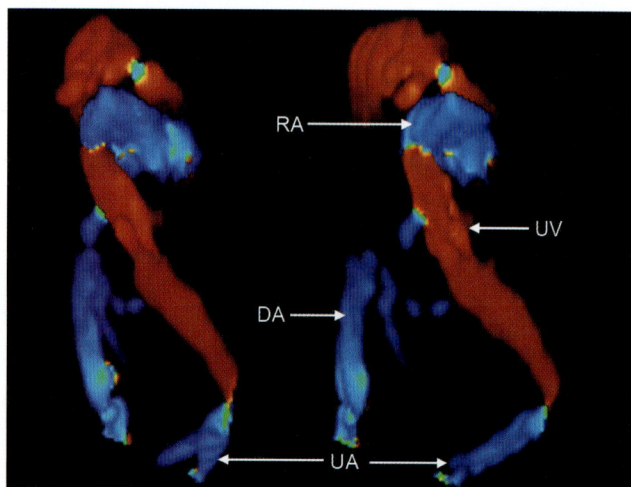

Fig. 48.6: The same patient as in Figure 48.5, but the volume has been rendered in a 3D color Doppler again without the gray scale information. The information provided from 3D color Doppler is similar to the one provided by 3D power Doppler, but in color Doppler, we have additional information regarding the direction of flow

Abbreviations: RA, right atrium; DA, ductus venosus; UV, umbilical vein; UA, umbilical arteries

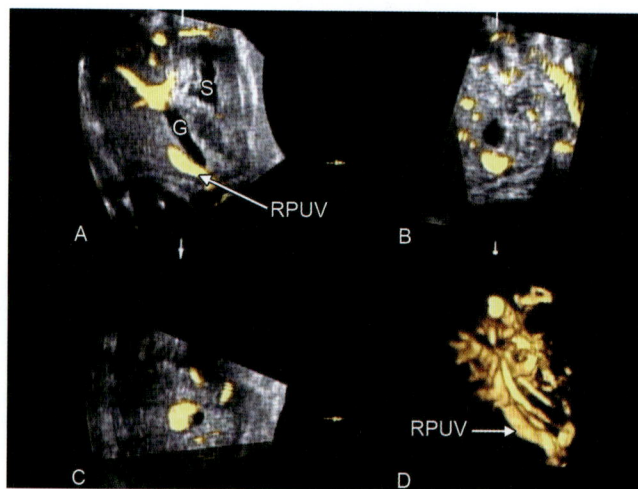

Figs 48.7A to D: Multiplanar display and a rendered display of a fetus at 25 weeks of gestation with persistent right umbilical vein. (A) Transverse plane through the fetal abdomen at the level obtained to measure the abdominal circumference. The right umbilical vein passes lateral and to the right side of the gallbladder connecting with the left portal vein. (λ) This is the intrahepatic form of the right umbilical vein. (B) A perpendicular view to plane A. (C) A coronal view to plane A. (D) The rendered 3D power Doppler view with the arrow pointing at the persistent right umbilical vein. Note that all these four windows are interactive with each other. Window A and D can be correlated to identify the right umbilical vein both in cross-sectional and rendered view

Abbreviations: S, stomach; G, gallbladder; RPUV, right persistent umbilical vein

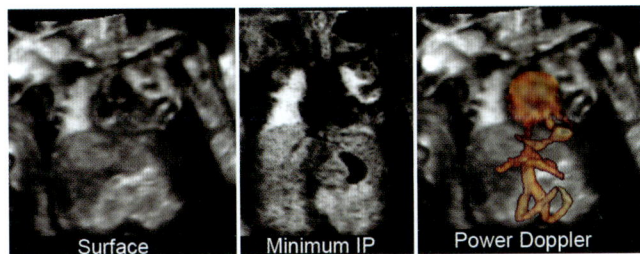

Fig. 48.8: A composite image of a frontal view through the fetal body of a normal fetus at 20 weeks of gestation. The volume was acquired with and without power Doppler. The volumes are displayed in 3D surface rendering to visualize tissue interfaces of heart, lung, liver and bowel (first to the right), minimum intensity projection to visualize fluid filled structures such as heart and stomach, and in surface and 3D power Doppler to visualize the relationships between vascular orientation and the fetal body

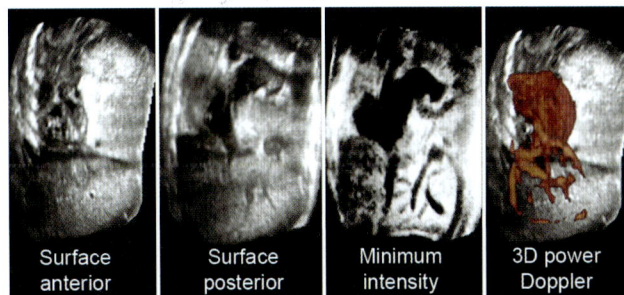

Fig. 48.9: A composite image of several different volumes of a frontal view through the fetal body of a fetus at 22 weeks of gestation with congenital diaphragmatic hernia. In surface anterior view, the volume has been rendered with surface rendering settings at a very anterior level right behind the sternum to show the fetal liver, the diaphragm and the heart displaced in the right. In surface posterior view, the volume has been rendered again with surface rendering settings but at a posterior level to show the fetal stomach up in the chest, the disappearance of the diaphragm posteriorly and to the left, as well as the left lobe of the liver going up in the chest. In minimum intensity view, the volume has been rendered with minimum intensity settings (good for fluid filled structures) at a posterior level to better display the fetal stomach up in the chest as well as left lobe of the liver vessels up in the chest. In 3D power view, the volume has been rendered with both surface and 3D power Doppler to better visualize the fetal heart and liver vessels in relationship to the chest wall and the diaphragm. Note the distorted angioarchitecture as compared to the normal fetus in Figure 48.8

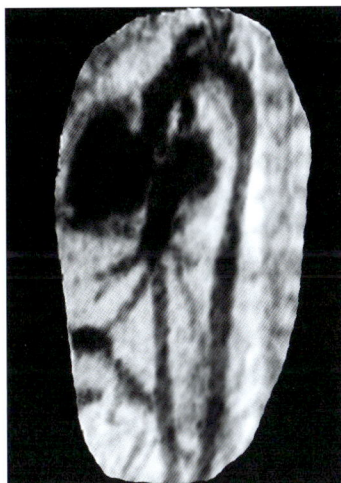

Fig. 48.10: A 3D volume of the fetal heart and vessels of a normal fetus at 22 weeks rendered with minimum intensity projection. This is a unique and very helpful view that visualizes the vessels in gray scale without any color or power Doppler information. This rendering parameter can be employed in all acquisition modes (3D, 4D and STIC) and can be a useful addition to the information provided by the 3D color or power Doppler

Fetal Echocardiography

Three dimensional volume acquisition speed has been improved significantly over the last 5 years. In the past, it was generally believed that increase in acquisition speeds will have a great impact in 3D fetal echocardiography. While the Voluson 730 Expert (GE MEDICAL, Milwaukee, USA) can achieve speeds of acquisition up to 32 frames per second, in acquiring fetal heart volumes these high speeds do not necessarily translate into higher quality volumes. Indeed, the opposite is true. Slower volumes yield higher quality information as there are more 2D frames incorporated in the volume. To overcome this obstacle, a new volume acquisition technology was introduced. This technology is called STIC. With STIC an extra slow (by 3DUS standards) acquisition from 7.5–15 seconds is performed over a preselected area of the fetal heart,

typically at the level of the four-chamber view. The acquisition angle varies from 15° to 40° and again is user selectable. The same image optimization criteria apply just as the ones mentioned above. After the acquisition, post processing of spatial and temporal data is performed so the 2D acquired images are correlated in time and space. This information is displayed in a classic multiplanar view and/or in a cine sequence depicting heart motion with total control on interactive reslicing and/or rendering the same as you would in a static 3D volume. Typically, in gray scale, this acquisition has a very high b-mode frame rate (approximately 150 frames/sec) due to the relatively small region of interest.

STIC technique was initially introduced only in gray scale, but latter the acquisition of fetal heart volumes with STIC could be achieved with color and/or power Doppler information. This development opened up a whole new area in evaluating the fetal heart with 3DUS. STIC represents the first significant development in 3D fetal heart scanning that has the potential to perform a full fetal echo examination out of a single fetal heart volume at the level of the four-chamber view. Studies done prior and post the introduction of STIC were able to demonstrate that a volume of the fetal heart can provide all the standard imaging views for a fetal echo (Figs 48.13 to 48.15).[4,18,19]

Several reports have been demonstrating the value of STIC to the evaluation of the fetal heart with 3DUS.[20-24] Recently Chaoui published a comprehensive prospective study in which he examined the potential of color Doppler STIC in the evaluation of normal and abnormal fetal hearts. He included 35 normal fetuses and 27 fetuses with congenital heart defects (CHD) examined between 18 weeks and 35 weeks of gestation. Volume acquisition was achieved

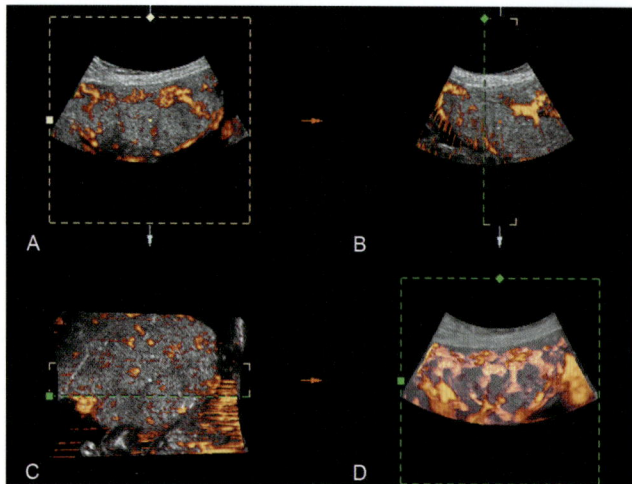

Figs 48.11A to D: Multiplanar and rendered display of a placental volume acquired with 3D color Doppler at 20 weeks of gestation. In (A) We see the acquisition plane, in this case along the long axis of the placenta, in (B) we see the short axis and (C) the coronal view. In (D) we see the 3D color Doppler and gray scale rendered view of the placenta. Note that the rendered view represents a rather thin slice through the placenta and not the whole placental volume. That thickness of this particular volume can be judged and appreciated at window B where you can see the green interrupted lines

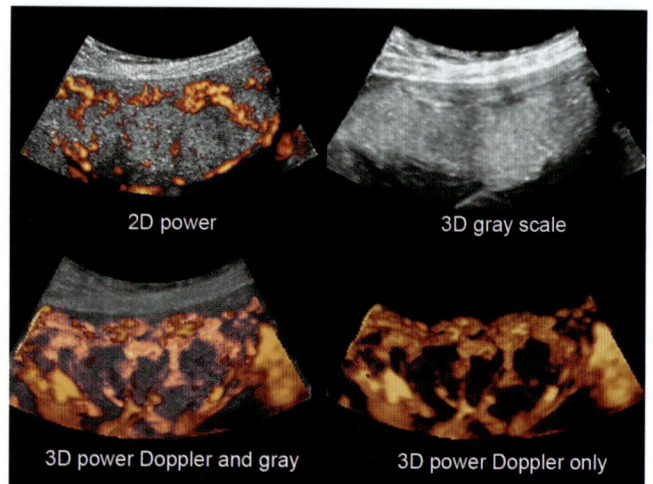

Fig. 48.12: A composite image of four different image displays of the placenta. In 2D power Doppler view in the upper right we see scattered power Doppler signal in a thin 2D ultrasound slice. In 3D gray scale, we see a rendered view through the placenta in gray scale. In 3D power Doppler and gray scale, we see the great depth perception and detail of placental vasculature provided by 3D power Doppler in a 3D volume. In 3D power Doppler only we can see more clearly the vascular anatomy of the placenta without the gray scale superimposed in it

by initiating the image capture sequence from the transverse four-chamber view. Volumes were stored for later offline evaluation using a personal computer-based workstation in a multiplanar mode and as spatial volume rendering. Successful acquisition was possible in all 62 cases. Spatial volume rendering was attempted in 18 fetuses with CHD. In the four normal fetuses had inadequate visualization using color Doppler STIC, as the region of interest was perpendicular to the ultrasound beam. In two fetuses with CHD inadequate visualization was related to an enlarged heart in late gestation, in which the entire cardiac volume could not be acquired. The third case was an 18-week fetus with complex CHD and transposed great vessels in which artifacts were related to confluent color signals as a result of low resolution in the reconstructed plane. He concluded that STIC in combination with color Doppler ultrasound is a promising new tool for multiplanar rendering of the fetal heart.[24]

While the potential of this technique is clear, there are a number of potential pitfalls that are worth mentioning. The acquisition is still relatively slow, from 7.5 seconds to 15 seconds and as such fetal breathing and gross body movement do commonly occur. Careful evaluation of the windows B and C in the multiplanar display after the acquisition is crucial to ensure that no artifacts are present. Adjusting the volume box tightly around the region of interest helps as it generally increases the frame rate. The best frame rates recommended are the ones above 15 Hz, typically with higher rates in smaller hearts and slower rates in bigger hearts. Important adjustment is the acquisition angle, as the default settings tend to be very narrow. Optimal angles vary from 15° to 30° and are related to the gestational age. The earlier the gestational age the narrower the angle.

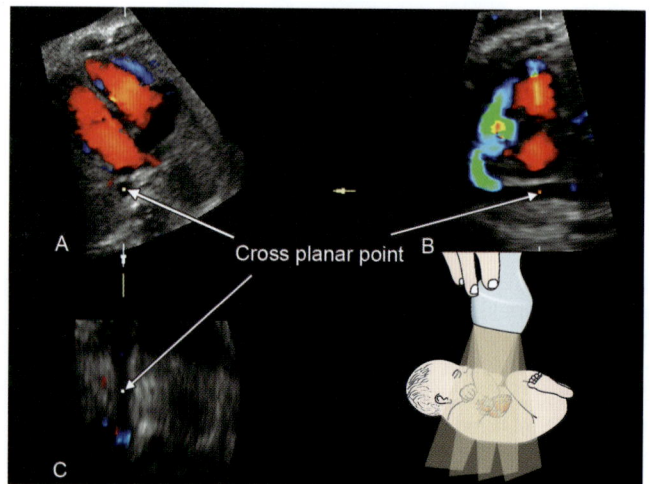

Figs 48.13A to C: A composite image of a multiplanar view of the fetal heart acquired with 3D STIC color Doppler at the four-chamber view level. In the lower left, there is a diagram illustrating the acquisition of a fetal heart volume with a dedicated volume transducer where the transducer is kept stationary and the mechanically steered transducer elements sweep through the volume of the heart at a predetermined angle and speed. After the acquisition of the volume, the cross-planar center point is placed at the descending aorta in plane A and oriented at 6 o'clock position. This rotation will ensure that we can obtain the ductal arch at B and the descending aorta in C. A STIC volume with color Doppler depicts in red the atrioventricular flow (see A) and in blue the outflow tracts (see B)

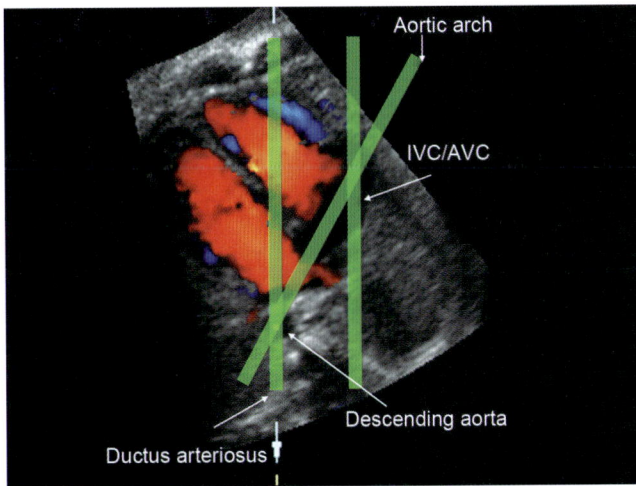

Fig. 48.14: This image shows the four-chamber view image with color Doppler extracted from a STIC 3D color Doppler volume. The green lines represent the scan planes where the additional views of the heart, such as inferior vena cava/superior vena cava (IVC/SVC) or aortic arch can be obtained. The vertical axis of the display can be aligned with these scan planes by rotating the image plane and simultaneously maintaining the descending aorta as the pivot point by placing the cross-planar point in it. Typically, the ductus arteriosus plane is the plane that goes through the descending aorta (placed at 6 o'clock) upward intersecting the left atrium, right ventricle and the sternum. The IVC/SVC plane is a plane parallel to the plane of ductus arteriosus and to the right of it close to the level of right atrium. Aortic arch is a plane that can be found by rotating the four-chamber view plane around 35–40° from the ductus arteriosus plane and maintaining the descending aorta as the pivot point by keeping the cross-planar point there

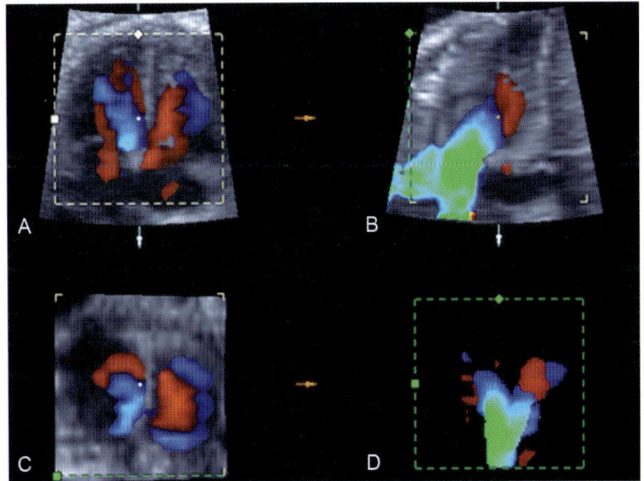

Figs 48.15A to D: This image is a multiplanar and rendered view of a fetal heart volume obtained with STIC and color Doppler at the level of the four-chamber view in a patient with transposition of the great arteries. In (A) the heart is seen at the level of the four-chamber view and the atrioventricular flow is seen in red. In (B) we see a plane through the fetal heart that is perpendicular to A that shows a cross-section of the outflow tracts in blue. In (C) we see a cross-sectional view of the heart tight under the atrioventricular valves. In (D) there is a rendered view of the outflow tracts (in blue color). Note the fact that the outflow tracts do not crisscross as normally expected do but they exit the ventricle in a parallel fashion indicative of a d-transposition of the great vessels

NETWORKING

A potential benefit of 3DUS lies in ultrasound documentation, storage and networking. Digitally saved volumes of patient data can be readily transferred to a remote site for interpretation or second opinion consultation. Further research is needed to define the indications, the potential advantages and limitations of volume data transfer across networks, but it is clear that this is a better method for sharing ultrasound information as you do not rely only on still 2D images or videotapes but have the whole anatomy that can be manipulated at any plane. Using this technology one would expect that in the future primary clinical sites in remote areas would have access to expert consultation and offline interpretation, enabling high quality and cost-effective medical care. The digitally stored patient volumes can be accessed and analyzed by physicians and sonographers in training facilitating training in ultrasound. As this information is digital, it can be encrypted for patient data safety considerations, and efficiently compressed with loss-less algorithms to be shared across hospital networks.

CONCLUSION

It is important to emphasize that 3DUS color and power Doppler information is based on acquisition and reformatting of conventional 2DUS data. Therefore, it is not surprising that 3DUS is prone to the same problems that affect 2DUS, such as unfavorable body habitus, motion and shadowing artifacts and poor scanning technique. Although, 3DUS with color and power Doppler may improve overall comprehension of the vascular anatomy, it does not make up for poor scanning technique. Poor resolution in 2DUS will very likely result in sub-optimal image quality in the volume data as well. Imaging the vessels in perpendicular planes with the beam will also result in poor imaging as the best results are achieved with parallel vessel orientation to the ultrasound beam. The resolution of the three perpendicular planes in the multiplanar display varies according to their deviation from the plane during acquisition. Typically, the coronal reconstructed plane, which is unique to 3DUS, has the lowest resolution of the three planes in the multiplanar display. There definitely is a learning curve associated with the adequate use of this technology. Professionals contemplating the introduction of this modality into their practices should consider dedicating time and effort for additional training in its principles. As this technology improves and becomes more widely available, clinical indications for its use will continue to emerge. There is a great need for comprehensive and rigorous research studies that would hopefully standardize optimal acquisition and analysis of 3D color and power Doppler studies for specific fetal indications.

REFERENCES

1. Nelson T, Downey D, Pretorius D, et al. Three-Dimensional Ultrasound. Philadelphia: Lippincott Williams and Willkins; 1999.
2. Riccabona M, Pretorius DH, Nelson TR, et al. Three-dimensional ultrasound, display modalities in obstetrics. J Clin Ultrasound. 1997;25(4):157-67.
3. Kavic MS. Three-dimensional ultrasound. Surg Endoscopy. 1996;10(1):74-6.
4. Bega G, Kuhlman K, Lev-Toaff A, et al. Application of three-dimensional ultrasonography in the evaluation of the fetal heart. J Ultrasound Med. 2001;20:307-13.
5. Ota T, Kisslo J, Von Ramm OT, et al. Real-Time, Volumetric Echocardiography: Usefulness of Volumetric Scanning for the Assessment of Cardiac Volume and Function. J Cardiol. 2001;37 (Suppl 1):93-101.
6. Kisslo J, Firek B, Ota, T et al. Real-time volumetric echocardiography: The technology and the possibilities. Echocardiography. 2000;17:773-9.
7. Sklansky MS, DeVore GR, Wong PC. Real-time threedimensional fetal echocardiography with an instantaneous volume-rendered display: early description and pictorial essay. J Ultrasound Med. 2004;23(2):283-9.
8. Liang RI, Chang FM, Yao BL, et al. Predicting birth weight by upper-arm volume with use of three-dimensional ultrasonography. Obstet Gynecol. 1997;1773:632-8.
9. Lee W, Comstock CH, Kirk J, et al. Birthweight prediction by three-dimensional ultrasonographic volumes of the fetal thigh and abdomen. J Ultrasound Med. 1997;16:799-805.
10. Pohls UG, Rempen A. Fetal lung volumetry by three-dimensional ultrasound. Ultrasound Obstet Gynecol. 1998;11(1):6-12.
11. Laudy J, Janssen M, Struyk P, et al. Three dimensional ultrasonography of normal fetal lung volume: a preliminary study. Ultrasound Obstet Gynecol. 1998;11:13-6.
12. Lee A, Kratochwil A, Stumpflen I, et al. Fetal lung determination by three dimensional ultrasonography. Am J Obstet Gynecol. 1996;175(3):588-92.
13. Matijevic R, Kurjak A. Three dimensional color and power imaging: experience in prenatal diagnosis. In Kurjak A ed. Clinical Application of 3D Sonography. New York: Parthenon Publishing. 2000:155-60.
14. Chaoui R, Kalache K. Three dimensional color power imaging: principles and first experience in prenatal diagnosis. In: Merz E, (Ed). 3D Ultrasound in Obstetrics and Gynecology. Philadelphia: Lippincot Williams and Wilkins; 1998. pp. 135-41.
15. Lee W, McNie B, Chaiworapongsa T, et al. Three-dimensional power Doppler ultrasonography during pregnancy. J Ultrasound Med. 2003;22:91-7.
16. Kalache K, Romero R, Goncalves L, et al. Three-dimensional color power imaging of the fetal hepatic circulation. Am J Obstet Gynecol. 2003;189(5):1401-6.
17. Hull AD, Pretorius DH. Three-dimensional power Doppler in the study of placental and umbilical cord abnormalities. In: Kurjak A (Ed). Clinical Application of 3D Sonography. New York: Parthenon Publishing. 2000. pp 167-70.
18. DeVore GR, Polanco B, Sklansky MS, et al. The "spin" technique: a new method for examination of the fetal outflow tracts using three-dimensional ultrasound. Ultrasound Obstet Gynecol. 2004;24(1):72-82.
19. Devore GR, Falkensammer P, Sklansky MS, et al. Spatiotemporal image correlation (STIC): New technology for evaluation of the fetal heart. Ultrasound Obstet Gynecol. 2003;22:380-7.
20. Vinals F, Poblete P, Giuliano A. Spatiotemporal image correlation (STIC): a new tool for the prenatal screening of congenital heart defects. Ultrasound Obstet Gynecol. 2003;22:388-94.
21. Goncalves LF, Lee W, Espinoza J, et al. Four dimensional fetal echocardiography with spatiotemporal image correlation (STIC): a systematic study of standard cardiac views assessed by different observers. Ultrasound Obstet Gynecol. 2003;22(Suppl): 50.
22. Chaoui R, Kalache K, Heling KS. Potential of off-line 4D fetal echocardiography using new acquisition and rendering technique (STIC). Ultrasound Obstet Gynecol. 2003;22(Suppl):50.
23. Chaoui R, Schneider MBE, Kalache KD. Right aortic arch with vascular ring and aberrant left subclavian artery: prenatal diagnosis assisted by three-dimensional power Doppler ultrasound. Ultrasound Obstet Gynecol. 2003;22:661-3.
24. Chaoui R, Hoffmann J, Heling KS. Three-dimensional (3D) and 4D color Doppler fetal echocardiography using spatio temporal image correlation (STIC). Ultrasound Obstet Gynecol. 2004;23:535-45.

49

Noninvasive Detection of Fetal Anemia by Doppler Ultrasonography

L Pereira

INTRODUCTION

Cases of hemolytic disease of the newborn have been described as early as 1609 in France,[1] however it was not until 1932, over 300 years later, that the association of erythroblastosis with fetal hydrops, jaundice and hemolytic anemia was characterized by Diamond, Blackfan, and Baty.[2] Shortly thereafter, the discovery of the Rhesus blood group by Landsteiner and Weiner in 1940, and their demonstration of agglutination when rhesus monkey's red blood cell antiserum was mixed with Rh-positive, but not Rh-negative blood, stands as one of the most important hematologic discoveries of the twentieth century.[3] From this landmark achievement, treatment of hemolytic disease of the newborn with transfusion therapy and ultimately prevention of Rh sensitization with anti-D immune globulin became possible. However, despite the availability of postnatal transfusion therapy, the medical practice of this era was limited by an inability to screen for hemolytic disease antenatally.

The discovery that Rh sensitization could be quantified by assessing the spectral absorption curve of amniotic fluid 450 nm (ΔOD_{450}) was first described by Bevis and Walker and then further characterized by Liley in 1961.[4-6] From this important observation, successful antenatal management strategies were developed for Rh alloimmunized patients and for those alloimmunized with non-Rh antigens as well. Years of experience have taught us that amniocentesis ΔOD_{450} assessment is a reliable predictor of fetal anemia in most cases of alloimmunization. However, because amniocentesis ΔOD_{450} assessment is limited to hemolytic causes of fetal anemia and because it has the potential to cause fetal-maternal hemorrhage and worsen sensitization, active research for nearly 30 years has focused on attempts to detect fetal anemia noninvasively.

ULTRASONOGRAPHIC EVALUATION OF FETAL ANEMIA

Serial ultrasound evaluations for fetal hydrops in cases of suspected anemia have become a routine component of perinatal medicine. The observation of hydrops on ultrasound is highly specific for severe anemia, with most hydropic fetuses having hemoglobin levels which are less than 5 g $\times$ dL^{-1}. The finding of fetal hydrops in cases of suspected anemia should lead directly to therapeutic interventions aimed at restoring blood volume. However, basing treatment on the presence of hydrops alone may miss over 50% of fetuses with hemoglobin concentrations below 6.0 g $\times$ dL^{-1}.[7]

Partially because of this shortcoming, many investigators have attempted to detect fetal anemia prior to the onset of hydrops. Rightmire et al. published one of the first successful endeavors at noninvasive diagnosis of fetal anemia in non-hydropic fetuses in 1986. The authors developed a model of combined Doppler measurements of the fetal aorta, inferior vena cava, and umbilical vein, which was able to predict fetal anemia with a mean error of only 3.8 hematocrit units in a retrospective study.[8] Nicolaides et al. prospectively measured six different ultrasonographic parameters, including umbilical vein diameter and placental thickness, but concluded that in the absence of hydrops, none of these successfully distinguished mild from severe fetal anemia.[9] This observation was confirmed by Whitecar et al. who reported on a variety of parameters including amniotic fluid volume, intrahepatic and extrahepatic umbilical vein diameters, hepatic length, and splenic perimeter.[10] Most of these parameters have proven unreliable clinically. Attempts to accurately predict fetal anemia by measurement of the mean blood velocity in the fetal aorta have likewise not been clinically applicable.[11]

Measurement of peak systolic velocity as opposed to mean blood velocity seems to have improved the clinical utility of Doppler velocimetry. One author has reported on the utility of measuring peak systolic velocity in the splenic artery for the detection of fetal anemia in cases of Rhesus factor alloimmunization[12] and no fewer than 7 prospective studies have reported on the reliability of peak systolic velocity measurements in the middle cerebral artery for detection of fetal anemia in pregnancies complicated by red cell alloimmunization (including Kell sensitization) and *Parvovirus* B19 infection.[13-19]

Evidence Supporting Middle Cerebral Artery Peak Systolic Velocity Measurements for Fetal Anemia

In 1995, Mari et al. reported that middle cerebral artery peak systolic velocity Doppler measurements could accurately predict fetal anemia in a prospective series of 16 pregnancies complicated by maternal red cell alloimmunization.[13] This report was followed in 2000 by a larger multi-centered study in which 111 fetuses at risk for anemia were followed prospectively.[15] In this cohort, 23 fetuses had moderate to severe anemia without hydrops and in all 23 middle cerebral artery peak systolic velocities were above 1.5 multiples of the median (MoM). In this study, 83 women were RhD alloimmunized, 18 were Kell sensitized and another 9 were alloimmunized to non-RhD antigens. The authors also published reference tables for fetal hemoglobin levels and middle cerebral artery peak systolic velocities, which have served as the basis for further research studies and are useful reference guides for current clinical management (Tables 49.1 and 49.2).

Teixeira et al. in 2000 published results from a prospective cohort study of 26 fetuses (24 cases of RhD and 2 cases of RhC alloimmunization), and using a peak systolic velocity above 1 standard deviation (SD) reported a sensitivity of 73% and

Table 49.1: Middle cerebral artery peak systolic velocity as a function of gestational age

Weeks of gestation	MCA-PSV (multiples of the median)			
	1.00 cm × sec⁻¹	1.29 cm × sec⁻¹	1.50 cm × sec⁻¹	1.55 cm × sec⁻¹
18	23.2	29.9	34.8	36.6
20	25.5	32.8	38.2	39.5
22	27.9	36.0	41.9	43.3
24	30.7	39.5	46.0	47.5
26	33.6	43.3	50.4	52.1
28	36.9	47.6	55.4	57.2
30	40.5	52.2	60.7	62.8
32	44.4	57.3	66.6	68.9
34	48.7	62.9	73.1	75.6
36	53.5	69.0	80.2	82.9
38	58.7	75.7	88.0	91.0
40	64.4	83.0	96.6	99.8

Abbreviations: MCA-PSV, middle cerebral artery peak systolic velocity; cm: centimeters; sec, seconds
Source: From reference no 15.

Table 49.2: Fetal hemoglobin as a function of gestational age

Weeks of gestation	Fetal Hb (multiples of the median)				
	1.16 g × dL⁻¹	1.00 g × dL⁻¹	0.84 g × dL⁻¹	0.65 g × dL⁻¹	0.55 g × dL⁻¹
18	12.3	10.6	8.9	6.9	5.8
20	12.9	11.1	9.3	7.2	6.1
22	13.4	11.6	9.7	7.5	6.4
24	13.9	12.0	10.1	7.8	6.6
26	14.3	12.3	10.3	8.0	6.8
28	14.6	12.6	10.6	8.2	6.9
30	14.8	12.8	10.8	8.3	7.1
32	15.2	13.1	10.9	8.5	7.2
34	15.4	13.3	11.2	8.6	7.3
36	15.6	13.5	11.3	8.7	7.4
38	15.8	13.6	11.4	8.9	7.5
40	16.0	13.8	11.6	9.0	7.6

Abbreviations: Hb, hemoglobin; g, grams; dL, deciliter
Source: From reference no. 15.

specificity of 93% for fetal hematocrit values below 3 SD.[14] A large prospective, intent to treat trial of 125 cases of red cell alloimmunization was published by Zimmermann et al. in 2002 and confirmed the findings of previous authors.[17] This trial reported that for the detection of moderate to severe fetal anemia, middle cerebral artery peak systolic velocities over 1.5 MoM had a sensitivity of 88% and specificity of 87%.

Further studies have provided evidences that middle cerebral artery peak systolic velocity Doppler can be used to estimate actual hemoglobin concentrations[18] and to predict the timing of a second in utero blood transfusion.[20]

In addition to cases of red cell alloimmunization, two studies have found that, in a total of 42 cases of *Parvovirus* B19 infection, middle cerebral artery peak systolic velocity assessment could detect fetal anemia with sensitivity between 94% to 100% and specificity between 93% and 100%.[16,19]

Technique for Measuring the Middle Cerebral Artery Peak Systolic Velocity

Measurement of peak systolic velocity in the middle cerebral artery should be technically straightforward in most cases. Obtain an axial view of the fetal calvarium, as if one were measuring the biparietal diameter. Center and magnify the image until the fetal calvarium fills the image window. Following identification of midbrain structures, including the thalami and cavum septum pellucidum, move the transducer in a slight caudal direction and identify the circle of Willis using color Doppler. The bilateral middle cerebral arteries should then be visualized flowing anteriorly and outward just behind the orbits. The sample volume line should be parallel to the walls of the vessel, as close to a 0° angle of insonation as possible (Fig. 49.1). Either the ipsilateral or contralateral middle cerebral artery can be measured, but angle correction should not be used. The peak systolic velocity should be measured in the proximal middle cerebral artery, 2 mm after its origin from the internal carotid artery. Placement

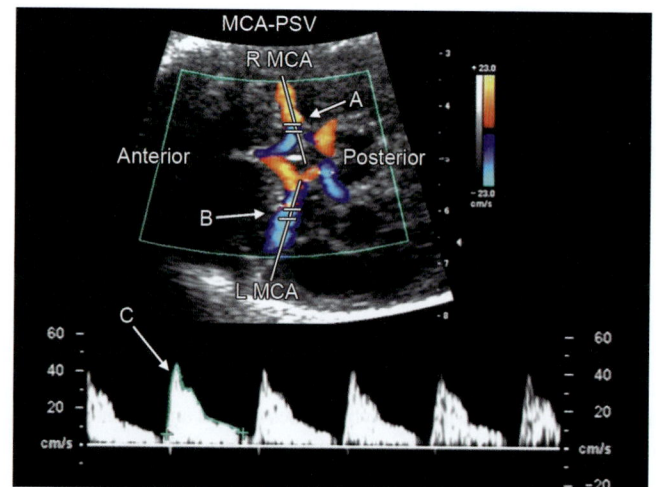

Fig. 49.1: Doppler assessment of the fetal middle cerebral artery; A arrow (correct position of Doppler cursor over anterior MCA); B arrow (correct position of Doppler cursor over posterior MCA); C arrow (correct measurement of the PSV)

Abbreviations: MCA, middle cerebral artery; PSV, peak systolic velocity; R, right; L, left; cm, centimeters; sec, seconds

of the sample volume line in the proximal middle cerebral artery (MCA) is crucial since systolic velocity decreases with distance from the point of origin of the MCA.[15,21]

The sample volume should be made relatively small so that the Doppler signal does not incorporate the internal carotid artery. The peak systolic velocity should be measured at the highest point of the Doppler waveform. The measurement should be repeated multiple times during periods of fetal apnea, while the fetus is relatively stationary. The highest Doppler measurement obtained should be recorded. When performed in this fashion, multiple sources have previously reported low intraobserver and interobserver variability rates between 2.3% and 4.0%.[13, 21-22]

Management with Middle Cerebral Artery Peak Systolic Velocity Compared to Conventional Management with Amniocentesis ΔOD_{450}

Based on the results of the previously mentioned studies,[13-19] clinical reliance upon serial middle cerebral artery peak systolic velocity Dopplers is becoming more common. However, few studies have compared Doppler velocimetry to conventional management with amniocentesis. At time of publication of this chapter, only two published trials had compared the two management strategies.

The first study, published by Nishie et al. followed 28 non-hydropic fetuses and found that conventional management and middle cerebral artery peak systolic velocity Doppler were both accurate predictors of fetal anemia in cases of red cell alloimmunization.[23] The authors suggested in their conclusion that management with middle cerebral artery peak systolic velocity Doppler could decrease the number of invasive procedures performed in their population. A second study, by Pereira et al. also reported outcomes on 28 cases of red cell alloimmunization followed with both middle cerebral artery peak systolic velocity Doppler and conventional management with amniocentesis.[24] In this study, management by middle cerebral artery peak systolic velocity Doppler compared favorably to conventional management, with a sensitivity of 91% and a specificity of 100% for moderate to severe fetal anemia. The authors concluded that compared to conventional management, management by middle cerebral artery peak systolic velocity Doppler may have a better predictive value for moderate to severe anemia in red cell alloimmunization, eliminate the need for amniocentesis, and reduce the number of percutaneous umbilical cord blood samplings (PUBS) performed on non-anemic fetuses.

The main benefit to management with middle cerebral artery peak systolic velocity Doppler is a reduction in invasive procedures and avoidance of potential complications. Transplacental fetal hemorrhage, which may worsen sensitization, occurs following 2–11% of amniocenteses.[25-27] Another 1–2% of amniocenteses are complicated by rupture of amniotic membranes, premature labor, vaginal bleeding, or infection, while fetal loss occurs in approximately 0.5% of cases.[28] Complications associated with PUBS are even more common, with at least 50% of procedures complicated by umbilical cord vessel bleeding and a procedure-related loss rate of 2-3%.[29]

In the USA, there are approximately 14,000 cases of allo-immunization annually.

Extrapolating from published trends, management with middle cerebral artery peak systolic velocity Doppler could avoid 24,500 amniocenteses and over 1500 PUBS per year in the USA population.[24] With a complication rate of 0.5% for amniocentesis and a conservative estimate of 2% for PUBS, one pregnancy loss or preterm delivery per 100 patients (over 140 annually) could be avoided by using middle cerebral artery peak systolic velocity Doppler over conventional management, and these would likely occur in a mildly anemic or non-anemic fetuses. Furthermore, an additional benefit would occur from avoiding procedure related bleeding complications which increase sensitization and worsen disease.

Limitations of Middle Cerebral Artery Peak Systolic Velocity

Management of suspected fetal anemia by middle cerebral artery peak systolic velocity Doppler has limitations. The accuracy of middle cerebral artery peak systolic velocity Doppler appears to diminish after 35 weeks of gestation, leading to higher false positive rates for prediction of anemia.[17, 30] Furthermore, multiple intrauterine transfusions increase fetal blood viscosity, which may alter the predictive accuracy of middle cerebral artery peak systolic velocity Doppler.[20, 31] The reliability of middle cerebral artery peak systolic velocity Doppler to predict fetal anemia in fetuses after three or more transfusions has not been tested prospectively, and false negative cases have been reported.[17, 20] At present, serial amniocenteses for ΔOD_{450} assessment should be considered in fetuses greater than 35 weeks of gestation, and in those who have received three or more in utero transfusions. This will also allow for fetal lung maturity, which will assist in planning perinatal management.

The predictive accuracy of middle cerebral artery peak systolic velocity Doppler in fetuses with compromised left-sided cardiac output from structural heart disease has not yet been established. Anomalies such as mitral stenosis or hypoplastic left heart syndrome that compromise left ventricular cardiac output may result in decreased middle cerebral artery peak systolic velocities. Amniocentesis ΔOD_{450} measurements should not be affected by the presence of congenital heart disease and may be superior to Doppler in this setting.

Another limitation of middle cerebral artery peak systolic velocity Doppler occurs in the setting of fetal hydrops. The middle cerebral artery peak systolic velocity in hydropic fetuses may be diminished by compromised cardiac output. In these cases, the fetus may not be able to maintain adequate cardiac output resulting in a lower middle cerebral artery peak systolic velocity than would be expected for the degree of anemia. False negative middle cerebral artery Dopplers have been previously reported in hydropic fetuses with severe anemia.[17, 32]

Potential Pitfalls in Measuring Middle Cerebral Artery Peak Systolic Velocity

Serial middle cerebral artery peak systolic velocity Doppler measurements must be conducted in strict adherence with proper technique as previously discussed to maintain diagnostic accuracy. Measurements taken in the distal middle cerebral artery or with an angle of insonation above 20° may underestimate the peak systolic velocity and decrease sensitivity.

Intermittent vascular constriction of the middle cerebral artery can occur and may explain several reported cases where an elevated middle cerebral artery peak systolic velocity measurement has not been reproducible.[17, 19]

Multiple factors influence fetal cerebral hemodynamics and can influence middle cerebral artery Doppler studies. Variations in fetal heart rate, both bradycardia[33-34] and tachycardia[35] alter flow through the middle cerebral artery. Fetal behavioral state and activity level also result in dynamic changes in middle cerebral artery perfusion.[36] For these reasons, the middle cerebral artery peak systolic velocity should be measured during periods of fetal apnea and when fetal activity is minimal.

Alterations in middle cerebral artery Doppler waveforms should be anticipated during active labor and in fetuses with severe intrauterine growth restriction. The reliability of middle cerebral artery peak systolic velocity to detect anemia during active labor has not been established, and Yagel et al. reported a 40% reduction in middle cerebral artery blood flow impedance during labor.[37] Fetuses with severe intrauterine growth restriction display similar reductions in cerebral blood flow impedance independent of hematocrit.[38-39] This is likely due to "brain-sparing," which has been characterized by a decrease in the middle cerebral artery pulsatility index as a cephalization of blood flow in response to fetal hypoxemia.[39-41]

Algorithm for Fetal Surveillance Using Middle Cerebral Artery Peak Systolic Velocity

For clinical purposes, a sample algorithm for management of suspected fetal anemia using middle cerebral artery Doppler velocimetry is shown in (Flow chart 49.1) and can be summarized as follows:

- Identify pregnancies at risk for fetal anemia, such as, patients with prior affected pregnancies, antibody titers which have reached a critical threshold level, anti-Kell antibodies, congenital *Parvovirus*, suspected fetomaternal hemorrhage (e.g. strongly positive Kleihauer-Betke test or unexplained elevated maternal serum alphafetoprotein level). Beginning at 18–20 weeks of gestation, perform weekly sonograms to measure the middle cerebral artery peak systolic velocity and evaluate for evidence of fetal hydrops. If the middle cerebral artery peak systolic velocity is less than 1.5 MoM then repeat it weekly for the next 3 weeks. If over that time, the middle cerebral artery peak systolic velocity remains stable and is under 1.29 MoM then it is probably safe to follow the middle cerebral artery peak systolic velocities on every 10–14 days.

- If serial middle cerebral artery peak systolic velocities remain between 1.29 and 1.5 MoM or are increasing in MoM values, then repeat the middle cerebral artery peak systolic velocity measurement in 7 days or less. If at any time the middle cerebral artery peak systolic velocity is greater than or equal to 1.5 MoM, then plan to repeat the measurement in 12–18 hours and plan for a cordocentesis with preparations for a possible in utero transfusion at that time.

If there is sonographic evidence of fetal hydrops then plan for a cordocentesis and transfusion even if the middle cerebral artery peak systolic velocity is less than 1.5 MoM.

Continue to follow at risk fetuses as outlined above until the fetus reaches 35 weeks of gestation or has received greater than or equal to 3 in utero transfusions, then revert back to conventional management by amniocentesis ΔOD_{450} measurements.

Areas for Future Research with Middle Cerebral Artery Peak Systolic Velocity

Areas for future research include studies to determine how well middle cerebral artery Dopplers predict anemia in fetuses with genetic syndromes (thrombocytopenia-absent radius, Fanconi syndrome), hemoglobinopathies (alpha-thalassemia), or viral infections which can cause a myocarditis as well as anemia. There have been case reports of fetuses with hydrops due to *Parvovirus* B19 that were not anemic at time of umbilical cord sampling and recovered without transfusion.[42-43] In these cases, hydrops may be due to the myocarditis caused by the tropism of *Parvovirus* B19 for myocardial cells. Perhaps in these cases, middle cerebral artery peak systolic velocity will prove a valuable modality for avoiding an unnecessary cordocentesis.

The possibility of measuring middle cerebral artery peak systolic velocity Dopplers in fetuses with platelet or neutrophil

Flow chart 49.1: Antenatal surveillance for fetal anemia using MCA-PSV

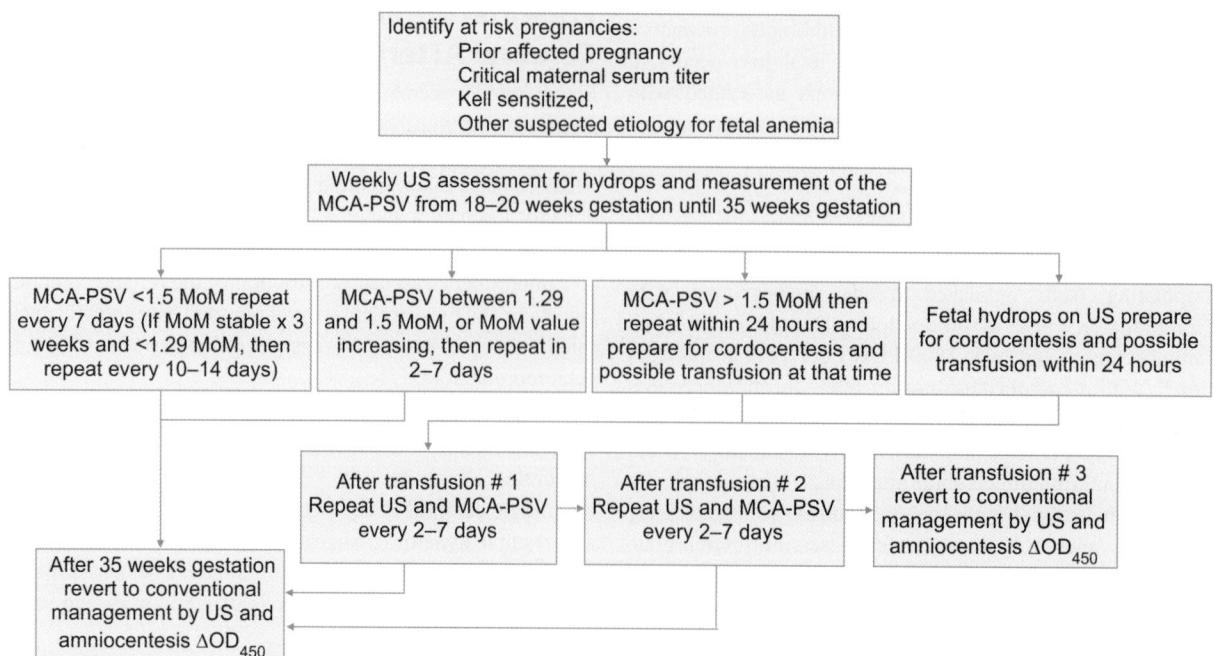

Abbreviations: MCA, middle cerebral artery; PSV, peak systolic velocity; US, ultrasound; MoM, multiples of the median

disorders, such as neonatal alloimmune thrombocytopenia, should be explored remembering that the basis for elevated middle cerebral artery peak systolic velocities is not actual hematocrit but decreased blood viscosity.

Suspected Fetal Hemorrhage

Acute or chronic fetomaternal hemorrhage may lead to anemia, hydrops and intrauterine death. In suspected cases, the diagnosis of fetomaternal hemorrhage is typically made by demonstration of fetal erythrocytes in maternal circulation by Kleihauer-Betke acid-elution stain. Measurement of the maternal serum alpha-fetoprotein level may also be useful in cases of suspected fetomaternal hemorrhage.

As in cases of red blood cell alloimmunization, the appearance of hydrops in the setting of fetomaternal hemorrhage remote from term should generally be treated with intrauterine transfusion as these fetuses are at risk for in utero demise.[44-46] Based on limited data, it appears that middle cerebral artery peak systolic velocities may be useful for detection of fetal anemia in these cases. Baschat et al. in 1998, reported a case of acute fetomaternal hemorrhage in which the middle cerebral peak systolic velocity was elevated at presentation (hematocrit < 11%) and then normalized after in utero transfusion (hematocrit 27%).[47]

Some authors have reported that intraplacental Dopplers may be useful in predicting adverse pregnancy outcomes (IUGR, preeclampsia) in cases of fetomaternal hemorrhage. In 1996, Jaffe and Woods reported results from 32 patients followed due to abnormal first trimester Doppler studies. In these patients, an abnormal ratio of intraplacental resistive index (RI) to umbilical artery RI (defined as > 1) between 22 and 25 weeks of gestation was associated with adverse pregnancy outcomes in 17/21 women compared to 2/11 controls.[48] A second study in 1997, Haberman and Friedman compared intraplacental pulsatility index (PI) to umbilical artery PI and reported a higher rate of IUGR and preeclampsia when the intraplacental PI to umbilical artery PI ratio was over 1.[49]

In rare cases, fetal anemia may be due to fetal intracranial hemorrhage, usually subdural hematomas.[50,51] Coagulation deficiencies such as neonatal alloimmune thrombocytopenia should be suspected when a fetal intracranial hemorrhage is identified in the absence of antecedent trauma.[52] The reliability of middle cerebral artery Doppler assessment in the setting of intracranial hemorrhage has not been established at this time.

CONCLUSION

The clinical management of fetuses at risk for anemia is currently evolving. Based on the results of several prospective trials, the accuracy of middle cerebral artery peak systolic velocity Doppler has been established for the prediction of fetal anemia in cases of red cell alloimmunization. Limited evidence seems to support its accuracy in cases of *Parvovirus* B19 infection as well. When conducted in strict adherence with proper technique, the reliability and accuracy of middle cerebral artery peak systolic velocity Doppler is high, and intraobserver variability uniformly low. In the near future, evidence may support the application of middle cerebral artery peak systolic velocity Doppler to a broad spectrum of conditions, which may cause fetal anemia. At the present time, however, reliance solely on middle cerebral artery peak systolic velocity Doppler should be limited to cases where its accuracy has been established and normal left ventricular cardiac output preserved. In cases where the accuracy of middle cerebral artery peak systolic velocity Doppler has not been established, and in centers in which middle cerebral artery peak systolic velocity Dopplers are not performed regularly, simultaneous management by conventional amniocentesis ΔOD_{450} measurements should probably be continued. Exciting research in the field of Doppler velocimetry is ongoing, and in the near future further advances in our ability to detect fetal anemia noninvasively are certain to emerge.

REFERENCES

1. Bowman J. Hemolytic Disease (Erythroblastosis Fetalis). In: Creasy RK, Resnik R (Eds). Maternal-fetal medicine. Philadelphia: WB Saunders. 1999. pp. 736-67.
2. Diamond LK, Blackfan KD, Baty JM. Erythroblastosis fetalis and its association with universal edema of the fetus, icterus gravis neonatorum and anemia of the newborn. J Pediatr. 1932;1:269-76.
3. Landsteiner K, Weiner AS. An agglutinable factor in human blood recognized by immune sera for rhesus blood. Proc Soc Exp Biol Med. 1940;43:223-4.
4. Bevis DCA. Blood pigments in hemolytic disease of the newborn. J Obstet Gynecol Br Emp. 1956;63:68-75.
5. Walker AHC. Liquor amnii studies in the prediction of haemolytic disease of the newborn. Br Med J. 1957;2:376-8.
6. Liley AW. Liquor amnii analysis in the management of the pregnancy complicated by rhesus sensitization. Am J Obstet Gynecol. 1961;82:1359-70.
7. Nicolaides KH, Rodeck CH, Mibashan RS, et al. Have Liley charts outlived their usefulness? Am J Obstet Gynecol. 1986;155:90-4.
8. Rightmire DA, Nicolaides KH, Rodeck CH, et al. Fetal blood velocities in Rh-isoimmunization: Relationship to gestational age and to fetal hematocrit. Obstet Gynecol. 1986;68:233-6.
9. Nicolaides KH, Fontanarosa M, Gabbe SG, et al. Failure of ultrasonographic parameters to predict the severity of fetal anemia in rhesus isoimmunization. Am J Obstet Gynecol. 1988;158:920-6.
10. Whitecar PW, Moise KJ Jr. Sonographic methods to detect fetal anemia in red blood cell alloimmunization. Obstet Gynecol Surv. 2000;55:240-50.
11. Nicolaides KH, Bilardo CM, Campbell S. Prediction of fetal anemia by measurement of the mean blood velocity in the fetal aorta. Am J Obstet Gynecol. 1990;162:209-12.
12. Bahado-Singh R, Oz U, Deren O, et al. Splenic artery Doppler peak systolic velocity predicts severe fetal anemia in rhesus disease. Am J Obstet Gynecol. 2000;182:1222-6.
13. Mari G, Adrignolo A, Abuhamad AZ, et al. Diagnosis of fetal anemia with Doppler ultrasound in the pregnancy complicated by maternal blood group immunization. Ultrasound Obstet Gynecol. 1995;5:400-5.
14. Teixeira JMA, Duncan K, Letsky E, et al. Middle cerebral artery peak systolic velocity in the prediction of fetal anemia. Ultrasound Obstet Gynecol. 2000;15:205-8.
15. Mari G, Deter RL, Carpenter RL, et al. Noninvasive diagnosis by Doppler ultrasonography of fetal anemia due to maternal red-cell alloimmunization. N Eng J Med. 2000;342:9-14.

16. Delle Chiaie L, Buck G, Grab D, et al. Prediction of fetal anemia with Doppler measurements of the middle cerebral artery peak systolic velocity in pregnancies complicated by maternal blood group alloimmunization or *Parvovirus* B19 infection. Ultrasound Obstet Gynecol. 2001;18:232-6.

17. Zimmermann R, Durig P, Carpenter RJ Jr, et al. Longitudinal measurement of peak systolic velocity in the fetal middle cerebral artery for monitoring pregnancies complicated by red cell alloimmunisation: A prospective multicentre trial with intention-to-treat. Br J Obstet Gynecol. 2002;109:746-52.

18. Mari G, Detti L, Oz U, et al. Accurate prediction of fetal hemoglobin by Doppler ultrasonography. Obstet Gynecol. 2002;99:589-93.

19. Cosmi E, Mari G, Delle Chiaie L, et al. Noninvasive diagnosis by Doppler ultrasonography of fetal anemia resulting from *Parvovirus* infection. Am J Obstet Gynecol. 2002;187:1290-3.

20. Detti L, Oz U, Guney I, et al. Doppler ultrasound velocimetry for timing the second intrauterine transfusion in fetuses with anemia from red cell alloimmunization. Am J Obstet Gynecol. 2001;185:1048-51.

21. Akiyama M, Detti L, Abuhamad A, et al. Is the middle cerebral artery peak systolic velocity measurement affected by the site of vessel sampling? Presented at the Twenty-third annual meeting of the society for maternal-fetal medicine, San Francisco, CA. 2003;7:381.

22. Mari G, Abuhamad A, Brumfield J, et al. Doppler ultrasonography of the middle cerebral artery peak systolic velocity in the fetus: reproducibility of measurement. Presented at the twenty-second annual meeting of the society for maternal-fetal medicine, New Orleans, LA.2002;14:669.

23. Nishie EN, Brizot ML, Liao AW, et al. A Comparison between middle cerebral artery peak systolic velocity and amniotic fluid optical density at 450 nm in the prediction of fetal anemia. Am J Obstet Gynecol. 2003;188:214-9.

24. Pereira L, Jenkins T, Berghella V. Conventional management of Fetal Alloimmunization compared to management by middle cerebral artery peak systolic velocity. Am J Obstet Gynecol. 2003;189(4):1002-6.

25. Bowman JM, Pollock JM. Transplacental fetal hemorrhage after amniocentesis. Obstet Gynecol. 1985;66:749-54.

26. Woo Wang MYF, McCutcheon E, Desforges JF. Fetomaternal hemorrhage from diagnostic transabdominal amniocentesis. Am J Obstet Gynecol. 1967;97(8):1123-8.

27. Peddle LJ. Increase of antibody titer following amniocentesis. Am J Obstet Gynecol. 1968;100(4):567-9.

28. Simpson JL. Incidence and timing of pregnancy losses: relevance to evaluating safety of early prenatal diagnosis. Am J Med Genet. 1990;35:165-73.

29. Ghidini A, Sepulveda W, Lockwood CJ, et al. Complications of fetal blood sampling. Am J Obstet Gynecol. 1993;168:1339-44.

30. Moise Jr KJ. Management of rhesus alloimmunization in Pregnancy. Obstet Gynecol. 2002;100:600-11.

31. Stefos T, Cosmi E, Detti L, et al. Correction of fetal anemia on the middle cerebral artery peak systolic velocity. Obstet Gynecol. 2002;99:211-5.

32. Abdel-Fattah SA, Soothill PW, Carroll SG, et al. Noninvasive diagnosis of anemia in hydrops fetalis with the use of middle cerebral artery Doppler velocity. Am J Obstet Gynecol. 2001;185:1411-5.

33. Gembruch U, Baschat AA. Circulatory effects of acute bradycardia in the human fetus as studied by Doppler ultrasound. Ultrasound Obstet Gynecol. 2000;15:424-7.

34. Mari G, Moise KJ Jr, Deter RL, et al. Fetal heart rate influence on the pulsatility index in the middle cerebral artery. J Clin Ultrasound. 1991;19:149-53.

35. Gokay Z, Ozcan T, Copel JA. Changes in fetal hemodynamics with ritodrine tocolysis. Ultrasound Obstet Gynecol. 2001;18:44-6.

36. Shono M, Shono H, Sugimori H. Dynamic changes in the middle cerebral artery perfusion in normal full-term human fetuses in relation to the timing of behavioral state. Early Hum Devlop. 2000;58:57-67.

37. Yagel S, Anteby E, Lavy Y, Ben Chetrit A, et al. Fetal middle cerebral artery blood flow during normal active labour and in labour with variable decelerations. Br J Obstet Gynecol. 1992;99:483-5.

38. Wladimiroff J, Tonge H, Stewart P, et al. Severe intrauterine growth retardation: Assessment of its origin from fetal arterial flow velocity waveforms. Eur J Obstet Gynecol Reprod Biol. 1986;22:23-8.

39. Vyas S, Nicolaides KH, Bower S, et al. Middle cerebral artery flow velocity waveforms in fetal hypoxaemia. Br J Obstet Gynaecol. 1990;97:797-803.

40. Mari G, Deter R. Middle cerebral artery flow velocity waveforms in normal and small-for-gestational age fetuses. Am J Obstet Gynecol. 1992;166:1262-70.

41. Johnson P, Stojilkovic T, Sarkar P. Middle cerebral artery Doppler in severe intrauterine growth restriction. Ultrasound Obstet Gynecol. 2001;17:416-20.

42. Humprey W, Magoon M, O'Shaughnessy R. Severe nonimmune hydrops secondary to *Parvovirus* B19 infection: spontaneous reversal in utero and survival of a term infant. Obstet Gynecol. 1991;78:900-2.

43. Pryde PG, Nugent CE, Pridjian G, et al. Spontaneous resolution of nonimmune hydrops fetalis secondary to human *Parvovirus* B19 infection. Obstet Gynecol. 1992;79:859-61.

44. Cardwell MS. Successful treatment of hydrops fetalis caused by fetomaternal hemorrhage: a case report. Am J Obstet Gynecol. 1988;158:131-2.

45. Thorp JA, Cohen GR, Yeast JD, et al. Nonimmune hydrops caused by massive fetomaternal hemorrhage and treated by intravascular transfusion. Am J Perin. 1992;9:22-4.

46. Montgomery LD, Belfort MA, Karolina A. Massive fetomaternal hemorrhage treated with combined intravascular and intraperitoneal fetal transfusions. Am J Obstet Gynecol. 1995;173:234-4.

47. Baschat AA, Harman CR, Alger LS, et al. Fetal coronary and cerebral blood flow in acute fetomaternal hemorrhage. Ultrasound Obstet Gynecol. 1998;12:128-31.

48. Jaffe R, Woods JR. Doppler velocimetry of intraplacental fetal vessels in the second trimester: Improving the prediction of pregnancy complications in high-risk patients. Ultrasound Obstet Gynecol. 1996;8:262-6.

49. Haberman S, Friedman ZM. Intraplacental spectral Doppler scanning: Fetal growth classification based on Doppler velocimetry. Gynecol Obstet Invest. 1997;43: 11-9.

50. Bose C. Hydrops fetalis and in utero intracranial hemorrhage. J Pediatr. 1978; 93:1023-4.

51. Hanigan WC, Ali MB, Cusack TJ, et al. Diagnosis of subdural hemorrhage in utero. J Neurosurg. 1985;63:977-9.

52. Daffos F, Forestier F, Muller JY, et al. Prenatal treatment of alloimmune thrombocytopenia. Lancet. 1984;2(8403):632.

50 Doppler Ultrasound Studies in the Fetal Pulmonary Circulation

DC Wood Jr, JP Räsänen

INTRODUCTION

The fetal lungs may be quickly evaluated for size and function by observation using real time ultrasound. There should be adequate amniotic fluid but there should be no thoracic fluid spaces, cysts or echo dense areas. The size of the lungs should occupy about two-thirds the area of the thoracic cavity in a transverse plane at the level of the four-chamber view of the heart. The heart should have a normal 45° axis from the sternal/spine axis in the levocardia position and occupy the other third of the chest cavity. The pulmonary outflow tract should emerge from the heart aiming toward the left shoulder and cross anteriorly over the aortic outflow tract that aims toward the right shoulder. While these observations of normality in the first half of the second trimester will typically rule out most forms of congenital heart disease, pulmonary obstructions and anomalous venous connections will typically be missed at anatomic fetal ultrasound. In the second half of pregnancy, diaphragmatic fetal breathing movements may reassure the observer of normal physiologic growth of the lungs, but this does not rule out lethal pulmonary hypoplasia. However, changes in lung size and heart position may be signs of potential neonatal pulmonary hypoplasia and hypertension problems (Fig. 50.1).

The fetal pulmonary circulation consists of the pulmonary arteries, ductus arteriosus and pulmonary veins, all of which may be identified with ultrasound by 16 weeks of gestation. However, subtle differences in the circulation of the fetal lungs and the vascular connections to the heart require interrogations of the venous and arterial Doppler color and spectral flow patterns. These investigations may be both difficult and time consuming because of fetal position and movement, maternal habitus and the presence of fetal breathing and may require an advanced ultrasound system. It is important to remember that normal appearing of fetal lungs and normal cardiac situs can be seen with any major structural cardiac abnormality including pulmonary atresia and totally anomalous pulmonary venous connection.

PULMONARY ANGIOGENESIS

The cardiovascular system is the first organ developed in the embryonic period. Primitive blood vessels are in place to accommodate the output of the heart, which begins to beat in the human fetus as early as 19 gestational days. Endothelial cells are the earliest specialized cells. They form endothelial tubes and recruit precursors to smooth muscle cells that form the arteries, arterioles, veins and venules. Proliferation, migration, matrix production and contractile protein expression characterize early circulatory development.[1] Vasculogenesis within the primitive lungs may be considered to be of constant capillary production, fusion and regression. During the embryonic period, the lung appears as a ventral diverticulum of the foregut that becomes separated in a caudocranial direction from the future esophagus by the laryngotracheal grooves. By day 26, that developing bud divides and grows into the surrounding mesenchyme into right and left lungs.[2] Blood is pumped from the heart into the common truncus arteriosus, which divides into paired right and left branches which connect to the dorsal aorta via various arches, most of which will regress and disappear. The sixth or most proximal arch connection to the distal aorta is maintained throughout fetal life, typically on the left side, as the ductus arteriosus. The sixth arch vessel gives rise to the main branches of the pulmonary arteries, and, with the helical

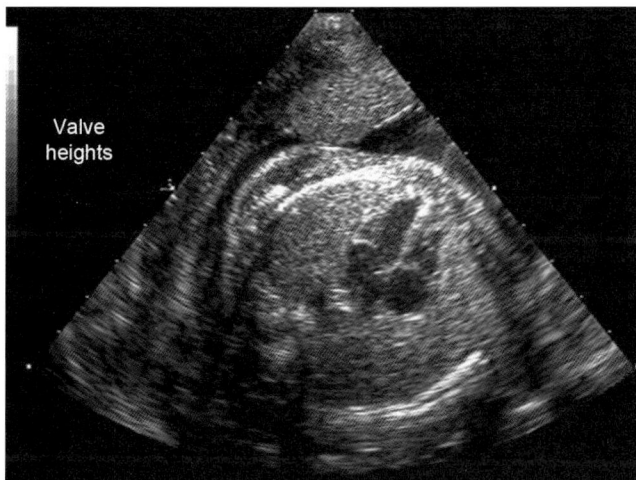

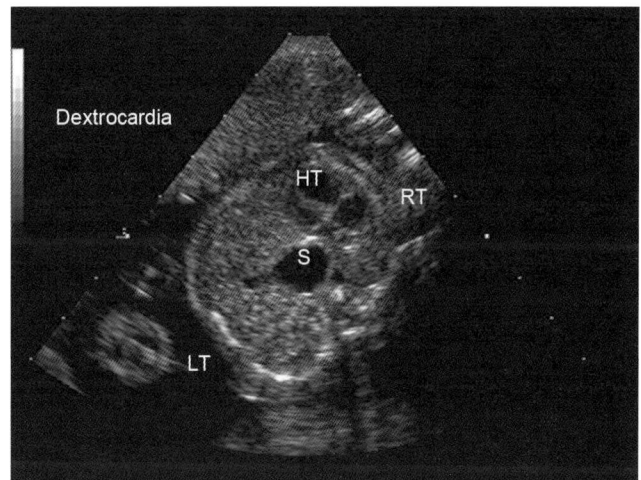

Fig. 50.1: Four-chamber heart in the transverse thorax view with normal size lungs and diaphragmatic hernia with small lungs

division of the truncus and muscular division of the conotruncus, becomes the main pulmonary artery, the anterior vessel originating from the right ventricular outflow tract. At the same time, a bud develops from the dorsal surface of the sinoatrial part of the heart, which divides and connects with the pulmonary plexus. As the atria expand, this single pulmonary vein is carried into the right atrium but eventually becomes absorbed into the left atrium as four separate ostia. Therefore, the pulmonary veins actually drain into the systemic venous system until about day 30, when they become the proximal pulmonary veins of the left atrium. In anomalous migratory patterns, the pulmonary veins can continue with their connection as a common venous sack, draining to the ascending vein of Marshall to the innominate vein to the superior vena cava, to a connection below the diaphragm to the hepatic veins, or continue in part or completely attached to the right atrium or the vena caval connections to the right atrium.

Pulmonary development in the postembryonic fetus has been studied extensively in various animal models and has generally divided into three overlapping morphological stages: (1) the pseudoglandular lung, (2) the canalicular lung and (3) the sacular stage of the viable lung.[3] Development of the human pulmonary vasculature is closely timed to cardiac development. In the human embryo at 5 weeks, it has been shown that the upper poles of the right and left lungs are supplied by primitive pulmonary arteries, which arise from the sixth aortic arch between the pulmonary trunk and the dorsal aorta. The lower poles are supplied from the dorsal aorta via intersegmental arteries that penetrate through the diaphragm. Anomalous growth at this connection leads to pulmonary sequestration. As the branching bronchi develop, so do the aligned pulmonary veins and arteries.

During the early pseudoglandular period (5–17 weeks), the bronchial system has formed such that at each airway generation, there is an accompanying artery, in addition to supernumerary bronchial arteries which supply the major airways and pulmonary arteries.[4] The lung, therefore, possesses two vascular systems: (1) a low pressure pulmonary system and (2) a high pressure bronchial system. By the end of the pseudoglandular period, Kitaoka counted twenty generations of airways with their accompanying arteries; the adult human lung averages 24 generations.[5] During this period, the growth in veins and arteries is enormous, not in total length or volume, but in the number of generations.

The canalicular stage (16–26 weeks) represents the development of the gas exchange tissues. During this period, pulmonary capillary expansion corresponds to epithelial cell differentiation that permits the formation of thin air-blood barriers and surfactant production. The tremendous growth of the capillary system into the lung parenchyma gives rise to the concept of "canals" and gives the lungs a spongy appearance. Arteries and veins develop both in length and diameter as they follow the growth of the preacinar airways.

The saccular stage of lung development (24 weeks to birth) is demarcated by the expansion of the alveolar spaces. The interstitium between the airspaces contain the capillary system and the development of a network of elastic fibers where the postnatal interalveolar wall will be located. The arterial pathways increase in length and diameter. It has been shown that the diameter of the artery is a function of the distance from the previous branching such that the diameters are constant at a given distance from the end of the alveolar tree.[6] Arterial growth is faster centrally than in the periphery. Distally, the number of additional branches grows exponentially. The intrapulmonary veins begin to grow the circular

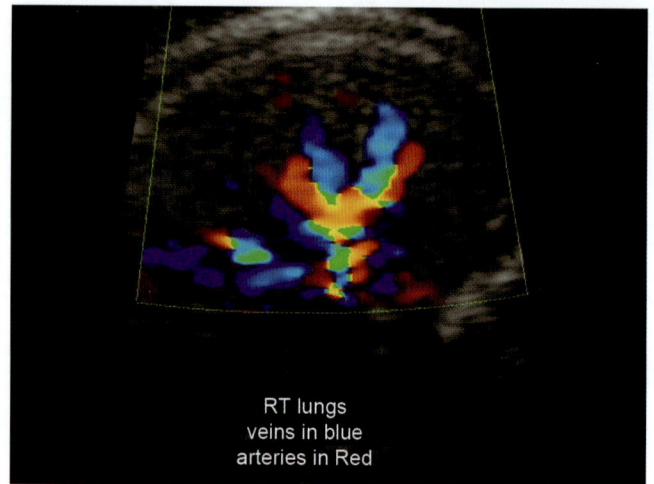

Fig. 50.2: Color Doppler image of pulmonary vascularity

muscular layer of mature vessels during the saccular period. The function of the lung tissue changes dramatically with birth, but the structure is not radically altered (Fig. 50.2).

PULMONARY VASCULAR RESISTANCE (IMPEDANCE)

Fetal pulmonary arterial vascular impedance decreases significantly during the second half of pregnancy. The linear decrease in the vascular impedance during the second trimester and in the beginning of the third trimester may be related to the growth of the lung and to the increase in the number of resistance vessels. During the latter part of the third trimester pulmonary vascular impedance does not decrease further. In a cross-sectional study of 100 uncomplicated singleton pregnancies, we evaluated human fetal pulmonary blood flow by Doppler techniques to analyze the relationships between proximal and distal pulmonary arterial blood velocity waveforms and to determine normal pulmonary arterial vascular impedance and physiologic parameters in proximal and distal branch pulmonary arteries. We found that high resistance, high pressure and low blood flow characterize the fetal pulmonary circulation throughout pregnancy.[7]

Using color Doppler to identify and align the vessel in a position parallel to the pulsed Doppler beam, a narrow sample volume was placed into the proximal part of the branch pulmonary artery immediately after the bifurcation of the main pulmonary artery. Using color Doppler guidance in a high resolution magnification imaging mode, distal pulmonary arteries beyond the first bifurcation of the branch pulmonary artery were identified and waveforms were obtained during fetal apnea and in the absence of fetal body movements (Fig. 50.3). Waveforms were also measured at the aortic and pulmonary valve levels and at the ductus arteriosus. Proximal left and right pulmonary artery diameters were measured from captured real-time images. In each fetus, a sagittal section right lung length was measured from the tip of the apex to the base of the lung on the dome of the diaphragm during fetal apnea, as described by Roberts and Mitchell.[8] Proximal right pulmonary artery Doppler measurements were obtained successfully in 98% of cases and proximal left pulmonary artery Doppler measurements in 96% of cases, respectively. In the distal pulmonary artery, success rate on the right side was 88% and on the left side 94%.

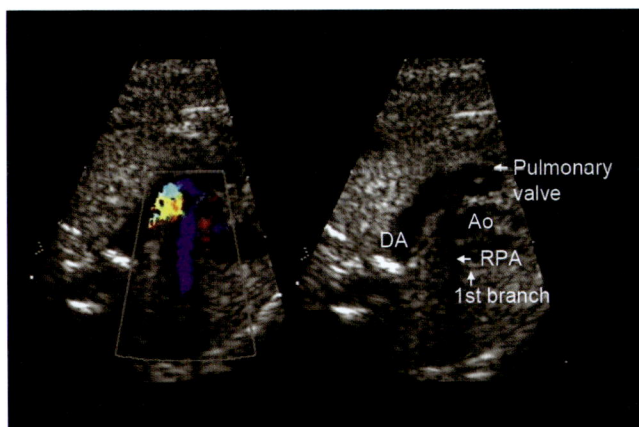

Fig. 50.3: Site of pulmonary Doppler imaging

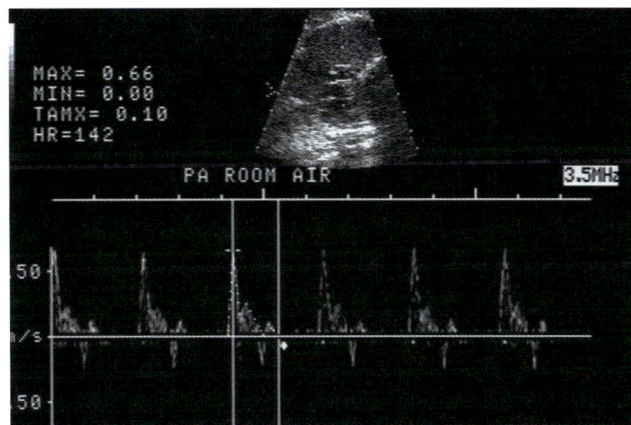

Fig. 50.4: Distal pulmonary artery waveforms

During the second half of pregnancy the pulsatility index (PI) values in both proximal and distal left and right pulmonary arteries decreased and the systolic peak velocities and time to peak (TTP) velocity intervals increased significantly. In the proximal branch pulmonary arteries, a near linear decrease in the PI values was detected until 34–35 weeks of gestation, while in the distal pulmonary arteries, after 31 weeks of gestation there was no significant decrease in the PI value. Respectively, peak systolic velocities in the proximal branch pulmonary arteries increased in a linear fashion until 30 weeks of gestation and remained unchanged until term. Proximal and distal pulmonary arterial TTP-intervals were significantly shorter at 18–22 weeks of gestation and at term (36–40 weeks) than at the pulmonary valve. The TTP-interval at the ductus arteriosus was shown to be significantly longer than at the pulmonary or aortic valves. TTP-intervals at the aortic valve were significantly longer than at the pulmonary valve. In this study, the fetal heart rate did not change significantly during the second half of pregnancy. There were no significant differences in PI values, peak systolic velocities, TTP-intervals or pulmonary artery diameters between right and left proximal and distal pulmonary arteries. Both proximal right and left pulmonary arterial diameters, as well as the right lung length, increased significantly during the second half of pregnancy, demonstrating a 2.5-fold increase in their respective measurements.

In the proximal pulmonary arteries, the PI values and peak systolic velocities were significantly higher and TTP-intervals were significantly longer when compared with the distal pulmonary arteries. The ratio between the peak systolic velocities in proximal and distal pulmonary arteries decreased significantly with advancing gestational age. However, the ratio between the proximal and distal branch pulmonary artery PI values did not vary significantly during the study period. This study demonstrated that ultrasound techniques may be used to evaluate human fetal pulmonary circulation as early as 18 weeks of gestation. The shape of the proximal branch pulmonary arterial Doppler velocity waveform profile is unique in the fetal circulation (Fig. 50.4). It is characterized by rapid initial flow acceleration followed by a very early and rapid deceleration phase, producing a needle-like systolic peak followed by a short, but relatively stable systolic flow segment culminating in a gradual decay in systolic flow. At the beginning of diastole, proximal branch pulmonary artery blood flow patterns demonstrate a short reverse flow interval following either no or a small amount of diastolic flow. The fetal branch pulmonary artery

Doppler tracing is similar to that obtained by direct invasive blood flow recordings in fetal lambs.[9] Fetal growth during the second half of pregnancy is characterized by a 2.5-fold increase in the lung length, as well as in the diameters of proximal pulmonary arteries. The significant decrease in the PI values in both proximal and distal pulmonary arteries during the study period suggests a significant decrease in the pulmonary vascular impedance. There is no difference in changes in the pulmonary vascular impedance between the right or left lungs during the second half of pregnancy.

It is assumed that the phenomenon of wave reflection in a vascular bed is closely related to impedance. From the heart to the periphery, the pulsatility of pressure waves progressively increases while the flow velocity waves decline. This explains the difference between the proximal and distal branch pulmonary artery PI values. The forward propagating waves of pressure and flow demonstrate the same configuration, but after wave reflection, the retrograde flow waves are inverted, while the retrograde pressure waves are not. Wave reflections occur mainly in arterial system at the level of arterial-arteriolar junctions.[11]

Vasodilatation decreases the wave reflection and impedance while increasing flow.[12] The changes in the branch pulmonary arterial vascular impedance are similar to changes in the fetoplacental vascular impedance during the same pregnancy period. The continuing angiogenesis in both the fetoplacental unit and fetal lung causes diminished wave reflections associated with progressively declining vascular impedance. If the angiogenesis or angiomorphology is abnormal in the fetoplacental unit this vascular pathology results in increased vascular impedance associated with enhanced wave reflections (increased systolic to diastolic ratio).[13] We speculate that the failure of angiogenesis in fetal lungs could cause similar changes in vascular impedance, increasing the pulsatility of the Doppler waveform. The plateau stage, especially in the distal pulmonary artery vascular impedance during the third trimester, could be explained by acquired vasoconstriction in the pulmonary circulation, even though the number of resistance vessels is increasing in a linear fashion during this period according to animal studies.[14] However, other factors affect the regulation of the pulmonary circulation. For example, prostaglandin I_2 production is increased after lung distention, distortion or spontaneous ventilation of fetal lungs without changes in O_2 environment producing pulmonary vasodilatation.[15]

The changes in the peak systolic velocities support the concept that during the last trimester, the decrease in pulmonary vascular impedance reaches the plateau stage. Fetal lamb studies have revealed that an increase in the pulmonary vascular resistance due to hypoxia reduces the magnitude and duration of the forward flow in pulmonary arteries, while acetylcholine, which is a potent pulmonary vasodilator, produces a marked increase in the magnitude and duration of systolic flow and reduces or eliminates backflow.[16] However, peak systolic velocities are not only affected by changes in afterload or vascular impedance, but also by fetal cardiac contractility, compliance, size of the vessels, and the distance between the point of measurement and the fetal heart will affect peak systolic velocities.

TTP-intervals increased significantly from 18–22 weeks of gestation to term in all the vessels examined, while the fetal heart rate was unchanged. At the pulmonary valve level the TTP-interval was significantly longer than in the proximal and distal pulmonary arteries and significantly shorter than in the aortic valve level and ductus arteriosus. These findings are partially in agreement with Machado et al., concerning difference between aortic and pulmonary TTP-intervals[17] and with Choi et al. and Hata et al. demonstrating significant increases in aortic, pulmonary and ductal TTP-intervals with increasing gestation.[18,19] Invasive animal studies have shown significant increase in both mean systemic and pulmonary arterial pressures with advancing gestation. Mean pulmonary arterial pressure is higher than mean systemic pressure throughout gestation.[20] These findings are parallel, i.e. significant increases in cardiac output, peak systolic velocities, vessel size and by significant decrease in the placental vascular impedance. The difference in the mean arterial pressures and TTP-intervals may therefore be explained by the differences in end organ impedance: the placenta for the systemic circulation and the lung parenchyma for the pulmonary circulation. There is a structural obstruction in the ductus arteriosus that accelerates outflow into the descending aorta and increase the PI above that of the main pulmonary artery.[21] We speculate that during the latter part of the second trimester and in the beginning of the third trimester, the decrease in the vascular impedance may be related to the growth of the lung and especially to the increase in the number of resistance vessels. During the latter part of the third trimester, the pulmonary vascular impedance does not decrease further.

Pulmonary Blood Flow Effects on Fetal Combined Cardiac Output

The human fetal pulmonary circulation has an important role in the distribution of the cardiac output.[22] The latter part of the second and the beginning of the third trimester is characterized by a decrease in the pulmonary vascular resistance and an increase in the proportion of pulmonary blood flow of the fetal combined cardiac output (CCO). This proportion is higher in human fetuses than suggested by previous animal studies. The proportion of blood flow across the foramen ovale decreases. Later during the last trimester, the pulmonary vascular resistance increases again. The proportion of pulmonary blood flow of the fetal CCO remains about 20% during this period, and is proportionate to that of the foramen ovale blood flow. Right ventricular dominance persists and even increases toward the end of pregnancy (Fig. 50.5).

We studied 63 normal singleton fetuses in uncomplicated pregnancies referred for fetal echocardiography in a cross-sectional manner between 19 and 39 weeks of gestation (median 28 weeks) to establish the relative outputs of the left and right ventricles. The normal distribution of human fetal CCO from the left and right ventricles was determined and the weight-indexed pulmonary (R_{Pi}) and systemic (R_{Si}) vascular resistances and the changes during the second half of pregnancy were established.

Volumetric blood flow was calculated by using the formula: Q = fetal heart rate × valve area × time velocity Integral. Left ventricular cardiac output (LVCO) equals the blood flow through aortic valve. Right ventricular cardiac output (RVCO) equals the blood flow through the pulmonary valve. CCO is the sum of LVCO and RVCO. Total pulmonary artery blood flow (Q_p) was calculated by combining right and left pulmonary artery blood flows. We calculated blood flows across the aortic and pulmonary valve annuli, right and left pulmonary arteries and ductus arteriosus. Foramen ovale blood flow was estimated by the formula Q_{FO} = LVCO - Q_p.

Biometric weight-indexed pulmonary and systemic vascular resistances were calculated by using the formula: $R_i = P / Q_i$, where P is blood pressure (mm Hg) and Q_i is weight indexed volume blood flow (mL/min/kg). These indexes were analyzed at 20, 30 and 38 weeks of gestation. Systemic blood flow (Q_{Si}) was calculated by pulmonary volume blood flow from CCO. The mean transpulmonary pressure gradient was assumed to be equal to mean systemic blood pressure. At 20 weeks of gestation human fetal blood pressure is about 30–35 mm Hg.[23] At 30 and 38 weeks of gestation fetal blood pressure values were assumed from values in newborns at the same gestational age.[24]

From 20 to 30 weeks of gestation the proportion of pulmonary blood flow (Q_p) of the CCO doubled (13–25%), while the proportion of flow across the foramen ovale (Q_{FO}) decreased by half (34% to 18%). After 30 weeks of gestation the proportions

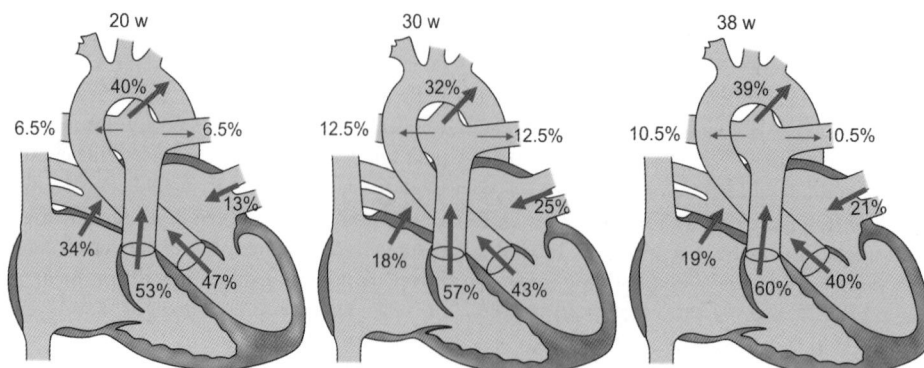

Fig. 50.5: Distribution of fetal cardiac output

of Q_P and Q_{FO} remained unchanged. At 38 weeks of gestation, the proportion of RVCO (60%) was higher than that of LVCO (40%). The proportion of flow across the ductus arteriosus (Q_{DA}) did not change significantly. The correlation between RVCO calculated from blood flow across the pulmonary valve to the combined Q_{DA} and Q_P was excellent. R_{Pi} decreased from 20 to 30 weeks of gestation but increased from 30 to 38 weeks of gestation. However, R_{Si} continuously increased from 20 to 38 weeks of gestation. Thus, the R_{Pi}/R_{Si} decreased from 20 to 30 weeks of gestation and later remained unchanged. The area and TVI of aortic and pulmonary valves, ductus arteriosus and branch pulmonary arteries increased significantly with advancing gestational age as did right and left ventricular stroke volumes. RVSV/LVSV-ratio was greater at term of pregnancy than at 20 weeks of gestation. Fetal CCO, RVCO and LVCO increased more than 10-fold from 20 weeks to term, and Q_{DA}, Q_{FO} and Q_P increased also significantly with advancing gestation. The PV area, RVSV and RVCO were greater than AV area, LVSV and LVCO. The ratio between diameters of the pulmonary valve and the ductus arteriosus increased significantly from 20 weeks of gestation toward the term of pregnancy. The DA area was always greater than LPA or RPA area, but the ratio of LPA or RPA to DA area increased significantly with advancing gestation. There were no significant differences in the area, TVI or volume blood flow between right and left pulmonary arteries. The proportions of Q_P and Q_{FO} of the CCO remained unchanged from 30 to 38 weeks of gestation.

During the third trimester, the proportion of Q_P of the LVCO is about 50% suggesting that the Q_P contribution to the LVCO increases with advancing gestation. These measurements concur with previously published estimates.[25] Our results show that the proportion of Q_P of the human fetal CCO is clearly higher than suggested in previously published animal studies, where the proportion of Q_P of the CCO was estimated at less than 10%.[26,27]

Volume blood flow across the FO is very difficult to assess directly. The cross-sectional area of the FO is difficult to calculate accurately because of the shape and relative size and position of the flap tissue of the septum primum and the fact that the blood velocity waveform is multiphasic during the cardiac cycle.[28] However, our measurements correlated with published diameters of the foramen ovale and showed linear increase with advancing gestation.[29] In our study, the Q_{FO} increased 4-fold, but its proportion of the CCO decreased by half from 20 weeks to term. At 20 weeks of gestation, it represents about 73% of the LVCO, but after 30 weeks of gestation its proportion has decreased to about 50% of the LVCO. In the human fetus, the Q_{FO} has an important role, because highly oxygenated blood returning from the placenta is directed via the ductus venosus across the FO to the left atrium.[30] Thus, the most oxygenated blood from the placenta is supplied to the fetal coronary and cerebral circulations. Our findings suggest that during the third trimester, the FO becomes relatively restrictive and therefore unable to increase its proportion of the CCO. This supports proportional right ventricular dominance in the human fetus during the last trimester of pregnancy. After 20 weeks of gestation, the right ventricular output becomes dominant. At 38 weeks of gestation RVCO (60%) significantly exceeds LVCO (40%) as a proportion of the CCO, which may explain the appearance of relative RV>LV disproportion seen in late third trimester fetuses.

Effects of Indomethacin Treatment on Pulmonary Circulation

Maternally administered indomethacin used as tocolysis is transferred across the placenta to the fetus.[31] Maternal and fetal serum levels of indomethacin are identical after few hours of maternal oral administration of indomethacin.[32] Indomethacin is known to reduce fetal urine output leading to decreased amniotic fluid volume.[33] Another well-known effect of indomethacin on the fetus is the constriction or even occlusion of the ductus arteriosus.[34] It is evident that the prevalence of indomethacin-induced fetal ductal constriction increases with advancing gestational age.[35,36] These fetal side effects of indomethacin are usually reversible after either reducing the indomethacin dose or stopping the indomethacin therapy.[37] Maternal indomethacin therapy affects human fetal pulmonary arterial vascular impedance.[38]

In a cross-sectional study, we compared Doppler echocardiographic findings in three groups of fetuses between 24 and 34 weeks of gestation. Fifty-two normal fetuses were without maternal medication, while 33 fetuses without constriction of the ductus arteriosus, 15 fetuses with mild to moderate and 8 fetuses with severe ductal constriction occlusion during maternal indomethacin therapy. The indication for maternal indomethacin therapy was preterm labor; the daily indomethacin dose varied between 50 and 200 mg. Blood velocity waveforms across the ductus, aortic and pulmonary valves, and proximal right or left pulmonary artery were obtained. The constriction of the ductus arteriosus was defined as mild to moderate when the PI of the ductus arteriosus varied between 1.0 and 1.9. The ductal constriction was defined as severe if the PI value was less than 1.0. During the second half of pregnancy normal values for the PI of the ductus arteriosus are between 1.9 and 3.0.[39] Occlusion of the fetal ductus arteriosus was diagnosed when no blood flow across the ductus arteriosus could be identified by color, continuous or pulsed Doppler techniques but tricuspid regurgitation was identified (Fig. 50.6).

Pulsatility indices were measured in the peripheral pulmonary arteries and left and right ventricular outflows. CCOs were calculated. The pulsatility of the peripheral pulmonary arteries was constantly greater in the indomethacin fetuses than in the control group. After 26 weeks of gestation, the values in the mild to moderate group were significantly higher than in the control group. In the study groups I and II, LVCO, RVCO and CCO were similar to the control group. In the study group III, RVCO and CCO were lower than in the control group. Only LVCO did not differ from the control group. Human fetal pulmonary arterial vascular impedance is increased by maternal indomethacin therapy even without ductal constriction. In the presence of mild to moderate DC, the magnitude of the increase, in the vascular impedance is related to the gestational age. In the group with severe ductal constriction or occlusion of DA pulmonary vascular impedance is similar to the control group. In this group, decreased RVCO and CCO without significantly increased LVCO show that these fetuses were unable to redistribute the cardiac output from the right to left ventricle. Interestingly, the newborns with ductal occlusion in utero did not show any signs of pulmonary hypertension during the neonatal period.

Prostaglandins are potent vasoactive substances, which have a role in the pulmonary vascular changes occurring after birth. Prostaglandins D_2, E_1, and I_2 have been shown to be fetal pulmonary vasodilators in near term animal models.[40] Indomethacin, which is a prostaglandin synthetase inhibitor, may affect fetal pulmonary

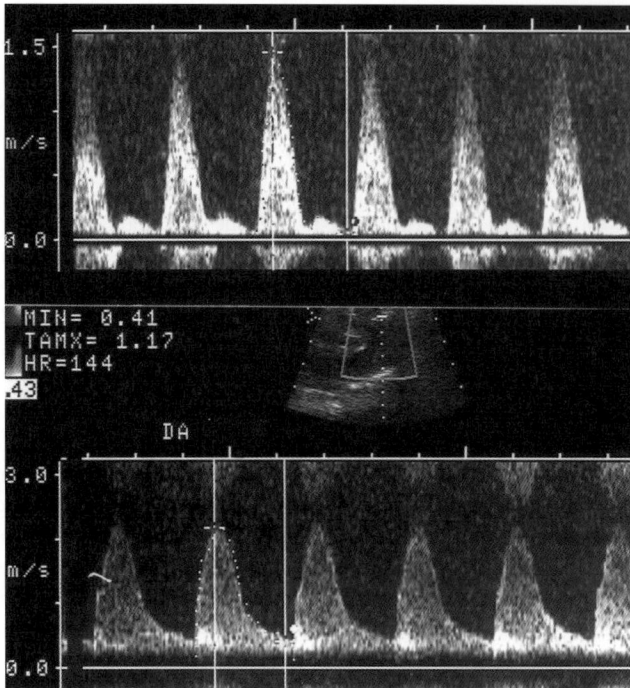

Fig. 50.6: Ductal constriction with high velocity and increased diastolic flow

function by decreasing lung liquid production and altering pulmonary hemodynamics. During rhythmic distention of the lungs in the fetal lambs, prostaglandin synthetase inhibitors have been demonstrated to abolish the 4-fold decrease in pulmonary vascular resistance seen without prostaglandin inhibitors.[41,42] However, indomethacin has not been shown to change the pulmonary vascular response to increased oxygen tension in fetal lambs.[43] In the presence of indomethacin induced ductal constriction in fetal lambs the smooth muscle has been found to be significantly increased and the external diameter decreased in the fifth generation resistance vessels in the lung tissue compared to control fetuses.[44] Also, in fetal lambs, the acute mechanically induced occlusion of the ductus arteriosus decreases the total fetal cardiac output by about 34%.[45] We have earlier demonstrated that pulmonary vascular impedance decreases significantly during the second half of pregnancy until 34–35 weeks of gestation and thereafter it remains unchanged. Likewise, weight-indexed pulmonary vascular resistance decreases significantly from 20 to 30 weeks of gestation and increases again from 30 to 38 weeks of gestation.[22] Maternal indomethacin therapy without constriction of the fetal ductus arteriosus is associated with higher PI values in the branch pulmonary arteries than in the control fetuses. This finding suggests that prostaglandins have a role in the regulation of the human fetal pulmonary circulation. In fetuses with mild to moderate ductal constriction, the PI values were higher and the average weekly change in the PI values was significantly different from the control group. This suggests that after 27–28 weeks of gestation the human fetus is able to regulate branch pulmonary arterial vascular tone in response to increased pulmonary arterial pressure. In the group with severe constriction or occlusion of the ductus arteriosus the PI values of the branch pulmonary arteries were not different from the control group showing that further increase in the pulmonary arterial pressure overcomes the regulatory capacity of the pulmonary circulation. In these fetuses right ventricular and CCOs were less than in the

control group, while the LVCO remained similar to the control group demonstrating that these fetuses were not able to redistribute the cardiac output from the right to the left ventricle.

The Effects of Right Ventricular Loading Conditions on Pulmonary Circulation

The equation for ventricular ejection force (EFo) estimates the energy transferred from the ventricular myocardial shortening to work done by accelerating blood into the circulation. This information can be used for the assessment of the ventricular systolic function. Ventricular EFo does not require estimation of ventricular volumes and is independent of ventricular configuration. Newton's second law of motion defines force as the product of mass and acceleration: Force = mass × acceleration. The mass of blood accelerated across the aortic and pulmonary valves over a time interval is calculated by multiplying the density of blood, which is 1.055, with the cross-sectional area and the TVI at the valve. The acceleration component is calculated by dividing peak systolic velocity by the TTP velocity interval.[46] Ventricular EFo is calculated by using the formula: $EFo = (1.055 \times CSA \times TVI_{ac}) \times (PSV/TTP)$. In adults, a close correlation has been found between the mean left ventricular ejection force (LVEF) and ejection fraction suggesting that Doppler echocardiography can be used for the noninvasive assessment of right and left ventricular performance. The mean LVEF has been shown to be more sensitive for the diagnosis of mild to moderate left ventricular systolic dysfunction than the peak aortic blood velocity or mean acceleration.[47]

Human fetal right ventricular ejection force (RVEF) and LVEF both increase 10-fold during the second half of gestation.[48,49] There is no significant difference between the RVEF and the LVEF in utero. Right ventricular performance is modified by abnormal loading conditions: It is increased by a chronic volume overload and decreased by an acute pressure overload. These findings demonstrate that the human fetal right ventricle is able to adapt its systolic function when it is facing chronically increased volume load. Pressure overload against the right ventricle must be dramatically increased as in severe ductal constriction or occlusion before the right ventricular ejection force (RVEF) decreases demonstrating the capability of the right ventricle to maintain its systolic performance.[50] In growth-retarded fetuses both ventricular ejection forces are reduced compared to normal fetuses as related to the severity of fetal compromise. Animal studies have suggested that early systolic flow is less affected by changes in afterload and preload than flow during late systole.[51,52]

To determine whether abnormal loading conditions can modify human fetal RVEF, we studied 73 normal fetuses, 27 fetuses with hypoplastic left heart syndrome, 14 fetuses with mild to moderate constriction of the ductus arteriosus and 7 fetuses with severe constriction or occlusion of the ductus arteriosus. In the normal and ductal constriction/occlusion groups, blood velocity waveforms were recorded at the level of the aortic and pulmonary valves, and in the group with hypoplastic left heart syndrome at the level of the pulmonary valve. The ventricular ejection forces were calculated. In the HLHS group, 7 patients terminated the pregnancy after diagnosis and there was one stillborn fetus. Except for one newborn, who had a heart transplant operation, others underwent three-stage palliative cardiac surgery. All the fetuses in the HLHS group had a normal karyotype. In the ductal occlusion or constriction groups, there were no perinatal or neonatal deaths.

In the normal group, RVEF and LVEF increased and were equal during the second half of gestation. The average weekly increases were greater in the hypoplastic left heart syndrome group than in the normal group. In the group with mild to moderate ductal constriction, both ventricular ejection forces were similar to those of the normal group. The average weekly increase was lower in the group with severe ductal constriction or occlusion than in the normal group, but the LVEF did not differ from that of the normal group. This study showed that chronic volume overload increases and relatively acute pressure overload decreases human fetal RVEF.

Increased chronic volume load (HLHS group) was associated with increased EFo developed by the right ventricle. This demonstrates the capacity of the right ventricle to adapt its systolic performance and to maintain adequate cardiac output. This also shows that chronic volume overload of the RVEF rises with other parameters of ventricular size, i.e. mass, end-diastolic volume and stroke volume. In fetuses with anemia due to red cell alloimmunization, intravascular transfusion, which represents acute volume overload transiently, decreases fetal cardiac output with a recovery to baseline levels by the day following the correction of the anemia.[53,54] It has been proposed that relative hyperviscosity secondary to the acute correction of anemia during the transfusion increases afterload. The transient decrease in the cardiac output could also represent the time period needed for the adaptation of the ventricles to the acute volume overload.

Severe ductal constriction or occlusion significantly decreased RVEF, possibly because of tricuspid regurgitation in this group. However, RVEF was similar in fetuses with holosystolic tricuspid regurgitation to those without tricuspid regurgitation. Rizzo[55] showed that in fetal intrauterine growth restriction secondary to uteroplacental insufficiency, both ventricular ejection forces were symmetrically decreased. A direct relationship was present between EFo and umbilical vein pH values, suggesting that decreased EFo was primarily caused by myocardial dysfunction. In ductal constriction or occlusion groups, there were no signs of placental insufficiency and the growth of the fetuses was appropriate for gestational age in all cases. Also during fetal ductal constriction the umbilical artery PI is similar to or even significantly less than without constriction suggesting that fetal ductal constriction and indomethacin therapy itself are not detrimentally affecting placental impedance.[56,57] It seems that the human fetus with normal placental function is able to maintain RVEF development until there is a dramatic increase in the right ventricular afterload. This demonstrates the capability of the right ventricle to maintain its systolic function, which seems to be disturbed only after the pulmonary artery diastolic pressure is significantly increased. We believe that in cases of severe ductal constriction or occlusion, which develops in a short time interval, the right ventricular systolic pressure is increased without myocardial hypertrophy leading to increased systolic wall tension and myocardial oxygen consumption. During that period, the foramen ovale becomes relatively restrictive because its fixed dimension and ability to increase blood flow is limited, which results in a decreased CCO.

Effects of Maternally Administered Oxygen on Fetal Pulmonary Circulation

Maternal hyperoxygenation decreases human fetal pulmonary arterial vascular impedance and increases pulmonary blood flow between 31 and 36 weeks of gestation. Earlier in pregnancy, between 20 and 26 weeks of gestation, maternal hyperoxygenation does not alter human fetal pulmonary circulation. These findings shows that the reactivity of the human fetal pulmonary circulation to oxygen develops between these two study periods and oxygen tension in the fetus has a role in the regulation of the fetal pulmonary circulation. Fetal oxygen tension has a role in the regulation of the pulmonary circulation and in the distribution of fetal cardiac output during the later part of the third trimester when the human fetal pulmonary arterial bed is under acquired vasoconstriction, directing RVCO from the pulmonary circulation to the systemic circulation. Maternal hyperoxygenation, at least after 31–36 weeks of gestation, mimics the changes in the fetal central hemodynamics, which occur after birth.[58]

To determine the role of oxygen tension on the human fetal pulmonary arterial circulation during the second half of gestation, we studied 20 women between 20 and 26 weeks of gestation and 20 women between 31 and 36 weeks of gestation with normal singleton pregnancies. They were randomized to receive either 60% humidified oxygen or medical compressed air (room air) by face mask. Fetal aortic and pulmonary valve, ductus arteriosus, and right, left and distal pulmonary artery blood velocity waveforms were obtained by Doppler ultrasound before, during and after maternal administration of either 60% oxygen or room air. Left and RVCO, and DA (Q_{DA}), RPA and LPA (Q_p) volume blood flows were calculated. Foramen ovale blood flow was estimated. PI values of DA, RPA, LPA and DPA were calculated. Maternal hyperoxygenation did not change any of the measured fetal parameters between 20 and 26 weeks, while between 31 and 36 weeks, the PI values of RPA, LPA and DPA decreased and the PI of DA increased. Q_p increased, and Q_{DA} and Q_{FO} decreased. LVCO and RVCO were unchanged. All changes returned to baseline after maternal hyperoxygenation was discontinued. Reactivity of the human fetal pulmonary circulation to maternal hyperoxygenation increases with advancing gestation.

The mean increase in the Q_p was 24.5% and the mean decrease in the Q_{DA} was 17.1% from the baseline values. One fetus at 36 weeks of gestation developed a reversal of diastolic blood flow in the DA during maternal hyperoxygenation (from the aorta to the pulmonary artery). The estimated Q_{FO} remained stable in groups 1, 2 and 4 during the study period whereas maternal hyperoxygenation after 30 weeks of gestation decreased foramen ovale blood flow significantly. The foramen ovale blood flow decreases because the pulmonary volume blood flow increases significantly without any change in the LVCO. In fetal lambs, the foramen ovale blood flow decreases by an average of 50% during maternal hyperbaric oxygenation at near term gestation.[59] Both distal and proximal pulmonary arteries showed a similar decrease in the PI values during maternal hyperoxygenation suggesting that both sampling sites gave the same information about the pulmonary vascular reactivity.

This study supports the concept that in the human fetus the reactivity of the pulmonary arterial bed to changes in the fetal oxygen tension develops after 21–26 weeks of gestation and is detectable by noninvasive Doppler ultrasound techniques between 31 and 36 weeks of gestation. This suggest that human fetal pulmonary circulation is under acquired vasoconstriction at least after 31–36 weeks of gestation with blood flow directed from the pulmonary circulation to the systemic circulation. The reactivity of the pulmonary arterial circulation to oxygen with advancing gestation has been explained by an increasing amount of smooth muscle in small pulmonary arteries.[14] The decrease in the pulmonary vascular resistance is mainly caused by the release of endothelium derived nitric oxide, which leads to vasodilatation of the pulmonary arterial bed.[60,61]

The decrease in the pulmonary vascular impedance and the increase in the pulmonary blood flow by maternal hyperoxygenation between 31 and 36 weeks of gestation were accompanied by opposite changes in the fetal ductus arteriosus. The decrease in the DA PI has been associated with the constriction of the DA and the increase in the DA PI has been found in the cases with increased RVCO.[39] This study shows that the changes in the DA PI may also reflect fetal pulmonary vascular impedance. The decrease in the pulmonary vascular impedance directs blood flow from the systemic circulation to the pulmonary circulation. Mainly this affects the diastolic flow component in the DA by decreasing it or even reversing the direction of the blood flow during diastole. This leads to increased PI in the DA, because the end-diastolic velocity and the mean velocity during the cardiac cycle decrease. In normal circumstances, the direction of the blood flow in the human fetal DA during the diastole is from the pulmonary artery to the aorta. This study supports previous animal data that the increase in the pulmonary blood flow and the decrease in the pulmonary vascular impedance during maternal hyperoxygenation are not caused by the constriction of the ductus arteriosus.[7,27,62] In the presence of the ductal constriction peak systolic, end-diastolic and mean velocities across the ductus arteriosus are increased in the human fetus leading to decreased PI value. These findings agree with those of Burchell et al. where children and adults with patent ductus arteriosus and pulmonary hypertension when breathing of a low oxygen mixture either initiated or increased the blood flow from the pulmonary artery to the aorta whereas the breathing of 100% oxygen caused opposite changes.[63]

PULMONARY HYPOPLASIA

Pulmonary hypoplasia is a term that describes lungs that are sufficiently small enough to impede the exchange of respiratory gases leading to severe neonatal pulmonary disease or death.[64] It occurs secondarily to other fetal anomalies that restrict volumetric lung expansion. It can be associated with mediastinal shift or cardiac malposition. However, pulmonary hypoplasia is different from pulmonary agenesis where there is complete absence of a lung and from pulmonary aplasia where there is absence of a bronchus or bronchiolar pathway as survival is likely with either of those two malformations. As gas exchange does not occur in the fetal lung, it is difficult to prove that fetal lungs may be functionally hypoplastic. Pulmonary hypoplasia is defined as incomplete or under-development of lung tissue present at autopsy as determined by the wet lung to body weight ratio, reduced alveoli count or by reduced lung DNA content.[65] Fetal detection of pulmonary hypoplasia is based on ultrasound imaging techniques based on a reduced chest size for gestational age. The thoracic to abdominal ratio of 0.89 is relatively constant throughout gestation and a ratio of less than 0.77 is consistent with pulmonary hypoplasia.[66]

The association between pulmonary hypoplasia and reduced amniotic fluid volume was first observed in infants with bilateral renal agenesis.[67] Abnormalities that result in oligohydramnios include renal agenesis, renal dysplasia and those that restrict urinary flow into the amniotic sac. Urethral atresia or stenosis, urethral valve and bladder outlet obstructions also restrict urinary

flow. In pregnancies with prolonged leakage of amniotic fluid or premature rupture of the membranes may also be subject to pulmonary hypoplasia. With these conditions, it has been proposed that compression or forced flexion of the fetal trunk secondary to restricted movement.[68] It has been shown that fetal lung expansion becomes restricted within 48 hours of diminution of amniotic fluid but the process may be reversed by amnioinfusion.[69] A reduction in fetal breathing patterns in patients with reduced amniotic fluid may also contribute to pulmonary hypoplasia, although, there are conflicting reports.[70-72]

Fluid in the fetal thorax either as primary hydrothorax or from hydrops fetalis is one of the most common causes of pulmonary hypoplasia with overall mortality reported at over 50%.[73] If fluid is drained from the chest in fetal hydrothorax by catheter or needle aspiration, lung growth may be restored.[74] Other "space occupying lesions" of the fetal thorax include cardiomegaly (mitral valve insufficiency associated with giant left atrium and aortic stenosis, Ebstein's anomaly of the tricuspid valve and tricuspid valve dysplasia), pericardial effusion and neuroblastoma.

The incidence of congenital diaphragmatic hernia is estimated at 1 in 3,000–5,000 births. As a result of incomplete closure of the pleuroperitoneal membranes, the abdominal contents may enter the thorax and result in a mediastinal shift. This may affect the growth of the effected side and the contralateral lung, and may cause esophageal obstruction resulting in polyhydramnios. Postnatal survival is approximately 50% depending upon the degree of pulmonary hypoplasia.[75] In the absence of a congenital closure defect, the diaphragm may be affected by abnormal development of function as in phrenic nerve agenesis and Pena Shokeir syndrome leading to an elevation or eventration of the dome of the diaphragm.[76] Central neural defects that as associated with absent fetal breathing movements may also lead to pulmonary hypoplasia including anencephaly, microcephaly and encephalocele.[77]

Congenital cystic adenomatoid malformation (CCAM) of the lung is a failure of maturation of certain bronchial structures during the pseudoglandular stage of development. The lesion is typically unilobar and consists of cystic areas that may be identified on ultrasound. Type I lesions have a single or multiple large cysts and represent 50% of CCAMs. Type II has multiple smaller cysts and may be associated with gastrointestinal or renal anomalies. Type III lesions are large with cysts often too small to measure and carry a poor prognosis. When associated with developing hydrops fetalis, preterm surgical intervention has been offered.[78]

Pulmonary hypoplasia is also associated with skeletal dysplasias because of a narrowed or constricted fetal thorax.[79,80] These anomalies may include Jeunes Syndrome (asphyxiating thoracic dystrophy), achondrogenesis, achondroplasia, osteogenesis imperfecta, thanatophoric dwarfism and hypophosphasia. Ultrasound measurements of fetal lung or chest size as a ratio to normal gestational biometric measurements have been advanced as predictors of pulmonary hypoplasia.[81-84] Yoshimura et al. analyzed several methods of prediction for fetal lung hypoplasia, concluding that the lung area against gestational age and the ratio of the thoracic circumference to the abdominal circumference were the most clinically useful.[85] Recently, estimates of lung volumes from three-dimensional ultrasound have been used in an attempt to estimate lung maturity and predict hypoplasia.[86-89] We and others believe that a method that evaluates function as well as relative size may prove to be a more reliable predictor of postnatal pulmonary dysfunction from pulmonary hypoplasia. Pulmonary blood flow parameters may be measured by the methods previously mentioned. We have seen in the fetus later found to have lethal pulmonary hypoplasia that the proximal and distal pulmonary artery flow patterns are reduced in peak velocity while pulsatility indices are increased. Those patients with space occupying lesions such as diaphragmatic hernias may have a blunted or no response to a maternal hyperoxia test after 32 weeks of gestation.[90] One of the most easily obtained waveform patterns recorded during these studies has been the proximal pulmonary venous flow, which normally increases significantly with maternal hyperoxia. Mitchell et al. showed a high resistance pattern quite different from that of normal fetuses in the peripheral pulmonary arteries in ten fetuses with bilateral multicystic dysplastic kidney disease all of whom died from associated pulmonary hypoplasia.[91] Yoshimura et al. made similar observations in the proximal pulmonary artery flow patterns with lethal pulmonary hyperplasia in hydrops fetalis, thanatophoric dwarfs and Potter syndrome.[92] Roth et al. has found an association with lethal pulmonary hypoplasia with the lack of pulmonary artery flow patterns with power color Doppler techniques.[93] Chaoui et al. has shown that abnormal pulmonary artery flow patterns may be seen as early as 19–23 weeks of gestation in fetuses with lung hypoplasia.[94]

A Test for the Prediction of Lethal Pulmonary Hypoplasia

To determine the predictive accuracy of our test for neonatal death from pulmonary hypoplasia we measured the Doppler changes in fetal pulmonary artery blood flow in room air and during maternal hyperoxygenation. Women carrying fetuses with those congenital anomalies as illustrated above or with prolonged oligohydramnios often associated with pulmonary hypoplasia were offered participation in the study as part of a comprehensive fetal echocardiogram. Each fetus at more than or equal to 30 weeks of gestation had the Doppler blood flow pattern in the first branch of either the right or the left pulmonary artery measured before and again during at least 10 minutes exposure to maternal breathing of 60% oxygen by mask. An increase in the relative fetal pulmonary blood flow with oxygen (a decrease of at least 25% of the PI) was considered a reactive test. A change of less than 20% in the flow pattern during maternal hyperoxygenation was a non-reactive test and suggested pulmonary hypoplasia. The primary outcome for this study was neonatal outcome of death from pulmonary hypoplasia. In the 29 pregnancies that met criteria for our study, 14 fetuses who had a non-reactive hyperoxygenation test, 11 (79%) died of pulmonary hypoplasia. Of the 15 that had a reactive hyperoxygenation test, only 1 (7%) died in the neonatal period. Sensitivity, specificity, positive, and negative predictive values were 92%, 82%, 79%, and 93%, respectively, with an odds ratio of 51 (95% CI 4.6-560).[95] We have now performed over one hundred of these oxygen challenge tests with excellent results in sensitivity and specificity.

The oxygen challenge method evaluates fetal pulmonary function and therefore may prove to be a more reliable predictor of postnatal pulmonary dysfunction from pulmonary hypoplasia as compared to those that evaluate relative anatomic size. Maternal hyperoxygenation increases fetal pulmonary blood flow by decreasing pulmonary arterial vascular impedance. The changes we have observed between 31 and 36 weeks of gestation mimics the changes in the fetal hemodynamics after birth.[15] During normoxia,

when the human fetal pulmonary arterial bed is under acquired vasoconstriction, RVCO is directed away from the lungs and into the systemic circulation via the ductus arteriosus. Increased blood oxygen content decreases pulmonary vascular resistance and thus increases pulmonary blood flow in the normal fetus. The reactivity of the pulmonary arterial circulation to oxygen with advancing gestation has been explained by an increasing amount of smooth muscle in small pulmonary arteries.[14] The decrease in the pulmonary vascular resistance is mainly caused by the release of endothelium-derived nitric oxide, which leads to vasodilatation of the pulmonary arterial bed.[60,61]

The method to accurately predict those fetuses who will die from pulmonary hypoplasia is important for parental counseling and subsequent decision-making regarding obstetric and neonatal management. As the oxygen challenge is an extension of our comprehensive fetal echocardiogram, we also measure the cardiac circumference to thoracic circumference ratio (CC/TC) and the thoracic circumference to the biometric abdominal circumference ratio (TC/AC) as well as M-mode measurements of the ventricles in systole and diastole. These measurements typically show normal size heart for gestational age, but the CC/TC and TC/AC are widely divergent relative to the cause of the small lungs. For example, oligohydramnios may show a relative cardiomegaly whereas a diaphragmatic hernia will have a relatively small heart to thoracic size. Likewise, we have seen exaggerated fetal breathing movements in fetuses who have lethal pulmonary hypoplasia and an absence of such movements in fetuses with long standing oligohydramnios who have a normal physiologic response to maternal oxygen and go on to a normal neonatal course. Difficulty in performing the examination occurs, especially in the fetuses with diaphragmatic hernia, who has hard to image lungs and who typically increases both its gross body movements and breathing movements when exposed to an increased oxygen environment.

Intrauterine growth restricted (IUGR) fetuses with oligohydramnios can have a negative response to maternal hyperoxygenation. Those fetuses may present in extremis with abnormal Doppler measurements in the MCA, FLUA and DV, suggesting redistribution of cardiac output by cephalization, placental insufficiency and congestive heart failure with increased central venous pressure. The blunted or absent response to oxygen appears to be an extension of redistribution of cardiac output as these fetuses, who were delivered within hours of their oxygen tests, did reasonably well in the newborn period and were eventually discharged home (Figs 50.7 and 50.8).

CYSTIC ADENOMATOID MALFORMATION

Probably the most common lung lesion detected in-utero by ultrasound is cystic adenomatoid malformation. This appears as an echo bright portion within a lobe of the lung and may be associated with large, small mixed or micro cysts, appearing as a solid mass. It is characterized by dysplastic or hamartomatous tissue often mixed with normal tissue and typically confined to a single lobe. Regression is common, but when large and/or associated with hydrops it may be lethal because of pulmonary hypoplasia. As it is likely to be the result of early maldevelopment of terminal brochiolar structures, color or power Doppler in the area of the lesion may show pulmonary arterial flow around but not into the lesion (Fig. 50.9).

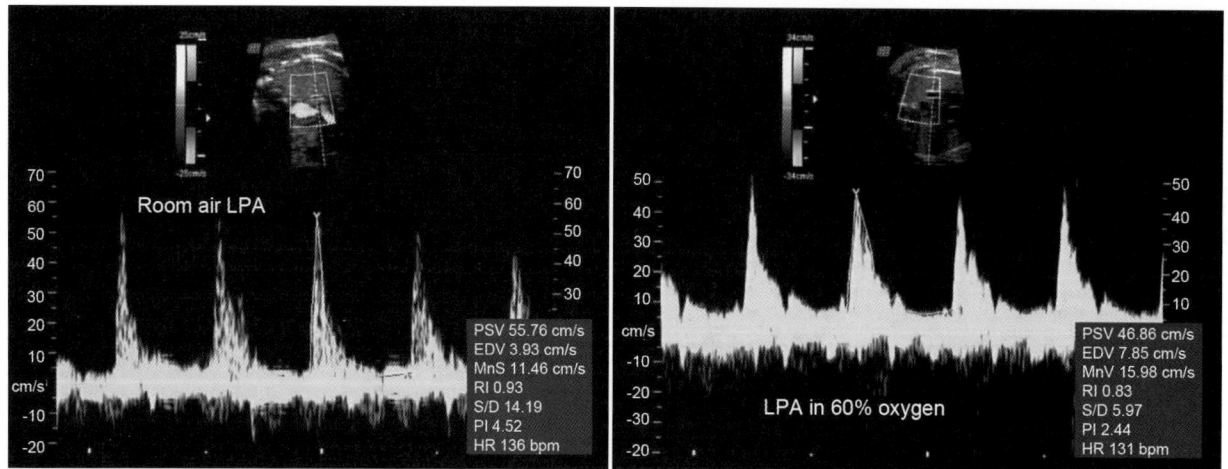

Fig. 50.7: Positive change in Doppler flow patterns of pulmonary vascular reactivity with oxygen
Abbreviation: LPA, left pulmonary artery

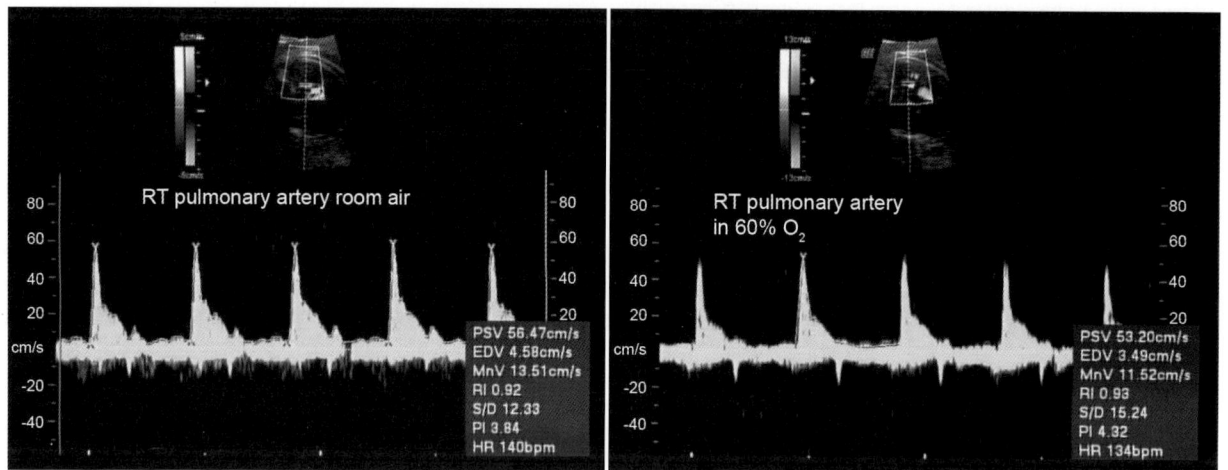

Fig. 50.8: Negative change in Doppler flow patterns of pulmonary vascular reactivity with oxygen
Abbreviation: RT, right

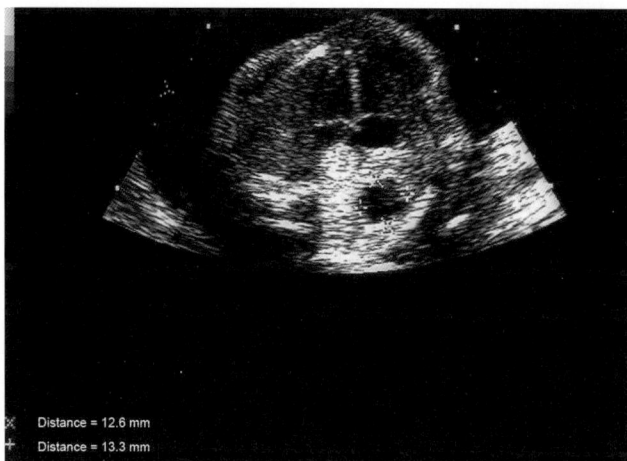

Fig. 50.9: Cystic adenomatoid malformation

PULMONARY SEQUESTRATION

Pulmonary sequestration is a rare anomaly identified in-utero by a difference in echo density of a particular lobe of the lung. It is seen as either above or below the diaphragm and is defined as either intra-pulmonary or extrapulmonary depending on its position relative to the visceral pleura. It may present with mediastinal shift or cardiac malposition and occasionally with hydrops from impingement or torsion of the inferior vena cava. The sequestered lobe receives its blood supply from the aorta rather than the pulmonary artery with venous return usually to the right atrium via the inferior vena cava. The majority of sequestrations are extrapulmonary and occupy the lower portion of either hemithorax. Color directed pulsed Doppler may be used to identify the arterial origin from the descending aorta and thereby differentiate sequestration from cystic adenomatoid malformation. Most subdiaphragmatic sequestration as identified in-utero regress and may not require neonatal surgical resection (Fig. 50.10).

CONGENITAL PULMONARY BLOOD FLOW ABNORMALITIES

Observable abnormalities of fetal pulmonary circulation may be related to structural congenital heart disease or, to thoracic space occupying lesions. The pulmonary artery should be superior and anterior to, and slightly larger than the aorta in the four-chamber view of the fetal heart. The pulmonary artery blood flow is directed toward the fetal left shoulder and ductus

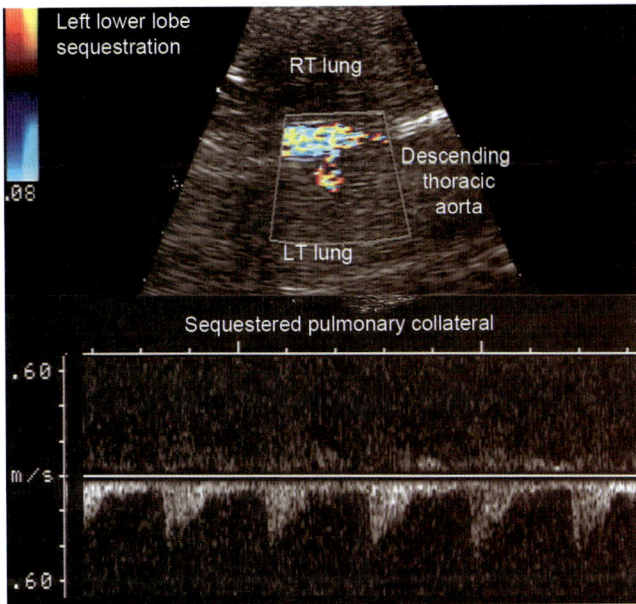

Fig. 50.10: Color Doppler of sequestration flow pattern

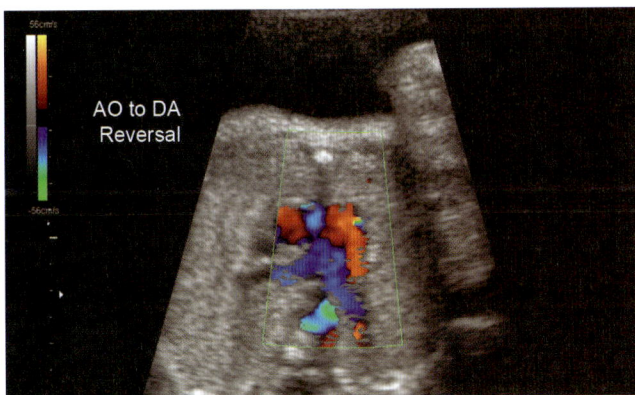

Fig. 50.11: Color Doppler of normal pulmonary artery bifurcation with pulmonary valve atresia and reversed ductus arteriosus flow pattern

Abbreviations: AO, aorta; DA, ductus arteriosus

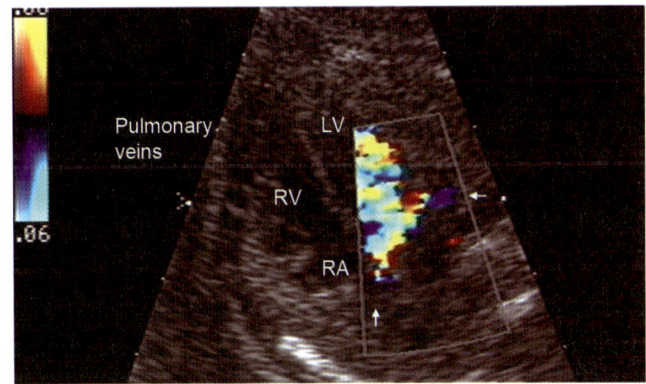

Fig. 50.12: Color Doppler of normal pulmonary venous connections

Abbreviations: LV, left ventricle; RV, right ventricle; RA, right atrium

arteriosus. Likewise, the normal connections of the pulmonary veins are easily identified from the four-chamber image, just as the LVOT comes into view. Anomalous connection of the pulmonary veins should be ruled out when major structural congenital heart defects are identified. By combining high resolution ultrasound magnification with the color flow and narrow sample size pulsed Doppler techniques we have described, blood flow connection abnormalities of the veins and arteries including sequestered lobes of the fetal lung may be identified. However, hydrothorax, cystic masses and diaphragmatic hernias may impede pulmonary blood flow to the extent that the flow may be difficult or impossible to observe or measure in one or both of the fetal lungs. Congenital malformations of pulmonary circulation should be considered in the presence of other forms of congenital heart disease. Direction of the fetal ductus arteriosus should be evaluated with both color and pulsed Doppler when arterial connection or obstruction is suggested in order to identify a ductal dependent lesion (Fig. 50.11).

Major pulmonary venous abnormalities can generally be ruled out by imaging the right and left venous ostia as they connect into the left atrium on either side of the descending aorta when seen in the four-chamber view of the heart in a transverse image of the thorax (Fig. 50.12). Exceptions to expect are when there is visceral heterotaxy when the stomach and heart may be on opposite sides of the fetus and/or when there is a common atrium or large atrial septal defect. Ipsilateral venous connections may be seen in these diagnoses but may be difficult to identify by fetal echocardiography. Both partially anomalous and totally anomalous pulmonary venous connection are typically associated with a disproportion of right sided chambers larger than the left sided structures. More obvious is total anomalous pulmonary venous connection (TAPVC) to the coronary sinus where a dilated coronary sinus can be identified as an eccentric line parallel to the mitral valve annulus in the four-chamber view. However, a dilated coronary sinus may also be seen with normally connected pulmonary veins when the left superior vena cava drains into the coronary sinus behind the lower left corner of the left atrium. The extra line in the left atrium may also signify the membrane in cor triatriatum (triatrial heart) where the common pulmonary venous sack is attached to the posterior left atrial wall but may drain anomalously into the right atrium or via restricted fenestrations into the left atrium. The most common type of TAPVC is when the common pulmonary venous sac is not attached to the left atrium but to a vein that ascends to join the innominate vein which then flows into the right superior vena cava and right atrium. The form of TAPVC most likely to become obstructed in the early newborn period is when the common pulmonary venous sack is attached to a vein that descends below the diaphragm and connects to a hepatic venous structure. Partially anomalous pulmonary venous veins are difficult to identify as they may enter the right atrium, coronary sinus, the right or left superior vena cava, the inferior vena cava or into the azygous venous system as single attachments with otherwise normally connecting pulmonary veins. In cases of hypoplastic left heart syndrome, the pulmonary veins may appear dilated for gestational age, but may be anomalously connected and associated with pulmonary venous stenoses. Stenosis of pulmonary veins may be difficult to identify in fetal life from ultrasound because of the relative paucity of pulmonary blood flow. Pulmonary venous dimensions can usually be measured successfully after 22 weeks of gestation. Pulmonary venous blood flow is best measured with color directed pulsed Doppler techniques in a lateral approach to the four-chamber view.

We believe that all fetal ultrasound anatomic survey examinations should include identification and relative quantification of the outflow tracts of the heart. The pulmonary artery should arise above the anterior right ventricle aiming toward the left shoulder at the ductus arteriosus, while the aorta arises centrally from the left ventricle aiming toward the right shoulder in a 90° crossing fashion relative to the main pulmonary artery. The ascending aorta and the main pulmonary artery should be about the same size. Pulmonary outflow obstructions may not become obvious on fetal ultrasound until the third trimester. A form of hypoplastic right heart where there is pulmonary atresia with intact ventricular septum may have a normal four-chamber view in the second trimester and normal sized pulmonary arteries at birth. In these cases, the pulmonary valve may acquire more severe obstruction with fetal growth resulting in a reversal of flow through the ductus arteriosus. We have seen this in the recipient twin-in-twin to twin transfusion syndrome as well as in singleton pregnancies. In these situations, the left ventricle begins to become disproportionately larger than the right ventricle during the second trimester as blood flow patterns change. Color Doppler is useful in proving a normal pulsed Doppler flow pattern into the main pulmonary artery. Normally, the forward flow pattern from the right ventricle into the pulmonary artery is a hollow envelope rarely exceeding 0.7 meters per second. Pulmonary stenosis can be recognized by a course spectral flow pattern measuring greater than 1.0 meter per minute and often associated with tricuspid valve regurgitation. Pulmonary outflow obstruction should be considered with presumptive fetal diagnoses of Ebstein's malformation of the tricuspid valve, double outlet right ventricle (DORV), transposition of the great arteries (d or l-TGA), ventricular septal defect, tetralogy of Fallot and in cases of early diagnosis of transient cystic hygroma associated with Noonan's syndrome. In those cases with the physiology of tetralogy of Fallot with pulmonary atresia, color Doppler is useful in identifying collateral arterial vessels feeding the lungs form the aorta. It is important to differentiate this disease from truncus arteriosus. Collateral vessels can also be seen using color Doppler in cases of pulmonary sequestration.

We use a team approach of prenatal counseling by the perinatologist, neonatologist, pediatric cardiologist and cardiothoracic surgeon for the family of any fetus with congenital heart disease that may require prenatal or early neonatal intervention. Any suggestion of a fetal anomaly of venous or arterial connection or obstruction must be confirmed after deliver by newborn echocardiography or at cardiac catheterization.

REFERENCES

1. Morrell NW, Weiser MCM, Stenmark KR. Development of the pulmonary vasculature. In: Gaultier, Bourbon and Post (Eds). Lung Development. New York: Oxford University Press; 1999.
2. Burri PH. Lung development and angiogenesis. In: Gaultier, Bourbon and Post (Eds). Lung Development. New York: Oxford University Press; 1999.
3. Kikkawa, Yutaka. Morphology and morphologic development of the lung. In: Scarpelli, Emile (Eds).Pulmonary Physiology of the Fetus, Newborn and Child. Philadelphia: Lea and Fibiger; 1975.
4. Rabinovitch M. Developmental Biology of the Pulmonary Vasculature. In: Polin RA, Fox WW (Eds). Fetal and Neonatal Physiology, 2nd edition. Philadelphia: Saunders; 1998.
5. Kitaoka Y, Burri PH, Weibel ER. Development of the human fetal airway tree: analysis of the numerical density of airway endtips. Anatomical Record. 1996;244:207-13.
6. Hislop A, Reed I. Growth and development of the respiratory system-anatomic development. In: Davis JA, Dobbing J (Eds). Scientific Foundations of Pediatrics. London: Heinemann; 1972.
7. Rasanan J, Huhta JC, Weiner S, et al. Fetal branch pulmonary artery vascular impedance during the second half of pregnancy. Am J Obstet Gynecol. 1996;174:1441-9.
8. Roberts AB, Mitchell JM. Direct ultrasonographic measurement of fetal lung length in normal pregnancies and pregnancies complicated by prolonged rupture of membranes. Am J Obstet Gynecol. 1990;163:1560-6.
9. Lewis AB, Heymann MA, Rudolph AM. Gestational changes in pulmonary vascular responses in fetal lambs in utero. Circ Res. 1976;39:536-41.
10. Tessler FN, Kimme-Smith C, Sutherland ML, et al. Inter- and intra-observer variability of Doppler peak velocity measurements: an in-vitro study. Ultrasound Med Biol. 1990;16:653-7.
11. O'Rourke MF. Vascular impedance in studies of arterial and cardiac function. Physiol Rev. 1982;62:571-621.
12. Downing GJ, Maulik D, Phillips C, et al. In vivo correlation of Doppler waveform analysis with arterial input impedance parameters. Ultrasound Med Biol. 1993;19:549-9.
13. Giles WB, Trudinger BJ, Paird PJ. Fetal umbilical artery flow velocity waveforms and placental resistance: pathological correlation. Br J Obstet Gynaecol. 1985;92:31-8.
14. Levin DL, Rudolph AM, Heymann MA, et al. Morphological development of the pulmonary vascular bed in fetal lambs. Circulation. 1976;53:144-51.
15. Heymann MA. Regulation of the pulmonary circulation in the perinatal period and in children. Intensive Care Med. 1989;15:S9-12.
16. Eik-Nes SH, Brubakk AO, Ulstein M. Measurement of human fetal blood flow. Br Med J. 1980;1:283-4.
17. Machado MVL, Chita SC, Allan LD. Acceleration time in the aorta and pulmonary artery measured by Doppler echocardiography in the midtrimester normal human fetus. Br Heart J. 1987;58:15-8.
18. Choi JY, Noh CI, Yun YS. Study on Doppler waveforms from the fetal cardiovascular system. Fetal Diagn Ther. 1991;6:74-83.
19. Hata T, Senoh D, Makihara K, et al. Fetal cardiac time intervals determined by Doppler echocardiography. J Perinat Med. 1989;17:85-92.
20. Morin FC III, Egan EA. Pulmonary hemodynamics in fetal lambs during development at normal and increased oxygen tension. J Appl Physiol. 1992;73:213-8.
21. Huhta JC, Moise KJ, Fisher DJ, et al. Detection and quantitation of constriction of the fetal ductus arteriosus by Doppler echo-cardiography. Circulation. 1987;75:406-12.
22. Rasanen J, Wood DC, Weiner S, et al. The role of the pulmonary circulation on the distribution of human fetal cardiac output during the second half of pregnancy. Circulation. 1996;94:1068-73.
23. Schmidt KG, Di Tommaso M, Silverman NH, et al. Doppler echocardiographic assessment of fetal descending aortic and umbilical blood flows. Validation study in fetal lambs. Circulation. 1991;83:1731-7.
24. Versmold HT, Kitterman JA, Phibbs RH, et al. Aortic blood pressure during the first 12 hours of life in infants with birth weight 610 to 4220 grams. Pediatrics. 1981;67:607-13.
25. St John M, Groves A, MacNeill A, et al. Assessment of changes in blood flow through the lungs and foramen ovale in the normal

human fetus with gestational age: a prospective Doppler echocardiographic study. Br Heart J. 1994;71:232-7.

26. Rudolph AM, Heymann MA. Circulatory changes during growth in the fetal lamb. Circ Res. 1970;26:289-99.

27. Morin FC III, Egan EA, Ferguson W, et al. Development of pulmonary vascular response to oxygen. Am J Physiol. 1988;254:H542-6.

28. Soyeur D, Schaaps JP, Kulbertus H. Pulsed Doppler assessment of fetal blood flow across the foramen ovale and pulmonary vascular bed. Eur Heart J. 1990;11:90.

29. Phillipos EZ, Robertson MA, Still KD. The echocardiographic assessment of the human fetal foramen ovale. J Am Soc Echocardiogr. 1994;7:257-63.

30. Kiserud T, Eik-Nes SH, Blaas HG, et al. Foramen ovale: an ultrasonographic study of its relation to the inferior vena cava, ductus venosus and hepatic veins. Ultrasound Obstet Gynecol. 1992;2:389-96.

31. Traeger A, Noschel H, Zaumseil J. The pharmacokinetics of indomethacin in pregnant and parturient women and their newborn infants. Zentralbl Gynaekol. 1973;95:635-41.

32. Moise KJ, Ou CN, Kirshon B, et al. Placental transfer of indomethacin in the human pregnancy. Am J Obstet Gynecol. 1990;162:549-54.

33. Kirshon B, Moise KJ, Wasserstrum N, et al. Influence of short-term indomethacin therapy on fetal urine output. Obstet Gynecol. 1988;72:51-3.

34. Moise KJ, Huhta JC, Sharif DS, et al. Indomethacin in the treatment of premature labor. Effects on the fetal ductus arteriosus. N Engl J Med. 1988;319:327-31.

35. Tulzer G, Gudmundsson S, Tews G, et al. Incidence of indomethacin-induced human fetal ductal constriction. J Matern Fetal Invest. 1992;1:267-9.

36. Moise KJ. Effect of advancing gestational age on the frequency of fetal ductal constriction in association with maternal indomethacin use. Am J Obstet Gynecol. 1993;168:1350-3.

37. Huhta JC, Cohen AW, Wood DC. Premature constriction of the ductus arteriosus. Journal of the American Society of Echocardiography. 1990;3(1):30-4.

38. Rasanen J, Debbs RH, Wood DC, et al. The effects of indomethacin on pulmonary arterial vascular impedance and cardiac output. Ultrasound in Obstetrics and Gynecology. 1999;13(2):112-6.

39. Tulzer G, Gudmundsson S, Sharkey AM, et al. Doppler echocardiography of fetal ductus arteriosus constriction versus increased right ventricular output. J Am Coll Cardiol. 1991;18:532-6.

40. Cassin S. Role of prostaglandins and thromboxanes in the control of the pulmonary circulation in the fetus and newborn. Semin Perinatol. 1980;4:101-7.

41. Wlodek ME, Harding R, Thorburn GD. Effects of inhibition of prostaglandin synthesis on flow and composition of fetal urine, lung liquid, and swallowed fluid in sheep. Am J Obstet Gynecol. 1994;170:186-95.

42. Velvis H, Moore P, Heymann MA. Prostaglandin inhibition prevents the fall in pulmonary vascular resistance as a result of rhythmic distension of the lungs in fetal lambs. Pediatr Res. 1991;30:62-8.

43. Morin FC, Egan EA, Norfleet WT. Indomethacin does not diminish the pulmonary vascular response of the fetus to increased oxygen tension. Pediatr Res. 1988;24:696-700.

44. Levin DL, Mills LJ, Weinberg AG. Hemodynamic, pulmonary vascular, and myocardial abnormalities secondary to pharmacologic constriction of the fetal ductus arteriosus. A possible mechanism for persistent pulmonary hypertension and transient tricuspid insufficiency in the newborn infant. Circulation. 1979;60:360-4.

45. Tulzer G, Gudmundsson S, Rotondo KM, et al. Acute fetal ductal occlusion in lambs. Am J Obstet Gynecol. 1991;165:775-8.

46. Kenny JF, Plappert T, Doubilet P, et al. Changes in intracardiac blood flow velocities and right and left ventricular stroke volumes with gestational age in the normal human fetus: a prospective Doppler echocardiographic study. Circulation. 1986;74:1208-16.

47. Isaaz K, Ethevenot G, Admant P, et al. A new Doppler method of assessing left ventricular ejection force in chronic congestive heart failure. Am J Cardiol. 1989;64:81-7.

48. St. John Sutton M, Gill T, Plappert T, et al. Assessment of right and left ventricular function in terms of force development with gestational age in the normal human fetus. Br Heart J. 1991;61:285-9.

49. Rizzo G, Capponi A, Rinaldo D, et al. Ventricular ejection force in growth-retarded fetuses. Ultrasound Obstet Gynecol. 1995;5:247-55.

50. Rasanen J, Debbs RH, Wood DC, et al. Human fetal right ventricular ejection force under abnormal loading conditions during the second half of pregnancy. Ultrasound in Obstetrics and Gynecology. 1997;10(5):325-32.

51. Noble MIM, Trenchard D, Guz A. Left ventricular ejection in conscious dogs: II. Determinants of stroke volume. Circ Res. 1966;19:148-52.

52. Noble MIM. The contribution of blood momentum to left ventricular ejection in the dog. Circ Res. 1968;23:663-70.

53. Copel JA, Grannum PA, Green JJ, et al. Fetal cardiac output in the isoimmunized pregnancy: a pulsed Doppler-echocardiographic study of patients undergoing intravascular intrauterine transfusion. Am J Obstet Gynecol. 1989;161:361-5.

54. Moise KJ, Mari G, Fisher DJ, et al. Acute fetal hemodynamic alterations after intrauterine transfusion for treatment of severe red blood cell alloimmunization. Am J Obstet Gynecol. 1990;163:776-84.

55. Rizzo G, Nicolaides KH, Arduini D, et al. Effects of intravascular fetal blood transfusion on fetal intracardiac Doppler velocity waveforms. Am J Obstet Gynecol. 1990;163:1231-8.

56. Moise KJ, Mari G, Kirshon B, et al. The effect of indomethacin on the pulsatility index of the umbilical artery in human fetuses. Am J Obstet Gynecol. 1990;162,199-202.

57. Khowsathit P, Tian ZY, Wood DC, et al. Indomethacin-induced placental vasodilation: association with fetal ductal constriction. J Matern Fetal Inves. 1995;5:30-2.

58. Rasanen J, Wood DC, Debbs R, et al. Reactivity of the human fetal circulation to maternal hyperoxygenation increases in the second half of pregnancy a randomized study. Circulation. 1998;97:257-62.

59. Assali NS, Kirschbaum TH, Dilts PV. Effects of hyperbaric oxygen on uteroplacental and fetal circulation. Circ Res. 1968;22:573-88.

60. Mital S, Konduri GG. Vascular K+ ATP channels mediate O2 induced pulmonary vasodilation in fetal lambs. Pediatrics. 1996;98:527. Abstract.

61. Mital S, Konduri GG. Oxygen causes pulmonary vasodilation by stimulating synthesis and release of ATP in fetal lambs. Pediatrics. 1996;98:533. Abstract.

62. Heymann MA, Rudolph AM, Nies AS, et al. Bradykinin production associated with oxygenation of the fetal lamb. Circ Res. 1969;25:521-34.

63. Burchell HB, Swan HJC, Wood EH. Demonstration of differential effects on pulmonary and systemic arterial pressure by variation in oxygen content of inspired air in patients with patent ductus arteriosus and pulmonary hypertension. Circulation. 1953;8:681-94.

64. Harding R, Hooper SB. Regulation of lung expansion and lung growth before birth. Journal of Applied Physiology. 1996;81:209-24.

65. Askenazi SS, Perlman M. Pulmonary hypoplasia: lung weight and radial alveolar count as critical diagnosis. Arch Dis Child. 1979;54:614-8.

66. Chitkara U, Rosenberg J, Chervenak FA, et al. Prenatal sonographic assessment of the fetal thorax: normal values. Am J Obstet Gynecol. 1989;156:1069-74.

67. Potter EL. Bilateral renal agenesis. J Pediatrics. 1946;29:68-76.

68. Rotschild A, Ling EW, Puterman ML, et al. Neonatal outcome after prolonged preterm rupture of the membranes. Am J Obstet Gynecol. 1990;162(1):46-52.

69. Savich RD, Guerra FA, Lee CC, et al. Effects of acute oligohydramnios on respiratory system of fetal sheep. J Appl Physiol. 1992;73(2):610-7.

70. Roberts AB, Mitchell J. Pulmonary hypoplasia and fetal breathing in preterm prmature rupture of membranes. Early Human Development. 1995;41(1):27-37.

71. Fisk NM, Talbert DG, Nicolini U, et al. Fetal breathing movements in oligohydramnios are not increased by aminoinfusion. Br J Obstet Gynaecol. 1992;99(6):464-8.

72. Ohlsson A, Fong K, Hannah M, et al. Prediction of lethal pulmonary hypoplasia and chorioamnionitis by assessment of fetal breathing. Br J Obstet Gynaecol. 1991;98(7):692-7.

73. Longaker MT, Laberge JM, Dansereau J, et al. Primary fetal hydrothorax: natural history and management. J Pediatr Surg. 1989;24(6):573-6.

74. Blott M, Nicolaides KH, Greenough A. Pleuroamniotic shunting for decompression of fetal pleural effusions. Obstetrics and Gynecology. 1988;71(5):798-800.

75. Harrison MR, Adzick NS, Estes JM, et al. A prospective study of the outcome for fetuses with diaphragmatic hernia. JAMA. 1994;271(5):382-4.

76. Persutte WH, Lenke RR, Kurczynski TW, et al. Antenatal diagnosis of Pena-Shokeir syndrome (type I) with ultrasonography and magnetic resonance imaging. Obstetrics and Gynecology. 1988;72(3Pt2):472-5.

77. Dornan JC, Ritchie JW, Meban C. Fetal breathing movements and lung maturation in the congenitally abnormal human fetus. Journal of Developmental Physiology. 1984;6(4):367-75.

78. Adzick NS, Harrison MR, Crombleholme TM, et al. Fetal lung lesions: management and outcome. Am J Obstet Gynecol. 1998;179(4):884-9.

79. Merz E, Miric-Tesanic D, Bahlmann F, et al. Prenatal sonographic chest and lung measurements for predicting severe pulmonary hypoplasia. Prenatal Diagnosis. 1999;19(7):614-9.

80. Lachman RS, Rappaport V. Fetal imaging in the skeletal dysplasias. Clinics in Perinatology. 1990;17(3):703-22.

81. Ohlsson A, Fong K, Rose T, et al. Prenatal ultrasonic prediction of autopsy proven pulmonary hypoplasia. Am J Perinatol. 1992;9(5-6):334-7.

82. Nimrod C, Davies D, Iwanicki S, et al. Ultrasound prediction of pulmonary hypoplasia. Obstetrics and Gynecology. 1986;68(4):495-8.

83. D'Alton M, Mercer B, Riddick E, et al. Serial thoracic versus abdominal circumference ratios for the prediction of pulmonary hypoplasia in premature rupture of the membranes remote from term. Am J Obstet Gynecol. 1992;166(2):658-63.

84. Songster GS, Gray DL, Crane JP. Prenatal prediction of lethal pulmonary hypoplasia using ultrasonic fetal chest circumference. Obstetrics and Gynecology. 1989;73(2):261-6.

85. Yoshimura S, Masuzaki H, Gotoh H, et al. Ultrasonographic prediction of lethal pulmonary hypoplasia: comparison of eight different ultrasonographic parameters. Am J Obstet Gynecol. 1996;175(2):477-83.

86. Laudy JA, Janssen MM, Struyk PC, et al. Three-dimensional ultrasonography of normal fetal lung volume: a preliminary study. Ultrasound in Obstetrics and Gynecology. 1998;11(1):13-6.

87. Pöhls UG, Rempen A. Fetal lung volumetry by threedimensional ultrasound. Ultrasound Obstet Gynecol. 1998;11(1):6-12.

88. D'Arcy TJ, Hughes SW, Chiu WS, et al. Estimation of fetal lung volume using enhanced 3-dimensional ultrasound: a new method and first result. Br J Obstet Gynaecol. 1996;103(10):1015-20.

89. Lee A, Kratochwil A, Stumpflen I, et al. Fetal lung volume determination by threedimensional ultrasonography. Am J Obstet Gynecol. 1996;175(3 Pt 1):588-92.

90. Rasanen J, Wood DC, Debbs RH, et al. Diagnosis of lung hypoplasia by Doppler ultrasound in human fetuses. Miami: Abstract Society of Perinatal Obstetricians; 1998.

91. Mitchell JM, Roberts AB, Lee A. Doppler waveforms from the pulmonary arterial system in normal fetuses and those with pulmonary hypoplasia. Ultrasound Obstet Gynecol. 1998;11(3):167-72.

92. Yoshimura S, Masuzaki H, Miura K, et al. Diagnosis of fetal pulmonary hypoplasia by measurement of blood flow velocity waveforms of pulmonary arteries with Doppler ultrasonography. Am J Obstet Gynecol. 1999;180(2 Pt 1):441-6.

93. Roth P, Agnani G, Arbez-Gindre F, et al. Use of energy color Doppler in visualizing fetal pulmonary vascularization to predict the absence of severe pulmonary hypoplasia. Gynecologic and Obstetric Investigation. 1998;46(3):153-7.

94. Chaoui R, Kalache K, Tennstedt C, et al. Pulmonary arterial Doppler velocimetry in fetuses with lung hypoplasia. European Journal of Obstetrics, Gynecology and Reproductive Biology. 1999;84(2):179-85.

95. Broth RE, Wood DC, Rasanen J, et al. Prediction of lethal pulmonary hypoplasia: the hyperoxygenation test for pulmonary artery reactivity. Am J Obstet Gynecol. 2002;187(4):940-5.

51

Uteroplacental and Umbilical Circulation: Physiologic Changes in Pregnancy

AK Ertan, HA Tanriverdi, W Schmidt

INTRODUCTION

Doppler sonography in obstetrics is a widely accepted functional method of examining the uteroplacental and fetal unit. It is a noninvasive means and became almost a standard technique in antenatal care. This method became an important tool for qualifying high risk pregnancies. Color Doppler ultrasound represents blood flow changes as a color image, superimposed on the real-time ultrasound image being examined. In this way different vessels of the uteroplacental circulation can be accurately identified. Also, by identifying the vessel at a fixed point, e.g. where the uterine artery crosses the external iliac artery, it is possible to examine the same point in the circulation. Endovaginal color Doppler transducers allow easy and quick visualization of even the smallest vessels in the uteroplacental and fetal circulation. This, in turn, has enabled us to build a picture of the physiological changes in uteroplacental and fetal blood flow before and during the early stages of pregnancy.[1]

One of the first steps toward realizing the potential of Doppler ultrasound is to gain a clear understanding of the physiological changes that occur in the uteroplacental circulation during normal pregnancy. With this knowledge, we can obtain a clearer understanding of the pathophysiological changes that occur in the presence of disease.

INDICES

Although measurement of volume flow changes in an organ would be ideal, in vivo the current methods for determining true flow are too inaccurate to derive meaningful conclusions which can be of clinical value. Consequently we rely on indices of resistance and velocity derived from the flow velocity waveforms (FVW) of a vessel.

Blood flow velocity in the fetal circulating system depends on the type of vessel. The arteries always have a pulsatile pattern (Fig. 51.1), whereas veins have either a pulsatile or continuous pattern (Fig. 51.2).

Analysis of Doppler sonographic FVWs quantitatively is more difficult than analyzing qualitatively. Qualitative analysis also overcomes erroneous measurements in small vessels. There are plenty of indices for qualitative analysis. Following are the most frequently used indices:

- Systolic/Diastolic ratio (S/D ratio, Stuart 1980)
- Resistance index (RI, Pourcelot 1974)
- Pulsatility index (PI, Gosling and King 1977).

In analyzing sonographic results and calculating indices, following characters are used:

S = Temporal peak of maximum frequency

D = End-diastolic maximum frequency

C = Temporal average of maximum frequency, F_{mean}

I = Instantaneous spatial average frequency

E = Temporal average of spatial average frequency

Calculations of formulas are as follows (Fig. 51.3):

$$S/D \text{ ratio} = S/D$$
$$RI = (S-D)/S$$
$$PI = (S-D)/C$$

The above presented indices overcome a very serious problem involved with the angle between the ultrasound beam and the direction of blood flow (insonation angle). These indices are relatively angle independent and are therefore easily applied in clinical practice.

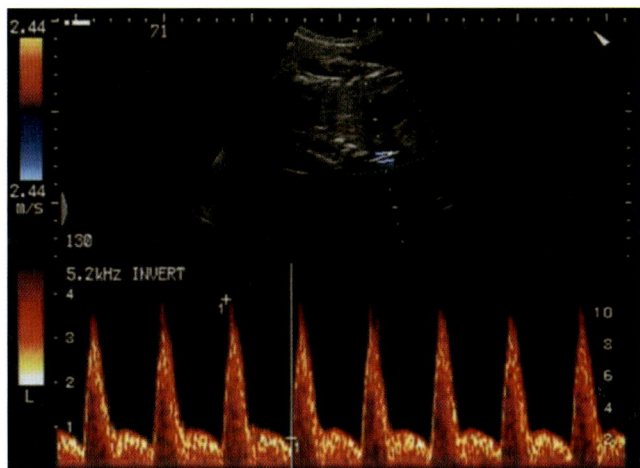

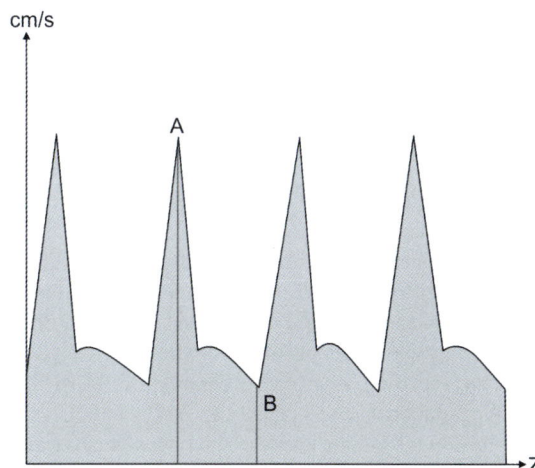

Fig. 51.1: Doppler sonography of fetal aorta with a pulsatile pattern

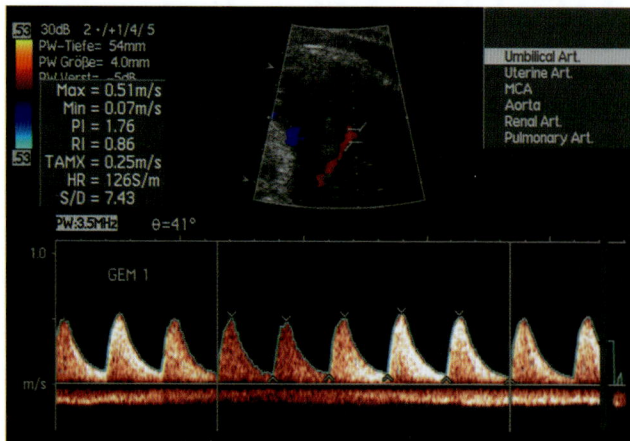

Fig. 51.2: Umbilical artery with a pulsatile (upper line) and umbilical vein with a continuous pattern (lower line)

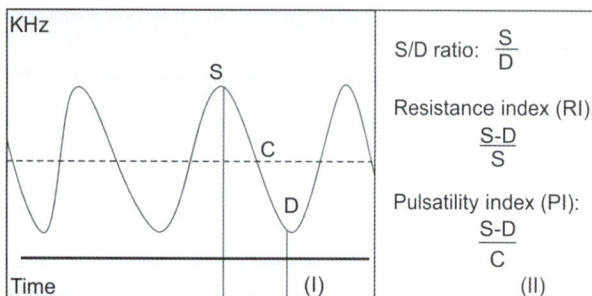

Fig. 51.3: Scheme of the Doppler curve (I). S = systolic, D = diastolic, C = temporal average of maximum frequency. Calculation of formulas of the main Doppler sonographic indices (II)

In practice, none of the indices is superior to the other[2-4] and any index may be used. Although S/D ratio is easily calculated, RI is the easiest to interpret. RI values approach to zero if the resistance decreases and approach to one if resistance increases. If end-diastolic flow is absent, PI is the only index making evaluation of blood flow possible, because in this situation S/D will equal to infinite and RI to one. The PI is more complex because it requires the calculation of the mean velocity, but modern Doppler sonographic devices provide those values in real time.

PHYSIOLOGIC COLOR DOPPLER SONOGRAPHIC CHANGES OF THE EMBRYONIC AND UTEROPLACENTAL VESSELS IN EARLY PREGNANCY

Results of a recent study performed by Ertan et al.[5] evaluating the uteroplacental and fetal circulation during early pregnancy in non-complicated pregnancies showed that vascular impedance to blood flow in all examined vessels decreased significantly throughout the first gestational trimester. Resistance to flow was highest in the main uterine artery and decreased toward the spiral artery. When the flow velocity waveform patterns of the arteries under investigation were analyzed, specific changes were observed. In all of the cases during early gestational development, an early diastolic notching was determined in the uterine arteries. The flow velocity waveforms of the fetal aorta and umbilical arteries were similar, until week 10 the arteries were typically without a diastolic flow. From week 16

onward, diastolic velocities were present in all signals at the fetal aorta and umbilical arteries.

Changes in Uterine Artery Circulation in Early Pregnancy

The uterine artery FVW was characterized by an early diastolic notch and a gradually increasing flow velocity during early pregnancy. The peak systolic velocities (PSV) increase, whereas the S/D and RI decrease progressively during early pregnancy. The end-diastolic velocity increases progressively. In all of the cases during early gestational development, an early diastolic notching was determined, but there was a gradually flattening in the depth of the notch (Fig. 51.4). At the third trimester of pregnancy this "notch" disappeared. The RI of the uterine arteries decreased gradually, which means that the resistance of the arteries lessens during pregnancy progression.

Changes in Umbilical Circulation in Early Pregnancy

The color signal of the umbilical artery was recorded for the first time at 7 weeks of gestation.

From week 10 onward it was able to show the end diastolic velocity and from week 16 onward diastolic signals were present in all cases (Figs 51.5 and 51.6). The PSV between week 7 and week 9 remained constant and from week 9 onward it increased, while S/D and RI decreased progressively during the first 16 weeks of gestation.

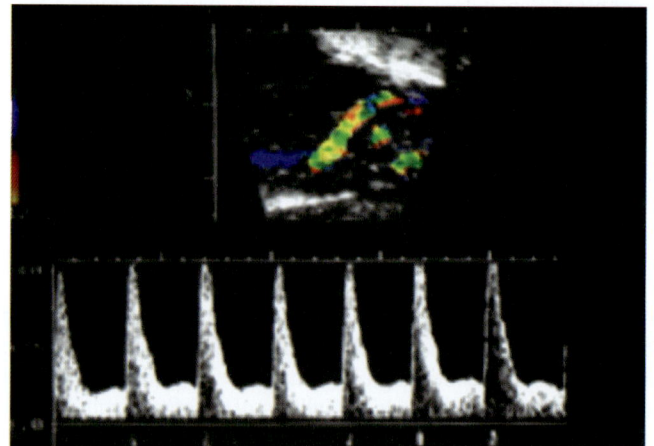

Fig. 51.4: Doppler sonography of uterine artery in first trimester of pregnancy (7 + 6 weeks) with early notch

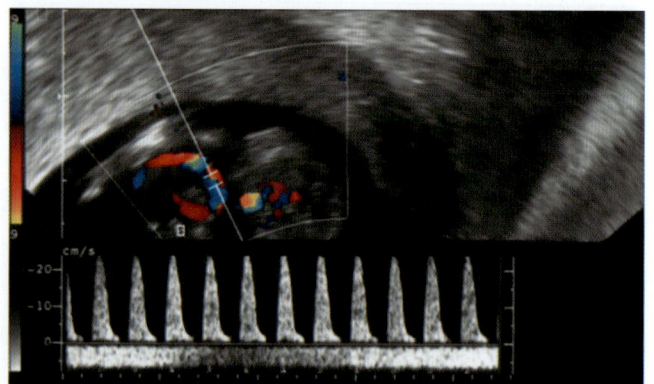

Fig. 51.5: Doppler velocity waveforms of umbilical artery (end-diastolic zero flow) and continuous venous blood flow of umbilical vein in 11 + 4 weeks of pregnancy

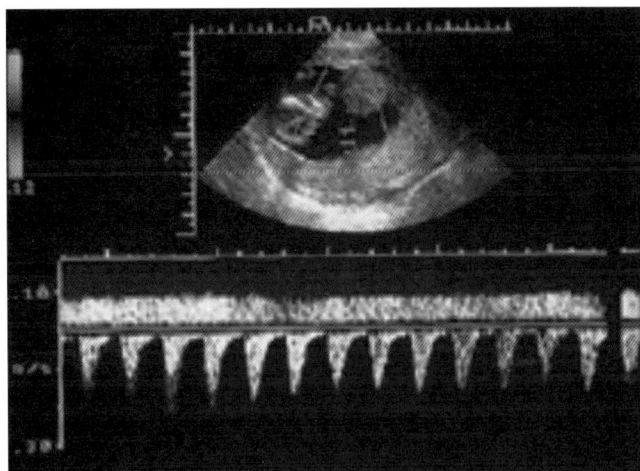

Fig. 51.6: Doppler velocity waveforms of umbilical artery with an end-diastolic flow (lower line) in 13 + 4 weeks of pregnancy

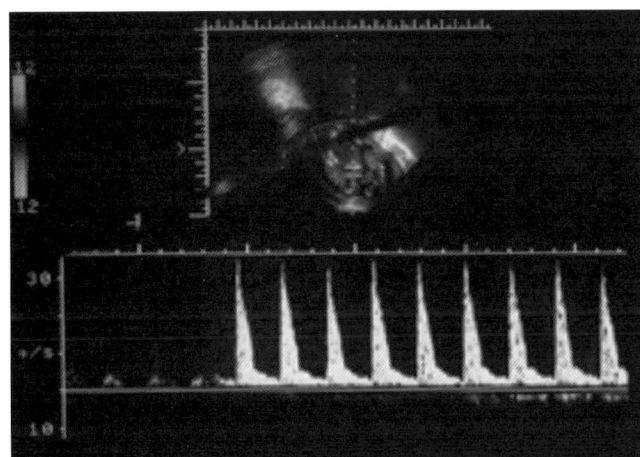

Fig. 51.7: Doppler velocity waveforms of fetal aorta with an end-diastolic flow in 15 + 4 weeks of pregnancy

Changes in Fetal Aorta Circulation in Early Pregnancy

The color signal of the fetal aorta was possible to be recorded for the first time at 7 weeks of gestation. The main problem in achieving Doppler signals of the aorta were fetal body movements and to make measurements with a correct angle, less than 60°.

The FVW was similar to the umbilical artery. Until week 10 of gestation the FVW was typically without a diastolic flow (end-diastolic zero flow). From week 16 onward, diastolic velocities were present in all aortic signals (Fig. 51.7). The PSV increases and the S/D and RI decreases progressively during the first 16 weeks of gestation.

UTEROPLACENTAL AND FETAL CIRCULATION AFTER MIDPREGNANCY

The Maternal Side: Uterine Circulation

The uterine artery is a branch of the internal iliac artery. It courses along the lateral wall of the pelvis before crossing the external iliac artery and reaching the uterus at the level of the cervix. After giving off a cervical branch, it ascends along the lateral wall of the body of the uterus in a tortuous manner, before

anastomozing with the Fallopian branch of the ovarian artery. As it passes along the body of the uterus it gives off the arcuate arteries, which encompass the uterine body. These in turn give off radial arteries that penetrate into the inner third of the myometrium, where they become the basal arteries. The spiral arteries, a continuation of the basal arteries, supply the endometrium, their coiled form allowing contraction during menstruation (Fig. 51.8).[1]

Using transvaginal color Doppler sonography, it is possible to identify the uterine artery in early pregnancy at the level of the cervical os, as it enters the uterus, and as it ascends into the uterine body (Fig. 51.9). It is possible to examine the uterine artery by the transabdominal approach after 12 weeks of gestation, when the uterus becomes an abdominal organ. The FVWs obtained from the uterine artery do not significantly change from when it enters the cervix up to the point that it reaches the body of the uterus. It is important to measure at this level, before the uterine artery enters the uterus and branches into the arcuate arteries. An arcuate artery can exhibit a relatively low resistance pattern even when the uterine artery has high resistance with persistent notching present (Fig. 51.10). It is therefore necessary to ensure that the uterine artery is examined as it reaches the uterus at the level of cervix, if the changes in the uterine circulation are to be interpreted as a whole. Similarly, if the sample site is too low on the cervix, the cervical branch of the uterine artery will be examined; this can show high resistance when the main uterine artery waveform is normal.[1]

Blood flow velocities in the uterine artery depends on the localization of placenta and gestational age.[6] If the placenta is laterally located, blood flow velocities in the ipsilateral uterine

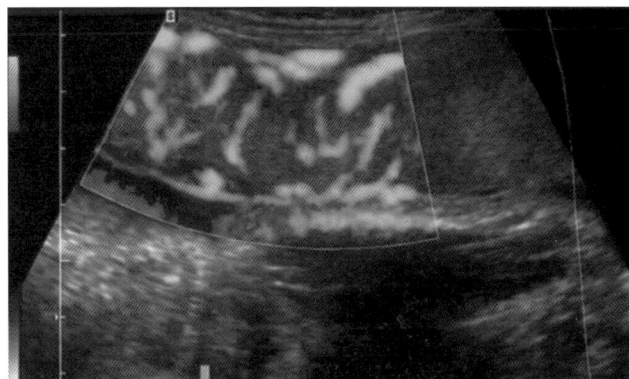

Fig. 51.8: Power Doppler of arcuate and intraplacental arteries

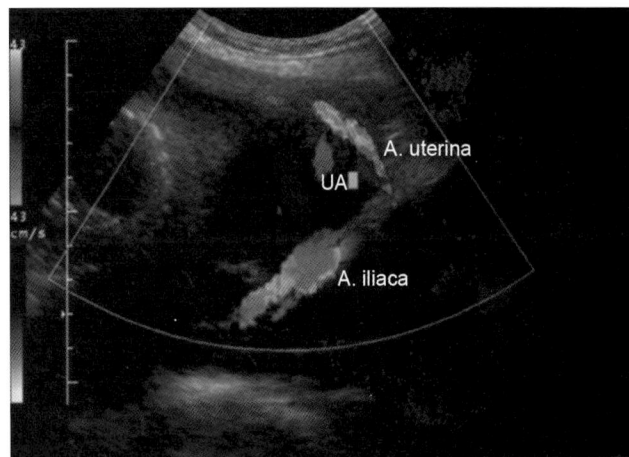

Fig. 51.9: Color Doppler sonographic view of the main uterine artery crossing the iliac artery

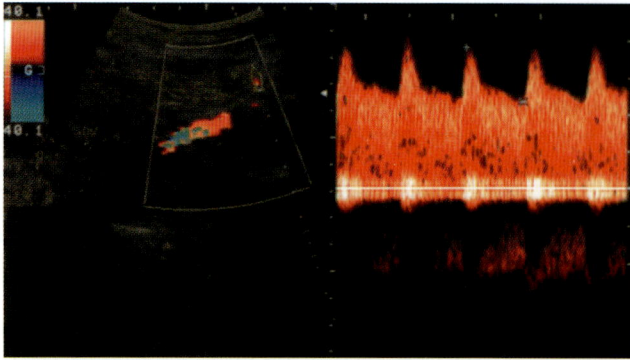

Fig. 51.10: Flow in different parts of the uteroplacental circulation can be measured with color Doppler technology, here the relatively low resistance pattern of the uteroplacental arteries

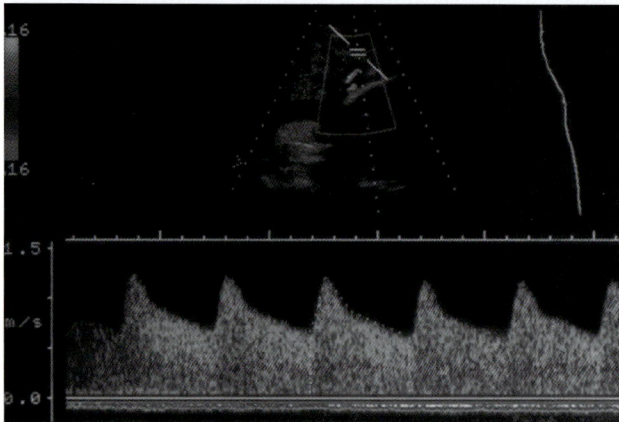

Fig. 51.11: Normal Doppler flow velocity waveform of the uterine artery in the third trimester

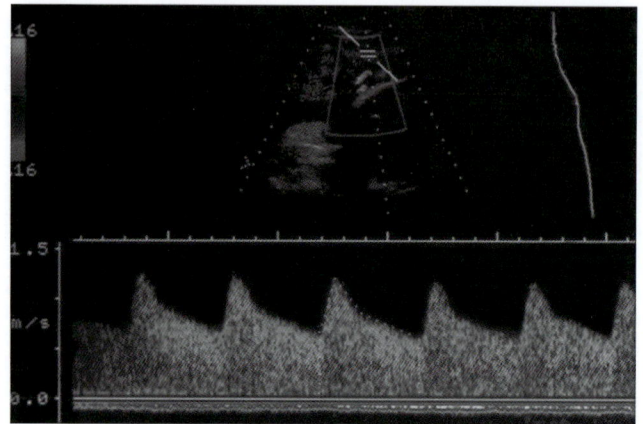

Fig. 51.12: Pathological waveforms of uterine artery in 29 + 3 weeks of pregnancy with IUGR and preeclampsia

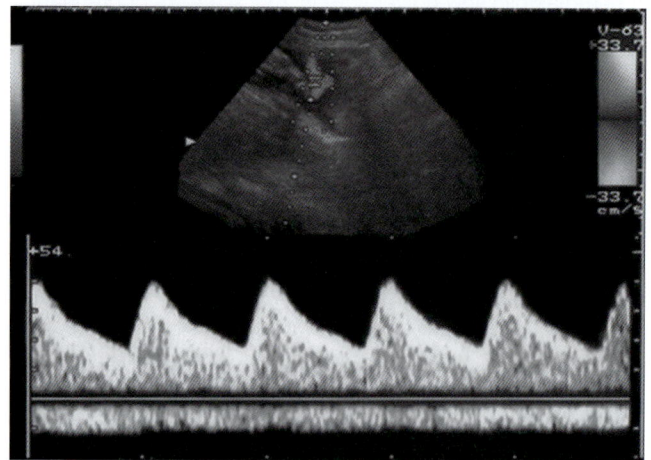

Fig. 51.13: Blood velocity waveform in umbilical artery in the late pregnancy

artery are more important than the flow velocities of the contralateral vessel. Differences between flow velocities of the right and left uterine artery are evident at early stages of pregnancy. But in the third trimester, the difference between the S/D ratio of the vessels decrease up to 0.3–0.4.[2] If an abnormal flow pattern is observed in the uterine arteries in midpregnancy, this most probably indicates the defective perfusion of fetoplacental unit, which predicts a high probability for developing preeclampsia and/or intrauterine growth restriction.[7]

At early stages of pregnancy end diastolic flow velocities in placental arteries are low, but systolic flow is evident.[2] With trophoblastic invasion and maturation of the uteroplacental vessels, beyond the second trimester the high pressure system is converted to a low pressure system, and vascular resistance declines.[8] The biologic variability after the middle of the second trimester becomes almost stable.

Before 24 weeks of gestation early diastolic notching, due to the immature uteroplacental vascular system, is normally observed. Beyond this gestational age, persistent early diastolic notching is associated with preeclampsia (Figs 51.11 and 51.12).[9-11]

The Fetal Side: Umbilical Arteries, Fetal Aorta and Middle Cerebral Artery

Umbilical Arteries

Blood flow velocity in the umbilical arteries increases with the progressing gestational age (Fig. 51.13). As a result, S/D ratio

continuously decreases due to increasing arterial blood flow. With progressing gestational age end-diastolic flow becomes evident during the whole heart cycle, matching with previous longitudinal studies of Fogarty et al.[2] and Hünecke et al.[12] as with many cross-sectional studies.[13-16]

Trudinger et al.[17] put forth the following mechanisms to explain this development:

- Continuous maturation in placental villi
- Continuous widening of placental vessels cause a continuous decrease in vascular resistance
- Continuous increase in fetal cardiac output
- Continuous changes in the vessel compliance
- Continuous increase in fetal blood pressure.

Especially in the third trimester of pregnancy, depending on the above factors normal values become scattered on nomograms. This scattering is more prominent in the S/D ratio than the PI. Resistance index is not affected by above factors after 28 weeks of gestation.

Descending Fetal Aorta

Beside the umbilical arteries, routine Doppler sonographic measurements on the descending fetal aorta are possible. As the gestational age increases S/D ratio of fetal aorta decreases insignificantly, paralleling to the results of Hecher et al.[18] The FVW of the fetal aorta shows a continuous forward stream during the whole heart cycle, but when compared to the FVW of the umbilical arteries, the end-diastolic flow is less than the systolic component. Due to this reason the S/D ratio in the fetal aorta is greater than the S/D ratio in the umbilical arteries. As pregnancy progresses, the diameter of the vessel gets wider and as a result peripheral resistance decreases, and diastolic flow increases. Nevertheless, this does not cause a significant S/D ratio decrease in the fetal aorta. Resistance and pulsatility indices are not affected significantly, and show a similar course as in the umbilical arteries.

Middle Cerebral Artery

The most favorably positioned vessel for Doppler sonographic examination of the fetal brain perfusion is the middle cerebral artery (MCA). Biologic variability of vessels perfusing the fetal brain is excessive due to the fetal activity status. As pregnancy progresses the vascular resistance decreases.[19] During the early stages of pregnancy, end diastolic flow velocities in cerebral vessels are weak, but velocities increase toward the end of gestation. Hyperactivity of fetus, increase of intrauterine pressure (e.g. polyhydramnios) and external pressure to the fetal head (e.g. by the probe) might erroneously increase end-diastolic flow velocities.[20] Different investigators have undertaken studies utilizing data obtained from umbilical arteries and MCA to develop indices for evaluation of intrauterine risk.

DEPENDENCY OF DOPPLER FLOW VELOCITY WAVEFORMS ON GESTATIONAL AGE

The amount of perfusion in trophoblastic tissue is related to gestational age. For this reason, in interpreting the Doppler sonographic findings, gestational age should be taken into account as well. In general, the accepted time for starting Doppler sonographic examinations is the beginning of the second trimester. This is the right time that allows for modifications in antenatal care in a high-risk pregnancy. For specific conditions, earlier timing of measurements may be considered.[21]

The main objective in using fetomaternal Doppler sonographic nomograms is to improve perinatal outcome in high-risk pregnancies. Curves presented in Figures 51.14 to 51.25 depict normal fetal and maternal Doppler sonographic values standardized according to gestational age, and can be used in routine practice.

Doppler sonographic nomograms are used for differentiation of normal and abnormal blood FVWs, which helps to determine high risk pregnancies. By taking threshold values of pathologic pregnancies into consideration, nomograms are capable of differentiating between normal and abnormal.[22] While using these nomograms, it must always kept in mind that the values on these nomograms should not be taken as mathematical equations, and that limitations of sensitivity and specificity exist.

Using Nomograms in Practice

Just like the defense mechanism of peripheral vasoconstriction in an adult in the face of hemorrhagic shock, the "brain sparing" mechanism (brain-sparing effect) becomes active in a fetus with hypoxia or chronic placental insufficiency. As a result of the brain

sparing effect, resistance either in the umbilical artery (UA) and fetal descending aorta (FDA) increases. As a consequence Doppler indices related to these vessels increase. The end diastolic blood flow increases in MCAs by the same effect. Doppler indices for this vessel decreases consequently.

Some points should be considered while using Doppler sonographic nomograms:

1. Among the measurements performed on the UA and FDA, values between 90–95th percentiles should be considered as borderline and repeat follow-ups should be planned. Values exceeding the 95th percentile are considered abnormal.

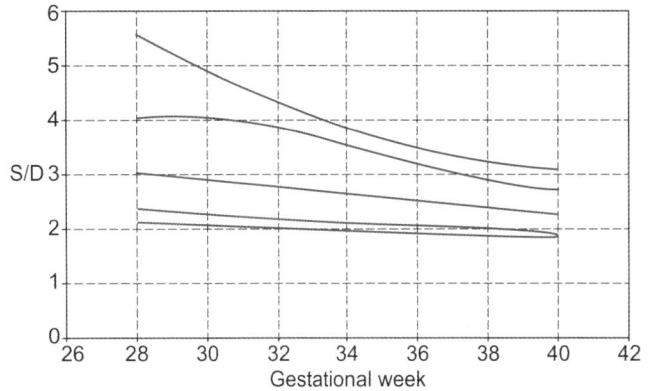

Fig. 51.14: Umbilical artery systolic/diastolic (S/D) ratio nomogram

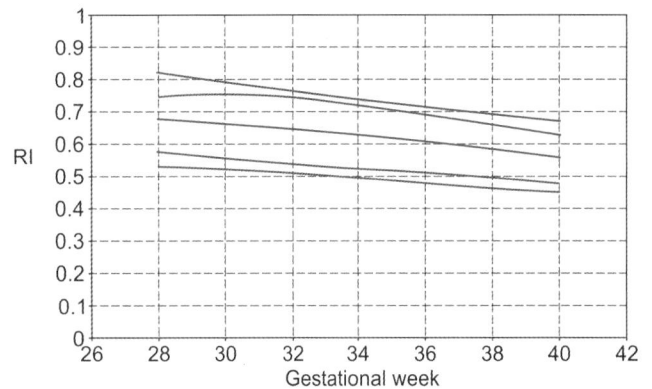

Fig. 51.15: Umbilical artery resistance index (RI) nomogram

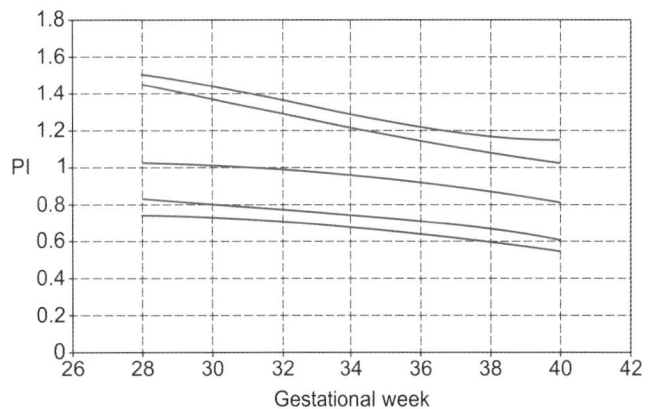

Fig. 51.16: Umbilical artery pulsatility index (PI) nomogram

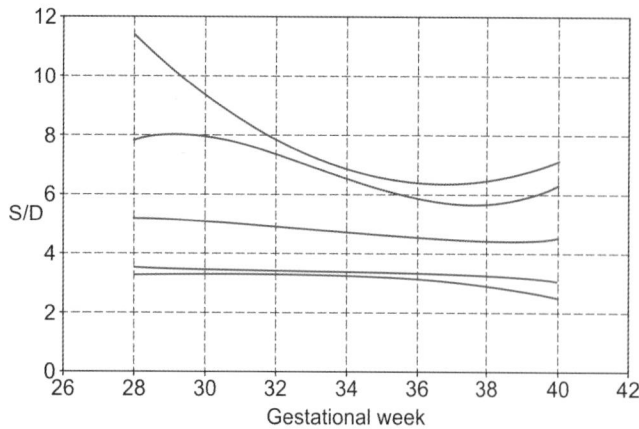

Fig. 51.17: Descending fetal aorta S/D ratio nomogram

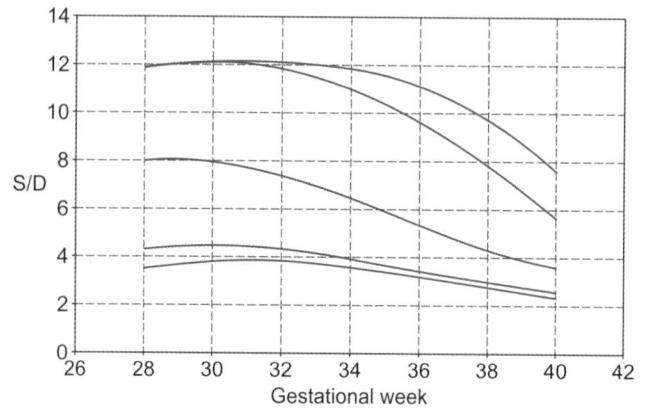

Fig. 51.20: Middle cerebral artery S/D ratio nomogram

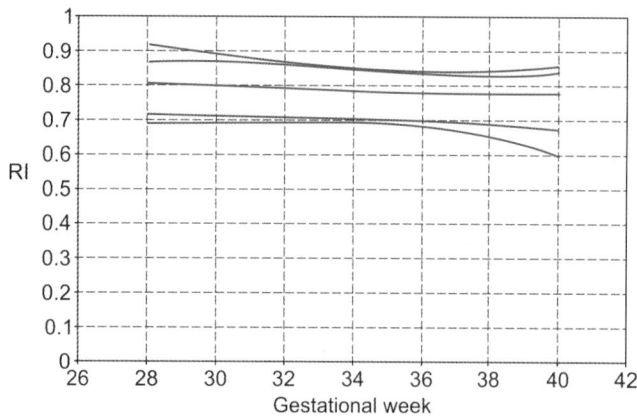

Fig. 51.18: Descending fetal aorta RI nomogram

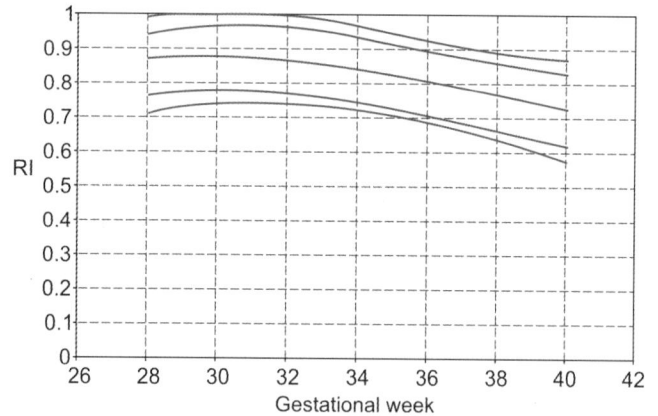

Fig. 51.21: Middle cerebral artery RI nomogram

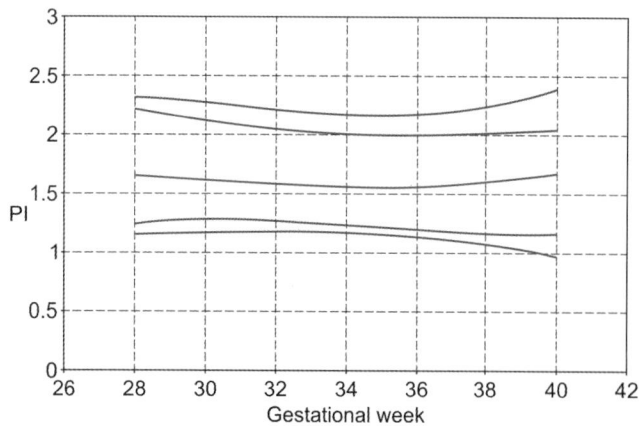

Fig. 51.19: Descending fetal aorta PI nomogram

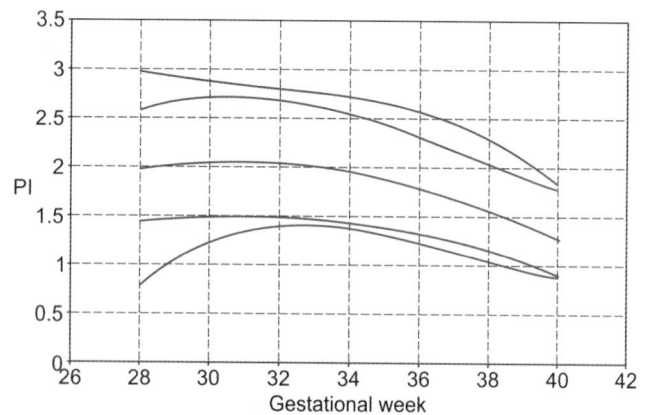

Fig. 51.22: Middle cerebral artery PI ratio nomogram

2. Doppler values between 5–10th percentiles in MCA should be considered as borderline and repeat follow-ups should be planned. Values below the 5th percentile are considered abnormal.

3. Measurements taken after 24 weeks of gestation from uterine arteries are more valuable. The early diastolic notching of and values exceeding the 95th percentile are considered as abnormal. One point to remember is that notching by itself predicts an elevated risk of preeclampsia.

CONCLUSION

In normal pregnancies, uteroplacental flow velocities become almost stable after the middle second trimester, meanwhile fetal

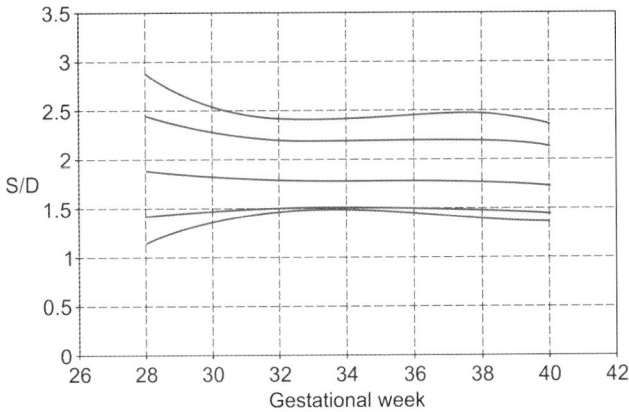

Fig. 51.23: Uterine artery S/D ratio nomogram

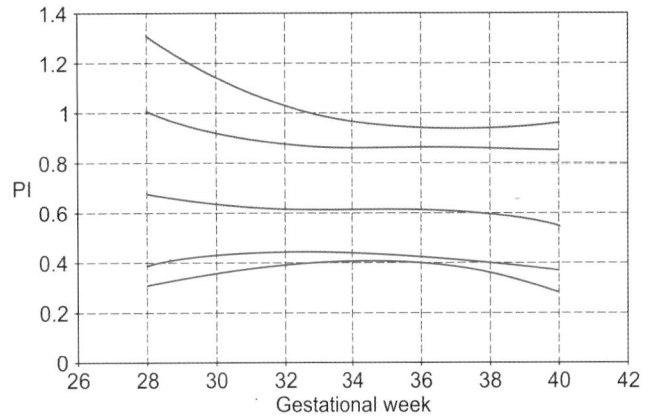

Fig. 51.25: Uterine artery PI nomogram

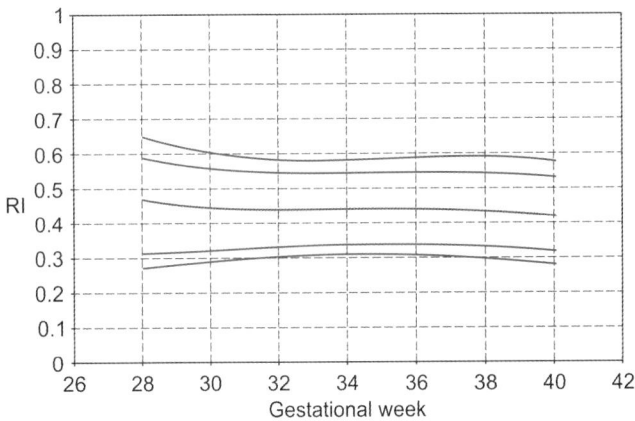

Fig. 51.24: Uterine artery RI nomogram

blood flow velocities also alter. With advancing gestational age, S/D ratio in the umbilical artery and MCA decreases. Although the S/D ratio in the descending aorta is almost stable during pregnancy, advancing gestational age narrows the biologic variability of the flow spectrum. Accordingly, it is recommended to use gestational age matched nomograms to define threshold values, and to differentiate and predict pathologic pregnancies.

The key points relating to physiological changes in the uteroplacental and fetal circulation can be summarized as follows:

- The technique of Doppler ultrasound is a noninvasive method of examining the uteroplacental and fetal circulation. Color

Doppler sonography allows the uteroplacental and fetal circulation to be investigated throughout pregnancy.

- The main changes in FVW in the fetal and uteroplacental vessels happen in the first trimester of pregnancy and go on slowly in the remaining periods. Fetal and uteroplacental velocities increase gradually during early pregnancy and velocimetric indices show a progressive decrease of the uteroplacental resistances. In early pregnancy, the umbilical artery and fetal aorta FVWs are initially of high resistance, with absent end diastolic flow. Resistance falls rapidly toward the end of the first trimester; and end diastolic flow is usually present by the 16th week of gestation. Resistance continues to fall throughout the remainder of the pregnancy.

- In normal pregnancy there is a gradual fall in resistance, an increase in diastolic flow and a disappearance of the diastolic notch in the uterine artery FVW.

- Preeclampsia, intrauterine growth retardation and placental abruption are associated with inadequate placentation/function, and a relationship exists between these complications and a failure of physiological change in the uteroplacental circulation.

ACKNOWLEDGMENTS

The authors acknowledge Mr Aykut Barut, MD (Zonguldak, Turkey), Hakan Sade, MD (Zonguldak, Turkey), and Mehmet Vural, MD (Zonguldak/Turkey) for their technical and editorial assistance in the preparation of this manuscript.

REFERENCES

1. Harrington K, Thompson O, Aquilina J. Uteroplacental and umbilical circulation: physiological changes in pregnancy. In: Kurjak A (Ed). Textbook of Perinatal Medicine. New York: Parthenon Publishing; 1998. pp. 422-6.
2. Fogarty P, Beattie B, Harper A, et al. Continuous wave Doppler flow velocity waveforms from the umbilical artery in normal pregnancy. J Perinat Med. 1990;18:51-7.
3. Deutinger J. Physiology of Doppler blood flow in maternal blood vessels in pregnancy. Gynakologe. 1992;25:284-91.
4. Fendel H, Fendel M, Pauen A, et al. Doppler studies of arterial blood flow in the uterus during labor. Z Geburtshilfe Perinatol. 1984;188:64-7.
5. Ertan AK, Wagner A, Tanriverdi HA, et al. Physiologic color Doppler sonographic changes of the embryonic and uteroplacental vessels in early pregnancy. Ultrasound Review Obstet Gynecol. 2003;3:219-22.
6. Schneider KT. Standards in der Perinatalmedizin -Doppler sonographie in der Schwangerschaft. Frauenarzt. 1997;38:452-8.

7. Bower S, Schuchter K, Campbell S. Doppler ultrasound screening as part of routine antenatal scanning: prediction of pre-eclampsia and intrauterine growth retardation. Br J Obstet Gynecol. 1993;100:989-94.

8. Brosens I, Dixon HG, Robertson W. Fetal growth retardation and the arteries of the placental bed. Br J Obstet Gynecol. 1977;84:656-64.

9. Campbell S, Pearce JM, Hackett G, et al. Qualitative assessment of uteroplacental blood flow: early screening test for high-risk pregnancies. Obstet Gynecol. 1986;68:649-53.

10. Hoffmann H, Chaoui R, Bollmann R, et al. Potential clinical application of Doppler ultrasound in obstetrics. Zentralbl Gynakol. 1989;111:1277-84.

11. Trudinger BJ, Giles WB, Cook CM. Uteroplacental blood flow velocity-time waveforms in normal and complicated pregnancy. Br J Obstet Gynecol. 1985; 92:39-45.

12. Huneke B, Holst A, Schroder HJ, et al. Normal values for relative Doppler indices. A/B ratio, resistance index and pulsatility index of the uterine artery and umbilical artery in normal pregnancy. A longitudinal study. Geburtshilfe Frauenheilkd. 1995;55: 616-22.

13. Arabin B, Bergmann PL, Saling E. Simultaneous assessment of blood flow velocity waveforms in uteroplacental vessels, the umbilical artery, the fetal aorta and the fetal common carotid artery. Fetal Ther. 1987;2:17-26.

14. Arduini D, Rizzo G. Normal values of pulsatility index from fetal vessels: A cross-sectional study on 1556 healthy fetuses. J Perinat Med. 1990;18:165-72.

15. Schulman H, Fleischer A, Stern W, et al. Umbilical velocity wave ratios in human pregnancy. Am J Obstet Gynecol. 1984;148:985-90.

16. Thompson RS, Trudinger BJ, Cook CM. Doppler ultrasound waveform indices: A/B ratio, pulsatility index and Pourcelot ratio. Br J Obstet Gynecol. 1988;95:581-8.

17. Trudinger BJ, Ishikawa K. Use of Doppler ultrasound in the high-risk pregnancy. Clin Diagn Ultrasound. 1990;26:119-37.

18. Hecher K, Spernol R, Szalay S, et al. Reference values for the pulsatility index and the resistance index of blood flow curves of the umbilical artery and fetal aorta in the 3d trimester. Ultraschall Med. 1989;10:226-9.

19. Vetter K. The significance of Doppler blood flow measurement in recognizing placental insufficiency. Arch Gynecol Obstet. 1988;244 (Suppl):S12-S8.

20. Vyas S, Nicolaides KH, Bower S, et al. Middle cerebral artery flow velocity waveforms in fetal hypoxemia. Br J Obstet Gynecol. 1990;97:797-803.

21. Mires GJ, Christie AD, Leslie J, et al. Are 'notched' uterine arterial waveforms of prognostic value for hypertensive and growth disorders of pregnancy? Fetal Diagn Ther. 1995;10:111-8.

22. Ertan AK, Hendrik HJ, Tanriverdi HA, et al. Fetomaternal Doppler sonography nomograms. Clin Exp Obstet Gynecol. 2003;30:211-6.

52 Doppler Sonography in High-risk Pregnancy

AK Ertan, HA Tanriverdi, W Schmidt

INTRODUCTION

One of the main aims of routine antenatal care is to identify the "at risk" fetus in order to apply clinical interventions which could result in reduced perinatal morbidity and mortality.[1] Doppler sonography in obstetrics is a widely accepted functional method of examining the utero-feto-placental unit.

Doppler ultrasound is a noninvasive technique whereby the movement of blood (usually in a vessel) is studied by detecting the change in frequency of reflected sound. Doppler ultrasound has been used in obstetrics since 1977 to study the fetoplacental (umbilical) circulation,[2] and since the 1980s to study the uteroplacental (uterine) circulation[3] and fetal circulation.[4] Recently, this method became an important tool for qualifying high-risk pregnancies.

Information obtained with Doppler sonography helps obstetricians managing patients in situations like pregnancies complicated by intrauterine growth restriction (IUGR), Rhesus alloimmunization, multiple pregnancies and anamnestic risk factors. Examination of the uteroplacental and fetomaternal circulation by Doppler sonography in the early second trimester helps predicting pregnancy complications like preeclampsia, IUGR and perinatal death.[5-13]

This chapter aims to introduce Doppler sonographic examinations in high-risk pregnancies. Doppler blood flow velocity waveforms (FVWs) of the fetal side (umbilical artery, descending aorta and middle cerebral artery) are discussed.

THE SAFETY OF DOPPLER ULTRASOUND IN OBSTETRICS

The safety of Doppler ultrasound in Obstetrics remains a concern. The data available to date suggests that diagnostic ultrasound has no adverse effects on embryogenesis or fetal growth. In addition, ultrasonographic scanning has no long-term effects on cognitive function or noted changes of visual or hearing functions. However, although B and M mode scans are safe during pregnancy, color, power and pulsed Doppler procedures should be performed with caution due to possible thermal effects. Lastly, a new method, the three-dimensional technique, was introduced. While there are no studies regarding the safety of this new technique, the short acquisition time and the post-processing analysis may decrease exposure and thus reduce the risk of possible effects of the ultrasound waves on fetal development.[14]

In particular the use of pulsed Doppler involves the use of higher intensities compared to diagnostic ultrasound, and hence may cause significant tissue heating and thermal effects. However these thermal effects depend on the presence of a tissue/air interface and may therefore not be clinically significant in obstetric ultrasound examinations.[15] Clearly, while there is continuing concern regarding the safety of Doppler ultrasound, it should only be used in cases of proven value or controlled investigational circumstances.

INDICATIONS OF DOPPLER SONOGRAPHY IN OBSTETRICS

Prospective randomized studies of fetal vessels and their collective evaluation have shown no benefit of Doppler sonography in screening the nonselected population.[16] In high-risk pregnancies, however, there is definitive evidence that the use of Doppler studies can significantly reduce the number of antenatal examinations and the number of necessary inductions of labor and cesarean deliveries for fetal distress. Doppler sonography reduces the perinatal mortality, the number of elective deliveries, the incidence of intrapartum distress and the occurrence of hypoxic encephalopathy.[17] A definite benefit has been established for Doppler sonography in selected cases (Table 52.1).

Table 52.1: Indications for Doppler sonography in obstetrics

- Suspicion of intrauterine growth restriction (IUGR)
- Pregnancy induced hypertension (PIH)/preeclampsia/ eclampsia
- Suspicion for a fetal malformation or disease
- Multiple pregnancy with discordant growth
- Investigation of fetal cardiac anomaly or heart disease
- Fetal heart rate abnormalities/arrhythmia
- Preexisting maternal diseases with vascular relevance
- Prior history of IUGR or intrauterine fetal death
- Prior history of (PIH)/preeclampsia/eclampsia

CHANGES IN DOPPLER SONOGRAPHIC RESULTS DURING THE COURSE OF PREGNANCY AND COMPLICATED PREGNANCIES

During the course of pregnancy and in some specific pregnancy complications, Doppler sonographic results of fetomaternal vessels display changing values. Chronic placental insufficiency is a major research application for Doppler sonography in high-risk pregnancies. Various fetal vessels are examined to determine/diagnose perinatal problems.

Umbilical Artery

It has been shown in a longitudinal, observational study that Doppler ultrasound of the umbilical artery (UA) is more helpful than other tests of fetal wellbeing (e.g. heart rate variability and biophysical profile score) in distinguishing between the normal small fetus and the "sick" small fetus.[18] However, its exact role in

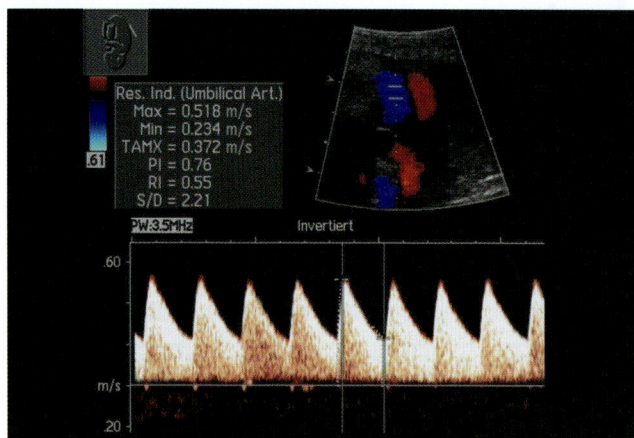

Fig. 52.1: Normal flow velocity waveforms of the umbilical artery in the third trimester

optimizing management, particularly timing of delivery, remains unclear, and is currently being investigated by many study groups. The optimal timing of delivery in pregnancies complicated by highly pathological Doppler flow findings is still an issue to be resolved. The established approach to resolve this question and to improve the perinatal morbidity and mortality by the use of Doppler examination is being investigated in multicenter clinical trials,[19] e.g. the Trial of Umbilical and Fetal Flow in Europe Group (TRUFFLE-Protocol, unpublished data).

Blood flow velocity in the UA increases with the advancing gestation. As a result impedance to blood flow continuously decreases due to increasing arterial blood flow in the systole and diastole. End-diastolic velocity is often absent in the first trimester[2,20] and the diastolic component increases with advancing gestation (Fig. 52.1).[21] With advancing gestational age end-diastolic flow becomes evident during the whole heart cycle (Fig. 52.1), proven with previous longitudinal studies of Fogarty et al.[22] and Hünecke et al.[23] as with many cross-sectional studies.[21,24]

Trudinge et al.[25] explained this phenomenon with the following mechanisms:

- Continuous maturation in placental villi
- Continuous widening of placental vessels cause a continuous decrease in vascular resistance
- Continuous increase in fetal cardiac output
- Continuous changes in the vessel compliance
- Continuous increase in fetal blood pressure.

Especially in the third trimester of pregnancy, depending on the above factors normal values become scattered on nomograms. This scattering is more prominent in the S/D ratio than the PI. Resistance index is not affected by above factors after 28 weeks of gestation.

Flow velocity waveforms of the UA are slightly different at the abdominal wall and the placental site, with indices higher at the fetal abdominal wall than the placental insertion.[26] The difference, however, is minimal, and therefore in clinical practice it is not important to obtain the FVWs always at the same level. FVWs must always be obtained during fetal apnea periods because fetal breathing affects the waveforms.

In case of an abnormal test, clinical experience and randomized controlled trials showed significant association with an adverse perinatal outcome.

Intrauterine Growth Restriction

The IUGR fetus is a fetus that does not reach its potential growth. Environmental factors responsible may be due to maternal, uteroplacental and fetal factors. Many authors have reported on the association between an abnormal UA Doppler FVW and IUGR.

Differentiating the fetus with pathologic growth restriction that is at risk for perinatal complications from the constitutionally small but healthy fetus has been an ongoing challenge in obstetrics. Not all infants whose birth weight is below the 10th percentile have been exposed to a pathologic process in utero; in fact, most small newborns are constitutionally small and healthy. Doppler sonography has become the most important investigation method to differentiate between these fetuses.

It should be noted that Doppler sonography is not suitable for the primary diagnosis of fetal growth restriction, but it provides an excellent adjunctive method for risk differentiation in suspicious cases.

Pathophysiology of Abnormal FVWs in Placental Insufficiency[27]

In the presence of placental insufficiency, there is greater placental resistance, which is reflected in a decreased end-diastolic component of the UA FVWs.[28-32] An abnormal UA FVW has an S/D ratio above the normal range. As their placental insufficiency worsens, the end-diastolic velocity decreases (Fig. 52.2), then become absent (Fig. 52.3), and finally it is reversed (Fig. 52.4). Some fetuses have decreased end-diastolic velocity that remains constant with advancing gestation and never become absent or reversed, which may be due to a milder form of placental insufficiency (Fig. 52.2). Pitfalls can be caused due to, for example, fetal breathing (Fig. 52.5).

Abnormal UA Doppler studies, but not normal results were found to be associated with lower arterial and venous pH values, an increased likelihood of intrapartum fetal distress, more admissions to the neonatal intensive care unit (NICU) and a higher incidence of respiratory distress in IUGR fetuses.[33]

Therefore, intensive antenatal surveillance in fetuses with suspected IUGR if the UA Doppler FVWs are normal was not recommended by the authors. Conflicting data were presented by

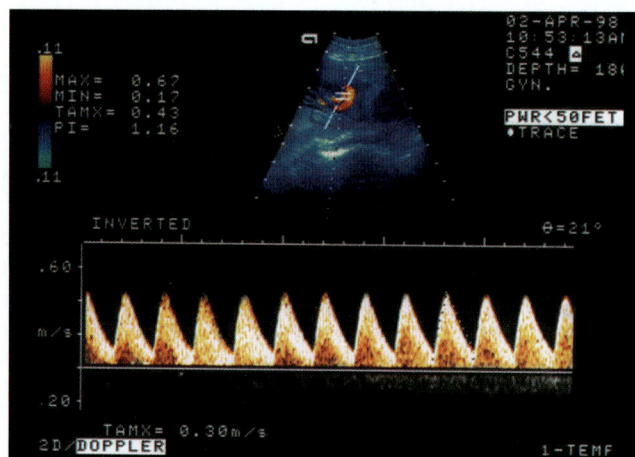

Fig. 52.2: Abnormal flow velocity waveforms of the umbilical artery in the third trimester (high resistance index)

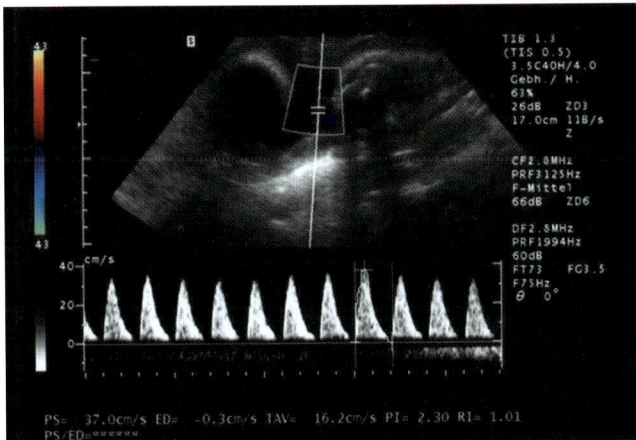

Fig. 52.3: Absent end-diastolic flow (AEDF) of the umbilical artery in the third trimester

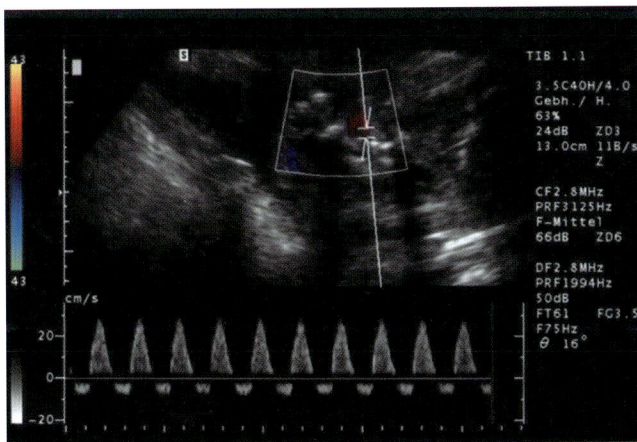

Fig. 52.4: Reverse flow (RF) of the umbilical artery

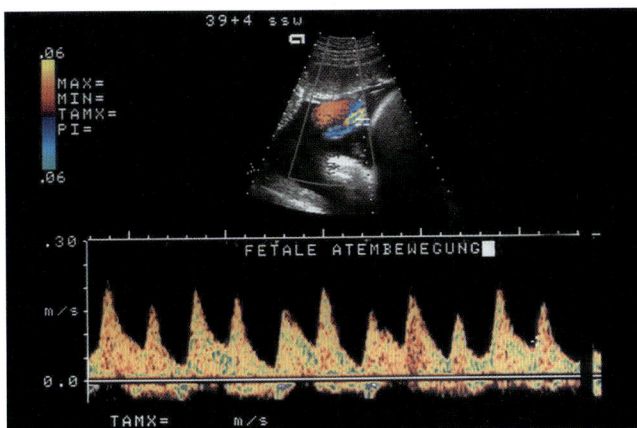

Fig. 52.5: Pitfalls in umbilical artery Doppler velocimetry (fetal breathing)

McCowan et al.[34] They confirmed that abnormal UA Doppler studies are associated with a poor perinatal outcome in IUGR fetuses but also concluded that the perinatal outcome in small for gestational age fetuses with normal UA Doppler studies is not always benign (i.e. low ponderal index, postnatal hypoglycemia, admission to the NICU). Recently, Ertan et al.[35] suggested that reversed flow should be seen as a particular clinical entity with higher incidences

of perinatal and overall mortality, and severe intrauterine growth restriction compared to absent end-diastolic flow (Figs 52.3 and 52.4).

In our clinical experience, when an IUGR fetus is suspected, the UA, FDA and MCA are the first fetal vessels to be assessed. The ductus venosus (DV), umbilical vein, inferior vena cava Doppler examinations are secondary vessels to be examined, only when an abnormal FVW is detected on the arterial vessels. Adding serial Doppler evaluation of the UA, MCA and DV to IUGR surveillance will enhance the performance of the biophysical score in the detection of fetal compromise and therefore optimizing the timing of intervention.[36]

COMPARISON OF PERINATAL OUTCOME IN FETUSES WITH REVERSE OR ABSENT END-DIASTOLIC FLOW IN THE UMBILICAL ARTERY/FETAL DESCENDING AORTA[35]

An abnormal flow velocity waveform (FVW) is a good predictor for poor perinatal outcome in high-risk pregnancies.[37-41] The absence or reversal of end-diastolic flow in the umbilical artery (UA) and fetal aorta is widely accepted as an ominous sign of fetal compromise, with a very high perinatal mortality (from 35% to 100%) and morbidity.[27,39,42,43]

The incidence of absent end-diastolic flow is low, and of reversed flow it is even lower (reverse flow/absent end-diastolic flow ratio = 1:10).[27,42,43] Studies so far analyzed the fetal outcome in reversed and absent end-diastolic flow cases together as one clinical entity. The difference between the prognosis of fetuses with reversed flow and absent end-diastolic flow is still unknown.

We undertook a study, in which the highly pathologic flow profiles, consisting of absent end-diastolic flow and reverse flow at the umbilical artery and fetal aorta were compared for perinatal outcome. The aim of this study was to clarify whether reverse flow at the umbilical artery and fetal aorta worsens perinatal outcome more than absent end-diastolic flow at the same vessels and to assess the possibility of making predictions about the further course of pregnancy.

Materials and Methods

During a 10-year period, 30 cases with reverse flow in the umbilical artery and/or fetal aorta (Group I) were detected. We selected matched pairs of 30 cases with absent end-diastolic velocities (Group II). The selection criterion into the groups was an absent or reverse flow at the time of delivery. Fetal malformations and chromosomal anomalies were excluded from both groups. For matching of the absent end-diastolic flow group fetuses to the reversed flow group, same gestational ages, estimated fetal weights and gestational ages at delivery were stipulated.

Results

Maternal complications were similar in both groups. Intrauterine growth retardation and oligohydramnios incidences were significantly more common ($p<0.05$, Table 52.2) in the reverse flow group (83% and 70% vs 73% and 43%). The median time interval between the registration of reverse flow and death of fetuses was 2.5 days. After diagnosis of reverse flow, 11 fetuses (91.7%) died within a week (three on the same day, two on the next day, three on the second day, and the remaining four cases on day 3–8).

The mean gestational age at live birth was 31 weeks in both groups. Of the 18 survivors in group I, 17 (94.4%) were delivered by cesarean section. This was not significantly different from group II. The main indication for the cesarean section was fetal distress. The mean birth weight [1071(112 g) versus, 1214(82 g)] was not statistically different between the groups.

The mean values and the frequency of pathological Apgar scores (7) at 1, 5 and 10 minutes, the arterial cord blood pH values, and the mean values of umbilical arterial PO_2, PCO_2 and HCO_3 were not different among the groups.

All the fetuses with absent and reversed end-diastolic flow were admitted to the NICU, and there was no difference in the duration of NICU treatment required. The rates (83% versus 86%, respectively for group I and II) and duration of mechanical ventilation were not different among the groups.

Neonatal cerebral hemorrhage occurred more often in group I, but without statistical significance (27.8% versus 17.2%). Neonatal morbidity (Table 52.3) included infections, hyaline membrane

Table 52.2: Antenatal complications of the reversed ($n = 30$) and absent end-diastolic flow cases ($n = 30$)

Type of complication	Reverse flow n (%)	Absent flow n (%)
Pregnancy Induced hypertension	19 (63.3)	19 (63.3)
HELLP syndrome	1 (3.3)	6 (20)
Gestational diabetes	1 (3.3)	2 (6.7)
Fetal infection	1 (3.3)	0
Abruptio placenta	0	4 (13.3)
Birth weight in g (M ± SD)	1,071 ± 112	1,214 ± 82
Intrauterine growth retardation* (< 5 percentile)	25 (83.3)	19 (63.3)
Oligohydramnios*	21 (70)	13 (43.3)

HELLP = Hemolysis, elevated liver enzymes, low platelets (*= p<0.05)

Table 52.3: Perinatal and neonatal parameters of the reverse ($n = 18$) and absent end-diastolic ($n = 29$) flow cases (live-born)

	Reverse flow n (%)	Absent end-diastolic flow n (%)
5' Apgar ≤ 7	7 (39)	13 (45)
pH ≤ 7.2	6 (33)	9 (31)
Cerebral hemorrhage	5 (27.8)	5 (17.2)
Infections	8 (44.4)	8 (27.6)
Anemia	8 (44.4)	9 (31.0)
Hypocalcemia	3 (16.7)	0
Hyaline membrane syndrome	12 (67)	19 (66)
Icterus	8 (44.4)	12 (41.4)
Shock lung	3 (16.7)	2 (6.9)
Lung emphysema	2 (11.1)	0
Retinopathy	1 (5.6)	3 (10.4)
Muscle hypotony	1 (5.6)	3 (10.4)

syndrome, icterus, and anemia and shock lung, without statistical difference between the groups. Only hypocalcemia was found more often in group I (p<0.05).

There was a significantly higher overall and per natal mortality in the reversed end-diastolic flow group (53% and 27%) as compared to the absent end-diastolic flow group (10% and 7%) (p<0.05).

Discussion

Reverse flow in umbilical velocimetry is associated with dismal perinatal outcome. Perinatal mortality ranges from 35% to 100%, and postnatal morbidity is significant.[37,43-45] As per the presented study, 35 confirmed the adverse fetal outcome in fetuses with reversed end-diastolic flow in the umbilical artery and/or fetal aorta with a high overall mortality (53.3%) and perinatal mortality (26.8%).

Because of the low incidences of reverse flow cases, most authors have studied the effect of both reverse flow and absent end-diastolic flow velocity, often referred to an "ARED-Flow", on the fetal outcome together as one entity.[46] Reverse flow was considered to be the last phenomenon preceding fetal death.[37,47,48]

Absent or reversed end-diastolic flow in the umbilical artery or fetal aorta is closely associated with intrauterine growth retardation due to uteroplacental insufficiency and higher rates of pre-eclampsia.[39,40,43] On the other hand, fetuses with intrauterine growth retardation have a high risk of developing absent or reversed end-diastolic flow.[44]

These fetuses with reverse flow had a very high incidence of oligohydramnios, intrauterine growth retardation and maternal pregnancy induced hypertension. Therefore, pregnant women with these complications should be evaluated with Doppler sonography to detect the compromised fetuses.

Several authors found an increasing association between reversed flow of the umbilical artery and the rate of fetal malformations, especially congenital heart anomalies, ranging from 12% to 50%.[43,49] These malformations of fetuses were associated with a low growth potential, not only for the fetus (intrauterine growth retardation) but also for the placenta, regardless of whether the placenta/neonatal weight was normal or below normal.[39] For a better understanding of this correlation, an additional study of subgroups with fetal malformations including more cases would be required.[49]

A close association between the reversed flow and neonatal cerebral hemorrhage has been reported.[44] The inappropriate autoregulation of the cerebral blood flow which is induced by extreme prematurity is the major risk factor for intracerebral hemorrhage.[50]

Normal fetal blood velocity values are considered reassuring and are generally believed to characterize a normal fetal oxygenation.[51] Absent or reversed end-diastolic flow velocity in the umbilical artery is associated with fetal hypoxia.[47,52,53] Although normal results of blood gas analysis from umbilical vessels were observed in some cases with reversed or absent end-diastolic flow velocities, infants with this severe Doppler flow pathologies are at a high risk for neonatal asphyxia.[51] It was further suggested that fetuses with reverse flow should immediately be delivered after diagnosis.[48] "Once the diastolic component of umbilical artery flow velocity waveforms becomes absent or reversed, the fetus is in a state of hypoxia and acidosis, and fetal death is impending."[49] Our results showed almost the same frequency of neonatal acidosis in 33%

(pH≤7.2) in the reverse flow group, compared to 31% in cases with absent end-diastolic flow velocities. As significant reduction in the proportion of villous tissue occupied by the peripheral villi in pregnancies with absent or reversed end-diastolic flow was well documented previously,[54,55] in our presented cases the higher intrauterine death rates in the reverse flow group denotes an extreme placental insufficiency.

The incidence of infection, hyaline membrane syndrome and icterus was not influenced by reverse or absent end-diastolic flow. The incidence of anemia and shock lung was especially high, and hypocalcemia occurred statistically more frequent in the neonates with reversed end-diastolic flow. There was no difference in NICU-admission and mechanical ventilation rates and duration of NICU stay. The overall neonatal morbidity was not significantly different between the groups. This suggests that both highly pathological Doppler findings are affecting the surviving neonates adversely. However, the higher rates of intrauterine and neonatal deaths in the reversed flow cases should be noticed.

The highly pathological Doppler findings (absent and reverse end-diastolic flow) of the umbilical artery and fetal aorta, which are attributable to severe impairment of placental circulation, are representing compromised fetal condition with high incidence of perinatal and neonatal mortality. In our opinion, the finding of a reverse flow spectrum of the umbilical arteries or fetal aorta should be accepted as a more abnormal Doppler finding, compared to absent end-diastolic flow. If absent or reversed end-diastolic flow is detected, a very close antenatal follow-up is advised and delivery should be considered if biophysical parameters and venous Doppler indices become abnormal.

Chromosomal Abnormalities

It was shown that absent end-diastolic flow in the UA is associated with chromosomal abnormalities like trisomies, triploidies or chromosomal deletions.[56] Setting out from the point that structural anomalies are more frequent in fetuses with chromosomal aberrations, the authors recommended a rapid acquisition of a karyotype in fetuses with congenital anomalies and an absent end-diastolic flow in the UA.[35]

Impact on Perinatal Consequences

Abnormal UA FVWs are associated in IUGR fetuses with one of the following outcomes: early delivery, reduced birth weight, oligohydramnios, NICU admission, and prolonged hospital stay.[27,57] In a meta-analysis it was shown that the use of UA Doppler sonography in pregnancies complicated by IUGR reduces perinatal mortality up to 38% and improves perinatal outcome.[17] A review consisting of 7,000 high-risk pregnancies[58] found that Doppler ultrasound was associated with a trend toward reduction in perinatal death especially in pregnancies complicated with preeclampsia or IUGR. The Doppler ultrasound use was also associated with fewer inductions of labor and fewer hospital admissions, without reports of adverse perinatal effects. The reviewers concluded that the use of Doppler ultrasound in high-risk pregnancies is likely to reduce perinatal mortality.

Neonatal Intraventricular Hemorrhage

Fetal status as well as neonatal complications of prematurity in IUGR both contribute to adverse perinatal outcome and increase the risk for the development of intraventricular hemorrhage (IVH). Data suggest that absent and reversed end-diastolic flow in the UA early in gestation carries a high risk of subsequent neonatal IVH.[59] However, this observation is not independent of other perinatal variables; prematurity and difficult births remain the most important determinants of this complication.

Neuromotor Outcome

Valcomonico et al.[57] evaluated the association of UA Doppler velocimetry with long term neuromotor outcome in IUGR fetuses with normal ($n = 17$), reduced ($n = 23$) and absent or reversed ($n = 31$) UA end-diastolic flow. The infants who survived the neonatal period were observed for a mean of 18 months. Their postural, sensorial and cognitive functions were evaluated at 3, 6, 9, 12 and 18 months of age. Although, due to small number of cases the results did not reach statistical significance, the incidence of permanent neurological sequelae increased as the UA end-diastolic flow decreased (35% with absent or reversed flow, 12% with reduced flow and 0% with normal flow). Recently, in another study[60] 23 IUGR fetuses with absent or reversed UA end-diastolic flow were matched with fetuses with appropriate growth. All children were followed for 6 years, and intellectual development, neuromotoric development was significantly diminished in fetuses with abnormal FVWs. Only social development was not impaired in fetuses with abnormal UA FVWs. Similar results were previously published by our working group too.[38,61]

Intrapartum Studies

A review of intrapartum UA Doppler velocimetry for adverse perinatal outcome gave disappointing results.[62] Out of 2,700 pregnancies, which were evaluated for the intrapartum use of Doppler velocimetry, the technique proved to be a poor predictor for outcome measures like low Apgar scores, intrapartum fetal heart rate abnormalities, umbilical arterial acidosis and cesarean section for fetal distress.

Umbilical Artery Doppler Ultrasound in Unselected Patients

Theoretically, the use of routine UA Doppler ultrasound in unselected or low risk pregnancies would be to detect those pregnancies in which there has been failure to establish or maintain the normal low-resistance umbilical and uterine circulations (a pathological process leading to placental dysfunction and associated with intrauterine growth retardation and preeclampsia) before there is clinical evidence of fetal compromise. In practice, observational and longitudinal studies of Doppler ultrasound in unselected or low risk pregnancies have raised doubts about its application as a routine screening test, and authors have cautioned against its introduction into obstetric practice without supportive evidence from randomized trials.[63-65] The relatively low incidence of significant, poor perinatal outcomes in low risk and unselected populations presents a challenge in evaluating the clinical effectiveness of routine UA Doppler ultrasound, as large numbers are required to test the hypothesis.

Multiple Gestation

The S/D ratio of twins at the UA are in agreement with singleton pregnancies in the third trimester.[66] Twins with an abnormal UA FVW tend to be born earlier, have a higher perinatal mortality and morbidity, and have more frequent structural anomalies than fetuses without abnormal Doppler results.[67]

In cases of twin-twin transfusion syndrome, a poor placental implantation site or chromosomal anomalies discordant growth between the twins may occur. This is a very high-risk situation, with a high perinatal mortality and morbidity. The diagnosis is made mainly by ultrasound biometry. The best predictor for diagnosis of discordant twins appears to be the presence of either a difference in the UA S/D ratio greater than 15% or a different estimated fetal weight greater than 15%.[68] Recently it has been reported that abnormal UA velocimetry can be observed in small twins more often in monochorionic than dichorionic twins.[69] Doppler ultrasound abnormalities of the UA in either twin are associated with poor perinatal outcome in twin-twin transfusion syndrome.

The Biophysical Profile and Multivessel Doppler Ultrasound in IUGR

Biophysical profile scoring (BPS) and Doppler surveillance are the primary methods for fetal assessment in IUGR. As placental insufficiency worsens, the fetus adapts by progressive compensation. Previously it has been suggested that the sequential changes in arterial and venous flow occur before some biophysical parameters (fetal tonus, movement, breathing, amniotic fluid volume and nonstress test) decline.[70,71] Baschat et al.[36] evaluated whether multivessel Doppler parameters (UA, UV, MCA, DV and inferior vena cava) precede biophysical fetal parameters in fetuses with severe IUGR. They found that combining multivessel Doppler and composite BPS will provide significant early warning and a definitive indication for action in the management of severe IUGR, and suggested that delivery timing may be based on this new gold standard.

Fetal Descending Aorta (FDA)

Beside the UA, routine Doppler sonographic examination at the descending fetal aorta is possible. FVWs of the FDA are usually recorded at the level of the diaphragm. In fact, FVWs at the level of the diaphragm and distally to the origin of the renal arteries are different.[72] Normal blood FVWs in the FDA is highly pulsatile, with a minimal diastolic component (Fig. 52.6). The descending

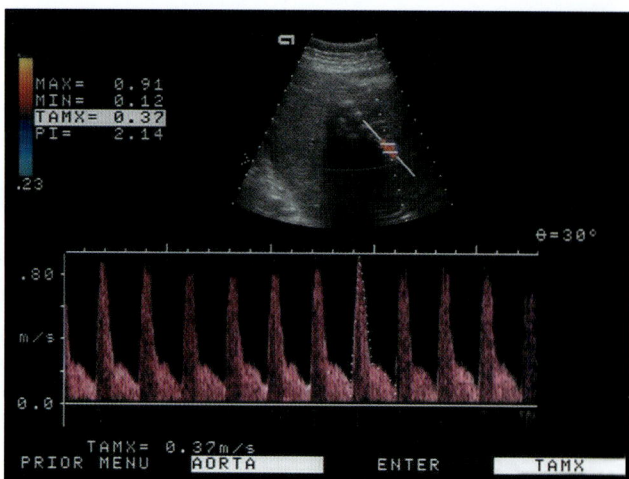

Fig. 52.7: Abnormal flow velocity waveforms of the fetal descending aorta in the third trimester (high resistance index)

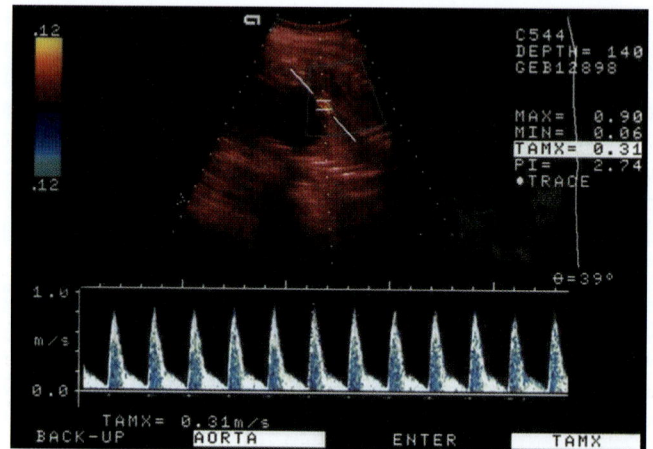

Fig. 52.8: Absent end-diastolic flow (AEDF) of the fetal descending aorta (FDA) in the third trimester

part of the aorta provides perfusion to the fetal abdominal organs, umbilical-placental circulation and lower extremities. The flow velocity waveform of the FDA shows a continuous forward stream during the whole heart cycle, but when compared to the FVW of the UA, the end-diastolic flow is less than the systolic component. Due to this reason the S/D ratio in the fetal aorta goes far than the S/D ratio in the UA. As pregnancy advances, the fetal aortic diameter gets wider, which decreases peripheral resistance and increases diastolic flow component. Nevertheless, this does not cause a significant S/D ratio decrease in the FDA.[73] Resistance and pulsatility indices in the last trimester are also not affected significantly, and show a similar course as in the UA.

Increased placental impedance combined with redistribution of blood flow from nonvital to vital organs may result in changes in the aortic FVWs. An elevated S/D-ratio, RI and PI (Fig. 52.7) is associated with both IUGR and adverse perinatal outcomes, such as severe growth restriction, necrotizing enterocolitis, fetal distress and perinatal mortality.[74-81] Absent end-diastolic flow at the FDA is also a predictor of fetal heart rate abnormalities (Fig. 52.8). It was shown that absent flow in the FDA were detected 8 days prior to the onset of decelerations at fetal heart rate monitoring.[78] The sensitivity and specificity of absent end-diastolic flow in the FDA for prediction of IUGR with fetal heart rate abnormalities are 85% and 80% respectively.[80,81]

Abnormal FVWs of the FDA were also evaluated for intellectual function and minor neurological dysfunction.[38,61,82,83] At 7 years

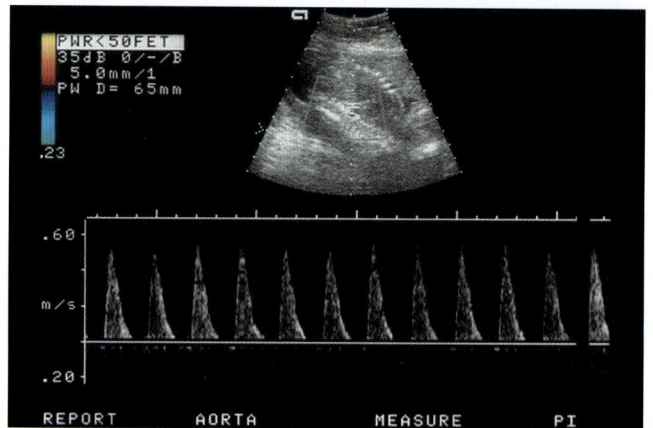

Fig. 52.6: Normal flow velocity waveforms of the fetal descending aorta in the third trimester

of age, verbal and global performances as well as neurological examination were significantly better in the fetuses with normal aortic FVWs.

Albeit, most of the studies showed Doppler velocimetry abnormalities of the FDA is a predictive test for the onset of decompensation due to placental insufficiency in the IUGR fetuses (Figs 52.8 and 52.9); it cannot be recommended as a screening or diagnostic test for IUGR in an unselected obstetric population.[84]

Middle Cerebral Artery (MCA)

The circle of Willis is composed anteriorly of the anterior cerebral arteries (branches of the internal carotid artery that are interconnected by the anterior communicating artery) and posteriorly of the two posterior cerebral arteries (branches of the basilar artery that are interconnected on either side with internal carotid artery by the posterior communicating artery).[85] These two trunks and the MCA, another branch of the internal carotid artery, supply the hemispheres on each side (Fig. 52.10). All of the defined arteries have different FVWs, therefore, it is important to know which artery is being examined during clinical practice.[86]

The most favorably positioned vessel for Doppler sonographic examination of fetal brain perfusion is the MCA. As the pregnancy advances, the vascular resistance in the MCA decreases (Fig. 52.11),[87] and the Doppler indices change. During the early stages of pregnancy, end-diastolic flow velocities in cerebral vessels are small or absent, but velocities increase toward the end of gestation. In the normal developing fetus, the brain is an area of low vascular impedance and receives continuous forward

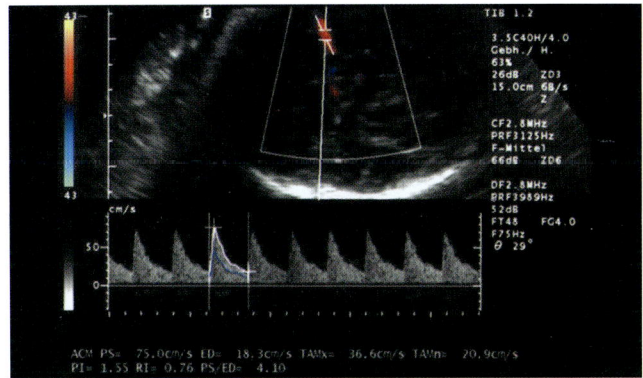

Fig. 52.11: Normal flow velocity waveforms of the middle cerebral artery in the third trimester

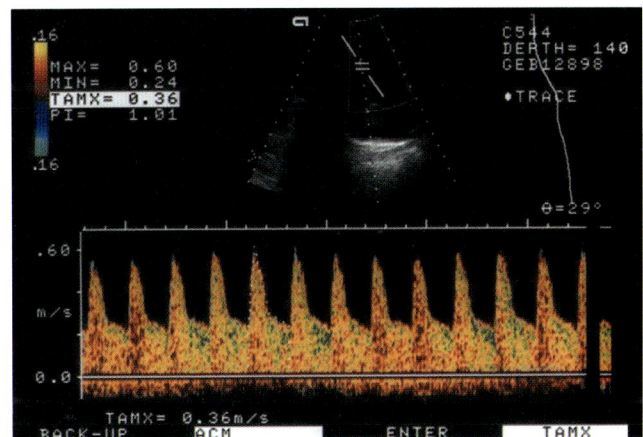

Fig. 52.12: Abnormal flow velocity waveforms of the middle cerebral artery in the third trimester (brain-sparing effect)

flow throughout the cardiac cycle. IUGR due to placental insufficiency is likely to be caused by redistribution of fetal blood flow in favor of the fetal brain and "stress organs", at the expense of less essential organs such as subcutaneous tissue, kidneys and liver. Finally, the already low resistance to blood flow in the brain drops further to enhance brain circulation (Fig. 52.12). This results with increased end-diastolic velocities, and a decrease in the S/D ratio of the MCA (brain-sparing effect).[88]

Abnormalities of the UA flow correlated with fetal compromise better than intracerebral artery blood flow impairment. This suggests that high placental impedance precedes the onset of the "brain sparing effect". In a study, in which 576 high-risk pregnancies were evaluated for the UA and MCA velocimetry, neither test was able to predict adverse perinatal outcome in the normal growing fetus.[89] Results showed that simultaneous assessment of UA and MCA velocimetry in IUGR fetuses did not improve the perinatal outcome. When the UA velocimetry was normal, the MCA velocimetry did not improve the prediction of IUGR or adverse perinatal outcome. However, when both arteries velocimetric values were abnormal, the risk of being growth restricted and having an adverse perinatal outcome was doubled.

It has been reported that the MCA PI is below the normal range when pO_2 is reduced.[90] Maximum reduction in PI is reached when the fetal pO_2 is 2-4 standard deviations below normal for gestation. When the oxygen deficit becomes greater, there is a tendency for the MCA PI to rise; this presumably reflects the prefinal stage due to development of brain edema (Fig. 52.13).

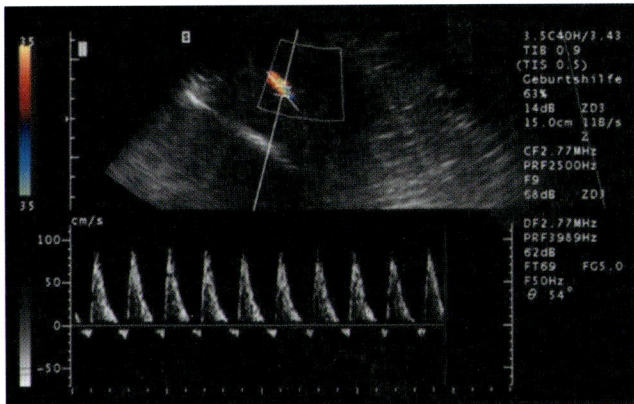

Fig. 52.9: Reverse flow (RF) in the fetal descending aorta

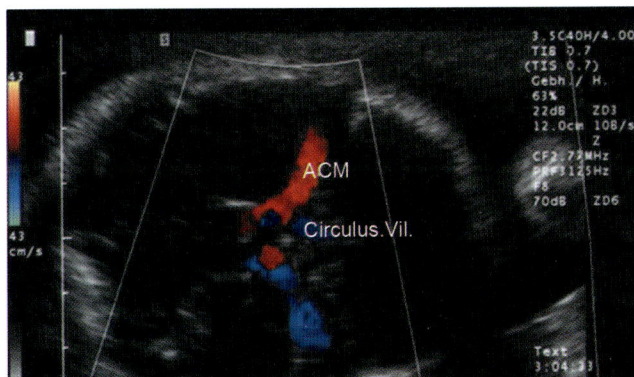

Fig. 52.10: Circle of Willis and middle cerebral artery visualized with color Doppler

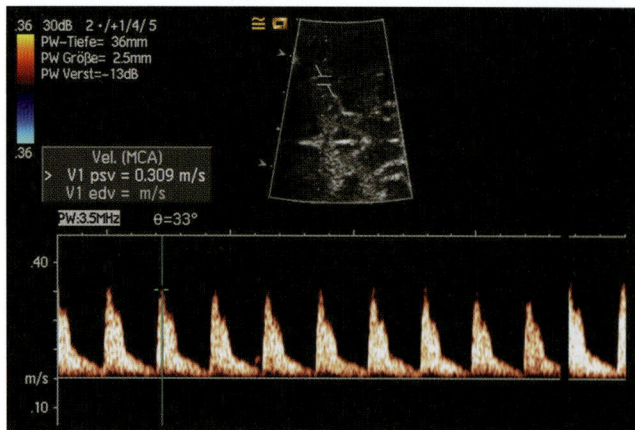

Fig. 52.13: Low end-diastolic flow (normal PI) after the brain sparing effect (de-centralization). This presumably reflects the preterminal stage due to development of brain edema

Hyperactivity of fetus, increase of intrauterine pressure (e.g. polyhydramnios) and external pressure to the fetal head (e.g. by the probe) might erroneously increase end-diastolic flow velocities in the MCA.[91] Different investigators have undertaken studies utilizing data obtained from the UA and MCA to develop indices for evaluation of intrauterine risk.[85]

Prediction of Fetal Hemoglobin in Red Cell Alloimmunization

Fetal anemia caused by red cell alloimmunization can be detected noninvasively by Doppler ultrasound on the basis of an increase in the peak systolic velocity in the MCA.[92,93] Although there is not a strong correlation between these two parameters when the fetus is nonanemic, the correlation becomes stronger as the hemoglobin levels decrease.[93] Prospective evaluation of the MCA peak systolic velocity to detect fetuses at risk for anemia in red cell alloimmunization showed that 90 of the 125 anticipated invasive procedures could be avoided.[94]

In anemic fetuses, change in hematocrit leads to a corresponding alteration in blood viscosity and to an impaired release of oxygen to the tissues. Increased cardiac output and vasodilatation are the main mechanisms by which the fetus attempts to maintain the oxygen and metabolic equilibrium in various organs. It is likely that when the fetus is nonanemic or mildly anemic, there are only minor or insignificant hemodynamic changes. Therefore, the blood velocity does not change. When the fetus becomes more anemic, various mechanisms compensate to maintain the oxygen and metabolic equilibrium in the various organs. The MCA peak systolic velocity changes proportionally to the hemoglobin deficiency.

Doppler measurements appear to be valuable for estimating hemoglobin concentration in fetuses at risk for anemia. Doppler sonography of the MCA has the potential to decrease the need for invasive testing (amniocentesis, cordocentesis) and its potential risks.[95]

Table 52.4: Indications for fetal venous Doppler sonography

- Fetal arrhythmias
- Suspected twin-twin transfusion syndrome
- Nonimmune hydrops fetalis (NIHF)
- Suspected stenosis in the cardiac outflow tract
- Congenital heart disease
- Severe centralization of the fetal circulation (brain sparing)
- Suspicious fetal heart rate tracings

Fetal Venous Circulation

In recent years research on the fetomaternal circulation has focused more on the venous side of the fetal circulation. Physiologically, blood flow velocities in the umbilical vein (UV) and the portal circulation are steady and nonpulsatile. However, it has been shown that both fetal body and breathing movements can interrupt the FVWs. In a recent review, it was concluded that several pathologic conditions such as nonimmune hydrops, severe IUGR and cardiac arrhythmias also result in an abnormal, pulsatile venous blood flow.[96] However, the relationship between fetal venous blood flow patterns and imminent fetal asphyxia or fetal death is still unknown. Recently, studies on venous circulation in the fetal brain[97] and pulmonary venous circulation in the diagnosis of pulmonary hypoplasia were performed.[98] Venous Doppler has also applications in several other disorders (Table 52.4).

An understanding of the fetal venous circulation provides a platform for the clinical management of perinatal problems, especially timing of delivery in high-risk pregnancies, a subject that is dealt with later in this section.

CONCLUSION

Doppler ultrasound is a noninvasive technique that is commonly used in high-risk pregnancies. Examination of fetomaternal vessels using Doppler sonography has been subject of intensive investigation in recent years. However, to date, randomized controlled trials were able to establish only limited clinical value of Doppler velocimetry to improve perinatal outcome in high-risk situations. Umbilical artery, fetal descending aorta and middle cerebral artery Doppler velocimetric studies are acceptable tools in the diagnosis and management of intrauterine growth restricted fetuses, and in the reduction of perinatal mortality in high-risk pregnancies. The majority of severely compromised fetuses also show pathological venous velocimetry, which might give valuable clinical information for surveillance in high-risk pregnancies and their optimal perinatal management. In addition, Doppler sonography might have a role in predicting long term neuromotor outcome. Large scale randomized controlled trials are needed to establish the clinical utility of Doppler ultrasound in obstetrics.

ACKNOWLEDGMENT

The authors acknowledge Mr. Aykut Barut, MD (Zonguldak, Turkey), Hakan Sade, MD (Zonguldak, Turkey), and Mehmet Vural, MD (Zonguldak, Turkey) for their technical and editorial assistance in the preparation of this manuscript.

REFERENCES

1. Ertan AK, Tanriverdi HA, Schmidt W. Doppler sonography in Obstetrics. In: Kurjak A, Chervenak FA (Eds). Donald School Textbook of Ultrasound in Obstetrics and Gynecology. New Delhi, India: Jaypee Brothers; 2003. pp. 395-421.
2. FitzGerald DE, Drumm JE. Non-invasive measurement of human fetal circulation using ultrasound: A new method. Br Med J. 1977;2:1450-1.
3. Campbell S, Diaz-Recasens J, Griffin DR, et al. New Doppler technique for assessing uteroplacental blood flow. Lancet. 1983;1:675-7.
4. Eik-Nes SH, Marsal K, Brubakk AO, et al. Ultrasonic measurement of human fetal blood flow. J Biomed Eng. 1982;4:28-36.
5. Bower S, Schuchter K, Campbell S. Doppler ultrasound screening as part of routine antenatal scanning: prediction of pre-eclampsia and intrauterine growth retardation. Br J Obstet Gynecol. 1993;100:989-94.
6. Caforio L, Testa AC, Mastromarino C, et al. Predictive value of uterine artery velocimetry at midgestation in low- and high-risk populations: A new perspective. Fetal Diagn Ther. 1999;14:201-5.
7. Campbell S, Pearce JM, Hackett G, et al. Qualitative assessment of uteroplacental blood flow: early screening test for high-risk pregnancies. Obstet Gynecol. 1986;68:649-53.
8. Harrington K, Cooper D, Lees C, et al. Doppler ultrasound of the uterine arteries: The importance of bilateral notching in the prediction of pre-eclampsia, placental abruption or delivery of a small-for-gestational-age baby. Ultrasound Obstet Gynecol. 1996;7:182-8.
9. Harrington K, Goldfrad C, Carpenter RG, et al. Transvaginal uterine and umbilical artery Doppler examination of 12-16 weeks and the subsequent development of pre-eclampsia and intrauterine growth retardation. Ultrasound Obstet Gynecol. 1997;9:94-100.
10. Irion O, Masse J, Forest JC, et al. Prediction of pre-eclampsia, low birthweight for gestation and prematurity by uterine artery blood flow velocity waveforms analysis in low risk nulliparous women. Br J Obstet Gynecol. 1998;105:422-9.
11. Hoffmann H, Chaoui R, Bollmann R, et al. Potential clinical application of Doppler ultrasound in obstetrics. Zentralbl Gynakol. 1989;111:1277-84.
12. Trudinger BJ, Giles WB, Cook CM. Uteroplacental blood flow velocity-time waveforms in normal and complicated pregnancy. Br J Obstet Gynecol. 1985;92:39-45.
13. Zimmermann P, Eirio V, Koskinen J, et al. Doppler assessment of the uterine and uteroplacental circulation in the second trimester in pregnancies at high risk for pre-eclampsia and/or intrauterine growth retardation: comparison and correlation between different Doppler parameters. Ultrasound Obstet Gynecol. 1997;9:330-8.
14. Hershkovitz R, Sheiner E, Mazor M. Ultrasound in obstetrics: A review of safety. Eur J Obstet Gynecol Reprod Biol. 2002;101:15-8.
15. Barnett S, Kossoff G, Edwards M. Is diagnostic ultrasound safe? Current international consensus on the thermal mechanism. Med J Aust. 1994;160:33-7.
16. Schneider KT. Doppler ultrasound: patient safety and incorporation of the method into clinical management. Gynakol Geburtshilfliche Rundsch. 1993;33 (Suppl 1):113-5.
17. Alfirevic Z, Neilson JP. Doppler ultrasonography in high-risk pregnancies: Systematic review with meta-analysis. Am J Obstet Gynecol. 1995;172:1379-87.
18. Soothill PW, Ajayi RA, Campbell S, et al. Prediction of morbidity in small and normally grown fetuses by fetal heart rate variability, biophysical profile score and umbilical artery Doppler studies. Br J Obstet Gynecol. 1993;100:742-5.
19. Romero R, Kalache K, Kadar N. Timing the delivery of the preterm severely growth-restricted fetus: venous Doppler, cardiotocography or the biophysical profile? Ultrasound Obstet Gynecol. 2002;19:118-21.

20. Stuart B, Drumm J, FitzGerald DE, et al. Fetal blood velocity waveforms in normal pregnancy. Br J Obstet Gynecol. 1980;87:780-5.
21. Thompson RS, Trudinger BJ, Cook CM. Doppler ultrasound waveform indices: A/B ratio, pulsatility index and Pourcelot ratio. Br J Obstet Gynecol. 1988;95:581-8.
22. Fogarty P, Beattie B, Harper A, et al. Continuous wave Doppler flow velocity waveforms from the umbilical artery in normal pregnancy. J Perinat Med. 1990;18:51-7.
23. Huneke B, Holst A, Schroder HJ, et al. Normal values for relative Doppler indices. A/B ratio, resistance index and pulsatility index of the uterine artery and umbilical artery in normal pregnancy. A longitudinal study. Geburtshilfliche Frauenheilkd. 1995;55:616-22.
24. Schulman H, Fleischer A, Stern W, et al. Umbilical velocity wave ratios in human pregnancy. Am J Obstet Gynecol. 1984;148:985-90.
25. Trudinger BJ, Giles WB, Cook CM, et al. Fetal umbilical artery flow velocity waveforms and placental resistance: clinical significance. Br J Obstet Gynecol. 1985;92:23-30.
26. Maulik D, Yarlagadda AP, Youngblood JP, et al. Components of variability of umbilical arterial Doppler velocimetry—A prospective analysis. Am J Obstet Gynecol. 1989;160:1406-9.
27. Ertan A, Hendrik H, Schmidt W. Hochpathologische Doppler-Flow-Befunde und perinatale Auffälligkeiten. In: Schmidt W, Kurjak A (Eds). Farbdopplersonographie in Gynäkologie und Geburtshilfliche. Stuttgart: Thieme Verlag; 2000. pp.177-87.
28. Fleischer A, Schulman H, Farmakides G, et al. Umbilical artery velocity waveforms and intrauterine growth retardation. Am J Obstet Gynecol. 1985;151:502-5.
29. Devoe LD, Gardner P, Dear C, et al. The significance of increasing umbilical artery systolic-diastolic ratios in third-trimester pregnancy. Obstet Gynecol. 1992;80:684-7.
30. Rochelson B, Schulman H, Farmakides G, et al. The significance of absent end-diastolic velocity in umbilical artery velocity waveforms. Am J Obstet Gynecol. 1987;156:1213-8.
31. Trudinger BJ, Cook CM, Giles WB, et al. Fetal umbilical artery velocity waveforms and subsequent neonatal outcome. Br J Obstet Gynecol. 1991;98:378-84.
32. Gudmundsson S, Marsal K. Umbilical and uteroplacental blood flow velocity waveforms in pregnancies with fetal growth retardation. Eur J Obstet Gynecol Reprod Biol. 1988;27:187-96.
33. Baschat AA, Weiner CP. Umbilical artery doppler screening for detection of the small fetus in need of antepartum surveillance. Am J Obstet Gynecol. 2000;182: 154-8.
34. McCowan LM, Harding JE, Stewart AW. Umbilical artery Doppler studies in small for gestational age babies reflect disease severity. BJOG. 2000;107:916-25.
35. Ertan AK, He JP, Tanriverdi HA, et al. Comparison of perinatal outcome in fetuses with reverse or absent end-diastolic flow in the umbilical artery/fetal descending aorta. J Perinat Med. 2003;31:307-12.
36. Baschat AA, Gembruch U, Harman CR. The sequence of changes in Doppler and biophysical parameters as severe fetal growth restriction worsens. Ultrasound Obstet Gynecol. 2001;18:571-7.
37. Brar H, Platt L. Reverse enddiastolic flow velocity on umbilical artery velocimetry in high-risk pregnancy: An ominous finding with adverse pregnancy outcome. Am J Obstet Gynecol. 1988;159:559-61.
38. Ertan A, Jost W, Hendrik H, et al. Perinatal events and neuromotoric development of children with zero flow in the fetal vessels during the last trimester. In: Cosmi EV DRG (Ed). 2nd World Congress of Perinatal Medicine. Bologna: Monduzzi Editore Spa; 1993. pp.1049-52.

39. Jacobson S, Imhof R, Manning N, et al. The value of Doppler assessment of the uteroplacental circulation in predicting pre-eclampsia or intrauterine growth retardation. Am J Obstet Gynecol. 1990;162:110-4.

40. Trudinger B, Cook C, Giles W, et al. Thompson R. Umbilical artery flow velocity waveforms in high-risk pregnancy. Randomized controlled trial. Lancet. 1987;8526:188-90.

41. Marsal K. Rational use of Doppler ultrasound in perinatal medicine. J Perinat Med. 1994;22:463-74.

42. Rühle W, Ertan A, Gnirs J, et al. Dopplersonographie in der Geburtshilfe-Beitrag zum Verständnis des Reverse Flow in der Arteria umbilicalis. Ultraschall in Med. 1991;12:134-8.

43. Schmidt W, Rühle W, Ertan A, et al. Doppler-sonographische-Perinatologische Daten bei Fällen mit enddiastolischem Block bzw. Reverse Flow. Geburts Frauenheilk. 1991;51:288-92.

44. Karsdorp V, Vugt J, Van Geijin H, et al. Clinical significance of absent or reversed end-diastolic velocity waveforms in umbilical artery. Lancet. 1994;344:1664-8.

45. Zelop C, Richardson D, Heffner L. Abnormal umbilical artery Doppler velocimetry in structurally normal singleton fetuses. Obstet Gynecol. 1996;87:434-8.

46. Montenegro N, Santos F, Tavares E, et al. Outcome of 88 pregnancies with absent or reversed end-diastolic blood flow (ARED flow) in the umbilical arteries. Eur J Obstet Gynecol Reprod Biol. 1998;79:43-6.

47. Illyes M, Gati I. Reversed flow in the human fetal descending aorta as a sign of severe fetal asphyxia preceding intrauterine deaths. J Clin Ultrasound. 1988;16: 403-7.

48. Woo J, Liang S, Lo R. Significance of an absent or reversed end-diastolic flow in Doppler umbilical artery waveforms. J Ultrasound Med. 1987;6:291-7.

49. Hsieh F, Chang F, Ko T, et al. Umbilical artery flow velocity waveforms in fetuses dying with congenital anomalies. Br J Obstet Gynecol. 1988;95:478-82.

50. Weindling A, Wilkinson A, Cook J, et al. Perinatal events which precede periventricular hemorrhage and leukomalacia in the newborn. Br J Obstet Gynecol. 1985;92:1218-23.

51. Bilardo C, Nicolaides K, Campbell S. Doppler measurements of fetal and uteroplacental circulations: relationship with umbilical venous blood gas measured at cordocentesis. Am J Obstet Gynecol. 1990;162:115-20.

52. Gudmundsson S, Dubiel M. Doppler velocimetry in the evaluation of fetal hypoxia. J Perinat Med 2001;29:399-407.

53. Campbell S, Vyas S, Nicolaides K. Doppler investigation of the fetal circulation. J Perinat Med. 1991;19:21-6.

54. Biagiotti R, Sgambati E, Brizzi E. Placental morphometry in pregnancies complicated by intrauterine growth retardation with absent or reversed end-diastolic flow in the umbilical artery. Ital J Anat Embryol. 1999;104:201-7.

55. Kingdom J, Huppertz B, Seaward G, et al. Development of the placental villous tree and its consequences for fetal growth. Eur J Obstet Gynecol Reprod Biol. 2000;92:35-43.

56. Rizzo G, Pietropolli A, Capponi A, et al. Chromosomal abnormalities in fetuses with absent end-diastolic velocity in umbilical artery: analysis of risk factors for an abnormal karyotype. Am J Obstet Gynecol. 1994;171:827-31.

57. Valcamonico A, Danti L, Frusca T, et al. Absent end-diastolic velocity in umbilical artery: risk of neonatal morbidity and brain damage. Am J Obstet Gynecol. 1994;170:796-801.

58. Neilson JP, Alfirevic Z. Doppler ultrasound for fetal assessment in high-risk pregnancies. Cochrane Database Syst Rev. 2000; CD000073.

59. Baschat AA, Gembruch U, Viscardi RM, et al. Antenatal prediction of intraventricular hemorrhage in fetal growth restriction: What is the role of Doppler? Ultrasound Obstet Gynecol. 2002;19:334-9.

60. Wienerroither H, Steiner H, Tomaselli J, et al. Intrauterine blood flow and long-term intellectual, neurologic, and social development. Obstet Gynecol. 2001;97:449-53.

61. Ertan AK, Jost W, Mink D, et al. Neuromotoric development of children after AED-Flow during pregnancy. In: Kurjak A, Latin V, Rippmann E (Eds). Advances on the Pathophysiology of Pregnancy. Milano: CIC Edizioni Internazionali; 1995. pp.55-62.

62. Farrell T, Chien PF, Gordon A. Intrapartum umbilical artery Doppler velocimetry as a predictor of adverse perinatal outcome: A systematic review. Br J Obstet Gynecol. 1999;106:783-92.

63. Sijmons EA, Reuwer PJ, van Beek E, et al. The validity of screening for small-for-gestational-age and low-weight-for-length infants by Doppler ultrasound. Br J Obstet Gynecol. 1989;96:557-61.

64. Beattie RB, Dornan JC. Antenatal screening for intrauterine growth retardation with umbilical artery Doppler ultrasonography. BMJ. 1989;298:631-5.

65. Goffinet F, Paris-Llado J, Nisand I, et al. Umbilical artery Doppler velocimetry in unselected and low risk pregnancies: A review of randomised controlled trials. Br J Obstet Gynecol. 1997;104: 425-30.

66. Giles WB, Trudinger BJ, Cook CM, et al. Umbilical artery flow velocity waveforms and twin pregnancy outcome. Obstet Gynecol. 1988;72:894-7.

67. Gaziano EP, Knox H, Ferrera B, et al. Is it time to reassess the risk for the growth-retarded fetus with normal Doppler velocimetry of the umbilical artery? Am J Obstet Gynecol. 1994;170:1734-41.

68. Divon MY, Girz BA, Sklar A, et al. Discordant twins—a prospective study of the diagnostic value of real-time ultrasonography combined with umbilical artery velocimetry. Am J Obstet Gynecol. 1989;161:757-60.

69. Gaziano E, Gaziano C, Brandt D. Doppler velocimetry determined redistribution of fetal blood flow: correlation with growth restriction in diamniotic monochorionic and dizygotic twins. Am J Obstet Gynecol. 1998;178:1359-67.

70. Hecher K, Campbell S, Doyle P, et al. Assessment of fetal compromise by Doppler ultrasound investigation of the fetal circulation. Arterial, intracardiac, and venous blood flow velocity studies. Circulation. 1995;91:129-38.

71. Senat MV, Schwarzler P, Alcais A, et al. Longitudinal changes in the ductus venosus, cerebral transverse sinus and cardiotocogram in fetal growth restriction. Ultrasound Obstet Gynecol. 2000;16: 19-24.

72. Lingman G, Marsal K. Fetal central blood circulation in the third trimester of normal pregnancy—a longitudinal study. I. Aortic and umbilical blood flow. Early Hum Dev. 1986;13:137-50.

73. Hecher K, Spernol R, Szalay S, et al. Reference values for the pulsatility index and the resistance index of blood flow curves of the umbilical artery and fetal aorta in the 3d trimester. Ultraschall Med. 1989;10:226-9.

74. Soothill PW, Nicolaides KH, Bilardo K, et al. Utero-placental blood velocity resistance index and umbilical venous pO_2, pCO_2, pH, lactate and erythroblast count in growth-retarded fetuses. Fetal Ther. 1986;1:176-9.

75. Jouppila P, Kirkinen P. Blood velocity waveforms of the fetal aorta in normal and hypertensive pregnancies. Obstet Gynecol. 1986;67:856-60.

76. Laurin J, Lingman G, Marsal K, et al. Fetal blood flow in pregnancies complicated by intrauterine growth retardation. Obstet Gynecol. 1987;69:895-902.

77. Hackett GA, Campbell S, Gamsu H, et al. Doppler studies in the growth retarded fetus and prediction of neonatal necrotising enterocolitis, hemorrhage, and neonatal morbidity. Br Med J (Clin Res Ed). 1987;294:13-6.

78. Arabin B, Siebert M, Jimenez E, et al. Obstetrical characteristics of a loss of end-diastolic velocities in the fetal aorta and/or umbilical artery using Doppler ultrasound. Gynecol Obstet Invest. 1988;25:173-80.

79. Tonge HM, Wladimiroff JW, Noordam MJ, et al. Blood flow velocity waveforms in the descending fetal aorta: comparison between normal and growth-retarded pregnancies. Obstet Gynecol. 1986;67:851-5.

80. Bonatz G, Schulz V, Weisner D, et al. Fetal heart rate (FHR) pathology in labor related to preceeding Doppler sonographic results of the umbilical artery and fetal aorta in appropriate and small for gestational age babies. A longitudinal analysis. J Perinat Med. 1997;25:440-6.

81. Marsal K, Laurin J, Lindblad A, et al. Blood flow in the fetal descending aorta. Semin Perinatol. 1987;11:322-34.

82. Ley D, Tideman E, Laurin J. Abnormal fetal aortic velocity waveform and intellectual function at 7 years of age. Ultrasound Obstet Gynecol. 1996;8:160-5.

83. Ley D, Laurin J, Bjerre M, et al. Abnormal fetal aortic velocity waveform and minor neurological dysfunction at 7 years of age. Ultrasound Obstet Gynecol. 1996;8:152-9.

84. Divon MY, Ferber A. Doppler evaluation of the fetus. Clin Obstet Gynecol. 2002;45:1015-25.

85. Mari G, Detti L. Doppler ultrasound application to fetal medicine. In: Fleischer A, Manning F, Jeanty P, Romero R (Eds). Sonography in Obstetrics and Gynecology (Principles and Practice). New York, USA: McGraw Hill; 2001. pp. 247-83.

86. Mari G, Moise KJ Jr, Deter RL, et al. Doppler assessment of the pulsatility index in the cerebral circulation of the human fetus. Am J Obstet Gynecol. 1989;160:698-703.

87. Vetter K. The significance of Doppler blood flow measurement in recognizing placental insufficiency. Arch Gynecol Obstet. 1988;244 (Suppl):S12-S8.

88. Arabin B, Bergmann PL, Saling E. Simultaneous assessment of blood flow velocity waveforms in uteroplacental vessels, the umbilical artery, the fetal aorta and the fetal common carotid artery. Fetal Ther. 1987;2:17-26.

89. Strigini FA, De Luca G, Lencioni G, et al. Middle cerebral artery velocimetry: different clinical relevance depending on umbilical velocimetry. Obstet Gynecol. 1997;90:953-7.

90. Sepulveda W, Shennan AH, Peek MJ. Reverse end-diastolic flow in the middle cerebral artery: An agonal pattern in the human fetus. Am J Obstet Gynecol. 1996;174:1645-7.

91. Vyas S, Nicolaides KH, Bower S, et al. Middle cerebral artery flow velocity waveforms in fetal hypoxemia. Br J Obstet Gynecol. 1990;97:797-803.

92. Mari G, Adrignolo A, Abuhamad AZ, et al. Diagnosis of fetal anemia with Doppler ultrasound in the pregnancy complicated by maternal blood group immunization. Ultrasound Obstet Gynecol. 1995;5:400-5.

93. Mari G, Deter RL, Carpenter RL, et al. Noninvasive diagnosis by Doppler ultrasonography of fetal anemia due to maternal red-cell alloimmunization. Collaborative Group for Doppler Assessment of the Blood Velocity in Anemic Fetuses. N Engl J Med. 2000;342:9-14.

94. Zimmerman R, Carpenter RJ Jr, Durig P, et al. Longitudinal measurement of peak systolic velocity in the fetal middle cerebral artery for monitoring pregnancies complicated by red cell alloimmunisation: A prospective multicentre trial with intention-to-treat. BJOG. 2002;109:746-52.

95. Mari G, Detti L, Oz U, et al. Accurate prediction of fetal hemoglobin by Doppler ultrasonography. Obstet Gynecol. 2002;99:589-93.

96. Huisman TW. Doppler assessment of the fetal venous system. Semin Perinatol. 2001;25:21-31.

97. Laurichesse-Delmas H, Grimaud O, Moscoso G, et al. Color Doppler study of the venous circulation in the fetal brain and hemodynamic study of the cerebral transverse sinus. Ultrasound Obstet Gynecol. 1999;13:34-42.

98. Yoshimura S, Masuzaki H, Miura K, et al. Diagnosis of fetal pulmonary hypoplasia by measurement of blood flow velocity waveforms of pulmonary arteries with Doppler ultrasonography. Am J Obstet Gynecol. 1999;180:441-6.

53

Effect of Exercise on Fetoplacental Doppler Flow

HA Tanriverdi, AK Ertan, W Schmidt

THE EFFECTS OF MATERNAL EXERCISE ON PLACENTAL BED BLOOD FLOW

Sustained bouts of maternal exercise have both acute and chronic effects on placental bed blood flow. During exercise, blood flow is diverted away from the viscera to the exercising muscle and skin.[1] The magnitude of the reduction in flow is directly proportional to exercise intensity and the muscle mass used (which varies with the type of exercise), and with common types of exercise performed at usual exercise intensities, the reduction usually exceeds 50%. This exercise-induced decrease in visceral flow persists throughout pregnancy but, in late-pregnancy, the magnitude of the decrease is blunted in women who continue to exercise regularly.[2-4] Once the exercise ceases, flow rapidly returns to normal. Thus, during a routine exercise session both glucose and oxygen delivery to the placental site are acutely reduced and the magnitude of the decrease varies with exercise type and intensity, maternal fitness and the time point in pregnancy when the exercise is carried out.[4,5]

However, women who perform weight-bearing exercise regularly during pregnancy augment the pregnancy-associated increases in plasma volume, intervillous space blood volume, placental volume and cardiac output.[5,6] The fact that regular weight-bearing exercise augments the changes in these parameters by between 10% and 50% also suggests that it increases the rate of placental bed blood flow at rest. If this inference is correct then exercise training during pregnancy should actually increase the glucose and oxygen delivery to the placental site throughout mid- and late-pregnancy.

The main concern about exercise in pregnancy is that reduced uterine blood flow may cause hypoxia in the fetus.[7] Recent studies using Doppler ultrasonography found an increase in the systolic/diastolic (S/D) ratio of uterine circulation, indicating an increase in resistance of the main vessels that supply the uterus.[8,9]

Although uteroplacental blood flow may decrease with exercise, compensatory mechanisms may exist to ensure adequate fetal oxygenation. In studying ewes, Chandler reported an increase in uterine extraction of oxygen that occurred with the decreased uterine blood flow after maternal exercise.[10] Curet et al. reported altered distribution of uterine blood flow in favor of the placenta in ewes.[11]

COMPLICATED PREGNANCIES AND EXERCISE

Two worrisome antenatal complications of pregnancy are intrauterine growth restriction and preterm labor. Strenuous exercise in pregnancy has been assessed and is not harmful to the mother or the fetus in healthy women if it is of limited duration. Heavy work or exercise also does not appear to increase the risk of a preterm delivery or intrauterine growth restriction in women at low risk for an adverse pregnancy outcome.[12]

The influence of exercise during pregnancy and its effect on birth weight and pregnancy outcome remains uncertain. The most recent technical bulletin from the ACOG[13] suggests that lower birth weights are observed among vigorously exercising women, but there is no information linking exercise with an adverse outcome of the fetus. The effect of maternal exercise on prenatal complications is also unknown. A recent review from the Cochrane Database was unable to demonstrate important benefits or risks to the mother or fetus with exercise in pregnancy.[12]

Small patient numbers or failure to take into consideration the confounding variables in larger samples hampers the studies assessing exercise with birth weight and pregnancy outcome. Because the labor force is composed of more working women, many who exercise at conception and continue during pregnancy, the impact of exercise on pregnancy outcome in working women is very important. Influences of exercise, stress and occupation on pregnancy outcome are difficult to examine because of confounding variables not taken into account in large investigations and the lack of an adequate sample size in smaller studies.

As physical stress is relatively easy to standardize, several groups have studied changes in pregnant women as a result of sporting exertion, particularly the measurable physiological changes in the organisms of the mother and child. Although using different types of exercise—produced by ergometer, treadmill and running tests—all authors came to the conclusion that light and medium physical exercise has no significant adverse effect on the mother or the fetus.[14-16]

Doppler flow measurements of the fetoplacental unit after physical exercise of the mother have been performed with varying results by several investigators.[16-30] Only one study compared Doppler flow in uncomplicated and complicated pregnancies after physical exercise of the mother.[31] In this study, Hackett et al. studied 34 women (12 uncomplicated and the other 22 complicated by hypertension, IUGR fetus, or both) in the third trimester of singleton pregnancies. The patients underwent a bicycle exercise test during which pulsed Doppler sonographic assessment of the uteroplacental circulation was performed. Exercise appeared to increase the pulsatility of the uteroplacental Doppler waveform in all cases. The changes in the waveforms were more exaggerated in the complicated pregnancies, particularly when the resting waveform had been abnormal. These changes indicate an increase in uteroplacental vascular resistance with exercise, suggesting a deleterious effect of physical exertion in the third trimester, particularly in the presence of hypertension or IUGR fetus.

The effect of physical exertion on the fetoplacental unit in pregnancies complicated by intrauterine growth retardation or hypertensive disorders is of special clinical interest, because these fetuses are known to be at risk for long-term neurological morbidity.

Clinical Study on Exercise During Complicated Pregnancy and Doppler Sonography[32]

The authors conducted a study including measurements of the fetal aorta, fetal middle cerebral artery, umbilical artery and uteroplacental vessels in appropriate-for-gestational-age fetuses (AGA) and intrauterine growth retarded fetuses (IUGR) to investigate changes of the fetoplacental unit after defined maternal exercise in the third trimester of pregnancy.

Materials and Methods

A total of 33 pregnant women with AGA fetuses and 10 patients with IUGR fetuses in the third trimester were examined. Multiple pregnancies, cases with maternal renal disease, maternal diabetes, maternal cardiovascular pathology other than hypertension and fetuses with chromosomal or structural anomalies were excluded from evaluation. IUGR was defined as a fetal abdominal circumference <5th percentile for gestational age of our reference ranges.[33]

The exercise period began with an acclimatization period of 3 minutes (30 W), followed by 10 minutes of moderate exertion (1.25 W/kg body weight for each women). A bicycle ergometer from Mijnhardt (Mijnhardt-Jäger bv, Bunnik, The Netherlands) was used.

Immediately after the exercise period Doppler flow measurements were performed. The test period was 35 minutes. In the IUGR group, fetal heart rate monitoring (FHR) was performed for additional 15 minutes before and after the exercise.

Doppler flow recordings of the umbilical arteries, fetal aorta, middle cerebral and the uterine arteries were performed. During all Doppler examinations, the patients were positioned semi-recumbent to avoid "vena cava syndrome".

Doppler flow velocity waveforms were obtained from a free-floating central part of the umbilical artery in the absence of body movements, fetal breathing or cardiac arrhythmia with the sample volume covering the whole vessel. Care was taken to keep the insonation angle in the umbilical artery at the lowest possible angle. The fetal aorta was localized in its abdominal part at the origin of the renal arteries. The angle between ultrasound beam and fetal aorta was kept below 55°. The middle cerebral artery was visualized at about 1 cm of its origin in the circle of Willis in an axial view. The insonation angle in the middle cerebral artery was always below 15°. Care was taken to minimize fetal head compression, because this is known to influence the flow velocity waveforms of the middle cerebral arteries.

For uterine artery, the Doppler transducer was placed in the right or left lower part of the abdomen. Color Doppler imaging was used to localize the main uterine artery cranial to the crossing of the external iliac artery. The examination was repeated on the opposite side. The insonation angle was kept below 55° at the uterine arteries.

Abnormal umbilical, uterine and fetal aorta Doppler results were those >2 SD above the mean for gestational age of our local reference ranges.[34] Fetal brain sparing was supposed when the RI was <2 SD below the mean of our local reference ranges for the middle cerebral artery.[34]

Glucose and lactate levels were measured in capillary blood samples taken from the finger pad before and after exercise ("Monotest-Lactat in Halbmicro-Technik", Boehringer Mannheim). The pulse and blood pressure of the mother was automatically registered at 3-minute intervals during the test (Dinamap, Critikon).

The Wilcoxon pair difference test for associated random samples was used for statistical evaluation.

Results

Normal pregnancies: The mean performance on the bicycle ergometer was 79 W (±11 W). Gestational age at delivery was 40.0 weeks (±8 days). The mean birth weight was 3,270 g (± 383 g).

Mode of delivery: Twenty four (73%) women delivered vaginal spontaneously, one (3%) vaginal operative and eight (24%) by cesarean section.

Doppler Flow Results of Normal Pregnancies (*n = 33*) (*Table 53.1*)

Umbilical artery: The observed RI was within the normal range before and after exertion. However, in four (12%) fetuses the measurements reached the threshold range after exercise.

Table 53.1: Changes of RI during exercise in AGA pregnancies (*n* = 33)

	RI (Mean ± SD)			
	Before exertion (baseline)	**1–6 min**	**After exertion 7–12 min**	**13–18 min**
Fetal aorta	0.8 ± 0.21	0.82 ± 0.29	0.81 ± 0.22	0.82 ± 0.26
p value		<0.01	ns	<0.05
Middle cerebral artery	0.82 ± 0.48	0.77 ± 0.32	0.84 ± 0.54	0.83 ± 0.41
p value		<0.01	ns	ns
Umbilical artery	0.62 ± 0.12	0.6 ± 0.12	0.62 ± 0.12	0.62 ± 0.1
p value		ns	ns	ns
Uterine artery	0.44 ± 0.15	0.41 ± 0.1	0.44 ± 0.12	0.44 ± 0.1
p value		ns	ns	ns

Abbreviations: RI: Resistance index; ns, difference not significant; SD, Standard deviation

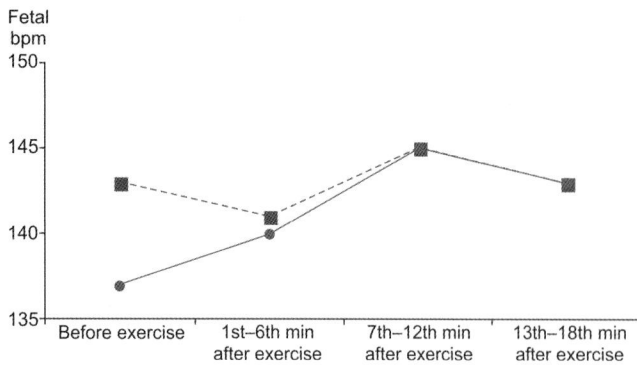

Fig. 53.1: Fetal heart rate during the test period (mean ± SD) in AGA (squares) and in IUGR (circles) pregnancies

Fetal aorta: The mean RI before exercise was 4.9 (±1.3). In eight (24%) fetuses, the RI was at the threshold range (RI between 0.83 and 0.86) and in one (3%) fetus at the pathological range (RI > 0.86). A significant increase in the RI was determined following exertion ($p < 0.01$). However, the mean value did not reach the pathological level. An increase in the RI of the aorta shortly after exertion was observed in 21 (63%) fetuses [In 5 (24%) within the threshold range, in 16 (76%) in the pathological range].

Middle cerebral artery: Before exercise, RI was in the normal range in all cases. A significant reduction in the RI was determined shortly after the exertion phase ($p < 0.01$). Twenty minutes after exertion, the results were almost the same as the baseline records.

Uterine artery: The observed RI was within the normal range before and after exertion.

FHR: The fetal heart rate remained nearly unchanged before and after exertion (Fig. 53.1). In one case, fetal bradycardia (lasting approximately 2 minutes at the end of the exertion phase) was observed. This patient developed preeclampsia in the last 2 weeks of pregnancy.

Maternal parameters: The maternal blood pressure and the maternal heart rate increased during the exertion phase but returned to the initial values at the end of the test.

The maternal glucose levels decreased by 21% ($p < 0.001$) after exercise, while the lactate values increased almost two-fold from 14.6 mg% to 27.6 mg% ($p < 0.001$).

IUGR pregnancies: The mean performance on the bicycle ergometer was 68 W (±10 W). Gestational age at delivery was 37.6 weeks (±19 days). The mean birth weight was 2,065 g (± 526 g).

Mode of delivery: Five (50%) women delivered vaginal spontaneously and 5 (50%) by cesarean section.

Doppler Flow Results of IUGR Pregnancies (n = 10) (Table 53.2)

Umbilical artery: In three (30%) fetuses, the baseline value was in the threshold and in another three (30%) fetuses it was pathological. After exercise the RI was in the threshold range in one (10%) fetus and pathological in four (40%) fetuses.

The RI in the umbilical artery was pathologic in three fetuses already before exercise. This had a marked influence on the mean RI value, because of the very small sample size. Thus, the calculated mean values of all measurements were in the pathological range from the beginning. After exclusion of these three cases, the RI became normal and no significant changes in the RI of umbilical arteries occurred during the test.

Fetal aorta: RI before exercise was within the pathological range in three (30%) fetuses and in two (20%) fetuses within the threshold range. The RI following exertion increased significantly ($p < 0.05$).

Four (40%), five (50%) and six (60%) fetuses Doppler values were within the pathological range, respectively for measurements after exertion between minutes 1–6 minutes 7–12 and minutes 13–18.

The mean values of fetal aortic RI values in IUGR fetuses were higher than in AGA fetuses ($p < 0.05$). In contrast to the AGA group, in the IUGR group all RI values after exercise were within the threshold or the pathologic range and did not return to normal values after exercise.

Middle cerebral artery: The RI revealed a stepwise reduction until 7–12 minutes after exertion ($p < 0.05$) and made a "plateau" until 13–18 minutes after exertion. In six (60%) fetuses, the RI following exertion was lower than the baseline values.

Table 53.2: Changes of RI during exercise in IUGR pregnancies (n = 10)

	RI (Mean ± SD)			
	Before exertion (baseline)		**After exertion**	
	1–6 min	**7–12 min**	**13–18 min**	
Fetal aorta *p* value	0.85 ± 0.37	0.87 ± 0.42 <0.05	0.89 ± 0.51 <0.05	0.89 ± 0.51 <0.05
A. cerebri media *p* value	0.8 ± 0.38	0.77 ± 0.29 <0.05	0.74 ± 0.11 <0.05	0.76 ± 0.33 <0.05
A. umbilicalis (all) *p* value	0.82 ± 0.82	0.83 ± 0.81 ns	0.84 ± 0.72 ns	0.77 ± 0.39 ns
A. umbilicalis (without extremes) *p* value	0.64 ± 0.11	0.66 ± 0.18 ns	0.64 ± 0.09 ns	0.69 ± 0.17 ns
A. uterinae *p* value	0.41 ± 0.19	0.52 ± 0.2 ns	0.47 ± 0.12 ns	0.47 ± 0.07 ns

Abbreviations: RI, Resistance index; ns, difference not significant; SD, Standard deviation

In growth retarded fetuses, the RI returned to normal levels more slowly than in AGA fetuses. In contrast to AGA fetuses, at the end RI in IUGR fetuses remained well below the values registered at baseline ($p < 0.05$).

Uterine artery: There were no significant changes in RI of the uterine vessels during the test.

FHR: The FHRs before and after exercise remained unchanged (Fig. 53.1).

Maternal parameters: Maternal blood pressure and heart rate increased during exercise but regained normal values rapidly after exercise. The maternal glucose levels decreased about 24% ($p < 0.001$), while the lactate concentrations doubled from 11.6 mg% to 24.2 mg% ($p < 0.001$).

Discussion

This study reports Doppler flow measurements of the placental vascular bed, the fetal aorta, umbilical artery together with the fetal cerebral arteries in the human AGA and IUGR fetus after physical exercise of the mother.

There is conflicting data regarding the question of uteroplacental supply during and after physical exercise of the mother in uneventful pregnancies and pregnancies at risk. The main hypothesis for guiding this study was that maternal exercise has both acute and chronic effects on placental bed blood flow. During the exercise, maternal blood flow is diverted away from the viscera to the exercising muscle and skin (fetoplacental blood steal effect). The magnitude of the reduction in flow is directly proportional to exercise intensity and the muscle mass used (which varies with the type of exercise), and with common types of exercise performed at usual exercise intensities, the reduction usually exceeds 50%. This exercise-induced decrease in visceral flow persists throughout pregnancy.[35]

The present Doppler flow results of the fetal aorta and fetal middle cerebral arteries in normal pregnancies showed significant differences before and after exertion. The RI in the aorta increased following exertion and remained higher for a considerable time (approximately 20 minutes), although the findings did not become pathological. In IUGR fetuses, the increase of the RI in the fetal aorta was more important with resistance indices being in the pathological range during the time period of the test.

The RI in the cerebral artery reduced significantly following exercise and returned very quickly approximately to its initial value in AGA fetuses. In IUGR cases, reduction of the RI could be observed until the end of the test without return to pre-test values, thus, indicating an initially decreased fetal cerebral circulation in IUGR cases after maternal exercise. RI of the placental vascular bed and the umbilical arteries remained unchanged throughout the test period. In three cases of IUGR, the authors found elevated RI values in the umbilical artery prior to maternal exercise. After exclusion of those cases, RI values in the umbilical artery were in the physiological range during the test in AGA and IUGR fetuses. These findings are in good accordance to results reported in the literature.[30,36-41] Furthermore, fetal heart rate remained unchanged after maternal exercise in AGA and IUGR fetuses. This is partly in accordance with previous studies.[30,42-47] Differences in study protocols might account for these differences.

The presented results support evidence of fetal cerebral vasodilatation leading to redistribution of fetal blood volume to the cerebrum as a physiologic answer after moderate maternal exercise during the third trimester of pregnancy. In IUGR fetuses, cerebral vasodilatation (brain sparing phenomenon) lasted longer than in AGA fetuses and did not return to initial levels during the test period, pointing toward an altered fetal oxygenation under these circumstances. Furthermore, our results suggest that maternal exercise does not significantly alter uterine and umbilical perfusion in AGA and IUGR pregnancies suggesting absence of change in the uterine vascular bed resistance.

OTHER STUDIES CONCERNED WITH DOPPLER SONOGRAPHY DURING EXERCISE IN PREGNANT WOMEN

In 1956, Morris et al.[48] already studied changes in uterine circulation following physical exertion by the mothers. The authors found a statistically significant lengthening of the uterine clearance half-time of NaCl and hence a reduction in circulation during exertion.[48] At rest, by contrast, the clearance half-time was shorter and uterine circulation improved. The main critic point to the results of this study was that during examination procedure, the patient rested in supine position, thus, inducing possible vena cava occlusion syndrome.

Several investigators reported of unchanged uteroplacental blood flow and umbilical perfusion after bicycle stress test in the third trimester.[30,49-52] Morrow et al. found higher resistance indices in the uterine arteries and elevated fetal heart rates after exercise of the mother in the third trimester. The RI in the umbilical artery, however, was unaltered.[53] Erkkola et al. demonstrated in a series of uncomplicated pregnancies an increase in RI of the uterine arteries and the maternal blood pressure after exercise, whereas no change in the RI occurred in the umbilical artery. Of note, the fetal heart rate increased significantly after exercise.[54]

The predictive value of maternal aerobic exercise for pregnancy-induced hypertension was studied by Hume et al. in a small series.[55] Preeclampsia developed in four patients with RI values being elevated in the umbilical artery after recovery in these four patients. It was concluded, that aerobic exercise of the mother might be a valuable tool in predicting hypertensive pregnancy complications.[56] On the other hand, decreased umbilical artery RI values were reported after maternal exercise in the third trimester, thus, indicating an improved placental circulation following exercise in healthy women.[28]

Hackett et al.[57] performed a bicycle exercise test in 34 women in the third trimester. Twelve pregnancies were uncomplicated, whereas 22 of the cases were complicated by small-for-gestational-age fetuses or maternal hypertension. Increase in pulsatility indices was more prominent in complicated pregnancies than in uncomplicated gestations, thus, indicating an important reduction of uteroplacental blood flow by maternal exercise in complicated pregnancies.[58] In a more recent study a fetal cerebral vasodilatation with decrease in umbilical resistance induced by submaximal maternal dynamic exercise was reported. Fetal heart rate remained unchanged in this study.[18]

CONCLUSION

1. In *healthy pregnant women* without obstetric or medical complications, the benefits of exercise seem to outweigh the risks. Therefore, pregnant women should continue to exercise, provided careful guidelines are followed. However, pregnant

women may have to modify their exercise regimens because of the physiologic changes associated with pregnancy. Although lower birth weights are noted among offspring of women who exercise during pregnancy, these birth weights are still within normal ranges. Currently there are no data to confirm that exercise during pregnancy has deleterious effects on the fetus.

2. Maternal exercise does not significantly alter uterine and umbilical perfusion in AGA and IUGR pregnancies suggesting absence of change in the uterine vascular bed resistance. However, submaximal maternal exercise was followed by a fetal cerebral vasodilatation and an increase of resistance in the fetal aorta which was more evident in IUGR fetuses. This might be due to a slight fetal hemoglobin desaturation in those cases. These findings underline the need of close antenatal surveillance of IUGR fetuses by Doppler flow measurements in order to detect circulatory deterioration in those fetuses and to reduce long-term morbidity. This is an important and relevant task of modern perinatal medicine.

APPENDIX

Guidelines for Exercise During Pregnancy

The American College of Obstetricians and Gynecologists (ACOG) has published a set of guidelines for exercise during pregnancy and the postpartum period. The most recent ACOG guidelines are listed in Table 53.3. These recommendations are made for women who do not have any additional risk factors for adverse maternal or perinatal outcome.[13]

Contraindications to Exercise

According to ACOG[13], conditions that should be considered contraindications to exercise during pregnancy include the following:

Table 53.3: American College of Obstetricians and Gynecologists' guidelines for exercise during pregnancy and postpartum

1. Regular exercise (at least three times per week) is preferable to intermittent activity
2. Avoid exercise in the supine position after the first trimester. This position is associated with decreased cardiac output in most pregnant women, causing a decreased distribution of blood to splanchnic beds including the uterus
3. Pregnant women should stop exercising when fatigued and not exercise to exhaustion.
4. Non-weight-bearing exercises such as cycling or swimming will minimize the risk of injury and facilitate the continuation of exercise during pregnancy
5. Adequate diet should be ensured
6. Avoid types of exercise in which loss of balance could be detrimental to maternal or fetal well-being, especially in the third trimester. Further, any type of exercise involving the potential for even mild abdominal trauma should be avoided
7. Adequate hydration, appropriate clothing and optimal environmental surroundings during exercise should be ensured
8. The physiologic and morphologic changes of pregnancy persist 4–6 weeks postpartum. Thus, prepregnancy exercise routines should be resumed gradually based on a woman's physical capability

Absolute Contraindications to Aerobic Exercise During Pregnancy

- Hemodynamically significant heart disease
- Restrictive lung disease

- Incompetent cervix/cerclage
- Multiple gestation at risk for premature labor
- Persistent second- or third-trimester bleeding
- Placenta previa after 26 weeks of gestation
- Premature labor during the current pregnancy
- Ruptured membranes
- Preeclampsia/pregnancy-induced hypertension.

Relative Contraindications to Aerobic Exercise During Pregnancy

- Severe anemia
- Unevaluated maternal cardiac arrhythmia
- Chronic bronchitis
- Poorly controlled type 1 diabetes
- Extreme morbid obesity
- Extreme underweight (BMI <12)
- History of extremely sedentary lifestyle
- Intrauterine growth restriction in current pregnancy
- Poorly controlled hypertension
- Orthopedic limitations
- Poorly controlled seizure disorder
- Poorly controlled hyperthyroidism
- Heavy smoker.

Warning Signs to Terminate Exercise While Pregnant

- Vaginal bleeding
- Dyspnea prior to exertion
- Dizziness
- Headache
- Chest pain
- Muscle weakness
- Calf pain or swelling (need to rule out thrombophlebitis)
- Preterm labor
- Decreased fetal movement
- Amniotic fluid leakage.

Conclusions and Recommendations of ACOG for Exercise During Pregnancy[13]

- Recreational and competitive athletes with uncomplicated pregnancies can remain active during pregnancy and should modify their usual exercise routines as medically indicated. The information on strenuous exercise is scarce; however, women who engage in such activities require close medical supervision

- Previously inactive women and those with medical or obstetric complications should be evaluated before recommendations for physical activity during pregnancy are made. Exercise during pregnancy may provide additional health benefits to women with gestational diabetes

- A physically active woman with a history of or risk for preterm labor or fetal growth restriction should be advised to reduce her activity in the second and third trimesters.

ACKNOWLEDGMENTS

The authors acknowledge Mr. Aykut Barut, MD (Zonguldak, Turkey), Hakan Sade, MD (Zonguldak, Turkey), and Mehmet Vural, MD (Zonguldak, Turkey) for their technical and editorial assistance in the preparation of this manuscript.

REFERENCES

1. Rowell LB. Human cardiovascular adjustments to exercise and thermal stress. Physiol Rev. 1974;54:75-159.
2. Clapp JF III, Capeless EL. The changing glycemic response to exercise during pregnancy. Am J Obstet Gynecol. 1991;165:1678-83.
3. Clapp JF III, Little KD, Capeless EL. Fetal heart rate response to sustained recreational exercise. Am J Obstet Gynecol. 1993;168:198-206.
4. Clapp JF III, Stepanchak W, Tomaselli J, et al. Portal vein blood flow-effects of pregnancy, gravity, and exercise. Am J Obstet Gynecol. 2000;183:167-72.
5. Clapp JF III. Exercise during pregnancy. A clinical update. Clin Sports Med. 2000;19:273-86.
6. Clapp JF III. The effects of maternal exercise on fetal oxygenation and feto-placental growth. Eur J Obstet Gynecol Reprod Biol. 2003;110(Suppl 1):S80-S5.
7. Ezmerli NM. Exercise in pregnancy. Prim Care Update Ob Gyns. 2000;7:260-5.
8. Hackett GA, Cohen-Overbeek T, Campbell S. The effect of exercise on uteroplacental Doppler waveforms in normal and complicated pregnancies. Obstet Gynecol. 1992;79:919-23.
9. Morrow RJ, Ritchie JW, Bull SB. Fetal and maternal hemodynamic responses to exercise in pregnancy assessed by Doppler ultrasonography. Am J Obstet Gynecol. 1989;160:138-40.
10. Chandler KD, Bell AW. Effects of maternal exercise on fetal and maternal respiration and nutrient metabolism in the pregnant ewe. J Dev Physiol. 1981;3:161-76.
11. Curet LB, Orr JA, Rankin HG, et al. Effect of exercise on cardiac output and distribution of uterine blood flow in pregnant ewes. J Appl Physiol. 1976;40:7258.
12. Magann EF, Evans SF, Weitz B, et al. Antepartum, intrapartum, and neonatal significance of exercise on healthy low-risk pregnant working women. Obstet Gynecol. 2002;99:466-72.
13. ACOG Committee opinion. Number 267, January 2002: Exercise during pregnancy and the postpartum period. Obstet Gynecol. 2002;99:171-3.
14. Van Hook JW, Gill P, Easterling TR, et al. The hemodynamic effects of isometric exercise during late normal pregnancy. Am J Obstet Gynecol. 1993;169:870-3.
15. Pijpers L, Wladimiroff JW, McGhie J. Effect of short-term maternal exercise on maternal and fetal cardiovascular dynamics. Br J Obstet Gynecol. 1984;91:1081-6.
16. Revelli A, Durando A, Massobrio M. Exercise in pregnancy: A review of maternal and fetal effects. Obstet Gynecol Survey. 1992;47:355-63.
17. Manders MA, Sonder GJ, Mulder EJ, et al. The effects of maternal exercise on fetal heart rate and movement patterns. Early Hum Dev. 1997;48:237-47.
18. Bonnin P, Bazzi-Grossin C, Ciraru-Vigneron N, et al. Evidence of fetal cerebral vasodilatation induced by submaximal maternal dynamic exercise in human pregnancy. J Perinat Med. 1997;25:63-70.
19. Veille JC. Maternal and fetal cardiovascular response to exercise during pregnancy. Semin Perinatol. 1996;20:250-62.
20. Erkkola RU, Pirhonen JP, Kivijarvi AK. Flow velocity waveforms in uterine and umbilical arteries during submaximal bicycle exercise in normal pregnancy. Obstet Gynecol. 1992;79:611-5.
21. Ruissen C, Jager W, Von Drongelen M, et al. The influence of maternal exercise on the pulsatility index of the umbilical artery blood velocity waveform. Eur J Obstet Gynecol Reprod Biol. 1990;37:1-6.
22. Hume RF Jr, Bowie JD, McCoy C, et al. Fetal umbilical artery Doppler response to graded maternal aerobic exercise and subsequent maternal mean arterial blood pressure: predictive value for pregnancy-induced hypertension. Am J Obstet Gynecol. 1990;163:826-9.
23. Veille JC, Bacevice AE, Wilson B, et al. Umbilical artery waveform during bicycle exercise in normal pregnancy. Obstet Gynecol. 1989;73:957-60.
24. Morrow RJ, Ritchie JW, Bull SB. Fetal and maternal hemodynamic responses to exercise in pregnancy assessed by Doppler ultrasonography. Am J Obstet Gynecol. 1989;160:138-40.
25. Baumann H, Huch A, Huch R. Doppler sonographic evaluation of exercise-induced blood flow velocity and waveform changes in fetal, uteroplacental and large maternal vessels in pregnant women. J Perinat Med. 1989;17:279-87.
26. Moore DH, Jarrett JC, Bendick PJ. Exercise-induced changes in uterine artery blood flow, as measured by Doppler ultrasound, in pregnant subjects. Am J Perinatol. 1988;5:94-7.
27. Steegers EA, Buunk G, Binkhorst RA, et al. The influence of maternal exercise on the uteroplacental vascular bed resistance and the fetal heart rate during normal pregnancy. Eur J Obstet Gynecol Reprod. Biol. 1988;27:21-6.
28. Rafla N, Beazely J. The effects of maternal exercise on fetal umbilical artery waveforms. Eur J Obstet Gynecol Reprod Biol. 1991;1:119-23.
29. Durak E, Jovanovic-Peterson L, Peterson C. Comparative evaluation of uterine response to exercise on five aeorobic machines. Am J Obstet Gynecol. 1990;162:279-84.
30. Drack G, Kirkinen P, Baumann H, et al. Doppler ultrasound studies before and following short-term maternal stress in late pregnancy. Z Geburtshilfe Perinatol. 1988;192:173-7.
31. Hackett GA, Cohen-Overbeek T, Campbell S. The effect of exercise on uteroplacental Doppler waveforms in normal and complicated pregnancies. Obstet Gynecol. 1992;79:919-23.
32. Ertan AK, Schanz S, Tanriverdi HA, et al. Doppler examinations of fetal and uteroplacental blood flow in AGA and IUGR fetuses before and after maternal physical exercise with the bicycle ergometer. J Perinat Med. 2004;32:260-5.
33. Schmidt W, Hendrik H, Gauwerky J, et al. Diagnosis of intrauterine growth retardation by intensive ultrasound biometry. Geburtsh Frauenheilk. 1987;42:543-8.
34. Ertan A, Hendrik H, Tanriverdi H, et al. Fetomaternal Doppler sonography nomograms. Perinatoloji. 2001;9:174-80.
35. Clapp J. The effects of maternal exercise on fetal oxygenation and feto-placental growth. Eur J Obstet Gynecol Reprod Biol. 2003;110:80-5.
36. Erkkola RU, Pirhonen JP, Kivijarvi AK. Flow velocity waveforms in uterine and umbilical arteries during submaximal bicycle exercise in normal pregnancy. Obstet Gynecol. 1992;79:611-5.
37. Ruissen C, Jager W, Von Drongelen M, et al. The influence of maternal exercise on the pulsatility index of the umbilical artery blood velocity waveform. Eur J Obstet Gynecol Reprod Biol. 1990;37:1-6.
38. Veille JC, Bacevice AE, Wilson B, et al. Umbilical artery waveform during bicycle exercise in normal pregnancy. Obstet Gynecol. 1989;73:957-60.
39. Morrow RJ, Ritchie JW, Bull SB. Fetal and maternal hemodynamic responses to exercise in pregnancy assessed by Doppler ultrasonography. Am J Obstet Gynecol. 1989;160:138-40.
40. Moore DH, Jarrett JC, Bendick PJ. Exercise-induced changes in uterine artery blood flow, as measured by Doppler ultrasound, in pregnant subjects. Am J Perinatol. 1988;5:94-7.
41. Steegers EA, Buunk G, Binkhorst RA, et al. The influence of maternal exercise on the uteroplacental vascular bed resistance and the fetal heart rate during normal pregnancy. Eur J Obstet Gynecol Reprod Biol. 1988;27:21-6.
42. Erkkola RU, Pirhonen JP, Kivijarvi AK. Flow velocity waveforms in uterine and umbilical arteries during submaximal bicycle exercise in normal pregnancy. Obstet Gynecol. 1992;79:611-5.

43. Ruissen C, Jager W, Von Drongelen M, et al. The influence of maternal exercise on the pulsatility index of the umbilical artery blood velocity waveform. Eur J Obstet Gynecol Reprod Biol. 1990;37:1-6.

44. Veille JC, Bacevice AE, Wilson B, et al. Umbilical artery waveform during bicycle exercise in normal pregnancy. Obstet Gynecol. 1989;73:957-60.

45. Morrow RJ, Ritchie JW, Bull SB. Fetal and maternal hemodynamic responses to exercise in pregnancy assessed by Doppler ultrasonography. Am J Obstet Gynecol. 1989;160:138-40.

46. Moore DH, Jarrett JC, Bendick PJ. Exercise-induced changes in uterine artery blood flow, as measured by Doppler ultrasound, in pregnant subjects. Am J Perinatol. 1988;5:94-7.

47. Steegers EA, Buunk G, Binkhorst RA, et al. The influence of maternal exercise on the uteroplacental vascular bed resistance and the fetal heart rate during normal pregnancy. Eur J Obstet Gynecol Reprod Biol. 1988;27:21-6.

48. Morris N, Osborn S, Wright H, et al. Effective uterine blood flow during exercise in normal and preeclpamtic pregnancies. Lancet. 1956;361:481-3.

49. Veille JC. Maternal and fetal cardiovascular response to exercise during pregnancy. Semin Perinatol. 1996;20:25062.

50. Ruissen C, Jager W, von Drongelen M, et al. The influence of maternal exercise on the pulsatility index of the umbilical artery blood velocity waveform. Eur J Obstet Gynecol Reprod Biol. 1990;37:1-6.

51. Moore DH, Jarrett JC, Bendick PJ. Exercise-induced changes in uterine artery blood flow, as measured by Doppler ultrasound, in pregnant subjects. Am J Perinatol. 1988;5:94-7.

52. Steegers EA, Buunk G, Binkhorst RA, et al. The influence of maternal exercise on the uteroplacental vascular bed resistance and the fetal heart rate during normal pregnancy. Eur J Obstet Gynecol Reprod Biol. 1988;27:21-6.

53. Morrow RJ, Ritchie JW, Bull SB. Fetal and maternal hemodynamic responses to exercise in pregnancy assessed by Doppler ultrasonography. Am J Obstet Gynecol. 1989;160:138-40.

54. Erkkola RU, Pirhonen JP, Kivijarvi AK. Flow velocity waveforms in uterine and umbilical arteries during submaximal bicycle exercise in normal pregnancy. Obstet Gynecol. 1992;79:611-5.

55. Hume RF, Jr, Bowie JD, McCoy C, et al. Fetal umbilical artery Doppler response to graded maternal aerobic exercise and subsequent maternal mean arterial blood pressure: predictive value for pregnancy-induced hypertension. Am J Obstet Gynecol. 1990;163:826-9.

56. Hume RF Jr, Bowie JD, McCoy C, et al. Fetal umbilical artery Doppler response to graded maternal aerobic exercise and subsequent maternal mean arterial blood pressure: predictive value for pregnancy-induced hypertension. Am J Obstet Gynecol. 1990;163:826-9.

57. Hackett GA, Cohen-Overbeek T, Campbell S. The effect of exercise on uteroplacental Doppler waveforms in normal and complicated pregnancies. Obstet Gynecol. 1992;79:919-23.

58. Hackett GA, Cohen-Overbeek T, Campbell S. The effect of exercise on uteroplacental Doppler waveforms in normal and complicated pregnancies. Obstet Gynecol. 1992;79:919-23.

54 Doppler Velocimetry in Intrauterine Growth Restriction: A Practical Clinical Approach

GP Mandruzzato, YJ Meir, G Maso

INTRODUCTION

Intrauterine growth restriction (IUGR) according to the current definition is that of a fetus that fails to reach his potential growth. The term IUGR should be only used in regard to the fetus, while SGA (small for gestational age) should be used only in regard to the newborn.[1] This distinction must be kept in mind very clearly. It is true that perinatal mortality and morbidity are significantly increased in cases presenting a birth weight inferior to the 10th percentile for gestational age (therefore defined as SGA) and also inferior to the 15th percentile[2] but it has been shown that symptoms of hypoxemia are observable in cases presenting a birth weight also superior to the 50th percentile, but showing a restriction of growth by ultrasound biometry during fetal life, with the same frequency as in SGA newborns.[3] IUGR can be associated to many conditions (malformations, karyotype aberrations, infections, maternal diseases) but the most frequent and most dangerous complications is represented by chronic fetal hypoxemia. This is the consequence of obliterative placental vasculopathy that reduces first maternal-fetal supply of nutrients and later on of oxygen. This ominous condition is encountered in about 30% of IUGR fetuses and is the cause of the poor perinatal outcome (intrauterine death or damage, acute hypoxemia in labor, neonatal death and morbidity early and late as well). Moreover, it has been postulated that intrauterine growth restriction can be responsible also of diseases occurring in adult life.

Chronic fetal hypoxemia induces changes in many fetal vital functions (hemodynamics, heart activity, fetal movements and behavior, amniotic fluid turnover) and one of the first to be observable is blood flow redistribution. As Doppler technology enables us to study in a noninvasive way of these changes, it has become a fundamental tool for assessing the fetal oxygenation and the fetal response to hypoxemia thus becoming a useful guide in clinical management of IUGR fetuses.

CHARACTERISTICS OF DOPPLER VELOCITY WAVEFORM (DVWF)

The DVWF reflects the velocities of blood during a cardiac cycle. The so called "angle independent parameters" are commonly used for studying the characteristics of the DVWF. The velocities of the systolic phase are compared to that of the diastolic one according to different formulas. The most simple is the S/D ratio obtained by dividing the two. The resistance index (RI) is obtained by dividing the systolic velocity for the systolic minus the diastolic. Probably the most comprehensive parameter is the pulsatility index (PI) because it takes into consideration not only systolic and diastolic velocities but also the mean of the velocities. Anyway the characteristics of the DVWF and so the different parameters are mainly influenced

by the diastolic phase therefore reflecting the peripheral resistance downstream the explored segment of the vessels, especially in case of investigation performed on arteries. When the peripheral resistance is markedly increased the forward blood flow can be absent or also reverted. These particular patterns of the DVWF are called ARED flow (absent/reverse end-diastolic flow). After the introduction of color flow mapping (CFM) technique it became possible to identify also very tiny vessels and vascular structures that can be sampled by Doppler technique. As a consequence it has been possible to build a map of fetal hemodynamic patterns in normally evolving pregnancies and in those affected by hypoxemia as well.

FETAL AND UMBILICAL HEMODYNAMICS IN NORMAL PREGNANCIES

In case of normally evolving pregnancy, Doppler investigation on somatic and cerebral fetal arteries shows a fairly constant pattern of the DVWF indicating an almost stable peripheral resistance or a small progressive reduction. When studying with the same technology the umbilical arteries a significant progressive reduction of peripheral resistance is observable possibly related to the increasing need of nutrients and oxygen for the growing fetus.

Object of the studies have been first umbilical arteries and fetal thoracic descending aorta. With the progress of the ultrasound imaging technology and the use of CFM, allowing to identify and sample also tiny vessels, many other arteries like cerebral (internal carotid, and middle and anterior cerebral), renal, mesenteric, adrenal, splenic, iliac aortic arch and coronary have been object of investigation.

As a consequence a very comprehensive overview of the fetal physiologic hemodynamics has been obtained that is a fundamental basis for studying and understanding the possible changes occurring in pathologic pregnancies.

ARTERIAL DOPPLER CHANGES IN HYPOXEMIC IUGR

As already said the most frequent and severe complication of IUGR is represented by the chronic fetal hypoxemia, consequence of the placental obliterative vasculopathy. Due to the capacity of Doppler technology, it is possible to study the hemodynamic changes occurring in this condition in umbilical arteries and those occurring in fetal arteries.

The first step of the fetal adaptation to hypoxemia is represented by blood flow redistribution inducing vasoconstriction in somatic arteries and vasodilatation in the cerebral arteries. This phenomenon is called "brain sparing effect" and is finalized to preserve sufficient oxygenation to the central nervous system. It has been postulated that such a "sparing effect" occurs also at the level of adrenal and coronary arteries. Therefore peripheral resistance is increased in somatic and splanchnic arteries, and reduced in cerebral arteries.

When placental obliterative vasculopathy occurs the peripheral resistance is also increased in umbilical arteries. It has been shown that PI elevation is proportional to the obliteration of the placental vascular bed.[4]

From the clinical point of view by using Doppler investigation, it is possible to assess both the cause (umbilical arteries) and the effect (fetal arteries) of hypoxemia.

DOPPLER PATTERNS OF IUGR

Doppler study on umbilical arteries and fetal thoracic descending aorta has been performed in 653 IUGR fetuses. In all the cases, gestational age has been established on the basis of ultrasonic biometry carried out in early pregnancy (by measuring CRL) and not later than 20 weeks of gestation (by measuring the biparietal diameter). IUGR has been diagnosed if the fetal biometry (abdominal circumference) showed a discrepancy in defect major than 2 weeks from the expected curve of growth that have been established in our institute. Cases presenting fetal abnormalities (anatomical and/or chromosomal) have been excluded from this study. After IUGR recognition Doppler investigation has been applied at a weekly or minor interval according to the severity of the growth restriction and of the maternal clinical conditions by measuring the PI values. Cases presenting PI values superior to the second standard deviation were considered as abnormal. Fetal biometry has been performed weekly if severe restriction was observed and/or abnormal PI were present, and at 14-day interval in cases presenting normal Doppler values. Computer assisted cardiotocography (CTG) according to the Oxford System 8002 has been performed for monitoring fetal conditions.

The IUGR cases have been divided in four groups according to the characteristics of Doppler patterns. In the first group 71 cases presenting absent or reverse diastolic flow (ARED) have been included (10.8%). In the second group, the collected cases are ($n = 64$, 9.8%) presenting abnormal PI (over the second SD) in both vascular district. In the third group, the cases are ($n = 85$, 13%) presenting abnormal PI only in aorta while still depicting normal values in umbilical arteries. The fourth group is represented by cases showing normal PI values in both aorta and umbilical arteries ($n = 433$, 66.3%).

The prevalence of fetal distress (FD) has been calculated for each group. FD has been diagnosed on the basis of short term variation (ST) below 3 ms in pregnancy and on the presence of late decelerations or bradycardia and/or fetal acidemia on FBS during labor requiring cesarean delivery. Overall the prevalence of FD was 31% but with a statistically significant difference in the four groups.

FD has been observed in 100% of the cases in the first group. This prevalence is reduced to 74% in the second group and even more, 33% in the third. In the fourth group, this figure is 12%.

Sensitivity and specificity of Doppler for predicting FD has been calculated separately for FA and UA. The sensitivity is 62.69 for FA and 35.18 for UA. The specificity is 81.56 for FA and 96.71 for UA. The reason for that difference depends on the pathophysiological background of hemodynamics changes of the two vascular districts. Fetal vessels, like aorta, changes represent the adaptation to hypoxemia while umbilical arteries changes are the consequence of increased peripheral resistance provoked by placental obliterative vasculopathy.

Practically by studying hemodynamics on umbilical arteries, we can assess the cause of chronic fetal hypoxemia while studying fetal vessels we can assess the phenomenon of fetal adaptation to the reduced oxygen supply.

As already said it has been shown that PI values are proportional to the obliteration of the placental vascular bed but evidence has also been given that DVWF becomes altered only when at least 60% of the placental vascular bed is obliterated[5] and oxygen supply to the fetus strongly reduced. As a consequence the specificity of PI on UA is much higher than that observable on FA.

Therefore, according to the Doppler patterns, the first group (ARED) represents a condition of restriction of oxygen supply to the fetus inducing a severe hypoxemia. Unfavorable perinatal outcome (death or handicaps in survivors) has been observed only in this group. The second and third groups represent a condition of reduced oxygen supply and fetal adaptation and possible FD. The fourth group represents IUGR fetuses not affected by chronic hypoxemia.

The clinical consequences can be indicated as follows:

Group 1   Timing of prompt delivery should be taken into consideration.

Group 2 and 3 Close surveillance and timing of the delivery according to fetal monitoring. Maternal corticosteroids administration if gestational age is lower than 34 weeks. Vaginal delivery after spontaneous onset of labor is possible in about 50% of the cases.

Group 4   Clinical and instrumental control at weekly or 14-days interval. In the majority of the cases vaginal delivery after spontaneous onset of labor occurs.

A particular attention should be deserved to IUGR cases when ARED flow is observed. This hemodynamic condition is encountered in about 10 of IUGR fetuses and is usually associated with a low gestational age, as a mean 30 weeks.

As the outcome is largely different in case of end-diastolic flow absent (EDFA) as compared to reverse flow (RF), being better in the first condition, the characteristics of the management should be different. In fact, it has been shown that perinatal mortality and handicaps rates are significantly higher in case of RF.[6]

CONCLUSION

IUGR can be associated with many fetal adverse conditions (malformations, chromosomal aberrations, infections) but the most important cause of both restriction of growth and poor perinatal outcome is represented by chronic fetal hypoxemia (CFH). This condition is the consequence of placental obliterative vasculopathy that affects the maternal-fetal supply of nutrients first and later on of oxygen. As a consequence hemodynamic changes occur in umbilical arteries and fetal as well. These modifications are easily observable by using Doppler technology by analyzing the characteristics of the DVWF.

As CFH occurs in about 30% of IUGR, therefore requiring close control and possibly active management, the crucial point, after IUGR recognition, is represented by identification or exclusion of CFH. By studying DVWF on umbilical and fetal arteries it is possible to assess the characteristics of the blood flow from mother to the fetus, and to monitor the aspects of the fetal adaptation if CFH is present. Fetal thoracic descending aorta is easy to be identified and sampled by using pulsed Doppler.

According to the patterns of the DVWF and PI values, it is possible to distinguish the IUGR fetuses affected by CFH from those that are not. As a consequence the characteristics of the control can be differentiated.

Moreover, if CFH is present, it is possible to monitor its evolution obtaining information of clinical practical validity in order to optimize the management and the timing of the delivery, if necessary.

REFERENCES

1. ACOG practice bulletin intrauterine growth restriction 2000. Int J Gynecol Obstet. 2001;72:85-96.
2. Seeds JW, Peng T. Impaired growth and the risk of fetal death: Is the tenth percentile the appropriate standard? Am J Obstet Gynecol. 1998;178:658-67.
3. De Jong CL, Francis A, Van Geijn HP, et al. Fetal growth rate and adverse perinatal events. Ultrasound Obstet Gynecol. 1999;13:86-9.
4. Giles W, Trudinger B, Baird P. Fetal umbilical artery flow velocity waveforms and placental resistance: Pathological correlation. Br J Obstet Gynecol. 1985;92:31-8.
5. Trudinger BJ, Cook CM. Doppler umbilical and uterine flow waveforms in severe pregnancy hypertension. Br J Obstet Gynecol. 1990;97:142-8.
6. Mandruzzato GP, Bogatti P, Fisher-Tamaro L, et al. The clinical significance of absent or reverse end diastolic flow in the fetal aorta and umbilical arteries. Ultrasound Obstet Gynecol. 1991;1:192-6.

55 Doppler Evaluation of Fetal Venous System

G Maso, G Conoscenti, GP Mandruzzato

INTRODUCTION

Fetal blood flow measurements have become an important tool in the surveillance of high risk pregnancies. There is a vast amount of literature on umbilical arteries and fetal arterial system, but fetal venous circulation has only recently been evaluated.

The introduction of high-resolution ultrasonography, combined with color-Doppler imaging (CDI), offered a breakthrough in the study of the fetal venous system, considerably enhancing our understanding in normal physiologic conditions, as well as in abnormal circumstances.

This review will focus on the embryologic, anatomic and physiological characteristics of the fetal venous circulation. The knowledge of the development and physiology represents the basis to understand the structural anomalies and the hemodynamic changes that occur in the venous district in pathological conditions.

EMBRYOLOGY OF THE FETAL VENOUS SYSTEM

In a 4-week embryo three pairs of veins are found.

The vitelline veins run from the yolk sac to the sinus venosus via liver sinusoid, and are connected to each other via anastomoses around the duodenum.

The umbilical veins transport oxygenated blood from the chorion to the sinus venosus, by-passing the liver. They merge with the cardinal veins, the third pair of embryonic veins, which originate from the body of the embryo and open into the right and left horns of the sinus venosus of the primitive heart.

The fetal liver and its development in the septum transversus play an important role in modifying the primitive vitelline and umbilical veins into their final morphology.

With the rapid growth of the liver, the umbilical veins connect with the liver sinusoids. The asymmetric development of the heart and the rotation of the intestinal tract cause a major change in the venous circulation by forming a single venosus blood stream from left to right.

In the 6 mm embryo, the complete right umbilical vein, the cranial part of the left umbilical vein, the left vitelline vein and part of the anastomoses obliterate and a new vessel, the ductus venosus (DV) develops. This is a shunt vessel between the left umbilical vein and the right hepatocardinal channel, which will become the upper inferior vena cava (IVC). At this stage all the placental blood enters the right atrium through the left distal umbilical vein (UV), DV and proximal right vitelline vein, which by pass the liver sinusoids. The upper two anastomoses of the distal vitelline veins fuse to form the portal vein, whereas the distal anastomoses form the superior mesenteric and splenic veins, and the proximal parts become the hepatic veins (Fig. 55.1).

Inferior vena cava and superior vena cava (SVC) originate from the cardinal veins that are the main drainage system of the embryo's body (Fig. 55.2). The anterior and posterior cardinal veins drain the cranial and caudal part of the body of the embryo, respectively. The left brachiocephalic vein is formed during the eighth week from the right anterior and right common cardinal veins, through left to right anastomoses, whereas the left anterior cardinal vein disappears. Azygos and hemiazygos veins originate from the upper portion of the division of the supracardinal veins, whereas the caudal part becomes the caudal part of the IVC.[1-4]

ANATOMY OF THE FETAL VENOUS SYSTEM

Two venous systems can be identified within the fetal liver— an afferent system, or umbilical-portal system, taking blood from the placenta and gut to the liver, and an efferent system, given by the hepatic veins, taking blood from the liver to the heart (Fig. 55.3). The DV shunts oxygenated blood from the umbilical-portal system directly to the heart.

In the afferent venous system, the UV enters the abdomen within the falciform ligament, ascending steeply toward the liver and runs along its surface in cephalad direction. It then joins a confluence of vessels termed the portal sinus. This is a wide L-shaped vessel at the distal part of the UV, connecting the right and left intrahepatic portal veins. These perfuse the right and left hepatic lobes, respectively. There are two main left (superior and inferior) intrahepatic portal veins. The right intrahepatic portal vein shows a more abundant branching pattern. The vein originating from the confluence of the splenic and superior mesenteric veins outside the liver represents the extrahepatic portal vein.

The DV originates from the portal sinus as the latter turned at an almost right angle into the right lobe of the liver. The diameter of the DV is approximately one-third that of the UV. This is a branchless, hourglass-shaped vessel ascending in the direction of the diaphragm, which joins distally with the hepatic left vein and the IVC, just proximal to the entrance into the right atrium (Fig. 55.4). The existence of a "sphincter" that regulates the blood flow through the DV to the heart has been postulated, and it has been supposed that the control of this anatomic structure is oxygen concentration-dependent.

The efferent system is represented by a number of vessels arising from the right and left hepatic lobes (right, middle and left hepatic veins), which drains into the subdiaphragmatic vestibulum. The hepatic veins, DV and IVC, open into the subdiaphragmatic

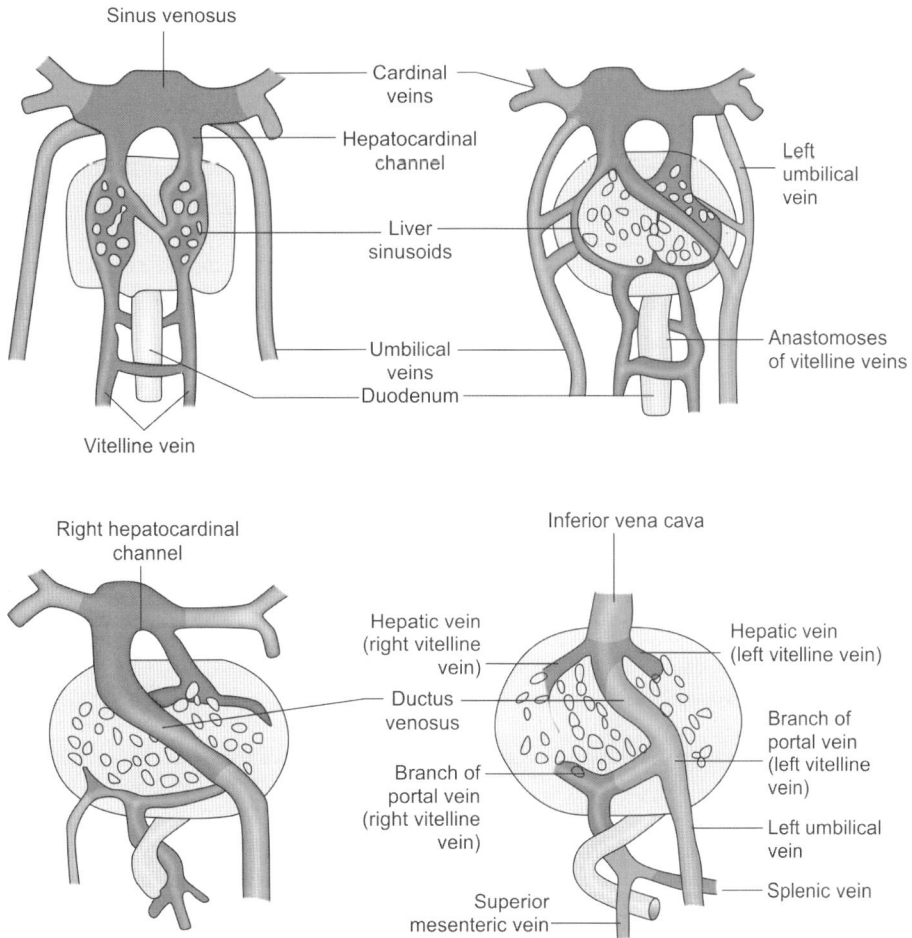

Fig. 55.1: Embryology of umbilical, portal and hepatic venous system
(*Source:* Reprinted with permission from Hoffstetter et al.[2])

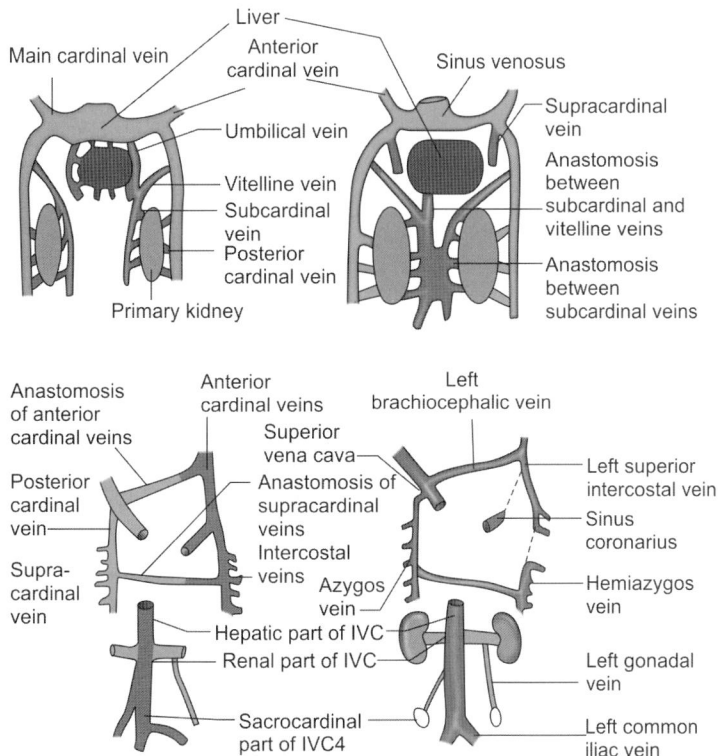

Fig. 55.2: Embryology of inferior and superior vena cava
(*Source:* Reprinted with permission from Hoffstetter et al.[2])

vestibulum, an inverted funnel-shaped, vascular space just below the diaphragm, ending into the right atrium.[3-5]

PHYSIOLOGY OF THE FETAL VENOUS SYSTEM

The anatomical relationship in the hepatic afferent venous system supports the well established concept that oxygenated blood flow from the placenta is distributed through the UV to the portal sinus, which supplies the left and right intrahepatic portal veins and the DV. Deoxygenated blood from the extrahepatic portal veins is diverted almost exclusively to the right hepatic lobe. The alignment of UV and DV, although not in anatomical continuity for the interposed portal sinus, favors the preferential streaming of oxygenated blood to the DV and consequently to the heart (Figs 55.3 and 55.4). Approximately 50% of the UV blood flow enters the DV and accounts for 98% of the blood flow through the DV. The portal blood is mainly directed to the right lobe of the liver.

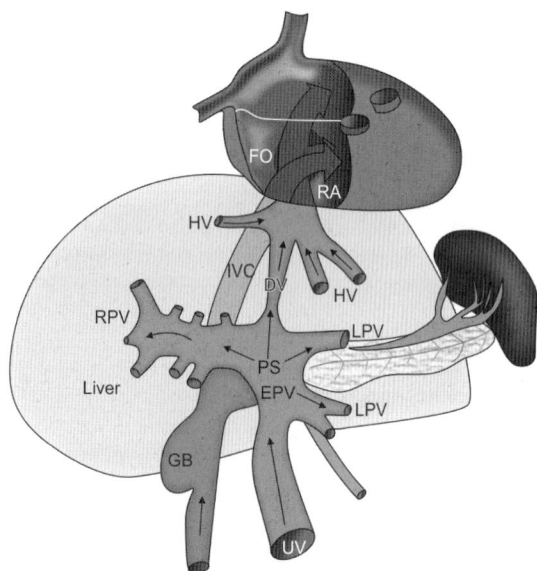

Fig. 55.3: Representation of fetal umbilical and hepatic venous system. The arrows indicate the direction of flow. The colors show the degree of oxygenation (red, high; purple, medium; blue, low)
Abbreviations: FO, foramen ovale; RA, right atrium; DV, ductus venosus; UV, umbilical vein; HV, hepatic vein; IVC, inferior vena cava; PS, portal sinus; LPV, left portal vein; RPV, right portal vein; EPV, extrahepatic portal vein; GB, gallbladder
(*Source:* Reprinted with permission from Mavrides et al.[5])

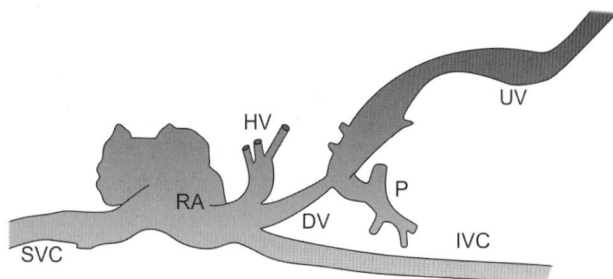

Fig. 55.4: Sagittal view of the fetal venous system
Abbreviations: RA, right atrium; DV, ductus venosus; UV, umbilical vein; HV, hepatic vein; IVC, inferior vena cava; P, portal system; SVC, superior vena cava

As far as the vessels of the efferent venous system is concerned, it is possible to observe that the right hepatic vein runs parallel to the IVC, while the left and middle hepatic veins run parallel to the DV. It has been postulated that this spatial rearrangement is the consequence of distribution of more oxygenated blood flow. The left hepatic lobe, in fact, is primarily supplied with the blood flow from the UV via the left portal vein.

Moreover it has been shown that there is streamlining of blood flow within the thoracic IVC: blood from DV and left hepatic vein flows in the dorsal and leftward part, whereas blood from the right lobe, distal IVC and right hepatic lobe flows in the ventral and rightward stream part of IVC. The ventral and rightward stream, together with blood from SVC, is directed to the right atrium and through the tricuspid valve into the right ventricle, ejected into the main pulmonary artery and shunted, via ductus arteriosus, into the descending aorta. The dorsal and leftward stream is directed toward the foramen ovale thereby delivering well-oxygenated blood flow directly to the left heart and, via ascending aorta, to the myocardium and the brain.[3,6,7]

NORMAL DOPPLER FINDINGS

The application of high resolution and color Doppler ultrasonography has allowed the structural and functional evaluation of fetal venous system.

At sonography, the UV can be detected in a sagittal or transverse section of the abdomen. In the transverse section it curves toward the right side of the upper abdomen (Fig. 55.5).

The DV can be visualized in its full length in a midsagittal longitudinal section of the trunk or in an oblique transverse section through the upper abdomen. Its origin from the UV can be found where CDI indicates higher velocities compared with the flow in UV, and sometimes this produces an aliasing effect. The blood flow velocities accelerate due to the narrow lumen of the DV, the maximum inner width of the narrowest portion being 2 mm (Figs 55.6 and 55.7).

The IVC could be well evaluated either in the longitudinal and coronal section; it runs anterior, to the right of and nearly parallel to the descending aorta (Fig. 55.8).

The hepatic veins can be visualized either in a transverse scan section through the upper abdomen or in a sagittal-coronal section through the hepatic lobes (Fig. 55.9).

The typical waveform for blood flow in the venous vessels, excluding the UV and portal veins, consists in three phases related to the cardiac cycle (Fig. 55.10). The highest pressure gradient between the venous vessel and the right atrium occurs during ventricular systole (S), resulting in the fastest blood flow velocities forward the fetal heart. Early diastole (peak D) with opening of the atrioventricular valves and passive early filling of the ventricles (peak E of the biphasic atrioventricular flow waveform) is associated with a second forward peak flow. The lowest velocities (a) in fetal venous vessels can be observed during the atrial contraction of the late diastole (peak A of the biphasic atrioventricular flow waveform).

The DV flow pattern is characterized by a triphasic forward flow (Fig. 55.11); it is directed toward the heart through the whole cardiac cycle. Even in early pregnancy, there is no retrograde flow during atrial contraction.

In the IVC and hepatic veins (Figs 55.12A and B) a physiological reverse flow during atrial contraction is observed. The percentage of reverse flow in IVC decreases with advancing gestational age.

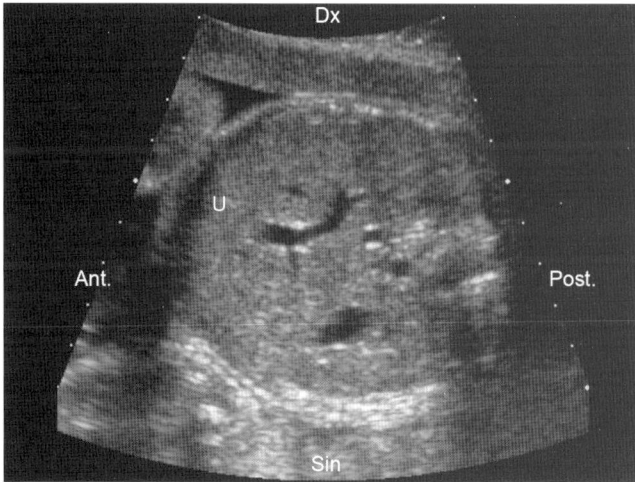

Fig. 55.5: Transverse view of the fetal abdomen. The UV curves forward the right side

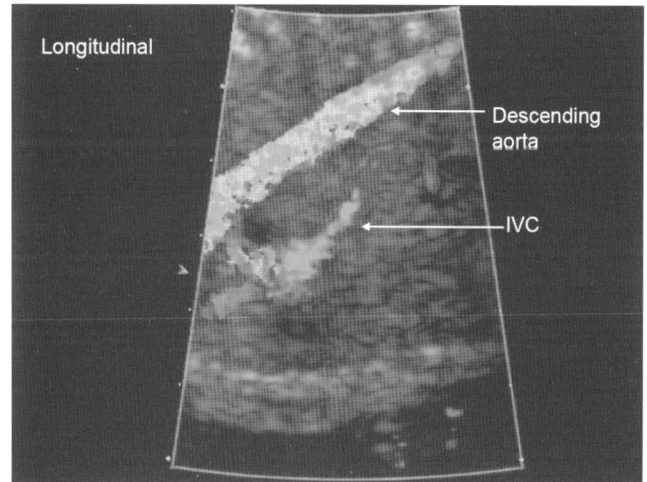

Fig. 55.8: Coronal plane of the upper abdomen: the IVC runs anterior to the right of and nearly parallel to the descending aorta

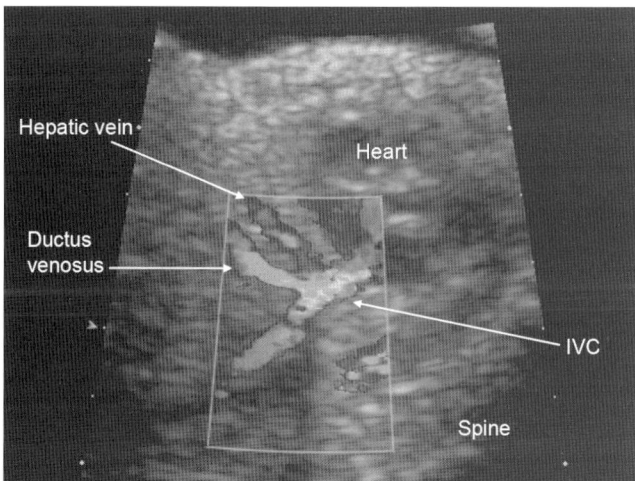

Fig. 55.6: Midsagittal view of the fetal upper abdomen. DV and hepatic vein merge into the IVC forming the subdiaphragmatic infundibulum, a funnel-shaped, vascular space just below the diaphragm, ending into the right atrium

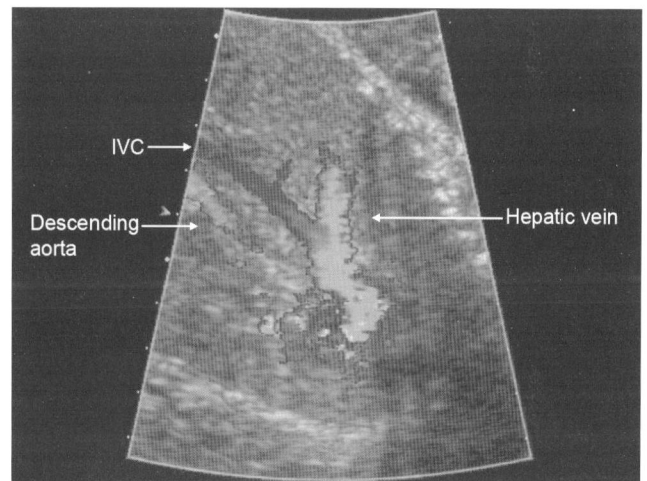

Fig. 55.9: Coronal section through the right hepatic lobe. The right hepatic vein and IVC merge into the subdiaphragmatic infundibulum

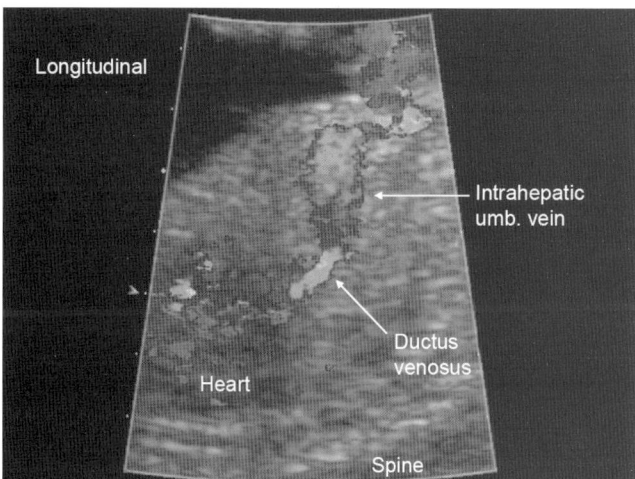

Fig. 55.7: Midsagittal section of the fetal trunk: DV is visualized in its full length arising from UV. The CDI indicates higher velocities compared with the flow in the UV—aliasing effect is present

As for the site of sampling, this is of main importance in the evaluation of fetal venous system. It has been shown that the highest velocities of the DV are at the inlet, immediately above the UV, respect to the outlet into IVC. It has been established that the inlet part of DV should be evaluated for Doppler waveform analysis.

As for the IVC, large standard deviations for various Doppler waveform variables and a mixture of overlapping signals from different bloodstreams have been shown at the subdiaphragmatic venous infundibulum. It has been established that the site of sampling is between the renal vein and DV; this is the place of the highest reproducibility.[6-9]

More than ten different angle—independent indices of the IVC and DV have been proposed and references ranges have been built (Fig. 55.13). Pulsatility index for veins and peak velocity index for vein are now commonly used for the highest correlation with adverse outcome variables such as fetal acidemia and perinatal mortality.[9-11] Even if flow volume and absolute velocity measurements can be

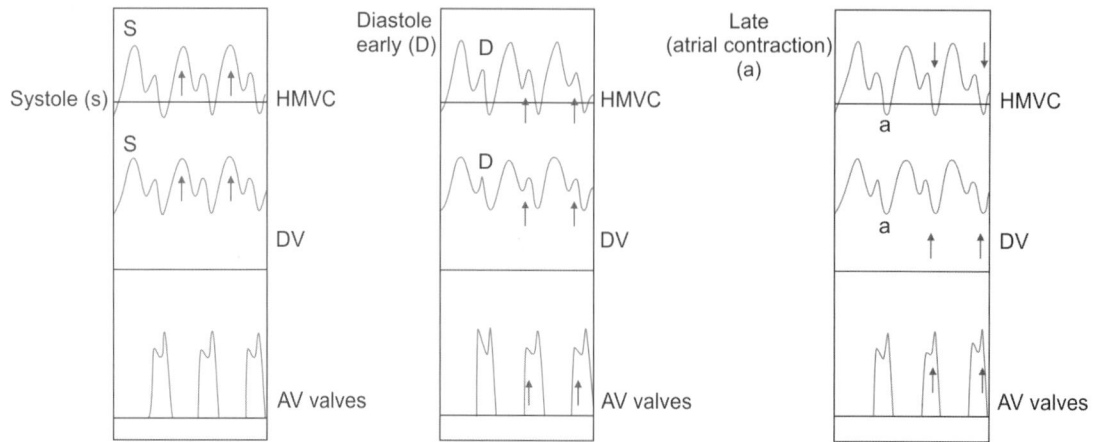

Fig. 55.10: Doppler waveform patterns in the DV, HV and IVC, and their relationship with the cardiac cycle (AV, atrioventricular valves; S, systole; D, early diastole). A physiologic reverse flow is evident in IVC/HV during atrial contraction (a).
(*Source:* With permission from Hecher K. The fetal venous circulation. In: Harrington K, Campbell S (Eds). A Color Atlas of Doppler ultrasonography in Obstetrics. pp. 71-9)

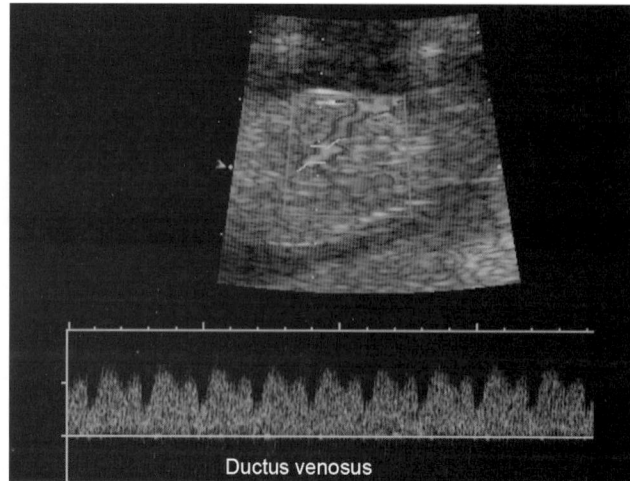

Fig. 55.11: Triphasic forward Doppler flow waveform in the DV. It is directed toward the heart through the whole cardiac cycle. A nadir of forward flow is observed during atrial contraction

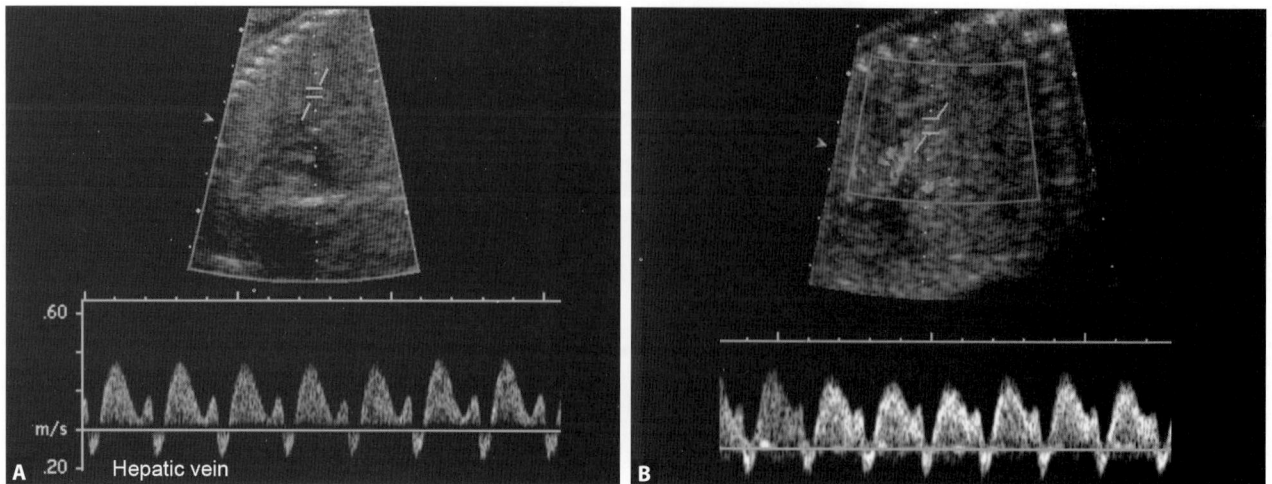

Figs 55.12A and B: Doppler flow waveforms in the HV and IVC: A physiological slight reversal flow is recorded during atrial contraction

Inferior vena cava

Ductus venosus

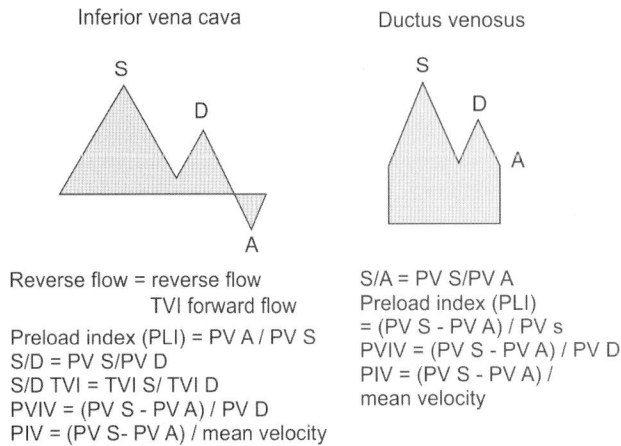

Fig. 55.13: Angle-independent indices reported in the literature for the IVC and DV.
Abbreviations: S, systole; D, diastole; A, atrial contraction; TVI, time velocity integral; PV, peak velocity; PLI, preload index; PVIV, peak velocity index for vein; PIV, pulsatility index for vein

evaluated, it has been demonstrated to have higher inaccuracy and intraobserver variation compared to qualitative ratios. This is mainly due to vulnerable errors of the evaluation of vessel diameter measurements, and unreliable or high angle of insonation.

The mean and peak velocities increase significantly in venous vessels with advancing gestational age. The highest and lowest velocities are found in the DV and right hepatic vein, respectively.

Conversely, the angle-independent indices decrease during gestation and this is consistent with a reduction in cardiac afterload due to the decrease in placental resistance. It may also reflect increased ventricular compliance. The reduction in cardiac afterload causes a decrease in end-diastolic ventricular pressure and therefore an increase in venous blood flow velocity toward the heart during atrial contraction.[10,11] As shown for arterial Doppler evaluation, from a methodological point of view, it is essential to avoid measurements during fetal breathing movements. Changes in intrathoracic pressure during breathing movements have significant effects on Doppler waveforms. Inward movement of the abdominal wall during inspiration is accompanied by an increase of blood flow velocities, whereas a decrease in velocities is evident during expiration. As the shape of Doppler waveforms shows changes during the breathing movements, indices or velocity ratios should be evaluated during fetal apnea (Figs 55.14A and B).[6,7,12]

The easiest vessel to investigate is the UV. Reference ranges for quantitative umbilical vein blood flow has been also built, according to the formulas: UV volume flow (mL/min) = Time Averaged Velocity (mm/s) × Cross-sectional vessel area (mm^2); UV absolute flow (mL/min) = vessel cross-sectional area (mm^2) × Mean velocity × 60. However, methodological differences in blood flow study have limited the quantitative evaluation of the UV in clinical practice. Qualitative analysis of the UV waveform in normal conditions shows a continuous forward flow without pulsations after the first trimester (Fig. 55.15). Mild sinusoidal pulsations synchronous with the fetal heart rate have been described in some normal fetuses between 34 weeks and 38 weeks and during fetal breathing movements (20% of the cases in the free-loop portion). These have to be distinguished

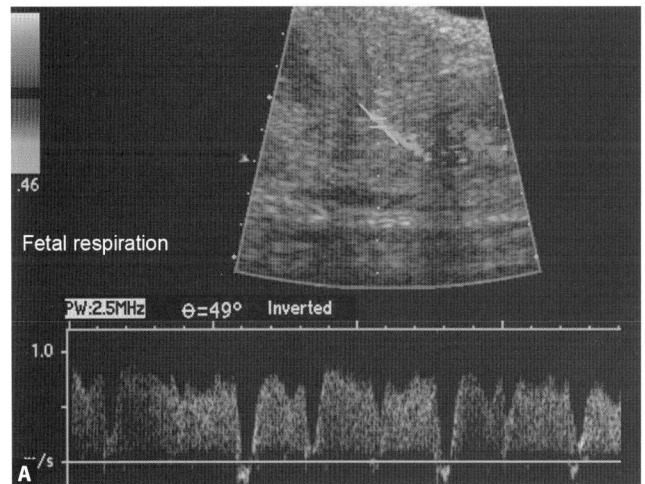

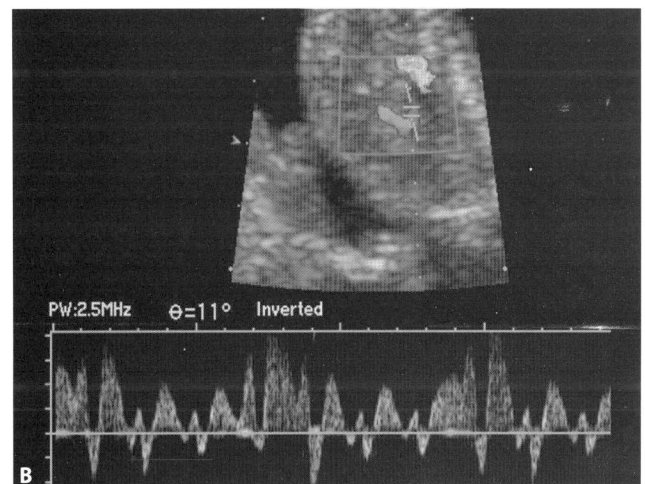

Figs 55.14A and B: Doppler flow waveforms during breathing movements in the DV and IVC

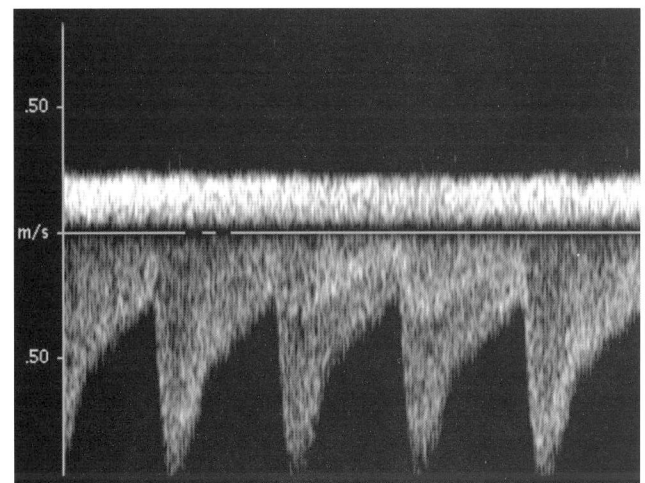

Fig. 55.15: Qualitative analysis of the UV waveform: A physiologic continuous forward flow without pulsations is observed after the first trimester

from the pathological pulsations in cases of severe fetal compromise and nonimmune hydrops (Fig. 55.16).[6,13-15]

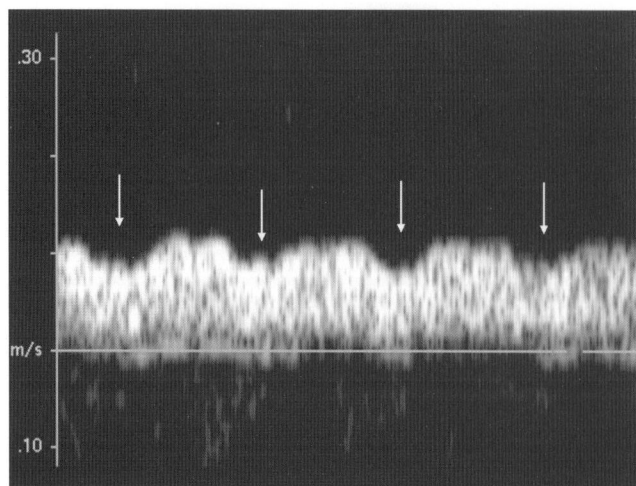

Fig. 55.16: Umbilical vein pulsations with notches synchronous with atrial contractions. Diphasic pulsations due to the increased central venous pressure and/or opening of the DV may be secondary to congestive heart failure or imminent fetal hypoxemia/acidemia

STRUCTURAL ANOMALIES OF THE FETAL VENOUS SYSTEM

A short review of the embryologic landmarks has been given in order to understand the fetal venous system structural anomalies (section 2 of this chapter).

The abnormal development of fetal venous vessels may be related to either of two different pathogenesis: the primary failure to transform or to form the critical anastomoses and the secondary occlusion of an already transformed system.

Four major groups of anomalies can be identified on the basis of the etiology (primary or secondary), the vessel involved and the embryologic precursor (Table 55.1):

1. Abnormal connection of the cardinal veins
2. Abnormalities of the UV
3. Abnormalities of the vitelline veins
4. Anomalous pulmonary venous connection (not discussed in this chapter).

Table 55.1: Classification of fetal venous system anomalies

A. *Cardinal Veins*
   a. Complex malformations, heterotaxy syndrome
   b. Isolated malformation
B. *Umbilical veins*
   a. Primary failure to create critical anastomoses
     • Complete: Abnormal connection of UV (venosus shunts) into iliac vein, IVC, SVC and right atrium
     • Partial: Persistent of right umbilical vein (PRUV) with or without DV
   b. Secondary occlusion
C. *Vitelline veins*
   a. Primary failure to create critical anastomoses
     • Complete agenesis of portal system
     • Partial agenesis of right or left portal branch (portosystemic shunt)
D. *Anomalous pulmonary venous connection (total or partial)*

(*Source:* Reprinted with permission from Fasouliotis et al.[3])

Anomalies of the fetal venous system may be also classified simply considering either:

1. The abnormalities of the caval venous system, or
2. The anomalies of umbilical, portal and hepatic veins.

The abnormal connections of the cardinal veins are part of the heterotaxy syndromes.

An interrupted or absent IVC with azygos vein continuation or the persistence of left SVC are the result of primary failure to create the anastomoses in embryologic period and may be a sign of cardiosplenic syndromes.

The anatomical correlations of aorta to IVC and the spine, and the venous connections to the atria are very helpful to diagnose left and right atrial isomerism. In situs solitus the aorta is located to the left of the spine, whereas in situs inversus the location is reversed. In right isomerism the aorta and IVC are on the same side of the spine, either right or left. Aplasia of the spleen should be a sign of right isomerism. In the left isomerism the aorta runs medial to the spine, the IVC is not identified and the azygos vein runs dorsal and lateral to the aorta, either on the right or on left side. In this subtype of heterotaxy syndrome, multiple spleens are usually present. A situs ambiguus is a common finding in both types of isomerism: the stomach can be in a left or right, or medial position. The position of the liver can be variable, as well.[2-4,6,16,17]

Abnormalities of the IVC and SVC are often associated with major impairments of the heart development, intestinal tract and body symmetry, influencing significantly the prognosis.[2-4,6]

The anomalies of the umbilical veins represent the major and most common group of the fetal venous system structural anomalies.

Primary failure to form the critical anastomoses results with an aberrant vessel that shunts the blood flow from the placenta to the systemic veins. This spectrum of anomalies may involve the iliac vein, the IVC or SVC, or the direct connection with the right atrium. Agenesis of DV is a common feature of these groups of anomalies. Two forms may be identified.

The first one is represented by the direct connection of the UV with the systemic venous circulation, by passing the liver. This is often associated with Noonan syndrome, pleural effusion and hydrops.

The second form includes cases in which the UV is adequately connected with the portal vein, but fails to establish a communication with the persistent proximal part of the right vitelline vein. The result is a prolonged hypoperfusion of the liver that may lead to portal hypertension.[2-4,17-19]

Partial failure to form critical anastomoses in left and right veins is quite common. Persistence of the right umbilical vein (PRUV) is the most common anomaly observed. Three types may be identified:

1. The intrahepatic form (the UV is connected with the right portal vein instead of the left portal vein)
2. The RUV is connected directly to the iliac vein, IVC or right atrium
3. Both the UVs persist.[16,17]

The first type is commonly identified as an isolated finding, and is considered a benign variant, whereas the other two are often associated with complex structural anomalies, especially cardiac malformations, or signs of congestive heart failure.

The pathophysiologic mechanisms of PRUV, primary or secondary, seem to be related to occlusion by thromboembolic events arising from the placenta. Teratogenic agents have been advocated as inducing primary failure of the critical anastomoses.

The anomalies of the vitelline veins are extremely rare and only few cases have been reported in prenatal literature. Primary failure to form the critical anastomoses may lead to complete agenesis of the portal system or to partial agenesis of the right or left portal vein. In the complete form, enterohepatic circulation is shunted systemically.

Partial forms of absence of the portal system might represent a more benign form of the vitelline veins abnormalities.[2-4]

VENOUS SYSTEM DOPPLER AND FETAL DISEASES

Umbilical vein pulsations with moderate to severe notches synchronous with atrial contraction have been described as an ominous sign. They are associated with various fetal pathological conditions such as nonimmune hydrops (NIH), fetal arrhythmia, fetal congestive heart failure, placental anomalies, fetal growth restriction (FGR), absent/reverse end diastolic flow (ARED) in umbilical artery (UA) and abnormal fetal heart rate patterns.

Different pathophysiological mechanisms may lead to UV pulsations. Single pulsation, caused by changes in forward flow from the placenta, might be related to ARED flow in UA during diastole or bradycardia, umbilical cord occlusion and true knot on the cord during systole. Diphasic pulsations, due to increased central venous pressure and/or opening of the DV, can be secondary to congestive heart failure or imminent fetal hypoxemia/acidemia (Fig. 55.18).[20]

Nonimmune hydrops fetalis (NIHF) is a severe clinical condition of varying etiologies with poor prognosis. Differentiating between NIHF caused by congestive heart failure and other non-cardiac causes is essential to formulate a prognosis.

In presence of NIHF and umbilical pulsations, the right ventricular shortening fraction is significantly decreased, and abnormal venous return to the heart is consistent with decreased cardiac output, leading to congestive heart failure and poor fetal outcome.

Structural heart diseases involving ventricular outflow, with or without hydrops, are frequently associated with abnormal venous blood flow. Altered pump function with increased workload causes a decrease or even reversal blood flow during atrial contraction. In cases with tricuspid regurgitation, increased reversed phase in IVC is frequently associated to fetal hydrops. Increased central venous pressure due to regurgitant flow into the atrium can cause hydrops, which implies poor prognosis.

The diagnosis of the different types of fetal arrhythmias is possible by simultaneous waveform recordings from abdominal aorta and IVC. High-velocity reverse flow due to increased right pressure is found either in atrial contraction against a closed tricuspid valve or in tricuspid regurgitation. The first occurs during premature atrial contraction and with complete atrioventricular block, and the second during premature ventricular contraction.

Premature beats of supraventricular or ventricular origin can be differentiated depending on the characteristic differences in blood flow velocity waveforms of the venous vessels (IVC) during atrial contraction. During premature beats of atrial origin an exaggerated reverse flow is recorded earlier than expected during the heart cycle. In cases of premature beats of ventricular origin, the reverse flow is evident at the moment of end-diastole, with a typical lag pattern in blood flow velocity after ventricular premature beat.[6-20]

Venous Doppler analysis is also essential to manage supraventricular tachycardia. From the observation of venous flow patterns (IVC, DV), it is possible to delay antiarrhythmic treatment if the heart rate is below 210 beats/min. Above this critical heart rate frequency, an abnormal monophasic forward flow is observed in DV and IVC. This pattern is related to direct impediment of diastolic filling causing elevation of atrial and venous pressure. Due to the presence of a parallel fetal flow circuitry, the increase of the left atrial pressure leads to right side congestive heart failure and ventricular dysfunction.[6,21,22]

Fetuses with intrauterine growth restriction (IUGR) are usually delivered on the basis of abnormal results of nonstress tests such as fetal heart rate (FHR) monitoring, biophysical profile or the presence of maternal pathological conditions. Although introduction of arterial Doppler ultrasound evaluation has resulted in a significant decrease in perinatal mortality and morbidity, the transition between adaptation and decompensation due to fetal hypoxemia/acidemia is difficult to identify accurately.

The decision regarding the optimal time of delivery, to avoid iatrogenic delivery of a mild affected premature neonate before irreversible asphyxia-related damage, is still a dilemma. The arterial multivessel evaluation (umbilical artery, descending aorta, middle cerebral artery) is commonly used in clinical practice to assess fetal well-being in high risk pregnancy. However, this assessment has a limited value in determining the time of delivery.[6,23-28]

Although maximal decrease in vascular cerebral resistance has been found to precede the onset of late decelerations by an average of 2 weeks, it has been insuitable to monitor IUGR fetuses closely during the last 2 weeks preceding the occurrence of acute distress or intrauterine death.

The Doppler study of the fetal venous blood flow in IVC and DV, and other venous vessels (sinus transversus, right hepatic vein) have raised new expectations by investigating fetal hemodynamic changes more accurately.

Two mechanisms can be considered for the onset of abnormal venous Doppler waveform: the increase of right ventricular afterload, and the myocardial failure. As long as the fetus is able to compensate for reduced placental supply by redistribution, preferential myocardial oxygenation delays the development of right heart failure, despite an increasing afterload. Progressive changes in fetal venous circulation may indicate failure of the compensatory mechanism and herald the development of right heart failure due to myocardial hypoxemia.[6,9,10]

It has been shown that evaluation of Doppler venous waveforms are correlated to computerized analysis of FHR monitoring; reverse flow in DV is significantly correlated with values of short term variation below 3.5 ms, ominous sign of hypoxemia/acidemia (Fig. 55.17).[29,30]

Recent studies are focusing on the role of fetal venous Doppler evaluation, combined or integrated with other methods of fetal surveillance, such as biophysical profile and computerized cardio-tocography, in the timing of delivery and the physiopathological sequence of the deterioration. Besides promising results, it has not been yet assessed what is the best method for timing the delivery of preterm severe IUGR fetuses.[30-32]

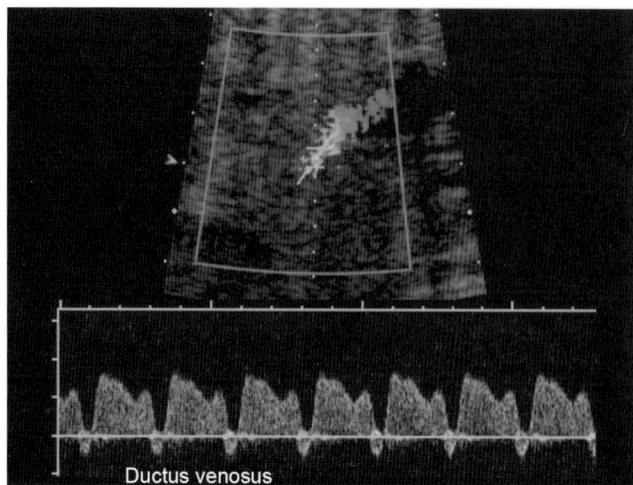

Fig. 55.17: Abnormal DV waveform: reversal flow during atrial contraction is the consequence of increased end-diastolic pressure

The widely held view that, in any case, venous Doppler abnormalities would precede deterioration of biophysical parameters has not been observed.

Ferrazzi et al.[30] reported that more than 50% of the fetuses delivered because of an abnormal FHR pattern did not have venous Doppler abnormalities.

Hecher et al.[31] observed that among fetuses born before 32 weeks of gestation, persistent abnormalities in FHR tracings preceded the occurrence of an abnormal DV pulsatility index in about 53% of the cases, and simultaneous anomalies were detected in 5% of the cases.

Muller et al.[27] found that absent/reverse flow in DV in a group of cases with umbilical artery ARED flow was significantly predictive of poor outcome. Delivery was indicated by nonreassuring status defined as either cardiotocographic (CTG) pathological pattern or when suspicious FHR traces were associated with absent or reverse in DV flow during atrial contraction. However it is not indicated how many cases of normal DV Doppler flow waveforms were delivered for abnormal CTG pattern.

Baschat et al.[32] reported that the deterioration of arterial/venous parameters occurred before an abnormal biophysical profile within 24 hours in the majority of the cases.

This data shows that hemodynamic changes of blood flow and decompensation, as detected by an abnormal FHR trace, biophysical profile or venous Doppler, are widely variable among fetuses and do not follow a predictable physiopathological cascade. It has been postulated that many variables have to be considered in the clinical practice. It has been shown that gestational age has a significant impact on the predictive value of venous Doppler for the timing of delivery. Moreover, in managing cases of severe preterm IUGR it has to be considered the high risk for the sequelae of prematurity.[33]

Probably the combination of Doppler evaluation of the fetal circulation, to assess cardiac function, and biophysical parameters/computerized CTG, as reflection of central nervous system involvement, should allow more precise information about the pathophysiology and assessment of fetal growth restriction. A multicenter randomized clinical trial should be addressed to assess what is the best method of monitoring and timing the delivery of severe premature growth restricted fetuses, and actually two ongoing trials, GRIT (Growth Restriction Intervention Trial) and TRUFFLE (Trial of Umbilical and Fetal Flow in Europe) studies, might clarify this issue.[33-35]

CONCLUSION

In recent years, high resolution sonography, combined with CDI has advanced our ability to investigate the fetal venous system. These noninvasive techniques have enhanced our understanding of the fetal venous circulation in physiologic condition and provide us the possibility to evaluate circulatory changes in abnormal circumstances.

From the literature, it can be speculated that fetal venous Doppler may be a helpful diagnostic tool and may influence the management of fetal diseases such as cardiovascular pathologies, hydrops and fetal growth restriction.

As for the latter condition, the longitudinal Doppler analysis of fetal arterial and venous districts provides us essential information about the progressive deterioration that occurs in chronic hypoxemia. Even though abnormal venous Doppler has a high likelihood of perinatal mortality/morbidity, further studies are needed to clarify the role of fetal venous Doppler in the timing of delivery. The understanding of the variables that affect the physiopathological changes in severely compromised fetuses should provide us this crucial information.

REFERENCES

1. Hamilton WJ, Mossman HW. Human Embryology, 4th edition. Cambridge: Heffer; 1972. pp. 272-82.
2. Hoffstetter C, Plath H, Hansmann M. Prenatal diagnosis of abnormalities of the fetal venous system Ultrasound Obstet Gynecol. 2000;15(3):231-41.
3. Fasouliotis SJ, Achiron R. The Human fetal venous system: Normal embryologic, anatomic, and physiologic characteristics and developmental abnormalities. J Ultrasound Med. 2002;21(10):1145-58.
4. Achiron R, Hegesh J, Yagel M, et al. Abnormalities of the central veins and umbilicoportal system: Prenatal ultrasonographic diagnosis and proposed classification. Ultrasound Obstet Gynecol. 2000;16:539-48.
5. Mavrides E, Moscoso G, Caravalho JS, et al The anatomy of the umbilical, portal and hepatic venous systems in the human fetus at 14-19 weeks of gestation. Ultrasound Obstet Gynecol 2001;18(6):598-604.
6. Hecher K, Campbell S. Characteristics of fetal venous blood flow under normal and during fetal disease. Ultrasound Obstet Gynecol. 1996;7:68-83.
7. Moll W. Venous return in the fetal-placental cardiovascular system. Eur J Obstet Gynecol. 1999.
8. Hecher K, Campbell S, Snijders R, et al. Reference ranges for fetal venous and atrioventricular blood flow parameters. Ultrasound Obstet Gynecol. 1994;4:381-90.

9. Hecher K, Snijders R, Campbell S, et al. Fetal venous, intracardiac, and arterial blood flow velocities in intrauterine growth restriction: Relationship with fetal blood gases. Am J Obstet Gynecol. 1995;173:10-5.

10. Rizzo G, Capponi A, Arduini D, et al. The value of fetal arterial, cardiac and venous flows in predicting pH and blood gases measured in umbilical blood at cordocentesis in growth retarded fetuses. Br J Obstet Gynecol. 1995;102(12):963-9.

11. DeVore GR, Horenstein J. Ductus venosus index: A method for evaluation of right ventricular preload in the second trimester. Ultrasound Obstet Gynecol. 1993;3:338-42.

12. Gardiner H, Brodszki J, Marsal K. Ventriculovascular physiology of the growth-restricted fetus. Ultrasound Obstet Gynecol. 2001;18(1):47-53.

13. Ferrazzi E, Rigano S, Bozzo M, et al. Umbilical vein blood flow in growth-restricted fetuses. Ultrasound Obstet Gynecol. 2000;16(5):432-8.

14. Reed KL, Anderson CF. Changes in umbilical venous velocities with physiologic perturbation. Am J Obstet Gynecol. 2000;182(4):738-40.

15. Boito S, Struijk PC, Ursen NT, et al. Umbilical venous volume flow in the normally developing and growth-restricted human fetus. Ultrasound Obstet Gynecol. 2002;19(3):229-34.

16. Volpe P, Marasini M, Caruso G, et al. Prenatal diagnosis of ductus venosus agenesis and its association with cytogenetic/congenital anomalies. Prenatal Diagn. 2002;22(11):995-1000.

17. Jaeggi ET, Fouron JC, Hornberger LK, et al. Agenesis of the ductus venosus that is associated with extrahepatic vein drainage: Prenatal features and clinical outcome. Am J Obstet Gynecol. 2002;187(4):1031-7.

18. Cohen SB, Lipitz S, Mashiach S, et al. In utero ultrasonographic diagnosis of an aberrant umbilical vein associated with hepatic hyperechogenicity. Prenatal Diagn. 1997;17(10):978-82.

19. Baz E, Zikulnig L, Hackeloer BJ, et al. Abnormal ductus venosus blood flow: A clue to umbilical cord complication. Ultrasound Obstet Gynecol. 1999;13(3):204-6.

20. Gudmunsson S. Importance of venous flow assessment for clinical decision-making. Eur J Obstet Gynecol Reprod Biol. 1999;84(2):173-8.

21. Gembruch U, Krapp M, Germer U, et al. Venous Doppler in the sonographic surveillance of fetuses with supraventricular tachycardia. Eur J Obstet Gynecol Reprod Biol. 1999;84(2):187-92.

22. Gembruch U, Krapp M, Baumann P. Changes of venous blood flow velocity waveforms in fetuses with supreventricular tachycardia. Ultrasound Obstet Gynecol. 1995;5(6):394-9.

23. Ozcan T, Sbracia M, d'Ancona RL, et al. Arterial and venous Doppler velocimetry in the severely growth-restricted fetus and associations with adverse perinatal outcome. Ultrasound Obstet Gynecol. 1998;12(1):39-44.

24. Baschat AA, Gembruch U, Reiss I, et al. Demonstration of fetal coronary blood flow by Doppler ultrasound in relation to arterial venous and flow velocity waveforms and perinatal outcome "the heart sparing effect". Ultrasound Obstet Gynecol. 1997;9(3):162-72.

25. Tchirikov M, Rybakowski C, Huneke B, et al. Umblical vein blood volume flow rate and umbilical arterial pulsatility as "venous-arterial index" in the prediction of neonatal compromise. Ultrasound Obstet Gynecol. 2002;20(6):580-5.

26. Hofstaetter C, Gudmundsson S, Hansmann M. Venous Doppler velocimetry in the surveillance of severely compromised fetuses. Ultrasound Obstet Gynecol. 2002; 20(3):233-9.

27. Muller T, Nanan R, Rehen M, et al. Arterial and ductus venosus Doppler in fetuses with absent or reverse end-diastolic flow in the umbilical artery: Correlation with short-term perinatal outcome. Acta Obstet Gynecol Scand. 2002;22(9):786-91.

28. Baschat AA, Gembruch U, Reiss I, et al. Relationship between arterial and venous Doppler and perinatal outcome in fetal growth restriction. Ultrasound Obstet Gynecol. 2000;16(5):407-13.

29. Senat MV, Schwarzler P, Alcais A, et al. Longitudinal changes in the ductus venosus, cerebral transverse sinus and cardiotocogram in fetal growth restriction. Ultrasound Obstet Gynecol. 2000;16(1):19-24.

30. Ferrazzi E, Bozzo M, Rigano S, et al. Temporal sequence of abnormal Doppler changes in the peripheral and central circulatory systems of the severely growth-restricted fetus. Ultrasound Obstet Gynecol. 2002;19:140-6.

31. Hecher K, Bilardo CM, Stigler RH, et al. Monitoring of fetuses with intrauterine growth restriction: A longitudinal study. Ultrasound Obstet Gynecol. 2001;18 (6):564-70.

32. Baschat AA, Gembruch U, Harman CR, et al. The sequence of changes in Doppler and biophysical parameters as severe growth restriction worsens. Ultrasound Obstet Gynecol. 2001;18(6):598-604.

33. Bilardo CM, Wolf H, Stigter RH, et al. Relationship between monitoring parameters and perinatal outcome in severe, early intrauterine growth restriction. Ultrasound Obstet Gynecol. 2004;23:119-25.

34. Romero R, Kalache KD, Kadar N. Timing the delivery of the preterm severely growth-restricted fetus: Venous Doppler, cardiotocography or the biophysical profile? Ultrasound Obstet Gynecol. 2002;19(2):118-21.

35. Baschat AA. Integrated fetal testing in growth restriction: combining multivessel Doppler and biophysical parameters. Ultrasound Obstet Gynecol. 2003;21:1-8.

SECTION 6

Basic Science

H Nakano, Y Murata

56 Immunological Basic Aspects during Pregnancy: Implantation

S Saito

INTRODUCTION

Human pregnancy represents a semi allograft to the maternal host.[1] However, the semi allogeneic embryo/fetus is not rejected by the mother. When a donated embryo is transplanted to a surrogate mother, the fetus is an allograft to the mother, but the allogeneic fetus is not rejected by the mother. Pregnancy is thus a mysterious biological phenomenon. Recent studies suggest that endometrial (maternal) lymphocytes play some roles in the maintenance of pregnancy via immune mediators such as cytokines.[2] It has been postulated that tolerance to paternal antigens must be present during pregnancy. Some regulatory lymphocytes and regulatory cytokines play very important roles for preventing allograft rejection. However, these mechanisms are not so rigid. The absence of these regulatory factors is involved in multiple implantation failure, pregnancy loss and preeclampsia. The low rate of successful implantation in humans suggests that the expression of these cytokines and their biologic signals should be optimal, precise and synchronized. In recent years, accumulating evidence has emerged that many factors, including cytokines, growth factors and maternal lymphocytes, contribute to the success of embryo implantation and maintenance of pregnancy.

UNIQUE HUMAN LEUKOCYTE ANTIGEN (HLA) EXPRESSION ON TROPHOBLASTS

The mechanism for maintenance of pregnancy has been proposed (Table 56.1). Cytotoxic T cells, which induce rejection, recognize antigeneic peptides expressed on major histocompatibility antigen (MHC) class I or class II on target cells. Interestingly, villous trophoblasts lack MHC class I and class II molecules on their surface. As a result, villous trophoblasts cannot be recognized by maternal T cells, resulting in prevention of rejection.

Table 56.1: Proposed mechanism for maintenance of pregnancy

- Absence of classical MHC class I and class II molecules on trophoblasts
- Expression of HLA-C, HLA-G, and HLA-E on trophoblasts
- Expression of complement regulatory proteins on trophoblasts (CD46, CD55, and CD59)
- Fas ligand, Fas receptor system
- Immunosuppressive factors (α_2 glycoprotein, AFP, and TGF-β)
- uNK (CD16-CD56^{bright} NK cells) (GMG cells in mice)
- Cytokines (Th2-type cytokines) and hormones
- Regulatory T cells (CD4$^+$CD25$^+$ T cells, Th3, Tr1)
- Regulatory NK cells (NK3, NKr1)

Natural killer (NK) cells are lymphocytes of the innate immune system that are involved in the early defences against foreign cells.[3] NK cell activation is controlled by a dynamic balance between complementary and antagonistic pathways. NK cells express an array of activating cell surface receptors that can trigger cytolytic programs, as well as cytokine or chemokine secretion. NK cells also express cell surface inhibitory receptors that antagonize activating pathways through protein tyrosine phosphatases. The classical MHC class I molecules HLA-C, and the nonclassical class I molecules HLA-E and HLA-G, interact with inhibitory receptors, such as killer-cell immunoglobulin-like receptors (KIRs) and CD94/NKG2. A wide range of MHC class I molecules such as HLA-G also bind ILT2 and ILT4, which are members of the immunoglobulin-like transcript (ILT) family. Interestingly, extravillous trophoblasts, which invade the uterus, express HLA-C, HLA-E and HLA-G.[3] Maternal NK cell-cytotoxic activity is suppressed by inhibitory receptors resulting in the fetus being protected from maternal NK cell attack. A unique characteristic of HLA-G is the generation of multiple spliced variants. Alternative splicing of the HLA-G mRNA yields different membrane-bound and soluble isoforms. Interestingly, soluble HLA-Gs which is produced by villous trophoblasts, is an immunosuppressive molecule inducing apoptosis of activated CD8$^+$ T cells and down-modulating CD4$^+$ T cell proliferation.[4] Therefore, soluble HLA-G probably plays very important roles in the maintenance of pregnancy at the feto-maternal interface. Soluble HLA-G may also contribute to the control of implantation. It has been reported that human implantation was strictly related to soluble HLA-G secretion by pre-implantation embryos.[5] Fuzzi et al. reported that after in vitro fertilization (IVF) or intracytoplasmic sperm injection (ICSI), only transfer of embryos secreting HLA-G could lead to pregnancies. In contrast, no pregnancy occurred after transfer of soluble HLA-G-negative embryos. Soluble HLA-G appears to be a key molecule at the time of implantation, and in early and late placentation.

EXPRESSION OF COMPLEMENT REGULATORY PROTEINS ON TROPHOBLASTS

Activation of a complement promotes cell lysis mediation by the membrane attack complex (MAC). Complements also bind and attack self tissues, especially in areas of inflammation. However, cells are protected from the deleterious effects of complement activation by complement regulatory proteins such as CD46 (MCP), CD55 (DAF), CD59 and Crry. Crry, present only in rodents, regulates the deposition of activated C3 and C4 on the surface of autologous cells. Decreased expression of complement regulatory molecules has been found in different inflammatory disorders. Complement activation is regulated by excessive expression of complement regulatory proteins on trophoblasts. However, complement deposition is recognized at the feto-maternal interface in miscarriage cases. Survival of Crry[-/-] embryos was compromised because of complement deposition and concomitant placental inflammation.[6] Interestingly, breeding with C3[-/-] mice rescued Crry[-/-] mice from lethality, suggesting that the regulation of complements is critical in fetal control of the maternal process that mediates tissue damage.[6]

In humans, antiphospholipid syndrome (APS) is characterized clinically by fetal loss and thrombosis, and serologically by the presence of autoantibodies to lipid-binding protein. Recent data suggested that complement activation, especially C5a and C5R interaction, is necessary for thrombosis of the placental vasculature.[7] APS is generally treated with anticoagulation therapy. Recent studies demonstrated that treatment with heparin prevented complement activation in vivo and in vitro and protected mice from pregnancy complications induced by antiphospholipid antibodies.[8] These data suggest that inhibition of complement activation is essential for maintenance of pregnancy.

FAS/FAS LIGAND (FAS L) SYSTEM

The Fas/Fas L pathway plays a critical role in promoting apoptosis and regulation of immune responses. The Fas/Fas L system appears to contribute to the immune privilege of the maternal-fetal interface. The maternal decidua and fetal trophoblasts express Fas L, and expression might prevent trafficking of reactive maternal cells into the fetal circulation and vice versa. T cells specific for fetal antigens (Ags) decrease in an Ag-specific manner during pregnancy, consistent with clonal deletion in the maternal immune system. Placental trophoblasts which express Fas L can induce Fas-mediated death of maternally activated T cells, and this clonal deletion is one mechanism of tolerance to the fetal allograft.[9] The Fas/Fas L system also plays important roles in implantation. Embryonic trophoblasts and maternal decidua produce corticotropin-releasing hormone (CRH) and CRH induces Fas L expression.[10,11] Female rats treated with a CRH receptor type 1 antagonist, antalarmin, showed a marked decrease in implantation sites and live embryos, along with diminished endometrial Fas L expression. Embryos from mothers that lacked T cells or from syngeneic matings were not rejected when the mothers were given antalarmin.[10] These data suggest that locally produced CRH promotes implantation and maintenance of early pregnancy by killing activated T cells.

TH1/TH2 BALANCE DURING PREGNANCY

The blastocyst and maternal endometrium develop an exquisite dialogue during the implantation window. Successful embryo implantation requires the synchronization of embryo development and uterine preparation. In mice, this period begins at day 3 and is complete by day 5 (Fig. 56.1). Pseudopregnancy at day 2 in mice does not represent the receptive phase for implantation of embryos. Takabatake et al. reported that in recipient pseudopregnant mice injected intravenously with splenocytes or culture supernatant on day 2, blastocyst transfer was formed on day 2.[11] The successful implantation rate was markedly higher in the pregnancy day 4- and day 8 splenocytes-injected groups. They further clarified that a significant increase in the implantation rate was observed when pregnancy day 4- CD4[+] T cells were injected into the uterus. These data suggest that CD4[+] T cells during early pregnancy could contribute to changing the implantation window and increase the chance of implantation.

T cells can be classified into CD4[+] T cells and CD8[+] T cells by their surface markers (Fig. 56.2). CD4[+] T cells are also classified into Th1 cells, which produce IL-2, IFN-g and TNF-b, and Th2 cells which produce IL-4, IL-5 and IL-13. Th1 cells are involved in cellular immunity such as rejection or cytotoxic T cell responses. On the other hand, Th2 cells are involved in immunoglobulin production. Based on these findings, Wegmann et al. hypothesized that physiological protection from maternal rejection is due to a Th2-type response at the materno-fetal interface.[12] In a mouse model, Th1 cells induced miscarriage and implantation failure. However, in humans, the peripheral blood Th1/Th2 balance in normal pregnancy is controversial, because the amplitude of this balance is very small in peripheral blood. On the other hand, the Th1/Th2 ratios in the endometrium or decidua change dramatically during the menstrual cycle and pregnancy. For example, it has been reported that the Th1/Th2 ratio was 147.5 during the proliferative phase of the endometrium, 37.4 during the secretory phase and 1.3 in early pregnancy decidua.[13] Furthermore, the numbers and population of Th2 cells are increased at the decidua basalis compared to those at the decidua parietalis, suggesting that Th2 cells accumulate at the implantation site.[14]

Hill et al. first reported that Th1 type immunity is present in women with recurrent pregnancy loss, and Piccinni et al. first reported defective production of Th2 cytokines by decidual T cells in unexplained recurrent spontaneous abortion. Michimata et al. first reported decreased Th2 cells in the decidua basalis in recurrent spontaneous abortion with normal embryo, although accumulation of Th2 cells was observed in the decidua basalis in recurrent

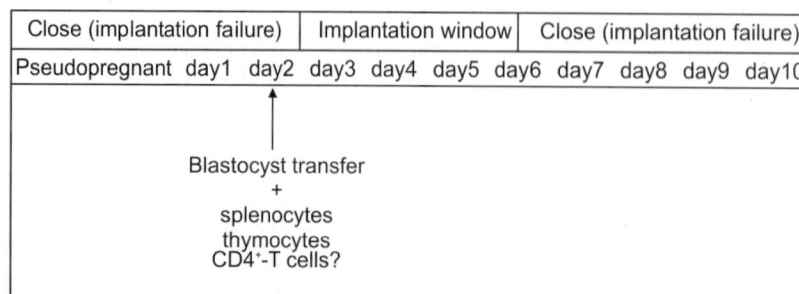

Close (implantation failure)	Implantation window	Close (implantation failure)
Pseudopregnant day1 day2 day3 day4 day5	day6 day7 day8	day9 day10

Blastocyst transfer
+
splenocytes
thymocytes
CD4[+]-T cells?

Fig. 56.1: Implantation window in mice

spontaneous abortion with abnormal chromosomal content.[15] These data suggested that accumulation of Th2 cells at the decidua basalis is important in maintaining pregnancy.

REGULATORY T CELLS IN PREGNANCY

Recent data demonstrated that immunoregulatory activity specific for donor alloantigens is enriched in the CD4+CD25+ regulatory T (Treg) cell population (Fig. 56.2). CD4+CD25+ Treg cells play a critical role in peripheral tolerance, transplantation tolerance and maternal tolerance to the fetus. The population of CD4+CD25+ Treg cells increase in iliac lymph nodes, inguinal lymph nodes, in the spleen, in decidua, and in blood, and these cells suppress alloreactive proliferation in vitro.[16,17] Alubihare et al. injected 2×10^7 lymphocytes or an equal numbers of cells from a CD25-depleted cell preparation (CD25-) into BALB/C nu/nu mice that lacked T cells.[16] All recipient BALB/C nu/nu female mice were mated with C57BL/6 male mice on the day after adoptive transfer. As a result, all the fetuses were aborted in allogeneic pregnancy when CD25-cells were injected, while this treatment did not induce fetal resorption in syngeneic pregnancy. These findings suggest that CD25+ cells, perhaps CD4+CD25+ T cells, mediate maternal tolerance to the fetus.

In human pregnancy, CD4+CD25bright Treg cells are increased in the early pregnancy decidua, but this elevated CD4+CD25bright Treg cell ratio decreases to a non-pregnancy level in miscarriage cases.[17] Therefore, CD4+CD25+ Treg cells are crucial to the maintenance of tolerance in pregnancy. Recently, Polanczyk et al. reported that estrogen augmented Foxp3 expression, which is an essential factor for the development of CD4+CD25+ Treg cells, and that treatment with estrogen increased the CD4+CD25+ Treg cell number in mice.[18] Estrogen might promote maternal tolerance to the fetus by increasing the number of CD4+CD25+ Treg cells.

INDOLEAMINE 2,3-DIOXYGENASE (IDO) EXPRESSION DURING PREGNANCY

Indoleamine 2,3-dioxygenase (IDO) is an enzyme for tryptophan catabolism and it is expressed in the blastocyst, syncytiotrophoblasts, extravillous trophoblasts, macrophages and endometrial gland cells. Pharmacologic inhibition of IDO activity resulted in dramatically decreased rates of successful allogeneic pregnancy due to maternal T cell response to fetal alloantigens.[19] IDO is a key immunosuppressive mechanism in normal pregnancies, although IDO-deficient mice can become pregnant and do not abort.

Cytotoxic T lymphocyte-associated antigen 4 (CTLA-4) plays a critical role in peripheral tolerance, and it is well known that CD4+CD25+ Treg cells express CTLA-4 on their surfaces. Interestingly, CTLA-4 induces IDO enzyme activity in dendritic cells and regulates tryptophan catabolism.[20] These findings suggest that decidual CD4+CD25+ Treg cells, which express CTLA-4 on their surface, interact with dendritic cells. As a result, these signals enhance IDO activity resulting in maintenance of pregnancy. The cross talk between CD4+CD25+ Treg cells and the IDO enzyme may induce successful pregnancy.

CYTOKINE PROFILE IN DECIDUAL NATURAL KILLER (NK) CELLS

The Th1/Th2 paradigm has been further developed. T cell subsets which produce the immunoregulatory cytokines IL-10 and TGF-b have been clarified. Th3 cells predominantly produce TGF-b, while Tr1 cells predominantly produce IL-10. They achieve immunoregulation via their cytokine production. NK cells also classified into NK1, NK2, NK3 and NKr1 cells by their cytokine profiles (Fig. 56.3).

It is well known that NK cells are the main population of lymphocytes in early pregnancy decidua. NK cells can be classified into CD16+CD56dim NK cells and CD16–CD56bright NK cells. The main population of peripheral blood NK cells is CD16+CD56dim NK cells, whereas the main population of endometrial and decidual NK cells is CD16–CD56bright NK cells. In the peripheral blood of non-pregnant subjects, IFN-g-producing CD16+CD56dim NK cells and CD16-CD56bright NK cells are the main populations. After pregnancy, the populations of IL-10-producing NKr1 cells in peripheral blood CD16+CD56dim NK cells and CD16- CD56bright NK cells increase, although, these populations decrease in miscarriage cases.[21] In the early pregnancy decidua, the main populations of CD16+CD56dim NK cells and CD16-CD56bright NK cells are TGF-b-producing NK3 cells, and NK3 cells in decidua are decreased in miscarriage cases.[21] Decidual CD16-CD56bright NK cells produce a variety of cytokines such as M-CSF, GM-CSF, G-CSF, LIF and angiopoietin. M-CSF and GM-CSF induce the DNA synthesis of trophoblasts, and LIF is an essential cytokine for implantation. Angiopoietin play an important role in angiogenesis. These findings suggest that NK cells in the decidua play some important roles in the maintenance of pregnancy by regulation of maternal immune function, placental growth and angiogenesis at the feto-maternal interface.

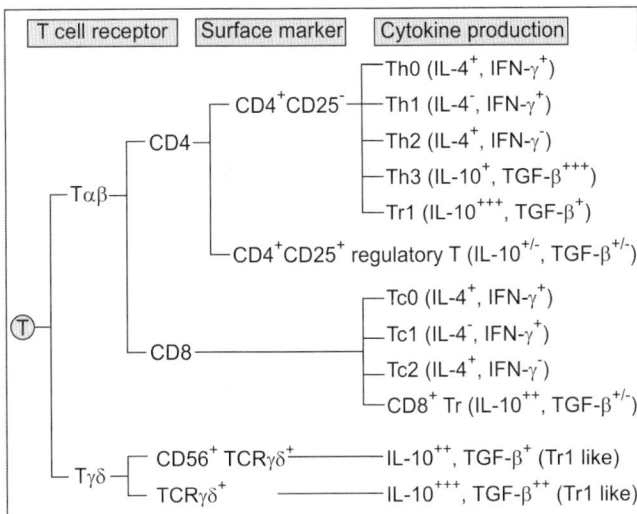

Fig. 56.2: T cell subsets classified by their surface markers and cytokine profiles

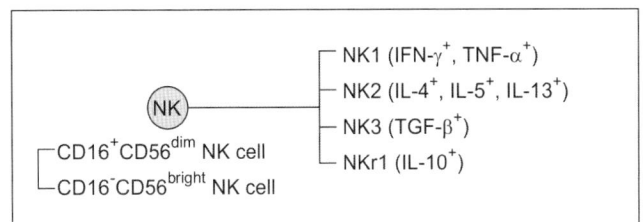

Fig. 56.3: NK cell subsets by their cytokine profiles

CONCLUSION

The immune environment, including the cytokine profile or lymphocyte subsets in the endometrium, clearly change during implantation and pregnancy. These dramatic and synchronized changes are present at the local implantation site. A better understanding of these sequential events could improve clinicians' ability to treat disorders related to these processes, including infertility and early pregnancy loss.

REFERENCES

1. Medawar PB. Some immunological and endocrinological problems raised by the evolution of viviparity in vertebrates. Symp Soc Biol. 1953;7:320-38.
2. Saito S. Cytokine cross-talk between mother and the embryo/placenta. J Reprod Immunol. 2001;52:15-33.
3. Moffett-King A. Natural killer cells and pregnancy. Nat Rev Immunol. 2002;2:656-63.
4. Bouteiller PL, Legrand-Abravanel F, Solier C. Soluble HLA-G1 at the materno-fetal interface. Placenta. 2003;24(Suppl A):S10-S5.
5. Fuzzi B, Rizzo R, Criscuoli L, et al. HLA-G expression in early embryos is a fundamental prerequisite for the obtainment of pregnancy. Eur J Immunol. 2002;32:3113-5.
6. Xu C, Mao D, Holers VM, et al. A critical role for murine complement regulator Crry in fetomaternal tolerance. Science. 2000;287:498-501.
7. Girardi G, Berman J, Redecha P, et al. Complement C5a receptors and neutrophils mediate fetal injury in the antiphospholipid syndrome. J Clin Invest. 2003;112:1644-54.
8. Girardi G, Redecha P, Salmon JE. Heparin prevents antiphospholipid antibody-induced fetal loss by inhibiting complement activation. Nat Med. 2004;10:1222-6.
9. Jiang SP, Vacchio MS. Multiple mechanisms of peripheral T cell tolerance to the fetal "allograft". J Immunol. 1998;160:3086-90.
10. Makrigiannakis A, Zoumakis E, Kalantaridou S, et al. Corticotropin-releasing hormone promotes blastocyst implantation and early maternal tolerance. Nat Immunol. 2001;2:1018-24.
11. Takabatake K, Fujiwara H, Goto Y, et al. Intravenous administration of splenocytes in early pregnancy changes the implantation window in mice. Hum Reprod. 1997;12:583-5.
12. Wegmann TG, Lin H, Guilbert L, et al. Bidirectional cytokine interactions in the maternal-fetal relationship: Is successful pregnancy a TH_2 phenomenon? Immunol Today. 1993;14:353-6.
13. Saito S, Tsukaguchi N, Hasegawa T, et al. Distribution of Th1, Th2 and Th0 and the Th1/Th2 cell ratios in human peripheral and endometrial T cells. Am J Reprod Immunol. 1999; 42:240-5.
14. Michimata T, Tsuda H, Sakai M, et al. Accumulation of CRTH2-positive T-helper 2 and T-cytotoxic 2 cells at implantation sites of human decidua in a prostaglandin D_2-mediated manner. Mol Hum Reprod. 2002;8:181-7.
15. Michimata T, Sakai M, Miyazaki S, et al. Decrease of T-helper 2 and T-cytotoxic 2 cells at implantation sites occurs in unexplained recurrent spontaneous abortion with normal chromosomal content. Hum Reprod. 2003;18:1523-8.
16. Alubihare VR, Kallikourdis M, Betz AG. Regulatory T cells mediate maternal tolerance to the fetus. Nat Immunol. 2004;5:266-71.
17. Sasaki Y, Sakai M, Miyazaki S, et al. Decidual and peripheral blood CD4+CD25+ regulatory T cells in early pregnancy subjects and spontaneous abortion. Mol Hum Reprod. 2004;10:347-53.
18. Polanczyk MJ, Carson BD, Subramanian S, et al. Estrogen drives expansion of the CD4+CD25+ regulatory T cell compartment. J Immunol, 2004;173:2227-30.
19. Munn DH, Zhou M, Attwood JT, et al. Prevention of allogeneic fetal rejection by tryptophan catabolism. Science. 1998;281:1191-3.
20. Grohmann U, Orabone C, Fallarino F, et al. CTLA-4-Ig regulates tryptophan catabolism in vivo. Nat Immunol. 2002;3:1097-101.
21. Higuma-Myojo S, Sasaki Y, Miyazaki S, et al. Cytokine profile of natural killer cells in early human pregnancy. Am J Reprod Immunol in press.

57 Placenta and Trophoblasts: Endocrinological Aspect

N Sagawa

INTRODUCTION

The production of steroid and protein hormones by human trophoblasts is the largest in amount and diversity among endocrine organs in all mammalians. A unique and obligatory interrelationship is present between the hyperestrogenic state of human pregnancy and the fetal adrenal secretion of large amount of C_{19} steroids, which serve as precursors for estrogen synthesis in the placenta. Human syncytiotrophoblast takes up maternal plasma low-density lipoprotein (LDL) cholesterol as a substrate for progesterone biosynthesis in the placenta.

The human placenta also synthesizes an enormous amount of protein and peptide hormones including human chorionic gonadotropin (hCG), human chorionic somatomammotropin (hCS), chorionic adrenocorticotropin (ACTH) and others.

STEROIDOGENESIS IN THE FETOPLACENTAL UNIT

Steroid Formation

Estrogen

The placenta is an incomplete steroid-producing organ. It must rely on precursors reaching it from the fetal and maternal circulations. The unique interdependence of fetus, placenta and mother arose the concept of an integrated fetoplacental-maternal unit.[1] The individual adult steroid-producing glands are capable of the formation of progestins, androgens and estrogens, but this is not true of the placenta. There is a constant interplay of fetus, placenta and mother to form the bulk of the sex steroids in pregnancy.[1] For estrogen formation by the placenta to occur, precursors must reach it from both the fetal and maternal compartments, whereas placental progesterone formation is accomplished in large part from circulation maternal low-density lipoprotein cholesterol.[2] In the placenta, cholesterol is first converted to pregnenolone and then rapidly and efficiently to progesterone.[3] Production of progesterone reaches approximately 250 mg/day by the end of pregnancy, when the circulating levels are on the order of 130 ng/mL.[4] The placenta also produces estrogens by aromatization of circulating androgens. The major precursor in placental estrogen formation is dehydroepiandrosterone sulfate (DHEA-S), mainly from the fetal adrenal gland. The abundant sulfatase enzyme in the placenta converts DHEA-S to free (unconjugated) DHEA, when it reaches the placenta. DHEA is further converted to androstenedione, thereafter to testosterone, and finally to estrone and 17β-estradiol. However, the major estrogen formed in the human pregnancy is neither estrone nor estradiol but another estrogen, estriol. Estriol is not secreted by the ovary of nonpregnant women but constitutes more than 90%

of the known estrogen in pregnancy urine. Concentrations increase with advancing gestation and reach to 35–45 mg/24 hr at term.[5] Estriol is also found in the amniotic fluid and maternal circulation.[6] The concentration of estriol in the maternal circulation is between 8 ng/mL and 13 ng/mL at term.[7]

Estriol is produced by a unique biosynthetic process, which forms the interdependence of three compartments: fetus, placenta and mother (Fig. 57.1). Maternal cholesterol is transported as LDL-cholesterol to the placenta. Cholesterol is converted to pregnenolone in the placenta and fetal adrenal. Fetal adrenal further metabolizes pregnenolone to dehydroepiandrosterone sulfate (DHEA-S), which is metabolized to 16α-hydroxy DHAS by 16α-hydroxylase in the fetal liver. DHAS and 16α-hydroxy DHAS are hydrolyzed by placental sulfatase in the placenta and resulting DHA is further metabolized to estrone and estradiol, and 16α-hydroxy DHA to estriol by placental aromatase. The precursor of placental estrone and estradiol is derived from both maternal and fetal adrenals. In contrast, the precursor of estriol, 16α-hydroxy DHAS is predominantly originated from fetus reflecting fetal adrenal and liver function. Thus, increase in the maternal plasma estriol concentration in late pregnancy is the reflection of total functions and development of fetal adrenal, fetal liver and the placenta.

Sulfatase deficiency occurs in male babies at the incidence of 1/15,000 pregnancies, in which 16α-hydroxy DHAS is not hydrolyzed and is not further converted to estriol. The infant with sulfatase deficiency later develops X-linked ichthyosis.[8] Anencephalus-lacking pituitary does not secrete ACTH and then estriol production is very low, approximately 10% of normal fetus. When the fetus dies in utero the precursor of estriol is not provided from fetal adrenal and the estriol levels declines significantly.[1] However, changes in the maternal plasma or urinary estriol levels are too slow and do not reflect real time fetal viability. In Down

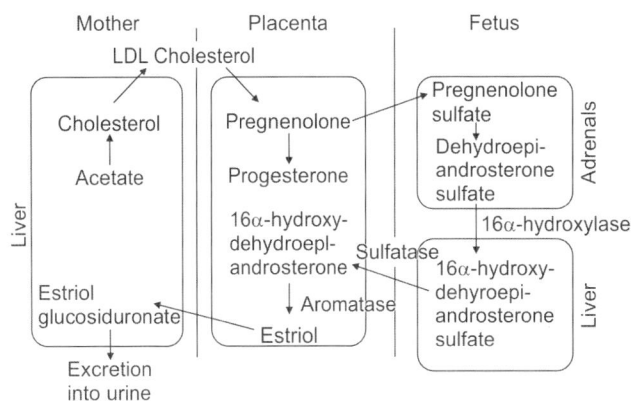

Fig. 57.1: Estriol biosynthesis in fetoplacental-maternal unit

syndrome, maternal plasma unconjugated estriol levels are low, because the production of precursor of estriol synthesis in the fetal adrenal is not adequate. Based on this fact, serum estriol levels in the late first trimester are utilized as one of serum markers of Down syndrome. Glucocorticoid administration suppresses placental estrogen synthesis because glucocorticoid suppresses ACTH secretion in both mother and fetus, and consequently decreases DHAS secretion from both maternal and fetal adrenals.

Progesterone

Placenta is the main source of progesterone in the maternal plasma.[9] Precursor of progesterone synthesis, cholesterol is predominantly derived from maternal plasma LDL cholesterol, since cholesterol synthesizing enzymes are not expressed in the placenta. Thus, progesterone synthesis is dependent on maternal and placental bioactivities but not on fetal viability.[10] This is the reason why the progesterone levels in maternal sera do not reflect acute fetal compromise as compared to that of estrogen. Placenta does not metabolize progesterone. Major part of placental progesterone is secreted to fetal circulation and further metabolized to glucocorticoids such as cortisol and aldosterone. Rest of the placental progesterone is secreted to maternal plasma. Plasma concentration of progesterone in the late first trimester is approximately 30–40 ng/mL and further increases to 130 ng/mL (secretion: 250 mg/day) which is approximately 10 times of corpus luteum production. Progesterone production in the syncytiotrophoblast during early first trimester is still low and is not enough to maintain the pregnancy. Thus, corpus luteum is necessary for the maintenance of pregnancy until 6–7 weeks of gestation. Half-life of progesterone is much more shorter than that of hCG. Therefore, plasma level of progesterone decreases much earlier than that of hCG when spontaneous termination of pregnancy occurs in early pregnancy.

Corticoids

Progesterone produced in the placenta is metabolized to either cortisol or aldosterone because fetal adrenal lacks 3β-hydroxysteroid dehydrogenase (3bHSD). Cortisol is further converted to cortisone by 11b-hydroxysteroid dehydrogenase (11bHSD) in the placenta. Cortisol level in the amniotic fluid increases as fetus maturates due to cortisol excretion into fetal urine. Maternal plasma cortisol level increases secondary to the increase in cortisol binding globulin (CBG) in maternal plasma. When uteroplacental blood flow decreases in the pregnant women complicated with pre-eclampsia, chronic hypertension or severe diabetes mellitus, blood flow in the placental intervillous space decreases resulting in the diffusion of placental steroid hormone to the fetus, increase in the steroid hormone levels in the umbilical cord. The increased cortisol might accelerate fetal lung maturation in case of fetal compromise associated with impaired uteroplacental perfusion.

Biological Function of Steroid

Estrogens

The functional role of placental estriol in pregnancy has caused a great deal of speculation. In many biologic systems, estriol is a weak estrogen. Its potency is approximately 0.01 times of estradiol and 0.1 times of estrone on a weight basis. However, estriol is reported to be as effective as other estrogens in one function—its ability to increase uteroplacental blood flow. Therefore, this may be a primary function of large amount of placental estriol. Its relatively weak estrogenic function on other organ systems may be beneficial to specifically increase uteroplacental blood flow. Although acute administration of estriol is ineffective as an estrogen and does not demonstrate extensive binding to estrogen receptors, prolonged exposure to estriol does produce estrogen effects and binding occurs. Estrogens exert their biological effect on blood flow by stimulating prostaglandin biosynthesis.[11]

Estradiol stimulates protein synthesis, cell proliferation in the endometrium, myometrium and mammary gland. It is also involved in the regulation of vascular permeability and fluid balance. The increase in blood volume and extracellular fluid volume is mediated by estrogen. Fetus is also the target of placental estrogen, and its growth and development are affected by estrogen.

Estrogens are also important for initiation of parturition at an appropriate time. Estrogen stimulates phospholipids synthesis and turnover, prostaglandin production and lysosome formation in the uterine endometrium, and modulates adrenergic mechanisms in uterine myometrium, thereby contributing to the onset of labor.[12]

Progesterone

Progesterone induces the secretory endometrium, which is required for implantation. Progesterone is also important in maintaining uterine quiescence during pregnancy by suppressing uterine smooth muscle contractility.[13] It also inhibits prostaglandin synthesis in the uterus.[14] Progesterone has also been proposed to be essential hormone of mammalian pregnancy because it inhibits T lymphocyte cell-mediated responses involved in tissue rejection.[15] In this theory, it is suggested that a high local (intrauterine) concentration of progesterone can effectively block cellular immune responses to foreign antigens. Therefore, progesterone has been aptly called the "hormone of pregnancy" because it appears to be essential for maintenance of pregnancy in all mammals examined, and its presence has been detected in species representing all classes of vertebrates. The essential nature of progesterone for pregnancy maintenance has been demonstrated by experiments in which abortion was induced after the administration of drugs that either inhibit progesterone synthesis or compete with progesterone for receptor binding or the administration of progesterone antibodies. The specificity of the abortifacient effect was demonstrated by the concurrent administration of progesterone in some of those experiments.

HUMAN CHORIONIC GONADOTROPIN

Human chorionic gonadotropin (hCG) is the earliest product of the cells which form embryo representing the first signal of the embryo even prior to implantation.[16] hCG is a glycoprotein of heterodimer with molecular weight of 36.7 kDa. It is composed of two subunits, 92-amino acids α-subunit and 145-amino acid β-subunit. The α-subunit is homologous to thyroid-stimulating hormone (THS), luteinizing hormone (LH) and follicle-stimulating hormone (FSH). The α-subunit gene is localized to chromosome 6. The β-subunit is similar to LH and the β-subunit gene is located on the chromosome 19, fairly close to the LH-β gene. In contrast to LH, hCG contains sialic acid residues, which account for its half-life (24 hours) longer than that of LH (2 hours).

Clinically, hCG can be detected in either the serum or urine 7–8 days after fertilization and is the earliest biochemical marker for pregnancy. Studies during in vitro fertilization cycle suggest that embryos expressed hCG mRNA as early as eight-cell stage but that intact hCG was not present until 8 days after egg retrieval. The increase in hCG levels between days 5 and 9 after ovum collection is principally due to free β-hCG production, while by day 22 most of the circulating hCG is in the dimmer form. After implantation, hCG is produced principally by the syncytiotrophoblast layer of chorionic villi and is secreted into the intervillous space. Cytotrophoblasts also can produce hCG.

These observations are in accordance with the in vitro studies that suggest dimmer hCG synthesis is controlled in a two-phase manner through a supply of subunits. In contrast to LH secretion in the pituitary gland, hCG is secreted constitutively as subunits are available and is not stored in secretory granules as in the case of pituitary LH.[17] The immature syncytiotrophoblast produces free β-hCG subunit while the ability to produce the α-subunit by cytotrophoblast appears to lag by several days.[18] As the trophoblast matures, the ratio of α-subunit to β-subunit reaches a 1:1 ratio, and the hCG concentration reaches a peak value of 100,000 mIU/mL around the 9–10 weeks of pregnancy. Placenta produces more α-subunit as gestation advances, and the ratio of α-subunit to hCG is approximately 10:1 at term.[19]

The doubling time of serum hCG levels during early gestation is approximately 30 hours.[20] The hCG doubling time has been utilized as a clinical marker to differentiate normal from abnormal pregnancies such as ectopic pregnancy or spontaneous abortions. When vaginal ultrasonography cannot detect intrauterine gestational sac even after the hCG levels reach 1,100–1,500 mIU/mL, an ectopic pregnancy is strongly suggested. On the other hand, higher hCG levels suggest the presence of molar pregnancy or multiple gestations.

The major biologic function of hCG during early pregnancy is to rescue corpus luteum from its premature demise while maintaining progesterone production. Until the luteal-placental shift in progesterone synthesis occurs at seventh week of pregnancy, hCG is required for rescue and maintenance of the corpus luteum. This is supported by the report that immunoneutralization of hCG results in early pregnancy failure.[21] In the explant experiment with first trimester chorionic tissue, intermittent administration of gonadotropin releasing hormone (GnRH) enhanced the pulsatile secretion of hCG from the explant tissue, implicating placental GnRH as a paracrine regulator of hCG secretion.[22] When pregnancy is not established, the corpus luteum is preprogrammed to undergo luteolysis. hCG also stimulate the production of estradiol, 17-hydroxyprogesterone and other peptides, such as relaxin, inhibin, from corpus luteum.

Ovarian progesterone is essential for maintenance of early pregnancy. When progesterone action is blocked with a competitive progesterone antagonist, such as mifepristone (RU 486), pregnancy is terminated. Removal of corpus luteum before, but not after seventh week of gestation resulted in subsequent abortion.[23,24] Removal of corpus luteum after ninth week of pregnancy had little or no influence on pregnancy. Thus, progesterone supplementation is required when corpus luteum function is compromised prior to ninth to tenth weeks of pregnancy. During later pregnancy, progesterone production in placenta is sufficient for the maintenance of pregnancy.

HUMAN CHORIONIC SOMATOMAMMOTROPIN (HCS), HUMAN PLACENTAL LACTOGEN (HPL)

Human chorionic somatomammotropin (hCS) was initially isolated in 1962 as human placental lactogen (hPL).[25] hCS has structural similarity to both pituitary human growth hormone (hGH) and prolactin (PRL). hCS is consisted of 191 amino acids with molecular weight of approximately 22 kD, and contains two disulfide bonds. It shares up to 96% homology with hGH and 67% homology with PRL.[26,27] hCS and hGH genes locate on the same portion of chromosome 17, which is consisted of five genes, two coding for hGH and three coding for hCS.[28] hCS is produced only in the syncytiotrophoblast and at a constant rate throughout gestation.[29,30] Consequently, serum hCS concentration correlate well with placental mass and viability. At term, placenta produces hCS approximately 1–4 g/day and maternal serum hCS levels range from 5 mg/mL to 15 mg/mL.

Despite the large amount of production during pregnancy, the physiological function of hCS has not fully clarified. hCS has been suggested to have major metabolic effect on the mother to ensure that the nutritional demands of the fetus are met, functioning as a growth hormone of pregnancy.[31] During pregnancy, maternal plasma glucose levels are decreased, plasma free fatty acids (FFAs) are increased, and insulin secretion is increased with resistance to endogenous insulin as a consequence of the GH-like and contra-insulin effects of hCS. Peripheral glucose uptake is suppressed in the mother but it crosses the placenta freely by a facilitated diffusion mechanism. Amino acids are transported across the placenta by an active transport mechanism against the concentration gradient. Transplacental passage of fatty acids is slow. Consequently, when the mother is in the unfed or starved state, glucose should be reserved largely for the fetus and the mother would use free fatty acids preferentially. Insulin and other protein hormones do not cross the placenta.

Regulation of placental secretion of hCS is poorly understood. Factors that regulate pituitary GH secretion are not effective in placenta. Although hCS has structural homology to hGH and PRL, it does not have growth promoting or lactogenic activity in humans.[31] There are several case reports on the healthy newborn from hCS deficient pregnancy.[32,33] Thus, it is possible that hCS is not essential for pregnancy but may serve as an evolutionary redundancy for pituitary GH and PRL. However, it remains to be clarified whether pregnancies without hCS production would have a good outcome even in the state of nutritional deprivation.

OTHER PLACENTAL PROTEIN HORMONES
Chorionic Adrenocorticotropin (ACTH)

A protein similar to pituitary adrenocorticotropic hormone (ACTH) has been isolated from the placenta. ACTH, lipotropin and β-endorphin are recovered from placental extract, presumably, from the same or similar 31 kDa precursor proopiomelanocortin (POMC).[34] It is also reported that ACTH is secreted from dispersed placental cells.[35] Dexamethasone treatment does not alter the production of ACTH in the placenta.

The physiological significance of placental ACTH is unclear. ACTH plasma levels during pregnancy are lower than in nonpregnant women; nonetheless, the concentration increases as gestation advances.[2] Placenta secretes ACTH into both maternal and fetal circulations, but it does not cross the placenta. The administration of dexamethasone to pregnant women does not suppress urinary free cortisol levels as effectively as it does in men or nonpregnant women. Corticotropin releasing hormone stimulates the synthesis and release of ACTH from chorionic tissue in vitro.[36]

Parathyroid Hormone-related Protein (PTH-rP) and Other Protein Hormones

PTH-rP is synthesized in various tissues including pregnant uterus, myometrium, endometrium and placenta. The rate of PTH secretion by the adult parathyroid is modulated by plasma Ca^{2+} concentration. PTH-rP secretion from the placenta is regulated by calcium concentration.[37]

Relaxin is also expressed in the human placenta.[38] Relaxin is synthesized as a single 105 amino acids preprorelaxin which is cleaved to form two chains A and B. Relaxin is structurally similar to insulin and nerve growth factor. Relaxin acts on myometrial smooth muscle to stimulate adenylate cyclase and to promote uterine relaxation.

Placenta produces chorionic thyrotropin, but its biological significance in normal human pregnancy is yet to be clarified.

The human growth hormone-variant (hGH-V) is expressed in the placenta but not in the pituitary.[39] The gene is located in the growth hormone-prolactin gene cluster. The variant of hGH, sometimes referred to as placental growth hormone, is a 191-amino acid protein that differs in 15-amino acids from hGH. hGH-V is synthesized in placenta, presumably in the syncytiotrophoblasts. hGH-V is present in the maternal plasma by 21–26 weeks of pregnancy, increases in concentration to about 36 weeks of pregnancy and remains relatively constant thereafter. The maternal plasma levels of hGH-V correlate well with those of insulin-like growth factor 1. Secretion of hGH-V from trophoblast is inhibited by glucose in a dose-dependent manner.[40] The biological activity of hGH-V is similar to that of hCS.

HYPOTHALAMIC-LIKE RELEASING HORMONES

Gonadotropin-releasing Hormone (GnRH)

Placenta secretes relatively large amount of GnRH.[41] GnRH is present only in the cytotrophoblast but not in the syncytiotrophoblast. Placental GnRH is suggested to act as hCG releasing hormone.[42] First trimester chorionic tissue secretes hCG in response to GnRH much more than that of term placenta.[43] Receptor for GnRH is expressed in both cytotrophoblast and syncytiotrophoblast. Trophoblast secretes inhibin and activin, and regulates GnRH production in a paracrine manner. Human placenta can also synthesize thyrotropin releasing hormone (TRH) in vitro.[44,45]

Corticotropin-releasing Hormone (CRH)

The same CRH gene expressed in hypothalamic tissues is also expressed in the trophoblast, amnion, chorion leave and decidua. Plasma levels of CRH in nonpregnant women are 15 pg/mL. Maternal plasma CRH levels increase to 250 pg/mL at early third trimester, and to 1,000 pg/mL abruptly during the last 5–6 weeks

of pregnancy.[46] After labor onset, maternal plasma CRH levels increase further to about two- to three-folds.[47] The biological function of uterine CRH including placental CRH is not clear yet. Receptors for CRH are present in many tissues including fetal adrenal, placenta and myometrium. Only very small amount of placental CRH can enter fetal circulation suggesting relatively insignificant role in fetal adrenal steroidogenesis. Large amount of CRH is secreted into maternal circulation, however, there is also a large amount of CRH-binding protein in maternal plasma. The bound form of CRH is biologically inactive and targeted for degradation. The possible biological function of placental CRH is the relaxation of both uterine and vascular smooth muscles, and immunosuppression. Physiological reverse of CRH function, the induction of myometrial contraction (i.e. the initiation of parturition by CRH) has been proposed.[48] CRH increases prostaglandin synthesis in placenta, amnion, chorion leave and decidua.[49] In the hypothalamus, glucocorticoids inhibit CRH release, however, in the trophoblast, glucocorticoids do stimulate the expression of the CRH gene, two- to three-fold increases in CRH mRNA and protein expression after treatment of human trophoblast in culture.[50] Thus, in the placenta, positive feedback loop of CRH, ACTH and glucocorticoids is proposed.[36]

Growth Hormone-releasing Hormone (GHRH)

The mRNA for GHRH has been identified in the human placenta.[51] The biological function of placental GHRH is not known.

OTHER PLACENTAL PEPTIDE HORMONES
Neuropeptide Y (NPY)

NPY, 36-amino acid peptide is originally isolated in the brain. It is also present in sympathetic neurons innervating the cardiovascular, respiratory, gastrointestinal and genitourinary systems. NPY is also expressed in the placenta and localized in cytotrophoblasts.[47] Receptors for NPY are also present in the placenta, which secrete CRH by stimulation with NPY.

Inhibin and Activin

Inhibin is a glycoprotein hormone that acts on the pituitary and inhibit FSH release. Inhibin is a heterodimer with dissimilar α- and β-subunits. The inhibin β-subunit is composed of one of two distinct peptides, βA or βB. Activin is closely related to inhibin and is formed by the combination of two β-subunits. This peptide hormone is produced by various tissues including testis, granulosa cells of the ovary and corpus luteum. The placenta can produce inhibin α-, βA-, and βB-subunits at the maximal rate at term.[52,53] Placental inhibin, in conjunction with large amount of sex steroid hormones produced in the placenta, may serve to inhibit FSH secretion and thereby block ovulation during pregnancy. Serum activin levels decline rapidly after delivery.[54] Receptors for activin are present in placenta and amnion. Inhibin may act via GnRH to regulate hCG production in placenta.[52]

Natriuretic Peptides

Atrial natriuretic peptide (ANP), 28-amino acid peptide is predominantly produced in the atrial myocytes, but is also produced in the placental trophoblast.[55] Brain natriuretic peptide (BNP), predominantly produced in the heart is also secreted from amnion cells.[56] These natriuretic peptides induce natriuresis, diuresis, and relaxation of smooth muscle. The receptors for natriuretic peptides are also expressed in the human placenta as well as in the myometrium suggesting a possible role of ANP and BNP in the uterine relaxation during pregnancy.[57]

Leptin

Maternal insulin sensitivity is regulated by various factors including placenta-derived hormones (Fig. 57.2). Several placenta-derived hormones, such as prolactin, human chorionic somatomammotropin (hCS or placental lactogen; hPL) and steroid hormones, have been considered to decrease insulin sensitivity.[58] Placental production of these hormones is increased in accordance with the increasing size of the placenta. Recently, novel peptide hormones, leptin and resistin, originally identified as adipocytokines and regulate glucose and energy metabolism have been reported to express in the human placenta.[59,60]

Leptin is initially identified as an adipocyte-derived hormone that decreases food intake and body weight via its receptor in the hypothalamus.[61] Subsequent animal studies revealed various physiological function of leptin.[62,63] Leptin plays an essential role in reproduction by regulating GnRH secretion from the hypothalamus.[64,65] It also modulates glucose metabolism by increasing insulin sensitivity and activates sympathetic nervous system.[66,67] In humans, leptin is also produced by placental trophoblasts and is secreted into both maternal and fetal circulations.[59] Leptin production in the placenta is increased in pregnancies complicated with several pathologic conditions.[68-70] Plasma leptin levels are significantly elevated in molar pregnancy.[68] Leptin gene expression in the placenta is augmented in severe preeclampsia, and maternal plasma leptin levels in severe preeclampsia are significantly higher than those in normotensive pregnant women.[69] Leptin production in the placenta is also increased in diabetic pregnancy with insulin treatment.[70] Leptin is also proposed to play a functional role in implantation by virtue of its stimulatory effect on matrix metalloproteinase expression in cytotrophoblast.[71]

Resistin

Resistin is a newly identified adipocyte-derived hormone that decreases insulin sensitivity and increases plasma glucose concentration, thus contributing the development of type II diabetes mellitus.[71] Resistin is proposed to link obesity to insulin resistance.[72]

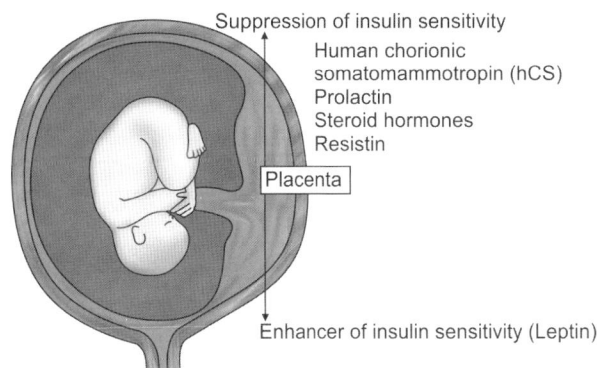

Fig. 57.2: Regulation of maternal insulin sensitivity by placental hormones

Adipocyte secretes various substances that modulate insulin sensitivity, such as free fatty acid, TNF-α and leptin. Resistin is recently cloned by Steppan et al. (2001) as a substance whose expression in the adipose tissue decreases by the treatment with thiazolidinedione, an antidiabetic drug. Thus, resistin is proposed to be a major factor that induces insulin resistance and hyperglycemia in obese person.

Northern blot analysis revealed resistin mRNA expression in term placenta as well as in the amniotic membrane.[60] Resistin mRNA expression was also detected in a trophoblastic cell line (BeWo cells) and a very faint band was detected in decidua vera tissue. In situ hybridization and immunohistochemistry suggest the expression of resistin in placental villi, mainly in syncytiotrophoblast. Resistin protein was secreted from cultured placental tissue.[60] Resistin gene expression in term placental tissue was significantly larger than that in chorionic villous tissue in the first trimester. By contrast, the resistin gene was expressed to a lesser degree in adipose tissue than in term placental tissue. Moreover, resistin gene expression in the adipose tissue of pregnant women at term did not differ from that of nonpregnant women. As resistin is supposed to induce insulin resistance and increase the plasma glucose level,[72,73] it is possible that placental resistin may contribute to regulation of maternal glucose metabolism in concert with various placental hormones including leptin (Fig. 57.2).

However, the regulatory mechanism of resistin gene expression in the human placenta is not yet elucidated. Further investigation on the effects of these hormones on the maternal glucose metabolism and insulin sensitivity may provide better understanding of the placental role in the maternal energy metabolism and fetal growth.

REFERENCES

1. Jaffe RB. Neroendocrine–metabolic regulation of pregnancy. In: Yen SS, Jaffe RB, Barbieri RL (Eds). Reproductive Endocrinology-Physiology, Pathophysiology, and Clinical Management. Philadelphia, PA: WB Saunders Company; 1999. pp. 751-84.
2. Carr BR, Parker CR Jr, Madden JD, et al. Maternal plasma adrenocorticotropin and cortisol relationship throughout human pregnancy. Am J Obstet Gynecol. 1981;139:416-20.
3. Pion R, Jaffe RB, Erickson G, et al. Studies on the metabolism of C-21 steroids in the human feto-placental unit 1. Formation of alpha, beta-unsaturated 3-ketones in midterm placentas perfused

in situ with pregnenolone and 17a-hydroxypregnenolone. Acta Endocrinol (Copenh). 1965;48:234-41.
4. Johanson EN. Plasma levels of progesterone in pregnancy measured by a rapid competitive protein binding technique. Acta Endocrinol (Copenh). 1979;61:607-15.
5. Frandsen VA, Stakeman G. The clinical significance of oestriol estimators in late pregnancy. Acta Endocrinol (Copenh). 1963;44:183-91.
6. Schindler AE, Siiteri PK. Isolation and quantitation of steroids from normal human amniotic fluid. J Clin Endocrinol Metab. 1968;28:1189-95.

7. Goebelsmann U, Chen LC, Saga M, et al. Plasma concentration and protein binding of oestriol and its conjugates in pregnancy. Acta Endocrinol (Copenh). 1973;74:592-8.

8. Bradshaw KD, Carr BR. Placental sulfatase deficiency: Maternal and fetal expressions of steroid sulfatase deficiency and X-linked ichthyosis. Obstet Gynecol Srv. 1986;68:505-9.

9. Simpson ER, MacDonald PC. Endocrine physiology of the placenta. Ann Rev Physiol. 1981;43:163-85.

10. Liu JH, Rebar RW. Endocrinology of pregnancy. In: Cresy RK, Resnik R (Eds). Maternal-Fetal Medicine, 4th Edition. WB Saunders Company, Philadelphia, PA. 1999. pp. 379-91.

11. Resnik R, Killam AP, Battablia FC, et al. Stimulation of uterine blood flow by various estrogens. Endocrinology. 1974;94:1192-8.

12. Casey ML, Winkel CA, Porter JC, MacDonald PC. Endocrine regulation of the initiation and maintenance of parturition. Clin Perinatol. 1983;10:709-25.

13. Roberts JM, Lewis VL, Riemer RK. Hormonal control of uterine adrenergic response. In: Bottari J, Thomas P, Vokser A, Vokser R (Eds). Uterine Contractility. Masson, New York, NY; 1984. pp. 161-85.

14. Cane EM, Villee CA. The synthesis of prostaglandin F by human endometrium in organ culture. Prostaglandins. 1975;281-90.

15. Siiteri PK, Ferbers F, Clemens LE, et al. Progesterone and maintenance of pregnancy: Is progesterone nature's immunosuppression? Ann NY Acad Sci. 1997;286:384-98.

16. Hay DL, Lopata A. Chorionic gonadotropin secretion by human embryo in vitro. J Clin Endocrinol Metab. 1988;67:1322-9.

17. Muyan M, Boime I. Secretion of chorionic gonadotropin from human trophoblast. Placenta. 1997;18:237-43.

18. Hay DL. Discordant and variable production of human chorionic gonadotropin and its free alpha- and beta-subunits in early pregnancy. J Clin Endocrinol Metab. 1995;61:1195-9.

19. Takemori M, Nishimura R, Ashitaka Y, et al. Release of human chorionic gonadotropin (hCG) and its alpha-subunit (hCGa) from perifused human placenta. Endocrinol Jpn. 1981;28:757-63.

20. Lenton EA, Woodward AJ. The endocrinology of conception cycles and implantation in women. J Reprod Fertil. 1988;36(Supl):1-12.

21. Stevens VG. Antifertility effects from immunization with intact subunits and fragments of hCG. In: Edwards RG, Johnson MG (Eds). Physiological Effects of Immunity against Reproductive Hormones. London: Cambridge University Press; 1975. pp. 249-64.

22. Barnea ER, Kaplan M, Naor Z. Comparative stimulatory effect of gonadotropin-releasing hormone (GnRH) and GnRH agonist upon pulsatile human chorionic gonadotropin secretion in superfused placental explants: Reversible inhibition by a GnRH antagonist. Hum Reprod. 1991;6:1063-9.

23. Csapo AI, Pulkkinen MO, Wiest WG. Effect of luteectomy and progesterone replacement therapy in early pregnant patients. Am J Obstet Gynecol. 1973;115:756-62.

24. Csapo AI, Pulkkinen MO. Indispensability of the human corpus luteum in the maintenance of early pregnancy: Luteectomy evidence. Obstet Gynecol Srv. 1978;33:69-75.

25. Josinovich JB, MacLaren JA. Presence in the human placenta and term serum of a highly lactogenic substance immunologically related to pituitary growth hormone. Endocrinology. 1962;71:209-16.

26. Bewley TA, Dixon JS, Li CH. Sequence comparison of human pituitary growth hormone, human chorionic somatomammotropin, and ovine pituitary growth and lactogenic hormones. Int J Pept Protein Res. 1972;4:281-9.

27. Cooke NE, Coit D, Shine J. Human prolactin cDNA structural analysis and evolutionary comparisons. J Biol Chem. 1981;256:4007-15.

28. Owerbach D, Rutter WJ, Martial JA. Genes for growth hormone chorionic somatomammotropin and growth hormone-like gene on chromosomes 17 in humans. Science. 1980;209:289-95.

29. McWilliams D, Boime I. Cytological localization of placental lactogen messenger ribonucleic acid in syncytiotrophoblast layers of human placenta. Endocrinology. 1980;107:761-9.

30. Hoshina M, Boothby M, Boime I. Cytological localization of chorionic gonadotropin a and placental lactogen mRNAs during development of the human placenta. J Cell Biol. 1982;93:190-8.

31. Grumbach MM, Kaplan SL, Abrams CL, et al. Plasma free fatty acid response to the administration of chorionic "growth hormone-prolactin". J Clin Endocrinol Metab. 1966;26:476-85.

32. Nielsen PV, Pedersen H, Kampmann EM. Absence of human placental lactogen in an otherwise uneventful pregnancy. Am J Obstet Gynecol. 1984;135:322-5.

33. Parks JS, Nielsen PV, Sexton LA, et al. An effect of gene dosage on production of human chorionic somatomammotropin. J Clin Endocrinol Metab. 1985;60:9948.

34. Odagiri E, Sherrill BJ, Mount CD, et al. Human placental immunoreactive corticotropin, lipotropin, and beta-endorphin: Evidence for a common precursor. Proc Natl Acad Sci USA. 1979;16:2027-35.

35. Liotta A, Osathanondh R, Ryan KJ, et al. Presence of corticotropin in human placenta: Demonstration of in vitro synthesis. Endocrinology. 1977;101:1552-8.

36. Riley SC, Walton JC, Herlick JM, et al. The localization and distribution of corticotropin-releasing hormone in the human placenta and fetal membranes throughout gestation. J Clin Endocrinol Metab. 1991;72:1001-8.

37. Hellman P, Ridefelt P, Juhlin C, et al. Parathyroid-like regulation of parathyroid hormone-related protein release and cytoplasmic calcium in cytotrophoblast cells of human placenta. Arch Biochem Biophys. 1992;293:174-81.

38. Bogic LV, Mandel M, Bryant-Greenwood GD. Relaxin gene expression in human reproductive tissues by in situ hybridization. J Clin Endocrinol Metab. 1995;80:130-9.

39. Cunningham FG, Gant NF, Leveno KJ, et al. The placental hormones. In: Williams' Obstetrics, 21st edition. New York, NY. McGraw-Hill, 2001. pp. 109-28.

40. Patel N, Alsat E, Igout A, et al. Glucose inhibits human placenta GH secretion, in vitro. J Clin Endocrinol Metab. 1995;80:1743-50.

41. Siler-Khodr TM. Chorionic peptides. In: McNellis D, Challis JR, MacDonald PC, Nathanielsz PW, Roberts JM (Eds). The Onset of Labor: Cellular and Integrative Mechanisms. An NICHD Workshop. Ithaca: Perinatology Press; 1988. pp. 213-31.

42. Siler-Khodr TM. Hypothalamic-like peptides of the placenta. Semin Reprod Endocrinol. 1983;1:321-40.

43. Currie WD, Steele GL. Luteinizing hormone-releasing hormone (LHRH) and LHRH-stimulated human chorionic gonadotropin secretion from perfused first trimester placental cells. Recent Prog Horm Res. 1993;97:71-4.

44. Gibbons JM, Mitnick M, Chieffo V. In vitro biosynthesis of THS- and LH-releasing factors by human placenta. Am J Obstet Gynecol. 1975;121:127-31.

45. Khodr GS, Siler-Khodr TM. Placental luteinizing hormone-releasing factor and its synthesis. Science. 1980;207:315-20.

46. Goland RS, Wardlaw SL, Blum M, et al. Biologically active corticotropin-releasing hormone in maternal and fetal plasma during pregnancy. Am J Obstet Gynecol. 1988;159:884-90.

47. Petraglia F, Calza L, Giardino L, et al. Identification of immunoreactive neuropeptide (gamma) in human placenta: Localization, secretion, and binding sites. Endocrinology. 1989;124:2016-20.

48. Wadhwa PD, Porto M, Garite JJ, et al. Maternal corticotropin-releasing hormone levels in the early third trimester predict length of gestation in human pregnancy. Am J Obstet Gynecol. 1998;179:1079-85.

49. Jones SA, Challis JRG. Local stimulation of prostaglandin production by corticotropin-releasing hormone in human fetal membranes and placenta. Biochem Biophys Res Commun. 1989;159:192-9.

50. Robinson BG, Emanuel RL, Frim DM, et al. Glucocorticoid stimulates expression of corticotropin-releasing hormone gene in human placenta. Proc Natl Acad Sci USA. 1988;85:5244-50.

51. Berry SA, Srivastava CH, Rubin LR, et al. Growth hormone releasing hormone-like messenger ribonucleic acid and immunoreactive peptide are present in human testis and placenta. J Clin Endocrinol Metab. 1992;75: 281-8.
52. Petraglia F, Sawchenko P, Lim AT, et al. Localization, secretion, and action of inhibin in human placenta. Science. 1987;237:187-91.
53. Petraglia F, Garuti GC, Calza L, et al. Inhibin subunits in human placenta: Localization and messenger ribonucleic acid levels during pregnancy. Am J Obstet Gynecol. 1991;165:750-5.
54. Petraglia F, Gallinelli A, De-Vita D, et al. Activin at parturition: Changes of maternal serum levels and evidence for binding sites in placenta and fetal membranes. Obstet Gynecol. 1994;84:278-82.
55. Lim AT, Gude NM. Atrial natriuretic factor production by the human placenta. J Clin Endocrinol Metab. 1995;80:30916.
56. Itoh H, Sagawa N, Hasegawa M, et al. Brain natriuretic peptide is present in the human amniotic fluid and is secreted from amnion cells. J Clin Endocrinol Metab. 1993;76:907-11.
57. Itoh H, Sagawa N, Hasegawa M, et al. Expression of biologically active receptors for natriuretic peptides in the human uterus during pregnancy. Biochem Biophys Res Commun. 1994;203: 602-7.
58. Abrams B, Pickett KE. Maternal nutrition. In: Creasy RK, Resnik R (Eds). Maternal-Fetal Medicine, 4th edition. Philadelphia, PA: WB Saunders Compan; 1999. pp. 122-31.
59. Masuzaki H, Ogawa Y, Sagawa N, et al. Nonadipose tissue production of leptin: Leptin as a novel placenta-derived hormone in humans. Nat Med. 1997;3:1029-33.
60. Yura S, Sagawa N, Itoh H, et al. Resistin is expressed in the human placenta. J Clin Endocrinol Metab. 2003;88:1394-7.
61. Zhang Y, Proenca R, Maffei M, et al. Positional cloning of the mouse obese gene and its human homologue. Nature. 1994;372:425-32.
62. Campfield LA, Smith FJ, Guisez Y, et al. Recombinant mouse OB protein: Evidence for a peripheral signal linking adiposity and central neural networks. Science. 1995;269:546-9.
63. Halaas JL, Gajiwala KS, Maffei M, et al. Weight-reducing effects of the plasma protein encoded by the obese gene. Science. 1995;269:5436.
64. Chehab FF, Lim ME, Lu R. Correction of the sterility defect in homozygous obese female mice by treatment with the human recombinant leptin. Nat Genet. 1996;12:318-20.
65. Yura S, Ogawa Y, Sagawa N, et al. Accelerated puberty and late onset hypothalamic hypogonadism in female transgenic skinny mice overexpressing leptin. J Clin Invest. 2000;105:749-55.
66. Ogawa Y, Masuzaki H, Hosoda K, et al. Increased glucose metabolism and insulin sensitivity in transgenic skinny mice overexpressing leptin. Diabetes. 1999;48:1822-9.
67. Shek EW, Brands MW, Hall JE. Chronic leptin infusion increases arterial pressure. Hypertension. 1998;31(At 2):40914.
68. Sagawa N, Mori T, Masuzaki H, et al. Leptin production by hydatidiform mole. Lancet. 1997;350:1518-9.
69. Mise H, Sagawa N, Matsumoto T, et al. Augmented placental production of leptin in pre-eclampsia: Possible involvement of placental hypoxia. J Clin Endocrinol Metab. 1998;83:3225-9.
70. Lepercq J, Cauzac M, Lahlou N, et al. Overexpression of placental leptin in diabetic pregnancy—A critical role for insulin. Diabetes. 1998;47:847-50.
71. Castellucci M, Matteis R, Meisser A, et al. Leptin modulates extracellular matrix molecules and metalloproteinases: Possible implications for trophoblast invasion. Mol Hum Reprod. 2000;6:951-8.
72. Steppan CM, Bailey ST, Bhat S, et al. The hormone resistin links obesity to diabetes. Nature. 2001;409:307-12.
73. Flier JS. The missing link with obesity? Nature. 2001;409:2923.

58 Regulation of Extravillous Trophoblast Differentiation

K Fukushima, K Tsukimori, H Nakano

INTRODUCTION

During early development, cytotrophoblast (CT) differentiation contributes to organization of the fetomaternal interface. One layer of the differentiated trophoblast, which is marked by an invasive phenotype is called extravillous trophoblast (EVT). EVT invades decidual tissue and the maternal uterine wall. Recent evidence shows that EVT invasion has a crucial role in organizing and maintaining fetoplacental circulation. In this chapter, we focus on interstitial and endovascular invasion and their regulatory mechanisms during EVT differentiation.

DIFFERENTIATION OF CYTOTROPHOBLAST

During the early phase of human pregnancy, CT cells are derived from trophoectodermal cells of the blastocyst and contribute to organization of the fetomaternal interface through cell proliferation and differentiation. Differentiation of CT proceeds by two pathways that result in morphologically and functionally distinct trophoblast populations (Fig. 58.1). One population consists of multinucleated, nonreplicating syncytiotrophoblast cells (ST), beneath which lie immature, replicating, mononuclear villous cytotrophoblast. After the blastocyst attaches to the endometrium, mononuclear CT cells that surround the embryonic disc fuse to ST to form a syncytial layer. This layer covers the intravillous space and transports nutrients, wastes, and gases between fetal and maternal blood.[1]

The other population is the extravillous trophoblast (EVT), and these cells have invasive properties. EVT cells leave the cellular column to intrude into the decidua and uterine wall, and they are observed as cytokeratin-positive cells in the decidua, the intima of the spiral arteries, and the proximal third of the myometrium. It is thought that interstitial invasion of the placental bed by EVT promotes placental anchorage. Interstitial invasion is accompanied by endovascular invasion, in which some invading EVT cells interact, resulting in replacement of endothelium and the muscular tunica of maternal vessels, including the spiral arteries. This replacement substantially decreases vascular resistance and results in increased blood flow toward the intervillous space.[2,3]

ALTERATION OF ADHESION MOLECULES DURING INTERSTITIAL INVASION

Examination of tissue sections of human placental bed biopsies shows that EVT cells switch integrin phenotype during differentiation and invasion.[4] The CT stem cells, which are anchored to the basement membrane, express α6β4 integrin. Formation of the cell column is accompanied by α5β1 up-regulation, and as EVT cells intrude into the uterine wall they express the α1β1 subunit as well as the α5β1 subunit. Generally, α6b4 staining is weak and discontinuous at the uterine wall.[4] During this normal trophoblast invasion, the extracellular matrix (ECM) undergoes a transition from laminin (Ln) to fibronectin (Fn) and collagen type IV (C4). Ln is abundant in the superficial areas that face the villous trophoblast. In contrast, C4 and Fn are more abundant at deeper sites.[4,5] Thus, it can be assumed that EVT cells alter their integrin expression in parallel with the variation in ECM distribution during invasion. Not only integrin adhesion receptors, but also E-cadherin expression, are altered during the invasive pathway.[6] Expression of E-cadherin, the cell-cell adhesion molecule, is strong in CT stem cells and weak in differentiating and invading EVT cells.[7] These findings are summarized in Figure 58.2.[7,8]

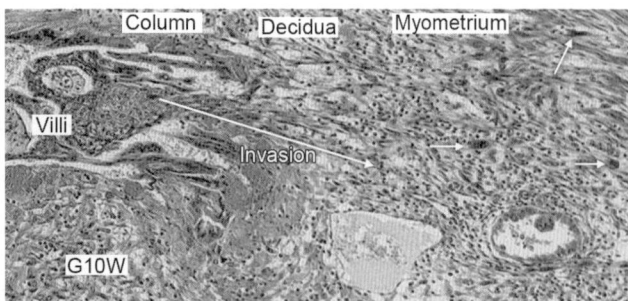

Fig. 58.1: Microscopic appearance of extravillous trophoblast in placenta in early gestation during invasion. H&E stained placental tissue from patients with cervical cancer who underwent radical hysterectomy at 10 weeks of gestation. Arrow, invaded extravillous trophoblast, arrow head, maternal vessel replaced by trophoblast

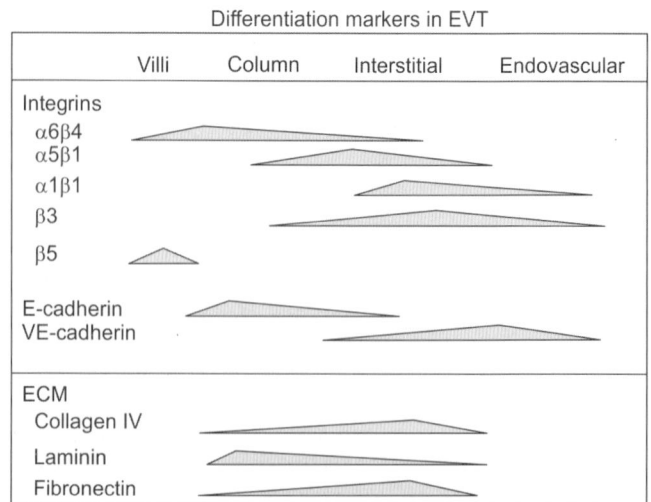

Fig. 58.2: Alteration of adhesion molecules expressed in EVT during invasion. Scheme of the alteration of integrin and cadherin expression and distribution of extracellular matrix at each placental site during invasion[8,9]

Extravillous trophoblast invasion is a biochemically active process because invading cells have to secrete proteases including serine protease, cathepsin and metalloproteinases. Matrix metalloproteinases (MMPs) have 15 family members that are classified by substrates and structure into four subgroups. The MMPs are inactivated by tissue inhibitor of metalloproteinases (TIMP). The TIMP family consists of four members: TIMP-1, -2, -3 and -4. Among all of these enzymes, MMP-2 and MMP-9 are considered to be the most important for EVT invasion.[10,11] Several pieces of evidence have shown that ECM and integrin can affect the activity of MMPs and behavior of EVT cells.[12,13] MMP-9 is upregulated at deeper sites as in the case of integrin α1β1.[14] Damsky et al.[5] investigated the effect of integrin-ECM interaction on EVT invasive properties using antibody-inhibition to matrigel invasion assay. Antibodies against Ln and C4 blocked EVT invasion. The anti-α6 antibody did not inhibit EVT invasion, whereas anti-α1 antibody did inhibit invasion. When combined, these antibodies acted synergistically. In contrast, anti-Fn antibodies stimulated rather than blocked invasion. Thus, the EVT-ECM interaction that subsequently arouses integrin conversion seems to be important in controlling EVT phenotype.

The significance for normal placentation of CT differentiation is highlighted by the fact that in preeclampsia, in which both interstitial and endovascular invasion are abnormally shallow, CT cells show significant defects in differentiation.[8,14-16] Furthermore, CT cells in women with preeclampsia increase expression of the α5β1 subunit, but fail both to upregulate α1β1 and to downregulate α6β4.[5,16] Thus, the cells appear arrested in their differentiation and express an ECM receptor phenotype that may not be optimal for invasion.[9] Taking all of these findings together, it is likely that expression of these integrin subunits is involved in regulation of normal EVT differentiation.

ALTERATION OF ADHESION MOLECULES DURING ENDOVASCULAR INVASION

Angiogenesis plays a crucial role both in normal physiological and pathological conditions including placental development. During invasion, EVT finally replaces the endothelial cells in uterine vessels. Moreover, EVT cells also intrude into the vascular muscles. This endovascular differentiation induces remodeling of spiral arteries to increase blood flow toward the intervillous space, which is covered by syncytiotrophoblast, the other form of differentiated CT. As in the case of interstitial invasion, integrin subunits expressed in EVT dramatically change. Along with endovascular differentiation, the adhesion molecule repertories change in a comprehensive manner that mimics the pattern for endothelial cells.[9] Zhou et al.[9] reported that EVT in vivo showed reduced staining for adhesion receptors characteristic of stable monolayer epithelial cells and showed enhanced staining for adhesion molecules characteristic of endothelial cells. CT in cell columns show reduced E-cadherin staining and express VE-cadherin, PECAM-1, VCAM-1 and α4-integrins. EVT cells in the uterine interstitium and maternal vessels start to express αVβ3 integrin. These molecules (αVβ3 and VE-cadherin) enhance CT invasiveness.[16] In a later report, Zhou et al. showed that preeclamptic CT does not stain for most of the endothelial-type adhesion molecules that are expressed by control CT cells.[17] Inhibitors of αVβ3 or αVβ5 show anti-angiogenic activity in many models.[18] Indeed, a humanized version of LM609, a monoclonal antibody that blocks αVβ3 signaling, has entered clinical trials for use in treatment.[19] Although genetic studies in

mice have provided several controversial points, it is believed that these integrins play an important role in angiogenesis.[20] Thus, these endothelial cell-related molecules are considered to play important roles in endovascular differentiation in EVT.

The vascular endothelial growth factor (VEGF) family members and their receptors (VEGFR) seem to have important actions during the initial stages of angiogenesis.[21] EVT cells in early gestation express VEGF-A, VEGF-C, placental growth factor (PlGF), VEGFR-1 and VEGFR-3. When binding of VEGF-A, PlGF and VEGF-PlGF heterodimer to VEGFR-1 is inhibited, tube-like formation on matrigel is impaired and expression of integrin α1β1 is decreased. This effect is enhanced when VEGF-C binding to endogenous VEGFR-3 is blocked. This result suggests that the signal from VEGFR1/3 is involved in alteration of integrin switching. The same research group also reported that CT responds to VEGF ligands by the autocrine system.[22] Dunk et al.[23] reported that angiopoietin 1 and angiopoietin 2 can act as a mitogen and stimulate nitric oxide release from first trimester trophoblast, as well as VEGF.[23-26] These angiogenic factors also influence the angiogenic state of maternal blood vessels.[27]

EFFECT OF CYTOKINES AND GROWTH FACTOR ON EVT INVASION (TABLE 58.1)

Interleukins

Interleukin-1(IL-1) increases MMP-9 secretion and stimulates MMP-9 activities.[28,29] IL-1 or its receptors are important for implantation of the blastocyst.[30] Thus, IL-1 is a positive regulator of trophoblast differentiation along the invasive pathway.[31] IL-6 activates MMP-2 and MMP-9 in trophoblasts.[32] Circulating levels of IL-6 are increased in patients with preeclampsia.[33,34] IL-10 down-regulates MMP-9 activity and EVT invasiveness. IL-15 increases EVT invasion and migration, as well as MMP-1 production by Jeg-3 cells.[35] IL-10 and IL-15 seem to regulate trophoblast invasiveness by autocrine mechanisms.[35-37] Wang et al. reported lower levels of expression of IL-8 and IL-15 in preeclamptic placentas.[38]

Transforming Growth Factor Beta (TGFβ)

Transforming growth factor beta (TGFβ) stimulates synthesis of matrix glycoproteins[39] and TIMP secretion through down-regulation of urokinase, plasmin and plasminogen activator.[40-42] TGFα inhibits cellular proliferation and migration,[37,43,44] whereas TGFα promotes EVT differentiation through the invasive pathway.[42]

Tumor Necrosis Factor Alpha (TNFα)

TNFα levels are elevated in patients with preeclampsia,[45,46] and TNFα has been shown to regulate progesterone, estradiol and human chorionic gonadotropin (hCG) production in cytotrophoblasts.[47] TNFα stimulates trophoblastic MMP-9, MMP-1 and MMP-3 production in human chorionic cells,[48] whereas TNFα decreases TIMP secretion.[32,49] TNFα induces apoptosis,[50] integrin subunit conversion and functional activation in EVT cell lines.[51]

Insulin-like Growth Factors and Relatives

Insulin-like growth factor (IGF-II) promotes trophoblast differentiation along the invasive pathway. Hamilton et al.[52] showed that IGF-II promotes cell migration. IGFBP-1 increases trophoblast cell migration,[42] invasion,[52] TIMP-1 secretion and gelatinolytic activity.[53]

Table 58.1: Summary of biological effects of soluble factors on cytotrophoblast

	Biological effect on cytotrophoblast (and/or EVT)	References
IL1	Promote invasion Increase MMP9 secretion Promote differentiation in invasive pathway	Lala, 1994; Librach, 1994 Meisser, 1999a
IL6	Increased circulating level in preeclamptic patients Activate MMP2 and 9	Conrad, 1997:98 Meisser, 1999b
IL8	Lower level of expression in preeclamptic placenta	Wang, 1999
IL10	Inhibit invasion	Roth, et al.,1998:99
IL15	Lower level of expression in preeclamptic placenta Increase invasiveness	Wang, 1999 Zygmunt, 1998
TNF	Progesterone, hCG, estradiol synthesis Stimulates MMP1, 3, 9, decrease TIMP Induces integrin subunit conversion Induces apoptosis Elevated circulating level and expression in preeclamptic patients and placenta	Li, 1994 So,1992; Takahashi, 1993; Meisser, 1994b Fukushima, 2003 Levy R, 2000 Hamai, 1997; Rinehart, 1999
TGF β	Stimulates matrix glycoproteins Inhibits cellular proliferation and migration Stimulate TIMP secretion by downregulate urokinase, plasmin, plasminogen activator	Feinbearg, 1994 Graham CH, 1992; Khoo NK, 1998; Roth 1999 Graham and Lala, 1991, Graham, 1994, Irving and Lala, 1995
TGF α	Promotes differentiation	Irving and Lala, 1995
LIF	Inhibibs gelatinolytic activity	Bischof, 1995
IGF2	Stimulates differentiation and migration	Irving and Lala, 1995
IGFBP1	Increase cell migration, invasion, TIMP-1 secretion and gelatinolytic activity	Irving and Lala, 1995; Hamilton, 1998; Bischof, 1998
VEGF	Increase proliferation and NO release Involved in tube-like formation in matrigel (VEGFR)	Charmock-Jones, 1994; Athanassiades, 1998; Ahmed 1997 Zhou, 2002
Ang2	Increase proliferation and NO release	Dunk, 2000

Abbreviations: IL, interleukin; TNF, tumor necrosis factor; TGF, transforming growth factor; LIF, leukemia inhibitory factor; IGF, insulin-like growth factor; IGFBP, IGF binding protein; VEGF, vascular endothelial growth factor; Ang, angiopoietin.

Other Soluble Factors

Leukemia inhibitory factor (LIF) is important for implantation of the blastocyst.[30] LIF inhibits the gelatinolytic activity of trophoblasts bearing an Ln receptor.[54]

TNF, VEGF AND ECM AS COLLABORATIVE REGULATORS IN EVT DIFFERENTIATION

As discussed above, many growth factors and cytokines have been shown to have an ability to produce certain effects on trophoblast function; however, the mechanism to regulate integrin subunit conversion has been unclear. Fukushima et al.[51] reported that TNFα suppressed α6 integrin expression and enhanced α1 integrin expression in a dose-dependent manner in a human EVT cell line; TNFα also induced apoptosis, which is suppressed by signals via integrin β1, with aggregation also induced by TNFα (Figs 58.3A and B). Because integrins comprise a large family of cell surface receptors that recognize a variety of ECM components,[55] these results suggest that TNFα and ECM might collaboratively regulate EVT differentiation through integrin signaling (Fig. 58.4). EVT cells alter their integrin expression in parallel with varied ECM distribution during invasion.[4,5] Thus, it has been suggested that alteration of integrin expression during differentiation of EVT may be responsible for mediating distinct signals to EVT upon adhesion to ECM. In other words, ECM regulates EVT differentiation; however, at the same time, this is an adaptation for EVT.

We should note physiological microenvironments surrounding EVT during early pregnancy. Hypoxia and oxidative

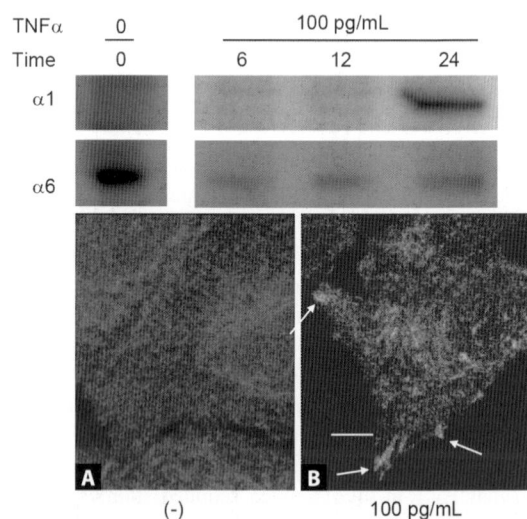

Figs 58.3A and B: TNFα induces integrin subunit switching in TCL-1 cells. (A) Immunoblot analysis using anti-α1 and -α6 integrin subunits. TCL-1 cells were seeded and grown at 37°C. After 1 day of incubation, the medium was replaced with fresh, complete medium containing 10% fetal calf serum and 20 or 100 pg/mL TNFα for the indicated times. Cellular proteins were extracted then analyzed by immunoblotting.[51] (B) TNFα strengthens integrin adhesive functions. TCL-1 cells were seeded on collagen type I-coated cover-slips. The cells were incubated with or without 100 pg/mL TNFα for 24 hours. Cells were then fixed and stained with an anti-α1 integrin subunit monoclonal antibody. The white arrows indicate integrin α1 subunit aggregation[51]

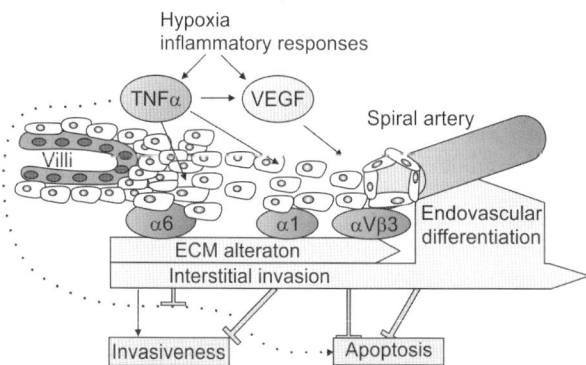

Fig. 58.4: A hypothetical paradigm for TNFα/VEGF/ECM collaboration during EVT differentiation. See text for detail

Abbreviations: ECM, extracellular matrix; VEGF, vascular endothelial growth factors; TNFα, tumor necrosis factor alpha; EVT, extravillous trophoblast.

stress caused by hypoperfusion and transient ischemia affect cytokine production.[56-58] Placental VEGF expression is up-regulated by hypoxia.[59] Hypoxia also induces proinflammatory cytokines including TNFα.[60] TNFα plays a pivotal role in pregnancy[61] and seems to be necessary for fetal development because it is expressed in normal tissues of a wide range of organs in the human fetus.[62] Zhou et al.[22] suggested that the signal from VEGF-VEGFR is involved in alteration of integrin switching. We have found that TNFα and VEGF induce integrin αVβ3 expression and aggregation in an immortalized human EVT cell line (Fukushima et al).[51] It might be assumed that signals via αVβ3 integrin receptor and VEGFR are involved in endovascular differentiation. TNFα induces expression of VEGF in several kinds of cells.[63,64] Thus, there could be sequential and synergistic effects

between TNFα and VEGF together with ECM in physiological regulation of EVT differentiation. This hypothesis might explain biological communication between maternal microenvironment and fetal trophoblast. As an immunological defending response, maternal cells secrete TNFα. Although, some trophoblast cells are eliminated by apoptosis, at the same time, ECM could act as a survival factor for trophoblast cells through integrin signaling if they can successfully convert phenotype. TNFα also enhances formation of a number of endothelial cell molecules.[65] If excessive hypoxia and/or inflammation develop, such regulation might be impaired with induction or failure of both cellular survival and EVT differentiation. Indeed, when cultured under hypoxic conditions, CT cells fail to differentiate.[66]

In this chapter, we have presented research findings along with EVT invasion, which has been implicated as one of the "key phenomena" in the normal placentation and hypothec paradigm. TNFα together with VEGF-systems might be key players in this differentiation adaptation with ECM. Of course, there have been suggestions that many other soluble factors could be involved in regulation of trophoblast phenotype, and there are probably other key molecules that are essential for invasive phenotype, e.g. regulation of MMP secretion and activity. It is necessary to take into account cross-talk among these molecules in the course of a normal pregnancy. Much more data is needed in order to integrate the current pieces of research evidence for this very interesting field.

ACKNOWLEDGMENT

This work was supported in part by a grant-in-aid from the Ministry of Education, Japan (16790609), Kanzawa Medical Research Foundation and Inamori Foundation.

REFERENCES

1. Vicovac L, Aplin JD. Epithelial-mesenchymal transition during trophoblast differentiation. Acta Anat. 1996;156: 202-16.
2. Brosens IA, Robertson WB, Dixon HG. The role of spiral arteries in the pathogenesis of pre-eclampsia. Obstet Gynecol Annu. 1972;1:177-91.
3. Robertson WB, Brosens IA, Dixon HG. Placental bed vessels. Am J Obstet Gynecol. 1973;117:294-5.
4. Damsky CH, Fitzgerald ML, Fisher SJ. Distribution patterns of extracellular matrix components and adhesion receptors are intricately modulated during first trimester cytotrophoblast differentiation along the invasive pathway, *in vivo*. J Clin Invest 1992;89:210-22.
5. Damsky CH, Librach C, Lim KH, et al. Integrin switching regulates normal trophoblast invasion. Development. 1994;120:3657-66.
6. Damsky CH, Sutherland AE, Fisher SJ. Adhesive interactions in early mammalian embryogenesis, implantation, and placentation. FASEB J. 1993;7:1320-9.
7. Fisher SJ, Cui TY, Zhang L, et al. Adhesive and invasive interactions of human cytotrophoblast cells *in vitro*. J Cell Biol. 1989;109:891-902.
8. Zhou Y, Damsky CH, Fisher SJ. Pre-eclampsia is associated with abnormal expression of adhesion molecules by invasive cytotrophoblast cells. J Clin Invest. 1993;91:950-60.

9. Zhou Y, Fisher SJ, Janatpour M, et al. Human cytotrophoblasts adopt a vascular phenotype as they differentiate. A strategy for successful endovascular invasion? J Clin Invest. 1997;99:2139-51.
10. Bischof P, Meisser A, Campana A. Involvement of trophoblast in embryo implantation: Regulation by paracrine factors. J Reprod Immunol. 1998;39(1-2):167-77.
11. Bischof P, Meisser A, Campana A. Paracrine and autocrine regulators of trophoblast invasion—a review. Placenta. 2000;21:S55-60.
12. Werb Z, Tremble PM, Behrendtsen O, et al. Signal transduction through the fibronectin receptor induces collagenases and stromelysin gene expression. J Cell Biol. 1989;109:877-89.
13. Kliman HJ, Feinberg RF. Human trophoblast-extracellular matrix (ECM) interactions in vitro. ECM thickness modulates morphology and proteolytic activity. Proc Natl Acad Sci. USA. 1990;87:3057-61.
14. Lim KH, Zhou Y, Janatpour M, et al. Human cytotrophoblast differentiation/invasion is abnormal in pre-eclampsia. Am J Pathol. 1997;151(6):1809-18.
15. Genbacev O, DiFederico E, McMaster M, Fisher SJ. Invasive cytotrophoblast apoptosis in pre-eclampsia. Hum Reprod. 1999;14:56-66.
16. Redline RW, Patterson P. Pre-eclampsia is associated with an excess of proliferative immature intermediate trophoblasts. Hum Pathol. 1995;26:594-600.

17. Zhou Y, Damsky CH, Fisher SJ. Pre-eclampsia is associated with failure of human cytotrophoblasts to mimic a vascular adhesion phenotype. One cause of defective endovascular invasion in this syndrome? J Clin Invest. 1997;99:2152-64.

18. Charnock-Jones DS, Sharkey AM, Boocock CA, et al. Localization and activation of the receptor for vascular endothelial growth factor on human trophoblast and choriocarcinoma cells. Biol Reprod. 1994;51:524-30.

19. Vuckovic M, Ponting J, Terman BI, et al. Expression of vascular endothelial growth factor receptor, KDR, in human placenta. J Anat. 1996;188:361-6.

20. Hynes RO. A re-evaluation of integrins as regulators of angiogenesis. Nature Medicine. 2002;8:918-21.

21. Shibuya M. Structure and function of VEGF/VEGF-receptor system involved in angiogenesis. Cell Struct Funct. 2001;26:25-35.

22. Zhou Y, McMaster M, Woo K, et al. Vascular endothelial growth factor ligands and receptors that regulate human cytotrophoblast survival are dysregulated in severe pre-eclampsia and hemolysis, elevated liver enzymes, and low platelets syndrome. Am J Pathol. 2002;160:1405-23.

23. Dunk C, Shams M, Nijjar S, et al. Angiopoietin-1 and angiopoietin-2 activate trophoblast Tie-2 to promote growth and migration during placental development. Am J Pathol. 2000;156:2185-99.

24. Charnock-Jones DS, Sharkey AM, Boocock CA, et al. Localization and activation of the receptor for vascular endothelial growth factor on human trophoblast and choriocarcinoma cells. Biol Reprod. 1994;51:524-30.

25. Athanassiades A, Hamilton GS, Lala PK. Role of vascular endothelial growth factor (VEGF) in human extravillous trophoblast proliferation, migration and invasiveness. Placenta. 1998;19:465-73.

26. Ahmed A, Dunk CE, Kniss D, et al. Role of VEGF Receptor (Flt-1) in mediating calcium dependent nitric oxide release and limiting DNA synthesis in human trophoblast cells. Lab Invest. 1997;76:779-91.

27. Zhou Y, Bellingard V, Feng KT, et al. Human cytotrophoblasts promote endothelial survival and vascular remodeling through secretion of Ang2, PlGF, and VEGF-C. Dev Biol 2003;263(1):114-25.

28. Meisser A, Chardonnens D, Campana A, et al. Effects of tumour necrosis factor alpha, interleukin-1 alpha, macrophage colony stimulating factor and transforming growth factor beta on trophoblastic matrix metalloproteinases. Mol Hum Reprod. 1999;5:252-60.

29. Librach CL, Feigenbaum SL, Bass KE, et al. Interleukin-1 beta regulates human cytotrophoblast metalloproteinase activity and invasion in vitro. J Biol Chem 1994;269:17125-31.

30. Simon C, Frances A, Lee BY, et al. Immunohistochemical localization, identification and regulation of the interleukin-1 receptor antagonist in the human endometrium. Hum Reprod. 1995;10:2472-7.

31. Lala P, Lysiak J. Role of locally produced growth factors in human placental growth and invasion with special reference to transforming growth factors. New York: Springer-Verlag; 1994.

32. Meisser A, Cameo P, Islami D, et al. Effects of interleukin-6 (IL-6) on cytotrophoblastic cells. Mol Hum Reprod. 1999;5:1055-8.

33. Conrad KP, Benyo DF. Placental cytokines and the pathogenesis of pre-eclampsia. Am J Reprod Immunol. 1997;37:240-9.

34. Conrad KP, Miles TM, Benyo DF. Circulating levels of immunoreactive cytokines in women with preeclampsia. Am J Reprod Immunol. 1998; 40:102-111.

35. Zygmunt M, Hahn D, Kiesenbauer N, et al. Invasion of cytotrophoblastic (Jeg-3) cells is up-regulated by interleukin-15 in vitro. Am J Reprod Immunol. 1998;40:326-31.

36. Roth I, Corry DB, Locksley RM, et al. Human placental cytotrophoblasts produce the immunosuppressive cytokine interleukin 10. J Exp Med. 1996;184:539-48.

37. Roth I, Fisher SJ. IL-10 is an autocrine inhibitor of human placental cytotrophoblast MMP-9 production and invasion. Dev Biol. 1999;205:194-204.

38. Wang Y, Baier J, Adair CD, et al. Interleukin-8 stimulates placental prostacyclin production in pre-eclampsia. Am J Reprod Immunol. 1999;42:375-80.

39. Feinberg RF, Kliman HJ, Wang CL. Transforming growth factor beta stimulates trophoblast oncofetal fibronectin synthesis in vitro: Implications for trophoblast implantation in vivo. J Clin Endocrinol Metab. 1994;78:1241-8.

40. Graham CH, Lala PK. Mechanism of control of trophoblast invasion in situ. J Cell Physiol. 1991;148:228-34.

41. Graham CH, Connelly I, MacDougall JR, et al. Resistance of malignant trophoblast cells to both the anti-proliferative and anti-invasive effects of transforming growth factor beta. Exp Cell Res. 1994;214:93-9.

42. Irving JA, Lala PK. Functional role of cell surface integrins on human trophoblast cell migration: Regulation by TGF beta, IGF-II, and IGFBP-1. Exp Cell Res. 1995;217:419-27.

43. Graham CH, Lysiak JJ, McCrae KR, et al. Localization of transforming growth factor-beta at the human fetal-maternal interface: Role in trophoblast growth and differentiation. Biol Reprod. 1992;46:561-72.

44. Khoo NK, Zhang Y, Bechberger JF, et al. SV40 Tag transformation of the normal invasive trophoblast results in a premalignant phenotype II. Changes in gap junctional intercellular communication. Int J Cancer. 1998;77:440-8.

45. Hamai Y, Fujii T, Yamashita T, et al. Evidence for an elevation in serum interleukin 2 and tumor necrosis factor a levels before the clinical manifestations of pre-eclampsia. Am J Reproduct Immunol. 1997;38:89-93.

46. Rinehart BK, Terrone DA, Lagoo-Deenadayalan S, et al. Expression of the placental cytokines tumor necrosis factor a, interleukin 1 and interleukin 10 is increased in pre-eclampsia. Am J Obstet Gynecol. 1999;181:915-20.

47. Li Y, Matsuzaki N, Masuhiro K, et al. Trophoblast-derived tumor necrosis factor-alpha induces release of human chorionic gonadotropin using interleukin- 6 (IL-6) and IL-6-receptor-dependent system in the normal human trophoblasts. J Clin Endocrinol Metab. 1992;74:184-91.

48. So T, Ito A, Sato T, et al. Tumour necrosis factor stimulates the biosynthesis of matrix metalloproteinases and plasminogen activator in cultured human chorionic cells. Biol Reprod. 1992;46:772-8.

49. Takahashi S, Sato T, Ito A, et al. Involvement of protein kinase C in the interleukin 1 alpha induced gene expression of matrix metalloproteinases and tissue inhibitor 1 of metalloproteinases (TIMP-1) in human uterine cervical fibroblasts. Biochim Biophys Acta. 1993;57-65.

50. Levy R, Nelson DM. To be, or not to be, that is the question. Apoptosis in human trophoblasts. Placenta. 2000;21:1-13.

51. Fukushima K, Miyamoto S, Komatsu H, et al. TNF-alpha-induced apoptosis and integrin switching in human extravillous trophoblast cell line. Biol Reprod. 2003; 68(5):1771-8.

52. Hamilton GS, Lysiak JJ, Han VK, et al. Autocrine-paracrine regulation of human trophoblast invasiveness by insulin-like growth factor (IGF)-II and IGF-binding protein (IGFBP)-1. Exp Cell Res. 1998;10:147-56.

53. Bischof P, Meisser A, Campana A, et al. Effects of decidua conditioned medium and insulin-like growth factor binding protein-1 on trophoblast matrix metalloproteinases and their inhibitors. Placenta. 1998;19:457-64.

54. Bischof P, Haenggeli L, Campana A. Effect of leukemia inhibitory factor on human cytotrophoblast differentiation along the invasive pathway. Am J Reprod Immunol. 1995;34:225-30.

55. Yamada KM, Geiger B. Molecular interactions in cell adhesion complexes. Curr Opin Cell Biol. 1997;9:187.

56. Wang Y, Walsh SW, Kay HH. Placental lipid peroxides and thromboxane are increased and prostacyclin is decreased in women with pre-eclampsia. Am J Obstet Gynecol. 1992;167:946-9.

57. Walsh SW, Wang Y, Jesse R. Peroxide induces vasoconstriction in the human placenta by stimulating thromboxane. Am J Obstet Gynecol. 1993;169:1007-12.

58. Nelson DM, Johnson RD, Smith SD, et al. Hypoxia limits differentiation and up-regulates expression and activity of prostaglandin H synthase 2 in cultured trophoblast from term human placenta. Am J Obstet Gynecol. 1999;180:896-902.

59. Shore VH, Wang TH, Wang CL, et al. Vascular endothelial growth factor, placenta growth factor and their receptors in isolated human trophoblast. Placenta. 1997;18:657-65.

60. Chung IB, Yelian FD, Zaher FM, et al. Expression and regulation of vascular endothelial growth factor in a first trimester trophoblast cell line. Placenta. 2000; 21:320-4.

61. Hunt JS, Chen HL, Miller L. Tumor necrosis factors: Pivotal components of pregnancy? Biol Reprod. 1996; 54:554-62.

62. Yui J, Garcia-Lloret M, Wegmann TG, et al. Cytotoxicity of tumour necrosis factor-alpha and gamma-interferon against primary human placental trophoblasts. Placenta. 1994;15:819-35.

63. Yoshida S, Ono M, Shono,T, et al. Involvement of interleukin-8, vascular endothelial growth factor, and basic fibroblast growth factor in tumor necrosis factor alpha-dependent angiogenesis. Mol Cell Biol. 1997;17:4015-23.

64. Ko Y, Totzke G, Gouni-Berthold I, et al. Cytokine-inducible growth factor gene expression in human umbilical endothelial cells. Mol Cell Probes. 1999;13:203-11.

65. Doukas J, Pober JS. IFN-gamma enhances endothelial activation induced by tumor necrosis factor but not IL-1. J Immunol 1990;145:1727-33.

66. Genbacev O, Zhou Y, Ludlow JW, et al. Regulation of human placental development by oxygen tension. Science. 1997;277:1669-72.

59

Trophoblast Dysfunction and Maternal Endothelial Cell Dysfunction in the Pathogenesis of Preeclampsia

K Tsukimori, K Fukushima, H Nakano

INTRODUCTION

The etiology and pathogenesis of preeclampsia remain poorly understood. Several investigators have suggested that poor placentation is an important predisposing factor of preeclampsia and that endothelial cell dysfunction underlies disease manifestations.[1-4] In response to reduced placental perfusion due to poor placentation, the placenta may promote release of various factors that initiate systemic endothelial cell dysfunction, leading to an increase in both vascular resistance and arterial pressure and activation of the coagulation cascade associated with preeclampsia. In this chapter, we focus on functional abnormalities of the placenta and trophoblast in preeclampsia, as well as the potential cellular and molecular mechanisms that contribute to the maternal endothelial cell dysfunction seen in this disorder.

POOR PLACENTATION

During early pregnancy, cytotrophoblast (CT) cells invade the uterus and its spiral arteries (in interstitial and endovascular invasion, respectively). As a result of endovascular invasion, CT cells replace the endothelial layers of spiral arteries with destruction of the medial elastic, muscular and neural tissue. This replacement substantially decreases vascular resistance, resulting in increased blood flow toward the intervillous space.[5,6] In preeclampsia, extravillous trophoblast (EVT) cell invasion of the uterus is shallow, and endovascular invasion does not progress beyond the terminal portion of the spiral arteries (Fig. 59.1).[5] Myometrial segments of

these arteries remain anatomically intact and undilated; in addition, adrenergic nerve supply to the spiral arteries is not affected. The mean external diameters of the uterine spiral arteries in women with preeclampsia are less than one-half the diameters of similar vessels from uncomplicated pregnancies. The failure of EVT invasion in preeclampsia results in a reduction in uteroplacental perfusion. Because the process of EVT invasion of spiral arteries is normally completed by weeks 20–22 of gestation,[7] a critical underlying lesion in preeclampsia is the failure of EVT to invade the myometrial portion of the muscular spiral arteries. Normal trophoblast invasion requires meticulously regulated expression of specific adhesion molecules for both cell-cell interacctions as well as cell-extracellular matrix (ECM) interactions.[8] In preeclampsia, CT cells increase expression of adhesion molecules present in the initial proliferative phenotype, $\alpha5\beta1$, but fail both to upregulate adhesion molecules that promote invasion, $\alpha1\beta1$, and to downregulate molecules that inhibit invasion, $\alpha6\beta4$ (Table 59.1).[9-12] Thus, the cells appear arrested in their differentiation and express an ECM receptor phenotype that may not be optimal for invasion.[12] In addition, endovascular invasion seems to require the ability of endovascular trophoblast cells to alter phenotype to resemble vascular endothelial cells.[13] In preeclampsia, trophoblast cells in decidual vessels do not express the endothelial antigens vascular adhesion molecule-1 (VCAM-1) and platelet endothelial adhesion molecule-1 (PECAM-1).[12] When these data are considered together, this overall dysfunctional expression of adhesion molecules may be responsible for the pathological findings of impaired interstitial and endovascular invasion in preeclampsia.

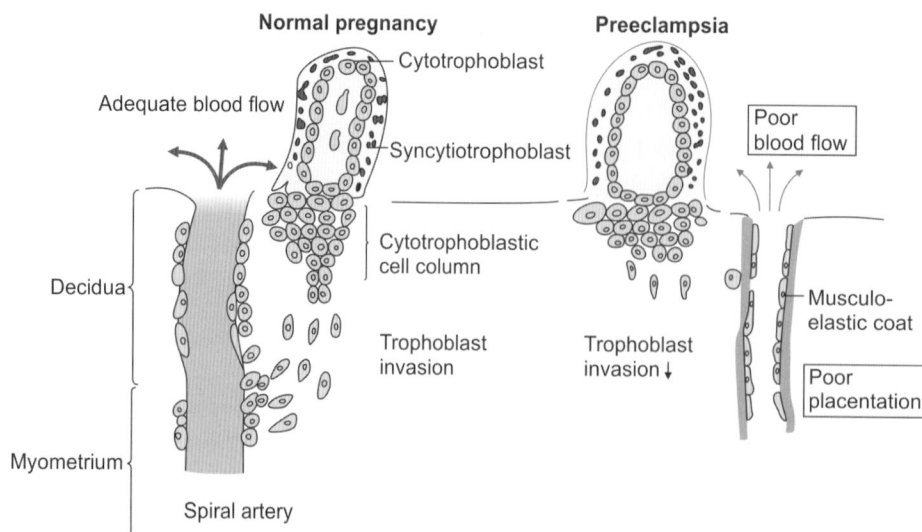

Fig. 59.1: Trophoblast invasion in normal and preeclamptic pregnancies
Source: Modified from Saito et al.[23]

Table 59.1: Integrin expression by cytotrophoblasts in normal and preeclamptic pregnancies

Integrin receptor	ECM ligands	Functional link	Change from villus to placental bed	
			Normal pregnancy	Preeclampsia
α6β4	BM ligand (Ln ?)	Inhibit invasion	Downregulated	Unchanged
α5β1	Fn	Initial proliferation	Upregulated	Upregulated
α3β1	Ln, Fn, Col	Proliferation	Uniformly expressed	Uniformly expressed
α1β1	Ln, Col IV, Col I	Promote invasion	Upregulated	Not expressed (weakly expressed)

Abbreviations: ECM, extracellular matrix; BM, basement membrane; Ln, laminin; Fn, fibronectin; Col, collagen.
(Modified from Zhou et al. 1993[12])

FACTORS INVOLVED IN POOR PLACENTATION

Hypoxic Environment

Several studies suggest that oxygen tension can modulate trophoblast differentiation. Fox and Path reported that placental villi cultured under hypoxic conditions showed variable syncytial degeneration and a marked increase in the number and growth-promoting activity of CT cells.[14] More recently, using an in vitro organ culture model, CT maintained under hypoxic conditions failed to express integrin α1 and VE-cadherin.[15,16] These findings suggest that under hypoxic conditions CT cells enter a proliferative pathway and do not differentiate to the invasive phenotype. The adhesion molecule phenotype of these cells mimics that of CT from women with preeclampsia.[12]

In vitro, hypoxia stimulates production of inflammatory cytokines and other mediators such as tumor necrosis factor-α (TNF-α), interleukin (IL)-1α, IL-1β,[17] and transforming growth factor-β (TGF-β)[18] by trophoblasts. TNF-α induces apoptosis,[19] integrin subunit conversion and functional activation in an EVT cell line.[20] TGF-β also inhibits cellular proliferation and migration.[21-23] In addition, trophoblasts under hypoxic conditions increase production of soluble fms-like tyrosine kinase 1 (sFlt-1), an antagonist for both vascular endothelial growth factor (VEGF) and placental growth factor (PlGF).[24] The enzyme sFlt-1 is involved in an alteration of integrin switching that decreases cell invasiveness.[25] In placentas from women with preeclampsia, there is increased production of TNF-α,[17] TGF-β,[18] and sFlt-1,[25,26] as well as decreased production of VEGF.[25] Taken together, this evidence suggests that hypoxia induces production of inflammatory cytokines and/or growth factors and then modulates cytotrophoblast differentiation and adhesion antigen expression, resulting in the inadequate invasion seen in preeclampsia.

Immunologic Factors

Epidemiological evidence indicates that first pregnancy, change of partner, donor insemination and use of barrier contraceptives all increase the risk of preeclampsia, suggesting that a prior immune response to foreign or paternal antigens protects against development of preeclampsia.[27-29] In preeclampsia, human leukocyte antigen (HLA-G), a surrogate autoantigen known to prevent recognition by natural killer (NK) cells, is not expressed in trophoblasts.[30,31] HLA-G downregulates NK cell-mediated cytotoxicity[32] and suppresses IL-2-induced cell damage.[33] The soluble HLA-G1 isoform also downregulates CD8-positive T cell (cytotoxic T cell) reactivity.[34] These findings suggest that invasive trophoblast lacking HLA-G is attacked by NK cells and cytotoxic T cells, resulting in the inadequate trophoblast invasion seen in preeclampsia. Recently, Saito and colleagues reported that preeclampsia is associated with a Th1 predominant immunity.[35] Th1type cytokines such as IL-2, IFNβ, TNFα and TNFβ activate cytotoxic T cells and NK cells. Activated cytotoxic T cells and NK cells can attack invading trophoblasts, causing a failure of trophoblast invasion.

Genetic Factors

There is evidence of an increased incidence of preeclampsia among sisters, mothers and daughters. Some studies have implicated several genes as risk factors for preeclampsia including angiotensin,[36] endothelial nitric oxide synthase (eNOS),[37] TNF-α,[38] the factor Leiden mutation[39] and hyperhomocysteinemia.[40] Recent data focused on fetoplacental rather than maternal acting genes suggest that fetoplacental genes may carry an associated risk. These could be genes encoding factors associated with CT invasion. The risk of preeclampsia increases with a change in partner,[41] implying the importance of paternal genes. By following both men and women who were products of preeclamptic pregnancy, it has been suggested that both maternally and paternally inherited genes play a contributory role,[42] possibly by contributing to the genetic constitution of the placenta.

BIOLOGICAL CHANGES OF PLACENTAL FUNCTION

Poor placentation causes a reduction in uteroplacental perfusion, causing placental ischemia/hypoxia. Placental ischemia/hypoxia is known to induce several mediators such as reactive oxygen species (ROS) and inflammatory cytokines. Several biochemical abnormalities have been reported in placentas obtained from women with preeclampsia (Table 59.2).

Increased Oxidative Stress

Increased superoxide (O_2^-) synthesis rates have been noted in placentas from women with preeclampsia.[43,44] The expression of xanthine oxidase, which is an important source of O_2^- generation, is also enhanced in placentas from women with preeclampsia.[45] As an indirect indication of excessive generation of ROS, nitrotyrosine content, a stable marker for peroxynitrite $(ONOO^-)$, is increased in placentas from women with preeclampsia.[46,47] When oxygen free radicals are not eliminated by antioxidants, lipid peroxide formation

Table 59.2: Biological changes in preeclamptic placenta

Marker or activity	Location	Reference nos
Increased oxidative stress		
• Increased superoxide synthesis	• Placental tissue and trophoblast cells	43, 44
• Increased xanthine oxidase expression	• Invasive cytotrophoblast	45
• Increased nitrotyrosine immunostaining	• Invasive cytotrophoblast	46, 47
• Increased MDA level	• Placental homogenate	49, 50
• Increased 8-isoprostane level and production	• Placental tissue pieces	51
• Increased protein carbonyl level	• Placental and decidual homogenate	52
• Increased lipid peroxide production	• Trophoblast cells and villous tissue	51, 53, 54
• Decreased glutathione peroxidase activity	• Placental homogenate	55
• Decreased vitamin E level	• Placental homogenate	55
• Decreased Cu/Zn-SOD activity and mRNA expression	• Trophoblast cells	44
Altered cytokine production		
• Increased TNF-α production and mRNA expression	• Placental tissue	56, 57
• Increased IL-1β mRNA expression	• Placental tissue	56
• No change for inflammatory cytokine (TNF-α, IL-1α, IL-1β, IL-6) mRNA expression	• Placental homogenate	58
• Decreased IL-8 production	• Placental villous tissue	59
• Decreased IL-10 immunostaining	• Villous trophoblast cells	60
• Decreased IL-15 production	• Placental tissue and trophoblast cells	61
Increased vasoconstriction		
• Increased thromboxane production	• Placental tissue and cytotrophoblast	62, 63
• Increased ET-1 production and mRNA expression	• Trophoblast cells	64, 65
• Increased NKB mRNA expression	• Outer syncytiotrophoblast	68
• Decreased prostacyclin production	• Placental tissue and cytotrophoblast	62, 63
• Decreased iNOS mRNA expression	• Trophoblast cells	64

Abbreviations: MDA, malondialdehyde; TNF, tumor necrosis factor; IL, interleukin; ET, endothelin; NKB, neurokinin B; iNOS, inducible nitric oxide synthase

is induced.[48] Placental levels of lipid peroxidation products, as well as other markers of oxidative stress such as malondialdehyde (MDA),[49,50] 8-iso-PGF2α[51] and protein carbonyl[52] are increased. In vitro production of lipid peroxides is also increased in trophoblasts from women with preeclampsia.[51,53,54] Placental antioxidant levels such as vitamin E, as well as the activities of glutathione peroxidase,[55] and both mRNA expression and enzyme activity for Cu/Zn-superoxide dismutase (SOD), are decreased in preeclampsia.[44] Thus, the placenta represents a state of oxidative stress in preeclampsia.

Altered Cytokine Production

Expression of inflammatory cytokines such as TNF-α and IL-1β is increased in pre-eclamptic placentas.[56,57] However, Benyo and colleagues failed to observe increased mRNA levels of both TNF-α and IL-1β in pre-eclamptic placenta.[58] Placental levels of IL-8,[59] IL-10,[60] and IL-15[61] are decreased in preeclampsia. Thus, although the picture is not entirely clear, placental cytokine production is altered in preeclampsia.

Increased Vasoconstriction

Placental thromboxane production is increased, whereas placental PGI$_2$ production is decreased in preeclampsia.[62,63] Endothelin (ET-1) expression and production are increased in trophoblasts obtained from women with preeclampsia.[64,65] Regarding nitric oxide (NO) production, Napolitano and colleagues reported that inducible nitric oxide synthase (iNOS) expression, which represents the main source of NO, is decreased; conversely, endothelial nitric

oxide synthase (eNOS) expression is increased in trophoblasts obtained from women with preeclampsia.[64] In contrast, other investigators have failed to observe increased eNOS activity[66] and eNOS immunostaining levels.[67] Page and colleagues reported that expression of neurokinin (NK) B is increased in trophoblasts from women with preeclampsia.[68] Thus, in preeclampsia placental vasoconstrictor production is increased, whereas placental vasodilator production is decreased.

MATERNAL ENDOTHELIAL CELL DYSFUNCTION IN PREECLAMPSIA

Several pieces of evidence indicate that adverse changes in structure and function of the maternal vascular endothelium account for the altered vascular reactivity, activation of the coagulation cascade, and multisystem damage that occurs in preeclampsia.[69,70] Pathologic changes in endothelial cells that line the renal glomerular capillaries (glomerular endotheliosis) are a consistent feature in women with preeclampsia.[71-73] Structural changes of the endothelium have been found in uteroplacental vessels.[74] In addition, functional evidence of endothelial alteration has been reported. The level of the endothelial prostanoid prostacyclin (PGI$_2$) is reduced weeks before as well as during clinically evident preeclampsia.[75-77] Vessels removed from women with preeclampsia manifest reduced endothelial-mediated vasodilator function.[78-80] A variety of substances indicative of endothelial dysfunction are increased in the blood of women with preeclampsia including cellular fibronectin (cFN),[81-83] von Willebrand Factor,[84,85] thrombomodulin[86,87] and vascular cell adhesion molecule-1 (VCAM-1).[88,89] Many of these substances including serum soluble VCAM-1[90] and cFN[83] are elevated weeks before preeclampsia becomes clinically evident.

LINKAGE BETWEEN PLACENTAL DYSFUNCTION AND MATERNAL ENDOTHELIAL DYSFUNCTION

To link placental dysfunction with the generalized endothelial dysfunction seen in preeclampsia, the existence of factor X, released from the placenta into the maternal circulation, was proposed. Indeed, we and other investigators have reported that serum from women with preeclampsia has a cytotoxic effect on cultured endothelial cells.[91,92] The factor seems to modulate endothelial cell function rather than damage the cells directly. In response to serum or plasma from women with preeclampsia, production of PGI_2[93,94] and NO[95-97] is altered, and increases are seen in cFN production,[98,99] mitogenic activity,[100,101] uptake of fatty acids[102] and expression of platelet-derived growth factor (PDGF).[103] Many of these activities are not only elevated weeks before preeclampsia becomes clinically evident, but, as with the clinical signs of the syndrome, they disappear shortly after delivery.[91,99-101] Initially, Factor X was thought to be a single factor, but increasing evidence suggests the presence of several interacting factors. Several candidate factors have been proposed, including oxidative damage products, proinflammatory cytokines, syncytiotrophoblast microvesicles (STBM) and angiogenic factors.

Oxidative Damage Products

Circulating levels of lipid peroxidation products such as MDA[104-106] and 8-iso-PGF2α[50,107] are increased in preeclampsia. As described above, these products are elevated in concentration in trophoblasts from women with preeclampsia. Increased lipid peroxidation increases endothelial monolayer permeability to protein[108] and increases incorporation of fatty acids into endothelial cell membranes.[109] Free 8-iso-PGF2α is also a biologically active vasoconstrictor in vivo.[110] Nitrotyrosine staining, a stable marker for ONOO⁻ is increased in sera from women with preeclampsia[111] and in preeclamptic placenta.[46,47] The free radical ONOO⁻ is one of the most potent reactive species, and it can lead to increases in lipid peroxides and direct or indirect cellular damage.[112]

Proinflammatory Cytokines

Proinflammatory cytokines such as TNF-α and IL-1β can produce endothelial dysfunction either directly or by activating maternal leukocytes.[3,113,114] In preeclampsia, circulating levels of IL-6, TNF-α[115-117] and its two soluble receptors (p55 and p75 TNF-R)[117] are increased. Expression of placental cytokines including TNF-α and IL-1β is also increased in preeclampsia.[56,57] In contrast, Benyo and colleagues demonstrated that placental levels of inflammatory cytokines (e.g. TNF-α, IL-1α, IL-1β and IL-6) are not altered,[58] suggesting that tissues other than the placenta, such as activated leukocytes or endothelium, may be involved in the elevation of inflammatory cytokines found in the circulation of women with preeclampsia. Hung and colleagues reported that hypoxia—reoxygenation of placental tissue in vitro increases production of TNF-α and causes endothelial dysfunction,[118] suggesting that a local inflammatory response can induce systemic endothelial

dysfunction either directly or by activating maternal leukocytes during their passage through the placenta.

Syncytiotrophoblast Microvesicles

Circulating syncytiotrophoblast microvesicles (STBM) are detected in the plasma of normal pregnant women, but they are present in significantly increased amounts in women with preeclampsia.[119] STBM induce ultrastructural endothelial cell injury[120,121] and reduce endothelial cell-mediated vasodilation in isolated human arteries.[122] Hung and colleagues reported that in vitro hypoxia-reoxygenation stimulates apoptotic changes within syncytiotrophoblasts in normal third-trimester placentas, suggesting that aponecrotic processes secondary to reduced placental perfusion can lead to deportation of STBM into the maternal circulation.[123]

Angiogenic Factors

VEGF is a well-known promoter of angiogenesis, and it also induces nitric oxide and vasodilatory prostacyclins in endothelial cells suggesting a role in decreasing vascular tone and blood pressure.[124,125] Decreased concentrations of circulating free VEGF have been noted in women with clinical preeclampsia,[26] and decreases have even been detected before clinically evident preeclampsia developed.[126,127] Recent studies have demonstrated that sFlt-1, an antagonist for VEGF, is increased in serum[26,128-130] and placenta[25,26] in women with preeclampsia. Levine and colleagues reported that increased levels of sFlt-1 predict subsequent development of preeclampsia.[129] In addition, animal model experiments have recently demonstrated that exogenous sFlt-1 administered to pregnant rats induces hypertension, proteinuria, and glomerular endotheliosis.[26] Nagamatsu and colleagues reported that trophoblasts under hypoxic conditions in vitro increase production of sFlt-1.[24] Interestingly, recent evidence suggests that TNF-α also stimulates release of sFlt-1 from placental explants.[131]

MATERNAL AND PLACENTAL INTERACTIONS IN PATHOGENESIS OF PREECLAMPSIA

Abnormal placentation is not uniquely associated with preeclampsia. For example, infants with intrauterine growth restriction[132] and one-third of infants with preterm birth[133] manifest abnormal features of placentation identical to those seen in preeclampsia. It has been proposed that abnormal placentation must interact with maternal factors to cause the clinical features of preeclampsia. Maternal constitutional factors, such as genetic, behavioral and environmental factors, would predispose to preeclampsia. These constitutional factors, likely influenced by the unique physiological changes of pregnancy, would interact with placental factors induced by placental ischemia/hypoxia to bring about the pathophysiological changes of preeclampsia.[1,134]

Constitutional Factors

Preexisting hypertension, diabetes obesity and increased insulin resistance, as well as African descent and increased blood homocysteine concentration, are already known to be predisposing factors.[135] Interestingly, these are also risk factors for other endothelial diseases, in particular atherosclerosis. The concept of common risk factors for the two disorders is supported by the relationship of

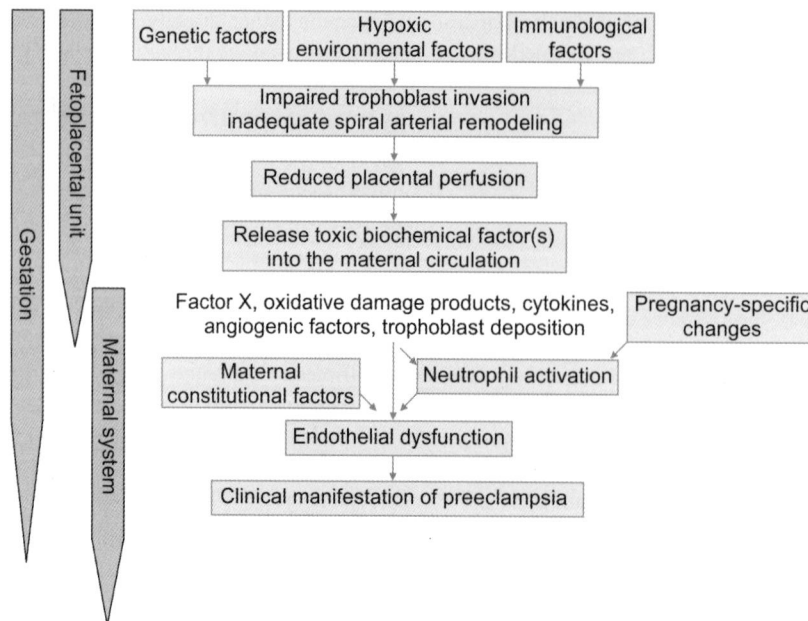

Fig. 59.2: Proposed linkage between poor placentation and maternal endothelial dysfunction in pathogenesis of preeclampsia (See text for detail)

preeclampsia to cardiovascular disease in later life.[136,137] In addition, preeclampsia and atherosclerosis share common alterations of lipid profile including elevated triglycerides,[104] reduced HDL-cholesterol[138] and increased small dense LDL-cholesterol.[139] LDL particles are smaller than those of normal controls, which may facilitate their oxidation.[140,141]

Pregnancy-specific Changes

It is well known that a neutrophilic leukocytosis occurs in pregnancy.[142] Sacks and colleagues used whole blood flow cytometric techniques to report that normal third-trimester pregnancy is characterized by remarkable activation of peripheral blood leukocytes, an activation that is further increased in preeclampsia.[143] We and other investigators have demonstrated that isolated neutrophils from women with preeclampsia synthesize more superoxide than those of normotensive pregnant women.[144-146] In an investigation of the mechanism of extreme neutrophil activation in preeclampsia, Aly and colleagues demonstrated that STBM, which are present in blood in elevated levels in preeclampsia,[119] lead to activation of maternal neutrophils.[147] Maternal neutrophils could also be locally activated during passage of maternal blood through the placenta.[117] In addition, we have reported that sera from women with preeclampsia enhance superoxide production of neutrophils in vitro.[144] The interaction of these activated neutrophils with endothelium would then result in release of reactive oxygen species and endothelial injury. Taken together, this evidence suggests that activated neutrophils, occurring as a usual component of maternal response to pregnancy, could

provide a link between the placental dysfunction and maternal endothelial cell dysfunction seen in preeclampsia.

CONCLUSION

The two central pathophysiological themes of preeclampsia are placental trophoblast dysfunction and endothelial cell dysfunction within the maternal systemic vasculature. As discussed above, it has been proposed that multiple factors (e.g. hypoxic environmental, genetic and immunological factors) may lead to impaired trophoblast invasion and inadequate spiral arterial remodeling (Fig. 59.2). This, in turn, results in reduced placental perfusion. In response to this ischemic and/or hypoxic state, affected placentas secrete or elaborate substances into the maternal circulation that directly or indirectly cause systemic vascular endothelial cell dysfunction. In addition, pregnancy-specific changes (e.g. activation of neutrophils) combined with maternal constitutional factors (e.g. genetic disposition and circulating lipoproteins) are also involved in development of preeclampsia. It is necessary to clarify the mechanisms involved in placental and maternal endothelial dysfunction and to identify the factor(s) connecting them in order to understand, treat and eventually prevent preeclampsia.

ACKNOWLEDGMENT

This work was supported in part by a grant-in-aid from the Japanese Ministry of Education (16790609 and 16591666).

REFERENCES

1. Roberts JM, Lain KY. Recent insights into the pathogenesis of pre-eclampsia. Placenta. 2002;23:359-72.
2. Redman CW, Sargent IL. Pre-eclampsia, the placenta and the maternal systemic inflammatory responses—A review. Placenta. 2003;24:S21-S7.
3. Roberts JM, Hubel CA. Is oxidative stress the link in the two-stage model of pre-eclampsia? Lancet. 1999;354:788-9.
4. Wang Y, Alexander JS. Placental pathophysiology in pre-eclampsia. Pathophysiology. 2000;6:261-70.

5. Brosens IA, Robertson WB, Dixon HG. The role of spiral arteries in the pathogenesis of pre-eclampsia. Obstet Gynecol Annu. 1972;1:177-91.

6. Robertson WB, Brosens IA, Dixon HG. Placental bed vessels. Am J Obstet Gynecol. 1973;117:294-5.

7. Pijnenborg R, Robertson WB, Brosens I, et al. Trophoblast invasion and the establishment of hemochorial placentation in man and laboratory animals. Placenta. 1981;2:71-92.

8. Damsky CH, Fitzgerald ML, Fisher SJ. Distribution patterns of extracellular matrix components and adhesion receptors are intricately modulated during first trimester cytotrophoblast differentiation along the invasive pathway, in vivo. J Clin Invest. 1992;89:210-22.

9. Damsky CH, Librach C, Lim KH, et al. Integrin switching regulates normal trophoblast invasion. Development. 1994;120:3657-66.

10. Redline RW, Patterson P. Pre-eclampsia is associated with an excess of proliferative immature intermediate trophoblasts. Hum Pathol. 1995;26:594-600.

11. Zhou Y, Damsky CH, Chiu K, et al. Pre-eclampsia is associated with abnormal expression of adhesion molecules by invasive cytotrophoblasts. J Clin Invest. 1993;91:950-60.

12. Zhou Y, Damsky CH, Fisher SJ. Preeclampsia is associated with failure of human cytotrophoblasts to mimic a vascular adhesion phenotype—One cause of defective endovascular invasion in this syndrome? J Clin Invest. 1997;99:2152-64.

13. Zhou Y, Fisher SJ, Janatpour M, et al. Human cytotrophoblasts adopt a vascular phenotype as they differentiate. A strategy for successful endovascular invasion? J Clin Invest. 1997;99:2139-51.

14. Fox H, Path MC. Effect of hypoxia on trophoblasts in organ culture. A morphologic and autoradiographic study. Am J Obstet Gynecol. 1970;107:1058-64.

15. Genbacev O, Zhou Y, Ludlow JW, et al. Regulation of human placental development by oxygen tension. Science. 1997;277:1669-72.

16. Zhou Y, Genbacev O, Damsky CH, et al. Oxygen regulates human cytotrophoblast differentiation and invasion—implications for endovascular invasion in normal pregnancy and in pre-eclampsia. J Reprod Immunol. 1998;39:197-213.

17. Benyo DF, Miles TM, Conrad KP. Hypoxia stimulates cytokine production by villous explants from the human placenta. J Clin Endocrinol Metab. 1997;82:1582-8.

18. Caniggia I, Grisaru-Gravnosky S, Kuliszewsky M, et al. Inhibition of TGF-beta 3 restores the invasive capability of extravillous trophoblasts in pre-eclamptic pregnancies. J Clin Invest. 1999;103:1641-50.

19. Levy R, Nelson DM. To be, or not to be, that is the question. Apoptosis in human trophoblasts. Placenta. 2000;21:1-13.

20. Fukushima K, Miyamoto S, Komatsu H, et al. TNF-alpha-induced apoptosis and integrin switching in human extravillous trophoblast cell line. Biol Reprod. 2003;68:1771-8.

21. Graham CH, Lysiak JJ, McCrae KR, et al. Localization of transforming growth factor-beta at the human fetal-maternal interface: Role in trophoblast growth and differentiation. Biol Reprod. 1992;46:561-72.

22. Khoo NK, Zhang Y, Bechberger JF, et al. SV40 Tag transformation of the normal invasive trophoblast results in a premalignant phenotype II. Changes in gap junctional intercellular communication. Int J Cancer. 1998;77:440-8.

23. Roth I, Fisher SJ. IL-10 is an autocrine inhibitor of human placental cytotrophoblast MMP-9 production and invasion. Dev Biol. 1999;205:194-204.

24. Nagamatsu T, Fujii T, Kusumi M, et al. Cytotrophoblasts upregulate soluble fms-like tyrosine kinase-1 expression under reduced oxygen: An implication for the placental vascular development and the pathophysiology of pre-eclampsia. Endocrinology. 2004;145:4838-45.

25. Zhou Y, McMaster M, Woo K, et al. Vascular endothelial growth factor ligands and receptors that regulate human cytotrophoblast survival are dysregulated in severe pre-eclampsia and hemolysis, elevated liver enzymes, and low platelets syndrome. Am J Pathol. 2002;160:1405-23.

26. Maynard SE, Min JY, Merchan J, et al. Excess placental soluble fms-like tyrosine kinase 1 (sFlt1) may contribute to endothelial dysfunction, hypertension, and proteinuria in pre-eclampsia. J Clin Invest. 2003;111: 649-58.

27. Robillard PY, Hulsey TC. Association of pregnancy induced hypertension, pre-eclampsia, and eclampsia with duration of sexual cohabitation before conception. Lancet. 1996;347:619.

28. Robillard PY, Dekker GA, Hulsey TC. Primipaternities in families—Is the incidence of pregnancy-induced hypertensive disorders in multigravidas an anthropological marker of reproduction. Aust NZJ Obstet Gynaecol. 1998;38:284-7.

29. Smith GN, Walker M, Tessier JL, et al. Increased incidence of pre-eclampsia in women conceiving by intrauterine insemination with donor versus partner sperm for treatment of primary infertility. Am J Obstet Gynecol. 1997;177:455-8.

30. Colburn GT, Chiang MH, Main EK. Expression of the nonclassic histocompatibility antigen HLA-G by preeclamptic placenta. Am J Obstet Gynecol. 1994;170:1244-50.

31. Lim KH, Zhou Y, Janatpour M, et al. Human cytotrophoblast differentiation/invasion is abnormal in pre-eclampsia. Am J Pathol. 1997;151:1809-18.

32. Marchal-Bras-Goncalves R, Rouas-Freiss N, Connan F, et al. A soluble HLA-G protein that inhibits natural killer cell-mediated cytotoxicity. Transplant Proc. 2001;33:2355-9.

33. Hamai Y, Fujii T, Yamashita T, et al. The expression of human leukocyte antigen-G on trophoblasts abolishes the growth-suppressing effect of interleukin-2 toward them. Am J Reprod Immunol. 1999;41:153-8.

34. Solier C, Aguerre-Birr M, Lenfant F, et al. Secretion of pro-apoptotic soluble HLA-G1 by human villous trophoblast. Eur J Immunol. 2002;32:3576-86.

35. Saito S, Sakai M. Th1/Th2 balance in pre-eclampsia. J Reprod Immunol. 2003;59:161-73.

36. Ward K, Hata A, Jeunemaitre X, et al. A molecular variant of angiotensinogen associated with pre-eclampsia. Nat Genet. 1993;4:59-61.

37. Arngrimsson R, Hayward C, Nadaud S, et al. Evidence for a familial pregnancy-induced hypertension locus in the enos gene region. Am J Hum Genet. 1997;61:354-62.

38. Masse J, Giguere Y, Kharfi A, et al. Pathophysiology and maternal biologic markers of pre-eclampsia. Endocrine. 2002;19:113-25.

39. Morgan T, Ward K. New insights into the genetics of pre-eclampsia. Semin Perinatol. 1999;23:14-23.

40. Dekker GA, de Vries JI, Doelitzsch PM, et al. Underlying disorders associated with severe early-onset preeclampsia. Am J Obstet Gynecol. 1995;173:1042-8.

41. Trupin LS, Simon LP, Eskenazi B. Change in paternity: A risk factor for pre-eclampsia in multiparas. Epidemiology. 1996;7:240-4.

42. Esplin MS, Fausett MB, Fraser A, et al. Paternal and maternal components of the predisposition to pre-eclampsia. N Engl J Med. 2001;344:867-72.

43. Sikkema JM, van Rijn BB, Franx A, et al. Placental superoxide is increased in pre-eclampsia. Placenta. 2001;22:304-8.

44. Wang Y, Walsh SW. Increased superoxide generation is associated with decreased superoxide dismutase activity and mRNA expression in placental trophoblast cells in pre-eclampsia. Placenta. 2001;22:206–12.

45. Many A, Hubel CA, Fisher SJ, et al. Invasive cytotrophoblasts manifest evidence of oxidative stress in pre-eclampsia. Am J Pathol. 2000;156:321-31.

46. Myatt L, Rosenfield RB, Eis AL, et al. Nitrotyrosine residues in placenta: Evidence of peroxynitrite formation and action. Hypertension. 1996;28:488-93.
47. Norris M, Todeschini M, Cassis P, et al. L-arginine depletion in pre-eclampsia orients nitric oxide synthase toward oxidant species. Hypertension 2004;43:614-22.
48. Walsh SW. The role of fatty acid peroxidation and antioxidant status in normal pregnancy and in pregnancy complicated by pre-eclampsia. World Rev Nutr Diet. 1994;76:114-8.
49. Cester N, Staffolani R, Rabini RA, et al. Pregnancy-induced hypertension: A role for peroxidation in microvillous plasma membranes. Mol Cell Biochem. 1994;131:151-55.
50. Gratacos E, Casals E, Deulofeu R, et al. Lipid peroxide and vitamin E patterns in pregnant women with different types of hypertension in pregnancy. Am J Obstet Gynecol. 1998;178:1072-6.
51. Walsh SW, Vaughan JE, Wang Y, et al. Placental isoprostane is significantly increased in pre-eclampsia. FASEB J. 2000;14:1289-96.
52. Zusterzeel PL, Rutten H, Roelofs HM, et al. Protein carbonyls in decidua and placenta of pre-eclamptic women as markers for oxidative stress. Placenta. 2001;22:213-9.
53. Walsh SW, Wang Y. Secretion of lipid peroxides by the human placenta. Am J Obstet Gynecol. 1993;169:1462-6.
54. Walsh SW, Wang Y. Trophoblast and placental villous core production of lipid peroxides, thromboxane, and prostacyclin in preeclampsia. J Clin Endocrinol Metab. 1995;80:1888-93.
55. Wang Y, Walsh SW. Antioxidant activities and mRNA expression are increased in preeclamptic placentas. J Soc Gynecol Investig. 1996;3:179-84.
56. Rinehart BK, Terrone DA, Lagoo-Deenadayalan, et al. Expression of the placental cytokines tumor necrosis factor α, interleukin 1α, and interleukin 10 is increased in pre-eclampsia. Am J Obstet Gynecol. 1999;181:915-20.
57. Wang Y, Walsh SW. TNFβ concentrations and mRNA expression are increased in pre-eclamptic placentas. J Reprod Immunol. 1996;32:157-69.
58. Benyo DF, Smarason A, Redman CW, et al. Expression of inflammatory cytokines in placentas from women with pre-eclampsia. J Clin Endocrinol Metab. 2001;86:2505-12.
59. Wang Y, Baier J, Adair CD, et al. Interleukin-8 stimulates placental prostacyclin production in pre-eclampsia. Am J Reprod Immunol. 1999;42:375-80.
60. Hennessy A, Pilmore HL, Simmons LA, et al. A deficiency of placental IL-10 in pre-eclampsia. J Immunol. 1999;163:3491-5.
61. Agarwal R, Loganath A, Roy AC, et al. Expression profiles of interleukin-15 in early and late gestational human placenta and in pre-eclamptic placenta. Mol Hum Reprod. 2001;7:97-101.
62. Walsh SW. Pre-eclampsia: An imbalance in placental prostacyclin and thromboxane production. Am J Obstet Gynecol. 1985;152:335-40.
63. Ding ZQ, Rowe J, Sinosich MJ, et al. In vitro secretion of prostanoids by placental villous cytotrophoblasts in pre-eclampsia. Placenta. 1996;17:407-11.
64. Napolitano M, Miceli F, Calce A, et al. Expression and relationship between endothelin-1 messenger ribonucleic acid (mRNA) and inducible/endothelial nitric oxide synthase mRNA isoforms from normal and pre-eclamptic placentas. J Clin Endocrinol Metab. 2000;85:2318-23.
65. Ding Z, Rowe J, Sinosich MJ, et al. Serum from women with pre-eclampsia partially corrects the abnormal in vitro prostacyclin secretion of pre-eclamptic villous cytotrophoblasts but not that of prostaglandin E2 or endothelin-1. Am J Obstet Gynecol. 1997;177:1491-5.
66. Conrad KP, Davis AK. Nitric oxide synthase activity in placentae from women with pre-eclampsia. Placenta. 1995;16:691-9.
67. Ghabour MS, Eis AL, Brockman DE, et al. Immunohistochemical characterization of placental nitric oxide synthase expression in preeclampsia. Am J Obstet Gynecol. 1995;173:687-94.
68. Page NM, Woods RJ, Gardiner SM, et al. Nature. 2000; 15;405(6788):797-800.
69. Clinical-pathological correlations and remote prognosis. Medicine. 1981;60:267-76.
70. McCartney CP, Spargo BH, Larincz AB, et al. Renal structure and function in pregnant patients with acute hypertension. Am J Obstet Gynecol. 1964;90:579-90.
71. Spargo B, McCartney C, Winemuller R. Glomerular capillary endotheliosis in toxemia of pregnancy. Arch Pathol. 1959;68:593-9.
72. Shanklin DR, Sibai BM. Ultrastructural aspects of pre-eclampsia I. Placental bed and uterine boundary vessels. Am J Obstet Gynecol. 1989;161:735-41.
73. Fitzgerald DJ, Entman SS, Mulloy K, et al. Decreased prostacyclin biosynthesis preceding the clinical manifestation of pregnancy-induced hypertension. Circulation. 1987;75:956-63.
74. Mills JL, DerSimonian R, Raymond E, et al. Prostacyclin and thromboxane changes predating clinical onset of pre-eclampsia: A multicenter prospective study. JAMA. 1999;282:356-62.
75. Remuzzi G, Marchesi D, Zoja C, et al. Reduced umbilical and placental vascular prostacyclin in severe pre-eclampsia. Prostaglandins. 1980;20:105-10.
76. Ashworth JR, Warren AY, Baker PN, et al. A comparison of endothelium-dependent relaxation in omental and myometrial resistance arteries in pregnant and nonpregnant women. Am J Obstet Gynecol. 1996;175:1307-12.
77. McCarthy AL, Woolfson RG, Raju SK, et al. Abnormal endothelial cell function of resistance arteries from women with pre-eclampsia. Am J Obstet Gynecol. 1993;168:1323-30.
78. Pascoal I, Lindheimer M, Nalbaltian-Brandt C, et al. Pre-eclampsia selectively impairs endothelium-dependent relaxation and leads to oscillatory activity in small omental arteries. J Clin Invest. 1998;101:464-70.
79. Friedman SA, deGroot CJM, Taylor RN, et al. Plasma cellular fibronectin as a measure of endothelial involvement in pre-eclampsia and intrauterine growth retardation. Am J Obstet Gynecol. 1994;170:838-41.
80. Lockwood C, Peters J. Increased plasma levels of ED1+ cellular fibronectin precede the clinical signs of pre-eclampsia. Am J Obstet Gynecol. 1990;162:358-62.
81. Taylor RN, Crombleholme WR, Friedman SA, et al. High plasma cellular fibronectin levels correlate with biochemical and clinical features of pre-eclampsia but cannot be attributed to hypertension alone. Am J Obstet Gynecol. 1991;165:895-901.
82. Redman CWG, Denson KWE, Beilin LJ. Factor-VIII consumption in pre-eclampsia. Lancet. 1977;2:1249.
83. Thorp J, White G, Moake J, et al. Von Willebrand factor multimeric levels and patterns in patients with severe pre-eclampsia. Obstet Gynecol. 1990;75:163-7.
84. Boffa MC, Valsecchi L, Fausto A, et al. Predictive value of plasma thrombomodulin in pre-eclampsia and gestational hypertension. Thromb Hemost. 1998;79:1092-5.
85. Minakami H, Takahashi T, Izumi A, et al. Increased levels of plasma thrombomodulin in pre-eclampsia. Gynecol Obstet Invest. 1993;36:208-10.
86. Lyall F, Greer IA, Boswell F, et al. Suppression of serum vascular endothelial growth factor immunoreactivity in normal pregnancy and in pre-eclampsia. Br J Obstet Gynaecol. 1997;104:223-8.
87. Higgins JR, Papayianni A, Brady HR, et al. Circulating vascular cell adhesion molecule-1 in pre-eclampsia, gestational hypertension, and normal pregnancy—evidence of selective dysregulation of vascular cell adhesion molecule-1 homeostasis in pre-eclampsia. Am J Obstet Gynecol. 1998;179:464-9.
88. Krauss T, Kuhn W, Lakoma C, et al. Circulating endothelial cell adhesion molecules as diagnostic markers for the early identification of pregnant women at risk for development of pre-eclampsia. Am J Obstet Gynecol. 1997;177:443-9.

89. Rogers GM, Taylor RN, Roberts JM. Pre-eclampsia is associated with a serum factor cytotoxic to human endothelial cells. Am J Obstet Gynecol. 1988;159:908-14.

90. Tsukimori K, Maeda H, Shingu M, et al. The possible role of endothelial cells in hypertensive disorders during pregnancy. Obstet Gynecol. 1992;80:229-33.

91. Baker PN, Davidge ST, Barankiewicz J, et al. Plasma of pre-eclamptic women stimulates and then inhibits endothelial prostacyclin. Hypertension. 1996; 27:56-61.

92. DeGroot DJM, Davidge ST, Friedman SA, et al. Plasma from pre-eclamptic women increases human endothelial cell prostacyclin production without changes in enzyme activity or mass. Am J Obstet Gynecol. 1995;172:976-85.

93. Baker PN, Davidge ST, Roberts JM. Plasma from women with pre-eclampsia increases endothelial cell nitric oxide production. Hypertension. 1995;26:244-8.

94. Davidge ST, Baker PN, Roberts JM. NOS expression is increased in endothelial cells exposed to plasma from women with pre-eclampsia. Am J Physiol. 1995;269: H1106-12.

95. Davidge ST, Signorella AP, Hubel CA, et al. Distinct factors in plasma of pre-eclamptic women increase endothelial nitric oxide or prostacyclin. Hypertension. 1996;28:758-64.

96. Roberts JM, Edep ME, Goldfine A, et al. Sera from pre-eclamptic women specifically activate human umbilical vein endothelial cells in vitro: morphological and biochemical evidence. Am J Reprod Immunol. 1992; 27:101-8.

97. Taylor RN, Casal DC, Jones LA, et al. Selective effects of pre-eclamptic sera on human endothelial cell procoagulant protein expression. Am J Obstet Gynecol. 1991;165:1705-10.

98. Musci TJ, Roberts JM, Rodgers GM, et al. Mitogenic activity is increased in the sera of pre-eclamptic women before delivery. Am J Obstet Gynecol. 1988;159:1446-51.

99. Taylor RN, Heilbron DC, Roberts JM. Growth factor activity in the blood of women in whom pre-eclampsia develops is elevated from early pregnancy. Am J Obstet Gynecol. 1991;163:1839-44.

100. Endresen MJ, Morris JM, Nobrega AC, et al. Serum from pre-eclamptic women induces vascular cell adhesion molecule-1 expression on human endothelial cells in vitro—a possible role of increased circulating levels of free fatty acids. Am J Obstet Gynecol. 1998;179:665 70.

101. Taylor RN, Musci TJ, Rodgers GM, et al. Pre-eclamptic sera stimulate increased platelet-derived growth factor mRNA and protein expression by cultured human endothelial cells. Am J Reprod Immunol. 1991;25:105-8.

102. Hubel CA, McLaughlin MK, Evans RW, et al. Fasting serum triglycerides, free fatty acids, and malondialdehyde are increased in pre-eclampsia, are positively correlated, and decrease within 48 hours post partum. Am J Obstet Gynecol. 1996;174:975-82.

103. Hubel CA. Dyslipidemia, iron and oxidative stress in pre-eclampsia: Assessment of maternal and feto-placental interactions. Semin Reprod Endocrinol. 1998;16:75-92.

104. Wang Y, Walsh SW, Guo J, et al. The imbalance between thromboxane and prostacyclin in pre-eclampsia is associated with an imbalance between lipid peroxides and vitamin E in maternal blood. Am J Obstet Gynecol. 1991;165:1695-700.

105. Barden A, Beilin LJ, Ritchie J, et al. Plasma and urinary 8-iso-prostane as an indicator of lipid peroxidation in pre-eclampsia and normal pregnancy. Clin Sci. 1996;91:711-8.

106. Granger DN, Rutili G, McCord JM. Superoxide radicals in feline intestinal ischemia. Gastroenterology. 1981;81:22-9.

107. Endresen MJ, Lorentzen B, Henriksen T. Increased lipolytic activity and high ratio of free fatty acids to albumin in sera from women with pre-eclampsia leads to triglyceride accumulation in cultured endothelial cells. Am J Obstet Gynecol. 1992;167:440-7.

108. Roberts LJ, Morrow JD. The isoprostanes: Novel markers of lipid peroxidation and potential mediators of oxidant injury. Adv Prostaglandin Thromboxane Leukot Res. 1995;23:219-24.

109. McCord N, Ayuk PT, Sargent IL, et al. Evidence of increased oxidative stress in pre-eclampsia. Placenta. 2002;23(A39):114.

110. Lowe DT. Nitric oxide dysfunction in the pathophysiology of pre-eclampsia. Nitric Oxide. 2000;4:441-58.

111. Pober JS, Cotran RS. Cytokines and endothelial cell biology. Physiol Rev. 1990;70:427 51.

112. Redman CWG, Sucks GP, Sargents IL. Pre-eclampsia, an excessive maternal inflammatory response to pregnancy. Am J Obstet Gynecol. 1999;180:499-506.

113. Conrad KP, Benyo DF. Placental cytokines and the pathogenesis of pre-eclampsia. Am J Reprod Immunol. 1997;37:240-9.

114. Conrad KP, Miles TM, Benyo DF. Circulating levels of immunoreactive cytokines in women with pre-eclampsia. Am J Reprod Immunol. 1998;40:102-11.

115. Vince GS, Starkey PM, Austgulen R, et al. Interleukin-6, tumor necrosis factor and soluble tumour necrosis factor receptors in women with pre-eclampsia. Br J Obstet Gynaecol. 1995;102:20-5.

116. Hung TH, Charnock-Jones DS, Skepper JN, et al. Secretion of tumor necrosis factor-alpha from human placental tissues induced by hypoxia-reoxygenation causes endothelial cell activation in vitro: A potential mediator of the inflammatory response in pre-eclampsia. Am J Pathol. 2004;164:1049-61.

117. Knight M, Redman CWG, Linton EA, et al. Shedding of syncytiotrophoblast microvilli into the maternal circulation in pre-eclamptic pregnancies. Br J Obstet Gynaecol. 1998;105:632-40.

118. Smarason AK, Sargent IL, Starkey PM, et al. The effect of placental syncytiotrophoblast microvillous membranes from normal and pre-eclamptic women on the growth of endothelial cells in vitro. Br J Obstet Gynaecol. 1993;100:943-9.

119. Smarason AK, Sargent IL, Redman CWG. Endothelial cell proliferation is suppressed by plasma but not serum from women with pre-eclampsia. Am J Obstet Gynecol. 1996;174:787-93.

120. Cockell AP, Learmont JG, Smarason AK, et al. Human placental syncytiotrophoblast microvillous membranes impair maternal vascular endothelial function. Br J Obstet Gynaecol. 1997;104: 235-40.

121. Hung TH, Skepper JN, Charnock-Jones DS, et al. Hypoxia-reoxygenation: A potent inducer of apoptotic changes in the human placenta and possible etiological factor in pre-eclampsia. Circ Res. 2002;90:1274-81.

122. Morbidelli L, Chang CH, Douglas JG, et al. Nitric oxide mediates mitogenic effect of VEGF on coronary venular endothelium. Am J Physiol. 1996;270:H411-5.

123. He H, Venema VJ, Gu X, et al. Vascular endothelial growth factor signals endothelial cell production of nitric oxide and prostacyclin through flk-1/KDR activation of c-Src. J Biol Chem. 1999;274:25130-5.

124. Polliotti BM, Fry AG, Saller DN, et al. Second-trimester maternal serum placental growth factor and vascular endothelial growth factor for predicting severe, early-onset pre-eclampsia. Obstet Gynecol. 2003;101:1266-74.

125. Taylor RN, Grimwood J, Taylor RS, et al. Longitudinal serum concentrations of placental growth factor: evidence for abnormal placental angiogenesis in pathologic pregnancies. Am J Obstet Gynecol. 2003; 88:177-82.

126. Koga K, Osuga Y, Yoshino O, et al. Elevated serum soluble vascular endothelial growth factor receptor 1 (sVEGFR-1) levels in women with pre-eclampsia. J Clin Endocrinol Metab. 2003;88:2348-51.

127. Levine RJ, Maynard SE, Qian C, et al. Circulating angiogenic factors and the risk of pre-eclampsia. N Engl J Med. 2004;350:672-83.

128. Tsatsaris V, Goffin F, Munaut C, et al. Overexpression of the soluble vascular endothelial growth factor in preeclamptic patients: Pathophysiological consequences. J Clin Endocrinol Metab. 2003;88:5555-63.

129. Ahmad S, Ahmed A. Elevated placental soluble vascular endothelial growth factor 1 receptor-1 inhibits angiogenesis in pre-eclampsia. Circ Res. 2004;95:884-91.

130. Khong TY, De Wolff, Robertson WB, et al. Inadequate maternal vascular response to placentation in pregnancies complicated by pre-eclampsia and by small-for-gestational age infants. Br J Obstet Gynaecol. 1986;93:1049-59.

131. Arias F, Rodriquez L, Rayne SC, et al. Maternal placental vasculopathy and infection: Two distinct subgroups among patients with preterm labor and preterm ruptured membranes. Am J Obstet Gynecol. 1993;168:585-91.

132. Ness RB, Roberts JM. Heterogeneous causes constituting the single syndrome of pre-eclampsia: A hypothesis and its implications. Am J Obstet Gynecol. 1996;175:1365-70.

133. Roberts JM, Cooper DW. Pathogenesis and genetics of pre-eclampsia. Lancet. 2001;357:53-6.

134. Chesley LC, Annitto JE, Cosgrove RA. The remote prognosis of eclamptic women: Sixth periodic report. Am J Obstet Gynecol. 1976;124:446-59.

135. Sibai B, El-Nazer A, Gonzalez-Ruiz A. Severe pre-eclampsia eclampsia in young primigravid women: Subsequent pregnancy outcome and remote prognosis. Am J Obstet Gynecol. 1986;155:1011-6.

136. Kaaja R, Tikkanen M, Viinikka L, et al. Serum lipoproteins, insulin, and urinary prostanoid metabolites in normal and hypertensive pregnant women. Obstet Gynecol. 1995;85:353-6.

137. Sattar N, Bendomir A, Berry C, et al. Lipoprotein subfraction concentrations in pre-eclampsia: Pathogenic parallels to atherosclerosis. Obstet Gynecol. 1997;89:403-8.

138. Hubel CA, Shakir Y, Gallaher MJ, et al. Low density lipoprotein particle size decreases during normal pregnancy in association with triglyceride increases. J Soc Gynecol Investig. 1998;5: 244-50.

139. Ogura K, Miyatake T, Fukui O, et al. Low-density lipoprotein particle diameter in normal pregnancy and pre-eclampsia. J Atheroscler Thromb. 2002;9:42-7.

140. Brinkman CR. Biological adaptation of pregnancy. In: Creasy RK, Resnik R (Eds). Maternal fetal medicine, 2nd edn. Philadelphia. WB Saunders. 1989;734-45.

141. Sacks GP, Studena K, Sargent K, et al. Normal pregnancy and pre-eclampsia both produce inflammatory changes in peripheral blood leukocytes akin to those of sepsis. Am J Obstet Gynecol. 1998;179:80-6.

142. Tsukimori K, Maeda H, Ishida K, et al. The superoxide generation of neutrophils in normal and pre-eclamptic pregnancies. Obstet Gynecol. 1993;81:536-540.

143. Crocker IP, Wellings RP, Fletcher J, et al. Neutrophil function in women with pre-eclampsia. Br J Obstet Gynecol. 1999;106:822-8.

144. Lee VM, Quinn PA, Jennings SC, et al. Neutrophil activation and production of reactive oxygen species in pre-eclampsia. J Hypertens. 2003;21:395-402.

145. Aly AS, Khandelwal M, Zhao J, et al. Neutrophils are stimulated by syncytiotrophoblast microvillous membranes to generate superoxide radicals in women with pre-eclampsia. Am J Obstet Gynecol. 2004;190:252-8.

146. Mellembakken JR, Aukrust P, Olafsen MK, et al. Activation of leukocytes during the uteroplacental passage in pre-eclampsia. Hypertension. 2002;39:155-60.

147. Palluy O, Morliere L, Gris JC, et al. Hypoxia/reoxygenation stimulates endothelium to promote neutrophil adhesion. Free Radic Biol Med. 1992;13:21-30.

60 Basic Aspects of Trophoblastic Disease

N Wake, K Asanoma, T Matsuda

GENETICS OF HYDATIDIFORM MOLES

Hydatidiform moles that have grossly swollen villi are divisible into two entities: the classical complete mole and the partial mole. The complete mole presents as a rapidly progressing hydatidiform change affecting the whole placenta, with widespread and gross trophoblastic hyperplasia in the absence of an embryo and its covering amnion. The majority of complete moles have a 46, XX karyotype. Inspection of karyotype from a mole and its parents readily discloses that both members of chromosome pairs of the complete mole are traceable to one paternal chromosome. Thus, these moles result from duplication of a paternal haploid set in a functionally empty ovum, a process called androgenesis. Most probably these moles develop from fertilization of an empty ovum by a haploid sperm followed by the duplication of its chromosomes.[1-6] The maternal nuclear complement is either eliminated or inactivated in an empty ovum. This mechanism would account for the preponderance of XX moles, because their YY counterparts are probably lost during early cleavage stages.

The rare 46, XY moles can also be found.[7-9] Estimates for the total number of these moles range from 4% to 20% in a small series. Southern blots of polymerase chain reaction (PCR) products clearly demonstrate that both alleles shown in the mole derive from the two paternal alleles in some gene loci, whereas the allele derives from one of two paternal alleles in the remaining loci. The genetic features shown in these moles are compatible with fertilization of an empty egg by two spermatozoa. Dispermy would result in an XX, XY or YY sex chromosome constitution, in a 1:2:1 ratio. Again, YY moles are lethal.

In addition to androgenesis, occasional complete moles that are diploid but biparental in origin have been described. While androgenetic complete moles are usually sporadic, biparental complete moles are associated with a predisposition to recurrent molar pregnancies and frequently occur in more than one member of a family. Women with biparental complete mole have a much greater risk of further complete mole than woman with androgenetic complete mole or partial mole and have an appreciable risk of persistent trophoblastic disease. Biparental complete mole arises from an unusual pregnancy associated with a failure to set maternal imprints within the ovum. The gene, mutated in woman with biparental complete mole, shows an autosomal recessive mode of inheritance and has been mapped to chromosome 19q 13.4.

In the partial moles there is a slow hydatidiform change that affects only some of the villi. There is focal, moderate, trophoblastic hyperplasia, irrespective of the survival of the embryo. An accumulation of cytogenetic data has shown that dispermic triploids that were products of an intact ovum fertilized by two spermatozoa were responsible for these partial moles.[10-13]

We have encountered unusual cases of partial moles in the course of systematic cytogenetic studies of partial moles each with a tetraploid karyotype. These rare partial moles result from the combination of a haploid ovum with three paternal haploid sets as a result of trispermic fertilization.[14-16] The majority of partial moles result from dispermic triploids. Tetraploids with one maternal and three paternal haploid sets provide unequivocal morphological examples of partial moles. In addition to these, complete moles that involve the whole placenta in hydatidiform changes are androgenetic in origin. These findings illustrate an intriguing correlation between a molar phenotype and the ratio of paternal to maternal genome in the conceptus. In this connection, the fact that benign ovarian teratomas are parthenogenetic in origin leads to the possibility that the maternal and paternal genome are not functionally equivalent. The teratoma that consists of embryonic tissue elements in the absence of extra-embryonic tissues has two maternally derived haploid sets. These findings point to some dependence of the extra-embryonic tissues, notably trophoblast, on the paternal genome, while some maternal genes are apparently required for the development of the embryo proper. Only male plus female diploid combinations of pronuclei would give rise to normal embryos. Particular sets of genes undergo a separate specific imprinting during oogenesis and spermatogenesis, respectively. Most probably, disruption of imprinted regulation for a particular set of genes in complete and partial moles contributes to the formation of molar phenotypes, but these remain to be identified. Histopathological criteria to differentiate partial and complete moles are inconsistent among countries. In addition, histological features overlap significantly between these moles especially when the moles are evaluated in early gestational stage. These indicate the necessity of genetic demonstration of each class of moles.

MALIGNANT TROPHOBLASTIC NEOPLASMS WITH DIFFERENT MODES OF ORIGIN

It is well-known that the complete mole has a propensity to malignancy. However, there has been no direct proof in the majority of patients that choriocarcinoma indeed derive from a complete mole. The androgenetic origin of complete moles provides us with a method for determining the origin of choriocarcinomas. The genome of choriocarcinoma should reflect that of the pregnancy from which the tumor arose. After a live birth or spontaneous abortion, both maternal and paternal contributions to the genome should be present in the tumor genome. Choriocarcinoma after complete mole conceptions should carry only the paternal genome. The absence of a paternal contribution in the tumor genome is a feature of non-gestational choriocarcinoma. Based on these genetic backgrounds, a small number of choriocarcinomas have been examined so far.[17-23] However, the number of cases reported is too small to show whether there is a predominant association of complete mole with choriocarcinoma or not. Thus, we examined the genetic origin of a relatively large number of trophoblastic tumors in order to demonstrate the propensity to malignancy of complete mole.

Genomic DNAs obtained from 24 fresh or paraffin-embedded tumors were successfully amplified by PCR.[24] Based on pregnancy history, these tumors included: (i) 9 post-molar trophoblastic tumors, (ii) 12 tumors preceded by live birth or abortion, and (iii) 3 non-gestational tumors. PCR polymorphism data revealed the absence of a maternal genome in 8 post-molar trophoblastic tumors (Table 60.1). This was contrasted with the presence of a maternal genome in all 12 tumors preceded by live birth or abortion and in the 3 non-gestational tumors. Thus, these 8 post-molar trophoblastic neoplasms developed from malignant transformation of complete moles. Six tumors were homozygous at three or more gene loci in which the partners were heterozygous. A female sex

chromosome constitution was anticipated because PCR failed to amplify any fragment specific to the *SRY* (which is specific to the Y chromosome) gene sequence in these tumors. These genetic features may be compatible with those of the complete mole that results from fertilization of an empty egg by an X-bearing sperm. The heterozygosity was recognized in two tumors at a few gene loci. The 240-base-pair (bp) PCR product specific to the *SRY* gene sequence was present in one tumor but not in the other. It seemed likely that the two tumors originated from an XX or XY dispermic, androgenetic mole (Fig. 60.1).

The remaining choriocarcinoma contained an allele derived from the patient at a few gene loci. This finding is compatible with the assumption that the tumor did not arise from a complete mole conception would explain this tumor development.

All 12 tumors in class (ii) had alleles of both paternal and maternal contribution. However, discordance of sex between the antecedent pregnancy product and the tumor was recognized in

Table 60.1: PCR-polymorphism analysis of choriocarcinomas and invasive mole (antecedent pregnancies were complete moles) and parents

Patients	DNA	D1S80	ApoB	D5S107	DRB	D9S43	RB	D17S30	DMD	SRY
1	P	f/g	a/–	a/b	4/–	a/–	a/b	c/–	(+)	(+)
	T	f/g	a/c	b/c	4/12	a/b	a/b	c/–		
	M	e/f	b/c	b/c	9/12	b/–	b/–	c/–		
2	P	b/d	a/c	a/b	2/3,6	a/c	a/b	c/f	(+)	(–)
	T	b/d	a/c	a/–	2/–	a/–	a/b	c/f		
	M	a/–	a/c	b/c	2/4	a/–	b/–	a/e		
3	P	b/g	a/b	c/d	4/–	b/–	a/–	b/e	(+)	(–)
	T	b/–	a/–	d/–	4/–	b/–	a/–	b/–		
	M	a/g	a/c	c/d	2/4	c/d	a/b	e/f		
4	P	d/h	a/c	c/–	2/3,6	a/b	c/–	c/e	(+)	(–)
	T	d/–	a/–	c/–	ND	b/–	c/–	e/–		
	M	c/–	a/c	e/f	3,6/–	b/c	a/b	d/–		
5	P	a/b	a/b	e/f	4/–	c/d	a/b	d/f	(+)	(–)
	T	a/–	b/–	f/–	4/–	c/–	b/–	d/–		
	M	d/e	a/–	b/d	2/–	d/e	a/d	f/g		
6	P	d/e	a/–	b/d	4/2	b/f	c/–	d/–	ND	ND
	T	i/–	a/–	b/–	4/–	b/–	c/–	d/–		
	M	i/j	a/–	b/c	3,6/–	b/g	a/b	c/d		
8	P	a/b	a/–	a/b	1/–	f/g		d/f	(+)	(–)
	T	b/–	a/–	a/–	1/–	g/–	ND	f/–		
	M	c/d	a/c	c/–	4/12	h/–		a/b		
9	P	h/i	a/–	a/b	11/9			b/–	(+)	(–)
	T	h/–	a/–	a/–	11/–	ND	ND	b/–		
	M	h/–	a/c	b/	4/9			b/c		
10*	P	d/–	a/c	a/b	4/8	b/h	a/–	b/d	(+)	(+)
	T	d/–	a/–	b/–	4/8	b/–	a/–	b/d		
	M	a/b	a/c	a/b	4/9	b/f	a/–	a/–		

P, paternal DNA; T, tumor DNA; M, maternal DNA; ND, not determined. Bold type indicates a heterozygous pattern in the tumor DNA.
*Invasive mole

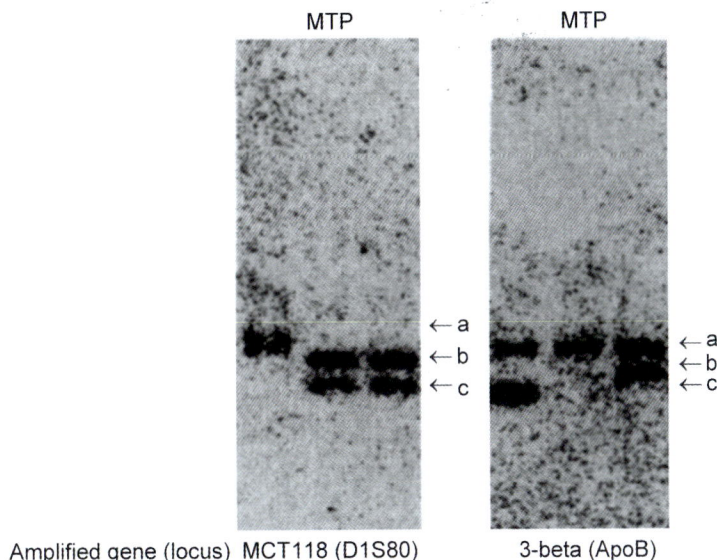

Fig. 60.1: PCR-polymorphism of two choriocarcinomas. The tumor showed two bands that were absent in maternal DNA, suggesting androgenic in origin. P = PCR products from paternal DNA; T = PCR products from tumor DNA; M = PCR products from maternal DNA; VNTR = variable number of tandem repeat

three choriocarcinomas. The absence of a paternal contribution suggested a parthenogenetic origin for the three non-gestational choriocarcinomas. The findings that PCR polymorphisms were either homozygous in certain loci or heterozygous in others may mean that the tumor was derived from a germ cell after meiosis I. As a result, at least three subtypes with different modes of origin were demonstrated in the 24 trophoblastic tumors. Although more than half of the trophoblastic tumors collected here had a maternal contribution to their genomes, the data still support the suggestion that of all forms of pregnancy that predispose patients to choriocarcinoma, the most likely is the complete mole.

MOLECULAR MECHANISMS ASSOCIATED WITH TROPHOBLASTIC DISEASES

Gene Expression Profile in Complete Mole

Kato et al. (2002)[25] used microarray analysis to investigate the expression profiles of 589 genes committed to cell growth control, in order to characterize the regulatory circuitry for cell proliferation in complete moles. Complete moles are characterized by hyperplastic trophoblast and have a high propensity to give rise to choriocarcinoma. Characteristic alterations in gene expression profiles were observed when compared with normal villi. A total of 57 genes were significantly upregulated in complete moles. These involved the Ras/MAP kinase III, JAK/STAT5 and Wnt signal pathways, implicating growth factor- or cytokine-mediated signal pathways in the trophoblastic hyperplasia of complete moles. Several genes associated with antiapoptosis, cell structuring and/or cell attachment were also upregulated in complete moles. In contrast, relatively fewer genes were downregulated and these involved insulin growth factor binding proteins (IGFBPs), Versican, Interleukin-1, tumor necrosis factor receptor, CD44 and Rad 52. The genes identified as being up or downregulated may help to elucidate the regulation mechanisms of trophoblastic proliferation and the mechanisms causing a pathological phenotype in complete moles (Fig. 60.2).[25]

Silencing of NECC1/Hop Expression in Choriocarcinoma

Choriocarcinoma is a highly invasive tumor consisting of markedly anaplastic trophoblasts totally lacking in residual villous structures. Demonstration of a predominant association between complete mole and choriocarcinoma suggests that the molecular events of mole and choriocarcinoma development are related, since the putative forerunner carries unique genetic features (as mentioned previously). The monoallelic contribution shown in the complete mole would render a certain gene susceptible to functional inactivation by "one-hit" kinetics. Alternatively, uniparental transmission of genes that are subject to parental imprinting in humans would impair their regulation. Thus, the features exhibited by complete mole would be associated with inactivation of particular tumor suppressor genes, contributing to the propensity to malignancy.

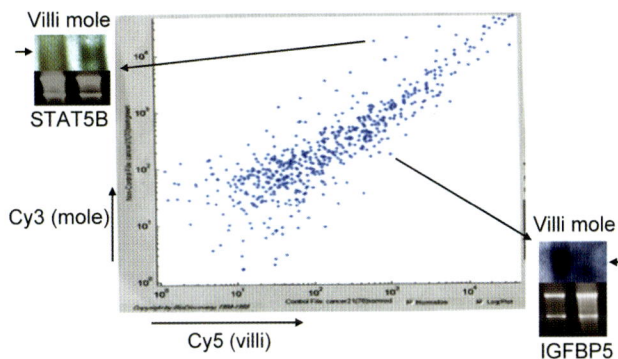

Fig. 60.2: A log plot of microarray experiment demonstrating distribution of 425-gene expression in normal and molar villi. Fluorointensity of Cy-3, which labeled to mRNA from complete mole, is plotted vertically. That of Cy-5, from normal villi, is horizontally plotted. Upregulation of STAT5B expression and downregulation of 1GFBP5 expression in mole were shown. x: control file: mole red Cy3; y: noncontrol file: normal villi green Cy5

Many tumor suppressor genes are inactivated by intragenic mutations in one allele, accompanied by the loss of a chromosomal region containing the remaining allele; this is termed loss of heterozygosity. Mapping such deleted regions has been used to identify sequences involved in malignancies. However, the monoallelic contribution exhibited by the complete mole and its transformant would mask the chromosomal region where the allelic loss frequently occurs. To resolve this difficulty, Asanoma et al.[26] constructed a PCR-subtracted fragmentary cDNA library between normal placenta villi and the choriocarcinoma cell line (CC1) and isolated a candidate choriocarcinoma suppressor gene. This gene comprised an open reading frame of 219 nucleotides (nt) encoding 73 amino acid residues and contained a homeodomain as a consensus motif, being identical with homeodomain only protein (HOP), which is essential for cardiomyocyte development.[27,28] This gene, designated as *not* expressed in *choriocarcinoma clone 1 (NECC1)*[26] is located on human chromosome 4q11-q12. *NECC1* expression is ubiquitous in the brain, placenta, lung, smooth muscle, uterus, bladder, kidney and spleen. Normal placental villi expressed *NECC1*, but all of the choriocarcinoma cell lines examined and most of the surgically removed choriocarcinoma tissue samples failed to express it. Asanoma et al.[26] transfected this gene into choriocarcinoma cell lines and observed remarkable alterations in cell morphology and suppression of in vivo tumorigenesis. Induction of chorionic somatomammotropin hormone 1 (CSH1) and remarkable alteration in cell morphology including multinucleation by *NECC1* expression suggested differentiation of choriocarcinoma cells to syncytiotrophoblasts (Fig. 60.3).

The tumor suppressive ability of *NECC1* does not require the 3rd/4th helix and the C-terminal domain. The inhibitory effect of mutant *NECC1*, which deletes the 3rd/4th helix and the C-terminal domain, on choriocarcinoma cell growth properties, is analogous to that of wild-type *NECC1*. The results imply that the DNA binding capability of *NECC1* is not required for choriocarcinoma cell differentiation and the resultant tumorigenic suppression. This unexpected finding may be supported by the previously reported evidence that several homeobox genes exhibit their biological functions in the absence of DNA binding. The data suggest that loss of *NECC1* expression is involved in the malignant conversion of placental trophoblasts.

Human chromosome 7 carries a putative tumor suppressor gene involved in choriocarcinoma.

To determine which chromosome carries a putative tumor suppressor gene, microcell hybrids were isolated following fusion of choriocarcinoma cells with microcells from mouse A9 cells containing a single human chromosome, 1, 2, 6, 7, 9 or 11. Microcell hybrids with the introduction of chromosome 7 were suppressed or modulated for tumorigenicity and exhibited altered in vitro growth properties. Introduction of chromosomes 1, 2, 6, 9 or 11 had no effect. Tumorigenic revertants isolated from microcell hybrids with the introduced chromosome 7 contained reduced numbers of chromosome 7. These findings suggest that chromosome 7 contains a putative tumor suppressor gene for choriocarcinoma. Changes in the phenotypes seen in microcell hybrids were not associated with the presence of either the *ERV3* or the *H-plk* locus on the introduced chromosome 7, indicating that the putative tumor suppressor gene is outside the *ERV3* and *H-plk* gene loci. Furthermore, we obtained evidence for defining a critical region on chromosome 7 (7p12-7q11.23) that was frequently lost in surgically removed choriocarcinoma tissues and cell lines. Using a panel of microsatellite markers, biallelic deletions were observed, which strongly suggests the presence of a tumor suppressor gene within this critical region (Fig. 60.4).[29]

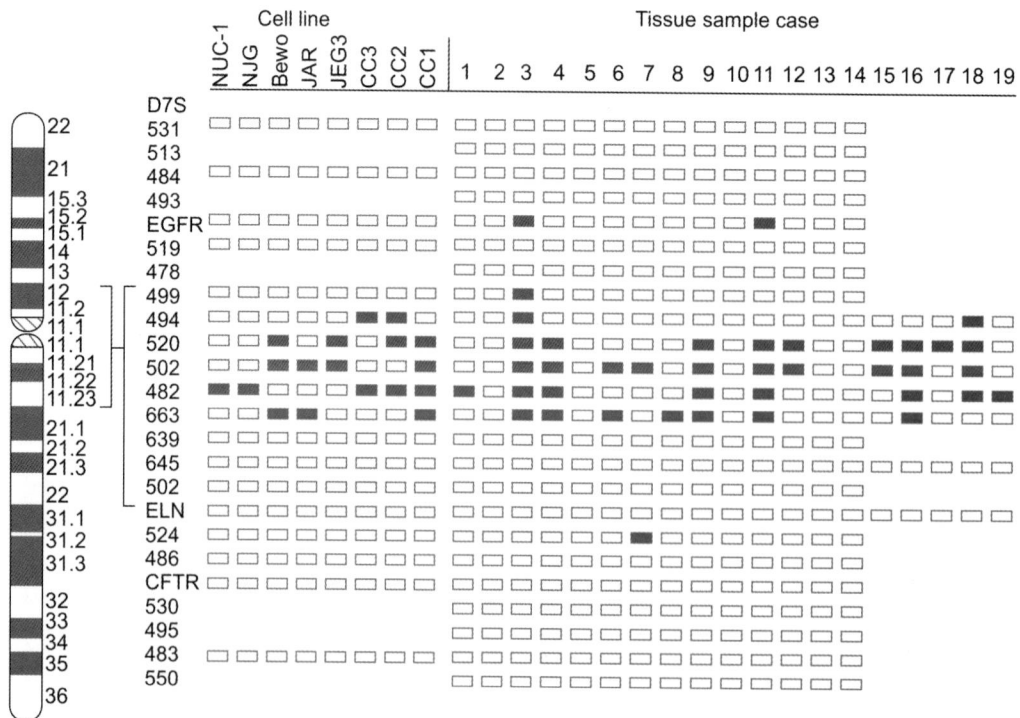

Fig. 60.3: Map of homozygous deletions on chromosome 7. Close squares represent homozygous deletions. Open squares mean the retention of a single or both alleles

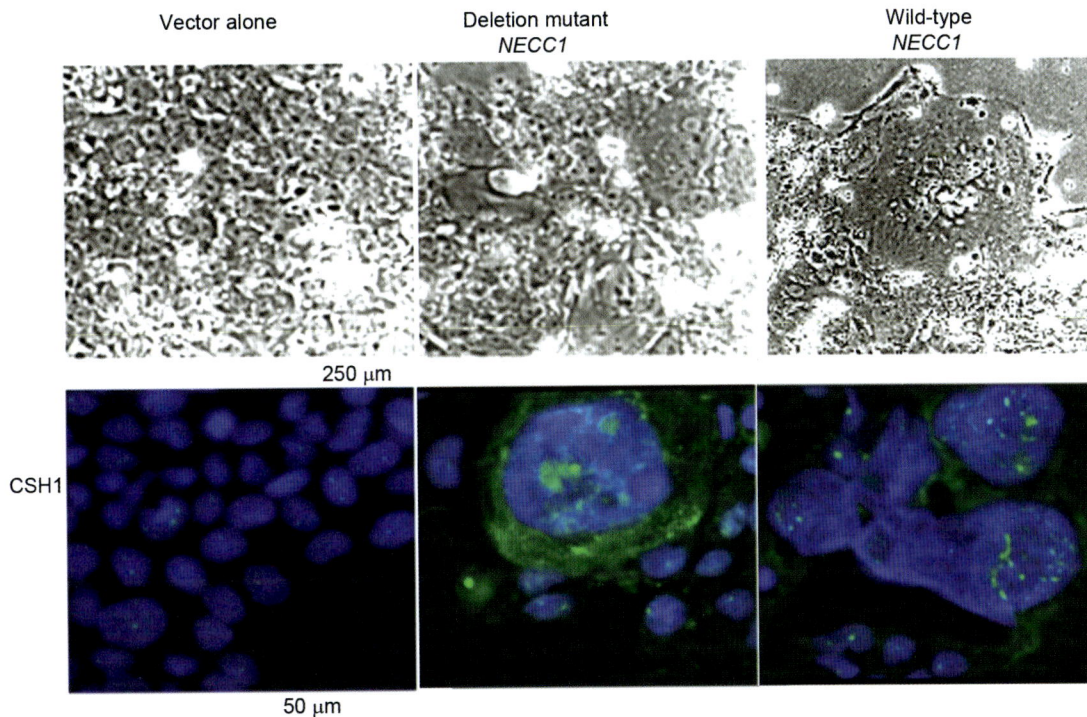

Fig. 60.4: Morphology and immunofluorescent staining of *NECC1* transfected BeWo cells. BeWo cells transfected with vector only, deletion mutant *NECC1*, and wild-type *NECC1* were photographed using phase-contrast microscopy at 40. Lower photographs were immunofluorescent staining of CSH1. *NECC1* deletion mutant and wild-type transfectants expressed abundant CSH1. CSH1, choriomammotropin hormone 1

Genome Imprinting

It has been clearly established that both paternal and maternal contributions are necessary for maintaining a balanced development of both embryonic and extra-embryonic tissues, and the disruption of such a balance may lead to hyperplastic proliferation of the trophoblast, which characterizes molar pregnancies. Based on this hypothesis, it is likely that genomic imprinting, which is disrupted in the androgenetic mole, may play a pivotal role in the development of choriocarcinoma. *H19* and *IGF2* are two classic examples of related imprinted genes. A high level of *H19* expression, in contrast to a considerably lower level of *IGF2* expression, was demonstrated in choriocarcinoma.[30] P57^{KIP2} may also play a role in the pathogenesis of gestational trophoblastic disease (GTD).[31] P57^{KIP2} is a cyclin-dependent kinase inhibitor and is imprinted with the maternal allele being expressed. *P57*^{KIP2} was found to be highly expressed in proliferating trophoblast of normal placenta, but expressed at a low level in complete mole and choriocarcinoma. This is in accordance with what is expected, on the basis of the imprinting of the maternal allele. However, at present, their exact role and diagnostic usefulness are not clear.

Other Molecular Events Involved in Trophoblastic Diseases

Malignant transformation in hydatidiform mole is a multistep process involving the accumulation of several genetic events, including activation of oncogene and/or loss of tumor suppressor genes. A small number of oncogenes and tumor suppressor genes have been found to play putative roles in the pathogenesis of GTD. For example, the oncogenes *c-myc*, *c-erb-B-2*, *bcl-2* and *mdm-2*,[32] the guanosine triphosphatase-activating (GTPase-activating)

protein genes, *p53*, *p21WAF1/KIP1* and *Rb*, and the tumor suppressor gene *DOC-2/hDab2*[33] have all been listed as candidates.

There are reports of increased *c-fms* RNA in complete mole compared with normal placentas,[34] and *c-myc* and *ras* RNA in choriocarcinomas.[35] The significance of such simple quantitative changes in proto-oncogene expression by abnormal trophoblast is hard to evaluate since several proto-oncogenes are already expressed at high levels in normal placentas.

Epidermal growth factor receptors (EGFR) are expressed more strongly in molar placenta than in normal placenta of similar gestational age. Tumors with a histological diagnosis of invasive mole and choriocarcinoma show very strong binding of EGFRs. EGFR expression has been associated with the secretion of human chorionic gonadotropin (hCG). Following exposure to chemotherapy, EGFR binding sites have been noted to be diminished in choriocarcinoma cells.[36]

SUMMARY

The complete mole is androgenetic in origin. The vast majority of complete moles results from the fertilization of an egg devoid of nuclei (an empty egg) by a haploid spermatozoon. Fertilization of an empty egg by two spermatozoa is responsible for a rare class of complete mole. The genome of choriocarcinoma should reflect that of the pregnancy from which the tumor arose. Thus, the predominant association of complete mole with choriocarcinoma suggests that the molecular events for the formation of a complete mole and the malignant conversion of trophoblasts are related. The monoallelic contribution shown in complete mole would render a certain gene susceptible to functional inactivation by "one-hit" kinetics. Alternatively, uniparental transmission of genes that are subject to parental imprinting in humans would impair their regulation. Loss of *NECC1* expression, biallelic deletions at the critical (7p12-7q11.23) region and enhanced *H19* expression in choriocarcinoma would reflect the genetic features

exhibited by the putative forerunner, complete mole. In addition, alterations in gene expression profiles accompanied by malignant conversion of trophoblasts would facilitate choriocarcinogenesis from complete mole. In future, identification of molecular targets down or upregulated in choriocarcinoma will provide us with the management tools for gestational trophoblastic diseases.

REFERENCES

1. Kajii T, Ohama K. Androgenetic origin of hydatidiform mole. Nature. 1977;268:633-4.
2. Wake N, Takagi N, Sasaki M. Androgenesis as a cause of hydatidiform mole. Journal of the National Cancer Institute. 1978;60:51-7.
3. Wake N, Shina Y, Ichinoe K. A further cytogenetic study of hydatidiform mole, with reference to its androgenetic origin. Proceedings of the Japan Academy. 1978;54:533-7.
4. Lawler SD, Pickthall VI, Fisher RA, et al. Genetic studies of complete and partial hydatidiform moles. Lancet. 1979;2:580.
5. Yamashita K, Wake N, Araki T, et al. Human lymphocyte antigen expression in hydatidiform mole/: Androgenesis following fertilization by a haploid sperm. Am J Obstet Gynecol. 1979;135:597-600.
6. Jacobs PA, Wilson CM, Sprenkle JA, et al. Mechanism of origin of complete hydatidiform moles. Nature. 1980;268:714-6.
7. Ohama K, Kajii T, Ikamoto E, et al. Dispermic origin of XY hydatidiform moles. Nature. 1981;292:551-2.
8. Wake N, Seki T, Fujita H, et al. Malignant potential of homozygous and heterozygous complete moles. Cancer Research. 1984;44:1226-30.
9. Wake N, Fujino T, Hoshi S, et al. The propensity to malignancy of dispermic heterozygous moles. Placenta. 1987;8:319-26.
10. Vassilakos P, Riotton G, Kajii T. Hydatidiform mode: two entities. A morphologic and cytogenetic study with some clinical considerations. Am J Obstet Gynecol. 1977;127:167-70.
11. Szulman AE, Surti U. The syndromes of hydatidiform mole. I. Cytogenetic and morphologic correlations. Am J Obstet Gynecol. 1978;131:665-71.
12. Szulman AE, Philippe E, Bou'e JG, et al. Human triploidy: Association with partial hydatidiform moles and non molar conceptuses. Human Pathology. 1981;12:016-21.
13. Lawler SD, Fisher RA, Pickthall VJ, et al. Genetic studies on hydatidiform moles. I. The origin of partial moles. Cancer Genetics and Cytogenetics. 1982;5:309–20.
14. Sheppard DM, Fisher RA, Lowler SD, et al. Tetraploid conceptus with three paternal contributions. Human Genetics. 1982;62:371-4.
15. Sutri U, Szulman AE, Waquer K, et al. Tetraploid partial hydatidiform moles: Two cases with a triple paternal contribution and a 92, XXXY karyotype. Human Genetics. 1986;72:15-21.
16. Vejerslev LO, Ficher RA, Surti U, et al. Hydatidiform mole: Cytogenetically unusual cases and their implications for the present classification. Am J Obstetr Gynecol. 1987;157:180-4.
17. Wake N, Tanaka K, Chapman V, et al. Chromosomes and cellular origin of choriocarcinoma. Cancer Research. 1981;41:3137-43.
18. Fisher RA, Lawler SD, Povey S, et al. Genetically homozygous choriocarcinoma following pregnancy with hydatidiform mole. Brit J Cancer. 1988;58:788-92.
19. Chaganti RS, Koduru PR, Chakraborty R, et al. Genetic origin of a trophoblastic choriocarcinoma. Cancer Research. 1990;50:6330-3.
20. Fisher RA, Paradinas FJ, Newland ES, et al. Genetic evidence that placental site trophoblastic tumours can originate from a hydatidiform mole or a normal conceptus. Brit J Cancer. 1992;65:355-8.
21. Fisher RA, Newlands ES, Jeffreys AJ, et al. Gestational and nongestational trophoblastic tumors distinguished by DNA analysis. Cancer. 1992;69:839-45.
22. Arima T, Imamura T, Amada S, et al. Genetic origin of malignant trophoblastic neoplasms. Cancer Genetics and Cytogenetics. 1994;73:95-102.
23. Sasaki S, Katayama PK, Roesler M. Cytogenetic analysis of choriocarcinoma cell lines. Acta Obstetricia et Gynecologica Japonica. 1982;34:2253-6.
24. Arima T, Imamura T, Sakuragi N, et al. Malignant trophoblastic neoplasms with different modes of origin. Cancer Genetics and Cytogenetics. 1995;85:5-15.
25. Kato H, Terao Y, Ogawa M, et al. Growth-associated gene expression profiles by microarray analysis of trophoblast of molar pregnancies and normal villi. Int J Gynecol Pathol. 2002;21:255-60.
26. Asanoma K, Matsuda T, Konda H, et al. NECC1, a candidate choriocarcinoma suppressor gene that encodes homeodomain consensus motif. Genomics. 2003;81:15-25.
27. Shin CH, Liu ZP, Passier R, et al. HOP, an unusual homeodomain protein. Cell. 2002;110:725-35.
28. Chen F, Kook H, Milewski R, et al. Hop is an unusual homeobox gene that modulates cardiac development. Cell. 2002;110:713-23.
29. Matsuda T, Sasaki M, Kato H, et al. Human chromosome carries a putative tumour suppressor gene(s) involved in choriocarcinoma development. Oncogene. 1997;15:2773-81.
30. Arima T, Matsuda T, Takagi N, et al. Association of IGF2 and H19 imprinting with choriocarcinoma development. Cancer Genetics and Cytogenetics. 1997;93:39-47.
31. Chilosi M, Piazzola E, Lestani M, et al. Differential expression of p57^{KIP2}, a maternally imprinted cdk inhibitor, in normal human placenta and gestational trophoblastic disease. Laboratory Investigation. 1998;78:269-76.
32. Fulop V, Mok SC, Genest DR, et al. c-myc, c-erbB-2, cfms and bcl-2 oncoproteins. Expression in normal placenta, partial and complete mole, and choriocarcinoma. Journal of Reproductive Medicine. 1998;43:101-10.
33. Fulop V, Colitti CV, Genest D, et al. DOC-2/hDab2, a candidate tumor suppressor gene involved in the development of gestational trophoblastic diseases. Oncogene. 1998;17:419-24.
34. Maruo T, Mochizuki M. Immunohistochemical localization of epidermal growth factor receptor and myc oncogene product in human placenta: Implication for trophoblast proliferation and differentiation. Am J Obstet Gynecol. 1987;156:721-7.
35. Cheung AN, Srivastava G, Pittaluga S, et al. Expression of c-myc and c-fms oncogenes in trophoblastic cells in hydatidiform mole and normal human placenta. J Clin Pathol. 1993;46:204-7.
36. Sarkar S, Kacinski BM, Kohorn EI, et al. Demonstration of myc and ras oncogene expression by hybridization in situ in hydatidiform mole and in the BeWo choriocarcinoma cell line. Am J Obstet Gynecol. 1986;154:390-3.

C H A P T E R

61 The Placenta

K Benirschke

THE NORMAL PLACENTA

In the idealized menstrual cycle of 28 days, fertilization takes place on day 14, the developing blastocyst develops in the fallopian tube, travels through the tube to the endometrial cavity and implants on approximately day 6½.[1] It usually implants on the anterior or posterior surface of the upper endometrium, invades the decidualizing endometrium by ingesting its cells through trophoblastic activity and becomes interstitially implanted; that is to say, it becomes completely surrounded by endometrium. At first, mostly trophoblastic proliferation takes place around a large cavity, the blastocystic cavity that contains a gel and the tiny embryo. From the gradually developing embryo, the three layers (ectoderm, mesoderm and endoderm) develop; the mesoderm expands into the future umbilical cord, and then comes to line the blastocystic cavity, thus making it the future chorionic membrane, and hence the mesoderm proliferates into the gradually developing villi, from inside outward. The trophoblast, initially polyploid, differentiates into cytotrophoblast from which the syncytiotrophoblast develops on the villous surfaces. The cytotrophoblast differentiates into two components, the villous cytotrophoblast (also called "Langhans' layer") that underlies the syncytium, and the extravillous trophoblast. It is the latter group of cells that assumes the infiltrative arm of the expanding shell; it infiltrates the decidua and, somewhat later, the endometrial (spiral) arterioles. This infiltration stops before the myometrium is reached, thus, it normally leaves a thin layer of decidua basalis to remain between villi and myometrium. It is at this interface where the Nitabuch and Rohr fibrinoid layers are produced, eosinophilic substances that are produced by the extravillous trophoblast. The latter cells, because of their formerly uncertain origin (maternal or fetal) have also been called the "X-cells"; they often produce small cysts containing major basic protein (MBP). The MBP is similar to that found in the granules of eosinophilic polymorphonuclear cells, and it is secreted into the maternal circulation, like hCG. Its function is completely unknown.

The embryo then lengthens and folds. From the edges of its ectodermal plate the amnionic cavity forms which then gradually fills with clear fluid. As the embryo folds in all directions, the edges of the ectoderm and amnion come to meet over the developing umbilical cord mesenchyme and the amnion fuses with this mesenchyme tightly. As the amnion fills with fluid (perhaps derived from that contained in the extraembryonic coelom), it expands and gradually becomes passively attached to the inner surface of the chorionic membrane. It completely fuses with this membrane at about 12 weeks of gestation.[2] Prior to that fusion, it is being held in position by the gel of the extraembryonic coelom (Fig. 61.1).

It is important to realize that the amnion has an inner epithelial layer that sits on a complex connective tissue layer, but it does not ever contain blood vessels. Moreover, the amnion can usually be dislodged from the chorionic surface of the placenta and is thus often so disrupted by the manipulations at delivery. Furthermore, if the amnion were to disrupt prior to it is becoming affixed to the chorion (before 12 weeks), then amnionic bands may form that ultimately can disrupt parts of the fetus.[3]

From the endodermal layer of the embryo develops the yolk sac. Its epithelium provides the precursors for liver, hematopoietic cells and germ cells, aside from producing the intestines after the embryo has folded. Having folded, the rotation of the intestines inside the embryo gradually pulls the yolk sac into the fetal abdominal cavity; it is there connected to possible remains of Meckel's diverticulum. Also, from the distal part of the yolk sac a small, temporary extension develops into the developing umbilical cord, the primitive allantoic diverticulum. It is very transitory in humans while a true sac develops in many other mammals and serves as a receptacle for fetal urine. In human placentation the fetal urine accumulates in the amnionic cavity. Blood vessels infiltrate the villi and establish the fetal circulation somewhat later in the expansion of the villous tissue. It is not quite certain whether these vessels also differentiate in situ in the placental villi or whether they progress only from the fetus toward the periphery. Thus, ultimately two umbilical arteries progress from the fetus through the umbilical cord to the villous circulation, ramifying over the chorionic plate of the placenta. They are readily distinguished as arteries or veins by their position: The major arterial branches pass over the veins. They are virtually indistinguishable histologically. The vessels can be followed toward the periphery where they are seen to dip

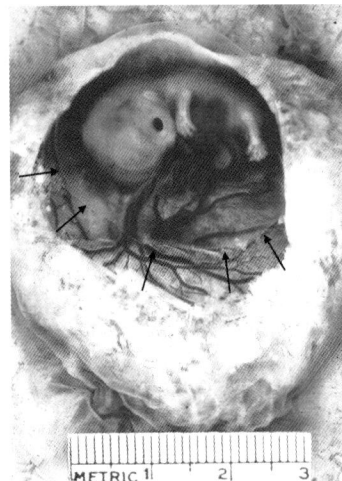

Fig. 61.1: Eight weeks conceptus in utero. The arrows denote the edge of the expanding amnion. Note that the dome of the placental membranes is not attached to the opposite side of the uterus

into the villous tissue and, generally, a single vein returns to the same location as the arterial branch. Each such branch establishes a single fetal cotyledonary district whose circulation does not merge with adjacent cotyledons.[4]

The extravillous cytotrophoblast arrodes the maternal arterioles, grows into them and there causes the "physiologic change", altering these maternal arterial blood vessels by removing their musculature and depositing fibrinoid. At first thick columns virtually occlude the lumens, later they hollow out and the complete intervillous circulation is then established (Figs 61.2 and 61.3). Needless to say, fetal and maternal circulations are separated by the trophoblast and a thin layer of connective tissue.

GROSS EXAMINATION

The placenta should be inspected after the baby is delivered and some minimal observations should be charted. It is our practice also to save the placenta in a refrigerator for several days as its examination may be valuable for pathologists in cases where the infant is abnormal or fails to thrive. The important observations to be made at the time of delivery are the following features: (1) the length and insertion of the umbilical cord should be ascertained;

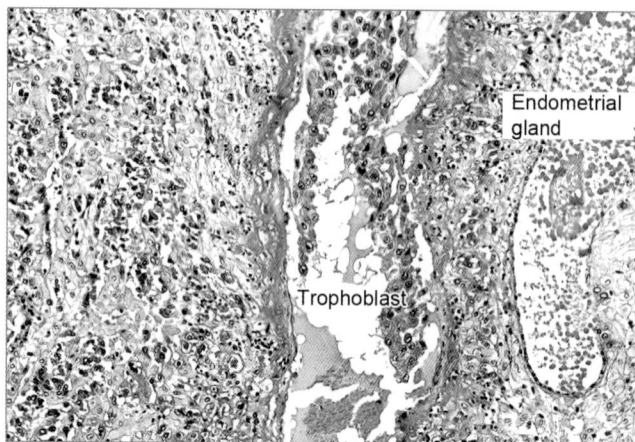

Fig. 61.2: Extravillous trophoblast growing within a decidual spiral arteriole

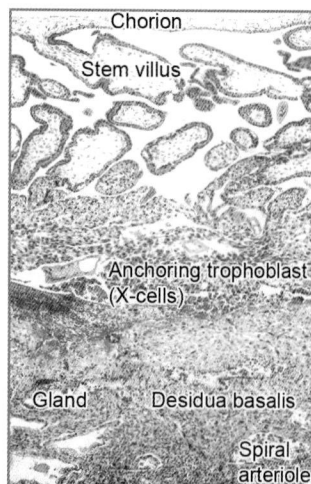

Fig. 61.3: The placental floor in early implantation. The darker cells are extravillous trophoblast that intermingle with the decidual cells

(2) the presence or absence of retroplacental clot (abruptio placentae) needs to be looked for; (3) the color of the fetal surface (meconium staining or opacification from chorioamnionitis) need to be charted, and (4) the color of the villous tissue should be inspected. The latter observation is important as it can denote whether a baby has lost blood through transplacental hemorrhage. The color of the villous tissue is almost totally a reflection of the fetal hemoglobin content. Thus, an anemic neonate has a very pale villous tissue that may reflect erythroblastosis, parvovirus B19 infection, hemoglobinopathy or, importantly, significant fetal blood loss. If it is unusually pale (and the obstetrician of course needs to be acquainted with the normal colors), then a maternal blood film should be made immediately and it needs to be studied by the Kleihauer-Betke technique.[3] If infarcts or other unusual findings are made, the placenta should be sent for pathologic examination. Special circumstances are to be observed in multiple pregnancy and these are discussed in a subsequent section.

UMBILICAL CORD

The normal cord insertion is somewhere near the center of the placental disk. In about 5% of normal gestations it inserts at the placental margin, and in ~1% of placentas it is located in the membranes ("velamentous insertion"). The latter is of significance in that it is often a cause of fetal growth restriction and also, because the fetal vessels ramifying in the membranes have lost their protection by Wharton's jelly and may become disrupted, leading to massive fetal hemorrhage. The length of the umbilical cord is important and it can rarely be reassessed after the placenta is sent for study. Thus, it should at least be estimated, if not measured, at the time of delivery. In the normal-term gestation, the umbilical cord is approximately 55 cm long, and 85% have a counterclockwise (left) twist. The reason for this "chirality" is unknown but I suspect that it relates to the fetal movements because immobile fetuses, such as found with osteogenesis imperfecta cases which have usually no twists. The cord in those cases is also unusually short (Fig. 61.4). In contrast, when knots in the cord exist or when there are nuchal cords, it is often significantly lengthened. This may be the result of excessive fetal movements. It is also important to ascertain in unusually long cords whether there is excessive twisting of the cord on the surface of the fetus, the place where it inserts on the abdomen. It is not uncommon that excessive twisting leads to fetal demise, even abortions (Fig. 61.4). In addition, one may find "false knots" which represent redundancies of vessels or excess Wharton's jelly, unimportant features.

The normal umbilical cord contains three blood vessels, two arteries and one vein. In some 1% of neonates, only one artery is found (SUA) and this is frequently associated with congenital anomalies (~45%) and also with fetal trisomies. While the presence of SUA may signal to the neonatologist that special attention should be paid to possible internal anomalies (heart, kidney), it is important to realize that many babies with SUA are entirely normal. True knots in the umbilical cord usually form early during development and they are now often recognized sonographically. They may lead to complete obstruction of blood flow and to fetal demise. In other cases, true knots have so impeded the venous (oxygenated blood) return from the placenta that surface thrombi will be observed on the placenta which can even be calcified. Obviously, such features

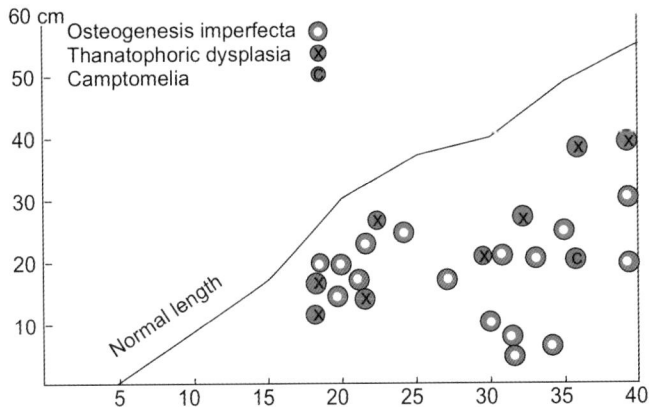

Fig. 61.4: Length of umbilical cord in excessively short cord syndromes. The line represents the normal length

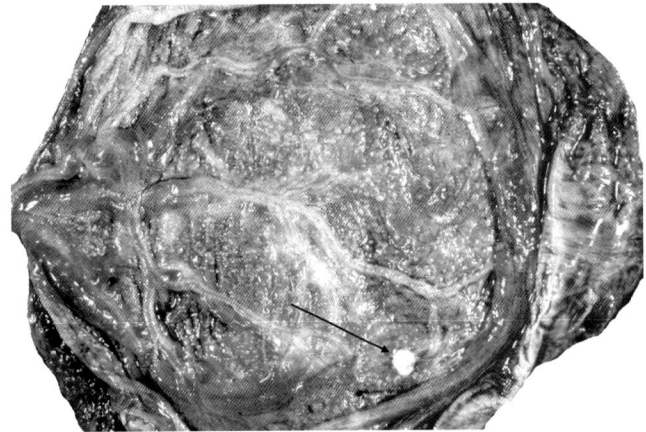

Fig. 61.5: Placental surface in renal agenesis with amnion nodosum; at the arrow is the degenerated, calcified remains of the yolk sac (a normal feature)

may determine whether major sequelae develop in the fetus such as CNS destruction and cerebral palsy.

THE MEMBRANES

The free membranes are referred to as the chorion leave but, in the older placental literature, all of the placenta and its membranes were referred to as the "membranes" or "secundines". The "free" membranes as we know them now have an outer layer of deciduas capsularis which is followed by atrophied villi in between extravillous trophoblast, then comes the chorion and innermost is the amnion. When the membranes have a measurable portion between the site of rupture and the placental disk, then it cannot be a placenta previa if it is delivered vaginally.

At the site of rupture one often finds blood clot and some inflammation can occur here from the processes of labor. Histologically, there is then deciduitis, and thrombosis may be present in the decidual blood vessels. While, this may be grossly interpreted as representing an abruptio placentae, that is not quite correct, as the blood is accumulated only behind the membranes, not behind the villous tissue. Of course, since chorioamnionitis is so much more common in immature placentas, these features are much more frequently found in such births. For the pathologist, the study of the deciduas capsularis is best undertaken when a membrane roll is made so as to increase the chances of finding abnormalities. These are principal findings of "atherosis" (alterations of decidual arteries in preeclampsia to be discussed below) aside from the inflammation. Since atherosis is so frequently found in these vessels, this has raised the question of where the vascular supply of the deciduas capsularis originates. It is usually assumed that the expanding membranes are merely pressed against the deciduas vera of the opposite side of the uterus and that there is perhaps no ingrowth of decidua vera into the decidua capsularis, but definitive studies have not been made. Macroscopic findings of early placentas negate this suggestion of true ingrowth from the deciduas vera (Fig. 61.1). It is important for the pathologist to recognize that the amnion consists of a single layer of epithelial cells (that occasionally have patches of squamous metaplasia) which are situated on a dense, avascular connective tissue membrane. When the amnion disrupts spontaneously before it attaches to the chorion in early pregnancy, the amnion fails to grow subsequently and may become

entangled in fetal extremities when the fetus moves about. This is the mechanism for amnionic bands and its many complications, primarily digital amputations. The cause of such disruptions is unknown but does not usually relate to trauma or any antecedent event that has been elucidated. In such cases, one can invariably find a rim of amnion at the reflection of the umbilical cord, as it is here firmly affixed to the mesenchyme of the cord. Amnion nodosum is the other pathological condition worthy of note. In the absence of amnionic fluid (as in renal agenesis, polycystic kidneys, urethral obstruction, etc.) fetal urine fails to fill the sac and focal degeneration of the amnionic epithelium takes place. Amnion nodosum is most pronounced on the placental disk, never on the cord and only rarely on the free membranes. At the sites of this epithelial disruption, vernix caseosa embeds and forms microscopic nodules, the amnion nodosum. This is of course possible only after the fetus has made sufficient vernix to be embedded, and it is thus not found in very immature fetuses with renal agenesis (Fig. 61.5).

Meconium staining of the membranes is common. It occurs in nearly 15% of our placentas and is usually the result of post-term gestations. Numerous clinical impressions have suggested that meconium discharge is the result of fetal hypoxia, but other studies indicate that this may not be so. For instance, most stillborn fetuses, assuredly having died from hypoxia, are not stained. Moreover, elevated levels of motilin (the GI hormone that regulates bowel movements) are present. Meconium can be recognized histologically in the macrophages of amnion and chorion by their yellow pigmentation and enlargement. It must be cautioned also that this pigment disappears quickly when slides are exposed to light. Slides must thus be examined soon after their preparation. Moreover, the pigment may also be due to hemosiderin from chronic bleeding somewhere in the gestational sac; it must therefore be critically appraised.

VILLOUS TISSUE

The villous tissue changes with the maturation of the placenta. In young organs, the villi are relatively large, have numerous cells and the fetal capillaries are dispersed peripherally beneath the trophoblast. The villi look "edematous" and this changes with maturity as more villi sprout peripherally (Fig. 61.6). In the term placenta the most peripheral villi are small and contain mostly

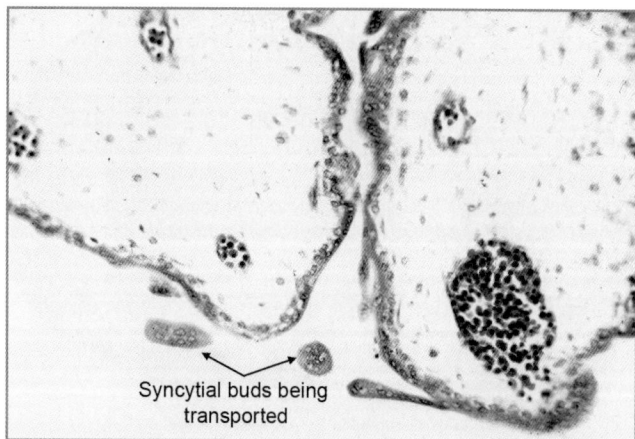

Fig. 61.6: Immature villi with numerous nucleated red blood cells within the capillaries. The stroma is "loose" and appears edematous, but that is normal. A few syncytial buds are in the process of detaching. The cytotrophoblastic Langhans' layer is visible beneath the superficial syncytium

3-4 capillaries with few connective tissue elements. There are also some macrophages within the villi, the so-called Hofbauer cells, and they are more readily seen in immature organs. They are important cells in the elimination of antigens and assist in the removal of focal hemorrhage as they occur for instance in CMV infections. They may then contain hemosiderin.

The surface of villi is covered by trophoblast. There is an inner layer of cytotrophoblast (the "Langhans" layer) in which mitoses occur that produce the cytoplasm and the nuclei for the covering syncytiotrophoblast. The syncytium, however, is the actual organ of exchange. It is a single, uninterrupted membrane covering all villi, has no cell borders and the nuclei have become incapable of mitosis. The syncytiotrophoblast has a fine brush border of microvilli and its cytoplasm possesses numerous transport vesicles, and its surface has many receptor sites for nutrient exchange. Importantly, the syncytium expresses no HLA antigens that could potentially excite a maternal rejection process. So far as is now known, only HLA-G is expressed and this is not antigenic to the mother. The cytotrophoblast is easily visible in young placentas but it is difficult to recognize these cells at term, although they are always there when studied by the electron microscope. Since cytotrophoblast continues to produce new syncytium, the cells and cytoplasm of the latter bunch up and form so-called knots or sprouts. These increase in number toward term and then they are recognized on about 30% of peripheral villi. They also often detach and are carried away in the intervillous (maternal) circulation and swept to the maternal lung. Here they die, as they have no reproductive capacity. When the villi shrink, as is the case in preeclampsia because of deficient water transfer to the fetus, there is more "buckling" of the syncytium and more knots are found; this is referred to as the "Tenney-Parker" change.

A number of conditions cause histologically recognizable changes in villi, the most important and frequent of which is infarction. Death of villi, usually of larger districts, is caused by the obliteration of spiral (decidual) arterioles. This occurs most commonly in preeclampsia and may be associated with abruption of the placenta from bleeding into the deciduas basalis. But infarcts are also common at the edge of the placenta and then they are usually without consequence. Edema of villi is a frequent finding in

fetal anemia (erythroblastosis, hemoglobinopathy) and of course in hydatidiform moles. In addition, one may find inflammatory cells within villi in the condition known as "villitis of unknown etiology (VUE)", in CMV infections and in syphilis.

Finally, there may be too many capillaries within the terminal villi. This condition, known as chorangiosis, is seen in chronic hypoxia (e.g. in placentas from high altitude), in the Beckwith-Wiedemann syndrome, associated with chorangiomas, and a few other conditions (diabetes). When such alterations are found one should also look for the presence of nucleated red blood cells (NRBCs) in the fetal capillaries; they are not present in placentas after about 25 weeks and, when present, they may also signal prolonged intrauterine hypoxic states.

INFECTIONS

One of the most important aspects of obstetrics today is ascending infection with chorioamnionitis and premature birth ensuing. This is an especially important feature for the 20–30 week gestations as the often associated severe prematurity may lead to fetal infection and, most importantly, to CNS damage with cerebral palsy as the outcome. Chorioamnionitis is common and it often recurs in subsequent pregnancies. I believe that it results mainly from the deficiency of endocervical mucus that normally protects the intrauterine environment from vaginal organisms. This, in turn, probably reflects severe chronic endocervicitis. While septic distribution of some maternal organisms occurs (listeriosis, cytomegalovirus infection, toxoplasmosis) these are, numerically speaking, unimportant entities.

The endocervical canal produces copious amounts of dense mucus in normal pregnancy that contains abundant antibodies and protective immunocytes. The canal is also normally closed and narrow until labor commences. When organisms are allowed to cause endocervicitis and proliferate here, the inflammatory process generates enzymes (mainly a phospholipase) that lead to the local production of prostaglandin with dilatation of the cervix and lower uterine segment following. This, in turn, leads to deciduitis of the "forelying" decidua capsularis and the organisms may then enter the amnionic cavity, with or without the rupture of membranes. Once they are in the amnionic cavity, the leukotactic property of the organisms leads to a series of inflammatory sequelae, first on the surface of the placenta, then the umbilical cord and, when inhaled, the infection may cause fetal pneumonia (Fig. 61.7). The first effect is the emigration of maternal leukocytes from the intervillous space beneath the chorionic surface of the placenta, then inflammation of surface vessels follows, thereafter umbilical phlebitis and finally umbilical arteritis takes place. This pus that obscures the fetal surface of the placenta and makes it to be "cloudy" (opaque) is thus of mixed origin, maternal and fetal. Studies of gastric aspirates and lung exudate have shown this admixture definitively. In time, after days of aspiration of this infective material, the fetal lung reacts with infiltration of a lymphocytic response. Often it is possible to identify some bacterial organisms, but this is generally uncommon. The reason for our inability to recognize organisms histologically lies in the nature of the inciting antigens. They are frequently not visible in histologic sections (such as *Trichomonas, Mycoplasma, Ureaplasma, Chlamydia*) but they can be cultured if efforts are made. An exception is found in the infections with group B streptococci. Because of their toxins (hemolytic and cytolytic), one may identify numerous organisms but find only relatively little inflammation with this common infection.

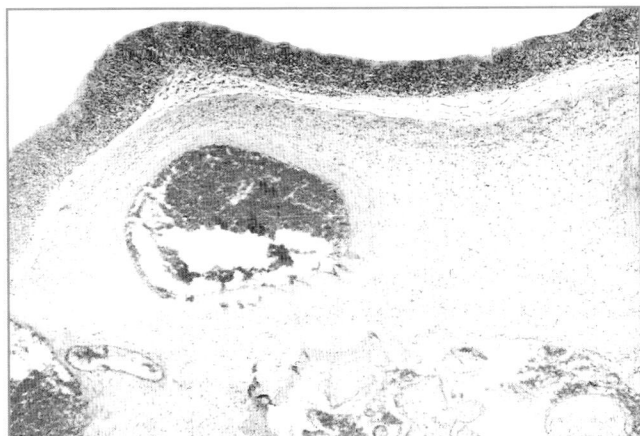

Fig. 61.7: Placental surface in marked, long-standing chorio-amnionitis.The dense leukocytic infiltrate is seen beneath the amnion

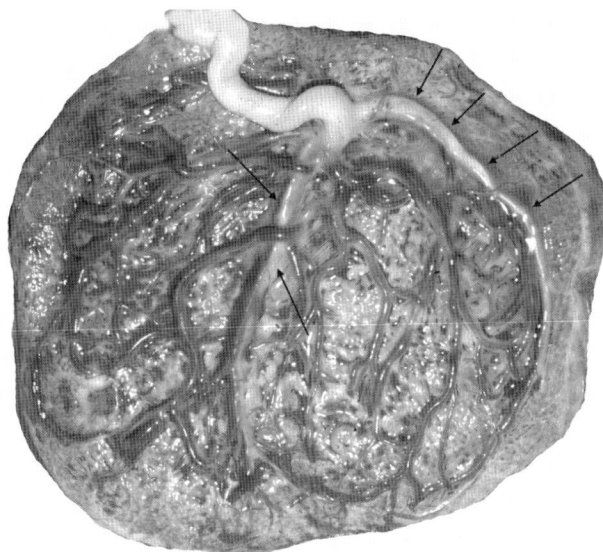

Fig. 61.8: Placenta in severe CMV infection with extensive venous thromboses at arrows. The thrombi were at least partially calcified

Numerous attempts have been made to treat this ascending infection when it is recognized by a dilating cervix or by maternal fever, but that is usually too late in the course of the disease. Moreover, most efforts to treat the fetus in utero with administration of antibiotics to the mother have been unsuccessful.

Thus, it becomes more important to anticipate the infection, especially its recurrent nature, and treat with antibiotics *prior* to the dilatation of the cervix. The pathologist observes placentas with an opacified (cloudy) fetal surface and, histologically, by the presence of numerous polymorphonuclear leukocytes in chorion and amnion (Fig. 61.7). Later, there is exudation from the umbilical vein and then the arteries. The remainder of the placenta, especially its villous structures, is entirely normal, but usually immature. The membranes, however, are markedly altered. The deciduitis and often decidual necrosis are severest near the point of membrane rupture which is so close to the endocervical canal. There may be fresh clot attached at this site and it is occasionally mislabeled as representing an abruption. In twin gestations, it is invariably twin A, lying closest to the endocervix that has the infection and severest inflammation. Chlamydial organisms are the commonest cause of genital infection nowadays, causing urethritis, salpingitis (with infertility ensuing), cervicitis and occasionally a disseminated infection. Since, this organism is not visible in routine preparations of histologic slides, it must be considered when chorioamnionitis is present.

Disseminated infections represented by lesions in the placenta are found in listeriosis. This gram positive *Coccobacillus* causes maternal sepsis and disseminates into the fetus probably most commonly via abscess formation in the placenta. Numerous epidemics have been described that have usually been of a food-borne origin, as the organism is widespread and proliferates well in the refrigerated state. The placenta may show small abscesses and many organisms are commonly found on the placental surface. When the fetus is thus infected, the condition known as "granulomatosis infantiseptica' may result, with disseminated abscesses, meningitis, dermatitis and other sequelae. Since, the organism is highly susceptible to ampicillin, early diagnosis is essential. Toxoplasma organisms of placenta and fetus are commonly acquired parenterally from the

fecal contamination originating from cats. In felines, the intestines propagate the organism and, when feces are dry and subject to dust contamination, the pregnant mother may become infected. That is an important reason for cleaning litter boxes while the fecal material is still moist. Toxoplasma cysts of a congenital infection may be seen in the chorion and even more commonly in Wharton's jelly of the umbilical cord, but they are sparse. The fetus may develop hydrocephalus and a variety of other pathologic states. The infection is easily preventable but difficult to treat once it is diagnosed.

Cytomegalovirus infection is also common and it may be sexually transmitted at times. It infects the villi of the placenta and can then disseminate into the fetus. The outcome is highly variable but is often associated with growth restriction, cerebral manifestations, jaundice and other complications. The usually small placenta may show characteristic changes. In early infections one finds inclusion bodies within villi, thrombosis of capillaries and occasional villous hemorrhages. Plasma cells then infiltrate which are otherwise very unusual features of normal placentas; eventually the villus atrophies and hemosiderin pigment deposits in Hofbauer cells. The antigen is easily demonstrated with modern techniques of antibody-marked histologic staining, as is of course the case also with the determination of serum antibodies. When the infection is longstanding and when it is severe, thrombi may develop even in the larger surface vessels (Fig. 61.8), and these may be calcified as well.

Only a few other disseminated infections are of importance. Thus, varicella infection has been described rarely, hepatitis antigens can cross the placenta, Coxsackie viruses have been transmitted with few placental lesions visible, and the placenta may also contain numerous intervillous malaria organisms during a malaria attack. Transmission to the fetus transplacentally, however, of the widespread malaria infection is extremely rare.

A final comment must be made about a reasonably common condition known as "villitis of unknown etiology (VUE)". This condition is frequently found in the placenta of growth-restricted fetuses and in stillbirths. Worse, it often recurs in subsequent pregnancies. When large districts of the placenta are so affected, fetal demise is common but there are no abnormal findings of any infectious nature in the fetal tissues. The villi in VUE are probably infiltrated by maternal T-cells and macrophages. They here cause an obliteration of the capillary beds and the restrictive cause of fetal growth is therefore readily understood. But the precise cause of why the maternal lymphocytes invade the placenta is yet unknown. It has been speculated that this is akin to a "rejection" phenomenon but why the fetal HLA type should be recognized by the mother's immune cells is so far obscure.

TUMORS AND MICROCHIMERISM

The commonest tumor of the placenta is the chorangioma.[6] It is frequently found only accidentally in sections prepared at random. Angiomas occur in villi as an expansion of the fetal capillary and mesenchymal cells; they form nodules that can be seen grossly and which are easily shelled out of their beds. Interestingly, their surface is usually covered by a single layer of trophoblast that suggests the expansion of fetal vessels being very focal in nature. Chorangiomas occur more frequently at high altitude and are often also associated with "chorangiosis", an increase of the normal number of capillaries in the peripheral villi. They are benign tumors despite their frequently great cellularity. In fact, chorangiomas have been mislabeled in the past as being sarcomas, mesenchymomas or have been assigned other appellations, but they have never metastasized. Large chorangiomas may protrude on the fetal surface (Fig. 61.9); they may be one cause of hydramnios and they may also infarct from thrombosis with cessation of the hydramnios resulting. Recent studies have shown that they are at least in part the result of increased angiopoietin expression.[7] On rare occasions the angioma may be associated with an excessive degree of trophoblastic proliferation. This condition has been labeled "chorangiocarcinoma", but its true nature and degree of malignancy are still poorly defined.

Maternal tumors are also been found to have set metastases in the placenta occasionally, perhaps most commonly the carcinoma of the breast. They may focally destroy placental tissue but most of them do not disseminate into the fetus. This only contrasts with the occasional metastatic melanomas which can travel into the fetus but here, the metastases are usually

"rejected" in neonatal life. Maternal B-cells lymphomas have been described recently as having disseminated into villi and they have caused neonatal deaths from tumor dissemination. Most maternal leukemias, however, do not spread to villi or the fetus.

The situation differs with *fetal* cells disseminating into the *mother* transplacentally. It is now recognized that fetal cells often traverse the placenta in small numbers. These are mostly red blood cells but nucleated elements have also reached the maternal circulation, perhaps even fetal stem cells. In the maternal organism, these elements may live for many years and, perhaps as determined by their antigenic expression, they may be destroyed in the mother. Recent studies, however, have also shown that some of these fetal cells themselves may impart an antibody/rejection response against the mother. This "microchimerism" is now thought to be the cause of some maternal autoimmune diseases such as systemic sclerosis and postpartum thyroiditis. Indeed, it has been shown that the maternal thyroid epithelium may on occasion be replaced by fetal cells when postpartum thyroiditis has occurred.

Choriocarcinoma in situ has been described a few times in otherwise normal placentas and this tumor has even been disseminated into the mother. Macroscopically such tumors have given the impression of being infarcts, and only histologic preparations have shown them to be malignant neoplasms. In some cases, the tumor has caused villous destruction with exsanguination of the fetus into the mother. This entity is completely unrelated to the usual cause of choriocarcinoma that may follow the presence of a hydatidiform mole, and its chromosomes have not yet been studied. The reason for their occurrence is obscure.

MOLES

When the villi swell up with much fluid from the intervillous space by transport through the syncytium, they swell and may become so swollen as to take on a grape-like configuration that is grossly visible. We refer to this as hydatid swelling and it is doubtlessly related to the deficient movement of the accumulated fluid to the fetus because the fetus has died and the fetal placental circulation has ceased. The result is the formation of a) "hydatid degeneration" of the placenta in abortion, and b) hydatidiform moles ("mole" merely means mass). Because not the entire placental tissue may have become transformed into grape-like masses, we speak of "partial hydatidiform moles (PHM)" and also of "complete hydatidiform moles (CHM)". The former may represent a variety of conditions; triploidy of the conceptus is the commonest antecedent condition but "PHM" may also be due to a set of twins, the placenta of one having become truly molar, i.e. a CHM.

The differentiation of these two types of moles is not always easy but it should be attempted. When two separate masses or a distinctly divided placenta is present, twinning is the most likely origin. But the differentiation of PHM and CHM may often present difficulties for the pathologist and the strong recommendation has been made to submit some of the abnormal tissue for ploidy analysis that is most efficiently done by flow cytometry or for cytogenetic study. Flow cytometry is the easiest and quickest way for this differential diagnosis. It quickly identifies triploidy (3n) from diploidy (2n) and this is relevant primarily because triploid moles are only exceptionally rarely followed by gestational trophoblastic neoplasms (GTNs).

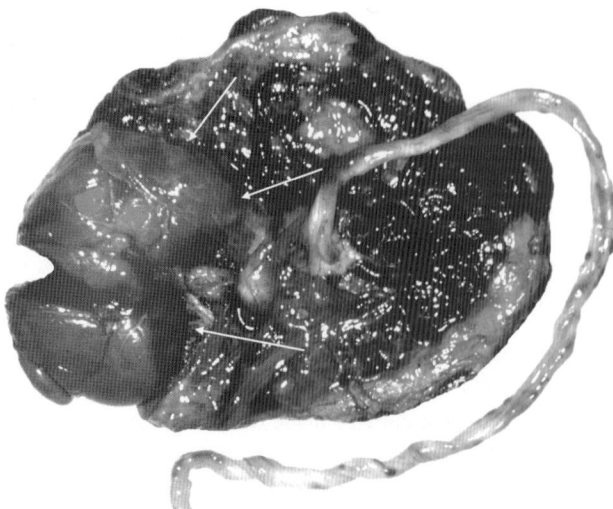

Fig. 61.9: Large chorioangioma bulging from the placental surface at left

Partial moles (PHM) are most commonly the result of fertilization of one oocyte by two spermatozoa. This imbalance leads to defective fetal development and, usually, the embryo dies early while the placenta continues to grow and accumulates fluid. It is much less common that a polar body (two maternal components—gynogenic) provides the additional set of chromosomes. In such pregnancies, there is considerably better fetal development. Nevertheless, the embryo develops somewhat abnormally and shows numerous anomalies that are invariably lethal soon after birth. One of the more characteristic anomalies is the fusion of two fingers and often also of toes. The placentas of PHM are enlarged, irregularly molar and the villi have scalloped borders that often lead to trophoblastic inclusions. These inclusions are not truly invasive features but represent tangential sections through infolded surfaces.

The CHM is similarly enlarged but more uniformly (Fig. 61.10).

The distension is mostly within the terminal villi and these can often be traced to thinner and firmer structures represented by the former stem villi that do not participate so much in the swelling. The amount of trophoblastic development varies greatly in CHM; at times it is massive and suspicious of tumor development. But the former method of "grading moles", depending on the amount and nature of trophoblastic proliferation, has been abandoned as it has proven to have little prognostic significance. The villi of CHM have no capillaries, in contrast to what is often the case in PHM. Since the revolutionary insight gained by Kajii and Ohama,[8] it is now accepted that CHM are "androgenetic". That is to say, their chromosomes are *only* derived from the spermatozoon. They are also 2n = 46,XX because a Y-bearing sperm would lead to a 2n = 46,YY conceptus and those cells are not viable. Thus, one can easily understand the development of a CHM by visualizing the fertilization by an X-bearing spermatozoon of an "empty" egg, i.e. an oocyte that has lost its nucleus. The 23,X chromosomes (from the spermatozoon) of the newly fertilized oocyte would then duplicate. But, because of imprinting features, an ovum fertilized by *only* male chromosomes does not develop a functional embryo; it can only produce a placenta. When early complete moles have been carefully examined, diminutive embryos are found occasionally; they are severely stunted and would soon have vanished. Thus, CHMs have generally no fetus and no vasculature, and there is also no recognizable amnionic cavity. For completeness sake, it must be mentioned that a few exceptions have been reported. Thus, a rare gynogenic mole has been found; also rarely, a diploid spermatozoon has led to the formation of moles and, equally amazing, a small portion of CHMs fertilized by two sperms was found to be 2n = 46,XY. These aberrations from the usual, however, have not had different sequelae.

Because the swelling of terminal villi and the enlargement of a molar placenta obviously take time to develop, really early CHMs may be difficult to identify; they may appear to be spontaneous abortions, i.e. "blighted ova". In addition, spontaneous intermixtures of normal villi and molar villi have been observed in chimeras. All of these are uncommon features; however, they merely indicate that detailed study may be needed to unravel what is otherwise a great biologic complexity. Furthermore, nobody has described an "empty egg" that we hypothesize as being the starting point for molar development. We thus assume that some abnormality in the maternal oocyte nucleus exists that prevents it from participating in embryonic development. What this is, that is being studied. Occasional chromosomal errors and genetic defects have thus been identified, but that is in a minority of cases so far. We may need more information on the reasons for the great geographic/racial differences in the occurrence of CHMs to attain a better understanding of its real causes. Genetic errors have been identified on occasion as the basis for familial moles. But why it is that CHMs occur in European/American stock with a frequency of ~1:2,000 and in the Japanese population for instance as commonly as in ~1:350 that is not known now.

TROPHOBLASTIC TUMORS

Choriocarcinoma is the most malignant, albeit uncommon outcome of hydatidiform moles. But other neoplastic entities are now recognized (epithelioid trophoblastic tumor; placental site nodule; exaggerated placental site) so that they have now all been comprised as "gestation trophoblastic neoplasias (GTNs)". Nevertheless, the choriocarcinoma is the best recognized and the most frequent of these tumors. It is composed solely of trophoblast, cytotrophoblast and syncytiotrophoblast, and most commonly it follows complete moles. Because the choriocarcinoma continues to produce chorionic gonadotropin, it is easily screened for and the follow-up of moles is usually undertaken with serial determination of gonadotropin levels. The other unusual feature of these tumors, especially the choriocarcinoma, is that it is highly susceptible to methotrexate and actinomycin D therapy. Even metastatic lesions are mostly treated successfully now when they are recognized early enough.

While choriocarcinoma most commonly follows a CHM, it may also arise from abortions, even from ectopic pregnancies. It may be present accidentally in an otherwise normal placenta and is then referred to a "choriocarcinoma in situ". It then looks like some bland infarct but may of course have serious sequelae. What causes choriocarcinoma to develop is uncertain, although it would appear that excessive proliferation of trophoblast is a precursor, as it is engendered often in moles. The tumor is usually very hemorrhagic and metastases occur anywhere but they are most feared when they occur in the brain.

The other tumorous lesions referred to above are more characteristically produced by the extravillous trophoblast, the

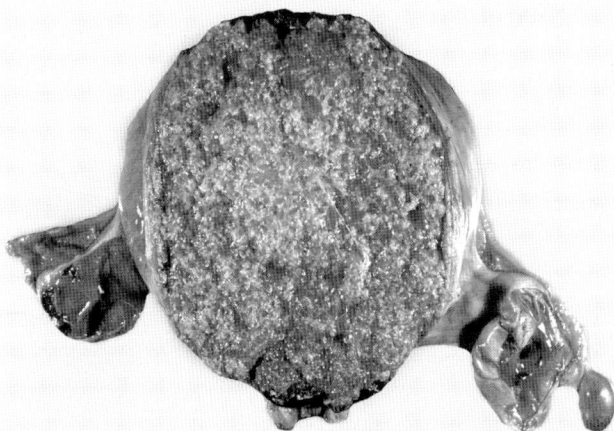

Fig. 61.10: Uterus filled with a "complete hydatidiform mole". The ovaries are enlarged because of gonadotropin stimulation

"X-cells" whose main purpose is the invasion of the uterus and the modulation of the uterine vessels. By and large, these tumors are much less common; they usually behave in a less malignant fashion and can often be treated by excision.

MULTIPLE PREGNANCIES

Twinning is common and monozygotic (MZ) "identical" and dizygotic (DZ)—"fraternal"—twins occur (Fig. 61.11). When higher multiple pregnancies take place, MZ and DZ multiples may be admixed. In order to understand the placenta of monozygotic twins, it is necessary that one visualizes the stages at which the "splitting" of the developing embryo can occur (Fig. 61.12). Thus, when segregation of blastomeres takes place very early (during the first 3 days), then two entirely separate placentas may develop; but when it occurs later, a single chorion and two amnions develop; and when it occur later still, a monoamnionic sac can be produced. Eventually, after 13 days of development, twinning becomes impossible or else conjoined twins would develop. Therefore, the placenta of MZ twins may be dichorionic (~20%) or monochorionic (~80%). This is what is actually found and it is important as the classification of twins may depend on this, and so does the formation of blood vessels that may connect the two fetal circulations. The anastomotic connections then occur only in MZ and monochorionic twins; DZ twins virtually never have such anastomoses and are worthy of being reported.

The frequency of DZ twins depends largely on genetic factors that control polyovulation. Polyovulation is controlled by maternal FSH levels; it is very high in the Nigerian Yoruba tribe, but much lower in Oriental people. Therefore, the percentage of MZ twins is much higher in Japan than it is in African or European populations. The consequences of this are significant also as most problems in the placentation of twins occur with monochorionic (MZ) twins.

The placenta of *dichorionic twins* is easy to understand (Figs 61.11 to 61.13). The two blastocysts implant either side-by-side in the uterus or on opposite surfaces. Two fused placentas may thus arise which have a diamnionic, dichorionic "dividing membrane". Sonographically this is commonly recognized by the thickness of the membrane and by a small elevation of placental tissue at the meeting point of the chorionic surface. The pathologist observes that these membranes are thicker, less translucent and that atrophied blood vessels may be apparent in the dividing membranes. Anastomoses between the two fetal circulations do not occur or are so rare that they warrant a case report. The umbilical cords of both types of twins are much more often marginally (or membranous-velamentous) inserted. That is also the case of occasional singleton placentas but in twins it may be the consequence of competition for space in an expanding placenta. Alternatively, it may be the result of improper early central implantation but the precise mechanics are undetermined. Importantly, such abnormal cord insertion may also be found on the dividing membranes and the velamentous vessels then represent a danger of disruption when these are ruptured during delivery.

Monochorionic placentas in contrast nearly always have blood vessel connections on the fetal surface. These take essentially three forms: Most common is an artery-to-artery communication (Fig. 61.14); next most commonly artery-to-vein connections occur, and vein-to-vein anastomoses are least often found. The connections are readily identified in the delivered placenta. One may stroke blood back and forth in an A-A anastomosis; the recognition of A-V connections is much more difficult and it is also the most important and troublesome connection. Injection with milk or other fluids makes it easy to recognize the type of anastomosis, and it is usually necessary to undertake such injections if the A-V anastomosis of the twin-to-twin-transfusion syndrome (TTTS) is to be understood. As has been said earlier, arteries generally cross over the veins, especially in the larger vessels. They are thus easily recognized and their course can be followed by careful gross inspection. Generally speaking, in the normal placenta an arterial branch distributes blood to a single cotyledon. When this branch is followed to its end, the artery suddenly stops, bends down into the villous and then perfuses one cotyledon. Nearby, a vein emerges from this cotyledon and sends blood back to the umbilical vein. In the TTTS, however, this vein sends blood back to the other twin, thus establishing the basis for the TTTS. One needs to inject these suspect terminal arterial branches, fill the cotyledon completely and see the injected material emerge in the vein of the "recipient" twin in order to establish the basis for the TTTS. There may be several such "common districts"

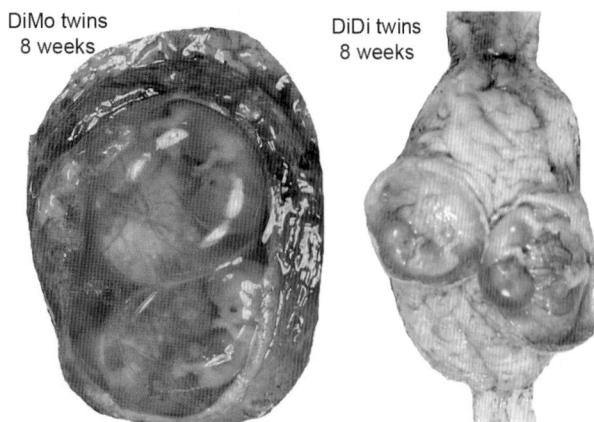

Fig. 61.11: Two uteri within which are 8-week-old twin fetuses. At left are monochorionic (identical) twins with their amnionic sacs. At right are two fraternal, dichorionic twins within adjacent placental implantations

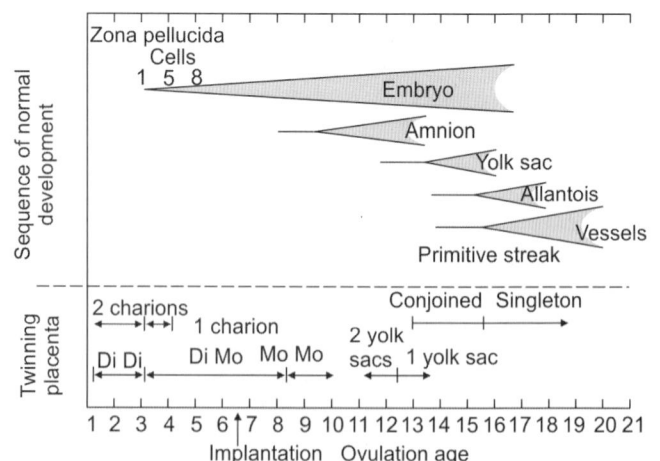

Fig. 61.12: Conceptual drawing of early splitting of embryos/placentas in the process of producing monozygotic twins

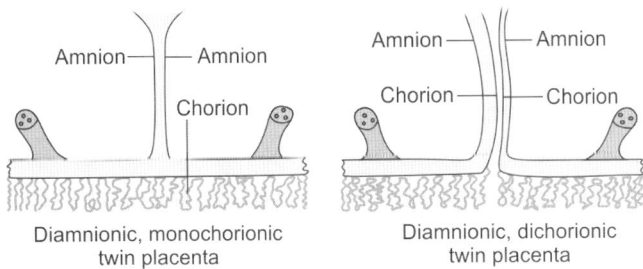

Fig. 61.13: Diagram to show the membrane relationship in monochorionic twin placentas (left) and dichorionic twin placentas (right)

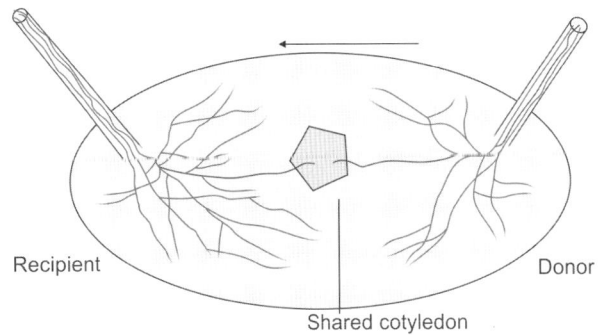

Fig. 61.15: Drawing to show the "shared cotyledon" in a monochorionic twin placenta with the twin-to-twin transfusion syndrome

DiMo (diamnionic-monochorionic), MZ twins with A-A anatomosis

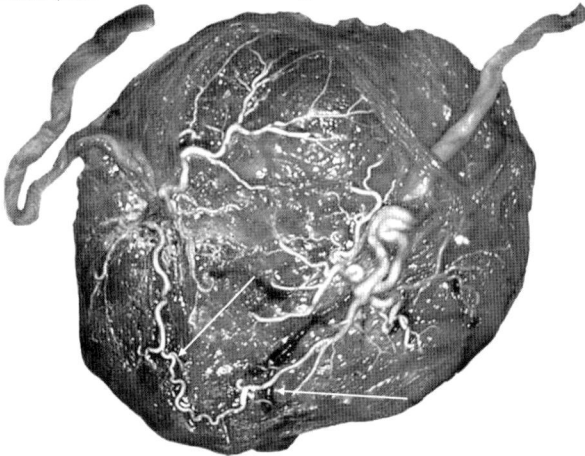

Fig. 61.14: Monochorionic twin placenta with a single large artery-to-artery anastomosis (at arrows)

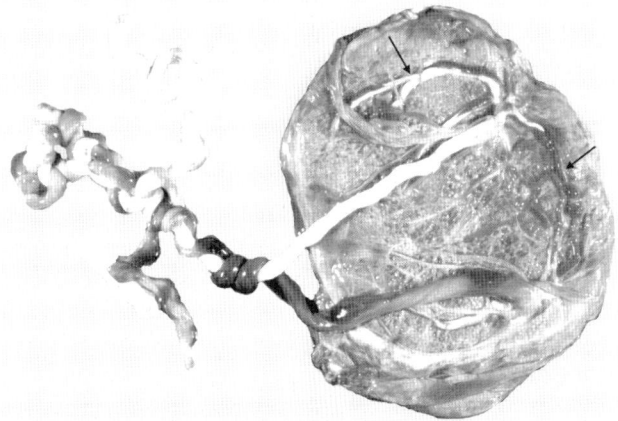

Fig. 61.16: Monoamnionic twin placenta with extensive entangling of umbilical cords that led to fetal demise

(they have been referred to as the "third circulation") and they may even have different directions. Their net size determines the severity of the TTTS; it is generally held now that the co-existence of an A-A communication prevents this syndrome in its worst states.

In such monochorionic twin placentas (the majority is diamnionic, monochorionic–DiMo), the dividing membranes are composed of two amnions; they are translucent and lack remnants of former vessels.

The most important and frequent complication of MZ twinning is the twin-to-twin transfusion syndrome (TTTS). It then comes about by the presence of a single "shared (common) cotyledon" (Fig. 61.15). An artery from the donor enters one cotyledon and this is drained to the "recipient" who becomes fluid-overloaded and because of excessive urination that recipient develops hydramnios. That is how the syndrome usually becomes symptomatic, most frequently between 20 weeks and 30 weeks of gestation. The donor urinates little or not at all and becomes the "stuck twin". Hydramnios usually terminates the pregnancy unless it is treated by the modern method of laser obliteration of the offending vessels. In order to do this surgery, one requires considerable DiMo twin dies in utero, blood may be transferred rapidly from the surviving twin back into the now dead fetus. This can lead to at least temporary deficient CNS perfusion in the survivor and thus, cerebral palsy in one of surviving twins is relatively common. Such a mechanism is also implored in understanding

the death of the later-dying original "Siamese" twin pair (Eng).

Monoamnionic twins are always monochorionic (MZ) and thus suffer the possibility of entangling of their umbilical cords. Complex knots may develop early in fetal life and they may become constrictive and cause fetal demise (Fig. 61.16). At times one find thrombi in such umbilical cords or in blood vessels of the chorionic surface from the chronically restricted blood flow during intrauterine life. Moreover, chorangiosis is often observed in such placentas.

Acardiac twins occur in many forms; some are nearly perfectly formed babies, but most are severely abnormal and they may even grossly appear as though they were skin-covered teratomas. Most acardiacs also have a single umbilical artery. They are always monozygotic, or "identical", although they represent the worst-possible congenital abnormality imaginable. The formation of acardiacs is best explained by the presence of both, an A-A and V-V anastomosis in the surface of the placenta (Fig. 61.17). We believe that in very early embryonic development the normal twin causes a reversal of blood flow through the A-A connection and the V-V thus returning the blood in the opposite direction; perhaps they were then already of different sizes. Because blood from the artery now enters the developing acardiac fetus at its abdomen, the legs develop more adequately, while the cephalic end is usually most deficiently developed. And, because of the reversal of flow, the heart of the "acardiac" develops poorly (it may be two-chambered) or not at all.

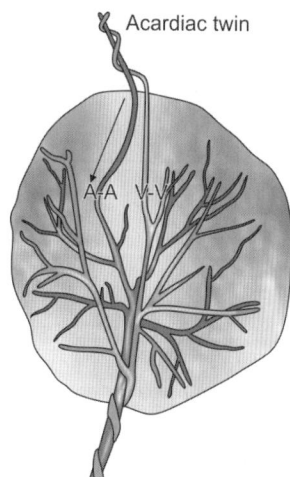

Fig. 61.17: Drawing to show the set-up of the vascular connections that lead to the development of an acardiac twin

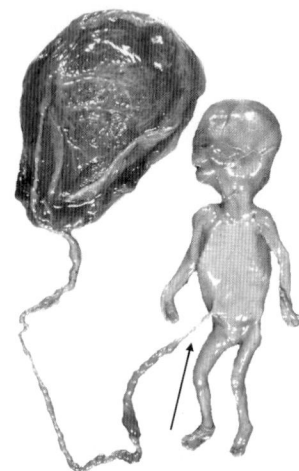

Fig. 61.18: Abortus with an excessively long and heavily twisted umbilical cord and the even more excessive twisting on the abdominal surface of the fetus (arrow)

These acardiac fetuses are chromosomally generally normal and of the same sex as the cotwin. It might be mentioned also that such acardiacs have been reported quite accidentally in many different species. When many more fetuses are implanted, a condition that is now much more common with the practice of assisted reproductive technology (ART), the placentas may be closely packed and have no blood vessel connections. They generally have abnormal cord insertions and, depending on their number, many are born prematurely. It has also been our observation that frequently one or more of the fetuses are surgically eliminated by KCl injection and a fetus papyraceus is then found in the membranes with a markedly atrophied placenta. What is amazing in such specimens is the marked spiraling of their cords, as this must have originated very early in development. Finally, the placentas of such ART pregnancies present challenging problems in that more fetuses and placentas may be found than embryos originally implanted into the uterus. Thus, monochorionic twins are admixed and can only be explained by assuming that one embryonic precursor has split early in gestation. Perhaps the practice of embryonic culture in vitro for several days is responsible for this spontaneous MZ twinning event.

ABORTIONS

Spontaneous abortions are very common in human development; they are much more common than in most species that have been studied in detail. The vast majority occurs during the first 3 months of gestation and the majority is due to chromosomal errors. Generally, a deformed or macerated embryo is found on examination of the specimen but equally often, especially in the earliest abortions, the amnionic sac is empty and the fetal vasculature of the placenta has atrophied; these specimens are often referred to as "blighted ovum". The placenta is otherwise atrophied and may have focal hydatid changes of the villi. The trophoblast is unremarkable or atrophied. Occasional retroplacental hemorrhages accompany these specimens. A frequent cause of spontaneous abortion is the presence of an excessive long umbilical cord with severe twisting (Fig. 61.18). The causes of the twisting and excessive length of the

cord are unknown but I speculate that this is the result of excessive movements in early life. It often leads to severe twisting on the surface of the umbilical cord insertion on the abdominal surface which must be observed to understand this cause of embryonic demise.

PLACENTAL AND FETAL HYDROPS

The placenta of hydropic fetuses is much enlarged and most commonly it is very water-logged. The villi are swollen and often contain prominent Hofbauer cells (macrophages). There are many causes for hydrops and depending on their nature, the histopathology differs. In erythroblastosis and in the placentas of the fetal thalassemias, the capillaries contain nucleated red blood cells in profusion; in transplacental infection with parvovirus B19, one may find characteristically nuclear inclusion bodies that are found most often within the nucleated red cells. But, at later stages, they may be inconspicuous and identification of the etiology of hydrops will commonly depend on serologic findings or on staining the tissue with specific antibodies. When the hydrops is caused by fetal anomalies such as left heart hypoplasia, cystic adenomatous malformation of the lung, sacrococcygeal teratoma, etc. then the placenta is merely large, edematous and pale. Some of the other fetal conditions that lead to hydrops are summarized below.

MATERNAL AND FETAL DISEASES AFFECTING THE PLACENTA

Preeclampsia

The cause of preeclampsia [or pregnancy-induced hypertension (PIH)] is still unknown, but speculations about its origin abound. Less controversial are the placental sequelae in PIH. Generally speaking, the placenta is smaller and exhibits what is called "advanced maturation". This is a misnomer, however, and merely applies to the histologic features of such placentas as having smaller villi; they *appear* to be more mature than would be expected at the usually immature gestational age. The villi are not only smaller but also, they have less mesenchymal fluid content. As a consequence, the superficial cover of trophoblast buckles and more "knots" or "sprouts" of syncytium become apparent. This is referred to as the Tenney-Parker change after the first authors to describe this feature. This increased number of sprouts (more than 30% of terminal villi) also leads to their more frequent deportation in the maternal circulation and was thus witnessed as a peculiarity of women dying in eclampsia as they had more such elements in their pulmonary capillaries.

Preeclampsia is associated characteristically with the presence of "atherosis" in the maternal, decidual spiral arterioles. It is conceived that the normal transformation of these blood vessels does not occur because of inadequate extravillous trophoblastic infiltration in early development. The atherosis is reasonably characteristic for PIH and may be found in the decidua basalis and also (often easiest) in the decidua capsularis of the membranes. But, not in all cases of even severe PIH can one find this change; it can also be associated with thrombosis. Atherosis affects only the maternal arterial bed; it spares the veins. Characteristically, it consists of the deposition of foam cells (cholesterol-laden macrophages) in the lumen and wall of the arterioles (Fig. 61.19). This lesion may obstruct blood flow, as thrombosis would also do and thereby lead to placental/fetal hypoxia and typically to placental infarcts. When infarcts are of recent origin, they still have fetal blood remaining and they are red. As infarcts age, they lose the fetal hemoglobin and become pale and, eventually white. They are firm and sharply delimited from the spongy adjacent placenta tissue. In contrast to the more common marginal infarcts seen in normal placentas, infarcts of PIH are distributed centrally. They also may surround focal intervillous thrombi which are characterized by a laminated appearance due to the "lines of Zahn" in a thrombus. The occlusion of maternal spiral arterioles also causes the degeneration of decidua basalis and destruction of maternal veins. This may lead to hemorrhages and the condition known as abruptio placentae (Fig. 61.20). While abruption is commonest in PIH, it also can occur in traumatic injuries to the placenta. For instance, amniocentesis occasionally needs to be done by trespassing the placental tissue and that can disrupt major blood vessels. More common though is abruption of the placenta in automobile accidents, for instance when a seat belt injures the pregnant uterus. Very rarely an abruption was caused by external version of a breech presentation thus it needs to be borne in mind that such can occur when versions are attempted. It

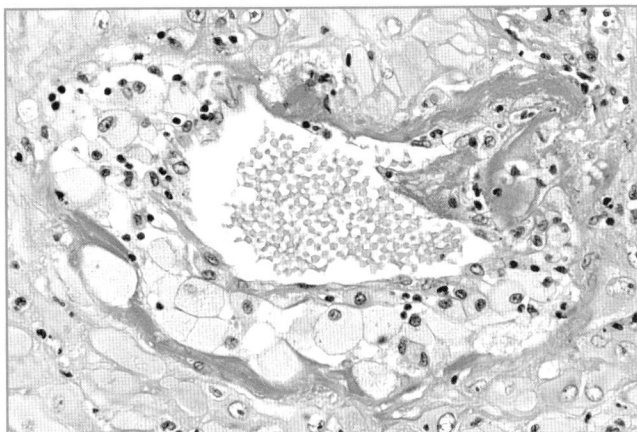

Fig. 61.20: Abruptio placentae with fetal demise in pre-eclampsia. Note the compression of nearly one-half of the placenta. Infarcts are also present

is not uncommon that small retroplacental hematomas are found on careful examination, especially adjacent to placental infarcts. When they are large and sudden as shown in Figure 61.20, they are lethal for the fetus.

One feature of placental infarcts differs from infarcts occurring in other organs (e.g. the kidney), namely, the dead tissue does not become "organized" in the usual sense. That is to say, blood vessels from the adjacent tissues do not enter the infarct and the dead tissue is also not removed by macrophage activity.

Placenta Percreta

It is normal for placentation that a small amount of decidua basalis separates the villi from the myometrium. It is not fully understood why it is that the trophoblast stops invading or destroying the endometrium at that point, as one can readily find "X-cells" in the myometrium underlying most placental sites and they are found in myometrial blood vessels beneath the placenta. Only when there is insufficient decidua present does the villous portion of the placenta attach itself to the myometrium and then forms a placenta accreta. I believe that this occurs most commonly because prior disease (e.g. tuberculosis or chronic endometritis) has destroyed the endometrium and endometrial repair does not take place by *lateral* growth of endometrium. Thus, when a placenta implants over a prior curettage site, the development of focal placenta accreta may occur. It is generally witnessed only by the disruption of the placenta floor when the placenta is examined or clinically by postpartum bleeding. When thus placental tissue remains attached to a focus of myometrium, a placental "polyp" may form that is composed of fragments of placental tissue enmeshed in blood clot and it is occasionally accompanied by inflammation. Also, because of insufficient decidualization of the higher endocervical canal, placenta previa is often associated with focal placenta accreta.

When deeper infiltration of the myometrium by placental tissue has occurred, we speak of placenta increta and when it has penetrated, we refer to it as "placenta percreta". These terms are frequently misinterpreted to mean that the placenta has actually *invaded* the myometrium to destroy it and "grow through the endometrium", to emerge on the peritoneal surface. This is really true only of ectopic pregnancies in the fallopian tube. When they rupture, this is due to placenta percreta but primarily, so because there is only minimal or absent decidualization, thus assuring that a placenta percreta can form; because of the thinness of the tubal wall, rupture may occur when the conceptus enlarges. It must be said, however, that ever so rarely a full term gestation takes place in the tube. Moreover, all abdominal implantations are placentas accreta and it is for that reason that the placenta will not detach

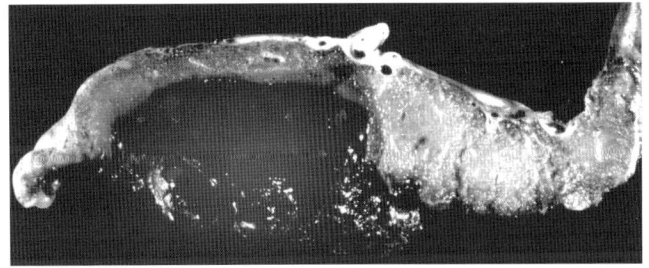

Fig. 61.19: Atherosis in the spiral arteriole of a patient with severe preeclampsia

upon delivery. It has also recruited an enormous blood supply from the neighborhood. *Placenta percreta* has become more common in recent years and it is now often diagnosed sonographically. Virtually invariably, this is the result of a prior cesarean section. When the uterus is sutured, usually by a single layer of resorbable fibers, the edges of the prior incision are poorly aligned and since there is no new growth of myometrium to connect the edges, repair occurs by connective tissue. When a new pregnancy takes place, this scar widens and thins; when a placenta is attached directly over the site, it may *appear* as though it has penetrated the uterus, but that occurs only by separating the myometrial edges from the prior cesarean section. Thus, having implanted on connective tissue (instead of the normal decidua), the placenta may even attach itself to the posterior surface of the urinary bladder. On occasion some bladder wall is removed at the excision of such specimens and it appears as though a true invasion has taken place. But that is no more than the usual infiltration of extravillous trophoblast into the uterine musculature that occurs in all pregnancies. In other words, while it is theoretically possible that an occasional placenta may truly invade, the common placenta percreta is the result of insufficient healing of a prior section scar. It might be mentioned parenthetically that, when a pathologist has the opportunity to examine the hysterectomy specimens of such percretas, the endocervical canal is tough to cut, it is firmly closed, and it is filled with that sticky mucus that normally prevents ascending infection of the amnionic cavity.

Fetal Storage Diseases

Numerous storage diseases of the fetus, the so-called "errors of metabolism", affect the placental morphology. One of the first to be recognized was "I-cell disease" in which the trophoblastic cells show diffuse vacuolation. The same is true for many other storage diseases and, to differentiate among them, it is necessary to undertake enzyme studies. Fetal leukemia occurs occasionally and can be recognized by the circulating nucleated cells but care must be taken not to over-interpret these as they may be transitory phenomena for instance in Down's syndrome. More important are fetal neuroblastoma and sacrococcygeal teratoma; both may present as hydrops with typical swelling and edema of the villi. In neuroblastoma, however, the neuroblasts are seen to plug many capillaries and occasional rosettes may be identified.

REFERENCES

1. Hertig AT. Human Trophoblast. Springfield: Charles C Thomas; 1968.
2. Boyd JD, Hamilton WJ. The Human Placenta. Cambridge: W Heffer; 1970.
3. Benirschke, Kaufmann P. The Pathology of the Human Placenta, 4th edition. New York: Springer-Verlag; 2000.
4. Wigglesworth JS. Vascular anatomy of the human placenta and its significance for placental pathology. J Obstet Gynecol Br Common. 1969;76:979.
5. Landing BH. Amnion nodosum: A lesion of the placenta apparently associated with deficient secretion of fetal urine. Am J Obstet Gynecol. 1950;60:1339.
6. Benirschke K. Recent trends in chorangiomas, especially those of multiple and recurrent chorangiomas. Pediatr Developm Pathol. 1999;2:264.
7. Guschmann M. Solitary and multiple chorangiomas—clinical consequences, expression of growth factors and differences in the growth rate. Z Geburtsh Neonatol. 2003;207:6.
8. Kajii T, Ohama K. Androgenetic origin of hydatidiform mole. Nature. 1977;268:633.

62 Clinically Significant Pathology of the Placenta

B Hargitai, T Marton

INTRODUCTION

Histopathological examination of the placenta can contribute to determine the causes of fetal demise, growth restriction, or neonatal condition. Recently several guidelines[1-3] and books have been published in the subject of placenta pathology.[4,5] The ever-growing evidence based knowledge requires recapitulation of the clinicopathologic correlation. The benefits of placenta examination include recognition of maternal conditions having effect on subsequent pregnancies (autoimmune disease, antiphospholipid syndrome, thombophylia) or may have medicolegal implications (e.g. concerning the etiology of long-term neurodevelopmental sequelae or the approximate timing of an intrauterine death).[6,7] Timing of the lesions and fetal damage can be estimated and possibly vital clues obtained concerning the etiology of the fetal or neonatal condition. Many features of the placenta can be judged only in the clinicopathological context, partly because of the occasionally loose correlation between the histological changes and the clinical symptoms and partly because of the large reserve capacity of the placenta. It is also apparent that satisfactory clinical information improves the rate of recognized histological features, which underlines the importance of the submitted clinical information to the pathologist.[8]

This chapter attempts to highlight clinicopathological associations bearing great importance in the everyday obstetrical and neonatal care.

PLACENTA REFERRAL TO THE HISTOPATHOLOGY LABORATORY

The increased workload of perinatal pathology departments would not allow examination of all placentas, which is not even necessary, except those well-defined conditions when placenta referral is indicated. This "minimal list" can be extended in selected centers with specific research project. Referral is decided at the delivery suit. The indications of placenta referral are as follows:[1]

Fetal conditions, when referral is indicated: Intrauterine growth restriction—(IUGR) (birthweight below 2.5 kg or 3rd centile), prematurity (less than 37 weeks of gestation), placental abruption, fetal hydrops, fetal developmental abnormality, chromosome aberration, stillbirth, severe fetal distress requiring admission to NNU, Rhesus (and other) isoimmunisation, morbidly adherent placenta, twins/other multiple pregnancy (complicated or uncomplicated), abnormal placental shape (if clinically relevant, including placental tumors) or other postnatally diagnosed disorders of the placenta (hematoma, too large or too small placenta, infarction, discoloration of membranes), umbilical cord, containing two vessels, premature rupture of membranes (PROM) (more than 36 hours).

Diseases of the neonate with possible IU origin: These include neonatal infection (pneumonia or sepsis within 72 hours) and neonates with neurological signs.

It is also recommended to examine the placentas from pregnancies with maternal diseases that might have consequences in the neonate: These are, maternal pyrexia and maternal group B streptococcus, preeclampsia, hypertension, severe diabetes including gestational diabetes, maternal thrombopathies -thrombophilias, other metabolic disease, maternal autoimmune disease, maternal tumor and storage disease.

Generally referral is *not indicated for* cholestasis of pregnancy (with no further complication), Hepatitis B, HIV infection (seropositivity with no manifest disease), other maternal disease with normal pregnancy outcome, normal pregnancy, placenta previa, postpartum hemorrhage.

In the pathology laboratory, placentas are selected for pathologic examination: A full examination of the placenta includes macrosocopic and histological examination of representative samples of the placenta, membrane and umbilical cord. The indications for examination of the placentas are as follows.[1]

Rhesus isoimmunization with admission to the neonatal unit, in any intrauterine death/stillbirth (even if a postmortem examination of the baby does not take place), anemia requiring intrauterine transfusion, morbidly adherent placenta, maternal pyrexia, neonatal infection, prematurity [<34 weeks and not PET (preeclamptic toxemia)/IUGR], severe fetal distress, any admission to the neonatal unit, IUGR, prematurity (<34 weeks) due to PET/IUGR, severe PET, abruption, hydrops and fetal anomaly. The goal in this group is to demonstrate the placental consequences of the clinical condition, in other instances to identify the etiology.

The rest of placentas belong to a risk group for neonatal disease, so storage is recommended (in unfixed state, for 2 weeks, 4°C, urgent examination on clinical request). These placentas are from pregnancies with PROM (premature rupture of membranes), prematurity (34–36 weeks), uncomplicated gestational diabetes, rhesus negative mother, maternal group B streptococcus and uncomplicated preeclampsia.

THE NORMAL PLACENTA

Normal human placenta has a range of features that are dependent on many factors including maternal size, ethnic origin, geographic area, age, parity, etc.

All placentas are examined at the delivery suit after birth macroscopically.

The *membranes* can loose the transparency, become mat/murky and thickened in chorioamnionitis and subchorionic hemorrhage. Small, white-gray granular nodules appear in oligohydramnios and this alteration referred as amnion nodosum can be mixed up with squamous metaplasia macroscopically, but the latter is a normal variant.

Circumvallate placenta presents with a yellow-whitish rim on the fetal surface. The significance of it is uncertain; some correlate it with IUGR.

The normal *placenta* is ovoid, and the fetus/placenta weight ratio is 7 at term, growing gradually from 1 at 14/40 weeks of gestation. Normal thickness is approximately 1.5–2.5 cm. Irregular placental shape, multilobed placenta can be a sign of disturbed implantation, or developmental abnormality of the uterus. The placenta weight correlates with the fetal weight and a small placenta is prone to result in placenta insufficiency and subsequent fetal demise. Large placenta is usually associated with fetal overgrowth syndromes and genetic disorders (Beckwith-Wiedeman syndrome, congenital nephrosis syndrome of the fetus). Other underlying conditions are maternal diabetes, maternal and fetal anemia, and fetoplacental hydrops.[9]

The fetal surface has to be searched for vessels leaving the disc, but not returning to it, because that can be a sign of a retained cotyledon. Generally the fetal surface reflects the changes that can be seen in the membrane or on the subchorionic surface. The color of the normal placenta varies between red and dark red, which depends on the time of clipping the umbilical cord. In a normal placenta palpation is spongy and homogenous, and does not suggest any focal lesions (except for small, peripheral infarcts or perivillous fibrin deposition in term placentas).

After turning the placenta, the maternal side has to be checked for completeness. The *umbilical cord* length is 40–70 cm at term, with one coil over 5 cm in average.[10] The normal umbilical cord has three vessels and is inserted on the placental disc, preferably in central or paracentral position.

TWIN PLACENTAS

It is essential to determine the chorionicity of twin placentas, because of the increased morbidity and mortality rate of the monochorionic gestation. The commonest type is the dichorionic placenta. It can have both a single disc (either fused or non-separated), or two separated discs. While dichorionic twins can be both di- and monozygotic, monochorionic twins are always monozygotic. Monochorionic, diamniotic twins represent the second most frequent twinning. There is always a single placenta disc. Chorionicity can be easily identified with the help of two forceps; The septum needs to be separated into two layers. In case of two thin, equally translucent webs the twin placenta is monochorionic, whereas in uneven separation, having one smooth, opaque, thin layer and a thicker one with uneven surface, the pregnancy is dichorionic.

The rarest finding is the monochorionic, monoamniotic twin placenta (with a single placenta disc).

CLINICOPATHOLOGICAL CORRELATIONS

Umbilical Cord

The umbilical cord is short by definition, if measures less than 40 cm. Short umbilical cord carries an increased risk for fetal/neonatal morbidity or mortality and there is an increased rate of neurological abnormality. The cord is considered to be long, if it is longer than 70 cm. Long umbilical cord has a correlation with maternal factors, such as systemic diseases, delivery complications and increased maternal age. According to Baergen et al. fetal factors included non-reassuring fetal status, respiratory distress, vertex presentation, cord entanglement, male sex, increased birth weight. Other frequently observed placental features were increased placental weight, overcoiled cord, true knots and congestion. Cord prolapse causing fetal distress occurred also more often with a long umbilical cord.[11]

Marginal cord insertion shows correlation with IUGR, stillbirth, neonatal death, premature birth and low birth weight. A possible explanation is that a disturbed implantation is behind the atypical cord insertion. The same is true for velamentous cord insertion.

Over- or undercoiling of the cord has an increased risk for fetal demise, fetal intolerance to labor, IUGR and chorioamnionitis.[10] It is apparent that extremely overcoiled umbilical cord has an elevated vascular resistance and vascular obstruction is often behind the fetal loss in these cases.

A true knot can cause fetal death (associated with perinatal mortality of 10%), whereas loose knot *per se* does not cause harm to the fetus (Fig. 62.1.) Long umbilical cord is a risk factor of both knot and increased coiling.

Single umbilical artery[12] has an association with fetal malformation chromosome aberration in 25–50%. In normally formed infants IUGR is frequent and there is also an increased perinatal mortality.

Thrombosis of the umbilical vessels has a very poor prognosis,[4] but survival can also occur.

Beside the well-known consequences of intrauterine infection (see the paragraph below), umbilical cord vessel vasculitis and funisitis are associated with cord vessel thrombosis and vasospasm of cord vessels.[5] Necrotising funisitis is usually seen with acute chorioamnionitis. Candida, streptococci, herpes and syphilis are reported to play role in the pathogenesis of necrotising funisitis (Fig. 62.2.).[4]

Membranes

Acute chorioamnionitis (including "subchorial intervillositis") has a strong association with premature rupture of the membranes and preterm delivery.[13] Fetal intrauterine infection may occur. Maternal pyrexia and tachycardia are described as maternal effects, but may

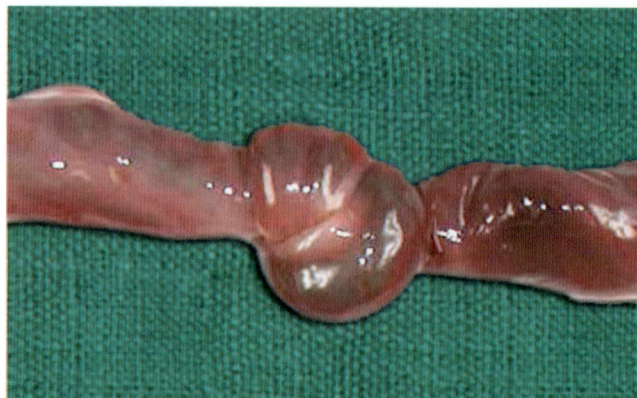

Fig. 62.1: Tight knot of the umbilical cord

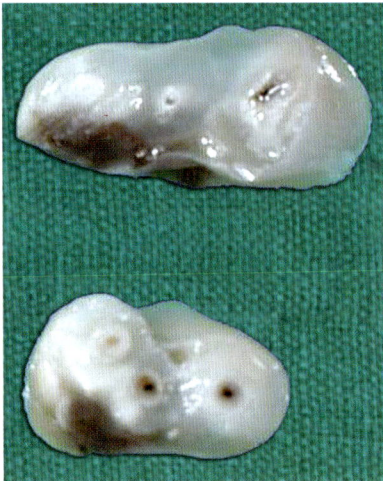

Fig. 62.2: Necrotizing funisitis. See the whitish necrotic areas in the umbilical cord

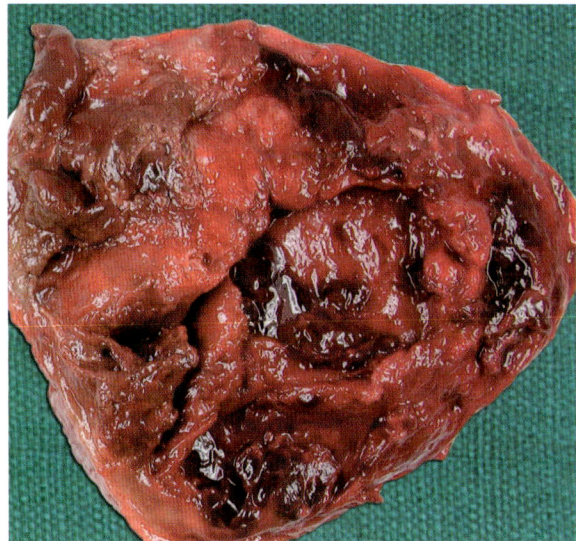

Fig. 62.3: The crater in the middle of the placenta was caused by a retroplacental hemorrhage

be asymptotic. Recently chorioamnionitis has been implicated as a risk factor for periventricular leukomalacia and cerebral palsy.[14]

Chronic chorioamnionitis has been observed in prolonged rupture of membrane and herpes virus infection.[4]

Amnion epithelial vacuolization can be artifact, but lipid containing droplets in the epithelium are specific for gastroschisis.[4]

In contrast to the common belief, pigmented macrophages and the presence of meconium staining are not necessarily associated with adverse fetal outcome. Meconium staining indicates the danger of meconium aspiration and with other histologic signs of fetal distress may underline the diagnosis. Vasospasm of cord vessels and fetal chorionic vessels are reported as a consequence of meconium exposure.[15]

Acute and chronic deciduitis and decidual necrosis in the parietal decidua are frequently associated with ascending infiltrations of the placental membranes; they may be non-significant in isolation. In retroplacental hematoma severe, necrotising acute deciduitis is a common finding. The significance of chronic deciduitis with scattered infiltration of lymphocytes is uncertain.[4]

Placenta

Macroscopic Alterations of the Placenta

Low placenta weight, below 10th centile for gestational age occurs in IUGR, preeclampsia, increased intervillous fibrin deposition, villitis of unknown origin and trisomies.[9] Placental weight shows correlation with the fetal weight, a small fetus has generally smaller placenta than a large fetus, but a small placenta may lead to growth restriction.

The placenta is thin (the medical term is placenta annulare or placenta membranacea) by definition if the average thickness is less than 2 cm and the placenta has a large membranous area. While the fetal outcome is usually favorable, there is a risk of maternal bleeding, placenta previa and placenta accreta. Often premature delivery occurs and possibly it is more frequent in IUGR.[16]

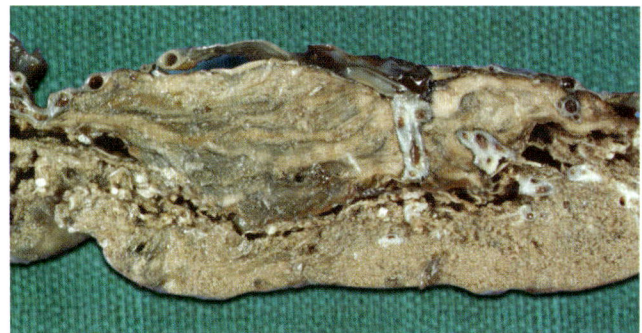

Fig. 62.4: Lamellated subchorionic hematoma can be seen on the fetal surface of this placenta

The hemorrhages of the placenta include retroplacental hematoma. A large retroplacental hematoma causes a crater (Fig. 62.3) and extensive infarction involving sufficient proportion of villous tissue with secondary fetal hypoxia and/or perinatal death. An early separation (placental abruption) can be lethal, if extensive. An elevated maternal serum AFP level can be associated with old hematomas.

Subchorionic hematoma (Fig. 62.4) usually has no clinical significance when patchy, focal or present as a thin diffuse layer. Although rarely, in extreme cases, a massive hematoma (massive subchorial thrombosis, Breus' mole) can result in abortion.

Placenta previa is usually diagnosed by ultrasound before delivery. If undetected and causes bleeding, it can be life threatening for both mother and fetus.

Placenta accreta, increta and percreta are potentially life threatening clinical conditions, causing uterine rupture and massive postpartum hemorrhage, or leading to cesarean section if prenatally diagnosed. Placenta creta is often an indication of postpartum hysterectomy because of the excessive bleeding. To make the pathologic diagnosis of placenta accreta, examination of the entire uterus is necessary as a posthysterectomy specimen.

Microscopic Alterations of the Placenta

Abnormalities of the placental chorionic villi, the intervillous space and chorionic vessels that result in a reduced functional capacity of the placenta:

1. *A placental infarct* (Figs 62.5A and B) has no significance if it is single, marginal and/or involves less than about 5% of the villous tissue. If a placental infarction involves more than 10% of the placental volume, it is regarded as extensive infarct and can have serious clinical consequences such as fetal hypoxia, IUGR, stillbirth, pregnancy induced hypertension, abruptio placentae, neurological abnormalities because of the reduced size villous tree.[4]

2. *Extensive perivillous fibrin deposition*, involving more than 20–30% of the villous tissue and functional placenta, is an important histological entity, associated with IUGR and fetal death. In these cases often 70–80% of villous population is enveloped by fibrin. The maternal serum AFP can be extremely elevated.[17,18]

There are two special patterns of the fibrin deposition; massive basal plate perivillous fibrin deposition is termed as "*maternal floor infarct*" and known to be associated with high mortality and IUGR.[4,5,19,20]

The massive perivillous fibrin deposition in a netlike pattern (Figs 62.6A and B) is the "*gitter infarct*". "Gitter infarct" and "maternal floor infarct" are historical names, none of them a true infarct, but a special type of perivillous fibrin deposition.

3. *Abnormalities of the fetal vessels*: Fetal chorionic vessels and fetal stem vessels of the placenta may contain fresh or organized thrombus. The organized thrombus can calcify, or contains small vascular spaces if recanalized. Obstruction of fetal vessels (Fig. 62.7) is associated with groups or fields of hyalinized, *avascular villi*. These villi can not take

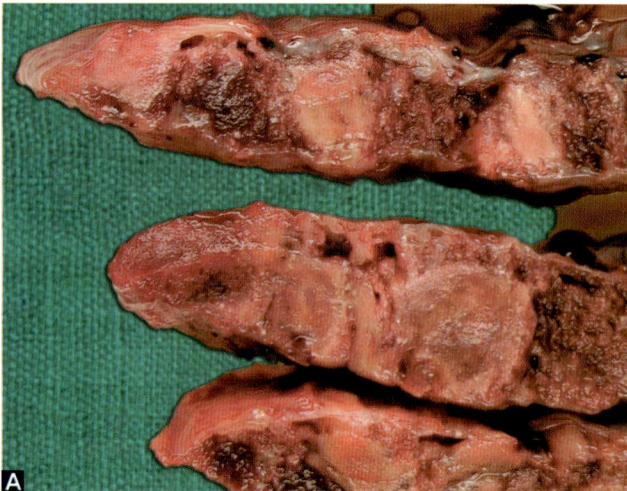

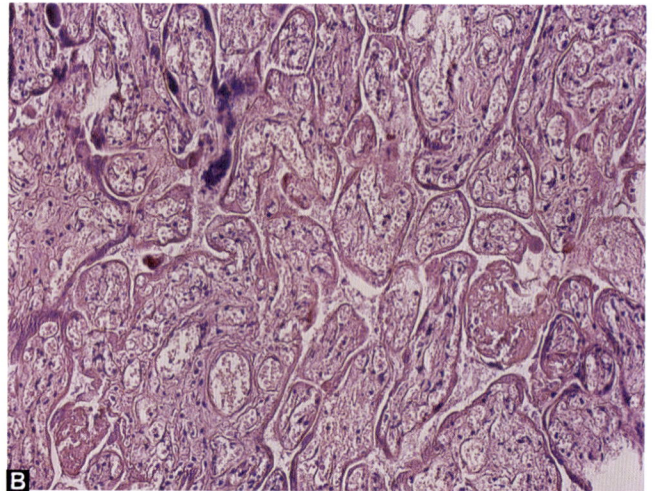

Figs 62.5A and B: Multiple fresh infarcts in a term placenta: (A) Macroscopic picture; (B) Microscopic image representing necrotic villi

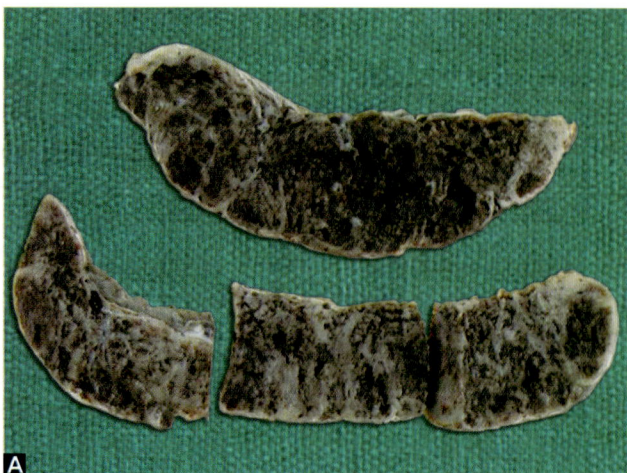

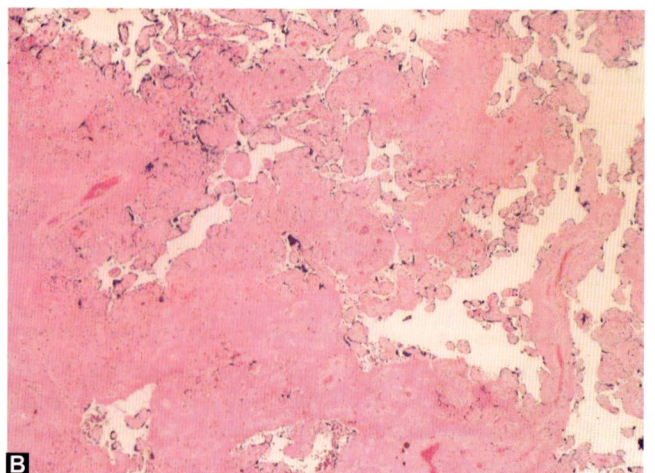

Figs 62.6A and B: Net-like fibrin deposition in the placenta: (A) Macroscopic picture; (B) Microscopic image shows villi entrapped by fibrin

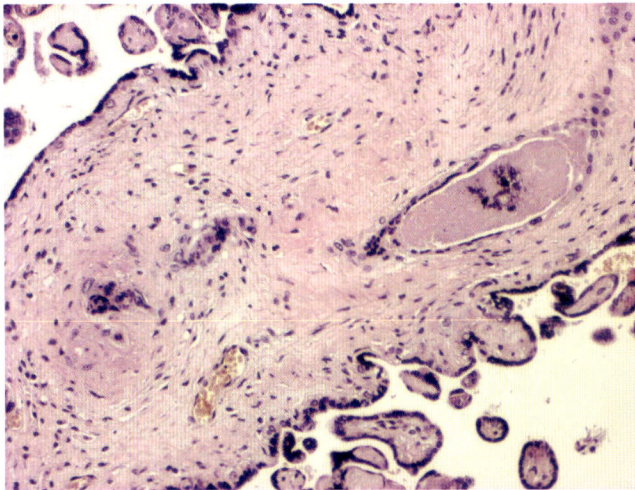

Fig. 62.7: Stem vessel occlusion with the small avascular villi

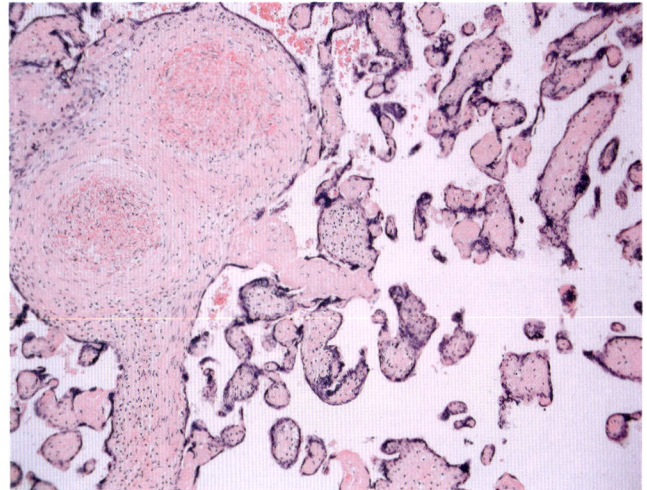

Fig. 62.8: A group of avascular villi around a stem villus. The stem villi shows hemorrhagic endovasculitis

a part in the blood gas exchange for the complete lack of capillaries. Presence of extensive avascular villi (Fig. 62.8), due to fetal vessel thrombosis, was reported in association with stillbirth, IUGR, maternal and fetal coagulopathy, and fetal thromboembolic disease leading to cerebral palsy.[7] *Intimal fibrin cushion*, a non-symmetric intimal swelling with endothelial disruption, is described in neonatal asphyxia, in association with disseminated capillary thrombi of fetal vessels. The severity of the fetal consequences depends more on the accompanying vascular lesions, mainly on fetal vessel thrombosis.[15] If there are large areas of avascular villi, the prognosis is dependent on the proportion of the placenta as described above.

Hemorrhagic endovasculitis (HEV) is a controversial entity, which was reported to be a postmortem artifact and was doubted as being a specific disease. The histological appearance is characterized by thrombotic-recanalized stem vessels and extravasated, fragmented red blood cells. HEV was found to be associated with meconium staining and postmaturity. Earlier report revealed association with stillbirth, IUGR, neurological disability and maternal hypertension. HEV was reported also in livebirths and associated with perinatal complications, fetal distress and IUGR.

Interlesional relationships exist between thrombotic, chronic inflammatory and chronic vaso-occlusive lesions.[4]

4. Most frequently *intervillous hemorrhage and thrombus* are related to maternal vessel lesion and are of maternal origin. Small and focal lesions have no clinical importance. Large and multiple lesions may cause fetal compromise or demise depending on the functional placenta parenchyma loss and the rest of the unaffected placenta. Quite often it can be seen in preeclamsia and is surrounded by infarct as a rim. In some cases intervillous hemorrhage and thrombus is sign of fetal bleeding into the maternal circulation as described by Kline. Only a minority of these alterations lead to large amount of fetal blood loss and stillbirth or severe anemia followed by ischemic lesions of parenchymal organs.

Changes of the chorionic villi secondary to preeclampsia, intrauterine hypoxia or fetal conditions and maternal spiral artery changes:

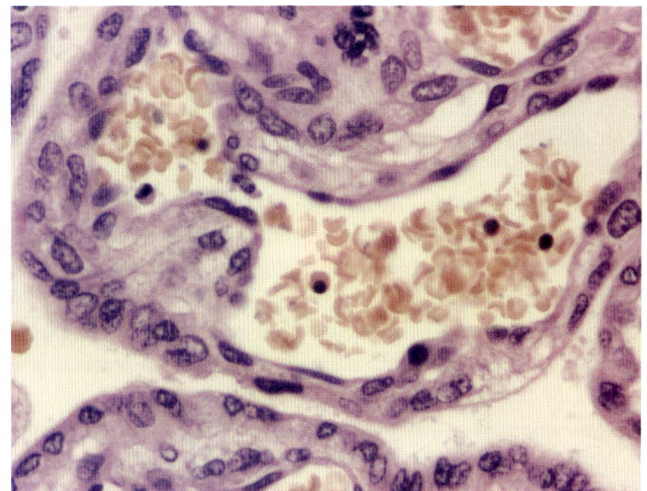

Fig. 62.9: Nucleated red blood cells in a terminal villus

1. Increased number of *syncytial knots* occurs in preeclampsia, hypertension, diabetes mellitus, maternal anemia, pregnancy at high altitude. It can also be seen in a thick histologic section (artifact). Despite of the fact that it occurs in preeclampsia, correlation between increased syncytial knotting and fetal hypoxia has not been proved. Excessive increase of syncytial knotting may be due to reduced fetal perfusion and placental hypoxia or can be the sign of accelerated maturation if the duration of pregnancy was less than 40 weeks.

2. *Elevated number of nucleated red blood cells* (NRBCs) may occur in many causes of chronic hypoxia (Fig. 62.9), IUGR, stillbirth, acute and chronic fetal blood loss or anemia, maternal diabetes and erythroblastosis fetalis.[4]

3. An increase of VSM (vasculosyncytial membrane) is described in pregnancies at high altitude, preeclampsia, maternal heart failure and maternal anemia. *VSM deficiency* was reported in pre-eclampsia, maternofetal rhesus incompatibility, maternal diabetes, low birthweight and stillbirths.[4,5]

4. *Extensive stromal fibrosis* occurs in terminal villous deficiency, in IUGR, and in avascular villi due to fetal stem vessel thrombosis.

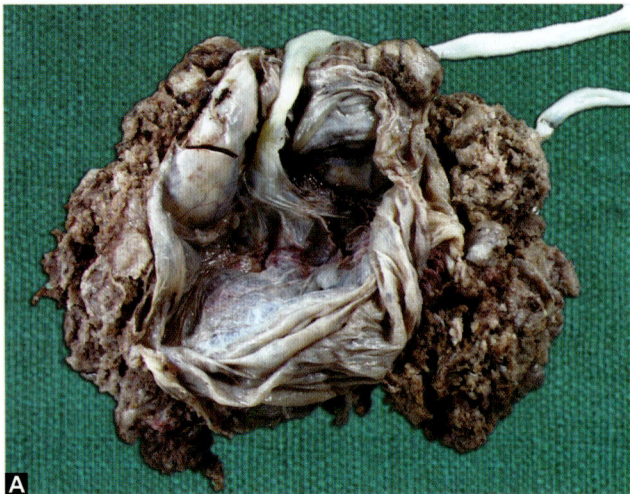

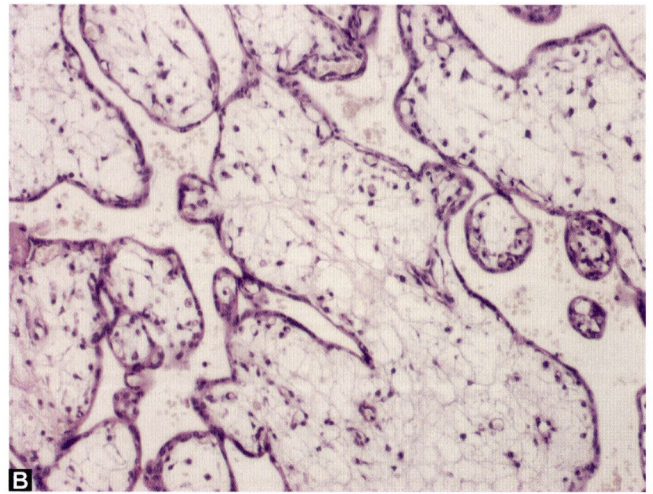

Figs 62.10A and B: Placenta edema: (A) Macroscopic picture—the placenta bulky; (B) Edematous terminal villi

5. Placentas from pregnancies with hydrops fetalis may show a combination of immaturity and edema. *Villous edema* occurs also in infections [syphilis, cytomegalovirus (CMV), toxoplasma, parvovirus] (Figs 62.10A and B) and in hydatidiform moles. Edema may be within normal limits, when focal.[4]

6. A *failure of villous maturation* was found to be associated with fetal hypoxia, IUGR, maternal diabetes and materno-fetal Rhesus incompatibility. Maturation failure may lead to intrauterine death.[5,21]

7. *Accelerated villus maturation* (maturitas precox)[4] can be observed in prematurely delivered placentas in preeclampsia and the features are related to chronic ischemia.

8. *Abnormalities of the maternal vessels* are usually associated with preeclamptic toxemia. *Uteroplacental or decidual arteriopathy* is a failure of physiological adaptation of maternal vessels. Uteroplacental vessel fibrinoid necrosis, acute atherosis and uteroplacental vessel thrombosis is closely related with pregnancy induced hypertension, maternal essential hypertension, preeclampsia and resulting in fetal complications such as IUGR, small for gestational age (SGA) and stillbirth. It is associated with APA, systemic lupus erythematosus (SLE) and thrombophilia.[4,5,22]

Inflammatory processes involving the placental villi or intervillous space

1. *Acute villitis* is usually associated with severe maternal infection, preterm delivery and might lead to intrauterine infection and intrauterine device (IUD).[4]

2. The etiology of *chronic villitis* is usually not known (villitis of unknown origin (VUO) or villitis of unknown etiology (VUE). (Fig. 62.11.) In about 15% of cases CMV, toxoplasma, syphilis infection is the underlying cause of chronic villitis. Chronic villitis is associated with IUGR and/or stillbirth. Chronic villitis of unknown etiology is associated with IUGR and preterm birth, and tends to recur during subsequent pregnancies.[4]

3. *Chronic histiocytic intervillositis*, (chronic perivillositis) is characterized by dense histiocytic intervillous infiltrate, and is reported in association with elevated maternal serum

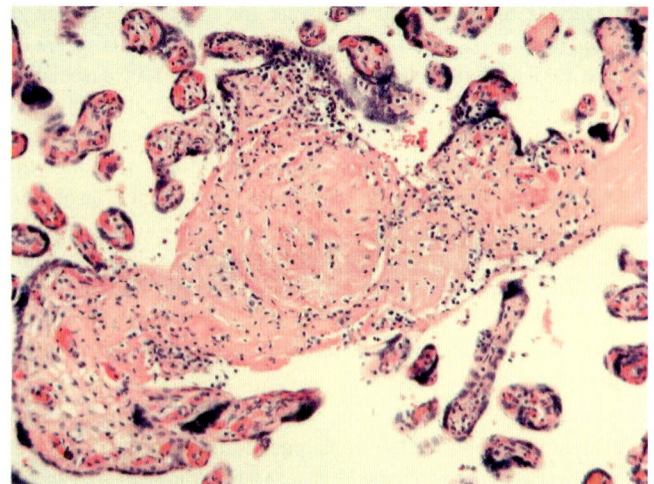

Fig. 62.11: Villitis of unknown etiology (VUE). Chronic inflammatory cells infiltrate the villus, the chorionic epithelium is damaged

AFP (alpha-fetoprotein), recurrent abortion, IUGR, preterm delivery. Malaria infection should be excluded.[23]

Miscellaneous conditions of the chorionic villi:

1. *Mesenchymal dysplasia* is the hallmark of Beckwith-Wiedeman syndrome.[24]

2. Perinatal death, congenital malformation and cerebral palsy were found to be associated with *chorangiosis* as a response to low-grade tissue hypoxia. Although others have supported this observation, it still remained a question how does the chronic hypoxia result in increased vascularization. The significance of this alteration needs further investigation.[25]

3. *Chorangioma* is a tumor-like lesion, resembling infantile hemangiomas. (Fig. 62.12.) It is most likely of hyperplastic origin, arising from the subtrophoblastic reticular tissue of the immature stem villi. Large lesions can lead to cardiac failure, hydrops and death of the fetus due to high output cardiac failure. Other possible complications are transplacental bleeding, and fetomaternal transfusion leading to anemia. Chorangioma was

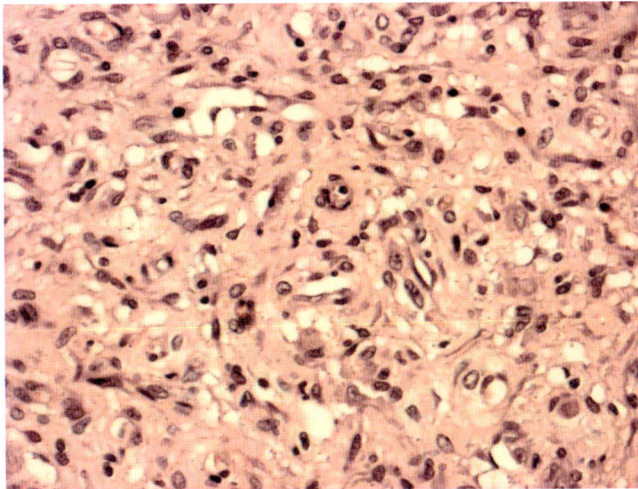

Fig. 62.12: Microscopic appearance of chorangioma with small capillary-like vessels and sinusoids

reported to be associated with preeclampsia, multiple gestation, premature delivery, fetal thrombocytopenia and fetal angiomas (Kasabach-Merritt syndrome).[4]

4. *Umbilical cord hemangioma* is a rare entity and its complications are related to the size of the lesion. It can be associated with elevated AFP level, fetal disseminated intravascular coagulation (DIC), fetal hydrops as well as fetal demise.[26]

CONCLUSION

In conclusion we would like to emphasize the importance of placental referral to the pathology laboratory and the placenta examination. We also would like to encourage communication between clinicians and pathologists to discover further clinico-pathological correlations for the benefit of the patients.

REFERENCES

1. Hargitai B, Marton T, Cox PM. Examination of the human placenta. Best practice no. 178. J Clin Pathol. 2004.
2. Khong TY. A topographical and clinical approach to examination of the placenta. Pathology. 2001;33(2):174-86.
3. Langston C, Kaplan C, Macpherson T, et al. Practice guideline for examination of the placenta: Developed by the Placental Pathology Practice Guideline Development Task Force of the College of American Pathologists. Arch Pathol Lab Med. 1997;121(5):449-76.
4. Benirschke K, Kaufmann P. Pathology of the human placenta, 4th edition. New York, Berlin, Heidelberg: Springer-Verlag; 1999.
5. Fox H. Pathology of the placenta, 2nd edition. London, Philadelphia, Toronto, Sydney, Tokyo: WB Saunders Company Ltd; 1997.
6. Altshuler G. Placenta within the medicolegal imperative. Arch Pathol Lab Med. 1991;115(7):688-95.
7. Kraus FT. Cerebral palsy and thrombi in placental vessels of the fetus: insights from litigation. Hum Pathol. 1997;28(2):246-8.
8. Redline RW, Boyd T, Campbell V, et al. Maternal vascular underperfusion: Nosology and reproducibility of placental reaction patterns. Pediatr Dev Pathol. 2004;7(3):237-49.
9. Naeye RL. Do placental weights have clinical significance? Hum Pathol. 1987;18(4):387-91.
10. Machin GA, Ackerman J, Gilbert-Barness E. Abnormal umbilical cord coiling is associated with adverse perinatal outcomes. Pediatr Dev Pathol. 2000;3(5):462-71.
11. Baergen RN, Malicki D, Behling C, et al. Morbidity, mortality, and placental pathology in excessively long umbilical cords: Retrospective study. Pediatr Dev Pathol. 2001;4(2):144-53.
12. Chow JS, Benson CB, Doubilet PM. Frequency and nature of structural anomalies in fetuses with single umbilical arteries. J Ultrasound Med. 1998;17(12):765-8.
13. Gibbs RS, Romero R, Hillier SL, et al. A review of premature birth and subclinical infection. Am J Obstet Gynecol. 1992;166(5):1515-28.
14. Wu YW, Colford JM Jr. Chorioamnionitis as a risk factor for cerebral palsy: A meta-analysis. JAMA. 2000;284(11):1417-24.
15. Altshuler G. Some placental considerations related to neurodevelopmental and other disorders. J Child Neurol. 1993;8(1):78-94.
16. Ahmed A, Gilbert-Barness E. Placenta membranacea: A developmental anomaly with diverse clinical presentation. Pediatr Dev Pathol. 2003;6:201-3.
17. Redline RW, O'Riordan MA. Placental lesions associated with cerebral palsy and neurologic impairment following term birth. Arch Pathol Lab Med. 2000;124(12):1785-91.
18. Görbe É, Rigó J Jr, Marton T, et al. Maternal floor infarct, gleichzeitiges Auftreten von intrauteriner Fetusretardierung und hohem mütterlichen AFP-Spiegel. Z Geburtshilfe Neonatol. 1999;203(5):218-20.
19. Bane AL, Gillan JE. Massive perivillous fibrinoid causing recurrent placental failure. BJOG. 2003;110(3): 292-5.
20. Naeye RL. Disorders of the placenta, fetus and neonate: Diagnosis and clinical significance. St Louis: Mosby Year Book; 1992.
21. Stalmach T, Hebisch G, Meier K, et al. Rescue by birth: Defective placental maturation and late fetal mortality. Obstet Gynecol. 2001;97(4):505-9.
22. Magid MS, Kaplan C, Sammaritano LR, et al. Placental pathology in systemic lupus erythematosus: A prospective study. Am J Obstet Gynecol. 1998;179(1):226-34.
23. Boyd TK, Redline RW. Chronic histiocytic intervillositis: A placental lesion associated with recurrent reproductive loss. Hum Pathol. 2000;31(11):1389-96.
24. Jauniaux E, Nicolaides KH, Hustin J. Perinatal features associated with placental mesenchymal dysplasia. Placenta. 1997;18:701-6.
25. Altshuler G. Chorangiosis: An important placental sign of neonatal morbidity and mortality. Arch Pathol Lab Med. 1984;108(1):71-4.
26. Kamitomo M, Sueyoshi K, Matsukita S, et al. Hemangioma of the umbilical cord: Stenotic change of the umbilical vessels. Fetal Diagn Ther. 1999;14(6):328-31.

Fetal Diagnosis and Therapy

W Holzgreve, M Evans

63 Noninvasive Prenatal Diagnosis: Maternal Blood

O Lapaire, B Zimmermann, X Yan Zhong

ABSTRACT

One of the major topics of prenatal research today is the genetic analysis of fetal cells or fetal DNA/RNA, which can be accumulated from the blood of pregnant women. It is the intention of the clinician and scientists of the laboratory to offer a risk-free diagnostic method for pregnant women in order to reduce the number of invasive interventions [e.g. amniocentesis (AC), chorionic villi sampling (CVS)] and the procedure related risk of fetal loss, as well as to provide additional new markers in prenatal screening programs. Up to now the technical problems of cell enrichment have prevented a routine use of fetal cell sampling in the clinics. In contrast, fetal cell-free DNA in maternal plasma can now be used for the extremely reliable identification of fetal genetic traits, clearly distinct from maternal sequences (e.g. the fetal rhesus status) or inherited polymorphism. Only recently, a new field of investigation has been opened by the demonstration of the cell free form of fetal RNA in maternal plasma, which is surprisingly stable and holds promise for noninvasive screening for fetal aneuploidies or pregnancy associated disorders.

INTRODUCTION

A routine clinical prenatal diagnosis with a view to identify fetal genetic disorders started in the 1970s. Since its inception, the reason for prenatal diagnosis is the detection of fetal aneuploidy and malformations. The overall risk of fetal chromosomal disorders is continuously rising due to the increasing average age of pregnant women in the western world, especially in Europe. The maternal age alone as a screening marker has a low sensitivity of 30%–40% for trisomy 21 (M. Down), dependent on the age distribution of the studied population. Down syndrome is the most common chromosomal abnormality among live births and is the most frequent form of mental retardation caused by a chromosomal aberration. Prenatal protocols for Down syndrome screening have been introduced for several reasons:

- Trisomy 21 has a high prevalence (1 in 700 births in the absence of prenatal intervention)
- The morbidity and mortality in affected fetuses and the consecutive socioeconomic burdens
- The area-wide availability of diagnostic tests to detect this chromosomal abnormality
- The availability of all over the country of safe and accessible interventions to introduce abortions of affected fetuses.

There is the existent desire of the society for Down syndrome screening to be done as early as possible in pregnancy, despite of the effectiveness of second trimester serum screening. First or early second trimester diagnosis of fetal abnormalities allows more time for decision making, greater privacy (the neighborhood may not be aware of the pregnancy), and, if chosen by the couple, safer methods of pregnancy termination. However, a number of issues must be addressed before earlier screening can be offered on a general population basis. These issues include the availability and acceptability of early invasive diagnostic methods (e.g. chorionic villus sampling[1]), and clinical effectiveness.

Three screening markers, two serum, and one fetal ultrasound marker have been shown to be effective for first trimester screening for Down syndrome.[2,3] The two serum markers in combination with the maternal age constitute a first trimester maternal serum screening test that achieves a sensitivity of 63% at a 5% false positive rate.[2]

An improved performance can be attained by the addition of sonographic analysis for increased fetal nuchal translucency (NT). NT by itself is a strong marker of Down syndrome and is associated with detection rates between 60%–70% and at a 5% false positive rate.[4] When it is combined with the pregnancy associated plasma protein A (PAPP-A), free beta-hCG and the maternal age, an overall sensitivity rate of approximately 85% at a 5% false positive rate can be obtained.[5-7]

The combination of serum and ultrasound markers at the end of the first trimester is better than any of the second trimester serum tests, that are nowadays available and, at least in a hypothetical model, are more cost effective (screening plus liveborn costs).[8] However, the performance of NT as a screening marker has not been consistent from study to study, probably because of the variability of operator's expertise and different qualities of the equipment.[9] Further studies as well as proper training and ongoing quality management are necessary before a noncritical widespread use of this screening regimen can be implemented.[10]

In case of a suspicious result (in Switzerland: overall risk for trisomy 21 > 1:380), an invasive testing, either with AC or CVS, is advised during a profound genetic counseling. Amniocentesis is the commonly used ultrasound guided technique for withdrawing amniotic fluid from the uterine cavity, using a needle via a transabdominal approach. CVS refers also to the invasive procedures for prenatal diagnosis of genetic disorders, in which small specimens of the placenta are achieved for chromosome or DNA analysis. Two approaches are available for obtaining chorionic tissue: a transcervical or a transabdominal CVS, depending on the routine of the performer and of the location of the placenta. However, due to the procedure related risk of fetal loss, that is estimated to be 0.5–1% of all interventions, a rising percentage of pregnant women opt not to have any invasive diagnostic procedures. Thus, the rate of procedure-related unaffected fetal loss is estimated to be 44–45 per 100,000 women screened when either first trimester screening (NT, free beta hCG and PAPP-A) or a second trimester quadruple test has been performed.

For that reason, international projects in the field of prenatal medicine research for effective, risk free and reliable alternative methods and additional markers. Object of the research is to obtain fetal tissue, either with the enrichment of fetal cells or cell-free DNA and recently RNA, extracted from the maternal blood. Fetal cells have been found in the maternal blood, though in very low quantity. Therefore, the primary step was their detection, enrichment and characterization with molecular-biologic methods.[11] Beside fetal cells, also fetal cell-free DNA and as mentioned above, fetal RNA, independent of fetal gender and genetic polymorphism status, was found in the maternal plasma. With the progress in prenatal research and technical advances, some results of noninvasive prenatal medicine research have already come into the clinical setting; as a diagnostic tool, fetal DNA, extracted from maternal plasma can now be used for the extremely reliable identification of fetal genetic traits, that are absent in the maternal genome (e.g. the fetal rhesus status or patients with an elevated risk for 'X'-chromosomal inherited disorders e.g. hemophilia, fragile X-syndrome).

To examine fetal DNA, nowadays a polymerase chain reaction (PCR) is normally used for the first step in the vast majority of DNA analysis. In a few hours, an automated PCR can amplify a single DNA molecule a million-fold. The greatly amplified target DNA is subsequently analyzed via other techniques.

The recent detection of fetal RNA in the plasma of pregnant women has led to new opportunities. Unlike fetal DNA, quantitative analysis of fetal RNA with PCR methods has the advantage of being applicable to all gravidae, irrespective of fetal gender and genetic polymorphism.[12]

To analyse fetal RNA, a reverse-transcriptase polymerase chain reaction (RT-PCR) is used for transforming messenger RNA (mRNA) into complementary DNA (cDNA) by an RNA-dependent DNA polymerase, specified as reverse transcriptase. The cDNA complex is then changed into a double-stranded DNA, and becoming so the template for a subsequent PCR reaction.

The main source of fetal RNA is thought to be the placenta. Fetal RNA is surprisingly stable in the maternal plasma. Data indicate that the measurement of circulating placental RNA may provide a new method for noninvasive prenatal diagnosis and monitoring. The futural clinical application of this technology would be the application of RNA as an additional screening tool for chromosomal aneuploidies and other pregnancy associated disorders.

NONINVASIVE CLINICAL DIAGNOSTICS USING FETAL CELLS IN MATERNAL BLOOD SAMPLES

A long sought goal of prenatal medicine has been the reduction of invasive diagnostic procedures for fetal cell sampling, and its procedurerelated risk of miscarriage, by isolating fetal cells from the maternal blood.

In the 90s of the last century, for the first time successful enrichment of fetal cells, extracted from maternal blood, was published. The cells could be checked for possible aneuploidies by fluorescent in situ hybridization (FISH).[13] FISH can identify different chromosomal mutations including deletions, duplications, aneuploidy and the presence of derivative chromosomes. However, small mutations, including small deletions and insertions as well as point mutations, cannot be identified with the FISH technique. When the DNA probes are designated with a fluorochrome, a fast detection of the fluorescent signal is possible via fluorescence microscopy. The main difficulty of this method has been the very low concentration of fetal cells in the maternal serum. It could be shown, that only 2–6 cells/mL of maternal blood are present.[14] Fetal cells can be found in the blood of pregnant women from the first trimester on. However, a rapid, simple and consistent procedure for their isolation for prenatal noninvasive testing has not been found. Almost any procedure available in experimental cell research for cell enrichment has been used to isolate fetal cells out of maternal blood. For the multistep enrichment, the density gradient centrifugation is always used as the first step,[15] fluorescent activated cell sorting (FACS),[16] or magnetic activated cell sorting (MACS), (Fig. 63.1)[17] follow as second step. A major effort has been made during the last years to standardize and validate these processes among different laboratories.

The later method is easy to perform and has a higher turnover of samples, as well as a higher sensitivity than FACS (Fig. 63.2). The third step includes either FISH, culture or PCR. However, the cell culture, with or without enrichment, as well as the multistep

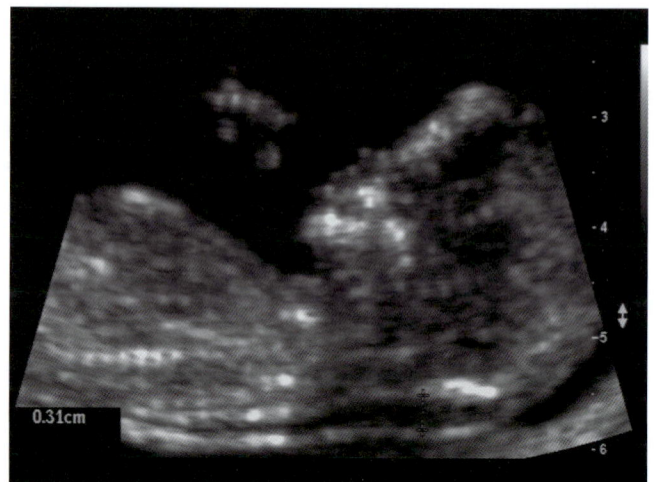

Fig. 63.1: Transabdominal measurement of the fetal nuchal translucency (0.31 cm) at the end of the first trimester

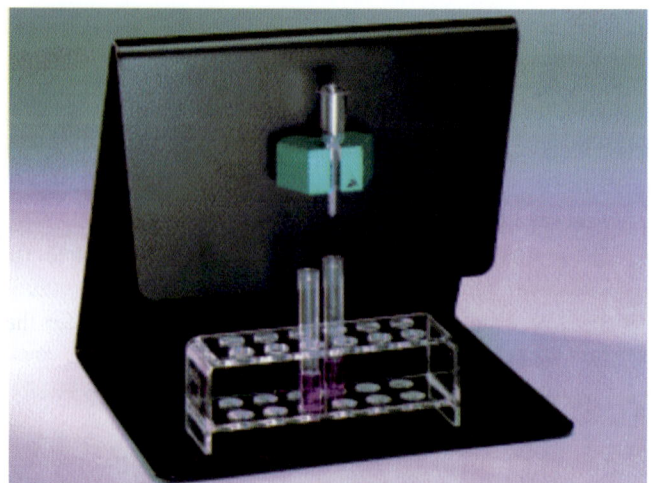

Fig. 63.2: Aspect of a MACS system, used in our laboratory

enrichment procedure itself require many manipulations in which a certain amount of cells are lost. New methods, such as automatic scanning, are needed to install the cell enrichment in the routine clinical use. Each of these cell lines has some specific disadvantages. For example, it is not possible to cultivate nuclear erythrocytes. This fact does not allow a metaphase analysis for chromosomal testing. On the other hand CD34+ cells can be cultivated. However, they persist postpartum in the maternal blood circulation and make a prenatal testing in the next pregnancy more difficult. Furthermore, cells are not constantly present in the maternal circulation. The isolated cells have been investigated using either cytochemistry, soret band absorption microscopy, monoclonal antibodies for e- and g-chain hemoglobin, monoclonal antibody for i-antigen and by FISH. For all those reasons, up to now the enrichment of fetal cells from the maternal blood is too laborious to be a serious alternative in the clinic and to supersede prenatal invasive diagnostic procedures. Today, the international research has partially turned its attention to the free fetal DNA and RNA.

NONINVASIVE PRENATAL DIAGNOSTIC TESTS WITH FETAL DNA

The first publication about fetal DNA, extracted from maternal blood dated from 1997.[18] Quantitative investigations showed, that the concentration of fetal DNA during pregnancy is much higher than that of fetal cells.[18] Quantitative levels can be measured with real time PCR. Real time PCR has several advantages over conventional PCR; the data collection occurs during amplification. The accumulation of PCR products over time is measured directly, without post-PCR modifications. Therefore, it is less prone to contamination, as the results are analyzed automatically without having to open the PCR reaction vessel and there is no post-PCR work. It also permits the rapid analysis of numerous samples in one analytic run and is, therefore, better for automation.

The quantitation of fetal DNA may obtain additional knowledge regarding the pregnancy outcome. Fetal DNA is elevated in specific pregnancy associated disorders, like preeclampsia,[13] hyperemesis gravidarum[19] or trisomy 21.[20] In case of preeclampsia, it could be demonstrated that the severity of the disease correlates with the level of fetal DNA in the blood of affected pregnant women.[21] These studies suggested, that an elevated concentration of fetal DNA may be a valuable marker for pregnancy associated diseases.[22] Because the majority (more than 90%) of free DNA in maternal serum derives from the mother, it has been difficult to differentiate the origin. Previously, it was possible only to examine genetic traits, that are not present in the maternal genome. However, with this noninvasive and risk free method, it is now possible to detect y-specific sequences in pregnancies with an elevated risk for X-chromosomal inherited disorders (e.g. hemophilia, fragile X-syndrome). Approximately, 15% of Caucasian pregnancies are potentially at risk for severe intrauterine hemolytic disease, mainly due to Rhesus D incompatibility. The need to know the Rhesus constellation, as well as the large number of X-linked disorders, has prodded several groups to develop noninvasive risk free methods for diagnostic tests.

With the highly specific real time PCR method, it is nowadays possible to detect these fetal genetic traits with an almost 100% sensitivity and specificity. A few laboratories offer routinely the

detection of the fetal rhesus status. This is a success in the 15-year old international research on this topic.

A recently published work of our laboratory demonstrated that fetal DNA can be separated from maternal DNA, due to the difference of its size.[23] A majority of fetal DNA has a size of <0.3 KB, whereas the maternal DNA, that constitutes more than 90% of the amount of circulating DNA in the maternal blood, shows a size of > 1 KB.[24] The difference in size may account for the different origin. Fetal DNA derives predominantly from the placenta, whereas maternal DNA has its main origin in the hematopoietic system.[25,26] After size separation of the fetal DNA, it is possible to detect fetal microsatellite markers with fluorescent PCR.[24] Up to now, this new technology has been used for the determination of many disorders like myotonic dystrophy,[23] achondroplasia[27] and beta-thalassemia.[28]

NONINVASIVE PRENATAL SCREENING TESTS WITH FETAL DNA

The current focus in research on fetal DNA investigates its use as a maternal serum marker in the second-trimester for fetal Down syndrome and other pregnancy associated disorders. The quantitative measurement of fetal DNA could complement the second trimester serum markers. By increasing the specificity of the screening it could help to prevent a considerable amount of unnecessary invasive procedures. The median of fetal DNA concentration is reported to be approximately twofold higher in pregnancies with Down syndrome, compared with unaffected pregnancies, but the data is disputed by other reports, and larger sample numbers and meticulously accurate, standardized quantification are demanded to allow final conclusions.

In order to use the fetal DNA as a screening marker, a gender-independent fetal DNA marker that can be assayed by real-time PCR is needed. Polymorphic sequences are presently used in the clinical samples that are investigated for fetal rhesus status to ascertain the presence of adequate amounts of fetal DNA. Although, a number of sequences has to be examined in each pregnancy to ascertain distinction between fetal and maternal, this approach is still relatively facile to implement.

The presence of fetal DNA in maternal plasma has revealed significant clinical potential for the prenatal diagnosis of fetal genetic diseases and pregnancy-associated complications.

A caveat of the approach is that the DNA present in the circulation is predominantly of maternal origin and interferes with molecular analysis of the fetal DNA. Hence, paternally inherited fetal loci that are clearly distinct from maternal genomic sequences can be readily examined. Paternally inherited mutant genes in compound heterozygous genetic disorders may also be detected if the paternal mutation is dissimilar from the maternal allele. In general, the detection of fetal single gene disorders is at least cumbersome and often impossible with current methods. Likewise does the determination of chromosomal abnormalities require further advancement in the technology before it is feasible in a non-invasive manner.

Most studies generate data from pregnancies with male fetuses as sequences on the Y-chromosome are unique DNA markers absent in the maternal genome. This approach is only applicable to approximately 50% of the pregnancies, but straightforward to perform. An impediment in the generation of accurate data is the low number of fetal sequences in the plasma, such that the samples quantified by the real-time PCR have copy numbers close to the detection limit and quantitative value of the results is reduced by increased variability of method and sampling.

NONINVASIVE PRENATAL DIAGNOSTIC AND SCREENING WITH FETAL RNA FROM MATERNAL PLASMA, EXPRESSED FROM THE PLACENTA

A new development in prenatal screening research constitutes the measurement of fetal RNA in the maternal blood. It gives the possibility to screen for sex—unspecific for disorders.[12] Fetal RNA in maternal plasma is surprisingly stable and holds promise

for noninvasive gene expression profiling.[12,29-31] Unlike fetal DNA, extracted from maternal serum or plasma, fetal RNA can be used for prenatal testing irrespective of fetal gender and genetic polymorphism status. To date only a few reports present quantitative data on this phenomenon. They indicate maternal plasma RNA as a gender independent marker group that may by noninvasive gene-expression profiling be a suitable screening tool for pregnancy associated pathologies. It could be demonstrated, that not only fetal DNA, but also fetal RNA was present in elevated concentrations in pregnant women with preeclampsia.[32] The presence of fetal RNA in the maternal serum gives the possibility to investigate the expression of certain genes in analogy with nowadays used RNA markers in oncology.[33]

The fast progresses and success in noninvasive prenatal research may give a futural prospect for valuable alternatives in regard to the prenatal invasive diagnostics.

REFERENCES

1. Stranc LC, Evans JA, Hamerton JL. Chorionic villus sampling and amniocentesis for prenatal diagnosis. Lancet. 1997;349:711-4.
2. Canick JA, Kellner LH. First trimester screening for aneuploidy: serum biochemical markers. Semin Perinatol. 1999;23:359-68.
3. Wald NJ, Hackshaw AK. Combining ultrasound and biochemistry in first-trimester screening for Down's syndrome. Prenat Diagn. 1997;17:821-9.
4. Stewart TL, Malone FD. First trimester screening for aneuploidy: nuchal translucency sonography. Semin Perinatol. 1999;23:369-81.
5. Crossley JA, Aitken DA, Cameron AD, et al. Combined ultrasound and biochemical screening for Down's syndrome in the first trimester: a Scottish multicentre study. BJOG. 2002;109:667-76.
6. Wapner R, Thom E, Simpson JL, et al. First-trimester screening for trisomies 21 and 18. N Engl J Med. 2003;349:1405-13.
7. Muller F, Benattar C, Audibert F, et al. First-trimester screening for Down syndrome in France combining fetal nuchal translucency measurement and biochemical markers. Prenat Diagn. 2003;23:833-6.
8. Cusick W, Buchanan P, Hallahan TW, et al. Combined first-trimester versus second-trimester serum screening for Down syndrome: a cost analysis. Am J Obstet Gynecol. 2003;188(3):745-51.
9. Haddow JE, Palomaki GE, Knight GJ, et al. Screening of maternal serum for fetal Down's syndrome in the first trimester. N Engl J Med. 1998;338:955-61.
10. Mennuti MT, Driscoll DA. Screening for Down's syndrome—too many choices?. N Engl J Med. 2003; 349:1471.
11. Holzgreve W, Hahn S. Prenatal diagnosis using fetal cells and free fetal DNA in maternal blood. Clin Perinatol. 2001;28:353-65.
12. Poon LL, Leung TN, Lau TK, et al. The presence of fetal RNA in maternal plasma. Clin Chem. 2000;46:1832-4.
13. Hahn S, Sant R, Holzgreve W. Fetal cells in maternal blood: current and future perspectives. Mol Hum Reprod. 1998;4:515-21.
14. Krabchi K, Gros-Louis F, Yan J, et al. Quantification of fetal nucleated cells in maternal blood between the 18th and 22nd weeks of pregnancy using molecular cytogenetic techniques. Clin Genet. 2001;60:145-50.
15. Oosterwijk JC, Mesker WE, Ouwerkerk MC. Fetal cell detection in maternal blood: a study of 236 samples using erythroblasts morphology. DAB and HbF staining, and FISH analysis. Cytometry. 1998;32:178-85.
16. Bianchi DW, Williams JM, Sullivan LM, et al. PCR quantification of fetal cells in maternal blood in normal and aneuploid pregnancies. Am J Hum Genet. 1997;61:822-9.
17. Gaenshirt AD, Burschy M, Garritsen HS, et al. Magnetic cell sorting and the transferrin receptor as potential means to prenatal diagnosis from maternal blood. Am J Obstet Gynecol. 1992;166:1350-56.
18. Lo YMD, Corbetta N, Chamberlain PF, et al. Presence of fetal DNA in maternal plasma and serum. Lancet. 1997;350:485-7.
19. Sugito Y, Sekizawa A, Farina A, et al. Relationship between severity of hyperemesis gravidarum and fetal DNA concentration in maternal plasma. Clin Chem. 2003;49:1667-9.
20. Zhong XY, Burk MR, Troeger C, et al. Fetal DNA in maternal plasma is elevated in pregnancies with aneuploid fetuses. Prenat Diagn. 2000;20:795-8.
21. Swinkels DW, de Kok JB, Hendriks JC, et al. Hemolysis, elevated liver enzymes, and low platelet count (HELLP) syndrome as a complication of preeclampsia in pregnant women increases the amount of cell-free fetal and maternal DNA in maternal plasma and serum. Clin Chem. 2002;48:650-3.
22. Farina A, LeShane ES, Lambert-Messerlian GM, et al. Valuation of fetal cell free DNA as a second-trimester marker of Down syndrome pregnancy. Clin Chem. 2003;49:239-42.
23. Li Y, Zimmermann B, Rusterholz C, Kang A, et al. Size separation of circulatory DNA in maternal plasma permits ready detection of fetal DNA polymorphisms. Clin Chem. 2004;50:1002-11.
24. Lo YM, Tein MS, Lau TK, et al. Quantitative analysis of fetal DNA in maternal plasma and serum: implications for non-invasive prenatal diagnosis. Am J Hum Genet. 1998;62:768-75.
25. Guibert J, Benachi A, Grebille AG, et al. Kinetics of SRY gene appearance in maternal serum: detection by real time PCR in early pregnancy after assisted reproductive technique. Hum Reprod. 2003;18:1733-6.
26. Lui YY, Chik KW, Chiu RW, et al. Predominant hematopoietic origin of cell free DNA in plasma and serum after sex-mismatched bone marrow transplantation. Clin Chem. 2002;48:421-7.
27. Amicucci P, Gennarelli M, Novelli G, et al. Prenatal diagnosis of myotonic dystrophy using fetal DNA obtained from maternal plasma. Clin Chem. 2000;46:301-2.

28. Saito H, Sekizawa A, Morimoto T, et al. Prenatal DNA diagnosis of a single-gene disorder from maternal plasma. Lancet. 2000;356:1170.

29. Chiu RW, Lau TK, Leung TN, et al. Prenatal exclusion of beta thalassaemia major by examination of maternal plasma. Lancet. 2002;360:998-1000.

30. NG EK, Tsui NB, Lau TK, et al. mRNA of placental origin is readily detectable in maternal plasma. Proc Natl Acad Sci. 2003;100:4748-53.

31. Lo YMD, Chiu RWK. The biology and diagnostic applications of plasma RNA. Ann N Y Acad Sci. 2004;1022:135–9.

32. NG EK, Leung TN, Tsui NB, et al. The concentration of circulating corticotrophin-releasing hormone mRNA in maternal plasma is increased in preeclampsia. Clin Chem. 2003; 49:727-31.

33. Hasselmann DO, Rappl G, Rossler M, et al. Detection of tumour-associated circulating mRNA in serum, plasma and blood cells from patients with disseminated malignant melanoma. Oncol Rep. 2001;8:115-8.

64 Multiple Gestations: Pregnancy Evaluation by Ultrasonography

S Tercanli, DV Surbek, R Zanetti-Dallenbach

INTRODUCTION

Since, the introduction of ultrasound in prenatal medicine, the prognosis of multiple pregnancies has improved dramatically. Early and appropriate diagnosis of multiplicity and chorionicity, detection of discordant fetal growth, evaluation of fetal well-being by biophysical scoring and Doppler sonography as well as planning of delivery mode by determination of fetal presentation are some of the most important diagnostic advances which represent the basis of the adequate clinical management. Multiple pregnancies are at increased risk for several complications during pregnancy and childbirth like prematurity, fetal growth retardation, twin-twin transfusion syndrome (TTS), preeclampsia, stillbirth and malpresentation. Therefore, early diagnosis of multiple pregnancy and in particular chorionicity is mandatory for the appropriate assessment of risk factors for intensive prenatal care and early detection as well as treatment of complications. Before the introduction of prenatal ultrasound, detection rate of twin pregnancies before delivery was lower than 50%,[1] while in countries where routine ultrasound in pregnancy is performed, the rate is close to 100%.[2] Consequently, this has led to decreased perinatal morbidity and mortality in twin and higher multiple gestations in the past 30 years.

In the following chapter, the authors will give an overview of the most important clinical issues of multiple pregnancy where ultrasonography plays a major role in the diagnostic procedure.

EARLY DIAGNOSIS OF MULTIPLE PREGNANCY

Why should a multiple pregnancy be diagnosed early? First, the number of fetuses, which can be confirmed by ultrasound, is a strong determinator of prognosis of a pregnancy, which is generally best for singletons and gets worse with higher order multiplicity. As in singleton pregnancies, gestational age can be confirmed by an early ultrasound during the first trimester using growth charts of crown-rump length corresponding to gestational age.[3] In the first and second trimester of pregnancy, growth charts for singleton pregnancies can be used appropriately for twin pregnancies.[4] More importantly, early ultrasound allows for definitive diagnosis of chorionicity, which itself is also a strong predictor of fetal outcome.

Usually, early diagnosis of multiple pregnancy by transvaginal sonography is easy.[5] After the fifth week of pregnancy (from the last menstrual period), different gestational sacs are visible in multichorionic gestations, whereas in monochorionic twins only one chorionic cavity is visible. From the sixth or seventh week of pregnancy, it is possible to identify the number of embryos and yolk sacs in multichorionic as well as in monochorionic gestations (Figs 64.1A and B). As soon as two or more embryos with heart activity are discernible, the diagnosis of multiple gestation is confirmed. Although, a false diagnosis of a singleton pregnancy may happen if a hurried scan is performed by an inexperienced examiner, the diagnosis at this stage is virtually error-free. Possible pitfalls may be chorial hematomas or a decidual pseudosac mimicking a second or third gestational sac, or conjoined twins mimicking a singleton pregnancy (Figs 64.2A and B).

Another issue in early diagnosis is the phenomenon of vanishing twins, which seems to happen in a significant proportion twin gestations[6,7] and might be the reason for discordant diagnosis in subsequent ultrasound examinations. This phenomenon of "vanishing embryos" is especially well established from in vitro programs such as shown in Table 64.1, which summarizes data

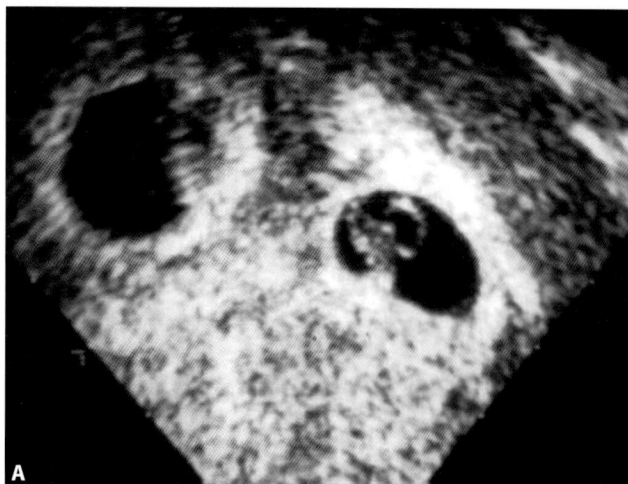

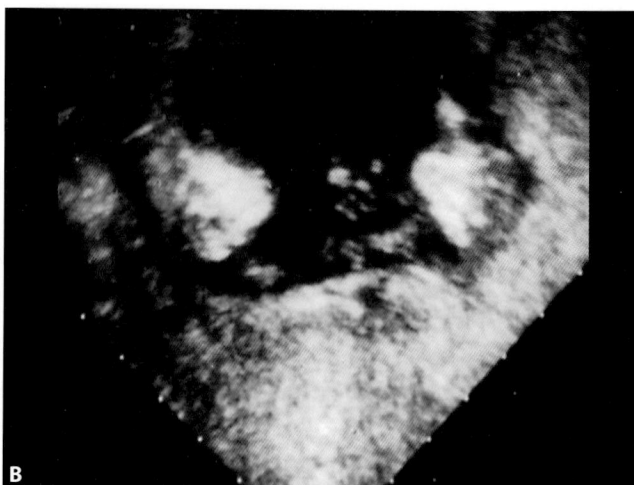

Figs 64.1A and B: Transvaginal sonograms of pregnancies in the first trimester. (A) Dichorionic twin pregnancy with clear separation of the chorionic cavities. (B) Monochorionic twin pregnancy with both embryos anencephalic

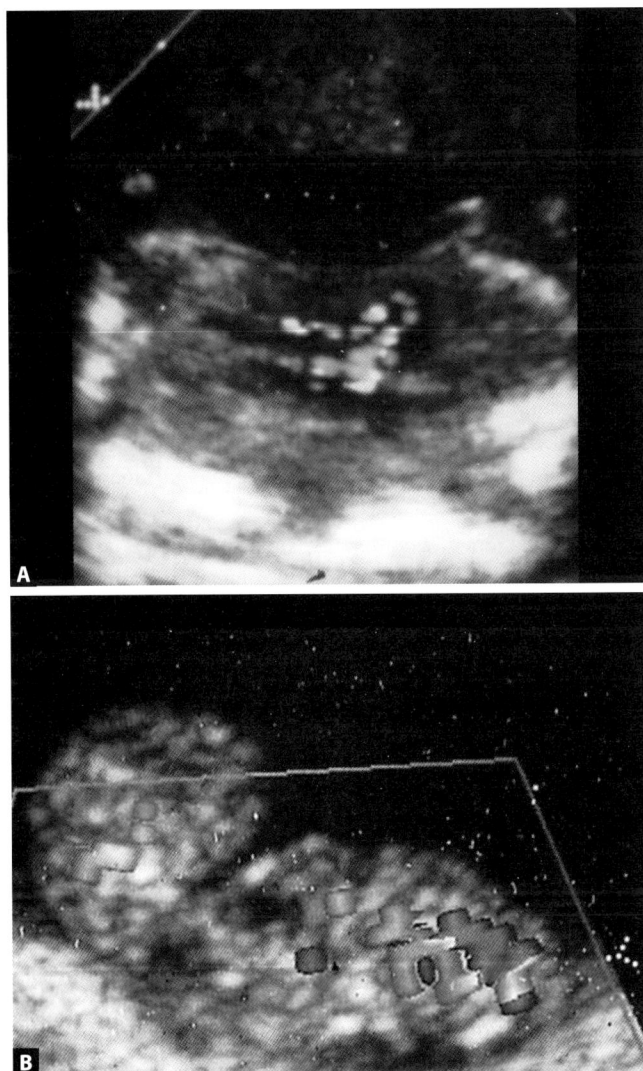

Figs 64.2A and B: Conjoined twins mimicking a singleton pregnancy. Color-coded Doppler sonography. (A) A common fetal heart. (B) Two independent fetal hearts

Table 64.1: Vanishing embryos in pregnancies with multiples. The "intake criterium" was intact heart action. All pregnancies are from the in vitro fertilization program of Dr Robert Fischer, Hamburg

Initial scan	Cases	2nd trimester
Twins	52	34 twins 18 singletons
Triplets	22	8 triplets 11 twins 3 singletons
Quadruplets	4	2 quadruplets 2 triplets

obtained in pregnancies after in vitro fertilization (IVF) where intact heart action of the embryos was the intake criterium for the prospective study. "Vanishing embryos" represent the spontaneous abortion of a multiple gestation member in the first trimester either by expulsion or—more often—by complete resorption of the embryo (Fig. 64.3). In many cases it remains asymptomatic, although sometimes it is accompanied by vaginal bleeding.

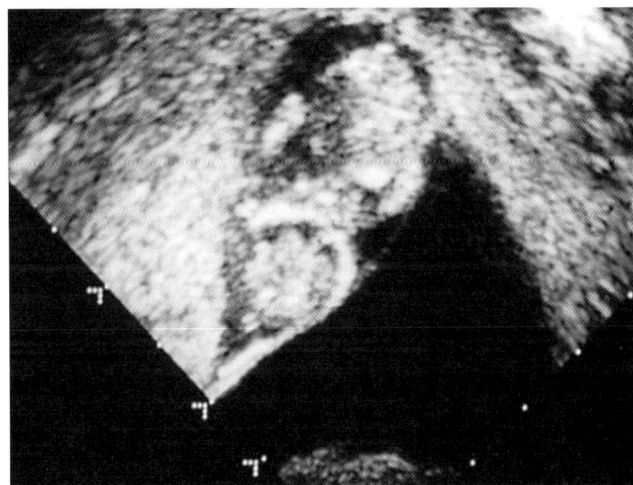

Fig. 64.3: Dichorionic twin pregnancy with a 'vanishing embryo'. After spontaneous abortion of the twin in the upper left corner of the uterus, the amniotic fluid in this sac has almost disappeared and the embryo is getting almost 'resorbed'

Prognosis for the surviving twin seems excellent, although recently it has been hypothesized that unexplained cerebral palsy might be the consequence in the survivor of a vanishing twin pair.[7-9]

PRENATAL DIAGNOSIS OF ZYGOSITY, CHORIONICITY AND AMNIONICITY

Dizygotic twinning results in dichorionic-diamniotic pregnancies, even though the placentae may be fused (Fig. 64.4). In contrast, monozygotic twinning may result in dichorionic-diamniotic, monochorionic-diamniotic or monochorionic-monoamniotic placentation, depending on the age of division. The division of the embryo results in the following constellations: from day 1 to day 3 after fertilization—dichorionic-diamniotic twins; from day 4 to day 6—dichorionic-monoamniotic twins; and from day 7 to day 9—monochorionic-monoamniotic twins. If the division happens after day 9, conjoined twins result. Dichorionic placentation is found in 30% of monozygotic pregnancies.[10] As a rule, dizygous twins are always dichorionic, although, this dogma has recently been disproven.[11,12]

Virtually all monochorionic twins, which represent about 20% of all twin pregnancies, have vascular anastomoses in the placenta, whereas almost none of dichorionic (fused) placentas shows such cross-circulation.[13] These vascular shunts usually remain balanced, but occasionally, they might become functional, leading to typical monochorionic twin complications like discordant growth (Fig. 64.5A) and TTS.[14] Alternatively, in situations with one intrauterine fetal demise (Fig. 64.5B) complications from vascular anastomoses might arise in the surviving twin. These include severe conditions like multicystic encephalomalacia and renal infarctions. In earlier publications, several authors postulated that embolization of thromboplastin-like material across the shared circulation followed by disseminated intravascular coagulation is the cause of this phenomenon, which is also called the twin disruption syndrome. More recent evidence, however, suggest another pathophysiological mechanism, which is based on the assumption that a sudden blood pressure gradient may occur at the moment of fetal demise, followed

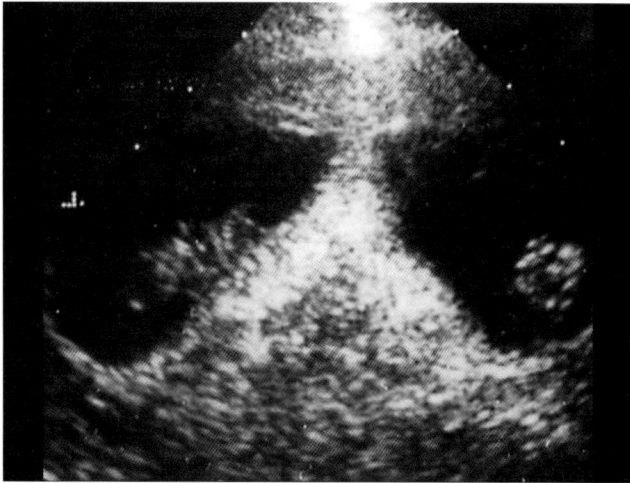

Fig. 64.4: Dichorionic twin pregnancy where both chorion frondosum areas are so close to one another that the two placentae seems to be "fused"

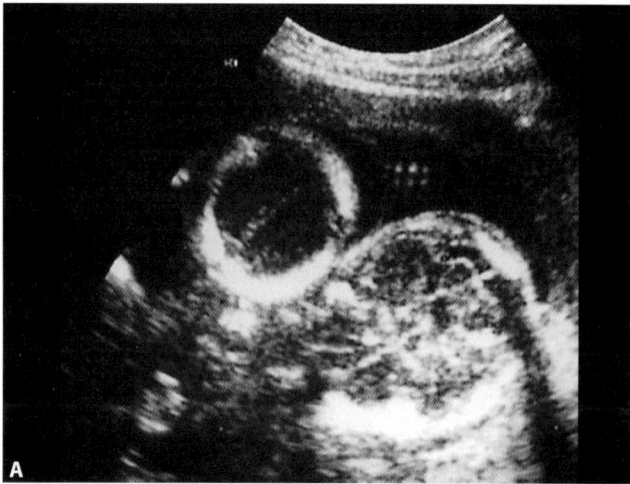

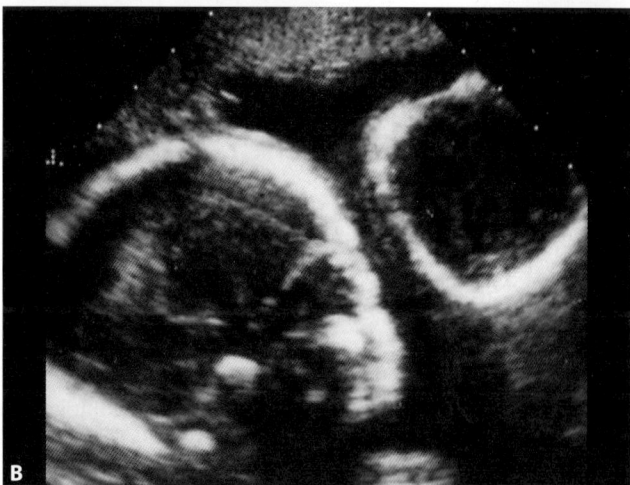

Figs 64.5A and B: Twin pregnancy with (A) discordant growth and (B) intrauterine fetal demise. The sonogram shows the head of the survivor in the lower left and the dead fetus in the upper right corner

by severe hypotension and exsanguination in the surviving fetus, leading to acute hypoxic organ damage predominantly in the brain in up to 20% of survivors.[15] This phenomenon could be called an acute TTS.[16]

These complications do only occur in monochorionic gestations (Fig. 64.6). In particular, the fetal loss rate in monochorionic pregnancies is up to four times higher in monochorionic as compared to dichorionic twin pregnancies. Chorionicity is thus the most important factor influencing outcome of twin pregnancies. Consequently, accurate prenatal diagnosis of chorionicity is of predominant importance for the clinical management of twin pregnancies.

As outlined above, monochorionic twins usually have a seperating membrane, thus being diamniotic. Fewer than 2% of twins are monoamniotic. Besides complications of monochorionicity, these pregnancies are at high risk for cord accidents during pregnancy and birth, resulting in an extremely high fetal loss rate of 50–75%. Delivery by early elective cesarean section is, therefore, one of the important features of the management of monoamniotic twins.

Determination of chorionicity and amnionicity before birth is made by ultrasonography. In early pregnancy during the first trimester, it is usually easy to differentiate the type of placentation by transvaginal sonography. If two gestational sacs with two embryos are identified, the diagnosis of dichorionic twins can be made with certainty (Fig. 64.7). On the other hand, if there is only one gestational sac with two embryos, monochorionic twins are diagnosed. To seperate monoamniotic from diamniotic gestation, it is necessary to discern two amniotic membranes surrounding the embryos (Fig. 64.8), or, at a later stage, to identify a partition membrane between the fetuses (Fig. 64.9). If there is no membrane visible, the sonographer has to be cautious as a seperating membrane might exist but might be hardly visible on ultrasound scan (Fig. 64.10A), particularly in cases of severe oligohydramnios or anhydramnios of one twin combined with polyhydramnios in the other (Fig. 64.10B), as it is typically present in twin-twin transfusion syndrome ("stuck twin").

Later in the first trimester, from about 10–14 weeks of gestation, the key to the differentiation of mono- and dichorionic diamniotic twins is that the "twin peak" sign or lambda sign (Fig. 64.11) was used to predict dichorionic twins if present.[17] This latter finding consists of chorionic tissue extending between layers of the interfetal septum close to the placenta.

In the second or third trimester of gestation, other criterias become important in determination of chorionicity. A reliable diagnosis of chorionicity can only be made if the fetuses are of opposite sex (dizygotic) or there are clearly two separated placentae visible, which is often not the case in dichorionic twins (Fig. 64.12). Entanglement of umbilical cords represents a reliable sign confirming the presence of a single amniotic cavity in monoamniotic gestation.[18] In cases with the same fetal sex, with one nonseperated placenta and with a dividing membrane between the fetuses, determination of chorionicity is difficult after the first trimester of gestation and requires other criteria. Thickness of the dividing membrane (Fig. 64.13) measured by ultrasound is one criterium, which is able to predict chorionicity, using a cutoff-level of 2 mm.[19] Another important sonographic feature is the number of layers identified in the dividing membrane.[20] While not always technically possible, it remains a reliable criteria of dichorionic placentation if three or more layers are present. Probably the best approach is the combination of these criterias, reaching excellent predicting values in the determination of chorionicity.[21]

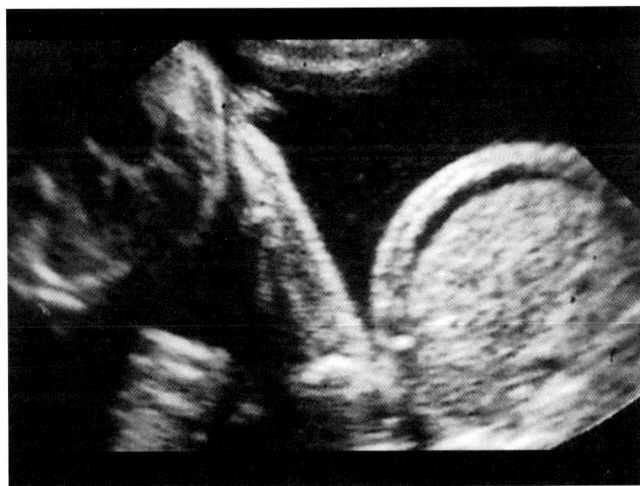

Fig. 64.6: Twin–twin transfusion sequence in monochorionic and monoamniotic twin pregnancy. The right fetus has a beginning ascites in the abdomen as a sign of cardiac failure

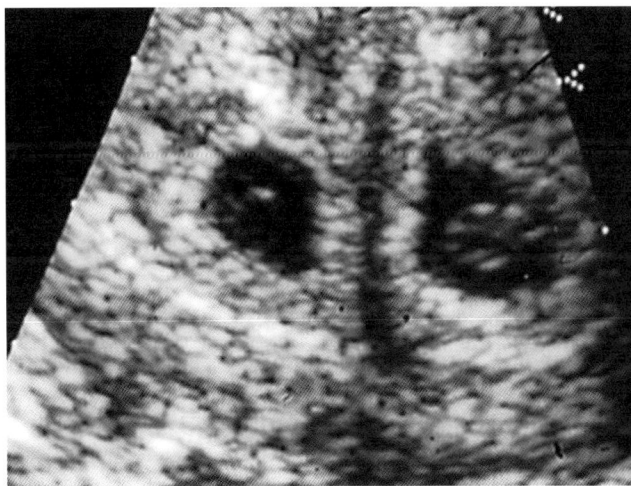

Fig. 64.7: Dichorionic twin pregnancies. The two sacs are clearly separated

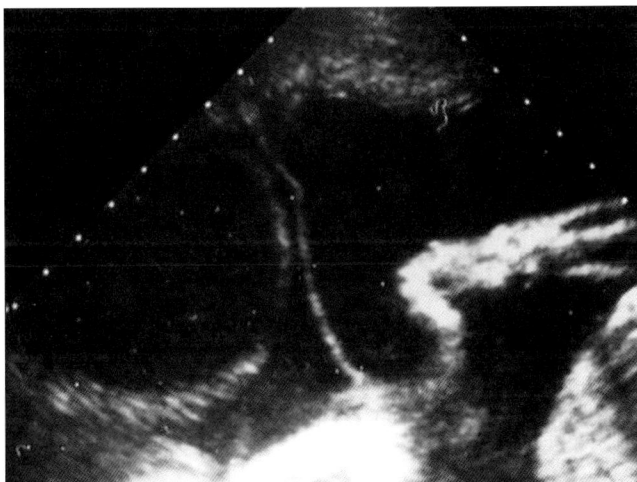

Fig. 64.8: Biamniotic twin pregnancy with two discernable amniotic membranes surrounding the embryo

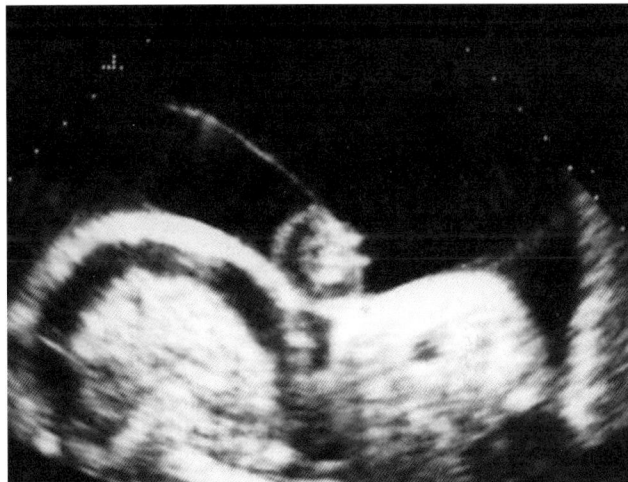

Fig. 64.9: Biamniotic twin pregnancies with the partition membrane between the fetuses. A twin–twin transfusion syndrome is indicated by severe ascites in the left twin

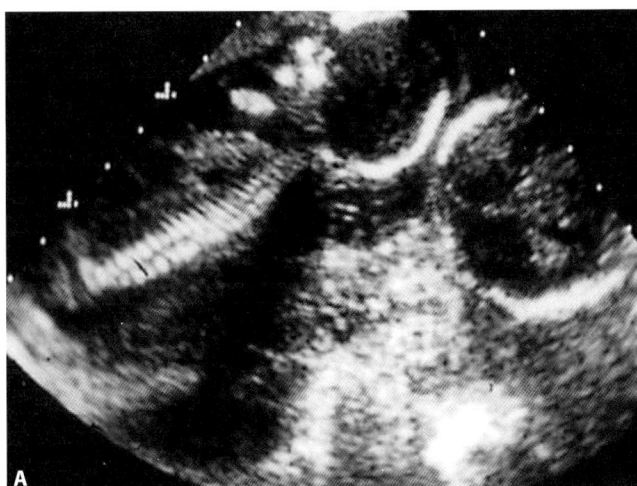

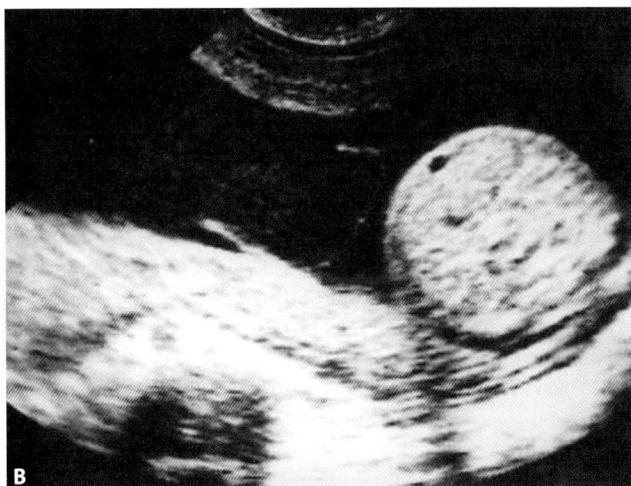

Figs 64.10A and B: Biamniotic twin pregnancies. (A) The separating membrane can hardly be seen on top of the head of the left, smaller fetus. (B) Polyhydramnios is visible in the left, oligohydramnios in the right sac

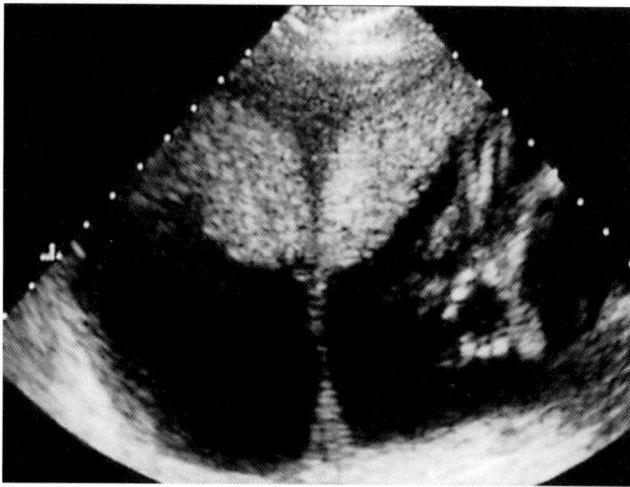

Fig. 64.11: "Twin peak" sign in dichorionic twin pregnancy

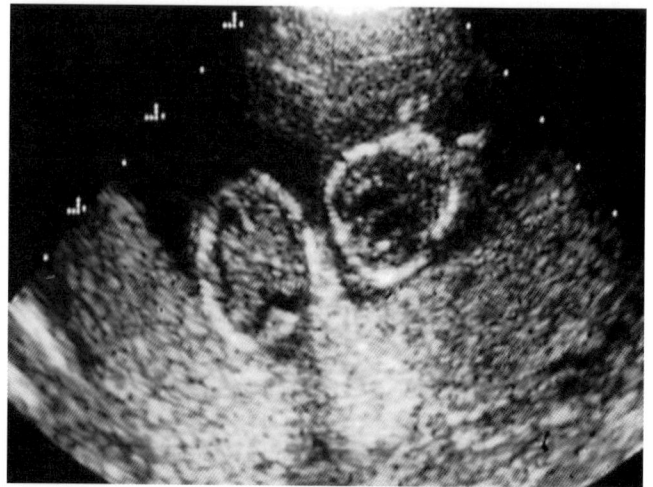

Fig. 64.12: Dichorionic twin pregnancies. Although the two placentae are in close proximity to one another, they are separated

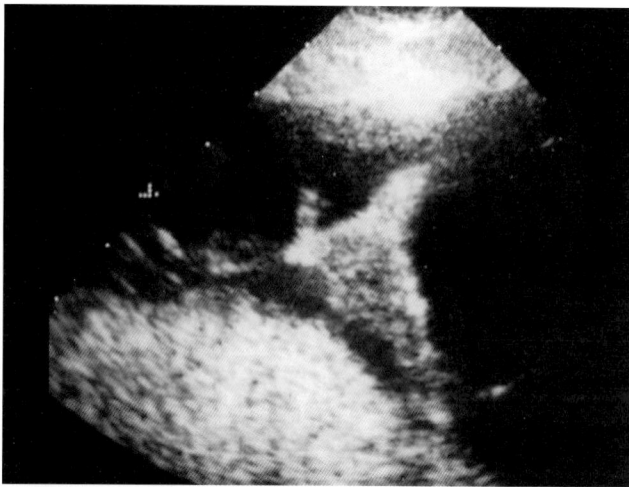

Fig. 64.13: Dichorionic twin pregnancies. The thickness of the dividing membrane is more than 2 mm

FETAL MALFORMATIONS AND CHROMOSOMAL ANOMALIES IN MULTIPLE PREGNANCY

Twins, above all monozygotic twins, are known to be at increased risk for malformations—not only because the presence of two fetuses in one pregnancy doubles the chance of a defect.[19] The incidence of malformations is higher in monochorionic than in dichorionic twins and the highest in monoamniotic twins. Furthermore, the incidence of chromosomal aneuploidy seems to be higher in twin gestations as compared to singletons.[22-24] A detail study of fetal morphology in multiple pregnancy by ultrasound is time consuming and sometimes much more difficult than in singletons, but it should be done during routine ultrasound surveillance. Emphasis should be put not only on typical anomalies unique to the twinning process, but also on other anomalies known to be increased in twin pregnancies.

Congenital anomalies specific to multiple gestation occur infrequently but are usually severe. The rate of conjoined twins (Fig. 64.14) is 1 in 50,000 birth.[25] Prenatal diagnosis by ultrasonography including determination of type of anomaly and of shared organs (Fig. 64.15) is important for the optimal management of those pregnancies in terms of appropriate determination of prognosis and plan of delivery route (cesarean section) and postnatal care. In severe cases diagnosed early, termination of pregnancy is an option which many parents choose. Ultrasonographic criteria for the detection of conjoined twins have been proposed: a missing seperating membrane, a fixed position of the twins toward each other and a lack of separate visualization of the fetuses in a specific anatomical region. Different patterns of physical joining exist, resulting in different prognosis of the pregnancies. The symmetric complete form of conjoined twinning is present when two fetuses are anatomically almost "complete" except the part of the body where they share a certain amount of tissue. These "diplopagi" are described after the body structure which is joined, namely craniopagi, thoracopagi (accounting for 57% of diplopagi), (Fig. 64.16) omphalopagi and pygopagi. Postnatal seperation is often possible in diplopagi except in cases where gross parts of the heart or central nervous system are shared. The symmetric incomplete forms are represented by twins with one trunk and a single lower part of the body together with two heads (dicephalus), or by twins with one head and upper trunk and a double lower body (dipygus). Asymmetric forms are conjoined twins one of which is severely malformed and often rudimentary (parasitic twin) while the other is normally developed.

An extreme form of twin-specific asymmetric malformation is acranius-acardius, also known as chorangiopagus parasiticus, or TRAP-sequence (twin reversed arterial perfusion sequence). Numerous theories about pathogenesis of this syndrome, which occurs in a frequency of 1 in 35,000 birth, have been subject of discussion in the literature. Typical features are functional vascular anastomoses between not-joined twins with reverse arterial perfusion of the lower part of the malformed twin leading to varying degrees of upper body reduction including acardia and acranius.[26] Doppler sonography may be helpful in identifiing cardiac structures, reversed perfusion and vascular anastomoses.[27] A different theory of pathogenesis is the primary existence of acranius- acardius malformation, which is supported by the fact that the malformed twin has been found to have a high prevalence of chromosomal anomalies. Mortality in the reversely perfused twin

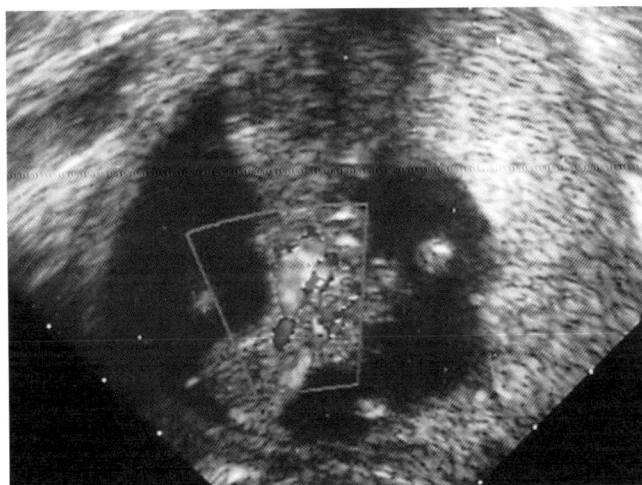

Fig. 64.14: Sonogram of conjoined twins with two separate hearts

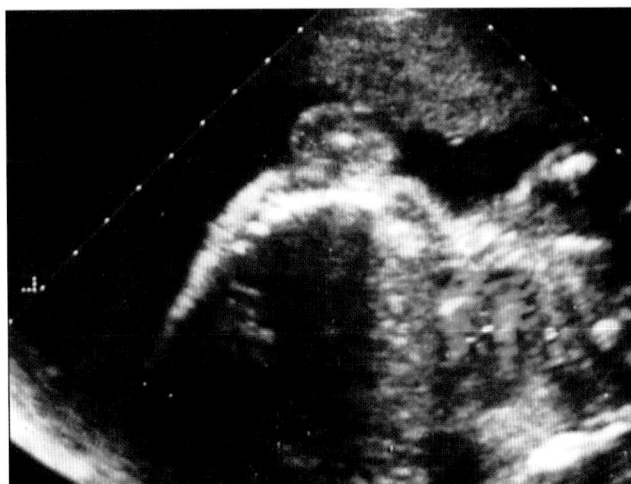

Fig. 64.15: Sonogram of conjoined twins with one heart

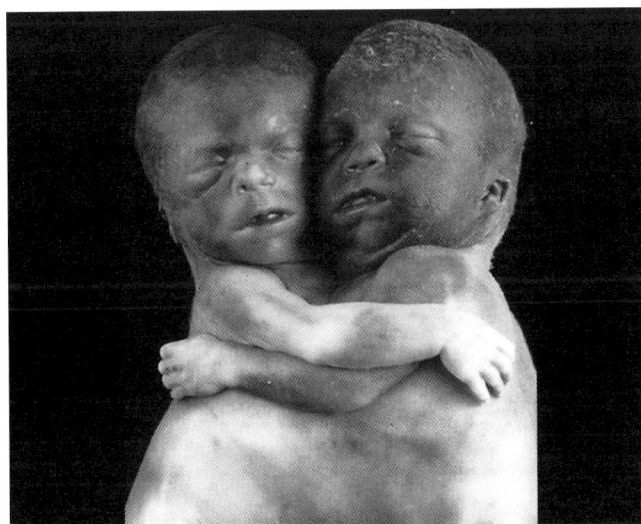

Fig. 64.16: Almost completely conjoined twins. Thoracopagus anomaly

is 100%. The other fetus, the so-called "pump-twin", is usually severely compromised by a high-output heart failure which leads to a mortality of 50%. An intervention might be necessary and indicated, which includes ligation/coagulation of the cord or of intra-abdominal blood vessels of the acranius-acardius twin.

Congenital anomalies not specifically related to multiple gestation have the same ultrasonographic features like in singleton pregnancies. These malformations affect mainly the tracheoesophageal anatomy, the genitourinary and central nervous system (neural tube defects), and the cardiovascular system.

Chromosomal anomalies are also increased in multiple gestations. The risk of chromosomal anomalies in a twin pregnancy can be calculated using maternal age, zygosity and nuchal translucency of the twin fetuses. In dichorionic twins, the detection rate of nuchal translucency measurements for chromosomal anomalies is similar as in singletons, whereas in monochorionic twins there are more false positives due to placentation-specific alterations of the nuchal translucency. In particular, care must be taken if a large difference in nuchal translucency is found in

monochorionic twins because this could be an early manifestation of TTS and not of a karyotype anomaly. In monozygous twins, the karyotype is the same in both twins, and calculations are used for both. In dizygous twins, the risk must be calculated separately for each of the twins. Biochemical parameters such as free β-hCG and PAPP-A (in the first trimester) or α-fetoprotein, free β-hCG, estriol and inhibin (in the second trimester) can be used but are less useful yielding a lower detection rate of chromosomal anomalies in twins.[24] Simple use of normative values from singleton pregnancies is not possible as medians are different. Current studies are evaluating the validity of twin pregnancy-adjusted normative values.

If the parents wish prenatal karyotyping, both chorionic villus sampling (CVS) or amniocentesis can be performed as possible options.[28-32] The parents though must be informed in detail about the difficulties and risks of karyotyping in multiple pregnancies. The procedure might be technically difficult, leading to incomplete results (i.e. karyotyping of only one fetus in twins). On the other hand, difficulties might arise if one fetus turns out to be healthy while the other is affected by a severe chromosomal anomaly. In multiple gestations, CVS imposes specific problems due to a missing safeguard in proving that identical karyotypes represent monozygotic twins rather than sampling from the same chorion frondosum. In multichorionic gestations, the placentas might be close to each other, leading to difficulties in separate sampling (Fig. 64.17). Furthermore, contamination of one sample with the villi of the other might happen. If fetal sex is different, it could be safely determined that both fetuses have been karyotyped. When suspicion arises, "follow-up" amniocentesis should be offered. Consequently, CVS in twins should only be performed if individual samples can be guaranteed. Amniocentesis is the alternative procedure, often preferred in multiple gestation. After the puncture and retrieval of amniotic fluid of one amniotic sac, indigo carmine is injected before the needle is retracted. In the following puncture of the second amniotic cavity, the aspirated amniotic fluid is checked in color to exclude reentry of the amniotic cavity of the same fetus. With this technique, amniocentesis in twins with a correct diagnosis of fetal karyotypes is feasible in most twin pregnancies[33] and has a somewhat lower loss rate as CVS. As a rule, the higher the risk for chromosomal anomaly in a twin, the earlier the diagnosis should be made, ideally by CVS. The reason for this is that if one twin is

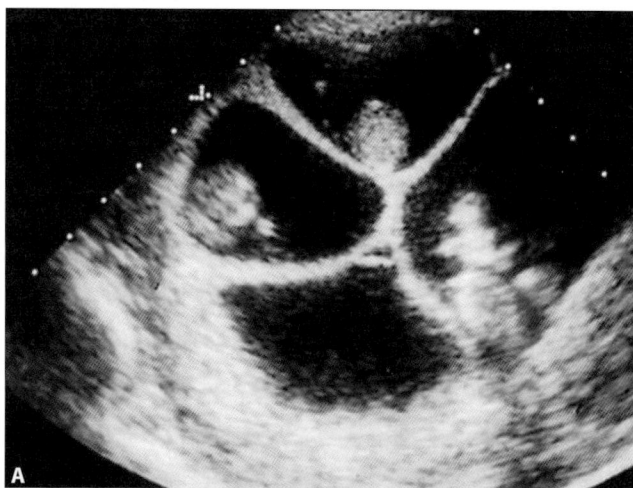

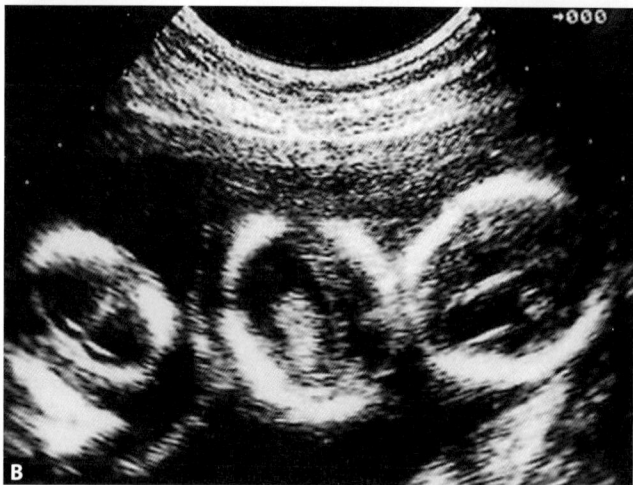

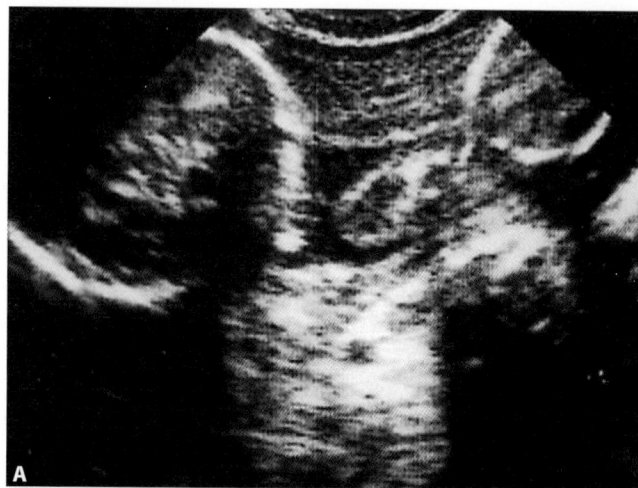

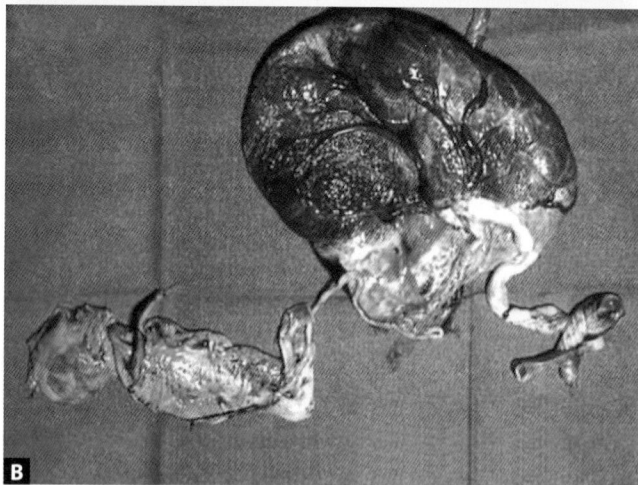

Figs 64.17A and B: High multiple pregnancies. (A) Quadruplet pregnancy in the first trimester. The placentae are so close to each other that they cannot be easily sampled separately. (B) Triplet pregnancy in the third trimester. The separating membranes are more difficult to be seen than in the first trimester

Figs 64.18A and B: Situation after selective feticide. (A) Sonogram shows the small dead fetus in the upper right corner of the picture. (B) After delivery the "fetus papyraceus" and the "dead part" of the placenta can easily be seen

affected and the parents opt for selective termination, the risk of the latter procedure for the surviving twin is lower the earlier the selective fetocide of the co-twin is performed.

If in a multiple pregnancy, one child is proven by prenatal diagnosis to be affected with an untreatable condition, e.g. trisomy 18 or 13 or a severe malformation, a selective fetocide can be performed by applying KCL directly to the fetal heart.[34] This technique, however, may exclusively be used if monochorionic placentation is excluded. The selective fetocide is ethically not much different from and termination of a whole pregnancy in singletons, except for the fact that the pregnancy per se continues and the dead fetus usually follows after the livebirth of the co-twin together with the placenta (Figs 64.18A and B).[35]

In pregnancies with very high multiples, e.g. octuplet pregnancies (Figs 64.19A and B), these would be bound to fail (Figs 64.20A and B), so that a "reduction" of the number of living twins has been performed in order to avoid loss of the whole pregnancy spontaneously or through termination. This procedure is called multifetal pregnancy reduction and is performed by intra-cardiac injection of KCL in "multichorionic" multiples; again, monochorionicity must be excluded. The outcome of the pregnancy

after this procedure depends significantly on the starting number of fetuses, the finishing number and the operators experience.[36] The primary aim, however, must be to avoid iatrogenic higher order multiple pregnancy, e.g. by controlled use of ovulation inducing drugs or by restriction of the number of transferred embryos to two during IVF procedure.

FETAL GROWTH IN MULTIPLE PREGNANCY

As in all pregnancies, appropriate dating of pregnancy is important in terms of determination of fetal growth to differentiate growth restriction from normal growth. Dating is best done in the first or early second trimester by combining the date of the last menstrual period with fetal ultrasound measurements.

We mentioned before that in twin pregnancies, growth charts of singletons can be used at least up to the beginning of the third trimester, because normal growth in twins is the same as in singletons. Only after 28–30 weeks of pregnancy, intrauterine growth gradually decreases compared to singletons.[4,37] It has been estimated that after 32 weeks of pregnancy, weight gain of both fetuses in twin pregnancy equals the weight gain of one singleton.

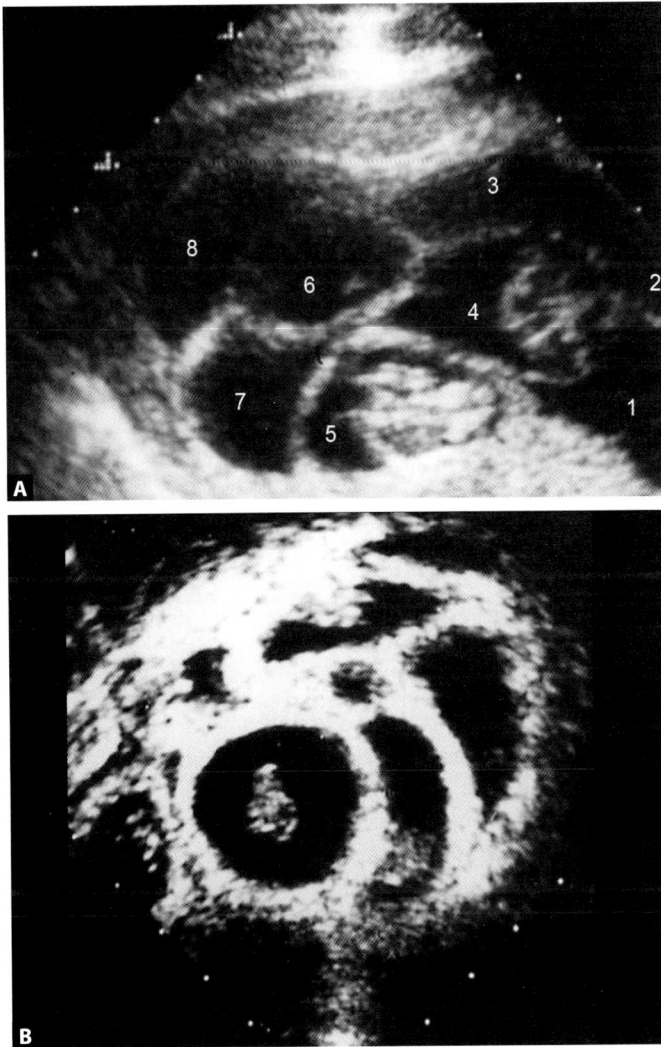

Figs 64.19A and B: Two independent octuplet pregnancies which both occurred after ovulation induction by gynecologic practitioners

Figs 64.20A and B: Complication of high multiple pregnancies. (A) Triplet pregnancy at 26 weeks of gestation. (B) Placenta of sextuplet pregnancy after spontaneous abortion

Assessment of fetal growth in twin pregnancies has been performed initially by measurements of biparietal diameter,[38] though it has been shown later, that biparietal diameter is not an appropriate measurement for detection of discordance in twins.[39] Possible explanations for these difficulties might be different fetal positions and overlaying fetal parts of the other twin. Better estimates of fetal growth and prediction of discordance are accomplished by femur length and abdominal circumference[40-43] where technical difficulties in measuring seem to be of minor importance.

If discordant growth in twin pregnancy (defined by an estimated weight difference of 20–25% between the fetuses) is diagnosed by prenatal ultrasound, several possibilities exist. The most common cause for the weight discordance is a constitutional weight difference in normal dizygotic twins. In contrast, pathologic causes might result in often severe growth difference between twins. The prevalence of intrauterine growth restriction is up to 10 times higher in twins than in singletons, in particular in monochorionic twins. Pathologic conditions include intrauterine growth retardation

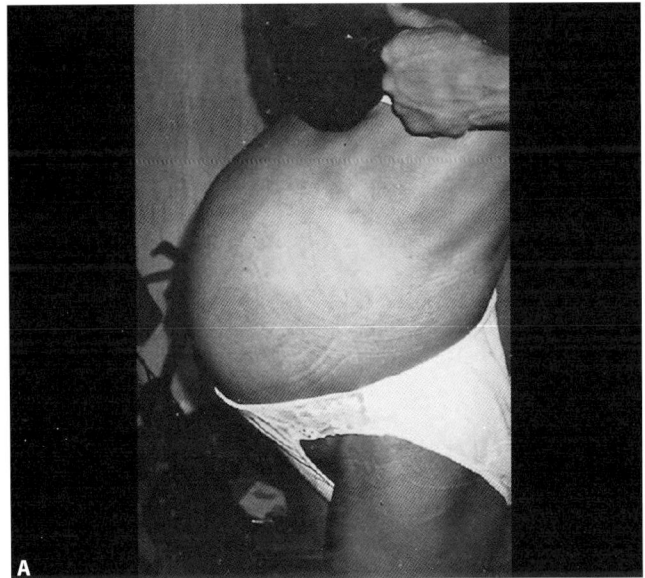

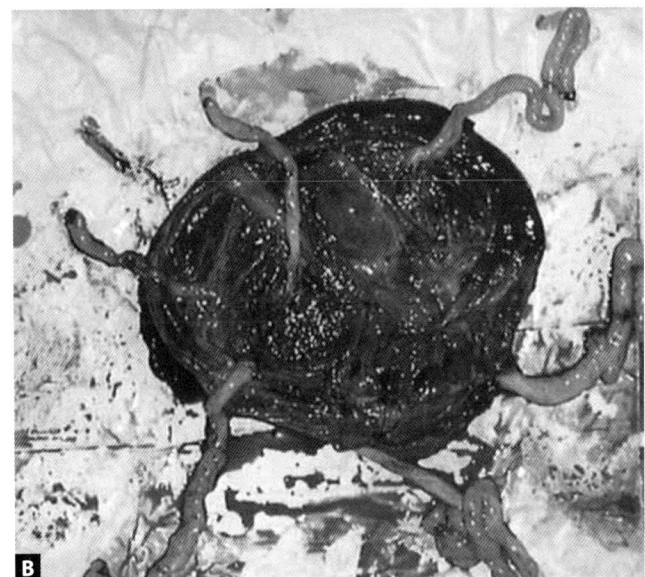

affecting one or both twins, because of local uteroplacental factors (which might happen in dichorionic or monochorionic pregnancies), or twin-twin transfusion syndrome (Figs 64.21A and B). In some cases, congenital anomaly of only one fetus might also lead to discordant growth. An important question in discordant twins is chorionicity and amniotic fluid amount. Overall, perinatal morbidity and mortality besides later intellectual sequelae are increased in twin pregnancies irrespective of the underlying cause.[44]

Doppler velocimetry has proved to be predictive of fetal hypoxia in growth-retarded singletons.[45] Similarly, this technique might be used in twins as additional measure for detection of growth discordance and fetal compromise.[46,47] Furthermore, with color Doppler placental anastomoses in twin-twin transfusin syndrome can be detected, which might be helpful for intrauterine treatment by fetoscopic laser-ablation of placental vessels (see below).[48]

As in singletons, an individual biophysical profile including nonstress testing should be applied in both twins in growth restricted twin pregnancies as an important tool for assessment of fetal well-being.[40]

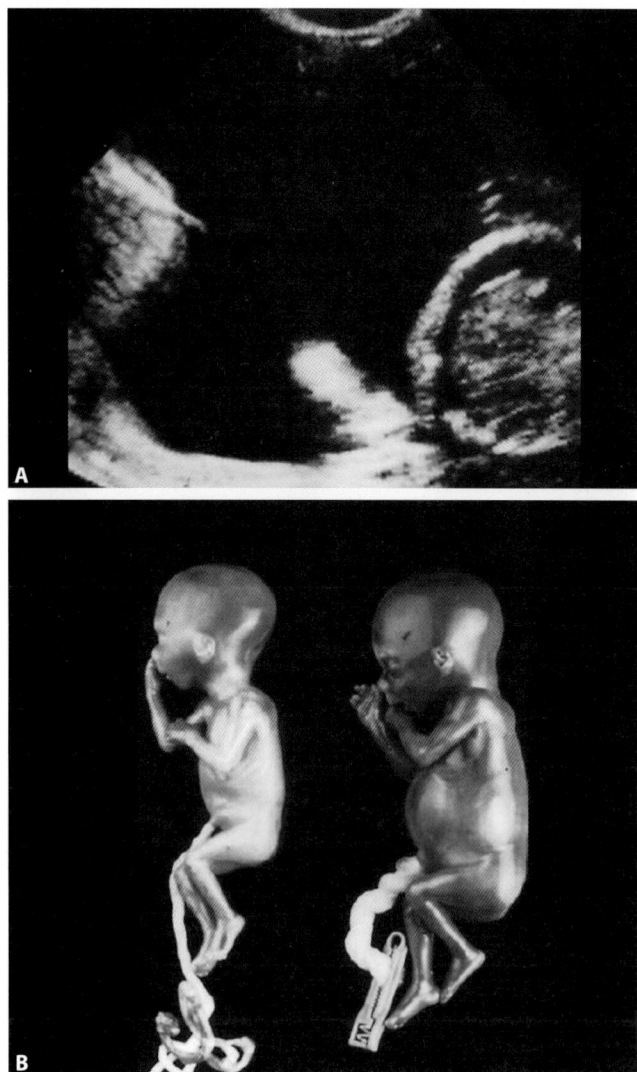

Figs 64.21A and B: Twin–twin transfusion syndrome. (A) Sonogram showing severe polyhydramnios and non-immune hydrops in the pumping twin. (B) Fetus after spontaneous abortion. The right one is plethoric, whereas the left one is anemic and smaller

TWIN-TWIN TRANSFUSION SYNDROME

Twin-twin transfusion syndrome (TTS) is a condition which develops in about 10–25% of monochorionic twin pregnancies. The underlying cause for this syndrome is imbalance of vascular anastomoses between the placental circulation of both twins within the single (monochorionic) placenta. This imbalance leads to decreased fetopacental blood volume in the donor and increased volume in the recipient. The definition of TTS includes polyhydramnios-oligohydramnios sequence. Typical sonographic features include in the donor fetus oligohydramnios or anhydramnios ("stuck twin" phenomenon), small or absent bladder and growth restriction, whereas the recipient shows polyhydramnios and a large bladder. In both twins, the condition can lead to cardiac decompensation, detectable by ultrasound (including tricuspid regurgitation and negative ductus venosus A-wave in the recipient, pericardial effusion, hydrops). Doppler flow measurements in umbilical arteries can be pathologic in both twins (absent or reversed end-diastolic flow). Ultimately, fetal death in one or both twins can occur. Severe TTS has a 90% mortality and a high rate of neurologic long-term morbidity (handicap) in survivors if untreated.

The severity of TTS can be assessed by ultrasound, which correlates with the prognosis. Several criteria for classification have been proposed; the Quintero staging system being the most widely used.

Management options depend on severity of TTS, gestational age and women's preference and include expectant management with close follow-up (in mild TTS), repetitive amniodrainage, needle septostomy or endoscopic laser coagulation of anastomoses. Cohort studies and a recent multicenter randomized trial suggest that laser treatment in severe TTS is superior to repetitive amniodrainage regarding neonatal mortality as well as morbidity. With regard to the current evidence, laser treatment seems to be the treatment of choice in severe TTS, but long-term neurologic outcome results of the randomized trial must yet be awaited.

ULTRASONOGRAPHY FOR PREDICTION OF PRETERM DELIVERIES IN MULTIPLE PREGNANCY

Twin gestations are known to have a significantly increased risk of preterm delivery as compared to singletons. Early diagnosis of preterm contractions and individual preterm delivery risk assessment is therefore particularily important. Cervical ultrasound has recently been shown to be predictive of preterm delivery. Initial studies measuring cervical length by transabdominal ultrasonography found a significant correlation of a shortened cervix with preterm delivery. As shown by different examiners, transabdominal measurement of cervical length has the disadvantage of being biased by the degree of bladder filling, which led to the increased use of transvaginal ultrasound probes in pregnancy. Beside the cervical length, dilatation of the internal cervical os, protrusion of membranes in the cervical canal, length of funneling and thickness of the wall of the lower uterine segment have been used more or less seccessfully to diagnose cervical incompetence and to predict preterm birth. Ultrasonographic determination of cervical morphology has been shown to be superior to digital examination of the cervix for the prediction of preterm birth if there is no overt cervical dilatation of 2 cm or more. While some studies have used transvaginal ultrasound for the prediction of the likelihood of preterm delivery in patients with preterm labor, a recent multicenter study proved a correlation of cervical length measured in the second trimester in asymptomatic patients with the risk of preterm delivery. A major finding in this study was that cervical length did seem to be a continuous variable rather than a dichotomous variable, suggesting that cervical function might be a continuum, in contrast to the earlier belief that the cervix is either "competent" or "incompetent". Other studies have shown that ultrasonography of the cervix might be used as well in the follow-up after cervical cerclage, measuring the distance between the cerclage suture and the internal cervical os.

Though some of these studies have excluded multiple pregnancies, others have specifically determined the predictive value in twin pregnancies. One may conclude that ultrasonographic determination of the cervix and the lower part of the uterus is an important additional tool in predicting preterm delivery in multiple gestation, where the risk of prematurity is especially high.

INTRAPARTUM ULTRASONOGRAPHY IN MULTIPLE GESTATION

There is considerable controversy in the literature around intrapartum management of multiple gestation. Multiple pregnancies of higher order are usually delivered by cesarean section. In twins, the single most important question is the route of delivery in different subsets of twins and, additionally, in different clinical situations like prematurity, growth retardation or preeclampsia. Above all, the management plan for delivery has to take presentation of the twins into consideration, which include all possible combinations of vertex, breech, transverse and oblique presentation of the first and second twin. Ultrasonography can be reliably used for detection of these different presentations before onset of labor, during labor, after delivery of the first twin or after interventions like external or internal version of the second twin. Again, ultrasound examination is a most important tool in the peripartum management of twin pregnancies.[49]

CONCLUSION

The aim of this chapter was to discuss the most important clinical applications of ultrasonography in multiple gestation. Beginning with early gestation, diagnosis of multiplicity, zygosity, chorionicity and amnionicity are predominant tasks for determination of the risk of complications later in pregnancy. Typical complications of monochorionic twins with vascular anastomoses are being explained. Fetal congenital anomalies in multiple gestation are different in many ways from singletons and represent another problem of primary importance in the routine medical care. Multiple gestation-specific anomalies like conjoining can be discerned from nonspecific congenital malformations which exist as well in singletons. Invasive procedures for prenatal chromosomal analysis are briefly discussed, being more difficult than in singletons as one has to deal with more than one maternal and one fetal karyotype.

Discordant fetal growth is a major complication in multiple gestation. The diagnosis is usually confirmed by ultrasonography; at the same time the underlying pathology like growth restriction based on fetal malformation of one twin or twin-twin transfusion syndrome might be evaluated. Cervical change assessed by vaginal ultrasonography has been shown to be predictive of spontaneous preterm delivery in singletons; similarly this might be applicable in multiple gestation. Finally, peripartum ultrasonography for the detection of presentation is crucial in planning delivery and possible intrapartum intervention in twins.

REFERENCES

1. Grennert L, Persson PH, Gennser G, et al. Ultrasound and human-placental-lactogen screening for early detection of twin pregnancies. Lancet. 1976;1(7949):4-6.
2. Wenstrom KD, Gall SA. Incidence, morbidity and diagnosis of twin gestations. Clin Perinatol. 1988;15:1.
3. Daya S. Accuracy of gestational age estimation using fetal crown-rump length measurements. Am J Obstet Gynecol. 1993;168:903.
4. Reece AE, Yarkoni S, Abdalla M, et al. A prospective longitudinal study of growth in twin gestations compared with growth in singleton pregnancies. I. The fetal head. II. The fetal limbs. J Ultrasound Med. 1991;10:439-45.
5. Holzgreve W, Westendorp J, Tercanli S. First trimester ultrasound. In: Evans MI (Ed). Reproductive Risks and Prenatal Diagnosis. Norwalk, USA: Appleton and Lange; 1992. pp. 121-50.
6. Sampson A, de Crespigny LC. Vanishing twins: the frequency of spontaneous fetal reduction of a twin pregnancy. Ultrasound Obstet Gynecol. 1992;2(2):107-9.
7. Newton R, Casabonne D, Johnson A, et al. A case-control study of vanishing twin as a risk factor for cerebral palsy. Twin Res. 2003;6(2):83-4.
8. Benirschke K, Chung KK. Multiple pregnancy. N Engl J Med. 1973;288:1276-329.
9. Souter VL, Kapur RP, Nyholt DR, et al. A report of dizygous monochorionic twins. N Engl J Med. 2003;349(2):154-8.
10. Robertson EG, Neer KJ. Placental injection studies in twin gestation. Am J Obstet Gynecol. 1983;147:170.
11. Blickstein I. The twin-twin transfusion syndrome. Obstet Gynecol. 1990;76:714.
12. Pharoah PO, Adi Y. Consequences of in-utero death in a twin pregnancy. Lancet. 2000;355(9215):1597-602.
13. Fusi L, McParland P, Fisk N, et al. Acute twin-twin transfusion: a possible mechanism for brain damages survivors after intrauterine death of a monochorionic twin. Obstet Gynecol. 1991;78:517.
14. Finberg HJ. The twin peak sign: reliable evidence of dichorionic twinning. J Ultrasound Med. 1992;11:571.
15. Nyberg DA. Entangled umbilical cords: A sign of monoamniotic twins. J Ultrasound Med. 1984;3:29.
16. Townsend RR, Simpson GF, Filly RA. Membrane thickness in ultrasound prediction of chorionicity of twin gestations. J Ultrasound Med. 1988;7:326.
17. D'Alton ME, Dudley DK. The ultrasonographic prediction of chorionicity in twin gestation. Am J Obstet Gynecol. 1989;160:557.
18. Scardo JA, Ellings JM, Newman RB. Prospective determination of chorionicity, amnionicity and zygosity in twin gestations. Am J Obstet Gynecol. 1995;173:1376.
19. Bryan E, Little J, Burn J. Congenital anomalies in twins. Baillières Clin Obstet Gynecol. 1987;1:697.
20. Lubs HA, Ruddle F. Chromosomal abnormalities in the human population: estimation of rates based on New Haven newborn study. Science. 1970;169:495.
21. Hanson JW. Incidence of conjoined twinning. Lancet. 1975;2(7947):1257.
22. Ash K, Harman CR, Gritter H. TRAP sequence successful outcome with indomethacin treatment. Obstet Gynecol. 1990;76:960.
23. Pretorius DH, Leopold GR, Moore TR, et al. Acardiac twin. Report of Doppler sonography. J Ultrasound Med. 1988;7:413.
24. Spencer K, Nicolaides KH. Screening for trisomy 21 in twins using first trimester ultrasound and maternal serum biochemistry in a one-stop clinic: a review of three years experience. BJOG. 2003;110(3):276-80.
25. Jackson LG, Wapner RJ, Barr MA. Safety of chorionic villus biopsy. Lancet. 1986;1(8462):874-5.
26. Librach CL. Genetic amniocentesis in seventy twin pregnancies. Am J Obstet Gynecol. 1984;148:585.

27. Wapner RJ, Johnson A, Davis G, et al. Prenatal diagnosis in twin gestations: A comparison between second-trimester amniocentesis and first-trimester chorion villous sampling. Obstet Gynecol. 1993;82:49-56.

28. Pruggmayer MR, Jahoda MG, Van der Pol JG, et al. Genetic amniocentesis in twin pregnancies: results of a multicenter study of 529 cases. Ultrasound Obstet Gynecol. 1992;2:6-10.

29. Westendorp A, Holzgreve W, Miny P. Selective fetocide of a twin with trisomy 18 by intracardial KCL application. Arch Gynecol. 1988;244:59-62.

30. Evans MI, Goldberg JD, Dumez Y, et al. Efficacy of second trimester selective termination (ST) for fetal abnormalities: International collaborative experience among the world's largest centers. Am J Obstet Gynecol. 1993;168:307.

31. Evans MI, Berkowitz RL, Wapner RJ, et al. Improvement in outcomes of multifetal pregnancy reduction with increased experience. Am J Obstet Gynecol. 2001;184(2):97-103.

32. McKeown T, Record RG. Observations on fetal growth in multiple pregnancy in man. J Endocrinol. 1952;8:386.

33. Grennert L, Persson PH, Genser G. Intrauterine growth of twins judged by BPD measurements. Acta Obstet Gynecol Scand. 1978;78:28.

34. Erkkola R, Ala-Mello S, Piiroinen O. Growth discordancy in twin pregnancies. A risk factor not detected by measurements of biparietal diameter. Obstet Gynecol. 1985;66:203.

35. Brown CE, Guzick DS, Leveno KJ. Prediction of discordant twins using ultrasound measurement of biparietal diameter and abdominal perimeter. Obstet Gynecol. 1987;70:677.

36. Babson SG, Philips DS. Growth and development of twins dissimilar in size at birth. N Engl J Med. 1973;289:937.

37. Soothill PW. Relation of fetal hypoxia in growth retardation to mean blood velocity in the fetal aorta. Lancet. 1986;2(8516):1118-20.

38. Giles WB. Doppler assessment in multiple pregnancy. Semin Perinatol. 1987;11:369.

39. DeLia JE, Cruikshank DP, Keye WR. Fetoscopic neodymium:YAG laser occlusion of placental vessels in severe twin-twin transfusion syndrome. Obstet Gynecol. 1990;75:1046.

40. Lodeiro JG, Vintzileos AM, Feinstein SJ. Fetal biophysical profile in twin gestations. Obstet Gynecol. 1986;67:824.

41. Quintero RA, Morales WJ, Allen MH, et al. Staging of twin-twin transfusion syndrome. J Perinatol. 1999;19:550-5.

42. Hecher K, Plath H, Bregenzer T, et al. Endoscopic laser surgery versus serial amniocenteses in the treatment of severe twin-twin transfusion syndrome. Am J Obstet Gynecol. 1999; 180:717-24

43. Senat MV, Deprest J, Boulvain M, et al. Endoscopic laser surgery versus serial amnioreduction for severe twin-to-twin transfusion syndrome. N Engl J Med. 2004;351(2):136-44.

44. Anderson HF, Nugent CE, Wanty SD, et al. Prediction of risk of preterm delivery by ultrasonographic measurement of cervical length. Am J Obstet Gynecol. 1990;163:859.

45. Iams JD, Goldenberg RL, Meis PJ, et al. The length of the cervix and the risk of spontaneous premature delivery. N Engl J Med. 1996;334:567.

46. Guzman ER, Houlihan C, Vintzileos A, et al. The significance of transvaginal ultrasonographic evaluation of the cervix in women treated with emergency cerclage. Am J Obstet Gynecol. 1996;175:471.

47. Vayssiere C, Favre R, Audibert F, et al. Cervical length and funneling at 22 and 27 weeks to predict spontaneous birth before 32 weeks in twin pregnancies: a French prospective multicenter study. Am J Obstet Gynecol. 2002;187(6):1596-604.

48. Cetrulo C. The controversy of mode of delivery in twins: the intrapartum management of twin gestation. Semin Perinatol. 1986;23:533.

49. Chervenak FA. Intrapartum management of twin gestation. Obstet Gynecol. 1985;65:119.

Chromosomal Abnormality Screening

MI Evans, JN Macri, R Snijders

PRINCIPLES OF SCREENING TESTS

Screening for any disease process requires a fundamental understanding of the differences between diagnostic and screening tests. Diagnostic tests are meant to give a definitive answer to the question—does the patient have this particular problem? They are often complex and require sophisticated analysis and interpretation. They are usually performed only on patients felt to be "at risk". Because, they tend to be expensive, in contrast, screening tests are typically performed on healthy patients and are often offered to the entire relevant population. They, therefore, need to be cheap, easy to use and interpretable by everyone; their function is only to help define who, among the low risk group is, in fact, at high risk (Table 65.1) Screening test results are, by definition, not pathognomonic for the disease.[1] Their role is to delineate who needs further testing.

There are four key measures used in the evaluation of screening tests (sensitivity, specificity, positive predictive value and negative predictive value) (Fig. 65.1). Sensitivity and specificity fundamentally address the question from an epidemiologic viewpoint. For example, of all the people with the disease, what percentage were identified by the test? This is the definition of sensitivity. Specificity is the converse, i.e. of all the people who do not have the disease process, what percentage of the patients test negative. Physicians are generally more interested in different questions, however, because only after a positive test does the patient usually get interested. Of all patients, who have a positive test, what percentage of them actually have the disease? This is the positive predictive value. The negative predictive value is just the opposite, i.e. of all the people who have a negative test, what percentage of them are actually negative?

A key point to remember is that, in general, sensitivity and specificity do not vary as a function of prevalence, unless there is an influence of other factors on the equation. However, positive and negative predictive values do vary (Figs 65.2 and 65.3). In a population in which the prevalence is very low, the proportion of positives that will be false positive will be much higher than in a population in which the prevalence is very high. In the former case, the vast majority of positives will, in fact, be false positives. In both high and low prevalence areas, the sensitivity and specificity of the tests should be the same. However, the positive and negative predictive values will be widely different. If a test is absolutely

Sensitivity—A/A+C
Specificity—D/B+D

Positive predictive value—A/A+B
Negative predictive value—D/C+D

Fig. 65.1: 2 × 2 table of disease and tests

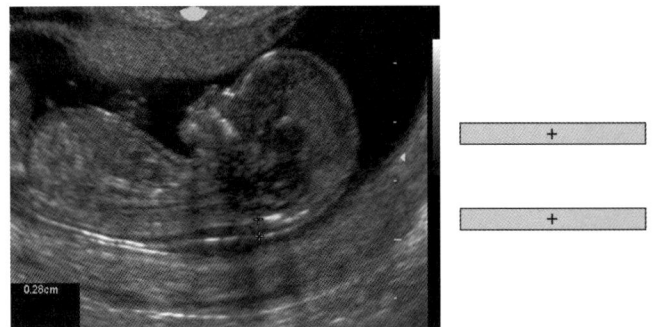

Fig. 65.2: Ultrasound measurement of the fetal neck at 12 week

Sensitivity—180/200 = 90%
Specificity—780/800 = 98%
Positive Predictive Value—180/200 = 90%
Negative Predictive Value—780/800 = 98%

Fig. 65.3: 2 × 2 table in high risk population for sensitivity and predictive values

Table 65.1: Screening tests vs. diagnostic tests

Diagnostic Tests
  Performed only on "at risk" population
  Commonly expensive
  Commonly have risk
  Give definitive answer
Screening Tests
  Offered to general population of patients
  Healthy patients
  Cheap
  Easy
  Reliable
  Quick
  Define "at risk" population
  Do not give definitive answer

useless (no better than chance) then the predictive value after testing will be the same as the population risk (prevalence) before testing. When this occurs, the test performs no better than a coin flip, and the sensitivity and specificity add to 100%.

The past few years have seen continued advancement in attempts to refine the sensitivity and specificity of chromosomal screening, and to reduce the overall costs of the screening programs per se.[2,3] The goal is to reduce the need for expensive costs of invasive testing that follow a positive screening, and also, although not commonly mentioned, to reduce the cost of the care of abnormal newborns who might as a result of screening be detected and terminated at the wishes of the parents.[1-5]

SCREENING FOR CHROMOSOMAL ABNORMALITIES

Merkatz et al. first published the association of low maternal serum alpha-fetoprotein with an increased risk of chromosomal abnormalities, particularly Down syndrome in 1984.[6] Subsequently, there was a gradual acceptance of the association, as well as an eventual understanding that Down syndrome is not the only aneuploid condition associated with low maternal serum alpha-fetoprotein. For example, Trisomy 18, usually, has even lower alpha-fetoprotein values.[7]

The adoption of wide scale screening with maternal serum alpha-fetoprotein effectively doubled the potential detection of chromosome abnormalities in the population. Before the massive explosion of infertility therapies, only about 20% of Down syndrome babies were born to women over age 35 (Fig. 65.4). More recent data suggest that the proportion of births to women over 35 has gone from about 5% to nearly 15%, and the proportion of Down syndrome cases in women over 35 is now more than 30%.[8] The addition of a well-coordinated maternal serum alpha-fetoprotein screening program as developed in the late 1980s could detect approximately 30% of the 75% of cases that are born to women under age 35. The detailed mechanics of biochemical screening, i.e. with adjustments for gestational age, race, diabetic status, multiple gestation status, maternal weight, and adjustments via a different database or correction factors for maternal race, have been published previously and will not be repeated here.[9]

In 1988, Wald et al. suggested that a combination of parameters including alpha-fetoprotein (AFP), beta-human chorionic gonadotropin (β-hCG) and unconjugated estriol (uE3) could significantly increase the detection frequency of Down syndrome

HIV testing in high risk big city STD clinic

Sensitivity—180/200 = 90%
Specificity—780/800 = 98%
Positive Predictive Value—180/200 = 90%
Negative Predictive Value—780/800 = 98%

Fig. 65.4: 2 × 2 table in low risk population for sensitivity and predictive values

to approximately 60% of the total.[10] Multiple studies have corroborated the increased efficacy of multiple marker screening as opposed to AFP alone in detecting chromosomal abnormalities, particularly Down syndrome.[11-14]

Despite overwhelming data and recommendations of national organizations such as the American College of Obstetricians and Gynecologists that multiple numbers be offered, by the millennium still nearly 20% of patients in the United States who had screening were still just having AFP alone.[15]

Evans, et al. have investigated many of the "dogmas" of three decades of biochemical screening and found that many of these are no longer valid. We believe that the wide variance in results reported from around the world is largely due to subtle and sometimes not so subtle differences in laboratory methodologies.[16-20] For example, the bitter arguments about double versus triple screening are in part explained by wide differences in assays among laboratories that particularly affect estriol. When the methods are "standardized", much of the variability disappears and will allow for an "apples vs. apples" as opposed to "apples vs. oranges" comparison.[20] Similarly, much of the other reported variations in the literature likewise disappear with standardization, and the diabetic correction factor becomes unnecessary with proper accounting for the fact that diabetic patients are of higher maternal weight,[16] and maternal weight correction, per se, continues to be important.[17,18]

Over the past several years, there have been numerous papers that have attempted to refine methodologies of sample collection[21,22] and more precisely explored the impact of various factors such as more precise dating or the efficacy of Down syndrome detection rates[23,24] likewise with an ever increasing proportion of pregnancies resulting from infertility therapies, questions have risen as to whether modifications of risk or screening strategies are required.[25]

A number of papers have suggested dimeric inhibin A as an excellent marker that may raise the sensitivity by 3–7% for a given screen positive rate.[26-29] Out of this data have come calls for "quadruple" screening, and various combinations of biochemical and biophysical (ultrasound) data. There are also paradigms that include different parameters at different times combined. While preliminary data do suggest a high sensitivity with improved specificity,[30,31] hiding results from patients for up to a month is ethically problematic in our opinion. No doubt there will be multiple approaches to screening that emerge, and there will be no one uniform standard approach.[32]

A two-step approach has been the so called "integrated" test.[29-32] This is a combination of first trimester blood and ultrasound. The first trimester results are not communicated to the patient, who then waits for second trimester blood results before a risk assessment is completed. Two studies, the "SURUSS" trial and the "FASTER" trial have data that suggest a reduced false positive rate for comparable sensitivity, but the trade off is the need for patients to wait as much as 6 weeks for start to finish of the screening process.[30,31] For patients, who do not particularly care about the results, the delay may be fine, but our experience suggests that many anxious patients would find such delay intolerable.[33-36] As reproductive techniques have dramatically increased the proportions of multiple pregnancies, questions about the efficacy of screening tests have emerged. We and others have debated the data of biochemical screening on twins or more. There have been several papers that have promoted "pseudorisks" for twins by biochemical data. We continue to be concerned about the accuracy of these tests and believe that in multiples biophysical data are more likely to be accurate.[37-40]

First Trimester

The future of screening for Down syndrome (and other anomalies) lies in the first trimester. Substantial evidence now shows that free β-HCG is reliably elevated and PAPP-A is diminished in Down's pregnancies.[40-41] Data from multiple laboratories have been consistent in suggesting 70% to even 90% detection rates. In combination with ultrasound nuchal translucency measurements, almost all publications in which the ultrasound component was performed in a technically sound fashion have shown at least a 70% sensitivity.[42]

Several large scale studies, particularly, the King College group in London and the NICHD funded "BUN" and "FASTER" trials all essentially confirmed that first trimester data will be at least equal to routine second trimester double or triple screening.[30,41]

Measurement of Fetal Nuchal Translucency Thickness

Guidelines for measurement of fetal NT thickness have been drafted by the fetal medicine foundation (FMF). More than 300 centers around the world have adopted the FMF guidelines and they take part in the quality control scheme. Quality control of ultrasound scans involves assessment of the distribution of NT measurements and assessment of randomly selected images in terms of magnification, section (sagittal or oblique), caliper placement, skin line (nuchal only or nuchal and back) and visualization of the amnion separate from the nuchal membrane.[35]

The ability to measure NT and obtain reproducible results improves with training; good results are achieved after 80 scans for the transabdominal route and 100 scans transvaginally.[42] The ability to achieve a reliable measurement of NT is dependent on the motivation of the sonographer. Results were compared from hospitals that used NT in clinical practice (interventional) to those obtained in hospitals that recorded the measurements but did not act on the results (observational). In the interventional group successful measurement of NT was achieved in 100% of cases and the measurement was >2.5 mm in 2.3% of cases; the respective percentages in the observational group were 85% and 12%.[43,44]

Guidelines

- Equipment to measure up to 0.1 mm and time allocated for each scan at least 10 minutes.
- Transabdominal or transvaginal route: The transabdominal route gives a success rate of 95%; in 5% of cases it is necessary to perform vaginal sonography.
- Gestational age between 10 + 3 weeks and 13 + 6 weeks (CRL 38-84 mm, BPD < 27 mm): At these gestations, the success rate for obtaining a measurement is more than 98%. From 14 weeks onward the fetal position (vertical) makes it more difficult to obtain measurements.[45]
- Good sagittal section of the fetus, as for measurement of fetal crown-rump length: An optimal measurement is obtained when the fetus is in a neutral position (neither in flexion nor in extension).
- Magnification so that the fetus occupies at least 3/4rd and that each increment in the distance between callipers is only 0.1 mm.

- Distinguish between fetal skin and amnion (both appear as thin membranes!) by waiting for spontaneous fetal movement away from the amniotic membrane.

  Alternatively, the fetus may be bounced off the amnion by asking the mother to cough and/or by tapping the maternal abdomen.

- Measure the maximum thickness of the subcutaneous translucency between the skin and the soft tissue overlying the cervical spine by placing the calipers on the lines as shown in the Figure 65.5.

  The umbilical cord may be round the fetal neck in 5–10% of cases and this can produce an increased NT as it adds about 0.8 mm to the measurement.[46] Measurements of NT above and below the cord will be different and in the calculation of risk, it is appropriate to use the smaller measurement. It is well established that NT normally increases with gestational age.[47-51] Therefore, the difference from the normal median for gestation is used to determine the factor by which the age-related risk is adjusted.

Increased Nuchal Translucency and Chromosome Defects

Studies that report on first trimester fetal NT thickness and chromosome defects can be divided in four groups. Initial observational studies examined the prevalence of chromosome defects in fetuses with increased NT. Subsequent observational studies examined in (high risk) pregnancies prior to invasive testing the proportion of Down syndrome and normal fetuses that present with increased NT. Implementation studies then reported on the feasibility of introducing screening by NT in routine practice and, finally, centers that introduced the test reported experience with screening based on the combination of maternal age, gestational age and fetal NT thickness.

Observational Studies

In the early 1990s, several reports on fetuses with increased NT demonstrated a possible association between NT and chromosome defects in the first trimester of pregnancy (Table 65.2).[52-65] The mean prevalence of chromosome defects in 14 series involving 1,457 patients was 28%. However, the percentage ranged from 19% to 88%. This variation in results presumably reflects differences in the maternal age distributions and differences in the definition of minimum thickness of the abnormal translucency, ranging from 2 mm to 10 mm.

In subsequent studies NT thickness was assessed immediately before fetal karyotyping, mainly for advanced maternal age (AMA). Detection rates for trisomy 21 varied from 30% to 84% (Table 65.3).[66-71] with false positive rates ranging from 1% to 6%. Detection rates were relatively low if measurements were taken before 10 weeks of gestation, and/or machines measured whole mm only.[50,51]

Increased Nuchal Translucency and Normal Karyotype

Souka et al.[72] recently presented findings in 4,116 chromosomally normal fetuses with increased NT together with a review of the literature. There are at least five conditions that may underlie increased NT and these include heart defects or heart failure, intrathoracic compression, altered composition of the dermis, abnormal lymphatic system and neuromuscular abnormalities.

Table 65.2: Summary of reported series on first trimester fetal nuchal translucency (NT) providing data on gestational age (GA) in weeks, criteria for diagnosis of increased NT thickness and the presence of associated chromosomal defects (T21 = trisomy 21, T18 = trisomy 18, T13 = trisomy 13)

Author		GA (wk)	NT (mm)	N	Abnormal karyotype					
					Total	T21	T18	T13	45,X	Other
Johnson 1993	-52	10–14	>2.0	68	41 (60%)	16	9	2	9	5
Hewitt 1993	-53	10–14	>2.0	29	12 (41%)	5	3	1	2	1
Shulman 1992	-54	10–13	>2.5	32	15 (47%)	4	4	3	4	0
Nicolaides 1992	-55	10–13	>3.0	88	33 (38%)	21	8	2	0	2
Pandya 1995	-56	10–13	>3.0	1,015	193 (19%)	101	51	13	14	15
Szabo and Gellen 1990	-57	10–12	>3.0	8	7 (88%)	7	0	0	0	0
Wilson et al. 1992	-58	8–11	>3.0	14	3 (21%)	0	0	0	1	2
Ville et al. 1992	-59	9–14	>3.0	29	7 (28%)	4	3	1	0	0
Trauffer et al. 1994	-60	10–14	>3.0	43	21 (49%)	9	4	1	4	3
Nadel et al. 1993	-61	10–15	>4.0	63	43 (68%)	15	15	1	10	2
Schulte-Valentin 1992	-62	10–14	>4.0	8	7 (88%)	7	0	0	0	0
Van Zalen-Sprock1992	-63	10–14	>4.0	18	5 (28%)	3	1	0	1	1
Cullen et al. 1990	-64	11–13	>6.0	29	15 (52%)	6	2	0	4	3
Suchet 1992	-65	8–14	>10.0	13	8 (62%)	0	0	0	7	1
				1,457	413 (28%)	198	100	24	56 (55-56)	35

Table 65.3: Summary of reported series on first trimester fetal NT before amniocentesis or CVS providing data on gestational age (GA) in weeks, criteria for diagnosis of increased NT thickness, false positive rate (FPR), detection rate (DR) and odds of an affected pregnancy (OAP) for trisomy 21

Author		GA (wks)	NT cut-off	N	FPR	DR for trisomy 21	OAP for trisomy 21
Nicolaides et al. 1994	67	10–13	>3 mm	1,273	4%	84% (21/25)	1 in 4
Zimmerman et al. 1996	68	10–13	>3 mm	1,151	2%	67% (2/ 3)	1 in 12
Hewitt et al. 1996	54	10–14	>3 mm	1,312	4%	57% (12/21)	1 in 5
Comas et al. 1995	69	9–13	>3 mm	487	1%	57% (4/ 7)	1 in 13
Salvodelli et al. 1993	70	9–12	>3 mm	1,400	<1%	54% (15/28)	1 in 2
Borell et al. 1997	71	10–13	>3 mm	479	6%	44% (8/18)	1 in 5
Haddow et al. 1998	51	9–15	95th	3,308	5%	31% (18/58)	1 in 10
Brambati et al. 1995	52	8–15	>3 mm	1,819	2%	30% (8/26)	1 in 7
Scott et al. 1996	72	9–13	95th	445	5%	30% (3/10)	1 in 8

Heart Defects

Two fetal echocardiographic studies at 10–16 weeks of gestation reported that 16 (80%) of the 20 fetuses with cardiac defects had abnormal collection of nuchal fluid.[73,74] In addition, a study of 29,154 pregnancies demonstrated that the prevalence of cardiac defects increases with increasing NT. In fetuses with a NT <95th percentile was 0.8 per 1,000 compared to 15 per 1,000 in the group with increased NT thickness (Table 65.4).[75-76] Examination of chromosomally normal pregnancies with an NT of 3.5 mm or more (1% of the population) at 15–20 weeks by an echocardiographer identifies approximately 40% of significant cardiac defects.

Public Policy

Why then has not first trimester screening already replaced the second trimester testing? The answers are complex, but can be divided into several different categories. Firstly many patients do not come for prenatal care until the second trimester. It is well known that there are universal correlation between socioeconomic status and gestational age at first visit for prenatal care. No matter how good a first trimester test is, it is not good for a patient first seen at 24 weeks.[77]

Secondly, even in 2001 with voluminous articles and college opinions touting multiple markers, 20% of patients were still getting the 1980s model of AFP alone.[15] Significant professional education will be needed to leapfrog the practice in first trimester screening.

Thirdly, until immediate invasive testing is readily available and accepted, first trimester screening results would be worse than none if the patient then had to wait a month to have an amniocentesis for a definitive answer.[35-66] We see this as very problematic for the "integrated" test that combines first and second trimester laboratory results and ultrasound. CVS has long since proven to be safe and effective in experienced hands. As the so-called limb reduction defect scare has been shown to be false at appropriate gestational

Table 65.4: Prevalence of major cardiac defects in chromosomally normal fetuses with increased NT thickness

NT thickness	N	Cardiac defects		
<95th centile	27,332	0.8/1,000	(~1 in	1,250)
95th centile–3.4 mm	1,507	5/1,000	(~1 in	200)
3.5-4.4 mm	208	29/1,000	(~1 in	35)
4.5–5.4 mm	66	91/1,000	(~1 in	10)
>5.5 mm	41	195/1,000	(~1 in	5)
Total	**29,154**	**1.7/1,000**		

ages hopefully the availability of CVS and acceptance will swing the pendulum back toward the desire for first trimester screening for testing which has many advantages in the patient. We actually expect the concept of maternal age as a stand alone variable to be phased out over the next several years.[77]

Trisomy 18

Although, screening has generally focused on Trisomy 21, our data, and those of others has always shown a varied pattern of anomalies detected by screening.[78] A different pattern of analyte levels has been observed in Trisomy 18. The values of AFP, hCG and uE3 appear to be very low.[79] This suggests a different pathophysiology than for Down syndrome. In Down syndrome, the low AFP and uE3, and high hCG can be explained as reflecting inappropriate immaturity or dysmaturity of the fetus, i.e. all values are consistent with a younger gestational age. In Trisomy 18, however, that explanation does not work.[80] We have previously shown that there are different patterns of genomically directed intrauterine growth retardation in different aneuploidies[78] but how this translates into serum markers is unclear. Nevertheless some reports have shown that an algorithm can be used to identify the majority of Trisomy 18 cases while adding about 0.75% to the population being offered amniocentesis.[80,81]

THE END OF "ADVANCED MATERNAL AGE"

The association of advanced maternal age (AMA) with increasing risks of chromosomal abnormalities particularly Down syndrome has been appreciated for decades (Fig. 65.5).

The choice of age 35 at least in the United States of America (USA) was an arbitrary compromise determined in part by naivety in data collection.

Cohorts of Down syndrome risk were usually reported in 5 year groupings, and there was clearly a big jump from the 30–34 and 35–39 age group. It was only later when data were reported on a year age specific curve that the slope of the curve was shown to be changing before age 35. Furthermore, the difference from 1 year to the next was obviously no where as dramatic as suggested in the 5-year cohorts.[9]

Another dramatic development of the 1970s was changing laws in the USA concerning a woman's right to end a pregnancy. New York and California were among the first states to repeal laws that made abortion virtually impossible to obtain legally. In 1973, the US Supreme Court ruled that in the first trimester a state had very little rights to interfere with a woman's defined right of privacy in terminating a pregnancy.[82-84] In the second trimester, the state's interests were primarily only in ensuring the safety of the

procedure. It was only the third trimester that the state could exert a compelling interest in protecting the "rights" of the fetus over the mother's wishes.

The combination of new technology plus the ability to terminate abnormal pregnancies led to a surge of interest in prenatal diagnosis. As with most of the new technologies, utilization was initially highest among patients of upper socioeconomic status who had the knowledge of the availability of the technology as well as the means to travel to far off centers to obtain such services.[85]

The evidence is clear that first trimester screening followed by first trimester diagnosis by CVS can bring about a substantially higher sensitivity and specificity within the same time frame as AMA offered CVS is overwhelming. The question thus reduces to how and when to update the accepted "culture" in the United States to be consistent with the current scientific knowledge base.

There has to be the understanding that age is not being discarded, but will merely become one of a number of variables that can be assessed to give the most accurate assessment of risk possible. With education, the ultrasound portion of the equation will become more standardized to laboratory levels of quality assurance. Nonprofit organizations such as the Fetal Medicine Foundation in London, and the Fetal Medicine Foundation in America as well as certainly others will help coordinate the transition and training needed to make such a reality.

It is also not realistic to expect a shift of "standards" and practice to change on a single day. Thus, there will have to be a short phase in period, under which either the old or the new approach will be considered acceptable. However, it is also reasonable to expect that the insurance companies who will have to pay for such to vociferously and clearly articulate to their subscribers and physicians, that they are not about to vastly increase the numbers of patients having tests. Thus, the right will be likely the "right" to pay out of one's own pocket for testing for AMA, per se.

It is time for advance maternal age, as a stand alone criteria, for having invasive testing to go the way of the buggy whip. The principal objection to screening as entry to testing has been removed. It can all now be done in the first trimester. The science has evolved. It is now time for the culture and the standards to follow.

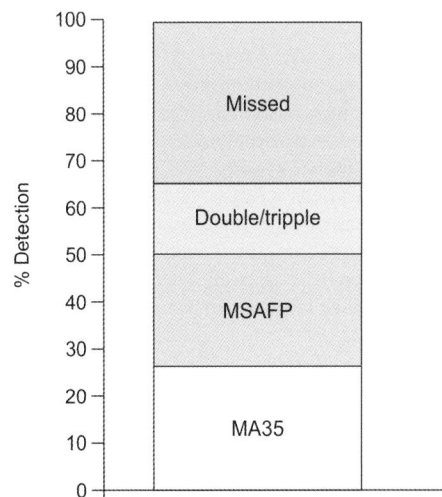

Fig. 65.5: Maternal age 35 identifies about 25% of Down syndrome pregnancies. Low AFP brings the total to about 50%. Double or triple screening raises that number to about 60%. Half of the 80% of cases occurring to women under 35 are detectable

REFERENCES

1. Evans MI, Krivchenia EL, Yaron Y. Screening In: Evans MI, Bui (Eds). Genomic Revolution and Obstetrics and Gynecology. Balliere's Clinical Obstetrics and Gynecology. 2002;16:645-58.
2. Evans MI, Chik L, O'Brien JE, et al. MOMs and DADS: improved specificity and cost effectiveness of biochemical screening for aneuploidy with DADS. Am J Obstet Gynecol. 1995;172:1138-47.
3. Evans MI, Chik L, O'Brien JE, et al. Logistic regression generated probability estimates for trisomy 21 outcomes from serum AFP and BHCG: Simplification with increased specificity. Mat Fetal Med. 1996;5:1-6.
4. Evans MI, Sobecki MA, Krivchenia EL, et al. Parental decisions to terminate/continue following abnormal cytogenetic prenatal diagnosis: "What" is still more important than "when. Am J Med Genet. 1996;61:353-5.
5. Pryde PG, Odgers AE, Isada NB, et al. Determinants of parental decision to abort or continue for non-aneuploid ultrasound detected abnormalities. Obstet Gynec. 1992;80:52-6.
6. Merkatz IR, Nitowsky FM, Macri JN et al. An association between low maternal serum alpha-fetoprotein and fetal chromosome abnormalities. Am J Obstet Gynecol. 1984;148:886-94.
7. Nyberg DA, Kramer D, Resta RG, et al. Prenatal monographic findings of trisomy 18: review of 47 cases. J Ultrasound Med. 1993;2:103-113.
8. Martin JA, Hamilton BE, Ventura SJ, et al. Births: Final data for 2001. National Vital Statistics Report 51, #2. National Center for Health Statistics. Hyattsville, MD: 2002.
9. Evans MI, Krivchenia EL, Yaron Y. Screening. In: Evans MI, Bui TH, (Eds). The Genome Revolution and Obstetrics and Gynecology. Balliere's Best Practice and Research in Clinical Obstetrics and Gynecology. London: Harcourt Brace Publishing. Co; 2002;16:624-57.
10. Wald NJ, Cuckle HS, Densem JW, et al. Maternal serum screening for Down syndrome in early pregnancy. Br Med J. 1988;297:883-7.
11. Cheng EY, Luthy DA, Zebelman AM, et al. A prospective evaluation of a second-trimester screening test for fetal Down syndrome using maternal serum alpha-fetoprotein, hCG, and unconjugated estriol. Obstet Gynecol, 1993;81:72-7.
12. Aitken DA, McCaw G, Crossley JA, et al. First-trimester biochemical screening for fetal chromosome abnormalities and neural tube defects. Prenat Diagn. 1993;13:681-3.
13. Wald N, Densem J, Stone R, Cheng R. The use of free 1993, β-hCG -in antenatal screening for Down's syndrome. Br J Obstet Gynaecol. 1993;100:550-7.
14. Goodburn SF, Yates JRW, Raggatt PR, Caff C, Ferguson-Smith ME, Kershaw Ai, et al. Second-trimester maternal serum screening using alpha-fetoprotein, human chorionic gonadotrophin, and unconjugated oestriol: experience of a regional programme. Prenat Diagn. 1994;14:391-402.
15. Evans MI Harrison HH, O'Brien JE et al. Correction for insulin dependent diabetes in maternal serum alpha fetoprotein testing has outlived its usefulness. Am J obstet Gynecol. 2002;87:1084-6.
16. Evans MI, Harrison HH, O'Brien JE, et al. Maternal weight correction for alpha-fetoprotein: mathematical truncations revisited. Genetic Testing. 2002;6:221-3.
17. Spencer K, Bindra R, Micolaides KH. Maternal weight correction of maternal serum PAPP-A and free beta-hCG MoM when screening for trisomy 21 in the first trimester pregnancy. Prenat Diagn. 2003;23(10):851-5.
18. Evans MI, O'Brien JE, Dvorun E, et al. Standardization of methods reduces variability: explanation for the historical discrepancies in biochemical screening. Genetic Testing. 2003;7:81-3.
19. Spencer K. The influence of different sample collection types on the levels of markers used for Down's syndrome screening as measured by the Kryptor Immunosassay system. Ann Clin Biochem. 2003;40(Pt 2):166-8.
20. Spencer K, Crossley JA, Aitken DA, et al. Temporal changes in maternal serum biochemical markers of trisomy 21 across the first and second trimester of pregnancy. Ann Clin Biochem. 2002;39(Pt 6):567-76.
21. Ghisoni L, Ferrazzi E, Castagna C, et al. Prenatal diagnosis after ART success: The role of early combined screening tests in counseling pregnant patients. Placenta Suppl. 2003;B:S99-S103.
22. Donnenfeld AE, Icke KV, Pargas C, Dowman C. Biochemical screening for aneuploidy in ovum donor pregnancies. Am J Obstet Gynecol. 2002;187(5):1222-5.
23. Canick JA, Saller DN Jr, Lambert-Messerlian GM. Prenatal screening for Down syndrome: Current and future methods. Clin Lab Med. 2003;23(2):395-411.
24. Silver HM, Lambert-Messerlian GM, Reis FM, et al. Mechanism of increased maternal serum total activin a and inhibin a in preeclampsia. J Soc Gynecol Investig. 2002;9(5):308-12.
25. Wald NJ, Huttly WJ, Hackshaw AK. Antenatal screening for Down's syndrome with the quadruple test. Lancet. 2003;8;361(9360):835-6.
26. Benn PA, Fang M, Egan JF, et al. Incorporation of inhibin-A in second-trimester screening for Down syndrome. Obstet Gynecol. 2003;102(2):413; author reply 413-4.
27. Spencer K, Liao AW, Ong CY, et al. Maternal serum levels of dimeric inhibin A in pregnancies affected by Trisomy 21 in the first trimester. Prenat Diagn. 2001;21(6):441-4.
28. Malone. Faster trial. NEJM (In press). 2004.
29. Wald NJ, Rodeck C, Hackshaw AK, et al. First and second trimester antenatal screening for Down's syndrome: the results of the Serum, Urine and Ultrasound Screening Study (SURUSS). J Med Screen. 2003;10(2):56-104.
30. Cuckle HS. Growing complexity in the choice of Down's Syndrome screening Policy. Ultrasound Obstet Gynecol. 2002;19:323-6.
31. Souter VL, Nyberg DA, Benn PA, et al. Correlation of second-trimester sonographic and biochemical markers. J Ultrasound Med. 2004;23(4):505-11.
32. Cusick W, Buchanan P, Hallahan TW, et al. Combined first-trimester versus second-trimester serum screening for Down syndrome: A cost analysis. Am J Obstet Gynecol. 2003;188(3):745-51.
33. Muller F, Benattar C, Audibert F, et al. First-trimester screening for Down syndrome in France combining fetal nuchal translucency measurement and biochemical markers. Prenat Diagn. 2003;23(10):833-6.
34. Nicolaides KH, Bindra R, Heath V, et al. One-stop clinic for assessment of risk of chromosomal defects at 12 weeks of gestation. J Matern Fetal Neonatal Med. 2002;12(1):9-18.
35. Crossley JA, Aitken DA, Cameron AD, et al. Combined ultrasound and biochemical screening for Down's syndrome in the first trimester: A Scottish multicentre study. BJOG. 2002;109(6):667-76.
36. Drugan A, O'Brien JE, Dvorin E, et al. Multiple marker screening in multifetal gestations: prediction of adverse pregnancy outcomes. Fetal Diagnosis and Therapy. 1996;11:16-19.
37. O'Brien JE, Dvorin E, Yaron Y, et al. Differential increases in AFP, HCG, and uE3 in twin pregnancies: Impact upon attempts to quantify Down syndrome screening calculations. Am J Med Gen. 1997;73:109-12.
38. Wald N, Cuckle H, Wu TS, et al. Maternal serum unconjugated oestriol and human chorionic gonadotrophin levels in twin pregnancies: implications for screening for Down's syndrome. Br J Obstet Gynaecol. 1991;98(9):905-8.
39. Cuckle H. Down's syndrome screening in twins. J Med Screen. 1998;5(1):3-4.
40. Wald NJ, Rish S, Hackshaw AK. Combining nuchal translucency and serum markers in prenatal screening for Down syndrome in twin pregnancies. Prenat Diagn. 2003;23(7):588-92.

41. Wapner R, Thom E, Simpson JL, et al. First trimester maternal serum biochemistry and fetal nuchal translucency screening (BUN) study group. First-trimester screening for trisomies 21 and 18. N Engl J Med. 2003;349(15):1405-13.
42. Braithwaite JM, Morris RW, Economides DL. Nuchal translucency measurements: Frequency distribution and changes with gestation in a general population. Br J Obstet Gynaecol. 1996;103:1201-4.
43. Bower S, Chitty L, Bewley S, et al. First trimester nuchal translucency screening of the general population: data from three centres [abstract]. 27th British Congress of Obstetrics and Gynaecolology. 1995.
44. Roberts LJ, Bewley S, Mackinson AM, et al. First trimester fetal nuchal translucency: Problems with screening the general population 1. Br J Obstet Gynaecol. 1995;102:381-5.
45. Whitlow BJ, Economides DL. The optimal gestational age to examine fetal anatomy and measure nuchal translucency in the first trimester. Ultrasound Obstet Gynecol. 1998;11:258-61.
46. Schaefer M, Laurichesse-Delmas H, Ville Y. The effect of nuchal cord on nuchal translucency measurement at 10-14 weeks. Ultrasound Obstet Gynecol. 1998;11(4):271-3.
47. Pandya PP, Goldberg H, Walton B, et al. The implementation of first trimester scanning at 10-13 weeks of gestation and the measurement of fetal nuchal translucency thickness in two maternity units. Ultrasound Obstet Gynaecol. 1995a;5:20-5.
48. Pajkrt E, de Graaf IM, Mol BW, et al. Weekly nuchal translucency measurements in normal fetuses. Obstet Gynecol. 1998;91(2):208-11.
49. Yagel S, Anteby EY, Rosen L, et al. Assessment of first-trimester nuchal translucency by daily reference intervals. Ultrasound Obstet Gynecol. 1998;11:262-5.
50. Haddow JE, Palomaki GE, Knight GJ, et al. Screening of maternal serum for fetal Down's syndrome in the first trimester. N Eng J Med. 1998;338:955-61.
51. Brambati B, Cislaghi C, Tului L, et al. First-trimester Down's syndrome screening using nuchal translucency: a prospective study. Ultrasound Obstet Gynecol. 1995;5:9-14.
52. Johnson MP, Johnson A, Holzgreve W, et al. First-trimester simple hygroma: Cause and outcome. Am J Obstet Gynecol. 1993;168:156-61.
53. Hewitt BG, de Crespigny L, Sampson AJ, et al. Correlation between nuchal thickness and abnormal karyotype in first trimester fetuses. Med J Aust. 1996.7;165(7):365-8.
54. Shulman LP, Emerson D, Felker R, et al. High frequency of cytogenetic abnormalities with cystic hygroma diagnosed in the first trimester. Obstet Gynecol. 1992;80:80-2.
55. Nicolaides KH, Azar G, Snijders RJ, et al. Fetal nuchal oedema: associated malformations and chromosomal defects. Fetal Diagn Ther. 1992;7:123.
56. Pandya PP, Altman D, Brizot ML, et al. Repeatability of measurement of fetal nuchal translucency thickness. Ultrasound Obstet Gynaecol. 1995a;5:334-7.
57. Szabo J, Gellen J. Nuchal fluid accumulation in trisomy-21 detected by vaginal sonography in first trimester. Lancet. 1990;336:1133.
58. Wilson RD, Venir N, Faquharson DF. Fetal nuchal fluid-physiological or pathological?-in pregnancies less than 17 menstrual weeks. Prenat Diagn. 1992;12:755-63.
59. Ville Y, Lalondrelle C, Doumerc S, et al. First-trimester diagnosis of nuchal anomalies: significance and fetal outcome. Ultrasound Obstet Gynecol. 1992;2:314-6.
60. Trauffer PL, Anderson CE, Johnson A, et al. The natural history of euploid pregnancies with first-trimester cystic hygromas. Am Obstet Gynecol. 1994;170:1279-84.
61. Nadel A, Bromley B, Benacerraf BR. Nuchal thickening or cystic hygromas in first- and early second-trimester fetuses: prognosis and outcome. Obstet Gynecol. 1993;82:43-8.
62. Schulte-Vallentin M, Schindler H. Non-echogenic nuchal oedema as a marker in trisomy 21 screening. Lancet. 1992;339:1053.
63. Van Zalen-Sprock MM, Van Vugt JM, Van Geijn HP. First-trimester diagnosis of cystic hygroma-course and outcome. Am J Obstet Gynecol. 1992;167:94-8.
64. Cullen MT, Gabrielli S, Green JJ, et al. Diagnosis and significance of cystic hygroma in the first trimester. Prenat Diagn. 1990;10:643-51.
65. Suchet IB, Van der Westhuizen NG, Labatte MF. Fetal cystic hygromas: Further insights into their natural history. Can Assoc Radiol. J 1992;6:420-4.
66. Nicolaides KH, Azar G, Byrne D, et al. Fetal nuchal translucency: ultrasound screening for chromosomal defects in first trimester of pregnancy. Br Med J. 1992;304:867-9.
67. Zimmerman R, Hucha A, Savoldelli G, et al. Serum parameters and nuchal translucency in first trimester screening for fetal chromosomal abnormalities. Br J Obstet Gynaecol. 1996;103:1009-14.
68. Comas C, Martinez JM, Ojuel J, et al. First-trimester nuchal edema as a marker of aneuploidy. Ultrasound Obstet Gynecol. 1995;5:26-9.
69. Savoldelli G, Binkert F, Achermann J, et al. Ultrasound screening for chromosomal anomalies in the first trimester of pregnancy. Prenat Diagn. 1993;13:513-8.
70. Borell A, Costas D, Martinez JM, et al. Criteria for fetal nuchal thickness cut-off: A re-evaluation. Pren Diagn. 1997;17:23-9.
71. Scott F, Boogert A, Sinosich M, et al. Establishment and application of a normal range for nuchal translucency across the first trimester. Pren Diagn. 1996;16:629-34.
72. Souka AP, Nicolaides KH. Diagnosis of fetal abnormalities at the 10-14 week scan. Ultrasound Obstet Gynecol. 1997;10:429-42.
73. Souka AP, Snijders RJ, Novakov A, et al. Defects and syndromes in chromosomally normal fetuses with increased nuchal translucency thickness at 10-14 weeks of gestation. Ultrasound Obstet Gynecol. 1998;11:391-400.
74. Gembruch U, Knopfle G, Bald R, et al. Early diagnosis of fetal congenital heart disease by transvaginal echocardiography. Ultrasound Obstet Gynecol. 1993;3:310-7.
75. Achiron R, Rotstein Z, Lipitz S, et al. First-trimester diagnosis of fetal congenital heart disease by transvaginal ultrasonography. Obstet. Gynecol. 1994;84:69-72.
76. Hyett J, Perdu M, Sharland G, et al. Using fetal nuchal translucency to screen for major congenital cardiac defects at 10-14 weeks of gestation: population based cohort study. BMJ. 1999;318:81-5.
77. Hyett JA, Perdu M, Sharland GK, et al. Increased nuchal translucency at 10-14 weeks of gestation as a marker for major cardiac defects. Ultrasound Obstet Gynecol. 1997;10(4):242-6.
78. Evans MI, Macri JN, Galen RS, et al. Biochemical Screening. In: Evans MI, Johnson MP, Yaron Y, Drugan A (Eds). Prenatal Diagnosis. New York: McGraw Hill (In press).
79. Johnson MP, Barr Jr M, Qureshi F, et al. Symmetrical intrauterine growth retardation is not symmetrical: The ontogeny of organ specific gravimetric deficits in midtrimester and neonatal trisomy 18. Fetal Diagn and Ther. 1989 (released 1990);4:110-9.
80. Drugan A, Dvorin E, Koppitch FC, et al. Counseling for low maternal serum alpha-fetoprotein should emphasize all chromosome anomalies, not just Down Syndrome! Obstet Gynecol. 1989;73:271-4.
81. Palomaki GE, Haddow JE, Knight GJ, et al. Risk-based prenatal screening for trisomy 18 using alpha-fetoprotein, unconjugated estriol, and human chorionic gonadotropin. Prenat Diagn. 1995;15:713.
82. Leporrier N, Herrou M, Morello R, et al. Fetuses with Down's syndrome detected by prenatal screening are more likely to abort spontaneously than fetuses with Down's syndrome not detected by prenatal screening. BJOG. 2003;110(1):18-21.
83. US Supreme Court: Roe vs. Wade 410 US, 113 (1973).
84. US Supreme Court: Doe vs. Bolton 410 US, 179 (1973).
85. Evans MI, Hanft RS. The introduction of new technologies. ACOG Clin Semin. 1997;2:1-3.

66 Amniocentesis

S Tercanli, P Miny, W Holzgreve

INTRODUCTION

Midtrimester amniocentesis is the most commonly performed invasive technique in prenatal diagnosis. Valenti et al. reported the first successful diagnosis of Down's syndrome in 1968.[1] Since that time, the number of midtrimester amniocentesis has increased dramatically and amniocentesis is nowadays an established standard tool in the assessment of pregnancies that are at risk for a variety of chromosomal disorders, single gene defects, biochemical analysis and fetal infections, etc. Chromosome analysis and tests related to risk of screening for aneuploidy remain worldwide by far the most common laboratory procedures in prenatal diagnosis. Conventional chromosome analysis has maintained its role as a gold standard for the primary exclusion of aneuploidy from amniotic fluid cells. Frequent indications listed in Table 66.1 for offering second trimester amniocentesis are pregnancies considered to be at an increased risk.

Prior to any prenatal invasive test, patients should be counseled. The risks and benefits of all invasive and non-invasive tests must be discussed as well as the limitations of any procedure. In the cases of specific risk factors or abnormal ultrasound findings, the information should be as complete and appropriate as possible. Considering the current developments in prenatal diagnosis by performing advanced methods for individual risk calculation, e.g. nuchal translucency measurement and biochemical serum marker screening, counseling of pregnant women will become more and more

Table 66.1: Common indications for amniocentesis

- Advanced maternal age (= 35 years old)
- Family history for chromosome anomalies, single gene defects, etc.
- Abnormal maternal serum screening in the second trimester
- Increased risk for chromosomal anomalies following first trimester screening—if chorionic villus sampling is not available
- Abnormal ultrasound findings
- Maternal infections potentially affecting the fetus

important. It can be assumed that in this context, a more selective approach to invasive testing may result in the next years. One of the significant problems in counseling of pregnant women is still how to explain women (e.g. social, economical, ethical and cultural variability), the complex implications of risk calculation. Own experiences showed that appropriate individual counseling is more time-consuming and requires more appropriate methods.

TECHNIQUE

Midtrimester amniocentesis is commonly performed between 15 weeks and 16 weeks of gestation (Figs 66.1 and 66.2). Prior to the procedure of ultrasound, evaluation of the uterus (e.g. exclusion of fibroids), the fetus, amniotic fluid volume and position of the placenta are recommended, because the failure rate can be reduced by avoiding the removal of bloody fluid or multiple injections.[2-4] Patients anxiety may be reduced if adequate information is given to the patients during the procedure at each step. After disinfection of the maternal abdomen, amniocentesis is performed under direct ultrasound guidance, generally, using a 18–20 gauge needle. The obtained amniotic fluid volume should be not more than 1 mL per gestational week. The first 2 mL of amniotic fluid should be rejected in order to avoid maternal cell contamination. If bloody amniotic fluid is aspirated, the analysis of the chromosomes from cultured cells will take longer time and there might be a slightly higher risk for misdiagnosis due to the risk of culturing maternal cells from any other tissue other than blood cells. In women with Rh-negative blood group Rh-immune globuline must be administered, if the father of the

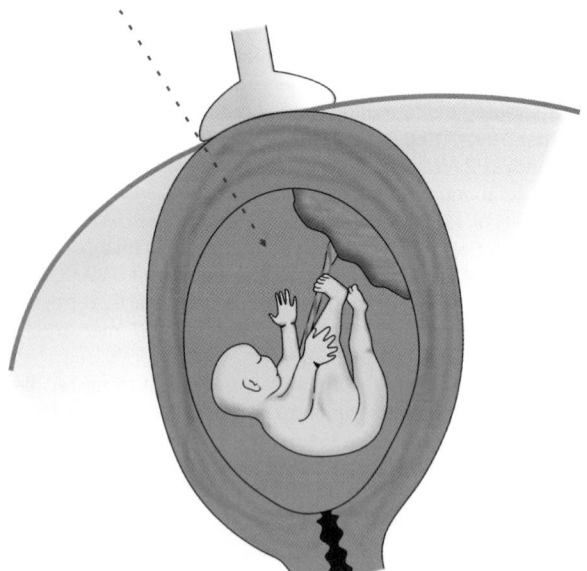

Fig. 66.1: Diagram of amniocentesis. Transplacental perforation should be avoided if possible

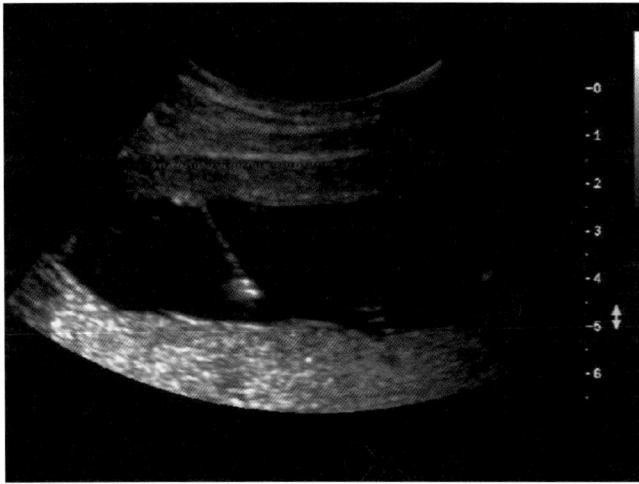

Fig. 66.2: Second trimester amniocentesis under ultrasound guidance

child is Rh-positive or his blood group is unknown. Following the procedure, it seems helpful to demonstrate the fetus again to the mother by ultrasound evaluation. There is no clear evidence in the literature that ultrasound guidance itself will reduce the fetal loss rate, but these may lower the maternal fears. In contrast, it is assumed that the abortion rate increases if the placenta is perforated.[5] Operator experience may also prejudice the fetal loss rate but this has not been definitively determined.[6] However, there is a general agreement that the number of genetic amniocentesis needed to be trained and maintaining stable ongoing expertise is recommended.[7-9] Exceptionally in multiple pregnancies, amniocentesis should be performed by trained investigators. Amniocentesis in twin pregnancies consists of obtaining of amniotic fluid from both cavities. As recommended in the past, dye injection into the first punctured sac was performed routinely.[10] Advanced ultrasound technology allows the evaluation of both fetuses and makes dye injection obsolete in experienced hands. Controversy is ongoing whether both amniotic sacs should be injected in cases of monochorionic diamniotic twins. In dichorionic twins, a single needle insertion technique is often favored, but may result in cytogenetic problems. On the other hand, it is unknown whether a single needle technique may induce a rupture of the membrane.

CYTOGENETIC ASPECTS

Compared to other methods for prenatal karyotyping, the benefits of an amniocentesis are the simplicity of the implementation of the procedure and the convenience of the analysis for the cytogenetic laboratory. In clinical practice, the level of α-fetoprotein (AFP) in amniotic fluid is determined routinely. Currently, it is debated that these may not longer be needed because high resolution ultrasound is able to detect neural tube defect and abdominal wall defects. However, the detection of spina bifida is depending on the experiences of the sonographer. Therefore, evaluation of AFP in the amniotic fluid is still recommended.

Cell culture as a prerequisite for conventional chromosome analysis on amniocytes causes a turn around time of atleast 1 week.

In practice, the average processing time is probably close to 2 weeks in most of the laboratories. Ongoing trends in prenatal diagnosis aim at early and rapid diagnosis as well as at the improvement of risk-screening for aneuploidy. Flourescent in situ hybridization (FISH) on interphase amniocytes and quantitative fluorescence polymerase chain reaction (QF-PCR) are efficient tools for the rapid exclusion of selected aneuploidies.[11] Regarding the overall detection rate of unbalanced chromosome anomalies the same limitations apply for both techniques with current approaches. It is suggested that QF-PCR is advantageous at least in all centers with access to the necessary hardware or those with large sample numbers. We believe, however, that for rapid karyotyping if available, direct preparation from chorionic villi should be the method of first choice when there is an increased risk for unbalanced chromosome anomalies, i.e. after the ultrasound diagnosis of fetal malformations. This method carries a false negative rate of below 1% as compared to up to 35% with interphase FISH or QF-PCR.[13] In conclusion, it can be stated that FISH and QF-PCR should be used as additional tests.

Particularly in blood-stained probes, maternal cell contamination of amniotic fluid cell is rare but well known cause of diagnostic error in the prenatal diagnosis of fetal disorders (< 3/1,000).[14] Using flourescent labeled microsatellites permits the differentiation between maternal and fetal cells. Mosaicism is one other remaining problem and is seen in 1/1,000 of samples.[15]

COMPLICATIONS

The risks which may be associated with second trimester amniocentesis include leakage of amniotic fluid, vaginal bleeding, contractions, chorioamnionitis, failure to obtain a sample, pregnancy loss and possible fetal injury.[5,16-23]

Actual fetal loss rates related to genetic amniocentesis vary among randomized studies and may be comixed by transplacental needle passage, multiple needle insertion and use of larger needles sizes.[17-19]

The total fetal loss rate related to the procedure is often calculated to be around 0.5%.[24] But in many studies the source for this reported level of risk was nondistinctive, and the background risk for miscarriage was unaccounted. In the three larger multicenter studies, the risk for fetal loss following amniocentesis was approximately 1%, but bias because of selection cannot be excluded.[3,7,22] These results were comparable with the former findings in the only randomized controlled trial reported by Tabor.[5] Recently, Seeds reviewed 68,119 amniocenteses from both controlled and uncontrolled studies providing straightforward arguments for several conclusions.[25]

Currently midtrimester amniocentesis under ultrasound guidance is associated with a procedure-related rate of excess pregnancy loss of 0.33% (95% CI, 0.09, 0.56). Among only controlled studies, this risk is 0.6% (95% CI, 0.31, 0.90). Adding the natural loss risk of about 1.08% among control groups the total rate of losses can be determined around 1.6%.

Application of ultrasound guidance may reduce the number of injections and may also lower the incidence of blood stained fluid. Analysis of only controlled studies shows that this trend remains, but not statistically significant.

Injury of the fetus is rare and cannot be perfectly prevented by using ultrasound guidance, but may occur more frequently.

Former reported experience of higher risks due to placental perforation does not support an increased rate of miscarriage. As shown in the comprehensive overview other complications (such as vaginal bleeding, infection or leakage of amniotic fluid) could not be analyzed due to the limited number of described terms or were not comparable. Following the improvement of the technique and the laboratory methods, there has been attempts in bringing forward the time of amniocentesis in the past by performing early amniocentesis, which is technically more demanding (Fig. 66.3). The both randomized studies designed to assess the safety and cytogenetic accuracy of early amniocentesis showed increased rate of fetal losses as well as higher rates of talipes equinovarus and oligohydramnios. Furthermore, multiple needle insertions were performed in early pregnancies compared to midtrimester amniocentesis. The rate of laboratory failures following early investigations was arised. Comparing early vs late amniocentesis, it is suggested that the procedure in the second trimester is more favorable.[26,27]

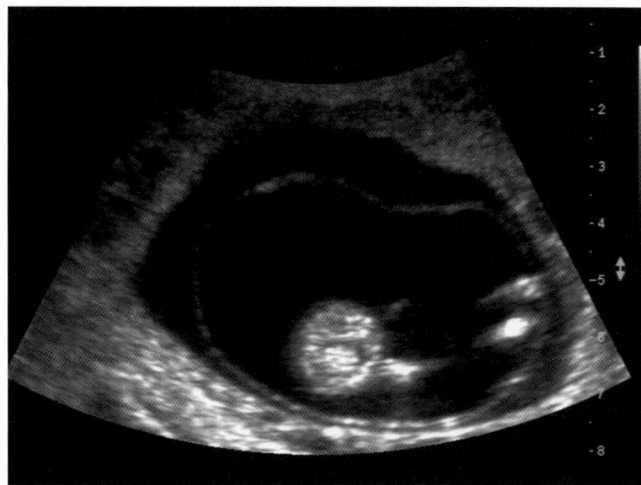

Fig. 66.3: Gestational and amniotic sac at 12 weeks demonstrating absence of fusion between amniotic membranes and the surrounding cavitiy

REFERENCES

1. Valenti C, Schutta EJ, Kehaty T. Prenatal diagnosis of Down's syndrome. Lancet. 1968;2(7561):220.
2. Romero P, Jeanty EA, Reece P, et al. Berkowitz, et al. Sonographically monitored amniocentesis to decrease intraoperative complications, Obstet Gynecol. 1985;65:426-30.
3. Simpson NE, Dallaire L, Miller JR, et al. Prenatal diagnosis of genetic disease in Canada: report of a collaborative study. Can Med Assoc J. 1976;115:793-6.
4. NICHD National Registry for Amniocentesis Study Group. Midtrimester amniocentesis for prenatal diagnosis. Safety and accuracy. J Am Med Assoc. 1976;236:1471-6.
5. Tabor A, Madsen M, Obel E, et al. Randomized controlled trial of genetic amniocentesis in 4606 low-risk women, Lancet. 1986;1:1287-93.
6. William B, Blessed MD, Helene Lacoste MD, et al. Obstetrician-gynecologists performing genetic amniocentesis may be misleading themselves and their patients. Am J Obstet Gynecol. 2001;184:1340-4.
7. National Institute of Child Health and Human Development. National Registry for Amniocentesis Study Group. Midtrimester amniocentesis for prenatal diagnosis: safety and accuracy. JAMA. 1976;236:1471-6.
8. Mennuti MT, Brummond W, Crombleholme WR, et al. Fetal-maternal bleeding associated with genetic amniocentesis. Obstet Gynecol. 1980;55:48-54.
9. Porreco RP, Young PE, Resnik R, et al. Reproductive outcome following amniocentesis for genetic indications. Am J Obstet Gynecol. 1982;143:653-60.
10. Pijpers L, Jahoda MG, Vosters RP, et al. Genetic amniocentesis in twin pregnancies. Br J Obstet Gynaecol. 1988;95(4):323-6.
11. Kuo WL, Tenjin H, Segraves R, et al. Detection of aneuploidy involving chromosomes 13, 18 or 21 by fluorescence in situ hybridization (FISH) to interphase and metaphase amniocytes. Am J Hum Genet. 1991;49:112-9
12. Fauth C, Speicher MR. Classifying by colors: FISH-based genome analysis. Cytogenet Cell Genet. 2001;93:1-10.
13. Miny P, Tercanli S, Holzgreve W. Developments in laboratory techniques for prenatal diagnosis. Curr Opin Obstet Gynecol. 2002;14(2):161-8.
14. Benn PA, Hsu LY. Maternal cell contamination of amniotic fluid cell cultures: results of a US nationwide survey. Am J Med Genet. 1983;15:297-305.
15. Bui TH, Iselius L, Lindsten J. European collaborative study on prenatal amniotic fluid cell cultures. Prenat Diagn. 1984;4:145-62.
16. Jeanty P, Rodesch F, Romero R, et al. How to improve your amniocentesis technique, Am J Obstet Gynecol. 1983;146:593-6.
17. Carpenter RJ, Hinkley CM, Carpenter AF. Midtrimester genetic amniocentesis: use of ultrasound direction vs. blind needle insertion. J Reprod Med. 1983;28:35-40.
18. Williamson RA, Varner MW, Grant SS. Reduction in amniocentesis risks using a real-time needle guide procedure. Obstet Gynecol. 1985;65:751-5.
19. Romero R, Jeanty P, Reece EA, et al. Sonographically monitored amniocentesis to decrease intraoperative complications, Obstet Gynecol. 1985;65:426-30.
20. Simpson NE, Dallaire L, Miller JR, et al. Prenatal diagnosis of genetic disease in Canada: report of a collaborative study, CMAJ. 1976;115:739-46.
21. Philip J, Bang J. Outcome of pregnancy after amniocentesis for chromosome analysis. BMJ. 1978;2:1183-4.
22. United Kingdom Medical Research Council. An assessment of the hazards of amniocentesis: report of the MRC Working Party on Amniocentesis, BJOG. 1978;85:(Suppl 2):1-41.
23. Antsaklis A, Papantoniou N, Xygakis A, et al. Genetic amniocentesis in women 20-34 years old: associated risks. Prenat Diagn. 2002;20:247-50.
24. Centers for Disease Control and Prevention. Chorionic villus sampling and amniocentesis: recommendations for prenatal counseling, MMWR Morb Mortal Wkly Rep. 1995;44:1-4.
25. Seeds JW. Diagnostic mid trimester amniocentesis: How safe? Am J Obstet Gynecol. 2004;191(2):607-15.
26. Randomised trial to assess safety and fetal outcome of early and midtrimester amniocentesis. The Canadian Early and Mid-trimester Amniocentesis Trial (CEMAT) Group. Lancet. 1998;351(9098):242-7.
27. Sundberg K, Bang J, Smidt-Jensen S, et al. Randomised study of risk of fetal loss related to early amniocentesis versus chorionic villus sampling. Lancet. 1997;350(9079):697-703.

67

Cordocentesis

CP Weiner

INTRODUCTION

The development of high resolution ultrasound made it feasible to clearly image the umbilical cord. Daffos performed in the early 1980s the first intentional percutaneous umbilical blood sampling (cordocentesis) under ultrasound guidance spurred by a desire to accurately diagnose fetal toxoplasmosis.[1] The procedure rapidly gained favor with demonstration of its safety[2-4] and directly spurred the development of fetal medicine. A wide range of fetal norms (hematological, endocrinological, immunological, biochemical, and biophysical)[5] were developed, a crucial step in the evolution of fetal medicine. And while many early indications for cordocentesis have been supplanted by less invasive techniques, there remain several indications for fetal blood sampling. The most common techniques are the assessment and treatment of red cell and platelet alloimmunization, the antenatal diagnosis of inherited blood or metabolic diseases, rapid karyotyping of malformed or severely growth restricted fetuses in some countries, and rarely the determination of fetal acid-base status.

METHODS

Cordocentesis is performed in the outpatient setting by a single operator with or without an assistant. There is no benefit of maternal fasting, sedation, prophylactic antibiotics or tocolysis. Though, it is technically more difficult prior to 20 weeks, and the loss rate is much higher prior to 16 weeks, cordocentesis can be performed as early as 12 weeks. The patient's partner is encouraged to attend both the counseling session preceding the procedure, and the procedure itself. The limitations and potential complications must be stated unambiguously before written informed consent obtained, and a targeted ultrasound examination performed.

There are two methods for cordocentesis: freehand and the use of a fixed needle guide. The preferred location for umbilical cord puncture is the placental origin where it is relatively fixed, regardless of technique. The first few centimeters of the fetal origin of the umbilical cord are innervated, and puncture there causes pain. The umbilical vein is the preferred target rather than the umbilical artery because of its lower association with complications discussed subsequently. A "no touch" philosophy is essential. If you do not touch the shaft of the needle, you cannot contaminate it.

The freehand technique employs an 18–20 gauge spinal needle 8–12 cm long.[1] The subcutaneous and deep layers are infiltrated with a local anesthetic agent. The needle course is tracked by imaging the tip and shaft with the ultrasound transducer held either in the opposite hand of the operator or by the assistant. Since, the needle is not fixed, the tip can move several centimeters in all axes should either the site of insertion be suboptimal or the fetus move during the procedure. The operator secures the needle after the vessel has

been punctured and the assistant aspirates a series of 1 mL syringes. Preheparinization of the syringe is unnecessary unless a fetal blood gas is needed. The freehand technique remains most popular because of the flexibility it allows to the operator.

The author, however, prefers to perform cordocentesis using a fixed needle guide[2] attached to the base of the ultrasound transducer. Typically, the transducer is held by the operator's assistant. The predicted course of the needle, which can travel only in the vertical plane, is displayed on the ultrasound screen, allowing the operator to select a precise target for puncture. Deviation from the predicted path occurs when there is an abrupt change in the relationship between the puncture site in the maternal abdominal wall and the uterus as the needle traverses between the two. The most common causes are abrupt patient movement or inspiration and failure to hold the transducer surface flat against the maternal abdomen. Fetal movement is rarely an issue because of the speed of the procedure. A smaller gauge needle such as a 22 or 25 is used because lateral movement of the needle is not possible. He prefer to target the umbilical cord longitudinally at the "easiest" site for a direct approach. More than 50% of the time, he target a free loop. Placental puncture is avoided whenever possible when the indication is alloimmunization (RBC or platelet) just as for amniocentesis. Local anesthesia is unnecessary for diagnostic procedures using a 22 gauge needle. A local anesthetic should be used when the procedure is lengthy (e.g. intravascular transfusion). Prophylactic antibiotics are not indicated for either cordocentesis or intravascular transfusion. In his experience, amnionitis complicates less than 1 in 800 diagnostic procedures when the "no touch" philosophy is rigorously adhered to and a needle guide is used (1 in 1,200 procedures).

Fetal movement while the needle is intraluminal increases the risk of umbilical cord trauma; it may also either prevent a successful puncture or shorten the access time available regardless of technique.

He prepared a neuromuscular antagonist such as pancuronium (0.3 mg/kg EFW) on the sterile field for every procedure, and routinely use it to eliminate fetal movement when performing a midloop puncture. The pancuronium is given either intramuscular into the fetal buttock, or preferably, intravenously as soon as the vein is punctured; the effect here is evident within seconds. Vercuronium is preferred over pancuronium for simple diagnostic procedures because its shorter half-life allows a more rapid return of fetal movement and heart rate variability.[6] In contrast, pancuronium is preferred for fetal transfusion because it maintains fetal cardiac output despite the volume load.

The volume of blood removed depends on the gestation and indication for sampling. Five milliliters is typical, and adequate for a karyotype, umbilical venous blood gas, and complete blood profile with Kleihauer-Betke testing with 2 mL remaining for use.

Table 67.1: Complications of cordocentesis

1. Bradycardia or asystole
2. Premature rupture of membranes
3. Premature labor
4. Umbilical hemorrhage
5. Placental hemorrhage
6. Chorioamnionitis
7. Umbilical thrombosis
8. Fetal to maternal hemorrhage

Table 67.2: Risk factors for cordocentesis

1. Umbilical artery puncture (associated with bradycardia)
2. Fetal hypoxemia (associated with bradycardia)
3. Technique (freehand versus needle guide)
4. Gestational age—prior to 20 weeks, both techniques
5. Number of punctures (freehand technique only)
6. Duration of procedure (freehand technique only)
7. Experience (freehand technique only, presumably because of # 4, 5)

MAJOR COMPLICATIONS AND RISK FACTORS FOR CORDOCENTESIS

The major complications of cordocentesis are listed in Table 67.1. They include all complications associated with amniocentesis plus fetal bradycardia, umbilical cord laceration and thrombosis. Risk factors for cordocentesis are noted in Table 67.2.

Bradycardia is the major complication of cordocentesis. Essentially all emergency cesarean deliveries and most perinatal losses are associated with a fetal bradycardia. Umbilical artery puncture and hypoxia are the major risk factors for bradycardia. In the absence of profound anemia or fetal heart failure, fetal hypoxia is associated with an elevated umbilical artery resistance index and it can be used as a risk marker. The incidence of bradycardia with absent and/or reversed diastolic flow approaches 25%. Umbilical artery puncture increases the risk of fetal bradycardia 5–10 fold.[3,7] The presence of either oligohydramnios or a two-vessel cord increases the risk of arterial puncture.

The observation of the bradycardia is associated with an elevated resistance index in one but not both umbilical arteries suggests localized vasospasm is the cause. Pancuronium reduces the prevalence of bradycardia in appropriately grown but not growth restricted fetuses[7]. It is possible that some episodes of bradycardia may occur when fetal movement tugs on the umbilical cord causing needle trauma and irritation to the underlying vascular smooth muscle. Bradycardia after umbilical vein puncture may reflect disruption of the adjacent umbilical artery smooth muscle as the tip traverses the cord. In the event of a bradycardia, vigorous fetal stimulation by palpation is beneficial as the heart will speed up and then slow again if the manual stimulation is stopped too early. A variety of chronotropes (e.g. atropine) and bicarbonate have also been given as part of the fetal resuscitation without predictable effect.

Umbilical cord laceration and thrombosis are associated with freehand procedures and not to date reported when a needle guide was used. Though bleeding from the umbilical puncture site is common, prolonged bleeding with sequelae is uncommon.

Even when performed at a midloop, the fetus does "react" to the cordocentesis. Umbilical artery resistance typically declines after either a diagnostic procedure or a fetal intravascular transfusion.[8] The higher the "normal" baseline resistance index, the greater the decline. The decrease is associated with prostacyclin release from the vascular endothelium.[9,10] Endothelial adaptation to hypoxia also explains why hypoxemia is a risk factor for bradycardia.[7] Rizzo et al. demonstrated that endothelin is released upon umbilical vein puncture of growth restricted but not appropriately grown fetuses.[11] Fetuses who develop bradycardia release more endothelin.

It was generally accepted that the technique selection was a matter of operator preference and had no impact on outcome. There is now evidence to challenge that concept. The first line of evidence is indirect. The often stated "advantage" of the freehand technique, its flexibility, may also increase risk. Analogous to a lever, a small movement at the hub of the needle amplifies the distance the tip moves. In association with this inescapable fact, freehand cordocentesis produces a significantly greater increase in the maternal serum alpha-fetoprotein (MSAFP) than amniocentesis after controlling for placental puncture.[12] In contrast, the incremental change in MSAFP when a needle guide is used is similar to amniocentesis.[13] Further, the association between fetal thrombocytopenia and bleeding from the umbilical puncture site after a freehand cordocentesis is high enough to have prompted a recommendation that all fetuses at risk for alloimmune thrombocytopenia receive a prophylactic platelet transfusion at cordocentesis.[14] Yet, there is no relationship between the fetal platelet count and the bleeding time from the puncture site when a needle guide is used.[15] The latter may reflect either less lateral movement of the needle after puncture or the thinner gauge needle, or both. The loss rates reported after second trimester amniocentesis are lower when thinner needles are used.[16] Not surprising, there are also reports which suggest that an amniocentesis performed with a needle guide is safer than one performed freehand.[17]

Though no single center has adequate volume for a randomized trial, and comparisons of loss rates sustained by groups using the freehand and needle guide techniques are problematic since it is hard to separate procedure related losses from those secondary to the natural progression of disease, there is evidence to suggest many losses are technique dependent. He examined the role of technique by combining our experience with Professor Okamura of Tokohu University, who also uses a fixed needle guide for all procedures. Over 25 operators with varying levels of experience performed 1,260 diagnostic cordocenteses at a mean gestational age of 29 weeks. The umbilical vein (confirmed by the blood pressure reading) was punctured in 90% demonstrating the desired vessel can be targeted. A procedure related loss was defined as any loss within 2 weeks of the procedure except those resulting from elective pregnancy termination. Overall, there were 12 losses (0.9%) (Table 67.3).

Though there are more recent studies, Ghidini et al. provided adequate information for stratification and the low level of experience reported by the involved centers may be more reflective of today's reality.[18] After deleting his experience from the analysis, the overall loss rate was 7.2% (96/1,328) with the freehand method.[18] This rate was significantly higher than the overall loss rate when a needle guide was used (0.9%, 12/1, 260; p < 0.00001). But this is a superficial comparison.

To exclude the contribution of the underlying pathology to the loss rate, procedures may be divided into high and low risk with the later excluding chromosomal abnormalities, non-immune

Table 67.3: Frequency of major complications of cordocentesis when a needle guide is used

Final diagnosis	GA (weeks) at cordocentesis	*Percent emergency delivery	**Percent death within 2 weeks
RBC alloimmunization	28 ± 4	0.2	0.2
Uteroplacental dysfunction	32 ± 4	5.0	0.9
Chromosome abnormality	29 ± 6	7.7	9.9
All others	28 ± 6	0.3	0.2

* Weiner, unpublished
**from Weiner and Okamura.[40] Fetuses with a chromosome abnormality delivered by cesarean section were delivered before the karyotype was completed

hydrops, intrauterine growth restriction and fetal infection. Such exclusions virtually eliminate all abnormal fetuses that might be at risk for a loss unrelated to the procedure. The perinatal loss rate for these low risk procedures using the freehand technique was 3% (20/660). This rate is 15 times the needle guide rate (0.2%, 2/1021; $p < 000001$) which includes fetuses with infection, hydrops and structural malformations.

Donner et al. reported 759 diagnostic cordocenteses with a known outcome using the freehand technique.[19] Acknowledging several limitations (final diagnoses were not necessarily reported and 87% (34/39) of their perinatal losses were excluded as being unrelated to the procedure), their stated loss rate was 0.8% including 94 therapeutic terminations in the denominator. Subtracting the terminations from their total yields a loss of 1.1% (7/665). Of these pregnancies, 160 were sampled because of severe early IUGR. We can identify their low-risk group by excluding the IUGR fetuses and assume all fetuses with chromosomal abnormalities were either in the growth restriction group, therapeutic termination group, or the 1 fetus with trisomy 18 noted in the paper. This leaves a low risk group of 504 in which there were 6 fetal/neonatal losses (1.2%). This rate is significantly higher than that achieved in a similar group using a needle guide (p=0.03).

These findings strongly suggest that many of the procedure related losses associated with cordocentesis are technique dependent. And while a few skilled operators might duplicate the results obtained with a needle guide, the majority of practitioners who perform only a few cordocenteses per year would benefit from the use of a guide.

INDICATIONS AND APPLICATIONS

Antenatal Diagnosis of Blood Disorders

The use of recombinant DNA techniques on placental biopsy material in the first trimester of pregnancy or amniocytes in the second trimester for the diagnosis has supplanted cordocentesis for the diagnosis of many of these conditions.[20] Cordocentesis is still needed for a phenotype diagnosis, in those patients requiring confirmation of normality based on a linked probe, those who lack key affected relatives, those who are not informative by any of the available probes, and those in whom DNA analysis is not feasible because of late referral.

Antenatal Diagnosis of Metabolic Disorders

Antenatal diagnosis of over 100 of these disorders is now possible by the analysis of amniotic fluid, placental tissue or fetal blood.

Cordocentesis is particularly useful when the gestational age is close to the local limit for abortion, as with late prenatal care or after failed chorionic villus or amniotic fluid techniques.

Red Blood Cell Alloimmunization

Cordocentesis is not indicated in most instances of maternal RBC alloimmunization for fetal blood typing. Accurate typing can now be accomplished by applying PCR to either trophoblast or amniocytes obtained in the early second trimester when the risk of exacerbating sensitization is lower.[21,22]

Fetal blood sampling made it possible to better understand the pathophysiology of this disease and allows for an improved method of assessment and treatment.[23-28] The net result of improved understanding is a improved perinatal outcome. The most important advancement in the noninvasive management of RBC alloimmune disease was the recognition that most severely anemic fetuses have an elevated peak flow velocities in the middle cerebral artery.[29,30] Previously, the severity of fetal hemolysis was estimated from (1) the history of previously affected pregnancies; (2) the level of maternal hemolytic antibodies in a first sensitized pregnancy; (3) the amniotic fluid bilirubin concentration; (4) the altered morphometry of fetus and placenta; and (5) the presence of pathological FHR patterns. However, the scatter of values around the regression lines describing the relationships between fetal anemia and the data obtained from these indirect methods of assessment was wide.[31] And though the vast majority of fetuses with an elevated peak velocity in the middle cerebral artery are anemic, a sizable percentage of anemic fetuses have normal velocities, and the relationship between velocity and the magnitude of the hemoglobin deficit varies greatly among fetuses.

The only accurate method for determining severity is blood sampling by cordocentesis with the measurement of fetal hemoglobin concentration, reticulocyte count, blood type, strength of the direct Coombs test and total bilirubin concentration. However, the timing of the first cordocentesis remains less than concrete. Invasive procedures should be minimized not only because of the fetal risk but also because transplacental puncture enhances the risk of fetomaternal hemorrhage,[13,32] increases maternal antibody titer and worsens disease. I prefer to avoid cordocentesis until the peak middle cerebral artery flow velocities are abnormal in those pregnancies under 20 weeks of gestation. However, since as many as half the fetuses with mild to moderate anemia have normal velocities, it is reasonable depending on referral patterns and distances to consider sampling all women with a history of severe disease, those with high antibody titers, and fetuses with pathological FHR patterns.

A fetal blood sample is obtained, the hemoglobin concentration measured, and an intravascular blood transfusion given as necessary.[33] The goal of the first transfusion is to correct the hemoglobin deficit completely unless there is hydrops. Immune hydrops in the human fetus is almost always characterized by an elevated umbilical venous pressure which is consistent with high output heart failure or left ventricular dysfunction perhaps secondary to the low oxygen carrying capacity.[34] These fetuses tolerate the first intravascular transfusion poorly, and should be corrected initially to a hemoglobin level of not more than 8–9 g/dL (We routinely monitor the fetal umbilical venous pressure to avoid over transfusion.) The second transfusion is performed a few days later at which time the target hemoglobin for this and all subsequent transfusions is 18 g/dL. Subsequent transfusions are given at 3–4 week intervals until 34–36 weeks of gestation, their timing based on the findings in the middle cerebral artery and the knowledge that following a fetal blood transfusion, the mean rate of decrease in fetal hemoglobin is approximately 0.3 g/dL/day.[33] Currently, the survival rate of red cell isoimmunized pregnancies treated with cordocentesis exceeds 90% in experienced hands, and virtually all losses are associated with immune hydrops fetalis.[33] As important, we have demonstrated normal long-term neurodevelopment despite the profound anemia prior to treatment.[35]

How often to repeat cordocentesis in the occasional affected fetus who is not anemic is determined by the change in the peak flow velocity in the middle cerebral artery and by the "hemolysis pattern" determined at the first sampling.[36] This prospectively validated grading scheme is based on the reticulocyte count and the strength of the positive direct Coomb's test. Most fetuses do not require a second sampling. That said, nonanemic sensitized fetuses remain at risk for postnatal hyperbilirubinemia that is in direct correlation to their antenatal bilirubin levels.[37,38]

Platelet Alloimmunization

Immune thrombocytopenia (ITP) is not an indication for cordocentesis.[39] The assumed risk of fetal intracranial hemorrhage during labor is not supported by the aggregate experience of the last two decades. There is no more than one fetal loss documented in the literature secondary to an intrapartum fetal hemorrhage.[39] Most losses attributed to ITP were associated with a maternal connective tissue disorder or a neonatal bleed. In almost all other instances, either the cause of death or the timing of death is either not stated or not known. ITP is the most common autoimmune disorder of reproductive age women; if true, there should be no controversy that thrombocytopenia secondary to ITP posed a significant fetal risk during labor. Yet, the loss rate from cordocentesis in the best hands for a "low risk" fetus is 0.2%.[40] Further, there is no direct or indirect evidence that cesarean section for autoimmune thrombocytopenia improves neonatal outcome.

There has been significant progress in the management of severe fetal alloimmune thrombocytopenia.[41,42] It is clear that medical therapy consisting of primarily high doses of intravenous immunoglobulin (IVIG) (1–2 g/kg/week) with a prednisone rescue for suboptimal responders is effective treatment for the majority of affected pregnancies.[43] At risk pregnancies begin the weekly infusion between 10 weeks and 20 weeks depending on past history. Most undergo a single cordocentesis around 28 weeks to confirm normal platelet counts. When secondary to Pl(A1) platelet antigen incompatibility, fetuses with platelet counts > 20,000 at the initiation of therapy are predicted to maintain their platelet count at the second fetal blood sampling at > 20,000. The history of the previous sibling does not predict the initial fetal blood sampling, the second fetal blood sampling, or the response to treatment.[44] Even suboptimal fetal responders have a dramatic decrease in the risk of antenatal hemorrhage. Fetal platelet transfusion is associated with a high loss rate when used for primary therapy (up to 17%).[45] Its role is now secondary, indicated for those fetuses with extremely low platelet counts or those with a count < 50,000 prior to a planned vaginal delivery. There is no relationship between the fetal platelet count and bleeding from the puncture site when a needle guide is used.[15]

Evaluation of Nonimmune Hydrops Fetalis

Cordocentesis is central for the complete evaluation of nonimmune hydrops since it allows the separation of cardiac from noncardiac etiologies.[46] The umbilical venous pressure (UVP) is a surrogate for the central venous pressure. Studies of human fetuses[47] indicate that it is very similar to right sided heart pressure. An elevated UVP is consistent with myocardial dysfunction whether caused by anemia (e.g. parvovirus infection, hemolytic disease) or myocarditis, or obstructed cardiac return (thoracic mass effect). Successful treatment of cardiogenic hydrops is associated with normalization of the UVP before the hydrops resolves. Hydrops that is responsive to shunting is caused by a shift of the mediastinum which then obstructs cardiac return. An elevated UVP also predicts the fetus with hydrothorax and hydrops will be cured by a thoracoamniotic shunt. If the UVP is neither elevated nor normalizes after draining the chest, a shunt will not help. The underlying problem lies elsewhere.

Miscellaneous

Not yet accepted but a likely valid indication for cordocentesis is presence of maternal thyroid stimulating antibody (TSiG) or active maternal Graves disease.[48,49] Emerging evidence suggests even mild degrees of thyroid dysfunction is associated with impaired long-term neurodevelopment.[50-52] While there is a relationship between the degree of maternal and fetal thyroid suppression with such agents as propylthiouracil, it is common to find that the fetus is significantly over or under treated despite the mother being euthyroid. For fetal hyperthyroidism, the maternal PTU dose is increased and the woman given thyroxine replacement. For hypothyroidism, the fetus can be given thyroxine intraamniotically on a weekly basis.[53] Women with a history of Graves disease who have undergone thyroid ablation should be screened for the presence of TSiG. The fetus is at minimal risk if the TSiG study is negative.

REFERENCES

1. Daffos F, Capella-Pavlovsky M, Forestier F. A new procedure for fetal blood sampling in utero: preliminary results of fifty-three cases. Am J Obstet Gynecol. 1983;146:985 7.

2. Weiner CP. Cordocentesis for diagnostic indications two years experience. Obstet Gynecol. 1987;70:664-8.

3. Daffos F. Access to the other patient. [Review] Seminars in Perinatology. 1989;13:252-9.

4. Maxwell DJ, Johnson P, Hurley P, et al. Fetal blood sampling and pregnancy loss in relation to indication. Br J Obstet Gynaecol. 1991;98:892-7.

5. Ramsay MM, James DK, Steer PJ (Eds). Normal Values in Pregnancy. 3rd edition. Philadelphia: WB Saunders; 2005.

6. Mouw RJ, Hermans J, Brandenburg HC, et al. Effects of pancuronium or atracurium on the anemic fetus during and directly after intrauterine transfusion (IUT): A double blind randomized study. Am J Obstet Gynecol. 1997;176(2):S18.

7. Weiner, CP, Wenstrom KD, Sipes SL, et al. Risk factors for cordocentesis and fetal intravascular transfusions. Am J Obstet Gynecol. 1991;165:1020-3.

8. Weiner CP, Anderson T. The acute effect of cordocentesis with or without fetal curarization and of intravascular transfusion upon umbilical artery waveform indices. Obstet Gynecol. 1989;73:219-24.

9. Weiner CP, Robillard JE. Effect of acute intravascular volume expansion upon human fetal prostaglandin concentrations. Am J Obstet Gynecol. 1989;161:1494-7.

10. Capponi A, Rizzo G, Pasquini L, et al. Indomethacin modifies the fetal hemodynamic response induced by cordocentesis. Am J Obstet Gynecol. 1997;176(2):S19.

11. Rizzo G, Capponi A, Rinaldo D, et al. Release of vasoactive agents during cordocentesis: differences between normally grown and growth-restricted fetuses. Am J Obstet Gynecol. 1996;175:563-70.

12. Nicolini U, Kochenour NK, Greco P, et al. Consequences of fetomaternal hemorrhage after intrauterine transfusion. BMJ. 1988;297:1379-81.

13. Weiner CP, Grant SS, Hudson J, et al. Effect of diagnostic and therapeutic cordocentesis upon maternal serum alpha fetoprotein concentration. Am J Obstet Gynecol. 1989;161:706-8.

14. Paidas MJ, Lynch L, Lockwood CJ, et al. Alloimmune thrombocytopenia: Fetal and neonatal losses related to fetal blood sampling. Am J Obstet Gynecol. 1995;172: 475-9.

15. Weiner CP. Fetal blood sampling and fetal thrombocytopenia. Fetal Diagn Therapy. 1995;10:173-7.

16. Tabor A, Philip J, Bang J, et al. Needle size and risk of miscarriage after amniocentesis [letter]. Lancet. 1988;1(8578):183-4.

17. Weiner CP, Williamson RA, Varner MW, et al. Safety of second trimester amniocentesis. Lancet. 1986;ii: 226.

18. Ghidini A, Sepulveda W, Lockwood CJ, et al. Complications of fetal blood sampling. Am J Obstet Gynecol. 1993;168:1339-44.

19. Donner C, Simon P, Karioun A, et al. Experience of a single team of operators in 891 diagnostic funipunctures. Obstet Gynecol. 1994;84: 827-31.

20. Boehm CD, Kazazian HH. Examination of fetal DNA for hemoglobinopathies. In: Alter BP (Ed). Perinatal Hematology. New York: Churchill Livingstone; 1989. pp. 30-63.

21. Yankowitz J, Li S, Murray JC. Polymerase chain reaction determination of RhD blood type: an evaluation of accuracy. Obstet Gynecol. 1995;86:214-7.

22. Yankowitz J, Li S, Weiner CP. Polymerase chain reaction determination of RhC, Rhc, and RhE blood types: an evaluation of accuracy and clinical utility. Am J Obstet Gynecol. 1997;176:1107-11.

23. Berkowitz RL, Chitkara U, Goldberg JD, et al. Intrauterine transfusion in utero: The percutaneous approach. Am J Obstet Gynecol. 1986;154:622.

24. Grannum PA, Copel JA, Plaxe SC, et al. In utero exchange transfusion by direct intravascular injection in severe erythroblastosis fetalis. N Engl J Med. 1986;314:1431.

25. Nicolaides KH, Rodeck CH, Kemp J, et al. Have Liley charts outlived their usefulness? Am J Obstet Gynecol. 1986;155:90.

26. Nicolaides KH. Studies on fetal physiology and pathophysiology in Rhesus disease. Semin Perinatol. 1989;13:328.

27. Weiner CP, Robillard JE. Atrial natriuretic factor, digoxin-like immunoreactive substance, norepinephrine, epinephrine, and plasma renin activity in human fetuses and their alteration by fetal disease. Am J Obstet Gynecol. 1988;159(6):1353-60.

28. Soothill PW, Lestas AN, Nicolaides KH, et al. 2,3 Diphosphoglycerate in normal, anaemic and transfused human fetus. Clin Sci. 1988;74:527.

29. Mari G, Moise KJ Jr, Deter RL, et al. Flow velocity waveforms of the umbilical and cerebral arteries before and after intravascular transfusion. Obstet Gynecol. 1990;75:584-9.

30. Mari G, Deter RL, Carpenter RL, et al. Noninvasive diagnosis by Doppler ultrasonography of fetal anemia due to maternal red-cell alloimmunization. Collaborative Group for Doppler Assessment of the Blood Velocity in Anemic Fetuses. N Engl J Med. 2000;342:9-14.

31. Nicolaides KH, Sadovsky G, Cetin E. Fetal heart rate patterns in red blood cell isoimmunized pregnancies. Am J Obstet Gynecol. 1989;161:35.

32. Nicolini U, Kochenour NK, Greco P. Consequences of fetomaternal haemorrhage after intrauterine transfusion. Br Med J. 1988;297:1379.

33. Weiner CP, Williamson RA, Wenstrom KD, et al. Management of fetal hemolytic disease by cordocentesis. II. Outcome of treatment. Am J Obstet Gynecol. 1991;165:1302-7.

34. Weiner CP, Pelzer GD, Heilskov J, et al. The effect of intravascular transfusion on umbilical venous pressure in anemic fetuses with and without hydrops. Am J Obstet Gynecol. 1989;161:1498-501.

35. Swingle HM, Harper DC, Bonthius D, et al. Long-term neurodevelopmental follow-up and brain volumes of children following severe fetal anemia with hydrops. American Academy of Cerebral Palsy and Developmental Medicine, Los Angeles. 1989;9:29-101.

36. Weiner CP, Williamson RA, Wenstrom KD, et al. Management of fetal hemolytic disease by cordocentesis. I. Prediction of fetal anemia. Am J Obstet Gynecol. 1991;165(3):546-53.

37. Weiner CP, Wenstrom KD. Outcome of alloimmunized fetuses managed solely by cordocentesis but not requiring antenatal transfusion. Fetal Diagn Ther. 1994;9(4):233-8.

38. Weiner CP. Human fetal bilirubin levels and fetal hemolytic disease. Am J Obstet Gynecol. 1992;166(5):1449-54.

39. Weiner CP. Why fuss over diagnosing fetal thrombocytopenia secondary to ITP? Contemp. OB/GYN. 1995;40:45-50.

40. Weiner CP, Okamura K. Diagnostic fetal blood sampling - technique related losses. Fetal Diagnosis and Therapy. 1996;11:169-75.

41. Radder CM, Brand A, Kanhai HH. Will it ever be possible to balance the risk of intracranial haemorrhage in fetal or neonatal alloimmune thrombocytopenia against the risk of treatment strategies to prevent it? Vox Sang. 2003;84(4):318-25.

42. Bussel JB. Alloimmune thrombocytopenia in the fetus and newborn. Semin Thromb Hemost. 2001;27(3):245-52.

43. Bussel JB, Berkowitz RL, Lynch L, et al. Antenatal management of alloimmune thrombocytopenia with intravenous gamma-globulin: A randomized trial of the addition of low-dose steroid to intravenous gamma-globulin. Am J Obstet Gynecol. 1996;174(5):1414-23.

44. Gaddipati S, Berkowitz RL, Lembet AA, et al. Initial fetal platelet counts predict the response to intravenous gammaglobulin therapy in fetuses that are affected by PLA1 incompatibility. Am J Obstet Gynecol. 200;185(4):976-80.

45. Overton TG, Duncan KR, Jolly M, et al. Serial aggressive platelet transfusion for fetal alloimmune thrombocytopenia: platelet dynamics and perinatal outcome. Am J Obstet Gynecol. 2002;186(4):826-31.

46. Weiner CP. Umbilical venous pressure measurement in the evaluation of nonimmune hydrops. Am J Obstet Gynecol. 1993;168:817-23.

47. Weiner Z, Efrat Z, Zimmer EZ, et al. Direct measurement of central venous pressure in human fetuses. Am J Obstet Gynecol. 1997;176:S19.

48. Wenstrom KD, Weiner CP, Williamson RA, et al. Prenatal diagnosis of fetal hyperthyroidism using funipuncture. Obstet Gynecol. 1990;75:1-5.

49. Yankowitz J, Weiner CP. Medical fetal therapy. Clin Obstet Gynaecol. 1995;9:553-70.

50. Salerno M, Di Maio S, Militerni R, et al. Prognostic factors in the intellectual development at 7 years of age in children with congenital hypothyroidism. J Endocrinol Invest. 1995;18:774-9.

51. Kooistra L, van der Meere JJ, Vulsma T, et al. Sustained attention problems in children with early treated congenital hypothyroidism. Acta Paediatrica. 1996;85:425-9.

52. Weber G, Siragusa V, Rondanini GF, et al. Neurophysiologic studies and cognitive function in congenital hypothyroid children. Ped Res. 1995;37:736-40.

53. Van Loon AJ, Derksen JT, Bos AF, et al. In utero diagnosis and treatment of fetal goitrous hypothyroidism, caused by maternal use of propylthiouracil. Prenatal Diagnosis. 1995;15:599-604.

68

Perinatal Rh Hemolytic Disease and Other Alloimmunizations: Screening and Treatment

LS Voto

INTRODUCTION

Severe hemolytic disease due to Rh-incompatibility still constitutes a source of concern for obstetricians and pediatricians. In Argentina, as well as in most developing countries, this disease is one of the main causes of fetoneonatal morbidity and mortality due to the lack of appropriate prophylaxis with postpartum anti-D gamma globulin and inadequate prenatal control.[1]

Perinatal hemolytic disease (PHD) represents one of the most significant examples in medicine of successful management of a disease and adequate prophylaxis.

By the first half of the century PHD accounted for 45% of all perinatal deaths. Nowadays, this rate has significantly decreased to 5%, as a result of in depth understanding of the etiology and pathogenesis of the disease, the advances in perinatal technology, the creation of sophisticated centers for high risk perinatal care and, mainly, from its prophylaxis.

Rh BLOOD GROUP ANTIGENS

Biochemistry and Molecular Genetics

A group of nonglycosylated hydrophobic transmembrane proteins of 30–32 kDa are known to carry the Rh blood antigens (D, Ce and Ee series). These proteins, which are not found in the red cells of rare Rh-null individuals with membrane defects, are erythroid specific and have a distinctive sequence homology. The Rh-D and non-D proteins show 92% sequence identity and a similar predicted membrane topology.

The Rh proteins D and Cc/Ee are encoded by the Rh-D and RHCE genes, respectively, these genes are arranged in tandem on chromosome 1p34-p36 and probably result from the duplication of a common ancestral gene.

The human Rh locus is considered a two-gene model where all Rh-D positive haplotypes have two structural genes (namely, Rh-D and RHCE) and most Rh-D negative ones have only one structural gene (namely, RHCE). D protein is encoded by the Rh-D gene, whereas the C/c and E/e proteins are encoded by the RHCE gene. The relationship between blood group D epitopes and the amino acid polymorphisms of the Rh proteins still remains unclear, but it has been found that the molecular basis for the C/c (Ser → Pro) and E/e (Pro → Ala) specificities result from aminoacid polymorphisms at positions 103 and 226, respectively. In the Rh system, polymorphism and gene diversity seem to be produced mainly by gene conversion. But cases of gene deletion have also been observed in the Rh system. Rh-null phenotypes have been found to be caused by a mechanism of transcriptional regulation, which has not been clearly described yet.

In the cells of the Rh-null individuals, morphological and functional abnormalities of cation transport as well as phospholipid asymmetry have been observed and are thought to lead to severe clinical conditions. Also, Rh proteins and other glycoproteins (such as Rh50 glycoprotein, CD47, glycophorin B, Duffy, LW) are either not present, or their quantity is markedly lower in the Rh-null individuals' cells, which might mean that Rh proteins form a multimeric complex with these glycoproteins.[2]

Etiology and Pathogenesis of Rh-Hr Incompability

The antigens of the Rh system are located on the surface of the erythrocyte, although, they are also thought to be part of the trophoblast.[3]

Rh system's anti-D antibodies are responsible for the majority of clinically detectable PHD cases. This situation is observed in Rh negative mothers whose husbands are Rh positive, and whose immunization occurred during pregnancy, abortion, postpartum or incompatible transfusion.

There are other Rh-Hr system's antibodies that are capable of producing a clinical disease.

They are listed below in order of frequency:

Anti-C (Hr's), anti-C (Rh'), anti-E (Hr'') or the combination of any of them with factor D.

In Argentina, 13% of couples are Rh incompatible, and it is estimated that there is 1 PHD case every 150 deliveries. On the other hand, according to different statistics, the immunization rate is between 7% and 14%.

Rh-sensitization Mechanism

The passage of fetal red blood cells to maternal circulation is considered normal during pregnancy. Using the Kleihauer-Betke technique it was established the passage of fetal red blood cells is not higher than 0.1–0.2 mL. In this case the competent immunological system would not be activated; however, the chances of it being stimulated are much higher if transplacental hemorrhage is greater than the established values.

There are certain obstetric events that can increase the risk, such as placenta previa, ruptured placental membranes, external version, cesarean section, manual removal of placenta, and in the early stages of pregnancy—abortion, and ectopic pregnancy.

All invasive procedures during pregnancy cause passage of fetal red blood cells. Chorionic villous sampling performed during the first trimester of pregnancy, which is frequently used nowadays, has been associated with very severe cases of hemolytic disease even with hydrops. Amniocentesis causes fetomaternal hemorrhage in 2–3% of the cases. Spontaneous or induced abortion if also associated with transplacental hemorrhage.

Antigen D has already developed by the 35th to 45th day of gestation, which explains why 4–5% of postabortion patients may become sensitized. Intravenous drug abuse can also lead to isoimmunization.

When an Rh-negative person receives Rh-positive blood an immunologic response takes place in 50% or more of the cases.

The primary immunologic response is usually weak. The initial antibodies are of IgM nature, with a high molecular weight and are unlikely to cross the placenta. As a result, they do not produce fetal hemolysis labely in pregnancy, the IgG antibodies, cross the placenta and produce hemolysis.

The IgG antibodies involved in the etiology and pathogenesis of PHD due to anti D, are mainly subtypes of IgG I and IgG III. The former crosses the placenta early in pregnancy, and therefore have a role in the most severe cases of PHD.

In our experience, the frequency of immunization in Rh-negative patients during their second pregnancy with compatible Rh-positive fetuses is 12–15%.

ABO incompatibility in an Rh-negative patient provides partial protection against primary anti-Rh isoimmunization, but not against a secondary immunologic response. In the former, the anti-A or anti-B incompatibility immunized blood cells are captured by the liver, which is not an immunologically active organ and does not produce anti-Rh antibodies.

On the other hand, in a secondary immunologic response, the spleen receives the blood cell stroma and produces anti-Rh antibodies. Therefore, there is a higher incidence of Rh hemolytic disease in children whose parents are HBO compatible.

PATHOGENESIS AND PHYSIOPATHOLOGY OF PERINATAL HEMOLYTIC DISEASE

According to different studies, the rate of active transport of human IgG varies in the course of normal gestation; before 12 weeks of pregnancy this transfer is very low, but it has been demonstrated that, in severe Rh disease, the direct antiglobulin test on the fetal (Rh-positive) red cells may be positive as early as 6–10 weeks. The IgG antibodies rise exponentially until term. Sometimes, IgG levels in the infants could be higher than in the mother. The placental transport of IgG1 and IgG3 in women with Rh (D) immunizations is not diminished compared with normal pregnancy. The placental transport of IgG3 is significantly higher in pregnancies at risk of hemolytic disease of the newborn with IgG3 concentrations in normal pregnancy.[4]

The pathogenesis of PHD lies in the hemolysis of fetal erythrocytes caused by maternal antibodies. Hemolysis then results in fetal anemia.

According to the severity of hemolysis, PHD will be anemic, ictero-anemic or hydropic. In hydropic PHD, the hepatic parenchyma is replaced partially with secondary erythropoiesis tissue, which causes a portal and umbilical venous hypertension syndrome, as well as alterations in the metabolism of proteins and decreased albumin. Both clinical conditions cause edema and ascites, which are characteristic of hydrops.

Frequently, fetal cardiac failure secondary to severe anemia is observed. Both other forms of PHD, anemic and ictero-anemic, are the result of a less severe hemolysis that does not compromise either the cardiocirculatory system or the protein metabolism.

EARLY FETAL GENE DIAGNOSIS

The use of polymerase chain reaction (PCR) for detection of the RHD gene can measure the RHD gene status for unborn babies at risk for hemolytic disease of the newborn. The occurrence of D gene variants has led to errors in prenatal typing. The effectiveness of using PCR in a clinical setting has been reported. It verifies the importance of testing more than one region of the gene and also the need for a testing strategy where both maternal and paternal testing for RHD gene dosages are performed.[5]

In present time, it is possible to determine the fetal DNA in maternal serum during the first trimester of pregnancy. The advantage of this method is its noninvasive nature.[6]

FOLLOW-UP OF THE Rh-NEGATIVE PATIENT

The anamnesis will focus on relevant data such as: number of previous deliveries, history of anti-D prophylaxis, history of perinatal morbidity and mortality attributable to hemolysis, history of previous transfusions, and history of neonatal exchange transfusions or luminotherapy in previous deliveries.

If an indirect Coombs test does not detect anti-D antibodies, it should be repeated every 4 weeks until immediate puerperium. If the test is positive we will proceed as follows:

- Study of husband's zygosity. If he is heterozygous, the fetus might not be Rh-positive.
- Serial titration of anti-D antibodies every 3 weeks with the purpose of drawing a curve.
- Serial ultrasonographic follow-up to evaluate fetal growth or detect characteristic signs of the disease: polyhydramnios, hepatomegaly, ascites, soft tissue edema, etc.
- MCA peak systolic velocity provides a noninvasive modality for determining moderate to severe fetal anemia. This technique does not differentiate between mild fetal anemia and no anemia. The sensitivity of an increased peak systolic velocity in the MCA for prediction of moderate to severe fetal anemia is 100% either in the presence or the absence of hydrops fetalis and the false positive is 12%.[7,8] On the contrary, amniotic fluid is more direct to predict the fetal status and it constitutes an intermediate step for cordocentesis when it is difficult to implement it.[9] The timing of the initial amniocentesis depends on the patient's history and antibody titer. If the patient's antibody titer is just at the critical level and the patient has not had a baby with EBF, the initial amniocentesis can be done at 28–29 week of gestation. If the titer or the history suggests that the EBF may be more severe, then amniocentesis can be performed earlier. In this way, a fetus that needs an intrauterine transfusion can be identified. Many methods have been used to evaluate AF by detecting fetal hemolysis. Liley plotted curves of AF DOD450 values based on gestational age and derived three zones of severity of fetal disease. Therefore, using the Liley curves, fetal condition can be predicted based on the AF DOD450 value.[10,11]
- Amniotic fluid spectrophotometry, in accordance with previous history of Rh disease and levels of anti-D antibodies in relation to the patient's gestational age.
- Cordocentesis for the prediction of the severity of fetal anemia through the analysis of fetal blood is used since the

development of high-resolution US. It is indicated in cases either requiring assessment of fetal anemia < 26 weeks of gestation (anti-D titers > 1/128) or showing amniotic fluid spectrophotometric analysis in the upper zone B or zone C of Liley's chart, anterior placenta and a poor obstetric history.[12]

- Antenatal fetal monitoring as soon as it is reliable to assess fetal vitality and specially esinusoid patterns.

TREATMENT OF SEVERE MATERNAL FETAL Rh-INCOMPATIBILITY

In 1963 Liley described intrauterine transfusion as the only possible way to prevent intrauterine fetal death of severely affected Rh-positive fetuses. When pregnancy interruption is indicated, fetal prematurity becomes an aggravating factor, which conspires against successful results.

The purpose of all the procedures described below is to allow the fetus to reach viability.

Intrauterine Fetal Transfusion

Intraperitoneal Route

It is estimated that the total amount of blood transfused into the peritoneal cavity flows into fetal bloodstream within 7–10 days after being injected.

This technique relies on the absorption capability of the fetal peritoneum and subdiaphragmatic lymphatic, and it is not usually indicated before the 24th week gestation. Ultrasound plays an essential role in this procedure: it locates the fetal abdomen and shows the precise point of entry.

The inferior portion of the peritoneal cavity is then accessed, considering the bladder as a reference point to prevent injury to the liver or spleen.

Type O, Rh-negative blood—compatible with maternal blood—with a hematocrit concentration not less than 75% should be transfused. Blood should have been recently extracted (not more than 48 hours before the procedure).

Ascites, if present, should be evacuated before the procedure, although in this case, the intravascular route is always preferred.

The use of uterine inhibitors is recommended, and the administration of antibiotics in order to prevent possible infections is controversial.

The procedure should be repeated, according to the patient's evolution, every 14 days or more, until fetal viability is achieved.

The amount of blood to be transfused should be estimated as follows—gestational age in weeks minus 20, multiplied by 10. For example, in a 28 weeks of pregnancy (28–20) × 10 = 80, a total of 80 mL of erythrocytes should be transfused.

Intravascular Fetal Transfusion

Indications to use this approach are—especially in case of fetal hydrops or very severe fetal anemia. This technique, which may be used as from 18 weeks of pregnancy, involves access to an umbilical vessel near its placental insertion, in the intrahepatic portion of the umbilical vein or in the fetal heart (fetal rescue operation).

Nowadays, this procedure is superior to the former because it allows the immediate reversal of fetal anemia as it is possible to obtain a sample of fetal blood and determine its hematocrit and hemoglobin values. Also, a faster remission of fetal hydrops is observed in most of the cases.

The amount of blood to be transfused depends on the patient's gestational age, and blood donor's and fetal blood's hematocrit. The procedure should be repeated according to post-transfusion hematocrit values, until fetal extraction is indicated.

If no complications occur, this technique allows the lengthening of intrauterine fetal life until the fetus is viable, which results in a marked decrease in perinatal mortality rates.

High-dose Intravenous IgG for the Treatment of Severe Rhesus Alloimmunization

Intrauterine fetal transfusion, either by the intraperitoneal or intravascular routes, has shown to be an effective treatment of Rh-hemolytic disease. However, some fetuses are already severely compromised at an early stage when it is technically impossible to indicate the procedure.

In agreement with other authors, we have found that repeated invasive techniques result in an important increase in anti-D titers owing to the variable amounts of fetomaternal bleeding inevitably caused by the procedure itself. As a result of this, a moderate Rh disease in a present pregnancy can often become a severe one in the subsequent gestation.

It has been reported that transfusional therapy before 32 weeks of gestation is associated with a higher fetal mortality rate.[13] The early treatment in the first weeks of pregnancy would reduce the severity of fetal anemia, decreasing the fetal morbidity and mortality. That is why we started a protocol of treatment with high doses of gammaglobulin.[1]

The use of high doses of intravenous immunoglobulin (IVIG) in the treatment of immunologic diseases both in children and adults and recurrent intrauterine fetal loss has been frequently reported in the literature with varying degrees of effectiveness.

Although the mechanisms of action of IVIG remain unclear, several explanations have been proposed during pregnancy—feedback inhibition of antibody synthesis, competition for macrophage or Fc receptors of target cells, and blockade of Fc-mediated antibody placental transport. We have used IVIG therapy in a prospective study in order to analyze its effectiveness in the antenatal treatment of severe Rh-hemolytic disease.

The only immunoglobulin, which is transferred into the fetal circulation is IgG; the other classes of maternal immunoglobulins are either not transferred or only cross the placenta in small quantities. The mechanisms involved in the active transfer of IgG across the human placenta are not yet known. Brambell et al's studies in rabbits suggest that the transport of IgG molecules across the placenta is mediated through a receptor for the Fc part of the molecule. Further studies have clarified the role of Fc as a placental Fc receptor for IgG. This receptor has been demonstrated on the surface of the trophoblast at 10 weeks and at term.

The mechanisms of placenta transfer of exogenous IgG infused into the mother are still to be elucidated. It must be emphasized that transplacental IgG transfer is a slow process and requires an intact

Fc portion of the IgG molecule. Gitlin et al's studies demonstrated that when labeled IgG was injected into pregnant women at various intervals before delivery, even after 12 days, the concentration in the infant's serum was only about 40% of that in the mother. Studies performed by Contractor et al. about IgG transport in perfused placentas suggest that the trophoblast absorbs a substantial amount of human IgG and all bovine IgG, both broken down in small fractions by a mechanism of nonspecific endocytosis, and transmits these fragments to the fetal circulation. A small amount of human IgG, however, would escape this process of lysosomal destruction by diverse protective mechanisms, and would be released intact on the fetal side.

There are very few cases in the literature reporting the treatment of severe Rh-hemolytic disease with high doses of IVIG and the findings are too dissimilar to allow for conclusive generalizations. Rewald and Berlin et al. obtained satisfactory results with the combined use of plasmapheresis and IVIG in four cases of severe Rh-hemolytic disease. De la Cámara et al. reported the successful treatment of two cases with repeated doses of IVIG throughout gestation. Scott et al., on the other hand, used a combined protocol of IVIG and repeated intrauterine transfusions in one case of hemolytic disease.

We have administered IVIG as the only treatment in 24 severely Rh-sensitized patients with a previous history of affected fetuses and/or neonates, with elevated anti-D titers, and a high degree of intrauterine hemolysis. Patients in group 1 (< 20 weeks, n = 8) fulfilled the first two of these inclusion criteria, whereas in groups 2 (20–28 weeks, n = 7) and 3 (> 28 weeks, n = 9), IVIG treatment was indicated on the basis of intrauterine hemolysis.

IVIG was infused at a daily dose of 0.4 g/kg maternal body weight for 4–5 consecutive days, and repeated every 21 days until delivery.

Group 3 also included those patients who attended the antenatal clinic very late in pregnancy; as a consequence of this delay, the fetuses in these cases were highly compromised because of the advanced stage of the hemolytic disease, and they evidenced major neonatal depression and severe fetal anemia at birth, requiring—in almost all cases—exchange transfusions.

Initial mean anti-D level was significantly higher in group 1 (25.9 ± 12.9 IU/mL) than in the other two groups, whose values were, however, higher than 10 IU/mL. Amniotic fluid total bilirubin levels before the onset of therapy were pathologic and in 55% of the cases they coincided with zone 3 of Liley's chart. Hydrops fetalis at the onset of treatment accounted for the only three fetal deaths in groups 1 and 2. None of the fetuses developed hydrops during treatment.

Six of the nine neonates in group 3 were depressed at birth (1-min Apgar below 7). However, at 5 minutes only 1 newborn showed an Apgar below 7. Mean birth weight was over 2,500 g in all the cases. Neonatal hematological condition in group 2 (50% of the babies required only phototherapy) was better than in the other two groups (transfusional therapy).

The decrease in pre- versus post-treatment anti-D antibody quantification, the reduction in intrauterine hemolysis, and the strongly positive direct antiglobulin test in all neonates may indicate that the mode of action of high doses of IVIG in Rh hemolytic disease is (1) feedback inhibition of antibody synthesis, and (2) partial blockade of Fc mediated antibody transport across the placenta. No adverse effects from the drug were observed in the mother or neonate.

Our findings show that IVIG treatment was effective in both groups 1 and 2, where IVIG was administered before the 28th week of gestation and the fetuses were not hydropic at the onset of therapy. In group 3, however, where fetal anemia was already advanced at the time of treatment, intrauterine transfusions and prompt fetal extraction should have been the treatment of choice.

The analysis of the series including only the 13 most severely affected cases as judged by their history of fetal/neonatal death, demonstrated again the effectiveness of IVIG treatment. It can be inferred from the results in this particular group of patients that— (1) after 28 weeks of gestation the administration of IVIG does not elicit significant reductions in anti-D titers and intrauterine hemolysis, thus intrauterine transfusion is the therapy of choice, and (2) IVIG treatment is not indicated in case of hydrops fetalis. Excepting these two indications, it is in this series with the poorest history, the highest antibody level, and failure of transfusional therapy in previous gestations, where we find the most encouraging therapeutical results of IVIG treatment.

The high cost of IVIG therapy is immediately outweighed by the highly satisfactory perinatal results obtained in our population of extremely severe Rh-sensitized patients. Moreover, babies born after treatment with intrauterine transfusions, as well as those prematurely delivered because of their severe disease, require a prolonged stay in the neonatal intensive care unit (a mean of 60 days in the latter case), the cost of which greatly exceeds that of IVIG therapy.

To conclude, the results of our study, which to the best of our knowledge is the largest reported in the literature, show the value of high doses of IVIG in the treatment of severe Rh incompatibility when administered repeatedly before 28 weeks of gestation and in the absence of hydrops fetalis.

High-dose Gammaglobulin (IVIG) Followed by Intrauterine Transfusions (IUTs): A New Alternative for the Treatment of Severe Fetal Hemolytic Disease

Intrauterine fetal transfusion is currently the therapy of choice in cases of severe anti-D isoimmunization. However, its efficacy is reduced in patients with early severe hydrops fetalis due to the technical difficulties in performing this procedure before 20 weeks of gestation and because the fetuses are already anemic at that term.

The purpose of this study was to determine whether early onset of high-dose gammaglobulin therapy followed by intrauterine transfusions (IUTs) is more effective than IUTs alone in the treatment of very severe isoimmunized fetuses.

The population studied in this retrospective clinical research was assigned to one of the following two groups: (1) Gamma group: 30 patients receiving gammaglobulin therapy before 21 weeks of gestation and IUTs after 20 weeks; or (2) IUT group: 39 patients receiving IUT treatment starting at a gestational age of 20–25 weeks.

Both groups were statistically similar regarding history of perinatal deaths and anti-D antibody titers. The number of hydropic fetuses at the first IUT and of fetal deaths were significantly higher in the IUT than in the Gamma group. No significant differences were observed between the groups in fetal hematocrit at first IUT and at birth. However, the percentage of severely anemic fetuses was higher in the IUT group. Fetal mortality rate was 36% less in the gamma group.

In summary, considering that in very severe cases of Rh-isoimmunization:

a. The development of fetal hemolysis in the first 20 weeks of gestation increases the risk of fetal death;
b. The early onset of invasive fetal therapy is only partially effective and potentially harmful; and
c. According to the present study, those patients who received high-dose intravenous gammaglobulin in the first 20 weeks of pregnancy, seem to have a better fetal outcome.

Our results show that high-dose gammaglobulin therapy followed by IUTs improves fetal survival in these severe cases.[14] Conventional treatment has also been modified by the administration of immunoglobulin to the neonate.[15]

Neonatal Treatment

Our studies suggest that the frequency of neonatal transfusion therapy can be reduced by a combination of conventional phototherapy with high-dose intravenous immunoglobulin (HDIVIG). Further studies are needed to determine the optimum timing and dosage of HDIVIG therapy.[16]

Other studies show that the intravenous immunoglobulin is effective in decreasing the maximum bilirubin levels and the need for repeated exchange transfusions in Rh hemolytic disease of the newborn. There is, however, an increased need of blood transfusions for late anemia in the babies treated with IVIG.[17]

Other Alloimmunizations

Routine antibody screening of Rh (D)-positive women is probably not warranted from a clinical cost-benefit perspective.[18]

Anti-C isoimmunization follow-up is similar to that of anti-D and, together with anti-E, they are the next in order of frequency as a cause of perinatal alloimmunization.[19]

The treatment for anti-E sensitization is similar to that of anti-D. Amniotic fluid is a weak indicator of the result, that is why the management of the disease remains questionable. It is not clear yet if the presence of anti-E implies the accummlation of a hemolytic effect with other antibodies.

Pregnancy Follow-up in Anti-Kell Alloimmunization

It is identified by the presence of anti-Kell antibodies in maternal serum or previous fetal anemia. The search for hemolysis in amniotic fluid through bilirubin concentration is not useful as the pathogenesis responds to fetal anemia due to the inhibition of erythroid progenitor and not to the destruction of the Kell-positive erythroid by the antibodies.

Therefore, cordocentesis should be chosen to obtain fetal blood and, in this way, be able to detect fetal anemia and make the Kell-serotyping by studying the fetal DNA when the father is K1 heterozygous.

Other studies show that fetal anemia due to anti-Kell isoimmunization might be due in part to erythropoietic suppression, but it is still largely a hemolytic process. The methods based on a hemolytic process, including use of a critical maternal serum titer of

1:32, serial amniotic fluid analyses when the titer was exceed and liberal use of venipuncture were successful in identifying severely affected fetuses.[20]

Natural and monoclonal anti-Kell antibodies inhibit the growth in the Kell-positive erythroid progenitor.

Fetal Hematology

It shows just a few reticulocytosis and normoblasts compared to fetuses affected by anti-D, which suggests that erythroid suppression would be the mechanism responsible for fetal anemia, mechanism that has been proved by Vaughan's studies.[21]

The treatment is similar to that of the anti-D. Needless to say, an ultrasound follow-up is very important.

SUMMARY: STEPS TO FOLLOW

Steps to follow for Rh-isoimmunization are shown in Flow charts 68.1 to 68.3.

Flow chart 68.1: Rh-isoimmunization: (non-immunized patients) Patients with no maternal and/or perinatal history of the disease

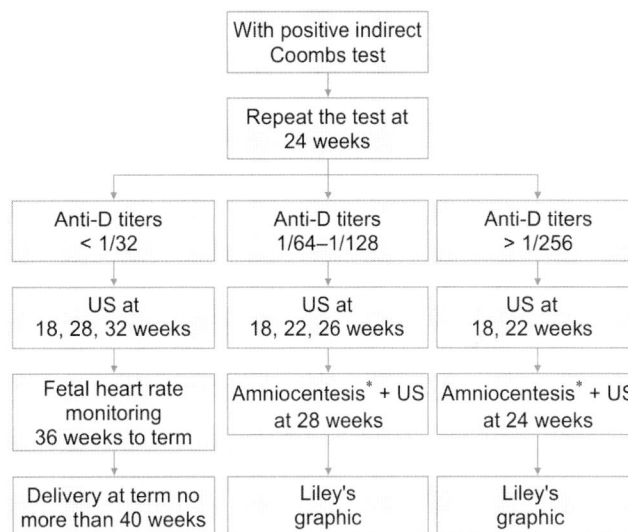

| With positive indirect Coombs test |
| Repeat the test at 24 weeks |

Anti-D titers < 1/32	Anti-D titers 1/64–1/128	Anti-D titers > 1/256
US at 18, 28, 32 weeks	US at 18, 22, 26 weeks	US at 18, 22 weeks
Fetal heart rate monitoring 36 weeks to term	Amniocentesis* + US at 28 weeks	Amniocentesis* + US at 24 weeks
Delivery at term no more than 40 weeks	Liley's graphic	Liley's graphic

*And/or MCA peak systolic velocity and conventional ultrasound

PROPHYLAXIS

In 40–50% of pregnancies, the passage of fetal red blood cells to maternal circulation usually takes place during the last trimester. In majority of the cases the amount of blood transferred is less than 0.1 mL.[22]

In 1977 there were 110 cases of still-births or postnatal deaths due to anti-D hemolytic disease in the UK. In 1992, the figure decreased to only 9 cases. This decrease came as a result of the introduction of anti-D gammaglobulin prophylaxis since 1969 but it is also subject to the application of public health policies for perinatal care, especially in developing countries.[23]

In 1969, the prophylaxis protocol consisted of anti-D gammaglobulin administration only after the birth of an Rh-positive child, or after certain pregnancy events such as antepartum hemorrhage. Most of the deaths resulted from maternal sensitization between 28 weeks and 40 weeks of the first pregnancy (third trimester) and during postpartum.

Flow chart 68.2: Rh-isoimmunization (immunized patients): Patients with no maternal and/or perinatal history of the disease

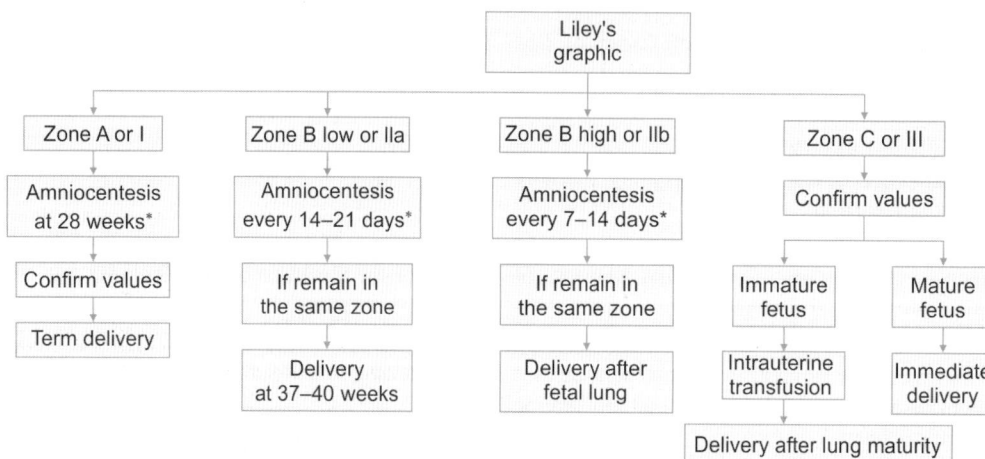

*And/or MCA peak systolic velocity and conventional ultrasound

Flow chart 68.3: Rh-isoimmunization: Patients with maternal and/or perinatal history of the disease

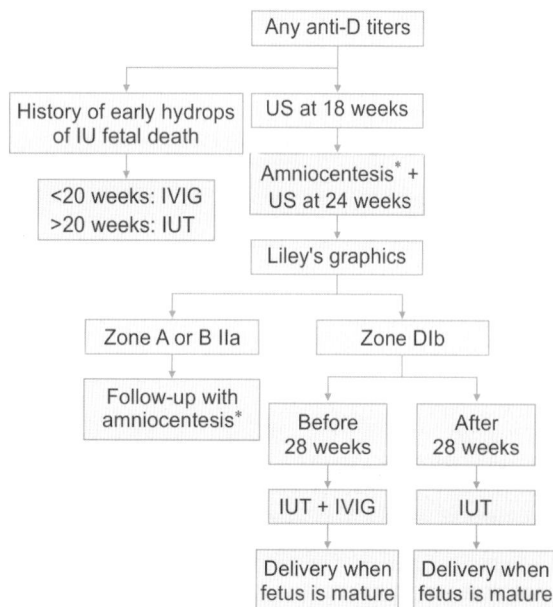

*And/or MCA peak systolic velocity and conventional ultrasound

Further studies have determined that the percentage of sensitization decreases from 1.2% to 0.28% if antenatal prophylaxis is carried out.

In practice, the combination of antenatal and postnatal prophylaxis will prevent immunization in 96% of the high risk cases. The remaining 4% corresponds to the absence or inappropriate administration of immunoglobulin when it is indicated.

Due to the fact that isoimmunization during pregnancy is caused by transplacental hemorrhage,[24] the risk of immunization increases after the following procedures:

1. Spontaneous or induced abortion
2. Amniocentesis
3. Chorionic villous sampling
4. Cordocentesis
5. Ectopic pregnancy
6. Fetal manipulation: external version
7. Antepartum hemorrhage
8. Antepartum fetal death
9. Positive blood transfusion.

The standard postpartum dose of 300 mg contains enough anti-D to neutralize atleast 15 mL of fetal red blood cells.

There are different methods to detect excessive fetomaternal hemorrhage:

- Kleihauer Betke if carried out correctly, is a very sensitive and specific method, but it is subject to laboratory and technological errors.
- Flow cytometry is also a very sensitive method, but difficult to perform and too expensive.
- The Rosette method is easy to carryout and very sensitive, but has low specificity and its results must be confirmed by Kleihauer or flow cytometry.
- A gel technology method has been reported for the assessment of fetomaternal hemorrhage and determination of minimum necessary dose of Rh-IG. This technique works well in determining the appropriate dose of anti-D required to treat D-patients with D+ newborns. There are potential cost savings in decreased use of Rh-IG, less direct technical time required and more rapid availability of results.[25]

Anti-D gammaglobulin has very few adverse effects. Some fetuses yield with a slightly positive direct Coombs test at birth after antenatal administration. The presence of anemia or hyperbilirubinemia is very rare. All plasma involved in the production of anti-D immunoglobulin is carefully checked for infectious diseases.

There have not been any HIV cases due to contaminated plasma.

The American College of Obstetricians and Gynecologists recommends both typifying the pregnant patient and looking for antibodies in her first visit, and again at 24–28 weeks, offering anti-D gammaglobulin to all Rh-negative, nonsensitized patients.

It has been found that transplacental hemorrhage occurs in 3%, 12% and 45% of the cases during the first, second and third trimesters, respectively.

The capacity of an antibody to eliminate D-red cells in vivo depends both on its avidity, and to a lesser degree, on its affinity for the D-antigen. Absorption is also a limiting factor.

Even though, antepartum gammaglobulin administration offers many additional benefits, some authors argue that, as the incidence of isoimmunization is relatively small, it makes medication 16 times less cost-effective than postpartum prevention programs. The Cochrane review states that anti-D, given within 72 hours after childbirth reduces the risk of RhD alloimmunization in Rhesus negative women who have given birth to a Rhesus positive infant. However, the evidence on the optimal dose is limited.[26]

Unit Equivalents

- 50 µg 250 IU
- 100 µg 500 IU
- 300 µg 1,500 IU
- 225 µg 1,250 IU.

Route of Administration

Intramuscular route, deltoids muscle. In the gluteal area, it only penetrates to subcutaneous tissue, thus absorption is prolonged.

Anti-D IgG Use Recommendations

- Dose: 500 IU or 100 µg every 4 mL of fetal red blood cells in maternal circulation.

- Indications:
  - Postpartum, within the first 72 hours = 300 mg
  - Prenatal:
    a. First trimester: Abortion, ectopic pregnancy, chorionic villous sampling or amniocentesis.
    b. Second trimester: Suspected fetomaternal hemorrhage, invasive procedures
    c. Third trimester: Prophylactic: 500 IU at 28 and 34 weeks or only one dose of 300 µg between above-mentioned weeks.[27]

GENERAL AND FUTURE MANAGEMENT OF Rh-D ISOIMMUNIZATION

Future therapy will involve selective modulation of the maternal immune system turning the need for intrauterine transfusions into a rarity.[28]

When RhD sensitization occurs, careful follow-up of these mothers and judicious intervention can result in good outcomes for most pregnancies. Both Doppler assessment of middle cerebral artery peak systolic velocity and spectral analysis of amniotic fluid at 450 nm (ΔOD_{450}) are useful in the diagnosis and management of fetal anemia.[29]

REFERENCES

1. Margulies M, Voto LS, Mathet E, et al. High-dose intravenous IgG for the treatment of severe alloimmunization. Department of Maternal-Fetal Medicine, Juan A. Fernández Hospital, University of Buenos Aires School of Medicine. Buenos Aires, Argentina. Vox Sang. 1991;61:181-9.
2. Carton JP. Defining the Rh blood group antigens. Biochemistry and molecular genetics. Blood Rev. 1994;8:199-212.
3. Hohlfeld P, Wirthner D, Tissot JA. Perinatal hemolytic disease: physiopathology. J Ginecol Obstet Biol Reprod. 1998;27(2):135-43.
4. Palfi M, Hilden JO, Gottvall T, et al. Placental transport of maternal immunoglobulin-G in pregnancies at risk of Rh (D) hemolytic disease of the newborn. Department of Transfusion Medicine and Clinical Immunology, University Hospital, Linkoping, Sweden. National Library of Medicine. Medline. Am J Reprod Immunol. 1998;39(5):323-8.
5. Chan FY, Cowley NM, Wolter L, et al. Prenatal RHD gene determination and dosage analysis by PCR: Clinical evaluation. Department of Maternal-Fetal Medicine, Mater Mother's Hospital, South Brisbane, Australia. National Library of Medicine. Prenat Diagn. 2001;21(4):321-6.
6. Costa JM, Giovangrandi Y, Ernault P, et al. Fetal RHD genotyping in maternal serum during the first trimester of pregnancy. Centre de Diagnostic Prenatal, American Hospital of Paris, Neuilly, France. Br J Haematol. 2002;119(1):25560.
7. Mari G, Deter RL, Carpenter RL, et al. Noninvasive diagnosis by Doppler ultrasonography of fetal anemia due to maternal red-cell alloimmunization. Collaborative Group for Doppler Assessment of the Blood Velocity in Anemia Fetuses. N Engl J Med. 2000; 342:914.
8. Queenan JT. Rh isoimmunization. Georgetown University School of Medicine, Washington DC, USA. Contemporary OB/GYN Archive. 2002.
9. Nishie EN, Brizot ML, Liao AW, et al. A comparison between middle cerebral artery peak velocity and amniotic fluid optical density at 450 nm in the prediction of fetal anemia. Department of Obstetrics, Hospital das Clinicas, Sao Paulo University Medical School, Sao Paulo, Brazil. Am J Obstet Gynecol. 2003;188(1):214-9.
10. Liley AW. Liquor amnii analysis in the management of the pregnancy complicated by rhesus sensitization. Am J Obstet Gynecol. 1961;82:1359.
11. Liley AW. Errors in the assessment of haemolytic disease from amniotic fluid. Am J Obstet Gynecol. 1969;86:485.
12. Voto LS. Ultrasonography in Rh hemolytic disease. Head, Maternal-Fetal Medicine Department, Juan A. Fernández Hospital, University of Buenos Aires, School of Medicine, Buenos Aires, Argentina.
13. Klumper FJ, van Kamp IL, Vandenbussche FP, et al. Benefits and risks of fetal red-cell transfusion after 32 weeks gestation. Department of Obstetrics and Fetal Medicine, Leiden University Medical Center, Leiden, The Netherlands. Eur J Obstet Gynecol Reprod Biol. 2000;92(1):91-6.
14. Voto LS, Mathet ER, Zapaterio JL, et al. High-dose gammaglobulin (IVIG) followed by intrauterine transfusions (IUTs): A new alternative for the treatment of severe fetal hemolytic disease. Maternal-Fetal Department, Juan A Fernández Hospital, University of Buenos Aires, Buenos Aires, Argentina. J Perinat Med. 1997;25:85-8.
15. Porter TF, Silver RM, Jackson GM, et al. Intravenous immune globulin in the management of severe RhD hemolytic disease. Obstet Gynecol Surv. 1997;52(3):193-7.
16. Voto LS, Sexer H, Ferreiro G, et al. Neonatal administration of high-dose intravenous immuno-globulin in rhesus hemolytic disease. Division of Obstetrics and Unit of Neonatology, Juan A. Fernández Hospital, University of Buenos Aires, Argentina. J Perinat Med. 1995;23:443-51.
17. Mukhopadhyay K, Murki S, Narang A et al. Intra-venouse immunoglobulins in rhesus hemolytic disease. Neonatal Unit, Department of Pediatrics, Postgraduate Institute of Medical Education and Research, Chandigarh, India. Indian J Pediatr. 2003;70(9):697-9.

18. Lurie S, Eliezer E, Piper I, et al. Is antibody screening in Rh (D)-positive pregnant women necessary? Women's Health Center, Netka, Tel Aviv, Israel. J Matern Fetal Neonatal Med. 2003;14(6):404-6.

19. Hackney DN, Knudtson EJ, Rossi KQ, et al. Management of pregnancies complicated by anti c isoimmunization. Department of Obstetrics and Gynecology, The Ohio State University, College of Medicine and Public Health, Columbus, Ohio, USA.

20. McKenna DS, Nagaraja HN, O'Shaughnessy R. Management of pregnancies complicated by anti-Kell isoimmunization. Department of Obstetrics and Gynecology, The Ohio State University, College of Medicine, Columbus, Ohio, USA.

21. Vaughan JI, Warwick R, Letsky E, et al. Erythropoietic suppression in fetal anemia because of Kell alloimmunization. Am J Obstet Gynecol. 1994;171:247-52.

22. Jorgensen J. Fetal-maternal bleeding during pregnancy and delivery. Acta Obstet Gynecol Scand. 1977;56:487-90.

23. Joseph KS, Kramer MS. The decline in Rh hemolytic disease: Should Rh prophylaxis get all the credit? Mc Gill University-Montreal Children's Hospital Research Institute, Quebec, Canada. Am J Public Health. 1998;88(2):209-15.

24. Quartier P, Floch C, Meier F, et al. Massive fetomaternal hemorrhage and prevention of fetomaternal Rhesus incompatibility. The failure of our present system of prevention. Service de Neonatologie, Hopital Louis-Mourier, Colombres. J Gynecol Obstet Biol Reprod (Paris). 1993;22(5):517-9.

25. Fernandes JR, Chan R, Coovadia As, et al. A gel technology system to determine postpartum RhIG dosage. Department of Laboratory Medicine and Pathobiology, University of Toronto. Immunohematol. 2000;16(3):115-9.

26. Crowther C, Middleton P. Anti-D administration after childbirth for preventing Rhesus alloimmunization. Cochrane Review. The Cochrane Library, Issue 4, 2004. Chichester, UK: John Wiley & Sons, Ltd.

27. Hartwell EA. Use of Rh immune globulin: ASCP practice parameter. American Society of Clinical Pathologists. Department of Pathology and Laboratory Medicine, University of Texas Health Science Center, Houston, USA. Am J Clin Pathol. 1998;110(3):281-92.

28. Moise KJ Jr. Management of rhesus alloimmunization in pregnancy. Division of Maternal-Fetal Medicine, University of North Carolina, School of Medicine, Chapel Hill, USA. Obstet Gynecol. 2002;100(4):833.

29. Harkness UF, Spinnato JA. Prevention and management of RhD isoimmunization. Division of Maternal Fetal Medicine, Department of Obstetrics and Gynecology, University of Cincinnati, Cincinnati, OH, USA. Clin Perinatol. 2004;31(4):721-42.

69 Prenatal Therapy of Endocrine and Metabolic Disorders

G Rosner, SB Shachar, Y Yaron

INTRODUCTION

Our understanding of molecular and genetic basis of disease is ever-incresing. This has resulted in more and better ways for primary prevention. This is often achieved by prenatal diagnosis and termination of affected pregnancies and more recently, preimplantation genetic diagnosis. Some metabolic and endocrine disorders however, such as congenital adrenal hyperplasia and cardiac arrhythmias are amenable to pharmacological interventions.[1,2] This chapter describes different modes of intrauterine pharmacological therapy in the fetus with an endocrine or metabolic disorder. The use of folic acid supplementation for the prevention of neural tube defects will also be discussed.

ENDOCRINE DISORDERS

Adrenal Disorders

Congenital Adrenal Hyperplasia

Treatment of congenital adrenal hyperplasia (CAH) in the fetus is an excellent example of pharmacological therapy during pregnancy. CAH is a group of autosomal recessive metabolic disorders characterized by an enzymatic defect in the steroidogenetic pathway. As a result of the enzymatic deficiency, there is a compensatory increase in ACTH secretion in order to maintain cortisol production. This leads to overproduction of the steroid precursors in the adrenal cortex, causing adrenal hyperplasia. The most common abnormality, responsible for > 90% of patients with CAH is caused by a deficiency of the 21-hydroxylase (21-OH) enzyme. Other, less common causes for CAH, include deficiencies in 11β-hydroxylase, 17α-hydroxylase and 3β-hydroxysteroid-dehydrogenase. Decreased 21-OH activity results in accumulation of 17-hydroxyprogesterone (17-OHP), which is converted via androstenedione to androgens, the levels of which increase by as much as several hundred-fold (Fig. 69.1). The excess of androgens cause virilization of the undifferentiated female external genitalia. The degree of virilization may vary from mild clitoral hypertrophy to complete formation of a phallus and scrotum. In contrast, genital development in males is normal. The excess androgens cause postnatal virilization in both genders and may manifest in precocious puberty.

The "classical" form of CAH involves a severe enzyme deficiency or even a complete block of enzymatic activity, which is associated in more than half of the cases with a life-threatening salt-lossing form. The classical form is easy to recognize in female newborns but may be overlooked in males, who ma y present at a later stage with severe dehydration and even demise. The "non-classical" attenuated form of 21-OH deficiency results in partial blockade of enzymatic activity and results in simple virilization in women only later in life. It is estimated to occur in ~ 3.5% in Ashkenazi jews and ~ 2% in Hispanics.[3]

The gene for 21-OH is in close linkage to the HLA major histocompatability complex on the short arm of chromosome 6.[4] The gene for 21-OH (CYP21B) has now been mapped, allowing direct mutation analysis in informative families.[5]

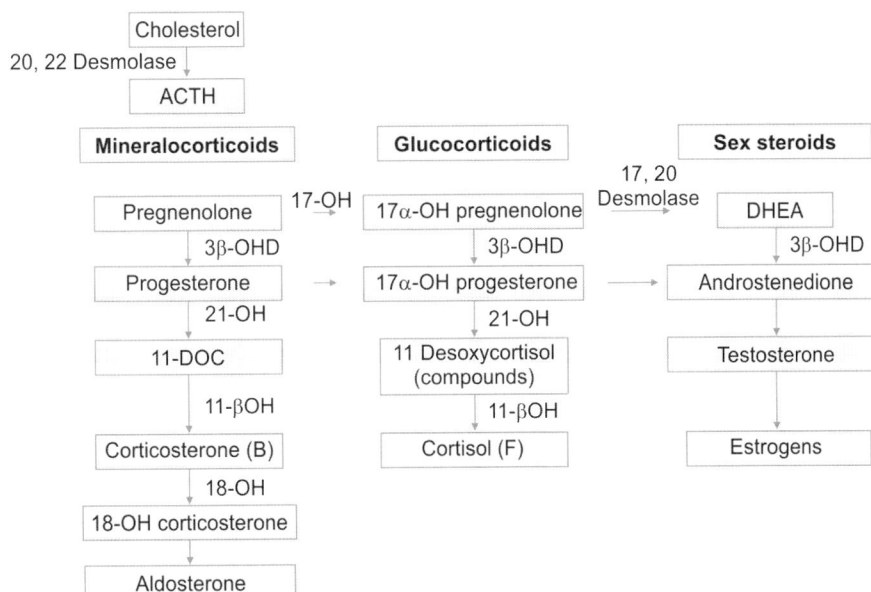

Fig. 69.1: Steroidogenic pathway: Androgen production in 21-hydroxylase deficiency (congenital adrenal hyperplasia)

In the past, diagnosis of CAH was made by the finding of elevated levels of 17-OHP in the amniotic fluid. With the development of chorionic villus sampling (CVS) in the 80s, linkage based molecular diagnosis in the first trimester became available. Since discovery and mapping of the gene, direct DNA mutation analysis has become the routine approach.

The fetal adrenal gland can be pharmacologically suppressed by maternal administration of dexamethasone.[6] The suppression can prevent masculinization of affected female fetuses in carriers couples. In the first attempt to prevent female genital birth defects in 1982, Evans et al. administered dexamethasone to a carrier mother beginning at 10 weeks of gestation.[6] Serial maternal estriol and cortisol levels indicated that adrenal gland suppression had been achieved. The female fetus was born at 39 weeks of gestation with normal external genitalia. Forrest and David then employed a similar protocol beginning at 9 weeks of gestation to treat several fetuses at risk for CAH.[7] Female fetuses subsequently confirmed to be affected with severe CAH were spared masculinization of the external genitalia. Several hundred pregnant women and their fetuses have since been treated with prevention of masculinization in more than 85% of affected females.[8] The differentiation of the external genitalia begins at about 7 weeks of gestation. Thus, diagnosis by amniocentesis or even CVS is too late to prevent masculinization. Therefore for carrier parents, pharmacological therapy has to be initiated prior to prenatal diagnosis. Therapy is administered to all patients at risk, despite the fact that the chance of an affected female fetus for carrier parents is only 1 in 8 (i.e. 1/4 affected × 1/2 female). Following molecular diagnosis, by CVS, in 7 out of 8 patients, therapy is discontinued if the diagnosis of a male is made or if CAH is ruled out. However, if the fetus is an affected female, therapy is continued throughout gestation. Stress dose corticosteroids should be given to the mother during labor and tapered gradually postpartum.

No consistent untoward effects on fetuses have been reported. Greater weight gain, edema and striae were noticed in treated mothers but no increased risk of hypertension or gestational diabetes was noted.[8]

Inclusion criteria of the European Society for Pediatric Endocrinology and Wilkins Pediatric Endocrine Society[9] for Prenatal Treatment of CAH include: (1) a previously affected sibling or first-degree relative with known mutation causing classical CAH proven by DNA analysis; (2) reasonable expectation that the father is the same as the proband's; (3) availability of rapid and quality genetic analysis; (4) therapy started less than 9 weeks following the last menstrual period; (5) lack of intent for therapeutic abortion; (6) reasonable expectation of patient's compliance.

There is an agreement that the treatment requires a professional team that includes an expert high risk obstetrician, a pediatric endocrinologist, genetic counselor and a molecular genetic laboratory.

Thyroid Disorders

Hypothyroidism

Congenital hypothyroidism affects about 1:3,000 to 1:4,000 infants.[10] About 85% of the cases are the result of thyroid dysgenesis, a heterogeneous group of developmental defects characterized by inadequate amount of thyroid tissue. Congenital hypothyroidism is only rarely associated with errors of thyroid hormone synthesis, TSH (thyroid-stimulating hormone) insensitivity or absence of the pituitary gland. Fetal hypothyroidism may not necessarily manifest in a goiter before birth since maternal thyroid hormones may cross the placenta. Congenital hypothyroidism presenting with a goiter can be found in only about 10–15% of cases, with an estimated prevalence of 1:30,000–1:50,000 livebirths.[11] Fetal goiterous hypothyroidism is caused in most instances by maternal exposure to thyrostatic agents used to treat maternal hyperthyroidism.[12] These drugs include propylthiouracil (PTU), the inadvertent use of radioactive ^{131}I in the pregnant women or iodide exposure. Maternal ingestion of amiodarone (antiarrhythmic drug) or lithium (drug for people with mood disorders may also cause hypothyroidism in the fetus. Finally, fetal hypothyroidism may result from transplacental passage of maternal blocking antibodies (known as TBIAb or TBII) or rarely due to rare defects in fetal thyroid hormone biosynthesis.[11]

Fetal goiterous hypothyroidism may lead to severe fetal and neonatal consequences. An enlarged goiter may cause esophageal obstruction which may lead to polyhydramnios, which may result in preterm delivery or premature rupture of membranes. Rarely, a goiter may even lead to high-output heart failure due to high vascular flow in the goiter.[13] A large fetal goiter can cause extension of the fetal neck leading to dystocia in labor. The effects of the fetal hypothyroidism itself may be devastating. Without treatment, postnatal growth delay and severe mental retardation may ensue. Even with immediate diagnosis and treatment at birth, long term follow-up of children with congenital hypothyroidism has demonstrated that they have lower scores on perceptual-motor, visuospatial and language tests.[14]

In suspicious cases, an extensive maternal and family history should be obtained. In patients with a positive history, maternal thyroid hormone levels, as well as blocking immunoglobulin levels should be measured. In addition, all women with a history of any thyroid disease (both hypothyroidism and hyperthyroidism) are advised to have monthly fetal ultrasound scans to screen for fetal goiter, polyhydramnios or fetal tachycardia.[15]

Occasionally, fetal goiterous hypothyroidism may be identified by and ultrasound performed due to increased uterine size caused by polyhydramnios secondary to esophageal obstruction and impaired swallowing. Sometimes, a fetal goiter may incidentally be discovered on a routine scan. Before the advent of cordocentesis, amniotic fluid levels of TSH and FT4 (free thyroxine) were used as potential indicators of fetal thyroid function. However, these proved to be inconsistent.[16] With cordocentesis, fetal thyroid status can be directly and accurately evaluated; fetal response to therapy can therefore, be reliably measured using available appropriate nomograms for fetal serum levels of FT4, total T4 (thyroxine), free T3 (triiodothyronine), total T3 and TSH.[15,17] In utero treatment was initially suggested by Van Herle et al. using intramuscular injection of levothyroxine sodium.[18] Subsequent studies however, have indicated that intra-amniotic administration of thyroxine may be superior and can lead to resolution of the polyhydramnios as well. The dose of the injected drug may be refined using the fetal thyroid profile in the amniotic fluid and the thyroid size.[19] The doses commonly used for treatment range from 200 mg to 500 mg intra-amniotic every week. With this regimen, fetal goiters have been shown to regress, the hyperextension of the fetal head have been shown to resolve, and fetal and newborn TSH levels have normalized.[19]

Hyperthyroidism

Neonatal hyperthyroidism is rare with an incidence of 1:4,000 to 1:40,000/live births.[10] Fetal thyrotoxic goiter is usually secondary to maternal autoimmune disease, principally Graves' disease or Hashimoto's thyroiditis. As many as 12% of infants of mothers with a known history of Graves' disease are affected with neonatal thyrotoxicosis, which may occur even if the mother is euthyroid.[20] As with hypothyroidism, inherent to the underlying mechanism is the transplacental passage of maternal IgG antibodies. In this case, the antibodies, known as TSAb or TSI, are predominantly directed against the TSH receptor.

Usually, the investigation of fetal hyperthyroidism begins only after the discovery of fetal goiter. Often, the goiter is diagnosed on ultrasound in patients referred due to elevated thyroid stimulating antibodies. In some cases, fetal goiters are realized serendipitously on routine ultrasonography. Others may be discovered in patients referred for scan because of polyhydramnios. Beside the risks related to the goiter itself, untreated fetal hyperthyroidism may be associated with a mortality rate of 12–25% due to high-output cardiac failure.[21] Once a fetal goiter is identified, biochemical evaluation is indicated. Historically, amniotic fluid levels of TSH and FT4 were used as potential indicators of fetal thyroid function. These, however, proved inconsistent in that amniotic fluid levels of these hormones do not always correlate with their serum levels. Some controversy still exists regarding their use, however, they may be of some benefit in centers that do not have available cordocentesis.[16] As previously stated, cordocentesis allows reliable assessment of fetal thyroid status TSH,[15,17] and treatment can be planned accordingly.

Once the diagnosis of fetal hyperthyroidism is confirmed, fetal treatment should be initiated. Authors have attempted treating fetal hyperthyroidism with maternally administered antithyroid drugs. Porreco has reported maternal treatment of fetal thyrotoxicosis with the antithyroid drug propylthiouracil (PTU), which lead to a good outcome.[22] The initial dose used was 100 mg PO three times a day, which was later decreased to 50 mg PO three times a day. Wenstrom et al. described a favorable outcome using maternal methimazole to treat fetal hyperthyroidism in a patient who could not tolerate PTU.[21] Hatjis also treated fetal goiterous hyperthyroidism with a maternal dose of 300 mg PTU. This patient however, required supplemental synthroid to remain euthyroid. There was good fetal outcome in this case as well.[23]

INBORN ERRORS OF METABOLISM
Methylmalonic Acidemia

The methylmalonic acidemias (MMA) are a group of enzyme-deficiency diseases inherited in an autosomal recessive manner resulting from one of several genetically distinct etiologies. Some cases are caused by mutations in the gene encoding methylmalonyl-coenzyme A mutase while others are due to a defect that reduces the biosynthesis of adenosylcobalamin from vitamin B_{12}. The disease is characterized by wide clinical spectrum ranging from a benign condition to a fatal neonatal disease. In the severe form, MMA is characterized by severe metabolic acidosis, developmental delay and biochemical abnormalities that include methylmalonic aciduria, long chain ketonuria and intermittent hyperglycinemia. Patients with defects in adenosylcobalamin biosynthesis may

respond to administration of large doses of vitamin B_{12}, which may enhance the amount of active holoenzyme (mutase apoenzyme plus adenosylcobalamin). A proposed mechanism for the neurological abnormalities observed in methylmalonic acidemia was suggested by a group of Brazilian investigators who administered methylmalonic acid to rats during the first month of their life.[24] A significant diminution of myelin content and of ganglioside N-acetylneuraminic acid were noted in the cerebrum.

More than 20 years ago, Ampola and colleagues were the first to attempt prenatal diagnosis and treatment of a B_{12}-responsive variant of MMA.[25] They followed the pregnancy of a patient who had previously suffered the loss of a child to severe acidosis and dehydration at the age of 3 months. The diagnosis of MMA was made posthumously by chemical analysis of blood and urine. In the subsequent pregnancy, amniocentesis at 19 weeks revealed elevated methylmalonic acid in the amniotic fluid. Cultured amniocytes also demonstrated defective propionate oxidation and undetectable levels of adenosylcobalamin. When adenosylcobalamin was added, normal succinate oxidation and methylmalonyl-coenzyme A mutase activity were noted. These studies established that the fetus also suffered from MMA apparently due to deficient synthesis of adenosylcobalamin. It was already been known that fetal MMA is associated with increased methylmalonic acid excretion in the maternal urine. Indeed, Ampola et al.[25] documented increased methylmalonic acidemia in maternal urine at 23 and 25 weeks of gestation. Late in the pregnancy, cyanocobalamin (10 mg/day) was orally administered to the mother in divided doses. The treatment only marginally altered the maternal serum B_{12} level. However, there was a slight reduction of maternal urinary methylmalonic acid excretion that remained several fold above normal. At approximately 34 weeks of gestation, 5 mg of cyanocobalamin per day was administered intramuscularly. The maternal serum B_{12} level then rose gradually to more than sixfold above normal and was accompanied by a progressive decrease in urinary methylmalonic acid excretion. Maternal urinary methylmalonate was only slightly above the normal range when delivery occurred at 41 weeks. Amniotic fluid methylmalonic acid concentrations were three times the normal mean at 19 menstrual weeks and four times the normal mean at term, despite prenatal treatment. Postnatally, the diagnosis of methylmalonic acidemia was confirmed. The infant suffered no acute neonatal complications and had an extremely high serum B_{12} level. Long-term postnatal management involved protein restriction; however, no continuous B_{12} treatment was required. In this instance, prenatal treatment certainly improved the fetal and, secondarily, the maternal biochemistry. Whether there was any significant clinical benefit to the fetus by in utero treatment cannot be assessed adequately. It seems likely that reducing the fetal burden of methylmalonic acid should have some beneficial effect on fetal development and could reduce the risks in the neonatal period.

Andersson et al.[26] followed a cohort of eight children with MMA for an average of 5.7 years. Congenital malformations were described, reinforcing the deleterious effects of prenatally abnormal cyanocobalamin metabolism. Growth was significantly improved in most cases after initiation of therapy postnatally and in one case microcephaly resolved. However, developmental delay of variable severity was always present regardless of treatment onset. These data suggest that prenatal therapy of MMA may be effective and perhaps ameliorate some of the prenatal effects. Evans et al. have documented the changing dose requirements necessary over the course of pregnancy to maintain adequate levels of B_{12}. They sequentially followed maternal plasma and urine levels in a prenatal treated pregnancy.[27] Data such as these suggest that modulation of maternal-fetal pharmacological interchange of therapeutic drugs will be difficult to precisely control.

Multiple Carboxylase Deficiency

Biotin-responsive multiple carboxylase deficiency is an inborn error of metabolism caused by diminished activity of the mitochondrial biotin-dependent enzymes (pyruvate carboxylase, propionyl-coenzyme A carboxylase and α-methylcrotonyl-coenzyme A carboxylase). The condition may arise from mutations in the holocarboxylase synthetase (HCS) gene on chromosome 21q22.1 or the biotinidase gene localized to chromosome 3p25.[28-32] Affected patients present as newborns or in early childhood with dermatitis, severe metabolic acidosis and a characteristic pattern of organic acid excretion. It has been demonstrated that metabolism in patients or in their cultured cells can be restored toward normal levels by biotin supplementation. Prenatal diagnosis can be made by demonstration of elevated levels of typical organic acids (3-hydroxyisovalerate, methylcitrate) in the amniotic fluid or in the chorionic villi. However, the existence of a mild form of HCS deficiency can complicate prenatal diagnosis as organic acids level in amniotic fluid might be normal.[33] Therefore, prenatal diagnosis must be performed by enzyme assay in cultured fetal cells in biotin-restricted medium.

Roth and colleagues treated a fetus without the benefit of prenatal diagnosis in a case in which two previous siblings had died of multiple carboxylase deficiency.[34] The first had died within 3 days of birth and in the second, the diagnosis of biotin-responsive carboxylase deficiency was made posthumously. Since the mother was first seen at 34 weeks of gestation, prenatal diagnosis was not attempted. Because of severe neonatal manifestations in previous offspring and due to the probable harmlessness of biotin oral administration was begun at a dose of 10 mg/day. There were no apparent untoward effects; maternal urinary biotin excretion increased by a factor of approximately 100 during biotin administration. Nonidentical twins were subsequently delivered at term. Cord blood and urinary organic acid profiles were normal, and cord blood biotin concentrations were four to seven times greater than normal. The neonatal course for both twins was unremarkable. Subsequent study of the cultured fibroblasts of both twins indicated that the cells of twin B (but not of twin A) had virtually complete deficiency of all three carboxylase activities. Genetic complementation studies confirmed that despite the normal clinical presentation during the newborn period, twin B was homozygous for the disease mutation. Packman and colleagues have also reported prenatal diagnosis and treatment of biotin-responsive multiple carboxylase deficiency for a mother who had previously given birth to a male with the neonatal-onset form of this disease.[35] In the subsequent pregnancy, maternal urine organic acid profiles were normal. Carboxylases activities were assayed in cultured amniotic fluid cells obtained by amniocentesis at 17 menstrual weeks. In biotin-restricted medium, the amniotic cells demonstrated the characteristic severe reduction in carboxylase activities. Since these initial reports of prenatal administration of biotin to fetuses affected with this disorder, other cases have been published,[33,36,37] further provided compelling evidence that biotin

administration antenatally is effectively taken up by the fetus and prevents functional deficiency of the carboxylases in an affected newborn. No toxicity from treatment was observed. However, because experience with this treatment is confined to a small number of cases, it is reasonabe to carry out prenatal diagnosis and only then to initiate treatment with biotin in any affected fetus.

Smith-Lemli-Optiz Syndrome (SLOS)

Smith-Lemli-Optiz syndrome (SLOS) is a dysmorphological syndrome first reported in 1964.[38] Features include characteristic facies, growth and mental retardation, and anomalies of the heart, kidneys, central nervous system and limbs. Cleft palate, postaxial polydactyly, 2–3 syndactyly of the toes and cataracts are often seen in affected patients.

The 2–3 syndactyly of the toes is very specific for this disorder and is seen in > 90% of affected patients. Affected patients typically present with a narrow forehead, ptosis, anteverted nares, low-set ears and micrognathia.

Males may present with ambiguous genitalia. In contrast with CAH, patients with SLOS are deficient in cholesterol and therefore lack steroid precursors. This leads to lack of androgens that results in under-masculinization of the male genitalia. Patients with the severe form of the syndrome present not only with these dysmorphological findings but also with a high rate of neonatal mortality.[39] The incidence of SLOS is estimated to be 1:20,000–1:40,000 live births,[40] and it appears to be most common in Caucasians population of North European origin, with an estimated carrier frequency of 1:70.[41] In 1993, the etiology of SLOS was discovered to be an inborn error of cholesterol biosynthesis due to a deficiency of the enzyme 7-dehydrocholesterol DD^7 reductase.[38,41-44] The gene for 7-dehydrocholesterol DD^7 reductase has been localized to chromosome 11q12-13.[44]

As a result of this enzymatic defect, there is a characteristic biochemical pattern of reduced cholesterol levels and elevated 7 and 8 dehydrocholesterol levels (7-DHC and 8-DHC respectively) in all body fluids and tissues including red blood cells, fibroblasts, amniotic fluid and chorionic villi. The values observed in affected patients may be extremely variable. The diagnosis is made primarily by the presence of the cholesterol precursor, 7-DHC and not by the deficiency of cholesterol. Unaffected individuals have levels of 7-DHC and 8-DHC of less than 1 mg/dL whereas patients with SLOS usually have levels of 7 to 20 or greater. Clinical manifestations correlate with cholesterol levels. Severely affected patients have very low levels of total cholesterol (usually < 10–15 mg/dL), while those with more mild manifestations may present with levels of 40–70 mg/dL. Prenatal diagnosis of SLOS has been available since 1994 by either amniocentesis or chorionic villus sampling.[45-47]

Since identification of the cholesterol metabolic defect in SLOS, a treatment protocol has been attempted providing exogenous cholesterol. This form of therapy has now been provided to many patients with SLOS for the past several years in many centers in the United States and internationally,[48-50] with the goal of raising cholesterol levels and decrease the precursors, 7-DHC and 8-DHC. It has been shown that dietary cholesterol supplementation can restore a normal growth pattern in children and adolescents with SLOS, alleviate behavioral abnormalities and improve general health.[48-50]

Fetal therapy strategies may theoretically include providing cholesterol to the mother or to the fetus. The former however, is not possible because cholesterol does not cross the placenta well in the second trimester and there is lack of evidence that it crosses the placenta in the third trimester. Moreover, cholesterol is available only in a crystalline form, which cannot be given intravenously or intramuscularly. Furthermore, it is impractical to inject cholesterol into the amniotic fluid because it would precipitate. However, cholesterol can be given to the fetus by giving fresh frozen plasma in the form of LDL-cholesterol. The group at Tufts University has attempted treatment antenatally in several affected fetuses. In cases where treatment was started late in pregnancy, the results were inconclusive. Although, few descriptions of fetal therapy for SLOS exist, the latest report of antenatal treatment comes from that same group of investigators.[51] Therapy was begun at 34 weeks of gestation and resulted in increased fetal cholesterol levels and red blood cell mean corpuscular volume with subtle improvement in fetal growth, as assessed by consequent fetal weight plots. However, no significant change in 7-DHC and 8-DHC levels was observed, further emphasizing the inconclusiveness of that treatment. However, the main point is that since significant development of the central nervous system and myelination occurs prior to birth it is a reasonable to assume that providing cholesterol to the fetus, as early as possible would result in the most clinical benefit.

Galactosemia

Galactosemia is an inborn error of metabolism caused by diminished activity of the enzyme galactose-1 phosphate uridyltransferase (GALT). This causes a defective metabolism of the sugar galactose which is the constituent of lactose, the main carbohydrate of milk, resulting in accumulation of galactose in the bloodstream. It is inherited in an autosomal recessive manner and results in cataract, mental deficiency, growth deficiency and ovarian failure. Clinical symptoms appear in the neonatal period and can be largely ameliorated by elimination of galactose from the diet. Cellular damage in galactosemia is thought to be mediated by accumulation of galactose-1 phosphate intracellularly and of galactitol in the lens. The GALT gene, localized to chromosome 9p13, is the only known gene to be associated with galactosemia. Several disease-causing mutations are commonly encountered in classical galactosemia, the most frequently observed is the Q188R classical mutation. Mutational analysis is available usefully for the six classical galactosemia alleles (Q188R, S135L, K285N, L195P, Y209C, F171S) and for the N314D Durate variant mutation.[52] In cases in which disease causing mutation are not identified (as observed in 10–29% of classic galactosemia), GALT sequence analysis may be performed to detect private mutations. Galactosemia can be diagnosed prenatally by study of cultured amniocytes and chorionic villi.

There are suggestions that even the early postnatal treatment of galactosemic individuals with a low galactose diet may not be sufficient to ensure normal development. Some have speculated that prenatal damage to galactosemic fetuses could contribute to subsequent abnormal neurological development and to lens cataract formation. Furthermore, it has been recognized that female galactosemics, even when treated from birth with galactose deprivation, have a high frequency of primary or secondary amenorrhea because of ovarian failure. This is because oocytes have already been damaged irreversibly long before birth. There also may be some subtle abnormalities of male gonadal function.

Exposure to a high-galactose diet has been considered to represent an animal model for human galactosemia. Chen and colleagues have observed a reduction in the oocyte content of rat ovaries after prenatal exposure to a 50% galactose diet.[53] No analogous alterations in the testes were observed in prenatally treated males. Experiments in rats suggest that toxicity to the female gonads from galactose or its metabolites is most obvious during the premeiotic stages of ovarian development. Recently, impaired germ cell migration leading to the development of gonads with deficient initial pools of germ cells was proposed as the causal link between galactosemia and premature ovarian failure.[54]

These observations in animals and human beings have led to speculation that galactose restriction during pregnancy may be desirable if the fetus is affected with galactosemia. In the human female, ovarian meiosis begins at 12 and is complete by 28 menstrual weeks. Thus, ovarian damage, and perhaps neurological or lens abnormalities, might occur prior to the usual time when prenatal diagnosis by amniocentesis can be accomplished. Thus, anticipatory treatment in pregnancies at risk for having a galactosemic fetus might best be initiated very early in gestation or even preconceptually.

Despite these experiments and speculations, we are unaware of studies that adequately assess the impact of prenatal administration of a low-galactose diet to galactosemic fetuses. However such data, especially controlled, will be difficult to obtain. Nevertheless, prenatal galactose restriction is probably desirable in galactosemia and should be harmless. There is little reason to suppose that galactose restriction would have adverse consequences, since galactosemic and normal fetuses are both capable of some endogenous galactose synthesis.

MULTIFACTORIAL DISORDERS
Neural Tube Defects

Neural tube defects (NTDs) are malformations secondary to abnormal neural tube closure between the third and fourth weeks of gestational age. The etiology is complex and imperfectly understood with both genetic and environmental factors involved. Animal studies suggest that NTDs can arise from a variety of vitamin or mineral deficiencies. There are historical data in humans suggesting increased NTD frequencies in subjects with poor dietary histories or with intestinal bypasses. Biochemical evidence of suboptimal nutrition is present in some women bearing infants with NTDs. Analysis of recurrence patterns within families and of twin-twin concordance data provides evidence of a genetic influence in nonsyndromal cases, although factors such as socioeconomic status, geographic area, occupational exposure and maternal use of antiepileptic drugs are also associated with variations in the incidence of NTDs.[55] In 1980, Smithells et al. suggested that vitamin supplementation containing 0.36 mg folate can reduce the frequency of NTD recurrence by sevenfold in women with one or more prior affected children.[56,57] For almost a decade, there has been a great deal of controversy regarding the benefit of folate supplementation for the prevention of NTDs.[58-61] Finally, in 1991, a randomized double-blinded trial designed by the Medical Research Council Vitamin Study Research Group demonstrated that preconceptual folate reduces the risk of recurrence in high risk patients.[62] Subsequently, it was shown that preparations containing folate and other vitamins also reduce the occurrence of first time NTDs.[63] In response to these findings, guidelines were issued calling for consumption of 4.0 mg/

day folic acid by women with a prior child affected with an NTD, for at least 1 month prior to conception through the first 3 months of pregnancy. In addition, 0.4 mg/day folic acid is recommended to all women planning a pregnancy to be taken preconceptually. The data on NTD recurrence prevention is now very well established, and became routine for high risk cases. As of January 1998, the United States Food and Drug Administration has mandated that breads and grains be supplemented with folic acid. The impact of food fortification with folic acid on NTDs birth prevalence during the years 1990–1999 was evaluated by assessing birth certificate reports before and after mandatory fortification.[64] It was found that the birth prevalence of NTDs reported decreased by 19% . It is important to note that the continuing decline in NTDs rates are estimated to be due to the introduction and increased utilization of prenatal diagnosis, recommendations for multivitamin use in women of childbearing age, and the population-wide increases in blood folate levels since food fortification was mandated.[65]

Folate plays a central part in embryonic and fetal development because of its role in nucleic acid synthesis mandatory for the widespread cell division that takes place during embryogenesis. Folate deficiency can occur because of low dietary folate intake or because of increased metabolic requirement as seen in particular genetic alterations such as the polymorphism of the thermolabile enzyme methyltetrahydrofolate reductase (MTHFR). A metabolic effect of folate deficiency is homocysteine elevation in blood. As mentioned, the thermolabile variant of MTHFR 677TT, is a known risk factor for NTDs. However, evidence regarding a second polymorphism in the same gene, 1298AàÐC, does not support its role in NTDs.[66] Additionally, numerous studies analyzing MTHFR variants have resulted in positive associations with increased NTD risk only in certain populations, suggesting that these variants are not large contributors to the etiology of NTDs.[67] Therefore, it seems less likely to advise parents prospectively to test for MTHFR variants. Reinforcement to the assumption that additional candidate genes other than MTHFR may be responsible for an increase risk to NTDs comes from the NTD collaborative group of Duke University.[68] About 175 American Caucasians NTD patients and their families were examined for the thermolabile variant of MTHFR. Although, a significant association has been found comparing patients and controls, no such association was found in patients' parents. Two other key enzymes in the metabolic pathway of homocysteine are methionine synthase (MTR) and methionine synthase reductase (MTRR). Recently reported, MTR and a specific (A66G) MTRR polymorphisms have been found to be associated with increased risk for NTDs. Interestingly, the NTDs risk was not influenced by maternal preconception folic acid intake at doses of 0.4 mg/day. However, due to limited sample size, further studies are needed in order to draw meaningful inferences.[69] Other candidate genes suggested as risk factor for NTDs (mainly spina bifida), are polymorphisms in the mitochondrial membrane transporter gene UCP2.[70] Despite previous studies suggesting zinc deficiency to play a role in the etiology of NTDs,[71,72] further studies found this observation inconclusive.[73,74] Methionine deficiency might be involved in NTDs as 30–55% reduction in the risk of having NTD associated pregnancy was reported when methionine intake was greater then the lowest quartile of intake, with further reduction in risk with greater methionine intake.[75] In conclusion, preconception intake of folic acid alone or as multivitamin supplementation reduces the risk of recurrence and first time NTDs. Additionally, folic acid-multivitamin supplementation reduces the occurrence of other congenital anomalies such as seen in the urinary tract (e.g. vesicorenal reflux, horseshoe kidney and others),in the cardiovascular system (e.g. conotruncal heart defects), and anomalies involving the limbs and face (orofacial clefting).

PHARMACOLOGIC APPROACHES

It might be appropriate to consider suppressing excessive cholesterol production prenatally in severe hypercholesterolemia when a safe and effective agent for accomplishing this becomes available (although, there is no clear evidence for hypercholesterolemic prenatal damage). If cysteamine or related agents were to prove an effective treatment for lethal variants of cystinosis, prenatal therapy might be considered, because excessive and possibly harmful cystine accumulation is evident even in cystinotic fetuses. Cysteamine levels have been detected in chorionic villi, and significant elevations even at 10 weeks of gestation have been hypothesized. Inhibitors of gammaglutamyl transpeptidase, if safe, would elevate intracellular glutathione levels and inhibit oxoproline production in glutathione synthase deficiency, thereby averting the characteristic neonatal acidosis. In theory, it would be desirable to minimize copper accumulation in Wilson disease as early as possible. If and when reliable prenatal diagnosis of Wilson disease is possible, cautious administration of penicillamine prenatally might be considered. This would be a double-edged sword, however, as the teratogenic potential of penicillamine would demand careful evaluation. Batshaw and colleagues[76] have treated certain urea cycle defects by administering arginine and benzoate. Since hyperammonemia in some of these entities develops very acutely after birth, it might be desirable to consider pretreating the fetus with these compounds just prior to or during labor to minimize postnatal hyperammonemia.[76] Conversely, it may be desirable to consider drug avoidance as an approach to fetal treatment. For example, fetuses with glucose-6-phosphate dehydrogenase deficiency are sensitive to a variety of drugs that induce hemolysis. It would probably be appropriate to avoid administering such agents to women carrying or known to be at risk for carrying fetuses deficient in glucose-6-phosphate dehydrogenase.

Umbilical cord catheterization under ultrasound guidance may lead to the development of other types of fetal treatment.[77] Systems such as gene replacement are being developed for certain lysosomal storage disorders. Progress is being made in postnatal experimental models on administration of thymic cells for certain immune deficiency states, bone marrow transplantation for a variety of genetic disorders and gene transfer. The development of better and earlier techniques for prenatal treatment will be complex, especially with regard to gene transfer, but progress will be made, and access to the fetal vasculature may be required for these methods to have a chance for success.

Bone marrow transplantation or thymic cell infusion is actually only a specialized example of organ transplantation. In the future, fetal organ transplantation may become possible and may open many prospects for surgical treatment of certain biochemical genetic disorders.

One can also speculate about the therapeutic possibilities involving compounds administered directly into the amniotic fluid or into the fetal intestinal tract. It might be possible, for example, to administer thyroid hormone in this fashion or to prevent meconium ileus in cystic fibrosis by instilling not yet determined enzymes into the fetal intestinal tract.

CONCLUSION

While a multitude of metabolic disorders exist, prenatal treatment for most has never been attempted or considered. The discovery of new disease associated genes and prenatal carrier testing may in the future allow preconceptual carrier detection, without the tragedy of first having an affected child. This may provide targeted therapy in families who chose to continue the pregnancy and offer the prospect of improved outcome by ameliorating at least some of the prenatal deleterious effects of the metabolic disease.

REFERENCES

1. Evans MI, Pinsky WW, Johnson MP, et al. Medical fetal therapy. In: Evans MI (Ed). Reproductive Risks and Prenatal Diagnosis. Norwalk: Appleton and Lange. 1992:236.
2. Johnson MP, Evans MI, Quintero RA, et al. In utero therapy of the fetus. In: Gleisher N, Buttino L Jr, Elkayam U, Evans MI, Galbraith RM, Gall SA, Sibai BM (Eds). Principles and Practice of Medical Therapy in Pregnancy, 3rd edition. Norwalk: Appleton and Lange; Chapter 25.
3. Speiser PW, Dupont B, Rubinstein P, et al. High frequency of nonclassical steroid 21-hydroxylase deficiency. Am J Hum Genet. 1985;37:650-67.
4. Dupont B, Oberfield SE, Smithwick EM, et al. Close genetic linkage between HLA and congenital adrenal hyperplasia (21-hydroxylase deficiency). Lancet. 1977;2:1309-12.
5. White PC, Grossberger D, Onufer Bj, et al. Two genes encoding steroid 21-hydroxylase are located near the genes encoding the fourth component of complement in man. Proc Natl Acad Sci. USA. 1985;82:1089-93.
6. Evans MI, Chrousos GP, Mann DL, et al. Pharmacologic suppression of the fetal adrenal gland *in utero*: attempted prevention of abnormal external genital masculinization in suspected congenital adrenal hyperplasia. JAMA. 1985;253:1015-20.
7. Forest M, David M. Prenatal treatment of congenital adrenal hyperplasia due to 21-hydroxylase deficiency. 7th International Congress of Endocrinology, Quebec, Canada. 1984, Abstract y11.
8. New MI, Carlson A, Obeid J, et al. Prenatal diagnosis for congenital adrenal hyperplasia in 532 pregnancies. Clin Endocrinol Metab. 2001;86:5651-7.
9. Clayton PE, Miller WL, Oberfield SE, et al. Consensus statement on 21-hydroxylase deficiency from the European Society for Pediatric. Endocrinology and the Lawson Wilkins Pediatric Endocrine Society. Horm Res. 2002;58:188-95.
10. Fisher DA. Neonatal thyroid disease of women with autoimmune thyroid disease. Thyroid Today. 1986;9:17.
11. Fisher DA, Klein AH. Thyroid development and disorders of thyroid function in the newborn. N Engl J Med. 1981;304:702-12.
12. Volumenie JL, Polak M, Guibourdenche J, et al. Management of fetal thyroid goitres: A report of 11 cases in a single perinatal unit. Prenat Diagn. 2000;20:799-806.
13. Morine M, Takeda T, Minekawa R, et al. Antenatal diagnosis and treatment of a case of fetal goitrous hypothyroidism associated with high-output cardiac failure. Ultrasound Obstet Gynecol. 2002;19:506-9.
14. Rovet J, Ehrlich R, Sorbara D. Intellectual outcome in children with fetal hypothyroidism. J Pediatr. 1987;110:700-4.
15. Thorpe-Beeston JG, Nicolaides KH, McGregor AM. Fetal thyroid function. Thyroid. 1992;2;207-17.
16. Sack J, Fisher DA, Hobel CJ, et al. Thyroxine in human amniotic fluid. J Pediatrics. 1975;87;364-8.
17. Ballabio M, Nicolini U, Jowett T, et al. Maturation of thyroid function in normal human fetuses. Clin Endocrinol. 1989;31:565-71.
18. Van Herle AJ, Young RT, Fisher DA, et al. Intrauterine treatment of a hypothyroid fetus. J Clin Endocrinol Metab. 1973;40;474-7.
19. Gruner C, Kollert A, Wildt L, et al. Intrauterine treatment of fetal goitrous hypothyroidism controlled by determination of thyroid-stimulating hormone in fetal serum. A case report and review of the literature. Fetal Diagn Ther. 2001;16:47-51.
20. Bruinse HW, Vermeulen-Meiners C, Wit JM. Fetal treatment for thyrotoxicosis in non-thyrotoxic pregnant women. Fetal therapy. 1988;3:152-7.
21. Wenstrom KD, Weiner CP, Williamson RA, et al. Prenatal diagnosis of fetal hyperthyroidism using funipuncture. Obstet Gynecol. 1990;76:513-7.
22. Porreco RP, Bloch CA. Fetal blood sampling in the management of intrauterine thyrotoxicosis. Obstet Gynecol. 1990;76:509-12.
23. Hatjis CG. Diagnosis and successful treatment of fetal goitrous hyperthyroidism caused by maternal Graves' disease. Obstet Gynecol. 1993;81:837-9.
24. Brusque A, Rotta L, Pettenuzzo LF, et al. Chronic postnatal administration of methylmalonic acid provokes a decrease of myelin content and ganglioside *N*-acetylneuraminic acid concentration in cerebrum of young rats. Braz J Med Biol Res. 2001;34:227-31.
25. Ampola MG, Mahoney MI, Nakamura E, et al. Prenatal therapy of a patient with vitamin B responsive methylmalonic acidemia. N Engl J Med. 1975;293:313.
26. Andersson HC, Marble M, Shapira E. Long-term outcome in treated combined methylmalonic acidemia and homocysteinemia. Genet Med. 1999;1:146-50.
27. Evans MI, Duquette DA, Rinaldo P, et al. Modulation of B12 dosage and response in fetal treatment of methylmalonic aciduria (MMA). Titration of treatment dose to serum and urine MMA. Fet Diag and Ther. 1997;12:21-3.
28. Leon Del Rio A, Leclerc D, Gravel RA. Isolation of a cDNA encoding human holocarboxylase synthetase by functional complementation of a biotinauxotroph of *E. coli*. Proc Natl Acad Sci, USA. 1995;92:4626-30.
29. Suzuki Y, Akoi Y, Ishida Y, et al. Isolation and characterization of mutations in the holocarboxylase synthetase cDNA. Nature Genet. 1994;8:122-8.
30. Akoi Y, Suzuki Y, Sakamoto O, et al. Molecular analysis of holocarboxylase synthetase deficiency: A missense mutation and a single base deletion are predominant in Japanese patients. Biochim Biophys Acta. 1995;1272:168-74.
31. Dupuis L, Leon-Del-Rio A, Leclerc D, et al. Clustering of mutations in the biotin-binding region of holocarboxilase synthetase in biotin responsive multiple carboxylase deficiency. Hum Mol Genet. 1996;5:1011-6.
32. Popmponio RJ, Hymes J, Reynolds TR, et al. Mutation in the human biotinidase gene that cause profound biothinidase deficiency in symptomatic children: molecular, biochemical, and clinical analysis. Pediatr Res. 1997;42:840-8.
33. Suormala T, Fowler B, Jakobs C, et al. Late onset holocarboxylase synthetase deficiency: pre- and postnatal diagnosis and evaluation of effectiveness of antenatal biotin therapy. Eur J Pediatr. 1998;157:570-5.

34. Roth KS, Yang W, Allen L, et al. Prenatal administration of biotin: biotin responsive multiple carboxylase deficiency. Pediatr Res. 1982;16:126-9.

35. Packman S, Cowan Mj, Golbus MS, et al. Prenatal treatment of biotin responsive multiple carboxylase deficiency. Lancet. 1982;1:1435-8.

36. Thuy LP, Belmont J, Nyhan W. Prenatal diagnosis and treatment of holocarboxylase synthetase deficiency. Prenat Diagn. 1999;19:108-12.

37. Thuy LP, Jurecki E, Nemzer L, et al. Prenatal diagnosis of holocarboxylase synthetase deficiency by assay of the enzyme in chorionic villus material followed by prenatal treatment. Clinica Chimica Acta. 1999;284:59-68.

38. Smith DW, Lemli L, Opitz JM. A newly recognized syndrome of multiple congenital anomalies. J Pediatr. 1964;64:210-7.

39. Curry CJ, Carey JC, Holland JS. Smith-Lemli-Opitz syndrome, type II: Multiple congenital anomalies with male pseudohermaphroditism and frequent early lethality. Am J Med Genet. 1987;26:45-57.

40. Opitz JM. RSH-SLO ("Smith-Lemli-Opitz") syndrome: historical, genetic, and development considerations. Am J Med Genet. 1994;50:344-6.

41. Kelley RI. Diagnosis of Smith-Lemli-Opitz syndrome by gas chromatography/mass spectrometry of 7 dehydrocholesterol in plasma, amniotic fluid and cultured skin fibroblasts. Clin Chim Acta. 1995;236:45-58.

42. Kelley RI. A new face for an old syndrome. Am J Med Genet. 1997;65:251-6.

43. Tint GS, Irons M, Elias E, et al. Defective cholesterol biosynthesis associated with the Smith-Lemli-Opitz syndrome. N Engl J Med. 1994;330:107-13.

44. Waterham HR, Wijburg FA, Hennekam RC, et al. Smith-Lemli-Opitz is caused by mutations in the 7-dehydrocholesterol reductase gene. Am J Hum Genet. 1998;63:329-38.

45. Gelman-Kohan Z, Nisani R, Chemke J, et al. Prenatal detection of recurrent SLOS type 2. Am J Hum Genet. 1990;47:A57.

46. Hobbins JC, Jones OW, Gottesfeld MD, et al. Transvaginal ultrasonography and transabdominal embryoscopy in the first trimester diagnosis of Smith-Lemli-Opitz syndrome, type II. Am J Obstet Gynecol. 1994;171:546-9.

47. Sharp P, Haan E, Fletcher JM, et al. First trimester diagnosis of Smith-Lemli-Opitz syndrome. Prenatal Diagnosis. 1997;17:4:355-61.

48. Irons M, Elias E, Tint GS, et al. Abnormal cholesterol metabolism in the Smith-Lemli-Opitz syndrome: Report of clinical and biochemical findings in 4 patients and treatment in 1 patient. Am J Med Genet. 1994;50:347-52.

49. Irons M, Elias ER, Abuelo D, et al. Treatment of Smith-Lemli-Opitz syndrome: Results of a multicenter trial. Am J Med Genet. 1997;68:311-4.

50. Elias ER, Irons MB, Hurley AD, et al. Clinical effects of cholesterol supplementation in six patients with the Smith-Lemli-Opitz syndrome (SLOS). Am J Med Genet. 1997;68:305-10.

51. Irons MR, Nores J, Stewart TL, et al. Antenatal therapy of Smith-Lemli-Opitz syndrome. Fetal Diagn Ther. 1999;14:133-7.

52. Elsas LJ. Prenatal diagnosis of galactos-1-phosphate uridyltransferase (GALT) deficient galactosemia. Prenat diagn. 2001;21:302-3.

53. Chen YT, Mattison DR, Feigenbaum L, et al. Reduction in oocyte number following prenatal exposure to a high galactose diet. Science. 1981;314:1145-7.

54. Bandyopadhyay S, Chakrabarti J, Banerjee S, et al. Prenatal exposure to high galactose adversely affects initial gonadal pool of germ cells in rats. Hum Reprod. 2003;18:276-82.

55. Frey L, Hauser WA. Epidemiology of neural tube defects. Epilepsia. 2003;44(Suppl 3):4-13.

56. Smithells RW, Nevin NC, Seller MJ, et al. Further experience of vitamin supplementation for prevention of neural tube defect recurrences. Lancet. 1983;1:1027-31.

57. Smithells RW, Sheppard S, Schorah CJ, et al. Possible prevention of neural tube defects by preconceptual vitamin supplementation. Lancet. 1980;1:339-40.

58. Younis JS, Granat M. Insufficient transplacental digoxin transfer in severe hydrops fetalis. Am J Obstet Gynecol. 1987;157:1268-9.

59. Mills JL, Rhoads GG, Simpson JL, et al. The absence of a relation between the periconceptional use of vitamins and neural-tube defects. N Engl J Med. 1989;321:430-5.

60. Mulinare J, Cordero JF, Erickson JD, et al. Periconceptional use of multivitamins and the occurrence of neural tube defects. JAMA. 1988;260:3141-5.

61. Schulman JD. Treatment of the embryo and the fetus in the first trimester: current status and future prospects. Am J Med Genet. 1990;35:197-200.

62. MRC Vitamin Study Research Group. Prevention of neural tube defects: results of the MRC vitamin study. Lancet. 1991;338:132-7.

63. Czeizel AE, Dudas I. Prevention of the first occurrence of neural-tube defects by preconceptional vitamin supplementation. N Engl J Med. 1992;327:1832-5.

64. Honein MA, Paulozzi LJ, Mathews TJ, et al. Impact of folic acid fortification of the US food supply on the occurrence of neural tube defects. JAMA. 2001;285:2981-6.

65. Olney RS, Mulinare J. Trends in neural tube defect prevalence, folic acid fortification, and vitamin supplement use. Semin Perinatol. 2002;26:277-85.

66. Parle-McDermott A, Mills JL, Kirke PN, et al. Analysis of MTHFR 1298A → C and 677 C → T polymorphisms as risk factor neural tube defects. J Hum Genet. 2003;48:190-3.

67. Finnell RH, Shaw GM, Lammer EJ, et al. Does prenatal screening for 5,10-methylenetetrahydrofolate reductase (MTHFR) mutations in high-risk neural tube defect pregnancies make sense? Genet Test. 2002;6:47-52.

68. Rampersaud E, Melvin EC, Siegel D, et al. Updated investigations of the role of methylenetetrahydrofolate reductase in human neural tube defects. Clin Genet. 2003; 63:210-4.

69. Zhu H, Wicker NJ, Shaw GM, et al. Homocysteine remethylation enzyme polymorphisms and increased risks for neural tube defects. Mol Genet Metab. 2003;78:216-21.

70. Volocik KA, Shaw GM, Zhu H, et al. Risk factors for neural tube defects: associations between uncoupling protein 2 polymorphisms and spina bifida. Birth Defects Res Part A Clin Mol Teratol. 2003;67:158-61.

71. Sever LE. Zinc deficiency in man. Lancet. 1973;I:887.

72. McMichael AJ, Dreosti IE, Gibson GT. A prospective study of serial maternal serum zinc levels and pregnancy outcome. Early Hum Dev. 1982;7:59-69.

73. Stoll C, Dott B, Alembik Y, et al. Maternal trace elements, vitamin B12, vitamin A, folic acid, and fetal malformations. Rep Toxicol. 1999;13:53-7.

74. Hambidge M, Hackshaw A, Wald N. Neural tube defects and serum zinc. Br J Obstet Gynecol. 1993;100:746-9.

75. Shoob HD, Sargent RG, Thompson SJ, et al. Dietary methionine is involved in the etiology of neural defect-affected pregnancies in humans. J Nutr. 2001;131:2653-8.

76. Batshaw M, Brusilow S, Waber L, et al. Treatment of inborn errors of urea synthesis: activation of alternative pathways of waste nitrogen synthesis and excretion. N Engl J Med. 1982;306:1387-92.

77. Nicolaides KH, Thorpe-Beeston JG, Noble P. Cordocentesis. In: Eden RD, Boehm H (Eds). Assessment and Care of the Fetus: Physiological, Clinical and Medicolegal Principles. Norwalk: Appleton and Lange; 1990. p. 291.

70

Fetal Surgical Interventions

MR Harrison, MI Evans

INTRODUCTION

Over the last two decades, fetal therapy has evolved into four major areas—open surgical approaches, "closed" endoscopic surgical approaches, pharmacologic therapy, and stem cell/gene therapy. Advances in the field have been characterized by dramatic successes, but also intense frustration at technical challenges and moving targets as ancillary therapies change risk/reward equations.[1]

If something can be treated safely postnatally, then there is no justification for prenatal intervention. However, for the conditions discussed below, profound and irreparable damage occurs before birth, making fetal intervention the best or sometimes only way to ameliorate the damage. Some procedures have been quite rare. Others are more common, but the expectation is that with improvements and increasing utilization of prenatal diagnosis, more women will choose and consider the opportunities to treat fetuses before birth.[2]

SURGICAL THERAPY

In Utero "Closed" Fetal Surgery

The most efficacious percutaneous in utero fetal surgery has been for the evaluation and treatment of obstructive uropathy. Lower urinary tract obstruction (LUTO) is a heterogeneous entity that affects 1:5,000–8,000 newborn males. Posterior urethral valves or urethral atresias are the most common causes for LUTO, although other etiologies such as stenosis of the urethral meatus, anterior urethral valves, ectopic insertion of a ureter and tumors of the bladder have been observed. LUTO can result in massive distention of the bladder with compensatory hypertrophy and hyperplasia of the smooth muscle within the bladder wall, leading to a loss of compliance and elasticity and poor postnatal function generally requiring surgical reconstruction.[3] Elevated intravesicular pressures prevent urine inflow from the ureters and eventual distortion of the ureterovesicle angles contribute to reflux hydronephrosis. Progressive pyelectasis and calyectasis compress the delicate renal parenchyma within the encasing serosal capsule, leading to functional abnormalities within the medullary and eventually the cortical regions. Focal compressive hypoxia likely contributes to the progressive fibrosis and perturbations in tubular function resulting in urinary hypertonicity which is observed. Obstructive processes can eventually lead to type IV cystic dysplasia and renal insufficiency.[4-7]

The effects extend beyond the genitourinary tract. Progressive oligo/anhydramnios leads to compressive deformations as seen in Potter sequence, including extremity contractures and facial dysmorphology. Absence of normal amniotic fluid volume also interferes with pulmonary growth and development. Constant compressive pressure on the fetal thorax leads to restriction of expansion of the chest through normal physiologic "breathing movements". Babies born with LUTO generally die secondary to pulmonary complications and not renal failure.

The prenatal sonographic diagnosis of LUTO includes dilated and thickened walls of the bladder, hydronephrosis and oligohydramnios (Fig. 70.1). Urethral strictures or atresia, urethral agenesis, megalourethra, ureteral reflux and cloacal anomalies may be present and have a very similar appearance on ultrasound. The typical "keyhole sign" of proximal urethral dilation is secondary to urethral obstruction present in PUV or atresia. However, the precise diagnosis can only be made after birth.[7]

The prenatal evaluation and management of fetuses with the sonographic findings of LUTO are complex.[4-6] Ruling out other congenital anomalies such as cardiac and neural tube defects is necessary before intervention can be considered.

Karyotyping is needed to confirm a normal male chromosomal status, as cases of LUTO have an increased incidence of aneuploidy. Female fetuses almost always have more complex syndromes of cloacal malformations which do not benefit from in utero shunt therapy. Because of the presence of oligo/anhydramnios, we commonly obtain karyotypes by transabdominal chorionic villus sampling which gives reliable results within 5 days during which the remainder of the prenatal evaluation is underway. Fluorencence in situ hybridization (FISH) can be used to get rapid status of chromosomes 13, 18, 21, X and Y.[8]

Essential to the prenatal workup is the evaluation of underlying renal status in the fetus. Over the past 15 years, we have developed a multicomponent approach for the analysis of fetal urine that evaluates proximal tubular and possible glomerular status using sodium, chloride, osmolality, calcium, β-2 microglobulin, albumin, and total protein concentrations.[5] Predictive reliability has been shown to be significantly improved by sequential samplings at 48–72 hour intervals.[6] Using such an approach, one can directly correlate the degree of impaired renal function and damage with the extent of urinary hypertonicity and proteinuria. As such, the ability to counsel patients about the renal status of their fetus and the long-term prognosis has been dramatically improved.

Vesicoamniotic catheter shunts bypass the urethral obstruction diverting the urine into the amniotic space to allow appropriate drainage of the upper urinary tract and prevention of pulmonary hypoplasia and physical deformations (Fig. 70.2). In fetuses with isolated LUTO, a normal male karyotype, and progressively improving urinary profile that meet threshold parameters (Table 70.1), intervention has been very successful in salvaging fetuses using percutaneous vesicoamniotic shunt therapy.

Experiencew in humans has been widely variable and appears to be related to the extent of prenatal evaluation prior to shunt placement, as well as the etiology of obstruction. Freedman

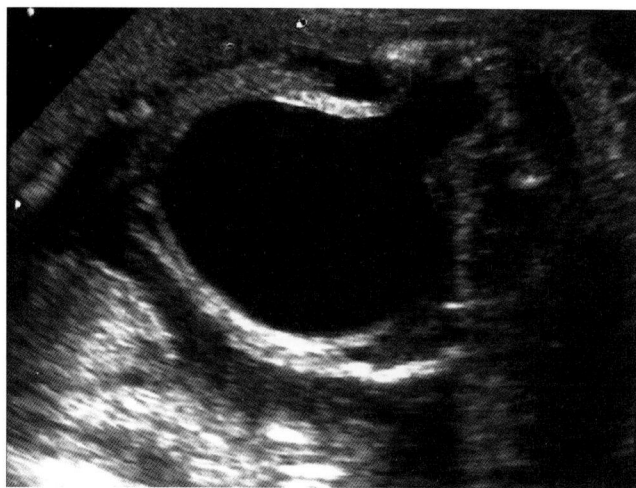

Fig. 70.1: Oligohydramnios and dilated bladder in a fetus at 17 weeks with good electrolytes

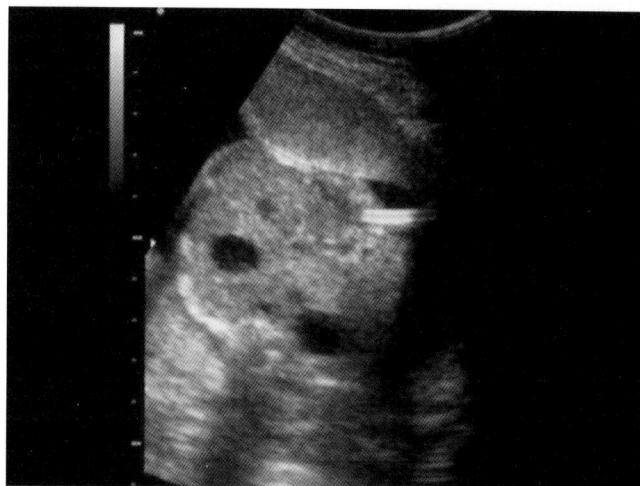

Fig. 70.2: Vesicoamniotic shunt with the proximal portion lying within the fetal bladder while the distal portion lies within the amniotic fluid space allowing diversionary draining of urine into the appropriate space

Table 70.1: Upper threshold values for selecting fetuses that might benefit from prenatal intervention

Sodium	< 100 mg/dL
Chloride	< 90 mg/dL
Osmolality	< 190 mOsm/L
Calcium	< 8 mg/dL
β-2 microglobulin	< 6 mg/L
Total protein	< 40 mg/dL

et al. confirmed that Prune Belly infants, without complete urethral obstructions have very good renal outcomes following vesicoamniotic shunt therapy.[7] They have also found significant improvement in survival and renal function in infants with posterior urethral valves treated by shunting, however, many have mild to moderate renal insufficiency at birth and several of these have progressed to renal failure, dialysis and transplantation. The worst group of infants appears to be those with urethral atresia. However, there have been survivors with urethral atresia following early shunt intervention. These findings support animal studies, which indicated that early onset, complete obstructions resulted in more severe renal damage than later onset or partial obstructions. Such data emphasize the necessity for early diagnosis, evaluation and intervention in such cases.

More recently, data from our experience over the past 15 years suggests that patients having bladder shunts had a 91% survival, but long-term renal function was not guaranteed. Just under half had "normal renal function", and about a quarter had mild impairments. The experience depended highly on the exact etiology of the disorder with posterior urethral value having the best outcomes and urethral atresia the worst. The experience suggests that close pediatric urologic/renal function assessment is essential. The Paris group has found that about 25% of children had serious, long-term renal impairments and about 15% actually developed end stage renal disease requiring transplant.[9]

Although vesicoamniotic shunting has clearly improved survival and renal function in cases of early obstructive uropathy, complications of this procedure remain unacceptably high. We

found in the 80s and 90s that in 40% of our cases, the shunts became physically displaced into the amniotic or intraperitoneal space, or have become obstructive with loss of drainage function, necessitating replacement. On balance, intervention for LUTO has saved fetuses who would otherwise have surely died. Many have normal to moderately impaired renal function. A carefully balanced approach in counseling is required for patients to determine what is right for them.

OTHER SHUNTS

In the late 1970s, shunting was attempted for obstructive hydrocephalus.[10] Attempts in the late 1970s and early 80s at in utero ventriculoperitoneal shunting were nearly uniformly disastrous. However, in retrospect, most operated patients were, in fact, very poor candidates for intervention. Many had multisystem syndromic disorders, including aneuploidy, and hopeless congenital anomalies such as holoprosencephaly.

Accordingly, ventriculoamniotic shunts were abandoned since the early 80s. With a better understanding of the poor natural history of the anomaly, and better, more accurate diagnostic techniques, we have speculated that there may eventually be limited applications for prenatal neurologic shunting in cases of early-onset, isolated, progressive obstructive hydrocephaly.

The other use of percutaneously placed shunts has been for thoracic abnormalities.[11,12] The macrocystic form of congenital cystic adenomatous malformation can present with a very large intrathoracic mass with a dominant macrocyst which causes cardiac and mediastinal shift and comes with its potential hemodynamic changes, as well as pulmonary compression and risk of lung hypoplasia. Such dominant cysts can be approached using pleuroamniotic shunts to chronically drain these structures, reducing their volume, and diminishing their space occupying effects within the thoracic cavity.

Isolated pleural effusions can also accumulate to the point of causing hemodynamic changes and onset of generalized hydrops as well as pulmonary compression, which interferes with normal lung development increasing the risk of hypoplasia. Small, unilateral effusions generally do not warrant intervention, but must be followed closely as they have the potential for rapid progression and development of generalized hydrops.[12]

As with all fetal interventions, prenatal evaluation prior to intervention is critical for appropriate case selection. Seemingly isolated effusions may be the first sign of a cardiac malformation, aneuploidy, anemia or an infectious process. Thoracoamniotic shunting is effective in carefully evaluated cases when the risk of pulmonary hypoplasia from large effusions early in gestation is present, or early signs of progressive hydrops (unilateral-bilateral effusion, skin or scalp edema, ascites, pericardial effusion) appear. Fetal anemia, per se, is not an indication for thoracoamniotic effusion shunting, as hydropic changes will usually resolve with timely fetal transfusion therapy. Also, if one waits to intervene until the fetus develops significant ascites, the prognosis even with successful shunt intervention diminishes considerably.[12] However, several cases with suddenly progressive pleural effusions and onset of generalized hydrops (skin/scalp edema, pericardial effusion and moderate ascites) have been treated with complete resolution of all hydropic complications and normal postnatal infants.

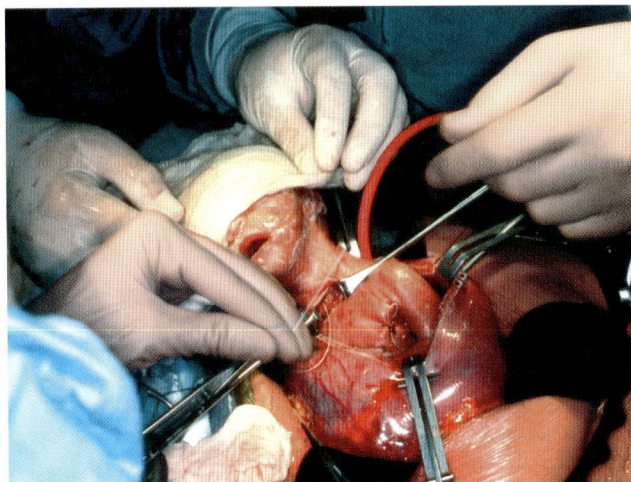

Fig. 70.3: Surgical isolation of the fetal trachea prior to placement of hemoclips in a tracheal occlusion procedure for congenital diaphragmatic hernia

OPEN SURGICAL APPROACHES

For a limited number of indications open fetal surgery has been performed for about 20 years.[2] Appropriate concerns for maternal risk, rigorous selection criteria and somewhat frustrating results have limited its use. There has been continuing innovation and development of instruments and techniques, motivated by the clinical necessity to improve the safety of open fetal surgery for both the fetus and the mother.

Congenital Diaphragmatic Hernia (CDH)

The fetal approach to CDH has undergone continuous evolution since the first attempted CDH repair in 1986 and the first success in 1989.[13-16] Definitive repair of CDH by reduction of viscera from the chest, diaphragmatic patch placement and abdominal silo construction (to reduce intraabdominal pressure) had unacceptable mortality, particularly after a clinical trial showed open fetal repair was no better than postnatal repair, when the liver was herniated into the chest.[17,18] The definitive repair was abandoned as an option for CDH; in utero tracheal occlusion took its place[18-25] (Fig. 70.3). Tracheal occlusion leads to an increase in lung size through accumulation of pulmonary secretions, which reduces the herniated viscera from the chest and decreases the risk for lung hypoplasia. The technique of achieving reliable, complete and reversible tracheal occlusion has evolved. Initially, it could only be accomplished by open fetal surgery and fetal neck dissection (taking care to avoid the recurrent laryngeal nerves) and placement of occlusive hemoclips. Next, a fetoscopic technique was developed to accomplish the same neck dissection and tracheal clip (the Fetendo Clip Procedure).[22-23] While successful, it proved difficult, with a significant learning curve. Attempts to simplify the procedure by developing an appropriate polymer to use as a tracheal plug inserted through the fetal mouth were unsuccessful. Experience quickly showed that unless there was complete occlusion, the pulmonary secretions would leak, thereby defeating the purpose of the plug. Finally, a relatively simple technique was developed in which a fetoscope passed through a single port is advanced into the fetal trachea (fetal

bronchoscopy) and a detachable silicone balloon is inflated to occlude the trachea.

CDH has been a classic example of rapid changes in technology clouding any simple attempts to understand the role for fetal surgery. With increasing sophistication of the surgical approach as well as concomitant improvements in neonatal care using extracorporeal membrane oxygenation (ECMO), it was impossible to accurately determine the relative benefits of each approach without a prospective, randomized comparison that held all other details constant. Thus, after much debate, a randomized trial of surgery for CDH versus optimal postnatal care was funded by NICHD.[18] The principle component of the trial was that patients in the postnatal care (control) arm would receive the same neonatal care by the same center as the surgical arm.

It was originally expected that patients having the surgery would have a survival rate of about 70% as compared to the best data on controls expecting about 35%. The surgically treated patients achieved expected survival. However, the trial was stopped prematurely, when by having the controls cared for at the same tertiary specialty centers as the surgical group, survival in the controls was essentially the same as the surgical group. Such data show conclusively the principle of "the moving target" and how our use of technology must continually adapt to changing conditions.[25]

Congenital Cystic Adenomatoid Malformation (CCAM)

CCAM is a space occupying congenital cystic lesion of the lung which may grow and induce hydrops by causing mediastinal shift and compromise venous return to the heart. When fetuses with CCAM develop hydrops, the fetal mortality approaches 100% (Fig. 70.4).[26-28] Fetal resection of CCAM reverses hydrops and has improved survival dramatically.[26-28] The fetal operation is performed by exposure of the arm and chest wall on the side of the lesion through the maternal hysterotomy. A large muscle sparing thoracotomy is performed through the midthorax of the fetus and the lobe containing the CCAM is isolated. The attachments of

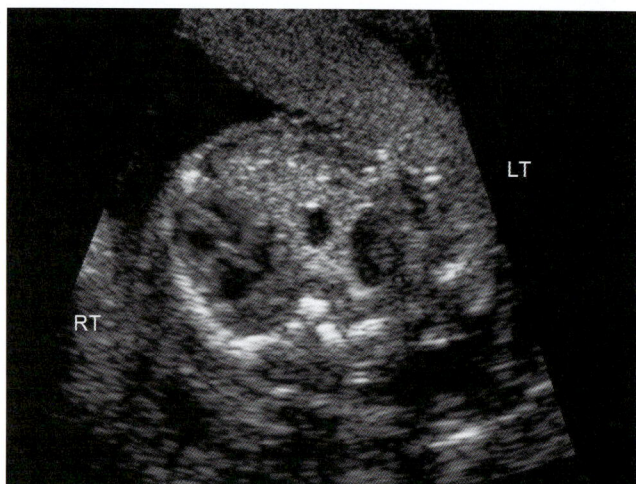

Fig. 70.4: Microcystic congenital cystic adenomatous malformation (microcystic) with beginnings of hydrops

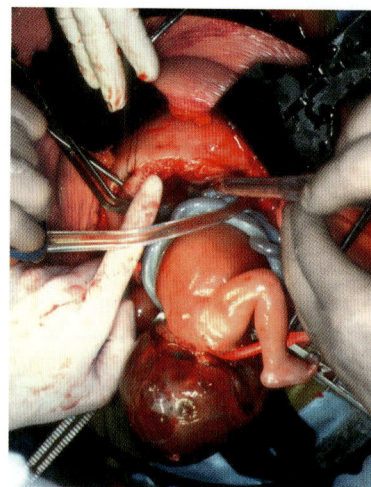

Fig. 70.5: Sacrococcygeal teratoma in a fetus

the lobe to adjacent lung tissue are bluntly divided and the lobar hilum is divided by use of a TIA stapler or a bulk ligature. During the remainder of the pregnancy, the remaining normal lung shows compensatory growth filling the space left showing mass removal.

Sacrococcygeal Teratoma (SCT)

Fetal SCT arises from the presacral space, which may grow to massive proportions and in some fetuses induce high output failure from tumor vascular steal. Fetal SCT with high output physiology with associated placentomegaly or hydrops uniformly result in fetal demise (Fig. 70.5).[29,30] The pathophysiologic rationale for fetal surgery is to ligate the vascular connections to the tumor, remove the vascular "sin", and reverse the high output physiology. The fetal operation is performed by exteriorization of the fetal buttocks with attached tumor.[29] Every attempt is made to keep the head, torso and lower extremities of the fetus in the uterus. Since, the tumor can sometimes be larger than the fetus, significant loss of uterine volume occurs, and the uterus may contract increasing the risk for placental abruption, placental dysfunction because of compression, or postoperative preterm labor. Once exteriorized, the anus is identified and the fetal skin incised posterior to the anorectal sphincter complex to avoid injury to the continence mechanism. A tourniquet is then applied to the base of the tumor and brought down gradually as the tumor is finger fractured down to its vascular pedicle. The vascular pedicle is then ligated with suture ligatures or TIA device stapled depending upon the width of the pedicle. The entire fetal procedure can be performed in less than 15 minutes with minimal blood loss. Because of the increase in afterload following ligation of the low resistance tumor circuit, the fetal hemodynamic status must be monitored by fetal echocardiography during and in the immediate period following the ligation.

The EXIT Procedure

The ex utero intrapartum treatment (EXIT) procedure is a modified cesarean delivery and may be applied to deliver fetuses after fetal surgical procedures such as tracheal ligation, or for fetuses with difficult airway problems such as massive cervical teratomas or cystic hygromas.[31,32] The most important component of the EXIT procedure is maintenance of uteroplacental perfusion until the fetal airway is secured and ventilation is established. In direct contrast

to cesarean section where uterine contraction for hemostasis is encouraged, uterine relaxation is maintained by deep general anesthesia. The fetal manipulations are then performed with maternal support via the placenta. Clips can be removed, chest masses removed, bronchoscopy performed and stable airway access established in otherwise very difficult circumstances with this approach. Once the fetus is ready for transport to the nursery or adjacent operating suite following these preliminary steps, the cord is clamped and cut, and the cesarean delivery completed.

Meningomyelocele

Babies with myelingomyeloceles have impaired lower motor function, and loss of bowel and bladder control. A significant percentage develop obstructive hydrocephalus which requires ventriculoperitoneal shunting.[33] Experience from the 1970s and 80s showed that babies with meningomyelocele delivered atraumatically by cesarean section had a better level of motor function for the given level of anatomic defect, than those babies delivered through the vaginal canal.[34] Such data suggest that compression and trauma to the cord in the delivery process can have permanent long-term sequelae to motor function. It therefore follows that trauma to the spinal cord in utero, either from banging into the uterine wall, or the toxic effects of the amniotic fluid in the third trimester, per se, could be detrimental to the function of the spinal cord. Furthermore, the traditional dogma that the pathogenesis of meningomyelocele was that an abnormally developed spinal cord, which did not in turn, engender the proper development of the bony spinal column, may not be the whole story. It is possible that the primary defect is in the bony spinal column, which exposes a presumptively undamaged spinal cord. The cord is then damaged by the toxic effects of amniotic fluid and trauma from the uterine environment and repeated contact with the uterine wall. Thus, the rationale for attempts to cover and protect the spinal cord in utero, to minimize the sequelae.[35]

Three groups have done most of the work in this area and have attempted to repair meningomyeloceles in utero, both as an open surgical procedure, and endoscopically, with the stated attempt to reduce long-term morbidity and mortality.[36–38]

The principal benefit of the surgery is likely secondary, i.e. a significant reduction in the number of babies requiring ventriculoperitoneal shunting for obstructive hydrocephalus.[39,40] There is still much controversy surrounding the data.[33] A randomized, prospective trial comparing fetal to postnatal neurosurgical closure began in 2003 but will take several years to be completed. A major milestone of this trial has been the agreement among the participating centers not to perform any cases outside the trial, and other centers around the country have agreed not to start programs until the trial is completed.

CONCLUSION

There are an increasing number of congenital and genetic abnormalities for which in utero treatment is possible, and in some cases, now relatively routine. Advances in therapies have progressed at different paces for different disorders, but there is great hope and enthusiasm that progress will continue to expand the number of disorders for which therapy can be effective.

REFERENCES

1. Evans MI, Bui TH (eds). The Genome Revolution and Obstetrics and Gynecology. Balliere's Best Practice and Research in Clinical Obstetrics and Gynecology. London: Harcourt Brace Publishing Co.; 2002. p. 16.
2. Harrison MR, Evans MI, Adzick NS, et al. The Unborn Patient. WB Philadelphia PA: Saunders; 2000.
3. Johnson MP, Flake AW, Quintero RA, et al. Shunt procedures. In: Evans MI, Johnson MP, Moghissi KS (Eds). Invasive Outpatient Procedures in Reproductive Medicine, New York: Raven Press; 1997.
4. Evans MI, Sacks AL, Johnson MP, et al. Sequential invasive assessment of fetal renal function, and the in utero treatment of fetal obstructive uropathies. Obstet Gynecol. 1991;77(4):545-50.
5. Wilson RD, Johnson MP. Prenatal ultrasound guided percutaneous shunt for obstruction, uropathy and thoracic disease. Seminars in Pediatric Surgery. 2003;12:182-9.
6. Johnson MP, Corsi P, Bradfield W, et al. Sequential fetal urine analysis provides greater precision in the evaluation of fetal obstructive uropathy. Am J Obstet Gynecol. 1995;173:59-65.
7. Freedman AL, Bukowski TP, Smith CA, et al. Fetal therapy for obstructive uropathy: Specific outcomes diagnosis. J Urology. 1996;156:720-4.
8. Feldman B, Aviram-Goldring A, Evans MI. Interphase FISH for prenatal diagnosis of common aneuploidies. Methods Mol Biol. 2002;204:219-41.
9. Dommergues M, Mueller F. Experience of 100 Obstructive Uropathies. International Fetal Medicine and Surgery Society (unpublished). 2003.
10. Drugan A, Krause B, Canady A, et al. The natural history of prenatally diagnosed ventriculomegaly. JAMA. 1989;261:1785-8.
11. Ahmad FK, Sherman SJ, Hagglund KH, et al. Isolated unilateral pleural effusion: The role of sonographic surveillance and in utero therapy. Fetal Diagn and Ther. 1996;11:383-9.
12. Nicolaides KH, Azar GB. Thoracoamniotic shunting. Fetal Diagn and Ther. 1990;5:153-64.
13. Adzick N, Harrison M, Flake A, et al. Automatic uterine stapling devices in fetal surgery: Experience in a primate model. Surgical Forum. 1985; XXXVI:479-81.
14. Jennings RW, Adzick NS, Longaker MT, et al. New techniques in fetal surgery. J Ped Surg. 1992;27:1329-33.
15. Jennings RW, Adzick NS, Longaker MT, et al. Radiotelemetric fetal monitoring during and after open fetal operation. Surgery, Gynecologic and Obstetrics. 1993;176:59-64.
16. Harrison MR, Longaker MT, Adzick NS, et al. Successful repair *in utero* of a fetal diaphragmatic hernia after removal of herniated viscera from the left thorax. NEJM. 1990;322:1582-4.

17. Harrison MR, Adzick NS, Flake AW, et al. Correction of congenital diaphragmatic hernia in utero: VI. Hard-learned lessons. J Ped Surg. 1993;28:1141-7; discussion. 1417-8.
18. Harrison MR, Keller RL, Hawgood SB, et al. A randomized trial of fetal endoscopic tracheal occlusion for severe fetal congenital diaphragmatic hernia. N Engl J Med. 2003;349:1916-24.
19. Harrison MR, Sydorak RM, Farrell JA, et al. Fetoscopic temporary tracheal occlusion for congenital diagphragmatic hernia: Prelude to a randomized, controlled trial. J Pediatr Surg. 2003;38(7):1012-20.
20. Heerema AE, Rabban JT, Sydorak RM, et al. Lung pathology in patients with congenital diaphragmatic hernia treated with fetal surgical intervention, including tracheal occlusion. Pediatr Dev Pathol. 2003.
21. Sydorak RM, Harrison MR. Congenital diaphragmatic hernia: Advances in Prenatal Therapy. Clin Perinatol. 2003;30(3):465-79.
22. Danzer E, Sydora RM, Harrison MR, et al. Minimal access fetal surgery. Eur J Obstet Gynecol Reprod Biol 2003;1;108(1):3-13.
23. Evans MI, Harrison MR, Flake AW, et al. Fetal Therapy. Best Pract Res Clin Obstet Gynecol. 2002;16(5):67-183.
24. Paek BW, Coakley FV, Lu Y, et al. Congenital diaphragmatic hernia: prenatal evaluation with MR lung volumetry. Preliminary Experience. 2000;220(1):63-7.
25. Wenstrom KD. Fetal surgery for congenital diaphragmatic hernia. N Engl J Med. 2003;13;349(20):1887-8.
26. Adzick NS, Kitano Y. Fetal surgery for lung lesions, congenital diaphragmatic hernia, and saccrococcygeal teratoma. Seminars in Pediatric Surgery. 2003;12:154-67.
27. Adzick NS, Harrison MR, Crombleholme TM, et al. Fetal lung: management and outcome. Am J Obstet Gynecol. 1998;179:884-9.
28. Crombleholme TM, Coleman BG, Howell LJ, et al. Elevated cystic adenomatoid malformation volume (CVR) outcome in prenatal diagnosis of cystic adenomatoid malformation of the Lung. J Pediatr Surg. 2002;37:331-8.
29. Hotterman AX, Filiatrault D, Lallier M, et al. The natural history of sacrococcygeal teratomas diagnosed through routine obstetric sonogram: A single institution experience. J Pediatr Surg. 2002;37:331-8.
30. Paek B. Vaezy S, Fujimoto V, et al. Tissue ablation using high-intensity focused ultrasound. Potential for Fetal Treatment. Am J Obstet Gynecol. 2003;1875-77.
31. Liechty KW, Crombleholme TM, Flake AW, et al. Intrapartum airway management for giant neck masses. The EXIT (ex utero intrapartum treatorus procedure. Am J Obstet Gynecol. 1997;177:870-4.
32. Hedrick HL. Ex utero intrapartum therapy. Seminars in Perinatology 2003;12:190-5.

33. Meningomyelocele: Prenatal diagnosis, pathophysiology and management. Seminars in Perinatology. 2003;12:168-74.
34. Lemire RJ. Neural tube defects. JAMA. 1988;259:558-62.
35. Meuli M, Meuli-Simmen C, Hutchins GM, et al. In utero surgery rescues neurological function at birth in sheep with spina bifida. Nature Med. 1995;1(4):342-6.
36. Bruner JP, Tulipan N, Paschall RL, et al. Fetal surgery for myelomeningocele and the Incidence of shunt-dependent hydrocephalus. JAMA. 1999;282(19):1819-25.
37. Sutton LN, Adzick NS, Bilaniuk LT, et al. Improvement in hind-brain herniation demonstrated by serial fetal magnetic resonance imaging following fetal surgery for myelomeningocele. JAMA. 1999;282:1826-31.
38. Tulipan N, Hermanz-Schulman M, Breniner JP. Reduced hind-brain herniation after intrauterine myelomingocele repair. A report of four cases. Pediatr Neurosurgery. 1998;29:4-278.
39. Bruner JP, Tulipan N, Paschall RL, et al. Intrauterine repair of myelomeningocele, "Hind-brain herniation", and the incidence of shunt dependent hydrocephalus. JAMA. 1999;282:1819-25.
40. Johnson MP, Adzick WS, Rintoul N, et al. Fetal meningocele repair: short-term outcomes. Am J Obstet Gynecol. 2003;189:482-7.

SECTION 8

Screening and Risk Assessment

G Monni, S Chasen

71

First Trimester Ultrasound Screening for Fetal Malformations

ST Chasen

INTRODUCTION

The most significant advance in first trimester ultrasound screening has been the recognition of nuchal translucency (NT) as a potent marker for fetal aneuploidy.[1] Abnormal NT in a euploid fetus is also associated with structural fetal abnormalities that can be diagnosed in the second trimester.[2] Thus, measurement of NT can lead to earlier and targeted screening in the second trimester.

While abnormal NT can suggest the possibility of a structural abnormality, advances in ultrasound imaging have made the direct diagnosis of some anomalies possible.[3,4] Evaluation of other anatomic structures in the first trimester can diagnose anomalies or identify useful markers for anomalies that may be diagnosed later in pregnancy. As more women will be presenting for NT measurement at 11–14 weeks of gestation, it is important to consider other anatomic structures amenable to evaluation at this time.

EVALUATION OF FIRST TRIMESTER ANATOMY

Fetal Head

Structures that can be well visualized in the first trimester include the calvarium and portions of the developing brain. Midline structures, including a falx cerebri and thalamic bodies, are easily visualized. Choroid-filled lateral ventricles can be identified as well. The cavum septum pellucidum and structures in the posterior fossa cannot be reliably evaluated in many cases, though visualization becomes more likely by 14 weeks.

Fetal Face

The profile is well imaged in most fetuses from 11 weeks to 14 weeks, and this has led to the use of nasal bone evaluation in Down syndrome screening.[5] The orbits can be identified as well. While the lips can be seen at these gestational ages in some fetuses, they cannot be reliably evaluated in a significant proportion of cases.

Fetal Spine

The cervical and cervical spines can be evaluated in the first trimester. Unfortunately, the lumbar and sacral spines, in which spina bifida are much more likely to occur, are often not well imaged prior to the second trimester.

Fetal Heart

Aside from cardiac axis, the structure of the fetal heart is generally not well evaluated at 14 weeks of gestation or earlier. Four-chamber view, outflow tracts, ductus arteriosus, and the aortic arch cannot be evaluated in many cases at these gestational ages.[6]

Abdomen

An intact diaphragm and stomach bubble are visible at 11–14 weeks in most cases. The umbilical cord insertion in the ventral wall and the urinary bladder just below the site of cord insertion can be seen in the vast majority of fetuses as well. The kidneys can usually be identified, though this is not possible in a small proportion of cases.

Extremities

By 11 weeks, high-resolution ultrasound can document the presence of all long bones in the extremities in most fetuses. Reference ranges for limb measurements early in pregnancy have been published.[7] The hands and feet are usually easily identified. Evaluation of the fingers is possible, though this may be limited prior to the second trimester.

DIAGNOSIS OF FETAL ANOMALIES AT 11–14 WEEKS

While we can identify many structures by the end of the first trimester, sonographic diagnosis of abnormalities in these structures is limited. Although first trimester sonographic diagnosis has been reported for a wide variety of anomalies,[4,8-10] relatively few can be reliably diagnosed or excluded with confidence. The following anomalies can be reliably diagnosed or excluded sonographically in most cases at the 11–14 weeks' scan.

Anencephaly/Acrania

Anencephaly and acrania are characterized by the absence of a cranial vault. Both conditions are easily identified or excluded after 10 weeks of gestation.[11] While anencephaly is characterized by absence of the cranial vault and the cerebral cortex, the latter structure can be seen in acrania (Fig. 71.1). Both conditions are uniformly lethal. While there is some controversy as to whether acrania is due to failed closure of the rostral portion of the neural tube (as is anencephaly), women should be counseled to take high doses of folic acid starting prior to conception in future pregnancies to prevent open neural tube defects.

Holoprosencephaly

This condition is due to the failure of the forebrain to cleave into hemispheres early in gestation. Alobar holoprosencephaly, in which no midline structures are noted and only a single ventricle is present, is the most severe variant. This condition should be strongly suspected when two separate choroid plexuses are not seen in a transverse view through the fetal brain. Alobar holoprosencephaly can be diagnosed or excluded after 10 weeks of gestation[12] (Fig. 71.2). Semilobar and lobar holoprosencephaly, in which some

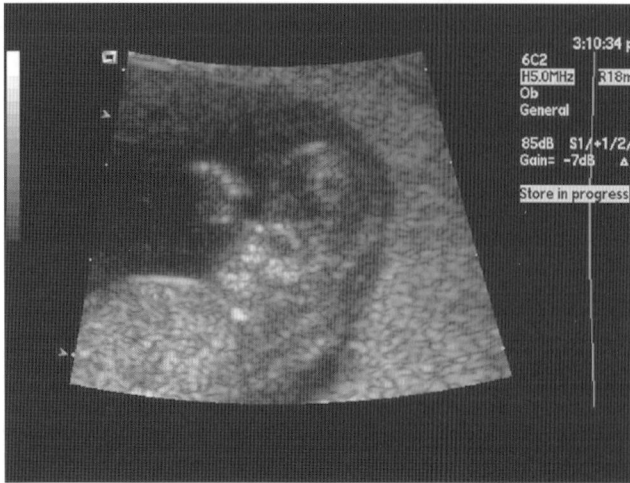

Fig. 71.1: Acrania at 11 weeks of gestation. No bony structures are seen above the level of the orbits. Brain tissue can be seen. This would not be visualized in the case of anencephaly

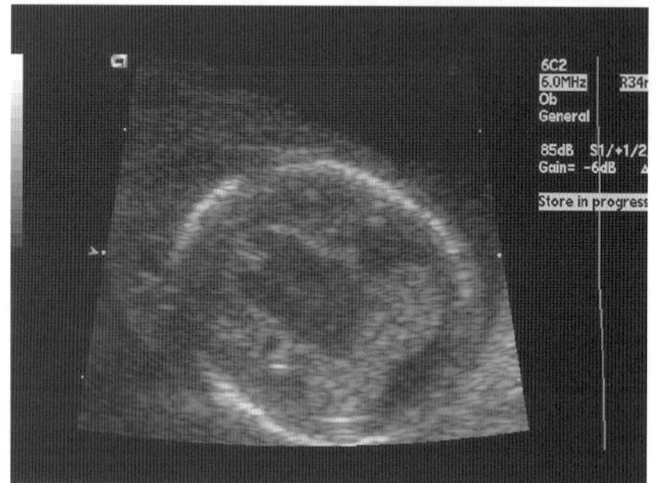

Fig. 71.2: Alobar holoprosencephaly at 12 weeks of gestation. A single, small crescent-shaped holoventricle is seen anteriorly. The thalami are large, and not divided by a third ventricle. Separate choroid plexuses are not seen

form of midline division has occurred, cannot always be detected prior to the second trimester.

While not lethal in all cases, alobar holoprosencephaly is associated with virtual absence of cognitive function. Cytogenetic studies are indicated, as this abnormality is associated with trisomy 13 as well as other less common forms of aneuploidy. As holoprosencephaly has been described to have autosomal recessive inheritance in some families,[13] recurrence can be excluded with identification of normal midline structures by the end of the first trimester.

Cephalocele

Cephalocele is characterized by a defect in the skull, with protrusion of the meninges. In most cases, there will be brain tissue in the meningeal sac (encephalocele). Most midline cephaloceles are open neural tube defects, though they are much less common than either anencephaly or spina bifida. When a non-midline cephalocele is detected, amniotic band syndrome may be present.

Ultrasound can detect cephalocele at 11–14 weeks (Fig. 71.3). Large cephaloceles are easily identified, though smaller ones may not be seen early in pregnancy. In patients with a prior fetus with Meckel-Gruber syndrome, which is characterized by cephalocele, multicystic kidneys, and polydactyly, first trimester ultrasound can be used to detect early signs of recurrence of this autosomal recessive condition.[14]

Omphalocele

Omphalocele is a midline ventral wall defect. All layers of the abdominal wall are absent at the site of the umbilical cord insertion, and a sac can be seen protruding from this site. The sac usually contains bowel and stomach. In larger lesions, liver may be present. The umbilical cord can be seen inserting into the sac.

It is important not to confuse physiologic midgut herniation, which occurs prior to 11–12 weeks of gestation, with omphalocele.[15] After 12 weeks of gestation, omphalocele, particularly if a large defect is present, is easily identified (Fig. 71.4). Omphalocele is frequently associated with trisomy 18 or trisomy 13.

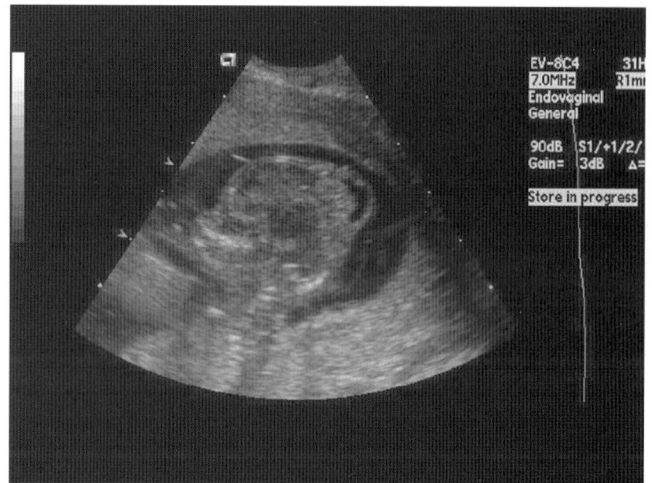

Fig. 71.3: Encephalocele at 12 weeks of gestation. In this profile view, a midline skull defect is seen above the level of the occiput

Skeletal Defects

Though fetal long bones can be identified and measured late in the first trimester, most skeletal dysplasias that are characterized by abnormal limb growth cannot be reliably detected or excluded early in pregnancy.[16] Limb reduction defects, which occur sporadically, are characterized by absence of all or a large part of an extremity can be identified at the 11–14 weeks' scan.

Megacystis

In this condition, the fetal urinary bladder is markedly enlarged (Fig. 71.5). A longitudinal diameter of >7 mm has been suggested to establish the diagnosis.[17] While the presence of megacystis does not indicate a specific diagnosis, high rates of fetal aneuploidy (especially when NT is abnormal) and obstructive uropathy have been reported.[18] The presence of megacystis is an indication to evaluate the genitourinary tract for obstructive uropathy early in the second trimester.

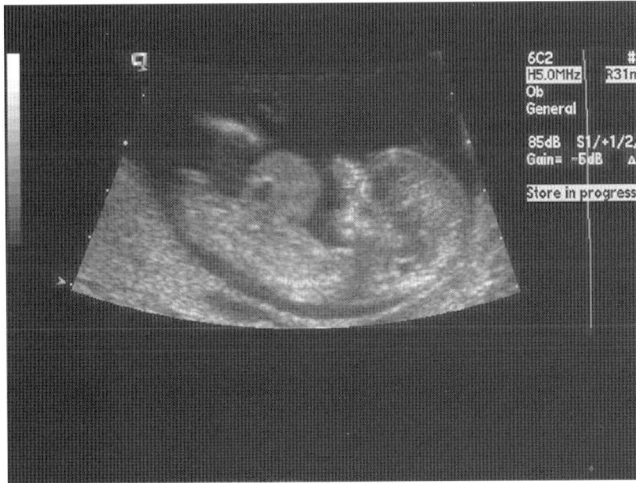

Fig. 71.4: Omphalocele at 13 weeks of gestation. A large sac containing bowel and liver is seen

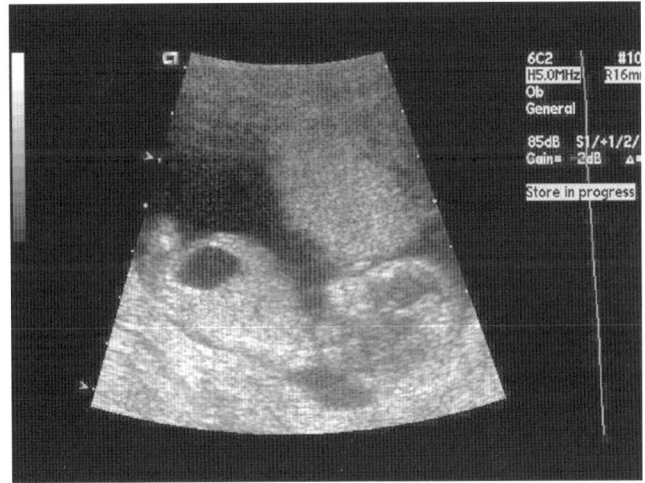

Fig. 71.5: Megacystis at 11 weeks of gestation. A cystic midline mass is seen in the pelvis

APPROACH TO SCREENING

In patients who present for ultrasound late in the first trimester, evaluation of fetal anatomy can provide valuable information. This information can be obtained in a relatively short amount of time in most patients.[4,6] While certain findings (such as nuchal edema or megacystis) are not diagnostic and require second trimester follow-up, some conditions can be diagnosed or excluded at this stage in pregnancy. This may be especially useful to those at high risk of having a fetus with malformations detectable in the first trimester.

Studies evaluating the detection rates for anomalies in the first trimester suggest that the majority of major structural anomalies can be identified or suspected.[4,8,9] As these studies have been done in large perinatal centers, however, it is not clear that similar outcomes can be achieved outside this setting. The experience of the examiner is important, as a learning curve for prenatal diagnosis in the first trimester has been demonstrated.[9]

While evaluation of anatomy at 11–14 weeks is recommended when NT is measured, this examination cannot replace routine second trimester ultrasound. Comparison of detection rates of fetal anomalies demonstrates higher sensitivity at 16–20 weeks.[9] This is particularly true for cardiac abnormalities, the most common category of malformations.

CONCLUSION

With the emergence of first trimester risk assessment for aneuploidy, many patients will be undergoing ultrasound late in the first trimester. If the sole objective of this examination is to measure NT, the opportunity to assess fetal anatomy will be lost. With experience, examination of the fetus at 11–14 weeks of gestation can be accomplished in a short amount of time, and patients will have the benefit of early diagnosis of certain anomalies.

REFERENCES

1. Nicolaides KH. Nuchal translucency and other first trimester sonographic markers of chromosomal abnormalities. Am J Obstet Gynecol. 2004;191:45-67.
2. Hyett JA. Increased nuchal translucency in fetuses with a normal karyotype. Prenat Diagn. 2002;22:864-8.
3. Whitlow BJ, Chatzipapas IK, Lazanakis ML, et al. The value of sonography in early pregnancy for the detection of fetal abnormalities in an unselected population. Br J Obstet Gynecol. 1999;106:929-36.
4. Souka AP, Nicolaides KH. Diagnosis of fetal abnormalities at the 10–14 week scan. Ultrasound Obstet Gynecol. 1997;10:429-42.
5. Cicero S, Curcio P, Papageorghiou A, et al. Absence of nasal bone in fetuses with trisomy 21 at 11–14 weeks of gestation: An observational study. Lancet. 2001;358:1665-7.
6. Timor-Tritsch IE, Bashiri A, Monteagudo A, et al. Qualified and trained sonographers in the US can perform early fetal anatomy scans between 11 and 14 weeks. Am J Obstet Gynecol. 2004;191:1247-52.
7. Zorzoli A, Kustermann A, Caravelli E, et al. Measurements of fetal limb bones in early pregnancy. Ultrasound Obstet Gynecol. 1994;4:29-33.
8. Chen M, Lam YH, Lee CP, et al. Ultrasound screening of fetal structural abnormalities at 12 to 14 weeks in Hong Kong. Prenat Diagn. 2004;24:92-7.
9. Taipale P, Ammala M, Salonen R, et al. Learning curve in ultrasonographic screening for selected fetal structural anomalies in early pregnancy. Obstet Gynecol. 2003;101:273-8.
10. Dugoff L. Ultrasound diagnosis of structural abnormalities in the first trimester. Prenat Diagn. 2002;22:316-20.
11. Johnson SP, Sebire NJ, Snijders RJ, et al. Ultrasound screening for anencephaly at 10-14 weeks of gestation. Ultrasound Obstet Gynecol. 1997;9:14-6.
12. Sepulveda W, Dezerega V, Be C. First trimester sonographic diagnosis of holoprosencephaly: Value of the "butterfly" sign. J Ultrasound Med. 2004;23:761-5.

13. Barr M Jr, Cohen MM Jr. Autosomal recessive alobar holoprosencephaly with essentially normal faces. Am J Med Genet. 2002;112:28-30.

14. Tanriverdi HA, Hendrik HJ, Ertan K, et al. Meckel Gruber syndrome: A first trimester diagnosis of a recurrent case. Eur J Ultrasound. 2002;15:69-72.

15. van Zalen-Sprock RM, Vugt JM, van Geijn HP. First trimester sonography of physiological midgut herniation and early diagnosis of omphalocele. Prenat Diagn. 1997;17:511-8.

16. Gabrielli S, Falco P, Pilu G, et al. Can transvaginal fetal biometry be considered a useful tool for early detection of skeletal dysplasias in high-risk patients? Ultrasound Obstet Gynecol. 1999;13: 107-11.

17. Sebire NJ, Von Kaisenberg C, Rubio C, et al. Fetal megacystis at 10-14 weeks of gestation. Ultrasound Obstet Gynecol. 1996;8: 387-90.

18. Sepulveda W. Megacystis in the first trimester. Prenat Diagn. 2004;24:144-9.

72 Fetal Nasal Bone in Screening for Down's Syndrome

S Cicero, JD Sonek, G Rembouskos

INTRODUCTION

The major cause of perinatal death and childhood disabilities are chromosomal abnormalities. Prenatal diagnosis of chromosomal defects necessitates invasive testing by chorionic villous sampling, amniocentesis or cordocentesis, which is associated with a risk of miscarriage of about 1%. For this reason, these techniques are reserved for pregnancies considered to be at high risk for chromosomal defects. The methods of screening to identify the high-risk group are described in Table 72.1. Screening using ultrasound is based on the fact that most fetuses with chromosomal abnormalities have structural defects that can be detected by sonographic examination, both in the first and the second trimesters of pregnancy. In order to calculate the individual patient-specific risk of chromosomal defects, it is necessary to take into account the background risk (which depends on maternal age and gestational age) and multiply this by a series of factors, which depend on the results of a series of screening tests carried out during the course of the pregnancy. Every time a test is carried out the background risk is multiplied by the test factor to calculate a new risk, which then becomes the background risk for the next test. This process is called *sequential screening*.[1]

BACKGROUND

The physical characteristic of the individuals affected by trisomy 21, were described for the first time in 1866 by the physician Langdon Down.[2] He reported that the skin is too large for their body, their face is flat and the nose is small.[2] In recent years, it has become possible to observe these features by ultrasound examination during the third month of intrauterine life. Extensive studies over the last decade have demonstrated that the most effective sonographic marker of trisomy 21, and other chromosomal abnormalities, is increased nuchal translucency (NT) at 11–13[+6] weeks of gestation. Another promising marker for trisomy 21, which has been extensively studied over the past 4 years, is the absence of the fetal nasal bones (NB), both in the first and in the second trimesters of pregnancy.

This chapter reviews the association between absence or hypoplasia of the fetal nasal bones (NB) Down's syndrome in the first and second trimester of pregnancy, and examine the value of incorporating this novel marker in screening policies.

DEVELOPMENT OF THE NASAL BONES

During the fourth week of gestation, collections of neural crest cells undergo proliferation, forming the nasal placodes. In the sixth week, the nasal placodes of the frontonasal prominence invaginate to form the nasal pits, and the lateral and medial processes. The medial nasal processes will fuse with the nasofrontal process to form the nasal septum, which in turn will grow toward the forming palate, defining the left and right nasal cavities. While this is occurring, the cartilaginous frame of the nose is developing. During the eighth week, initial centers of ossification of the NB will appear in the membrane covering the cartilaginous nasal capsule.[3-7]

In 1994, Sandikcioglu et al.[8] established normal prenatal development standards for the NB. This study showed that the two bilateral NB appear as a thin bony contour ventral to the cartilaginous nasal septum in the sagittal plane, and changes gradually during growth to a wedge-shaped bone. The initial appearance of the NB occurred at different developmental stages in normal fetuses. The smallest crown-rump length (CRL) at which NB was observed histologically was 42 mm corresponding to approximately 10.9 weeks of gestation. Furthermore, the NB increased in length with advancing gestation and their appearance changed morphologically, being wider and more pointed at the anterior tip in the most mature specimens.[8]

ANTHROPOMETRICS AND RADIOLOGICAL STUDIES

An anthropometric study in 105 patients with Down's syndrome at 7 months to 36 years of age reported that the nasal root depth was abnormally short in about 50% of cases.[9]

Sandikciolglu et al.[8] demonstrated the feasibility of post-mortem radiological evaluation of the NB in 62 chromosomally normal aborted fetuses at 9–24 weeks of gestational age, and a CRL ranging from 33 mm to 225 mm. Radiographically, the first appearance of the NB was documented in a specimen with a CRL of 50 mm.[8]

Keeling et al.[10] investigated the abnormal development of the NB in aborted Down syndrome fetuses. They examined the development of the axial skeleton in 31 human trisomy 21 aborted fetuses at 12–24 weeks of gestation and found a 60% incidence

Table 72.1: The screening performance of the various tests is compared by examining the detection rate (DR) for a fixed screen positive rate of 5%

Screening test	DR (%)
MA (≥ 37 years)	30
Maternal serum biochemistry at 16 weeks (AFP and β-hCG and uE3)	65
NT at 12 weeks	80
NT and β-hCG and P-APPA at 12 weeks	90
NT and NB and β-hCG and P-APPA at 12 weeks	96

Abbreviations: MA: maternal age; AFP: α-fetoprotein; β-hCG: free β-human chorionic gonadotropin; uE3: unconjugated estriol; NT: nuchal translucency; PAPP-A: pregnancy-associated plasma protein-A; NB: nasal bone.

of either NB absence (26%) or NB hypoplasia (34%).[10] Stempfle et al.[11] conducted a radiological study and found that the NB was absent in 23% of the 60 Down's syndrome aborted fetuses between 15 weeks and 40 weeks of gestation. The authors also observed that, when present, the NB in the Down syndrome fetuses were short.[11]

SONOGRAPHIC, RADIOLOGICAL AND HISTOLOGICAL CORRELATION

Tuxen et al.[12] conducted a postmortem radiological study to investigate the presence of the NB in 33 aborted Down's syndrome fetuses at 14–25 weeks of gestation. They found that 30% (10 of 33) of fetuses had either bilateral or unilateral absence of NB. They also performed a histological evaluation of the specimens, which confirmed a complete NB absence in 7 of 10 fetuses. Histological evaluation was not performed in the remaining 3, including the 2 that had unilateral absence of the NB. Presence of a NB was confirmed in all 23 fetuses that had a radiological evidence of NB formation.[12]

Minderer and his colleagues[13] compared prenatal sonographic findings on the NB in 17 Down's syndrome fetuses between 11 weeks and 14 weeks of gestation, to those obtained by histological study performed after termination of pregnancy. In this report, the NB could not be examined sonographically in 1 of the 17 cases, due to fetal position, and in the remaining 16 cases the NB was either absent or hypoplastic. By contrast, the histological evaluation of the NB area showed evidence of NB formation in 16 of the 17 cases. Armed with the knowledge of the results of the histological evaluation, the investigators reviewed the ultrasound images of the fetuses originally classified as having an absent NB. They claimed that they were able to now detect evidence of a NB albeit "smaller, less distinct, and less echogenic".[13]

A study by Larose et al.[14] compared sonographic and radiological findings on the NB in 21 aborted fetuses with trisomy 21. The ultrasonographic evaluations were done between 11^{+3} weeks and 13^{+5} weeks of gestation. The subsequent radiological studies on the aborted fetuses were performed between 13 weeks and 25^{+5} weeks of gestation. Interestingly, the incidence of NB absence on ultrasound was very similar to the one noted on X-ray. However, the ultrasound and X-ray findings were discordant in 9 of the 21 cases (43%). Four of the cases where the NB was present on ultrasound showed no evidence of an NB on X-ray, indicating a possible wrong assessment of the fetal profile by ultrasound. In the other 5 cases where the NB was noted to be absent on ultrasound, this resulted to be present on X-ray. However, radiological examinations were performed at a later gestational age than that of the ultrasound examination, suggesting that the NB could have developed in the period of time occurred between the two examinations.[14]

The apparent discrepancies in the NB identification among the three modalities (ultrasound, radiology and histology) have a number of possible explanations. It is likely that small areas of calcification can be seen on histological evaluation even if those cannot be detected on either ultrasonography or X-ray. The likelihood of picking these up will depend on the number of sections done. Different types of staining were used in the two studies mentioned above possibly contributing to the contradictory results. In the study by Larose et al.[14] the ultrasounds and the X-rays were done at very different gestational ages (11^{+3}–13^{+5} weeks for ultrasound and 13–25^{+5} weeks for X-ray). Since the prevalence of NB absence changes with gestational age, they are not truly comparable. Just

as is the case with the ultrasound examination, controlling for the gestational age and standardization of the technique for both the radiological and the histological examinations is crucial.

SONOGRAPHIC STUDIES

The observation that in fetuses affected by trisomy 21 sonographic examination may reveal absence of the NB was only made at the beginning of 2001. In the initial description,[15] three Down's syndrome fetuses were evaluated in the second trimester. Two of them had no identifiable NB and one had a hypoplastic NB. A review of the videotaped examination from the first trimester examination of one of the fetuses at the time of the NT evaluation revealed that the NB could not be identified at that point in pregnancy.[15] Armed with this information, observational studies were undertaken to investigate the role of NB examination in screening for Down syndrome.

First Trimester: The 11–13^{+6} Week Scan

Several studies have demonstrated that the fetal NB can be visualized by sonography in the first trimester of pregnancy, and that there is a high association between absent NB at 11–13^{+6} weeks and trisomy 21, as well as other chromosomal abnormalities.[16-25]

Cicero et al.[16] reported for the first time on the absence of the NB in trisomy 21 fetuses in the first trimester of pregnancy. In this observational study ultrasound examination of the fetal profile, for evaluation of absence or presence of the NB, was performed in 701 fetuses at 11–13^{+6} weeks of gestation following screening test by maternal age and NT, and immediately before chorionic villous sampling. In this series, the NB was absent in 73% (43 of 59) of Down's syndrome fetuses and in only 0.5% (3 of 603) of chromosomally normal fetuses. In this initial study, presence or absence of the NB was found to be independent of other fetal and maternal variables. It became clear that incorporation of the examination of the NB into the screening for trisomy 21 by maternal age and NT could increase the sensitivity of the test and reduce, at the same time, the false positive rate.[16]

In an extended series[18] of 5,818 fetuses undergoing prenatal diagnosis by chorionic villous sampling at 11–13^{+6} weeks, the fetal profile was successfully examined in 5,851 (98.9%) cases. Furthermore, the NB was absent in 129 of 5,223 (2.5%) chromosomally normal fetuses, in 229 of 333 (68.8%) fetuses with trisomy 21 and in 95 of the 295 (32%) with other chromosomal defects. An important finding of this study was that the incidence of absent NB is higher in fetuses of Afro-Caribbean origin than in Caucasians; it decreases with fetal CRL and increases with fetal NT. Consequently, in the calculation of an individual patient-specific risk for trisomy 21 it is necessary to take into account these demographic and ultrasound findings.[18]

The fact that ethnic origin of the mother may play a role on the evaluation of the fetal NB, was also suggested by Prefumo et al.[26] The authors conducted a prospective study in 4,492 fetuses. Due to chromosomal abnormalities or an unsatisfactory examination 500 cases were excluded from the analysis. In the remaining 3,992 fetuses, the failure to visualize the fetal NB was significantly higher in women of African but not Asian origin, compared to the Caucasian origin. In this study, it was demonstrated that having a mother of African origin is significantly associated with an increased likelihood of absent fetal NB compared with Caucasians, even after correcting for maternal age, parity and CRL length. The authors suggested that corrections for maternal ethnicity might be required to ensure equity of fetal NB screening in multiracial populations.[26]

There are seven additional studies[19-25] that support the high association between trisomy 21 and absent NB at 11–13[+6] weeks. In their combined data on 12,315 fetuses the fetal profile was successfully examined in 11,973 (97.2%) cases. The NB was absent in 56 of 9,825 (0.6%) chromosomally normal fetuses and in 53 of 79 (67.1%) fetuses with trisomy 21 (Table 72.2).

Malone et al.[27] reported that they were able to examine the fetal nose in only 4,796 of 6,316 (75.9%) fetuses scanned at 10–14 weeks and that the NB was apparently present in all nine of their trisomy 21 fetuses. Their results contrast significantly with the above published studies in a number of ways. In this study, the fetal nose could be examined in only 75.9% of the cases and the NB was reported as being present in all nine of the trisomy 21 fetuses. Issues regarding adequacy of training in this study remain to be elucidated. Furthermore, images published by the lead authors of this study suggest that their technique may not be consistent with that used by others.[28] Similarly, De Biasio and Venturini,[29] who examined retrospectively the photographs obtained for measurement of NT, reported that the NB was present in all five fetuses with trisomy 21. However, the five images that they published were inappropriate both for the measurement of NT and for examination of the NB, because they were either too small or the fetus was too vertical or too oblique.

Preliminary data of a prospective study conducted by the Fetal Medicine Foundation on a series of 18,636 fetuses,[30] who underwent screening by maternal age, NT, maternal serum free β-human chorionic gonadotropin (β-hCG) and pregnancy-associated plasma protein-A (PAPP-A) at 11–13[+6] weeks, the fetal profile was successfully examined in 18,405 (98.8%) cases. The NB was absent in 101 of 18,388 (0.5%) chromosomally normal fetuses, in 85 of 138 (61.6%) fetuses with trisomy 21 and in 34 of the 103 (33%) with other chromosomal defects.[30]

Based on the available data (Table 72.2), it can be concluded that at 11–13[+6] weeks the fetal profile can be successfully examined in about 95% of cases, and that the NB is absent in about 65% of trisomy 21 fetuses and in about 1% of chromosomally normal fetuses.

Consequently, absence of the NB is an important marker of trisomy 21. However, appropriate adjustments need to be made on the basis of maternal ethnic origin, fetal CRL and NT when calculation of individual patient-specific risk for trisomy 21 is performed.

Second Trimester: 15–24 Week Scan

Absence or hypoplasia of the NB represents a new ultrasound marker also in the second trimester of pregnancy, and it is likely to have a major impact on screening for trisomy 21 during the 16–24 week scan. Its role has now been confirmed in large trials.

Bromley et al.[31] assessed the NB using ultrasound in 239 fetuses between 15 weeks and 20 weeks of gestation. Six (37%) of the 16 Down's syndrome fetuses had no detectable NB. Among the fetuses with a normal karyotype, absence of the NB had a prevalence of 0.5%. In this study, absence of the NB was associated with a likelihood ratio for Down's syndrome of 83. Interestingly, in 2 of the 16 (13%) Down's syndrome fetuses, NB absence was the only abnormal finding. In addition, the NB length was found to play an important role. Biparietal diameter (BPD) to NB length (NBL) ratio was generated to control for the gestational age and the size of the fetus. This ratio increases as the NB becomes shorter. Using the BPD/ NBL ratio of 10 or greater as a cut off in screening for Down syndrome gives this test sensitivity of 81% with a false positive rate of 11%. This study confirmed that NB length increases linearly with gestation in chromosomally normal fetuses. However, the NB length in Down syndrome fetuses was found to be remarkably uniform over the gestational age investigated (3.5 ± 0.47 mm) suggesting the possibility that a single cut-off value for NB length may be appropriate in Down syndrome screening in the first half of the second trimester.[31]

Such approach was used in another study[32] looking at the utility of NB evaluation in the second trimester (15–22 weeks). The authors examined the fetal profile in 1,046 singleton pregnancies undergoing amniocentesis for fetal karyotyping at 15–22 weeks. The NB was absent or hypoplastic (<2.5 mm) in 21 of the 34 (61.8%) fetuses with Down syndrome, in 12 of 982 (1.2%) chromosomally normal fetuses, and in 1 of the 30 (3.3%) with other chromosomal defects.

Table 72.2: Summary of studies reporting on the incidence of absent nasal bone in first trimester trisomy 21 fetuses

Author(s)	Study	Successful examination; n (%)	Absent nasal bone	
			Normal; n (%)	Trisomy 21; n (%)
Cicero et al. 2001[16]*	Pre-CVS	701/701 (100)	3/603 (0.5)	43/59 (72.9)
Otano et al. 2002[19]	Pre-CVS	183/194 (94.3)	1/175 (0.6)	3/5 (60.0)
Zoppi et al. 2003[20]	Screening	5,525/ 5,532 (99.8)	7/3,463 (0.2)	19/27 (70.0)
Orlandi et al. 2003[21]	Screening	1,027/1,089 (94.3)	10/1,000 (1.0)	10/15 (66.7)
Viora et al. 2003[22]	Screening	1,752/1,906 (91.9)	24/1,733 (1.4)	8/10 (80.0)
Senat et al. 2003[23]	Retrospective	956/1,040 (91.9)	4/944 (0.4)	3/4 (75)
Wong et al. 2003[24]	Pre-CVS	119/143 (83.2)	1/114 (0.9)	2/3 (66.7)
Cicero et al. 2003[17]*	Pre-CVS	3,788/3,829 (98.9)	93/3,358 (2.8)	162/242 (67)
Cicero et al. 2004[18]	Pre-CVS	5,851/5,818 (98.9)	129/5,223 (2.5)	229/333 (68.8)
Orlandi et al. 2005[25]	Screening	2,411/2,411 (100)	9/2,396 (0.4)	8/15 (53)
FMF[30]	Screening	18,405/18,636 (98.8)	101/18,388 (0.5)	85/138 (61.6)
Total		36,229/36,769 (95.5)	286/33,436 (0.9)	367/550 (66.7)

* Included in Cicero et al. 2004[18]

It was noted that the prevalence of NB hypoplasia was higher in the euploid Afro-Caribbean population (8.8%) in comparison to the Caucasian population (0.5%), suggesting for the first time that adjustments based on ethnicity may need to be made when using the NB for screening. Furthermore, the overall likelihood ratio for trisomy 21 for hypoplastic NB was 50.5 (95% CI 27.1–92.7) and for present NB it was 0.38 (95% CI 0.24–0.56).[32]

Bunduki et al.[33] looked at the utility of NB measurement in the second trimester (16–24 weeks of gestation) in 1,631 patients. The association between hypoplasia of the NB and Down's syndrome was also demonstrated. Using the 5th percentile of the normal curves generated in the same study as a cut off for screening for trisomy 21, a sensitivity of 59% was achieved.[33]

Vintzileos et al.[34] looked retrospectively at profiles of 29 Down's syndrome fetuses between 17.7 weeks and 20.7 weeks of gestation. The nasal bone was absent in 12 of the 29 (41%) fetuses with trisomy 21 and in none of the 102 chromosomally normal fetuses.[34]

A prospective study involving ultrasound evaluation of the fetal NB between 19 weeks and 22 weeks of gestation[35] also looked at the utility of NB length and its presence or absence in screening for Down's syndrome. The normal NB ranges were based on examinations of 1,913 fetuses. All of the five Down's syndrome fetuses in the study had either an absent NB or an NB length below the 2.5th percentile. None of the fetuses with other chromosomal abnormalities had a short or absent NB.[35]

It is premature to speculate on the precise detection rates that could be achieved in the second trimester by a combination of maternal age, serum biochemistry and ultrasound examination for the fetal NB and other sonographic markers. Nevertheless, on the basis of currently available data, nasal hypoplasia is likely to be the single most sensitive and specific second trimester marker of trisomy 21.

ULTRASOUND EXAMINATION OF THE NASAL BONE: TECHNIQUE

Ultrasound evaluation of the NB requires strictly adherence to standard criteria and it is essential that the operators performing this examination undergo adequate training and gain extensive experience.[36,37]

The need for adequate training is highlighted by a study published in 2003,[37] which looked at the extent of training needed for 15 sonographers experienced in measuring fetal NT, to become competent in examining the fetal NB at $11^{+0}–13^{+6}$ weeks of gestation. The study demonstrated that the number of supervised scans required to achieve proficiency is on average 80 with a range of 40–120. However, evaluation of the NB does not appear to significantly impact the length of the ultrasound examination.[38]

This was confirmed in a study of 501 consecutively scanned fetuses by experienced sonographers. The authors reported that the fetal NB could be successfully examined and measured in all cases without extending the length of time required for scanning.[39]

With a few minor exceptions, the method of NB evaluation is very similar in both the first and second trimesters of pregnancy. The NB should be seen as an echogenic line within the nasal bridge, i.e. underneath the nasal skin. This is usually not a difficult task in the second trimester.

1. The gestation should be $11–13^{+6}$ weeks and the fetal CRL should be 45–84 mm. There is no value examining the fetal NB before this gestational age, as the NB first appear at a CRL of 42 mm and increase linearly with gestation.[8]

2. The image should be magnified so that the head and the upper thorax only are included in the screen (Figs 72.1 and 72.2).

3. A mid-sagittal view of the fetal profile should be obtained with the ultrasound transducer held in parallel to the direction of the nose (i.e. ultrasound beam perpendicular to longitudinal axis of the NB). The ultrasound transducer should then be gently tilted from side-to-side to ensure that the NB is seen separate from the nasal skin. The fetus should be facing the transducer.

4. When the correct view is obtained, three distinct lines will be visualized: the first two lines, which are proximal to the forehead, are horizontal and parallel to each other and resemble an "equal sign" (Fig. 72.1). The top line represents the skin and bottom one, which is usually thicker and more echogenic than the overlying skin, represents the NB. A third line, distal to the forehead, and almost in continuity with the skin, but at a higher level, represents the tip of the nose. Therefore, the absence of the bottom line of the equals sign represents the absence of the fetal NB (Fig. 72.2).

5. If the bottom line of the "equal sign" is absent, the diagnosis of nasal bone absence is fairly straightforward. Occasionally, a

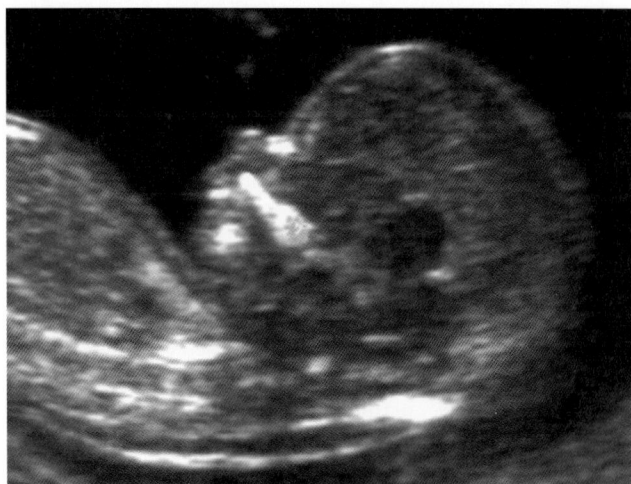

Fig. 72.1: Fetal profile at 12 weeks of gestation in a normal fetus showing the nasal bone

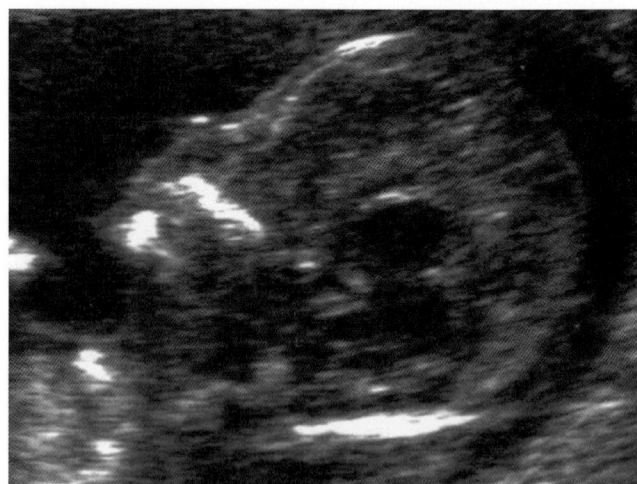

Fig. 72.2: Fetal profile at 12 weeks of gestation in a trisomy 21 fetus showing absence of the nasal bone

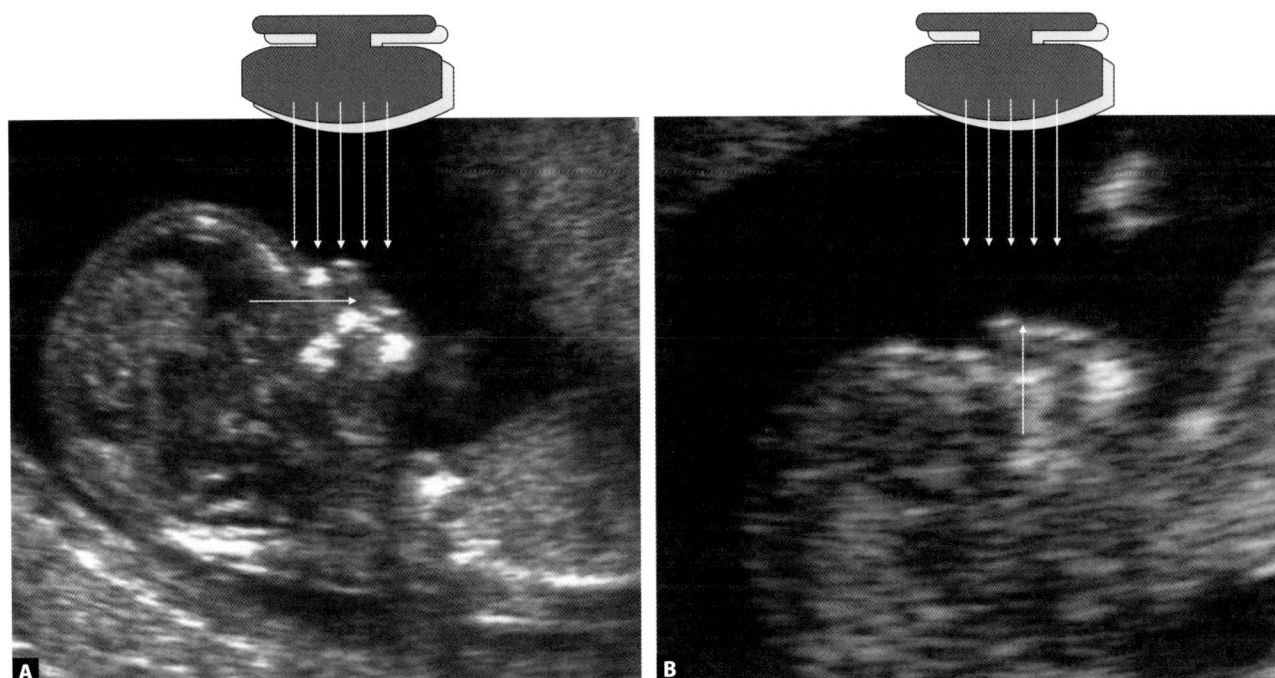

Fig. 72.3A and B: (A) The best angle of insonation to assess the nasal bone in the first trimester is 90° to the longitudinal axis of the nasal bone (i.e. the beam of the ultrasound perpendicular to the longitudinal axis of the nasal bone) (B). Evaluation of the nasal bone should not be attempted with either a 0° or 180° angle of insonation (i.e. with the ultrasound beam parallel to the longitudinal axis of the nasal bone)

line that is thinner and less echogenic than the skin line is noted within the nasal bridge. This may either represent a nasal bone that is not yet ossified or an unusually prominent cartilage. Either way, this finding should also be classified as nasal bone absence. Similarly, the presence of a tiny echogenic dot that can occasionally be seen in the area of the nasal bone should not be interpreted as nasal bone presence.

Two techniques for caliper placement have been employed to measure the NB in the first trimester of pregnancy: including the central hyperechogenic region only or including the entire length of the echogenic line.[21,40]

The angle of insonation used to evaluate the NB is extremely important. The best angle of insonation used to simply differentiate between the presence and the absence of the NB is 90° to the longitudinal axis of the NB (i.e. the beam of the ultrasound perpendicular to the longitudinal axis of the NB) (Fig. 72.3A). Evaluation of the NB should not be attempted with either a 0° or 180° angle of insonation (i.e. with the ultrasound beam parallel to the longitudinal axis of the NB) (Fig.72.3B). At this angle, the NB is insonated at its thinnest dimension and the lateral resolution of the ultrasound equipment available today is not sufficient to reliably detect the NB in this view. When the transducer is adjusted to an angle of insonation approaching 45° or 135°, the lateral scatter at the ends of the NB is reduced rendering the NB ends as more sharply delineated (Fig. 72.4). This is helpful in the second trimester to improve the accuracy of NB length measurement. Figures 72.5 to 72.7 show absence, hypoplasia and presence of NB in the mid-second trimester.

Several factors make the ultrasound examination challenging; the foremost of these are maternal habitus and an unfavorable fetal position such as hyperextension or vertical position. Others factors, such as large uterine fibroids or, early in pregnancy, retroflexion

of the uterus can also make the examination difficult. Fetal small parts, especially the hand, often lie in a close proximity to the fetal face, especially early in gestation. This can lead to erroneous results in two ways. If the digits are actually resting on the fetal face they can mimic the NB. Small parts in front of the fetal face, but not actually resting on it, can produce an obscuring effect and may create an erroneous impression of NB absence. Finally, fetal face contains other echogenic structures, which are located laterally to the NB, which can give the incorrect impression that the NB is present if the correct technique is not followed. These structures include the medial aspect of the orbis oculi and the maxilla. Being able to demonstrate either the presence or the absence of the NB from several different angles will make the correct diagnosis more certain.

Occasionally, the addition of transvaginal sonography can be a helpful adjunct. However, the directions and angles with which the fetus can be viewed using this approach are limited. Rarely, the patient may need to be asked to return for a follow-up if the initial examination is not satisfactory.

THREE-DIMENSIONAL ASSESSMENT OF THE NASAL BONES

The role of three-dimensional (3D) sonography and its potential benefit in the assessment of the fetal NB, has been investigated in the last 2 years in the first, second and third trimesters of pregnancy. The published studies have focused on trying to overcome the technical difficulties encountered during routine two-dimensional (2D) sonography, and on further investigating aspects of the NB development, by using different techniques such as multiplanar imaging and 3D rendering of the facial bones.

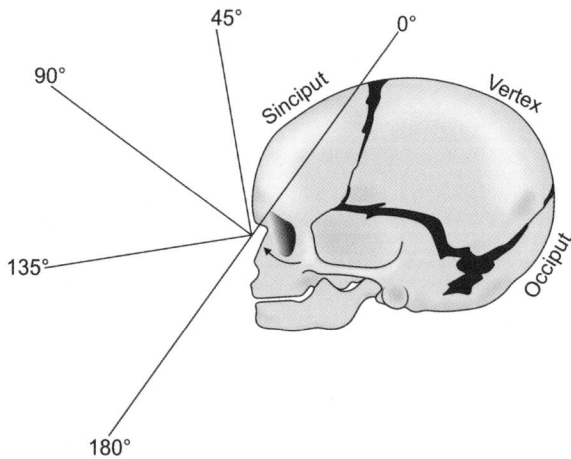

Fig. 72.4: Diagrammatic representation of the bony structures of the fetal face with angles of insonation

Source: Reprinted and adopted with permission from O'Brien W, Cefalo R. Simpson J (Eds). Obstetrics: Normal and Problem Pregnancies, 3rd edition. New York: Churchill Livingstone; 1996. p. 393.

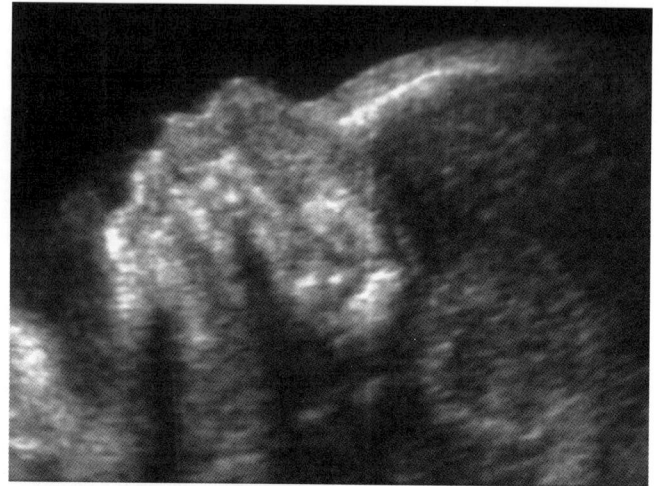

Fig. 72.5: Fetal profile at 20 weeks of gestation in a trisomy 21 fetus showing absence of the nasal bone

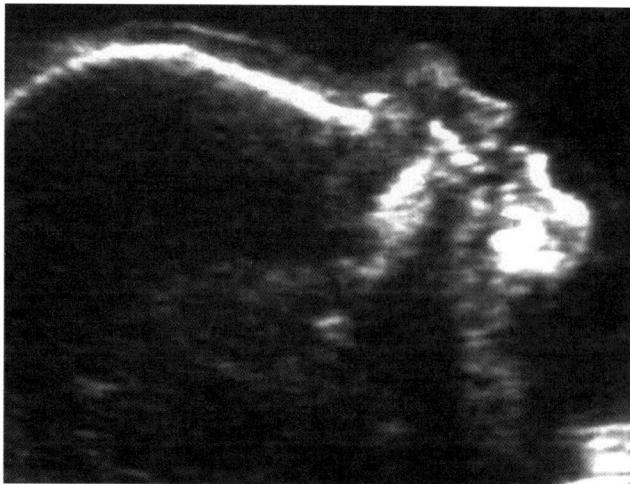

Fig. 72.6: Fetal profile at 20 weeks of gestation in a trisomy 21 fetus showing nasal bone hypoplasia

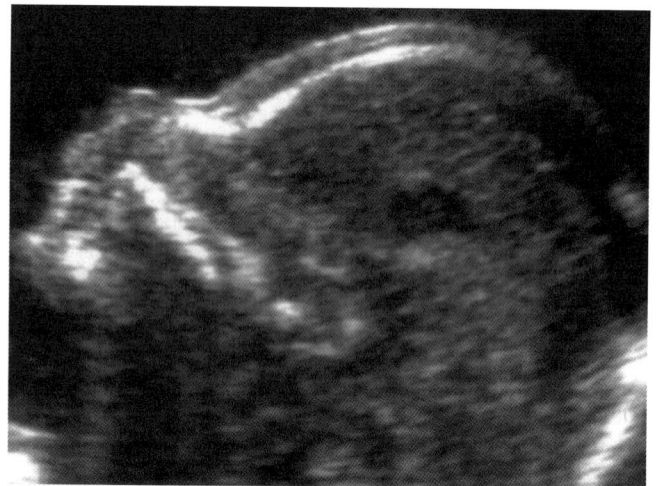

Fig. 72.7: Fetal profile at 20 weeks of gestation in a normal fetus showing presence of the nasal bone

First Trimester of Pregnancy

The two major technical problems in the assessment of the fetal NB during the 11–13^{+6} weeks scan are the need to obtain a mid-sagittal view of the fetal profile and the need for the angle between the ultrasound beam and the fetal profile to be about 45° (i.e. ultrasound beam perpendicular to the NB). In the acquired 3D volume, multiplanar imaging permits to obtain both a perfect midsagittal section and a perfect angle. However, in the first study published on 3D assessment of the NB in the first trimester of pregnancy, Rembouskos et al.[41] found that the visualization of the fetal NB in a perfect reconstructed view of the nasal bridge by 3D multiplanar imaging, is entirely dependent on the initial 2D section. In this study, the authors demonstrated that in order to obtain a good quality volume, the initial section should be taken with a sagittal view of the fetal profile facing upward, and that the angle between the fetal profile and the ultrasound beam should be in a range of 30°–60°, with maximum quality at 45°. In volumes obtained in any other initial 2D view, the visualization of the fetal NB was

poor at this gestation, and could lead to an erroneous diagnosis of absent NB. Consequently, the inability to examine the NB by 2D scanning because of the fetal position cannot be overcome by 3D ultrasound.[41]

In correctly acquired volumes, 3D multiplanar mode permits further assessment of both NB. Peralta et al.[42] used this technique to examine the gap between the two NB at 11–13^{+6} weeks of gestation, and compared the 3D findings to those obtained following 2D examination. The authors found that a gap between the NB is present in about 20% of the fetuses examined by 3D. When the gap measured 0.6 mm or more (40% of cases), it was possible to obtain a perfect mid-sagittal plane where the NB could erroneously be considered absent. By contrast, in all cases in which the gap was less than 0.6 mm, the NB was visualized in the perfect mid-sagittal plane. These findings can be explained by the limit of the lateral resolution of the ultrasound equipment. However, none of the cases with a gap was associated with a diagnosis of absent NB when the examination was performed with the 2D scan, and therefore the false positive rate would not increase. Furthermore, the authors observed that, when using the multiplanar mode, unilateral or bilateral absence of the NB could be demonstrated in about 1% of the chromosomally normal fetuses, and in 61% of the fetuses with trisomy 21. In about 10% of trisomy 21 fetuses, only one of the two NB was absent. However, all the cases with unilateral absence demonstrated with the 3D scan, were classified as "absent" NB during the 2D ultrasound examination, and therefore the sensitivity of the test, when performed by 2D sonography, would not decrease.[42]

In the original description of the technique for examination of the fetal NB by 2D ultrasound,[16] it was suggested that, once obtained the midsagittal section of the fetus, the transducer should be gently tilted from one side of the fetal profile to the other, in order to adequately examine the NB. Therefore, by using this technique, it is extremely unlikely that the presence of a gap can lead to a false positive diagnosis of absent NB when 2D sonographic assessment of the NB is undertaken.[16]

Second and Third Trimesters of Pregnancy

The role of multiplanar imaging and 3D rendering of the NB have also been evaluated in the second and third trimester of pregnancy. It has been suggested that 3D ultrasonography allows a better description of normal, absent, hypoplastic and unilaterally absent NB.[43-45]

Lee et al.[43] used the multiplanar mode to evaluate the NB of 20 fetuses with Down syndrome and 20 fetuses with normal karyotype, between 16 weeks and 30 weeks of gestation. Two examiners independently evaluated the same images. The incidence of absent NB in the fetuses with Down's syndrome was 40% (8 of 12) and 45% (9 of 11) by examiner #1 and examiner #2 respectively. These results were similar to those observed by 2D sonography. However, the prevalence of absent NB in the normal population was 20% (4 of 16) and 10% (2 of 18) by examiner #1 and examiner #2 respectively. These prevalences are much higher than those reported using 2D sonography during this gestational time period (<1.3%). These data suggest that routine application of 3D assessment of the NB in screening for trisomy 21 could increase the false positive rate.[43]

Benoit and Chaoui,[45] assessed the unilateral absence of NB by using 3D rendering of the facial bones. In their study, similarly to what Peralta et al.[41] found in the first trimester, in all Down's syndrome fetuses with unilateral absent NB, the two dimensional assessment of the nasal bridge had diagnosed "absent" NB.[45]

In conclusion, 3D ultrasound evaluation in those cases with suspicious findings of hypoplastic/absent NB may improve the accuracy of the test. However, the extent to which 3D ultrasound could be demonstrated essential in effective screening using the NB at 11–13[+6] weeks needs to be further investigated.

INTEGRATED FIRST TRIMESTER SONOGRAPHIC AND BIOCHEMICAL SCREENING

A retrospective case-control study,[46] comprising of 100 trisomy 21 and 400 chromosomally normal singleton pregnancies at 11–13[+6] weeks of gestation, and a subsequent study which extended the previous series of data,[47] examined the potential performance of screening for trisomy 21 by a combination of sonography for measurement of fetal NT and assessment of the presence or absence of the fetal NB, and measurement of maternal serum free β-hCG

and PAPP-A. It was concluded that, as no relationship between an absent fetal NB and the levels of maternal serum PAPP-A or free β-hCG in trisomy 21 fetuses was demonstrated, for a false positive rate of 5%, the detection rate of trisomy 21 would be 96%.[46,47]

NASAL BONE REFERENCE RANGES BY ULTRASOUND

First Trimester

Cicero et al.[40] reported that in the chromosomally normal group the fetal NB length increases significantly with CRL from a mean of 1.3 mm at a CRL of 45 mm to 2.1 mm at CRL of 84 mm. In the fetuses with Down's syndrome in which the NB was present, even though these were found to be shorter than in chromosomally normal fetuses, the difference in the NB lengths was not sufficiently great to be of clinical utility.[40]

Second Trimester

Guis et al.[48] published reference ranges for NB lengths, based on 376 cases, between 14 weeks and 34 weeks of gestation. Sonek et al.[49] provided reference range based on a larger number of patients (3,547) and for a wider gestational range (11–40 weeks) using the ultrasound technique described above was published in 2003.

IMPACT OF THE NASAL BONE IN SCREENING FOR TRISOMY 21 IN THE FIRST TRIMESTER OF PREGNANCY

In this chapter, the authors have already reported on the prospective study of 5,918 fetuses,[18] in which assessment of the fetal profile for absence or presence of the NB was performed during the routine ultrasound examination at 11–13[+6] weeks, carried out before chorionic villus sampling (CVS) for fetal karyotyping. In all cases, there was prior screening for chromosomal defects by a combination of maternal age and fetal NT[49] and after counseling the parents elected to have invasive testing. The NB was absent in 129 of 5,223 (2.5%) chromosomally normal fetuses and in 229 of 333 (68.8%) fetuses with trisomy 21. Logistic regression analysis was used to examine the effect of maternal ethnic origin, fetal CRL and NT on the incidence of absent NB in the chromosomally normal and trisomy 21 fetuses. This study demonstrated that the incidence of absent NB is higher in fetuses of Afro-Caribbean origin than in Caucasians; it decreases with fetal CRL and increases with fetal NT. Therefore, when calculating an individual patient-specific risk for trisomy 21, it is necessary to take into account these demographic and ultrasound findings. The likelihood ratio for trisomy 21 with absent NB is considerably higher in Caucasians than in those of Afro-Caribbean origin, it is lower at 11 than at 13 weeks and it is higher for low than high NT. The relationship between absent NB and ethnic group, fetal CRL and fetal NT are shown in Tables 72.3 to 72.5.

It has been estimated that if examination of the fetal profile for the absence/presence of the NB is incorporated in first trimester screening for trisomy 21 by fetal NT thickness or NT and maternal serum free β-hCG and PAPP-A the detection rates for trisomy 21 would increase substantially and the false positive rate would decrease.[16-18,46,47]

Very recently, the potential role of the NB in screening for trisomy 21 in the first trimester of pregnancy, has been further

Table 72.3: Incidence of absent nasal bone (NB) in chromosomally normal and trisomy 21 fetuses and likelihood ratio (LR) according to ethnic group

Ethnic group	Trisomy 21;	Normal karyotype;	LR (95% CI) for Trisomy 21	
	n (%)	n (%)	NB absent	NB present
Total (n = 5,851)	229/333 (68.8)	129/5,223 (2.5)	27.8 (23.1-33.5)	0.32 (0.27-0.37)
Caucasian (n = 5,384)	207/303 (68.3)	105/4,811 (2.2)	31.3 (25.5-38.4)	0.32 (0.27-0.38)
Afro-Caribbean (n = 170)	11/14 (78.6)	13/145 (9.0)	8.8 (4.7-15.5)	0.24 (0.08-0.52)
Asian* (n = 201)	10/14 (71.4)	9/179 (5.0)	14.2 (6.8-28.4)	0.30 (0.12-0.58)
Chinese/Japanese (n = 69)	1/2 (50.0)	2/61 (3.3)	15.3 (2.1-73.4)	0.52 (0.10-0.94)
Mixed (n = 27)	–	0/27 (–)	–	–

*People originating from India, Pakistan, Bangladesh, Sri Lanka and Philippines
Source: Adopted from Cicero et al.[18]

Table 72.4: Incidence of absent nasal bone (NB) in chromosomally normal and trisomy 21 fetuses and likelihood ratio (LR) according to crown-rump length (CRL)

CRL (mm)	Trisomy 21	Normal karyotype	LR (95% CI) for Trisomy 21	
	n (%)	n (%)	NB absent	NB present
Total (n=5,851)	229/333 (68.8)	129/5223 (2.5)	27.8 (23.1–33.5)	0.32 (0.27–0.37)
45–54	41/49 (83.7)	32/675 (4.7)	17.6 (12.3–25.2)	0.17 (0.09–0.30)
55–64	78/118 (66.1)	63/1,850 (3.4)	19.4 (14.7–25.5)	0.35 (0.27–0.44)
65–74	85/118 (72.0)	25/1,805 (1.4)	52.0 (34.8–77.8)	0.28 (0.21–0.37)
75–84	25/48 (52.1)	9/893 (1.0)	51.8 (25.8–102.8)	0.48 (0.35–0.62)

Source: Adopted from Cicero et al.[18]

Table 72.5: Incidence of absent nasal bone (NB) in chromosomally normal and trisomy 21 fetuses and likelihood ratio (LR) according to nuchal translucency thickness (NT)

NT (mm)	Trisomy 21;	Normal karyotype;	LR (95% CI) for Trisomy 21	
	n (%)	n (%)	NB absent	NB present
Total (n=5,851)	229/333 (68.8)	129/5223 (2.5)	27.8 (23.1–33.5)	0.32 (0.27–0.37)
<95th	23/38 (60.5)	53/3245 (1.6)	37.1 (25.0–52.5)	0.40 (0.26–0.56)
>95th–3.4	48/83 (57.8)	40/1500 (2.7)	25.1 (16.7–37.4)	0.45 (0.34–0.56)
3.5–4.4	49/67 (73.1)	16/294 (5.4)	13.4 (8.2–22.1)	0.28 (0.19–0.41)
4.5–5.4	26/41 (63.4)	5/84 (6.0)	10.7 (4.6–25.3)	0.39 (0.25–0.55)
≥5.5	83/104 (79.8)	15/100 (15.0)	5.3 (3.4–8.7)	0.24 (0.16–0.34)

Source: Adopted from Cicero et al.[18]

investigated in a large series by Nicolaides et al.[51] The authors proposed a new policy for first trimester screening, based on two-stage individual risk. After having evaluated the performance of first trimester screening for trisomy 21 by a combination of maternal age, fetal NT and maternal serum free β-hCG and PAPP-A (Combined test) in prospective study of 75,821 singleton pregnancies, they examined the potential impact of a new individual risk orientated two-stage approach to first trimester screening (Fig. 72.8), based on the additional examination of the fetal NB in the group of women who fell in an intermediate risk following the initial screening test. The detection and false-positive rates were calculated for different risk cut-offs and the screened population was then classified in three groups: a high-risk group, which included patients with a risk estimate of 1 in 100 or more; a low risk group, which included those with a risk estimate of less than 1 in 1,000; and the intermediate-risk category, with a risk estimate of between 1 in 101 and 1 in 1,000. The authors proposed that patients in the high-risk category

are offered karyotyping by CVS, and those in the low-risk category are reassured that their fetus is unlikely to be chromosomally abnormal. Those in the intermediate-risk category have further assessment of risk by first-trimester ultrasound examination to determine absence/presence of the NB, and CVS is offered if their adjusted risk becomes 1 in 100 or more.[51]

Following the combined screening test, for a false positive rate of 2% the detection rate was 80%. When the nasal bone examination is performed into the two-stage screening, for a risk cut-off of 1 in 100 the total false-positive rate would be 2.1%, and the detection rate would be 92.0%. The authors confirmed that first trimester combined screening for trisomy 21 is associated with a detection rate of about 90% for a false-positive rate of 5%[52-54] and concluded that individual risk-orientated two-stage screening for trisomy 21 can potentially identify, in the first trimester of pregnancy, more than 90% of affected fetuses for a false-positive rate of about 2%.

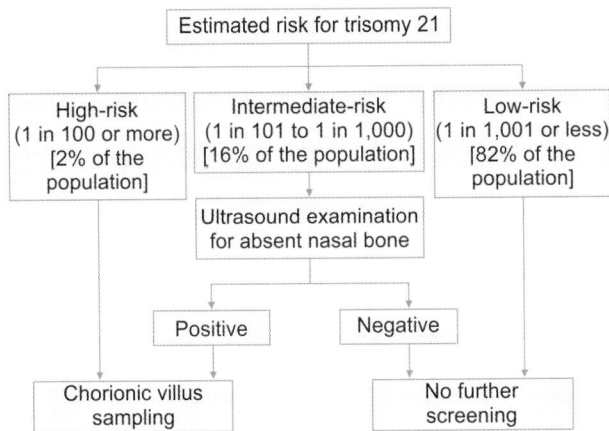

Fig. 72.8: New individual risk orientated two-stage approach to first trimester screening.[50] Screening by maternal age, fetal nuchal translucency and maternal serum free β-human chorionic gonadotropin and pregnancy-associated plasma protein-A

CONCLUSION

Trisomy 21 is the most common chromosomal abnormality found at birth, with an incidence of about 1:600. However, the sonographic appearance of individuals with Down's syndrome, is often quite similar to those with normal karyotype, making screening for Down syndrome more difficult compared to that of other chromosomal abnormalities. Hence, there is importance of a continued search for markers that would accurately discriminate between affected and unaffected fetuses.

The sonographic appearance of increased nuchal translucency and absent/hypoplastic nasal bone could be due to connective tissue abnormalities.[55-57] The increased thickness of subcutaneous tissues in association with Down syndrome has lead to the development of the NT measurement between 11 weeks and 13+6 weeks of gestation, which is the most sensitive and specific ultrasound marker for this condition.[58]

Several studies have demonstrated that the best screening test for trisomy 21 is given by the combination, in the first trimester of pregnancy, of maternal age, fetal NT thickness and maternal serum free β-hCG and PAPP-A. This test allows a detection rate of 90%

for a false positive rate of 5%.[51-54] By adding the ultrasonographic evaluation of the NB, a sensitivity of over 90% could be achieved for a false positive rate of about 2%.[46,47,51] Although extensive studies have demonstrated that absence of the NB is highly sensitive and specific marker of trisomy 21, its accurate examination requires highly skilled operators and at present it is unlikely that this assessment will be incorporated into the routine firs-trimester scan. Nevertheless, this sonographic marker could be used in specialist centers to re-evaluate the risk in patients with intermediate risk after screening by fetal NT and maternal serum biochemistry.[51] If the individual risk-orientated two-stage screening for trisomy 21,[51] which includes examination of the fatal NB in those women with a individual risk between 1:101 to 1:1,000, is to be introduced in the routine clinical practice, the detection rate could be potentially be increased to more that 90%, and the false positive rate could be decreased to about 2%. This aspect is extremely important for three main reasons: firstly such a screening test would reduce the economic costs due to unnecessary invasive testing; secondly, it would reduce the number of miscarriage of chromosomally normal fetuses due to the invasive testing;[59,60] and thirdly would provide an early reassurance to pregnant women, and at the same time, would allow them to have an early termination of pregnancy should they wish so in case their baby is found to be affected. However, in order to reproduce the same results, it is imperative that sonographers receive appropriate training and adhere to a standard technique for the measurement of NT and the assessment of the NB. Furthermore, the success of a screening program necessitates the presence of a system for regular audit of results and continuous assessment of the quality of images. The Fetal Medicine Foundation, which is a UK registered charity, has established a process of training and quality assurance for the appropriate introduction of NT screening into clinical practice.[61]

In conclusion, improvements in ultrasound resolution have allowed us to evaluate and measure very minute fetal structures with a concomitant decrease in the room for error. If they are to be included in prenatal screening protocols, their evaluation must be done with a high degree of precision and accuracy. This can be accomplished only through strict standardization of the fetal image and with appropriate training and an ongoing quality assurance. Just like the NT measurements, it is only by strictly adhering to these principles that the evaluation of the NB can be incorporated into any screening protocol using prenatal sonography.

REFERENCES

1. Snijders RJ, Nicolaides KH. Assessment of risk. Ultrasound Markers for Fetal Chromosomal Defects. Carnforth, UK: Parthenon Publishing; 1996.
2. Down LJ. Observations on an ethnic classification of idiots. Clinical Lectures and Reports. London Hospital. 1866;3:259-62.
3. Enlow DH. Facial Growth, 3rd edition. Philadelphia: WB Saunders; 1990.
4. Beck JC, Sie KC. The growth and development of the nasal airway. Functional Reconstructive Rhinoplasty. 1999:257-62.
5. Larsen WJ. Human Embryology, 3rd edition. Churchill Livingstone; 2001;368.
6. Sperber GH. Craniofacial Embryology, 4th edition, London. Wright, Butterworths; 1989. pp. 104-24.
7. Williams PL, Warwick R, Dyson M. Gray's Anatomy, 37th edition. London: Churchill Livingstone; 1989. pp. 386.
8. Sandikcioglu M, Molsted K, Kjaer I. The prenatal development of the human nasal and vomeral bones. J Craniofac Genet Dev Biol. 1994;14:124-34.
9. Farkas LG, Katic MJ, Forrest CR, et al L. Surface anatomy of the face in Down's syndrome: Linear and angular measurements in the craniofacial regions. J Craniofac Surg. 2001;12:373-9.
10. Keeling JW, Hansen BF, Kjaer I. Pattern of malformation in the axial skeleton in human trisomy 21 fetuses. Am J Med Genet. 1997;68:466-71.
11. Stempfle N, Huten Y, Fredouille C, et al. Skeletal abnormalities in fetuses with Down's syndrome: A radiologic postmortem study. Pediatr Radiol. 1999;29:682-8.
12. Tuxen A, Keeling JW, Reintoft I, et al. A histological and radiological investigation of the nasal bone in fetuses with Down syndrome. Ultrasound Obstet Gynecol. 2003;22:22-6.

13. Minderer S, Gloning KP, Henrich W, et al. The nasal bone in fetuses with trisomy 21: sonographic versus pathomorphological findings. Ultrasound Obstet Gynecol. 2003;22:16-21.

14. Larose C, Massoc P, Hillion Y, et al. Comparison of fetal nasal bone assessment by ultrasound at 11-14 weeks and by postmortem X-ray in trisomy 21: A prospective observational study. Ultrasound Obstet Gynecol. 2003;22:27-30.

15. Sonek J, Nicolaides K. Prenatal ultrasonographic diagnosis of nasal bone abnormalities in three fetuses with Down syndrome. Am J Obstet Gynecol. 2002;186:139-41.

16. Cicero S, Curcio P, Papageorghiou A, et al. Absence of nasal bone in fetuses with trisomy 21 at 11-14 weeks of gestation: An observational study. Lancet. 2001;358:1665-7.

17. Cicero S, Longo D, Rembouskos G, et al. Absent nasal bone at 11-14 weeks of gestation and chromosomal defects. Ultrasound Obstet Gynecol. 2003;22:31-5.

18. Cicero S, Rembouskos G, Vandecruys H, et al. Likelihood ratio for trisomy 21 in fetuses with absent nasal bone at the 11-14 weeks scan. Ultrasound Obstet Gynecol. 2004;23:218-23.

19. Otano L, Aiello H, Igarzabal L, et al. Association between first trimester absence of fetal nasal bone on ultrasound and Down's syndrome. Prenat Diagn. 2002;22:930-2.

20. Zoppi MA, Ibba RM, Axiana C, et al. Absence of fetal nasal bone and aneuploidies at first trimester nuchal translucency screening in unselected pregnancies. Prenat Diagn. 2003;23:496-500.

21. Orlandi F, Bilardo CM, Campogrande M, et al. Measurement of nasal bone length at 11-14 weeks of pregnancy and its potential role in Down syndrome risk assessment. Ultrasound Obstet Gynecol. 2003;22:36-9.

22. Viora E, Masturzo B, Errante G, et al. Ultrasound evaluation of fetal nasal bone at 11 to 14 weeks in a consecutive series of 1906 fetuses. Prenat Diagn. 2003;23:784-7.

23. Senat MV, Bernard JP, Boulvain M, et al. Intra- and interoperator variability in fetal nasal bone assessment at 11-14 weeks of gestation. Ultrasound Obstet Gynecol. 2003;22:138-41.

24. Wong SF, Choi H, Ho LC. Nasal bone hypoplasia: Is it a common finding amongst chromosomally normal fetuses of southern Chinese women? Gynecol Obstet Invest. 2003;56:99-101.

25. Orlandi F, Rossi C, Orlandi E, et al. First trimester screening for trisomy-21 using a simplified method to assess the presence or absence of the fetal nasal bone. Am J Obstet Gynecol. 2005;192:1107-11.

26. Prefumo F, Sairam S, Bhide A, et al. Maternal ethnic origin and fetal nasal bones at 11-14 weeks of gestation. BJOG. 2004;111:109-12.

27. Malone FD, Ball RH, Nyberg DA, et al. FASTER Research Consortium. First trimester nasal bone evaluation for aneuploidy in the general population. Obstet Gynecol. 2004;104:1222-8.

28. Welch KK, Malone FD. Nuchal translucency-based screening. Clinical Obstet Gynecol. 2003;46:909-22.

29. De Biasio P, Venturini PL. Absence of nasal bone and detection of trisomy 21. Lancet. 2002;13:1344.

30. Fetal Medicine Foundation. Screening study on absent nasal bone at 11-14 weeks of gestation: Preliminary results. (In press).

31. Bromley B, Lieberman E, Shipp T, et al. Fetal nasal bone length: A marker for Down syndrome in the second trimester. J Ultrasound Med. 2002;21:1387-94.

32. Cicero S, Sonek J, McKenna D, et al. Nasal bone hypoplasia in fetuses with Trisomy 21. Ultrasound Obstet Gynecol. 2003;21:15-8.

33. Bunduki V, Ruano J, Miguelez J, et al. Fetal bone length: Reference range and clinical application in ultrasound screening for Trisomy 21. Ultrasound Obstet Gynecol. 2003;21:156-60.

34. Vintzileos A, Walters C, Yeo L. Absent nasal bone in the prenatal detection of fetuses with trisomy 21 in a high-risk population. Obstet Gynecol. 2003;101:905-8.

35. Gamez F, Ferreiro P, Salmean JM. Ultrasonographic measurement of fetal nasal bone in a low-risk population at 19-22 gestational weeks. Ultrasound Obstet Gynecol. 2003;22:152-3.

36. Bouley R, Sonek J. Fetal nasal bone: the technique. Down's Screening News. 2003;10:33-4.

37. Sonek JD, Cicero S. Ultrasound evaluation of the fetal nasal bone: The technique (an update). Down's Screening News. 2004;11:25.

38. Cicero S, Dezerega V, Andrade E, et al. Learning curve for sonographic examination of the fetal nasal bone at 11-14 weeks. Ultrasound Obstet Gynecol. 2003;22:135-7.

39. Kanellopoulos V, Katsetos C, Economides DL. Examination of fetal nasal bone and repeatability of measurement in early pregnancy. Ultrasound Obstet Gynecol. 2003;22:131-4.

40. Cicero S, Bindra R, Rembouskos G, et al. Fetal nasal bone length in chromosomally normal and abnormal fetuses at 11-14 weeks of gestation. J Matern Fetal Neo Med. 2002;11:400-2.

41. Rembouskos G, Cicero S, Longo D, et al. Assessment of the fetal nasal bone at 11-14 weeks of gestation by three-dimensional ultrasound. Ultrasound Obstet Gynecol. 2004;23:232-6.

42. Peralta CF, Falcon O, Wegrzyn P, et al. Assessment of the gap between the fetal nasal bones at 11 to 13^{+6} weeks of gestation by three-dimensional ultrasound. Ultrasound Obstet Gynecol. 2005;25:464-7.

43. Lee W, DeVore GR, Comstock CH, et al. Nasal bone evaluation in fetuses with Down syndrome during the second and third trimesters of pregnancy. J Ultrasound Med. 2003;22:55-60.

44. Goncalves LF, Espinoza J, Lee W, et al. Phenotypic characteristics of absent and hypoplastic nasal bones in fetuses with Down syndrome: Description by 3-dimensional ultrasonography and clinical significance. J Ultrasound Med. 2004;23:1619-27.

45. Benoit B, Chaoui R. Three-dimensional ultrasound with maximal mode rendering: A novel technique for the diagnosis of bilateral or unilateral absence or hypoplasia of nasal bones in second trimester screening for Down syndrome. Ultrasound Obstet Gynecol. 2005;25:19-24.

46. Cicero S, Bindra R, Rembouskos G, et al. Integrated ultrasound and biochemical screening for trisomy 21 using fetal nuchal translucency, absent fetal nasal bone, free β-hCG and PAPP-A at 11 to 14 weeks. Prenat Diagn. 2003;23:306-10.

47. Cicero S, Spencer K, Avgidou K, et al. Maternal serum biochemistry at 11-14 weeks in relation to the presence or absence of the fetal nasal bone on ultrasonography in chromosomally abnormal fetuses: An updated analysis of integrated ultrasound and biochemical screening. Prenat Diagn (In press).

48. Guis F, Ville Y, Doumerc S, et al. Ultrasound evaluation of the length of the fetal nasal bones throughout gestation. Ultrasound Obstet Gynecol. 1995;5:304-7.

49. Sonek J, McKenna D, Webb D, et al. Nasal bone length throughout gestation: Normal ranges based on 3537 fetal ultrasound measurements. Ultrasound Obstet Gynecol. 2003;21:152-5.

50. Snijders RM, Noble P, Sebire N, et al. UK multicentre project on assessment of risk of trisomy 21 by maternal age and fetal nuchal translucency thickness at 10-14 weeks of gestation. Lancet. 1998;351:343-6.

51. Nicolaides KH, Spencer K, Avgidou K, et al. Multicenter study of first trimester screening for trisomy 21 in 75821 pregnancies: results and estimation of the potential impact of individual risk-orientated two-stage first trimester screening. Ultrasound Obstet Gynecol. 2005; 25:221-6.

52. Spencer K, Souter V, Tul N, et al. A screening program for trisomy 21 at 10–14 weeks using fetal nuchal translucency, maternal serum free β-human chorionic gonadotropin and pregnancy-associated plasma protein-A. Ultrasound Obstet Gynecol. 1999;13:231-7.

53. Bindra R, Heath V, Liao A, et al. One stop clinic for assessment of risk for trisomy 21 at 11–14 weeks: A prospective study of 15030 pregnancies. Ultrasound Obstet Gynecol. 2002;20:219-25.

54. Spencer K, Spencer CE, Power M, et al. Screening for chromosomal abnormalities in the first trimester using ultrasound and maternal serum biochemistry in a one stop clinic: A review of three years prospective experience. BJOG. 2003;110:281-6.

55. von Kaisenberg CS, Krenn V, Ludwig M, et al. Morphological classification of nuchal skin in human fetuses with trisomy 21, 18, and 13 at 1218 weeks and in a trisomy 16 mouse. Anat Embryol. 1998;197:105-24.

56. von Kaisenberg CS, Brand-Saberi B, Christ B, et al. Collagen type VI expression in the skin of trisomy 21 fetuses. Obstet Gynecol. 1998;91:319-23.

57. Bohlandt S, von Kaisenberg CS, Wewetzer K, et al. Hyaluran in the nuchal skin of chromosomally abnormal fetuses. Human Reprod. 2000; (5)15:1155-8.

58. Nicolaides KH. Nuchal translucency and other first trimester sonographic markers of chromosomal abnormalities. Am J Obstet Gynecol 2004;191:45-67

59. Tabor A, Philip J, Madsen M, et al. Randomized controlled trial of genetic amniocentesis in 4,606 low-risk women. Lancet. 1986; 287-93.

60. Smidt-Jensen S, Permin M, Philip J, et al. Randomized comparison of amniocentesis and transabdominal and transcervical chorionic villus sampling. Lancet. 1992;340:1238-44.

61. Fetal Medicine Foundation. Down's screening at 11-14 weeks. Available from www.fetalmedicine.com. [Accessed May 2005]

73 Second Trimester Ultrasound Screening of Fetal Anomalies

L Yeo, AM Vintzileos

INTRODUCTION

It is an unfortunate fact that birth defects sometimes occur in human development.

In fact, they are the single most common cause of perinatal mortality in many countries. It is important to detect fetal congenital anomalies prior to birth for various reasons, such as delivering at a tertiary care center, offering prenatal surgical correction, giving the option of invasive testing, and appropriately and accurately counselling parents.

While there are varying modalities that currently exist to screen for fetal anomalies (such as magnetic resonance imaging and fetoscopic examination), the most accepted method is ultrasonographic imaging. The concept of prenatal ultrasonography as a screening tool has received widespread acceptance among both physicians and patients. Unlike biochemistry screening, ultrasound is a very tangible and realistic tool that provides a visible assessment for patients. Accordingly, the second trimester is often utilized because fetal anatomic structures are readily assessed at this time of pregnancy. Once sonographic screening in the second trimester reveals the presence of abnormalities, further diagnostic testing may be offered to the patient such as amniocentesis or percutaneous umbilical blood sampling. Although, the advantage of performing sonography in patients at high-risk for fetal structural anomalies is clear, the benefits and cost-effectiveness of routine ultrasound screening in low-risk pregnant patients are not as clear.

This chapter focuses on the components of a normal fetal anatomic survey, second trimester sonographic markers for aneuploidy and describes the value of sonographic second trimester screening.

SECOND TRIMESTER FETAL ANATOMIC SURVEY AND ITS CONTENTS

Because ultrasonography utilizes sound waves to provide imaging capability, it has rapidly become the most commonly used method for imaging during pregnancy. Its major advantages include lack of adverse fetal effects,[1] ability to view the fetus in real-time mode (with capabilities of observing and studying fetal behavior/movements), and most recently the ability to acquire a volume of data to generate three-dimensional imaging. With the introduction of two-dimensional static scanning in the early 1970s, physicians were allowed to view the fetus for the first time. Subsequently in the late 1970s and early 1980s, real-time B-mode imaging became widespread as a clinical tool. However, despite its many technological advancements over the years, many in the United States still believe that the appropriate use of fetal sonography should be limited to only when there is an indication. This is despite the fact that detailed examination of the fetus for both aneuploidy markers and structural abnormalities has become a true reality. In contrast, many European countries perform ultrasound examinations routinely during pregnancy.

In order to screen for fetal abnormalities on a second trimester ultrasound, the sonographer must be able to recognize normal fetal anatomy first. Accordingly, we will describe the features of a targeted, complete fetal anatomic survey on ultrasound. There are many possible indications to undergo an obstetrical examination such as estimating gestational age and/or growth, vaginal bleeding, multiple gestation, history of prior congenital anomaly or syndrome, placental localization, adjunct to interventional or invasive procedures, biophysical profile, and evaluation of amniotic fluid quantity. In most cases, ultrasonography will provide reassurance of a normal and healthy fetus. Because most anomalies are sporadic and often occur in otherwise low-risk women, we believe that all patients regardless of risk should have uniform access to obstetrical sonography in the second trimester. Most importantly, this should be performed with a high level of expertise, since both false-positive and false-negative information can have a detrimental impact. A systematic fetal anatomic survey is able to detect the majority of fetal malformations,[2] and can also evaluate fetal growth, amniotic fluid, placenta and cervix. To be effective, the sonographic examination should be performed systematically, and with complete thoroughness.

Recently, we examined the value (from the patient's perspective) of a targeted ultrasound performed after an abnormal karyotype was discovered.[3] All patients valued the ultrasound because it provided visualization of anomalies, and this additional information influenced pregnancy management. Interestingly, all patients thought that the impact of sonography was superior to chromosomal diagnosis alone, and all believed that sonography should be utilized in patients facing likewise clinical situations. These patients found sonography invaluable because it provided more information and helped them to accept the diagnosis of fetal aneuploidy.

Published guidelines exist that describe the components of a complete obstetrical ultrasound. This involves both biometric measurements which reflect gestational age, growth or size, and evaluation of specific organ structures for the absence/presence of anomalies. In 1994, the American Institute of Ultrasound in Medicine published standards for the performance of obstetrical ultrasound.[4] In the first trimester, the requirements include evaluation of the uterus, adnexa, cul-de-sac, gestational sac, crown-rump length, fetal number, and presence/absence of cardiac activity. In the second and third trimesters, the requirements include fetal life/number/presentation/activity (with multiple gestations requiring additional documentation), amniotic fluid, placental location/appearance/relationship to the internal os, fetal biparietal diameter

(BPD) or head circumference (HC), limb measurement, estimated fetal weight (requires abdominal diameter or circumference), uterus, cervix, adnexa, cerebral ventricles, posterior fossa, four-chamber view of the heart and position, spine, stomach, kidneys, bladder, abdominal cord insertion site, and umbilical cord.

However, in order to increase the diagnostic sensitivity for fetal anomalies, a more comprehensive examination above and beyond what is required by the American Institute of Ultrasound in Medicine should be performed. Table 73.1 depicts the components of a second trimester fetal anatomic survey that we routinely perform via ultrasonography. Of course, to carry out this task, other criteria should also be met. For instance, proper sonographic equipment and transducers with the highest frequency probe should be utilized to maximize fetal anatomic resolution. The sonographers should be adequately and appropriately trained to ensure that these detailed examinations are performed at the highest level. To properly recognize fetal anomalies, one must have familiarity with normal fetal anatomy, normal variants and the various sonographic landmarks.

Factors that can limit the ability to adequately examine the fetus sonographically in the second trimester include sonographer expertise, quality of ultrasound equipment, length of time spent in scanning, incompletely filled or overfilled maternal bladder, maternal habitus, depth of penetration, tissue density, and other scanning characteristics, fibroids, early or advancing gestational age, ossification of fetal bony structures (later in the second trimester), fetal position and amniotic fluid abnormalities (increased or decreased). Techniques that can improve fetal visualization include using various probes (including transvaginal scanning, for instance, in the obese patient) and changing maternal position (which effectively changes the fetal position).

The timing of scans in the second trimester may vary, depending on the scanning center, indication for the examination (amniocentesis), or physician preference. Later scans (for example 23–24 weeks) can improve visualization of certain fetal anatomic structures such as the heart and improve overall sensitivity. However, scanning later in the second trimester of pregnancy may limit the window of opportunity for patients who desire termination of pregnancy for various reasons. On the other hand, patients who desire amniocentesis testing may choose to undergo a sonographic survey earlier such as 16–17 weeks of gestation. Some patients who have had a previous child affected with structural anomalies or genetic syndromes may choose to undergo an initial early scan for some reassurance, and then a more detailed repeat examination later in the pregnancy. At our own center, we schedule fetal anatomy surveys around 18–21 weeks in order to optimize anatomy assessment, and yet still provide patients the opportunity for amniocentesis, if necessary. Some studies suggest that among low-risk women, second trimester ultrasound screening is easier to perform and less likely to require an additional scan at 20–22 weeks than at 18 weeks.[5] Fetal echocardiograms are best performed between 22 weeks and 24 weeks when cardiac structures are large enough, and better visualization and assessment are possible.

With multiple gestations, not only should the fetal anatomy be evaluated, but the number, position of fetuses and type of dividing membrane should be delineated. In addition, when screening for fetal anomalies sonographically, the placenta and amniotic fluid volume must also always be assessed. Placental appearance, thickness, echogenicity, location and characteristics should be examined, along with amniotic fluid volume, to rule out polyhydramnios,

Table 73.1: Components of second trimester sonographic fetal anatomic survey (at Robert Wood Johnson Medical School)

Anatomic structures
Head
• Cranial shape, degree of mineralization
• Cerebral hemispheres, cavum septum pellucidum, thalami, cerebral peduncles, lateral ventricles, choroid plexus, third and fourth ventricles, cerebellum and vermis, cisterna magna
Face/neck
• Orbits, nasal bone, lips/palate, profile, nuchal fold, ear length
• Thoracic cavity
• Lungs
• Configuration of bony thorax, including ribs and clavicles
Heart
• Four-chamber views (apical and subcostal), both outflow tracts, aortic and ductal arches, inferior and superior vena cava, valves, atria and ventricular septums
Abdominal
• Situs
• Stomach
• Liver, gallbladder, spleen
• Umbilical vein, portal vein
• Bowel
• Wall/cord insertion site
Genitourinary system
• Kidneys
• Bladder
• Genitalia
Spine
Extremities
• Upper (including bilateral hands)
• Lower (including bilateral feet)
Umbilical cord
• Number of umbilical arteries
• Placental insertion site
Biometry measurements
• Biparietal diameter
• Head circumference
• Atria of lateral ventricles, cisterna magna, nuchal fold (when applicable)
• Cerebellum
• Thoracic circumference (when applicable)
• Abdominal circumference
• Femur lengths, humerus lengths, radius and ulna lengths, tibia and fibula lengths
• Foot length
• Nasal bone length
• Orbital diameters
Other
• Estimation of dates or evaluation of growth
• Number of fetuses, position
• Placenta
• Amniotic fluid
• Cervix/lower uterine segment

oligohydramnios or anhydramnios. These structures can provide clues to a potential anomalous fetus. For instance, polyhydramnios is associated with esophageal atresia, anhydramnios is associated with renal agenesis, and a thickened placenta can be seen with fetal hydrops.

At the beginning of the examination, the entire uterus should be imaged both transversely and longitudinally to assess fetal position, amniotic fluid volume, and placental location. Determining the right and left sides of the fetus is crucial. Situs solitus is the term used when there is the usual arrangement of organs and vessels within the fetal body. Finally, examination of the lower uterine segment and cervix is important.

The examination of the fetal intracranial anatomy is extremely important since the presence of central nervous system abnormalities can have a major and devastating impact on perinatal morbidity and mortality. From the late first trimester until delivery, the calvarium can be identified. Thus, the BPD and HC can be readily measured. The calvarium should not be hypomineralized (which can indicate a skeletal dysplasia), and should be elliptical in shape. Reverberation artifact from properly mineralized bone will usually obscure the proximal hemisphere. "Strawberry" or "lemon" shaped heads can indicate the presence of trisomy 18 or neural tube defects, respectively. Brachycephaly (anteroposterior shortening) can also be a sign of fetal trisomy 21 or trisomy 18 ("strawberry" head). Dolicocephaly (elongation of the anteroposterior length) can be a normal variant, or secondary to decreased amniotic fluid and compression of the fetal head. Tangential imaging through the fetal calvarium may identify cranial sutures (hypoechoic spaces between bones), which are best visualized early in gestation since ossification progresses with time. In certain syndromes (such as craniosynostosis and skeletal dysplasias), premature closure of the sutures can be seen.

The transthalamic view (Fig. 73.1) is an axial view through the cranium at the level of the thalami. At this level, the BPD and HC are obtained. Because of excessive variation in the BPD shape which can occur, when the head is either brachycephalic or dolicocephalic, the HC is the preferred measurement. The BPD is obtained with the cranial bones perpendicular to the ultrasound beam, and is measured from the outer margin of the near calvarium to the inner margin of the far calvarium. The HC is measured circumferentially at the outer margin of the calvarium. Other anatomic structures that should be assessed in the transthalamic view are the cavum septum pellucidum (fluid-filled midline structure anterior to the thalami and between the lateral ventricles), midline falx, third ventricle (located between the thalami) and frontal horns of the lateral ventricles. Visualization of the cavum septum pellucidum implies proper formation of midline intracranial structures. Its absence can be a sign of agenesis of the corpus callosum, holoprosencephaly, or other brain anomalies.

The transventricular view (Fig. 73.2) is found just superior to the transthalamic view, and is marked by the lateral ventricles, which contain sonolucent cerebrospinal fluid. Within this system is the echogenic choroid plexus, which normally fills the body of the lateral ventricle extending into the atrium. The frontal horns are seen as prominent sonolucent anterior components of the lateral ventricles. Through an axial plane of the atrium, the cerebral ventricle is measured. To rule out ventriculomegaly/hydrocephalus, normally it should be < 10 mm.

The transcerebellar view (Fig. 73.3) contains the biconvex cerebellar hemispheres and midline vermis, cisterna magna (between the dorsum of cerebellar hemispheres and inner calvarium) and nuchal fold. Importantly, the transcerebellar diameter can also be measured and utilized as a one-point estimate of gestational age. The transcerebellar view is obtained by angling the scan plane down posteriorly from the transthalamic view. This area is of vital importance in ruling out open spina bifida, since obliteration of the cisterna magna and a "banana" shape of the cerebellum may be seen with this disorder. Other anomalies that can be ruled out in this view include Dandy-Walker malformation/variant, cerebellar agenesis/hypoplasia and occipital encephaloceles. The cisterna magna normally ranges from 3 cm to 9 cm.[6] On occasion, this measurement may be increased, but is a usually normal finding if the transcerebellar diameter is normal for gestational age and the vermis is well seen and intact. An incorrect scan plane can lead to a false positive appearance of Dandy-Walker variant or to an abnormally large measurement of the cisterna magna.[7] An increased nuchal fold (greater than 6 mm) may be secondary to fetal aneuploidy [especially Down's syndrome (DS)] or may be falsely thickened due to breech presentation. In certain clinical scenarios, the intracranial major vessels (such as middle cerebral artery) can be identified with color and/or power Doppler imaging (Fig. 73.4). This information may be quite useful in assessing for anemia (Rh isoimmunization, Parvovirus infection) or intrauterine fetal growth restriction. On occasion, the fetal head may be low in the pelvis that it prohibits an adequate examination of the intracranial anatomy; transvaginal scanning may be quite useful and solve this dilemma.

Although examination of the fetal face is not required, we believe it should be examined routinely because it can add tremendous information when discriminating between genetic disorders/syndromes, including aneuploidy, and it completes the full examination of the fetus. Three distinct planes can be examined: axial, coronal (Fig. 73.5) and sagittal (profile) although a combination of these planes is the most optimal. In evaluating for cleft lip/palate (anterior palate), both axial and coronal images toward the anterior surface of the nose/upper lips provide the best visualization. The posterior or hard palate cannot be imaged sonographically, since it is obscured by overlying osseous structures. Other anatomic structures that should be evaluated include the chin (to rule out micrognathia), nasal bone (Fig. 73.6), nose, lower lips, tongue, orbits (and diameters if necessary, to exclude hyper/hypotelorism), and ear length (which can be shortened in both aneuploid and nonaneuploid fetuses). Multiple studies have found sonographically absent or short fetal nasal bone in both the first, and second trimesters to be sensitive for the detection of DS[8-10] Structures in the anterior neck that may have to be examined on occasion include the fetal thyroid, and the fluid-filled trachea and hypopharynx.

Examination of the fetal spine should be performed in three planes: sagittal, transverse and coronal. Each vertebral segment is composed of three echogenic ossification centers (two posteriorly, and one anteriorly, which is the vertebral body), which are positioned in a symmetric triangular shaped configuration in the transverse plane. In this plane, the posterior processes are also oriented toward the midline like the roof of a house. When these processes appeared splayed, a neural tube defect must be ruled out. Transverse imaging of the spine is perhaps the most sensitive method of examining for a spinal defect, since it allows a simultaneous examination of posterior ossification centers and overlying soft tissue. Sagittal imaging of the fetal spine (Fig. 73.7) should show two rows of approximately parallel ossification centers with overlying intact skin. Both sagittal and coronal views are useful to observe this "lining up" of the ossification centers, and should be able to rule out scoliosis or hemivertebrae (which can cause disorganization or absence of ossification centers). The sacrum normally should curve slightly upward. The overlying skin and soft tissues should also be examined carefully to rule out masses/tumors or open spina bifida.

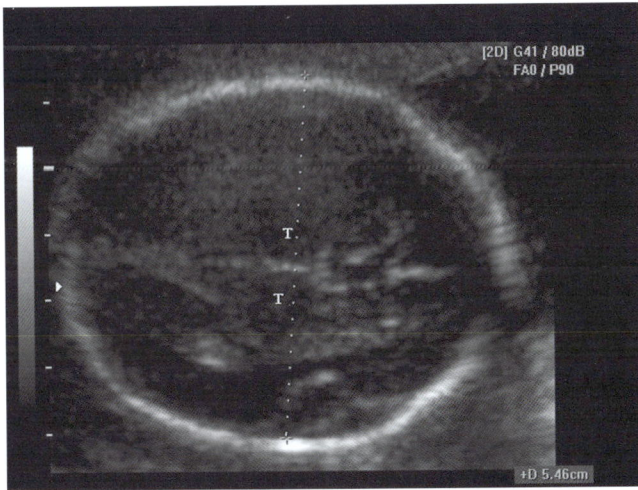

Fig. 73.1: Axial view through the fetal head with calipers demonstrating measurement of the biparietal diameter. This is also the view for measurement of the head circumference. Both thalami (T) are also depicted

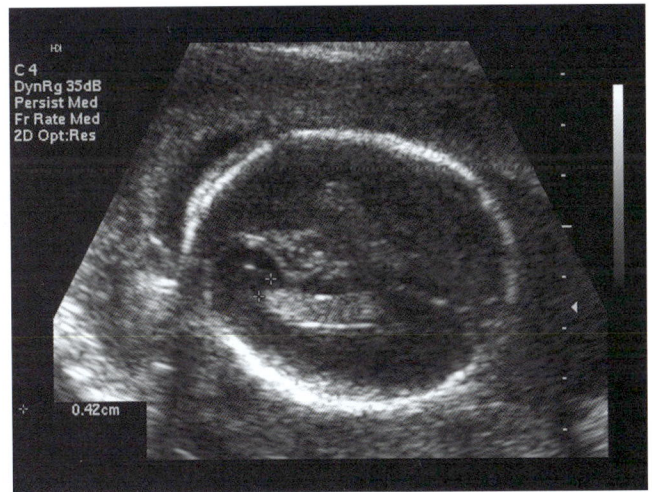

Fig. 73.2: Transventricular view of the fetal head demonstrating measurement of the atria of the lateral ventricle (0.42 cm) and the echogenic choroid plexus

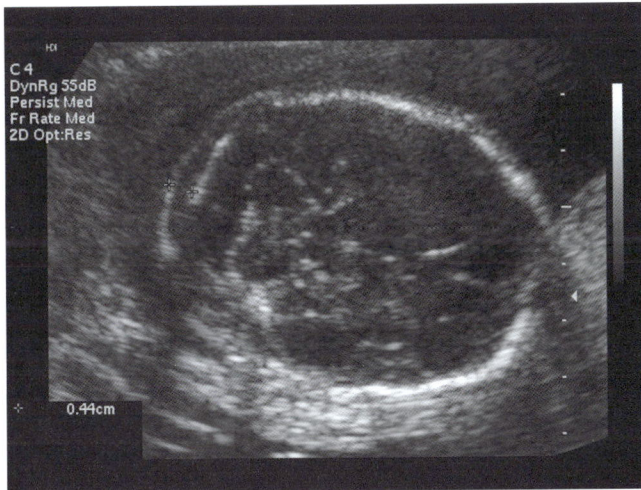

Fig. 73.3: Transcerebellar view demonstrating cerebellar hemispheres, cisterna magna and nuchal fold measurement (0.34 cm, normal)

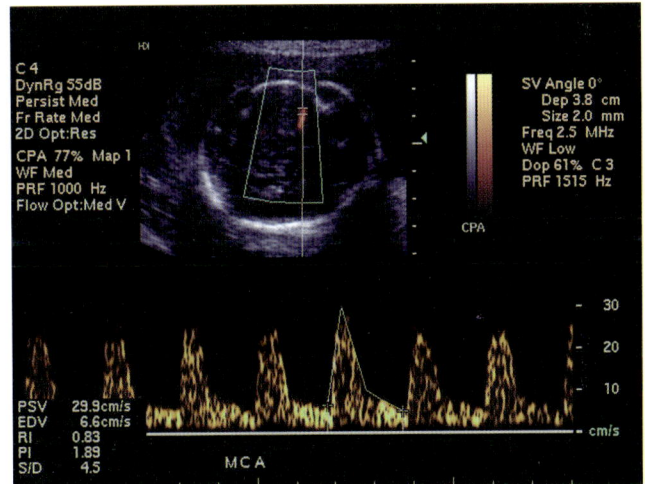

Fig. 73.4: Normal middle cerebral artery Doppler waveform. The systolic/diastolic ratio is high (6.47), consistent with normal high-resistance pattern

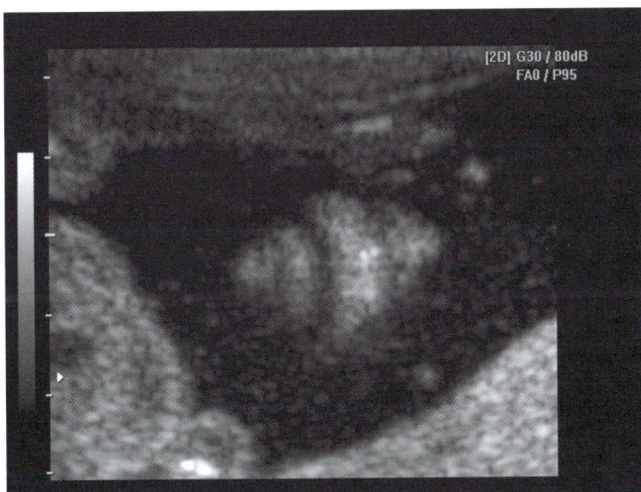

Fig. 73.5: Coronal view of fetal face showing nose, upper and lower lips

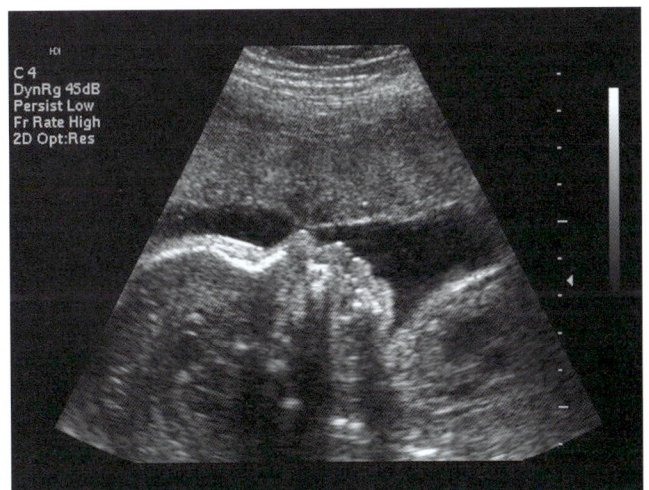

Fig. 73.6: Normal sagittal profile of fetus showing nasal bone

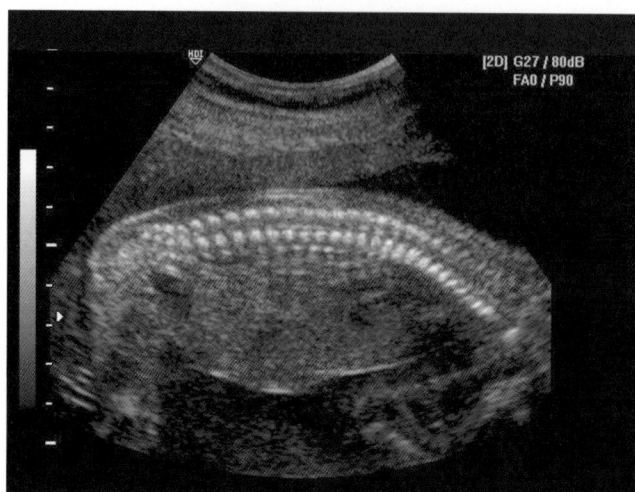

Fig. 73.7: Normal sagittal view of fetal spine. Note the overlying skin is intact, and the parallel features of the spinal centers

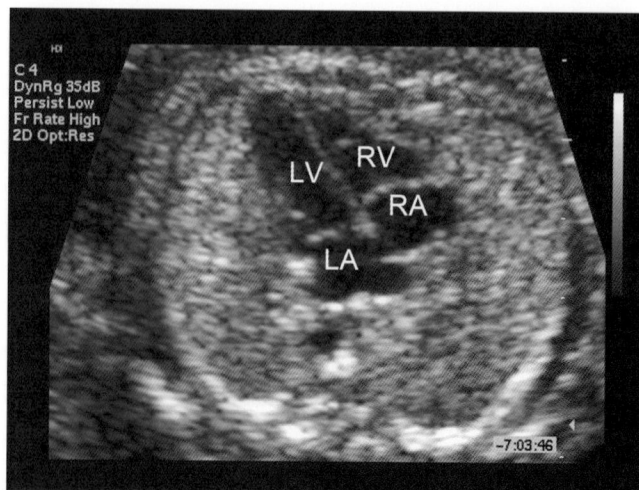

Fig. 73.8: Apical four-chamber view of the fetal heart, demonstrating left atrium and ventricle (LA, LV) and right atrium and ventricle (RA, RV)

In examining the fetal thorax, the scapulae, clavicles and ribs should be assessed, especially when ruling out certain types of skeletal dysplasias. Abnormal lung tissue and echogenicity (such as bronchopulmonary sequestration, cystic adenomatoid malformations), diaphragm, pleural effusions, and thoracic circumference (to rule out pulmonary hypoplasia) should all be examined.

Performing an adequate and detailed fetal cardiac examination on ultrasound can be one of the most difficult and challenging tasks, since it is dynamic, complex and can depend significantly on fetal position. First, the situs should be established along with the presence of a normal cardiac rate and rhythm. In a transverse image of the fetal chest, the heart should occupy about one-third of the fetal thorax, and its normal axis and position should be verified (apex points to the left, bulk of the heart occupies left side of chest, $45 \pm 20°$ angle of the heart relative to the midline). Any alterations in position, axis or both can suggest intrinsic malposition or an intrathoracic mass. In order to sufficiently rule out cardiac defects, multiple planes and views (in addition to the four-chamber view) should be examined in real-time imaging. A single static four-chamber view is no longer acceptable or adequate to completely examine the heart. Both outflow tracts should be evaluated to increase the sensitivity for cardiac defects, such as tetralogy of Fallot, transposition of the great vessels, truncus arteriosus, etc. In screening second trimester fetuses, we advocate visualization of the four-chamber apical (Fig. 73.8) and subcostal views, both outflow tracts, longitudinal parasternal arches (aortic and ductal), inferior/superior vena cava, valves, and the atria/ventricular septa. All chambers should have approximately equal sizes, the great vessels should cross each other, the pulmonary veins should be seen entering the left atrium, and there should be no pericardial effusion. Depending on the indication or clinical scenario, color, M-mode or pulsed Doppler sonography can also be performed of the fetal heart and its great vessels. In about 3–4% of normal second trimester fetuses,[11] an echogenic intracardiac focus can be seen, usually located in the left ventricle. It is caused by specular reflection from the papillary muscle and chordae tendinae. However, some studies have also confirmed an association between this and fetal DS in high-risk populations.[12]

Fetal abdominal organs that can be identified on second trimester ultrasonography include liver (majority of the upper abdomen), gallbladder (right upper quadrant at inferior edge of the liver and "teardrop" shaped), spleen (solid organ posterior to stomach), stomach, bowel, umbilical vein, and cord insertion site/adjacent anterior abdominal wall. The abdominal circumference (AC) is taken at the transverse level where stomach and spine are visualized, and the umbilical vein joins the right portal venous system, which should curve away from the stomach (Fig. 73.9). If, however, the curve is toward the stomach, persistence of the right umbilical vein should be suspected. The AC has its greatest value in evaluating fetal growth later in pregnancy, and also comprises a parameter used for fetal dating. This is because AC deviations are a result of changes in both liver size and subcutaneous fat. The stomach should always be located below the diaphragm as a fluid-filled structure in the left upper quadrant. An absent or small stomach in the usual location despite prolonged scanning to allow for filling, can be indicative of esophageal atresia with or without tracheoesophageal fistula, or diaphragmatic hernia (stomach located within the chest). The rest of the abdomen is filled with

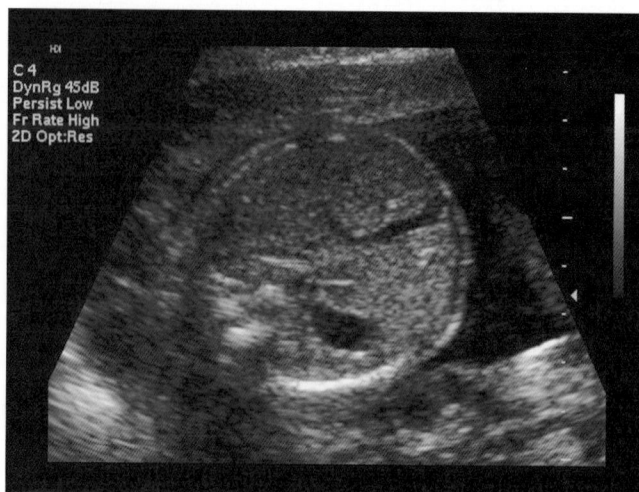

Fig. 73.9: Correct view of taking the abdominal circumference measurement

bowel, with the appearance changing with advancing gestational age. In the second trimester, the fetal bowel appears as midlevel to increased echogenicity filling the abdominal cavity; when using higher frequency transducers, it often appears mildly echogenic when compared to the liver.[13] True hyperechoic bowel is diagnosed when its echogenicity is similar to that of bone. It can be a normal variant, or associated with aneuploidy, infection, cystic fibrosis, fetus swallowing blood, intrauterine growth restriction and bowel malformations/atresias. To exclude ventral wall defects such as omphalocele or gastroschisis, the umbilical cord insertion site into the abdominal wall must be evaluated to confirm the cord penetrating the abdomen, with the adjacent abdominal wall intact. No fetal ascites or hydrops should be seen under normal circumstances.

The fetal genitourinary tract is a common site for fetal anomalies. The kidneys appear as bilateral, hypoechoic, paraspinal structures that contain the urine-filled renal pelvis and can sometimes be difficult to visualize. Dilation of the renal pelvis/calyx or ureter, renal masses, hyperechogenicity, parenchymal cysts, or enlargement/absence of the kidneys may reflect anomalies. To delineate the renal arteries, color or power Doppler imaging is frequently used. The fetal adrenals can be seen cephalad to their kidneys. While the right adrenal lies immediately posterior to the inferior vena cava, the left adrenal lies lateral to the aorta. The fetal bladder is sonolucent (contains urine) and located in the midline, anteriorly and low in the pelvis (Fig. 73.10). Absence of the bladder may be secondary to recent voiding or bladder/cloacal exstrophy, while a very enlarged bladder may be a sign of lower obstructive uropathy. Male genitalia is confirmed only if penis and scrotum are seen. Occasionally, the hypoechoic umbilical cord lying between the thighs can be mistaken for the solid penis. Also, a prominent clitoris seen during the early second trimester can also sometimes be confused for a penis. The echogenic testicles usually do not descend into the scrotum until the seventh month. Female genitalia are identified by the presence of several parallel linear echoes, which represent the margins of the labia, and not by the observed absence of penis/scrotum. One should never forget that ambiguous genitalia may also be present.

Although routine evaluation of all fetal upper and lower extremities is not a part of routine obstetrical sonographic guidelines,

it is our opinion that a complete survey of all extremities (including hands/feet) may provide important diagnostic information and can screen for abnormalities. Both of the hands should contain five fingers, should be open (full extension of all fingers in the same plane as the metacarpals), have normal movement and tone, and the middle phalanx of the fifth digit must be visualized (Fig. 73.11). The presence of clenched hands with overlapping digits is a highly sensitive (95%) sonographic marker of trisomy 18.[14] All the long bones (femur, humerus, radius, ulna, tibia, fibula) should be present and there should not be demineralized, shortened, fractured, contracted, or bowed bones. The ulna normally extends farther into the elbow, and the tibia extends farther into the patella. Routinely on our second trimester surveys, we measure all long bone lengths. These measurements should be obtained with the long bone located horizontally within the image, since vertical measurements can falsely "shorten" the actual length (Fig. 73.12). Also, only the ossified portions of the bone should be measured, with the hypoechoic cartilaginous epiphyses excluded. Both lower extremities should not be clubbed, nor the plantar surface appear "rocker-bottom". Five toes should be present, and they should not appear dysplastic. Foot length (Fig. 73.13) is also another biometric parameter than can be obtained.

Normally, the umbilical cord is comprised of three vessels: two smaller umbilical arteries and one larger umbilical vein; this can be confirmed by directly imaging the cord or by observing the umbilical arteries coursing around the fetal bladder. Depending on the clinical situation, an umbilical artery Doppler waveform can be obtained (Fig. 73.14). Its flow is a reflection mainly of the placental resistance, and to a certain extent, of the fetal systemic circulation. Once the umbilical vein enters the fetal abdomen, it turns superiorly, enters the liver, and communicates with the portal vein. The umbilical vein also continues into the ductus venosus, and then the inferior vena cava and right atrium.

SONOGRAPHIC ANEUPLOIDY MARKERS IN THE SECOND TRIMESTER

Aneuploid fetuses account for approximately 6–11% of all stillbirths and neonatal deaths.[15] Prenatal ultrasonography can

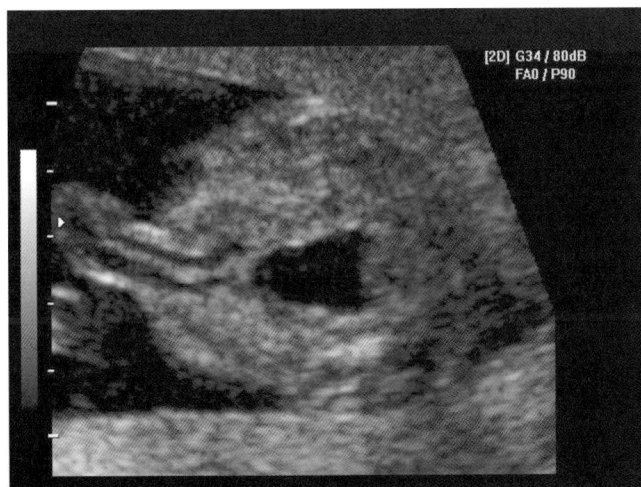

Fig. 73.10: Transverse view of fetus depicting abdominal wall cord insertion site. The sonolucent bladder is also visualized with each of the two umbilical arteries coursing around its periphery

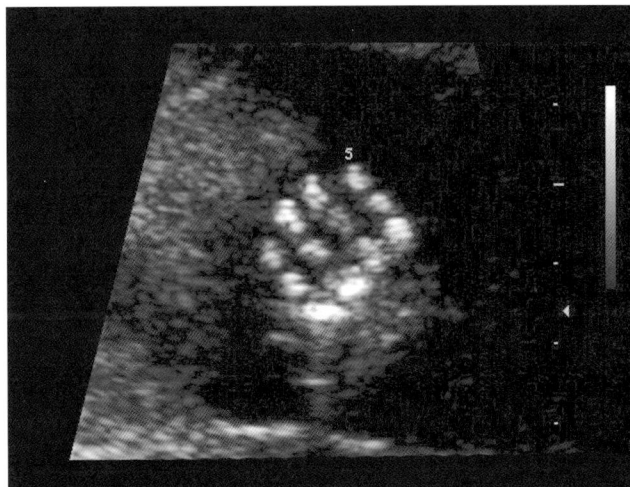

Fig. 73.11: Fetal hand demonstrating echogenic phalanges of four fingers, including the fifth digit

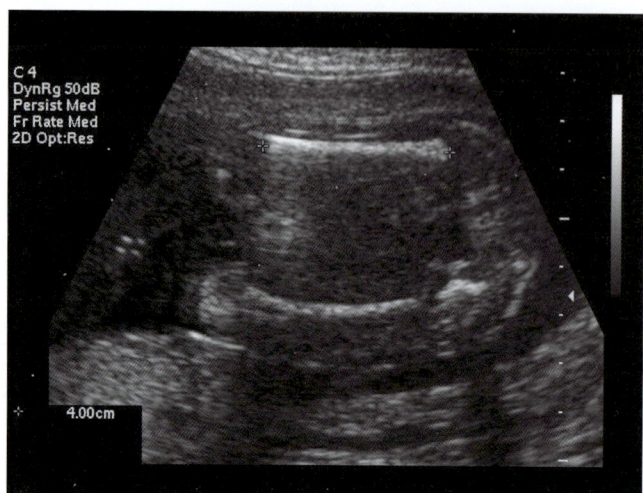

Fig. 73.12: Femur length measured from proximal end to distal metaphysis, including only the ossified portions. Note the other femur lying parallel and directly below the measured femur length

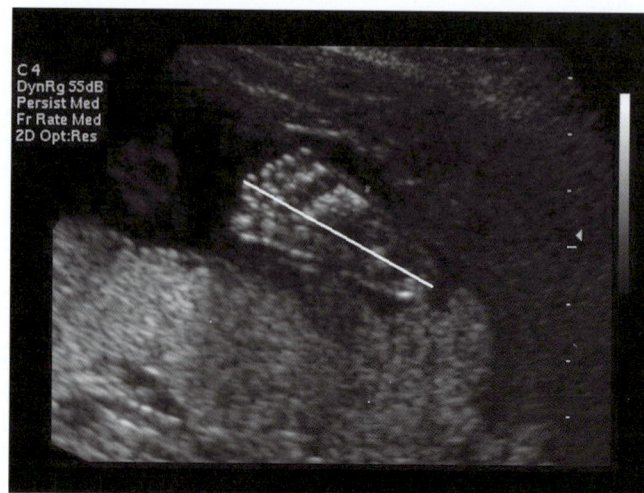

Fig. 73.13: Measurement of second trimester fetal foot length, with all five toes demonstrated

often detect many abnormalities in fetuses with aneuploidy. These can include major structural defects or other "soft" sonographic markers of aneuploidy. Aneuploidy "soft" markers are usually nonspecific, most commonly seen in normal fetuses, are often transient (such as choroid plexus cysts) and may not be significantly linked to perinatal outcome. The aneuploidy markers that we use in our institution include shortened long bones, pyelectasis, increased nuchal fold thickening, hyperechoic bowel, choroid plexus cysts, hypoplastic middle phalanx of the fifth digit, clinodactyly, sandal gap (wide space between first and second toes), two-vessel cord, echogenic intracardiac focus, short ear length and absent nasal bone. Each marker alone, has only low to moderate sensitivity for detecting fetal DS. Many of these sonographic findings when found in isolation in low-risk patients do not necessarily increase the risk for aneuploidy. However, when found in the context of multiple other sonographic abnormalities or markers (in low-risk patients), or when isolated markers are seen in high-risk patients, the risk for fetal aneuploidy may increase. In general, as the number of markers present increases, the risk for chromosomal abnormality also increases directly.

The presence of most fetal congenital abnormalities will increase the risk for underlying aneuploidy except for some disorders felt to be "acquired" (rather than inherent) from tissue or vascular disruption. Such disorders include hydranencephaly, gastroschisis, tumors, amniotic band syndrome, limb-body wall complex, etc. Examples of specific structural anomalies that can be associated with fetal aneuploidy are: cerebral ventriculomegaly, holoprosencephaly, agenesis of the corpus callosum, Dandy-Walker malformation/cerebellar hypoplasia, spina bifida, cleft lip/palate, ocular abnormalities, craniofacial anomalies, cystic hygroma, nonimmune hydrops, cardiac abnormalities, diaphragmatic hernia, duodenal atresia, omphalocele, genitourinary anomalies, clubfeet and extremity malformations.

The most common autosomal trisomy in live born infants is DS. Because only 25% of DS fetuses in the second trimester have a sonographically detectable major anomaly (unlike trisomies 18 and 13 where the majority will have anomalies visualized), several investigators have been searching to find aneuploidy

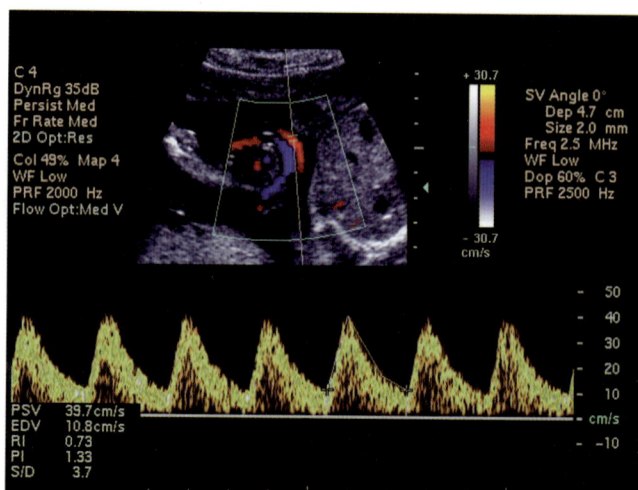

Fig. 73.14: Normal Doppler waveform of umbilical artery in a second trimester fetus. The systolic/diastolic ratio is 3:28

ultrasonographic markers in order to increase the sensitivity for fetal DS.[16] Genetic sonography is performed in the second trimester, ideally between 18 weeks and 20 weeks. It is a specific, targeted examination for fetal aneuploidy (most specifically for trisomy 21) where the examiner evaluates for abnormal fetal biometry, fetal structural anomalies, and other markers of aneuploidy. By combining multiple aneuploidy markers, the sensitivity for DS can be increased to > 80%, with false-positive rates of 10–15% (by defining as abnormal ultrasound exam with at least 1 abnormal marker present). Information derived from a normal genetic sonogram is used to generate an adjusted (lower) DS risk to guide a high-risk woman's decision on genetic amniocentesis. Thus far, many studies have been published that examine the accuracy of genetic sonography for detecting DS in high-risk populations.[17] By defining as abnormal the ultrasound with at least one abnormal marker, the overall sensitivity is 77% (50–93%) and the false-positive rate is 13% (7–17%).[17] In 1998, a large multicenter collaborative study involving 11 centers (including our own) examined the sensitivity of sonography in detecting fetal DS.[18] They found that 85% of DS fetuses (n = 241) had at least one abnormal finding on ultrasound. In 2003, an eight center study (including our own) evaluated the utility of second trimester genetic sonography among high-risk pregnancies, including 176 DS fetuses.[19] The sensitivity for DS was 72%, with a range from 64% to 80% at the various sites. Of significance, about half (47%) of DS fetuses had a thickened nuchal fold of 5 mm or more, making this marker the one with the highest sensitivity.

Nuchal fold thickening is the single most sensitive and specific marker for fetal DS (sensitivity 40% and false-positive rate of 0.1%),[20] although absent nasal bone has also recently been shown by us to have a 41% sensitivity and 100% specificity for fetal DS.[8] Short femur length (measured to expected length < 0.91) has been found in 24% of DS fetuses,[21] while a short humerus (measured to expected length < 0.90) identified 50% of DS fetuses, with a false-positive rate of 6.25%.[22] Unfortunately, there tends to be a large overlap in bone measurements between affected and normal fetuses. The sensitivity for pyelectasis (anteroposterior diameter renal pelvis > 4 mm in second trimester) for DS is 25%.[22] Echogenic bowel has a reported sensitivity of 7–12.5%, while echogenic intracardiac focus has a sensitivity of 18%.[22] Recently, we examined the sensitivity for fetal DS by sonographic ear length.[23] We found that of 51 DS fetuses, 41% (n = 21) had ear length < 10th percentile. However, short ear length was not as sensitive a marker for DS as it was for trisomies 18 (96%) and 13 (100%). Although an association between choroid plexus cysts and trisomy 18 has been established,[24] the association with fetal DS has been controversial, especially when isolated. When the choroid plexus cyst(s) are isolated, obstetrical management should not be altered in the absence of any other high-risk factors.[25] Single umbilical artery has been found to be associated with aneuploidy and congenital malformations. The risk for fetal aneuploidy depends on the presence of associated anomalies, the greater the number of anomalies, the greater the chances for aneuploidy. In a low-risk patient, an isolated single umbilical artery on ultrasound is probably not an indication for fetal karyotyping, provided that a search for additional malformations is negative.

In 1996, our group was the first to publish data on using second trimester genetic sonography to guide clinical management of women at high-risk for fetal DS.[26] Subsequently, once we analyzed our 1999 data, in the presence of a normal genetic ultrasound, we counseled patients that the likelihood for fetal DS was reduced by at least 80% from the *apriori* risk (triple or quadruple screen, or if unavailable, maternal age).[17] Over almost a 10-year-period (since November 1992), we have evaluated 5,299 fetuses by genetic sonography; the overwhelming majority (85%) had no markers seen (normal scan), 12% had one abnormal marker present, and 3% had two or more markers present. When one or more abnormal sonographic markers were present, the sensitivity, specificity, positive and negative predictive values for DS were 87% (52/60), 91% (4,395/4,831), 11% (52/4,88) and 99.8% (4,395/4,403), respectively. Approximately two-thirds of DS fetuses had two or more abnormal sonographic markers seen.

SECOND TRIMESTER ULTRASOUND SCREENING FOR FETAL ABNORMALITIES

While there are numerous acceptable indications for performing a second trimester sonographic examination during pregnancy, perhaps one of the most common indications is to rule out the presence of fetal abnormalities. While the advantages of performing a screening ultrasound in the pregnancies at high-risk for fetal anomalies is clear, the benefits and cost-effectiveness of routine sonographic screening in pregnancy are not as obvious. In the United States, approximately 60–70% of all pregnant women undergo an ultrasound at various times in the gestation.[27] However, the efficacy of routine sonographic screening for fetal abnormalities varies widely. One of the first studies to determine the diagnostic accuracy of ultrasonography in high-risk pregnancies was performed during the late 1970s and early 1980s in the United Kingdom.[28] It was around this time that real-time imaging became widespread as a clinical tool. This study found that 95% of malformations were correctly diagnosed.[28] Other published sensitivities have ranged broadly anywhere from 13.3% to 82.4%,[29] with the average collaborative world experience being 50%.[30] After reviewing these extremely wide and different detection rates, it becomes apparent why the reliability and utility of sonographic screening for fetal abnormalities has become very controversial in some countries. Even for those who already advocate routine sonographic screening, when to perform scans and the number of sonographic examinations are debatable and inconsistent. Since 75% of patients with abnormal fetuses will be "low-risk", it is reasonable to review data in the literature that assesses the impact of routine screening sonography.[29]

Diagnosing fetal anomalies prior to birth can provide many advantages. Prenatal sonographic diagnosis can lead to further diagnostic testing (such as amniocentesis), prepare parents for an adverse pregnancy outcome, alert the clinician to the possibility of other abnormalities, and can determine appropriate management choices (such as intrauterine therapy, early delivery, delivery at a tertiary care center or termination of pregnancy). However, all these advantages are achieved only if the ultrasound examination is performed by qualified, knowledgeable individuals who possess expertise performing ultrasonographic examinations. Sonographic screening done by individuals who are inexperienced and unqualified may not only increase the costs of healthcare, but can create high false-negative and false-positive results with significant consequences.

There are a multitude of biases and problems that can account for the sensitivity variation across various studies.[29] Fetal abnormalities that resolve, technical factors (obesity, fetal positioning), quality of sonographic equipment and undetectability of certain anomalies comprise some of the reasons. In addition, each center has differing criteria and interpretations as to what exactly constitutes a detailed sonographic examination. There is no doubt that the less detailed the examination, the higher the chances are for having a lower diagnostic accuracy. Selection bias can also play an important role in affecting diagnostic accuracy, depending on whether the patient source is a hospital or office practice-based. Perhaps the most important bias is the variation in sonographic skills, capability, and experience of individuals performing the ultrasound examination. In the Helsinki study that incorporated patient populations from two hospitals, the ultrasonographic sensitivity for detecting anomalies was more than twofold higher in the university hospital than in the city hospital (77% vs 36%).[31] A study in Vienna examined the influence of the experience of the investigator on the rate of sonographic diagnosis of fetal malformations.[32] Of 323 cases of fetal malformations, obstetricians in private offices detected 22%, hospital examiners detected 40%, and examiners in the prenatal diagnosis and therapy center detected 90% of all fetal malformations.[32] The selection of pregnant women is also significant. Screening high-risk women is likely to be much more effective. In this scenario, the chances of discovering an anomaly is higher, and the sonographers may be more attentively focused. For instance, in one study they found that the average sensitivity in low-risk populations is 55%, while in high-risk populations, it is 92%.[29]

The gestational age at the time of ultrasound screening also impacts sensitivity, since various anomalies are manifested at differing gestational weeks or may be easier to visualize/detect, and some anomalies may present only later in gestation (duodenal atresia). In general, the more sonographic examinations a patient undergoes during the pregnancy, the higher the rate of anomaly detection. Levi found that the average sensitivity from studies including scans performed once before 20 weeks was 45%; when scanning was done several times during the pregnancy, the sensitivity rose to 60%.[29] The prevalence of specific malformations within a given population may also have a significant impact on the overall sensitivity of ultrasound. A low frequency of anomalies in a certain population can introduce bias in diagnostic accuracy. Studies which exclude certain anomalies because they are felt to be "minor" or undetectable may have dramatically different sensitivities than when all fetal anomalies are included. In 1996, one study found that the sensitivity of sonography for diagnosing both minor/major anomalies was only 8.7%; however, if only major anomalies detectable by ultrasound were included, the sensitivity was increased up to 75%.[30] Finally, other factors that can affect the reported fetal abnormality detection rates in sonographic screening may be related to ascertainment biases, such as lack of autopsies (considered the "gold standard"), suboptimal or incomplete neonatal evaluation at birth, and insufficient length of neonatal follow-up since some abnormalities may not express themselves immediately after birth and can take time to manifest.[29]

In the United States, the RADIUS (Routine Antenatal Diagnostic Imaging with Ultrasound) study was the first randomized clinical trial of second trimester ultrasound.[33] This trial was performed to determine the benefits, if any, of routine sonograms among pregnant women at low risk. It compared routinely scanned pregnant women to those having ultrasounds only when indicated. An additional ultrasound exam was performed in the early third trimester in the study group. Although, the identification rate of anomalies was found to be three times better with routine ultrasound vs indicated ultrasound (35% vs 11%, respectively), the sensitivity in detecting anomalies by ultrasound performed between 15 weeks and 22 weeks was extremely low (17%). A possible source of bias was that practice-based patients were utilized, which may have created an inadvertent selection bias (rather than a community or hospital-based population). This study reported a relative detection rate of 2.7 (95% CI, 1.3–5.8) in tertiary vs non-tertiary ultrasound units.[33] Within a subgroup evaluated at tertiary care centers, the detection rate of anomalous fetuses was 35% vs. 13% in non-tertiary centers. This trial found that sonographic screening did not significantly influence the management or outcome of pregnancies complicated by congenital malformations. A 1998 study at a tertiary care center found that the sensitivity of anomaly detection in women at risk for anomalies was very high (89.7%).[34] In the screening group, or lower-risk population, although the sensitivity was less (47.6%), it was still sufficient to ensure cost-effectiveness for their patients.[34]

In 1999, the Eurofetus study was designed to evaluate the sensitivity of routine sonographic screening for fetal malformations.[35] In the largest among screening studies, ultrasound screening was applied to almost 200,000 pregnant women in 60 hospital laboratories and 14 European countries. They found a sensitivity rate of 64% (2,363/3,685), which at first glance, was much higher compared to the RADIUS study. However, for various reasons these two studies may not be exactly comparable. For example, patients studied in the RADIUS trial were low-risk (and probably not relevant to the average population), since very strict exclusion criteria had been applied prior to patient recruitment. The criteria used to designate major fetal anomalies (gold standard) was also very liberal, and both of these facts could have lowered the sensitivity. On the other hand, in the Eurofetus study, all patients were studied regardless of their risk status, and only "truly" major abnormalities were considered as endpoints. This could have artificially raised the sensitivity of the sonographic screening.

The Helsinki trial had patients who undergo one ultrasound screening exam within the second trimester; 40% of major fetal anomalies were detected.[36] Although screening did detect most anomalies of the central nervous system, genitourinary system and cases with multiple anomalies, it was less satisfactory in detecting cardiac and gastrointestinal tract anomalies.[36] The Belgian Multicentric Study found that of 381 structurally abnormal fetuses, 154 were correctly detected by ultrasound (sensitivity 40%).[37] The specificity, positive, and negative predictive values were 99.9% 95% and 98.6% respectively.

In 2002, we examined the value of our aforementioned complete anatomic sonographic survey in detecting fetal abnormalities, and correlated our sonographic findings with perinatal autopsy results.[38] Autopsy findings were considered the "gold standard". Of 88 abnormal autopsies, 85 fetuses had one or more abnormal structural sonographic findings, for a sensitivity of 97% (for anomalous fetuses). From autopsy, a total of 372 separate abnormalities were found; of the 299 major and 73 minor abnormalities, prenatal ultrasonography detected 75% and 18%, respectively. Thus, we found that the sensitivity for detecting minor abnormalities was poor, even when utilizing a complete sonographic survey. We found either complete agreement or only minor differences between sonographic and autopsy findings in 65% of the cases.[38]

In examining the literature, it is evident that there is a wide range in sensitivity of ultrasonography to detect fetal anomalies, and it depends highly on the clinical setting in which the examination is performed, along with the varying skills, expertise and experience of those performing the sonographic examination. Therefore, there appears to be insufficient evidence to comment on a single estimate of the sensitivity of routine ultrasound in screening for fetal anomalies. However, in many studies, the specificity of a fetal anatomic survey has been found to exceed 99%.[33,39-41] This fact indicates that in the low-risk population, sonography may be helpful in ruling out abnormalities and detecting the normal, but may not be equally reliable in detecting abnormalities. It is expected that with time, the sensitivity of sonographic screening programs should improve. This can be partly attributable to improvements in equipment quality, training, and experience of sonographers, along with the emergence of new technological advances such as 3- and 4-dimensional sonography. It is thought that uniform and detailed training for practitioners is the best guarantee for an efficient screening program.[29] In addition, standardization of the scanning process for each and every scan should also improve overall sensitivity. In a 1996 review article, Seeds argues that the diagnostic sensitivity of the screening obstetrical ultrasound examination appears to be highest in high-risk patients examined by highly specialized and experienced personnel.[42] However, diagnostic sensitivity may be quite good even in low-risk patients with a basic or routine examination if recognized guidelines for content are followed and referral to experienced referral resources for unclear or suspicious images is liberally practiced.[42]

A common and often touted benefit of the prenatal detection of fetal abnormalities, especially those that are life-threatening, is the delivery of these infants in tertiary care centers that are capable of providing immediate and appropriate care. A valid and legitimate question often asked is whether routine sonography improves the survival rates of anomalous neonates. Ten years ago, the RADIUS study examined this question.[33] Screening ultrasound was not found to have any impact on the detection, management and outcome of fetuses with anomalies. Although, survival rates for fetuses with anomalies were not affected by sonographic screening, in an analysis of infants with life-threatening anomalies, 75% (21/28) in the routinely screened group survived, vs 52% (11/21) in the routine-care group.[33] While this difference did not reach statistical significance, this may be attributed in part to the small sample sizes. At the current time, there is insufficient evidence to either refute or support the benefit of routine sonography in reducing mortality of those neonates with life-threatening anomalies, although this may not be intuitively apparent to those families affected with these problems. It is clear that further studies are required to address this issue.

A significant question regarding routine ultrasonography is whether this improves overall perinatal morbidity and mortality. It is known that routine diagnostic sonography can lead to accurate determination of gestational age, multiple gestations and placental abnormalities, thus theoretically improving perinatal risk. Three trials have examined perinatal morbidity and mortality in patients undergoing routine ultrasonography. In both the RADIUS and Stockholm trials, perinatal mortality rates were similar between the routine sonography and control groups.[27,43] However, the Helsinki trial found that the perinatal mortality rate was significantly improved in the routine ultrasound group (4.6/1,000 vs 9.0/1,000); this 49.2% reduction was mainly attributable to improved early detection of major malformations which led to termination of pregnancy.[31] In all three trials, no differences were found between the study and control groups in terms of perinatal morbidity.[27,31,43] Perinatal morbidity was defined as admission to the neonatal unit,[31,43] moderate morbidity (neonatal sepsis, grade I or II intraventricular hemorrhage, stay of >5 days in neonatal unit) or severe morbidity (ventilation >48 hours, stay of >30 days in neonatal unit).[27] In terms of birth weight and number of low birth weight (<2,500 grams) infants, the RADIUS and Helsinki trials found a similar birth weight distribution between the routine ultrasound and control groups.[27,31] However, the Stockholm trial found fewer births of <2,500 g (2.5% vs 4%) in the routine ultrasound group.[43] Finally, this same trial found that for women smokers, there was a higher mean birth weight (3,413 vs 3,354 g) in the routine ultrasound group, and the authors surmised that this improvement could be attributed to healthier maternal behaviors after women visualized their fetuses on ultrasound.[43] The RADIUS trial investigators concluded that adopting sonographic screening in the United States would increase healthcare costs without either improving perinatal outcome or providing any measurable benefit from early detection of fetal anomalies. By contrast, however, another group found that routine abnormality screening improves perinatal outcome by leading to termination of pregnancies for certain anomalies, and selected delivery at tertiary care centers for life-threatening malformations.[34]

An important issue to examine is the cost-benefit analysis of routine second trimester sonography. Our group recently performed a cost-benefit analysis based on the RADIUS results, and compared a policy of routine second trimester sonography in low-risk pregnant women vs. not offering such screening.[44] We concluded that routine second trimester sonographic screening is associated with net benefits only if the ultrasound was performed in tertiary care centers. Another tertiary center also assessed the cost-effectiveness of anomaly screening in their patient population, and found that routine screening appeared cost-effective.[34] Leivo and associates demonstrated that a one-stage second trimester screening ultrasound was cost-effective, and was associated with fewer perinatal deaths.[45] In the United Kingdom, a prospective study was performed to evaluate the cost-benefit of changing from selective to routine ultrasound screening for fetal anomaly.[46] They found that routine sonography was the sole method of detection for 11 major and 18 less severe congenital abnormalities found in low-risk pregnancies, which would not previously have qualified for selective ultrasound. They felt that routine fetal anomaly ultrasound would seem to be economically justifiable.[46] In 2002, Roberts reviewed evidence from the literature and found a need for more data on the costs and cost-effectiveness of routine sonographic screening for fetal anomalies.[47]

All published trials have shown that more twin pregnancies are diagnosed earlier with routine ultrasound. The Helsinki trial found that with the routine ultrasound group, 100% of twins were detected prior to 21 weeks, compared with 76% in the control group.[31] In addition, they found that the perinatal mortality for the twins was 27.8/1,000 vs. 65.8/1,000 respectively. The RADIUS trial also performed subgroup analyses for small for gestational age infants and neonates born at 42 weeks.[27] The data did not show improvement in overall outcome for these conditions when routine sonography was performed.

In conclusion, examination of the available evidence shows that in low-risk pregnancies, routine ultrasonography may reduce perinatal mortality because of induced abortions following the detection of fetal abnormalities. In the United States, the current standard of care remains at performing ultrasound only for specific indications. However, some would argue that every obstetrical patient should have an ultrasound examination only if it is competently performed, properly recorded, and if the patient is aware of appropriate goals and limitations.[42]

Although, ultrasonographic screening for fetal abnormalities may have widely varying sensitivities depending on the particular unit, in our opinion it still offers great value to both patients and physicians that may not be quantifiable. Psychological reassurance, referrals, genetic counseling, antepartum management, and preparation of families and healthcare providers are just some examples of the possible advantages. Overall, these reasons may outweigh the "risks" of ultrasound, such as false-positive diagnoses. If patients are given the choice and counseled regarding the diagnostic capabilities of present day sonography, most would choose to undergo fetal anomaly screening. It is important to remember that pregnant women often do not perceive ultrasonography as a "test", but rather utilize it as a tool to evaluate their fetus as a patient. We concur with this philosophy, and would also argue that examining the fetus as a patient via ultrasound should be offered routinely, as in all other aspects of adult medicine.

CONCLUSION

Second trimester sonographic screening for fetal anomalies and prenatal diagnosis is performed for many reasons. It can provide useful information and knowledge for patients, may give them reassurance regarding their pregnancy and the health of their fetus, provides the opportunity for further diagnostic testing such as amniocentesis, provides counseling regarding prognosis, and can modify management (such as location and method of delivery, termination, fetal surgery, etc.). Some patients will utilize this information to prepare ahead of the delivery date by consulting genetics, pediatric surgeons, neonatologists and other specialists. In addition, for the physician, information regarding specific abnormalities or aneuploidy can optimize pregnancy management, along with the labor and delivery process. Importantly, knowledge of anomalies can raise the possibility of genetic syndromes, can impact future pregnancies, and can influence counseling regarding genetics and prognosis. Therefore, because of its many advantages, it is our opinion that all patients should have access to sonographic screening within the second trimester of pregnancy, and a complete, targeted and thorough exam should be performed to increase sensitivity.

REFERENCES

1. American College of Obstetricians and Gynecologists. New Ultrasound Output Display Standard. 2003 Compendium of Selected Publications; 2003. pp. 69-70.
2. Grandjean H, Larroque D, Levi S. The performance of routine ultrasonographic screening of pregnancies in the Eurofetus Study. Am J Obstet Gynecol. 1999;181(2):446-54.
3. Yeo L, Vintzileos AM, Guzman ER, et al. Targeted ultrasound after an abnormal karyotype: The patient's perspective. Am J Obstet Gynecol. 2001;185:S233.
4. The American Institute of Ultrasound in Medicine. Standards for Performance of the Antepartum Obstetrical Ultrasound Examination. Laurel, MD: American Institute of Ultrasound in Medicine; 1994.
5. Schwarzler P, Senat MV, Holden D, et al. Feasibility of the second trimester fetal ultrasound examination in an unselected population at 18, 20 or 22 weeks of pregnancy: A randomized trial. Ultrasound Obstet Gynecol. 1999;14(2):92-7.
6. Mahony BS, Callen PW, Filly RA, et al. The fetal cisterna magna. Radiology. 1984;153:773-6.
7. Laing FC, Frates MC, Brown DL, et al. Sonography of the fetal posterior fossa: False appearance of mega-cisterna magna and Dandy-Walker variant. Radiology. 1994;192:247-51.
8. Vintzileos A, Walters C, Yeo L. Absent nasal bone in the prenatal detection of fetuses with trisomy 21 in a high-risk population. Obstet Gynecol. 2003;101:905-8.
9. Cicero S, Bindra R, Rembouskos G, et al. Fetal nasal bone length in chromosomally normal and abnormal fetuses at 11–14 weeks of gestation. J Matern Fetal Neonatal Med. 2002;11:400-2.
10. Bromley B, Liberman E, Shipp TD, et al. Fetal nose bone length; a marker for Down syndrome in the second trimester. J Ultrasound Med. 2002;21:1387-94.
11. Levy DW, Mintz MC. The left ventricular echogenic focus: A normal finding. Am J Roentgenol. 1988;150(1):85-6.
12. Sepulveda W, Cullen S, Nicolaidis P, et al. Echogenic foci in the fetal heart: A marker of chromosomal abnormality. Br J Obstet Gynaecol. 1995;102(6):490-2.
13. Vincoff NS, Callen PW, Smith-Bindman R, et al. Effect of ultrasound transducer frequency on the appearance of the fetal bowel. J Ultrasound Med. 1999;18(12):799-803.
14. Yeo L, Guzman ER, Day-Salvatore D, et al. Prenatal detection of fetal trisomy 18 through abnormal sonographic features. J Ultrasound Med. 2003;22:581-90.
15. Alberman ED, Creasy MR. Frequency of chromosomal abnormalities in miscarriages and perinatal deaths. J Med Genet. 1977;14:313-5.
16. Vintzileos AM, Egan JF. Adjusting the risk for trisomy 21 on the basis of second trimester ultrasonography. Am J Obstet Gynecol. 1995;172:837-44.
17. Yeo L, Vintzileos AM. The use of genetic sonography to reduce the need for amniocentesis in women at high-risk for Down syndrome. Semin Perinatol. 2003; 27:152-9.
18. Persutte WH, Hobbins JC, Nyberg DA, et al. Trisomy 21 multicenter collaborative project. Am J Obstet Gynecol. 1998;178:S22.
19. Hobbins JC, Lezotte DC, Persutte WH, et al. An eight center study to evaluate the utility of mid-term genetic ultrasounds among high-risk pregnancies. J Ultrasound Med. 2003;22:33-8.
20. Benacerraf BR, Barss BA, Laboda LA. A sonographic sign for the detection in the second trimester of the fetus with Down's syndrome. Am J Obstet Gynecol. 1985;151:1078-9.
21. Nyberg DA, Resta RG, Hickok DE, et al. Femur length shortening in the detection of Down syndrome: Is prenatal screening feasible? Am J Obstet Gynecol. 1990;162:1247-52.
22. Bromley B, Benacerraf BR. The genetic sonogram scoring index. Semin Perinatol. 2003;27:124-9.
23. Yeo L, Guzman ER, Ananth CV, et al. Prenatal detection of fetal aneuploidy by sonographic ear length. J Ultrasound Med. 2003;22:565-76.
24. Gross SJ, Shulman LP, Tolley EA, et al. Isolated fetal choroid plexus cysts and trisomy 18: A review and meta-analysis. Am J Obstet Gynecol. 1995;172:83-7.
25. Chitty LS, Chudleigh P, Wright E, et al. The significance of choroid plexus cysts in an unselected population: Results of a multicenter study. Ultrasound Obstet Gynecol. 1998;12:391-97.
26. Vintzileos AM, Campbell WA, Rodis JF, et al. The use of second trimester genetic sonogram in guiding clinical management of patients at increased risk for fetal trisomy 21. Obstet Gynecol. 1996;87:948-52.
27. Ewigman BG, Crane JP, Frigoletto FD, et al. Effect of prenatal ultrasound screening on perinatal outcome. RADIUS Study Group. N Engl J Med. 1993;329:821-7.
28. Campbell S, Pearce JM. The prenatal diagnosis of fetal structural anomalies by ultrasound. Clin Obstet Gynecol. 1983;10:475-506.
29. Levi S. Ultrasound in prenatal diagnosis: Polemics around routine ultrasound screening for second trimester fetal malformations. Prenat Diagn. 2002;22:285-95.
30. Skupski DW, Newman S, Edersheim T, et al. Fetus placenta-newborn: The impact of routine obstetric ultrasonographic screening in a low-risk population. Am J Obstet Gynecol. 1996;175:1142-5.
31. Saari-Kemppainen A, Karjalainen O, Ylostalo P, et al. Ultrasound screening and perinatal mortality: controlled trial systematic one-stage screening in pregnancy. The Helsinki Ultrasound Trial. Lancet. 1990;336:387-91.
32. Bernaschek G, Stuempflen I, Deutinger J. The influence of the experience of the investigator on the rate of sonographic diagnosis of fetal malformations in Vienna. Prenat Diagn. 1996;16:807-11.

33. Crane JP, LeFevre ML, Winborn RC, et al. A randomized trial of prenatal ultrasonographic screening: impact on the detection, management, and outcome of anomalous fetuses. The RADIUS Study Group. Am J Obstet Gynecol. 1994;171:392-9.

34. VanDorsten JP, Hulsey TC, Newman RB, et al. Fetal anomaly detection by second trimester ultrasonography in a tertiary center. Am J Obstet Gynecol. 1998;178:742-9.

35. Grandjean H, Larroque D, Levi S, et al. The performance of routine ultrasonographic screening of pregnancies in the Eurofetus study. Am J Obstet Gynecol. 1999;181:446-54.

36. Saari-Kemppainen A, Karjalainen O, Ylostalo P, et al. Fetal anomalies in a controlled one-stage ultrasound screening trial. A report from the Helsinki Ultrasound Trial. J Perinat Med. 1994;22:279-89.

37. Levi S, Hyjazi Y, Schaapst JP. Sensitivity and specificity of routine antenatal screening for congenital anomalies by ultrasound: The Belgian Multicentric Study. Ultrasound Obstet Gynecol. 1991;1:102-10.

38. Yeo L, Guzman ER, Shen-Schwarz S, et al. Value of a complete sonographic survey in detecting fetal abnormalities: correlation with perinatal autopsy. J Ultrasound Med. 2002;21:501-10.

39. Chitty LS, Hunt GH, Moore J, et al. Effectiveness of routine ultrasonography in detecting fetal structural abnormalities in a low-risk population. BMJ. 1991;303:165-9.

40. Levi S, Schaaps JP, De Havay P, et al. End-result of routine ultrasound screening for congenital anomalies: The Belgium Multicentric Study 1984-92. Ultrasound Obstet Gynecol. 1995;5:366-71.

41. Shirley IM, Bottomley F, Robinson VP. Routine radiographer screening for fetal abnormalities by ultrasound in an unselected low risk population. Br J Radiol. 1992;65:564-9.

42. Seeds JW. The routine or screening obstetrical ultrasound examination. Clin Obstet Gynaecol. 1996; 39:8148-50.

43. Waldenstrom U, Axelsson O, Nilsson S, et al. Effects of routine one-stage ultrasound screening in pregnancy: A randomized controlled trial. Lancet. 1988;2:585-8.

44. Vintzileos AM, Ananth CV, Smulian JC, et al. Routine second trimester ultrasonography in the United States: A cost benefit analysis. Am J Obstet Gynecol. 2000;182:655-60.

45. Leivo T, Tuominen R, Saari-Kemppainen A, et al. Cost-effectiveness of one-stage ultrasound screening in pregnancy: A report from the Helsinki ultrasound trial. Ultrasound Obstet Gynecol. 1996;7:309-14.

46. Long G, Sprigg A. A comparative study of routine versus selective fetal anomaly ultrasound scanning. J Med Screen. 1998;5:6-10.

47. Roberts T, Henderson J, Mugford M, et al. Antenatal ultrasound screening for fetal abnormalities: A systematic review of studies of cost and cost effectiveness. BJOG. 2002;109:44-56.

74 First Trimester Maternal Serum Markers of Fetal Anomalies

DA Krantz, TW Hallahan, JN Macri

INTRODUCTION

Historically, prenatal screening for Down syndrome and other chromosomal abnormalities had been conducted in the second trimester of pregnancy with results available between 16 weeks and 18 weeks of pregnancy. Such screening can detect 60–70% of Down syndrome cases with a false positive rate of 5%.[1] Now, first trimester Down syndrome screening has become an important option for prospective parents providing risk information as early as 11–12 weeks of pregnancy and detecting up to 90% of Down syndrome cases at the same 5% false-positive rate.[2-16]

The advantages of first trimester screening are that most patients (95%) receive very early reassurance that they are at low risk, the test provides a significantly higher detection efficiency compared to most second trimester screening methods, patients have more time and more diagnostic options to consider, and in cases where patients choose to terminate an affected pregnancy safer procedures are available in the first trimester. Further, pregnancies that may have ended in an unexplained fetal loss may now have karyotype information available.

First trimester Down syndrome and Trisomy 18 screening includes the biochemical analysis of free beta human chorionic gonadotropin (free beta hCG) and pregnancy-associated plasma protein-A (PAPP-A) combined with the ultrasound evaluation of nuchal translucency. This protocol has been studied extensively, and the first trimester risk estimates have been validated.[17]

FREE BETA hCG

During normal pregnancy free beta hCG rises to peak levels at 8–9 weeks of pregnancy and then steadily declines to about 20 weeks when concentrations begin to level off. In second trimester Down syndrome pregnancies free beta hCG is significantly elevated with a median MoM (multiple of the median) of 2.64.[18] By contrast, free alpha hCG has been observed to be unchanged (median MoM = 0.99)[19] or marginally elevated (median MoM = 1.31)[20] in cases of Down syndrome. This proportionally higher increase observed in the beta subunit relative to the alpha subunit observed at the protein level is reflected at the mRNA level. Indeed, Eldar-Geva et al. demonstrated that the beta subunit MRNA content was proportionally increased compared to the alpha subunit in cultured second trimester trophoblasts.[21] This suggests that the increase of the beta subunit in maternal serum may be due in part to increased synthesis. More recently, beta subunit MRNA has been detected in maternal serum and has also been demonstrated to be elevated in cases of Down syndrome.[22]

In the first trimester, free beta hCG is significantly elevated in Down syndrome pregnancies and is the only Down syndrome marker that is effective in both first and second trimester screening. In two recent studies, the median free beta hCG multiples of the median (MoM) in Down syndrome increased with increasing gestational age from about 1.5 MoM at 9 weeks of gestation to 2.1 MoM at 13 weeks 6 days gestation.[23,24] In the SURUSS (serum, urine and ultrasound screening study) case-control study the median MoM of free beta hCG in Down syndrome cases increased from 1.6 MoM at 10 weeks of gestation to 2.6 MoM at 13 weeks 6 days.[25] Therefore, free beta hCG becomes more effective with increasing gestational age. In trisomy 18 affected pregnancies, a study of 28 cases showed the median free beta hCG MoM to be 0.18 in the first trimester representing an 80% reduction from normal pregnancies.[7]

PREGNANCY ASSOCIATED PLASMA PROTEIN-A

Pregnancy associated plasma protein-A is a 750 kDa zinc metalloproteinase. It is produced by the trophoblast and exists in maternal circulation as a disulfide bridged dimeric glycoprotein and as a 2:2 complex with the proform of eosinophil major basic protein (proMBP). Circulating levels are detectable as early as 4 weeks in pregnancy and double approximately every 6 days throughout the first trimester. PAPP-A concentrations rise exponentially in the second trimester to reach approximately 50 mg/L in the third trimester.

In the first trimester, PAPP-A is significantly decreased in Down syndrome pregnancies. The discrimination between unaffected and Down syndrome pregnancy is greatest earlier in pregnancy. Our own data on 163 cases of Down syndrome showed a median MoM of 0.3 at 9 weeks and 0.8 MoM at 13 weeks 6 days.[23] Spencer et al.[24] showed a median MoM of 0.37 at 9 weeks and 0.70 at 13 weeks 6 days while the SURUSS study showed a median MoM of 0.29 at 9 weeks and 0.62 at 13 weeks 6 days.[25] Therefore, PAPP-A becomes less effective with increasing gestational age and by the second trimester is no longer a marker for Down syndrome. In trisomy 18 pregnancies, the median first trimester level of PAPP-A is 0.33 representing a 2/3 reduction from normal levels.[7]

COMBINING FREE BETA hCG AND PAPP-A

The levels of both free beta hCG and PAPP-A in Down syndrome affected pregnancies tend to increase with increasing gestational age. As a result, with increasing gestational age free beta hCG is becoming more effective while PAPP-A is becoming less effective. These two trends tend to offset each other, such that the combination is effective in screening for Down syndrome between 9 weeks and 13 weeks 6 days. However, the combined performance of free beta hCG and PAPP-A is optimized in the earlier gestations. For example, at a 5% false-positive rate, the detection rate is 69% if the blood is drawn at 10 weeks while it is 63% if the blood is drawn at 13 weeks.[26] These detection rates are as good as or better than those seen with second trimester triple test.

DRIED BLOOD COLLECTION

Maternal serum screening has largely involved venepuncture collection of whole blood into red-top tubes. Recently, whole blood sample collection using finger-stick lancets and filter paper has become more common. The ease of collection and transport of dried blood specimens allows for greater flexibility in screening logistics. Since no phlebotomist is required, the simple finger-stick procedure can easily take place in the physician's office, ultrasound laboratory or ultimately in the patient's home. Quantitative analysis of prenatal screening markers in dried blood samples is highly correlated with liquid serum samples.[27] In addition, dried blood technology stabilizes serum proteins and therefore provides better overall analyte precision leading to both higher detection rates and lower false positive rates.

COMBINED BIOCHEMISTRY AND ULTRASOUND SCREENING

In addition to maternal serum markers, the evaluation of fetal nuchal translucency in ultrasound has been demonstrated to be a highly effective marker for Down syndrome.[28] As a result, for the first time, biochemical and biophysical markers are combined in a single screening protocol for the detection of Down syndrome. The challenge has been to introduce nuchal translucency assessment in a standardized, quality-controlled fashion to allow for efficient population screening. Laboratories perform a significant number of quality control procedures prior to releasing the results of biochemical tests to the clinician. Nuchal translucency, as a quantitative marker in the screening process, must meet similar standards of quality control as biochemical markers. Therefore, sonographers must be specifically trained to perform nuchal translucency measurement using a standardized methodology and their results audited on a regular basis. The improved effectiveness of nuchal translucency screening when a quality control program is in place is dramatic (Table 74.1). In the study of Snidjers et al.[28] in which sonographers underwent training and quality review, nuchal translucency detected 77% of Down syndrome cases while in the study of Haddow et al.[29] in which there was no specific training or quality control, the detection was only 31%.

Currently, the standard first trimester Down syndrome and Trisomy 18 screening protocol combines the biochemical analysis of free beta hCG and PAPP-A with the ultrasound evaluation of nuchal translucency. A summary of 15 studies encompassing over 80,000 patients using the free beta hCG, PAPP-A and nuchal translucency protocol demonstrates a 88% detection rate for Down syndrome at a 5% false-positive rate (Table 74.2).[2-16]

Combined biochemical and biophysical screening significantly improves the detection and false positive rates for Down syndrome compared to either mode alone. The study by Krantz et al. for example, showed the additional detection rate attributable to each marker in the protocol. In that study, free beta hCG added 10%, PAPP-A added 11% and nuchal translucency added 28% detection beyond that achieved by the corresponding other two markers alone

Table 74.1: Impact of training and quality review of nuchal translucency measurements on first trimester Down syndrome screening detection rates

Study	Snidjers et al. 1998[28]	Haddow et al. 1998[29]
Training and quality review	Yes	No
Centers	22	11
Patients	96,127	3,991
False positive rate	5%	5%
Detection rate	77%	31%

Note: Results based on nuchal translucency only without biochemistry.

(Table 74.3). Therefore, to reach the optimal detection rate it is necessary to include all of these markers in the analysis.

Combined screening is also highly effective in detecting trisomy 18 and other chromosomal abnormalities. Using an independent algorithm for the calculation of patient specific trisomy 18 risk detects 97% of trisomy 18 cases with only an additional 1.2% false-positive rate.[7] In the BUN study, all 11 cases of trisomy 18 and 16 of 29 (55%) cases of other chromosomal abnormalities were detected.[12] Spencer et al. have shown that triploidy is associated with abnormal combined screening results with triploidy types I and II having different patterns of marker levels.[30] Type I triploidy, in which the additional chromosome is of paternal origin is associated with extremely high free beta hCG , mildly decreased PAPP-A and increased nuchal translucency. Type II triploidy, in which the additional chromosome is of maternal origin is associated with extremely low free beta hCG, extremely low PAPP-A and normal nuchal translucency.

OTHER PERINATAL RISKS

Abnormal free beta hCG and PAPP-A are both associated with increased perinatal risk. Low levels of PAPP-A are associated with increased risk of intrauterine growth restriction.[31-37] For example, Krantz et al.[31] found that PAPP-A values less than the 1st percentile were associated with a 5.4-fold increase in the odds of intrauterine growth restriction with a positive predictive value of 24.1%. Krantz et al.[31] also found that free beta hCG values less than the 1st percentile were associated with a 2.7-fold increase in the odds of intrauterine growth restriction with a positive predictive value of 14.3% while other studies that evaluated less extreme cut-offs for free beta hCG or treated free beta hCG as a continuous variable did not find an association with intrauterine growth restriction.[32-33,36-39] Goetzl et al.[40] have found that low levels of both free beta hCG and PAPP-A are associated with increased risk of spontaneous abortion. Free beta hCG levels below the 1st percentile were associated with an 8.5-fold increase in the odds of spontaneous abortion while levels below the 5th percentile were associated with a 4.3-fold increase in the odds ratio. PAPP-A levels below the first percentile were associated with a 5.4-fold increase, while PAPP-A levels below the 5th percentile were associated with a 2.4-fold increase in the odds of spontaneous abortion. Most importantly, patients with normal free beta hCG, PAPP-A and nuchal translucency (i.e. those with levels between the 5th and 95th percentiles) had a very low risk of fetal loss before 20 weeks (0.36%). Yaron et al.[34,38] found a similar association between free beta hCG and PAPP-A with fetal loss.

Table 74.2: Summary of first trimester Down syndrome screening studies using free beta hCG, PAPP-A and nuchal translucency

| Study | N | FPR | Down syndrome cases | | Detection rate (%) |
			Number detected	Total	
Orlandi 1997[7]	744	5.0	6	7	86
Biagiotti 1998[3]	232	5.0	24	32	75
De Biasio 1999[4]	1,467	3.3	11	13	85
De Graaf 1999[5]	300	5.0	31	37	84
Spencer 1999[6]	1,156	5.0	187	210	89
Krantz 2000[7]	5,718	5.0	30	33	91
Niemimaa 2001[8]	1,602	5.4	4	5	80
Schucter 2002[9]	4,939	5.0	12	14	86
Von Kaisenberg 2002[10]	3,864	6.6	16	19	84
Bindra 2002[11]	15,030	5.0	74	82	90
Wapner 2003[12]	8514	5.0	48	61	79
Spencer 2003[13]	10,458	5.0	23	25	92
Sheffield 2003[14]	18,140	5.0	60	64	94
Borrell 2004[15]	2,780	3.3	7	8	88
Stenhouse 2004[16]	5,084	5.9	14	15	93
Total	80,028	5.0	547	625	88

Abbreviation: FPR, false-positive rate

Table 74.3: Relative contribution of biochemistry and nuchal translucency in first-trimester Down syndrome screening at a 5% false-positive rate

Initial protocol	PAPP-A+NT	Free beta hCG + NT	Free beta hCG + PAPP-A	NT
A. % detected	81%	80%	63%	74%
B. % undetected	19%	20%	37%	26%
Additional marker(s)	Free beta hCG	PAPP-A	NT	Free beta hCG + PAPP-A
C. Combined detection (%)	91%	91%	91%	91%
D. Extra detection with inclusion of additional marker(s) = (C-A)	10%	11%	28%	17%
E. % of remaining undetected cases detected with inclusion of additional marker(s) = (D ÷ B)	53%	55%	76%	65%

Source: Krantz DA, Hallahan TW, Orlandi F, et al. First trimester Down syndrome screening using dried blood biochemistry and nuchal translucency. Obstet Gynecol. 2000;96(2):207-13.

MATERNAL FACTORS

As with second trimester screening, maternal factors play a role in first trimester Down syndrome screening. Several studies have shown that patients with increased maternal weight tend to have lower free beta hCG and PAPP-A levels.[41-43] Spencer et al.[42] showed that there can be a twofold difference in Down syndrome risk estimates if maternal weight is not accounted for. The effect on trisomy 18 risk can be even greater since heavier patients would have lower levels of both free beta hCG and PAPP-A which would increase the trisomy 18 risk based on both markers.

Ethnic differences in biochemical results have also been observed.[43] After weight adjustment, free beta hCG levels are higher for African Americans (15%) and Asians (6%) but lower for Hispanics (11%) compared to Caucasians. For PAPP-A, African Americans have 30% higher levels than Caucasians after weight adjustment.

The effect of assisted reproduction techniques on first trimester combined ultrasound and biochemical Down syndrome screening is minimal. Orlandi et al.[44] found that the false-positive rate for ICSI (5.2%) and IVF pregnancies (4.2%) was only slightly higher than the false-positive rate in naturally conceived pregnancies (3.3%). Similarly, Liao et al.[45] found that the false-positive rate increased by only 1.2% points in IVF pregnancies. Wojdemann et al.[46] found no significant difference in the false-positive rates among a group of naturally conceived pregnancies (4.9%), IVF pregnancies (4.7%) and ovulation induction pregnancies (5.1%).

SCREENING IN TWIN PREGNANCY

First trimester screening of twin pregnancies offers a distinct advantage over second trimester screening in that it can be used to evaluate the risk of each individual fetus. In second trimester screening, which is based on biochemical markers alone, the risk is pregnancy specific. For monozygotic twins, in which either both are affected or both are unaffected, second trimester detection efficiencies can be expected to be similar to that observed in singleton pregnancies. However, 67% of naturally conceived and 93% of assisted reproduction twin conceptions are dizygotic, and therefore the majority of Down syndrome affected twin pregnancies can be expected to be discordant. In such cases, since the observed maternal serum marker levels are the sum contribution from each fetus, not only is it impossible to determine which fetus is contributing abnormal analyte levels but the detection efficiency will be decreased due to a dilution effect from the contribution of the normal fetus. Indeed the detection of Down syndrome in twins by second trimester maternal serum screening is estimated at about 50%, significantly lower than that expected in singletons at a 5% FPR.[47]

In first trimester screening, nuchal translucency, a biophysical marker, is fetus specific. Fetus-specific risks can be calculated based on nuchal translucency and the detection rate should be similar to that observed in singleton pregnancy. However, each fetus will carry an approximate 5% false-positive rate and therefore the false-positive rate per twin pregnancy based on nuchal translucency only is significantly greater than in singleton pregnancy. For example, in a study by Sebire et al.[48] 7.3% of fetuses had an increased nuchal translucency. However, among pregnancies, 11.6% had at least one twin with an increased nuchal translucency.

Incorporating biochemistry into the first trimester protocol along with nuchal translucency can reduce the false-positive rate. In our own data on a group of 212 twin pregnancies the false-positive rate was reduced from 13.2% using maternal age and nuchal translucency to 6.6% by also including the biochemistry.[49] Detection efficiency in twin pregnancy is difficult to document because Down syndrome affected twin pregnancies are rare. However, modeling indicates that combining free beta hCG and PAPP-A with nuchal translucency can result in 80% detection rate for a 7% false-positive rate in twin pregnancy.[49] Therefore, it is feasible to screen twin pregnancies for Down syndrome in the first trimester. However until larger datasets of affected twin pregnancy are available a caution that risk estimates in twin pregnancy are less precise than in singleton pregnancy should be indicated on patient reports.

FREE BETA hCG VERSUS INTACT hCG

HCG is a non-covalently bound heterodimeric glycoprotein consisting of an alpha and beta subunit. It exists in maternal circulation predominantly as the biologically active intact dimer. It is also found in the unbound state as both the free alpha and free beta subunits (Fig. 74.1). The genes for the alpha and beta subunits of hCG are separate and distinct with the alpha subunit located on chromosome 6 and the beta subunit located on chromosome 19.[50] The separate synthesis and unbalanced secretion of subunits provides the rationale for monitoring levels of hCG subunits in obstetrical and gynecological disorders. Thus, assays for free beta hCG and intact hCG measure distinct proteins in the maternal blood.

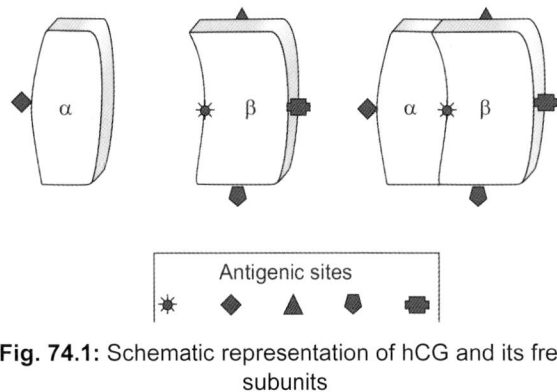

Fig. 74.1: Schematic representation of hCG and its free subunits

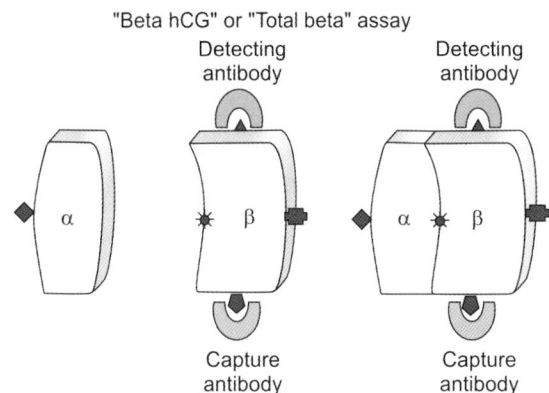

Fig. 74.2: Schematic representation of assay commonly used to measure intact hCG

Assays used to measure intact hCG are commonly called "total beta" or simply "beta hCG" assays. These assays use a capture antibody directed to the beta subunit of hCG and a detecting antibody directed to another epitopic site on the beta subunit (Fig. 74.2). As a consequence, these assays detect both intact hCG and free beta hCG. However, since the intact molecule is present in a 200-fold molar excess relative to the free beta subunit, these assays reflect the concentration of intact hCG. During pregnancy intact hCG is measurable as early as 5 weeks in pregnancy making it an excellent indicator of pregnancy. An immediate and steep increase is observed with hCG levels peaking at about 120 IU/mL at 9 weeks followed by a steady decline to about 20 weeks when concentrations level off at 10–20 IU/mL.

Free beta hCG exists in maternal blood at a level of about 1/200th that of intact hCG. Assays that measure free beta hCG utilize an epitopic site that is located at the interface with the alpha subunit such that it is covered in the intact hCG molecule (Fig. 74.3). As a result, antibodies directed toward this site capture free beta hCG but not intact hCG which is washed away in the assay procedure.

Prior to the prospective evaluation of the first trimester combined screening protocol free beta hCG and intact hCG were evaluated in a number of studies.[29,51-76] Overall, it was seen that intact hCG was not an effective marker in the first trimester of pregnancy with a median MoM in 463 cases of Down syndrome of just 1.30 while free beta hCG was an effective marker with a median MoM of 2.0 based on 858 cases of Down syndrome (Tables 74.4 and 74.5). Hallahan et al.[64] summarized seven case-control studies[57-60,64-66] in which both intact hCG and free beta hCG were measured in the same

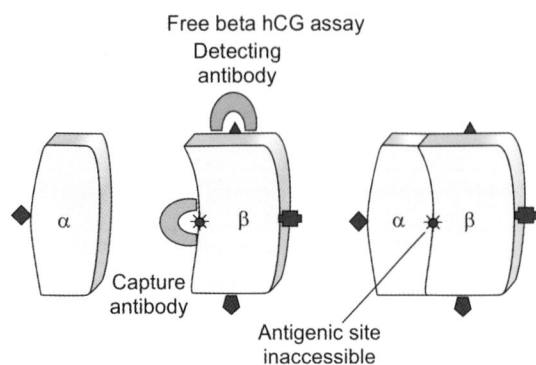

Fig. 74.3: Schematic representation of free beta hCG assay

Table 74.4: Median first trimester intact hCG multiples of the median (MoM) values in Down syndrome cases

Study	Cases	Median Down syndrome MoM
Cuckle '88[51]	22	1.10
Bogart '89[52]	6	1.14
Brock '90[53]	21	1.43
Johnson '91[54]	11	0.91
Kratzer '91[55]	17	1.23
Van Lith '92[56]	24	1.19
Aitken '93[57]	16	0.97
Macintosh '94[58]	20	1.45
Biagiotti '95[59]	41	1.12
Brizot '95[60]	41	1.50
Forest '95[61]	12	1.83
Cassals '96[62]	19	1.35
Aitken '96[63]	8	1.05
Wald '96[64]	77	1.23
Jauniaux '96[65]	17	0.96
Haddow '98[29]	48	1.54
Hallahan '00[66]	63	1.37
Overall	463	1.30

Table 74.5: Median first trimester free beta hCG MoM in Down syndrome cases

Study	N	Median down syndrome MoM
Spencer '92[67]	13	1.85
Aitken '93[57]	16	1.96
Macri '93[68]	38	2.20
Brambati '94[69]	13	1.13
MacIntosh '94[58]	21	2.10
Biagiotti '95[59]	41	2.00
Brizot '95[60]	41	2.00
Noble '95[70]	102	2.13
Forest '95[61]	12	1.60
Krantz '96[71]	22	2.09
Scott '96[72]	8	2.00
Wald '96[64]	77	1.79
Jauniaux '96[65]	17	1.46
Berry 97[73]	47	1.99
Spencer '97[74]	22	1.72
Haddow '98[29]	48	2.08
Wheeler '98[75]	17	2.06
Spencer '99[76]	210	2.15
Hallahan '00[66]	63	1.89
Overall	828	2.00

samples and showed that free beta hCG detected nearly twice as many cases of Down syndrome as intact hCG (Table 74.6). On the basis of these results prospective first trimester screening studies using the combined protocol have all included free beta hCG.

Recently, Spencer et al.[24,26] have suggested, that the evaluation of all the Down syndrome markers should be conducted on a week by week basis since the performance of the markers varies by gestational age. Spencer et al. showed that the combination of free beta hCG and PAPP-A had detection rates that were 7–11% better than the combination of intact hCG and PAPP-A at each gestational week from 10 weeks to 13 weeks at a corresponding 5% false-positive rate (Table 74.7).

In a case control study, Wald et al.[25] modeled the performance of free beta hCG and PAPP-A in combination with nuchal translucency. The model indicated that free beta hCG significantly

outperformed intact hCG within the combined protocol at 10 and 11 weeks of gestation but that at 12 weeks the two markers had similar performance and that at 13 weeks intact hCG performed better. However, Krantz et al.[77] determined that a more appropriate analysis would show that free beta hCG was better than intact hCG at 10, 11 and 12 weeks and that the two markers only appear similar in the model at 13 weeks. In response, Wald et al.[78] concluded that their data at 13 weeks were probably due to chance and that there was an advantage of using free beta hCG compared to intact hCG in the first trimester. An analysis[79] combining the results from Spencer et al.[72] and Wald, et al.[23] demonstrated that using free beta hCG was better than intact hCG in a protocol that includes PAPP-A and nuchal translucency at 10–13 weeks. When false-positive rates were evaluated the difference between the two markers was even more apparent. For example at 10 weeks, the false-positive rate with free beta hCG was half that of intact hCG (Table 74.8).

SCREENING STRATEGIES

First trimester screening is usually conducted between 11 weeks 1 day and 13 week 6 days, gestation. In general, the patient comes in for an ultrasound examination, CRL is measured for accurate gestational dating and a nuchal translucency value is obtained. At the time of the ultrasound examination a blood specimen is collected and forwarded to the laboratory along with the ultrasound information. The biochemical analytes are analyzed in the laboratory and risk results based on free beta hCG, PAPP-A and nuchal translucency are available usually within a few days.

Table 74.6: Meta-analysis of intact hCG vs. free beta hCG in case control studies in which both analytes were measured in the same sample set

| Study | N | | Intact hCG | | | | %DSA >95th percentile | Free beta hCG | | | | %DSA >95th percentile |
| | Unaff | DS | Unaffected | | DS cases | | | Unaffected | | DS cases | | |
			Median	SD	Median	SD		Median	SD	Median	SD	
Aitken et al. 1993[57]	320	16	1.0	0.2190	0.97	0.3150	11.8	1.0	0.2580	1.96	0.2560	30.3
Macintosh et al. 1994[58]	258	21	1.0	——	1.45	0.4512	——	1.0	——	2.10	0.4280	——
Biagiotti et al. 1995[59]	246	41	1.01	0.2458	1.12	0.2555	8.2	1.0	0.2208	2.00	0.2294	39.3
Brizot et al. 1995[60]	394	41	1.0	0.2054	1.50	0.1939	20.2	1.0	0.2911	2.00	0.3168	28.7
Wald et al. 1996[64]	383	77	1.0	——	1.23	0.1957	13.0	1.0	0.2833	1.79	0.2870	22.9
Jauniaux et al. 1996[65]	51	17	1.0	0.2375	0.96	0.1347	0.0	1.0	0.3474	1.46	0.1673	0.1
Hallahan et al. 2000[66]	400	63	1.0	0.1697	1.37	0.2158	25.5	1.0	0.2157	1.89	0.2322	36.8
Overall OSC	2052	276	1.0	0.2083	1.27	0.2421	16.2	1.0	0.2545	1.89	0.2782	30.4

Table 74.7: Comparison of the performance of free beta hCG vs. intact hCG in combination with PAPP-A and maternal age in first trimester screening using an overall 5% false-positive rate

| Gestational age | Intact-hCG + PAPP-A | | Free beta-hCG + PAPP-A | |
	FP	DR	FP	DR
10	4.7	58	4.7	69
11	4.9	56	4.8	67
12	5.1	56	5.0	65
13	5.2	56	5.3	63

Data from Spencer et al.[26]

Table 74.8: Free beta hCG vs. intact hCG within a Down syndrome protocol including PAPP-A and nuchal translucency and maternal age

| Gestational age | Detection rate at a 5% false-positive rate | | False-positive rate at a fixed 85% detection rate | |
	Intact hCG(%)	Free hCG(%)	Intact hCG(%)	Free beta hCG(%)
10	84	88	6.0	3.1
11	83	86	6.7	4.1
12	82	86	6.9	4.3
13	85	85	5.1	4.7

Analysis[79] performed using results from Spencer et al.[24,26] and Wald et al.[25]

One Stop Clinic for the Assessment of Risk (Oscar)

The OSCAR approach represents a procedural variation of first trimester screening in which the blood sample is collected and analyzed on a rapid assay instrument during the patient's ultrasound appointment. The advantage of this modality is that the biochemical result is ready during the patient's visit allowing her to have her combined risk result immediately with the option of having chronic villus sampling (CVS) the same day. This screening strategy is currently practiced very effectively in many European clinics.[11,13] The disadvantage is that in order to analyze the biochemistry specialized equipment and personnel are required at the ultrasound center. Therefore, this strategy is best suited for settings with high volume in order for the biochemical screening to be cost-effective. The rapid assays needed to provide a blood result in under a half hour have not yet been approved by the FDA and are therefore not currently available in the United States. Even with the rapid assays the total time required to interview the patient, draw a blood specimen, allow time for clotting and centrifugation, perform the biochemical assays and conduct the ultrasound examination could easily last more than 1 hour. Further the burdens of data entry, quality control and risk assessment in this modality are all the responsibility of the ultrasound clinic.

Finger Stick Blood Collection with Instant Risk Assessment (IRA)

IRA is a variation of the OSCAR approach that takes advantage of the simplified blood collection and transport of dried blood. In this approach, patients draw their own blood at home about 1 week before their ultrasound appointment using a sterile lancet and a dried blood collection card. The sample is mailed to the laboratory and the biochemical results are ready in time for the ultrasound examination. Like the OSCAR approach the risk results are available immediately at the conclusion of the ultrasound examination but with IRA the ultrasound center has no need for specialized equipment and personnel. Additional time is not required for drawing blood and waiting for a biochemical result. That time may be better spent performing more detailed ultrasound evaluations such as ductus venosus, nasal bone and tricuspid valve regurgitation for those specific patients that have a borderline risk.

Independent Sequential Screening

The first trimester combined screening test with free beta hCG, PAPP-A and nuchal translucency can detect approximately 90% of Down syndrome pregnancies with a 5% false-positive rate. In sequential testing both first trimester screening and second trimester multiple marker screening are performed independently.

In this case, the false-positive rate in first trimester is additive with the false-positive rate in second trimester. For example in the BUN study, a group that contained about 50% advanced maternal age patients, 9.9% of patients had increased risk results in the first trimester and another 9.0% had increased risk results in the second trimester.[80] Thus the overall false-positive rate for the screening program using data in both trimesters was nearly doubled.

Modified Sequential Screening

Alternatively, the Down syndrome risk can be calculated based on both the first and second trimester markers. Such an approach can reduce the increase in the false-positive rate compared to the independent sequential approach described above. However, sophisticated software is required to ensure that the patient's results in the second trimester are appropriately matched with those from the first trimester.

The modified sequential screening approach requires 95% of the population to return for second trimester multiple marker screening. A refinement to this approach could be to offer second trimester screening only to those patients with a borderline result.[81] For example, those patients with very high risks (e.g. greater than 1 in 100) in the first trimester can be immediately offered CVS. Those patients with low risk (e.g. less than 1 in 1,500) can be reassured that no further screening is necessary. Patients with borderline first trimester risks (e.g. between 1 in 100 and 1 in 1,500) could be offered second trimester multiple marker screening and have their final risk calculated based on the marker results in both the first and second trimester. This so-called "contingency" screening approach has the advantage of reducing by as much as 75% the number of second trimester screening tests that are performed, reducing the overall cost of the screening program and minimizing the number of added false positives generated by second trimester testing.[81]

The sequential screening approaches outlined above have been described with respect to multiple marker serum screening in the second trimester. Nyberg et al.[82] and Bromley et al.[83] have determined likelihood ratios for second trimester ultrasound markers. Any of the sequential screening methodologies described above could be conducted by substituting the second trimester serum markers with second trimester ultrasound markers. More data is needed to determine whether one approach is superior to the other. However, in settings where a second trimester anomaly scan is common practice, use of the ultrasound screen may provide significant logistical advantages.

FUTURE IMPROVEMENTS

Future goals are to improve upon the already excellent screening performance while still maintaining screening in the first trimester. The most promising advancement may be the inclusion of ultrasound assessment of fetal nasal bone. Cicero et al.[84] observed that 73% of Down syndrome cases had absent nasal bone while only 0.5% of unaffected cases had absent nasal bone in the first trimester of pregnancy. The results of Cicero et al. have been confirmed in several studies[23,85-90] but one study by Malone et al.[91] had divergent results. The promising results with the nasal bone marker open up the possibility of significantly reducing the false-positive rate of first trimester Down syndrome screening while maintaining a 90% detection rate or alternatively increasing the detection rate to better than 95%.

CONCLUSION

One of the first questions that expectant parents ask after discovering they are pregnant is "Will my baby be normal?". Although there are no guarantees that a baby will be healthy, screening can reassure the vast majority of couples that they are not likely to have a baby with a major birth defect. Along with the benefits of early reassurance and diagnosis, first trimester screening with free beta hCG, PAPP-A and nuchal translucency has raised the standards in terms of detection efficiency. As a result, the ability to screen for Down syndrome and trisomy 18 in the first trimester of pregnancy represents the most significant advancement in prenatal screening in the past 10 years.

REFERENCES

1. Wald NJ, Huttly WJ, Hackshaw AK. Antenatal screening for Down's syndrome with the quadruple test. Lancet. 2003;361:835-6.
2. Orlandi F, Damiani G, Hallahan TW, et al. First trimester screening for fetal aneuploidy: biochemistry and nuchal translucency. Ultrasound Obstet Gynaecol. 1997;10(6):381-6.
3. Biagiotti R, Brizzi L, Periti E, et al. First trimester screening for Down's syndrome using maternal serum PAPP-A and free beta hCG in combination with fetal nuchal translucency thickness. Br J Obstet Gynecol. 1998;05(8):917-20.
4. De Biasio P, Siccardi M, Volpe G, et al. First trimester screening for Down syndrome using nuchal translucency measurement with free beta hCG and PAPP-A between 10 and 13 weeks of pregnancy—the combined test. Prenat Diagn. 1999;19(4):360-3.
5. de Graaf IM, Pajkrt E, Bilardo CM, et al. Early pregnancy screening for fetal aneuploidy with serum markers and nuchal translucency. Prenat Diagn. 1999;19(5):458-62.
6. Spencer K, Souter V, Tul N, et al. A screening program for trisomy 21 at 10-14 weeks using fetal nuchal translucency, maternal serum free beta human chorionic gonadotropin and pregnancy-associated plasma protein-A. Ultrasound Obstet Gynecol. 1999;13(4):231-7.
7. Krantz DA, Hallahan TW, Orlandi F, et al. First trimester Down syndrome screening using dried blood biochemistry and nuchal translucency. Obstet Gynecol. 2000;96(2):207-13.
8. Niemimaa M, Suonpaa M, Perheentupa A, et al. Evaluation of first trimester maternal serum and ultrasound screening for Down's syndrome in Eastern and Northern Finland. Eur J Hum Genet. 2001;9(6):404-8.
9. Schuchter K, Hafner E, Stangl G, et al. The first trimester 'combined test' for the detection of Down syndrome pregnancies in 4939 unselected pregnancies. Prenat Diagn. 2002;22(3):211-5.
10. von Kaisenberg CS, Gasiorek-Wiens A, Bielicki M, et al. German speaking Down syndrome screening Group. Screening for trisomy 21 by maternal age, fetal nuchal translucency and maternal serum biochemistry at 11-14 weeks: A German multicenter study. J Matern Fetal Neonatal Med. 2002;12(2):89-94.
11. Bindra R, Heath V, Liao A, et al. One-stop clinic for assessment of risk for trisomy 21 at 11-14 weeks: A prospective study of 15030 pregnancies. Ultrasound Obstet Gynecol. 2002;20(3):219-25.
12. Wapner R, Thom E, Simpson JL, et al. First trimester maternal serum biochemistry and fetal nuchal translucency screening (BUN) study group. First-trimester screening for trisomies 21 and 18. N Engl J Med. 2003;349(15):1405-13.

13. Spencer K, Spencer CE, Power M, et al. Screening for chromosomal abnormalities in the first trimester using ultrasound and maternal serum biochemistry in a one-stop clinic: A review of three years prospective experience. BJOG. 2003;110(3):281-6.

14. Sheffield LJ, Williamson R, Halliday JL, et al. SLAMDUNC-a very successful new community program for first trimester combined screening for Down syndrome. Am J Human Genet. 2003;73(5 suppl):593.

15. Borrell A, Casals E, Fortuny A, et al. First trimester screening for trisomy 21 combining biochemistry and ultrasound at individually optimal gestational ages. An interventional study. Prenat Diagn. 2004l;24(7):541-5.

16. Stenhouse EJ, Crossley JA, Aitken DA, et al. First-trimester combined ultrasound and biochemical screening for Down syndrome in routine clinical practice. Prenat Diagn. 2004;24(10):774-80.

17. Spencer K. Accuracy of Down syndrome risks produced in a first trimester screening programme incorporating fetal nuchal translucency thickness and maternal serum biochemistry. Prenat Diagn. 2002;22:244-6.

18. Macri JN, Spencer K, Garver K, et al. Maternal serum free beta hCG screening: Results of studies including 480 cases of Down syndrome. Prenat Diagn. 1994;14:97-103.

19. Spencer K. Free alpha-subunit of human chorionic gonadotropin in Down syndrome. Am J Obstet Gynecol. 1993;168:132-5.

20. Wald NJ, Densem JW, Smith D, et al. Four-marker serum screening for Down's syndrome. Prenat Diagn. 1994;14:707-16.

21. Eldar-Geva T, Hochberg A, deGroot N, et al. High maternal serum chorionic gonadotropin level in Down's syndrome pregnancies is caused by elevation of both subunits messenger ribonucleic acid level in trophoblasts. J Clin Endocrinol Metab. 1995;80:3528-31.

22. Ng EK, El-Sheikhah A, Chiu RW, et al. Evaluation of human chorionic gonadotropin beta-subunit mRNA concentrations in maternal serum in aneuploid pregnancies: A feasibility study. Clin Chem. 2004;50:1055-7.

23. Orlandi F, Rossi C, Orlandi E, et al. Optimization of first trimester Down syndrome screening with simplified nasal bone assessment. Am J Obstet Gynecol (in press).

24. Spencer K, Crossley JA, Aitken DA, et al. Temporal changes in maternal serum biochemical markers of trisomy 21 across the first and second trimester of pregnancy. Ann Clin Biochem. 2002;39 (Pt 6):567-76.

25. Wald NJ, Rodeck C, Hackshaw AK, et al. First and second trimester antenatal screening for Down's syndrome: The results of Serum, Urine and Ultrasound Screening Study (SURUSS). Health technol Assess. 2003;7(11):1-87.

26. Spencer K, Crossley JA, Aitken DA, et al. The effect of temporal variation in biochemical markers of trisomy 21 across the first and second trimesters of pregnancy on the estimation of individual patient-specific risks and detection rates for Down's syndrome. Ann Clin Biochem. 2003;40:219-31.

27. Macri JN, Anderson RW, Krantz DA, et al. Prenatal maternal dried blood screening with alpha-fetoprotein and free beta human chorionic gonadotropin for open neural tube defect and Down syndrome. Am J Obstet Gynecol. 1996;174:566-72.

28. Snijders RJ, Noble P, Sebire N, et al. UK multicentre project on assessment of risk of trisomy 21 by maternal age and fetal nuchal-translucency thickness at 10-14 weeks of gestation. Fetal medicine foundation first trimester screening group. Lancet. 1998;352:343-6.

29. Haddow JE, Palomaki GE, Knight GJ, et al. Screening of maternal serum for fetal Down's syndrome in the first trimester. N Engl J Med. 1998;338:955-61.

30. Spencer K, Liao AW, Skentou H, et al. Screening for triploidy by fetal nuchal translucency and maternal serum free beta hCG and PAPP-A at 1014 weeks of gestation. Prenat Diagn. 2000;20:495-9.

31. Krantz D, Goetzl L, Simpson JL, et al. First trimester maternal serum biochemistry and fetal nuchal translucency screening (BUN) study group. Association of extreme first trimester free human chorionic gonadotropin-beta, pregnancy associated plasma protein- A, and nuchal translucency with intrauterine growth restriction and other adverse pregnancy outcomes. Am J Obstet Gynecol. 2004;191:1452-8.

32. Ong CY, Liao AW, Spencer K, et al. First trimester maternal serum free beta human chorionic gonadotrophin and pregnancy associated plasma protein- A as predictors of pregnancy complications. Br J Obstet Gynecol. 2000;107:1265-70.

33. Tul N, Pusenjak S, Osredkar J, et al. Predicting complications of pregnancy with first trimester maternal serum free beta hCG, PAPP-A and Inhibin A. Prenat Diagn. 2003;23:990-6.

34. Yaron Y, Heifetz S, Ochshorn Y, et al. Decreased first trimester PAPP-A is a predictor of adverse pregnancy outcome. Prenat Diagn. 2002;22:778-82.

35. Pedersen JF, Sorensen S, Ruge S. Human placental lactogen and pregnancy associated plasma protein-A in first trimester and subsequent fetal growth. Acta Obstet Gynecol Scand. 1995;74:505-8.

36. Smith GC, Stenhouse EJ, Crossley JA, et al. Early Pregnancy Origins of Low Birth Weight. Nature. 2002;417:916.

37. Smith GC, Stenhouse EJ, Crossley JA, et al. Early pregnancy levels of pregnancy associated plasma protein-A and the risk of intrauterine growth restriction, premature birth, preeclampsia, and stillbirth. J Clin Endocrinol Metab. 2002;87:1762-7.

38. Yaron Y, Ochshorn Y, Heifetz S, et al. First trimester maternal serum free human chorionic gonadotropin as a predictor of adverse pregnancy outcome. Fetal Diag Ther. 2002;17:352-6.

39. Morssink LP, Kornman LH, Hallahan TW, et al. Maternal serum levels of free beta hCG and PAPP-A in the first trimester of pregnancy are not associated with subsequent fetal growth retardation or preterm delivery. Prenat Diagn. 1998;18:147-52.

40. Goetzl L, Krantz D, Simpson JL, et al. Pregnancy associated plasma protein-A, free beta hCG, nuchal translucency, and risk of pregnancy loss. Obstet Gynecol. 2004;104:30-6.

41. de Graaf IM, Cuckle HS, Pajkrt E, et al. Co-variables in first trimester maternal serum screening. Prenat Diagn. 2000;20:186-9.

42. Spencer K, Bindra R, Nicolaides KH. Maternal weight correction of maternal serum PAPP-A and free beta-hCG MoM when screening for trisomy 21 in the first trimester of pregnancy. Prenat Diagn. 2003;23:851-5.

43. Krantz D, Hallahan T, Macri J. Weight correction and ethnic differences for first trimester Down syndrome biochemical Markers. Am J Hum genet. 2003;73(Suppl):411.

44. Orlandi F, Rossi C, Allegra A, et al. First trimester screening with free beta hCG, PAPP-A and nuchal translucency in pregnancies conceived with assisted reproduction. Prenat Diagn. 2002;22:718-21.

45. Liao AW, Heath V, Kametas N, et al. First trimester screening for trisomy 21 in singleton pregnancies achieved by assisted reproduction. Hum Reprod. 2001;16:1501-4.

46. Wojdemann KR, Larsen SO, Shalmi A, et al. First trimester screening for Down syndrome and assisted reproduction: No basis for concern. Prenat Diagn. 2001;21:563-5.

47. Spencer K, Salonen R, Muller F. Down's syndrome screening in multiple pregnancies using alpha-fetoprotein and free beta hCG. Prenat Diagn. 1994;14:53742.

48. Sebire NJ, Snijders RJ, Hughes K, et al. Screening for trisomy 21 in twin pregnancies by maternal age and fetal nuchal translucency thickness at 10-14 weeks of gestation. Br J Obstet Gynaecol. 1996;103:999-1003.

49. Orlandi F, Krantz DA, Hallahan TW, et al. First trimester Down syndrome screening in twins. Am J Hum Genet. 2000;67 (Suppl): Abstact 155.

50. Naylor SL, Chin WW, Goodman HM, et al. Chromosome assignment of genes encoding the alpha and beta subunits of glycoprotein hormones in man and mouse. Somatic Cell Genet. 1983;9:757-70.

51. Cuckle HS, Wald NJ, Barkai G, et al. First trimester biochemical screening for Down syndrome. Lancet. 1988;2:851-2.

52. Bogart MH, Golbus MS, Sorg ND, et al. Human chorionic gonadotropin levels in pregnancies with aneuploid fetuses. Prenat Diagn. 1989;9:379-84.

53. Brock DJ, Barron L, Holloway S, et al. First trimester maternal serum biochemical indicators in Down syndrome. Prenat Diagn. 1990;10:245-51.

54. Johnson A, Cowchock FS, Darby M, et al. First trimester maternal serum alpha-fetoprotein and chorionic gonadotropin in aneuploid pregnancies. Prenat Diagn. 1991;11:443-50.

55. Kratzer PG, Golbus MS, Monroe SE, et al. First trimester aneuploidy screening using serum human chorionic gonadotropin (hCG), free βhCG and progesterone. Prenat Diagn. 1991;11:751-63.

56. Van Lith JM. First trimester maternal serum human chorionic gonadotrophin as a marker for fetal chromosomal disorders: The Dutch working party on prenatal diagnosis. Prenat Diagn. 1992;12:495-504.

57. Aitken DA, McCaw G, Crossley JA, et al. First trimester biochemical screening for fetal chromosome abnormalities and neural tube defects. Prenat Diagn. 1993;13:681-9.

58. Macintosh MC, Iles R, Teisner B, et al. Maternal serum human chorionic gonadotrophin and pregnancy associated plasma protein A, markers for fetal Down syndrome at 8-14 weeks. Prenat Diagn. 1994;14:203-8.

59. Biagiotti R, Cariati E, Brizzi L, et al. Maternal serum screening for Down's syndrome in the first trimester of pregnancy. Br J Obstet Gynecol. 1995;102: 660-2.

60. Brizot ML, Snijders RJ, Butler J, et al. Maternal serum hCG and fetal nuchal translucency thickness for the prediction of fetal trisomies in the first trimester of pregnancy. Br J Obstet Gynaecol. 1995;102:127-32.

61. Forest JC, Masse J, Rousseau F, et al. Screening for Down syndrome during the first and second trimesters: Impact of risk estimation parameters. Clin Biochem. 1995;28:443-9.

62. Casals E, Fortunoy A, Grudzinskas JG, et al. First trimester biochemical screening for Down syndrome with the use of PAPP-A, AFP, and beta-hCG. Prenat Diagn. 1996;16:405-10.

63. Aitken DA, Wallace EM, Crossley JA, et al. Dimeric Inhibin A as a marker for Down's syndrome in early pregnancy. N Engl J Med. 1996;334:1231-6.

64. Wald NJ, George L, Smith D, et al. Serum screening for Down's syndrome between 8 and 14 weeks of pregnancy. International Prenatal Screening Research Group. Br J Obstet Gynaecol. 1996;103(5):407-12.

65. Jauniaux E, Nicolaides KH, Nagy AM, et al. Total amount of circulating human chorionic gonadotrophin alpha and beta subunits in first trimester trisomies 21 and 18. J Endocrinol. 1996;148:27-31.

66. Hallahan T, Krantz D, Orlandi F, et al. First trimester biochemical screening for Down syndrome: Free beta hCG versus Intact hCG. Prenat Diagn. 2000;20:785-9.

67. Spencer K, Macri JN, Aitken DA, et al. Free beta hCG as First trimester marker for fetal trisomy. Lancet. 1992;339:1480.

68. Macri JN, Spencer K, Aitken DA, et al. First trimester free beta hCG screening for Down syndrome. Prenat Diagn. 1993;13:557-62.

69. Brambati B, Tului L, Bonacchi I, et al. Serum PAPP-A and free beta hCG are first trimester screening markers for Down syndrome. Prenat Diagn. 1994;14:1043-7.

70. Noble PL, Abraha HD, Snijders RJ, et al. Screening for fetal trisomy 21 in the first trimester of pregnancy: maternal serum free beta hCG and fetal nuchal translucency thickness. Ultrasound Obstet Gynecol. 1995;6:390-5.

71. Krantz DA, Larsen JW, Buchanan PD, et al. First trimester Down syndrome screening: Free beta-human chorionic gonadotropin and pregnancy associated plasma protein-A. Am J Obstet Gynecol. 1996;174:612-6.

72. Scott F, Wheeler D, Sinosich M, et al. First trimester aneuploidy screening using nuchal translucency, free beta human chorionic gonadotropihin and maternal age. Aust NZ J Obstet Gynaecol. 1996;36:381-4.

73. Berry E, Aitken DA, Crossley JA, et al. Screening for Down's syndrome: Changes in marker levels and detection rates between first and second trimester. Br J Obstet Gynecol. 1997;104:811-7.

74. Spencer K, Noble PL, Snijders RJ, et al. First trimester urine free beta hCG, beta core, and total oestriol in pregnancies affected by Down's syndrome: Implications for first trimester screening with nuchal translucency and serum free beta hCG. Prenat Diagn. 1997;17:525-38.

75. Wheeler DM, Sinosich MJ. Prenatal screening in the first trimester of pregnancy. Prenat Diagn. 1998;18:537-43.

76. Spencer K, Souter V, Tul N, et al. A screening program for trisomy 21 at 10–14 weeks using fetal nuchal translucency, maternal serum free beta human chorionic gonadotropin and pregnancy associated plasma protein-A. Ultrasound Obstet Gynecol 1999;13:231-7.

77. Krantz DA, Hallahan TW, James Macri V, et al. Statistical flaw in SURUSS model (Letter). Prenat Diagn. 2004;24:753-4.

78. Wald N, Rodeck C, Hackshaw A, et al. Correlations between nuchal translucency and serum markers in SURUSS (Letter). Prenat Diagn. 2004;24:835-6.

79. Bloom P (Ed). Free beta or intact hCG. DS News. 2004;11:37.

80. Platt LD, Greene N, Johnson A, et al. First trimester maternal serum biochemistry and fetal nuchal translucency screening (BUN) study group. Sequential pathways of testing after first trimester screening for trisomy 21. Obstet Gynecol. 2004;104:661-6.

81. Wright D, Bradbury I, Benn P, et al. Contingent screening for Down syndrome is an efficient alternative to non-disclosure sequential screening. Prenat Diagn. 2004;24:762-6.

82. Nyberg DA, Souter VL, El-Bastawissi A, et al. Isolated sonographic markers for detection of fetal Down syndrome in the second trimester of pregnancy. J Ultrasound Med. 2001;20:1053-63.

83. Bromley B, Lieberman E, Shipp TD, et al. The genetic sonogram: A method of risk assessment for Down syndrome in the second trimester. J Ultrasound Med. 2002;21:1087-96.

84. Cicero S, Curcio P, Papageorghiou A, et al. Absence of nasal bone in fetuses with trisomy 21 at 11-14 weeks of gestation: An observational study. Lancet. 2001;358:1665-7.

85. Cicero S, Rembouskos G, Vandecruys H, et al. Likelihood ratio for trisomy 21 in fetuses with absent nasal bone at the 11–14 week scan. Ultrasound Obstet Gynecol. 2004;23:218:23.

86. Orlandi F, Bilardo CM, Campogrande M, et al. Measurement of nasal bone length at 11-14 weeks of pregnancy and its potential role in Down syndrome risk assessment. Ultrasound Obstet Gynecol. 2003;36-9.

87. Otano L, Aiello H, Igarzabal L, et al. Association between first trimester absence of fetal nasal bone on ultrasound and Down syndrome. Prenat Diagn. 2002;22:930-2.

88. Viora E, Masturzo B, Errante G, et al. Ultrasound evaluation of fetal nasal bone at 11 to 14 weeks in a consecutive series of 1906 fetuses. Prenat Diagn. 2003;784-7.

89. Zoppi MA, Ibba RM, Axianna C, et al. Absence of fetal nasal bone and aneuploidies at first trimester nuchal translucency screening in unselected pregnancies. Prenat Diagn. 2003;23:496-500.

90. Cicero S, Bindra R, Rembouskas G, et al. Integrated ultrasound and biochemical screening for trisomy 21 using fetal nuchal translucency, absent fetal nasal bone, free beta hCG and PAPP-A at 11–14 weeks. Prenat Diagn. 2003;23:306-10.

91. Malone FD, Ball RH, Nyberg DA, et al. First trimester nasal bone evaluation for aneuploidy in the general population. Obstet Gynecol. 2004;104:1222-8.

75 Influence of Ethnicity on Prenatal Screening

F Sethna, B Thilaganathan

INTRODUCTION

With each passing day, the western World becomes increasingly multicultural, multiethnic and multilingual. Statistics from the last census (2001) to be carried out in the UK revealed that 7.9% of the population (4.6 million people) were from a minority background, with the majority being from the Indian subcontinent or Africa and the Caribbean.[1] In comparison, in the United States, approximately 28% of the population at the present time are from a minority background (African Americans, Hispanics, Asians, Pacific Islanders, Native Americans and Alaskan Natives representing the majority).

It is anticipated that immigrants and their descendents will continue to shape and alter the demographic landscape for several years to come. Consequently, it can be predicted that women from the ethnic minorities will form a growing proportion of the obstetric populations of many health districts. As clinicians assume responsibility for caring of an increasingly diverse population, genetic and ethnic connections to disease will become clearer. All health professionals must be prepared to meet the challenges such diversity will pose, if a uniform standard of healthcare is to be provided for all patients. It is important to be aware of the variations in need between individuals within similar communities, and not just across the population as a whole.

Prenatal screening allows women to make informed decisions about their reproductive choices. The vast majority of structural and chromosomal abnormalities arise in pregnancies without any risk factors. Therefore, aneuploidy and anomaly screening is offered to all women. However, certain genetic disorders occur with an increased frequency, or are confined to certain ethnic groups, and in these cases screening will be targeted at these individuals. It is important to ensure that prenatal screening is available and accessible equally to all women regardless of their background. This chapter will be examining the influence of ethnicity on screening methods within the field of prenatal diagnosis, targeted screening in ethnic groups and finally at the effect of ethnicity on uptake of screening.

EFFECTS OF ETHNICITY ON SCREENING METHODS

Down Syndrome

Down syndrome is the commonest congenital cause of severe mental retardation.[2] In developed countries, there are approximately 100,000 deliveries per year, per 10,000,000 of the population. The birth incidence of trisomy 21 is about 1 in 500, and therefore in such a population the total number of affected neonates is about 200.[3] The incidence of Down syndrome rises sharply with increasing

maternal age,[4] however, as the majority of children are born to women in their twenties and early thirties, 75% of babies with Down syndrome are born to women in this age group. Screening women of all ages for Down syndrome is now common practice in the West.

There is substantial variation in screening services for Down syndrome throughout the world. Options for screening include nuchal translucency measurement (alone, in combination with first/second trimester biochemistry, fetal nasal bone assessment or ductus venous Doppler measurement), maternal serum screening in the second trimester, or ultrasound for the detection of fetal defects and markers at 16–23 weeks. The influence of ethnic origin on screening efficacy by each of these modalities will now be examined in turn.

Nuchal Translucency

Babies born with Down syndrome show a distinct set of physical characteristics. Langdon Down first reported in 1866 that the skin of individuals with trisomy 21 appeared to be too large for their bodies.[5] This excess skin, in the form of nuchal translucency thickness, has formed the basis of one of the main noninvasive prenatal tests for this disorder since the early 1990s. Since this time, the association between increased nuchal translucency at 11–14 weeks of gestation and chromosomal abnormality has been well established and documented.[6-8] For an invasive testing rate of 5%, about 75% of trisomic pregnancies can be identified using this method of screening alone. Two studies have shown that nuchal translucency screening can be effectively and equitably delivered to a multiethnic population. Thilaganathan et al. performed an observational study in a district general hospital with a large multiethnic population serving African, Asian, Caribbean and Caucasian women.[9] In comparison, Chen et al. examined the effect of ethnic origin on nuchal translucency in a multiethnic Asian population comprised of Chinese, Indian, Pakistani, Nepalese and Filipino women.[10] Significant differences in the nuchal translucency measurement were obtained between the different ethnic groups in both studies. The magnitude of the differences was small, ranging from 0.08 mm to 0.22 mm. However, when compared to reported nuchal translucency intraobserver and interobserver variabilities of 0.54 mm and 0.62 mm respectively,[11] the differences are clinically insignificant. No correction for ethnic origin is therefore required when first trimester nuchal translucency screening for Down syndrome is performed in multiethnic populations.

Ductus Venosus

There is a clear association between abnormal Doppler flow in the ductus venosus (absence/reversed) and fetal aneuploidy. The use of ductus venosus Doppler velocimetry in combination with nuchal translucency is better than either test alone, since it increases the sensitivity in the detection of Down syndrome to 94% and decreases the likelihood ratio of a negative test to 0.08.[12] Although, the effect of ethnicity on ductus venosus Doppler indices are unknown, this screening method is so technically demanding that it is only likely to be performed on selected high-risk populations.

Nasal Bone

In 2001, Cicero and colleagues demonstrated the possibility of using absence of the nasal bone at 11–14 weeks as a marker for Down syndrome. They examined 701 routine ultrasound scans performed on women about to undergo prenatal diagnosis because of positive results on nuchal translucency screening.[13] The same group subsequently reported that nasal bones were absent in about 3% of chromosomally normal fetuses, in two-thirds of those with trisomy 21 and in about one-third of babies with other chromosomal defects.[14] The estimated likelihood ratio for trisomy 21 in the latter study was over 120 when the nasal bone cannot be seen. Given the significance of this ratio, and before nasal bone assessment is integrated into routine screening programs, knowledge about how to correct for ethnicity is required if this test is to be used equitably in multiethnic populations.

It is known that morphometry of the splanchnocranium, and of nasal bones in particular, differs between adults of various ethnic origins.[15] Likewise, ethnicity is known influence whether the nasal bones are seen in second trimester fetuses. It has been shown that second trimester nasal bone hypoplasia is commoner in fetuses of Afro-Caribbean mothers than in Caucasian mothers.[16] More recently, studies have demonstrated a similar significant difference in the rate of visualization of the fetal nasal bones in the first trimester in chromosomally normal fetuses in mothers of different ethnic origins.[17]

In 2004 Cicero et al. produced data to update the likelihood ratio for trisomy 21 in fetuses with absent nasal bone at the 11–14 week scan. They examined 5,918 pregnancies undergoing first trimester karyotyping and found that the incidence of absent nasal bone was higher in fetuses of Afro-Caribbean and Asian origin than in Caucasians; it decreased with increasing fetal CRL and increased with increased fetal NT.[18] The authors provided data on the incidence of absent nasal bone in chromosomally normal and trisomy 21 fetuses and likelihood ratios according to ethnic group (Table 75.1).

These data suggest that appropriate corrections may be applied for maternal ethnic origin and the absence of the nasal bones. However, as both parents contribute to a baby's phenotypic appearance, it remains to be determined whether any correction is also required for the father's ethnic origin.

Second Trimester Maternal Serum Screening

In 1984, a major advance in screening for chromosomal defects was made by Merkatz et al. who reported low levels of maternal serum alpha-fetoprotein (AFP) in trisomy 21 pregnancies.[19] Since this time, prenatal screening for trisomy 21 based on the analysis of biochemical markers in maternal serum between 15 weeks and 22 weeks of pregnancy has become an established part of obstetric practice. The principal markers found to be of value are AFP, total human chorionic gonadotropin (hCG) (or its individual

Table 75.1: The prevalence of absent nasal bones (NB) in normal and aneuploid pregnancies and their associated likelihood ratios (LR) for trisomy 21

	Caucasian	Afro-Caribbean	Asian
Number	5,284	170	201
Absent NB in aneuploid fetuses	68.3%	78.6%	71.4%
Absent NB in normal fetuses	2.2%	9.0%	5.0%
LR for trisomy 21 with absent NB	31.3	8.8	14.2
LR for trisomy 21 with NB	0.32	0.24	0.3

(*Source:* Adapted from Cicero et al. 2004)

subunits: free β-hCG and free α-hCG), unconjugated estriol (uE_3) and dimeric inhibin A. On average, in Down syndrome affected pregnancies, the AFP and uE_3 levels are about three-quarters that of an unaffected pregnancy (MoM < 0.84), whereas inhibin A and free β-hCG levels are about double (MoM > 1.3 and > 1.6 respectively). Most screening programs use multiple markers in combination with maternal age to generate a risk. Performance is known to vary according to the choice of markers used and whether ultrasound has been used to determine the gestational age. When the latter is used in combination with maternal age, the detection rate for a 5% false-positive rate is estimated to be 59% for the double test (AFP and either total hCG or free β-hCG), 69% for the triple test (AFP, total hCG, uE_3) and 76% for the quadruple test (AFP, hCG, uE_3 and inhibin A).

The results of second trimester maternal serum biochemistry are expressed as multiple of the median (MoM) values for gestation. MoM values normalize results for gestation to provide an equivalent measure between laboratories. The majority of published population data used to derive median values for the individual markers relate to European and American Caucasian populations. The degree of risk to an individual pregnant woman relies on combining the results with maternal age in a complex mathematical algorithm using commercially available software programs. The test is interpreted as positive or negative according to whether or not risk exceeds a fixed cut-off point. It is known that smoking, maternal weight, parity, previous pregnancy results, multiple pregnancy and insulin dependent diabetes can influence the concentration of the markers. It has been proposed that adjusting the risk algorithm, by taking into account these factors, can lead to an improvement in detection efficiency, although to what extent is not clear.

Another factor known to have an impact on the biochemical marker levels is ethnic origin. Gilbert et al.[20] raised the issue that racial differences existed in both age ranges for Down syndrome and in the medians for biochemical markers. They proposed that outcome data on serum screening should be collected by ethnic groups, so that validated risk estimations could be formed, thereby making serum screening in ethnic groups more effective.

There have been several publications documenting differences in the marker levels in Afro-Caribbean, South Asian, Oriental and Hispanic women compared to White women. Maternal serum AFP and hCG levels have been shown to be approximately 10–15% higher in black women compared to Caucasian women. In contrast, uE$_3$ levels hardly differ, and dimeric inhibin A levels are about 8% lower in pregnancies in African women. One of the largest published studys[21] evaluated data from more than 21,000 pregnancies to determine the extent of race-specific differences in median concentrations of analytes used in the triple test. This study found that at most gestational ages, median AFP, hCG and uE$_3$ values for White, Black, Hispanic and other patients were all significantly different. Further, these differences remained significant even after the data was corrected for patient weight. For the individual analytes the extent of the variation was not the same at different gestational ages. It is important that screening laboratories follow the literature to keep abreast of new findings to ensure that they continue to provide the best possible screening service for women from minority backgrounds.

Correcting for ethnic origin has a small overall effect on screening performance. The detection rate increases by about 0.5% for a false-positive rate of 5%.[22] Having said that, the adjustment is worthwhile because it does not require resources and because of its established value in screening for open neural tube defects using serum AFP, where the false-positive rate is higher in Asian and Black women compared to white women for a fixed AFP cut off level. In fact, The American College of Medical Genetics recommends that a correction be made when also screening for NTD.[23] If Down screening is being carried out in isolation and no risk for NTD is being provided to the mother it could be argued that an adjustment for ethnicity need not be made because of the counterbalancing effect that of the different analytes used in combination. For example, a Hispanic patient screened at 16 weeks with median values (1.00 MoM) of AFP, hCG and uE$_3$ when interpreted against a Hispanic patient derived dataset. If a primary white population dataset had been used her AFP value would have remained the same, hCG would have been 1.06 MoM and the uE$_3$ value 1.12 MoM. Although the higher hCG MoM would increase the Down risk, the higher uE$_3$ MoM value would counteract to reduce the risk.

First Trimester Maternal Serum Screening

All the serum markers used or considered in the second trimester have been assessed in Down syndrome and unaffected pregnancies during the first trimester. Only two serum markers have stood out as being useful in screening at 11–14 weeks, namely, pregnancy-associated plasma protein-A (PAPP-A) and free β-hCG. Maternal serum PAPP-A levels are lower in pregnancies affected by trisomy 21, with the difference in PAPP-A levels between trisomy 21 and normal pregnancies decreasing with increasing gestational age. In comparison, the maternal serum free β-hCG level is higher in trisomy 21 pregnancies, and the difference in levels between unaffected and affected pregnancies increases with advancing gestation.[24]

The consensus estimate of screening performance by using PAPP-A and free β-hCG in combination with maternal age is a 60% detection rate with a 5% false-positive rate. This is similar to the screening performance of second trimester double markers, but not as good as the screening performance of second trimester triple or quadruple markers. However, there is a significant improvement in screening efficiency when biochemistry analysis is combined with ultrasound in the first trimester. This form of screening can be provided in the setting of a one-stop clinic for assessment of risk (OSCAR), and is associated with a detection rate of about 90%, when the fetal nuchal translucency is also measured.

In 2000, Spencer et al. examined the influence of ethnic origin on first trimester biochemical markers of chromosomal abnormalities. It was seen that the median maternal serum marker MoMs for free β-hCG and PAPP-A were 19% and 48% higher in Afro-Caribbean women, and 19% and 35% higher in Asian women compared to Caucasian women. Correcting for maternal weight made very little difference to the Afro-Caribbeans (21% and 57% higher after weight correction), but reduced the effect in Asians (4% and 17% higher after weight correction). Correcting first-trimester biochemical markers for maternal ethnicity and weight has little impact at the population level for detection rates (an increase in the overall detection rate by a mere 1.4%). However, the effect on the individual patient-specific risk can be substantial (up to a twofold increase), and can certainly make a difference to the patient's decision on whether to have an invasive test. For example, in a 67 Kg, 25-year-old Afro-Caribbean, with an uncorrected free β-hCG of 2.10 MoM, and a PAPP-A of 0.65 MOM, the risk for trisomy 21 without correction for weight and ethnicity would be 1 in 540. After correction the free β-hCG MoM would be 1.73, whilst the PAPP-A MoM would be 0.41, with a corrected screening risk of 1:260.[25]

It would appear that ethnic origin has a greater impact on first trimester biochemical markers than second trimester biochemical markers. However, further larger data sets are required to develop robust methods of correcting for ethnic origin and to assess the biological significance of such marker production between various ethnic groups.

16–23 Week Ultrasound Scan

If the midtrimester 16–23 week scan demonstrates major structural defects, it is advisable to offer fetal karyotyping, even if these defects are isolated. The prevalence of these defects is low and therefore the financial cost implications are relatively small. Even if the defect is potentially correctable by surgery, such as exomphalos, it would seem appropriate to exclude an underlying chromosomal abnormality. The management policy for major fetal structural abnormality is unlikely to require changing on an ethnic basis. The same does not follow for the so-called "minor" markers of chromosomal abnormality.

Minor defects or markers are common and they are not usually associated with any handicap, unless there is an associated chromosomal abnormality. Most practitioners adopt an individualized approach to the assessment of risk depending on the marker identified either using the appropriate likelihood ratio or a genetic sonogram score.[3] In high-risk populations as defined by advanced maternal age or positive maternal serum biochemistry, this approach has been shown to maintain a high sensitivity for fetal aneuploidy without significantly increasing the invasive prenatal testing rate.

However, routine karyotyping of all low-risk pregnancies with these markers would have major implications, both in terms of miscarriage and financial costs. As a general concern, this process of sequential screening assumes the unproven independence between the findings of different screening results. For example, second trimester intracardiac echogenic foci are known to increase in prevalence when first trimester nuchal translucency measurements are elevated in fetuses of normal karyotype.[26] Hence, prior screening test results should be followed until data evaluating the interdependence of such markers become available.

Additionally, only a few have attempted to evaluate ethnic variation in such minor markers for fetal aneuploidy. Despite this, they have all invariably established significant ethnic variations in prevalence of the markers such as nasal bone, intracardiac echogenic foci, humeral and femoral length.[27-33] Hence, if these markers are to be used for modulating the risk of fetal chromosomal abnormality, the ethnic influence of the exact markers used need to be evaluated. In the long-term, it would seem more reliable to use first trimester nuchal translucency and maternal serum biochemistry, where corrections are not required or are easily made.

Neural Tube Defects

Neural tube defects (NTDs) have a complex etiology in which both genetic and environmental factors appear to be involved. Analysis of recurrence patterns within families and of twin-concordance data provides evidence of a genetic influence in sporadic cases, but factors such as socioeconomic status and geographic area (independent of race or ethnicity) are also associated with variations in the incidence of NTDs. Furthermore, exposure in pregnancy to various drugs, most commonly antiepileptics, are associated with increased risk for NTDs. Recently, Rothenberg et al. demonstrated the increased prevalence of autoantibodies against folate receptors in serum of women with a current or previous pregnancy complicated by a fetal NTD.[34,35] It remains to be established whether there is a causative relationship between the presence of these antibodies and the development of NTDs.

Screening by midtrimester ultrasound appears to be superior to maternal serum AFP assessment, but the latter modality is still widely used as a prior screening modality before detailed ultrasound assessment. The ethnic variation in AFP levels are well established and corrective formulae may be applied to produce accurate risks for NTDs in various ethnic groups as recommended by the American College of Medical Genetics guidelines for the screening of NTDs.[23]

TARGETED SCREENING IN ETHNIC GROUPS

In every ethnic, demographic or racial group, there are certain inherited disorders that occur more frequently than in the general population. Small genetic differences are known to exist between individuals from different ethnic groups. Certain ethnic groups have a higher risk of certain genetic conditions, especially autosomal recessive disorders, than the general population. Prenatal diagnosis is available for many genetic conditions, and a growing number of women are seeking advice regarding prenatal testing for a present or planned pregnancy. Knowledge of a patient's ethnicity can therefore help make a diagnosis, or help to identify individuals or couples at an increased risk of having a child with a specific genetic condition. The American College of Obstetricians and Gynecologists (ACOG) recommends genetic counseling for couples at increased risk for birth defects. Counseling enables the couple to become more informed about the disorders involved, the current availability of prenatal and postnatal testing, the accuracy and limitations of such testing, and their reproductive options.[36]

"Jewish" Genetic Disorders

The "Jewish" genetic disorders are a group of disorders that occur at a higher frequency among Jews compared to the general population, yet are not exclusive to the Jewish population. There is no official list of conditions, however, it is known that Mendelian disorders, and diseases associated with predisposition genes occur at a higher incidence in an individual of Ashkenazi or Sephardic ancestry. As different Jewish groups are at risk for different disorders, it is important to establish not only a patient's religion, but also of their ethnicity and ancestral countries of origin.

Ancestors of the Ashkenazi Jews lived in Central and Eastern Europe (Germany, Poland, Lithuania and Russia). Approximately 95% of Jews living in North America are Ashkenazi. This population are more likely to carry genes for Tay-Sachs disease, Canavan disease, familial dysautonomia, Niemann-Pick (type A) disease, Fanconi anemia (group C), Bloom syndrome, Gaucher disease (the non-neuronopathic type), mucolipidosis type IV and cystic fibrosis (Table 75.2). As these conditions can be severely incapacitating, tragically debilitating or lead to death in infancy or early childhood, some orthodox communities encourage the use of premarital carrier screening to discourage the marriage of two carriers.

In comparison, the Sephardic Jews ancestry can be traced to Spain, Portugal, North Africa (Morocco and Tunisia) needs and the Middle East. This Jewish population are more likely to be carriers for beta-thalassemia, familial Mediterranean fever, glucose-6-phosphate dehydrogenase deficiency and Type III glycogen storage disease.

The Ashkenazi Jewish community is a unique and ideal population which needs to provide multiple diseases screening because detection rates are high (> 95%) by testing a limited number of mutations. The American College of Obstetricians and Gynecologists (ACOG) recommends screening couples with European-Jewish ancestry at a minimum for Tay-Sachs disease, Canavan disease and cystic fibrosis.[37,38] No standards of care have been set for the Sephardic population.

Hemoglobinopathies

Hemoglobinopathies are the commonest single gene recessive disorders in the world. They occur as a result of mutations in the globin gene and are primarily seen in populations whose ancestors are from Africa, the Middle East, the Caribbean, the Mediterranean, Asia and the Far East. These disorders have appeared in the West due to global migration. In the UK, the NHS Sickle Cell and Thalassemia Screening Program are working toward a policy of universal antenatal screening which will allow the offer of sickle cell and thalassemia screening to all women as an integral part of early antenatal care.

Table 75.2: Common genetic disorders and carrier frequency in the Ashkenazi Jewish population

Disease	Carrier frequency
Tay-Sachs disease	1 in 26
Canavan disease	1 in 38
Familial dysautonomia	1 in 30
Niemann-Pick disease (type A)	1 in 70
Fanconi anemia (group C)	1 in 89
Bloom syndrome	1 in 110
Gaucher disease	1 in 10
Mucolipidosis IV	1 in 100
Cystic fibrosis	1 in 25

The population of Cyprus (both Greek and Turkish) has one of the highest rates of beta-thalassemia carriers in the world, and in the past 1 of every 158 infants was born with the condition. Today in Cyprus, antenatal screening for thalassemia has been almost totally superseded by premarital screening. The religious authorities had ethical objections to screening during pregnancy, on the grounds that it excluded most options other than termination of affected pregnancies. The church in Cyprus therefore insists on testing as a formal prerequisite to church weddings. The certificate required states merely that the partners have been tested and appropriately advised. In this way the confidentiality of the test result is preserved and the couple can exercise an informed choice about reproduction. This societal approach to inherited genetic disorders is to be applauded and is would be a suitable model for other communities to adapt.

Cystic Fibrosis

Cystic fibrosis (CF) is a common inherited condition that affects many systems in the body, most often resulting in chronic, progressive lung disease, problems with digestion, and subsequent malnutrition. CF is the most commonly inherited disease in Caucasians affecting approximately 1:2500 individuals, but it has been identified in people of all races and ethnicities around the world. The incidence in other ethnic groups varies from 1:15,000 for African Americans to 1:90,000 in Asians. In 2001, the American College of Obstetricians and Gynecologists and the American College of Medical Genetics[38] recommended that CF carrier screening be offered to all Caucasian couples that are pregnant, or are considering pregnancy. These groups additionally recommended that carrier screening be made available to other ethnic populations with the understanding that the likelihood of being a CF carrier may be much lower in non-Caucasian populations (Table 75.3).[39]

Although, there have been over 1,000 mutations identified that cause CF, only 25 have been recommended for carrier screening as additional mutations are rare, not well understood, and have

Table 75.3: The detection rate for the cystic fibrosis ΔF508 mutation test in various populations, including carrier frequency before and after a negative ΔF 508 mutation test[39]

Ethnicity	Detection rate (%)	Before test	After negative test
Ashkenazi Jewish	97	1/29	1/934
Caucasian (Northern European)	90	1/25	1/241
Caucasian (Southern European)	70	1/25	1/81
African American	69	1/65	1/207
Hispanic American[a]	57	1/46	1/105
Asian	30[b]	1/90	1/128[b]

[a] This is a pooled set of data based on ΔF 508 deletion and requires additional information to accurately predict risk for specific Hispanic populations. Residual carrier risk after a negative test is further modified by the presence of a positive family history of CF and/or by mixed ethnicity.

[b] Source: Laboratory Standards and Guidelines for Population-based Cystic Fibrosis Carrier Screening. Genetics in Medicine. 2001;3:149-54.

minimal impact on the overall probability of affecting a child. Mutations of the CF also vary with ethnicity. The ΔF 508 mutation accounts for 70% of the CF mutations in Caucasians of Northern European descents but only 30% of CF mutations in individuals of Ashkenazi Jewish descent. A different mutation, W1282X, is more common in the Ashkenazi Jews.

Glucose-6-Phosphate Dehydrogenase Deficiency

Glucose-6-phosphate dehydrogenase (G6PD) deficiency is the most common human enzyme deficiency. G6PD deficiency can result in the rapid destruction of blood cells in the presence of infection or certain drugs. Different populations have different types of mutations, but within a specific population, common mutations are usually shared. There are a wide variety of normal genetic variants of the enzyme G6PD. The main races affected are in West Africa, the Mediterranean, the Middle East and South East Asia. The degree of deficiency varies, often being mild in Black Africans, more severe in Orientals and most severe in Mediterraneans. Severe deficiency also occasionally occurs in Caucasians. Antenatal screening is available for at risk patients.

EFFECTS OF SCREENING ON ETHNICITY

Knowledge

The uptake of any screening test is influenced by knowledge of the condition being screened for. Parents need appropriate knowledge of Down syndrome, what it is, and how it affects the child and adult, both mentally and physically. They also need appropriate knowledge of the screening test, together with the limitations of the test, so that they can decide whether they wish to be screened. A study by Chilaka et al.[40] at Leicester General Hospital in the UK looked at the knowledge of Down syndrome amongst pregnant women from different ethnic groups. The study showed that racial groups other than Caucasian had a poorer understanding of Down syndrome. Fifty one percent of Caucasians in the study had a good knowledge of Down syndrome compared to 8% of Asians born outside the UK. The factors affecting knowledge included the quality of spoken English, knowing an affected child, parity and religion. Only 5 women in the study could not speak English; however none of these women had any reasonable knowledge of Down syndrome compared to those who could speak English. The importance of the study results are highlighted by its main finding that knowledge of the condition was the most influential factor in the decision making process about accepting or declining a Down syndrome screening test. In addition, information retention about prenatal screening also varies significantly by ethnicity and level of education.[41]

Access and Equity

Women from ethnic minorities can experience financial, linguistic, and cultural barriers to access healthcare services, limiting utilization of genetic and other maternal child health services. Genetic conditions may go undetected with deleterious impact during prenatal, perinatal and newborn periods. Society has an ethical obligation to ensure equitable access to healthcare for all, yet there remains a persistence of health disparities across race, income and ethnicity.

The extent and quality of prenatal care is important for the health of women and their babies. Early prenatal care can encourage healthy habits during pregnancy, help to identify potential medical problems, facilitate screening and involvement with parenting support, nutrition and other educational resources. Women from ethnic groups have been shown to use antenatal services less intensely with a high proportion booking too late for screening to be useful. Although, the percentage of women receiving prenatal care during the first 3 months of pregnancy has increased over the past two decades for white, black, Asian and Hispanic women; white women are still the most likely to receive prenatal care in their first trimester. Sadly a significant proportion of women from the ethnic minorities still receive no care until the third trimester.

In some countries in the world, a substantial barrier to healthcare access for some people is the lack of either public or private health insurance. Another difficulty in accessing health services is problems of communication and language barriers. The difficulties for the patient if English is not the first language with respect to screening can be divided into problems of recruitment into a screening program, of giving the patients enough information to allow informed consent, and of problems arising if detailed information needs to be provided in follow-up. To counter language difficulties interpreters may be used and information leaflets can be produced in different languages. Interpreting skills continue to be a scare resource in any health service. One way round this problem has been the setting up of a language service which enables remote interpreting via a shared telephone line. Another is via asking relatives to act as interpreters. However, this can however be problematic as it is often assumed that they are knowledgeable in all aspects of both languages, and this may place them under a great deal of stress. Also, patients may feel uncomfortable with even close relatives knowing about their medical conditions, as it may have profound cultural implications such as impacting on marriage prospects for themselves or their close family.

In many cultures, the concept of having to go outside the family for health education or infant care is an alien concept, and would indicate an unacceptable lack of respect for the older women in the family who traditionally are an important part of the child care system, and who expect to instruct the young mother in the care of her baby. To be obliged to seek such education from members of another culture whose values and beliefs are different from one's own is almost bizarre. However, if the concept of instruction in parentcraft by a midwife is accepted, the actual attendance at parentcraft may present considerable difficulties. The "usual" inhibitions to attendance experienced by young women, e.g. child care, the need to take time off work, may be further complicated by the need for a young woman to be escorted (particularly in the evenings), or by difficulties with communication or socioeconomic issues.

Despite these constraints, with an ethnically-sensitive strategy, it is still possible to provide equal access to prenatal screening. For example, in a previous study on ethnic differences in nuchal translucency measurement, it was noted that the ethnic balance of the population accepting and declining prenatal Down syndrome screening was not significantly different in an obstetric population from one of the most socially deprived regions of the UK, where over 15% of the women did not speak English.[42]

Culture and Religion

Understanding and valuing cultural diversity is critical to ensure the best possible care. For example, a woman is likely to decline prenatal screening and diagnosis because of fears that she may be divorced by her partner or shunned by her in-laws in the event that a fetal abnormality is diagnosed. The difficulties such attitudes create are further amplified by the fact that such women may well have a poorer understanding of the local language, be financially insecure and be reliant on her partner for right of residency in the country. This maternal perception, often unbeknown to the clinician, may be interpreted by healthcare workers as denial or lack of knowledge.

It is also important not to make the assumption that all women from a particular community follow the same customs and religion. For example, attitudes to termination vary even within the Muslim community. Some Muslim parents do not see termination as "halal" (permitted) but as "haram" (not permitted). They know their child is diseased but they choose to keep it believing that God will (inshaallah) created that child and they expect to get their rewards in heaven. Even when termination of pregnancy is acceptable, there are different interpretations of the gestation up to which such a procedure may be carried out.[43]

Clinicians therefore need to develop an appreciation and respect for cultures and religions that differ hugely from their own. This may be often impossible to attain unless members of the local ethnic and religious communities are co-opted into health service delivery as healthcare workers of aides.

Consanguinity

In the West, our knowledge and understanding of consanguinity is limited. Whilst marriages between close biological kin are preferential in many parts of the world, such unions are not commonplace in the West. First cousin marriages are legal in countries such as the UK and Australia, but are against the law in others. The 1981 marriage law of the People's Republic of China prohibits marriage between couples related as first cousins or closer, and in the USA, consanguineous unions are prohibited in 30 States. Irrespective of prevailing legislation, a future decline in the prevalence of consanguineous unions can be predicted, accompanying the expected reduction in family sizes. Regardless, it is important that healthcare providers have an understanding of the potential genetic consequences of such unions. This was recognized by National Society of Genetic Counselors (NSGC) in America who developed guidelines providing recommendations on counseling and screening for consanguineous couples defined as being second cousins or closer.[44]

Most of the genetic fall-out of consanguinity is in the form of autosomal recessive disorders, which in fact adversely affect only a minority of such families. The more closely two people are related, the more genes they share, and the more likely that both will carry a copy for the same recessive mutation, thereby increasing their chances of having a child affected by that disorder. Although, it is not possible to come up with one number for all populations of consanguineous couples, the risk is not as high as was previously envisaged. It is estimated that the additional risk for significant birth defects, including mental retardation or genetic disorders, above the general population risk is about 1.7–2.8% for first cousin unions.

The consensus from the NSGC is that beyond a thorough medical family history, with follow-up of significant findings, no additional preconception screening is recommended for consanguineous couples. Consanguineous couples should be offered similar genetic screening as suggested for any couple of their ethnic group.

CONCLUSION

Ethnic differences in the delivery of healthcare are prevalent across various domains of health, including mortality, morbidity, behavior and utilization of health services. This chapter highlights some areas of ethnic differences and potential inequalities in access to prenatal testing. The elimination of health inequality will firstly require a reliable assessment of the disparity in care provision as well as a clear understanding of differences across populations identified in terms of race/ethnicity. Further research is required to improve our understanding of why testing may not be offered, the reasons for failure to take up testing when offered, and to identify whether there are other social inequalities in access to prenatal testing.

REFERENCES

1. Office of National Statistics. Census, 2001.
2. Matilainen R, Airasksinen E, Mononen T, et al. A population-based study on the causes of mild and severe mental retardation. Acta Paediatr. 1995; 84(3):261-6.
3. Nicolaides KH. Screening for chromosomal defects. Ultrasound Obstet Gynaecol. 2003;21:313-21.
4. Hook EB. Rates of chromosome abnormalities at different maternal ages. Obstet Gynaecol. 1987;94:387-402.
5. Down LJ. Observations on an ethnic classification of idiots. Clinical lectures and Reports, London Hospital. 1866;3:259-62.
6. Nicolaides KH, Brizot ML, Snijders RJ. Fetal nuchal translucency: ultrasound screening for fetal trisomy in the first trimester of pregnancy. Br J Obstet Gynaecol. 1994;101:782-6.
7. Pandya PP, Brizot ML, Kuhn P, et al. First trimester fetal nuchal translucency thickness and risk for trisomies. Obstet Gynaecol. 1994;84:420-3.
8. Pandya PP, Snijders RJ, Johnson SP, et al. Screening for fetal trisomies by maternal age and fetal nuchal translucency thickness at 10–14 weeks of gestation. Br J Obstet Gynaecol. 1995;102:957-62.
9. Thilaganathan B, Khare M, Williams B, et al. Influence of ethnic origin on nuchal translucency screening for Down syndrome. Ultrasound Obstet Gynaecol. 1998;12(2):112-4.
10. Chen M, Lam YH, Tang MH, et al. The effect of ethnic origin on nuchal translucency at 10-14 weeks of gestation. Prenat Diagn. 2002;22(7):576-8.
11. Pandya PP, Altman DG, Brizot ML, et al. Repeatability of measurement of fetal nuchal translucency thickness. Ultrasound Obstet Gynecol. 1995;5(5):334-7.
12. Mavrides E, Sairam S, Hollis B, et al. Screening for aneuploidy in the first trimester by assessment of blood flow in the ductus venosus. BJOG. 2002;109(9):1015-9.
13. Cicero S, Curuio P, Papageorghiou A, et al. Absence of nasal bone in fetuses with trisomy 21 at 11-14 weeks of gestation: An observational study. Lancet. 2001;358:1665-7.
14. Cicero S, Longo D, Rembouskos G, et al. Absent nasal bone at 11-14 weeks of gestation and chromosomal defects. Ultrasound Obstet Gynecol. 2003;22(1): 31-5.
15. Ofodile FA. Nasal bones and pyriform apertures in blacks. Ann Plast Surg. 1994;32(1):21-6.
16. Cicero S, Sonek JD, McKenna DS, et al. Nasal bone hypoplasia in trisomy 21 at 15-22 weeks' gestation. Ultrasound Obstet Gynecol. 2003;21(1):15-8.
17. Prefumo F, Sairam S, Bhide A, et al. Maternal ethnic origin and fetal nasal bones at 11-14 weeks of gestation. BJOG. 2004;111(2):109-12.
18. Cicero S, Rembouskos G, Vandecruys H, et al. Likelihood ratio for trisomy 21 in fetuses with absent nasal bone at the 11-14-week scan. Ultrasound Obstet Gynecol. 2004;23(3):218-3.
19. Merkatz IR, Nitowsky HM, Macri JN, et al. An association between low maternal serum alphafetoprotein and fetal chromosomal abnormalities. Am J Obstet Gynecol. 1984;148(7):886-94.
20. Gilbert L, Nicholl J, Alex S, et al. Ethnic differences in the outcome of serum screening for Down syndrome. BMJ. 1996;312:94-5.
21. Benn PA, Clive JM, Collins R. Medians for second trimester maternal serum alpha-fetoprotein, human chorionic gonadotropin, and unconjugated estriol; differences between races or ethnic groups. Clin Chem. 1997;43(2): 333-7.
22. Watt HC, Wald NJ, Smith D, et al. Effect of allowing for ethnic group in prenatal screening for Down syndrome. Prenat Diagn. 1996;16(8):691-8.
23. American College of Medical Genetics. Standards and guidelines for clinical genetics laboratories; 2004.
24. Spencer K, Souter V, Tul N, et al. A screening program for trisomy 21 at 10-14 weeks using fetal nuchal translucency, maternal serum free β-human chorionic gonadotropin and pregnancy-associated plasma protein-A. Ultrasound Obstet Gynecol. 1999;13(4):231-7.
25. Spencer K, Ong CY, Liao AW, et al. The influence of ethnic origin on first trimester biochemical markers of chromosomal abnormalities. Prenat Diagn. 2000;20(6): 491-4.
26. Prefumo F, Presti F, Thilaganathan B, et al. Association between increased nuchal translucency and second trimester cardiac echogenic foci. Obstet Gynecol. 2003;101(5 Pt 1):899-904.
27. Rebarber A, Levey KA, Funai E, et al. An ethnic predilection for fetal echogenic intracardiac focus identified during targeted midtrimester ultrasound examination: A retrospective review. BMC Pregnancy Childbirth. 2004 25;4(1):12.
28. Shipp TD, Bromley B, Lieberman E, et al. The frequency of the detection of fetal echogenic intracardiac foci with respect to maternal race. Ultrasound Obstet Gynecol. 2000;15(6):460-2.
29. Zelop CM, Borgida AF, Egan JF. Variation of fetal humeral length in second trimester fetuses according to race and ethnicity. J Ultrasound Med. 2003;22(7):691-3.
30. Mastrobattista JM, Pschirrer ER, Hamrick MA, et al. Humerus length evaluation in different ethnic groups. J Ultrasound Med. 2004;23(2):227-31.

31. Kovac CM, Brown JA, Apodaca CC, et al. Maternal ethnicity and variation of fetal femur length calculations when screening for Down syndrome. J Ultrasound Med. 2002;21(7):719-22.

32. Borgida AF, Zelop C, Deroche M, et al. Down syndrome screening using race-specific femur length. Am J Obstet Gynecol. 2003;189(4): 977-9.

33. Shipp TD, Bromley B, Mascola M, et al. Variation in fetal femur length with respect to maternal race. J Ultrasound Med. 2001;20(2):141-4.

34. Rothenberg SP, Da Costa MP, Sequeira JM, et al. Autoantibodies against folate receptors in women with a pregnancy complicated by a neural-tube defect. N Engl J Med. 2004;350(2):134-42.

35. Rothenberg SP, Da Costa MP, Sequeira JM, et al. Autoantibodies against folate receptors in women with a pregnancy complicated by a neural tube defect. Obstet Gynecol Surv. 2004;59(6):410-1.

36. Driscoll DA, Wenstrom KD, Williams J. Third ACOG Committee on Genetics. ACOG Technology Assessment in Obstetrics and Gynecology. Number 1, July 2002. Genetics and molecular diagnostic testing. Obstet Gynecol. 2002;00:193-211.

37. ACOG Committee on Genetics. Screening for Tay-Sachs disease— ACOG Committee Opinion 162. International Journal of Gynecology and Obstetrics. 1996;52(3):311-2.

38. American College of Obstetricians and Gynecologists, American College of Medical Genetics. Preconception and prenatal carrier screening for cystic fibrosis. Clinical and laboratory guidelines; 2001.

39. Grody WW, Cutting GR, Klinger KW, et al. Laboratory standards and guidelines for population-based cystic fibrosis carrier screening. Genet in Med. 2001;3(2):149-54.

40. Chilaka VN, Konje JC, Stewart CR, et al. Knowledge of Down syndrome in pregnant women from different ethnic groups. Prenat Diagn. 2001;21(3):159-64.

41. Browner CH, Preloran M, Press NA. The effects of ethnicity, education and an informational video on pregnant women's knowledge and decisions about a prenatal diagnostic screening test. Patient Educ Couns. 1996;27(2):135-46.

42. Thilaganathan B, Sairam S, Michalidis G, et al. First trimester nuchal translucency: effective routine screening for Down's syndrome. Br J Radiol. 1999;72(862):946-8.

43. Zlotogora J. Parental decisions to abort or continue a pregnancy with an abnormal finding after an invasive prenatal test. Prenat Diagn. 2002;22(12):1102-6.

44. Bennett RL, Motulsky AG, Bittles A, et al. Genetic counseling and screening of consanguineous couples and their offspring: recommendations of the National Society of Genetic Counselors. J Genet Counsel. 2002;11(2): 97-119.

76 Ultrasound Screening of Congenital Heart Defects

R Chaoui

INTRODUCTION

Congenital heart defects (CHD) are one of the most common anomalies in human fetuses (5/1,000 livebirths) and are the leading cause of death due to malformations in the first year of life. Heart abnormalities and soft markers are present in a substantial amount in fetuses with chromosomal aberrations and fetal echocardiography is thus intrinsic part of the genetic scan.[1]

A prenatal diagnosis can be reliably achieved by means of ultrasound during pregnancy and the accurate prenatal diagnosis improves in many conditions fetal outcome by delivering the baby at a specialized tertiary center. In this chapter, the examination of the fetal heart is reviewed, focusing on the role of screening and how to imply the heart into the genetic scan.

EXAMINATION TECHNIQUES OF THE FETAL HEART

No organ in the fetus can be examined with as many diagnostical techniques as the heart. Detailed information on structure, function and time-related events has become available thanks to the development of sophisticated tools.[1] However, this has not been accompanied by a significant increase in prenatal detection rate of anomalies, but rather in increasing reliability in precise diagnosis.

Real-time Gray-scale Ultrasound and Two-dimensional Echocardiography

Gray-scale two-dimensional ultrasound is still the gold standard for the structural evaluation of the fetal heart. Resolution has continuously increased over the last two decades in step with the huge progress in the development of computer technology and fast processors. In most sophisticated (and expensive) ultrasound machines, there is an ideal setting for fetal heart examination, which is based on a high image resolution (using scan heads with 250–1,012 acoustic lines), a high frame rate and good penetration. Visualization of very tiny structures like the coronary arteries using real-time ultrasound has become possible as well as of other structures such as the fetal thymus that has not been seen before. The increased resolution using 5–7 MHz transducers has also led to the identification of new details like the echogenic intracardiac focus with the discussion whether or not it is associated with chromosomal or other anomalies.

Two main features, however, have facilitated enormously the fetal heart examination and are now standard even on mid- to low-range machines: the cine-loop and the zoom functions. The magnification of the image allows better assessment of the structures of interest, and visualization of the different cardiac cycle phases image-by-image facilitates assessment of the structures during systole and diastole. In the recent years, image resolution in gray-scale was increased by completing the native image with harmonic and/or compound imaging.

Time Motion or M-Mode

Time motion application in the fetus was not possible until simultaneous real-time visualization became available. Cardiac biometry first performed with M-Mode was very soon abandoned since such measurements became easier using cine-loop technique to image selectively diastole and systole.[2,3] Two main fields of interest are still in the domain of M-Mode: one is the classification of fetal arrhythmia and the other is the calculation of indices used in cardiology to assess contractility, e.g. shortening fraction, ejection fraction, etc.

Spectral Doppler Flow Velocity Waveform

Doppler ultrasound enables a noninvasive quantification of perfusion across different fetal cardiac valves and vessels. Peak velocities can be assessed and indices calculated. By measuring the area of a valve the perfusion can then be calculated either as stroke volume or involving the heart frequency as cardiac output. The advent of color Doppler enabled a more reliable use over of spectral Doppler across the known valves, but also the evaluation of more difficult otherwise not assessable regions, as pulmonary arteries and veins, ductus arteriosus, foramen ovale and even coronary vessels.

Color Doppler

In addition to the gray-scale examination of the fetal heart, color Doppler is now considered as the second part of a complete cardiac evaluation. The method allows rapid orientation within the fetal heart and completes the evaluation supplied by gray-scale information. Once abnormal flow is suspected, quantification becomes mandatory using spectral Doppler. The advent of color Doppler did not contribute to a huge increase in detection rate of CHD but increased the reliability of screening when routinely applied and in the detailed fetal echocardiography in suspected heart diseases.

We described few years ago how most congenital heart anomalies could be detected in only three planes using color Doppler: the four-chamber view, the five-chamber view and the three-vessel-trachea view.[4] The exact examination in gray scale completed by the expected typical flow in color Doppler became the basis of diagnosis of fetal CHD.

Three-dimensional Fetal Echocardiography

As soon as the first three-dimensional (3D) ultrasound equipment became available an attempt to examine the fetal heart was undertaken. It was hoped that 3D information of the fetal heart could facilitate understanding of orientation especially the assessment of the great vessels' anatomy which is difficult for many examiners. However, since the heart is beating, the main challenge is still the gating of the signals and the acquisition of information during systole or diastole.[5] The advent of spatiotemporal image correlation (STIC) technology few years ago allowed a reliable acquisition of a 3D with systole and diastole as off-line 4D fetal echo.[6] STIC can be used in gray scale[6] or in combination with color or power Doppler mode.[7] A detailed description of 3D of heart and vessels is described elsewhere in this book and I refer to the reader to this chapter. The technique is however too young to be evaluated for its role in screening for fetal heart defects or in genetic scan.

SCREENING OF THE FETAL HEART OR TARGETED EXAMINATION BASED ON INDICATIONS

Chronic heart disease (CHD) have a multifactorial etiology and therefore prenatal detection cannot be achieved solely by concentrating on the high-risk population defined by patient history. Therefore, seeking for heart abnormalities should be part of the midtrimester ultrasound screening. In many countries such a general screening is not established (no insurance or mother care coverage), but is often performed either on risk indication or by the willingness of the patient.

Signs of cardiac disease are often subtle, necessitating careful targeted examination. In the 1980s, the four-chamber view was proposed as the most important plane for screening, allowing a greater detection rate for anomalies. Recently, however, incorporation of views of the great vessels has been recommended as part of the routine screening examination.

Many studies in the last 10 years have emphasized the importance of cardiac screening, but they have achieved widely divergent results, with reported detection rates varying from 5% to 92%.[8] However, it should be noted that these studies employed different approaches and are therefore not directly comparable.[8]

There is a list of indications, generally accepted as referral reason for fetal echocardiography, and were presented in another chapter. The percentage of detection of heart anomalies within single groups (the yield) differs between 3% and 5% (i.e. diabetes, drugs, genetic ultrasound) to more than 50% (i.e. suspicious four-chamber view). In some indications fetal echocardiography are performed rather to calm the pregnant woman (low recurrence risk in positive family history) whereas in other conditions to seriously rule out a heart anomaly (nonimmune hydrops, extracardiac malformations, etc.).

FETAL CARDIAC EXAMINATION IN A LOW-RISK POPULATION AND TARGETED FETAL ECHOCARDIOGRAPHY IN A HIGH-RISK POPULATION

It is generally agreed that the "four-chamber view" should be part of every routine ultrasound in pregnancy. However, there are different reasons why this plane was not successful in improving the detection rate of CHD in the recent past. In order to achieve an accurate assessment of this plane we recommend to follow a step-by-step checklist on every single cardiac examination, including the list in Table 76.1.

It is furthermore agreed that the assessment of the great vessels belongs rather to an extended fetal cardiac examination. We expect however that in future this will be part of a basic cardiac examination as well, since many anomalies of the great vessels are not detectable in the simple "four-chamber screening" and their detection has been demonstrated to improve children outcome in various CHD. Whereas the four-chamber view can be examined in a single plane, the great vessels can be only assessed by a dynamic scan, i.e. by tilting and moving the transducer.[9] The checklist for assessing the great vessels will include the list as presented in Table 76.2.

Targeted fetal echocardiography should be performed by those familiar with the prenatal diagnosis of CHD and the wide spectrum of possible anomalies. In such a chapter, I cannot recommend whether the examiner should be an obstetrician or a pediatric cardiologist, since this may be decided by the local specificities of the country. I recommend however a close cooperation between both groups, especially during counseling a pregnant woman with a suspected heart anomaly in the fetus.

Often the expectations are bigger and therefore the time, equipment and expertise needed for an examination are larger. In these conditions, the use of color and pulsed Doppler techniques increase the accuracy of the examination. In cases of arrhythmia, M-Mode or pulsed Doppler should be used to demonstrate the relationship between atrial and ventricular contractions.

The checklist in these conditions is longer and the dynamic examination of the heart in different planes[9] is mandatory as shown in Tables 76.1 and 76.2.

FETAL ECHOCARDIOGRAPHY AND THE DETECTION OF A CONGENITAL HEART DEFECT

There are two steps in the detection of a fetal heart defect, namely, first, the suspicion of an abnormality and second, the detailed precise description and classification of the heart defect. Generally, the first is easily achieved when the examiner is able to get the four-chamber view and the great vessels in nearly all patients as described in Tables 76.1 and 76.2, and he/she knows the typical hints for an abnormal heart in these planes. The second step can be solved chiefly by getting experience in many CHD and knowing the spectrum of the different diseases. In many countries, the latter examination is either achieved together with a pediatric cardiologist or by referring the pregnant to a pediatric cardiologist specialized in fetal echo examination.

It is important to know the most common "abnormalities" detected during fetal cardiac scan and leading to a referral. In my experience, the most common signs detected in the four-chamber view and the great vessel planes are summarized in Table 76.3. The differential diagnosis of most common suspicions of referrals are summarized in Table 76.4.

Table 76.1: Checklist for the basic cardiac examination and the targeted fetal echocardiography for the four-chamber view

	Basic examination	Targeted fetal echocardiography
Upper abdomen	Stomach and heart on the same side of the fetus	Same
Descending aorta/Inferior vena cava		– Aorta on the left side of the spine – Normal arrangement of aorta and inferior vena cava in the upper abdomen
Heart size	About 1/3 of the thoracic cavity	Same
Heart position	2/3 of the heart is in the left hemithorax	Same
		Same
Heart axis	Septum at an angle of about 45° to the midline	Same
Heart rhythm	120–180 beats/min, no arrhythmia	Same
Ventricles	Two equally contracting ventricles, of approximately equal cavity size and wall thickness	Right ventricle is shorter than the left and has the moderator band at the apex. Heart apex is build by the left ventricle
Atria	Two atria of approximately equal size with foramen ovale defect in middle third of atrial septum	Same
Valves	Two opening atrioventricular valves	Same
Crux of heart	Intact	Intact and slightly lower insertion of the tricuspid valve than to the mitral valve
Ventricular septum	Intact from apex to crux	Same
Pulmonary vein(s)		At least one should be seen by color flow mapping connecting to the left atrium
Color Doppler flow shows		– Antegrade perfusion across atrioventricular valves – No aliasing (turbulences) – No regurgitation – No crossing over the ventricular septum

Table 76.2: Examination of the great arteries as part of an extended basic cardiac examination or as targeted fetal echocardiography

	Extended basic examination	Targeted fetal echocardiography
Aorta	Arises from the left ventricle	Arises from the left ventricle continues toward the aortic arch
Ventricular septum	Continuous with ascending aorta	Same
	• Arises from the RV • Is slightly larger than aorta • Crosses over the ascending aorta • Bifurcates to give the left and right pulmonary arteries • Connects to the ductus arteriosus	
Duct and aortic arch		• Are of approximately equal size • Point to the left side of the spine • The trachea is on the right of both vessels • Thymus is present • No left superior vena cava on the left of the pulmonary trunk
Color flow shows		• Antegrade perfusion across both semilunar valves • No aliasing (turbulences) except in the ductus region in third trimester • No regurgitation • No reverse flow in either the ductus arteriosus or the aortic arch

Table 76.3: Common suspicions leading to referral to targeted fetal echocardiography

Common suspicions in the four-chamber view	• Cardiomegaly • Arrhythmia • Heart to the right/heart-stomach on different site • Single ventricle • One small ventricle (right or left) • Discrepant size of the ventricles • Defect in the ventricular septum, AV junction • One common AV valve • Echogenic focus in the LV • Tumors in the heart
Common suspicions in the great vessels assessment	• Perimembranous VSD in the five chamber view • VSD with overriding aorta • Dilated aortic root • Discrepant caliber of ascending aorta and pulmonary trunk • Hypoplastic or noncontinuing aorta or pulmonary trunk • Parallel great vessels arrangement • One single vessel only visualized • Aortic arch on the right side of the spine (and trachea)

Table 76.4: Differential diagnoses of some common suspicions

Single ventricle	• Mitral atresia • Tricuspid atresia • Double inlet ventricle • Large atrioventricular septal defect
Small left ventricle	• Hypoplastic left heart syndrome • Coarctation of the aorta • Mitral atresia with VSD • Double outlet right ventricle
Small right ventricle	• Pulmonary atresia with intact septum • Tricuspid atresia with VSD
Ventricular septum defect (VSD)	• Isolated VSD • Atrioventricular septal defect • Double inlet ventricle • Interrupted aortic arch • Aortic coarctation • Conotruncal anomalies (see overriding aorta)
Overriding aorta over the VSD	• Tetralogy of Fallot • Pulmonary atresia with VSD • Truncus arteriosus communis • Absent pulmonary valve syndrome • Double outlet right ventricle
Parallel vessels	• Double outlet right ventricle • Complete transposition of the great arteries • Congenitally corrected transposition of the great arteries
Tiny ascending aorta	• Hypoplastic left heart syndrome • Aortic coarctation • Tubular hypoplasia of the aortic arch • Interruption of the aortic arch
Two normal appearing ventricles, but one single great vessel recognized	• Double outlet right ventricle (vessels over each other) • Transposition of the great arteries (vessels over each other) • Truncus arteriosus communis • Dilated aorta (in pulmonary atresia with VSD)

FETAL ECHOCARDIOGRAPHY IN GENETIC SCAN

Fetal examination allows to detect fetuses at high-risk for chromosomal aberrations owing to malformations or signs called soft markers.[10] The latter increases the risk to a specific malformation, without being obligatory per se a structural malformation. The fetal heart belongs to the organs often evaluated carefully when seeking for a chromosomal anomaly, either the common numerical aberrations as trisomy 21,18,13 or monosomy X or more specific deletions as the microdeletion 22q11 involving often the heart. In numerical aberrations except Down syndrome, the other anomalies have many extracardiac signs leading to an invasive procedure independent from the heart finding.

Structural Heart Anomaly

Atrioventricular septal defect (AVSD) (Fig. 76.1) is the most common heart anomaly associated with a chromosomal aberration mainly trisomy 21 and 18. The diagnosis can be achieved by detecting the gap in the crux of the heart (the combination of defects within the interventricular and interatrial septa). The association with trisomy 21 or 18 is between 50% and 80%; however, when in AVSD the left ventricle is small as in combination with aortic coarctation, the rate of aneuploidy is lower (10% or less) and if there are signs of isomerism (i.e. stomach on the right side) there is no association with chromosomal aberrations.

We proposed recently a new simple cardiac measurement the atrial to ventricular length (AVL) ratio, in order to increase the detection rate for AVSD on routine scan. After a standardized four-chamber view, the ratio of the atrial length to the length of the ventricle in the midline is measured. Whereas the normal AVL-ratio during second trimester is constant around 0.5, almost all fetuses with AVSD had a ratio exceeding 0.6.[11]

Other anomalies which are found in association with trisomy 21 are the VSD and the tetralogy of Fallot. Typical anomalies for trisomy 18 are besides the VSD and AVSD, the overriding of the aorta (Fig. 76.2) with or without the pulmonary stenosis, a double outlet right ventricle and occasionally a left outflow tract obstruction. Trisomy 13 cardiac anomalies are besides the VSD, left outflow tract obstructions as aortic coarctation of the aorta and occasionally a hypoplastic left heart syndrome (HLHS). Turner syndrome has in almost all cases detected prenatally generally in combination with a cystic hygroma also the left ventricular outflow tract obstruction typically the aortic coarctation and also occasionally the HLHS.

Cardiac Soft Markers

Intracardiac Echogenic Focus

The debate on this unspecific sign will not be continued in this chapter. There are controversial data in the literature supporting the echogenic focus (EF) as a sign for Down syndrome[10] as well as a benign sign with no relationship to chromosomal anomalies.

Since most cases (around 90%) are found as isolated EF in the left ventricle (Fig. 76.3), it is to be emphasized that EF in the right ventricle or two EF either in the left (Fig. 76.3), right or in both ventricles increase significantly the risk for chromosomal anomalies. The isolated EF in the left ventricle was accepted in the last years as increasing the background risk of a factor of 1.5 or even only 1. This led recently to a debate whether the finding of an echogenic focus should be told to younger women or not.[12,13]

In an observation of a series with CHD we found that 11% of all cardiac defects were associated with an EF,[14] some with malformations not detectable in the four-chamber plane as the tetralogy of Fallot or a transposition of the great arteries (TGA). A total of 50% of all the cases were, however not isolated left ventricular EF. Therefore, not only chromosomal anomalies but also cardiac defects should be ruled out in fetuses with a detected EF. Since the use of nuchal translucency in the risk assessment for chromosomal anomalies, the importance of second trimester soft markers is reduced, especially the EF.

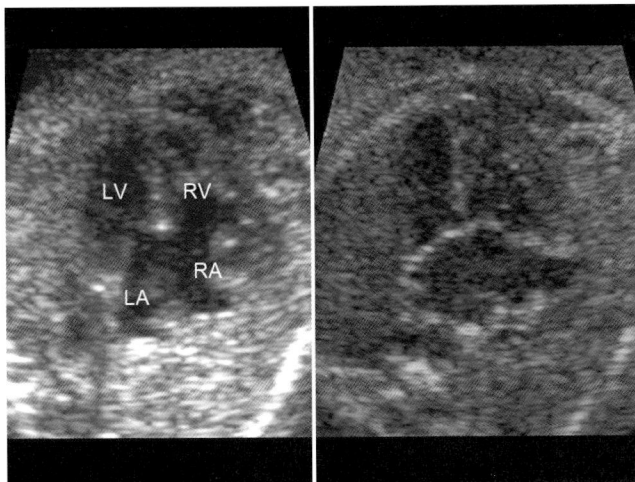

Fig. 76.1: Fetuses with atrioventricular septal defect (AVSD) during diastole (left) and systole (right). In the left image the gap in the crux of the heart is easily recognized. On the right side on one hand both AV valves are linear and on the other the measurement of atrial to ventricular length will reveal a ratio >0.6 suspicious for an AVSD

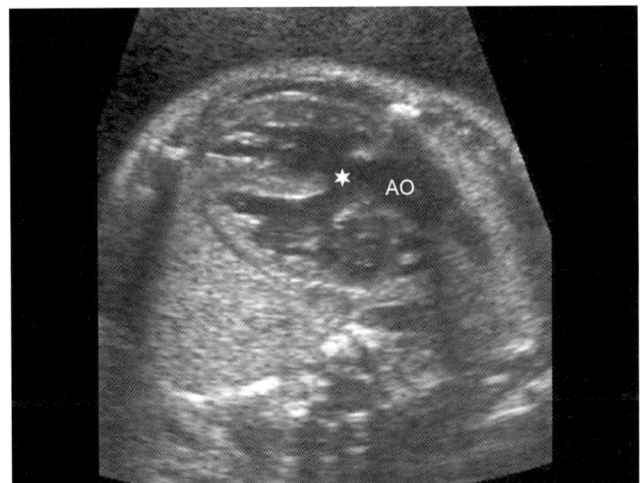

Fig. 76.2: This is an overriding of the aorta (AO) over a VSD (*), which can be detected in the visualization of the five-chamber view. This is a sign and its differential diagnosis is listed in Table 76.4

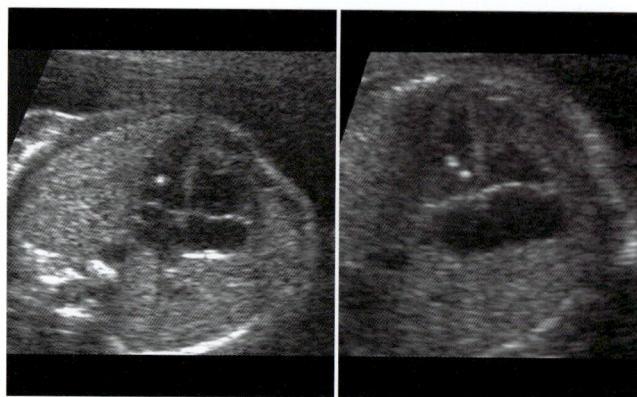

Fig. 76.3: Two fetuses with echogenic foci. On the left the echogenic focus is present in the left ventricle and is the most common condition found. In the right figure two echogenic foci are present in the left ventricle. This fetus had a heart defect associated with a del.22q11

Discrepant LV/RV Width

Devore[15] described an increased risk for trisomy 21 in early second trimester fetuses with a narrow left ventricle compared with the right ventricle, without the additional signs of an aortic coarctation.

Tricuspid Regurgitation

Isolated tricuspid regurgitation detected by the routine use of color Doppler is present in 4% of all normal fetuses at 20–22 weeks scan.[16] Tricuspid regurgitation was however also discussed as associated with Down syndrome when detected at 16–18 weeks[15] or at the 11–14 weeks scan.[17]

Pericardial Effusion

An isolated pericardial effusion was described to increase the risk of association with Down syndrome (Fig. 76.4).[18] It is not known whether in these cases, the effusion is the remaining of early

hydrops with a thickened nuchal translucency in early pregnancy. This sign was unfortunately not evaluated in the recent years in the age of NT measurement.

Linear Insertion of the AV Valves

This is an interesting new sign presented by a French group few years ago. Fredouille and coworkers[19] found on autopsy specimens of hearts from fetuses with Down syndrome that in some cases, even with the absence of structural heart anomalies both atrioventricular valves inserted at the same level and not the tricuspid valve inserting lower in the right ventricle as under normal conditions. This is a very subtle and interesting subtle sign, used also in the detection of AV-septal defect, but should be evaluated by other groups.

Aberrant Right Subclavian Artery (ARSA): The New Cardiac Sign for Down Syndrome

The normal right subclavian artery arises as a first vessel from the brachiocephalic artery and courses ventral of the trachea. An aberrant right subclavian artery arises separately from the aortic arch in the region of the junction of the aortic arch and the ductus arteriosus. It courses to the right arm behind the trachea and is thus detectable with color Doppler in the three-vessels-trachea view (Fig. 76.5).[20]

In few pediatric cardiology studies it was described that an ARSA (also called lusorian artery) is found in 1% of the normal population but as high as 35% in persons with Down syndrome with or without heart defects.

We were the first to describe this sign in fetuses with Down syndrome in a paper published recently,[20] where we found that 5/14 (36%) of consecutive fetuses with Down syndrome had this aberrant vessel, we detected prenatally. Only one had it as an isolated sign, three in association with an echogenic focus in addition to extracardiac signs, and in only one case, it was associated with an AVSD.

Personal experience and communication from pathologists support that this sign is also common in trisomy 13, 18 and recent

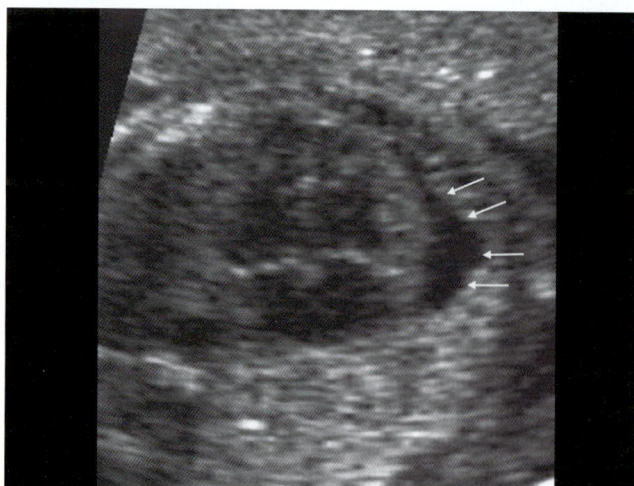

Fig. 76.4: In this fetus with Down syndrome there is a pericardial effusion at 20 weeks (arrows)

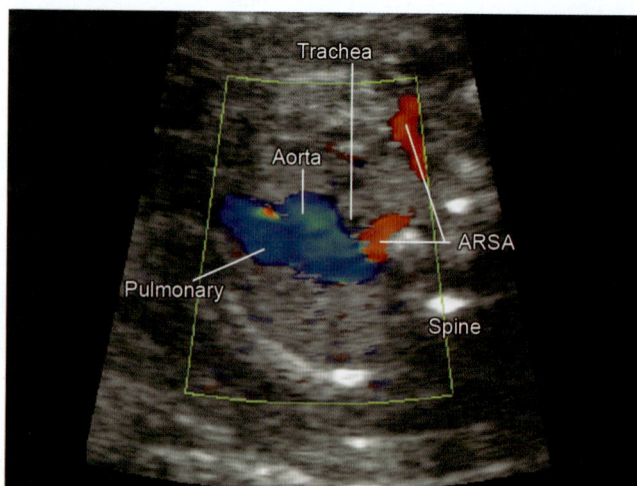

Fig. 76.5: In this fetus with Down syndrome at 20 weeks, an aberrant right subclavian artery is present. It is demonstrated in the three-vessel, tracheal view as a vessel with a course behind the trachea toward the right arm

reports emphasized the occurrence in Turner syndrome and in microdeletion 22q11.

Further observations from other groups are necessary to confirm our new finding.

Cardiac Signs for Microdeletion 22q11

The del 22q11 is reported to have a frequency of 1:4,000 livebirths and is considered to be after trisomy 21 the second most common chromosomal anomaly in live born children with a CHD. The earlier used and now abandoned acronym CATCH-22 summarizes the combination of finding in these patients: C = cardiac anomaly, A = abnormal facies, T = thymus hypo or aplasia, C = cleft palate, H = hypercalcemia, 22 for del.22q11. Prenatally, the clinical features of an abnormal facies are generally very subtle and we can mainly rely on the heart anomaly and as we showed few years ago also on the thymus sign.

Among the heart anomalies, conotruncal and aortic arch malformations are the leading defects permitting a concrete suspicion of a del.22q11. The occurrence of this deletion is present in 50% of all cases with interrupted aortic arch, 40% of absent pulmonary valve syndrome, 30% of truncus arteriosus communis, 20% of pulmonary atresia with VSD, 15% with tetralogy of Fallot, and in around 5% in other anomalies as complex transpositions, double outlet right ventricle and others.[21]

Few years ago, we examined a group of 147 fetuses with CHD including 76 with conotruncal defects. In this study, we examined the role of analyzing the absence or hypoplasia of the thymus in predicting a del.22q11. Ten of the 147 cases had a del.22q11, all being in the group with conotruncal anomaly. Nine of the ten fetuses with microdeletion had an abnormal thymus detected prenatally (sensitivity 90%, specificity 98.5%). In our experience,

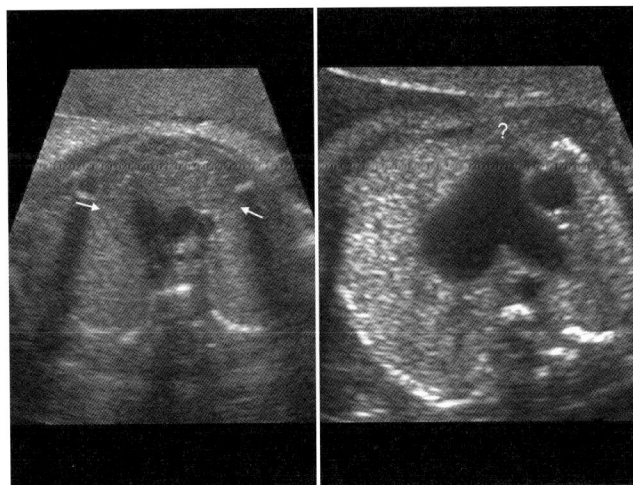

Fig. 76.6: Thymus sign in predicting fetuses with del.22q11. In the left figure the thymus is recognized (arrows) as a slightly echogenic structure in front of the three vessels and behind the sternum. In the right figure the fetus had a absent pulmonary valve syndrome with gross dilated pulmonary arteries. No thymus was visualized between the vessels and sternum (?) and FISH technique revealed the suspected del.22q11

the examination of the thymus region helps in defining a group at high risk for del.22q11[21] (Fig. 76.6).

According to other studies additional signs were described to increase the risk of 22q11 (in predefined high-risk groups) and some of these are increased NT in early pregnancy, intrauterine growth retardation, polyhydramnios, renal or facial abnormality, right aortic arch, aberrant right subclavian artery, aberrant pulmonary artery, etc.[22,23]

REFERENCES

1. Chaoui R. Fetal echocardiography: State of the art of the state of the heart. Ultrasound Obstet Gynecol. 2001;17:277-84.
2. Sharland GK, Allan LD. Normal fetal cardiac measurements derived by cross-sectional echocardiography. Ultrasound Obstet Gynecol. 1992;2:175-81.
3. Chaoui R, Heling KS, Bollmann R. Ultrasound measurements of the fetal heart in the 4-chamber image plane. Geburtsh. Frauenheilk. 1994;54:92-7.
4. Chaoui R, McEwing R. Three cross-sectional planes for fetal color Doppler echocardiography. Ultrasound Obstet Gynecol. 2003;21:81-93.
5. Chaoui R, Kalache KD, Hartung J. Application of three-dimensional power Doppler ultrasound in prenatal diagnosis. Ultrasound Obstet Gynecol. 2001;17:22-9.
6. DeVore GR, Falkensammer P, Sklansky MS, et al. Spatio temporal image correlation (STIC): New technology for evaluation of the fetal heart. Ultrasound Obstet Gynecol. 2003;22:380-7.
7. Chaoui R, Hoffmann J, Heling KS. Three-dimensional (3D) and 4D color Doppler fetal echocardiography using spatiotemporal image correlation (STIC). Ultrasound Obstet Gynecol. 2004;23:535-45.
8. Chaoui R. The four-chamber-view: four reasons why it seems to fail in screening for cardiac abnormalities and suggestions to improve detection rate. Ultrasound Obstet Gynecol. 2003;22:3-10.
9. Chaoui R. The examination of the normal fetal heart using two-dimensional echocardiography. In: Yagel S, Silvermann N, Gembruch U (Eds). London, New York: Martin Dunitz; 2003. pp. 141-9.
10. Bromley B, Lieberman E, Shipp TD, et al. The genetic sonogram—A method of risk assessment for Down syndrome in the second trimester. J Ultrasound Med. 2002;21:1087-96.
11. Machlitt A, Heling KS, Chaoui R. Increased cardiac atrial-to-ventricular length ratio in the fetal four-chamber view: A new marker for atrioventricular septal defects. Ultrasound Obstet Gynecol. 2004;24:618-22.
12. Filly RA, Benacerraf BR, Nyberg DA, et al. Choroid plexus cyst and echogenic intracardiac focus in women at low-risk for chromosomal anomalies. J Ultrasound Med. 2004;23:447-9.
13. Doubilet PM, Copel JA, Benson CB, et al. Choroid plexus cyst and echogenic intracardiac focus in women at low risk for chromosomal anomalies: The obligation to inform the mother. J Ultrasound Med. 2004;23:883-5.
14. Chaoui R , Bierlich A. Intracardiac echogenic focus and fetal heart defects. Ultrasound Obstet Gynecol. 2000;16:13-4 (abstract).
15. Devore GR. The role of fetal echocardiography in genetic sonography. Sem Perinatol. 2003;27:160-72.
16. Respondek ML, Kammermeier M, Ludomirsky A, et al. The prevalence and clinical significance of fetal tricuspid valve

regurgitation with normal heart anatomy. Am J Obstet Gynecol. 1994;171:1265-70.

17. Huggon IC, DeFigueiredo DB, Allan LD. Tricuspid regurgitation in the diagnosis of chromosomal anomalies in the fetus at 11-14 weeks of gestation. Heart. 2003;89:1071-3.

18. Sharland G, Lockhart S. Isolated pericardial effusion: An indication for fetal karyotyping? Ultrasound Obstet Gynecol. 1995;6:29-32.

19. Fredouille C, Piercecchi-Marti MD, Liprandi A, et al. Linear insertion of atrioventricular valves without septal defect: A new anatomical landmark for Down's syndrome? Fetal Diagn Ther. 2002;17:188-92.

20. Chaoui R, Heling KS, Sarioglu N, et al. Aberrant right subclavian artery (lusorian artery) as a new cardiac sign in second and third trimester fetuses with Down syndrome. Am J Obstet Gynecol. 2005 (in press).

21. Chaoui R, Kalache KD, Heling KS, et al. Absent or hypoplastic thymus on ultrasound: A marker for deletion 22q11.2 in fetal cardiac defects. Ultrasound Obstet Gynecol. 2002;20:546-52.

22. Boudjemline Y, Fermont L, Le Bidois J, et al. Prevalence of 22q11 deletion in fetuses with conotruncal cardiac defects: A 6-year prospective study. J Pediatr. 2001;138:520-4.

23. Volpe P, Marasini M, Caruso G, et al. 22q11 deletions in fetuses with malformations of the outflow tracts or interruption of the aortic arch: Impact of additional ultrasound signs. Prenat Diagn. 2003;23:752-7.

77

Ultrasound Screening of Chromosomal Abnormalities by Nuchal Translucency

MA Zoppi, G Monnia

INTRODUCTION

Nuchal translucency (NT) is the term that has been used for 10 years to describe the echo-free space behind the fetal neck visible by ultrasound in almost all fetuses at 10–14 weeks (Fig. 77.1).[1] Before this gestational age the NT is not clearly evident in all cases and after 14 weeks the NT reduces, becoming less transonic and turning into the nuchal fold space visible in the second trimester.

The NT is in fact the ultrasound image of some soft tissues that cover the occipital bone and cervical spine (muscles, connective tissue, lymphatic vessels, subcutaneous tissues and cutis).

In physiological condition, these tissues can accumulate more or less fluids and as a result the thickness of the NT is expected to individually differ among normal fetuses.

Moreover, during the 11–14 weeks period, the thickness of the NT increases with the crown-rump length (CRL) and with the age of the fetus. Tables of reference for NT thickness in normal fetuses have been generated by cross-sectional studies. Some studies have calculated the ranges by using linear regression formulas, however, quadratic regression approach seems to better fit the trend of the nuchal thickness.[2-5]

Other studies have shown that longitudinal assessments of NT in the same fetus showed a tendency toward a growth of the thickness to reach a peak that is achieved individually and differently by each fetus, mostly around 12 weeks and then it show a decrease.[6]

It is evident that some subtle differences can be achieved among different centers that perform the measurement of the NT, due to local contingent conditions (operators, machines, approach to the ultrasound technique, ethnicity, etc.). Therefore, it has been suggested to favor local reference ranges for normal NT, to assess the thickness, whenever it is possible.[7]

At 10 weeks, essentially, the NT thickness in normal fetuses most frequently measures around 1–1.2 mm and at 13–14 weeks, around 1.7–1.9 mm.

The visualization and measurement of the NT is not included among the main identified objectives for first trimester ultrasound as recommended in most guidelines issued by ultrasound scientific societies. The presence of the gestational sac in the uterine cavity, the number of fetuses, the visualization of embryonic or fetal heart beat, and the datation of pregnancy are the most frequent goals of the first trimester scan.[8-10]

Therefore, during the first trimester ultrasound examination, only if it is specifically requested, a normal NT is then visualized and measured. Because of the implications that the measurement of the NT can carry for the pregnancy (reducing or increasing the risk for chromosomal abnormalities, opening a scenario for invasive prenatal diagnosis), it is advisable to perform the measurement of the NT only in the right setting (after a conscious request for screening by the informed patient and measurement performed by a skilled operators and in a certificated screening program).[11]

THE ENLARGED NUCHAL TRANSLUCENCY

Sometimes a surplus accumulation of fluid in the nuchal tissues can occur (Fig. 77.2). The accumulation of nuchal fluid can be caused by either an increased amount of fluid directed in the nuchal region or by some difficulty in the drainage of the normal quantity of fluid present in the neck.

Regardless the underlying cause of the accumulation of fluids, what is apparent on the ultrasound is the increased thickness of the echo-free space behind the fetal neck, that has been labeled "enlarged nuchal translucency".[12] This space can be absolutely transonic or faintly echogenic, and can be limited to the neck or extended at the whole length of the fetus, as a "space suit" (Fig. 77.3).[13]

When the thickness of an NT is very enlarged at 10–14 weeks, it could easily be visualized during the scan without especially looking for it. This is a situation comparable with that occurs with some soft markers for chromosomopathies in the second trimester (hyperechogenic focus, hyperechogenic bowel, dilated renal pelvis, etc.),[14] where these signs could be obviously evident, without looking for them. While these signs are not malformations, and they could be visible during an ultrasound examination which has not been performed with the finality of chromosomopathies screening, the guidelines of some scientific societies that have

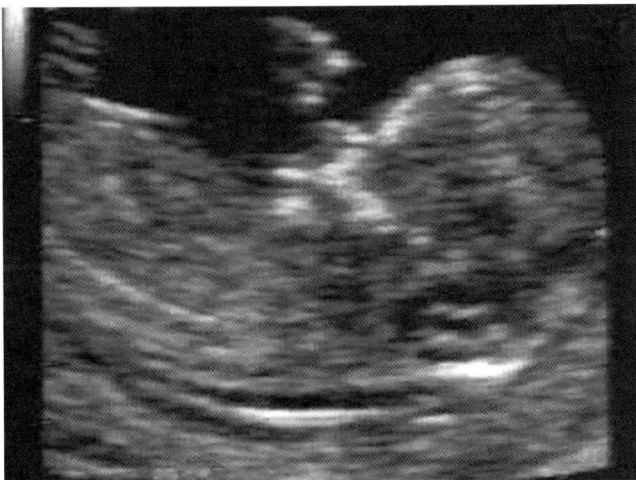

Fig. 77.1: Nuchal translucency

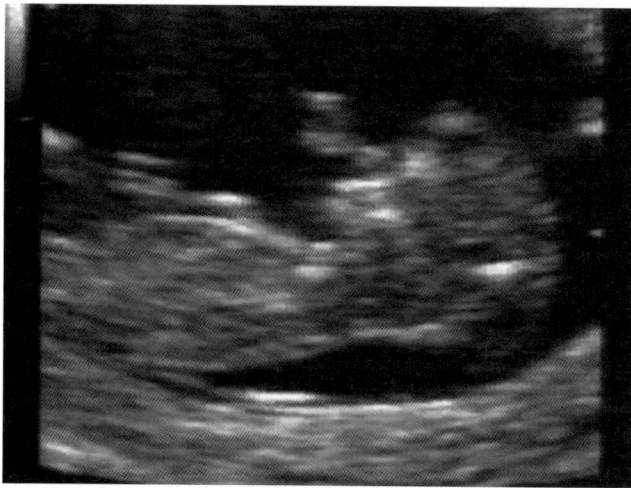

Fig. 77.2: Enlarged nuchal translucency

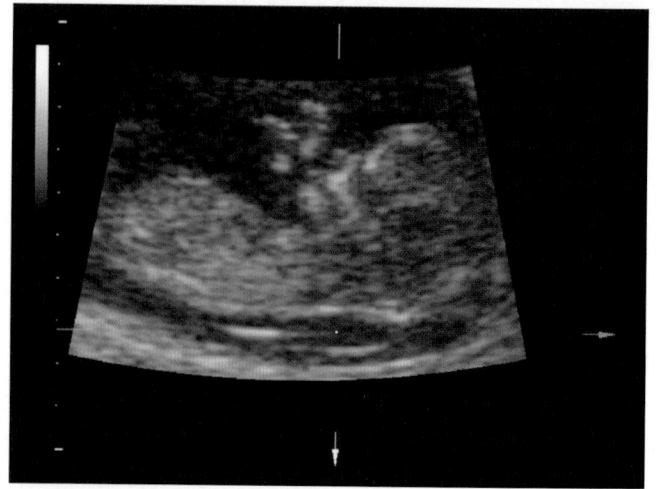

Fig. 77.4: Trisomy 21 fetus with enlarged nuchal translucency

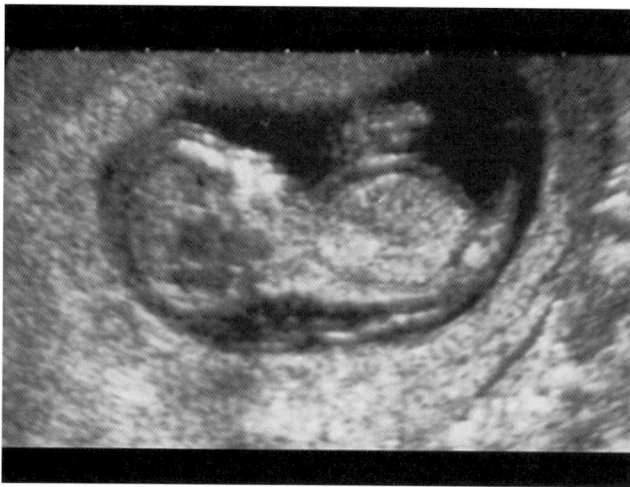

Fig. 77.3: "Space suit" nuchal translucency

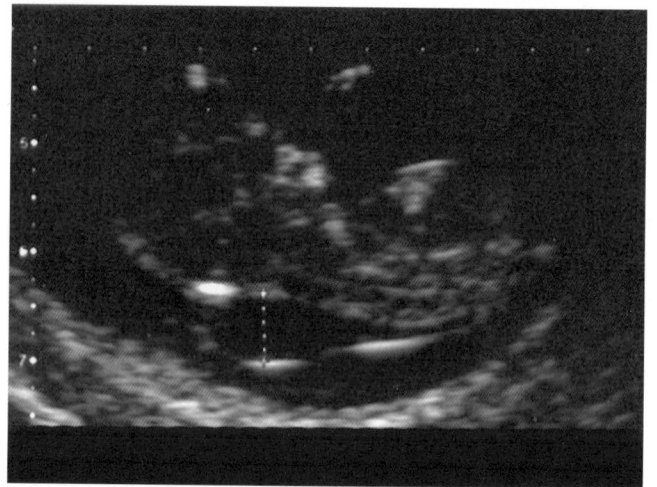

Fig. 77.5: Trisomy 18 with enlarged nuchal translucency

faced this problem, recommend to disclose the presence of evident soft markers to the patient, in order to offer the opportunity of an adequate genetic counseling.[8]

It has been noticed since the early 90s that fetuses with trisomy 21 can show an enlarged NT at first trimester examination (Fig. 77.4).[15]

When an ultrasound scan is performed with the specific intention to measure the NT it is essential to correctly visualize the fetus and to perform the NT measurement in adequate way in order to compare the actual measurement with the reference values. The range of NT thickness varies with CRL, so that the 95th centile for a CRL of 45 mm is quite different than for 82 mm of CRL, and it was evident that a fixed cut-off for NT measurement could not be used with efficiency to assess the enlargement of an NT.[16]

It has been noted that the majority of fetuses with trisomy 21 show an NT greater than the 95th percentile of ranges obtained for normal fetuses with a standard technique of NT measurement. Fetuses with chromosomal abnormalities other than trisomy 21 (trisomy 18, trisomy 13, Turner syndrome, Klinefelter syndrome and triploidy) can have an enlarged NT (Figs 77.5 to 77.7).[16]

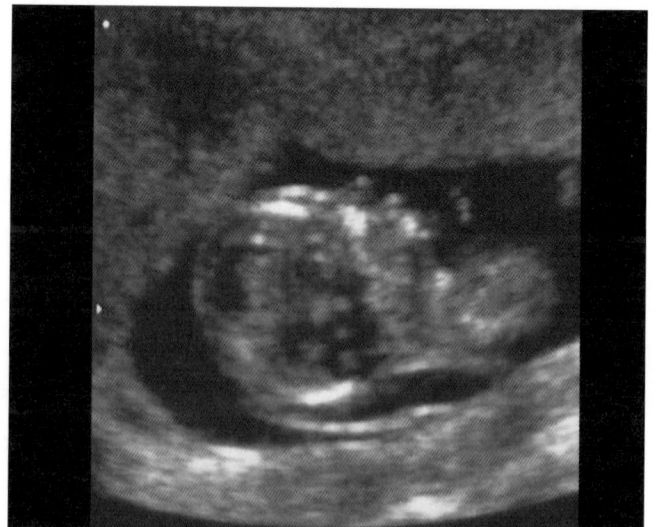

Fig. 77.6: Trisomy 13 with enlarged nuchal translucency

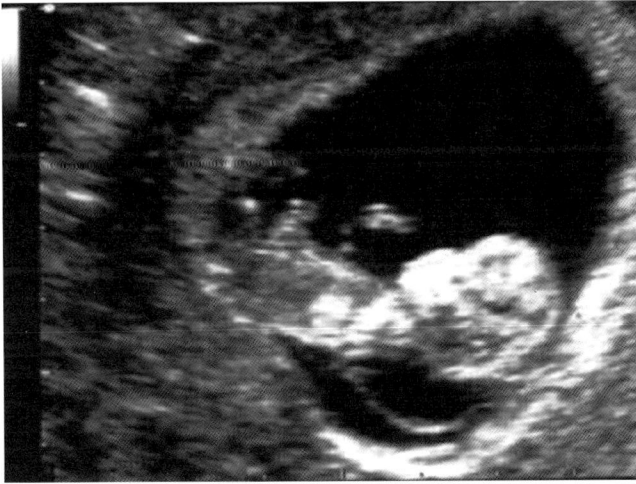

Fig. 77.7: Turner syndrome with enlarged nuchal translucency

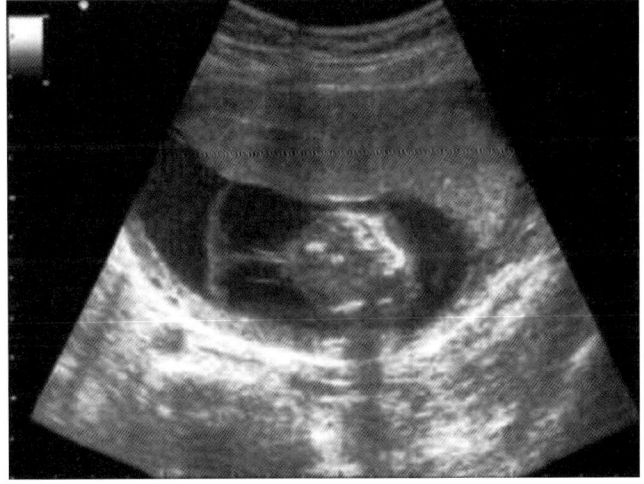

Fig. 77.8: Turner syndrome fetus at 16 weeks

In fetuses with normal and abnormal chromosomes the enlarged NT is frequently a transient sign. In an early study of trisomies 21, at the beginning of the second trimester, a reabsorption of the nuchal edema has been longitudinally described in six cases.[17] A study of the evolution of enlarged NT during the first trimester described a decrease in the thickness that occurred in both chromosomally normal and abnormal fetuses. At second measurement performed in the same fetus, the frequency of decreasing NT was greater in the normal than in the abnormal karyotype fetuses.[18]

In fetuses with Turner syndrome, the evolution of first trimester enlarged NT is frequently described into a cystic hygroma (cystic malformation of the lymphatic system) in the second trimester (Fig. 77.8).[19]

PATHOPHYSIOLOGY OF ENLARGED NUCHAL TRANSLUCENCY

The term of enlarged NT in the first trimester that is used in ultrasound practice may indicate many different background conditions.

An accumulation of fluids in the neck is presumed to come from either an abnormal local composition of the tissues that tend to capture more fluids, or from a situation of hampered reabsorption of a normal quantity of fluids regularly passed from the vessel to the interstitial spaces, or to a condition of increased passage of fluids from the vessel to the connective, due to an abnormal hydrostatic pressure as consequence of impairment of the arterial or venous circulation.[20-26]

In trisomy 21, some alteration in the composition of the skin, with an increased expression of type VI collagen and a raise in the quantity of hyaluronic acid could justify an increased entrapment of liquids, that for reasons not yet explained, in the first trimester fetus is evident only in the nuchal region.[23-24] An extra accumulation of fluid that overcome the normal capacity of mechanism deputate to the drainage may be the cause of enlarged NT in trisomy 21 fetuses.[26]

In Turner syndrome, the accumulation of fluid in the nuchal region seems to be related to a failure in the drainage by the lymphatic system, because of an abnormal structure, that involves either the minor lymphatic vessels in the skin, and the greater vessel,

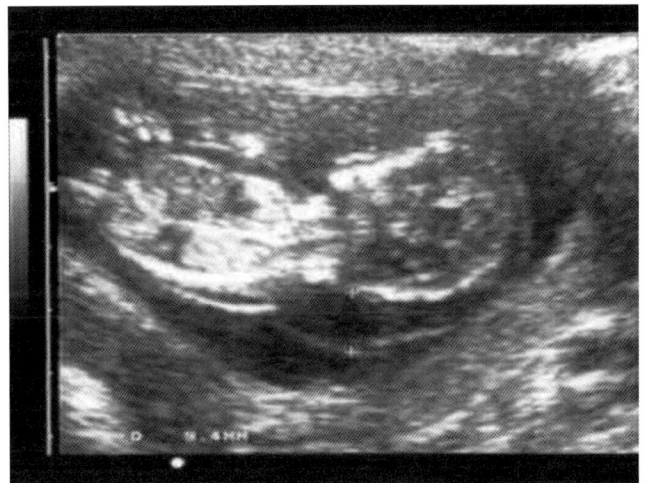

Fig. 77.9: Turner syndrome fetus at 12 weeks

with a lack of definitive connections between the jugular lymphatic sacs and jugular veins system, as an expression of a failure in the development of the lymphatic system, due to the underlying karyotype anomaly (Fig. 77.9).[22,26] In fetuses with Turner syndrome, the first trimester translucencies are typically large, bilateral and septated, occupying the lateral and posterior regions of the neck of the fetus. In Turner syndrome, the first trimester NT is in fact often not transient, with a tendency to evolve into a second trimester "cystic hygroma colli".[26]

A different mechanism related to a temporary lymphatic failure due to a delay in the connection with the venous system has been considered in trisomy 21 and normal fetuses. In these cases, the evolution toward a reabsorption in the second trimester is frequent.[26]

Pathological studies carried out on fetuses with enlarged NT with normal karyotype and trisomies 21 and 18, have in fact shown in the posterior side of the neck of the fetus, exactly where the NT is visualized by ultrasound, the presence of some cavities, negative for immunohistochemical markers for lymphatic vessel endothelium and arteries. These cavities seem to be the result of coalescence of edematous mesenchymal spaces (due to an edematous mesenchymal). In these cases, a lymphatic distension of jugular lymphatic sacs in the lateral side of the neck has been shown to occur prior to the manifestation of the nuchal edema (Figs 77.10 and 77.11). The hypothesis was that the first occurrence would be the delay in the lymphatic drainage, which may then cause the accumulation of mesenchymal fluid and nuchal edema. At 14 weeks, when jugular lymphatic sacs complete their development, making definitive connections with the venous system, both findings (nuchal edema and dilatation of lymphatic sacs) finally resolve.[26-27]

In trisomy 21, another mechanism has been postulated to cause the accumulation of fluids and enlargement of the NT, due to an increase of the perfusion of the vessel direct to the neck and the upper part of the fetus. In pathology studies, a narrowing of the isthmus of the aorta, associated with a dilatation of the supravalvular portion of the vessel has been described. An increased passage of fluids into the connective tissue for hydrostatic pressure factors could be involved in the enlargement of the NT.[28]

An accumulation of extravascular liquids, as it is present in adults with an impairment of cardiac function can also be present in fetuses with chromosomal abnormalities or normal karyotype fetuses, with structural heart abnormality. The subcutaneous edema depends on an impaired reabsorption of fluids due to an increase of the hydrostatic pressure in the venous system. A wide spectrum of heart defects has been described to be present in chromosomal abnormalities and normal fetuses with enlarged NT, but a clear connection between specific cardiac diseases and the development of the enlarged NT in the first trimester of pregnancy has not been demonstrated (Figs 77.12 to 77.15).[28-29]

A relationship between an impaired diastolic function and enlarged NT has been hypothesized on the grounds of some alteration signs on the velocimetry of the ductus venosus in fetuses with abnormal karyotype, cardiac defects and NT thickness.[30-31] The ductus venosus is a vessel that connects the umbilical circulation with the right atrium. In the first trimester of pregnancy the pulsed Doppler waveform of this vessel is characterized by a forward flow with a peak during systole, a second peak in diastole and a forward velocity during atrial contraction (Fig. 77.16). In cases when the pressure in the atrium at the end of diastolic phase is increased (that could be a sign of cardiac dysfunction due to a great number of factors, including some heart structural malformations), the velocity during the atrial contraction in the ductus venosus

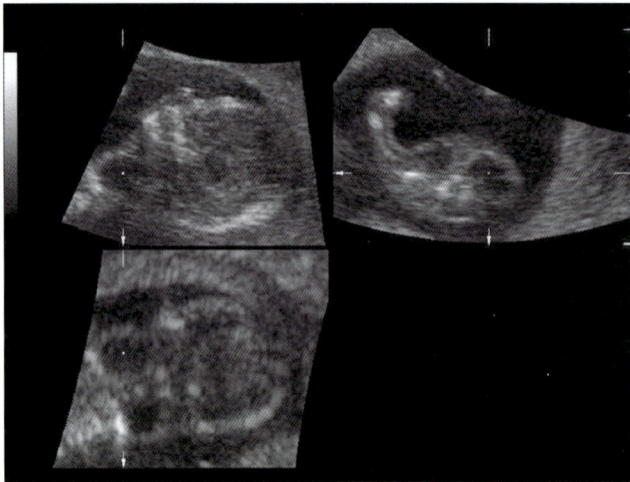

Fig. 77.10: Multiplanar view of a trisomy 21 fetus with enlarged jugular lymphatic sacs

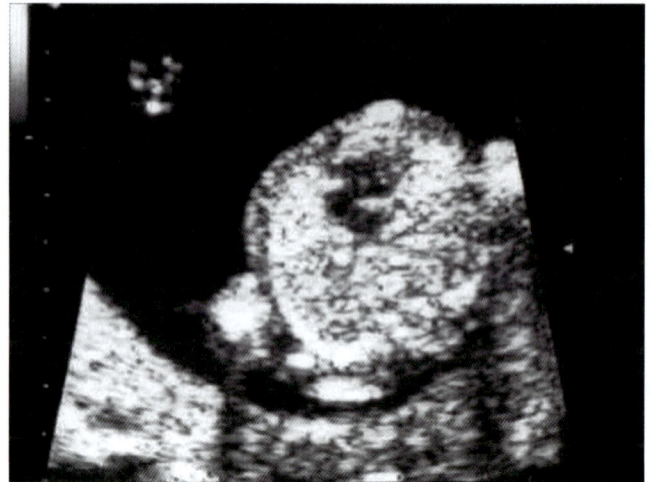

Fig. 77.12: Heart defect in a first trimester fetus with normal karyotype and enlarged nuchal translucency

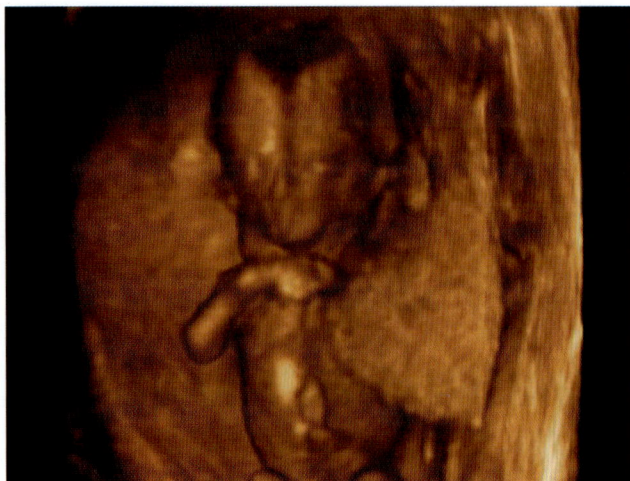

Fig. 77.11: Three-dimensional surface rendering of a trisomy 21 fetus with enlarged jugular lymphatic sacs

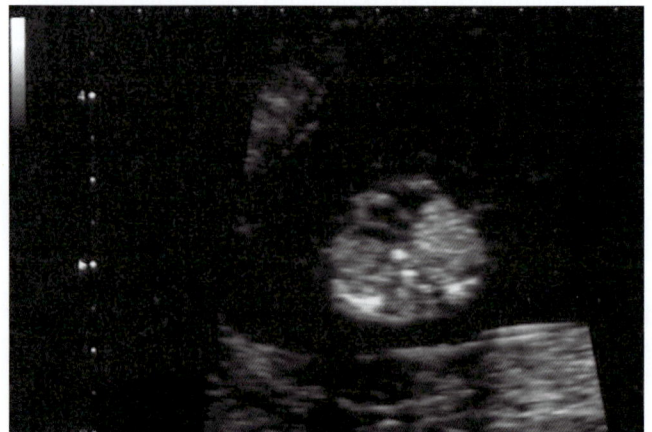

Fig. 77.13: Heart defect in a first trimester fetus with trisomy 21 and enlarged nuchal translucency

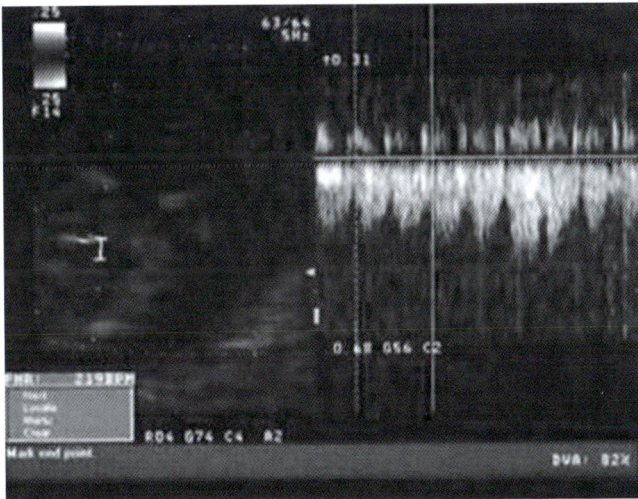

Fig. 77.14: First trimester tachycardia in a first trimester fetus with normal karyotype and enlarged nuchal translucency

decreases, it can be zero or inverted (Figs 77.17 and 77.18). In fetuses with chromosomal abnormalities, that are suspected to have a greater occurrence of cardiac abnormalities, and that show frequently an enlarged NT, the velocimetry of the ductus venosus is frequently altered (70–90%), with an atrial contraction velocity absent or inverted.

Another parameter that has been used to evaluate the alteration of the velocimetry in the ductus venosus is the pulsatility of the waveform, that in chromosomal abnormalities appears increased.[32] If there is a single cause that determines at the same time two parallel consequences as the altered ductus venosus flow and the enlarged nuchal thickness, or if there is a consequential connection between the two findings, and which of these findings happen first, needs to be demonstrated.

Impairment in the diastolic function has been shown in fetuses with enlarged NT in the first trimester and normal karyotype, that persist in the second trimester, and this is demonstrated by an alteration of the velocimetry of the atrium-ventricular valves.[33]

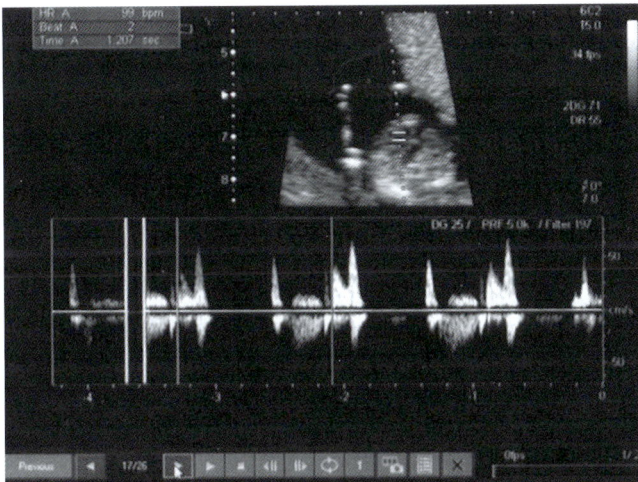

Fig. 77.15: First trimester second degree heart block in a normal karyotype fetus with enlarged nuchal translucency

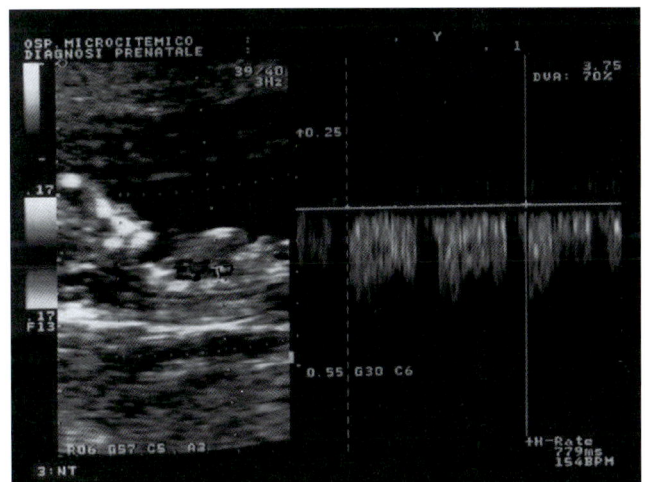

Fig. 77.17: Absent velocity during atrial contraction in the ductus venosus

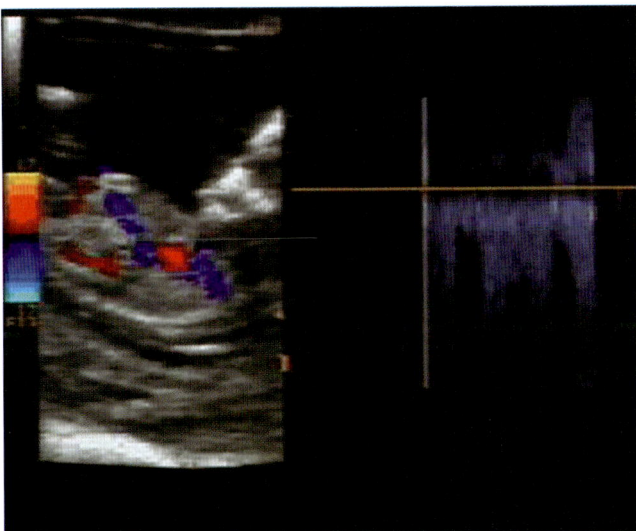

Fig. 77.16: Normal velocity flow in the ductus venosus in a first trimester fetus

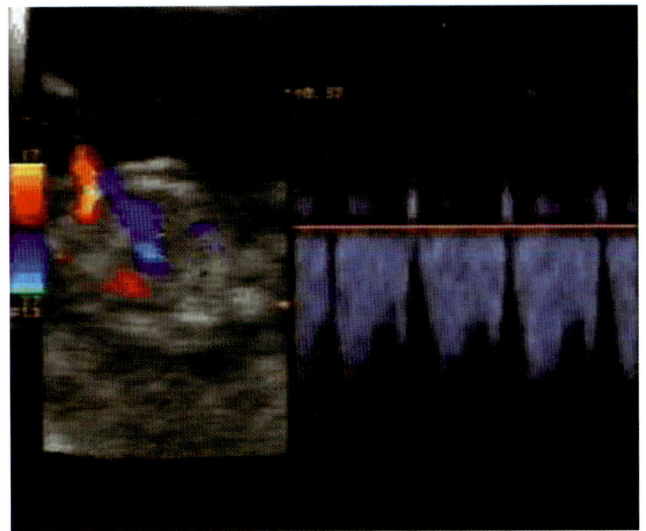

Fig. 77.18: Inverted velocity during atrial contraction in the ductus venosus

In fetuses with enlarged NT, no impairment in the ventricular systolic function has been described. In fact, no difference of umbilical pulsatility index in the first trimester, has been shown in normal karyotype fetuses with normal and enlarged NT, and in trisomy 21 fetuses with enlarged NT.[34]

A mechanism of increased hydrostatic pressure in the thorax has been postulated to be involved in cases of first trimester enlarged NT and venous congestion as in cases of diaphragmatic hernia and skeletal dysplasias.[21]

ENLARGED NUCHAL TRANSLUCENCY FOR TRISOMY 21 SCREENING

Amniocentesis or chorionic villus sampling (CVS) are invasive prenatal diagnosis techniques for fetal karyotype analysis that carry a procedure-related risk of abortion of about 1%. Since the introduction of invasive prenatal diagnosis, medical and financial reasons have pushed to offer karyotype analysis only to high-risk cases, and the maternal age-related risk Down syndrome was the older and most commonly used approach to prenatal screening. The aim of the screening is to select those women that are at high enough risk for Down syndrome to justify an invasive prenatal diagnosis procedure.[35]

In the last 20 years, prenatal ultrasound examination has been able to identify some of the malformations of trisomy 21 fetuses and other aneuploidies, and some of the anatomical features that slightly differ from normal fetuses. The ultrasound approach has been proposed for identification of cases at a higher risk.[14] In the middle 80s, the first finding of trisomy 21 that has been identified by ultrasound as a marker for trisomy 21 was the increased nuchal fold thickness in the second trimester fetuses.[36] Later, in the middle 90s, the association between first trimester increased NT thickness and trisomy 21 and other chromosomal abnormalities was described.[1]

For NT, an algorithm for the calculation of individualized risk and a specific quality control for the test has been proposed since its introduction, while for serum markers for trisomy 21 this is a consolidated approach, for ultrasound in prenatal diagnosis was relatively new.[2]

Frequencies of trisomy 21 cases and normal fetuses were compared for the deviation of the measured NT from the normal expected values, in order to calculate likelihood ratios.[2] Two principal methods have been used to calculate the deviation from the normality: the Delta value and MoM approach.[2,37] The Delta value approach is now considered more correct.[38] Delta value in millimeters indicates the difference from the measured NT and the expected median of NT calculated for normal fetuses given a determined CRL. An estimate of the risk for trisomy 21 was calculated by multiplying the maternal age related risk for trisomy 21 by the likelihood ratios obtained from the NT thickness, giving a new, individual numerical risk.[16] The risk estimate for trisomy 21 based on the ultrasound measurement of NT is based on few but important principles. First of all, the maternal background risk is the essential factor of the screening test for trisomy 21, and each time it needs to be considered in the calculation. Second, the results is given not as "test positive" or "test negative" on the

ground of an arbitrarily chosen cut-off, but the woman is faced with a numerical result, on which she can base her thoughts according to her wishes and anxieties. Third, a quality control method has been applied to ultrasound measurement (this is new for this field of medicine, while it has been used for decades for, i.e. laboratory serum markers). There is evidence that the NT test is reliable, because the inter-operators and inter-centers variability can be reduced and comparable results are obtained, in cases when the measurement is performed according to a defined technique, with adequate training of operators and constant audit of the results.[39] Using this approach, in a multicentric study (22 centers involved), performed over 100,000 cases, with an average maternal age of 28 years, for a risk greater than or equal to 1 in 300, the sensitivity for trisomy 21 has been estimated to be 82%, with 8% false-positive rate.[40] With this performance results the NT test was considered to be the most effective prenatal screening to identify cases at risk for trisomy 21. Comparable results were obtained by other centers where guidelines for NT screening were observed.[5]

Fetuses at higher risk for trisomy 21 because of enlarged NT were at the same time found to be at higher risk for other chromosomopathies as trisomies 18 and 13, triploidy and sex aneuploidies.[40]

CLINICAL IMPORTANCE OF NUCHAL TRANSLUCENCY SCREENING

The availability of an accurate screening test in the first trimester, such as NT, is useful to recognize cases at a higher risk for trisomy 21 at an early stage, in order to offer an early invasive prenatal diagnosis that could be performed preferably by CVS. It is true that when the performance of NT test is considered, the spontaneous intrauterine mortality of affected fetuses, from first trimester to term has to be taken into account. A number of those fetuses identified to be at high risk on the first trimester, and on which an invasive prenatal diagnosis procedure is performed, would be spontaneously demised in uterus before birth, without all the troubles and anxieties that the prenatal screening procedure can carry. In numbers, about 30% of trisomy 21 fetuses that are detected by first trimester NT screening are destined to die during the pregnancy. This percentage is about an extra 10% than the lethality of fetuses detected by a second trimester screening test, that is about 20% to term.[41]

However, there is evidence that for pregnant women there are some particular aspects of prenatal screening that are of value. A test that give the result early in pregnancy, that obviously has at the same time a low rate of false negatives and false positives, with a reduced number of invasive procedures and fetal demises because of procedure-related risk, is considered to be better.[42,43] Enlarged first trimester NT could identify, at the same time, fetuses at higher risk for abnormalities other than chromosomopathies. Cardiac defects, some structural abnormalities and genetic syndromes can occur more frequently in fetuses with enlarged NT than in the general population.[29]

Women at high risk for trisomy 21 because of advanced age can have some advantage to have the NT test offered. In fact, a more precise estimate of individual risk for trisomy 21 can be made, and therefore the opportunity to decide about prenatal diagnosis with more autonomy is given. Reduction of request for

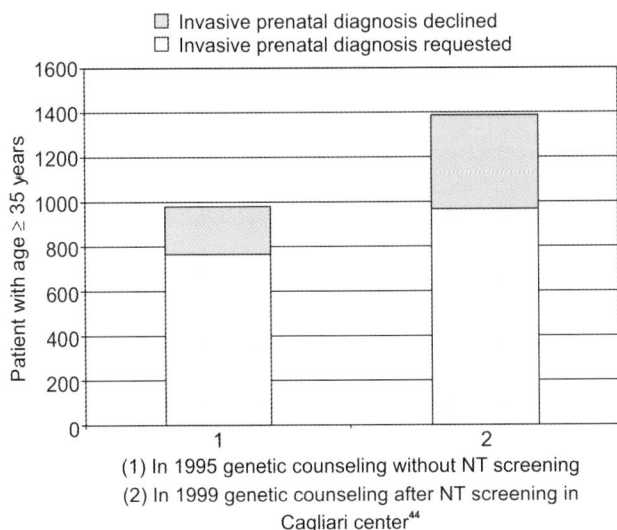

Fig. 77.19: Acceptance of invasive prenatal diagnosis

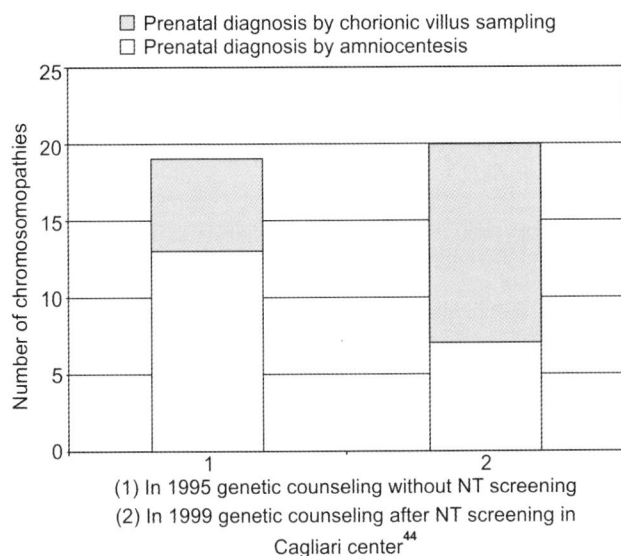

Fig. 77.20: Procedure used for prenatal diagnosis of chromosomopathies

invasive prenatal diagnosis in women aged 35 years or over and earlier detection of cases at risk by first trimester CVS has been underlined when NT screening test is performed in a contest where invasive prenatal diagnosis because of maternal age is offered.[44] (Figs 77.19 and 77.20).

NT screening can be used for chromosomal abnormalities screening with the same accuracy on twin and multiple pregnancies.[45,46]

RECENT DEVELOPMENT OF NUCHAL TRANSLUCENCY SCREENING

At its introduction in clinical practice, NT screening test has been proposed to be performed from 10 weeks plus 3 days (from a 38 mm of CRL). After evidence that around 12 week a better evaluation of fetal anatomy could be in most cases achieved, it was suggested to perform the screening after 45 mm of CRL, so that at the same time, an early detection of structural abnormalities can be obtained.[47]

In order to decrease the false negatives and the rate of invasive testing, the risk obtained by maternal age and NT has been combined with other markers, which occur more frequently in trisomy 21 cases than in normal fetuses, but are not related to the increase of the thickness of first trimester NT. First trimester maternal serum markers, PAPP-A and free β-hCG, combined with NT test, increase the sensitivity to 90% and decrease the false-positive rate to about 3%.[48]

The combination of NT test with the sign of absent nasal bone in the first trimester is still under assessment.[49-50] The integration of the NT test with maternal screening markers of the first and second trimester has been shown to improve the accuracy of the test, but it requires to wait until the second trimester to disclose the result and eventually to offer the diagnosis.[51]

Having the possibility to combine and integrate different tests, a new scenario for trisomy 21 prenatal screening for trisomy 21 is now appearing. Different tests can be performed at different time (one stop, two step, one step), the results can be disclosed after every single test or integrated, the successive test can be performed only in established cases, for example only in borderline cases (contingent test), and each test could obtain different performance.[35] Some tests carry a greater sensitivity, others a greater specificity. There are many options to screen for trisomy 21, but the choice on which direction to move is delicate. If the screening test for trisomy 21 is performed on a financial ground basis, and the national healthcare systems is the purchaser, it can offer a policy of screening that is more cost-effective after a rigorous cost-benefit analysis.

When a screening program regards a disease for which the definitive diagnosis exposes a human being to a potential lethal risk, and, in case of ascertained disease, there is no cure as there is for trisomy 21 at prenatal diagnosis, many ethical problems come into light and they put doctors and patients in front of great dilemmas.

In this specific case of screening, the principle of self determination for the patient, that for decades has been applied to the field of invasive prenatal diagnosis, should be the fundamental issue of the entire process, and should be the goal to be achieved.[52] From the start, all the steps of the screening procedure should be accurately considered, leaving nothing to chance, such as, for example, the first apparently innocent question on how old she is, that everyone asks, on the path to motherhood, to a completely unaware (about prenatal screening troubles) prospective mother.

REFERENCES

1. Nicolaides KH, Azar G, Byrne D, et al. Fetal nuchal translucency screening for chromosomal defects in first trimester of pregnancy. Br Med J. 1992;304:867-9.

2. Pandya PP, Snijders RJ, Johnson SP, et al. Screening for fetal trisomies by maternal age and fetal nuchal translucency thickness at 10 to 14 weeks of gestation. Br J Obstet Gynecol. 1995;102:957-62.

3. Snijders RJ, Nicolaides K. Ultrasound Markers for Chromosomal Defects. London, UK: Pathenon Publishing; 1996.

4. Braithwaite JM, Morris RW, Economides DL. Nuchal translucency measurements: frequency distribution and changes with gestation in a general population. Br J Obstet Gynecol. 1996;103(12):1201-4.

5. Zoppi MA, Ibba RM, Floris M, et al. Fetal nuchal translucency screening in 12,495 pregnancies in Sardinia. Ultrasound Obstet Gynecol. 2001;18:649-51.

6. Pajkrt E, De Graaf IM, Mol BW, et al. Weekly nuchal translucency measurements in normal fetuses. Obstet Gynecol. 1998;91:208-11.

7. Logghe H, Cuckle H, Sehmi I. Centre-specific ultrasound nuchal translucency medians needed for Down syndrome screening. Prenat Diagn. 2003;23:389-92.

8. SIEOG (Società Italiana Ecografia Ostetrica e Ginecologica); Cento. Linee Guida (FE), Italy: Editeam Publishing; 2002.

9. Antenatal care routine care for the healthy pregnant woman. Clinical Guideline. National Collaborating Centre for Women's and Children's Health. London, UK: RCOG press; 2003.

10. Practice guidelines for the Performance of an Antepartum Obstetric Ultrasound Examination. AIUM (American Institute of Ultrasound in Medicine); 2003.

11. Chasen ST, Skupsi DW, McCullogh LB, et al. Prenatal informed consent for sonogram: The time for first trimester nuchal translucency has come. J Ultrasound Med. 2001;20:1147-52.

12. Nicolaides KH. The 11-14 Weeks Scan. Fetal Medicine Foundation, London; 2004.

13. Shulman LP, Phillips OP, Emerson DS, et al. Fetal 'space-suit' hydrops in the first trimester: Differentiating risk for chromosome abnormalities by delineating characteristics of nuchal translucency. Prenat Diagn. 2000;20(1):30-2.

14. Benacerraf BR. The second-trimester fetus with Down syndrome: Detection using sonographic features. Ultrasound Obstet Gynecol. 1996;7:147-55.

15. Szabo J, Gellen J. Nuchal fluid accumulation in trisomy 21 detected by vaginosonography in first trimester. Lancet. 1990;336(8723):1133.

16. Nicolaides KH, Subire NJ, Snijders RJ, et al. The 11-14 Week's Scan Book. London, UK: Pathenon Publishing; 2001.

17. Pandya PP, Snijders RJ, Johnson S, et al. Natural history of trisomy 21 fetuses with increased nuchal translucency thickness. Ultrasound Obstet Gynecol. 1995;5:381-3.

18. Zoppi MA, Ibba RM, Floris M, et al. Changes in nuchal translucency thickness in normal and abnormal karyotype fetuses. Br J Obstet Gynecol. 2003;110:584-8.

19. Fukada Y, Yasumizu T, Takizawa M, et al. The prognosis of fetuses with transient nuchal translucency in the first and early second trimester. Acta Obstet Gynecol Scand. 1997;76:913-6.

20. Moscoso G. Fetal nuchal translucency: A need to understand the physiological basis. Ultrasound Obstet Gynecol. 1995;5:6-8.

21. Von Kaisenberg CS, Brand-Saberi B, Jonat W, et al. Pathophysiology of increased nuchal translucency in chromosomally abnormal fetuses. Prenat Neonat Med. 1999;4:431-40.

22. von Kaisenberg CS, Krenn V, Ludwig M, et al. Morphological classification of nuchal skin in human fetuses with trisomy 21, 18, and 13 at 1218 weeks and in a trisomy 16 mouse. Anat Embryol. 1998;197:105-24.

23. von Kaisenberg CS, Brand-Saberi B, Christ B, et al. Collagen type VI gene expression in the skin of trisomy 21 fetuses. Obstet Gynecol. 1998;91:319-23.

24. Bohlandt S, von Kaisenberg CS, Wewetzler K, et al. Hyaluronan in the nuchal skin of chromosomally abnormal fetuses. Hum Rep. 2000;15:1155-8.

25. Haak MC, van Vugt JM. Pathophysiology of incresed nuchal translucency: A review of the literature. Hum Reprod Update. 2003;2:175-84.

26. Haak MC, Bartelings MM, Jackson DG, et al. Increased nuchal translucency is associated with jugular lymphatic distension. Hum Reprod. 2002;17:1086-92.

27. Castelli E, Todros T, Mattutino G, et al. Light and scanning electron microscope study of nuchal translucency in a normal fetus. Ultrasound Obstet Gynecol. 2003;21:514-6.

28. Hyett J, Moscoso G, Nicolaides K. Abnormalities of the heart and great arteries in first trimester chromosomally abnormal fetuses. Am J Med Genet. 1997;17:207-16.

29. Hyett J, Perdu M, Sharland G, et al. Using fetal nuchal translucency to screen for major congenital cardiac defects at 10-14 weeks of gestation: Population based cohort study. Br Med J. 1999;318:70-71.

30. Matias A, Montenegro N. Ductus venosus blood flow in chromosomally abnormal fetuses at 11 to 14 weeks of gestation. Semin Perinatol. 2001;25:32-7.

31. Zoppi MA, Putzolu M, Ibba RM, et al. First trimester ductus venosus velocimetry in relation to nuchal translucency thickness and fetal karyotype. Fetal Diagn Ther. 2002;17:52-7.

32. Antolin E, Comas C, Torrents M, et al. The role of ductus venosus blood flow assessment in screening for chromosomal abnormalities at 10-16 weeks of gestation. Ultrasound Obstet Gynecol. 2001;17:295-300.

33. Rizzo G, Muscatello A, Angelini E, et al. Abnormal cardiac function in fetuses with increased nuchal translucency. Ultrasound Obstet Gynecol. 2003;21(6): 539-42.

34. Zoppi MA, Ibba RM, Putzolu M, et al. First trimester umbilical artery pulsatility index in fetuses presenting enlarged nuchal translucency. Prenat Diagn. 2000;20:701-4.

35. Cuckle HS. Growing complexity in the choice of Down's syndrome screening policy. Ultrasound Obstet Gynecol. 2002;19:323-6.

36. Benacerraf BR, Barss VA, Laboda LA. A sonographic sign for the detection in the second trimester of the fetus with Down's syndrome. Am J Obstet Gynecol. 1985;151:1078-9.

37. Biagiotti R, Periti E, Brizzi L, et al. Comparison between two methods of standardization for gestational age differences in fetal nuchal translucency measurement in first trimester screening for trisomy 21. Ultrasound Obstet Gynecol. 1997;9(4):248-52.

38. Spencer K, Bindra R, Nix AB, et al. Delta-NT or NT MoM: Which is the most appropriate method for calculating accurate patient-specific risks for trisomy 21 in the first trimester? Ultrasound Obstet Gynecol. 2003;22(2):142-8.

39. Monni G, Zoppi MA, Ibba RM, et al. Fetal nuchal translucency test for Down's syndrome. Lancet. 1997;350:1631.

40. Snijders RJ, Noble P, Sebire N, et al. UK multicentre project on assessment of risk of trisomy 21 by maternal age and fetal nuchal translucency thickness at 10-14 weeks of gestation. Lancet. 1998;352:343-6.

41. Snijders RJ, Sundberg K, Holzgreve W, et al. Maternal age and gestation-specific risk for trisomy 21. Ultrasound Obstet Gynecol. 1999;13:167-70.

42. Monni G, Ibba RM, Zoppi MA. Antenatal screening for Down's syndrome. Lancet. 1998;352:1631-2.

43. Mulvey S, Zachariah R, McIlwaine K, et al. Do women prefer to have screening tests for Down syndrome that have the lowest screen-positive rate or the highest detection rate? Prenat Diagn. 2003;23(10):828-32.

44. Zoppi MA, Ibba RM, Putzolu M, et al. Nuchal translucency and the acceptance of invasive prenatal chromosomal diagnosis in women aged 35 and older. Obstet Gynecol. 2001;97:916-20.

45. Sebire NJ, Snijders RJ, Hughes K, et al. Screening for trisomy 21 in twin pregnancies by maternal age and fetal nuchal translucency thickness at 10-14 weeks of gestation. Br J Obstet Gynecol. 1996;03: 999-1003.

46. Monni G, Zoppi MA, Ibba RM, et al. Nuchal translucency in multiple pregnancies. Croat Med J. 2000;41:266-9.

47. Souka AP, Krampl E, Bakalis S, et al. Outcome of pregnancy in chromosomally normal fetuses with increased nuchal translucency in the first trimester. Ultrasound Obstet Gynecol. 2001;18:5-8.

48. Spencer K, Souter V, Tul N, et al. A screening program for trisomy 21 at 10-14 weeks using fetal nuchal translucency, maternal serum free beta-human chorionic gonadotropin and pregnancy-associated plasma protein-A. Ultrasound Obstet Gynecol. 1999;13:231-7.

49. Cicero S, Curcio P, Papageorghiou A, et al. Absence of nasal bone in fetuses with trisomy 21 at 11-14 weeks of gestation: An observational study. Lancet. 2001;358:1665-7.

50. Monni G, Zoppi MA, Ibba RM. Absence of nasal bone and detection of trisomy 21. Lancet. 2002;359:1343.

51. Wald NJ, Watt HC, Hackshaw AK. Integrated screening for Down's syndrome on the basis of test performed during the first and second trimesters. N Engl J Med. 1999;12:461-7.

52. Chasen ST, Skupski DW, McCullough LB, et al. Prenatal informed consent for sonogram: the time for first trimester nuchal translucency has come. J Ultrasound Med. 2001; 20(11):1147-52.

78 First Trimester Ultrasound Screening for Down's Syndrome in Multiple Gestations

G Monni, MA Zoppi

INTRODUCTION

In the last decades, the older maternal age at conception and the more frequent use of assisted reproductive techniques, have moved to a constant increased rate of multiple pregnancies. Some specific prenatal and perinatal problems make these pregnancies at higher risk.[1-4] Neonatal mortality and morbidity is higher in multiple pregnancies, and maternal complications are more frequent.

Moreover, mostly because of the advanced maternal age, multiple pregnancies are at higher risk for chromosomal defects. At the same time, as these pregnancies (frequently obtained after years of infertility) are especially precious to the prospective parents, there is no unanimous acceptance of the need of invasive prenatal diagnosis procedures, which are more difficult to perform than in singleton pregnancies.[5,6]

Noninvasive screening test for chromosomal abnormalities in multiple pregnancies are more acceptable. Maternal serum biochemistry for trisomy 21 in multiple pregnancies has been proposed.[7,8] However, it may be difficult to interpretate because of the interference between the serum marker concentrations and assisted reproductive therapies, and a great concern is the identification of which of the fetuses is positive at the biochemical test.

For invasive prenatal diagnosis, the risk of miscarriage related to the procedure is increased, depending mostly on the number of needle insertions.[9,10] Prenatal diagnosis of a chromosomal abnormality in multizygotic multiples, allows an informed decision about the management of the pregnancy. Therefore, an accurate estimate of individual fetal risk for chromosomal abnormality is advisable in multiple pregnancies.

Ultrasound screening for trisomy 21 by first trimester nuchal translucency (NT) measurement is correctly applicable in twin and multiples.[11-13] The test gives an individual risk for each fetus and it is comparable in the accuracy to the screening test for trisomy 21 in singleton pregnancies.[14-17]

TYPE OF MULTIPLES

Zygosity depends on the type of conception.

Monozygotic pregnancies originate from the division of a single zygote, and account about 30% of twin pregnancies. The frequency of monozygotic pregnancy is stable in the world and among different populations at around 1 case on 250 deliveries. The origin of monozygotic pregnancy is unknown. Next to the theory of an accidental event, a delay in the implantation of the zygote, with a reduction of oxygen transport, has been hypothesized.[18]

Multizygotic pregnancies originate from the fertilization of two or more oocytes by two or more spermatozoa (Fig. 78.1). Dizygotic pregnancies account for about 70% of the total twin pregnancies.

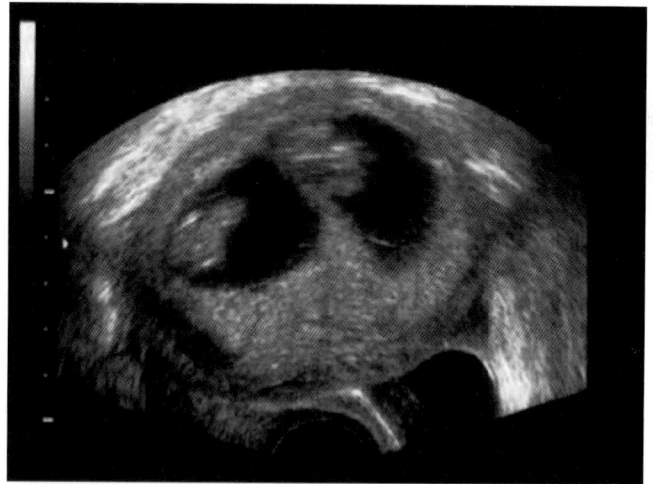

Fig. 78.1: A dichorionic diamniotic twin pregnancy at 9 weeks

The frequency of dizygotic pregnancy varies among population, and the origin appears to be multifactorial. High levels of follicle stimulating hormone (FSH), advanced maternal age, high grade of parity, tall maternal stature and proportionate maternal weight (reflecting a good nutritional maternal status and probably higher levels of FSH), ethnical and familiar inherited factors, seasonality (peak of those kind of conceptions in summer), the application of technologies of assisted reproduction and the use of drugs for the induction of ovulation, support an increased frequency of multiple conceptions.[1,2] The in vitro manipulation of embryos in techniques of assisted reproduction and the use of special culture mediums, seem to induce a greater frequency of iatrogenic monozygotic pregnancies (Fig. 78.2).[19]

The chorionicity depends on the type of placentation. Dizygotic and multizygotic pregnancies are always dichorionic and multichorionic (Fig. 78.3). Monozygotic pregnancies can be dichorionic or monochorionic, and the chorionicity depends on the time of the division of the conceptus (Fig. 78.4).

If the division occurs by the third day from fertilization (and this happen in about 30% of monozygotic pregnancies), two placentas are generated. If the division occurs between the fourth and the eighth day from fertilization (and this happens in about 70% of monozygotic pregnancies), the placenta will be single with two amniotic cavities (monochorionic, diamniotic pregnancy). If the division occurs between ninth day and thirteenth day from fertilization (it happens in less than 1% of monozygotic pregnancies), the placenta and the amniotic cavity will be only one (monochorionic, monoamniotic pregnancy). In very rare cases, the division occurs by fourteenth to sixteenth days from conception, and the result is the conjoined twins.

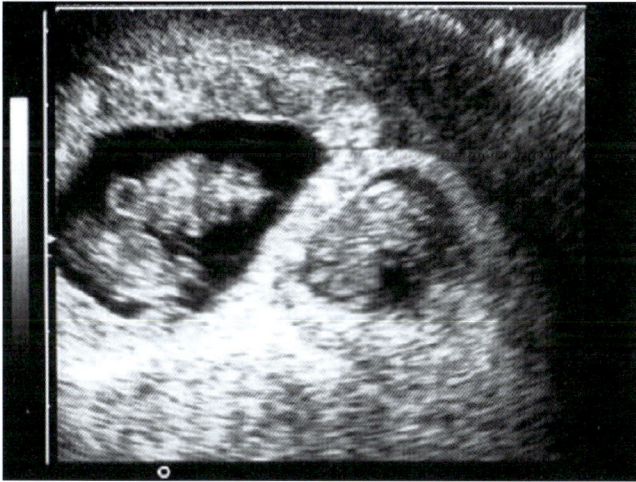

Fig. 78.2: A dichorionic triamniotic triplet pregnancy obtained by in vitro fertilization

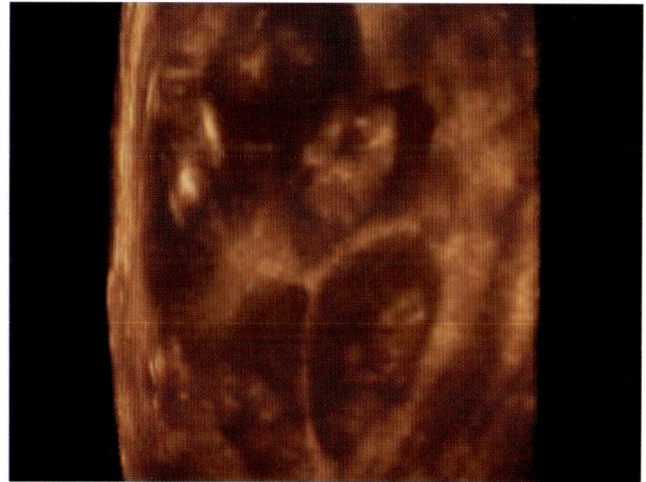

Fig. 78.3: 3D rendering of multizygotic pregnancy (9 fetuses)

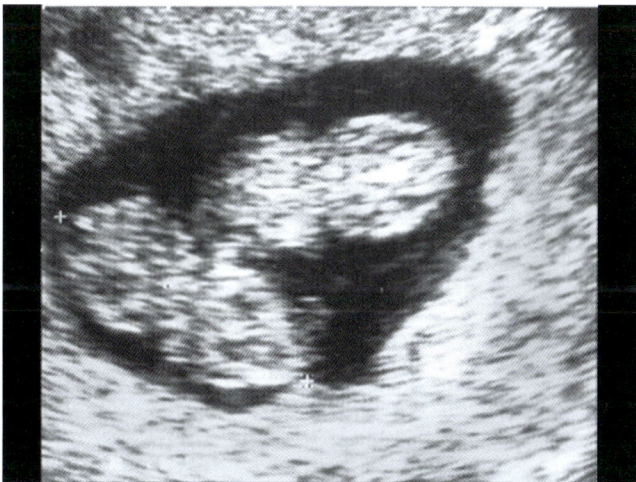

Fig. 78.4: A monochorionic diamniotic pregnancy at 9 weeks

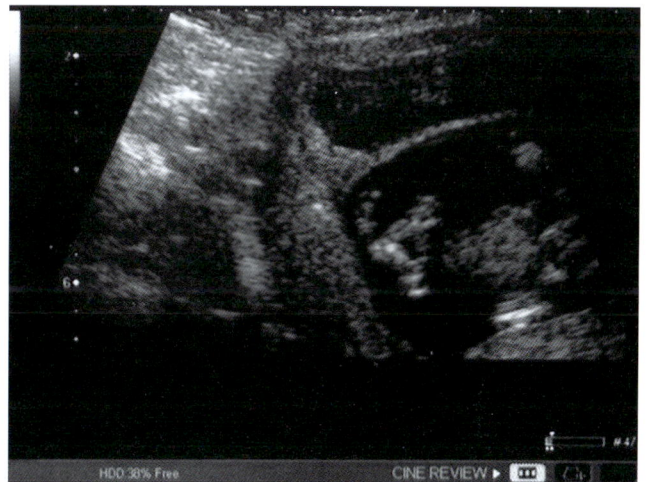

Fig. 78.5: First trimester lambda sign in a dichorionic pregnancy

Monozygotic twins are at higher risk for structural anomalies than multizygotic because of higher potential errors in the division of the zygote and pre-embryo.[1]

PRENATAL ULTRASOUND DETERMINATION OF CHORIONICITY

Prenatal diagnosis of chorionicity can be made easier by ultrasound in the first trimester. By transvaginal ultrasound, gestational sacs can be seen at 5 weeks of gestation (from 4 weeks plus 2 or 3 days), and the number of sacs indicates the number of placentas (monochorionic, dichorionic, trichorionic, etc.). As the gestation proceeds, the septum between the sacs become thinner, and only a triangular structure, the "lambda sign" or "twin-peak sign", remains from 10 weeks to 14 weeks (Fig. 78.5). In monochorionic pregnancy, there is no chorionic tissue between the two amniotic sacs, and the joint of membranes to the chorionic sac is called "T sign" (Fig. 78.6). In dichorionic pregnancies, later in pregnancy, the "lambda sign" is difficult to visualize in all case, and it can completely disappear around 20 weeks (Fig. 78.7).[20]

The visualization of the "lambda sign" is an unequivocal sign of dichorionicity, while the absence in the second trimester is not sufficient to exclude the presence of two placentas. In triplet trichorionic pregnancies, the junction of interfetal membranes is called "ipsilon zone" (Fig. 78.8).[21]

The accurate identification of chorionicity is one of most important goal of obstetrics ultrasound in multiple gestations, and in all cases it should be ideally performed by first trimester, so that the risk of each individual pregnancy can be assessed.

Monochorionic pregnancies are at higher risk than dichorionic pregnancies of prenatal and perinatal problems, as they are monozygotic, and because of the occurrence of specific problems due to transplacental circulation imbalance, which is the twin-to-twin transfusion syndrome. This complication occurs in about 20% of monochorionic pregnancies and frequently manifests itself at 16–22 weeks, by polyhydramnios in one sac and oligoanhydramnios in the other sac. If untreated, the mortality is about 90%. Amniodrainage or laser coagulation of arteriovenous connections in the placenta are the therapies proposed in the second trimester, allowing a survival of about 50% of cases.[22]

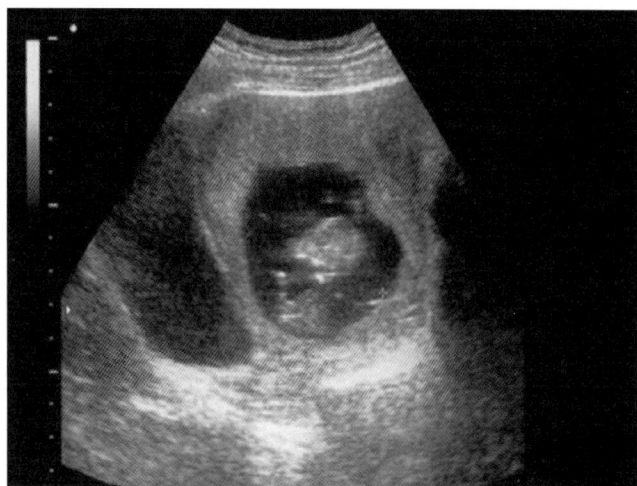

Fig. 78.6: Absence of lambda sign (T sign) in a monochorionic twin pregnancy

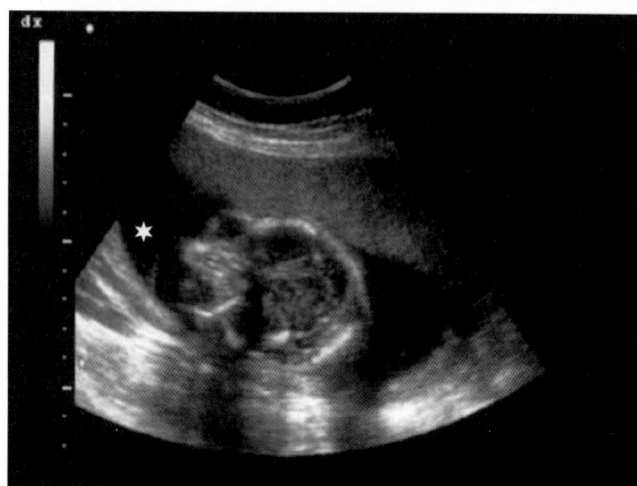

Fig. 78.7: Second trimester dichorionic pregnancy: the lambda sign has disappeared (*)

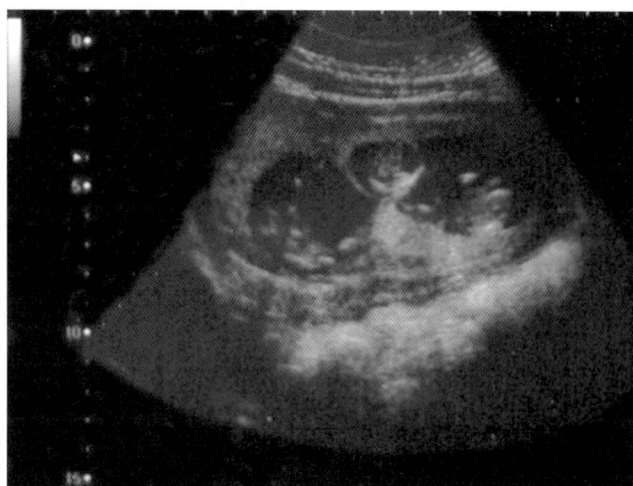

Fig. 78.8: The ipsilon sign in a trichorionic pregnancy

RISK OF CHROMOSOMAL ABNORMALITIES IN MULTIPLES

To calculate the risk of chromosomal abnormalities in multiple pregnancies, it is fundamental to estimate the zygosity.

For monozygotic pregnancies, if cases with mitotic nondisjunction are excluded that determine "heterokaryotypia", the karyotype in both fetuses would be the same.[23] Fetuses can be discordant for anomalies that are generated by the splitting phenomenon, but are concordant for anomalies genetically-determined. Both fetuses have the same karyotype either normal or abnormal.

For multiple pregnancies derived from multizygotic conception, discordant karyotypes are expected. Therefore, prenatal sonographic estimation of zygosity is fundamental in the process of risk calculation.[9,24] In prenatal life, ultrasonographic evaluation of the placentas can give information in this direction. DNA analysis of the fetal or neonatal sampling allows a definitive diagnosis of zygosity.

When a monochorionic pregnancy is diagnosed by prenatal ultrasound (whether monoamniotic or diamniotic), monozygosity can be supposed, and an equal risk for trisomy 21 for both fetuses, similar to the maternal age-related risk, can be calculated. When

dichorionic or multiple placentas are evidenced, a little probability of monozygotic pregnancy cannot be excluded, but the most frequent condition is multizygotic pregnancy. If the assessment is made in a period where it is possible to define by ultrasound the fetal gender, and the placentas are multiple, in cases with discordant sex, the probability of multizygosity is validated. The risk for the pregnancy of having one fetus with trisomy 21 is calculated by the sum of the risk for each fetus. For example, in a triplet trizygotic pregnancy, if the maternal trisomy 21 background risk is 1 in 150, the final risk for the entire pregnancy is 1 in 150 + 1 in 150 + 1 in 150. For calculations, risks can be expressed as odds (that is 1:149 + 1: 149+ 1:149), that is about 3:149, or 1:47, for a final risk for the pregnancy to have one fetus with trisomy 21 of 1 in 48. In multichorionic pregnancies, the risk for all fetuses to have trisomy 21 is very rare, this being calculated by multiplying the maternal age risk for one fetus for the risk of the other. For example, in a dichorionic and "hypothetical" dizygotic pregnancy, where the maternal age risk for trisomy 21 is 1 in 150, the background risk of the entire pregnancy is calculated by multiplying 1:149 X 1:149, then 1:22,201, that is a risk of 1 in 22,202.

A sort of uncertainty is originated by the presence of those cases of monozygotic dichorionic pregnancies that are unrecognized in prenatal life, where the background risk of the pregnancy would be the same as the age-related risk for trisomy 21 of the pregnant woman.

INVASIVE PRENATAL DIAGNOSIS PROCEDURES FOR KARYOTYPE ANALYSIS IN MULTIPLES

When a multiple pregnancy is discovered, extra counseling is due regarding procreative risks, pregnancy-related risk for the mother, prenatal management of the pregnancy, screening and prenatal diagnosis of fetal anomalies and chromosomal abnormalities is advisable.[9,10]

When an invasive procedure for prenatal diagnosis is planned, whatever is the approach considered (chorionic villus sampling, amniocentesis, fetal blood sampling), some fundamental conditions should be fulfilled.

The knowledge of the type of placentation is imperative (mono or multichorionic placenta). Each sample obtained from a distinct twin should be defined (or checked by biological tests that analyze the fetal phenotype or genotype); each fetus should be mapped carefully by ultrasound during the procedure to later allow the precise identification when the result from diagnosis becomes available. We should consider the increased risk of procedure-related abortions, of invasive diagnosis in multiples, compared to singles, which depends among others factors, mostly on multiple needle entrances through the uterus.

When the operators are faced with invasive procedures in multiple pregnancies, a specific experience and skill in this particular field of prenatal diagnosis is required.

SELECTIVE FETOCIDE AND MULTIFETAL EMBRYO REDUCTION

The diagnosis of a single affected twin after a procedure of invasive prenatal diagnosis, can consents to plan a selective termination of the affected fetus and to continue the pregnancy of the normal fetus.

Multifetal embryo reduction is an option that could be considered for therapeutical options in cases of high order multiple pregnancies. Maternal and fetal risk (related to high prematurity) are increased in these pregnancies. The neonatal and pregnancy outcome has been shown to improve in cases of four or higher multiples reduced to twin, because a significant increase of the gestational age at delivery, and a better maternal outcome. At present time, the role of embryo reduction for the management of triplet pregnancies is under discussion.[25,26]

Embryo reduction is usually performed in the first trimester, because it carries fewer complications than in the second, by intrathoracic or intracardiac injection of potassium chloride at 11–13 weeks, under ultrasonographic continuous guidance. When the number of fetuses is high, it is preferable to perform the reduction by steps.

At the beginning, when performing this procedure, the choice as to which fetus to reduce was based fundamentally on technical considerations (the fetus nearest to the uterine surface or the one easier to reduce for the operator). The likelihood to reduce a normal fetus while maintaining some abnormal cases (affected by structural anomalies or chromosomopathies) was considered. Therefore, it was proposed to offer in invasive prenatal diagnosis for karyotype by chorionic villus sampling in all cases before performing embryo reduction.[27] Because of the difficulties and costs of such invasive prenatal diagnosis in multiples, and the greater risk of miscarriage related to the numerous procedures carried out, this approach has not been universally approved and performed.

To avoid a nonselective reduction and to decrease the use of invasive procedures, it has been considered to offer the NT screening before embryo reduction. In fact, the finding of an enlarged NT, allowing the possibility to calculate the individual risk for trisomy in each fetus, can identify cases at higher risk for chromosomal abnormalities and for structural malformation in multiple pregnancies.[28]

NUCHAL TRANSLUCENCY IN MULTIPLES

The ultrasound measurement of the soft tissues behind the fetal neck (nuchal translucency thickness or NT) (Fig. 78.9), and the combination of the likelihood ratios obtained with the maternal

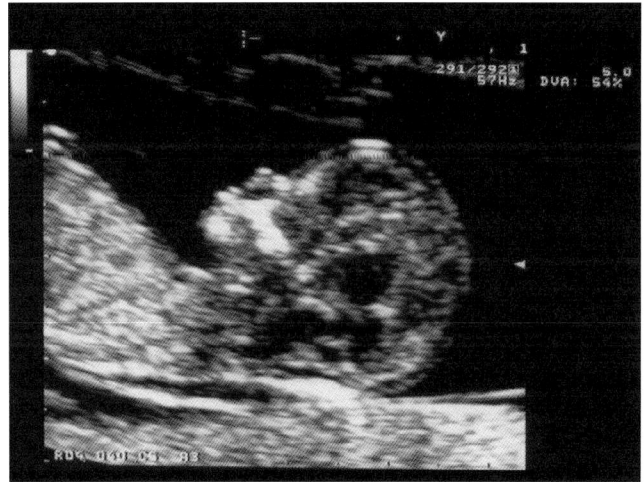

Fig. 78.9: Nuchal translucency

background risk for trisomy 21, is a valid test of screening to identify fetuses with chromosomal abnormalities.

In multiple pregnancies, an individual risk for trisomy 21 can be calculated for each fetus, and, as for the background risk due to maternal age, the risk for the entire pregnancy can be considered.

In twin and multiple pregnancies, screening for chromosomal abnormalities by NT can be performed and it is as accurate as in singleton pregnancies.[14-17]

In a large collaborative study on 448 twin pregnancies, Sebire et al. have found an enlarged NT in 7.3% of all cases and in 7 out of 8 cases of trisomy 21.[15]

NT measurement can be used in high-order multiple pregnancies, and in those cases obtained by assisted reproductive technologies, because no evident difference has been found in the rate of enlarged NT than in spontaneous multichorionic pregnancies, and the sensitivity was the same.[17]

The increased accumulation of fluid in the fetal nuchal, leading to the ultrasound finding of an enlarged NT, can be determined by several different mechanisms: cardiac failure, abnormal or delayed development of the lymphatic vessels, altered composition of the connective tissue of the skin or venous congestion due to an increased pressure in the fetal thorax.[29,30]

The presence of an enlarged NT is associated with an increased rate of chromosomal abnormalities, but moreover the risk for structural malformations and mostly cardiac defects in fetuses with normal karyotype is increased.[31,32]

It has to be considered that a higher frequency of fetal malformation per pregnancy is expected in multifetal pregnancies than in singleton pregnancies, and in a dizygotic twin pregnancy there is a slight chance of a double risk per pregnancy for fetal malformations (because of the independent probability that is carried by each fetus).

In multiple pregnancies, the absence of nasal bone visualization, which is another accurate soft marker for trisomy 21 in the first trimester, can be used with the same efficiency as in singleton pregnancies (Fig. 78.10). About 70% of trisomy 21 and an important percentage of other chromosomal abnormalities as trisomy 18 and 13, 45, X0, can manifest the sign of the absent nasal bone at ultrasound examination performed at 11–14 weeks (Figs 78.11 to 78.13).[33,34]

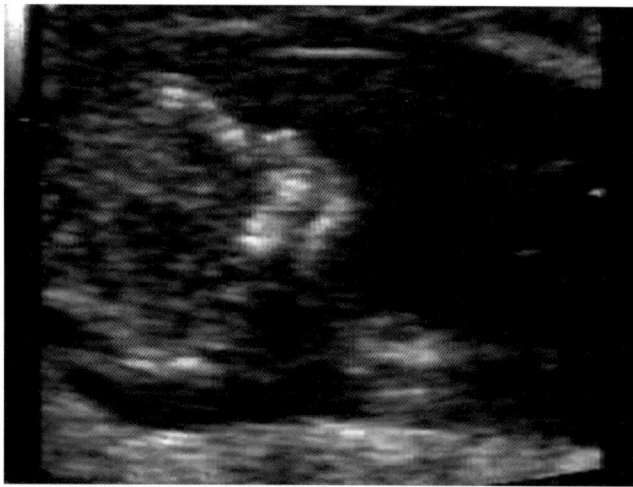

Fig. 78.10: Absent nasal bone in a trisomy 21 fetus

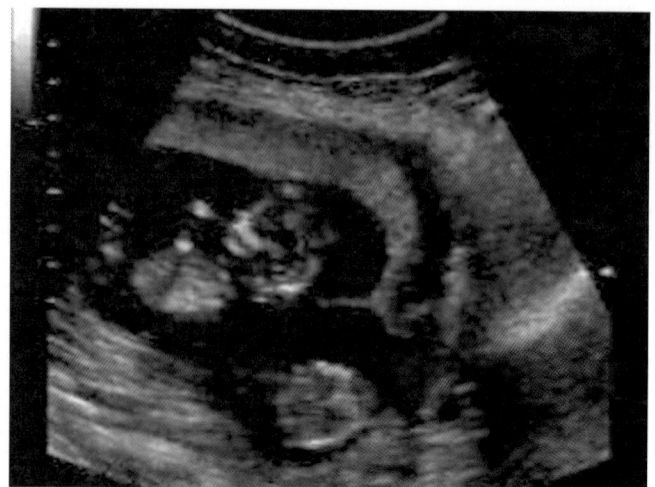

Fig. 78.11: Dichorionic pregnancy with a normal fetus and a fetus with trisomy 21

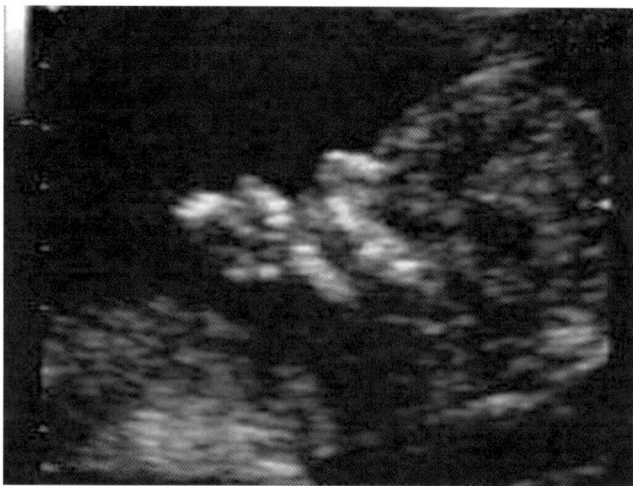

Fig. 78.12: Dichorionic pregnancy: the fetus with normal karyotype with normal nasal translucency and present nasal bone

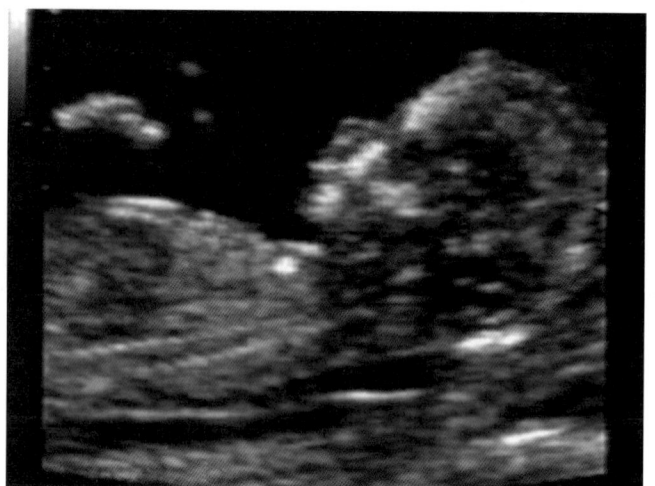

Fig. 78.13: Dichorionic pregnancy: the fetus with trisomy 21 with enlarged nasal translucency and absent nasal bone

THE CASE OF ENLARGED NT IN MONOCHORIONIC PREGNANCIES

In monozygotic pregnancies, the rate of Mendelian disorders and chromosomal abnormalities are identical to those of singleton pregnancies, while there is an increased risk of structural malformations. Malformations due to disruption mechanisms, as midline facial, heart and abdomen anomalies are more frequent.

A higher rate of enlarged NT has been described in monochorionic pregnancies. The enlarged NT has been described in both fetuses or in one. The enlarged NT in monochorionic pregnancies can indicate fetuses at higher risk for chromosomal abnormalities, or structural defects or can be a possible early manifestation of heart failure due to twin-to-twin transfusion.[35]

When in a monochorionic pregnancy, the enlarged NT is discordant between fetuses, a consideration should be made (Figs 78.14 to 78.18). Excluding the extremely rare case of heterokaryotypia, due to a mitotic nondisjunction, where a normal karyotype can co-exists with a 45, X0 or a trisomy fetus, it should be considered that the two fetuses should have the same karyotype.

The increased NT in one fetus may indicate a chromosomal abnormality in both fetuses. However, while the presence of a trisomy in both fetuses cannot be ruled out without kayrotype analysis, this finding can be associated to a normal karyotype in both fetuses. Moreover, it should be considered indicative for a structural anomaly that could be present in only one of the monozygotic fetuses. Concordance for the most common structural abnormalities that occur in monochorionic-monozygotic twins is rare.

In monochorionic diamniotic pregnancy, an enlarged NT could be caused by placental circulation problems, rather than chromosomal abnormalities. This early imbalance of fluids between the fetuses can anticipate in the first trimester the inter-twin-to-twin transfusion, that manifest the most important diagnostic sign only after 16 weeks.

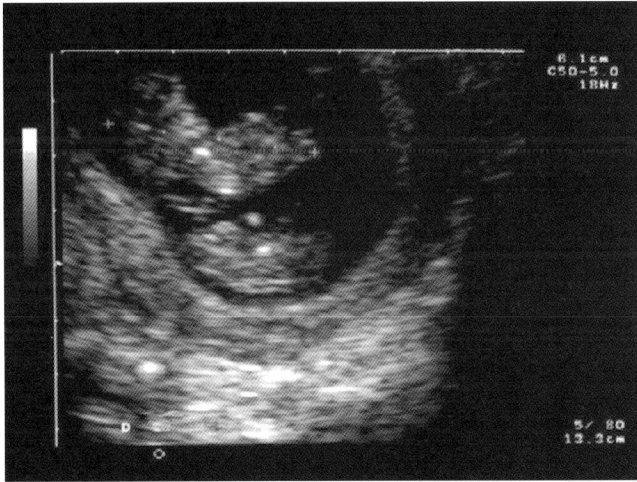

Fig. 78.14: Discordant nuchal translucency in a monochorionic diamniotic twin pregnancy

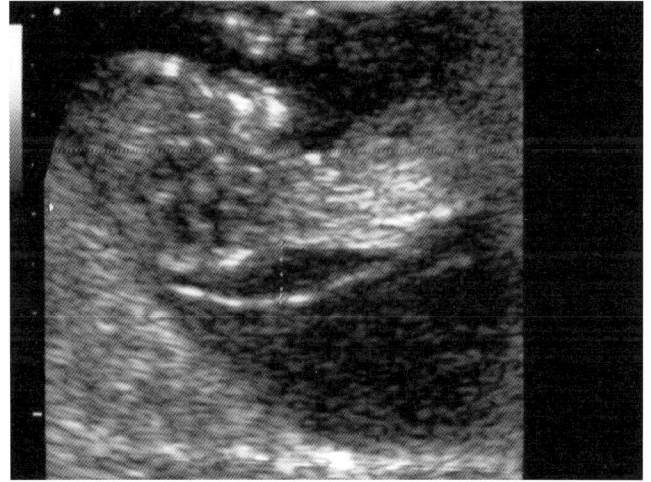

Fig. 78.15: The fetus with enlarged nuchal translucency (NT) in a monochorionic diamniotic twin pregnancy with discordant NT

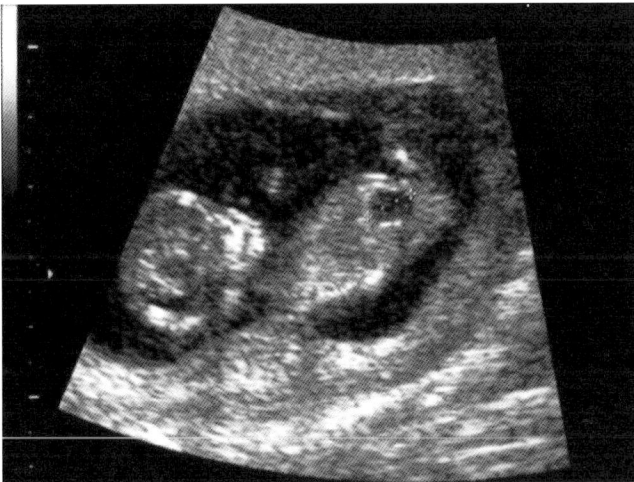

Fig. 78.16: The same fetus with enlarged NT in a monochorionic diamniotic twin pregnancy with discordant NT with an enlarged bladder

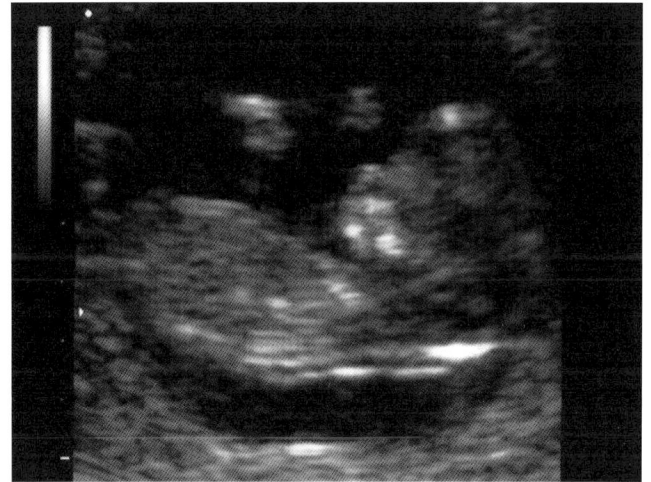

Fig. 78.17: The fetus with normal NT in a monochorionic diamniotic twin pregnancy with discordant NT

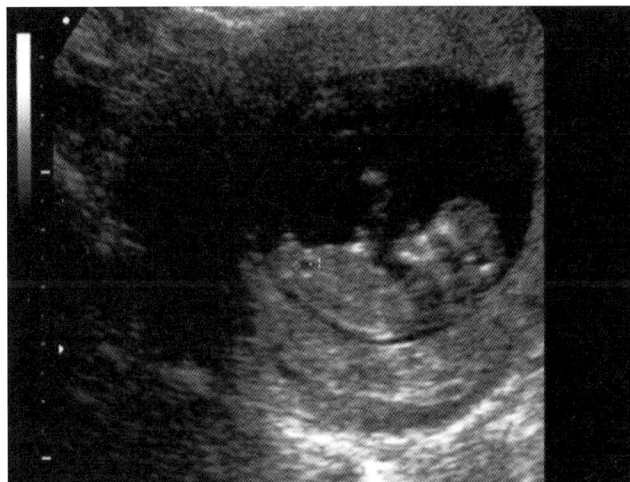

Fig. 78.18: The same fetus with normal NT in a monochorionic diamniotic twin pregnancy with discordant NT with an enlarged bladder

REFERENCES

1. Snijders RJ, Nicolaides K. Ultrasound Markers for Chromosomal Defects. London, UK: Parthenon Publishing; 1996.
2. Nicolaides KH, Sebire NJ, Snijders RJ, et al. The 11–14 Week's Scan Book. London, UK: Parthenon Publishing; 2001.
3. Dunn A, MacFarlane A. Recent trends in the incidence of multiple births and associated mortality in England and Wales. Arch Dis Child. 1996;75:10-9.
4. Callahan T, Hall J, Ettner S, et al. The economic impact of multiple-gestation pregnancies and the contribution of assisted-reproduction techniques to their incidence. N Engl J Med. 1994;331:244-9.
5. Meschede D, Lemcke B, Stussel J, et al. Strong preference for non-invasive prenatal diagnosis in women pregnant through intracytoplasmic sperm injection. Prenat Diagn. 1998;18:700-5.
6. Monni G, Cau G, Lai R, et al. Intracytoplasmic sperm injection and prenatal invasive diagnosis. Prenat Diagn. 1999;19:389-90.
7. Neveux LM, Palomaki GE, Knight GJ, et al. Multiple marker screening for Down syndrome in twin pregnancies. Prenat Diagn. 1996;16:29-34.
8. Spencer K. Screening for trisomy 21 in twin pregnancies in the first trimester using free beta-hCG and PAPP-A, combined with fetal nuchal translucency thickness. Prenat Diagn. 2000;20:91-5.
9. Wapner RJ. Genetic diagnosis in multiple pregnancies. Sem Perinat. 1995;19:351-62.
10. Monni G, Ibba RM. Invasive procedures in multiple pregnancies. In: Weiner S, Kurjak A (Eds). Interventional Ultrasound. New York: The Parthenon Publishing Group; 1999. pp. 105-15.
11. Nicolaides KH, Azar G, Byrne D, et al. Fetal nuchal translucency screening for chromosomal defects in first trimester of pregnancy. Br Med J. 1992;304:867-9.
12. Monni G, Zoppi MA, Ibba RM, et al. Fetal nuchal translucency test for Down's syndrome. Lancet. 1997;350:1631.
13. Snijders RJ, Noble P, Sebire N, et al. UK multicentre project on assessment of risk of trisomy 21 by maternal age and fetal nuchal translucency thickness at 10-14 weeks of gestation. Lancet. 1998;352:343-6.
14. Pandya PP, Hilbert F, Snijders RJ, et al. Nuchal translucency thickness and crown-rump length in twin pregnancies with chromosomally abnormal fetuses. J Ultrasound Med. 1995;14:565-8.
15. Sebire NJ, Snijders RJ, Hughes K, et al. Screening for trisomy 21 in twin pregnancies by maternal age and fetal nuchal translucency thickness at 10-14 weeks of gestation. Br J Obstet Gynecol. 1996;103: 999-1003.
16. Maymon R, Dreazen E, Tovbin Y, et al. The feasibility of nuchal translucency measurement in higher order multiple pregnancies achieved by assisted reproduction. Hum Reprod. 1999;14:2102-5.
17. Monni G, Zoppi MA, Ibba RM, et al. Nuchal translucency in multiple pregnancies. Croat Med J. 2000;41:266-9.
18. Keith LG, Papiernik E, Keith DM, Luke B (Eds). Multiple Pregnancy, Epidemiology, Gestation and Perinatal Outcome. New York: The Parthenon Publishing Group; 1995.
19. Wenstrom KD, Syrop CH, Hammitt DG, et al. Increased risk of monochorionic twinning associated with assisted reproduction. Fertil Steril. 1993;60:510-4.
20. Sepulveda W, Sebire NJ, Hughes K, et al. The lambda sign at 10-14 weeks of gestation as a predictor of chorionicity in twin pregnancies. Ultrasound Obstet Gynecol. 1996;7:421-3.
21. Sepulveda W, Sebire NJ, Odibo A, et al. Prenatal determination of chorionicity in triplet pregnancy by ultrasonographic examination of the ipsilon zone. Obstet Gynecol. 1996;88:855-8.
22. Senat MV, Deprest J, Boulvain M, et al. Endoscopic laser surgery versus serial amnioreduction for severe twin-to-twin transfusion syndrome. N Engl J Med. 2004;351:136-44.
23. Machin GA. Some causes of genotypic and phenotypic discordance in monozygotic twin pairs. Am J Med Genet. 1996;61:216-28.
24. Rodis JF, Egan JF, Craffey A, et al. Calculated risk of chromosomal abnormalities in twin gestations. Obstet Gynecol. 1990;76:1037-41.
25. Evans MI, Berkowitz RL, Wapner RJ, et al. Improvement in outcomes of multifetal pregnancy reduction with increases experience. Am J Obstet Gynecol. 2001;184:7-103.
26. Dodd JM, Crowther CA. Reduction of the number of fetuses for women with triplet and high order multiple pregnancies (Cochrane Review). In: The Cochrane Library 2003, Issue 4, Chicester, UK: John Wiley and Sons, Ltd.
27. Eddleman KA, Stone JL, Lynch L, et al. Chorionic villous sampling before multifetal pregnancy reduction. Am J Obstet Gynecol. 2000;183:1078-81.
28. Monni G, Zoppi MA, Cau G, et al. Importance of nuchal translucency in multifetal pregnancy reduction. Ultrasound Obstet Gynecol. 1999;13,377-8.
29. Moscoso G. Fetal nuchal translucency: A need to understand the physiological basis. Ultrasound Obstet Gynecol. 1995;5:6-8.
30. Von Kaisenberg CS, Brand-Saberi B, Jonat W, et al. Pathophysiology of increased nuchal translucency in chromosomally abnormal fetuses. Prenat Neonat Med. 1999;4:431-40.
31. Souka AP, Snijders RJ, Novakov A, et al. Defects and syndromes in chromosomally normal fetuses with increased nuchal translucency thickness at 10-14 weeks of gestation. Ultrasound Obstet Gynecol. 1998;11: 391-400.
32. Hyett J, Perdu M, Sharland G, et al. Using fetal nuchal translucency to screen for major congenital cardiac defects at 10-14 weeks of gestation: population based cohort study. Br Med J. 1999;318:81-5.
33. Cicero S, Curcio P, Papageorghiou A, et al. Absence of nasal bone in fetuses with trisomy 21 at 11-14 weeks of gestation: An observational study. Lancet. 2001;358:1665-7.
34. Monni G, Zoppi MA, Ibba RM. Absence of nasal bone and detection of trisomy 21. Lancet. 2002;359:1343.
35. Sebire NJ, D'Ercole C, Hughes K, et al. Increased nuchal translucency thickness at 10-14 weeks of gestation as a predictor of severe twin-to-twin transfusion syndrome. Ultrasound Obstet Gynecol. 1997;10: 86-9.

SECTION 9

Fetal and Maternal Physiology

B Arabin, DW Skupski

79

Maternal Hemodynamic Changes in Pregnancy

J Nizard

INTRODUCTION

Adaptation to pregnancy begins rapidly after conception. Most probably, all described modifications of maternal hemodynamics are triggered early every menstrual cycle, before conception, but are too small to be detected. These modifications are reversible, either at the end of the cycle with menstruations, or within the first weeks or months after delivery. Physiological modifications are only detectable when the amplitude of changes is sufficient, thus most of the time at the end of the first trimester of pregnancy. Functional as well as anatomical changes are observed in most systems, of which the cardiovascular and volume homeostasis systems are among the most important.

These changes in maternal physiology are asymptomatic in normal pregnant women, resulting from an adapted process. They are nevertheless important to know for their implications in pathology and its treatment. Most data we have are from time radioactive molecules and cells, or dye techniques that were used in pregnant women. Modern noninvasive techniques do not provide the same possible measurements. If echocardiography, for instance, can replace invasive measurements of cardiac output, we still lack noninvasive techniques for such parameters as plasma volume.

CARDIOVASCULAR SYSTEM

Blood Volume

Plasma volume increase starts as early as 6 weeks and reaches a maximum volume by the end of the third trimester of 5,200 mL, which represents an increase of 1,200–1,600 mL or 45% from nonpregnant values.[1,2] Although absolute volume values vary from individual to individual, and among studies, the overall percentage of increase is constant, between 45% and 50%.[3] It is not clear whether the importance of plasma volume is constant for an individual[2,3] or depends on parity.[4,5] Interestingly, plasma volume increases throughout pregnancy, even when indexed to weight.[2]

The plasma volume increase is greater in multiple gestations and the increase is proportional to the number of fetuses.[6-8] More fetuses also means more placental volume. It is probable that the amplitude of these changes is proportional to placenta volume since the plasma volume increase is greater, on average, in cases of molar pregnancy.[9] In the study from Pritchard on hemodilution in patients with molar pregnancies, after accounting for blood loss associated with the pathology, he describes in five out of eight patients anemia associated with significant hypervolemia.[9] The increase in blood volume ranged from 25% to 51% at 9–24 weeks when compared with nonpregnant values in the same patients. This is consistent with the increase in cases of multiple pregnancy or increased fetal weight where placenta volume is proportionally increased.

On the other hand, in cases where placenta volume is likely to be decreased, such as preeclampsia and intrauterine growth restriction, plasma expansion is reduced.[10-12]

What happens at the very end of the third trimester of pregnancy is largely debated in the literature. Contradictory data on whether maternal plasma volume declines in the last month of pregnancy seems related to maternal positioning. The increase in plasma volume seems to continue even in the last month of pregnancy when mothers are in the left lateral position, at least in twin pregnancies. According to some authors, plasma volume reaches a plateau at around 32 weeks in singleton pregnancies, but continues to increase in twin pregnancies.[6] This peculiarity explains the increased risks of pulmonary edema in twin pregnancies when using beta-mimetics or plasma expansion in the third trimester.

Why does plasma volume expand?

There are several theories to explain why plasma volume expands during pregnancy:

- *Hyperaldosteronism*: Physiologic hyperaldosteronism during pregnancy can be responsible for plasma increase. Primary hyperaldosteronism is responsible for hypervolemia in non-pregnant patients, with an increase in plasma volume in the two cases described by Briglier and Forsham of 48% and 76%, with no changes in total red blood cell volume.[13]

- *Influence of estrogens*: Estrogens affect plasma volume in many circumstances. Plasma volume expansion has been described in women using oral contraception or hormonal replacement therapy (i.e. estrogens in postmenopausal women).[14,15] Estrogens are responsible for an increase in renin levels, which are responsible for an increase in aldosterone level.

- Placental growth hormones implications are uncertain.

- *Placental circulation*: The placenta acts like a low pressure maternal arteriovenous shunt, affecting arterial blood pressure and cardiac output. Placental circulation could thus explain part of the plasma expansion by induced hyperaldosteronism.

Red Blood Cells

Total red blood cell mass increases by 20–40% by term, which represents an absolute increase of 250–450 mL. The rise is the consequence of greater production of red blood cells, not longer lifetime, since iron supplementation increases even more the red blood cell mass.[1] The increase in total red blood cell volume is proportional to weight gain in singleton pregnancies as opposed to plasma volume which increases more than the weight gain.[2] The lesser increase in total red blood cell volume than the physiologic plasma volume expansion is responsible for pseudoanemia (Fig. 79.1). Biologically, women have a hemoglobin at 1 standard

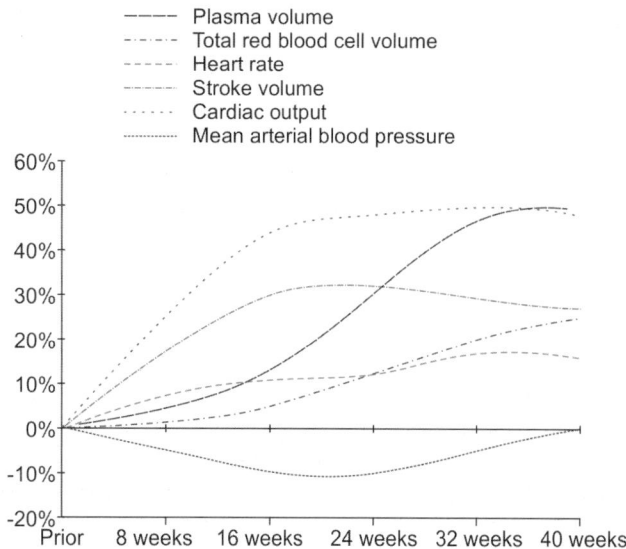

Fig. 79.1: Evolution of different parameters throughout pregnancy

Source: Adapted from Ayala et al.,[40] Capeless and Clapp,[36] Robson et al.,[33] Thomsen et al.[8] and Pitkin[17])

deviation (SD) below the mean, but the value should always be above 10.5 g/dL.[16] Hematocrit can physiologically go as low as 33%.[17] The increase in red blood cell mass starts, or is detectable, later than plasma volume, by the end of the first trimester. Twin pregnancy is responsible for an increase in total red blood cell mass but is not as proportional to weight gain as in singleton pregnancy. This increase in erythropoiesis is probably influenced by placental secretion of placental chorionic somatomammotropin, progesterone, or prolactin.[18] This increase in erythropoiesis increases maternal needs for iron by about 500 mg.[18] Moreover, maternal hemoglobin, by an increase in 2,3-diphosphoglycerate concentrations in red blood cells, has less affinity for oxygen to facilitate dissociation across the placenta to the fetus.[19]

This hemodilution, as a result of a greater increase in plasma volume than total red blood cell mass, has beneficial effects:

- It limits hemoglobin loss in cases of prepartum or postpartum hemorrhage
- It facilitates heart function by limiting the blood viscosity
- It facilitates placental microcirculation by limiting blood viscosity
- It facilitates venous circulation to limit thromboembolic events[16,20]
- It limits impaired venous return, reduction in cardiac output, and hypotension in the supine position.

Heart Anatomical Changes

Ventricles

End-diastolic ventricular volume and ventricular mass increase throughout pregnancy. These modifications, which include anatomical modification of the maternal heart during pregnancy, take place without end-systolic volume or end-diastolic pressure increasing.[21,22] The combination of increasing end-diastolic ventricular volume and stable end-systolic volumes and end-diastolic pressure are the consequences of an increased compliance of the myocardium. It is not clear when cardiac compliance starts to increase during pregnancy.

Ventricular mass increases as soon as the first trimester[23] and the end-diastolic volume increase and detectable only in the second trimester,[21] and although the changes are not detected at the same moment, they are part of a continuum.

Atria

Left atrial diameter increases during pregnancy to reach a plateau at around 30 weeks.[24] Left atrial diameter is related to vascular filling. The increase in left atrial diameter during pregnancy is in relation with physiologic plasma volume expansion.

Vessels

Changes are observed in large vessels during pregnancy. Aortic compliance increases, which combined with decreasing vascular tone, results in lower afterload and enhanced left ventricular performance.[25] Venous distensibility increases throughout pregnancy as soon as the first trimester.[26] Increasing capacity of the venous system is essential for the physiological adaptation to plasma volume increase. It allows stability in venous pressure and protects the right heart from too high preload pressure. The fall in vascular resistance occurs at the same time as increasing compliance of large arteries and veins as early as the fifth week of gestation.[27] The causal relation between increased vascular compliance, fall in vascular resistance, physiologic plasma volume expansion, and increasing cardiac output during pregnancy are yet to be determined.

Cardiac Output

Cardiac function was initially studied using invasive techniques. It has even been used in term pregnancies more recently.[28] Echocardiography combined with pulse- or continuous-wave Doppler measurements of cardiac output was validated against invasive techniques in nonpregnant patients.[29] These techniques were later validated in pregnant women.[30,31] Since then, most available data collected has used noninvasive techniques.

Cardiac output depends on heart rate and stroke volume. Stroke volume increases throughout pregnancy as demonstrated by mid twentieth century invasive procedures and more recent noninvasive ultrasound examinations.[32-34] The major parameters responsible for stroke volume increase are:

- A moderate increase in preload and greater venous return
- A decreased afterload, increased arterial compliance and fall in vascular resistance
- An increased cardiac compliance and an intrinsic myocardial contractility increase that is independent of loading conditions.[35]

Cardiac output increases by 30–50% during pregnancy.[28,30,32-35] The increase in cardiac output is detectable as early as the fifth week of gestation. Early in pregnancy, the cardiac output increase is mostly the result of a stroke volume increase.[33,36] Heart rate increase occurs later in pregnancy and contributes, then, to the increase in cardiac output observed in the second half of pregnancy (Fig. 79.1).[33,37]

Caval syndrome in pregnancy was described by Holmes in 1960.[38] Maternal position influences hemodynamics. When in the supine position, the uterus compresses the inferior vena cava, affecting venous return to the right atrium. The reduction in preload affects all hemodynamic parameters. Ueland et al. compared stroke volume, heart rate and cardiac output at three different intervals in pregnancy, 20–24 weeks, 28–32 weeks and 38–40 weeks.[39] They performed their measurements in the supine, lateral decubitus and sitting position. Their main findings were:

- In the lateral decubitus, there is a fall in cardiac output by the end of the third trimester, as a result of the fall in stroke volume.
- In the supine position, cardiac output values at the very end of pregnancies are lower than nonpregnant values, as a result of a major fall in stroke volume partly compensated by an increase in heart rate.

Evolution of cardiac output in late pregnancy was not coherent in the literature. This issue seems settled by the work of Clark et al. in 1989.[28] In a study on 10 healthy singleton pregnant patients between 36 weeks and 38 weeks of gestation, using invasive central hemodynamic assessment, they found a 44% increase in cardiac output, with a 17% increase in heart rate and 27% increase in stroke volume.[28] Cardiac output does not fall in late pregnancy.

The variations in cardiac output measurements in late pregnancy observed in older studies were probably related to maternal positioning during measurements.

Blood Pressure

Arterial Blood Pressure

Arterial blood pressure declines from seventh week.[36]

Using 24-hour mean blood pressure measurements in normal pregnancies, Ayala et al. found a steady decrease of systolic blood pressure, diastolic blood pressure and mean arterial pressure up to the 21st week of gestation, followed by an increase to near non-pregnant values by the end of pregnancy (Fig. 79.1).[40] When the circadian variations of blood pressure were studied, the lowest pressures were measured at 4–5 hours, and the highest at 12–21 hours.[41] The magnitude of the difference between highest and lowest blood pressure within the same circadian period is maximal in the second trimester. These modifications in blood pressure are influenced by maternal age, but not by parity.[42]

Vascular Systemic Resistance

The total vascular resistance drop early in pregnancy is probably due to low resistance placental vascularization. It seems actually to be the first parameter to be significantly modified in early pregnancy.[43] Duvekot et al. performed serial weekly measurements from 5 weeks to 8 weeks of gestation. They unfortunately did not have non-pregnant values and compared the results with the 5 weeks of gestation data. It is not clear if this drop in total vascular resistance, due to the placental low resistance effect on the maternal circulation, is a cause or a consequence of plasma expansion and hyperaldosteronism. The only significant changes observed from the sixth week to eighth week of gestation compared to the fifth week were a raise in plasma 17-estradiol and a drop in plasma 17β-hydroxyprogesterone. Interestingly, Walters and Lim described in 1969 a fall in total vascular resistance when estroprogestative contraceptives were given to women.[15] The total vascular resistance remains low throughout pregnancy and is still 21% lower than non-pregnant values at 36–38 weeks of gestation.[28]

CONCLUSION

Pregnancy is characterized by early modifications in most hemodynamic parameters. These modifications are a consequence of normal adaptation to pregnancy and serve as control values for inadequate adaptation of pathologic pregnancies.

REFERENCES

1. Pritchard JA. Changes in the blood volume during pregnancy and delivery. Anesthesiology. 1965;26:393-9.
2. Lund CJ, Donovan JC. Blood volume during pregnancy. Significance of plasma and red cell volumes. Am J Obstet Gynecol. 1967;98:394-403.
3. Pritchard JA, Rowland RC. Blood volume changes in pregnancy and the puerperium. III. Whole body and large vessel hematocrits in pregnant and non-pregnant women. Am J Obstet Gynecol.1964;88:391-5.
4. Adams JQ. Cardiovascular physiology in normal pregnancy: Studies with the dye dilution technique. Am J Obstet Gynecol. 1954;67:741-59.
5. Pirani BB, Campbell DM, MacGillivray I. Plasma volume in normal first pregnancy. J Obstet Gynecol Br Commonw. 1973; 80:884-7.
6. Rovinsky JJ, Jaffin H. Cardiovascular hemodynamics in pregnancy. I. Blood and plasma volumes in multiple pregnancy. Am J Obstet Gynecol. 1965;93:1-15.
7. MacGillivray I, Campbell D, Duffus GM. Maternal metabolic response to twin pregnancy in primigravidae. J Obstet Gynecol Br Commonw. 1971;78:530-4.
8. Thomsen JK, Fogh-Andersen N, Jaszczak P. Atrial natriuretic peptide, blood volume, aldosterone, and sodium excretion during twin pregnancy. Acta Obstet Gynecol Scand. 1994;73:14-20.
9. Pritchard JA. Blood volume changes in pregnancy and the puerperium. IV. Anemia associated with hydatidiform mole. Am J Obstet Gynecol. 1965;91:621-9.
10. Salas SP, Rosso P, Espinoza R, et al. Maternal plasma volume expansion and hormonal changes in women with idiopathic fetal growth retardation. Obstet Gynecol. 1993;81:1029-33.
11. Duvekot JJ, Cheriex EC, Pieters FA, et al. Severely impaired fetal growth is preceded by maternal hemodynamic maladaptation in very early pregnancy. Acta Obstet Gynecol Scand. 1995;74:693-7.
12. Brown MA, Gallery ED. Volume homeostasis in normal pregnancy and pre-eclampsia: Physiology and clinical implications. Baillieres Clin Obstet Gynecol. 1994;8:287-310.
13. Biglieri EG, Forsham PH. Studies on the expanded extracellular fluid and the responses to various stimuli in primary aldosteronism. Am J Med. 1961;30:564-76.
14. Luotola H, Pyorala T, Lahteenmaki P, et al. Hemodynamic and hormonal effects of short-term oestradiol treatment in postmenopausal women. Maturitas. 1979;1:287-94.
15. Walters WA, Lim YL. Cardiovascular dynamics in women receiving oral contraceptive therapy. Lancet. 1969;2:879-81.
16. Koller O. The clinical significance of hemodilution during pregnancy. Obstet Gynecol Surv. 1982;37:649-52.
17. Pitkin RM. Nutritional support in obstetrics and gynecology. Clin Obstet Gynecol. 1976;19:489-513.
18. Jepson JH, Lowenstein L. Role of erythropoietin and placental lactogen in the control of erythropoiesis during pregnancy. Can J Physiol Pharmacol. 1968;46:573-6.
19. Bille-Brahe NE, Rorth M. Red cell 2,3-diphosphoglycerate in pregnancy. Acta Obstet Gynecol Scand. 1979;58:19-21.

20. Peeters LL, Verkeste CM, Saxena PR, et al. Relationship between maternal hemodynamics and hematocrit and hemodynamic effects of isovolemic hemodilution and hemoconcentration in the awake late-pregnant guinea pig. Pediatr Res. 1987;21:584-9.

21. Rubler S, Damani PM, Pinto ER. Cardiac size and performance during pregnancy estimated with echocardiography. Am J Cardiol. 1977;40:534-40.

22. Laird-Meeter K, van de Ley G, Bom TH, et al. Cardiocirculatory adjustments during pregnancy—an echocardiographic study. Clin Cardiol. 1979;2:328-32.

23. Thompson JA, Hays PM, Sagar KB, et al. Echocardiographic left ventricular mass to differentiate chronic hypertension from pre-eclampsia during pregnancy. Am J Obstet Gynecol. 1986;155:994-9.

24. Vered Z, Poler SM, Gibson P, et al. Noninvasive detection of the morphologic and hemodynamic changes during normal pregnancy. Clin Cardiol. 1991;14:327-34.

25. Hart MV, Morton MJ, Hosenpud JD, et al. -Aortic function during normal human pregnancy. Am J Obstet Gynecol. 1986;154:887-91.

26. Sakai K, Imaizumi T, Maeda H, et al. Venous distensibility during pregnancy. Comparisons between normal pregnancy and pre-eclampsia. Hypertension. 1994;24:461-6.

27. Spaanderman ME, Willekes C, Hoeks AP, et al. The effect of pregnancy on the compliance of large arteries and veins in healthy parous control subjects and women with a history of pre-eclampsia. Am J Obstet Gynecol. 2000;183:1278-86.

28. Clark SL, Cotton DB, Lee W, et al. Central hemodynamic assessment of normal term pregnancy. Am J Obstet Gynecol. 1989;161:1439-42.

29. Loeppky JA, Hoekenga DE, Greene ER, et al. Comparison of noninvasive pulsed Doppler and Fick measurements of stroke volume in cardiac patients. Am Heart J. 1984;107:339-46.

30. Easterling TR, Carlson KL, Schmucker BC, et al. Measurement of cardiac output in pregnancy by Doppler technique. Am J Perinatol. 1990;7:220-2.

31. Easterling TR, Watts DH, Schmucker BC, et al. Measurement of cardiac output during pregnancy: validation of Doppler technique and clinical observations in pre-eclampsia. Obstet Gynecol. 1987; 69:845-50.

32. Bader RA, Bader ME, Rose DF, et al. Hemodynamics at rest and during exercise in normal pregnancy as studies by cardiac catheterization. J Clin Invest. 1955;34:1524-36.

33. Robson SC, Hunter S, Boys RJ, et al. Serial study of factors influencing changes in cardiac output during human pregnancy. Am J Physiol. 1989;256:H1060-5.

34. Walters WA, MacGregor WG, Hills M. Cardiac output at rest during pregnancy and the puerperium. Clin Sci. 1966;30:1-11.

35. Gilson GJ, Samaan S, Crawford MH, et al. Changes in hemodynamics, ventricular remodeling, and ventricular contractility during normal pregnancy: A longitudinal study. Obstet Gynecol. 1997; 89:957-62.

36. Capeless EL, Clapp JF. Cardiovascular changes in early phase of pregnancy. Am J Obstet Gynecol. 1989;161:1449-53.

37. Mabie WC, DiSessa TG, Crocker LG, et al. A longitudinal study of cardiac output in normal human pregnancy. Am J Obstet Gynecol. 1994;170:849-56.

38. Holmes F. The supine hypotensive syndrome. Its importance to the anesthetist. Anesthesia. 1960;15:298-306.

39. Ueland K, Novy MJ, Peterson EN, et al. Maternal cardiovascular dynamics. IV. The influence of gestational age on the maternal cardiovascular response to posture and exercise. Am J Obstet Gynecol. 1969;104:856-64.

40. Ayala DE, Hermida RC, Mojon A, et al. Blood pressure variability during gestation in healthy and complicated pregnancies. Hypertension. 1997;30:611-8.

41. Hermida RC, Ayala DE, Mojon A, et al. Blood pressure patterns in normal pregnancy, gestational hypertension, and pre-eclampsia. Hypertension. 2000;36:149-58.

42. Ayala DE, Hermida RC. Influence of parity and age on ambulatory monitored blood pressure during pregnancy. Hypertension. 2001;38:753-8.

43. Duvekot JJ, Cheriex EC, Pieters FA, et al. Early pregnancy changes in hemodynamics and volume homeostasis are consecutive adjustments triggered by a primary fall in systemic vascular tone. Am J Obstet Gynecol. 1993;169:1382-92.

80 Pathophysiology of Preeclampsia

T Podymow, P August, D Skupski

INTRODUCTION

Preeclampsia is a hypertensive condition unique to pregnancy with both maternal and fetal manifestations. The maternal disease is characterized by vasospasm, endothelial dysfunction, activation of the coagulation system and high blood pressure. The maternal pathophysiologic changes are systemic and are mainly ischemic, affecting the placenta, kidney, liver and brain. Preeclampsia is diagnosed in a woman with new onset hypertension >140/90 mm Hg after 20th gestational week accompanied by proteinuria >300 mg/day. Other common clinical and laboratory abnormalities include facial and peripheral edema, thrombocytopenia, elevated uric acid levels (>5.5 mg/dL) and elevated transaminase levels (greater than twice the normal). The greatest concern is that pre-eclampsia can progress to eclampsia, which are life-threatening convulsions associated with cerebral hemorrhage or to HELLP syndrome, which is Hemolysis, Elevated Liver enzymes and Low Platelets. Eclampsia is frequently preceded by severe headaches, visual disturbance (halos or auras) and hyper-reflexia, while HELLP syndrome is frequently preceded by right upper quadrant or epigastric pain. The consequences of preeclampsia for the fetus are a result of decreased placental perfusion and include intrauterine growth restriction and fetal loss. Delivery is the only definitive cure of preeclampsia/eclampsia, and in order to prevent serious maternal complications premature delivery is often necessary, as such hypertensive disorders in pregnancy are the leading cause of indicated premature delivery. In this chapter, the pathophysiology of preeclampsia and the pathogenesis of these manifestations will be examined.

PATHOPHYSIOLOGY

The pathophysiology of preeclampsia has been described divided into two stages:[1] alterations in placental perfusion (stage 1) and the maternal syndrome (stage 2).

Placenta

The pathophysiology of preeclampsia begins with abnormalities in the development of the placenta, leading to the production of abnormal vasculogenic substances, which upon reaching the maternal circulation produce the maternal clinical syndrome. There is considerable evidence for the importance of the placenta in the pathogenesis of preeclampsia; preeclampsia can develop without a fetus in the case of molar pregnancies (a rapidly growing placenta with trophoblastic tissue) and in multiple gestations (increased placental mass). There are also case reports of twin pregnancies where preeclampsia is reversed upon termination of the severely growth restricted twin and involution of the pathologic placenta.[2]

In normal gestation, the uterine artery's terminal branches, the spiral arteries, invade the placenta and are transformed from muscular arteries into relaxed flaccid vessels to accommodate an eventual 10-fold increase in uterine blood flow. This transformation is dependent on the placental trophoblasts which invade and surround the uterine spiral artery's vascular walls.[3] The placental trophoblasts, normally epithelial cells, replace their adhesion molecules with those of endothelial cells to assume vascular endothelial cell phenotype prior to invading the uterine arteries,[4] a process termed pseudovasculogenesis. This vascular remodeling results in increased blood flow and supply of nutrients and oxygen to the fetus by the end of the first trimester. In preeclampsia, pseudovasculogenesis is defective; cytotrophoblast invasion from the placenta is shallow, the arteries remain small and muscular,[5] and the ensuing placental ischemia is thought to trigger the release of placenta-derived factors. Of considerable interest is the increased incidence of preeclampsia in women with medical conditions associated with microvascular disease such as hypertension, diabetes and collagen vascular disease, as the impaired placental perfusion leading to ischemia may be the common source of this disease.[1]

The idea that impaired placental perfusion leads to release of "factors" into the maternal circulation to cause the clinical manifestations of preeclampsia is not new, although the precise nature of these "factors" awaits ultimate description. The placenta-derived preeclampsia factors causing systemic endothelial dysfunction have for decades been elusive. Maynard et al. have reported that angiogenic proteins such as placental growth factor (PlGF) and vascular endothelial growth factor (VEGF) are both required for normal angiogenesis and endothelial function in pregnancy, and are reduced in women with preeclampsia. Recent studies report elevated maternal serum levels of a protein which in preeclampsia appears to scavenge these factors and induce endothelial dysfunction: a soluble fms-like tyrosine kinase 1 (sFlt-1) (also called soluble vascular endothelial growth factor receptor 1; sVEGFR-1). This molecule is a circulating modified VEGF receptor, which functions to neutralize VEGF and PlGF, and is found in excess quantities in both the placenta and the serum of preeclamptic women.[6,7] When administered to pregnant rats, sFlt-1 has been shown to induce a preeclampsia-like phenotype with albuminuria, hypertension and renal pathologic changes of glomerular endotheliosis.[6] In human studies, increased serum levels of sFlt-1 and reduced levels of PlGF have been found to predict the subsequent development of preeclampsia,[7] and decreased urinary PlGF in the early second trimester is strongly associated with subsequent early development of preeclampsia (Fig. 80.1).[8] The mechanism for the upregulation of sFlt-1, and whether normalization of VEGF and PlGF levels might halt progression of preeclampsia are yet unknown.

Other factors that may be derived from the placenta, and are postulated to be related to preeclampsia are substances which increase oxidant stress, leptin and a variety of cytokines including TNF alpha. Oxidative stress due to hypoxia driven free-radical generation at the fetal-maternal interface has been suggested as a cause of preeclampsia. The byproducts of increased oxidative stress, possibly released by the placenta in response to hypoxia or ischemia, have been implicated in the genesis of endothelial cell damage in preeclampsia.[9,10] Small studies using antioxidants to prevent preeclampsia have been encouraging and vitamins E and C are currently being studied in larger trials to determine their potential role in prevention.[11]

Pathologically, the lesion of the placenta in preeclampsia is termed acute atherosis and is characterized by an accumulation of fat-laden macrophages and infiltrates in the arteries not invaded by trophoblast cells. In a study of 400 placentas from preeclamptic women, vascular lesions in the placenta correlated with the severity of clinical disease.[12] Preeclampsia is also associated with a greater degree of placental infarction than in normal gestation, however, the placenta has considerable reserve, explaining why some infants are growth restricted or die but more often are normal for gestational age.

Maternal Syndrome of Preeclampsia

Blood Pressure in Preeclampsia

High blood pressure in preeclampsia is mainly due to a reversal of the vasodilatation of normal pregnancy, replaced by a marked increase in peripheral vascular resistance.[13] Preeclamptics do not develop overt hypertension until late gestation (after week 20, and usually not until the third trimester), but vasoconstrictor influences may be present much earlier. For instance longitudinal and epidemiologic surveys show that women destined to develop preeclampsia have slightly higher "normal" blood pressure (e.g. diastolic levels >70 mm Hg) as early as the second trimester.[14-16]

The precise mechanism of preeclamptic hypertension is obscure. During normal pregnancy the renin-angiotensin system is stimulated, most likely in response to vasodilatation and lower blood pressure. In contrast with normal pregnancy, women with preeclampsia have suppressed plasma renin activity, aldosterone,

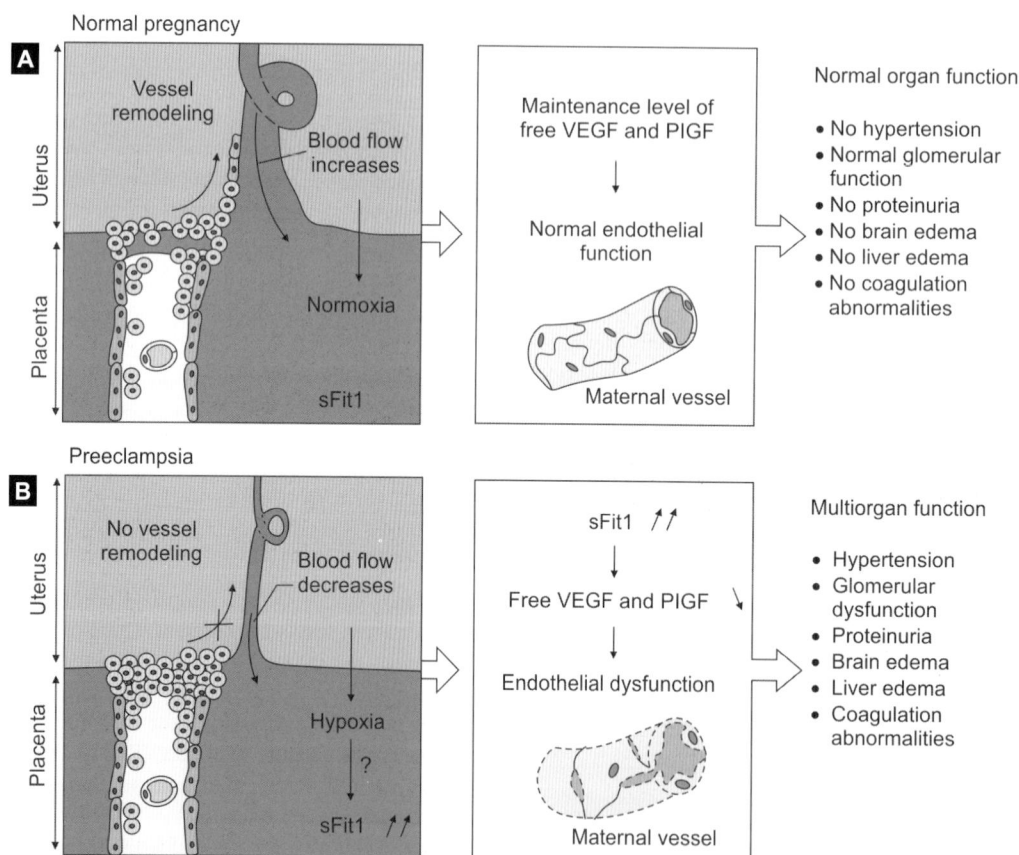

Fig. 80.1: Hypothesis on the role of sFlt1 in preeclampsia. (A) During normal pregnancy, the uterine spiral arteries are infiltrated and remodeled by endovascular invasive trophoblasts, thereby increasing blood flow significantly in order to meet the oxygen and nutrient demands of the fetus. (B) In the placenta of preeclamptic women, trophoblast invasion does not occur and blood flow is reduced, resulting in placental hypoxia. In addition, increased amounts of soluble Flt1 (sFlt1) are produced by the placenta and scavenge VEGF and PlGF, thereby lowering circulating levels of unbound VEGF and PlGF. This altered balance causes generalized endothelial dysfunction, resulting in multiorgan disease. It remains unknown whether hypoxia is the trigger for stimulating sFlt1 secretion in the placenta of preeclamptic mothers and whether the higher sFlt1 levels interfere with trophoblast invasion and spiral artery remodeling.

Source: Used with permission Luttun and Carmeliet[8]

urinary aldosterone excretion and angiotensin II levels. There is evidence that the renin-angiotensin system is stimulated early in pregnancy in women who later develop preeclampsia and that the developing vasoconstriction and hypertension turn off renin secretion. This decrease in renin has been used as a screening test to identify gravidas in midgestation who are at risk for the development of preeclampsia.[17]

Blood pressure in preeclampsia is also characteristically labile, and exaggerated responses to norepinephrine and angiotensin despite normal plasma levels have been noted.[18] There is a reversal of the normal circadian rhythm, with blood pressures often being higher at night.[19] In addition, increases in peripheral vascular resistance and blood pressure that characterize preeclampsia have been found to be mediated, at least in part, by a substantial increase in sympathetic vasoconstrictor activity which reverts to normal after delivery.[20] These observations lend mechanistic support for the use of methyldopa, which is metabolized to α-methylnorepinephrine and replaces norepinephrine to decrease sympathetic tone centrally.

Changes in eicosanoid metabolism occur in normal pregnancy, particularly prostacyclin (PGI_2) and thromboxane (TXA_2) production, and further alterations arise in preeclampsia. Prostaglandins such as PGI_2 are increased in normal pregnancy, particularly vasodilatory prostanoids (mostly PGI_2) by vascular endothelial cells,[21] and this may contribute to the generalized vasodilatation characteristic of pregnancy. Reduced PGI_2, but not TXA_2, has been found to occur months before the clinical onset of preeclampsia.[22,23] There is substantial literature suggesting that alterations in prostaglandin metabolism underlie the pathogenesis of preeclampsia.[21-25] Manifestations such as increments in vascular reactivity and blood pressure, as well as intravascular coagulation, have been proposed to be due to an imbalance between PGI_2 and TXA_2 synthesis, resulting in a relative or absolute PGI_2 deficiency. These findings are consistent with evidence that preeclampsia is characterized by generalized vascular endothelial cell dysfunction, leading to diminished production of PGI_2, as well as other vasodilatory endothelial cell products.

In spite of the large body of evidence supporting a role for alterations in prostaglandin metabolism in preeclampsia, it is important to emphasize that these substances are difficult to measure, and act locally, so measurements from peripheral blood may not reflect local effects. Nevertheless, the notion that preeclampsia is characterized by a deficiency of PGI_2 with stable or increased TXA_2 production has been the basis of several large multicenter randomized trials evaluating low-dose aspirin (which inhibits platelet TXA_2 generation but spares vascular PGI_2 production) in the prevention of preeclampsia. Despite early, relatively small studies that reported striking reductions in the risk of preeclampsia in women treated with low-dose aspirin, a recent Cochrane review including data from 36,500 women did not reveal overall beneficial effect of aspirin on pregnancy outcome.[26]

Endothelial Cell Function

In recent years, the role of the vascular endothelial cells in the modulation of vascular smooth muscle contractile activity, as well as in coagulation and regulation of blood flow, has increased understanding of endothelial cell function in the pathophysiology of preeclampsia, and other chronic cardiovascular conditions such as atherosclerosis and essential hypertension. Endothelial cells, which have receptors for numerous vasodilators and constrictors

produce hormones, autacoids and mitogenic cytokines, including PGI2, nitric oxide and endothelin. The pathophysiologic changes of preeclampsia, particularly those present before clinically apparent disease, support the hypothesis that altered endothelial function contributes to many of the changes observed in the preeclamptic syndrome.[27] Women with preeclampsia manifest increased circulating markers of endothelial activation (von Willibrand Factor, cellular fibronectin, thrombomodulin, endothelin, V-CAM).[28] Preeclamptic blood vessels demonstrate reduced endothelial mediated vasodilation in vitro,[28] and in vivo studies have shown that flow mediated (endothelium dependent) dilatation is impaired in women with previous preeclampsia.[25] Most recently, raised plasma concentrations of asymmetric dimethylarginine (ADMA), the endogenous inhibitor of endothelial nitric oxide synthase, has been shown to be elevated in women with evidence of abnormal endothelial function prior to the development of preeclampsia.[29]

There are numerous reports of a hypertensive syndrome produced by inhibiting nitric oxide synthase in various experimental models of gestation, with some features similar to human preeclampsia.[30,31] Results from women with preeclampsia are conflicting, with reports of increased as well as decreased serum and urinary metabolites of nitric oxide in preeclampsia.[32-34]

Endothelins represent another vasoactive endothelial cell product postulated to play a role in preeclampsia.[35-38] In this respect, circulating levels of endothelin-1 are generally (but not universally) reported as increased in this disorder, but it is unclear if such levels have pathogenic significance or are a byproduct of endothelial damage.

The evidence for endothelial cell dysfunction in the pathogenesis of the maternal manifestations of preeclampsia is strong and its cause continues to be actively investigated. As mentioned circulating factors of placental origin, e.g. sFlt 1, are likely involved. Indeed, sera from women destined to develop or manifest preeclampsia alter endothelial cell function or cause endothelial cell activation in vitro (assessed by nitric oxide and PGI_2 generation).[39] Sera from preeclamptic patients are also mitogenic and increase messenger RNA for, as well as production of, the growth factor PDGF-β in culture.[40] There is also a growing body of evidence implicating increased lipid peroxides as well as byproducts of increased oxidative stress, possibly released by the placenta in response to hypoxia or ischemia, in the genesis of endothelial cell damage in preeclampsia.[9,41-43]

Metabolic Disturbances in Preeclampsia

Hyperinsulinemia, obesity, glucose intolerance and dyslipidemia (e.g. increased triglycerides, reduced HDL) are associated with cardiovascular disease and essential hypertension. Insulin resistance and hyperinsulinemia (mediated by hormonal changes) are also characteristic of normal pregnancy, and are maximal in the third trimester.[44] Several laboratories have reported exaggerated metabolic disturbances in patients with preeclampsia, including hypertriglyceridemia, increased levels of free fatty acids, decreased levels of lipoprotein (a) increased insulin levels and glucose intolerance.[45-49] These observations are intriguing, particularly because they may be related to the evidence for increased oxidative stress in preeclampsia (lipid abnormalities may result in increased oxidative stress).

Obesity remains an important risk factor for preeclampsia, with strong positive association between maternal prepregnancy body mass index and the risk of preeclampsia.[50] Early pregnancy dyslipidemia[51] and gestational diabetes[52] are also associated with an increased 2–3 fold risks of preeclampsia. At this time it is uncertain if these are cause or markers for endothelial dysfunction, or if they may be cause or evidence of increased oxidative stress in preeclampsia.

Cardiac Function in Preeclampsia

Blood pressure normally declines in early pregnancy; systolic pressure changes little, while diastolic pressure falls by 10 mm Hg at 13–20 weeks, then rises again to prepregnancy levels in the third trimester. Normal pregnancy is characterized by primary vasodilatation and increased cardiac output is due in part to the decreased afterload. As noted high blood pressure in preeclampsia is due mainly to a reversal of the vasodilatation of normal pregnancy, replaced by marked increase in peripheral vascular resistance. Most studies of cardiovascular hemodynamics in women with preeclampsia have been performed in women with established disease and may be confounded by ongoing treatment. Invasive hemodynamic monitoring of untreated preeclamptics as well as limited careful echocardiographic studies demonstrate that women with preeclampsia have either normal or slightly decreased cardiac output in association with increased systemic vascular resistance and increased afterload. Serial echocardiographic studies throughout gestation have shown that in women who eventually developed preeclampsia, increased cardiac outputs and decreased peripheral vascular resistance were found early in pregnancy followed by high resistance low cardiac output states when preeclampsia developed.[53] Other studies of nulliparous gravidas with preeclampsia in the third trimester using pulmonary artery catheter, show decreased cardiac output in preeclamptic patients compared with controls.[13,54] Peripheral vascular resistance was increased and pulmonary capillary wedge pressure was low normal. This has been confirmed in other studies, and amounts to a normal ventricle contracting normally against a markedly increased afterload.[55] Peripartum heart failure can occur in this setting, though it is usually a complication of preexisting heart disease.[56]

Plasma volume and red blood cell mass are increased in normal pregnancy, as physiologic vasodilatation leads to stimulation of the renin-angiotensin system, and volume retention ensues. In preeclampsia, however, plasma volume is decreased, this is documented by measurement with Evans blue dye.[57,58] The decrease in plasma volume may be secondary to vasoconstriction and hypertension, although there are some reports that decrease in plasma volume may precede hypertension.[57,59,60] These latter reports have led to the use of volume expansion therapy with vasodilator drugs in the treatment of preeclampsia. In view of the suppressed renin-angiotensin system in preeclampsia, the decreased plasma volume seems likely secondary to vasoconstriction and a "smaller" intravascular compartment. Reports that the decreased plasma volume may have preceded hypertension[60] led to the experimental use of volume expansion therapy; although in Cochrane analysis, this treatment remains unproven.[61]

Renal Changes in Preeclampsia

Consistent with the effects of preeclampsia on the endothelium, the renal lesion characteristic of preeclampsia is glomerular endotheliosis.[18,62,63] The glomeruli are enlarged and swollen but not hypercellular, due primarily to hypertrophy of the intracapillary cells (mainly endothelial but mesangial as well), which encroach on the capillary lumina, giving the appearance of a bloodless glomerulus. The basement membrane is usually not thickened and foot process are usually well preserved, even when severe proteinuria is present. Interestingly sFlt-1, which is elevated in women with preeclampsia, has been administered to pregnant rats and induces hypertension, proteinuria, and glomerular endotheliosis, the classic lesion of preeclampsia.[6] Similarly, these renal alterations are also observed in experimental models that are characterized by reduced VEGF levels in the case of VEGF knockout mice.[64]

Localized lesions resembling those of focal and segmental glomerulosclerosis (FSGS) are present in about 20% of women with preeclampsia. The significance of this finding is not clear; some consider it to be a sequelae of preeclampsia, a form of secondary FSGS, whereas others consider that it may be a manifestation of preexisting subclinical nephrosclerosis.

In preeclampsia, both glomerular filtration rate and renal blood flow decrease, the former more than the later, leading to a decrease in filtration fraction.[18] The decrement is usually modest (25%) even when morphologic changes are pronounced. Because renal function normally rises 35–50% during pregnancy, creatinine levels are usually still below the upper limits of normal. The basis for the altered renal hemodynamics is not certain; renal histological and hormonal changes are probably involved. Recent evidence suggests that the hormone relaxin, a natural vasodilator produced by the corpus luteum and placenta, is reduced in women with preeclampsia and may contribute to the renal changes observed.[65,66] Fractional urate clearances decrease, often before overt disease is apparent, with a uric acid level greater than 5.5 mg/dL (327 mmol/L) being an important marker of preeclampsia. This appears to be a sensitive marker of decreased renal clearance and glomerular filtration. Proteinuria > 0.3 g/day (but in some cases nephrotic range i.e. >3 g/day) is another hallmark which may appear late in the clinical course of the disease. Rarely, renal insufficiency may develop due to acute tubular or cortical necrosis associated with preeclampsia.[67]

Sodium excretion appears to be impaired in preeclampsia, documented in studies of renal excretory ability after saline infusion,[68] though the reduction in intravascular volume and decreased placental perfusion are major reasons to avoid diuretics in preeclampsia.[18] Renal handling of calcium is also abnormal in preeclampsia, with hypocalciuria, low plasma 1,25-dihydroxyvitamin D3 and high parathyroid hormone noted.[69,70]

Coagulation System

Pregnancy is associated with an increase in hemostatic factors and decrease in fibrinolytic proteins: factors II, VII, X, VIII, XII, and fibrinogen increases 20–200% whereas the fibrinolytic protein S has a 40% decrease during pregnancy.[71] The inherited coagulopathies are major causes of thromboembolic disease in both pregnant and nonpregnant individuals; the most common are autosomal dominant deficiencies of antithrombin III, protein C, protein S, as well as activated protein C resistance due to the factor V Leiden mutation, and a function-enhancing mutation in the prothrombin gene (Prothrombin G20210A) and hyperhomocystinemia. The pregnancy associated changes in hemostatic and fibrinolytic proteins exacerbate the clinical effect of heritable coagulopathies. A postulated mechanism for preeclampsia in relation to the coagulopathies is the development of microthrombi in the placental circulation, with decreased placental perfusion leading to preeclampsia, hypertension and proteinuria.[72] Factor V Leiden mutation is the most common heritable coagulopathy, affecting 5–9% of European populations, though is rare in Asian and African populations.[73,74] A recent meta-analysis suggests that factor V Leiden is associated with a twofold increased risk for preeclampsia.[75] The risk of the Prothrombin 202210 polymorphism though suggestive as a risk factor is less clearly so, and the MTHFR genotype (leading to hyperhomocystinemia) does not appear to confer an increased risk.[75] Increased incidence of pregnancy-related complications including preeclampsia have been found for deficiencies in protein C, protein S, antithrombin III, but determination of the specific odds of developing preeclampsia with these thrombophilias is ongoing.[76] Clinically some advocate screening for thrombophilias in women with early (<34 weeks) or severe (>160/110 mm Hg) pre-eclampsia with consideration of heparin treatment in those found to be positive. Primary preventive treatment for women with known thrombophilic mutations but no clotting history is less certain until more trial data is available.

Falling platelet counts are a known manifestation of pre-eclampsia. The precise mechanism is unclear, but it appears that microangiopathy and endothelial cell damage stimulate platelet activation and consumption.[77,78] When severe, this may lead to disseminated intravascular coagulation.[79] Platelet activation may lead to increased generation of TXA_2 that may in turn increase vasoconstriction and platelet aggregation.[80] Increased release of platelet products such as serotonin may also contribute to vasoconstriction, and pharmacologic agents that inhibit serotonin such as ketanserin have been used successfully in the treatment of pre-eclampsia.[81]

Hepatic Abnormalities

The liver dysfunction that may accompany preeclampsia is correlated to the histological findings, which include periportal hemorrhages, ischemic lesions and fibrin disposition. These are consistent with both endothelial damage and activation of the coagulation system leading to some amount of liver tissue edema or necrosis. Involvement may range from mild enzyme abnormalities to HELLP with markedly elevated transaminase levels, to subcapsular bleeding or hepatic rupture. HELLP syndrome is well described in the clinical literature[82] and requires the presence of hemolysis on peripheral smear and platelet counts below 100,000/mm[3] and transaminase levels greater than twice the normal for diagnosis. Liver involvement in preeclampsia generally signifies more serious disease and is associated with an increased risk of maternal complications compared to preeclampsia alone.[83]

Central Nervous System

Eclampsia and seizures in preeclampsia which cannot be attributed another cause, are the most common central nervous system complication and are responsible for the most maternal deaths in this disease. In one small series, seizures were preceded by headache in 64% and by visual changes in 32%.[84] Visual disturbances include blurred vision, scotomas, and rarely, reversible cortical blindness (reversible posterior leukencephalopathy). In these cases, CT and MRI studies showed extensive bilateral white-matter abnormalities suggestive of vasogenic edema without infarction in the occipital and posterior parietal lobes of the cerebral hemispheres.[85,86]

Pathologic specimens postmortem of eclampsia reveal hemorrhages and petechiae, vasculopathy and ischemia with microinfarcts.[87] The cause of cerebral hemorrhage is debated; vasospasm, thrombosis and rupture have been postulated and transcranial Doppler studies document increased cerebral blood flow velocity consistent with vasospasm in women with pre-eclampsia and eclampsia.[88-90] Convulsions have been observed in women with only mild to moderate hypertension; the mechanisms for the seizures are not known, though by computed tomography and magnetic resonance imaging[91,92] cerebral edema has been described, as have hemorrhage and edema in the vascular watershed areas of the posterior hemispheres.[93] Predominance of posterior lesions may explain the increased incidence in preeclampsia—eclampsia of visual disturbances. Rarely, hemorrhages may be major and associated with permanent neurologic sequelae. Cerebral edema observed on some computed tomography studies may be a consequence of excess administration of fluids in patients with low oncotic pressure due to hypoalbuminemia. Rarely, reversible posterior leukoencephalopathy may develop in patients with eclampsia, which is transient blindness that resolves completely in most cases.[85] The findings on neuroimaging are characteristic of subcortical edema without infarction.

Long-term Sequelae of Preeclampsia

The pathophysiologic changes of preeclampsia appear to confer long-term risk for cardiovascular disease in the mother. In an analysis of follow-up of over 30,000 hypertensive pregnant women, gestational hypertension, mild preeclampsia and severe preeclampsia were associated with 2.8-, 2.2- and 3.3-fold greater risks for premature cardiovascular events,[94] a magnitude of excess risk which is on par with smoking. Severe preeclampsia was also associated with a 2.3 greater risk for thromboembolic events[94] and in a separate study the rate ratio for later death from stroke for the preeclampsia/eclampsia group was 3.59.[95,96] Whether this is a result of permanent endothelial injury or if preeclampsia is a manifestation of an underlying predisposition to vascular disease is not known.

REFERENCES

1. Roberts JM, Pearson G, Cutler J, et al. Summary of the NHLBI Working Group on research on hypertension during pregnancy. Hypertension. 2003;41(3):437-45.
2. Heyborne KD, Porreco RP. Selective fetocide reverses pre-eclampsia in discordant twins. Am J Obstet Gynecol. 2004;191(2):477-80.
3. Pijnenborg R, Dixon G, Robertson WB, et al. Trophoblastic invasion of human decidua from 8 to 18 weeks of pregnancy. Placenta. 1980;1(1):3-19.

4. Zhou Y, Damsky CH, Chiu K, et al. Pre-eclampsia is associated with abnormal expression of adhesion molecules by invasive cytotrophoblasts. J Clin Invest. 1993;91(3):950-60.
5. Brosens IA, Robertson WB, Dixon HG. The role of the spiral arteries in the pathogenesis of pre-eclampsia. Obstet Gynecol Annu. 1972;1:177-91.
6. Maynard SE, Min JY, Merchan J, et al. Excess placental soluble fms-like tyrosine kinase 1 (sFlt1) may contribute to endothelial

dysfunction, hypertension, and proteinuria in pre-eclampsia. J Clin Invest. 2003;111(5):649-58.

7. Levine RJ, Maynard SE, Qian C, et al. Circulating angiogenic factors and the risk of pre-eclampsia. N Engl J Med. 2004;350(7):672-83.

8. Lutten A, Carmeliet P. Soluble VEGF receptor Flt 1: The elusive pre-eclampsia factor discovered? J Clin Invest. 2003;111:600-2.

9. Levine RJ, Thadhani R, Qian C, et al. Urinary placental growth factor and risk of pre-eclampsia. JAMA. 2005;293(1):77-85.

10. Poranen AK, Ekblad U, Uotila P, et al. Lipid peroxidation and antioxidants in normal and preeclamptic pregnancies. Placenta. 1996;17(7):401-5.

11. Barden A, Ritchie J, Walters B, et al. Study of plasma factors associated with neutrophil activation and lipid peroxidation in pre-eclampsia. Hypertension. 2001;38(4):803-8.

12. Roberts JM, Speer P. Antioxidant therapy to prevent pre-eclampsia. Semin Nephrol. 2004;24(6):557-64.

13. Ghidini A, Salafia CM, Pezzullo JC. Placental vascular lesions and likelihood of diagnosis of pre-eclampsia. Obstet Gynecol. 1997;90(4 Pt 1):542-5.

14. Visser W, Wallenburg HC. Central hemodynamic observations in untreated pre-eclamptic patients. Hypertension. 1991;17(6 Pt 2):1072-7.

15. Fallis NE, Langford HG. Relation of second trimester blood pressure to toxemia of pregnancy in the primigravid patient. Am J Obstet Gynecol. 1963;87:1235.

16. Page EW, Christianson R. The impact of mean arterial pressure in the middle trimester upon the outcome of pregnancy. Am J Obstet Gynecol. 1976;125(6):740-6.

17. Kyle PM, Clark SJ, Buckley D, et al. Second trimester ambulatory blood pressure in nulliparous pregnancy: A useful screening test for pre-eclampsia? Br J Obstet Gynecol. 1993;100(10):914-9.

18. August P, Helseth G, Cook EF, et al. A prediction model for superimposed pre-eclampsia in women with chronic hypertension during pregnancy. Am J Obstet Gynecol. 2004;191(5):1666-72.

19. Lindheimer M, Katz A. Renal physiology and disease in pregnancy, 2nd edition. New York: Raven Press; 1992.

20. Ayala DE, Hermida RC, Mojon A, et al. Circadian blood pressure variability in healthy and complicated pregnancies. Hypertension. 1997;30(3 Pt 2):603-10.

21. Schobel HP, Fischer T, Heuszer K, et al. Pre-eclampsia—a state of sympathetic overactivity. N Engl J Med. 1996;335(20):1480-5.

22. Fitzgerald D, FitzGerald G. Eicosanoids in the pathogenesis of pre-eclampsia. In: Laragh J BBe (Ed). Hypertension: Pathophysiology, Diagnosis, and Management. New York: Raven Press; 1990. pp. 1789-807.

23. Fitzgerald DJ, Entman SS, Mulloy K, et al. Decreased prostacyclin biosynthesis preceding the clinical manifestation of pregnancy-induced hypertension. Circulation. 1987;75(5):956-63.

24. Mills JL, DerSimonian R, Raymond E, et al. Prostacyclin and thromboxane changes predating clinical onset of pre-eclampsia: A multicenter prospective study. JAMA. 1999;282(4):356-62.

25. Fitzgerald DJ, Rocki W, Murray R, et al. Thromboxane A2 synthesis in pregnancy-induced hypertension. Lancet. 1990;335(8692):751-4.

26. Chambers JC, Fusi L, Malik IS, et al. Association of maternal endothelial dysfunction with pre-eclampsia. JAMA. 2001; 285(12):1607-12.

27. Duley L, Henderson-Smart DJ, Knight M, et al. Antiplatelet agents for preventing pre-eclampsia and its complications. Cochrane Database Syst Rev. 2004;1:CD004659.

28. Roberts JM, Taylor RN, Musci TJ, et al. Pre-eclampsia: An endothelial cell disorder. Am J Obstet Gynecol. 1989;161(5):1200-4.

29. Sibai BM, Kustermann L, Velasco J. Current understanding of severe pre-eclampsia, pregnancy-associated hemolytic uremic syndrome, thrombotic thrombocytopenic purpura, hemolysis, elevated liver enzymes, and low platelet syndrome, and postpartum acute renal failure: Different clinical syndromes or just different names? Curr Opin Nephrol Hypertens. 1994;3(4):436-45.

30. Savvidou MD, Hingorani AD, Tsikas D, et al. Endothelial dysfunction and raised plasma concentrations of asymmetric dimethylarginine in pregnant women who subsequently develop pre-eclampsia. Lancet. 2003;361(9368):1511-7.

31. Baylis C, Beinder E, Suto T, et al. Recent insights into the roles of nitric oxide and renin-angiotensin in the pathophysiology of pre-eclamptic pregnancy. Semin Nephrol. 1998;18(2):208-30.

32. Molnar M, Suto T, Toth T, et al. Prolonged blockade of nitric oxide synthesis in gravid rats produces sustained hypertension, proteinuria, thrombocytopenia, and intrauterine growth retardation. Am J Obstet Gynecol. 1994;170(5 Pt 1):1458-66.

33. Seligman SP, Buyon JP, Clancy RM, et al. The role of nitric oxide in the pathogenesis of pre-eclampsia. Am J Obstet Gynecol. 1994; 171(4):944-8.

34. Begum S, Yamasaki M, Mochizuki M. Urinary levels of nitric oxide metabolites in normal pregnancy and pre-eclampsia. J Obstet Gynecol Res. 1996;22(6):551-9.

35. Silver RK, Kupferminc MJ, Russell TL, et al. Evaluation of nitric oxide as a mediator of severe pre-eclampsia. Am J Obstet Gynecol. 1996;175(4 Pt 1):1013-7.

36. Taylor RN, Varma M, Teng NN, et al. Women with pre-eclampsia have higher plasma endothelin levels than women with normal pregnancies. J Clin Endocrinol Metab. 1990;71(6):1675-7.

37. Nova A, Sibai BM, Barton JR, et al. Maternal plasma level of endothelin is increased in pre-eclampsia. Am J Obstet Gynecol. 1991;165(3):724-7.

38. Clark BA, Halvorson L, Sachs B, et al. Plasma endothelin levels in pre-eclampsia: Elevation and correlation with uric acid levels and renal impairment. Am J Obstet Gynecol. 1992;166(3):962-8.

39. Benigni A, Orisio S, Gaspari F, et al. Evidence against a pathogenetic role for endothelin in pre-eclampsia. Br J Obstet Gynecol. 1992;99(10):798-802.

40. Davidge ST, Signorella AP, Hubel CA, et al. Distinct factors in plasma of pre-eclamptic women increase endothelial nitric oxide or prostacyclin. Hypertension. 1996;28(5):758-64.

41. Taylor RN, Casal DC, Jones LA, et al. Selective effects of pre-eclamptic sera on human endothelial cell procoagulant protein expression. Am J Obstet Gynecol. 1991;165(6, Pt 1):1705-10.

42. Hubel CA, Roberts JM, Taylor RN, et al. Lipid peroxidation in pregnancy: New perspectives on pre-eclampsia. Am J Obstet Gynecol. 1989;161(4):1025-34.

43. Barden A, Beilin LJ, Ritchie J, et al. Plasma and urinary 8-iso-prostane as an indicator of lipid peroxidation in pre-eclampsia and normal pregnancy. Clin Sci (Lond). 1996;91(6):711-8.

44. Serdar Z, Gur E, Develioglu O, et al. Placental and decidual lipid peroxidation and antioxidant defenses in pre-eclampsia. Lipid peroxidation in pre-eclampsia. Pathophysiology. 2002;9(1):21.

45. Seely EW, Solomon CG. Insulin resistance and its potential role in pregnancy-induced hypertension. J Clin Endocrinol Metab. 2003;88(6):2393-8.

46. Sattar N, Bendomir A, Berry C, et al. Lipoprotein subfraction concentrations in pre-eclampsia: pathogenic parallels to atherosclerosis. Obstet Gynecol. 1997;89(3):403-8.

47. Murai JT, Muzykanskiy E, Taylor RN. Maternal and fetal modulators of lipid metabolism correlate with the development of pre-eclampsia. Metabolism. 1997;46(8):963-7.

48. Lorentzen B, Birkeland KI, Endresen MJ, et al. Glucose intolerance in women with pre-eclampsia. Acta Obstet Gynecol Scand. 1998;77(1):22-7.

49. Long PA, Abell DA, Beischer NA. Importance of abnormal glucose tolerance (hypoglycemia and hyperglycemia) in the aetiology of pre-eclampsia. Lancet. 1977;1(8018):923-5.

50. Solomon CG, Graves SW, Greene MF, et al. Glucose intolerance as a predictor of hypertension in pregnancy. Hypertension. 1994;23(6, Pt 1):717-21.

51. O'Brien TE, Ray JG, Chan WS. Maternal body mass index and the risk of pre-eclampsia: A systematic overview. Epidemiology. 2003;14(3):368-74.

52. Enquobahrie DA, Williams MA, Butler CL, et al. Maternal plasma lipid concentrations in early pregnancy and risk of pre-eclampsia. Am J Hypertens. 2004;17(7):574-81.

53. Ostlund I, Haglund B, Hanson U. Gestational diabetes and pre-eclampsia. Eur J Obstet Gynecol Reprod Biol. 2004;113(1):12-6.

54. Easterling TR, Benedetti TJ, Schmucker BC, et al. Maternal hemodynamics in normal and pre-eclamptic pregnancies: A longitudinal study. Obstet Gynecol. 1990;76(6):1061-9.

55. Groenendijk R, Trimbos JB, Wallenburg HC. Hemodynamic measurements in pre-eclampsia: Preliminary observations. Am J Obstet Gynecol.1984;150(3):232-6.

56. Lang RM, Pridjian G, Feldman T, et al. Left ventricular mechanics in pre-eclampsia. Am Heart J. 1991;121(6, Pt 1):1768-75.

57. Cunningham FG, Pritchard JA, Hankins GD, et al. Peripartum heart failure: Idiopathic cardiomyopathy or compounding cardio-vascular events? Obstet Gynecol. 1986;67(2):157-68.

58. Brown MA, Zammit VC, Mitar DM. Extracellular fluid volumes in pregnancy-induced hypertension. J Hypertens. 1992;10(1):61-8.

59. Silver HM, Seebeck M, Carlson R. Comparison of total blood volume in normal, pre-eclamptic, and nonproteinuric gestational hypertensive pregnancy by simultaneous measurement of red blood cell and plasma volumes. Am J Obstet Gynecol. 1998;179(1):87-93.

60. Chesley L. Hypertensive Disorders in Pregnancy. New York: Appleton-Century-Crofts; 1978.

61. Gallery ED, Hunyor SN, Gyory AZ. Plasma volume contraction: A significant factor in both pregnancy-associated hypertension (pre-eclampsia) and chronic hypertension in pregnancy. Q J Med. 1979;48(192):593-602.

62. Duley L, Williams J, Henderson-Smart DJ. Plasma volume expansion for treatment of women with pre-eclampsia. Cochrane Database Syst Rev. 2000;2:CD00 1805.

63. Packham DK, Mathews DC, Fairley KF, et al. Morphometric analysis of pre-eclampsia in women biopsied in pregnancy and post-partum. Kidney Int. 1988;34(5):704-11.

64. Gaber L, Lindheimer M. Hypertensive disorders in pregnancy. Stanford (CT): Appleton and Lange; 1999.

65. Eremina V, Sood M, Haigh J, et al. Glomerular-specific alterations of VEGF-A expression lead to distinct congenital and acquired renal diseases. J Clin Invest. 2003;111(5):707-16.

66. Jeyabalan A, Novak J, Danielson LA, et al. Essential role for vascular gelatinase activity in relaxin-induced renal vasodilation, hyperfiltration, and reduced myogenic reactivity of small arteries. Circ Res. 2003;93(12):1249-57.

67. Davison JM, Homuth V, Jeyabalan A, et al. New aspects in the pathophysiology of pre-eclampsia. J Am Soc Nephrol. 2004; 15(9):2440-8.

68. Pertuiset N, Grunfeld JP. Acute renal failure in pregnancy. Baillieres Clin Obstet Gynecol. 1994;8(2):333-51.

69. Brown MA, Gallery ED, Ross MR, et al. Sodium excretion in normal and hypertensive pregnancy: A prospective study. Am J Obstet Gynecol. 1988;159(2):297-307.

70. Taufield PA, Ales KL, Resnick LM, et al. Hypocalciuria in pre-eclampsia. N Engl J Med. 1987;316(12):715-8.

71. August P, Marcaccio B, Gertner JM, et al. Abnormal 1,25-dihydroxyvitamin D metabolism in pre-eclampsia. Am J Obstet Gynecol. 1992;166(4):1295-9.

72. Delorme MA, Burrows RF, Ofosu FA, et al. Thrombin regulation in mother and fetus during pregnancy. Semin Thromb Hemost. 1992;18(1):81-90.

73. Preston FE, Rosendaal FR, Walker ID, et al. Increased fetal loss in women with heritable thrombophilia. Lancet. 1996;348(9032):913-6.

74. Lockwood CJ. Heritable coagulopathies in pregnancy. Obstet Gynecol Surv. 1999;54(12):754-65.

75. Ridker PM, Miletich JP, Hennekens CH, et al. Ethnic distribution of factor V Leiden in 4047 men and women. Implications for venous thromboembolism screening. JAMA. 1997;277(16):1305-7.

76. Lin J, August P. Genetic thrombophilias and pre-eclampsia: A meta-analysis. Obstet Gynecol. 2005;105(1):182-92.

77. Kupferminc MJ, Eldor A, Steinman N, et al. Increased frequency of genetic thrombophilia in women with complications of pregnancy. N Engl J Med. 1999;340(1):9-13.

78. Ballegeer VC, Spitz B, De Baene LA, et al. Platelet activation and vascular damage in gestational hypertension. Am J Obstet Gynecol. 1992;166(2):629-33.

79. Konijnenberg A, Stokkers EW, van der Post JA, et al. Extensive platelet activation in pre-eclampsia compared with normal pregnancy: enhanced expression of cell adhesion molecules. Am J Obstet Gynecol. 1997;176(2):461-9.

80. Letsky EA. Disseminated intravascular coagulation. Best Pract Res Clin Obstet Gynecol. 2001;15(4):623-44.

81. Malatyalioglu E, Adam B, Yanik FF, et al. Levels of stable metabolites of prostacyclin and thromboxane A2 and their ratio in normotensive and pre-eclamptic pregnant women during the antepartum and postpartum periods. J Matern Fetal Med. 2000;9(3):173-7.

82. Steyn DW, Odendaal HJ. Randomized controlled trial of ketanserin and aspirin in prevention of pre-eclampsia. Lancet. 1997;350(9087):1267-71.

83. Sibai BM. Diagnosis, controversies, and management of the syndrome of hemolysis, elevated liver enzymes, and low platelet count. Obstet Gynecol. 2004;103(5,Pt 1):981-91.

84. Martin JN Jr. Rinehart BK, May WL, et al. The spectrum of severe pre-eclampsia: comparative analysis by HELLP (hemolysis, elevated liver enzyme levels, and low platelet count) syndrome classification. Am J Obstet Gynecol. 1999;180 (6, Pt 1):1373-84.

85. Katz VL, Farmer R, Kuller JA. Pre-eclampsia into eclampsia: toward a new paradigm. Am J Obstet Gynecol. 2000;182(6):1389-96.

86. Hinchey J, Chaves C, Appignani B, et al. A reversible posterior leukoencephalopathy syndrome. N Engl J Med. 1996;334(8):494-500.

87. Chambers KA, Cain TW. Postpartum blindness: Two cases. Ann Emerg Med. 2004;43(2):243-6.

88. Richards A, Graham D, Bullock R. Clinicopathological study of neurological complications due to hypertensive disorders of pregnancy. J Neurol Neurosurg Psychiatry. 1988;51(3):416-21.

89. Riskin-Mashiah S, Belfort MA, Saade GR, et al. Transcranial Doppler measurement of cerebral velocity indices as a predictor of pre-eclampsia. Am J Obstet Gynecol. 2002;187(6):1667-72.

90. Ohno Y, Kawai M, Wakahara Y, et al. Transcranial assessment of maternal cerebral blood flow velocity in patients with pre-eclampsia. Acta Obstet Gynecol Scand. 1997;76(10):928-32.

91. Qureshi AI, Frankel MR, Ottenlips JR, et al. Cerebral hemodynamics in pre-eclampsia and eclampsia. Arch Neurol. 1996;53(12):1226-31.

92. Dahmus MA, Barton JR, Sibai BM. Cerebral imaging in eclampsia: Magnetic resonance imaging versus computed tomography. Am J Obstet Gynecol. 1992;167(4 Pt 1):935-41.

93. Moodley J, Bobat SM, Hoffman M, et al. Electroencephalogram and computerized cerebral tomography findings in eclampsia. Br J Obstet Gynecol. 1993;100(11):984-8.

94. Drislane FW, Wang AM. Multifocal cerebral hemorrhage in eclampsia and severe pre-eclampsia. J Neurol. 1997;244(3):194-8.

95. Kestenbaum B, Seliger SL, Easterling TR, et al. Cardiovascular and thromboembolic events following hypertensive pregnancy. Am J Kidney Dis. 2003;42(5):982-9.

96. Wilson BJ, Watson MS, Prescott GJ, et al. Hypertensive diseases of pregnancy and risk of hypertension and stroke in later life: results from cohort study. BMJ. 2003;326(7394):845.

81 Physiological Changes of the Uterine Cervix in Pregnancy and Delivery

VNA Breeveld-Dwarkasing, FK Lotgering

INTRODUCTION

During most of human pregnancy, the uterine cervix is a dynamic anatomical structure that serves as a barrier between the fetus in its intrauterine environment and the vagina as the portal to the outside world. In the prelude to parturition a process called ripening takes place in which the cervix changes from a structure that is firm and rigid to one that is soft and elastic that can be pulled open by uterine contractions, allowing passage of the fetus. It functions reliably, but is not foolproof. In preterm delivery the cervix opens prematurely and in cervical dystocia it may fail to dilate adequately. Recent work has improved our understanding of the mechanisms that underlie these changes, but current knowledge still cannot truly explain its dysfunctions. From the many factors and cells that are involved it is now concluded that cervical ripening and softening are caused by an inflammatory-like mechanism. In this chapter we summarize what is known and not known about the physiological changes of the uterine cervix in pregnancy and delivery, with emphasis on the remarkable remodelling of its viscoelastic properties.

Anatomy

The cervix is positioned between the muscular body of the uterus and the vagina, connecting the uterine cavity with the vagina through its canal which can dilate during delivery. The cervix consists predominantly of fibrous connective tissue (collagen 80% of total protein content) and 10–15% smooth muscle fibers.[1] The proportion of smooth muscle cells is higher near the myometrium (28%) than near the vagina (6%).[1] Through most of gestation the cervix is a firm structure but the fibrous tissue which is responsible for this has to change its structure to become soft and pliable during delivery. This process of cervical ripening is characterized by a gradual phase which starts in the early third trimester, preparing the cervix for the second phase (during delivery) in which it becomes soft and pliable in a few hours time. During the first phase of cervical ripening both collagen synthesis and denaturation increase, with denaturation dominating the process. During this stage, the cervix may already feel soft to touch but the highly denatured collagen network still provides sufficient resistance against uterine contractions. During dilatation further digestion of denatured collagen leads to loss of collagen and, consequently, of firmness.[2] The cervical ripening takes place mainly in the deep stromal layer of the cervix, a fact that emphasizes the importance of tissue sampling sites in biochemical studies of cervical ripening.

The cervix receives its blood supply primarily from the cervical branch of the uterine artery and anastomoses with the vaginal arteries are common. Blood flow increases markedly in the first trimester, when blood flow of the portio vaginalis uteri in healthy pregnant women was found to be increased to 69 mL/min/100 g.[3] The cervix contains abundant autonomic and sensory nerves, and

they are derived from the hypogastric (T13-L4), splanchnic (L6-S2) and vagus nerves.[4] The sensory information transmitted through the vagus nerves includes pain and other reflex information from the cervix during labor and delivery that seems to bypass the spinal cord.[5] In addition, afferent unmyelinated C-fibers of these nerves which are associated with cervical vasculature and smooth muscle cells produce neuropeptides that play a role in the local neurogenic inflammatory processes associated with cervical ripening such as causing the vasculature to leak, edema and migration of inflammatory immune cells.[4] However, the cervix apparently functions normally to retain the fetuses during pregnancy even in the absence of neuronal connections, as in the transplanted uterus in the mouse,[6] and in women with a pre-existing spinal cord lesion.

Clinical Considerations

The readiness of the uterine cervix to dilate after pharmacological induction of labor, but also in spontaneous preterm or term labor, is traditionally assessed with the use of the modified Bishop score.[7] The score takes into account the dilatation, length, consistency and position of the cervix. The ripeness of the cervix increases with advancing dilatation, reduction in length, progressive softening and a more anterior position of the cervix. These changes are the result of the changes in viscoelastic properties, uterine contractions, and descent of the fetus. Although clinicians use these variables to predict the risk of preterm delivery and/or the chance of successful induction, the subjectivity of the assessment and interobserver variability limit their predictive value. As a consequence, investigators have sought methods to measure the same variables objectively.

Cervical dilatation has been measured with the use of ultrasound crystals attached to the vaginal surface of the cervix, close to the cervical canal in humans[8,9] and in cows.[10] Because the propagation velocity of the ultrasound pulse in cervical tissue is approximately 1,500 m/s and remains constant, the distance between the two ultrasound crystals can be calculated from the time it takes for the pulse to travel from one to another. The method is somewhat limited in that it measures dilatation at the external opening of the cervix, instead of at the internal os where softening and opening (funnelling) may begin. Both species demonstrate a similar picture, as represented in (Fig. 81.1) for nulliparous women.

Initially, during the latent phase, uterine contractions do not result in an increase in distance between the crystals attached to the vaginal cervix. The first measurable response, during the early dilatation phase, is an increase in distance during a contraction followed by an almost complete rebound after the contraction. During the acceleration phase, the distance increases with each contraction and does not return to its prior position, thus resulting in progressive dilatation. A deceleration phase, as originally reported by Friedman,[12] does not normally occur.[8,13] The initial

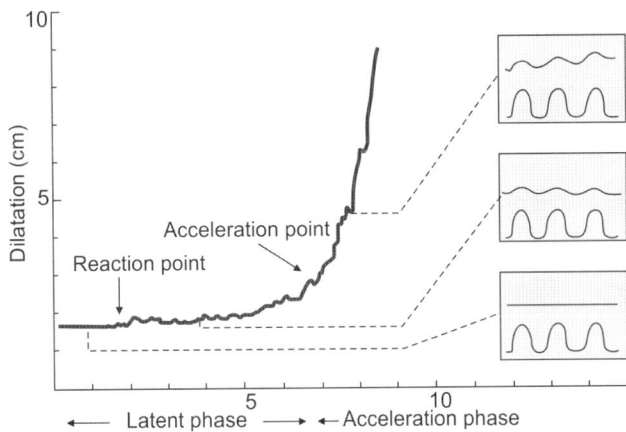

Fig. 81.1: Cervical dilatation in women as measured with ultrasound crystals attached to the cervix. In the early latent phase the cervix does not respond to contractions by dilatation, in the late latent phase dilatation increases temporarily with contractions, in the acceleration phase the cervix dilates progressively with contractions

Source: From van Dessel[11] with permission

cervical response to a uterine contraction as well as the onset of the acceleration phase occur at a smaller cervical diameter in parous than in nulliparous women. The initial response in parous women occurs at 2.9 cm and in nulliparous women it occurs at 3.6 cm. The onset of acceleration begins at 3.4 cm in parous and at 4.8 cm in nulliparous women respectively.[8] As a consequence, calculated myometrial work per cm of cervical dilatation in parous parturients is less than in nulliparous parturients, which means that less force is needed to dilate the cervix in parous than in nulliparous women.

Cervical length has been measured extensively in recent years with the use of transvaginal ultrasound transducers. The method is limited in that there is substantial intra and interobserver variability in measurements of cervical length, even when experienced observers perform the measurements under standardized conditions.[14] In singleton pregnancies, the uterine cervix on average is 40 ± 7 mm at midgestation and only slightly less at 30 weeks of gestation.[15] A short cervical length in asymptomatic women before 20 gestational weeks is a successful predictor of preterm delivery before 34 weeks of gestation, with a likelihood ratio of a positive test (cervical length < 25 mm) of 6.3 (CI 3.3–12.0) and that of a negative test of 0.8 (CI 0.65–0.95).[16] Likewise, a short cervical length is a useful predictor of successful labor induction, with a total rate of cesarean sections of 21% in women with a cervical length of ≤ 25 mm and 43% in women with a longer cervix.[17] Transvaginal sonographically measured cervical length itself was found to be a better predictor of successful labor induction than the traditional Bishop score,[17] with the notion however, that the differences were significant only in those women with an unripe cervix (Bishop score ≤ 5), which suggests that other factors, including the viscoelastic properties, are also important.

Softening of the cervix has been difficult to quantitate. However, light-induced fluorescence (LIF) of collagen has been used to investigate the changes in collagen content of the cervix during gestation and following labor induction with sodium nitroprusside, a nitric oxide donor, in the guinea pig[18] and in humans.[19] Collagen fluorescence decreased toward delivery and increased gradually postpartum, and treatment with sodium nitroprusside caused a

significant reduction in fluorescence. Collagen gives a characteristic fluorescence spectrum with a peak around 390 nm. One of the major cross-links of collagen, pyridinoline, is believed to be the intrinsic fluorophor. A decreased fluorescence suggests a reduction in collagen cross-links, associated with cervical ripening.

In the unripe cervix the cervical lips are positioned against the posterior fornix, and while ripening and softening, the cervix gradually moves forward so that the cervical canal lines up with the vagina. It has been attempted to study the position of the cervix with transvaginal ultrasound. However, the anterior cervical angle was found not to be either a useful predictor of induction success (sensitivity 22%, positive predictive value 40%) or of preterm birth.[20,21] The cervix is always involved in cases of preterm delivery, even if the primary cause is not the cervix. In the case of cervical insufficiency or cervical incompetence, a pre-existently weak cervix is unable to retain a pregnancy in the absence of uterine contractions. Historically, cervical incompetence is a clinical diagnosis based on a history of two or more second trimester pregnancy losses, after painless dilatation up to 4 cm.[22] The incidence of cervical incompetence has been estimated as 2/1,000 births in Denmark.[23] Such an intrinsic weakness of the cervix may be surgically treated by a cerclage. Cervical incompetence may be suspected in case of Mullerian abnormalities [cervical hypoplasia, as with in utero diethylstilbestrol (DES) exposure], surgical trauma as in prior late abortion, cone excision, trachelectomy, obstetrical trauma, or in the case of connective tissue disease (Ehlers-Danlos syndrome). A cervix which appears to be short by transvaginal sonography is also a risk factor for preterm delivery, but is not always caused by cervical incompetence. Therefore, the entities that could lead to preterm delivery should not be used interchangeably with cervical incompetence. Cervical incompetence may vary in degree and it may be expressed differently in subsequent pregnancies and although a short cervix may indicate a higher risk for preterm delivery it does not discriminate between underlying pathologies.[24] In normal pregnancies the cervix also shortens progressively between the 10th week and the 40th week.[25] That is why the American College of Obstetricians and Gynecologists recommends not to screen women at low risk routinely and to perform serial cervical length measurements only in women with a historical risk factor for preterm delivery.[26] These include bacterial vaginosis, placental and intra-amniotic infections, extreme uterine distension as in multiple pregnancies, blunt abdominal trauma leading to placental abruption, diabetes and smoking. When these causes lead to preterm delivery, irrespective of the etiology, a common biochemical pathway has to become active that will lead to cervical effacement and dilatation just as in normal delivery. Strategies to prevent preterm deliveries that are less invasive than cerclage, such as reduction of physical activities or even the application of vaginal pessaries are likely to be effective in the mere presence of risk factors, when clinical symptoms or a typical obstetrical history are absent.[27]

The change in cervical function from retaining the fetus in utero during pregnancy to allowing the fetus a smooth passage during delivery requires an extensive and intriguing remodelling of the viscoelastic properties of the cervix, as we will discuss in greater detail.

TISSUE REMODELING

Proper timing of the tissue remodeling in the cervix may make the difference between a severely premature, a healthy term or a post-term infant, and between spontaneous delivery, a cesarean section or a failed induction. Our understanding of the intriguingly complex mechanisms that underly this remodeling process is still far from complete. We will first describe the physiological changes that occur in the extracellular matrix (ECM) which is responsible for both the strength and plasticity of the cervix, subsequently the cellular events that are responsible for the changes in the ECM, and finally the hormonal changes that induce the invasion of cells and regulate the actions of both the resident and the invasive cells.

Extracellular Matrix

The cervix is not a static tissue but a dynamic organ, and the ECM plays a major role in dynamic changes in strength and plasticity of the cervix during pregnancy and parturition and the different phases of the menstrual cycle. The ECM constitutes collagens, proteoglycans and elastin, which are synthesized by the smooth muscle cells and fibroblasts that represent the majority of the cells that are usually present in the cervix. During ripening the structural integrity of the ECM changes as a result of structural changes in the collagen network, a shift in the composition of the total proteoglycan content and possibly a change in the arrangement of elastin fibers. During ripening the resident cells are mostly involved in releasing inflammatory mediators and proteolytic enzymes, while during labor an additional number of neutrophils and macrophages invade the cervix and release the enzymes stored in their granules, which are responsible for the much faster softening. We will discuss the dynamic regulation of collagen, elastin and other constituents of the ECM in more detail.

Collagen

The fibrous connective tissue of the cervix consists largely of collagen type I (70%) and type III (30%), and taken together they represent 80% of the total protein content of the cervix. Collagen molecules are three stranded molecules typically arranged in a triple helical configuration. Their strands are bound together by disulfide bridges and the molecules are cross-linked by pyridinoline side chains to form strong non-extendable fibers. The synthesis of collagen triple helices is complex in that it requires co-translational and post-translational steps in addition to the protein synthesis per se. Two relevant co-factors are vitamin C and copper. Copper is a co-factor for peptidyl-lysine oxidase, an enzyme involved in the cross-linking of collagen fibers that is inhibited by smoking.[28] Normally, the synthesis and degradation of collagen are in a dynamic balance, depending on the stage of pregnancy.

In the nonpregnant state, the collagen bundles are densely packed together. During pregnancy the collagen is gradually remodeled, during the process of ripening that prepares the cervix for labor and dilatation. Yet, even during the first trimester of pregnancy the collagen fibers become less tightly packed.[29] Through these changes, the pregnant cervix feels softer than the nonpregnant cervix, while a more parallel alignment of the fibers assures proper closing function.

As long as the helical conformation of the molecule remains intact, collagen is not readily accessible for proteolytic enzymes. Even when the collagen molecules are denatured, they can still maintain their three-dimensional network conformation through cross-bridges and still offer considerable resistance to physical stress, as is the case during cervical ripening.[2] Unwound, denatured,

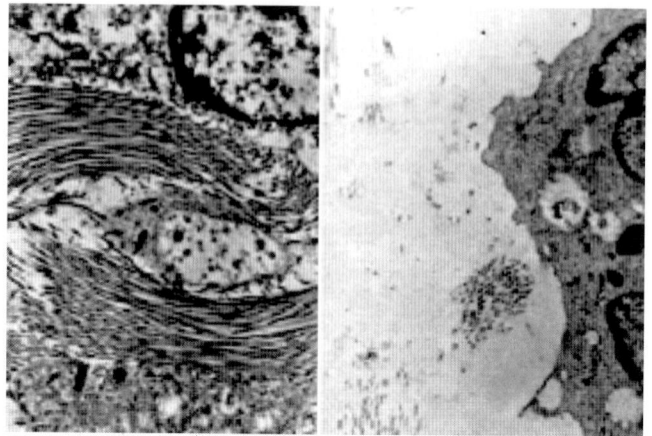

Fig. 81.2: Electron micrographs of cervix of pregnant guinea pigs obtained before term (left) and following ripening at term (right). Note the large number of collagen fibers present during early pregnancy and the decrease in fibers during ripening
Source: From Garfield et al.[31] with permission

collagen is subject to further digestion by proteolytic enzymes, including collagenases which may result in a greater solubility of collagen,[30] and this could be responsible for the decreased collagen content of the cervix shortly before delivery as observed in cows.[2] In pathologic conditions, including cervical incompetence and in utero diethylstilbestrol exposure, a too extensive ripening process may occur in mid-pregnancy.[29] The difference between an unripe and a maximally ripened cervix are clearly demonstrated in Figure 81.2. Subsequently, during parturition macrophages and neutrophils progressively invade the cervix, release their catabolic enzymes that dissolve the dispersed collagen fibers, and allow the cervix to dilate within hours.

Immediately after delivery, the involution of the cervix is accompanied by a two- to three-fold increase in the synthesis of collagen I and III,[32] thereby starting the repair that will allow the successful carrying of a subsequent pregnancy.

Elastin

Although elastin constitutes only 1% of the total connective tissue and its content does not appear to change with the stage of pregnancy, it is an important component of the extracellular matrix (ECM) of the cervix.[33] Elastin does not offer the same resistance against the mechanical forces of uterine contractions and the fetal presenting part as collagen does,[34] but it adds to the cervix the quality of elasticity. Added to the strength of the collagen, the elastic component may serve to keep the cervix closed during pregnancy, while allowing it to dilate during labor. But maybe even more importantly, it may enable the cervix to bounce back to its original diameter after delivery. Elastin is localized to specific regions of the cervix and is not dispersed through the cervical stroma. Elastin seems to be concentrated at the external os and from there on it spreads to the periphery in a band upward to the internal os where it becomes sparse in the muscular area below the internal os.[33] The elastin fibers of the cervix are made up of membranes and fibrils which are organized in a fishnet like structure[34] so they can be stretched in any direction. They are likely to be responsible for the dynamic changes in cervical length and temporary funneling at the internal os of the cervical canal that occur during pregnancy in response to maternal positional changes, fetal movements and uterine contractions as observed by ultrasound.[35] Biopsies from incompetent cervices have shown a reduction in total elastin, fragmented fibers and an abnormal arrangement of the elastin compared with those of uncomplicated term pregnancies.[36]

Proteoglycans and Hyaluronic Acid

Proteoglycans play an important but complex role in the spatial arrangements and stabilization of the ECM. In addition, they regulate the induction of cytokines. Proteoglycans are glycoproteins that contain one or more glycosaminoglycan (GAG) side chains in addition to a protein core. In the past, the nomenclature of the proteoglycans was based on these side-chains and studying the changes in content of the various GAGs during pregnancy showed a complex pattern (Fig. 81.3).

The changes in GAG concentrations (nmol/g dry weight) are most pronounced during late gestation and labor. The change in total GAGs content is already pronounced in the third trimester and is caused predominantly by an increase in chondroitin-6-sulfate, while the further increase during labor is largely caused by an increase in hyaluronic acid. From the functional point of view, however, the relevance of these changes in total and individual GAG concentrations may be questioned as the complete proteoglycan molecule and its spatial arrangement rather than the content of side chains is important with regard to their role as building blocks of the ECM. Thanks to modern gene technology,

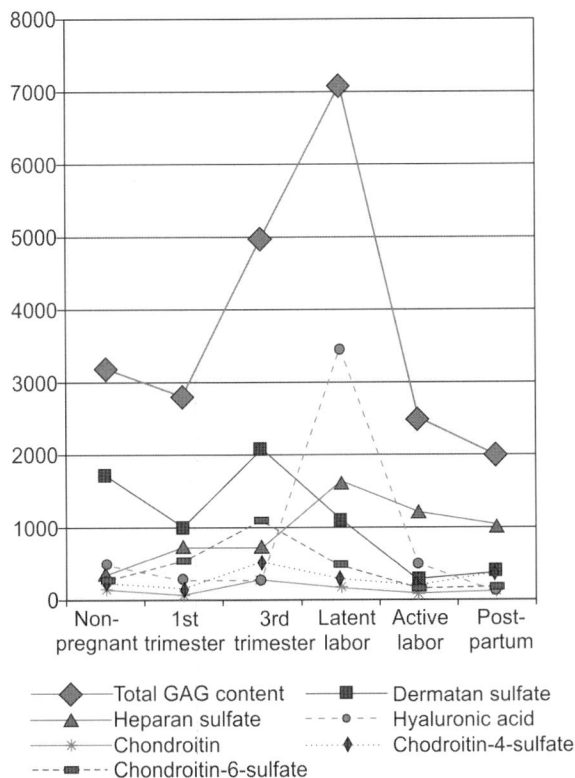

Fig. 81.3: Pregnancy-induced changes in the total glycosaminoglycans (GAG) content and the content of the individual GAGs (nmol/g dry weight) in the cervix of pregnant women at delivery and postpartum

Source: Adapted from Osmers et al.[37] with permission

a new appreciation of the molecular design has lead to a new and simplified nomenclature based on homologies of the protein core and to the grouping of distinct gene families and subfamilies, often with similar or identical structural and functional relationships.[38] Members of at least two proteoglycan subfamilies are present in the cervix, i.e. the small leucine-rich proteoglycans (formerly called small dermatan-sulfate proteoglycans) that include decorin and biglycan,[32,39] and the hyalectan (hyaluronan and lectin interacting) proteoglycans, that include versican (a large chondroitan/dermatan sulfate proteoglycan), aggrecan (a chondroitin sulfate proteoglycan) and a large (220 kDa) keratan sulfate proteoglycan.[40] Decorin seems relevant as it coats and stabilizes the collagen fibrils through a tight alignment of the fibrils, by binding its protein core with different sites of the collagen fibrils. The decorin concentration is lower in the cervix of term and parturient women than in nonpregnant and early pregnant women[41] and the decorin to collagen ratio correlates inversely with the softness of the cervix. This suggests that the dispersion of collagen near term is in part mediated by loss of decorin. Biglycan interacts with collagen via its GAG side chains and like decorin its concentration decreases during cervical ripening.[32] The hyalectans probably enhance the water binding capacity of hyaluronic acid. The concentrations of versican and the large keratin sulfate proteoglycan increase in the ECM during labor,[32,40] when a significant increase in the hyaluronic acid content also occurs.[37] Hyaluronic acid is a glycosaminoglycan which is produced by fibroblasts; it is hydrophilic and attracts water to the ECM, and helps to disrupt the collagen. In addition, it is involved in PGE_2 synthesis and cytokine production,[42] while its breakdown products have angiogenic, inflammatory, immune-stimulating, antiapoptotic and heat-shock protein-inducing properties,[43] all of which may contribute to accelerated ripening of the cervix in early labor. In the immediate postpartum period, uterine involution and cervical retraction are associated with a two- to threefold increase in the messages not only for collagen I and III but also of the small leucine rich proteoglycans, including decorin and biglycan, as part of the repair process.[32]

Mediators

Matrix Metalloproteinases

Matrix metalloproteinases (MMPs) are the primary mediators of extracellular matrix degradation in the cervix during pregnancy and parturition.[44-47] These zinc-dependant enzymes have been divided into four subgroups, collagenases, gelatinases, membrane type MMPs (MT-MMPs), and stromelysins. They are capable of degrading collagen and elastin, as well as other ECM components, including proteoglycans. All cell types present in the cervix are capable of producing MMPs. The physiologically important collagenases MMP-1 and MMP-8 are produced by the resident fibroblasts (MMP-1) and the invading neutrophils (MMP-8). They cleave the triple helices of the intact undenatured collagen, degrading it into smaller fragments. MMP-1 preferentially cleaves type III collagen and MMP-8 type I collagen.[48] MMP expression is regulated at several levels, including gene transcription, gene translation, latent enzyme secretion, pro-enzyme activation and, importantly, inactivation by endogenous inhibitors. Some MMPs, e.g. MMP1 are synthesized on demand in response to hormones, cytokines, growth factors and physical stress.[49] They may be secreted as latent enzymes into the ECM, or bound to the cell surface and become activated by proteinases, including other MMPs.[50]

Other MMPs such as MMP-8 are synthesized by leucocytes, such as neutrophils and macrophages, and stored in their granules as latent enzymes to be released when these cells are stimulated. At the onset of labor, neutrophils are attracted to the ECM. The MMPs present in neutrophil granules as well as in the ECM are activated, in response to increased cytokine activity resulting from hormone induction. As a consequence, during labor, MMP concentrations are increased both in the cervical tissue and in the circulation.

The ECM degrading activity of the MMPs is counterbalanced by the activity of tissue inhibitors of metalloproteinases (TIMPs). These inhibitors are present in the cervix throughout gestation[29] and prevent it from becoming too severely damaged by the MMPs. The synthesis of TIMPs varies with the level of MMP-activity, which in turn is dependant of the stage of cervical ripening and dilatation.[51] Other suppressive factors of MMP expression include TGF-β and glucocorticoid.[52]

Cytokines

Cytokines, including the interleukins (ILs) IL-1(α and β), IL-6, and IL-8, are causally linked to preterm and term labor. Cytokines attract neutrophils to the cervix, stimulate their extravasation, and the subsequent release of MMPs from their granules and also stimulate fibroblasts to synthesize and secrete MMPs. IL-1α stimulates MMP-1 secretion by human cervical fibroblasts and iNOS mRNA expression in these cells,[53] while IL-1β, IL-6, IL-8 and tumor necrosis factor alpha (TNFα) expression is linked to invading neutrophils.[54] When IL-1β or IL-8 are administered intracervically, they induce premature ripening and delivery.[55,56] IL-1β, IL- 6 and IL-8 are also found to be increased during bacterial vaginosis or intrauterine infections, and then they play a causal role in early cervical ripening and premature delivery.[57] Interleukin levels in the lower uterine segment,[58] placental blood, maternal serum and amnionic fluid[59] are also found to increase progressively with the increase of the cervical diameter in normal labor at term.

TGF-β is an immunosuppressant and a potent chemo-attractant for monocytes and neutrophils.[60] It stimulates fibroblasts to synthesize collagen and proteoglycans. TGF-β increases after delivery,[32] and may thereby contribute to the involution of the cervix.

Nitric Oxide

Nitric oxide (NO) is a short-lived free radical gas which is produced by nitric oxide synthases (NOS) in a reaction in which arginine, oxygen and NADPH are converted into citrulline, NO and NADP. There are three forms of nitric oxide synthases, all of them have been identified in the cervix. They are the constitutive calcium-dependent isoforms brainNOS (bNOS) and endothelial NOS (eNOS) and an inducible Ca-independent isoform (iNOS).

An important effect of NO is smooth muscle relaxation and therefore, it is believed to aid in myometrial relaxation during pregnancy and possibly in cervical relaxation during delivery,[61] as may be concluded from the observations in rats, where during active labor NO production is upregulated manyfold in the cervix, it is simultaneously downregulated in the myometrium.[62] Interestingly, the relaxing effect of NO on the myometrium appears to be mediated through an effect on calcium activated potassium channels and not through cGMP as has been previously assumed.[63,64]

The increase in cervical NO during labor is mediated mainly by the increased expression of inducible nitric oxide synthase (iNOS)[65]

in cervical stromal cells and invading neutrophils, macrophages and mast cells.[66] In addition to being a smooth muscle relaxant, and probably functionally more important, NO is also involved in the regulation of several inflammatory mediators that induce cervical softening. NO-donors such as sodium nitroprusside induce a rapid and significant softening of the cervix in early pregnant women, when it is applied into the cervical canal.[67] Sodium nitroprusside given intracervically to term pregnant guinea pigs induced changes in the ECM that were similar to those observed in guinea pigs that delivered spontaneously.[18] NO stimulates the release of prostaglandin (PG) E2 and PGF2α by human cervical fibroblast, through stimulating cyclo-oxygenase. It also stimulates the synthesis of proteoglycans, probably through a PGE2-dependent pathway. NO increases the production of MMP1 in human fibroblasts.[53] High concentrations in the cervical tissues may cause cell death.[68] The view that NO is actively involved in the pathways that lead to ECM degradation which contributes to cervical ripening is supported by the observation in pregnant rats that the NOS-synthesis inhibitor L-NAME significantly reduces the distensibility of the cervix.[62]

Endothelial NOS (eNOS) and brain NOS (bNOS) provide low background levels of NO in the cervix. The concentration of bNOS is significantly increased in active labor[69] while reports with regard to eNOS concentrations are contradictory. Both constitutive isoforms are believed to be more involved in smooth muscle relaxation, while the massive increase in NO synthesis which is caused through the greatly increased iNOS expression may be more important for its involvement in immune and inflammatory response.

Cellular Compartment

The cervix contains epithelial cells, smooth muscle cells and fibroblasts, as well as a variable population of migratory cells, neutrophils, macrophages and mast cells. All the various cell types in the cervix participate in one way or the other in the process of cervical ripening. The epithelial cells not only provide local protection against invading organisms, but secrete inflammatory modulators, including iNOS.[66] The resident fibroblasts and smooth muscle cells in the cervix are not only the source for collagens and proteoglycans and several growth factors, they also take part in the inflammatory-like response of the ripening cervix through the secretion of cytokines and proteolytic tissue-degrading enzymes. Early in gestation, smooth muscle cells and fibroblasts proliferate. Late in gestation, especially in early labor, the rate of proliferation is reduced, physiologic cell death (apoptosis) increases, and neutrophils and macrophages are attracted to the cervical stroma. Most of the information about the contribution of the individual cell types to the process of cervical ripening has been derived from in vitro studies, i.e. cell cultures and in a lesser amount from immuno-histochemical or in situ hybridization studies, so the possible effect of interactions between different cell types in most cases cannot be specified. Based on these studies, hormones or inflammatory mediators given to patients may not always induce the desired effect. In the following sections we will discuss what is known about the cellular components of the cervical stroma and their role in the physiological changes that occur during pregnancy and delivery.

Stromal Cells

Smooth muscle cells are present in the muscular outer layer of the cervix and in the stroma. Smooth muscle cells in the cervix may have two functions, one of muscle contraction and one of secretion of catabolic enzymes. Although the literature does not offer any clear guidance in this matter, it may be perceived as logical that muscle contractions may be the more important function in the outer layer, because of the arrangement of muscle fibers in bundles while in the stroma the more dispersed smooth muscle cells may contribute to the inflammatory-like mechanisms of the cervix. However, these two functions may not be completely separated because of the observation that an electromyogram (EMG) derived from the cervix is higher in women with a clinically unripe compared to a ripe cervix.[70,71] During parturition contractile activity of the cervix diminishes in response to increased levels of NO.[61]

The proposed mechanism by which NO exerts its relaxing effect on the myometrial smooth muscle cells has recently been revised. Previously it was thought that the relaxing effect of NO was mediated through soluble guanylyl cyclase (sGC) activation and cGMP accumulation, like in vascular and gastrointestinal smooth muscle cells. More recent studies, however, have shown that NO-induced relaxation is independent of this pathway.[64] It has been proposed that the NO-induced relaxation in the myometrium is mediated through the activation of calcium-activated potassium-[63] or PKG-independent regulation of myosin phosphatase.[64] Although it has been reported that an analog of the cGMP inhibits contractile activity of the cervix,[72] further studies are clearly needed to determine just how NO exerts its effect on cervical smooth muscle relaxation.

Besides contributing to the ECM by synthesizing collagens and proteoglycans,[38] cervical smooth muscle cells also participate in the inflammatory-like mechanism that leads to degradation of the ECM. They do so through the production of cytokines, including IL-1β and TNF-α, which in turn induce expression of MMP-1 and MMP-9.[73] They also produce IL-8, upon lipopolysaccharide- and cytokine-stimulation, which stimulates neutrophil invasion and degranulation and, consequently, the release of proteolytic enzymes, including MMPs.[74]

In some aspects cervical fibroblasts are similar to cervical smooth muscle cells in that they both contribute to the ECM by synthesizing collagens and proteoglycans, and they are both capable of producing cytokines, proteolytic enzymes such as MMPs and proteolytic enzyme inhibitors such as TIMPs. However, there are some fundamental differences in the way they react to stimulation by pro-inflammatory cytokines. For example, both cervical smooth muscle cells and fibroblasts increase their gene expression of MMP-1 and not of MMP-2 when stimulated by IL-1β or TNF-α, but fibroblasts also react by increasing TIMP expression, and cervical smooth muscle cells do not.[73] So fibroblasts have the primary function to provide the cervix with strength through the secretion of collagen and proteoglycans. Upon proper stimulation, they produce MMP-1, MMP-2 and MMP-9 as well as cytokines, including IL-6 and IL-8,[75,76] which are effective on the other side of the balance. Cultured human cervical fibroblasts respond to mechanical stress or the administration of PG-F2α, IL-1α or NO with the production or secretion of MMP-1.[49,53]

Invading Cells

Inflammatory cells of all kinds are present in cervical stroma throughout gestation[41] as they are in all organs that are in contact with the exterior. Shortly before the onset of labor the cervix is invaded by a large number of neutrophils, and to a lesser extent

by macrophages. They contribute to the increased levels of NO, cytokines and MMPs that are actively involved in cervical ripening and dilatation.

In pregnant women, neutrophils are thought to be the main source of the increased levels of collagenolytic enzymes, including MMPs.[77] During labor, neutrophilic infiltration of the lower uterine segment increases with cervical dilatation, as do the concentrations of MMP-8 and IL-8. At 2–3 cm dilatation, neutrophils are present close to the endothelium of the blood vessels but have not yet invaded the tissue. When dilatation progresses, the process of neutrophil invasion is associated with increased expression of adhesion molecules, including intercellular adhesion molecule-1, endothelial leucocyte adhesion molecule-1 and vascular cell adhesion molecule-1.[78] Shortly after delivery, the neutrophil concentration shows a marked further increase, and with it the expression of IL-1β and IL-8.[79] This may represent an anti-infectious property rather than being associated with cervical involution.

Macrophages are present in somewhat higher numbers in the cervical stroma of women during parturition,[79] while other inflammatory cells, including mast cells, T-cells and plasma cells that are present in small numbers during gestation, do not increase appreciably during labor.[41] Mast cells play a role in angiogenesis during the first half of gestation, through mast cell degranulation that causes the release of vascular endothelial growth factor (VEGF), basic fibroblast growth factor (bFGF), IL-1 and IL-6.[80] Macrophages and mast cells do not seem to play an important role in the initiation of labor.

HORMONAL REGULATION

Progesterone and Estrogen

Progesterone keeps the myometrium from contracting and the cervix from softening. Spontaneous labor is preceded by a reduction in the circulating concentration of progesterone and/or an increase in estrogen in several but not in humans, and premature labor can be induced successfully by estrogen injection in sheep.[81] This underlines the concept that progesterone dominance is important to maintain uterine quiescence, while estrogen dominance would lead to labor. The fact that parturition in humans is not preceded by a drop in serum progesterone concentration or a shift in serum progesterone/estrogen balance does not necessarily mean that the concept of the progesterone/estrogen balance is invalid in humans as circulating hormone concentrations are only part of the picture in which receptor quantity and sensitivity also plays a role. In the guinea pig, progesterone receptor expression decreases shortly before parturition, whereas estrogen receptor-α (ERα) remains high throughout late gestation and parturition.[82] Humans seem to be similar to guinea pigs in that the responsiveness of their cervix to progesterone and estrogen is likely not to be mediated through changes in circulating blood levels but by changes at the receptor level. The fact that progesterone antagonists effectively induce cervical ripening and labor in women supports the functional importance of progesterone blockade in the onset of labor.[83,84] In addition, progesterone may upregulate the production of TIMPs,[51] and inhibit the IL1- (α and β) mediated induction of MMP-9 in cervical fibroblasts of term pregnant rabbits,[85] by which it blocks the MMP-induced degradation of the ECM. Estrogen stimulates the infiltration of eosinophils in the rat[86] and the enzymatic activity of the procollagenases in cell cultures from the guinea pig cervix.[87,88]

Furthermore, estrogens enhance the cytokine-induced attraction of neutrophils to the cervix, an effect that is blocked by progesterone,[89,90] and the presence of ER-β in neutrophils suggests that estrogens may attribute to the release of MMPs from the neutrophils in the cervix.[91] Overall, the progesterone to estrogen ratio at the tissue and cellular level is likely to be of major importance for uterine quiescence and cervical closure during pregnancy as well as for the initiation of cervical ripening and delivery.

Prostaglandins

Prostaglandins (PGs) are unsaturated cyclic fatty acids derived from arachidonic acid in a reaction catalyzed by cyclo-oxygenase (COX)-1 and COX-2. COX-1 is expressed constitutively and COX-2 is induced by cytokines and growth factors.

Local (vaginal and intracervical) application and systemic administration of PGs (PGE_1, PGE_2 and $PGF_{2\alpha}$) and their synthetic analogs induce clinical ripening of the cervix and the onset of labor. In current obstetrical practice PGE_2-gel applied vaginally is routinely used to induce cervical softening. Collagen extractability from cervical biopsies of women treated with PG increased significantly compared to the cervix of non-pregnant women[92] or term pregnant women with an unfavorable cervix.[93] However, incubating biopsy samples with PGE_2 from pregnant women at different stages of pregnancy revealed that pregnancy stage has a major influence on the response of cervical tissues to PGE_2. For example, in the early first trimester collagen synthesis is stimulated, and proteoglycan synthesis is decreased, by PGE_2. In cervical tissues obtained from late first trimester pregnancy until term the effect of PGE2 on the synthesis of proteoglycans and collagen is reversed, while in tissues obtained at the start of labor, incubation with PGE2 causes a decrease in both collagen and proteoglycan synthesis.[94]

Several mechanisms are activated by PGs. PGE_2 enhances the effect of IL-8, a potent neutrophil chemoattractant,[95] which is abundantly present in the cervix and whose concentration in this tissue increases progressively with cervical dilatation.[96]

If endogenous PGs play a role in the physiological ripening and dilatation of the cervix it is to be expected that PG levels should rise in cervical tissue at late gestation and labor. However, analysis of cervical mucus samples shows no increase in PGE_2 and $PGF_{2\alpha}$ content during the period of cervical ripening.[97] This suggests that if PGE_2 and $PGF_{2\alpha}$ are active during normal labor, their levels are under tight temporal and spatial control and that they would be synthesized locally in the tissues, acting in a paracrine way. Incubated cervical tissues obtained from patients during the first trimester of pregnancy produced PGs and prostaglandin metabolites, an effect that may at least in part be mediated by NO.[98] Functional LH and hCG receptors have been localized in the cervix of women and treatment of endocervical tissue with hCG induced a significant decrease in COX-2 expression and thus could inhibit PG synthesis.

During the last few days prior to labor in the baboon, PGE_2 receptor expression in the cervix increases and thereby sensitizes the cervix to PGE_2.[99] The PGE_2 receptor, EP_4 is also present in human cervical fibroblasts and seems to mediate GAG synthesis.[100] PGE_2 may also cause an increase in cervical MMP-9 concentration in rats, by a cAMP-dependent mechanism.[101] Oxytocin infusion is widely used to augment labor by stimulating increased frequency and intensity of myometrial contractions, although in two randomized clinical studies intravenous infusion of low doses of oxytocin seemed to be as effective as local application of PGE_2 gel in inducing cervical effacement.[102,103] In cows, oxytocin-receptor expression in the cervix increases markedly during late gestation, predominantly in the mucosal cells.[104] In sheep, cervical oxytocin receptor levels during pregnancy are low[105] and remain low during late gestation and labor.[106] However, in sheep oxytocin is able to induce marked cervical softening in the estrus period because the oxytocin receptor is maximally present. The observations in sheep and the fact that in clinical practice oxytocin infusion is not always as effective in pre-labor ripening of the cervix of pregnant women, suggests that high oxytocin receptor levels are necessary to make the cervix sensitive to oxytocin. In cows it has been shown that oxytocin stimulates COX expression and by this way the release of PGE_2.[107] It could be possible that in women the effect of oxytocin is generated through an increased PGE_2 synthesis at the uterine level since oxytocin receptor expression in the uterus is increased during labor.[108] Preinduction with PGE_2, which is commonly practiced when oxytocin infusion is used to induce labor, may overcome the critical period when oxytocin receptors at the uterine or the cervical level have not yet increased to sufficiently high levels to induce endogenous PGE_2.

The conclusion is that although prostaglandins and oxytocin are able to induce cervical softening when used in labor induction, their role in cervical ripening and softening during physiological spontaneous deliveries at the cervical level is still disputed as the mechanisms that could possibly be involved have not yet been clearly established.

CONCLUSION

Since the concept of cervical ripening as a local inflammatory reaction has been introduced by Liggins,[109] the intriguingly complex remodeling of the uterine cervix in the onset of labor has shown to be an exciting field for continued research. Although many factors and mechanisms that could be involved in this process have been identified, mostly from animal models and in vitro studies, and have led to new concepts and ideas, not all of them have been shown to actually occur in the cervix of women that give normal birth. We have made a selection of those factors of which the clinical relevance is evident or could prove to be promising targets for pharmacological or mechanical interventions to prevent pre-term and post-term delivery as well as failure of ripening and dilatation in response to pharmacological induction of labor.

REFERENCES

1. Rorie DK, Newton M. Histologic and chemical studies of the smooth muscle in the human cervix and uterus. Am J Obstet Gynecol. 1967;99:466-9.
2. Breeveld-Dwarkasing VN, te Koppele JM, Bank RA, et al. Changes in water content, collagen degradation, collagen content, and concentration in repeated biopsies of the cervix of pregnant cows. Biol Reprod. 2003;69:1608-14.
3. Zubek L, Monos E, Csepli J. Significance of blood flow measurement in the cervix uteri in the 1st trimester of pregnancy. Zentralbl Gynakol. 1986;108:900-5.

4. Collins JJ, Usip S, McCarson KE, et al. Sensory nerves and neuropeptides in uterine cervical ripening. Peptides. 2002;23:167-83.

5. Whipple B, Komisaruk BR. Brain (PET) responses to vaginal-cervical self-stimulation in women with complete spinal cord injury: Preliminary findings. J Sex Marital Ther. 2002;28:79-86.

6. El Akouri RR, Kurlberg G, Dindelegan G, et al. Heterotopic uterine transplantation by vascular anastomosis in the mouse. J Endocrinol. 2002;174.

7. Bishop EH. Pelvic scoring for elective induction. Obstet Gynecol. 1964;24:266-8.

8. Van Dessel HJ, Frijns JH, Kok FT, et al. Ultrasound assessment of cervical dynamics during the first stage of labor. Eur J Obstet Gynecol Reprod Biol. 1994;53:123-7.

9. Eijskoot F, Storm J, Kok F, et al. An ultrasonic device for continuous measurement of cervical dilation during labor. Ultrasonics. 1977;15:183-5.

10. Breeveld-Dwarkasing VN, Struijk PC, Lotgering FK, et al. Cervical dilatation related to uterine electromyographic activity and endocrinological changes during prostaglandin F(2alpha)-induced parturition in cows. Biol Reprod. 2003;68:536-42.

11. Van Dessel HJ. The behavior of the uterine cervix during labor. Doctoral thesis, Erasmus, University, Rotterdam. 1992.

12. Friedman EA. Graphical analysis of labor. Am J Obstet Gynecol. 1954;68:1568-75.

13. Zhang J, Troendle JF, Yancey MK. Reassessing the labor curve in nulliparous women. Am J Obstet Gynecol. 2002;187:824-8.

14. Valentin LB. Intra and interobserver reproducibility of ultrasound measurements of cervical length and width in the second and third trimesters of pregnancy. Ultrasound Obstet Gynecol. 2002;20:256-62.

15. Dijkstra K, Janssen H, Kuczynski E, et al. Cervical length in uncomplicated pregnancy: A study of sociodemographic predictors of cervical changes across gestation. Am J Obstet Gynecol. 1999;180:639-44.

16. Honest H, Bachmann LM, Coomarasamy A, et al. Accuracy of cervical transvaginal sonography in predicting preterm birth: A systematic review. Ultrasound Obstet Gynecol. 2003;22:305-22.

17. Gabriel R, Darnaud T, Chalot F, et al. Transvaginal sonography of the uterine cervix prior to labor induction. Ultrasound Obstet Gynecol. 2002;19:254-7.

18. Fittkow CT, Shi SQ, Bytautiene E, et al. Changes in light-induced fluorescence of cervical collagen in guinea pigs during gestation and after sodium nitroprusside treatment. J Perinat Med. 2001;29:535-43.

19. Maul H, Olson G, Fittkow CT, et al. Cervical light-induced fluorescence in humans decreases throughout gestation and before delivery: Preliminary observations. Am J Obstet Gynecol. 2003;188:537-41.

20. Novakov-Mikic A, Ivanovic L, Dukanac J. Transvaginal ultrasonography of uterine cervix in prediction of the outcome of labour induction. Med Pregl. 2000;53:569-78.

21. Arabin B, van Eyck J. Sonographic diagnosis of cervical incompetence for prevention and management. Ultrasound Review. 2001;3:1-10.

22. Harger JH. Cerclage and cervical insufficiency: An evidence-based analysis. Obstet Gynecol. 2002;100:1313-27.

23. Lidegaard O. Cervical incompetence and cerclage in Denmark 1980-1990. A register based epidemiological survey. Acta Obstet Gynecol Scand. 1994;73:35-8.

24. Althuisius S, Dekker G, Hummel P, et al. Cervical Incompetence Prevention Randomized Cerclage Trial (CIPRACT): Effect of therapeutic cerclage with bed rest vs bed rest only on cervical length. Ultrasound Obstet Gynecol. 2002;20(2): 163-7.

25. Gramellini D, Fieni S, Molina E, et al. Transvaginal sonographic cervical length changes during normal pregnancy. J Ultrasound Med. 2002;21:227-32.

26. ACOG. ACOG Practice Bulletin Number 48. Cervical Insufficiency. Obstet Gynecol. 2003;102:1091-9.

27. Arabin B, Halbesma JR, Vork F, et al. Is treatment with vaginal pessaries an option in patients with a sonographically detected short cervix? J Perinat Med. 2003;31:122-33.

28. Kleissl HP, van der RM, Naftolin F, et al. Collagen changes in the human uterine cervix at parturition. Am J Obstet Gynecol. 1978;130:748-53.

29. Ludmir J, Sehdev HM. Anatomy and physiology of the uterine cervix. Clin Obstet Gynecol. 2000;43:433-9.

30. Uldbjerg N, Ekman G, Malmstrom A, et al. Ripening of the human uterine cervix related to changes in collagen, glycosaminoglycans, and collagenolytic activity. Am J Obstet Gynecol. 1983;147:662-6.

31. Garfield RE, Maul H, Shi L, et al. Methods and devices for the management of term and preterm labor. Ann NY Acad Sci. 2001;943:203-24.

32. Westergren-Thorsson G, Norman M, Bjornsson S, et al. Differential expressions of mRNA for proteoglycans, collagens and transforming growth factor-beta in the human cervix during pregnancy and involution. Biochimica et Biophysica Acta-Molecular Basis of Disease. 1998;1406:203-13.

33. Leppert PC, Cerreta JM, Mandl I. Orientation of elastic fibers in the human cervix. Am J Obstet Gynecol. 1986;155:219-24.

34. Leppert PC, Yu SY. Three-dimensional structures of uterine elastic fibers: scanning electron microscopic studies. Connect Tissue Res. 1991;27:15-31.

35. Yost NP, Bloom SL, Twickler DM, et al. Pitfalls in ultrasonic cervical length measurement for predicting preterm birth. Obstet Gynecol. 1999;93:510-6.

36. Leppert PC, Yu SY, Keller S, et al. Decreased elastic fibers and desmosine content in incompetent cervix. Am J Obstet Gynecol. 1987;157:1134-9.

37. Osmers R, Rath W, Pflanz MA, et al. Glycosaminoglycans in cervical connective-tissue during pregnancy and parturition. Obstet Gynecol. 1993;81:88-92.

38. Iozzo RV. Matrix proteoglycans: From molecular design to cellular function. Annual Review of Biochemistry. 1998;67:609-52.

39. Norman M, Ekman G, Malmstrom A. Changed proteoglycan metabolism in human cervix immediately after spontaneous vaginal delivery. Obstet Gynecol. 1993; 81:217-23.

40. Fischer DC, Kuth A, Winkler M, et al. A large keratan sulfate proteoglycan present in human cervical mucous appears to be involved in the reorganization of the cervical extra-cellular matrix at term. J Soc Gynecol Invest. 2001;8:277-84.

41. Winkler M, Rath W. Changes in the cervical extracellular matrix during pregnancy and parturition. J Perinat Med. 1999;27:45-60.

42. Kobayashi H, Sun GW, Terao T. Production of prostanoids via increased cyclo-oxygenase-2 expression in human amnion cells in response to low molecular weight hyaluronic acid fragment. Biochimica et Biophysica Acta (BBA)-General Subjects. 1998;1425:369-76.

43. Stern R. Devising a pathway for hyaluronan catabolism: Are we there yet? Glycobiology. 2003;13:105R-15.

44. Ledingham MA, Denison FC, Riley SC, et al. Matrix metalloproteinases-2 and -9 and their inhibitors are produced by the human uterine cervix but their secretion is not regulated by nitric oxide donors. Hum Reprod. 1999;14:2089-96.

45. Lenhart JA, Ryan PL, Ohleth KM, et al. Relaxin increases secretion of matrix metalloproteinase-2 and matrix metalloproteinase-9 during uterine and cervical growth and remodeling in the pig. Endocrinol. 2001;142:3941-9.

46. Lenhart JA, Ryan PL, Ohleth KM, et al. Relaxin increases secretion of tissue inhibitor of matrix metalloproteinase-1 and -2 during uterine and cervical growth and remodeling in the pig. Endocrinol. 2002;143:91-8.

47. Stygar D, Wang H, Vladic YS, et al. Increased level of matrix metalloproteinases 2 and 9 in the ripening process of the human cervix. Biol Reprod. 2002;67:889-94.

48. Balbin M, Fueyo A, Knauper V, et al. Collagenase 2á (MMP-8) expression in murine tissue-remodeling processes. Analysis of its potential role in postpartum involution of the uterus. J Biol Chem. 1998;273:23959-68.

49. Yoshida M, Sagawa N, Itoh H, et al. Prostaglandin F2(alpha), cytokines and cyclic mechanical stretch augment matrix metallo-proteinase-1 secretion from cultured human uterine cervical fibroblast cells. Mol Hum Reprod. 2002;8:681-7.

50. Curry TG, Osteen KG. The matrix metalloproteinase system: changes, regulation, and impact throughout the ovarian and uterine reproductive cycle. Endocr Rev. 2003;24:428-65.

51. Imada K, Ito A, Itoh Y, et al. Progesterone increases the production of tissue inhibitor of metalloproteinases-2 in rabbit uterine cervical fibroblasts. FEBS Letters. 1994;341:109-12.

52. Szabo KA, Ablin RJ, Singh G. Matrix metalloproteinases and the immune response. Clin Appl Immunol Rev. 2004;4:295-319.

53. Yoshida M, Sagawa N, Itoh H, et al. Nitric oxide increases matrix metalloproteinase1 production in human uterine cervical fibroblast cells. Mol Hum Reprod. 2001;7:979-85.

54. Young A, Thomson AJ, Ledingham M, et al. Immunolocalization of proinflammatory cytokines in myometrium, cervix, and fetal membranes during human parturition at term. Biol Reprod.2002; 66: 445-9.

55. El Maradny E, Kanayama N, Halim A, et al. Interleukin-8 induces cervical ripening in rabbits. Am J Obstet Gynecol. 1994;171:7783.

56. Chwalisz K, Benson M, Scholz P, et al. Cervical ripening with the cytokines interleukin-8, interleukin-1 beta and tumour necrosis factor alpha in guinea-pigs. Hum Reprod. 1994;9:217381.

57. Ito A, Hiro D, Ojima Y, et al. Spontaneous production of interleukin-1-like factors from pregnant rabbit uterine cervix. Am J Obstet Gynecol. 1988;159:261-5.

58. Maul H, Nagel S, Welsch G, et al. Messenger ribonucleic acid levels of interleukin-1 beta, interleukin-6 and interleukin-8 in the lower uterine segment increased significantly at final cervical dilatation during term parturition, while those of tumor necrosis factor alpha remained unchanged. Eur J Obstet Gynecol Reprod Biol. 2002;102:143-7.

59. Hebisch G, Grauaug AA, Neumaier-Wagner PM, et al. The relationship between cervical dilatation, interleukin-6 and interleukin-8 during term labor. Acta Obstet Gynecol Scand. 2001;80:840-8.

60. Parekh T, Saxena B, Reibman J, et al. Neutrophil chemotaxis in response to TGF-beta isoforms (TGF-beta 1, TGF-beta 2, TGF-beta 3) is mediated by fibronectin. J Immunol. 1994;152:2456-66.

61. Ekerhovd E, Brannstrom M, Weijdegard B, et al. Nitric oxide synthases in the human cervix at term pregnancy and effects of nitric oxide on cervical smooth muscle contractility. Am J Obstet Gynecol. 2000;183:610-6.

62. Buhimschi I, Ali M, Jain V, et al. Differential regulation of nitric oxide in the rat uterus and cervix during pregnancy and labor. Hum Reprod. 1996;11:1755-66.

63. Shimano M, Nakaya Y, Fukui R, et al. Activation of Ca^{2+}-activated K^+ channels in human myometrium by nitric oxide. Gynecol Obstet Invest. 2000;49:249-54.

64. Buxton IL, Kaiser RA, Malmquist NA, et al. NO-induced relaxation of laboring and non-laboring human myometrium is not mediated by cyclic GMP. Br J Pharmacol. 2001;134:206-14.

65. Ledingham MA, Thomson AJ, Young A, et al. Changes in the expression of nitric oxide synthase in the human uterine cervix during pregnancy and parturition. Mol Hum Reprod. 2000;6:1041-8.

66. Tschugguel W, Schneeberger C, Lass H, et al. Human cervical ripening is associated with an increase in cervical inducible nitric oxide synthase expression. Biol Reprod. 1999;60:1367-72.

67. Facchinetti F, Piccinini F, Volpe A. Chemical ripening of the cervix with intracervical application of sodium nitroprusside: A randomized controlled trial. Hum Reprod. 2000;15:2224-7.

68. Allaire AD, D'Andrea N, Truong P, et al. Cervical stroma apoptosis in pregnancy. Obstet Gynecol. 2001;97:399-403.

69. Bao S, Rai J, Schreiber J. Brain nitric oxide synthase expression is enhanced in the human cervix in labor. J Soc Gynecol Investig. 2001;8:158-64.

70. Rudel D, Pajntar M. Active contractions of the cervix in the latent phase of labour. Br J Obstet Gynaecol. 1999;106:446-52.

71. Pajntar M, Verdenik I. Electromyographic activity in cervices with very low Bishop score during labor. Int J Gynaecol Obstet 1995;49:277-81.

72. Ekerhovd E, Brannstrom M, Delbro D, et al. Nitric oxide mediated inhibition of contractile activity in the human uterine cervix. Mol Hum Reprod. 1998;4:915-20.

73. Watari M, Watari H, DiSanto ME, et al. Pro-inflammatory cytokines induce expression of matrix-metabolizing enzymes in human cervical smooth muscle cells. Am J Pathol. 1999;154:1755-62.

74. Watari M, Watari H, Fujimoto T, et al. Lipopolysaccharide induces interleukin- 8 production by human cervical smooth muscle cells. J Soc Gynecol Invest. 2003;10:110-7.

75. Sugano T, Narahara H, Nasu K, et al. Effects of platelet-activating factor on cytokine production by human uterine cervical fibroblasts. Mol Hum Reprod. 2001;7:475-81.

76. Sugano T, Nasu K, Narahara H, et al. Platelet-activating factor induces an imbalance between matrix metalloproteinase-1 and tissue inhibitor of metalloproteinases-1 expression in human uterine cervical fibroblasts. Biol Reprod. 2000; 62:540-6.

77. Osmers R, Rath W, Adelmann-Grill BC, et al. Origin of cervical collagenase during parturition. Am J Obstet Gynecol. 1992;166:1455-60.

78. Winkler M, Kemp B, Fischer DC, et al. Expression of adhesion molecules in the lower uterine segment during term and preterm parturition. Microsc Res Tech. 2003;60:430-44.

79. Osman I, Young A, Ledingham MA, et al. Leukocyte density and pro-inflammatory cytokine expression in human fetal membranes, decidua, cervix and myometrium before and during labour at term. Mol Hum Reprod. 2003;9:41-5.

80. Varayoud J, Ramos JG, Bosquiazzo VL, et al. Mast cells degranulation affects angiogenesis in the rat uterine cervix during pregnancy. Reproduction. 2004;127:379-87.

81. Wu WX, Ma XH, Coksaygan T, et al. Prostaglandin mediates premature delivery in pregnant sheep induced by estradiol at 121 days of gestational age. Endocrinology. 2004;145:1444-52.

82. Rodriguez HA, Kass L, Varayoud J, et al. Collagen remodelling in the guinea-pig uterine cervix at term is associated with a decrease in progesterone receptor expression. Mol Hum Reprod 2003;9:807-13.

83. Stjernholm YM, Sahlin L, Eriksson HA, et al. Cervical ripening after treatment with prostaglandin E2 or antiprogestin (RU486). Possible mechanisms in relation to gonadal steroids. Eur J Obstet Gynecol Reprod Biol. 1999;84:83-8.

84. Rechberger T, Abramson SR, Woessner JF. Onapristone and prostaglandin E2 induction of delivery in the rat in rate pregnancy: A model for the analysis of cervical softening. Am J Obstet Gynecol. 1996;175:719-23.

85. Imada K, Ito A, Sato T, et al. Hormonal regulation of matrix metalloproteinase 9/ gelatinase B gene expression in rabbit uterine cervical fibroblasts. Biol Reprod. 1997;56:575-80.

86. Luque EH, Ramos JG, Rodriguez HA, et al. Dissociation in the control of cervical eosinophilic infiltration and collagenolysis at the end of pregnancy or after pseudopregnancy in ovariectomized steroid-treated rats. Biol Reprod. 1996;55:1206-12.

87. Rajabi MR, Solomon S, Poole AR. Biochemical evidence of collagenase-mediated collagenolysis as a mechanism of cervical dilatation at parturition in the guinea pig. Biol Reprod. 1991;45:764-72.

88. Rajabi MR, Dodge GR, Solomon S, et al. Immunochemical and immunohistochemical evidence of estrogen-mediated collagenolysis as a mechanism of cervical dilatation in the guinea pig at parturition. Endocrinol. 1991;128:371-8.

89. Tanaka K, Nakamura T, Takagaki K, et al. Regulation of hyaluronate metabolism by progesterone in cultured fibroblasts from the human uterine cervix. FEBS Letters. 1997;402:223-6.

90. Ramos JG, Varayoud J, Kass L, et al. Estrogen and progesterone modulation of eosinophilic infiltration of the rat uterine cervix. Steroids 2000;65:409-14.

91. Stygar D, Wang H, Vladic YS, et al. Co-localization of oestrogen receptor (beta) and leukocyte markers in the human cervix. Mol Hum Reprod. 2001;7:881-6.

92. Norman M, Ekman G, Malmstrom A. Prostaglandin E2-induced ripening of the human Cervix involves changes in proteoglycan metabolism. Obstet Gynecol. 1993;82:1013-20.

93. Ekman G, Malmstrom A, Uldbjerg N, et al. Cervical collagen: An important regulator of cervical function in term labor. Obstet Gynecol. 1986;67:633-6.

94. Nostrӧm A. Influence of prostaglandin E_2 on the biosynthesis of connective tissue constituents in the pregnant human cervix. Prostaglandins. 1982;23:361-7.

95. Kelly RW. Pregnancy maintenance and parturition: The role of prostaglandin in manipulating the immune and inflammatory response. Endocr Rev. 1994;15:684-706.

96. Sennstrom MB, Ekman G, Westergren-Thorsson G, et al. Human cervical ripening, an inflammatory process mediated by cytokines. Mol Hum Reprod. 2000;6:375-81.

97. Hertelendy F, Zakar T. Prostaglandins and the myometrium and cervix. Prostag Leukotr Ess. 2004;70:20722.

98. Ledingham MA, Denison FC, Kelly RW, et al. Nitric oxide donors stimulate prostaglandin F2 (alpha) and inhibit thromboxane B2 production in the human cervix during the first trimester of pregnancy. Mol Hum Reprod. 1999;5:973-82.

99. Smith GCS, Wu WX, Nathanielsz PW. Effects of gestational age and labor on the expression of prostanoid receptor genes in pregnant baboon cervix. Prostag Other Lipid M. 2001;63:153-63.

100. Schmitz T, Dallot E, Leroy MJ, et al. EP4 receptors mediate prostaglandin E2-stimulated glycosaminoglycan synthesis in human cervical fibroblasts in culture. Mol Hum Reprod. 2001; 7:397-402.

101. Lyons CA, Beharry KD, Nishihara KC, et al. Regulation of matrix metallo proteinases (type IV collagenases) and their inhibitors in the virgin, timed pregnant, and postpartum rat uterus and cervix by prostaglandin E2-cyclic adenosine monophosphate. Am J Obstet Gynecol. 2002;187:202-8.

102. Jackson GM, Sharp HT, Varner MW. Cervical ripening before induction of labor: A randomized trial of prostaglandin E2 gel versus low-dose oxytocin. Am J Obstet Gynecol. 1994;171:1092-6.

103. Magann EF, Perry KG Jr, Dockery JR Jr, et al. Cervical ripening before medical induction of labor: A comparison of prostaglandin E2, estradiol, and oxytocin. Am J Obstet Gynecol. 1995;172:1702-6.

104. Fuchs AR, Ivell R, Balvers M, et al. Oxytocin receptors in bovine cervix during pregnancy and parturition: Gene expression and cellular localization. Am J Obstet Gynecol. 1996;175:1654-60.

105. Wathes DC, Smith HF, Leung ST, et al. Oxytocin receptor development in ovine uterus and cervix throughout pregnancy and at parturition as determined by in situ hybridization analysis. J Reprod Fertil. 1996;106:23-31.

106. Wu W, Nathanielsz PW. Changes in oxytocin receptor messenger RNA in the endometrium, myometrium, mesometrium, and cervix of sheep in late gestation and during spontaneous and cortisol-induced labor. J Soc Gynecol Investig. 1994;1:191-6.

107. Shemesh M, Dombrovski L, Gurevich M, et al. Regulation of bovine cervical secretion of prostaglandins and synthesis of cyclo oxygenase by oxytocin. Reprod Fertil Dev. 1997;9:525-30.

108. Fuchs AR, Fuchs F, Husslein P, et al. Oxytocin receptors in the human uterus during pregnancy and parturition. Am J Obstet Gynecol. 1984;150:734-41.

109. Liggins CG. Cervical ripening as an inflammatory reaction. In: Ellwood DA, Andersen AB (Eds). The cervix in pregnancy and labour: Clinical and Biochemical Investigations. Edinburgh, Scotland, UK: Churchill Livingstone; 1981.

82 Physiology of Maternal Sleep in Pregnancy

K Biedermann, R Huch

INTRODUCTION

Pregnancy involves fundamental readjustment of the maternal organism, often associated with unpleasant changes, notably fatigue and reduced energy.[1,2] It is popularly believed to impair sleep. Pregnant women try to sleep more, but are still often tired and perform less efficiently.[3] Those affected tend to account for their residual fatigue in terms of progressive sleep deprivation, due to altered and fragmented sleep in pregnancy.[4] By means of questionnaire, wrist actimetry in daily life and polysomnography in the sleep laboratory, we investigated the changes in sleep habit and quality in pregnancy and assessed their relationship to fatigue.

BACKGROUND

Methods of Sleep Research

Polysomnography—a combination of electroencephalography (EEG), electromyography (EMG) and electro-oculography (EOG)—is the gold standard for sleep investigation and arbiter of sleep stage division into rapid eye movement (REM) sleep and non-REM (NREM) sleep, itself subdivided into four stages of differing depth.[5]

The sleep EEG is the sum curve of the electrical vectors on the scalp produced by the discharge of thousands of neurons. This neuron activity consists of waves differing in frequency and amplitude. The sum curve is broken down by Fourier analysis into individual frequency bands. The proportion of waves at a given frequency (power density) is deduced from this spectrum; in particular, the slow waves (1–12 Hz frequency band) indicative of deep sleep are differentiated from intermediate (13–17 Hz, a-rhythm of the resting waking state) and rapid waves (18–25 Hz), which occur in NREM sleep stages 1 and 2. Whole-night spectral analysis shows waves of the whole frequency spectrum in all sleep stages, but with different power densities in the different frequency bands.

Figure 82.1 shows the different sleep stages (sleep structure) combined with Fourier analysis of the sleep EEG. The sleep stages are shown along the top, above the waves at different frequency bands over the entire sleep episode. Long-wave sleep (1–4 Hz) shows a marked increase in the first sleep cycles, with the maximum falling in NREM sleep stages 3 and 4. In the later sleep cycles long-wave activity decreases continuously until it eventually disappears almost completely.

Sleep Stages and Sleep Control

Non-rapid Eye Movement Sleep

In stage 1 sleep, there is a decrease in the high-frequency EEG waves, but muscle tone and autonomic function (blood pressure, heart rate, respiration) remain at their waking levels or only decrease insignificantly. Dream-like experiences occur frequently and mostly relate to the thought content of the preceding waking stage. Stage 2 sleep follows after approximately 5 minutes. The EEG shows the characteristic spindles and spontaneous and evoked K-complexes. Muscle tone is markedly reduced, the eyes are quiet, and movement artefacts absent. Autonomic function decreases further compared to stage 1; the arousal threshold is raised. Consciousness and receptivity to external events are absent. Stage 2 NREM sleep accounts for over 50% of total sleep time and is hence the chronologically dominant sleep stage. This protracted stage is followed by the transition to deep sleep (stages 3 and 4), with the first occurrence of distinct δ-waves (0.5–4 Hz). Muscle tone is lower than in stage 2; tendon reflexes are preserved. The eyes are actively closed; eye movement is absent. Consciousness is extinguished and autonomic function further reduced. Low-frequency d-waves dominate stage 4 NREM sleep (> 50%), and the EMG shows minimal muscle tone. Arousal from the deepest stage of sleep requires the strongest stimuli.

Rapid Eye Movement Sleep

REM sleep, characterized by salvoes of rapid eye movements[6] is also termed paradoxical sleep because the EEG is dominated by high-

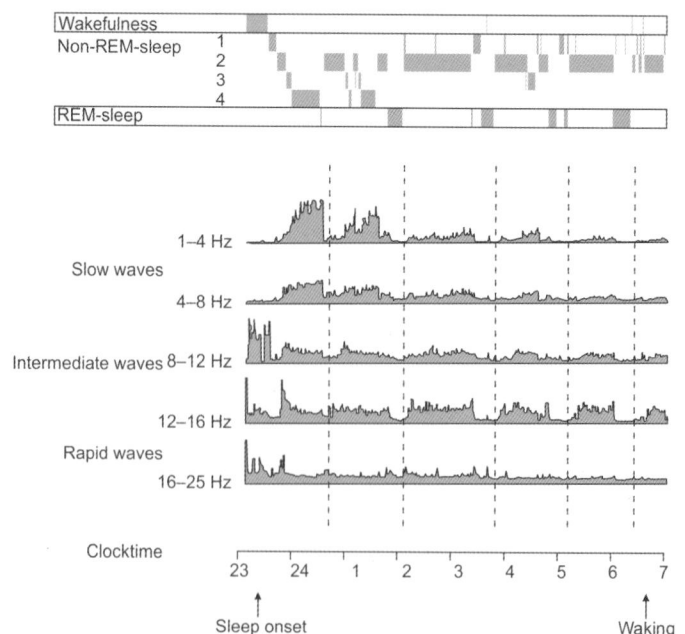

Fig. 82.1: Sleep stages (sleep structure) (top) and spectral analysis (sleep architecture) in a whole-night polysomnogram (bottom)

frequency waking waves. However, muscle tone is almost entirely absent. REM sleep is dream intensive and altogether accounts for approximately 20% of total sleep time; its share tending to decrease as the sleep episode progresses.

Internal Clock

Like many physical functions, the sleep-wake cycle is subject to a circadian rhythm. Under normal conditions this is set to a 24-h-day, but it also operates in experimental isolation where it is set to a 25-h-day.[7] Animal experiments have identified the oscillator of the internal clock as a small neuron nucleus lying above the optic chiasma: the suprachiasmatic nucleus.

Sleep Factors

Several sleep factors have been discovered to date, e.g. S factor,[8] sleep promoting substance (SPS)[7], d-sleep-inducing peptide (DSIP),[9,10] prostaglandin D_2,[11] immune polypeptides such as interleukin-1, interferon and tumor necrosis factor, and neuro-steroids.[12,13] None has yet been shown to play a central role. Sleep modulation and control is thus presumed to be multifactorial.[14]

Sleep and Fatigue in Pregnancy

Fatigue has been defined as a subjective and objective decrease in energy with respect to various spontaneous activities.[15] It is primarily the result of physical activity or more precisely of inadequate recovery from such activity. Many other factors can cause or increase fatigue, e.g. psychological[16] and hormonal influences, in addition to anemia, hypotension, obesity, magnesium deficiency and infectious disease. Fatigue in pregnancy is multifactorial, involving psychological and emotional factors, marked hormonal changes and obvious biological determinants such as weight gain, pregnancy anemia and the tendency to hypotension.

Sleep disturbance and decreased drive are common complaints throughout pregnancy, present in 20%–40% of women, respectively, in the first trimester, and increasing to 70% in the case of sleep disturbance at term.[17] A survey of 100 pregnant women at term found that mean sleep time increased in the first trimester and again in the third trimester; sleep was increasingly shallow and interrupted, while birth and baby themes came to dominate dream content at the expense of daytime experience.[18]

CLINICAL STUDY

Structure and Methods

A total of 189 women attending the Zurich University Hospital Obstetric Outpatients Clinic were recruited over 2.2 years. The inclusion criteria, in addition to informed consent, were a normal singleton pregnancy and the absence of sleep disturbance and relevant psychological or somatic complaints. At the booking visit, subjects were questioned by a (female) physician about their lifestyle and occupation, and sleep behavior before pregnancy. At the end of each trimester and 6 weeks postpartum, they were re-interviewed about any changes. The questionnaires were drafted with the aid of the Institute of Pharmacology, Zurich University and psychologists.

Activity was monitored in 70 of the subjects using wrist actigraphy:[19-21] a wrist-worn matchbox-sized monitor (Gähwiler Electronics, Zurich) converts movement to electrical signals via a piezoelectric transducer; the signals release an impulse if they exceed a set threshold (0.1 g/s^2). Epochs were set to 1 minute for optimal movement resolution compatible with the device's l-week storage capacity. Subjects were asked to wear the monitor as far as possible continuously for 1 week on the wrist of the nondominant hand, once per trimester and postpartum. They were also asked to record sleep times together with specific activities, e.g. driving, in a sleep and activity diary, to enable blank phases and passive vibration to be excluded from the analysis. Monitors were downloaded onto an IBM PC and the raw data, comprising 10,080 measurements over the 7 days, were edited according to the diary entries. It was these modified data sets which were then analyzed (Fig. 82.2).

In addition to interview and actigraphy, 10 subjects also underwent polysomnography (Grass, with on-line Fourier analysis) for two consecutive nights in each trimester (weeks 10, 20 and 30), commencing at lights out. Subjects could get up at their own discretion and were woken at the time they requested. The polygraphic data were manually scored according to the criteria of Rechtschaffen and Kales[5] for 20-s epochs and fed into the computer as data files for combined analysis of sleep stages and EEG spectra in addition to conventional sleep stage analysis.

The Mann-Whitney U rank test and Wilcoxon's signed rank test were used for statistical analysis, and the significance level for longitudinal changes through pregnancy adjusted with Bonferroni's correction. The Chi-Squared test and Fisher's exact test were used for multiple comparisons.

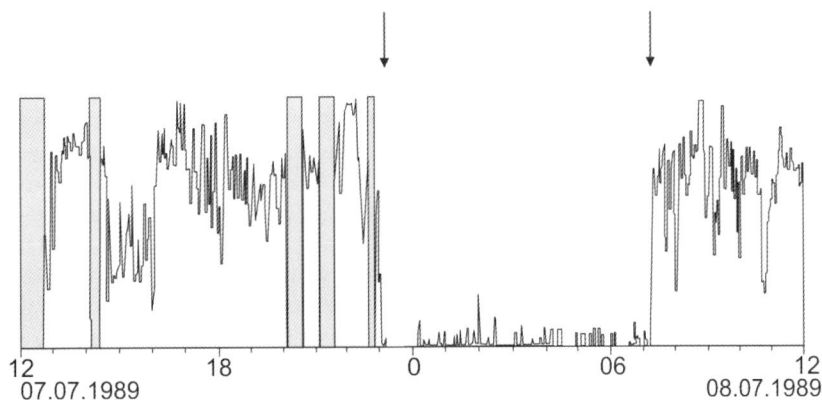

Fig. 82.2: Printout of modified 24-h (noon-noon) activity data files. Arrows, onset and end of sleep; hatched areas, erased recording phases (excluded from analysis)

Sleep Study Results

Population

Median age was 28 years (range 15–45 years). A total of 87 women (46.0%) were expecting their first child, 161 (85.2%) were married, and 47.1% were in full-time employment at the start of the pregnancy. Median booking visit body weight was 56 kg (range 40–93 kg); median weight gain during pregnancy was 13.9 kg (range –4 to +28.5 kg), equivalent to 25.4% of baseline body weight (range –9 to +53%).

Of the women 37.6% smoked until their pregnancy; 20% smoked more than 10 cigarettes daily. The remaining 62.4% described themselves as nonsmokers. Forty percent consumed virtually no alcohol before their pregnancy, while 11% had a weekly alcohol intake equivalent to 180 mL of 100% alcohol, for example in 1.5 L wine, 4.5 L beer or 0.5 L spirits, assuming a medium alcohol content (12%, 4% and 36%, respectively).

Sleep Times

The most reliable sleep-time data were obtained by actigraphy. These values were compared with the questionnaire answers provided by the same women and with control data for 20–40-year-old women from a representative 1983 Swiss population survey.[22]

Mean actigraphic time in bed in pregnancy was 8 h 22 min on weekdays and 8 h 42 min at weekends. These values deviated somewhat from the questionnaire responses: weekday time in bed was underestimated by 14 min, while weekend time in bed was overestimated by 25 min. The actigraphic weekday-weekend difference was only 20 min (8.42 vs 8.22) versus a subjective estimate of 59 min. Pregnant women reported 20 min more sleep during weekdays, and only 12 min more during weekends, than the reference population. When averaged over the week, time in bed was longer in pregnancy by 18 min/night (+3.3%). This difference is slight and illustrates the fact that pregnant women, like their non-pregnant counterparts, adjust their sleep time to their occupational and social commitments. A general finding was that the pregnant women generally went late to bed, thereby failing to use a possible means of sleep compensation.

Sleep times showed no significant changes during pregnancy, but actigraphic time in bed tended to be longer in the first trimester, due to an earlier bedtime than later in pregnancy. Bedtime differed significantly between first and third trimesters ($p < 0.01$). This was surprising in that many women (47.1%) were still working in the first trimester; their proportion decreased progressively during pregnancy (20% in the third trimester). Rising time, on the other hand, did not change during pregnancy, ranging from 07:34 to 07:44h.

Employment affected total sleep time. On weekdays housewives slept almost 1 h longer than employed women ($p < 0.001$), to bed at the same time but sleeping some 40 min longer in the morning (Fig. 82.3). However, they reported fatigue with the same frequency as their employed counterparts. At weekends employed women slept on average only 11 min longer than housewives (9 h 30 min vs 9 h 19 min; not significant).

Dreams

Dream activity is typically more intense in pregnancy, centered on themes of pregnancy, birth and baby,[18] and frequently tinged

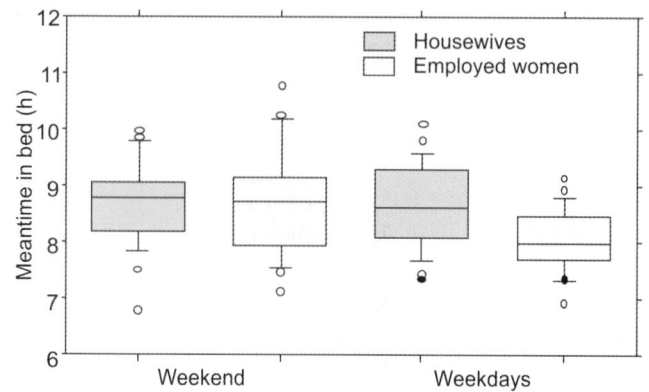

Fig. 82.3: Mean time in bed in housewives (n = 21) and full-time employees (n = 24) on weekdays and weekends. Housewives spent longer in bed than employees on weekdays (p = 0.008, Mann-Whitney test). Boxes. 25th, 50th and 75th centiles; T bars: 10th and 90th centiles

with anxiety.[23] A total of 22% of women reported more intense dreaming in the first trimester, rising to 30% in the second and third trimesters, and returning to pre-pregnancy levels days after delivery. The increase in dream activity in pregnancy and postpartum was unrelated to energy levels, despite nightmares being a frequent cause of waking in pregnancy. Pregnancy dream content is non-prognostic for pregnancy outcome or quality of subsequent mother-infant bonding.[24]

Daytime Naps

Before pregnancy only 37% of women took an occasional or regular daytime nap. During pregnancy the proportion increased to 41% in the first trimester (mean 42.6 min) and 50% in the third trimester (mean 31.3 min). Only 26% took no nap at any time during their pregnancy. Napping had little effect on sleep behavior. In fact total sleep time in 24-h periods that included a daytime sleep was approximately 1 h longer than in identical periods with no nap; nocturnal sleep times were therefore unchanged. Naps were more often associated with nocturnal sleep onset problems (21.7% vs 10.0%, $p < 0.05$). Napping had no effect on nocturnal motor activity (mean nil phase time and motor latency). Employment had no effect on napping.

Sleep Quality

Women reported sleep changes in early pregnancy in 85% of cases. Increases in sleep time and sleep latency were reported by 43% and 36%, respectively. Sleep was shallower (44%) and also disturbed by arousal stimuli, which had not caused waking before pregnancy. In the second trimester, 68% reported improved sleep quality, followed by further deterioration in the third trimester when sleep was more easily disturbed (52%) and more fragmented. These data were confirmed by very similar values in a Japanese study.[25] The main causes of sleep disturbance are bathroomtrips,[26] unaccustomed sleep position,[27,28] back pain,[29] fetal movement,[3] nightmares, hunger and thirst.

Sleep quality ran only partly in parallel with sleep time during pregnancy. Often the changes were mutually contradictory, greater fatigue being reported despite longer sleep or subjects describing themselves as more rested despite shorter sleep. Approximately 90% of women reported fatigue during pregnancy, from the first trimester onward; self-rated energy was lowest in the first and third trimesters, unaffected by the usual amplitude of sleep changes and unrelieved by longer sleep. Fetal sex did not affect maternal sleep behavior or energy. Hypnotics were taken only in exceptional cases (0.5%, mostly benzodiazepines); approximately 10% of women took 'natural' hypnotics (valerian, candy).

Sleep latency: Sleep latency (the interval between lights out and the first stage 2 sleep) can only be determined by polysomnography. However, we found a significant correlation between subjective sleep onset time and polysomnographic sleep latency. Difficulty in falling asleep was one of the commonest sleep disturbances, reported by 29%, including almost 10% reporting sleep latency exceeding 30 min. However, the great majority (63.7%) fell asleep in less than 10 min. Sleep latency decreased with increasing sleep pressure, i.e. the longer subjects had been awake the more quickly they fell asleep. Mean time in bed was longer in women taking longer to fall asleep: women falling asleep in $\leq$ 10 min slept 23 min less than those falling asleep in > 10 min (8 h 43 min vs 8 h 20 min, $p < 0.01$). The time taken to fall asleep showed only small changes throughout pregnancy but was longest (not significantly) at term.

Actigraphic motor latency was defined similarly to sleep latency as the interval between lights out and the first nil activity phase lasting $\geq$ 5 min. It was longer in pregnancy than postpartum (6 vs 5 min, $p < 0.01$), but unchanged during pregnancy itself. It was also longer on weekdays than at weekends (7 vs 6 min, $p < 0.01$), probably due to the earlier bedtime. Restless sleep was associated with a longer motor latency as motor activity in women with restless sleep was also increased during sleep onset.

Nocturnal waking: Sleep in pregnancy was fragmented by nocturnal waking, reported by at least 40% of subjects once per night even before pregnancy. The most frequent causes were "internal", e.g. bathroom trips or thirst (58%), external factors, e.g. noise and temperature (40%), and nightmares (21 %); 9% had no explanation.

In pregnancy, the proportion of women generally waking at night increased to 78% in the first trimester, fell to 69% in the second trimester, and increased again to 79% in the third trimester (vs 23% postpartum). The proportion of women waking up more than once increased steadily from 30% in the first trimester to 52% in the third trimester. Employed women awoke less often than housewives (1.4 vs 1.7 times per night, $p < 0.05$) who more frequently already had a young child to look after.

Nocturnal rising: Rising at night ran in parallel with waking at night during pregnancy, following 59-66% of waking episodes. Both sets of values were thus largely similar. Getting up at least once a night even before pregnancy was reported by 42.1% of women. In contrast to other studies,[16,30] this had no detectable impact on sleep quality. Fifty-eight percent and 51% of women rose at least once per night in the first and second trimesters, respectively (increases of 15% and 8%, respectively); the proportion then increased in the third trimester to 76% ($p < 0.0001$). Improvement was only partial after delivery when, mainly because of the baby, rising was still more frequent than in the first and second trimesters (Fig. 82.4). Bathroom trips were the commonest cause of rising at night even before pregnancy (43.8%), followed by caring for a small child (24.4%), hunger and thirst (14.6%), and uncomfortable environmental temperature and nervousness. Bathroom trips

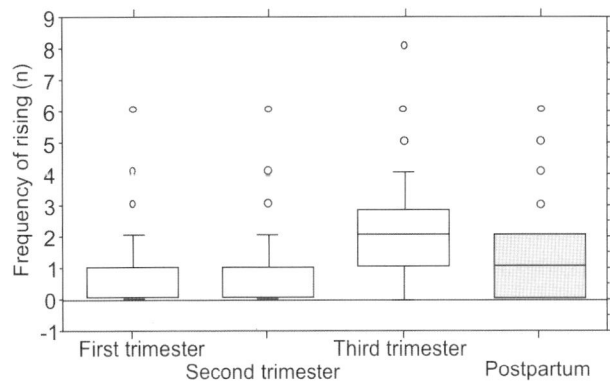

Fig. 82.4: Mean frequency of nocturnal rising in pregnancy and postpartum ($n = 70$), showing an increase from the second to third trimester ($p < 0.0001$)

remained the major cause throughout pregnancy, cited by 69.6% in the third trimester, with a proportionate decrease in risings caused by a small child. The baby was, as expected, the dominant cause after pregnancy.

Fatigue and energy: Fatigue has been defined as the subjective and objective decrease in energy.[15] Fatigue and energy thus represent opposite poles of the same spectrum, describing the same reality in inversely proportional terms. Only some 26% of women reported feeling rested on waking even before pregnancy; a good third described themselves as "tired" on waking. Physical and mental energy is known to be decreased early in pregnancy. A total of 70.9% of women reported fatigue/decreased energy at the end of the first trimester; 18.5% reported feeling marked fatigue/markedly reduced energy. Only a minority (3.7%) felt more energy in the first trimester than before pregnancy. Fatigue/decreased energy was thus a common complaint in early pregnancy, decreasing transiently to 34.6% in the second trimester before re-ascending in the third trimester to 65%. It improved postpartum in two-thirds of subjects, but was still reported in 31.6%.

Mean fatigue scores (1 = very tired, 6 = very energetic) were determined in the 70 subjects throughout pregnancy and used to divide the population into three groups. Sleep parameters and clinical findings were then analyzed separately for the three groups. Only one sleep parameter (bedtime) and two clinical parameters (basal hemoglobin and minimal diastolic blood pressure) correlated significantly with fatigue in pregnancy.

The mean difference in bedtime between tired and energetic women was 23 min ($p = 0.026$). There were no differences in rising time or time in bed. Nocturnal activity (nil activity time, % nil activity and mean nil phase length) and nocturnal waking were unrelated to fatigue. Motor latency appeared longer (not significantly) in the tired group. Daytime napping was equally frequent in all three groups.

The reasons advanced as possible causes of fatigue on waking differed throughout pregnancy and postpartum: the most frequent were bathroom trips, inadequate sleep or rest, evening coffee or tea, workload, personal problems, unaccustomed sleeping position, fetal movement and pregnancy complaints. Interestingly, pregnancy-specific effects on fatigue were not given; the causes were mostly those known to cause fatigue even outside pregnancy.

Employment had little impact on the fatigue reported by approximately 60% of housewives and employed women alike.

Energy was not therefore increased by a reduction in workload. Instead work was adjusted to energy as decreased energy in pregnancy leads to workplace stress and feelings of inadequacy. The increased emotional vulnerability in pregnancy also led many pregnant women to avoid such conflict by leaving their employment. The proportion of full-time employees fell from 47.1% in the first trimester to 20% in the third; the proportion of part-time employees stayed constant throughout pregnancy at 25%.

It is also interesting that performance was not improved by more sleep. Fatigue/decreased energy was no less frequent in women sleeping longer in the first trimester versus before pregnancy than in those not sleeping longer. The fact that pregnancy fatigue was not made good by longer sleep indicates that sleep disturbance was not the cause, provided it remained within the usual limits. Other complaints, e.g. nervousness, irritability and headache, were also often attributed to sleep disturbance, although they may themselves also be its cause.

Pregnant women are often worried that their decreased energy could affect the course of pregnancy, birth or the baby. These fears can be allayed; prematurity, birth weight and neonatal adjustment were identical in women with markedly decreased energy and those with high or only slightly reduced energy. Duration of labor and spontaneous delivery rates were also identical in both groups. We failed to confirm the association reported between birth weight and mean sleep time during pregnancy,[31] but confirmed the finding that employment does not affect the course of pregnancy or delivery.[32]

Motor activity during sleep: Like time in bed, the nocturnal nil activity time, i.e. the sum of minute measurement units showing nil activity, also remained largely unchanged throughout pregnancy (median 6 h 50 min). Individual fluctuation during pregnancy was slight, ± 18% in 80% of all subjects.

The percentage of nil activity of time in bed was 75–85% in most subjects, but fluctuated markedly (56–93%) in individual cases. It increased from the first to the second trimester ($p < 0.01$), evidencing more restless sleep in the first trimester. Other inter-trimester comparisons showed no differences. The percentage of nil activity did not differ between weekdays and weekends, or between housewives and employed women.

The number of nocturnal nil phases (intervals of uninterrupted nil activity) was maximal (median 57) in the first trimester, then decreased in the second trimester (median 54) ($p < 0.001$), remaining unchanged (median 55) in the third trimester before falling to a minimum postpartum (median 44). The postpartum value was lower than the pregnancy values ($p < 0.0001$). Since total nil activity time remained unchanged throughout pregnancy, it was broken during pregnancy into more individual nil activity phases by more frequent interruptions. Sleep was at its most restless and fragmented in the first trimester.

The increased number of nocturnal nil phases in pregnancy resulted in a shorter mean nil phase length (Fig. 82.5) in pregnancy versus postpartum (7.36-7.59 min vs 9.56 min, $p < 0.0001$). In addition, the increase in mean nil phase length from the first to the second trimester was significant ($p = 0.0002$), but not that to the third trimester ($p = 0.27$). Women with a low nocturnal percentage of nil activity had, as expected, a shorter mean nil phase length ($p = 0.0001$), also indicative of more restless sleep.

This means that during sleep in pregnancy, especially in the first trimester, motor activity was more frequent than in nonpregnancy.

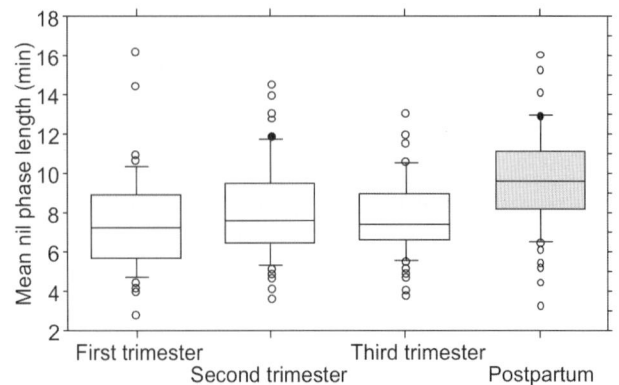

Fig. 82.5: Mean nil phase length (mNPL) in pregnancy and postpartum ($n = 70$), showing a longer mNPL postpartum than in any trimester ($p < 0.0001$, Wilcoxon's test with Bonferroni's correction for multiple comparisons)

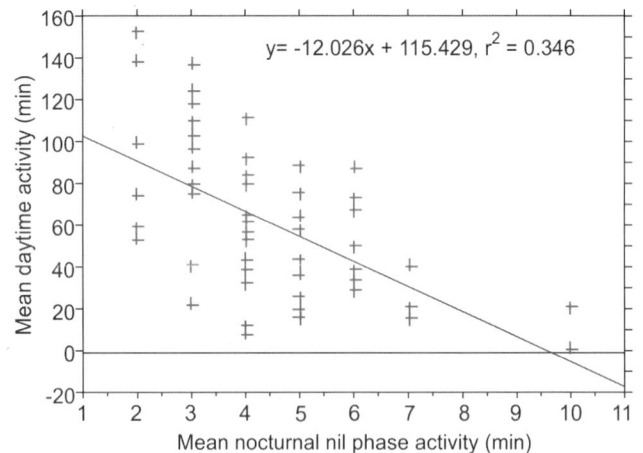

Fig. 82.6: Median daytime activity versus mean nocturnal nil phase length in first trimester pregnancies ($n = 63$), $r = 0.6$

However, such increased motor activity had no effect on sleep quality. Motor latency was also significantly increased throughout pregnancy, indicating increased motor activity during sleep onset.

Daytime activity decreased continuously during pregnancy, in parallel with nocturnal activity, reaching a minimum postpartum, which differed significantly from the first trimester. Women with high daytime activity had higher night-time motor activity. There was a negative correlation between median daytime activity and mean night-time nil phase length ($r = 0.6$), illustrated in Figure 82.6 (first trimester) and present in all recording periods.

Polysomnography

Conventional sleep analysis: Sleep structure, i.e. sleep stage distribution, remained largely unchanged over pregnancy. The only significant changes from the first to the third trimester were an increase in nocturnal wake phase time (from 32.5 min to 58.3 min) hence a decrease in sleep efficiency, defined as time asleep/time in bed (from 86.5% to 79.9%)—and a decrease in REM sleep time (from 79.7 min to 70.5 min) (Fig. 82.7).[33]

The same changes—decreased REM sleep and increased wake phase—had been found in previous studies.[34,35] An earlier report of an increase in paradoxical sleep during pregnancy[36] was based on

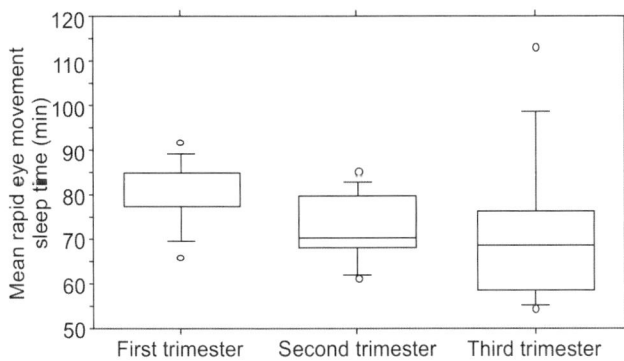

Fig. 82.7: Mean rapid eye movement (REM) sleep time in two nights per trimester (78, 70 and 69 min in trimesters 1, 2 and 3, respectively) in nine subjects, showing a significant decrease from the first to third trimester ($p < 0.05$)

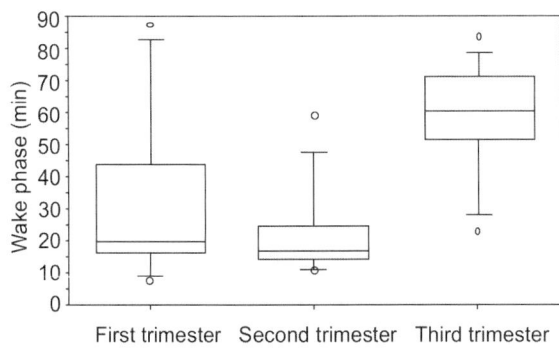

Fig. 82.8: Wake phase after sleep onset (mean of two nights) per trimester in nine subjects, showing a longer wake phase in the third versus first and second trimesters ($p < 0.05$, Wilcoxon's test)

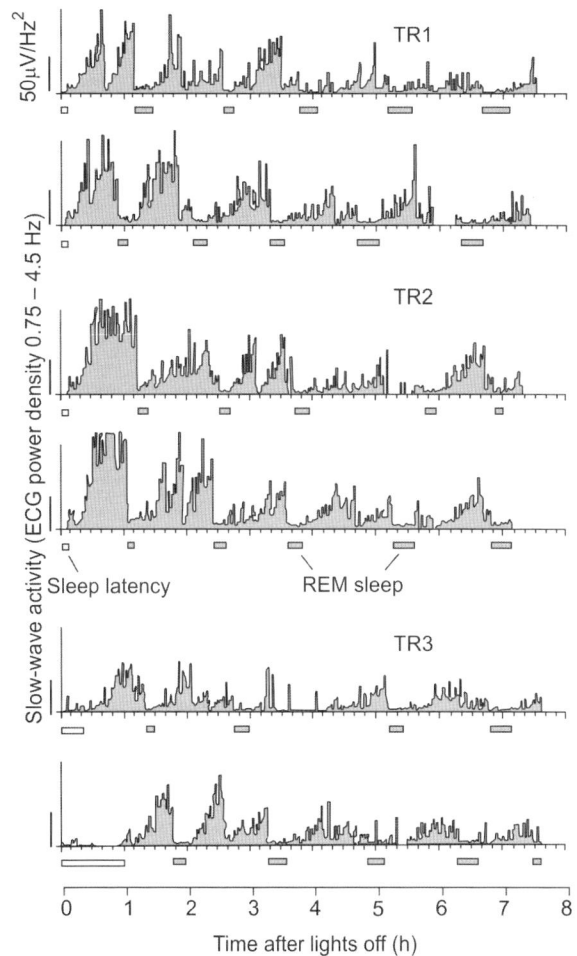

Fig. 82.9: Power density of slow-wave activity (0.75-4.5 Hz) over 6 nights in the same pregnant woman (two nights per trimester, chronological order from top to bottom) showing decrease of slow-wave activity during pregnancy.

Abbreviations: TR1, first trimester; TR2, second trimester; TR3, third trimester; REM, rapid eye movement[30]

the sleep staging criteria of Dement and Kleitman,[6] which differ from the Rechtschaffen and Kales criteria[5] in current use.

Median wake-phase time after sleep onset was longer in the third than in the first or second trimesters (60 vs 20 min, respectively; $p < 0.05$) (Fig. 82.8).

Whole-night spectral analysis: Sleep architecture analysis was focused on slow-wave EEG activity (0.75–4.5 Hz) as a measure of sleep depth. Slow-wave activity also occurs outside deep sleep but is not recorded by conventional sleep staging. The contribution of whole-night spectral analysis is that it records power densities in the different frequency bands independently of the conventional sleep stages.

Power density decreased significantly from first to third trimester in the long-wave frequency band in NREM and REM sleep[33] (Fig. 82.9), i.e. sleep was shallower overall in the third trimester versus the first, even though the proportion of deep sleep was unchanged in the third trimester.

The first trimester power density at each frequency band was used as the baseline (100%) in expressing the values in each subject during pregnancy; subsequent values were expressed as percentage deviations from this baseline. The collective deviations in the second and third trimesters (the mean of both nights in each trimester in nine subjects) are shown in Figure 82.10, which also shows the significant changes in power spectra during pregnancy as thick bars in the appropriate frequency band.

There was a clear correlation between decrease in power density at 10.5 Hz in NREM sleep and fatigue on waking from the first to the second trimester (Fig. 82.11). Thus, women with a decrease in power density at 10.5 Hz of 10% all reported greater fatigue in the second versus the first trimester, while all those feeling less tired in the second trimester showed a smaller decrease, or in some cases an increase, in power density in the same frequency band.

Hormonal Effects on Fatigue

The central depressant effect of progestagens causes symptoms such as fatigue, apathy, drowsiness, decreased libido, decreased drive, fluctuating mood, depressive mood and decreased energy,[37] i.e. many of the complaints typical of early pregnancy. But as serum progesterone levels up to 10 weeks of gestation do not differ significantly from luteal values,[38,39] additional mechanisms must be involved, notably changes in brain hormone metabolism (steroids in particular) and/or receptor status.

Neuroactive steroids or neurosteroids, are progesterone derivatives, which bind not to the cytoplasmic steroid receptor of the

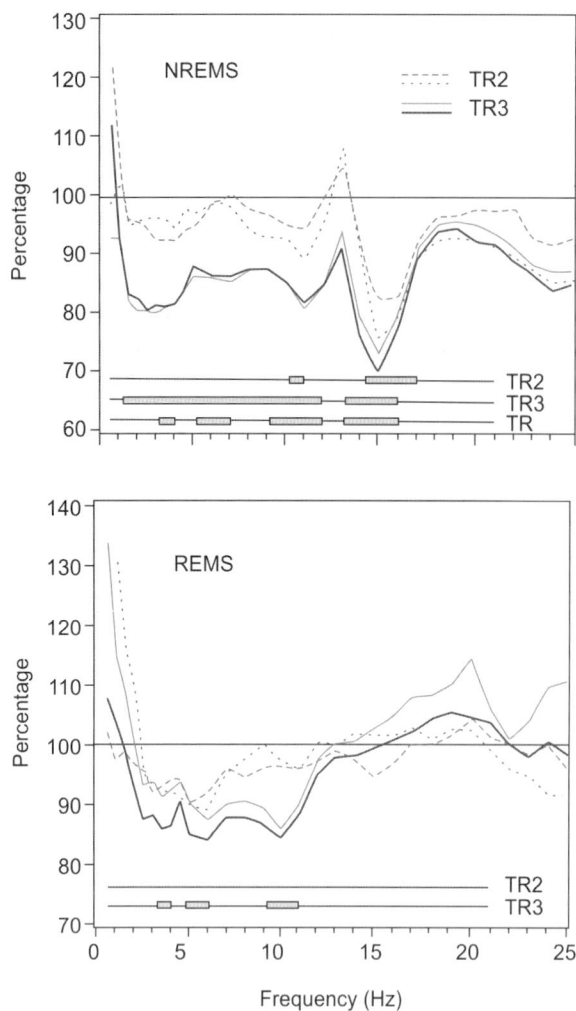

Fig. 82.10: Changes (collective mean % deviation per trimester from first trimester baseline (100%) in power density in NREMS and REMS in nine pregnant women. Bold, frequency bands with significant changes; TR2, second trimester; TR3, third trimester[30]

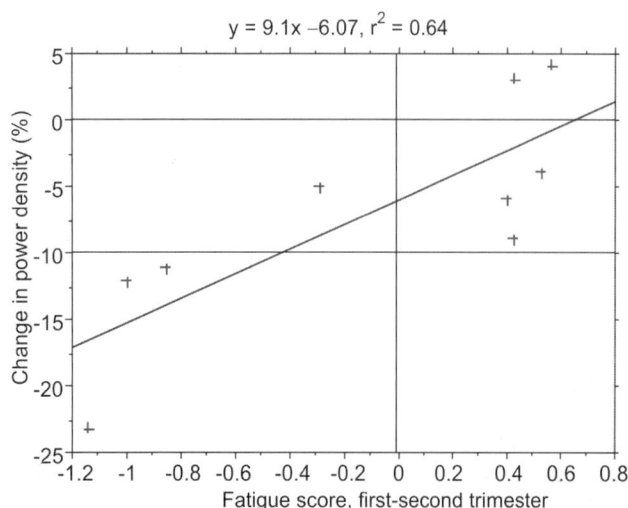

$$y = 9.1x - 6.07, r^2 = 0.64$$

Fig. 82.11: Correlation between fatigue and decrease in power density in 10.5 Hz frequency band from first to second trimester. $r = 0.8$

typical end organ but to neuron $GABA_A$ receptors where they exert benzodiazepine-like activity.[40,41] The result is marked fatigue, shown with several steroid hormones.[13,42-44] We used a binding assay [with the ionophore ligand (^{35}S)-t-butyl-bicyclophospho-rothionate (TBPS)] to screen for neurosteroids in a pilot study in 23 pregnant women between 10 weeks and 40 weeks of gestation.[45] The results showed a correlation between severe fatigue in pregnancy and the presence of neurosteroids in peripheral venous blood throughout pregnancy. Neurosteroid binding was present in six out of nine pregnant women with severe fatigue versus none out of eight women without fatigue. The correlation requires confirmation in further studies.

The sleep EEG changes seen toward the end of pregnancy—a significant decrease in power density in the slow-wave frequency band—have also been described in association with benzodiazepine use.[46-48] The physiological function of endozepines (diazepam binding inhibitors or endogenous ligands of the benzodiazepine receptors) remains to be elucidated, though they have a demonstrated role in some disease processes such as idiopathic recurring stupor[49] and hepatic encephalopathy.[50] No blood samples in the above neurosteroid pilot study showed any evidence of endozepine binding, making this an improbable explanation for pregnancy fatigue.[45]

Progesterone also contributes to the sleep changes in pregnancy. Experimental progesterone administration in men was associated with more frequent waking, decreased deep (stage 4) sleep and increased sleep latency.[51,52]

Pregnancy fatigue can be interpreted as a biological signal to the expectant mother to take things easy physically. Reduced physical activity reduces uterine contractions and increases uteroplacental blood flow.

CLINICAL IMPACT OF SLEEP IMPAIRMENT

Pregnancy, Sleep and Fatigue

The effects of pregnancy on sleep and fatigue can be summarized as follows:

1. Sleep changes during pregnancy: These changes show little relationship with fatigue. Some sleep parameters correlate with fatigue: later bedtime, increased waking after sleep onset, decreased power density in the low-frequency band.

2. As pregnancy fatigue does not respond to longer sleep or less work, sleep time and workload do not appear to be its principal determinants. More plausible candidates are endocrine causes, as in the case of neurosteroids.[45]

3. Sleep disturbance and fatigue do not affect the course of pregnancy. The most frequent pregnancy complications—prematurity, low birth weight for gestational age, intrapartum asphyxia and cesarean section rate—were no more frequent in the women with severely disturbed sleep or excessive fatigue than in the overall population.

Sleep Disturbance in Pregnancy: Management Guidelines

Pregnant women who complain about fatigue and sleep problems should be made aware that such complaints are not only frequent but have no demonstrable impact on the pregnancy or baby and are best viewed as the body's invitation to take things easy.

Symptomatic management is required for pregnancy complaints that may often cause sleep problems, e.g. restricted respiration (increase the number of pillows to leave the chest free), obstructed nasal respiration (humidifiers, vasoconstrictor nasal drops) or nocturnal carpal tunnel syndrome (splinting of the wrist overnight). Early morning nausea can be managed with drugs [vitamin B6; suppositories of meclozine dihydrochloride, pyridoxine hydrochloride and caffeine (Itinerol®, Vifor, Switzerland)], and nocturnal calf cramps with magnesium supplements. Nocturia may respond to compression stockings which reduce dependent fluid accumulation during the day and hence the diuretic response to recumbency.[53] Fatigue due to anemia can be treated with prophylactic iron.

Falling asleep and remaining asleep can also be assisted by further measures, such as discussing psychosocial problems and sensitizing the patient to the increased emotional vulnerability in pregnancy. A talk with the partner or employer may also be of benefit.

Tips for active sleep preparation include a regular bedtime, preceded by a short walk in the fresh air. Evening coffee and tea should be avoided, together with heavy meals and alcohol. It is also best to go to bed only when tired; otherwise reading or a similar activity can be recommended, and/or a warm bath.

Patients can also be helped by correcting their ideas about "enough" sleep. They need to understand that the body basically gets the sleep it needs, if not today then tomorrow or the day after.[54] It must be emphasized that it is not sleep so much as rest which is important.

Some nondrug remedies have been shown to be harmless in pregnancy, e.g. valerian drops, which have a documented hypnotic action,[55] herbal tea (e.g. lemon balm), alcohol-free beer, and milk and honey mixtures.

If none of the above are effective, a hypnotic can be prescribed in exceptional cases. All medication is contraindicated in principle during the first trimester. In the second or third trimester, benzodiazepines or barbiturates can be used as short-term symptomatic therapy. Both may have adverse neuropsychological effects on the child, above all with protracted use.[56-60] To reduce the risk of neonatal hemorrhage, vitamin K supplementation is recommended in the last 3 weeks of pregnancy in patients on long-term barbiturates (e.g. epileptics) because of increased vitamin K turnover due to hepatic enzyme induction.[61]

The fundamental message to get across is that women should be receptive and ready to respond positively to the signals which their bodies emit during pregnancy. The sleep problems and fatigue associated with pregnancy are transient in all cases and resolve shortly after birth.

CONCLUSION

The main pregnancy-associated changes in sleep are a decrease in depth and an increase in fragmentation, primarily due to nocturnal bathroom trips. Some 50–75% of study women got up at night during pregnancy versus only 8.5% of controls.[22] On average, pregnant women sleep approximately 18 min longer per night than nonpregnant women and do so throughout pregnancy with certain individual fluctuations. Yet despite longer sleep, significantly more pregnant than nonpregnant women rated their sleep quality as poor or very poor (40% and 27%, respectively, vs 4%).

More intense dream activity was reported by approximately one-fifth of the women in early pregnancy versus before pregnancy,

and by one-third in the further course of pregnancy. Dream content frequently revolved around birth and baby themes, often tinged with apprehension.

Sleep fragmentation was also shown by actigraphy. Nocturnal nil activity duration did not change through pregnancy; however, the number of nocturnal nil activity phases increased and mean nil activity phase length decreased. Motor latency was also significantly increased throughout pregnancy, confirming the more-marked motor activity during sleep onset. However, increased motor activity had no effect on the recuperative value of sleep.

Daytime sleep, reported by only 37% of women before pregnancy, increased during pregnancy to a maximum of 58% in the third trimester. Women who took a daytime nap did not differ from the others in sleep times or employment status. Daytime napping was not associated with the quality of waking or sleep fragmentation by waking and rising. In summary, there was no evidence that daytime napping was a response to poor nocturnal sleep quality; rather, it was taken if the opportunity arose.

Sleep structure showed two significant changes during pregnancy: first, a decrease in REM sleep (from 79.7 min to 70.5 min) and, second, an increase in nocturnal waking after sleep onset (from 32.5 min to 58.3 min). The longer waking phase reduced sleep efficiency, from 86.5% to 79.9%, i.e. one-fifth of total time in bed was spent awake, with α-EEG activity. The main casualty of the increased waking phase was REM sleep; NREM sleep stages did not change during pregnancy. Recuperative deep sleep decreased in pregnancy by approximately 10% (not significantly). These changes in sleep structure were only observed in late pregnancy and cannot account for fatigue in early pregnancy.

Whole-night spectral analysis during pregnancy showed a significant decrease in power density in the slow-wave frequency band (1–12 Hz) and intermediate band (13–17 Hz) in both REM and NREM sleep. The decrease in power density at 10.5 Hz in NREM sleep (from first to second trimester) correlated with increased fatigue. From the second to third trimester, we found a correlation between decreased power density in the 13–16 Hz frequency band and increased fatigue. These sleep changes need to be qualified by the fact that fatigue was already present early in the first trimester. The low grade sleep changes cannot explain the often marked fatigue. However, the correlation between fatigue and the decrease in power density in the slow-wave band suggests that changes in sleep architecture may be at least partial determinants of fatigue.

In our study population of 189 pregnant women, 89.4% complained of definite fatigue and decreased energy in the first trimester. The fatigue involved not just physical energy but also concentration ability and memory. Such complaints are common even before women know that they are pregnant, thereby largely excluding purely psychological causes triggered by the awareness of pregnancy onset.

Workload was reduced through to the third trimester by some 58% of full-time employees largely independently of fatigue. Fatigue did not decrease after the workload was reduced, indicating that the latter is not a major determinant of pregnancy fatigue. Complaints of fatigue were as frequent in housewives, despite being able to adjust their workload more easily and sleep a mean 27 min longer than their employed counterparts.

Pregnancy fatigue thus appears multifactorial and largely independent of sleep. Later bedtime, low basal hemoglobin and low diastolic blood pressure showed an individually significant association with fatigue. Frequent rising at night, restless sleep and increased weight gain in pregnancy were not significantly associated with fatigue. Only the endocrine changes can account for early pregnancy fatigue. Neurosteroids may play a major role in this regard,[44,45] in addition to the recognized sedative effects of progesterone.

ACKNOWLEDGMENTS

This study was supported by a grant of the Hartmann-Müller-Foundation (Zurich). The polysomnographies were carried out in the Institute of Pharmacology of the University of Zurich (Professor AA Borbely).

REFERENCES

1. Reeves N, Potempa K, Gallo A. Fatigue in early pregnancy. An exploratory study. Nurse Midwifery. 1991;36:303-9.
2. Sahota PK, Jain SS, Dhand R. Sleep disorders in pregnancy. Curr Opin Pulm Med. 2003;9:477-83.
3. Williams B. Sleep needs during the maternity cycle. Nurs Outlook. 1967;15:53-5.
4. Hedman C, Pohjasvaara T, Tolonen U, et al. Effects of pregnancy on mother's sleep. Sleep Med. 2002;3:37-42.
5. Rechtschaffen A, Kales A. A Manual of Standardized Terminology, Techniques and Scoring System for Sleep Stages of Human Subjects (Publication No. 204). Washington, DC: National Institutes of Health, US Government Printing Office; 1968.
6. Dement WC, Kleitman N. Cyclic variations in EEG during sleep and their relation to eye movements, body motility and dreaming. Electroencephalogr Clin Neuro Physiol. 1957;9:673-90.
7. Borbely AA. Das Geheimnis des Schlafs. Neue Wege und Erkenntnisse der Forschung. Ullstein-Sachbuch No. 34761. Frankfurt: Verlag Ullstein; 1991.
8. Pappenheimer JR. Sleep factor in CSF, brain and urine. Front Horm Res. 1982;9:173-8.
9. Schneider-Helmert D, Schönenberger GA. Effects of DSIP in man. Multifunctional psychophysiological properties besides induction of natural sleep. Neuropsychobiology. 1983;9:197-206.
10. Schoenenberger G, Maier PF, Tobler HJ, et al. A naturally occurring delta-EEG enhancing nonapeptide in rabbits. Final isolation, characterization and activity test. Pflügers Arch. 1977;369:99-109.
11. Hayaishi O. Molecular mechanisms of sleep-wake regulations: Roles of prostaglandins D2 and E2. FASEB J. 1991;5:2575-81.
12. McNeil RG, Gee KW, Bolger MB, et al. Neuroactive steroids that act at GABA-A receptors. Drug News Perspect. 1992;5:145-52.
13. Selye H. Anesthetic effect of steroid hormones. Proc Soc Exp Biol Med. 1941;46:116-21.
14. Borbely AA, Tobler I. Endogenous sleep-promoting substances and sleep regulation. Physiol Rev. 1989;69: 605-70.
15. Koella WP. Die Physiologie des Schlafes. Stuttgart: Gustav Fischer Verlag; 1988.
16. Lavidor M, Weller A, Babkoff H. How sleep is related to fatigue. Br J Health Psychol. 2003;8:95-105.
17. Schorsch E, Müller-Neff E. Psychiatrische Untersuchung an Wöchnerinnen. In: Bürger-Prinz H, Fischer PA (Eds). Psychiatrie und Neurologie der Schwangerschaft. Stuttgart: Enke Verlag; 1968.P.98.
18. Schweiger MS. Sleep disturbance in pregnancy. Am J Obstet Gynecol. 1972;114:879-82.
19. Borbely AA, Neuhaus HU, Mattmann P, et al. Langzeitregistrierung der Bewegungsaktivität: Anwendungen in Forschung und Klinik. Schweiz Wschr. 1981;111:730-5.
20. Mullaney DJ, Kripke DF, Messin S. Wrist-actigraphic estimation of sleep time. Sleep. 1980;3:83-92.
21. Sadeh A, Alster J, Urbach D, et al. Actigraphically based automatic bedtime sleep-wake scoring: Validity and clinical applications. J Ambulatory Monitoring. 1989;2:209-16.
22. Borbely AA. Schlafgewohnheiten, Schlafqualität und Schlafmittelkonsum der Schweizer Bevölkerung. Schweiz Aerztezeitung. 1984;65:1606-13.
23. Karacan I, Williams R, Webb WB, et al. Sleep and dreaming during late pregnancy and postpartum. Psychophysiology. 1968;4:378.
24. Gillman RD. The dreams of pregnant women and maternal adaptation. Am J Orthopsychiatr. 1968;38:68892.
25. Suzuki S, Dennerstein L, Greenwood KM, et al. Sleeping patterns during pregnancy in Japanese women. Psychosom Obstet Gynecol. 1994;15:19-26.
26. Lee KA, De Joseph JF. Sleep disturbances, vitality and fatigue among a select group of employed childbearing women. Birth. 1992;19:208-13.
27. Feinsilver SH, Hertz G. Respiration during sleep in pregnancy. Clin Chest Med. 1992;13:637-44.
28. Ogita S, Imanaka M, Takebayashi T, et al. Significance of exercise and bed rest in pregnancy—study on the lying postures of gravidas during sleep. Ann Physiol Anthropol. 1990;9:93-8.
29. Fast A, Hertz G. Nocturnal low back pain in pregnancy: polysomnographic correlates. Am J Reprod Immunol. 1992;28:251-3.
30. Levine B, Roehrs T, Stepanski E, et al. Fragmenting sleep diminishes its recuperative value. Sleep. 1987;10:590-9.
31. Rabkin CS, Anderson HR, Bland JM, et al. Maternal activity and birth weight: A prospective, population-based study. Am J Epidemiol. 1990;131:522-31.
32. Schramm WF, Stockbauer JW, Hoffman HJ. Exercise, employment, other daily activities, and adverse pregnancy outcomes. Am J Epidemiol. 1996;143:211-8.
33. Brunner DP, Münch M, Biedermann K, et al. Changes in sleep and sleep EEG across pregnancy. Sleep. 1994;17:576-82.
34. Driver HS, Shapiro CM. A longitudinal study of sleep stages in young women during pregnancy and postpartum. Sleep. 1992;15:449-53.
35. Hertz G, Fast A, Feinsilver SH, et al. Sleep in normal late pregnancy. Sleep. 1992;15:246-51.
36. Branchey M, Petre-Quadens O. A comparative study of sleep parameters during pregnancy. Acta Neurol Belg. 1968;68:453-9.
37. Kane FJ, Daly RJ, Ewing JA, et al. Mood and behavioral changes with progestational agents. Br J Psychiatr. 1967;13:265-8.
38. Yannone ME, McCurdy JR, Goldfien A. Plasma progesterone levels in normal pregnancy, labor and the puerperium. Am J Obstet Gynecol. 1968;101:1058-61.
39. Lee KA, Zaffke ME. Longitudinal changes in fatigue and energy during pregnancy and the postpartum period. J Obstet Gynecol Neonatal Nurs. 1999;28:183-91.
40. Baulieu EE. Neurosteroids: synthesis and function. In: Barnard EA, Costa E (Eds). Transmitter Amino Acid Receptors: Structures, Transduction and Models for Drug Development. Stuttgart: Thieme Verlag; 1991. pp. 185-201.
41. Simmonds MA. Modulation of the $GABA_A$ receptor by steroids. Semin Neurosci. 1991;3:231-9.

42. De Feudis FV. Modulation of GABA-A receptors by pregnane steroids—a new lead for developing anesthetics and anticonvulsants. Drug News Perspect. 1989;2:278-80.

43. Majewska MD, Ford-Rice F, Falkay G. Pregnancy-induced alterations of GABA$_A$ receptor sensitivity in maternal brain. An antecedent of post-partum 'blues'? Brain Res. 1989;482:397 401.

44. Marker RE, Kamm O, McGrew RV. Isolation of epipregnanol-3-one-20 from human pregnancy urine. J Am Chem Soc. 1937;59:616-8.

45. Biedermann K, Schoch P. Do neurosteroids or endozepines cause fatigue in pregnancy? Eur J Obstet Gynecol Reprod Biol. 1995;58:15-8.

46. Borbely AA, Mattmann P, Loepfe M, et al. A single dose of benzodiazepine hypnotics alters the sleep EEG in the following drug-free night. Eur J Pharmacol. 1983;89:157-61.

47. Borbely AA, Mattmann P, Loepfe M, et al. Effect of benzodiazepine hypnotics on all-night sleep EEG spectra. Hum Neurobiol. 1985;4:189-94.

48. Kubicki ST, Haag-Wüsthof C, Römmel J, et al. The pharmacodynamic influence of three bendzodiazepines on rapid eye movements, K-complexes and sleep spindles in healthy volunteers. Hum Psychopharmacol. 1988;3:247-55.

49. Rothstein JD, Guidotti A, Tinuper P, et al. Endogenous benzodiazepine receptor ligands in idiopathic recurring stupor. Lancet. 1992;340:1002-4.

50. Mullen KD, Szauter KM, Kaminsky-Russ K. 'Endogenous' benzodiazepine activity in body fluids of patients with hepatic encephalopathy. Lancet. 1990;336:81-3.

51. Heuser G, Kaies A, Jacobson A. Human sleep patterns after progesterone administration. Psychophysiology. 1968;4:378.

52. Kotorii T, Nokaka K, Nakazawa Y, et al. Effects of medroxyprogesterone acetate on sleep of healthy young male adults. Jpn J Psychol Neurol. 1987;41:261-7.

53. Biedermann K, Faisst K, Huch A, et al. Compression stocking prevention of pregnancy nocturia [Letter]. Prenat Neonat Med. 1996;1:159.

54. Schumacher W. Schlafstörungen in der Schwangerschaft. Ihre Diagnostik und Therapie aus psychiatrischer Sicht. Gynäkologe. 1987;20:176-81.

55. Balderer G, Borbely AA. Effect of valerian on human sleep. Psychopharmacology. 1985;87:406-9.

56. Bergman U, Rosa FW, Baum C, et al. Effects of exposure to benzodiazepine during fetal life. Lancet. 1992;340:694-6.

57. Blumenthal I, Lindsay S. Neonatal barbiturate withdrawal. Postgrad Med J. 1977;53:157-8.

58. Fishman RH, Yanai J. Long-lasting effects of early barbiturates on central nervous system and behavior. Neurosci Biobehav Rev. 1983;7:19-28.

59. Gillberg C. 'Floppy infant syndrome' and maternal diazepam. Lancet. 1977;2:244.

60. Weber LW. Benzodiazepines in pregnancy—academical debate or teratogenic risk? Biol Res Pregn. 1985;6:151-67.

61. Janz D. Antiepileptic drugs and pregnancy: altered utilization patterns and teratogenesis. Epilepsia. 1982; 23(Suppl):53-63.

83

Immunology at the Maternal-Fetal Interface

S Scherjon, F Class

INTRODUCTION

The maternal acceptance of the semi-allogeneic fetus seems to ignore the concepts of transplantation immunology. Elucidating the mechanism leading to this unique phenomenon is essential for our understanding of processes leading to normal and abnormal pregnancy, but may also result in important concepts in the field of transplantation, autoimmunity and possibly neoplasia control.

In 1953, Medawar explained the "immunological paradox of pregnancy" by considering pregnancy a state of "immunological neutrality".[1] One of the three possible mechanism he proposed was based on the idea that the fetus is antigenically immature. However, the idea of a complete absence of human leukocyte antigens (HLA) on fetal tissues appeared to be too simplistic. Billingham (a student of Medawar) showed in 1964 that nonclassical transplantation (HLA) antigens could be found on embryonic tissue from very early gestational ages onward.[2] It was later understood that the presence of these nonclassical HLA on trophoblasts are essential for the mother to recognize trophoblastic cells as "self" and to prevent the normal immune response to nonself tissues.[3,4] Nonclassical HLA were demonstrated—in direct contact with the decidua—both on extravillous trophoblast (EVT) and on the (amnion) chorion. The second possible explanation by Medawar was based on a diminished maternal responsiveness to pregnancy. A decreased ability to elicit both a humoral and cell-mediated immune response should lead to the acceptance of the "foreign" fetus. Indeed, antibody titers do decrease during pregnancy, but this decrease is caused by the physiological hemodilution occurring especially during the first trimester of pregnancy. The variety of the antibody profile remains unchanged during pregnancy. On the other hand, cellular immune responses seem to be decreased during pregnancy,[5] as reflected by the improvement of some T cell mediated autoimmune diseases and an increased incidence of infections. In contrast, the innate defense mechanism is more prominent during pregnancy.[6] This increase in function of the native immune system may be a compensatory mechanism for the decrease in specific T cell reactivity.[7] Wegmann challenged the idea of a systemic immune suppression in pregnant women and suggested that cellular interactions within the placenta lead to a local immune response.[8] Also the third possible explanation, that the uterus and especially the decidua is an immunologically privileged site, where mother and child are completely separated, cannot be the (only) explanation as even term pregnancies can be found outside the uterus with no decidua in place. Furthermore, it is now evident that during pregnancy there is cellular trafficking over the fetal-maternal interface.

Already very early after fertilization there is direct contact between the blastocyst and the maternal decidua. From those very early days onward the immunological balance between mother and fetus has to be established and maintained as there is no doubt that the maternal immune system is certainly able to recognize the paternal antigens inherited by the fetus.[9;10] The lack of a destructive immune response mounted by the mother seems to be related to the presence of an active immune process essential for normal pregnancy. This concept is supported by findings that an increase in the number of HLA differences between mother and child reduces the chance of getting certain complications of pregnancy. Sharing of HLA between mother and fetus is associated with increased incidence of preeclampsia and fetal growth retardation. This was confirmed by others suggesting that in women with a history of preeclampsia an unusual high degree of immunological compatibility with the fetus was found.[11-13] HLA-DR sharing between preeclamptic women and their partners is a risk factor for preeclampsia[14] and is also associated with a reduced birth weight, on average 200 g less.[15] Supporting this hypothesis is the observation that with more maternal-fetal HLA Class II disparities, an improvement in rheumatoid arthritis during pregnancy and in the period thereafter was found.[16] This improvement cannot be directly explained by the increase in Th2 cytokine bias occurring during normal pregnancy.[17] Also, priming of the mother by paternal antigens, e.g. by semen, might induce an immunological hyporesponsiveness specific immune regulation, essential for the process of maternal acceptance of her "foreign" fetus.[18,19] The studies by Robillard[20;21] showed that the immunological response to trophoblastic invasion is dependent on earlier confrontation with paternal antigens during sexual intercourse, suggesting that certain pregnancy complications might be related to "primi-paternity". Mucosal alloimmunization via repeated exposures to HLA occurring during unprotected sexual intercourse generates an active immune tolerance to paternal antigens.

It is becoming more and more clear that the immunological acceptance of the semiallogeneic or even fully allogeneic fetus– after oocyte donation—local immunomodulation at the maternal-fetal interface is of key importance.

IMPLANTATION

The endometrium has through every menstrual cycle a surprisingly high regenerating capacity. It constitutes many cell types including glandular epithelium, stromal (mesenchymal) cells and endothelial cells. Decidualization of the endometrium during the menstrual cycle implies the change of stromal cells of the endometrium into decidual cells. Although already in the 19th century William Hunter gave the first description of the *membrane decidua*, it was only recently accepted that the decidua is actually a maternal membrane surrounding the (two) fetal membranes.[22] The process of decidualization, initiated by the action of progesterone on estrogens induced endometrium, facilitates the apposition of the blastocyst and the acceptance and outgrowth of trophoblastic villi. Trophoblast cells by their production of human chorionic gonadotropin (HCG) support the persistence of the corpus luteum and by that the production of progesterone by the ovary. This system is also supported by the production of prolactin by the pituitary and by estrogen, inducing leukemia inhibiting factor (LIF) which enhances the effect on progesterone production.[23] From 8 weeks onward the main source of progesterone production becomes the syncythiotrophoblast. Although, decidualization is essential for implantation, it is independent of the blastocyst itself. The process depends on progesterone, but also cytokines as TGF-β and IGFBP[24,25] have a critical role in decidualization.[26]

Trophoblastic cells can be divided into two subtypes, i.e. villous trophoblast and EVT. Villous trophoblast is located around the villi and is in direct contact with maternal blood in the intervillous space. The cytotrophoblastic cells form the inner layer and are stem cells for the syncythiotrophoblast, which forms the outer layer of the villous. EVT has a proliferative and a migratory phenotype.[27] It invades the decidua and the uterine wall, and form the anchoring cytotrophoblast. At the decidual layer behind the placenta, the decidua basalis, there is direct contact between the ingrowing trophoblast, forming the anchor villi (interstitial trophoblast) and the endometrium surrounding the endometrial capillaries. The trophoblast which replaces the smooth muscle (intramural trophoblast) and endothelial cells (intra-arterial trophoblast) of these capillaries is called endovascular trophoblast.[27] At the other site of the developing fetus, villous structures will gradually disappear as the growing fetus and amniotic cavity will obliterate the endometrial cavity and the chorion will attach to the decidua, which at that side is called the decidua parietalis. The decidua is also considered of essential importance in the limitation of trophoblastic growth, which is necessary to prevent the occurrence of clinical features as placenta accreta and percreta.

Many biochemical active compounds are involved in the implantation process. Cytokines such as Il-1β induce the synthesis of prostaglandins and IGFBP-1, both needed for sufficient trophoblastic invasion. Invasion is also depending on cell adhesion molecules, as integrins[27,28] and on matrix metalloproteinases (MMPs).[29] The latter are produced by trophoblast cells. Fibronectin, produced upon promotion by TGF-β by the EVT and detectable in the extracellular matrix of the decidua has a critical role in the attachment of trophoblast cells to the decidua and supports the formation of cytotrophoblastic cell columns.[30]

IMPLANTATION AND THE NONCLASSICAL MHC-I MOLECULES

King and Loke described in 1991 an attractive model for a controlled permission of trophoblastic invasion and also of limiting this invasion— into the endometrium and myometrium of the uterus.[31] Trophoblastic cells express, besides the classical HLA class I molecule HLA-C, only the nonclassical class I antigens HLA-G, HLA-E and HLA-F, which have a very limited polymorphism. MHC class II antigens are completely absent on trophoblast.[32] HLA-G is only expressed on the invading extravillous cytotrophoblast and is not present on villous syncytiotrophoblast.[33,34] By the expression of the nonclassical HLA molecules, fetal trophoblastic cells, in their interaction with decidual leucocytes, are recognized as "self" and do not evoke an immunological response by NK cells. This allows the EVT to invade the uterus. HLAG is expressed in five different spliced, membrane bound or soluble isoforms.[35] Soluble

HLA-G (sHLA-G) is secreted by the syncytiotrophoblast and cytotrophoblast. HLA-G has the possibility to present peptides derived from classical HLA class I molecules and other intracellular molecules. Although some data suggest that HLA-G expression at the maternal-fetal junction is decreased in preeclampsia,[36,37] this is not confirmed by others.[38]

DECIDUA INFILTRATING CELLS

The decidua contains many different types of (immune) cells, of which the frequency changes throughout the menstrual cycle and during pregnancy.

Uterine NK Cells

In the early proliferative phase of the endometrium, many small, round agranular cells, with very little cytoplasm are found, which enlarge and become more granulated during the secretory phase. These cells, formerly called *uterine large granular lymphocytes*, turned out to be a special form of natural-killer (NK) lymphocytes: uterine NK-cells (uNK cells) with a different phenotype than NK cells found in peripheral blood. These cells do not express the classical NK marker CD16, while the CD56 surface density of these cells is more than 20 times higher compared to peripheral blood NK cells.[39,40] These uNK cells are bone marrow derived and replicate in situ in the endometrium.[41] Their number is maximal around ovulation and remain high around the period of implantation, accounting for at least 70% of the uterine lymphocytes.[40] uNK cells produce cytokines, like TGF-β, macrophage colony stimultating factor (M-CSF), tumor necrosis factor alpha (TNF-α), interferon gamma (IFN-γ), vascular, endothelial growth factor, angiopoietin 1 (Any 1), Any 2, IL-3 and LIf, IL-3 and LIF that are essential in trophoblast invasion and tissue remodeling.[40,42,43] On the other hand, appreciable amounts of granulocytes macrophage colony stimulating factor and IFN-β are produced by uNK cells, possibly stimulated by IL-2, a factor related to trophoblast apoptosis, limiting the invasiveness of trophoblast cells.[44] Although there is a significant decrease of the uNK cells during the second trimester of pregnancy, at term age uNK cells are still present in appreciable amounts in the endometrium.[45]

sHLA-G is able to block uNK cell function and cytolytic T lymphocyte action, the latter possibly by an increase in apoptosis of activated CD4[+] and CD8[+] T cells.[35] By this effect on uNK cells and eliminating harmful CD8[+] T cells, trophoblast invasion is facilitated and endothelial cell reactivity is diminished.[46] In this context, it is essential to realize the principle difference in allorecognition between CD8[+] T cells and NK cells. CD8[+] T cells are activated by foreign HLA, while NK cells are programmed to lyse cells that lack self HLA molecules. The absence of classical HLA would be a trigger for NK cells, but the interaction of HLA-G with KIR receptors on NK cells prevents such reactivity (Fig. 83.1).[47,48]

The interaction between uNK cells and HLA-G is basic for a normal, successful pregnancy, although it has been reported that women with a homozygous deletion in the HLA-G gene can have completely normal pregnancies. HLA-C is also expressed by the EVT cells and interacts with NK-cells possibly in the same way as HLA-G. Although the existence of a specific receptor for HLA-G on the uNK cell is still discussed, HLA-C —and most probably HLA-G also—is recognized by receptors belonging to the KIR family, e.g. ILT3 and KIR2DL1.[49] HLA-G might via binding of these receptors, influence cytokine secretion by T cells and modulate the Th1/

Target cell expressing

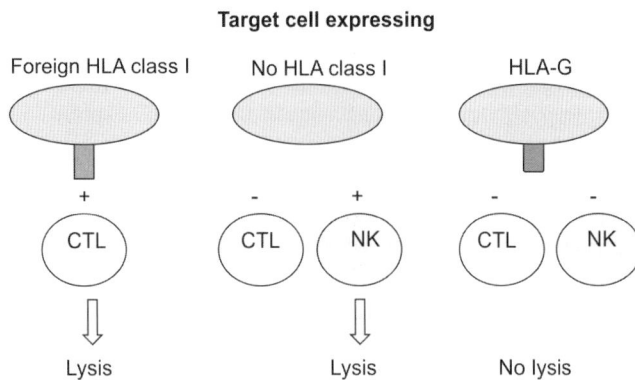

Fig. 83.1: Cytotoxic T cells will react against HLA-mismatched target cells. Downregulation of the surface expression of the foreign HLA molecules will prevent this reactivity but will lead to activitation of NK cells that are triggered by the lack of HLA class I molecules on the target cell. Expression of HLA-G will prevent activation of NK cells by its interaction with KIR receptors

Th2 balance.[46] HLA-E, also expressed by the EVT, is recognized by the NK cell by its CD94/NKG2A receptor. This interaction prevents cellular toxicity of the trophoblast.[50] It seems that HLA-E coexpression is at least necessary for the prevention of trophoblast lysis.[51] KIR receptors are expressed besides by uNK cells also by γδT cells.[52]

It seems that for implantation the cytokines produced as a result from the interaction between trophoblastic cells and uterine lymphocytes, especially uNK cells are essential. The process has many features in common with an inflammation like process, where cytokines play a pivotal role as well. In early pregnancy, the role of specific T cells is marginal as they seem not to be involved in the implantation process.

B and T Cells

B cells and plasma cells are considered irrelevant for the regulation of trophoblast invasion as they are nearly absent in the decidua.[40] T cells form around 10% of the decidual leukocytes.[40] The number of CD8[+] T-cells and CD4[+] (helper) T-cells may change during pregnancy.[53] Recently, it was found that activated T cells are present at the placental site (decidua basalis)[40] and even more numerous in the decidua aligning the fetal membranes (decidua parietalis).[54] Further functional characterization of T cells present in the decidua parietalis and basalis[45] should elucidate whether these cells play an active role in the (down) regulation of the maternal alloimmune response to the fetus.

Most in vitro studies of T cells isolated from maternal blood show a diminished T cell activity and a concomitant increase in B cell function. These findings are in line with clinical observations demonstrating an increased incidence of viral infections during pregnancy and the amelioration of T cell mediated autoimmune diseases such as rheumatoid arthritis. In contrast, the severity of antibody mediated autoimmune diseases, such as systemic lupus erythematosus, shows an increase during pregnancy.

In peripheral blood a reduction of T helper (Th) 1 cells is demonstrated, which is partly caused by progesterone, associated with a downregulation of NF-KB, which has an inhibitory effect on Th1 cell differentiation.[17] The consequence of this is that the balance of T helper cells is shifted to a Th2 bias, which is the reason why normal pregnancy is characterized by a dominance of the anti-inflammatory Th2 type cytokines such as IL-4, 6, 10 and 13. The Th1 pro-inflammatory cytokines, such as IL-2, IFN-γ and TNF-α, which activate cytotoxic T-cells, are thought to have a detrimental effect on pregnancy development. However, the relevance of a Th2 bias in pregnancy was disputed from the beginning as it cannot be excluded that the cytokines, beneficial for processes important during implantation like spiral artery development and local tissue remodeling process, are detrimental later during pregnancy.[55] Especially Th1 cytokines, as IFN-γ, are involved in the local inflammatory response during implantation.[56] Moreover, in the mouse IL-10 (Th2) knock out model, no negative effect on pregnancy outcome, on pregnancy rate, on litter size or on birth weight is observed. In contrast, uNK cell knockout mice showed that a maternal uNK cell-deficient decidua is associated with fetal demise and a reduction in birth weight.[57] These postpartum findings were related to abnormalities in the arterial and microvascular architecture of decidual vessels. Transplantation of these mice with normal bone marrow leads to the development of uNK cells preventing this pathology, whereby the decidual arterioles looked normal and the placental became larger again. uNK cells probably exert these effects in vascular modification (dilatation, elongation and branching) via the production of specific cytokines like IFN-γ.[41] The complex network of cytokines and the cells contributing to this balance even in time during pregnancy still have to be investigated, whereby it has to be considered that not only T-cells, but also uNK cells produce these cytokines.

During pregnancy, the adaptive immune system is activated, as shown by the development in 30% of the pregnancies of long persisting antibodies against paternal HLA and the activation of cytotoxic, T-lymphocytes specific for these HLA.[58] In the decidual environment T cells may be primed by paternal antigens, but the normally expected T-cell mediated cytotoxicity of trophoblastic cells does not occur. Through, both the elimination or suppression of fetus-reactive T cell clones and also because paternal antigens are presented via nonclassical HLA, the balance of T helper cells is shifted to a Th2 bias. For a successful pregnancy, the immunological acceptance of the fetus is essential. This acceptance is considered more and more an active process leading to the induction of immunological regulation, whereby the fetus is not attacked. The development of blocking antibodies may play a protective role by blocking HLA antibodies and potential fetus-reactive maternal lymphocytes. From the term placenta, activated alloreactive T cells can be isolated.[59] Locally at the level of the placenta, these activated T cells are probably downregulated by regulatory T cells. With a high level of HLA compatibility between partners this down-regulation might be less effective, explaining the higher change of pregnancy complications in these couples.

Macrophages

Macrophages are the second most numerous type of leucocytes present at the interface and are found in greater numbers in the decidua basalis as compared to the decidua parietalis.[45] They are the main producers of cytokine and growth factors, and contribute to an adequate balance between Th1 and Th2 cytokines in the placenta, either by producing cytokines as IL-4, IL-10 and IFN-γ or by indirectly stimulating the IFN-γ production by uNK cells.[60] Placental apoptosis, orchestrated by macrophages, is a normal occurring phenomenon in the placenta. Apoptosis is higher in third trimester placentas compared to first trimester placenta, and it might also be higher in abnormal pregnancies, complicated by

IUGR and/or preeclampsia.[61] Apoptosis is essential for the tissue remodeling occurring during implantation. The clearance of these apoptotic bodies is essential for placental homeostasis, preventing the release of potentially pro-inflammatory intracellular contents and of proteins which are foreign to the maternal immune system. The clearance of apoptotic debris is associated with the release of the anti-inflammatory TGF-β and possibly of other Th2 associated cytokines.

Recent evidence suggests that an even more important role for uNK cell lies in the production of cytokines (or other active substances), which prevent cytolytic actions by T cells, although, these T cells are already present in an activated state.[54] Leukemia inhibiting factor (LIF), but also IL-10, might control the transcription of HLA-G. In mouse, the absence of LIF is associated with total pregnancy failure. Also human data support a pivotal role for LIF.

Apoptosis of EVT is related to the number of CD56+ NK cells, while the number of uNK cells decline in parallel with apoptotic cells. The massive apoptosis of EVT is suggested to be the mechanism reducing invasiveness of the trophoblast.[62]

FAS-LIGAND INDUCED APOPTOSIS

Fas-Ligand (FasL) expression on the trophoblast induces apoptosis of T cells or NK cells, via their Fast receptors. In the trophoblast villi, FasL was only found on the cytotrophoblast, while the syncytiotrophoblast, which is in direct contact with the maternal blood, show no expression of FasL. This FasL-Fas receptor interaction eliminates maternal lymphocytes specific for fetal/paternal antigens.[63-66]

THE ACTIVE PROCESS OF TOLERANCE INDUCTION

Several mechanisms may lead to an active downregulation of a destructive alloimmunity by the maternal immune system toward the fetus.

Dendritic Cells and Regulatory T Cells

Dendritic cells (DCs) are important in the regulation of the immune response and have the unique opportunity to coordinate the innate and adaptive immune system. One can consider the endometrium as a mucosal surface, where DCs are confronted with trophoblastic antigens during pregnancy. DC process and present these antigens to the maternal immune system for the induction of regulatory cells (Treg),[67] which may lead to the induction of regulatory T cells and may explain some of the findings of specific maternal tolerance to paternal antigens during pregnancy.[68] In humans in early first trimester decidua DCs with a myeloid phenotype have been isolated,[69] although in low frequency (1%). The dominance of plasmacytoid DCs in the decidua might be essential for polarizing the T cell immune response to a Th2 bias.[70] DCs have been shown to produce TGF-β and also the T cell inhibiting factor IDO[71] (see further). In the mouse model immature DCs isolated from the decidua contain predominantly the pregnancy protective cytokine IL-10 and minor amounts of the Th1 type 1 cytokine IL-12.[72]

The family of regulatory T cells consists of the naturally occurring CD4+CD25+ T-regulatory cells (Treg) and the induced secondary Th3 cells and Treg type1 (T_R1) cells.[73,74] Treg cells are present in early pregnancy decidua.[75] Treg cells may develop after antigenic stimulation, under noninflammatory conditions. Treg cells inhibit CD4+ T cells to produce IL-2 and convert them into IL-10 producing T1-like cells and can also induce TGF-β producing Th3-like cells. This suppression is an important factor in the Th2 bias occurring during pregnancy.[76,77] IL-10 might be functional in three ways; suppression of cytotoxic T cells and their cytokines (IL-12 and IFN-γ), induction of regulatory T cells and inhibition of the maturation process of DCs leading to a more tolerogenic type of DC. Also IL-6 and IL-1β are produced by these cells.[78,79] TGF-β is involved in the inhibition of trophoblast invasion by downregulation of collagenases, and inhibition of metalloproteinases and integrins.[25,40] TGF-α is supposed to be a stimulator of trophoblast invasion. Some of these T helper cells express the regulatory T cell marker CTLA4 (Tilburgs 2004) and have already been shown to induce the production of IDO by DCs after interaction between CD80–CD86.[80] In the mouse, Treg cells, carrying the transcription factor FoxP3, are substantially increased in uterine tissue during pregnancy.[7] In venous blood during pregnancy, a doubling of CD4+CD25+ cells was found, which were increasing in parallel with the duration of pregnancy.[76] These expanding cells in the pregnant endometrium (both in mice and in human) are pivotal for the suppression of the maternal immune reaction against fetal derived paternal antigens.[7,81]

IDO

Recently, a role for Indoleamine 2,3-dioxygenase (IDO) regulating T cell immunity during pregnancy has been suggested.[82] As a mechanism to prevent trophoblast lysis, IDO secreted by EVT, decidual macrophages and possibly by dendritic cells, inhibits lymphocyte proliferation and survival via a decrease in extracellular tryptophan.[71,82,83] Its immunosuppressive effect might be exerted not only by a decrease of tryptophan but also by an increase of the tryptophan kynurenine metabolites. These metabolites might have a selective apoptotic effect on Th1 cells. IDO expression is induced by IFN-γ[84;85] and further stimulated by CTLA-4 expressing Treg cells.[76] It was shown that placental tissue, with a particularly high expression of IDO, made maternal CD8+ T cells specific tolerant for paternal class I MHC.[82]

Crry Protein

Crry protein, a murine protective cell surface protein and a component of the natural immunity system, is also expressed on trophoblast. This protein suppresses the ongoing complement activation, especially C3, after its deposition to the membranes at the feto-maternal interface. Complement activation, promoting inflammatory reactions to the placenta, resulting in embryonic lethality, is inhibited by the expression of the Crry protein.[86] It was shown in the Crry protein knock out mice, that Crry is necessary for embryonic development.[87] In human placenta, three other complement regulators, decay accelerating factor (DAF; CD 55), membrane cofactor protein (MCP; CD 46) and CD 59, are present in high concentrations. These regulators have the same function as Crry by preventing complement activation and placental inflammation at the interface.

Progesterone

Progesterone has immune modulatory activity because of its blocking effect on T cell activity.[88] Peripheral T cells from pregnant women have a much higher progesterone sensitivity compared to nonpregnant women, due to an increased number of progesterone receptors (PR).[89] There is an overlap between the PR-positive T cells and γδT cells.[90] PR receptors also exist on uNK cells.[91] PR-positive lymphocytes and uNK cells produce, on binding with progesterone, a progesterone inhibiting binding factor (PIBF). PIBF inhibits NK cells cytotoxicity by a failure in degranulation, to release perforin and granzymes,[92] and it might also induce the secretion of IL-10 by already activated lymphocytes.

Progesterone may also play an essential role in the local regulation of invasion. It regulates the genes, effecting an increase of factors essential for the local regulation of invasion like amphiregulin, insulin like growth factor binding protein 3 (IGFBP-3)[25] and immune response gene-1 (IRG-1).[23]

In animals, medroxyprogesterone rather than progesterone had the best anti-inflammatory properties by reducing the upregulation of type 2 cyclooxygenase (COX-2) mRNA.[93] COX-2 is essential for the production of the labor associated prostaglandins. Also other labor-associated genes are downregulated by progesterone: for example, IL-1β, IL-8, NF-KB,[93] and MMP8 and MMP9.

Recently, it has been shown that progesterone treatment results in a more than 40% reduction in the incidence of preterm delivery in a high-risk group.[94] Increased NF-KB levels have been found in preterm deliveries even without signs of an infection, whereas IL-10 has an inhibiting function on prostaglandin production. Even term delivery is associated with this inflammatory-like process.[95] There is no doubt that prolactin is produced by the decidua, partly controlled by the action of progesterone. Prolactin might have an immune modulatory role via receptors shown to be present on immunocompetent cells, e.g. the uNK cell.[96,97]

CELLULAR TRAFFICKING

There is a very intensive and reciprocal fetal-maternal trafficking, both actively and passively, of many different substances and cells through the placenta. This process is important for the maintenance and maternal adaptation to pregnancy but also for the maternal recognition and immunological acceptance of pregnancy. The placental supply of maternal blood, via the endometrial/decidual spiral arteries to the intervillous space, bathes the fetal syncythiotrophoblast in maternal blood and its constituent immunocompetent cells. Fetal villous tissue and fetal cells within the villous capillaries are only separated from the maternal blood by the capillary endothelial wall, the mesenchyme within the villous trophoblast and the syncytiotrophoblast. Also, at other locations there is a very near cell-to-cell contact. At the decidua parietalis there is a direct contact between the fetal membranes, e.g. the chorion leave and the maternal decidua. The consideration that fetal and maternal circulations, and by that the cells of fetus and mother were completely separated during pregnancy, has been challenged by the fact that chimerism, defined as long-term persistence of a small number of foreign cells, both within the mother (maternal microchimerism) and also within the fetus (fetal microchimerism) are regularly occurring processes. Chimerism is known to occur after solid organ transplantation, but especially after hematopoietic cell transplantation, it can result in a chronic graft-vs.-host disease, a disorder which has a profound resemblance with autoimmune diseases.

During pregnancy, these trafficking cells have a hematopoietic progenitor cell character.[98] In the third trimester, 80–90% of the mothers will have circulating fetal cells, with a proportion of around 1 fetal cell in 1,000 maternal cells. The occurrence of cellular trafficking over the fetomaternal interface results from a cellular imperfect placental barrier. This cellular trafficking confronts the mother with paternal antigens, resulting in activation of alloreactive T cells and HLA antibody formation but possibly also the induction of tolerance. HLA compatibility between mother and fetus supports the persistence of fetal cells in the maternal circulation. The migration of these cells into maternal tissues like thyroid and bone marrow have possible long standing consequences.[99,100] The suggestion has been made that the long-term persistence of fetal cells is associated with the development of autoimmune diseases including sclerodermia, rheumatoid arthritis, thyroiditis, primary biliary cirrhosis, Sjögren syndrome, systemic lupus erythematosus and neonatal lupus syndromes. However, microchimerism might also have positive effects. The induction of tolerance to non-inherited maternal HLA (NIMA) during pregnancy[101] leads to a better acceptance of NIMA mismatched transplantated organs[102] and a lower incidence of graft-versus-host disease.[103]

Also, a neonatally occurring tolerogenic effect of soluble maternal HLA resulting from breastfeeding was shown.[104] The presence of chimerism might be used therapeutically e.g. in bone marrow transplantation, where non, T cell depleted stem cells from haploidentical family donors were successfully used for transplantation provided that chimerism could be demonstrated.[105,106]

CONCLUSION

There are many immune mechanism playing together at the fetal-maternal interface. These mechanism are characterized by its redundancy and by its complexity. Any cytokine can be both down- and upregulated. The absence of B cells and the relative small numbers of T cells in the first trimester decidua suggests that the adaptive immune system is not as important in that period of gestation as the innate system. NK cells and macrophages, representing the innate system, are more apparent in this period. As the number of NK cells in interaction with nonclassical HLA (HLA-G) decreases substantially during pregnancy, other mechanisms resulting in maternal acceptance must become more important while pregnancy progresses.[107] Although trophoblast carries no HLA class II and no HLA-A and HLA-B, mother and fetus might interact via HLA-C, as suggested by the distribution of particular HLA-C allotypes and specific KIR receptors in the population.[108]

However, it is important to realize that a successful pregnancy cannot be based on only one mechanism. In a murine animal model with, e.g. class I expression on trophoblast and in the absence of Fas-L, a normal tolerance to histoincompatible pregnancies was shown, without an adverse effect on pregnancy outcomes.[109] Also, the recognition of HLA-G by the NK cell is not essential for repro-duction.[110] It is as Chaouat[111] stated that for a successful pregnancy, it is essential that there are "sequential windows and extreme complexity mixed with very precise timing and tuning".

The classical immunological model of the fetus being an allograft, which is not rejected, is less appropriate and newer models must be considered based on local immune regulation operating in parallel for the acceptance of the (semi) allogeneic fetal allograft.

REFERENCES

1. Medawar P. Some immunological and endocrinological problems raised by the evolution of viviparity in vertebrates. In: Pringle J (Ed). Cambridge University Press; 1953. pp. 320-38.

2. Billingham RE. Transplantation immunity and the maternal-fetal relation. N Engl J Med. 1964;270:667-72.

3. Head JR, Drake BL, Zuckermann FA. Major histocompatibility antigens on trophoblast and their regulation: Implications in the maternal-fetal relationship. Am J Reprod Immunol Microbiol. 1987;15:12-8.

4. Bazer FW, Vallet JL, Roberts RM, et al. Role of conceptus secretory products in establishment of pregnancy. J Reprod Fertil. 1986;76:841-50.

5. Krause PJ, Ingardia CJ, Pontius LT, et al. Host defense during pregnancy: neutrophil chemotaxis and adherence. Am J Obstet Gynecol. 1987;157:274-80.

6. Sacks G, Sargent I, Redman C. An innate view of human pregnancy. Immunol Today. 1999;20:114-8.

7. Aluvihare VR, Kallikourdis M, Betz AG. Regulatory T cells mediate maternal tolerance to the fetus. Nat Immunol. 2004;5:266-71.

8. Wegmann TG. Fetal protection against abortion: Is it immunosuppression or immunostimulation? Ann Immunol (Paris). 1984;135D:309-12.

9. Van Rood JJ, Eernisse JG, van Leeuwen A. Leucocyte antibodies in sera from pregnant women. Nature. 1958;181:1735-6.

10. Verdijk RM, Kloosterman A, Pool J, et al. Pregnancy induces minor histocompatibility antigen-specific cytotoxic T cells: Implications for stem cell transplantation and immunotherapy. Blood. 2004;103:1961-4.

11. Scott JS, Jenkins DM, Need JA. Immunology of pre-eclampsia. Lancet. 1978;1:704-6.

12. de LB I, Battini L, Simonelli M, et al. Increased HLA-DR homozygosity associated with pre-eclampsia. Hum Reprod. 2000;15:1807-12.

13. Daunter B. Immunology of pregnancy: Towards a unifying hypothesis. Eur J Obstet Gynecol Reprod Biol. 1992;43:81-95.

14. de LB I, Battini L, Simonelli M, et al. HLA-DR in couples associated with preeclampsia: Background and updating by DNA sequencing. J Reprod Immunol. 2003;59:235-43.

15. Ober C, Simpson JL, Ward M, et al. Prenatal effects of maternal-fetal HLA compatibility. Am J Reprod Immunol Microbiol. 1987;15:141-9.

16. Jansson R, Dahlberg PA, Winsa B, et al. The postpartum period constitutes an important risk for the development of clinical Graves' disease in young women. Acta Endocrinol (Copenh). 1987;116:321-5.

17. McCracken SA, Gallery E, Morris JM. Pregnancy-specific downregulation of NF-kappaB expression in T cells in humans is essential for the maintenance of the cytokine profile required for pregnancy success. J Immunol. 2004;172:4583-91.

18. Robertson SA, Bromfield JJ, Tremellen KP. Seminal 'priming' for protection from pre-eclampsia—a unifying hypothesis. J Reprod Immunol. 2003;59:253-65.

19. Dekker G. The partner's role in the etiology of pre-eclampsia. J Reprod Immunol. 2002;57:203-15.

20. Robillard PY, Hulsey TC, Perianin J, et al. Association of pregnancy-induced hypertension with duration of sexual cohabitation before conception. Lancet. 1994;344:973-5.

21. Clark DA. Does immunological intercourse prevent pre-eclampsia. Lancet. 1994;344:969.

22. Wewer UM, Faber M, Liotta LA, et al. Immunochemical and ultrastructural assessment of the nature of the pericellular basement membrane of human decidual cells. Lab Invest. 1985;53:624-33.

23. Sherwin J, Freeman T, Stephens R, et al. Identification of genes regulated by leukaemia inhibitory factor in the mouse uterus at the time of implantation. Mol Endocrinol. 2004;18(9):2185-95.

24. Ruoslahti E, Pierschbacher MD. New perspectives in cell adhesion: RGD and integrins. Science. 1987;238: 491-7.

25. Bell SC. Decidualization and insulin-like growth factor (IGF) binding protein: Implications for its role in stromal cell differentiation and the decidual cell in hemochorial placentation. Hum Reprod. 1989;4: 125-30.

26. Casey ML, MacDonald PC. The endothelin-parathyroid hormone-related protein vasoactive peptide system in human endometrium: modulation by transforming growth factor-beta. Hum Reprod. 1996;11(Suppl 2):62-82.

27. Kaufmann P, Castellucci M. Extravillous trophoblast in the human placenta—a review. Trophoblast Res. 2004;10:21-65.

28. Librach CL, Werb Z, Fitzgerald ML, et al. 92-kD type IV collagenase mediates invasion of human cytotrophoblasts. J Cell Biol. 1991;113:437-49.

29. Frenette PS, Wagner DD. Adhesion molecules—Part 1. N Engl J Med. 1996;334:1526-9.

30. Feinberg RF, Kliman HJ, Lockwood CJ. Is oncofetal fibronectin a trophoblast glue for human implantation? Am J Pathol. 1991;138:537-43.

31. King A, Loke YW. On the nature and function of human uterine granula lymphocytes. Immunol Today. 1991;12:432-5.

32. Zuckermann FA, Head JR. Expression of MHC antigens on murine trophoblast and their modulation by interferon. J Immunol. 1986;137:846-53.

33. Loke YW, King A, Burrows T, et al. Evaluation of trophoblast HLA-G antigen with a specific monoclonal antibody. Tissue Antigens. 1997;50:135-46.

34. Trundley A, Moffett A. Human uterine leukocytes and pregnancy. Tissue Antigens. 2004;63:1-12.

35. Le Bouteiller P, Legrand-Abravanel F, Solier C. Soluble HLA-G1 at the materno-fetal interface—A review. Placenta. 2003;24(Suppl) A-S10-S5.

36. Hara N, Fujii T, Yamashita T, et al. Altered expression of human leukocyte antigen G (HLA-G) on extravillous trophoblasts in pre-eclampsia: Immunohistological demonstration with anti-HLA-G specific antibody "87G" and anti-cytokeratin antibody "CAM5.2". Am J Reprod Immunol. 1996;36:349-58.

37. Colbern GT, Chiang MH, Main EK. Expression of the nonclassic histocompatibility antigen HLA-G by pre-eclamptic placenta. Am J Obstet Gynecol. 1994;170:1244-50.

38. Datema G, van Meir CA, Kanhai HH, et al. Pre-term birth and severe pre-eclampsia are not associated with altered expression of HLA on human trophoblasts. Am J Reprod Immunol. 2003;49:193-201.

39. Moffett-King A. Natural killer cells and pregnancy. Nat Rev Immunol. 2002;2:656-63.

40. Loke YW, King A, Burrows TD. Decidua in human implantation. Hum Reprod. 1995;10(Suppl)2:14-21.

41. Croy BA, Chantakru S, Esadeg S, et al. Decidual natural killer cells: Key regulators of placental development (a review). J Reprod Immunol. 2002;57:151-68.

42. Li XF, Charnock-Jones DS, Zhang E, et al. Angiogenic growth factor messenger ribonucleic acids in uterine natural killer cells. J Clin Endocrinol Metab. 2001;86:1823-34.

43. Saito S, Morii T, Enomoto M, et al. The effect of interleukin 2 and transforming growth factor-β2 (TGF-β2) on the proliferation and natural killer activity of decidual CD16$^-$CD56^{bright} natural killer cells. Cell Immunol. 1993;605-13.

44. Jokhi PP, King A, Loke YW. Production of granulocyte-macrophage colony-stimulating factor by human trophoblast cells and by decidual large granular lymphocytes. Hum Reprod. 1994;9:1660-9.

45. Sindram-Trujillo AP, Scherjon SA, van Hulst-van Miert PP, et al. Differential distribution of NK cells in decidua basalis compared with decidua parietalis after uncomplicated human term pregnancy. Hum Immunol. 2003;64:921-9.

46. Le Bouteiller P, Pizzato N, Barakonyi A, et al. HLA-G, pre-eclampsia, immunity and vascular events. J Reprod Immunol. 2003;59:219-34.

47. van der MA, Lukassen HG, van Lierop MJ, et al. Membrane-bound HLA-G activates proliferation and interferon-gamma production by uterine natural killer cells. Mol Hum Reprod. 2004;10:189-95.

48. King A, Hiby SE, Verma S, et al. Uterine NK cells and trophoblast HLA class I molecules. Am J Reprod Immunol. 1997;37:459-62.

49. Rouas-Freiss N, Goncalves RM, Menier C, et al. Direct evidence to support the role of HLA-G in protecting the fetus from maternal uterine natural killer cytolysis. Proc Natl Acad Sci USA. 1997;94:11520-5.

50. Huddleston H, Schust DJ. Immune interactions at the maternal-fetal interface: A focus on antigen presentation. Am J Reprod Immunol. 2004;51:283-9.

51. Llano M, Lee N, Navarro F, et al. HLA-E-bound peptides influence recognition by inhibitory and triggering CD94/NKG2 receptors: Preferential response to an HLA-G-derived nonamer. Eur J Immunol. 1998;28:2854-63.

52. Parham P. Killer cell immunoglobulin-like receptor diversity: Balancing signals in the natural killer cell response. Immunol Lett. 2004;92:11-3.

53. Luppi P. How immune mechanisms are affected by pregnancy. Vaccine. 2003;21:3352-7.

54. Sindram-Trujillo A, Scherjon S, Kanhai H, et al. Increased T-cell activation in decidua parietalis compared to decidua basalis in uncomplicated human term pregnancy. Am J Reprod Immunol. 2003;49:261-8.

55. Chaouat G, Ledee-Bataille N, Zourbas S, et al. Implantation: Can immunological parameters of implantation failure be of interest for pre-eclampsia? J Reprod Immunol. 2003;59:205-17.

56. Chaouat G, Ledee-Bataille N, Dubanchet S, et al. TH1/TH2 paradigm in pregnancy: Paradigm lost? Cytokines in pregnancy/early abortion: Reexamining the TH1/TH2 paradigm. Int Arch Allergy Immunol. 2004;134:93-119.

57. Croy BA, Ashkar AA, Minhas K, et al. Can murine uterine natural killer cells give insights into the pathogenesis of pre-eclampsia? J Soc Gynecol Investig. 2000;7:12-20.

58. van Kampen CA, Versteeg-van der Voort Maarschalk MF, Langerak-Langerak J, et al. Pregnancy can induce long-persisting primed CTLs specific for inherited paternal HLA antigens. Hum Immunol. 2001;62:201-7.

59. Sindram-Trujillo AP, Scherjon SA, van Hulst-van Miert PP, et al. Comparison of decidual leukocytes following spontaneous vaginal delivery and elective cesarean section in uncomplicated human term pregnancy. J Reprod Immunol. 2003;62:12537.

60. Lidstrom C, Matthiesen L, Berg G, et al. Cytokine secretion patterns of NK cells and macrophages in early human pregnancy decidua and blood: Implications for suppressor macrophages in decidua. Am J Reprod Immunol. 2003;50:444-52.

61. Abrahams VM, Kim YM, Straszewski SL, et al. Macrophages and apoptotic cell clearance during pregnancy. Am J Reprod Immunol. 2004;51:275-82.

62. von Rango U, Krusche CA, Kertschanska S, et al. Apoptosis of extravillous trophoblast cells limits the trophoblast invasion in uterine but not in tubal pregnancy during first trimester. Placenta. 2003;24:929-40.

63. Jiang SP, Vacchio MS. Multiple mechanisms of peripheral T cell tolerance to the fetal "allograft". J Immunol. 1998;160:3086-90.

64. Hunt JS, Vassmer D, Ferguson TA, et al. Fas ligand is positioned in mouse uterus and placenta to prevent trafficking of activated leukocytes between the mother and the conceptus. J Immunol. 1997;158:4122-8.

65. Guller S, LaChapelle L. The role of placental Fas ligand in maintaining immune privilege at maternal-fetal interfaces. Semin Reprod Endocrinol. 1999;17:39-44.

66. Hammer A, Blaschitz A, Daxbock C, et al. Fas and Fas-ligand are expressed in the uteroplacental unit of first-trimester pregnancy. Am J Reprod Immunol. 1999;41:41-51.

67. Sallusto F, Lanzavecchia A. Mobilizing dendritic cells for tolerance, priming, and chronic inflammation. J Exp Med. 1999;189:611-4.

68. Tafuri A, Alferink J, Möller P, et al. T cell awareness of paternal alloantigens during pregnancy. Science. 1995;270:630-3.

69. Gardner L, Moffett A. Dendritic cells in the human decidua. Biol Reprod. 2003;61:1438-46.

70. Ueda Y, Hagihara M, Okamoto A, et al. Frequencies of dendritic cells (myeloid DC and plasmacytoid DC) and their ratio reduced in pregnant women: Comparison with umbilical cord blood and normal healthy adults. Hum Immunol. 2003;64:1144-51.

71. Mellor AL, Munn DH. Tryptophan catabolism and T cell tolerance: Immunosuppression by starvation? Immunol Today. 1999;20:469-73.

72. Blois SM, Alba Soto CD, Tometten M, et al. Lineage, maturity, and phenotype of uterine murine dendritic cells throughout gestation indicate a protective role in maintaining pregnancy. Biol Reprod. 2004;70:1018-23.

73. Sakaguchi S, Sakaguchi N, Shimizu J, et al. Immunologic tolerance maintained by CD25+ CD4+ regulatory T cells: Their common role in controlling autoimmunity, tumor immunity, and transplantation tolerance. Immunol Rev. 2001;182:18-32.

74. Rutella S, Lemoli RM. Regulatory T cells and tolerogenic dendritic cells from basic biology to clinical applications. Immunol Lett. 2004;94:11-26.

75. Sasaki Y, Sakai M, Miyazaki S, et al. Decidual and peripheral blood CD4+CD25+ regulatory T cells in early pregnancy subjects and spontaneous abortion cases. Mol Hum Reprod. 2004;10:347-53.

76. Somerset DA, Zheng Y, Kilby MD, et al. Normal human pregnancy is associated with an elevation in the immune suppressive CD25+ CD4+ regulatory T cell subset. Immunology. 2004;112:38-43.

77. Ling EM, Smith T, Nguyen XD, et al. Relation of CD4+CD25+ regulatory T cell suppression of allergen-driven T cell activation to atopic status and expression of allergic disease. Lancet. 2004;363:608-15.

78. Nagaeva O, Jonsson L, Mincheva-Nilsson L. Dominant IL-10 and TGF-beta mRNA expression in gammadelta T cells of human early pregnancy decidua suggests immunoregulatory potential. Am J Reprod Immunol. 2002;48:9-17.

79. Costeas PA, Koumouli A, Giantsiou-Kyriakou A, et al. Th2/Th3 cytokine genotypes are associated with pregnancy loss. Hum Immunol. 2004;65:135-41.

80. Grohmann U, Orabona C, Fallarino F, et al. CTLA-4-Ig regulates tryptophan catabolism in vivo. Nat Immunol. 2002;3:1097-101.

81. Heikkinen J, Mottonen M, Alanen A, et al. Phenotypic characterization of regulatory T cells in the human decidua. Clin Exp Immunol. 2004;136:373-8.

82. Munn DH, Zhou M, Attwood JT, et al. Prevention of allogeneic fetal rejection by tryptophan catabolism. Science. 1998;281:1191-3.

83. Grohmann U, Fallarino F, Puccetti P. Tolerance, DCs and tryptophan: much ado about IDO. Trends Immunol. 2003;24:242-8.

84. Kudo Y, Hara T, Katsuki T, et al. Mechanisms regulating the expression of indoleamine 2,3-dioxygenase during decidualization of human endometrium. Hum Reprod. 2004;19:1222-30.

85. Kudo Y, Boyd CA, Spyropoulou I, et al. Indoleamine 2,3-dioxygenase: Distribution and function in the developing human placenta. J Reprod Immunol. 2004;61:87-98.

86. Xu C, Mao D, Holers VM, et al. A critical role for murine complement regulator crry in feto-maternal tolerance. Science. 2000;287:498-501.

87. Xu C, Mao D, Holers VM, et al. A critical role for murine complement regulator crry in feto-maternal tolerance. Science. 2000;287:498-501.

88. Mori T, Kobayashi H, Nishimoto H, et al. Inhibitory effect of progesterone and 20 alpha-hydroxypregn-4-en-3-one on the phytohemagglutinin-induced transformation of human lymphocytes. Am J Obstet Gynecol. 1977;127:151-7.

89. Szekeres-Bartho J, Hadnagy J, Pacsa AS. The suppressive effect of progesterone on lymphocyte cytotoxicity: unique progesterone sensitivity of pregnancy lymphocytes. J Reprod Immunol. 1985;7:121-8.

90. Barakonyi A, Polgar B, Szekeres-Bartho J. The role of gamma/delta T-cell receptor-positive cells in pregnancy: Part II. Am J Reprod Immunol. 1999;42:83-7.

91. van den HM, McBey BA, Hahnel AC, et al. An analysis of the uterine lymphocyte-derived hybridoma cell line GWM 1-2 for expression of receptors for estrogen, progesterone and interleukin 2. J Reprod Immunol. 1996;31:37-50.

92. Polgar B, Kispal G, Lachmann M, et al. Molecular cloning and immunologic characterization of a novel cDNA coding for progesterone-induced blocking factor. J Immunol. 2003;171: 5956-63.

93. Loudon JA, Elliott CL, Hills F, et al. Progesterone represses interleukin-8 and cyclo-oxygenase-2 in human lower segment fibroblast cells and amnion epithelial cells. Biol Reprod. 2003;69:331-7.

94. Meis PJ, Klebanoff M, Thom E, et al. Prevention of recurrent preterm delivery by 17 alpha-hydroxyprogesterone caproate. N Engl J Med. 2003;348:2379-85.

95. Simpson KL, Keelan JA, Mitchell MD. Labor-associated changes in interleukin-10 production and its regulation by immunomodulators in human choriodecidua. J Clin Endocrinol Metab. 1998;83:4332-7.

96. Pellegrini I, Lebrun JJ, Ali S, et al. Expression of prolactin and its receptor in human lymphoid cells. Mol Endocrinol. 1992;6: 1023-8.

97. Gubbay O, Critchley HO, Bowen JM, et al. Prolactin induces ERK phosphorylation in epithelial and CD56(+) natural killer cells of the human endometrium. J Clin Endocrinol Metab. 2002;87:2329-35.

98. Bianchi DW, Zickwolf G, Weil G, et al. Male fetal progenitor cells persist in maternal blood as long as 27 years postpartum. PNAS. 1996;93:705-8.

99. Srivatsa B, Srivatsa S, Johnson KL, et al. Maternal cell microchimerism in newborn tissues. J Pediatr. 2003;142:31-5.

100. O'Donoghue K, Chan J, de la Fuente J. Long-term consequenses of pregnancy: The persistence of fetal cells in maternal organs. J Soc Gynecol Invest. 2004;11:193A.

101. Claas F, Gijbels Y, VanderVelden-DeMunck J, et al. Induction of B cell unresponsiveness to noninherited maternal HLA during fetal life. Science. 1988,241.1815-7.

102. Burlingham W, Grailer A, Heisey D, et al. The effect of tolerance to noninherited maternal HLA on the survival of renal transplants from sibling donors. N Engl J Med. 1998;339:1657-64.

103. van Rood JJ, Loberiza FR Jr, Zhang MJ, et al. Effect of tolerance to noninherited maternal antigens on the occurrence of graft-versus-host disease after bone marrow transplantation from a parent or an HLA-haploidentical sibling. Blood. 2002;99:1572-7.

104. Molitor ML, Haynes LD, Jankowska-Gan E, et al. HLA class I noninherited maternal antigens in cord blood and breast milk. Hum Immunol. 2004;65:231-9.

105. Yoshihara T, Morimoto A, Inukai T, et al. Non-T-cell-depleted HLA haploidentical stem cell transplantation based on fetomaternal microchimerism in pediatric patients with advanced malignancies. Bone Marrow Transplant. 2004;34(4):373-5.

106. Monaco AP. Prospects and strategies for clinical tolerance. Transplant Proc. 2004;36:227-31.

107. Le Bouteiller P, Solier C, Proll J, et al. Placental HLA-G protein expression in vivo: Where and what for? Hum Reprod Update. 1999;5:223-33.

108. Hiby SE, Walker JJ, O'shaughnessy KM, et al. Combinations of maternal KIR and fetal HLA-C genes influence the risk of pre-eclampsia and reproductive success. J Exp Med. 2004;200:957-65.

109. Rogers AM, Boime I, Connolly J, et al. Maternal-fetal tolerance is maintained despite transgenedriven trophoblast expression of MHC class I, and defects in Fas and its ligand. Eur J Immunol. 1998;28:3479-87.

110. Gomez-Lozano N, de Pablo R, Puente S, et al. Recognition of HLA-G by the NK cell receptor KIR2DL4 is not essential for human reproduction. Eur J Immunol. 2003;33:639-44.

111. Chaouat G, Zourbas S, Ostojic S, et al. A brief review of recent data on some cytokine expressions at the materno-foetal interface which might challenge the classical Th1/Th2 dichotomy. J Reprod Immunol. 2002;53:241-56.

CHAPTER

84

Fetal Behavior

JG Nijhuis

INTRODUCTION

For many years, the fetus has been considered to be developing in a relatively safe surrounding. However, this view changed dramatically when the accessibility of the human fetus increased with the introduction of ultrasonography. This was the start of an avalanche into fetal behavioral research.[1] Increasing insight into the developing human fetus made it clear that the growing fetus could only be judged properly if one took gestational age into account, and it also became clear that intrauterine life was not so safe as one had always assumed: "after all, the fetus is but a human being, just as prone as a child or adult to have an accident, a disease or an iatrogenic problem!".[2]

In this chapter, we will review the most important data on fetal behavioral variables and behavioral states, and then discuss the clinical consequences of this knowledge.

BASIC STUDIES

Fetal Heart Rate Patterns

Electronic monitoring of the fetal heart rate in combination with contractions, if present, is used worldwide for the assessment of fetal condition [cardiotocography, (CTG)]. The technique was introduced for intrapartum use by Caldeyro-Barcia et al. in 1966,[3] Hammacher and Werners in 1968[4] and Hon in 1968.[5] In 1969, Kubli et al.[6] also introduced the technique for antepartum use. Although the intra- and interobserver variability is still large, the specificity is such that clinicians rely on the method.[7,8] The sensitivity, however, is rather poor. In general, good bandwidth or beat-to-beat variability in the presence of accelerations is indicative of a good fetal condition; a silent pattern (small bandwidth, no accelerations) is indicative for fetal distress, certainly in the presence of late decelerations. One of the problems is that many scores which were developed to improve the interpretation of the CTG did not take the age of the fetus into account, while Visser et al.[9] had already shown a clear developmental trend during gestation in the amplitude and duration of the accelerations. Timor-Tritsch et al.[10] pointed out that the fetal heart rate pattern (FHRP) was dependent on the fetal behavioral state. In 1982, we defined four different fetal heart rate patterns (FHRP), FHRP A to D respectively, which were then used to define behavioral states in combination with the presence or absence of body and eye movements (Figs 84.1A and B).[11] It was also found that not only the form of the accelerations changed during gestation but also that during gestation the length of silent heart rate patterns (FHRP A) increased, i.e. without any sign of fetal distress.[12,13] More recently, automated antepartum baseline fetal heart rate determination and detection of accelerations and decelerations has been introduced.[14]

Fetal Body Movements

"and the children struggled together within her"

Bible, Genesis 25:22

This is probably one of the first descriptions of fetal movements. In 1976, Reinold[15] was the first to show that the fetus was already moving spontaneously in the first trimester of pregnancy. He also showed that absence of body movements may indicate impending fetal death, while the presence of body movements is very reassuring. With modern ultrasound techniques the very first "fetal activity" that can be observed is fetal heart rate.[16] In 1982, de Vries and associates[17] published their results on the observation of fetal somatic activity in the first half of pregnancy. They introduced a categorization of movement patterns and described how the individual movements were performed in terms of speed, force and amplitude. This work clearly shows that the majority of the repertoire of movements that can be distinguished in the third trimester and after birth are already present at 14 weeks of gestation.[17]

In the second and third trimester much attention has been paid to the presence of gross body movements,[18] but only in the last weeks of pregnancy does the fetus exhibit quite clearly prolonged periods of presence and absence of fetal movements. As gestational age progresses, the periods during which body movements can be absent increase dramatically (Fig. 84.2).

This observation emphasizes again that the fetal age should be taken into account; what is normal in a fetus at 20 weeks may be abnormal in the same fetus at 38 weeks! Over the past decade it has also become clear that counting the number of movements is not very useful; even the mildly hypoxic growth-retarded fetus will still make body movements. It seems to be of much more importance to look at the quality of the movements, the speed and amplitude, etc. De Vries and associates[17,19] started to use the concept of quality in the first trimester and Bekedam and co-workers[20] looked for this aspect in 10 intrauterine growth-retarded fetuses between 29 weeks and 35 weeks.

Fetal Eye Movements

Bots and co-workers[21] published their first observation on fetal eye movements using ultrasound and they recorded them by means of M-mode ultrasonography in 1981. Their findings were confirmed in the same year by Birnholz.[22] The possibility of observing and recording eye movements created a change allowing the study of fetal motility in relation to a new variable. Of course, at this stage fetal and neonatal data appeared to be rather similar. It is, however, not always possible to compare the fetal data with those of the neonate, because in the neonate it is not the eye movements that are used in behavioral studies but rather the criterion "eyes open" or "eyes closed".[23]

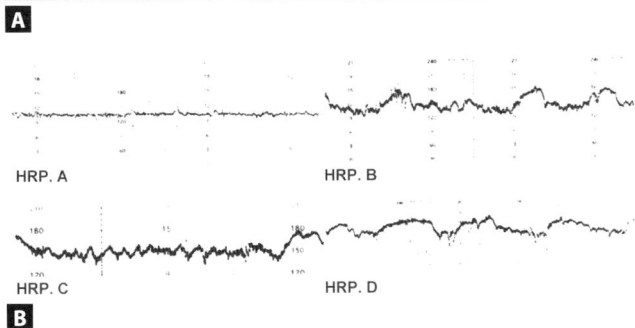

State criteria				
State criteria	State 1F	State 2F	State 1F	State 4F
Body movements	Incidental	Periodic	Absent	Continuous
Eye movements	Absent	Present	Present	Present
Heart rate pattern	A	B	C	D

A

HRP. A HRP. B

HRP. C HRP. D

B

Figs 84.1A and B: (A) Definition of the four behavioral states; (B) Examples given for each of the fetal heart rate patterns (HRP) A–D, at a recording speed of 3 cm/min

Source: Reproduced from van Vliet et al.[12] with permission

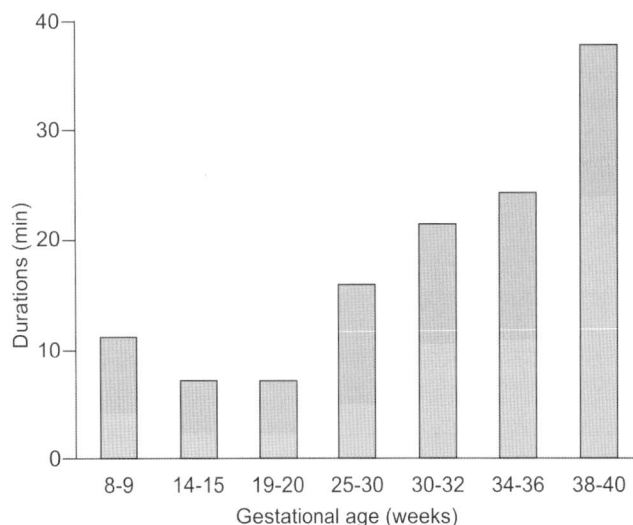

Fig. 84.2: Maximum and median duration (in minutes) of periods in which body movements can be absent at different gestational ages

Fetal Breathing Movements

It was Ahlfeld[24] in Germany who published the first observation of fetal breathing movements in 1888. His observations were almost unanimously neglected until the issue was re-introduced by Dawes and colleagues[25] in 1970 who described breathing movements in fetal lambs, and by Boddy and Robinson[26] in 1971 in the human fetus. Bots and associates[27] published a detailed analysis of human fetal breathing movements and described them as "paradoxic" because the ribcage made an inward movement during "inspiration" when the diaphragm made a downward movement. Originally, it was thought that breathing movements could be used as a perfect indicator for the detection of fetal distress, but soon it became apparent that breathing movements are not continuously present and are influenced by many conditions. A postprandial increase in breathing movements has already been described from 20 weeks to 22 weeks onward,[28] and Nijhuis and co-workers[29] showed an increase after glucose intake by the mother at 24 weeks. Furthermore, smoking diminishes the incidence of fetal breathing and breathing is not only much more likely to be absent during fetal rest periods,[30] but also much more regular.[31,32] During the last weeks of pregnancy, the incidence of fetal breathing decreases and breathing movements are absent during labor.[33] The duration of periods that breathing movements can be absent increases enormously during pregnancy, and near term it is not unusual for breathing movements to be absent for as long as 120 min.[34] In general, for behavioral studies, fetal breathing should not be studied as an independent variable but always in combination with other variables and preferably under highly standardized conditions.

Fetal Mouth Movements

With modern ultrasonographic equipment, the fetal mouth is easy to visualize. Specific mouthing or sucking behaviors can be observed; recurrent clusters of "regular mouthing movements" can be observed during quiet states (state 1F), while during state 3F "sucking movements" can be observed (for an overview, see van Woerden and van Geijn[35]). Both activities, regular mouthing and sucking, are able to entrain a fairly specific heart rate pattern, which may confuse the clinicians.[36,37]

Fetal Behavior

Certainly in the second half of pregnancy the observation of fetal activity can be combined with the simultaneous recording of the fetal heart rate and such a combined recording is then called the registration of "fetal behavior". In the beginning, it is as if all sorts of movements occur more or less independently of one another and they do not elicit specific FHRP. However, with the increase of gestational age, an increasing linkage can be observed between periods with "absence of eye movements", and periods with "absence of movements" and with a silent heart rate pattern, FHRP A.[38] This increasing linkage, which has been noticed by Drogtrop and colleagues[39] at 25–30 weeks and by Visser and associates[40] at 30–32 weeks, is crucial for the development of recognizable behavioral states.

Behavioral States in the Neonate

"Behavioral states are constellations of physiological and behavioral variables (e.g. eyes closed, regular breathing and no movements: quiet sleep) which are stable over time and recur repeatedly, not only in the same infant, but also in similar forms in all infants" (modified from Prechtl and co-workers[23]). In the neonate, Prechtl and co-workers[23] defined five behavioral states: state 1 [quiet sleep, similar to non-rapid eye movement (REM)-sleep], state 2 (active sleep, similar to REM-sleep), state 3 (quiet awake), state 4 (active awake) and state 5 (vocalization). Three major requirements have to be fulfilled before a behavioral state can be recognized. First of all, a specific combination of certain variables must occur at the same time ("coincidence", "linkage"), e.g. presence of body movements, eyes open and irregular breathing for state 2. Second, to be able to recognize this combination, it should be stable over time (by definition at least 3 min). Third, it must be possible to see a clear change from one state into another, a "state transition". If the transitional periods become too long (i.e. longer than 3 min of "no coincidence"), it is no longer possible to clearly distinguish behavioral states.[13]

Fetal Behavioral States

Following the concept of behavioral states in the neonate, Nijhuis and colleagues[11] described four fetal behavioral states. They recorded fetal behavior with two ultrasound scanners and a simultaneous registration of the FHRP. To emphasize the similarity with the neonatal states they were called 1F ("F" for fetal) to 4F, respectively.

State 1F (similar to state 1 in the neonate): Quiescence, which can be regularly interrupted by brief gross body movements, mostly startles. Eye movements are absent. The FHRP A is a stable pattern with a small oscillation bandwidth and no accelerations, except in combination with a startle (Fig. 84.1).

State 2F (similar to state 2 in the neonate): Frequent and periodic gross body movements—mainly stretches and retroflexions—and movements of the extremities. Eye movements are present. FHRP B has a wider oscillation bandwidth and frequent accelerations during movements (Fig. 84.1).

State 3F (similar to state 3 in the neonate): Gross body movements are absent. Eye movements are present. FHRP C is stable but with a wider oscillation bandwidth than FHRP A and no accelerations (Fig. 84.1).

State 4F (similar to state 4 in the neonate): Vigorous, continual activity including many trunk rotations. Eye movements are present. FHRP D is unstable, with large and long-lasting accelerations, often fused into a sustained tachycardia (Fig. 84.1).

After the introduction of the definitions, many other research groups were able to confirm the same findings.[41-43] The introduction of the concept of states had a great influence on the research that was performed in both animal and human research. As an example, it appeared to be the case that breathing movements were largely absent during state 1F,[30] but if they were present they were much more regular.[32] Therefore, to study the influence of a certain stimulus on breathing, it is now clear that such a study needs to be standardized for states. Otherwise one might think that the stimulus used abolishes breathing while, in fact, only a state transition from 2F (with breathing) into 1F (without breathing) has been induced.

Following the description of fetal behavior under normal conditions, many studies have been looking for changes in behavior in growth-retarded fetuses,[20,44,45] fetuses of diabetic mothers[46] and of mothers who used antiepileptic drugs,[47] cocaine,[48] methadone[49] and corticosteroids.[50] For reviews see Richardson,[51] Groome and Watson,[52] Koyanagi and associates,[53] and Romanini and Rizzo.[54] Furthermore, Doppler measurements in several fetal vessels also appeared to be state related, although in compromised fetuses this state dependency plays a minor role.[55]

CLINICAL EXPERIENCES

Studying fetal behavior is very time-consuming. This means that a behavioral study will only be performed, if simpler techniques do not answer the question that is posed. Fetal heart rate monitoring is the most frequently used method, but insight into fetal behavior has had a certain influence on the interpretation of CTGs. The two most important examples are the "silent" heart rate pattern and the "sinusoidal" heart rate pattern. Obviously, a silent FHRP may indicate fetal distress, but it may also reflect a physiological behavioral state 1F. It is therefore of crucial importance that one considers a differential diagnosis if a silent heart rate pattern is recorded (Table 84.1).[56] The most extreme example of a silent heart rate pattern is entrained by the "intrauterine brain death syndrome". In such a case the FHRP is silent over a long period of time, with a somewhat elevated baseline and the fetus does not move (Fig. 84.3). At birth—mostly via a Cesarean section because of "fetal distress"—a floppy infant is born and artificial ventilation will be needed. An electroencephalogram will be isoelectric and a diagnosis of "brain death" will then finally be made.[56,57] This "intrauterine coma" is probably the consequence of a hypoxic accident which is mostly not recorded. Hence, there has been a period of severe asphyxia during which the fetus almost died, but then recovered. In such a situation a cordocentesis would reveal a normal pH value.

We have already mentioned that a fetus makes regular mouthing movements during state 1F,[58] while sucking movements can be seen during 3F.[36,37] Both categories of mouth movements may entrain a "sinusoidal-like" FHRP, a heart rate pattern that can also be recorded in combination with severe fetal anemia. Again, also for this FHRP a differential diagnosis can be made (Table 84.1). We have only made a beginning with the understanding of the human fetus in its natural environment, but these examples make perfectly clear how important it is to be aware of these behavioral states.

Table 84.1: Differential diagnosis and proposed management in silent heart rate pattern and sinusoidal heart rate pattern

Differential diagnosis	Management
Silent heart rate pattern	
State 1F	Extension of recording time
Effect of drugs	Exclusion of use of drugs
Tachycardia	Inspection of baseline
Anomalies	Ultrasonographic examination, behavioral study
Hypoxia	Contraction stress test (CST)
Brain death	Cordocentesis
Sinusoidal heart rate pattern	
Fetal mouth movements	
• Sucking ("major" or "marked")	Behavioral study
• Regular mouthing ("minor")	Behavioral study
Effect of drugs	Exclusion of use of drugs
Congenital anomalies	Ultrasonographic examination
Fetal asphyxia	Biophysical profile testing
Fetal anemia	Cordocentesis

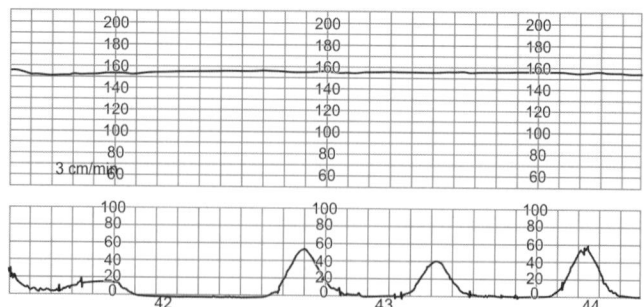

Fig. 84.3: An example of a persistently silent fetal heart rate pattern without decelerations, and absence of fetal activity. Note the relatively high baseline of 155 bpm, this recording indicates fetal brain death

Source: Reproduced with permission from Nijhuis et al.[56]

Another step forward was made by Mulder and co-workers,[50] who showed a clear effect of betamethasone on fetal behavior. This drug, which is used for the stimulation of lung maturation, decreases heart rate variability and the number of movements. Dexamethasone seems to have a similar effect, but to a much lesser degree.[58]

Visser and associates[60] have considered the change of consecutive variables in a deteriorating fetal condition, and proposed that changes in fetal behavior and quality of fetal movements are among the first signs, while a terminal heart rate pattern is of course the final step.

FUTURE CLINICAL ASPECTS

In normal post-term pregnancies, van de Pas and colleagues[61] showed that the fetus continues to mature further, similar to the neonate already born. In the post-term fetus the amount of states 3F and 4F increased significantly at the expense of state 2F, implying that the fetus is more "awake" in utero. If one accepts that the fetus exhibits clear behavioral states, similar to the neonate, then it is perfectly understandable that birth by itself does not seem to alter the developmental pathway of this output of the central nervous system. However, most neonatal tests are not applicable for the fetus. It has already been noticed that fetuses with congenital anomalies may show bizarre behavior[62] or dissociation of heart rate and movements.[63] Other authors have been studying state transitions rather than behavioral states,[64] but still it is difficult to draw conclusions from a single behavioral recording in a single fetus. Perhaps it would be more promising if we could develop a "neurological examination" for the fetus, knowing that we have limited possibilities. A first step has been made by Tas and associates,[65] who were able to evoke an intercostal-to-phrenic inhibitory reflex (IPIR); compression of the ribcage results in apnea. In a second series of experiments, they were not able to find a different result in a group of growth-retarded fetuses, defined as growth below the 10th centile.[66] Another possible approach is the study of fetal habituation, i.e. the fetal learning pattern. A normal fetus will habituate to a certain stimulus which means that

it will cease to respond to repeated exposure to the stimulus. For example, Hepper and Shahidullah[67] demonstrated that fetuses with Down's syndrome take longer to habituate than normal fetuses. Recently, Leader[68] concluded in a commentary "it seems likely that no single, isolated aspect of behavior alone will evolve but rather a combination of behaviors to form a prenatal neurological examination".[68]

CONCLUSION

The study of fetal behavior also plays an important role in the understanding of normal fetal well-being and in the evaluation of the possibly compromised fetus. It has introduced a completely different way of looking at the developing human being. It also has become more apparent that birth by itself is not the major cause for the neonatal neurological morbidity. Morbidity does not, in the majority of cases, originate from a (hypoxic) accident during birth, but rather from a (hypoxic) accident somewhere during gestation, or it may even be genetic. Most of these mild cases will not be detected at birth and may therefore be attributed to a "difficult birth, which is seldom the real cause.[69] It may well be that "difficult birth in itself in certain cases is merely a symptom of deeper effects that influenced the development of the fetus" (Sigmund Freud, 1897).[70]

The study of fetal behavior is still very time-consuming and therefore mostly used in research protocol. In the forthcoming years we should aim at the development of a more appropriate way to analyze fetal behavior because there is a definite need to get a better insight into the condition of the fetus before birth and in particular the condition of the fetal central nervous system. The development of an adequate and practical intrauterine neurological examination should have high priority in clinical perinatology. The fetus can no longer be regarded as a "growing organism" which will react independently of age and state. If one wants to say something about the condition of the fetus or to learn something about its development in its intrauterine environment, then one should start to do so under standardized conditions with respect to fetal age, time of the day, relation to maternal meals, etc. and last but not least certainly in the last trimester one should be aware of fetal behavioral states.

REFERENCES

1. Nijhuis JG (Ed). Fetal Behaviour, Developmental and Perinatal Aspects. Oxford: Oxford University Press; 1992.
2. Nijhuis JG. Physiological and clinical consequences in relation to the development of fetal behavior and fetal behavioral states. In: Krasnegor NA, Lecanuet P, Fifer WP (Eds). Fetal Development: A Psychobiological Perspective. New Jersey: Lawrence Erlbaum; 1995. pp. 67-82.
3. Caldeyro-Barcia R, Mendez-Bauer C, Poseiro JJ, et al. Control of human fetal heart rate during labor. In: Cassels DE (Ed). The Heart Rate and Circulation in the Newborn and Infant. New York: Grune and Stratton; 1966. pp. 122-8.
4. Hammacher K, Werners PH. Über die Auswertung und Dokumentation von CTG-Ergebnissen. Gynaecologia. 1968;166:410-23.
5. Hon EH. An Atlas of Fetal Heart Rate Patterns. New Haven: Harty Press Inc; 1968.
6. Kubli FW, Kaeser O, Hinselmann M. Diagnostic management of chronic placental insufficiency. In: Pecile A, Finzi C (Eds). The Foetoplacental Unit. Amsterdam: Excerpta Medica Foundation; 1969. pp. 323-39.

7. Trimbos JB, Keirse MJ. Observer variability in assessment of antepartum cardiotocograms. Br J Obstet Gynaecol. 1978;85:900-6.
8. Lotgering FK, Wallenburg HC, Schouten HJ. Interobserver and intraobserver variation in the assessment of antepartum cardiotocograms. Am J Obstet Gynecol. 1982;144:701-5.
9. Visser GH, Dawes GS, Redman CW. Numerical analysis of the normal human antenatal fetal heart rate. Br J Obstet Gynaecol. 1981;88:792-802.
10. Timor-Tritsch IE, Dierker LJ, Hertz RH, et al. Studies of antepartum behavioural states in the human fetus at term. Am J Obstet Gynecol. 1979;132:524-8.
11. Nijhuis JG, Bots RS, Martin CB Jr, et al. Are there behavioural states in the human fetus? Early Hum Dev. 1982;6:177-95.
12. van Vliet MA, Martin CB, Nijhuis JG, et al. The relationship between fetal activity and behavioral states and fetal breathing movements in normal and growth-retarded fetuses. Am J Obstet Gynecol. 1985;153:582-8.

13. Nijhuis JG, Martin CB Jr, Prechtl HF. Behavioural states of the human fetus. In: Prechtl HF (Ed). Continuity of Neural Functions from Prenatal to Postnatal Life. Clinics in Developmental Medicine. Oxford: Blackwell Scientific Publications Ltd; 1984. pp. 65-79.

14. Mantel R, Ververs I, Colenbrander G, et al. Automated antepartum baseline FHR determination and detection of accelerations and decelerations. In: Van Geijn HP, Copray FJA (Eds). A Critical Appraisal of Fetal Surveillance. Amsterdam: Elsevier Science BV; 1994. pp. 333-48.

15. Reinold E. Beobachtung fetaler Aktivität in der ersten Hälfte der Gravidität mit dem Ultraschall. Pädiatr Pädol. 1976;6:274-9.

16. van Heeswijk M, Nijhuis JG, Hollanders JM. Fetal heart rate in early pregnancy. Early Hum Dev. 1990;22:151-6.

17. de Vries JIP, Visser GH, Prechtl HF. The emergence of fetal behaviour. I. Qualitative aspects. Early Hum Dev. 1982;7:301-22.

18. Visser GH. The second trimester. In: Nijhuis JG (Ed). Fetal Behaviour, Developmental and Perinatal Aspects. Oxford: Oxford University Press; 1992. pp. 17-26.

19. de Vries JI, Visser GH, Prechtl HF. The emergence of fetal behaviour. II. Quantitative aspects. Early Hum Dev. 1985;12:99-120.

20. Bekedam DJ, Visser GH, de Vries JJ, et al. Motor behaviour in the growth-retarded fetus. Early Hum Dev. 1985;12:155-65.

21. Bots RS, Nijhuis JG, Martin CB Jr, et al. Human fetal eye movements: Detection in utero by ultrasonography. Early Hum Dev. 1981;5:87-94.

22. Birnholz JC. The development of human fetal eye movement patterns. Science. 1981;213:679-81.

23. Prechtl HF, Weinmann HM, Akiyama Y. Organization of physiological parameters in normal and neurologically abnormal infants. Neuropädiatrie. 1969;1:101-29.

24. Ahlfeld F. Ueber intrauterine Athembewegungen des Kindes. Ver Dsch Ges Gynäk. 1888;2:203-10. Kurjak-88.qxd 12/22/2005 6:29 PM Page 953.

25. Dawes GS, Leduc HE, Liggins GC, et al. Respiratory movements and paradoxal sleep in the foetal lamb. J Physiol. 1970;210:47-8.

26. Boddy K, Robinson JS. External method for detection of fetal breathing in utero. Lancet. 1971;2:1231-3.

27. Bots RS, Broeders GH, Farman DJ, et al. Fetal breathing movements in the normal and growth-retarded fetus: A multiscan/M-mode echofetographic study. Eur J Obstet Gynecol Reprod Biol. 1978;8:21-9.

28. de Vries JI, Visser GH, Mulder EJ, et al. Diurnal and other variations in fetal movement, and heart rate patterns at 20-22 weeks. Early Hum Dev. 1987;15:333-48.

29. Nijhuis JG, Jongsma HW, Crijns IJ, et al. Effects of maternal glucose ingestion on human fetal breathing movements at weeks 24, and 28 of gestation. Early Hum Dev. 1986;13:183-8.

30. van Vliet MA, Martin CB Jr, Nijhuis JG, et al. The relationship between fetal activity, and behavioural states and fetal breathing movements in normal and growth-retarded fetuses. Am J Obstet Gynecol. 1985;153:582-8.

31. Timor-Tritsch IE, Dierker LJ, Hertz RH, et al. Regular and irregular human fetal respiratory movements. Early Hum Dev. 1980;4:315-24.

32. Nijhuis JG, Martin CB Jr, Gommers S, et al. The rhythmicity of fetal breathing varies with behavioural state in the human fetus. Early Hum Dev. 1983;9:1-7.

33. Carmichael L, Campbell K, Patrick J. Fetal breathing, gross fetal body movements, and maternal and fetal heart rates before spontaneous labor at term. Am J Obstet Gynecol. 1984;148:675-9.

34. Patrick J, Campbell K, Carmichael L, et al. Patterns of human fetal breathing during the last 10 weeks of pregnancy. Obstet Gynecol. 1980;56:24-30.

35. van Woerden EE, van Geijn HP. Heart-rate patterns and fetal movements. In: Nijhuis JG (Ed). Fetal Behaviour, Developmental and Perinatal Aspects. Oxford: Oxford University Press; 1988. pp. 41-56.

36. Nijhuis JG, Staisch KJ, Martin CB Jr, et al. A sinusoidal-like fetal heart-rate pattern in association with fetal sucking - Report of 2 cases. Eur J Obstet Gynecol Reprod Biol. 1984;16:353-8.

37. van Woerden EE, van Geijn HP, Caron FJ, et al. Fetal mouse movements during behavioural states 1F and 2F. Eur J Obstet Gynecol Reprod Biol. 1988;29:97-105.

38. Nijhuis JG, van de Pas M. Behavioural states and their ontogeny: Human studies. Semin Perinatol. 1992;16:206-10.

39. Drogtrop AP, Ubels R, Nijhuis JG. The association between fetal body movements, eye movements, and heart rate patterns between 25 and 30 weeks of gestation. Early Hum Dev. 1990;23:67-73.

40. Visser GH, Poelman-Weesjes G, Cohen TM. Fetal behaviour at 30 to 32 weeks of gestation. Pediatr Res. 1987;22:655-8.

41. van Vliet MA, Martin CB Jr, Nijhuis JG, et al. Behavioural states in fetuses of nulliparous women. Early Hum Dev. 1985;12:121-35.

42. van Woerden EE, van Geijn HP, Caron FJ, et al. Automated assignment of fetal behavioural states near term. Early Hum Dev. 1989;19:137-46.

43. Arduini D, Rizzo G, Giorlandino C, et al. The fetal behavioural states: An ultrasonic study. Prenat Diagn. 1985;5:269-76.

44. van Vliet MA, Martin CB Jr, Nijhuis JG, et al. Behavioural states in growth retarded human fetuses. Early Hum Dev. 1985;12:183-97.

45. Arduini D, Rizzo G, Romanini C. Growth retardation. In: Nijhuis JG (Ed). Fetal Behaviour, Developmental and Perinatal Aspects. Oxford: Oxford University Press; 1992. pp. 181-208.

46. Mulder EJ, Leiblum DM, Visser GH. Fetal breathing movements in late diabetic pregnancy: Relationship to fetal heart rate patterns and Braxton Hicks' contractions. Early Hum Dev. 1995;43:225-32.

47. van Geijn HP, Swartjes JM, van Woerden EE, et al. Fetal behavioural states in epileptic pregnancies. Eur J Obstet Gynecol Reprod Biol. 1986;21:309-14.

48. Hume RF Jr, O'Donnell KJ, Stanger CI, et al. In utero cocaine exposure: Observations of fetal behavioural state may predict neonatal outcome. Am J Obstet Gynecol. 1989;161:685-90.

49. Archie CL, Milton IL, Sokol RJ, et al. The effects of methadone treatment on the reactivity of the nonstress test. Obstet Gynecol. 1989;74:254-5.

50. Mulder EJ, Derks JB, Zonneveld MF, et al. Transient reduction in fetal activity and heart rate variation after maternal betamethasone administration. Early Hum Dev. 1994;36:49-60.

51. Richardson BS. Fetal behavioural states. Semin Perinatol. 1992;16:4.

52. Groome LJ, Watson JE. Assessment of in utero neurobehavioural development. I. Fetal behavioural states. J Matern Fetal Invest. 1992;2:183-94.

53. Koyanagi T, Nabekura J, Nakano H. Brain function in utero unique to the developing fetus. Fetal Matern Med Rev. 1995;7:129-41.

54. Romanini C, Rizzo G. Fetal behaviour in normal and compromised fetuses. An overview. Early Hum Dev. 1995;43:117-31.

55. van Eyck J, Wladimiroff JW. Doppler flow measurements. In: Nijhuis JG (Ed). Fetal Behaviour, Developmental and Perinatal Aspects. Oxford: Oxford University Press; 1992. pp. 227-41.

56. Nijhuis JG, Crevels AJ, van Dongen PW. Fetal brain death: The definition of a fetal heart rate pattern and its clinical consequences. Obstet Gynecol Surv. 1990;46:229-32.

57. Nijhuis JG, Kruyt N, van Wijck JA. Fetal brain death. Two case reports. Br J Obstet Gynaecol. 1988;95:197-200.

58. van Woerden EE, van Geijn HP, Swartjes JM, et al. Fetal heart rhythms during behavioural state 1F. Eur J Obstet Gynecol Reprod Biol. 1988;28:29-38.

59. Mulder EJ, Derks JB, Visser GH. Antenatal corticosteroid therapy and fetal behaviour: A randomized study of the effects of betamethasone and dexamethasone. Br J Obstet Gynaecol. 1997;104:1239-48.

60. Visser GH, Ribbert LS, Bekedam DJ. Sequential changes in Doppler waveform, fetal heart rate and movements patterns in IUGR fetuses. In: Van Geijn HP, Copray FJ (Eds). A Critical Appraisal of Fetal Surveillance. Amsterdam: Elsevier Science; 1994. pp. 193-200.

61. van de Pas M, Nijhuis JG, Jongsma HW. Fetal behaviour in uncomplicated pregnancies after 41 weeks of gestation. Early Hum Dev. 1994;40:29-38.

62. Pillai M, Garrett C, James D. Bizarre fetal behaviour associated with lethal congenital anomalies: A case report. Eur J Obstet Gynecol Reprod Biol. 1991;39:215-18.

63. Tas BA, Nijhuis JG. Consequences for fetal monitoring. In: Nijhuis JG (Ed). Fetal Behaviour, Developmental and Perinatal Aspects. Oxford: Oxford University Press; 1992. pp. 258-69.

64. Arduini D, Rizzo G, Massacesi M, et al. Longitudinal assessment of behavioural transitions in healthy fetuses during the last trimester of pregnancy. J Perinat Med. 1991;1:67-72.

65. Tas BA, Nijhuis JG, Lucas AJ. The intercostal-to-phrenic inhibitory reflex in the human fetus near term. Early Hum Dev. 1990;22:145-9.

66. Tas BA, Nijhuis JG, Nelen W, et al. The intercostal-to-phrenic inhibitory reflex in normal and intra-uterine growth-retarded (IUGR) human fetuses from 26 to 40 weeks of gestation. Early Hum Dev. 1993,32.177-82.

67. Hepper P, Shahidullah S. Abnormal fetal behaviour in Down's syndrome fetuses. Q J Clin Psychol. 1992;44B:305-17.

68. Leader LR. Studies in fetal behaviour. Br J Obstet Gynaecol. 1995;102:595-7.

69. Nelson KB, Ellenberg JH. Intrapartum events and cerebral palsy. In: Kubli (Eds). Prenatal Events and Brain Damage in Surviving Children. Heidelberg: Springer-Verlag; 1988. pp. 139-48.

70. Freud S. Die infantile Cerebrallähmung. In: Nothnagel H (Ed). Specielle Pathologie und Therapie. Vienna: Holder; 1897. pp. 1-327.

85

Fetal and Neonatal Hearing

B Arabin, HLM van Straaten

INTRODUCTION

The phenomenon that the sensory development of the prenate is a quiet process of gradually responding to the extrauterine world has been anticipated by mythological and religious stories, artists, writers and many philosophers since ancient times.[1] Aristotle argued that the individual first acquires sensation during pregnancy and might experience the extrauterine environment. However, doubts remained about prenatal sensory capabilities. Jean Jacques Rousseau referred to the fetus as a "witless tadpole" and even the first scientific approaches by Preyer[2] in 1885 led to doubtful conclusions about fetal hearing capacities.

Hearing is one of the primary modalities of human beings for communicating and prerequisite for the development of language. Serious efforts to explore prenatal recognition began in the 1920s and 1930s. Peiper[3] performed sonic stimulation with the aid of a car horn to study movement responses of the fetus. Forbes and Forbes[4] were able to acknowledge the amodal link between movement and sound by stimulating a pregnant mother lying in a water bath which was struck with a metal object. Ray[5] attempted to measure fetal reactions to the smacking of two boards together. All these authors reported habituation responses following the stimulus presentations.

Habituation and conditioning became more focal as researchers attempted to tighten scientific controls for analysis. Sontag and Wallace[6] attempted to experiment involved variables orientated to a stimulus-response method by measuring physical responses toward external stimuli. It became obvious that auditory maturation does not solely function in isolation but is part of an integrated development. The hypothesis was put forward that intrauterine conditioning accounts for certain behavioral characteristics of the newborn and the refractory times of the habituation—dehabituation processes were studied.[7] Fetal movement (FM) responses to sound stimulation were observed as one major focus for fetal conditioning.[8-10] New methods of perinatal medicine such as Doppler registration of fetal heart rate (FHR) and FM, as well as ultrasound, became extremely helpful to objectify fetal responses to external stimuli.

The unborn is involved in a perceptual world with increasing specification and differentiation. During the first trimester self-generated movements are combined with somatosensory awareness resulting in coordination of early FM patterns. Later sensory challenges may derive from two environments. The "intrauterine world" includes the emotional state and daily rhythms of the mother, touch with the umbilical cord, the uterine wall and acoustic stimuli caused by maternal circulation, digestion, movements, breathing and, finally, with increased numbers and greater control of her voice. As birth approaches, stimuli from the "extrauterine world" are increasingly responded to. Neurological development allowing preparatory interaction involves a considerable number of genetic actions, which might be autoregulatory as well as activated or inhibited by positive- or negative-feedback mechanisms.

Different disciplines have therefore become interested in the field of prenatal maturation of the auditory system such as embryology, genetics, neurophysiology, psychoanalysis and developmental psychology. Since pregnant mothers and most of the current methods used to register immediate responses are in the hands of obstetricians, research and clinical investigations in perinatal medicine have been directed toward this field.

EMBRYOLOGY AND DEVELOPMENTAL ANATOMY

The special status of the ear is supported by the observation that the ossicles in the middle ear are of adult size by 8 months of gestation,[11] and thus the only bones to attain their final form in the prenatal period.[12] Conventionally, the ear is described in terms of the outer, middle and inner ear. Knowledge about the complex development of the ear helps in understanding its integrated function and disturbances of the auditory system.[13-28]

External Ear and Tympanic Membrane

The external ear is divided into the pinna and the external auditory canal. From 4 weeks of gestation onward the mesoderm from the first and second branchial arch gives rise to six outgrowths, the hillocks of His, condensing by 12 weeks to form the pinna. From 10 weeks onward the future ear can be visualized (Fig. 85.1). The external auditory canal develops from the first branchial groove. At 8 weeks, the cavum conchae deepens, growing toward the middle ear which can be demonstrated by ultrasound in advanced pregnancy (Figs 85.2A and B). Adult size of the external auditory canal is reached only by 9 years of age.

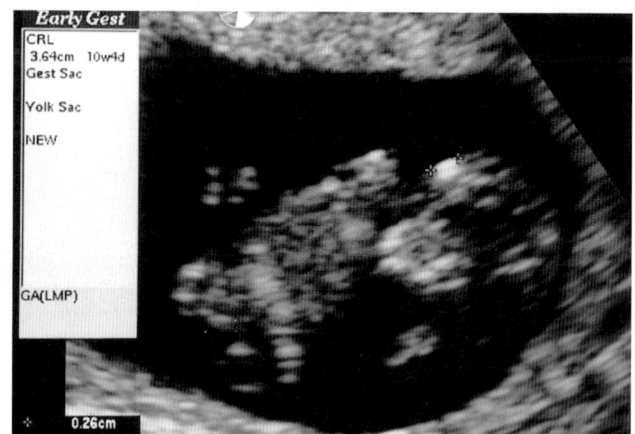

Fig. 85.1: Embryo of 10 weeks with a crown-rump length of 36 mm and an "ear length" of 2.6 mm

The tympanic membrane develops from structures associated with both the external and the middle ear. The completed tympanic membrane has three layers: an outer epithelial layer, a middle fibrous layer and an inner mucosal layer, continuous with the lining of the tympanic cavity. The tympanic membrane inserts into the tympanic ring which is complete at 16 weeks, and can be visualized by ultrasound at the end of the external auditory canal (Figs 85.2A and B). The maximal diameter is of adult size in the term fetus.

Middle Ear, Temporal Bone and Facial Nerve

The middle ear consists of the tympanic cavity, three ossicles (malleus, incus and stapes), the tensor tympani and the stapedius, tendons and the Eustachian tube.

The ossicles develop between 4 and 6 gestational weeks from the mesenchyme of the mandibular and the hyoid arches; full size is reached by 18 weeks. Only then do they become ossified and might be visualized located cranially of the mandible (Figs 85.3A and B). Extension of the first and second pharyngeal pouch, lined with endoderm, forms the tubotympanic recess. At week 7, constriction of the midportion leads to the formation of the Eustachian tube and the tympanic cavity. During further development, the tympanic cavity is filled with mucoid mesenchymal tissue becoming vacuolated. By 30–34 weeks the tympanic cavity is pneumatized.

The temporal bone derives from four separate elements: the tympanic bone, the squamous portion, the styloid process and the petromastoid. Only the first three parts have formed and ossified at birth. Postnatally, there is still no complete bony ear canal and no mastoid process. The facial nerve derives from the second branchial arch. At the end of the third gestational week the acousticofacial ganglion can be identified; by the end of the embryonic period its neuroblasts form the main trunk of the facial nerve and the chorda tympani nerve. The fully developed facial nerve transverses the internal acoustic meatus, the middle ear and, finally, exits superficially from the stylomastoid behind the tympanic membrane, where it can be injured by obstetric manipulations.

Inner Ear and Auditory Nerve

The inner ear lies in the petrous portion of the temporal bone consisting of a membranous labyrinth inside a bony labyrinth. The bony labyrinth includes the cochlea, three semicircular canals, the vestibule enclosing the utricle, the saccule and part of the cochlear duct, as well as the perilymphatic spaces. Development of the bony labyrinth occurs in three stages: cartilage formation, the formation of the perilymphatic spaces, the calcification and ossification. By 24 weeks, all centers have fused to form a complete bony capsule. Ossification of the inner ear does not occur until each portion has

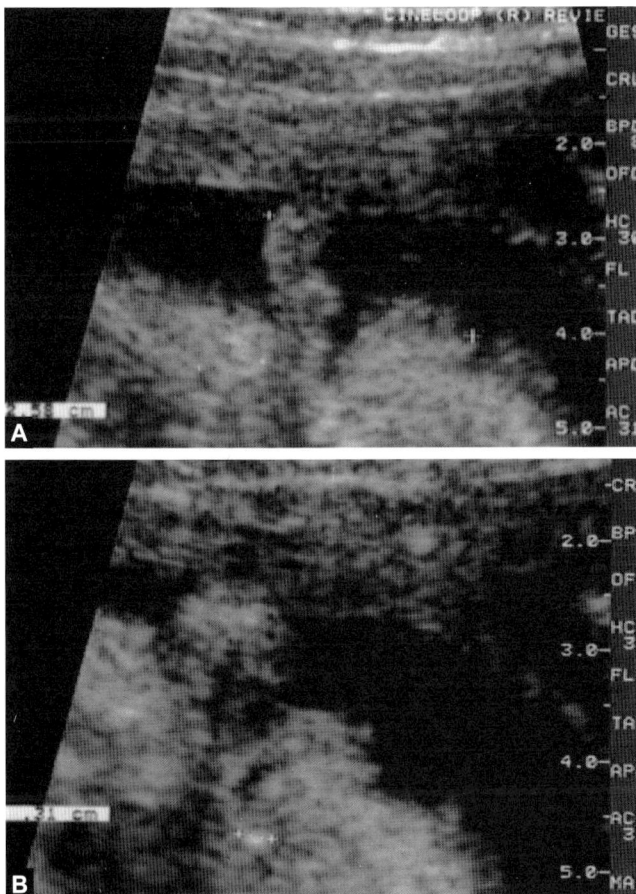

Figs 85.2A and B: (A) Pinna of a fetal ear at 34 weeks (2.6 cm) with external auditory canal. (B) The same external auditory canal obtained by scanning toward the midline with the tympanic membrane (ring) at the central end of 31 mm

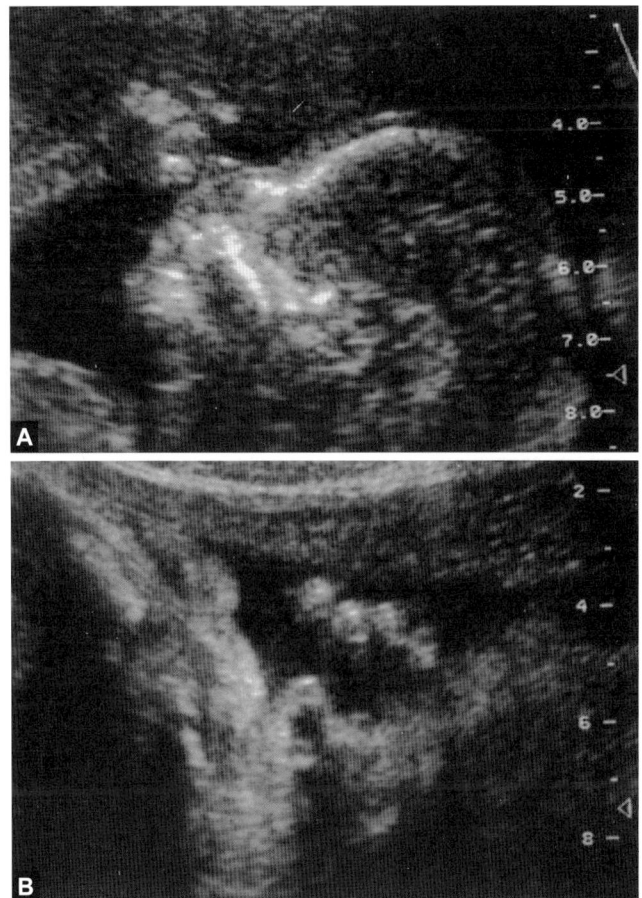

Figs 89.3A and B: (A) Sagittal view of a fetus. Note the three ossicles superior of the mandible in front of the pinna. (B) Frontal view of a fetus "attempting to listen", in spite of amniotic fluid in the outer ear canal, sound attenuation and internal background noise

attained adult size. The configuration of the membranous labyrinth is recognizable by 10 weeks and completed at around 24 weeks. Its neurosensory elements develop from the ectodermal otic placode in the 23-day-old human embryo giving rise to the otocyst. The differentiation of the vestibular and cochlear end organs takes place during the second month of pregnancy.

Light microscopy demonstrates that the first sign of differentiation of the organ of Corti in the wall of the cochlear duct starts at 10 gestational weeks. At 14 weeks, rows of inner and outer hair cells can be observed. At around 20 weeks, the human cochlear morphology is similar to what is considered the stage corresponding to the onset of cochlear function. The organ of Corti contains sensory and supporting cells. Ultrastructural development includes hair cell differentiation of inner and outer hair cells, synaptogenesis and ciliogenesis.

The eighth nerve ganglion also derives from the otocyst. After 4 weeks these cells form the auditory ganglion, dividing later into superior and inferior branches of the vestibular nerve and the cochlear nerve. The nerve cells remain bipolar throughout life, the peripheral processes terminating in the sensory areas of the inner ear and the central processes in the brainstem.

Auditory Pathways

In the auditory system the second neuron is the brainstem. Structures in the human auditory pathway, from the proximal end of the cochlear nerve to the inferior colliculus, undergo myelination between 26 and 29 gestational weeks. The density of myelination increases in all pathways up to 1 year of age. Though code transmission is improved in myelinated pathways, myelination is not prerequisite for transmission. Primary and secondary crossed and uncrossed pathways ensure that each ear is represented on both sides of the brain.

In mammals, the pathway proceeds to the auditory center in the cerebral cortex. The auditory pathway in human beings transforms the code represented by a mechanical response of the ear into a signal which can be utilized by higher centers. The codes are changed from level to level. Through maturation infants develop an information-processing capacity, the development of which has not yet been sufficiently studied. This knowledge, however, is essential for understanding how speech and language develop, and may have implications concerning auditory behavior, reaction to sound and diagnostic testing.

PHYSIOLOGICAL BASIS OF HEARING, ENCODING AND TRANSMISSION

Sound is created by a vibratory source that causes molecules to be displaced. It is designed for gaseous and liquid media, while oscillation in solids is mostly referred to as vibration. The quantification of sound requires measurement of the amplitude and the frequency. The amplitude is measured in units of sound pressure called pascals (Pa) proportional to the acoustic intensity or loudness. The measurement of sound pressure levels is given in decibels (dB), which are logarithmic numbers favored due to the inherent compression of the linear scales. The frequency of sound is measured in cycles/s, namely Hertz (Hz). The range of 20–20,000 Hz is accepted as the bandwidth of human hearing. Beyond these limits high sound pressure levels are required to evoke auditory

responses and there is also decreased discrimination ability. Frequency and magnitude components of sound form what is called spectrum analysis.

Physiological Acoustics

Knowledge of physiological acoustics can be obtained from selected references,[29-34] whereby most information is drawn from invasive recordings in nonhuman species.

The overall role of the outer ear is to collect sound energy and to shape it by the resonances of the concha and the external auditory canal toward the tympanic membrane. Acoustic energy is transformed into mechanical energy as vibrations of the tympanic membrane and the ossicular chain in the middle ear air, providing an energy gain of around 30 dB due to area differences between the tympanic membrane and the footplate of the stapes. The middle ear also protects the inner ear from high sound pressures.

The role of the cochlea and structures of the inner ear is to couple the vibratory energy delivered to the oval window by the stapes footplate to the hair cells. It was postulated in 1965 by Davis[35] that the binding of the sensory hairs of the organ of Corti depolarizes the hair-cell membrane by altering its resistance. The basis of the frequency-related regional displacement of the entire cochlear partition was revealed by the classic Nobel laureate von Bekesy[36] who described it as "traveling waves"; this was verified later by sophisticated methods.[37] The links between hair-cell receptors and the auditory system are primary auditory neurons with selective sensitivities for frequencies. With the entry of the acoustic nerve into the brainstem auditory neurons multiply. The frequency-to-place code is equally representative for the organization of central nuclei and the auditory cortex.[38,39] Many auditory abilities are attributable to subcortical processing. Decorticated animals are capable of detecting the intensity and frequency of sounds;[40-42] anencephalic fetuses demonstrate behavioral reactions to external stimuli (Fig. 85.4). Central neurons are sensitive to frequency modulation and sound features.[43] An efferent auditory pathway varies the input sensitivity at the level of the hair cells.[44]

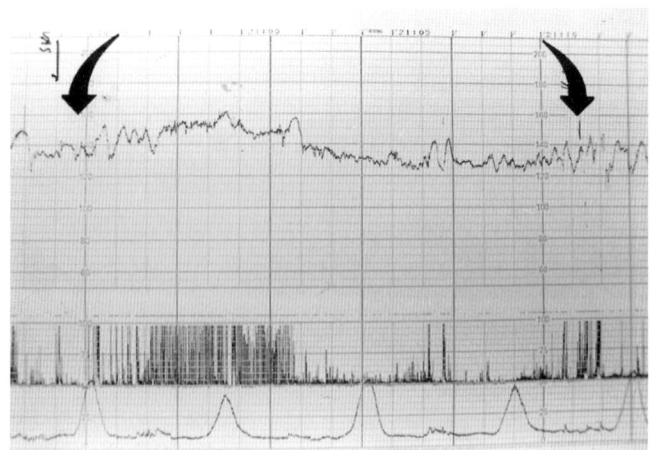

Fig. 85.4: Fetal heart rate (FHR, above)/fetal movement (FM, below) tracing after vibroacoustic stimulation in an anencephalic fetus of 34 weeks. There is a long reaction (>60s) with increased FM and FHR after the first stimulation (first arrow) and a weaker reaction after the second stimulation (second arrow)

Special Conditions Relating to the Fetus

Although perinatologists can occasionally observe gestures familiar from adult life, intrauterine hearing conditions are specific for the prenate. Information on fetal hearing has been obtained from invasive experiments on sheep or measurements in pregnancies with ruptured membranes.

Sound Conduction

Vibrational direct excitation of skin and tissue is more effective for developing an acoustic field than transmission across the air-skin interface.[45,46] The external auditory canal and the fetal middle ear are filled with amniotic fluid; the interface at the stapes footplate is a fluid medium prenatally as compared to an air medium postnatally. Sound pressures with the same phase are present at the two windows, which may reduce hair-cell activity. On the other hand, impedance similarities may cause pressure variations to be fairly well transformed.[47]

A bone conduction route is assumed for prenatal hearing based on measurements with round-window electrodes implanted after open fetal surgery in sheep. Cochlear microphonic recordings were registered toward broadband noise delivered by a loudspeaker and compared to input/output functions in the same lamb after delivery.[48] Sound energy is slightly diminished (10–20 dB) for frequencies < 250 Hz, yet significantly reduced for frequencies > 500 Hz (40–50 dB).[48,49] One reason for this "sound isolation" is the route of sound energy "underwater", described by bone conduction for adult and fetus.[50,51]

The effectiveness of sound transmission (outer and middle ear versus bone transmission) was tested by sheep experiments, proving that when the fetal head is covered with sound attenuating material, even though the pinna and the ear canal remain uncovered, sound levels must be greater than those necessary to evoke the same response from the bare head.[51] Both cochleae are equally stimulated, so that only one auditory image is likely to be formed.[52,53] This might have implications for lateralization in speech development.[54]

Sound Attenuation

A second reason for sound isolation is the sound pressure attenuation described for externally delivered pure tones.[55] A loudspeaker in a rubber annulus was attached to the maternal abdomen, a microphone placed in utero near the cervix. Transmission losses ranged from 39 dB at 500 Hz to 85 dB at 5,000 Hz,[56] and were 70 dB for frequencies above 2,000 Hz.[57] Since an impedance mismatch may bias the results, hydrophones (underwater microphones) were used in humans[58,59] and animals.[46,60-63]

It was shown that the mother's voice in the sheep uterus is louder when picked up by a hydrophone than by a microphone placed by the abdominal wall[62] and that sound attenuation decreases during the last weeks of gestation.[61,62] Further results were obtained by placing a pregnant ewe in a sound field produced by stereo speakers[46,63] recording simultaneous measurements with a microphone in the air and a hydrophone within the uterine cavity. There was sound enhancement of broadband noises in utero for frequencies below 250 Hz; transmission loss increased to an average of 20 dB at 4 kHz. The overall transmission loss was 6.7 dB for broadband noise, and 10–15 dB for pure tone at 1–10 kHz. In humans, exterior sound of at least 65–70 dB was transmitted to the intrauterine cavity with attenuation of 30 dB reduction in sound pressure levels for tones up to 12 kHz; frequencies below 200 Hz were enhanced.[58,59] All in all the results of hydrophone experiments were comparable in sheep and humans.

Sound Environment

The sound environment in utero might have an "imprinting" and a masking effect on external sounds as studied in humans[55,57-60,64,65] and in sheep.[61,62] Measurements in sheep have demonstrated that the basal noise is increased during labor.[62] Data in humans, all gathered after rupture of membranes, might underestimate the emergence of external sounds or overestimate background noise described as pulsations of uterine vessels,[66] intervillous injections,[67] or sounds associated with digestion,[68] maternal body movements and with the mother's breath and voice (see below). The intrauterine sound environment is dominated by frequencies below 500 Hz with mean sound pressures of 90 dB at 250 Hz.[58,59]

Sound Intelligibility

Intelligibility is based on the ability to distinguish complex sounds and thereby provide speech communication and musical abilities. The auditory sensitivity and prenatal sound attenuation characteristics are similar in sheeps and humans.[60,68-70] Language signals are comparable[50] as proven by simultaneous recordings from microphone, fetal cochlear microphone and intrauterine hydrophone recordings in sheep. Music and voices are distinguishable from the basal noise by 8–12 dB for exterior voices and 24 dB for the mother's voice, if all had an intensity of 60 dB. The male voice with an average frequency of 125 Hz is better transmitted, but emerges in the range where internal noise is highest. Female voices with an average frequency of 220 Hz receive a greater attenuation, but emerge in a range where internal noise is low.[58]

The fetus might detect speech and music, ideally low-frequency components below 500 Hz, when the airborne signals exceed 60 dB. Intrauterine sound levels of the mother's voice were enhanced by an average of 5.2 dB. Differences are not dependent on maternal abdominal-wall thickness or amniotic-fluid volume.[69] Intelligibility of directly transmitted maternal voice compared to airborne maternal, female or male voices did not differ if tapes from intrauterine devices were offered to adult observers.[47] While consonants are indistinguishable, vowel sounds, rhythms and melodic timbre of voices are recognizable. Though attenuation varies with frequency, a variety of music is easily recognized from intrauterine recordings.[64,71]

PRENATAL AUDITORY RESPONSIVENESS UNDER NORMAL CONDITIONS

To demonstrate the existence of prenatal sensory perception, one can empirically study electrophysiological, motor and cardiac auditory responsiveness.

Studies of fetal response to sound have chosen a variety of stimuli not always with apparent rationale such as car horns,[3] bicycle bells,[64] electric toothbrushes,[72] or pure tones of 100–2,000 Hz, sound pressure levels from 80 dB to 120 dB measured in air and with various durations.[73] Studies using airborne sounds should be differentiated from studies using vibroacoustic stimuli providing vibration and airborne sound. More recent studies have used the electronic artificial larynx with a vibrating disc attached to the maternal abdomen. It is portable and designed to propagate sound pressure more efficiently, matching impedances between tissue and fluid. The electronic artificial larynx output spectrum was measured by hydrophone fixed near to a lamb's ear in utero.[46] Most frequencies were between 0.5 kHz and 1 kHz with multiple harmonics up to 15,000 Hz in air. When the device was placed directly over the hydrophone, sound pressure levels averaged 135 dB, which was greater than predicted in humans.[65,74] In lambs with bilateral cochlear ablation no reactions toward vibroacoustic stimulation could be registered even with high intensities, indicating that in fetal sheep the auditory apparatus is necessary for the FHR and FM responses.[75]

Prenatal Responsiveness by Means of Electrophysiological Methods

Recordings of electrical potentials from levels of the auditory system by means of noninvasive techniques are based on compound potentials representing the activity of many cells. Noninvasive method to investigate the effects of early auditory stimulations are the stimulus-related electroencephalographic (EEG) and magnetoencephographic (MEG) methods. Human EEG responses toward acoustic signals[76-78] have been performed, with one exception,[77] only after ruptured membranes using scalp electrodes.[76,78]

In MEG recordings, sensitive magnetic-field detectors are used to measure neuromagnetic auditory brainstem responses, which can be performed prenatally with intact membranes.[79,80] Short auditory stimuli like clicks of 1 kHz and a duration of 100 ms up to 100 dB are performed, in a room guaranteeing electrical radiofrequency shielding, to evoke the activity of electromagnetic sources located in nuclei of the brainstem. In an experimental setting, we succeeded in recording stimulus-related auditory-evoked neuromagnetic fields through the mother's abdomen at 34 weeks by using a one-channel superconducting quantum interference device (SQUID) magnetometer (Fig. 85.5).[79,80] The tracings were comparable with postnatal recordings. Latency shifts of brainstem components are proposed to reflect early brain maturation[81] and decrease with advancing age. Although electromagnetic methods are more precise than indirect methods in reflecting the occurrence and latency of reactions, at this moment, the methods are not yet sufficiently developed to allow systematic conclusions to be drawn.

Prenatal Behavioral Responsiveness

The association of evoked potentials with heartbeat and motor responses implies the reception of the auditory signals up to subcortical levels (Fig. 85.4).[82] Due to the present lack of routine technology to record neural activity directly in the womb, fetal sensory abilities are examined by observing behavioral reactions. Appropriate methodology has to be used to ensure that stimulus and response are correlated. Problems arise when the fetus does not react, since we cannot say that the stimulus is not sensed.

Onset of Responsiveness

Relating to the onset of immediate fetal responses it was supposed that reactions toward acoustic stimuli do not occur before 24 weeks.[74,83] Using ultrasound, blink responses were first detectable between 24 weeks and 25 weeks, becoming consistent after 28 weeks.[74] Recently, responsiveness to sound was even described at 16 weeks of gestation.[1,84,85] Developmental origins were systematically

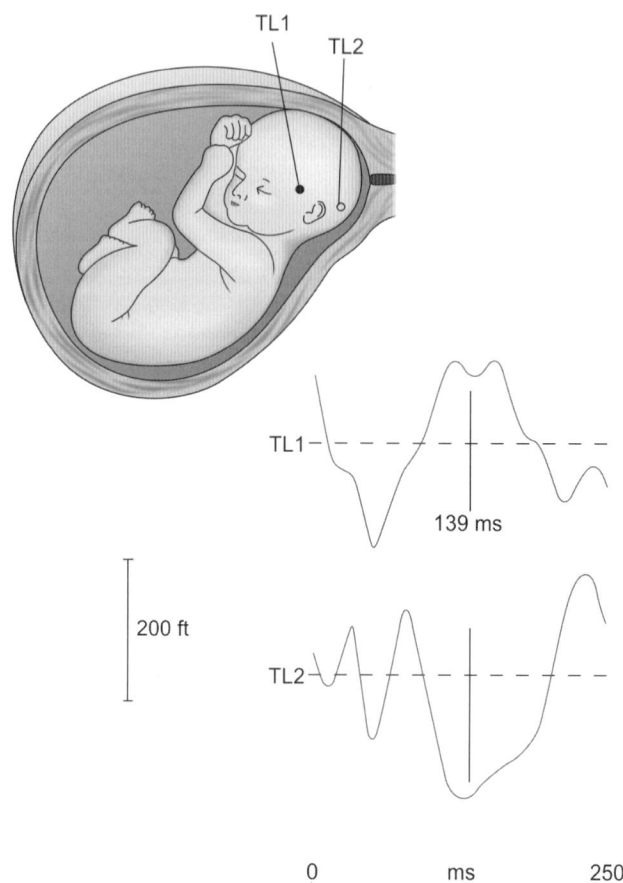

Fig. 85.5: Typical waveforms obtained from brainstem after click stimulation at 34 weeks by one-channel magnetoencephalography[79,80]

Abbreviations: TL1, temporal lateral1; TL2, temporal lateral2; Ft, femtotesla.

examined using 80–2,000 broadband stimuli between 15 and 25 gestational weeks. When changing the stimulus from a single sound to a series of ten 2-s pulses, an increased number of FM was found after stimulation at 20 weeks. Interpretation refers to hypotheses about the developing neural system prior to the formation of specific receptor cells as described for first reactions toward touch. Ultrasound observations also allow definition of motor responses such as body, head, arm and leg movements.[86] The methodology can be simplified by using Doppler services for the detection of FM which whilst unable to differentiate qualities of responses can differentiate quantities of FM responses with a high sensitivity and specificity.[87] Using this method to record fetal responses and external artificial larynx for stimulation we observed a first fetal reaction (FM) in singletons at 25 weeks[88] and simultaneous reactions of FM of both members of a twin pair at 27 weeks.

Developmental Aspects

The FM and FHR responses may be classified in immediate reactions such as startles, twinkling, accelerations or decelerations (reflexes) as well as long-term changes of either FM, FHR baseline or variability (changes of behavioral patterns). FHR/FM patterns including breathing movements were studied during 1 h after vibroacoustic stimulation.[89,90] Close company changes the development of reactions toward vibroacoustic stimuli in twins

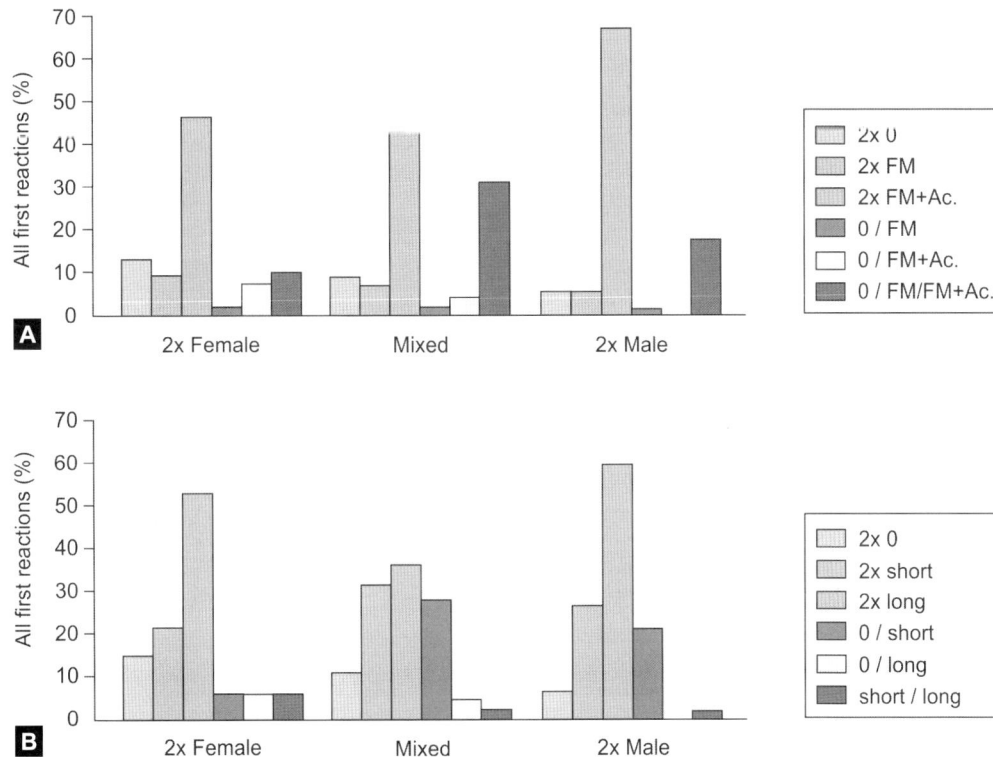

Figs 85.6A and B: Distribution of short (<60s) and long (>60s) behavioral reactions toward vibroacoustic stimuli in 74 healthy singletons (A) and 64 healthy twins (B) obtained by longitudinal weekly measurements between 26 weeks and 36 weeks. Note that there are significant changes with gestational age, Pearson χ2 test p <0.0005, and differences between twins and singletons, Pearson χ2 test p <0.0005

compared to singletons (Figs 85.6A and B). Reactions of longer duration become more frequent in twins compared to singletons. With increasing gestational age an increasing number of FM combined with FHR accelerations is observed in singletons and twins. Among reactions of long duration (>60s) FHR baseline changes more dramatically than FHR variability. We also found an increasing number of extreme changes from a very passive to a very active FHR/FM pattern in twin pregnancies. This is in accordance with findings in singletons that after vibroacoustic stimulation unusual changes of state 1F–4F occur, which rarely occur spontaneously.[91] More "physiologic" state changes from state 1F to 2F were found using a 100 Hz square-wave vibratory stimulus.[92] In any case, vibroacoustic stimulation with the external artificial larynx must have some quite dramatic influence on the fetus, since some gynecologists have even recommended it to induce a change of fetal position to improve visualization of fetal echocardiography (we do not!).[93]

Quality of Stimulus

Both the onset and development of auditory responsiveness also depend on qualities of the stimulus. Fetuses from 19 weeks onward were presented with pure-tone frequencies of 100–3,000 Hz. First responsiveness was detected at 23 weeks at 500 Hz, by 27 weeks responsiveness was found to 100, 250 and 500 Hz, and only at 31 weeks were responses observed to 1,000 and 3,000 Hz.[94] It was interpreted that the delayed responsiveness to high frequency is related to the development of phase-locked firing describing a cooperation of nerve fibers to encode high-frequency sound.[95] The sound pressure level required to elicit a response at 35 weeks is

20–30 dB less than at 23 weeks, indicating that the fetal auditory system becomes more sensitive with prenatal age.[94] However, changes in attenuation, maturing behavior and sensomotor neural connections might also have an impact. Even fetal intelligibility has developmental aspects.[95] Using a habituation-dishabituation technique, fetuses aged 35 weeks could discriminate between frequencies of 250 and 500 Hz and between different speech sounds, whereas fetuses of 27 weeks were unable to make this differentiation, although they were able to differentiate between a 250-Hz tone and 80–2,000-Hz broadband sound.

Specific or Momentary Disposition

Additional factors influence fetal acoustic responsiveness such as behavioral state before the stimulus,[96] gender,[72] position in utero and individual disposition (own data). Fetal responses to speech stimuli consisting of syllables ("ee" or "ah") were studied in healthy pregnancies at 26–34 weeks of gestation. During periods of low FHR variability, a decrease in FHR and an increase in the standard deviation of heart rate were found.[97] This is the only demonstration of prenatal responses to speech stimuli whereby the response is dependent on FHR variability which is the primary determinant of fetal state.[98] Female fetuses seem to respond earlier than males.[72] In our experience twins are ideal models to differentiate further the simultaneous influence of activity state before stimulation, individual disposition (zygosity), and position and sex of the prenates by analyzing intertwin differences of FHR/FM patterns toward external artificial larynx (Figs 85.7A and B). Similar reactions toward external artificial larynx were significantly increased in twins with the same sex and differences between sex-alike male compared to female groups can

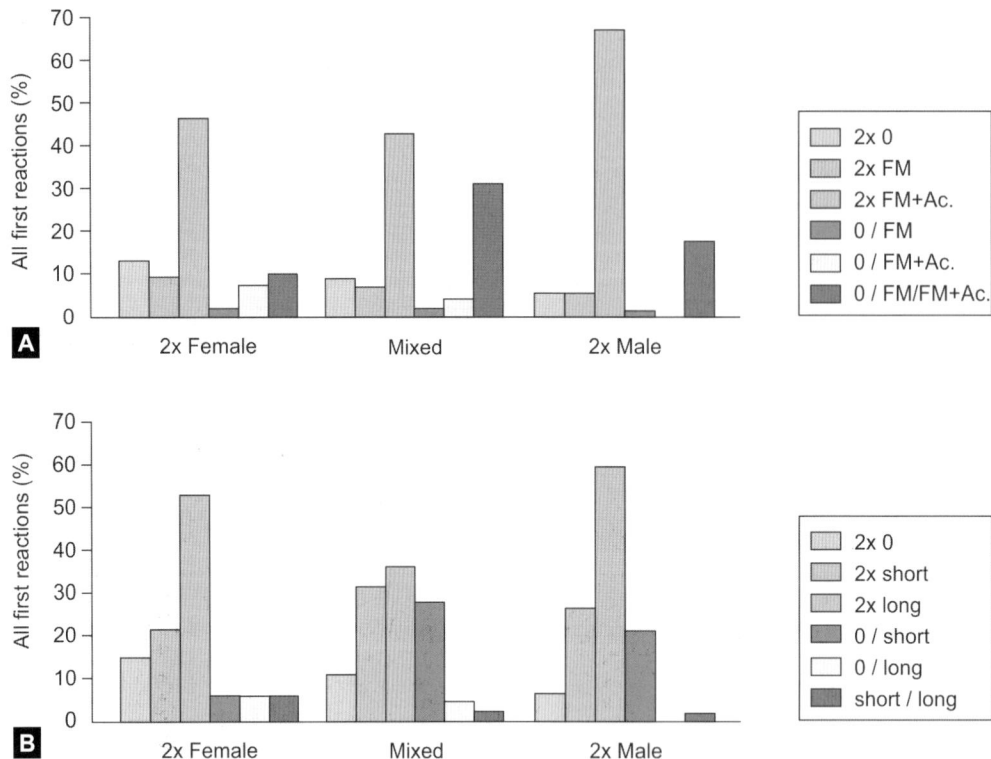

Figs 85.7A and B: Distribution of combinations of 390 fetal heart rate (FHR)/fetal movement (FM) reactions toward vibroacoustic stimuli within 32 twin pairs. (A) Classified relating to first short reactions, (B) classified relating to duration of reactions (0, no reaction; Ac, acceleration; long, >60s; short, <60s). Note the significantly higher intertwin differences (lighter columns) in twin pairs of different sex, Pearson $\chi 2$ test p <0.0001

be calculated. If all parameters are analyzed by multivariate analysis, age-dependent determinants of fetal responsiveness can be evaluated.

POSTNATAL AUDITORY RESPONSIVENESS UNDER NORMAL CONDITIONS

After delivery sound conduction and environment change significantly and the newborn is more directly accessible to behavioral[98,99] and electrophysiological examinations.[30-32,99]

Postnatal Responsiveness Assessed by Electrophysiological Methods

Auditory-evoked potentials reflect electrical activity from different anatomic levels of the auditory system; the earlier components from peripheral and brainstem levels, the later ones from midbrain and cortical levels. The cochlear (0–4 ms) and early components (4–12 ms) are used for assessing peripheral hearing in children by electrocochleography and auditory brainstem response. Whereas electrocochleography can only be used under anesthesia, auditory brain response has become the method of choice to estimate hearing sensitivity in newborns since it was first described.[100,101] It reflects the integrity of the outer, middle and inner ear, and the auditory pathway,[102,103] as described by Davis,[35] and is free from the effects of medication or state. Via headphones click stimuli are performed, and short-latency electroencephalographic waveforms are recorded by skull electrodes (Fig. 85.8). The detection of cortical potentials and auditory brainstem response as early as 25 weeks indicates functional maturity of the auditory pathway.[104] Electrophysiological responses from the cochlea, the eighth nerve

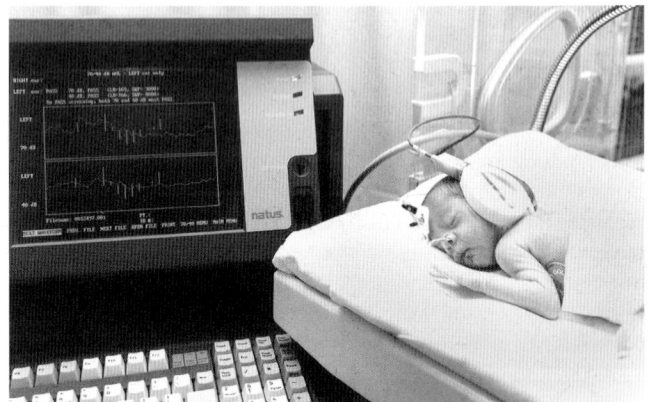

Fig. 85.8: Hearing screening in a preterm infant at the NICU with an automatic version (ALGO-1E automated auditory brainstem response infant hearing screener, Natus Medical, Inc.) detecting auditory brainstem responses

and the auditory brainstem are similar to those in the adult by 32–36 gestational weeks.[103,105] The responses continue to develop in wave components, shape and latency with myelinization[103,106] until the second year. The auditory brainstem response does not necessarily depend on the same neural events that are essential for perception of auditory capabilities.

Von Bekesy[36] postulated that some sound energy must be emitted from the cochlea back to the external auditory canal ("feedback from the inner ear"). Transiently evoked otoacoustic emissions can be measured, e.g. sounds generated and emitted by the outer hair cells of the cochlea in response to acoustic stimulation.[107] A small probe is placed in the external auditory canal and click stimuli are presented. Otoacoustic emission methods are candidates for application in the newborn permitting the acquisition of frequency-specific information, which can be drawn later from audiometry.

Postnatal Behavioral Responsiveness

Behavioral reactions toward acoustic stimuli are less suitable for preterm neonates, but they are of value to learn about what babies hear and about possible positive or negative influences. Responses and alertness to voices, bells and rattles, or the neonate's ability to shut down aversive reactions due to habituation toward repeated stimuli are used to score infants according to their "abilities".[97] Broadband sounds (speech) are more likely than narrowband sounds to elicit responses,[108] which also depend on physiological states of hunger and sleep/wakefulness.[98] A newborn infant can differentiate bandwidth, duration, interstimulus interval, frequency and sound pressure level.[109,110] Signals <4 kHz evoke responses three times more often than signals in the higher range. Lower frequencies generally evoke gross motor activity; high frequencies evoke freezing reactions. The newborn can respond to gross right-left changes, although sound localization is not purely auditory. Even soon after birth a blind infant is less likely to localize sound than a sighted infant. After 2 months, infants integrate auditory and visual space (e.g. voice and facial movements).[111]

Some methods have been introduced to objectify behavioral responsiveness. The auditory response cradle compares reactions with and without sound by a pressure sensitive mattress and a monitor for head movements. As in prenatal life high intensities of up to 85 dB are needed to elicit motor responses.[112] The observer-based psychoacoustic procedure controls for observer bias by documenting behavioral changes toward acoustic stimuli while the observer is "blinded" by earphones for all signals.[113] Using the observer-based psychoacoustic procedure infants of 2–5 weeks showed thresholds at 500 and 4,000 Hz of 55- and 60-dB sound pressure levels respectively.[114]

EFFECTS OF PRENATAL HEARING ON POSTNATAL DEVELOPMENT

By correlating morphological and neurofunctional results with perinatal observations, conclusions might be drawn for sensomotory, cognitive and emotional development.

Recognition or "Memorization"

Considerable attention is given by parents to the possibility that the fetus forms memories of speech and music that may influence the abilities postnatally. Habituation has primarily been described by Peiper[3] who reported a decrease in FM after repeated stimulation with a car horn. Since then a number of studies have demonstrated a decrement in response to repeated stimulation while using FHR/FM or ultrasound documentation. Habituation may be distinguished from adaptation or fatigue by several criteria, the most important being the recovery of response on presentation of a new stimulus ("dishabituation") and faster habituation upon representation of the stimulus.[115] The intensity of the stimulus influences habituation time (faster habituation to more intense stimuli).[115]

While habituation reflects short-term memory, there is also proof of long-term memory from pre to postnatal life. To demonstrate the existence of prenatal sensory perception, one can indirectly study behavioral modifications of a neonate presented with stimuli she or he has been confronted with during prenatal life ("memorization").[47] Prenatal sound experience might have an influence on postnatal sound preference and fine tune the developing auditory system.[116] Neonates have been taught that if they produce a specific sucking pattern they could listen to their mother's voice. Newborn babies showed a strong preference for the voice of their mother over that of other male or female talkers. Using the especially designed baby's dummy connected to a tape recorder, newborns are even able to distinguish between their mother speaking in her native versus in an unfamiliar language[117] (sucking with higher frequency). Using this "high-amplitude sucking procedure", 3-day-old newborns prefer a lullaby read twice a day by the mother during the last weeks of pregnancy to a new story.[118] All this suggests the possibility of prenatal acquisitions and antenatal discrimination, however elementary it might be.

Prenatal stimulation has an impact on temperament behavior. Settings of talking, music and meditation were performed during pregnancy and correlated with behavioral outcome.[119] Talking had a 65%, music a 34% and meditation a 31% correlation with all behaviors. For talking only 58% of behavioral variables were identified as positive (e.g. the child being easily comforted, contentment), 16% as ambiguous and 26% as negative (e.g. crying for obscure reasons, needing constant supervision). Music and meditation, however, correlated in 90% and 100%, respectively, with positive attitudes. Talking is known not only to express care, but also irritability, anger or anxiety experienced in pregnancy. It is speculated that not only variations of timbre, but also hormonal or physiological changes associated with the content of speech, may evoke associations in the infant. This hypothesis is supported by a study of infants whose excessive crying was in association with their mothers' depression scores.[120]

Implications for Language Development and Musical Expression

Hearing has a close relation to the kinetic system, i.e. "auditory-vocal-kinetic channel".[121] From embryology we know that the origins and innervation of hearing and language function are in close proximity, suggesting that there is also "crying in utero"—only we have not yet become sensitive for it. Vocal expression can be heard in fetuses from around 20 weeks onward. Uterine crying has been proposed following unpleasant maneuvers such as attaching electrodes, versions or catheter insertions.[122-124] The newborn's phonation is based on laryngeal coordination reflecting maturation processes and training. Newborn "cryprints" are as unique as fingerprints, and characterized by specific features such as fundamental frequency and variation in time (vibrato) using voice-signal recording.[125]

We suppose influences of nature and nurture on prespeech development. Monozygotic twins have synchronous cry patterns at birth.[126] By listening to the mother's speech the fetus obviously stores her speech features. Early spectrography of the first cries proved that even newborns born at 28 weeks had similar voice performance features to their mothers.[127,128] How far genetic influences or experience of the same sound environment are responsible for first hearing and cry patterns remains to be determined. Babies as young as 12-h-old react to rhythms of human speech.[129] This also might imply that learning of language begins soon after or even before birth. Newborns are able to distinguish between phones in any language and make all sounds of any language.[130] By 6 months linguistic experience has resulted in language-specific phonetic prototypes.[131] Adults can no longer distinguish between phones used in unfamiliar languages. In this context, experience seems paradoxically to diminish auditory skills. Somehow, babies even stimulate adults to speak to them in a stylized way.[132]

Music exists in the passage of time and cross-culturally. It is supposed that musicality is structured by an ensemble of protorhythms of biological inheritance.[133] The hypothesis that music has prenatal origins does not explain the survival value of music,[134] but might clarify its nature with cross-cultural features of rhythm and dancing comparable to rhythmic elements in utero, e.g. movements of maternal vessels felt and heard by the prenate. A summary of the up-to-date knowledge on the influence of music during pregnancy is meanwhile published by the main author.[135]

PRENATAL ACOUSTICAL RESPONSIVENESS AS A TEST FOR FETAL WELL-BEING

The understanding of pathophysiology has led to improvements in interpretation of behavioral and hemodynamic mechanisms. Fetal hypoxia is the condition studied most intensively. An arrest of muscular activity to reduce oxygen consumption and a redistribution of fetal blood flow to maintain oxygen delivery to essential organs were primarily described in sheep experiments[136,137] and later in humans.[138-140] Meanwhile correlations with antenatal blood gases have been performed.[141,142] Fetal activity and blood-flow redistribution have an impact on FHR patterns. FHR variability and the presence of FHR accelerations with FM are recognized as indicators of fetal health by noninvasive and invasive studies.[142,143] In this context, (vibro)acoustic stimulation was proposed mainly for the assessment of fetal well-being and to discriminate between "nonreactive" non-stress tests (NSTs) due to hypoxia or just to quiet state.[144,145] Using Medline we found more than 150 studies on vibroacoustic stimulation as a test of fetal well-being from 1980 to date; here we focus only on selected aspects.

Increase of "Efficiency" of Non-stress Testing and Biophysical Profile

To compare results, the frequency, duration and intensity of the stimulus as well as gestational age, FHR/FM criteria, habituation time and behavioral states in association with the response have to be analyzed. In general, a 3-s sound stimulus is adequate for a shift to an "awake" state.[146] In a review of 61 studies, the ability of vibroacoustic stimulation to elicit FHR accelerations has been established, decreasing false-positive rates of nonreactive NSTs.[147] Pregnancies with early-onset intrauterine growth retardation (IUGR) were studied after vibroacoustic stimulation between 26 weeks and 32 weeks of gestation. Accelerations, FHR variability and FM were reduced compared with age-matched normal fetuses.[148] The conclusion that nutritional deprivation is associated with delayed sensory maturation is not necessarily true, since similar FHR and FM patterns are recognizable in early NSTs. The result only proves that there is no reaction, though the stimulus might well be received. Vibroacoustic stimulation was performed in patients with low biophysical profile scores after 15 minutes. The results of patients whose biophysical profile score improved to normal were compared to normal scores without stimulation. Vibroacoustic stimulation was found to "improve" an abnormal or equivocal biophysical profile score to normal in 82% of cases

without increasing obstetric or neonatal complication rates or the false-negative rate of biophysical profile scores.[149]

Comparative Observational Studies and Clinical Trials

Some observational studies compare the vibroacoustic stimulation test concurrently with other tests. In most studies the prediction of poor outcome was comparable with results of the NST.[150,151] In the prediction of an abnormal contraction stress test (CST), a non-reactive vibroacoustic stimulation test had a sensitivity of 100% and a specificity of 91%; therefore vibroacoustic stimulation was slightly better able to diagnose fetal distress compared to the CST in pregnancies with a nonreactive NST at term.[152] After the introduction of Doppler velocimetry of fetal redistribution it has become possible to differentiate ambiguous results of NSTs noninvasively. Thus, we compared the clinical value of NST, Doppler ratio of cerebral versus umbilical blood flow, vibroacoustic stimulation test and CST to predict poor outcome using different cut-off values for all tests separately for IUGR and post-term pregnancies. Doppler velocimetry and NSTs had better prognostic capacities than vibroacoustic stimulation tests and CSTs (Figs 85.9A and B).[153,154] We therefore do not use CST or vibroacoustic stimulation tests in clinical routine, while Doppler studies, computerized FHR analysis, or real-time ultrasound of fetal behavior and amniotic fluid analysis can be performed without "unnatural stress" for mother and fetus. We admit that in units where skills in ultrasound examinations or sophisticated equipment are not available, vibroacoustic stimulation or CST might be of value. Clinical trials demonstrate that the introduction of vibroacoustic stimulation in combination with the NST[155] or with amniotic fluid assessment[156] has not led to an increased rate of mortality. Since in the Western world all of the currently used forms of antenatal surveillance are combined with low mortality rates, it is unlikely that vibroacoustic stimulation will ever lower perinatal mortality in any randomized or historic trial.[157] In the only controlled clinical trial, where vibroacoustic stimulation test was compared to NST,[145] false-positive tests were slightly lowered and performance reduced from a mean of 27 minutes to 23 minutes. Although it has been proved that vibroacoustic stimulation does at least not increase catecholamine release[158] or meconium passage in healthy fetuses,[159] the question remains whether 4 minutes justify frightening—or even awakening—an innocently sleeping fetus (it is recommended that vibroacoustic stimulation is performed during quiet sleep!). In other words, which parents would appreciate this postnatally?

Vibroacoustic Stimulation during Labor

The same holds true for studies during labor, where vibroacoustic stimulation was primarily applied to test attenuation via hydrophones. Data suggest that an intrauterine threshold of 94-dB sound pressure level is necessary to produce a consistent FHR response during active labor.[160] At the first stage of labor vibroacoustic stimulation was studied possibly to improve interpretation of ominous spontaneous FHR testing. Undoubtedly nonreactive responders to vibroacoustic stimulation were at significantly greater risk of subsequent abnormal FHR patterns, meconium staining and fetal distress; however, transient FHR decelerations occurred in 25% where fetal outcome was not impaired.[161] Although it was concluded that vibroacoustic stimulation differentiated compromised from noncompromised fetuses, we think that it might also confuse inexperienced staff. At the second stage of labor fetal blood sampling (FBS) has been

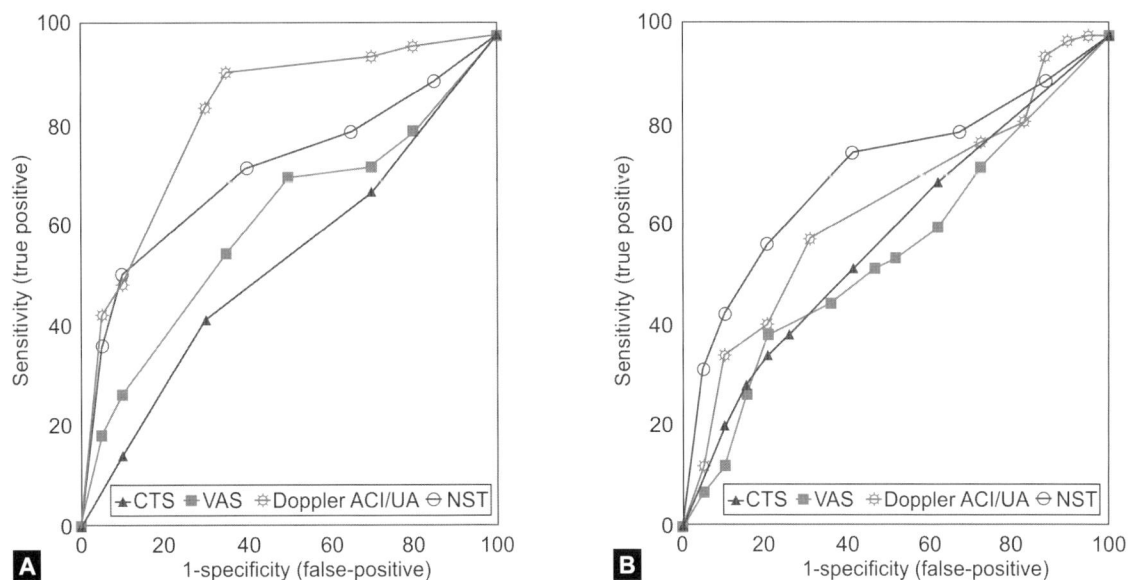

Figs 85.9A and B: Receiver-operator characteristics of antepartum tests to predict fetal distress requiring operative delivery (measurements 1–3 days antepartum; CTS, contraction stress test; VAS, vibroacoustic stimulation; Doppler ACI/UA, resistance index ratio of arteria carotis communis/umbilical artery; NST, nonstress test) in 103 intrauterine growth retarded (IUGR) (A) and 110 postterm (B) pregnancies[142,143]

correlated with vibroacoustic stimulation testing: vibroacoustic stimulation had a sensitivity of 100%, a specificity of 59.6% and a positive predictive value of 27.6% for the detection of fetal acidosis.[162] Although it was evident that mean fetal blood pH values obtained within 30 minutes of vibroacoustic stimulation were higher in reactive compared with decelerative or nonresponders; acidotic pH values were also found in fetuses with reactive FHR patterns after vibroacoustic stimulation.[163] In recent studies, it was concluded that the FHR response after vibroacoustic stimulation does not predict neonatal outcome and might not replace FBS.[164,165] There are even warning hints about using vibroacoustic stimulation as a routine procedure, such as an unknown influence on cerebral blood flow in quiet sleep,[166] false-negative results in fetal sepsis,[167] activation of swallowing[168] or micturation,[169] and provocation of unnecessary pathological FHR patterns in cases with nuchal cord.[170]

We conclude that many studies do not address the physiological changes of fetal responsiveness or habituation time by gestational age or standardize FHR/FM patterns before or after vibroacoustic stimulation. Appropriate implementation of vibroacoustic stimulation tests requires appropriate questions. In twin studies, we have found that prenatal reactiveness—either to touch of the co-twin or to external stimulation—is combined with larger interindividual variations than spontaneous behavior. For the time being, we recommend vibroacoustic stimulation as a challenge test only under controlled conditions, but not for routine use just to simplify antenatal surveillance. This has been proposed by other authors.[171]

EARLY HEARING DISTURBANCES

Compared with the vestibular part, the auditory system is phylogenetically young with a greater demand for oxygen and glucose, and can therefore be selectively damaged.

Early hearing is prerequisite for speaking, and for intellectual, social and emotional development.[172] Even a relatively mild hearing loss of 35–40 dB near hearing level means that a child misses approximately 50% of normal conversation.[173] Severe congenital hearing impairment affects 0.1% of live-born infants[104,174] and 1–4% of graduates of neonatal intensive care units (NICUs).[174,175] The prognosis is improved when the diagnosis is made early.[176] The fitting of hearing aids within the first 6 months improves speech and language development compared with placement at a later age. However, the age at diagnosis of hearing impairment was at least 18–30 months,[177] even in countries with a nationwide behavioral screening program starting at 9 months of age. However, the age of diagnosis is rapidly changing in those countries with a nationwide neonatal screening program. Using high-risk registers 50–75% of infants with hearing loss are identifiable.[178] Both the American Joint Committee on Infant Hearing and the European Consensus Development Conference postulated that universal hearing screening should be implemented within 3 months of life.[179,180] Habilitation should be started before 6 months of age. In those countries with limited financial facilities neonatal hearing screening may be limited to high-risk groups for hearing loss (Table 85.1). All infants admitted to neonatal intensive care units should be screened for hearing loss prior to discharge.

Electrophysiological Measurements for Screening

Auditory Brainstem Responses

The conventional auditory brainstem response (ABR) e.g. the ability to evoke and record a short-latency electroencephalographic waveform in response to a click stimulus is considered to be the gold standard in detecting the neonatal hearing threshold,[105,181,182] though it is not yet widely used because it is cost- and time-consuming. The click-evoked ABR may occur as early as at 25 gestational weeks but typically appears during the 27th week. Development of the infant ABR is usually complete by the end of the second year of life.

Automated ABR infant hearing screeners have been introduced as an alternative.[183] Based on a statistical model for the detection of a response (auditory brainstem response algorithm) and a dual

Table 85.1: Indicators associated with sensorineural and/or conductive hearing loss in the newborn (indications for hearing tests when universal screening is not available)

Indications
• Positive family history or hereditary childhood sensoneural hearing loss
• Congenital infections (toxoplasmosis, cytomegalovirus, rubella, syphilis, herpes)
• Craniofacial anomalies including those with morphological anomalies of pinna and ear canal
• Admission for ≥ 48 hours to a neonatal intensive care unit
• Stigmata or other findings associated with a syndrome known to include hearing loss

artifact rejection system for environmental noise and myogenic artifacts, the equipment provides a pass/fail outcome. Stimulation via headphones with 35 dB near hearing level clicks with frequencies of 700–5,000 Hz can be performed even under NICU conditions. No special training is necessary. Clinical trials proved the concordance between an automated version and conventional auditory brainstem response screening,[184] whereby a sensitivity of 100% and a specificity of 98.7%[185] was detected. Follow-up results support the value of automated auditory brainstem response screening.[185] The mean time needed to perform a screening has been reduced to 8 minutes.[186] To avoid ambiguous results in preterms, screening is advised from a post-conceptional age of 30 weeks onward.[185]

Otoacoustic Emissions

In transiently evoked otoacoustic emissions (TEOAE) measurements, "a pass" has been defined as the presence of emitted energy of at least 3 dB signal/noise ratio between 1.6 kHz and 4 kHz,[187] but until now no objective pass/fail criteria have been established. The response is frequency specific and does not provide an indication of audiometric threshold. Depending on the stimulus, TEOAE can be detected in up to 98% of humans with normal hearing and are absent in hearing impairment of 20–40 dB. TEOAE takes 7–9 minutes and can be administered by a trained nurse.[187,188] In NICU, infants screened with TEOAE at 3 months, there is a sensitivity of 93% and a specificity of 84% to detect absent auditory brainstem response.[189] Hypoxia or infection may result in a reversible reduction of the TEOAE spectrum. Children with hearing loss primarily due to involvement of the auditory pathway or CNS may have normal evoked otoacoustic emissions as a result of a normal functioning cochlea.[190]

Otoacoustic emissions (OAE) screening is less suitable for use on a NICU because of the ambient noise and the difficulty of placing the ear probe in preterms.[191] Besides, children with nonorganic hearing loss or hearing loss primarily due to involvement of the auditory pathway or central nervous system may have completely normal OAEs as a result of a functioning cochlea.[192] Therefore, children at risk for auditory neuropathy should be screened with ABR methods.

Several other types of otoacoustic emission (OAE) have been identified. These include spontaneous OAE, clicked evoked OAE, and distorsion product OAE. With future research and automated analysis, each of these methods will become increasingly available for hearing screening, especially in term neonates.

Behavioral Screening

Behavioral hearing screening methods such as the auditory response cradle and the crib-o-gram have been developed for term infants. Although easy to perform, they are not suitable for screening preterm or sick neonates and detect only severe hearing impairment. The sensitivity (75%) and specificity (71%) are too low compared to neurofunctional methods.[193] Behavioral observations remain the basis of the investigation of the harmful influences of high-intensity noise in neonatal intensive care units; prematures wearing earmuffs spent more time in quiet sleep states and had higher mean oxygen saturation levels compared to controls.[194]

Information about pediatric auditory research projects are available on Internet.[195]

Possible Damage from Environmental Hazards during Pregnancy

Children who have been exposed in utero to vibroacoustic stimulation for the assessment of fetal well-being have been evaluated at 4 years of age by auditory tests of 20–25 dB at frequencies between 500 Hz and 8,000 Hz in Sweden (n = 460)[196] and the USA (n = 465).[197] No hearing damage or neurodevelopmental abnormalities that could be connected to the vibroacoustic stimulation were found. Fetal noise-induced hearing loss has been a matter of concern regarding the working and living conditions of pregnant women.[198,199] Epidemiological and animal research suggest that noise can adversely change fetal hearing; however, studies in humans still lack control groups. Auditory brainstem response changes were examined in sheep suggesting that noise sources with low-frequency components and high-intensity impulses have temporary effects on auditory brainstem response waves, whereas long-term effects are still unknown.[200] In summary, the Committee on Hearing, Bioacoustics and Biomechanics,[201] attempting to protect fetal hearing, suggested that pregnant women should avoid noise exposures greater than 90 dB.

DIRECTION OF FUTURE RESEARCH

The phenomenon of prenatal perception and the implications for future life represent a wealth for ongoing and future research.

Methodological Aspects

Prenatal hearing reflects the complex neurological development of the early brain. Evaluation of fetal brain function is one of the most important objectives of basic and clinical research in perinatology. Imaging of the fetal brain only demonstrates a small part of its function and most functional approaches have been indirect. The introduction of magnetoencephalography in perinatal medicine was a pioneer step to evaluate prenatal brain function directly,[79,80] though the single-channel magnetometer did not allow high-quality auditory-evoked signals. By using multichannel magnetoencephalography[202] or detectors specifically designed for the prenate, the window of observation of early gestational age and various indications might be expected to be extended. The method might be used in newborns;[203] examinations in twins would enhance our knowledge about hereditary or environmental influences. The sophisticated method might have implications for prenatal neuroscience and clinical use. Prenatal training of laryngeal coordination is likely to occur during mouthing or breathing movements. Doppler combined with real-time ultrasound examinations might elucidate how far this is performed at a special rhythm. Correlations with postnatal cry spectroscopy might be of interest.

Aspects of Using Early Sensation for Developmental Support

Health is understood as the physical, mental and social well-being that goes further than just the absence of illness. As important as it is to teach children abilities at certain times creating integrated stimulations for the unborn might favor development or prevent sensory retardation. This should be a matter of concern in public health projects. In Venezuela, a program was introduced including weekly lectures to pregnant mothers about adequate stimulation and nutrition. Significant improvement was found at the 2nd and 25th days in orientation and autonomic stability of the infants in the experimental compared to the control group.[204] Perinatal auditory stimulation programs need the knowledge of critical developmental phases. Pilot studies have demonstrated an immediate reduction of fetal breathing and an increase of FM when mothers only listen to a preferred type of music via earphones,[205] or a reduction of fetal activity if fetuses only listen to rhythmic music.[64] The first study is proof that integrated programs for mother and fetus may even be regarded as conditioning (e.g. music, mother relaxed). Is the unborn more affected by the mother's preferences of listening—the same holds true for singing and talking to the unborn—than by the sound alone? Postnatal conditioning has a larger scale, e.g. sound stimulations recalling intrauterine noise can not only lull the newborn to sleep,[67] but also serve as a reinforcer during sucking.[206] Similarly, feeding may be enhanced by background music. The perception of music as pleasant might even be a process of conditioning from the parents.[71] Singing lullabies and simultaneously rocking cradles have been used to soothe babies by simultaneous stimulation of the vestibular and acoustic sensory system. The experience of rhythmic stimulations by a "breathing teddy bear" adapted to the child's individual breathing frequency has proven to facilitate neurobehavioral development.[207] Further studies relating to supportive perinatal conditioning are necessary whereby music stimulation might play an essential part.[135]

Aspects for Pathological Development

Working groups in Western countries are planning protocols for the evaluation of early hearing screening. Thereby it is a major goal of the Maternal Child Health grant in the USA to establish universal neonatal screening, to identify specific hearing loss by 3 months, to institute intervention by 6 months and to measure the impact of early identification on developmental outcome. Average costs were given as $25 per test,[208] and as $43,785 to identify a child with sensorineural hearing loss.[209] Considering the given incidence of hearing impairment further programs are needed. Future research of the use of acoustic therapy and shelter may provide measures positively to alter the critically ill newborn's environment.

CONCLUSION

Encouragement and avoidance of sound have to be considered and balanced in future analytical and interventional projects according to critical developmental phases. Whether we go so far as to found prenatal universities, as in California, is of secondary importance as long as we strive to understand the physiology and pathophysiology of early hearing and to create designs of adequate stimulation suitable to induce a comprehensive expression of our genetic potential, prevent unnecessary illness and to detect hearing loss as early as possible.

REFERENCES

1. Hepper PG. Fetal psychology: An embryonic science. In: Nijhuis JG (Ed). Fetal Behavior, Developmental and Perinatal Aspects. Oxford, New York: Oxford Medical Publications; 1992. pp. 129-56.
2. Preyer W. Spezielle Physiologie des Embryo. Leipzig: Grieben; 1885.
3. Peiper A. Sinnesempfindungen der Kinder vor seiner Geburt. Monat Kinderheilk. 1925;29:237-41.
4. Forbes HS, Forbes HB. Fetal sense reaction: hearing. J Comp Psychol. 1927;7:353-5.
5. Ray W. A preliminary report on a study of fetal conditioning. Child Dev. 1932;3:175-7.
6. Sontag W, Wallace R. The movement response of the human fetus to sound stimuli. Child Dev. 1939;6:253-8.
7. Spelt D. The conditioning of the human fetus in utero. J Exp Psychol. 1948;3:338-46.
8. Salk L. Mothers' heartbeat as an imprinting stimulus. Trans New Acad Sci. 1961/62;24:753-63.
9. Bench RJ. Sound transmission to the human fetus through the abdominal maternal wall. J Gen Psychol. 1968;113:86-7.
10. Sakabe N, Arayama T, Suzuki T. Human fetal evoked responses to acoustic stimulation. Acta Otolaryngol. 1969;252(Suppl):29-36.
11. Bast TH, Anson BJ. The Temporal Bone and the Ear. Springfield, IL: Charles C Thomas; 1949.
12. Anson BJ, Winch T. Vascular channels in the auditory ossicles. Ann Otol Rhinol Laryngol. 1974;83:142-58.
13. Anson BJ, Davies J, Duckert LG. Embryology of the ear. In: Paparella MM, Shumrick DA, Gluckman JL (Eds). Otolaryngology, 3rd edition. Philadelphia: Saunders; 1991. pp. 3-22.
14. Gasser RF, Shigihara S, Shimada K. The development of the facial nerve in man. Ann Otol Rhinol Laryngol. 1967;76:37-56.
15. Gasser RF, Shigihara S, Shimada K. Three-dimensional development of the facial nerve path through the ear region in human embryos. Ann Otol Rhinol Laryngol. 1994;103:395-403.
16. Pearson AA. Developmental anatomy of the ear. In: English GM (Ed). Otolaryngology, revised. New York: Harper Medical; 1988. pp. 1-68.
17. Gulya AJ. Developmental anatomy of the ear. In: Glasscock ME, Shambaugh GE Jr (Eds). Surgery of the Ear, 4th edition. Philadelphia: Saunders; 1990. pp. 5-33.
18. Kenna MA. Embryology and developmental anatomy of the ear. In: Bluestone CD, Stool SE, Kenna ME (Eds). Pediatric Otolaryngology. Philadelphia: Saunders; 1996;1:113-26.
19. Wright A. Anatomy and ultrastructure of the human ear. In: Kerr AG, Groves J (Eds). Scott-Brown's Otolaryngology, 5th edition. London, Boston: Butterworths; 1987. pp. 1-46.

20. Schulknecht HF, Gulya AJ. Phylogeny and embryology. In: Schulknecht HF, Gulya AJ (Eds). Anatomy of the Temporal Bone with Surgical Implications. Philadelphia: Lea and Febinger; 1986. pp. 235-73.
21. Bredberg G. Cellular pattern and nerve supply of the human organ of Corti. Acta Otolaryngol (Stockh). 1986;236(Suppl):1.
22. Pujol R, Lavigne-Rebillard M. Early stages of innervation and sensory cell differentiation in the human organ of Corti. Acta Otolaryngol. 1985;423(Suppl):43-50.
23. Pujol R, Uziel A. Auditory development: peripheral aspects. In: Meisami E, Tiniacas TS (Eds). Handbook of Human Growth and Developmental Biology. Boca Raton: CRC Press; 1988;1(Part 2): 109-30.
24. Pujol R, Hilding DA. Anatomy and physiology of the onset of auditory function. Acta Otolaryngol. 1973;76:1-10.
25. Lavigne-Rebillard M, Pujol R. Hair cell innervation in the human cochlea. Acta Otolaryngol. 1988;105:398-402.
26. Lavigne-Rebillard M, Pujol R. Development of auditory hair cell surface in human fetuses: A scanning electron microscopic study. Anat Embryol. 1986;174:369-72.
27. Moore JK, Perazzo LM, Braun A. Time course of axonal myelination in the human brainstem auditory pathway. Hearing Res. 1995;87:21-31.
28. Shido Y, Zhimin Q, Ningshen Z. Ultrastructure of the secondary tympanic membrane in the human fetus. Acta Anat. 1988;131: 332-7.
29. Fisch L. Integrated development and maturation of the hearing system. A critical review article. Br J Audiol. 1983;17:137-54.
30. Durrant JD, Lovrinic JH. Basis of Hearing Science, 2nd edition. Baltimore: Williams and Wilkins; 1984.
31. Haggard MP, Evans EF. Hearing. Br Med Bull. 1987;43:775-1042.
32. Jahn AF, Santos-Sacchi J. Physiology of the Ear. New York: Raven Press; 1988.
33. Ryan A, Dallos P. Physiology of the cochlea. In: Northern JJ (Ed). Hearing Disorders, 2nd edition. Boston: Little, Brown; 1984. pp. 253-66.
34. Oliver CC. Sound and vibration transmission in tissues. Semin Perinatol. 1989;13:3554-61.
35. Davis H. A model for transducer action in the human cochlea. Cold Spring Harb Symp Quant Biol. 1965;30:181-93.
36. von Bekesy G. Experiments in hearing. In: Wever EG (Ed). McGraw Hill Series in Psychology. New York: McGraw Hill; 1960. pp. 745-55.
37. Rhode WS. Basilar membrane motion: Results of Mossbauer motions. Scand Audiol Suppl. 1986;25:7-15.
38. Brugge JF, Geisler CD. Auditory mechanisms of the lower brainstem. Ann Rev Neurosci. 1978;1:363-94.
39. Merzenich MM, Knight PL, Roth GL. Representation of cochlea within primary auditory cortex in the cat. J Neurophysiol. 1975;38:231-49.
40. Canforth JL. Auditory cortex lesions and interaural intensity and phase-angle discrimination in cats. J Neurophysiol. 1979;42:1518-26.
41. Cassaday JH, Neff WD. Auditory localization: Role of auditory pathways in brain stem of the cat. J Neurophysiol. 1975;38:842-58.
42. Massopust LC, Wolin L, Frost V. Frequency discrimination thresholds following auditory cortex ablations in the monkey. J Aud Res. 1971;11:227-34.
43. Keidel WB. Information processing in higher parts of the auditory pathway. In: Zwicker E, Terhardt E (Eds). Facts and Models in Hearing. New York: Springer; 1974. pp. 216.
44. Warr WB, Guinan JJ. Efferent innervation of the organ of Corti: Two separate systems. Brain Res. 1979;173:152-5.
45. Busnel MC, Granier-Deferre C, Lacanuet JP. Fetal audition. In: Turkewitz G (Ed). Developmental Psychology. New York: New York Academy of Science; 1992. pp. 175-88.
46. Gerhardt KJ. Characteristics of the fetal sheep sound environment. Semin Perinatol. 1989;13:362-70.
47. Querleu D, Xavier R, Boutteville C, et al. Hearing by the human fetus? Semin Perinatol. 1989;13:409-20.
48. Gerhardt KJ, Otto R, Abrams RM, et al. Cochlear micro-phonics recorded from fetal and newborn sheep. Am J Otolaryngol. 1992;13:226-33.
49. Gerhardt KJ, Abrams RM. Fetal hearing: characterization of the stimulus and response. Semin Perinatol. 1996;20:11-20.
50. Hollien H, Feinstein S. Contribution of the external auditory meatus to auditory sensitivity underwater. J Acoust Soc Am. 1975;57: 1488-92.
51. Gerhardt KJ, Huang X, Arringtom KE, et al. Fetal sheep in utero hear through bone conduction. Am J Otolaryngol. 1995;17:374-9.
52. Dirks DD. Bone conduction threshold testing. In: Katz J (Ed). Handbook of Clinical Audiology, 4th edition. Baltimore: Williams and Wilkins; 1994. pp. 132-46.
53. Peters AJM, Gerhardt KJ, Abrams RM, et al. Three-dimensional intraabdominal sound pressures in sheep produced by airborne stimuli. Am J Obstet Gynecol. 1993;169:1304-15.
54. Previc FH. A general theory concerning the prenatal origins of cerebral lateralizations in humans. Psychol Rev. 1991;98:299-334.
55. Bench RJ. Sound transmission to the human fetus through the maternal abdominal wall. J Gen Psychol. 1968;113:85-7.
56. Grimwalde JC, Walker D, Wood C. Sensory stimulation of the human fetus. Aust J Ment Ret. 1970;2:63-4.
57. Walker DW, Grimwalde JC, Wood C. Intrauterine noise: A component of the fetal environment. Am J Obstet Gynecol. 1971;109:91-5.
58. Querleu D, Renard X, Crepin G. Preception auditive et reactivite foetale aux stimulations sonores. J Gynecol Obstet Biol Reprod (Paris). 1981;10:207-14.
59. Querleu Q, Xavier R, Fabienne V. Fetal hearing. Eur J Obstet Gynecol Reprod Biol. 1988;29:191-212.
60. Armitage SE, Baldwin BA, Vince MA. The fetal sound environment in sheep. Science. 1980;208:1173-4.
61. Vince MA, Armitage S, Baldwin BA. The sound environment in fetal sheep. Behavior. 1982;81:296-315.
62. Gerhardt KJ, Abrams RM, Oliver CC. Sound environment of the fetal sheep. Am J Obstet Gynecol. 1990;162: 282-7.
63. Vince MA, Billing AE, Baldwin BA, et al. Maternal vocalizations and other sounds in fetal lamb's sound environment. Early Hum Dev. 1985;11:179-90.
64. Saling E, Arabin B. Untersuchungen über akustische Einflüsse auf den Fetus. In: Stauber M, Diedrichs P (Eds). Psychosomatische Probleme in der Gynäkologie und Geburtshilfe. Berlin: Springer; 1987. pp. 19-28.
65. Benzaquen S, Gagnon R, Hunse C, et al. The intrauterine sound environment of the human fetus during labor. Am J Obstet Gynecol. 1990;163:484-90.
66. Henshall WR. Intrauterine sound levels. Am J Obstet Gynecol. 1971;112:576-8.
67. Wollak CH. The auditory activity of the sheep (ovis aries). J Aud Res. 1963;3:121-32.
68. Murooka H, Koie Y, Suda M. Analyse des sons intrauterins et leurs effects tranquillisants sur le nouveaué. J Gynecol Obstet Biol Reprod. 1976;5:367-76.
69. Richards DS, Frentzen B, Gerhardt KJ, et al. Sound levels in the human uterus. Obstet Gynecol. 1992;80:186-90.
70. Querleu D, Renard X, Versyp F, et al. La transmission intra-amniotique des voix humaines. Rev Fr Gynecol Obstet. 1988;83:43-50.
71. Woodward SC, Guidozzi F. Intrauterine rhythm and blues? Br J Obstet Gynecol. 1992;99:787-90.
72. Leader LR, Baille P, Martin B, et al. The assessment and significance of habituation to a repeated stimulus by the human fetus. Early Hum Dev. 1982;7:211-9.
73. Hepper PG, Shahidullah S. Habituation in normal and Down's syndrome fetuses. Q J Exp Psychol. 1992;44B:105-17.

74. Birnholz J, Benacerraf B. The development of fetal hearing. Science. 1983;222:516-8.
75. Parkes MJ, Moore PJ, Moore DR, et al. Behavioral changes in fetal sheep caused by vibroacoustic stimulation: The effects of cochlear ablation. Am J Obstet Gynecol. 1991;164:1336-43.
76. Barden TP, Peltzman P, Graham T. Human fetal electroencephalic response to intrauterine acoustic signals. Am J Obstet Gynecol. 1968;100:1128-34.
77. Sakabe N, Arayama T, Suzuki T. Human fetal evoked response to acoustic stimulation. Acta Otolaryngol Suppl. 1969;252:29-36.
78. Scribetta JJ, Rosen MG, Hochberg CJ, et al. Human fetal brain responses to sound during labor. Am J Obstet Gynecol. 1971;109:82-5.
79. Blum T, Saling E, Bauer R. First magnetoencephalographic recordings of the brain activity of a human fetus. Br J Obstet Gynaecol. 1985;92:1224-9.
80. Blum T, Bauer R, Arabin B, et al. Prenatally recorded auditory evoked neuro-magnetic fields of the human fetus. In: Barber C, Blum T (Eds). Evoked Potentials III. Boston: Butterworth; 1987;3:136-42.
81. Wilson LA, Wilson KS, Boros SJ. Gestational age as a factor in neonatal AEP screening. In: Nodar RH, Barber C (Eds). Evoked Potentials II. Boston: Butterworth; 1984;520-6.
82. Tuber D, Berntson CD, Brachman DS, et al. Associative learning in premature hydranecephalic and normal twins. Science. 1980;210:1035-7.
83. Crade M, Lovet S. Fetal response to sound stimulation: Preliminary report exploring use of sound stimulation in routine obstetrical ultrasound examination. J Ultrasound Med. 1988;7:499-503.
84. Hepper PG, White R, Shahidullah S. The development of fetal responsiveness to external auditory stimulation. Br Psychol Soc. 1991:Abstr 30.
85. Shahidullah S, Hepper PG. The developmental origins of fetal responsiveness to an acoustic stimulus. J Reprod Infant Psychol. 1993;11:135-41.
86. Arabin B, Riedewald S. An attempt to quantify characteristics of behavioral states. Am J Perinatol. 1992;9:115-19.
87. Arabin B, Riedewald S, Zacharias C, et al. Quantitative analysis of fetal behavioral patterns by means of real time sonography and the actocardiograph. Gynecol Obstet Invest. 1988;26:211-8.
88. Arabin B, Zacharias C, Riedewald S, et al. Analyse fetaler Reaktionen auf akustische Reize mit unterschiedlicher Registriertechnik. Geburtsh Frauenheilk. 1989;49:653-7.
89. Gagnon R, Hunse C, Carmichael L, et al. Effects of vibratory acoustic stimulation on human fetal breathing and gross fetal body movements near term. Am J Obstet Gynecol. 1986;155:1227-30.
90. Gagnon R, Hunse C, Patrick J. Fetal responses to vibratory acoustic stimulation: Influence of basal heart rate. Am J Obstet Gynecol. 1988;59:835-9.
91. Visser GH, Mulder HH, Wit HP. Vibro-acoustic stimulation of the human fetus: Effect on behavioral state organization. Early Hum Dev. 1989;19:285-96.
92. Gagnon R, Hunse C, Foerman J. Human fetal behavioral states after vibratory stimulation. Am J Obstet Gynecol. 1989;161:1470-6.
93. Lazebnik N, Hill LM, Costanino JP, et al. Vibroacoustic stimulation enhances visualization of the four-chamber cardiac view in the third trimester. Ultrasound Obstet Gynecol. 1996;8:309-14.
94. Hepper PG, Shahidullah S. Development of fetal hearing. Arch Dis Child. 1994;71:81-7.
95. Shahidullah S, Hepper PG. Frequency discrimination by the fetus. Early Hum Dev. 1994;36:13-26.
96. Devoe LD, Murray C, Faircloth D, et al. Vibroacoustic stimulation and fetal behavioral state in normal term human pregnancy. Am J Obstet Gynecol. 1990;163:1156-61.
97. Zimmer EZ, Fifer WP, Kim YI, et al. Response of the premature fetus to stimulation by speech sounds. Early Hum Dev. 1993;33:207-15.
98. Brazelton TB, Nugent KT. Neonatal Behavioral Assessment Scale, 3rd edition. Cambridge: Cambridge University Press; 1995.
99. Peck JE. Development of hearing III. Postnatal development. J Am Acad Audiol. 1995;6:113-23.
100. Sohmer H, Feinmesser M. Cochlear action potentials recorded from the external ear in man. Ann Otol Rhinol Laryngol. 1967;76:427-35.
101. Jewett DI, Romano MN, Williston JS. Human auditory evoked potentials: Possible brain stem components detected on the scalp. Science. 1970;167:1517-8.
102. Despland PA, Galambos R. The auditory brain stem response (ABR): A useful diagnostic tool in the intensive care nursery. Pediatr Res. 1980;15:154-8.
103. Starr A, Achor IJ. Auditory brain stem responses in neurological disease. Arch Neurol. 1975;32:761-6.
104. Martin WH, Schwegler JW, Gleeson AL, et al. New techniques of hearing assessment. Otolaryngol Clin North Am. 1994;27:487-510.
105. Galambos R, Wilson MJ, Silva PD. Identifying hearing loss in the intensive care nursery: A 20-year summary. J Am Acad Audiol. 1994;5:151-6.
106. Hecox KE. Neurologic application of the auditory brainstem response to the pediatric age group. In: Jacobson JE (Ed). The Auditory Brain Stem Response. San Diego: College Hill Press; 1985. pp. 287-95.
107. Kemp DT. Stimulated acoustic emissions from within the human auditory system. J Acoust Soc Am. 1978; 64:1386-91.
108. Eisenberg R. Auditory Competence in Early Life. Baltimore: University Park Press; 1976.
109. Eisenberg RB. Auditory behavior in the human neonate I. Methodological problems and the logical design of research procedures. J Audiol Res. 1965;5:159-77.
110. Eisenberg RB. Auditory behavior in the human neonate. Functional properties of sound and their ontogenetic implications. Int Audiol. 1969;9:34-45.
111. Muir DW. The development of infants' auditory spatial sensitivity. In: Trehub SE, Schneider BS (Eds). Auditory Development in Infancy. New York: Plenum; 1985. pp. 51-83.
112. Tucker SM, Bhatacharia J. Screening of hearing impairments in the newborn using the auditory reponse cradle. Arch Dis Child. 1992;67:911-9.
113. Olsho LW, Koch EG, Halpin CR, et al. An observer based psychoacoustic procedure for use with young infants. Dev Psychol. 1987;23:627-40.
114. Werner LA, Gillenwater JM. Pure-tone sensitivity of 2–5 week old infants. Infant Behav Dev. 1990;13:355-75.
115. Jeffrey WE, Cohen LB. Habituation in the human infant. Adv Child Dev Behav. 1971;6:63-97.
116. De Caspar AJ, Fifer WP. Of human bonding: newborns prefer their mothers' voices. Science. 1980;208:1174-6.
117. Mehler J, Jusczyk PW, Lambertz G, et al. A precursor of language acquisition in young infants. Cognition. 1988;29:143-78.
118. Spence MJ, de Caspar AJ. Prenatal experience with low frequency maternal voice sounds influence neonatal perception of maternal voice samples. Infant Behav Dev. 1987;10:133-42.
119. Sallenbach WB. A theoretical framework on prenatal cognition and bonding. Int J Prenat Perinat Stud. 1991;3:273-81.
120. Zuckerman B, Bauchner H, Parker S, et al. Maternal depressive symptoms during pregnancy and newborn irritability. J Dev Behav Pediatr. 1990;11:190-4.
121. Fisch L. The probability of response to test sounds in young children. Sound. 1971;5:7-10.
122. Ryder GH. Vagitus uterinus. Am J Obstet Gynecol. 1943;46:867-72.
123. Russell PM. Vagitus uterinus: crying in utero. Lancet. 1957;1:137-8.
124. Blair RG. Vagitus uterinus: crying in utero. Lancet 1965;2:1164-5.
125. Mende W, Wermke K, Schindler S, et al. Variability of the cry melody and the melody spectrum as indicators for certain CNS disorders. Early Child Dev Care. 1990;65:96-107.

126. Wermke K, Mende W, Borschberg H, et al. Voice characteristics of prespeech vocalizations of twins during the first year of life. In: Powell TW (Ed). Pathologies of Speech and Language. New Orleans: ICPLA Publication of the International Clinical Phonetics and Linguistics Association; 1996. pp. 1-7.

127. Truby HM, Lind J. Cry motions of the newborn infant. Acta Pediatr Scand. 1965;163(Suppl):61-92.

128. Truby HM. Prenatal and neonatal speech, pre-speech and an infantile speech lexicon. Child Language. 1975;27:1-3.

129. Condon WS, Sander WE. Neonate movement is synchronized with adult speech: interactional participation and language acquisition. *Science*. 1974;183:99-101.

130. Werker JF. Becoming a native listener. Am Scient. 1989;77:54-9.

131. Kuhl PK, Williams KA, Lacerda F, et al. Linguistic experience alters phonetic perception in infants by 6 months of age. Science. 1992;225:606-8.

132. Fernald A. Human maternal vocalizations to infants as biologically relevant signals: An evolutionary perspective. In: Barkow HJ, Cosmides L, Toby J (Eds). The Adapted Mind: Evolutionary Psychology and the Generation of Culture. New York: Oxford University Press; 1992. pp. 391-428.

133. Fridman R. Proto-rhythms: music in prenatal and postnatal life. In: Blum T (Ed). Prenatal Perception, Learning and Bonding. Berlin: Leonardo Publishers, 1993. pp. 247-52.

134. Roederer JG. The search for a survival value of music. Music Perception. 1984;1:350-6.

135. Arabin B. Music during pregnancy. Ultrasound Obstet Gynecol. 2002;20:425-30.

136. Natale R, Clelow F, Dawes GS. Measurement of fetal forelimb movements in lambs in utero. Am J Obstet Gynecol. 1981;140: 545-51.

137. Cohn HE, Sacks EJ, Heyman MA, et al. Cardiovascular responses to hypoxemia and acidemia in fetal lambs. Am J Obstet Gynecol. 1974;120:817-24.

138. Manning FA, Platt DA, Sipos L. Antenatal fetal evaluation. Development of a fetal biophysical profile. Am J Obstet Gynecol. 1980;136:787-95.

139. Wladimiroff JW, Wijngaard JA, Degani S, et al. Cerebral and umbilical blood flow velocity waveform in normal and growth-retarded pregnancies. Obstet Gynecol. 1987;69:705-9.

140. Arabin B, Bergmann PL, Saling E. Simultaneous assessment of blood flow velocity waveforms in uteroplacental vessels, the umbilical artery, the fetal aorta and the fetal common carotid artery. Fetal Diagn Ther. 1987;2:17-26.

141. Bilardo CM, Nicolaides KH, Campbell S. Doppler measurements of fetal uteroplacental circulations. Relationship with umbilical venous blood gases measured at cordocentesis. Am J Obstet Gynecol. 1990;162:115-20.

142. Visser GH, Sadovsky G, Nicolaides KH. Antepartum heart rate patterns in small-for-gestational age third trimester fetuses. Correlations with blood gas values obtained at cordocentesis. Am J Obstet Gynecol. 1990; 62:698-703.

143. Arabin B, Rüttgers H, Lorenz U, et al. Course and predictive value of heart rate parameters from the 27th to the 42nd week of gestation. Am J Perinatol. 1989;5: 272-7.

144. Read JA, Miller FC. Fetal heart rate acceleration in response to acoustic stimulation as a measure of fetal well-being. Am J Obstet Gynecol. 1977;149: 512-17.

145. Smith CV, Phelan JP, Platt LD, et al. Fetal acoustic stimulation testing II. A randomized clinical comparison with non-stress test. Am J Obstet Gynecol. 1986;155:131-4.

146. Pietrantoni M, Angel JL, Parsons MT, et al. Human fetal response to vibroacoustic stimulation as a function of stimulus duration. Obstet Gynecol. 1991;78:807-11.

147. Zimmer EZ, Divon MY. Fetal vibroacoustic stimulation. Obstet Gynecol. 1993;81:451-7.

148. Gagnon R, Hunse C, Carmichael L, et al. Vibratory acoustic stimulation in 26- to 32-week, small-forgestational-age fetus. Am J Obstet Gynecol. 1989;160:160-5.

149. Inglis SR, Druzin ML, Wagner WE, et al. The use of vibroacoustic stimulation during the abnormal or equivocal biophysical profile. Obstet Gynecol. 1993;82:371-4.

150. Trudinger MB, Boylan P. Antepartum fetal heart rate monitoring: Value of sound stimulation. Obstet Gynecol. 1980;55:263-8.

151. Jensen OH. Fetal heart rate response to a controlled sound stimulation as a measure of fetal well-being. Acta Obstet Gyneco Scand. 1984;63:97-101.

152. Schiff E, Lipitz S, Sivan E, et al. Acoustic stimulation as a diagnostic test: Comparison with oxytocin challenge test. J Perinat Med. 1992;20: 275-9.

153. Arabin B, Becker R, Entezami M, et al. Prediction of fetal distress and poor outcome combined with intrauterine growth retardation using FHR monitoring and Doppler ultrasound. Fetal Diagn Ther. 1993;8:234-40.

154. Arabin B, Becker R, Mohnhaupt A, et al. Prediction of fetal distress and poor outcome combined with prolonged pregnancy using FHR and Doppler monitoring. Fetal Diagn Ther. 1994;9:1-6.

155. Smith CV, Phelan JP, Nguyen HN. Continuing experience with the fetal acoustic stimulation test. J Reprod Med. 1988;33:365-8.

156. Clark SL, Sabey P, Jolley K. Nonstress testing with acoustic stimulation and amniotic fluid volume assessment. Am J Obstet Gynecol. 1989;160:694-7.

157. Richards DS. The fetal vibroacoustic stimulation test: An update. Semin Perinatol. 1990;14:305-10.

158. Fisk NM, Nicolaidis PK, Arulkumaran S, et al. Vibroacoustic stimulation is not associated with sudden fetal catecholamine release. Early Hum Dev. 1991;25:11-7.

159. Zimmer EZ, Talmon R, Makler-Shiran E, et al. Effect of vibroacoustic stimulation on fetal meconium passage in labor. Am J Perinatol. 1996;13:81-3.

160. Gagnon R, Benzaquen S, Hunse C. The fetal sound environment during vibroacoustic stimulation in labor: effect on fetal heart rate response. Obstet Gynecol. 1992;79:950-5.

161. Sarno AP, Ahn MO, Phelan JP, et al. Fetal acoustic stimulation in the early intrapartum period as a predictor of subsequent fetal condition. Am J Obstet Gynecol. 1990;162:762-7.

162. Ingemarsson I, Arulkumaran S. Reactive fetal heart rate response to vibroacoustic stimulation in fetuses with low scalp blood pH. Br J Obstet Gynecol. 1989;96:562-5.

163. Umstad M, Bailey C, Permezel M. Intrapartum fetal stimulation testing. Aust NZ J Obstet Gynecol. 1992;32:222-4.

164. Anyaegbunam AM, Ditchik A, Stoical R, et al. Vibroacoustic stimulation of the fetus entering the second stage of labor. Obstet Gynecol. 1994;83:963-6.

165. Irion O, Stuckelberger P, Moutquin JM, et al. Is intrapartum vibratory acoustic stimulation a valid alternative to scalp pH determination? Br J Obstet Gynecol. 1996;103:642-7.

166. Wladimiroff JW, Cheung K. Vibratory acoustic stimulation and the flow velocity waveform in the fetal internal carotid artery. Early Hum Dev. 1989;19:61-6.

167. Barford D. Fetal death from sepsis following a reassuring intrapartum fetal acoustic stimulation test [Letter]. Obstet Gynecol. 1990;75:307-8.

168. Petrikovsky BM, Schifrin B, Diana L. The effect of fetal acoustic stimulation on fetal swallowing and amniotic fluid index. Obstet Gynecol. 1993;81:548-50.

169. Zimmer EZ, Chao CR, Guy GP, et al. Vibroacoustic stimulation evokes human fetal micturition. Obstet Gynecol. 1993;81:178-80.

170. Sherer DM, Abramowicz JS, Hearn-Stebbins B, et al. Sonographic verification of a nuchal cord following VAS-induced severe variable FHR decelerations with abdominal delivery. Am J Perinatol. 1991;8:345-6.

171. Romero R, Mazor M, Hobbins HJ. A critical appraisal of fetal acoustic stimulations as an antenatal test for fetal well-being. Obstet Gynecol. 1988;71:781-6.

172. Elliott LL, Armbruster VB. Some possible effects of the delay of early treatment of deafness. J Speech Hear Res. 1967;10:209-24.

173. Bebout JM. Pediatric hearing aid fitting: A practical overview. Hear J. 1989;42:13-5.

174. Curnock DA. Identifying hearing impairment in infants and young children. Br Med J. 1993;307:1225-6.

175. Veen S, Sassen ML, Schreuder AM, et al. Hearing loss in very preterm and very low birth weight infants at the age of 5 years in a nationwide cohort. Int J Pediatr Otorhinolaryngol. 1993;26:11-28.

176. Yoshinaga-Itano C, Sedey AL, Coulter DK, et al. Language of early- and later-identified children with hearing loss. Pediatrics. 1998;102:1161-71.

177. Robertson C, Aldridge S, Jarman F, et al. Late diagnosis of congenital sensorineural hearing impairment: Why are detection methods failing? Arch Dis Child. 1995;72:11-5.

178. Mauk GW, White KR, Mortensen LB, et al. The effectiveness of screening programs based on high-risk characteristics in early intervention of hearing impairment. Ear Hear. 1991;12:312-9.

179. Joint Committee on Infant Hearing. Year 2000 Position Statement: Principles and Guidelines for Early Hearing Detection and Intervention Programs. Am J Audiol. 2000;9:9-29.

180. Oudesluys-Murphy AM, van Straaten HL, Bholasingh R, et al. Neonatal hearing screening. Eur J Pediatr. 1996;155:429-35.

181. Jacobson JT, Jacobson CA, Spahr RC. Automated and conventional ABR screening technics in high-risk infants. J Am Acad Audiol. 1990;1:187-95.

182. Cox LC. The current status of auditory brainstem response testing in neonatal populations. Pediatr Res. 1984;18:780-3.

183. Peters JG. An automated infant screener using advanced evoked response technology. Hearing J. 1986;9:1-4.

184. Herrmann BS, Thornton AR, Jospeh JM. Automated infant hearing screening using the ABR: Development and validation. Am J Audiol. 1995;4:6-14.

185. Van Straaten HL, Hille ET, Kok JH, et al. Dutch NICU Neonatal Hearing Screening Working Group. Implementation of a nation-wide automated auditory brainstem response hearing screening program in neonatal intensive care units. Acta Pediatr. 2003;92: 332-8.

186. Hall JW, Lamb MM, Freeman SD, et al. Infant hearing screening with automated ABR in the NICU. Presented at XXIII International Congress of Audiology, Bari, Italy, 1996.

187. Vohr BR, Maxon AB. Screening infants for hearing impairment. J Pediatr. 1996;128:710-4.

188. Kennedy CR, Kimm L, Cafarelli Dees D, et al. Otoacoustic emissions and auditory brainstem responses in the newborn. Arch Dis Child. 1991;66:1124-9.

189. Stevens JC, Webb HD, Hutchins J, et al. Click evoked otoacoustic emissions in neonatal screening. Ear Hear. 1990;11:128-33.

190. Baldwin M, Watkin P. The clinical application of otoacoustic emissions in pediatric audiological assessment. J Laryngol Otol. 1992;106:301-6.

191. Kok MR, Zanten GA, van Brocaar MP, et al. Click-evoked oto-acoustic emissions in very-low-birthweight infants: A cross-sectional data analysis. Audiology. 1994;33:152-64.

192. Doyle KJ, Sininger Y, Starr A. Auditory neuropathy in childhood. Laryngoscope. 1998;108:1374-7.

193. Prager DA, Stone DA, Rose DN. Hearing loss screening in the neonatal intensive care unit: auditory brainstem response versus Crib-O-Gram; a cost effectiveness analysis. Ear Hear. 1987;8:213-16.

194. Zahr LK, de Traversay J. Premature infant responses to noise reduction by earmuffs: effects on behavioral and physiologic measures. J Perinatol. 1995;15:448-55.

195. Sininger Y. Pediatric auditory research projects. Available at http://www.hei.org/pneonat.htm 1996.

196. Nyman M, Barr M, Westgren M. A four-year follow-up of hearing and development in children exposed in utero to vibro-acoustic stimulation. Br J Obstet Gynecol. 1992;99:685-8.

197. Arulkumaran S, Skurr B, Tong H, et al. No evidence of hearing loss due to fetal acoustic stimulation test. Obstet Gynecol. 1991;78:283-5.

198. Moss N, Carver D. Pregnant women at work. Am J Indust Med. 1992;23:1-7.

199. Pierson LL. Hazards of noise exposure on fetal hearing. Semin Perinatol. 1996;20:21-9.

200. Griffiths SK, Pierson LL, Gerhardt KJ, et al. Noise induced hearing loss in fetal sheep. Hear Res. 1994;74:221-30.

201. Joint Committee on Infant Hearing Position Statement. ASHA. 1982;24:1017.

202. Wakai RT, Leuthold AC, Martin CB. Fetal auditory evoked responses detected by magnetoencephalography. Am J Obstet Gynecol. 1996;174:1484-6.

203. Reite M, Scheuneman D, Gilger JW, et al. Auditory magnetic source localization in twins. Brain Res Bull. 1992;28:641-4.

204. Manrique B, Contasi M, Avarado MA, et al. Nurturing parents to stimulate their children from prenatal stage to three years of age. In: Blum T (Ed). Prenatal Perception, Learning and Bonding. Berlin: Leonardo Publishers; 1993. pp. 153-86.

205. Zimmer EZ, Divon MY, Vilensky A, et al. Maternal exposure to music and fetal activity. Eur J Obstet Gynecol Reprod Biol. 1982;13: 209-13.

206. De Caspar AJ, Sigafoos AD. The intrauterine heartbeat: A potent reinforcer. Infant Behav Dev. 1983;6:19-23.

207. Thoman EB, Ingersoll EW, Acebo C. Premature infants seek rhythmic stimulation and the experience facilitates neurobehavioral development. J Dev Behav Paediatr. 1991;12:11-8.

208. Downs MP. Universal newborn hearing screening. Int J Pediatr Otorhinolaryngol. 1995;32:257-60.

209. Maxon AB, White KR, Behrens TR, et al. Referral rates and cost efficiency in a universal newborn hearing screening program using transient evoked otoacoustic emissions. J Am Acad Audiol. 1995;6:271-7.

86 Fetal Responses to Placental Insufficiency

ML Kush, AA Baschat

INTRODUCTION

The placenta forms the interface for nutrient, fluid and gas exchange between mother and fetus. Successful placental development is of critical importance as it is permissive for the normal development of an individual. While the fetal growth potential is genetically predetermined[1] the ultimate neonatal weight, proportions and condition at birth are dependent on placental development, fetal health and maternal health. Normal placentation of a genetically normal fetus in a healthy mother is therefore most likely to end in fulfillment of the growth potential. However, if any of these factors is deficient a number of fetal and maternal adverse outcomes may be the consequence. Of these placental insufficiency is of particular interest because it may lead to fetal growth restriction (IUGR), a condition that is associated with an increased risk for adverse health events that manifest in fetal life and extend all the way into adult life.[2-6] There are several conditions, which are associated with fetal growth restriction (Fig. 86.1). Of these, placental vascular insufficiency is clinically the most relevant since it is most prevalent and potentially derives a benefit from intervention.

Because of its diverse impacts placental disease has been a constant research focus for decades. However, it is the multidisciplinary approach of multiple medical subspecialties that has elevated our level of understanding to a point where the diverse impacts of placental dysfunction on fetal health are being appreciated. While traditional antenatal surveillance examines a relatively narrow spectrum of fetal responses, utilization of more sophisticated research tools has uncovered responses in almost every organ system. Before expanding on these multiple effects of placental insufficiency an understanding of the normal maturational process of the placenta and fetus is essential.

Placental Development

Fetal growth is regulated at multiple levels, and requires successful placentation for the coordination of key components in the maternal, placental and fetal compartments for adequate maternal-fetal exchange throughout gestation. Successful placental adherence in the first trimester initiates a series of important milestones in the three overlapping gestational epochs. First trimester initiation of placental vascular development permits nutrient and oxygen delivery to the growing trophoblast beyond the capacity of simple diffusion. Maternal adaptations to pregnancy predominate in this epoch. Differentiation of placental transport mechanisms and paracrine and endocrine signaling pathways between the mother, placenta and fetus then continue throughout the second trimester. Successful initiation of these steps allows placental growth and establishment of efficient and coordinated nutrient transfer, waste and gas exchange by the second trimester. This is a prerequisite for exponential fetal growth and differentiation in the third trimester in preparation for extrauterine life.

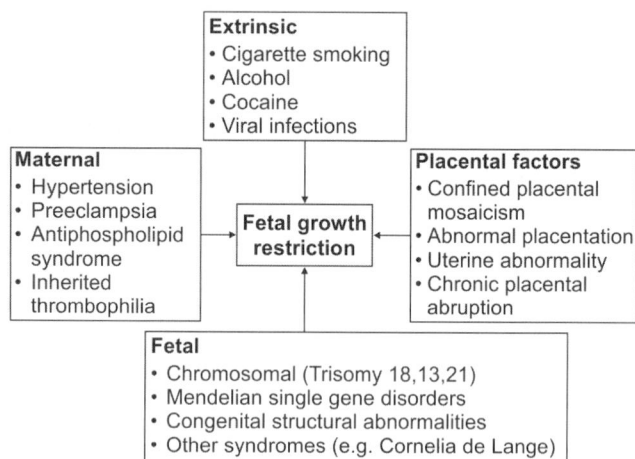

Fig. 86.1: The principal causes and most common conditions that are associated with fetal growth restriction

Following fertilization, the cytotrophoblast migrates to form anchoring sites through controlled breakdown of the extracellular matrix by metalloproteinases and localized expression of adhesion molecules. Placental adherence between the decidua and uterus is established by the formation of these anchoring villi that connect the decidua and uterus. Angiogenesis produces vascular connections to the maternal circulation that establishes maternal blood supply to the intervillous space. This high level of nutrient and oxygen supply is required to support the growing embryo and trophoblast.[7,8] With this nutritional and vascular support in place, the villous trophoblast, consisting of a maternal microvillous and fetal basal layer, is formed.[9] Increasing placental synthetic activity is now sufficiently supported and results in the appearance of several secretory substances in the maternal circulation (e.g. human chorionic gonadotrophin and placental lactogen). Some of these substances promote postprandial hyperglycemia, increased fasting levels of free fatty acids, triglycerides and cholesterol, fat deposition, maternal intravascular volume expansion and relative refractoriness to vasoactive agents. These maternal adaptations increase substrate availability and steadiness of nutrient delivery to the placenta and are permissive for ongoing placental development.[10] Several paracrine signaling substances also appear in the placenta (e.g. nitric oxide, endothelin) and active cellular transport systems for major nutrient classes (glucose, amino acids and fatty acids) differentiate. Initiation of fetal cardiac activity allows for the active distribution of nutrients between fetus and placenta, and completes the functionality of the feto-placental unit.[11] Ongoing development in the maternal and fetal compartments results in the formation of the villous trophoblast that consists of a maternal microvillous and fetal basal layer, and is the primary site of exchange. The efficiency of maternal-fetal exchange depends on four principal factors: (1) the thickness that has to be traversed by diffusible substances; (2)

the vascular throughput from the maternal and fetal circulations; (3) the surface area available for exchange; and (4) the elaboration of active transport mechanisms.

By the 16th week the villous trophoblast has progressively thinned down to 4 μ providing little resistance to diffusion. Vascular throughput through the placenta increases in both vascular compartments. Extravillous cytotrophoblast infiltration of the maternal spiral arteries results in progressive loss of the musculoelastic media, first in the decidual, then in the myometrial portion of these vessels.[12] This process is paralleled in the fetal compartment by continuous villous vascular branching.[13] Significant reduction in vascular resistance and a rapid increase in the exchange area are achieved by 26 weeks and then continue at a slower rate toward term. Through concurrent increases in fetal cardiac output, villous blood flow increases exponentially through the third trimester.[9,11] Under normal circumstances in the term placenta up to 600 mL/min of maternal cardiac output are delivered to an exchange area of up to 12 m[2]. In the fetal compartment this is matched with a blood flow volume of 200–300 mL/kg/min throughout gestation.[9,14,15] This magnitude of maternal blood flow is necessary since maintenance of placental function is energy intensive and consumes as much as 40% of O_2 and 70% of glucose supplied to the uterus.[16-18] Perfusion matching between the maternal and fetal compartments is further modulated and optimized through placental autoregulation, which is probably mediated through local paracrine factors such as nitric oxide (NO), endothelin, red blood cell (RBC) adenosine or cyclic guanosine monophoshate, and fetal atrial natriuretic peptide (ANP). Optimal fetal growth and development is achieved when nutrient and oxygen delivery is sufficient to allow ideal fetal substrate utilization. This is only possible when the magnitude of maternal nutrient and oxygen delivery to the uterus exceeds placental demands leaving sufficient surplus for the fetus and when perfusion matching between the maternal and fetal compartments is optimized through placental autoregulation. While these developments significantly enhance the efficiency of exchange for diffusible substances other substances such as glucose, amino acids, and fatty acids that cannot efficiently pass this bilayer by simple diffusion require additional elaboration of active transport mechanisms.

Transplacental transport systems optimize the transfer of glucose, amino acids and fatty acids.[19-21] Transmembrane ion pumps such as the Na/H+ pump also develop, maintaining cellular homeostasis and normal cellular function.[22] Each of the nutrient classes has different roles in the fetus. Glucose is the primary oxidative fuel while amino acids are incorporated into proteins. Fetal glucose and amino acids are the primary stimulants of insulin-like growth factors (IGF) I and II, and therefore stimulate longitudinal growth and differentiation.[23] Amino acids as major contributors to protein synthesis are also laid down as muscle bulk.[24] Fatty acids are precursors for bioactive compounds (including prostaglandins, thromboxanes, leukotrienes) and are also necessary for maintenance of cell membrane fluidity and permeability. In addition, long chain polyunsaturated fatty acids such as arachidionic and docosahexanoic acid are essential for normal brain and retinal development. Leptin coregulates transplacental amino acid and fatty acid transport and thereby modulates fetal body fat content and proportions.[25,26] With advancing gestation the magnitude and efficiency of transfer of these substances increases significantly to provide for placental and fetal growth requirements (Fig. 86.2).

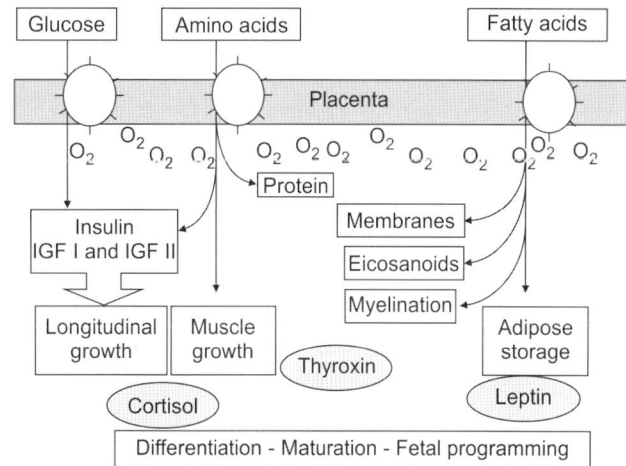

Fig. 86.2: In the presence of adequate oxygenation normal functioning of transplacental transport mechanisms for glucose, amino acids and fatty acids ensure availability of substrate for the fetus. Glucose and amino acids are the main stimulants of the insulin, IGF growth axis and stimulate longitudinal fetal growth. In addition amino acids are utilized for protein synthesis and contribute to muscle bulk. Fatty acids have roles at many levels serving as precursors for eicosanoids, and structural components of cell membranes and myelin sheaths. In the third trimester accumulation of adipose stores provides a reservoir for essential fatty acids. Endocrine axes—including hormones such as cortisol, thyroxin and leptin—modulate fetal maturation and differentiation according to substrate availability and may have significant impacts on adult life through fetal programming

Concurrent development of the fetal circulation as a conduit for nutrient and waste delivery is an important co-factor in the fetal growth process. With establishment of a functional circulation, nutrient and oxygen rich blood from the primitive villous circulation enter the fetus via the umbilical vein. The arrangement of the fetal circulation allows further preferential streaming of these nutrients. The ductus venosus is the first vascular conduit encountered. Through modulations in shunting through the ductus venosus, 68–82% of umbilical venous blood continues to the liver, while the remainder is distributed to the heart.[27] Differential directionality of blood streams entering the right atrium ensures that nutrient rich blood is distributed to the left ventricle, myocardium and brain, while low-nutrient venous return is distributed to the placenta for re-oxygenation, and nutrient and waste exchange.[28] In addition to this overall distribution of left and right-sided cardiac output, several organs can modify local blood flow to meet oxygen and nutrient demands by autoregulation.[29]

With achievement of these milestones the prerequisites for normal placental and fetal growth are met. The metabolic and vascular status of the mother promotes a steady and enhanced nutrient delivery to the uterus, and placental transport mechanisms allow for efficient bidirectional exchange of nutrient and waste. Under these circumstances placental and fetal growth remain closely related throughout gestation.[30] Their growth process across the three trimesters is characterized by sequential cellular hyperplasia, hyperplasia plus hypertrophy, and lastly hypertrophy alone. Placental growth follows a sigmoid curve that plateaus in midgestation preceding exponential third trimester growth of the fetus.[31,32]

During this exponential fetal growth phase of 1.5% per day initial weight gain is due to longitudinal growth and muscle bulk, and therefore correlates with glucose and amino acid transport. Throughout gestation essential fatty acids are deposited in the developing brain and retina, and account for up to 50% of dry brain weight.[33] After 20 weeks of gestation a notable increase in fatty acid transport and utilization initiate the deposition of significant fetal adipose tissue. From 24 weeks onward exponential fetal growth and adipose tissue deposition coincide with increasing conversion of glucose into fat, as well as increased utilization of fatty acids.[33,34] From 32 weeks to term fat stores increase from 3.2% of fetal body weight to 16% accounting for the significant reduction in body water content.[35,36] Throughout gestation relative serum concentrations of free fatty acids remain related to maternal dietary intake. However, enhanced transplacental transport of essential polyunsaturated fatty acids and especially their storage in adipose tissue occurs during the period of exponential fetal growth. Therefore third trimester increase in fetal size is characterized by longitudinal growth accompanied by accumulation of essential body stores in preparation for extrauterine life.

MECHANISMS OF PLACENTAL INSUFFICIENCY

The mechanisms by which various diseases affect placental function are the subject of much inquiry. In maternal hypertensive disorders, increased syncytial knot formation indicates premature placental aging and apoptosis. Occlusive vasculopathy affects both the maternal and fetal circulatory compartments of the placenta, and is most pronounced in antiphospholipid syndromes. Fetal causes may exert their effects on growth at multiple levels. Placental causes may result in decreased placental blood flow and/or altered transport mechanisms with resultant abnormal placental cellular homeostasis.

The majority of IUGR pregnancies are the result of conditions that interfere with placental vascular development.[37] Depending on the gestational age and on the extent of interference with placental development, various clinical scenarios may occur within the maternal, placental and fetal compartments. If interference with angiogenesis occurs early in the first trimester, successful placental adherence is unlikely to transpire and will likely result in miscarriage. If sufficient supply to the placenta can be established and maintained despite suboptimal vascular development, further placental differentiation is possible. However, suboptimal maternal pregnancy adaptation and deficient nutrient delivery pose limitations to placental metabolic and synthetic activity, which ultimately interfere with the differentiation of endocrine feedback loops and active transport mechanisms. If the trophoblast invasion remains confined to the decidual portion of the myometrium maternal spiral and radial arteries fail to undergo the physiologic transformation into low resistance vessels.[38,39] Altered expression of vasoactive substances may increase vascular reactivity, and if hypoxia stimulated angiogenesis cannot overcome these challenges, placental autoregulation becomes deficient. Eventually loss of this placental autoregulation promotes vascular occlusion, infarction and permanent structural damage.[40] Maternal placental floor infarcts, fetal villous obliteration and fibrosis both increase placental blood flow resistance, producing maternal-fetal placental perfusion mismatch that decreases the effective exchange area.[40-43] With progressive vascular occlusion feto-placental flow resistance is increased throughout the vascular bed and eventually the metabolically active placental mass is reduced. If adaptive mechanisms permit ongoing fetal survival early onset growth restriction with its many fetal manifestations develops.

The balance of compensatory and decompensatory responses determines the spectrum and degree of fetal manifestations in various organ systems. If compensatory mechanisms are unsuccessful, permanent fetal damage or stillbirth results. With successful compensation, the consequences of nutrient shortage may remain largely subclinical, only to be unmasked through the restrictive effect on exponential fetal growth in the second to third trimester. In these cases, vascular manifestations may be less pronounced and physical characteristics more apparent. A decrease in adipose tissue or abnormal body proportions at birth may be the only indication that placental insufficiency occurred. In addition, a sizeable proportion of subtle third trimester IUGR neonates may escape detection, particularly if population based, rather than customized, weight references are used.[44] An appreciation of the multiple manifestations of placental insufficiency provides the basis for the development of a uniform diagnostic approach to fetuses with suspected IUGR.

Fetal Metabolic Responses

In the setting of mild placental insufficiency, placental glucose and oxygen utilization initially remains unaffected, while fetal demands have to be met by increased fractional extraction. Only when uterine oxygen delivery falls below a critical value (0.6 mmol/min/kg fetal body weight in sheep) is fetal oxygen uptake and glucose transfer reduced.[45] When the levels of glucose transferred to the fetus fall, hypoglycemia ensues which results in a blunting of pancreatic insulin responses and allows gluconeogenesis from hepatic glycogen stores to begin.[46-49] A proportion of fetal glucose and lactate is then redirected to the placenta for nutrition. Since fetal hepatic glycogen stores are minimal, persistent or progressive nutrient scarcity results in worsening fetal hypoglycemia. Subsequently, the ability to maintain fetal oxidative metabolism and placental nutrition becomes limited.

At this point, the downregulation of active placental transport mechanisms and the fetal need to recruit other energy sources, result in widespread metabolic responses. Limitation of amino acid transfer and breakdown of endogenous muscle protein to obtain gluconeogenic amino acids results in depletion of branched chain and other essential amino acids.[50-52] Simultaneously, lactate accumulates due to the limited capacity for oxidative metabolism. The placental transfer capacity for fatty acids remains unaltered, unless there is a considerable loss of placental substance. However, despite maintaining the ability to transfer fatty acids, the selectivity of the transport mechanisms, especially for essential fatty acids, may decline. In the fetal circulation, free fatty acid and triglyceride levels increase secondary to reduced fetal utilization, which results in a failure to accumulate adipose stores. In this setting of advanced malnutrition, the liver metabolizes the majority of accumulating lactate. However, the fetal brain and heart can switch their primary nutrient source from glucose to lactate and ketones[53]—cardiac metabolism has the capacity to remove up to 80% of the circulating lactate.[54,55] Acid-base balance can be maintained as long as acid production is met by sufficient buffering capacity of fetal hemoglobin and a matching removal rate by these organs.

Table 86.1: Summary of metabolic responses to placental insufficiency

Substrate	Change
Glucose	Decreased proportional to the degree of fetal hypoxemia
Amino acids	Significant decrease in branched chain amino acids (valine, leucine, isoleucine) as well as lysine and serine. In contrast hydro-xyproline is elevated. The decrease in essential amino acids is proportional to the degree of hypoxemia. Elevated amniotic fluid glycine to valine ratio. Elevations in amniotic fluid ammonia with a significant positive correlation to the ponderal index.
Fatty acids and triglycerides	Decrease in long chain polyunsaturated fatty acids (docosahexanoic and arachidionic acid). Decrease in overall fatty acid transfer only with significant loss of placental substance. Hypertriglyceridemia due to decreased utilization. Lower cholesterol esters.
Oxygen and CO_2	Degree of hypoxemia proportional to villous damage and correlates significantly with hypercapnia, acidemia and hypoglycemia and hyperlacticemia.

These increasing degrees of metabolic compromise have been documented through cordocentesis in human fetuses. Hypoglycemia and hypoxemia with decreased levels of essential amino acids occurs first. As the placental dysfunction worsens, progressive hypoxemia and increasing lactate production are exponentially correlated to the degree of acidemia. Overt hypoaminoacidemia, hypercapnia, hyperlacticemia and triglyceridemia accompany the development of acidemia.[52,56-58]

Amniotic fluid elevation of the glycine/valine ratio and ammonia levels are additional indicators of this state of protein energy malnutrition (Table 86.1).[59,60] This degree of metabolic deterioration is associated with elevated transaminases as evidence of hepatic dysfunction, and may be precipitated by a significant decline of hepatic blood flow as a result of excessive shunting at the level of the ductus venosus.[61,62] Fetuses that manifest growth restriction early in gestation are more likely to have greater and broader metabolic derangements as compared to fetuses that manifest growth restriction in the third trimester, which are more likely to have less severe metabolic and acid-base disturbance and only subtle changes in lipid metabolism.[63]

FETAL ENDOCRINE RESPONSES

The immediate effect of decreased fetal glucose and amino acid levels is the downregulation of the principal endocrine growth axis involving insulin, IGF I, IGF II and transforming factor beta.[64,65] This may be further exacerbated by pancreatic cellular dysfunction that is evident through a decreased insulin/glucose ratio and impaired fetal glucose tolerance.[52,66] Elevations in serum glucagon and stimulation of the fetal adrenal axis promote the mobilization of hepatic glycogen stores and peripheral gluconeogenesis.[67] Corticotropin releasing hormone (CRH), adrenocorticotrophic hormone (ACTH) and cortisol levels are significantly elevated relating both to the level of hypoglycemia and the degree of placental vascular compromise.[52,68,69] However, elevations of cortisol downregulate IGF I activity and may therefore have additional negative impacts on linear growth as well as the potential to limit the capacity for postpartum catch-up growth.[70,71] In addition to the glucocorticoid axis significant elevations of adrenaline and noradrenaline levels are also found in IUGR fetuses, while aldosterone levels appear unchanged.[72-74]

Disturbances at all stages of thyroid function have been documented in IUGR fetuses and correlate with the degree of hypoxemia.[75,76] Glandular dysfunction, as denoted by low levels of thyroxine and T3 despite elevated thyroid stimulating hormone (TSH) levels, may develop. In other cases, central production of TSH may be responsible for fetal hypothyroidism.[77] Finally, downregulation of thyroid hormone receptors may limit the biologic activity of circulating thyroid hormones in specific target tissues such as the developing brain.[78]

IUGR fetuses also show evidence of disturbed endocrine regulation of bone formation. Serum levels of active vitamin D and osteocalcin are appreciably decreased and may be responsible for decreased bone mineralization as well as decreased bone growth.[79,80]

Hematologic Responses

Erythropoietin release and stimulation of red blood cell production, through both medullary and extramedullary sites, is triggered by fetal hypoxemia and results in polycythemia.[81-84] Extramedullary hematopoiesis may be physiologic until 28 weeks, but can occur in older fetuses by being induced by prolonged tissue hypoxia and/or acidosis. Extramedullary sites have larger capillary fenestrations that permit the escape of large nucleated red blood cells (NRBC). Thus, elevated NRBC counts correlate with metabolic and cardiovascular status and are independent markers for poor perinatal outcome.[85-88] With advancing compromise complex hematologic abnormalities suggest dysfunctional erythropoiesis. Fetal anemia despite increased NRBC release in conjunction with an overt decrease in red cell progenitors could reflect downregulation of proerythropoietic cytokines, vitamin B12 and ferritin deficiency, or a combination of these.[89-92]

Coinciding with the abnormalities in red cell indices, platelet counts also decrease. Although platelet-activating factor is inhibited,[93] abnormal villous vasculature is indicated by umbilical artery. Absence or reversal of end-diastolic velocities (AREDV) may pose on overwhelming stimulus for placental platelet activation and aggregation.[94] Under these circumstances the incidence of thrombocytopenia increases 10-fold.[95] As the anemia and hypoxemia progress, they become independent risk factors for declining platelet counts.[96] Elevation of whole blood viscosity,[97,98] decrease in red blood cell membrane fluidity[99] and platelet aggregation may be important cofactors for accelerating placental vascular occlusion and progressive dysfunction.

IUGR fetuses also show evidence of immune dysfunction at the cellular and humoral level. Decreases in immunoglobulin and absolute B-cell counts have long been recognized.[100] Reduction in total white blood cell counts and neutrophil, monocyte and lymphocyte subpopulations occur.[101] Selective suppression of T-helper and cytotoxic T-cells has been observed.[102] The extent of these abnormalities is related to the degree of acidemia and can explain the greater susceptibility to infection these fetuses experience as neonates.

Fetal Vascular Responses

Doppler ultrasound allows the assessment of vascular effects of placental dysfunction in the maternal (uterine arteries) and fetal (umbilical arteries) compartments. The presence of an early diastolic notch in the uterine arteries at 12–14 weeks is the earliest evidence of delayed trophoblast invasion of the maternal spiral arteries.[103] When the "notching" persists beyond 24 weeks of gestation, poor trophoblast invasion is almost certain.[39] These findings represent persistent elevated blood flow resistance in the maternal compartment, thus jeopardizing uterine perfusion. In the fetal circulation changes in blood flow are related to placental blood flow resistance, fetal oxygenation, organ autoregulation and vascular reactivity. A reduction of umbilical venous blood flow volume may be the earliest Doppler sign of subtle decreases in fetal villous perfusion.[104] Abnormal villous branching or progressive villous vascular occlusion results in elevated blood flow resistance that is reflected in the umbilical artery waveform. A decrease of the umbilical artery end-diastolic velocity becomes apparent when approximately 30% of the fetal villous vasculature is abnormal.[105] AREDV can occur after 60–70% of the villous vascular tree is damaged.[106] Progression of Doppler abnormalities in the maternal compartment identifies patients at risk for preeclampsia, abruption and IUGR,[107] while abnormal umbilical flow indicate increased risk for hypoxemia and acidemia proportional to the severity of Doppler abnormality (Figs 86.3 and 86.4).[108,109]

Fetal circulatory responses to placental insufficiency can be subdivided into early and late responses corresponding to the degree of fetal compromise.[110,111] These circulatory responses are in part passive and due to the effects of placental afterload on the distribution of cardiac output and in part due to active organ autoregulation. Through modulations in ductus venosus shunting, umbilical venous blood increasingly bypasses the liver and is preferentially directed toward the heart. At the same time, elevated placental blood flow resistance increases right ventricular afterload. Because of the parallel arrangement of the fetal circulation, changes in cardiac afterload determine how this increased blood volume is distributed in the downstream circulation.[112-114] The result is a relative increase in left-sided cardiac output.[113,114] Consequently, blood (and nutrient) supply to the coronary circulation and brain increase. This redistribution of cardiac output can be documented by a decrease in the ratio of Doppler indices in cerebral and umbilical arteries (cerebroplacental Doppler ratio).[115] This redistribution is achieved in two principal ways. First of all, peripheral arterial vasoconstriction in the fetal trunk in conjunction with elevated placental blood flow resistance lead to elevations in thoracic and descending aortic Doppler resistance indices (hind limb reflex) and therefore increased right ventricular afterload.[116,117] Next, cerebral blood flow may be actively enhanced during periods of perceived hypoxemia by a decrease in cerebral blood flow resistance with a subsequent decline in left ventricular afterload. This results in a decrease of the Doppler index in one of the cerebral vessels (brain sparing) (Fig. 86.5).[118,119] Fetuses that show these early Doppler changes are at increased risk for hypoxemia, while the pH is usually maintained in the normal range.[117,119,120] The shifting balance between right and left ventricular afterload accounts for decline of cerebroplacental Doppler index ratio and the measurable decline in end-diastolic velocities in the aortic isthmus.[121,122] At the same time, blood flow resistance in the peripheral pulmonary arteries,[123] celiac axis,[124] mesenteric vessels,[125,126] renal,[127,128] femoral and iliac arteries[129] may become elevated. Individual vital organs

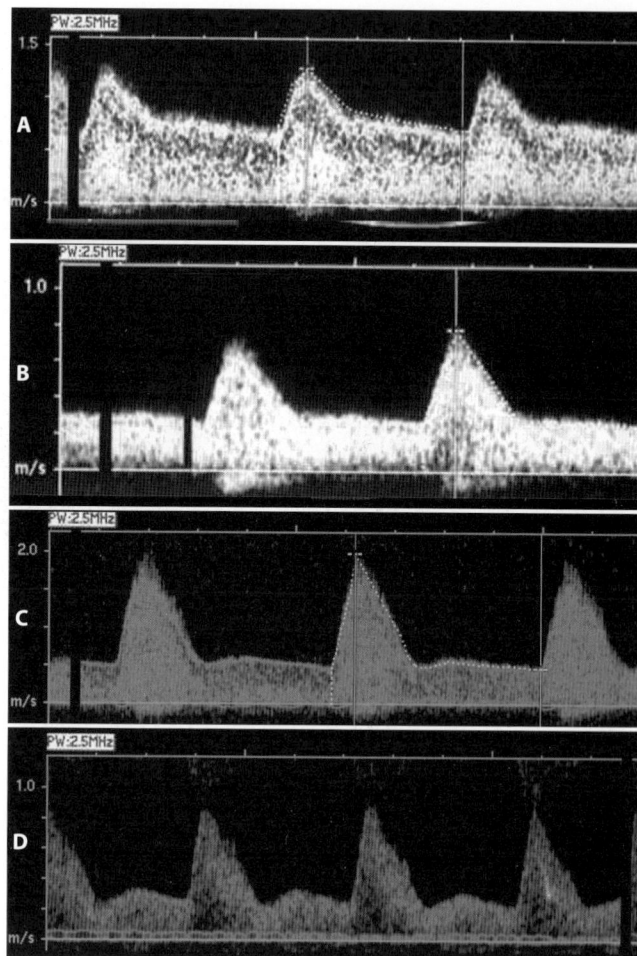

Figs 86.3A to D: Flow velocity waveforms obtained from the uterine artery beyond 24 weeks of gestation. In the first patient (A) high volume diastolic flow is established indicating successful trophoblast invasion. Elevated placental vascular resistance is associated with a decline in diastolic velocities and a subsequent rise in the Doppler index (B). Persistence of an early diastolic notch in the uterine artery flow velocity waveform is evidence of increased spiral artery blood flow resistance. Frequently "notching" is more subtle beyond 32 weeks (C) than in the late second or early third trimesters (D)

such as the adrenal glands[130] and spleen[131] may show evidence of enhanced blood flow. The overall impact of these changes is an improved distribution of well-oxygenated blood to the heart and brain with preferential streaming of descending aortic blood flow to the placenta for re-oxygenation (Table 86.2). These circulatory derangements are associated with elevations of endothelin, vasoactive intestinal peptide, vasopressin and renin-angiotensin levels.[132-134] A decrease of the thromboxane to prostacyclin ratio provides evidence of endothelial dysfunction, while elevations in NO production indicate a compensatory response.[135,136] It is likely that the degree of vascular reactivity is not only responsible for the high complication rate following invasive procedures, but also contributes to the clinical progression by impacting on blood flow resistance in many vascular beds.[137-140]

Late Doppler changes appear with further metabolic deterioration. Under these circumstances declining forward cardiac function, abnormal organ autoregulation and ductus venosus shunting away from the liver occur. The shunting of flow away

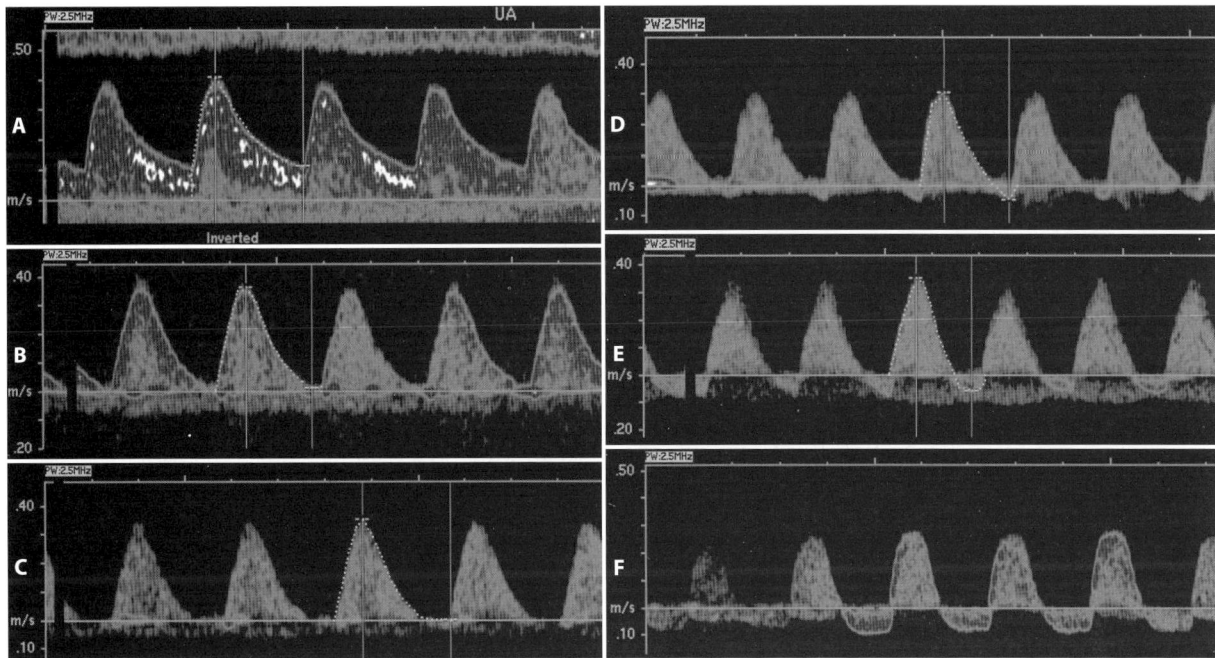

Figs 86.4A to F: The normal umbilical artery flow velocity waveform has marked positive end-diastolic velocity that increases in proportion to systole toward term (A). Moderate abnormalities in the villous vascular structure raise the blood flow resistance and are associated with a decline in end-diastolic velocities (B). When a significant proportion of the villous vascular tree is abnormal (50–70%), end-diastolic velocities may be absent (C) or even reversed (D). Depending on the magnitude of placental blood flow resistance and the fetal cardiac function reversal of end-diastolic velocities may be minimal (D) moderate (E) or severe (F). In the latter case precordial venous flows were universally abnormal

Table 86.2: Summary of fetal vascular responses to placental insufficiency

Response	Features	Doppler evidence
Hind limb reflex	Diversion of blood flow away from the carcass at the expense of the lower body. Achieved through increase in right ventricular afterload proximal to the umbilical arteries as well as increased blood flow resistance distally. In addition to centralization (see below), descending aortic blood flow is also preferentially distributed to the placenta.	Elevation of blood flow resistance in the thoracic aorta and iliac artery
Centralization	A measurable shift in the relationship between right and left ventricular afterload, that results in redistribution of cardiac output in favor of the left ventricle (i.e. the heart and the brain)	Decrease in the cerebroplacental Doppler ratio. Direct measurement of cardiac output. Reversal of end-diastolic velocity in the aortic isthmus. Inferred through absence or reversal of umbilical artery enddiastolic velocity
Brain sparing	Cerebral vasodilatation in response to perceived hypoxemia	Decrease in the carotid or middle cerebral artery Doppler index
Liver sparing	Preferential arterial blood supply to the fetal liver invoked when increased diversion of umbilical venous blood through the ductus venosus jeopardizes hepatic perfusion	Measured dilation of the ductus venosus with elevated Doppler index accompanied by a decreased hepatic artery Doppler index
Adrenal sparing	Enhanced adrenal perfusion is triggered as part of the fetal stress response to chronic or acute-on-chronic malnutrition	Decreased Doppler index in the adrenal artery flow velocity waveforms
Heart sparing	Marked augmentation of coronary blood flow in situations of acute on chronic hypoxemia that is achieved through up-regulation of coronary vascular reserve and vasodilatation	Sudden ability to visualize and measure coronary blood flow in a setting of deteriorating venous Doppler indices in a premature IUGR fetus

from the liver may compromise hepatic perfusion to a degree that interferes with organ function. In this condition, steep elevation in blood lactate and transaminases, as well as sudden compensatory hepatic artery vasodilatation have been reported.[61,62,141] When the increased metabolic demands of cardiac function cannot be met, myocardial dysfunction occurs. Declining cardiac function results in a failure to accommodate venous return and leads to increased venous Doppler indices indicating evidence of increased central venous pressure.[142] The venous flow velocity waveform is triphasic, and therefore more complex than the arterial waveform. It consists of systolic and diastolic peaks (the S- and D-waves) that are generated by the descent of the AV-ring during ventricular systole and passive diastolic ventricular filling, respectively. The sudden increase in right atrial pressure with atrial contraction in late diastole causes a

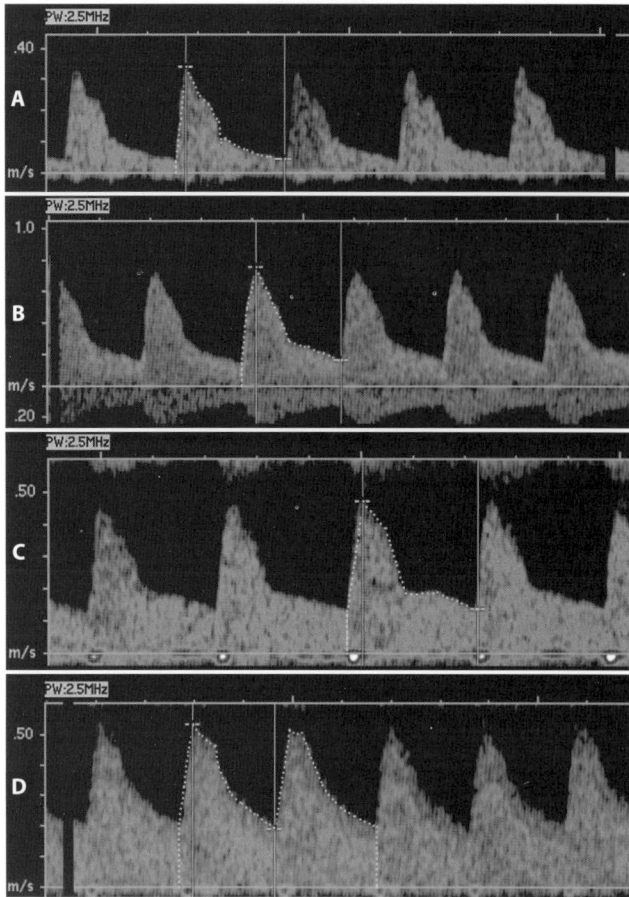

Figs 86.5A to D: The normal middle cerebral artery flow pattern has relatively little diastolic flow (A). With elevation of placental blood flow resistance the changes in the middle cerebral artery waveform may be subtle, although the cerebroplacental ratio may become abnormal (B). With progressive placental dysfunction there may be increase in the diastolic velocity resulting in a decrease in the Doppler index (Brain sparing, C). With marked brain sparing the systolic down slope of the waveform becomes smoother so that the waveform almost resembles that of the umbilical artery (D). The associated rise in the mean velocity results in a marked decline in the Doppler index

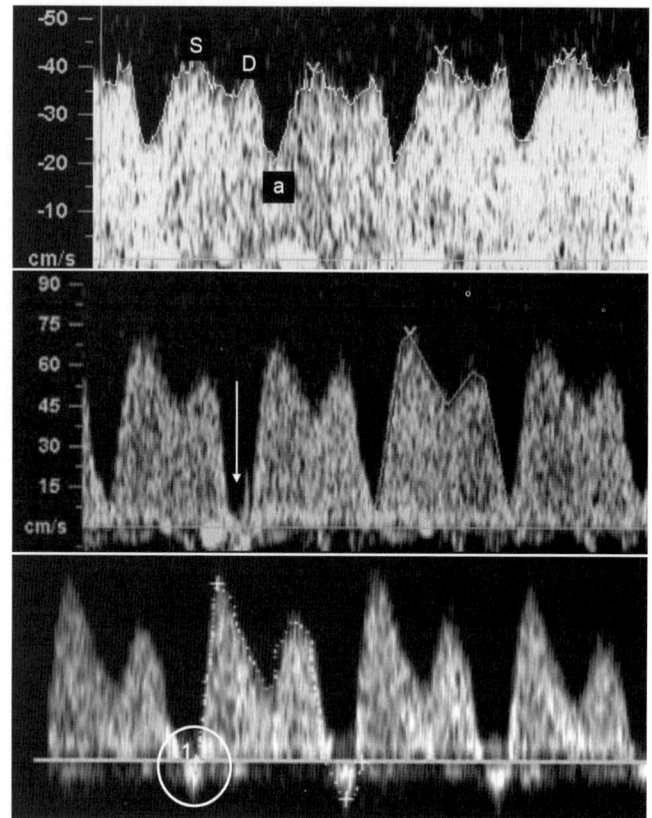

Fig. 86.6: Top panel: In the venous Doppler waveform systolic and diastolic peaks (the S- and D-wave) are generated by the descent of the AV-ring during ventricular systole and passive diastolic ventricular filling, respectively. A second late diastolic trough after the D-wave is the consequence of sharply increasing right atrial pressures during atrial systole (the a-wave). Middle Panel: With declining forward cardiac function forward velocity during atrial systole (arrow) and to a lesser degree during diastole decreased. This is associated with an increase in venous Doppler indices. Bottom panel: When ductus venosus Doppler indices escalate absence or reversal of forward flow during atrial systole (circle) may be observed as the most marked Doppler abnormality

variable amount of reverse flow producing a second trough after the D-wave (the a-wave) (Fig. 86.6). In extreme cases, atrial pressure waves may be transmitted all the way back into the free umbilical vein resulting in pulsatile flow.

When venous Doppler indices become elevated, a significant rise in ANP occurs, probably as a compensatory mechanism to regulate blood volume.[143,144] When forward cardiac function declines significantly, coronary vasodilatation becomes exaggerated to recruit all the available coronary blood flow reserve.[145] If these adaptations fail to support myocardial nutrition sufficiently, the amount of cardiac dysfunction may become critical. Cardiac dilatation with holosystolic tricuspid regurgitation and loss of cerebral autoregulation (normalizing cerebral Doppler indices) are observed at this level of compromise and indicate loss of cardiovascular homeostasis.[146] Elevations of troponin I, S100B protein levels and transaminases provide evidence of cellular

damage in the myocardium, brain and liver.[147-149] An increased risk for necrotizing enterocolitis in survivors has been attributed to bowel injury secondary to chronic underperfusion.[150] If the fetus remains undelivered, spontaneous late decelerations of the fetal heart rate and stillbirth ensue.[151,152]

Fetal Biophysical Responses

Normal fetal behavioral development proceeds sequentially with the appearance of movement, coupling, cycling of behavior and finally the integration of movement patterns into stable behavioral states. Autonomic reflexes originating from the brainstem are superimposed on intrinsic cardiac activity and determine fetal heart rate characteristics. As gestation advances, the interaction between the nervous system and the heart becomes more refined and is modulated by ambient oxygen tension, signals from higher brain centers and the reticular activating system as well as peripheral sensory inputs. Successful maturation of these connections is reflected by decreasing baseline heart rate, increasing heart rate, heart rate variability and variation, coupling of episodic accelerations with fetal movement and the superimposed impact of behavioral states. This level of central integration of fetal heart rate characteristics with fetal behavior is normally accomplished by 28 weeks of gestation.[153]

IUGR fetuses with chronic hypoxemia exhibit a delay in all aspects of central nervous system (CNS) maturation, which probably relates to altered myelination as well changes in central neurotransmitter availability.[154-158] The delayed development of behavioral milestones and their central integration with the fetal heart rate are primary determinants of lower short and long term variation (on computerized analysis), delayed decline in heart rate baseline and delayed development of heart rate reactivity in IUGR fetuses.[159-163] Despite the maturational delay of some aspects of CNS function, several centrally regulated responses to acid-base status are preserved.

Once fetal hypoxemia is perceived, a decline in global fetal activity precedes the loss of individual biophysical variables and is often also accompanied by a gradual decline in amniotic fluid volume.[164,165] With increasing hypoxemia, fetal breathing movement ceases. Gross body movements and tone decrease further and are lost as acidemia deepens.[166] Abnormal fetal heart rate patterns are generally also observed at this time (Fig. 86.7).[167,168] The effects of hypoxemia and vascular status on renal perfusion and fetal urine production affect amniotic fluid volume. As, progressive deterioration of acid-base and vascular status occurs, a progressive decline in amniotic fluid volume is observed. The decline of these biophysical variables is determined by the central effects of hypoxemia/acidemia independent of the cardiovascular status.[169-172]

The biophysical profile score (BPS) as a composite score applies categorical cutoffs for fetal tone, breathing movement, gross body movement, amniotic fluid volume as well as traditional fetal heart rate analysis. Although a gradual decline in all of these parameters precedes an overtly abnormal BPS analysis of the percentage change in these variables offers no advantage in the prediction of acidemia.[164] The five component BPS shows a reliable and reproducible relationship with the fetal pH irrespective of the underlying pathology and gestational age.[167,173] Concurrent evaluation of fetal cardiovascular and biophysical variables indicates that Doppler deterioration precedes an abnormal BPS in the majority of IUGR fetuses.[165] When the relationship between the various testing modalities and fetal acid base status is compared, biophysical parameters show a closer relationship with the pH while Doppler parameters have a wider variance (Fig. 86.8).

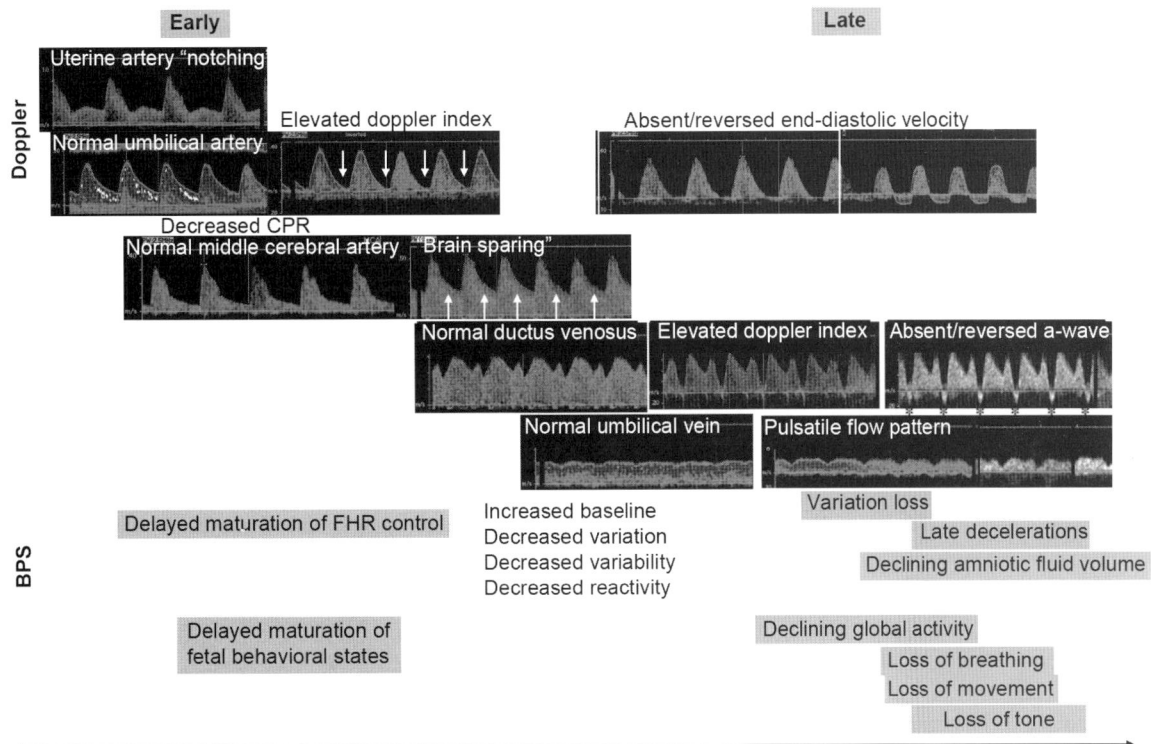

Fig. 86.7: This figure summarizes the early and late responses to placental insufficiency. Doppler variables in the placental circulation precede abnormality in the cerebral circulation. Biophysical parameters (BPS) are still normal at this time and computerized analysis of fetal behavioral patterns is necessary to document a developmental delay. With progression to late responses venous Doppler abnormality in the fetal circulation is characteristic often preceding the sequential loss of fetal dynamic variables and frequently accompanying the decline in amniotic fluid volume. The * in the ductus venosus flow velocity waveform marks reversal of blood flow during atrial systole (a-wave).The decline in biophysical variables shows a reproducible relationship with acid base status. If adaptation mechanisms fail stillbirth ensues

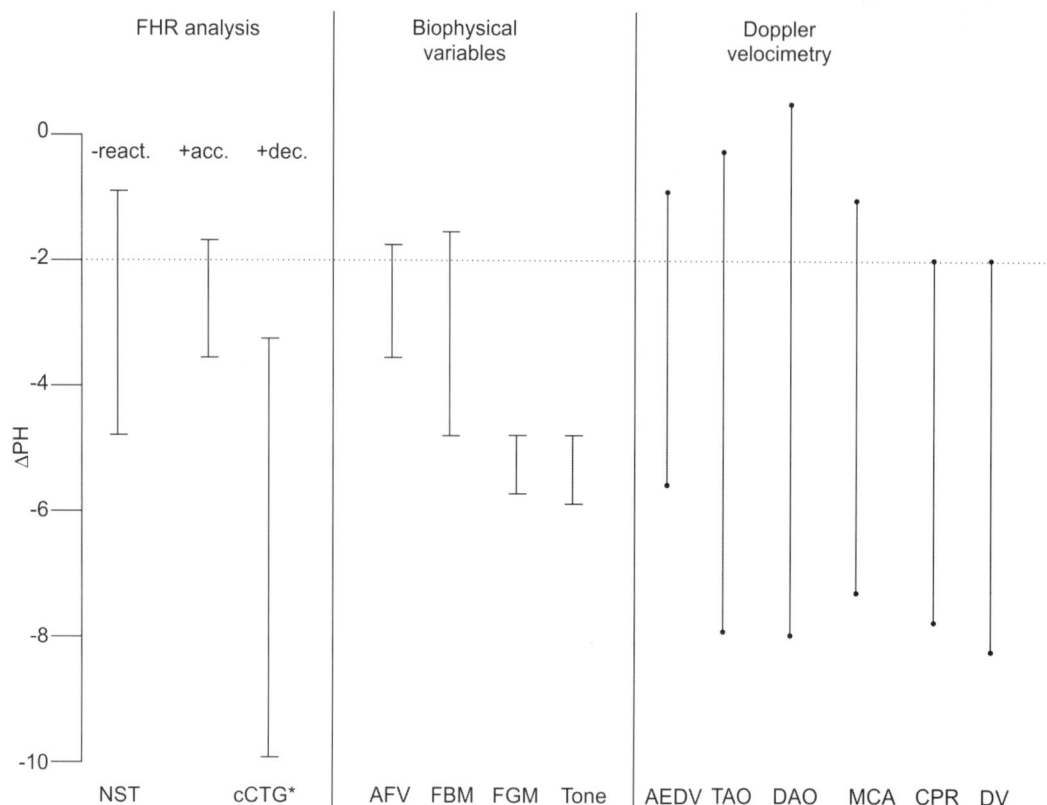

Fig. 86.8: This figure displays a diagrammatic representation of pH deviation from the gestational age mean (ΔpH) with abnormal test results in various antenatal tests. These include fetal heart rate (FHR) analysis using traditional nonstress testing (NST,– react = nonreactive) and the computerized cardiotocogram (cCTG, +acc = accelerations present, +dec = obvious decelerations present). Biophysical variables (AFV = amniotic fluid volume, FBM = fetal body movement, FGM = fetal gross movement). The same relationships are expressed for umbilical artery absent end-diastolic velocity (AEDV) and deviation of the arterial or venous Doppler index >2SD from the gestational age mean for the thoracic aorta (TAO), descending aorta (DAO), the middle cerebral artery (MCA), cerebroplacental ratio (CPR) and the ductus venosus (DV)

Source: Reproduced with permission from Baschat[120]

AN INTEGRATED APPROACH TO DIAGNOSIS AND MANAGEMENT OF FETAL GROWTH RESTRICTION

The many etiologies and presentations of fetal growth restriction require a diagnostic approach that integrates information from several diagnostic modalities. Only a complete evaluation of the maternal history, and the fetal, placental and amniotic fluid characteristics can direct an appropriate diagnostic workup and perinatal management. The accurate identification of fetuses that are truly at risk for adverse outcome requires exclusion of small fetuses that are normally grown and those in whom IUGR is due to an underlying condition not amenable to intervention. Conditions such as aneuploidy (especially trisomy 18, 13 and 21), skeletal dysplasia, nonaneuploid syndromes and viral infections should always be placed high on the list of differential diagnoses. Gray-scale ultrasound is the primary diagnostic tool allowing for a detailed fetal anatomic survey, biometric assessment of fetal growth, assessment of amniotic fluid volume and placental appearance. Although ultrasound provides important clues to the presence of IUGR the liability of preterm delivery and iatrogenic complications is large if the diagnosis and management is based only on biometry.[174] It is the complementary use of fetal biometry and Doppler assessment, which creates the best available tool

for the identification of small fetuses who are at risk for adverse outcome due to placental insufficiency.[175-178]

A detailed anatomic survey is mandatory in any fetus with suspected IUGR. Critical evaluation for aneuploidy markers such as echogenic bowel, nuchal thickening, abnormal hand positioning is necessary. Important anomalies that are associated with IUGR include gastroschisis, omphalocele, diaphragmatic hernia and congenital heart defects. Assessment of the thoracic shape may suggest the presence of a skeletal dysplasia. Markers for viral infection are nonspecific, but may include echogenicity and calcification in organs such as the brain and liver. Occasionally, hydrops may be present.[179] The amniotic fluid volume should be assessed at the same time as the fetal anatomic survey. The regulation of amniotic fluid volume is complex, but by the third trimester primarily dependent on fetal urine production. Placental dysfunction and fetal hypoxemia both may cause fetal oliguria and consequently oligohydramnios. However, the accuracy of ultrasound in the assessment of amniotic fluid volume is poor,[180] and serves as a poor screening tool for the prediction of IUGR and fetal acidosis.[181,182] Nonetheless, assessment of amniotic fluid volume by any method (four-quadrant AFI and maximum vertical pocket), especially if performed serially, provides an important diagnostic as well as prognostic tool. In the setting of small fetal size, abundant amniotic fluid volume is an indicator of aneuploidy or fetal infection while normal or decreased amniotic fluid is more compatible with placental insufficiency.

The actual quantification of growth is based on fetal biometry. Since almost all fetal measurements change with gestation, an accurate assessment of gestational age is a prerequisite for the calculation of percentile ranks of absolute measurements. An estimated date of confinement (EDC) is ideally based on a sure last menstrual period when the sonographic estimate of gestational age is within the predictive error (7 days in the first and 14 days in the second trimester, and 21 days in the third trimester). Once the EDC is set by this method or a first trimester ultrasound, it should not be changed. Later adjustments to the EDC will interfere with the ability to diagnose fetal growth abnormalities. Once the EDC has been assigned, selection of appropriate reference ranges that are based on uncomplicated pregnancies delivered at term is of importance. Individualized reference ranges of growth potential that account for maternal, ethnic and fetal variables provide the most accurate reference.[1,183] Once gestational age is assigned, the interpretation of the ultrasound examination is based on the fetal anatomic survey, amniotic fluid volume, percentile rank of fetal size measurements, the interval growth since the last study and a functional assessment of the fetoplacental unit with Doppler ultrasound.

Of all fetal biometric measurements the abdominal circumference (AC) is related to the liver size as a major indicator of fetal glycogen storage and therefore the single best measurement with the highest sensitivity and negative predictive value for the detection of IUGR.[184-186] Its sensitivity is further enhanced by serial measurements at least 14 days apart.[187] The most accurate AC is the smallest directly measured circumference obtained at the level of the hepatic vein between fetal respirations.[188] Using a reference range based on healthy women delivering appropriately nourished neonates at term, an AC <10th percentile for gestational age is consistent with IUGR. If cross-sectional population references including small, appropriately grown, preterm and term newborns are used the 2.5th percentile is more appropriate.[189] Compared to the AC, the biparietal diameter, head circumference (HC) and transverse cerebellar diameters are poor tools for the detection of IUGR. This is in part due to the inherent physiologic variation in skull shape,[190] and the relative sparing of the head growth and therefore delayed manifestation of placental insufficiency.[191] Ratios of fetal measurements do not improve the detection of growth delay,

but may be helpful pointers toward underlying aneuploidy.[192-194] Concurrent measurement of the HC, AC and femur length allows calculation of the sonographically estimated fetal weight (SEFW). An SEFW below the 10th percentile for gestational age has a lower sensitivity than the AC (85% vs. 98%) but a higher positive predictive value (51% vs. 36%).[186]

The next step in the diagnostic assessment of the suspected IUGR fetus is the evaluation of fetoplacental vascular function. Randomized trials and meta-analyses confirm that the use of umbilical artery Doppler in suspected IUGR results in a significant reduction in perinatal mortality and iatrogenic intervention since documentation of placental vascular insufficiency effectively separates constitutionally small fetuses from those in need for surveillance and possible intervention.[195-197] A more complete assessment of fetoplacental vascular status can be achieved if the uterine and middle cerebral arteries are examined in addition to the umbilical artery. For qualitative waveform analysis presence of uterine artery notching and umbilical artery end-diastolic velocity (positive, absent or reversed) should be noted. For clinical Doppler waveform analysis angle independent indices are used. Of these, the pulsatility index offers the advantage of a smaller measurement error, narrower reference limits and the possibility for ongoing numerical analysis even when end-diastolic velocity is absent.[198,199] In fetuses presenting with IUGR due to placental insufficiency before 34 weeks of gestation the umbilical artery Doppler waveform is frequently abnormal. Beyond this gestational age the umbilical artery Doppler waveform may be normal. At the same time cerebral artery Doppler responses to placental insufficiency still occur.[177,200] Therefore the middle cerebral-umbilical artery Doppler ratio (cerebroplacental ratio) may be abnormal in fetuses with mild placental disease.[175,201] Beyond 34 weeks of gestation a decrease in the middle cerebral artery Doppler index or the cerebroplacental ratio should therefore heighten suspicion for IUGR even if the umbilical artery blood flow is normal (Fig. 86.9).

Once the suspicion of IUGR is confirmed, fetal karyotyping should be offered and further specialized tests such as maternal serology (TORCH), thrombophilia studies or amniotic fluid viral DNA testing, may be indicated. Once nontreatable underlying fetal conditions and chromosome abnormalities have been ruled

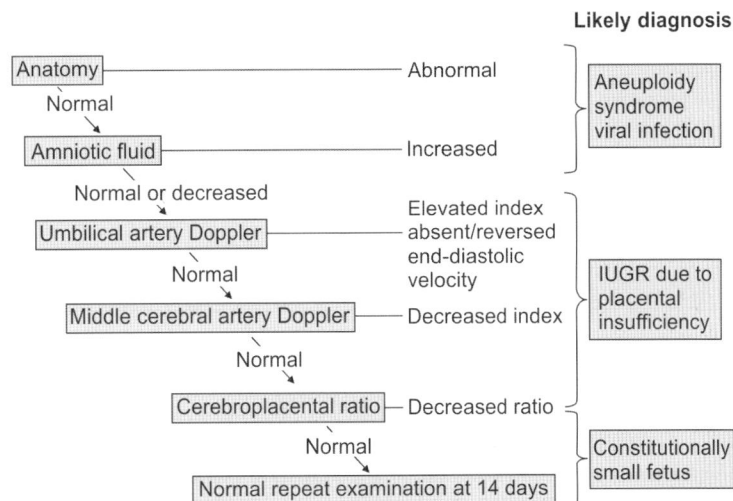

Fig. 86.9: This figure displays a decision tree following the evaluation of fetal anatomy, amniotic fluid volume, and umbilical and middle cerebral artery Doppler. The most likely clinical diagnosis is presented on the right hand side. A high index of suspicion for aneuploidy, viral and nonaneuploid syndrome needs to be maintained

Abbreviations IUGR = intrauterine growth restriction

out further antenatal surveillance should be instituted based on the severity of the maternal and/or fetal condition.

AN INTEGRATED APPROACH TO SURVEILLANCE IN FETAL GROWTH RESTRICTION

Antenatal surveillance in IUGR gestations aims to provide longitudinal assessment that is tailored to the severity of the fetal condition and is predictive of critical outcomes. Since, there are no effective therapies for in utero treatment of IUGR, management options include increasing the frequency of monitoring and delivery when fetal testing suggests that the intrauterine risks exceed neonatal risks of adverse outcomes. It is increasingly becoming apparent that IUGR fetuses are at particularly high risk for prematurity related complications and adverse outcomes, especially below 32 weeks of gestation.[4,202] Therefore, the delivery threshold is highest between viability and 32 weeks, placing the greatest demands on the precision of fetal assessment. This requirement for detailed assessment is offset by the need for practicability in order to facilitate generalized application. Utilizing knowledge about the fetal responses to placental insufficiency and

the limitations of antenatal testing modalities helps formulate an appropriate monitoring approach to IUGR fetuses at highest risk. In this context several principles are important.

In pregnancies that present with IUGR prior to 34 weeks of gestation, umbilical artery blood flow changes usually precede other cardiovascular responses.[201,203] Once the diagnosis of IUGR has been made by biometry and Doppler evaluation, continuing surveillance for deterioration of fetal cardiovascular status requires examination of the cerebral circulation and the precordial veins. When brain sparing develops, venous Doppler indices are frequently normal and biophysical abnormalities are generally not clinically observed. Development of abnormal venous Doppler indices indicates an acceleration of the deterioration.[204,205] At this time, abnormalities in biophysical parameters become clinically apparent. However, since the biophysical profile score is a composite of five variables the overall result may deteriorate relatively late in the disease process.[165] When Doppler and biophysical parameters show abnormalities, the information gained through their concurrent evaluation is complementary and offers the best prediction of fetal status and outcome.[120]

Taking these principles into account, a surveillance approach to pregnancies with IUGR due to placental disease that combines

IUGR unlikely		
Normal AC, AC growth rate and HC/AC ratio UA, MCA Doppler, BPS and AFV normal	Asphyxia extremely rare low risk for intrapartum distress	Deliver for obstetric, or maternal factors only, follow growth

IUGR		
AC<5th, low AC growth rate, high HC/AC ratio abnormal UA +/or CPR; normal MCA and venous Doppler, BPS ≥ 8/10, AFV normal	Asphyxia extremely rare Increased risk for intrapartum distress	Deliver for obstetric or maternal factors only, fortnightly Doppler Weekly BPS
with blood flow redistribution		
IUGR diagnosed based on above criteria, low MCA, normal venous Doppler, BPS ≥ 8/10, AFV normal	Hypoxemia possible, asphyxia rare Increased risk for intrapartum distress	Deliver for obstetric or maternal factors only, weekly Doppler BPS two times per week
with significant blood flow redistribution		
UA A/REDV, normal venous Doppler, BPS ≥ 6/10, oligohydramnios	Hypoxemia common, acidemia or asphyxia possible Onset of fetal compromise	>34 weeks—deliver 32–34 weeks consider delivery <32 weeks—antenatal steroids repeat all testing daily
with proven fetal compromise		
Significant redistribution present Increased DV pulsatility BPS ≥ 6/10, oligohydramnios	Hypoxemia common, acidemia or asphyxia likely	>32 weeks—deliver <32 weeks—admit, steroids, individualize testing daily vs. tid
with fetal decompensation		
Compromise by above criteria Absent or reversed DV a-wave, pulsatile UV BPS < 6/10, oligohydramnios	Cardiovascular instability, metabolic compromise, stillbirth imminent, high perinatal mortality irrespective of intervention	Deliver at tertiary care center with the highest level of NICU care

Fig. 86.10: The management algorithm for pregnancies complicated by fetal growth restriction is based on the ability to perform arterial and venous Doppler as well as a full five component biophysical profile score

Abbreviations: AC = abdominal circumference, AFV = amniotic fluid volume, A/REDV = absent/reversed end-diastolic velocity, BPS = biophysical profile score, CPR = cerebroplacental ratio, DV = ductus venosus, HC = head circumference, MCA = middle cerebral artery, NST = nonstress test, NICU = neonatal intensive care unit, tid = three times daily, UA = umbilical artery

Doppler ultrasound and biophysical profile scoring (integrated fetal testing) has been devised. The testing is always supplemented with maternal assessment of fetal movement (kick counts). Doppler examination includes evaluation of the umbilical artery, middle cerebral artery, ductus venosus and free umbilical vein flow velocity waveform. The traditional nonstress test component of the biophysical profile score is supplemented by computerized fetal heart rate analysis. Monitoring frequencies are adjusted to the fetal condition. Before 28 weeks, fetuses with isolated elevation of the umbilical artery Doppler index are followed with weekly biophysical profile scoring and repeat Doppler every fortnight. If umbilical artery end-diastolic velocity disappears, MCA Doppler meets criteria for centralization or amniotic fluid volume declines, all testing (Doppler and biophysical profile score) are repeated every 3–4 days. In patients with elevated ductus venous Doppler index with umbilical venous pulsations complete testing is repeated every 24 hours (Fig. 86.10).

The issue of optimal delivery timing for IUGR fetuses remains unresolved. In principle the decision for delivery always weighs fetal versus NICU risks. Typically, decline in neonatal mortality is greatest between 24 weeks and 28 weeks while morbidity declines progressively thereafter toward 32 weeks.[202] Perinatal mortality and morbidity is greatest among IUGR fetuses with abnormal venous Doppler indices irrespective of the umbilical artery Doppler waveform.[202,204] Therefore, basing delivery decision on the umbilical artery waveform alone appears no longer appropriate.[206] In preterm IUGR fetuses we consider abnormal venous Doppler indices and/or abnormal BPS as indicators for delivery. Beyond 34 weeks where the frequency of dramatically abnormal Doppler is lower reliance on BPS and obstetrical factors should guide delivery.

Since, the outlined surveillance approach requires multi-vessel Doppler as well as biophysical profile scoring it can only be performed at centers which are familiar with both techniques. Modifications of this surveillance protocol should address the limitations of such an approach. For example, the biophysical profile score alone offers little in the prediction of longitudinal progression. Thus, if biophysical profile scoring is the only surveillance tool, daily testing may be required to assure a good outcome.

Further investigation and evaluation of nutritional, metabolic, endocrine and hematologic responses at birth in growth restricted neonates and their relationship to fetal proportions, Doppler and behavioral parameters will refine our understanding of this condition. Neonatal management will become optimal when knowledge of the fetal status and an appreciation of the spectrum of fetal consequences of placental insufficiency are integrated to guide their evaluation and management. A uniform prenatal diagnostic standard and a comprehensive integrated management approach that bridges fetal and neonatal periods is most likely to impact adult health focusing on the small fetus at risk and sparing normally developed babies from iatrogenic interventions.

REFERENCES

1. Gardosi J, Chang A, Kalyan B, et al. Customised antenatal growth charts. Lancet. 1992;339:283-7.
2. Lubchenco LO, Hansman C, Boyd E. Intrauterine growth as estimated from live born birth-weight data at 24-42 weeks of gestation. Pediatrics. 1963;32:793.
3. Battaglia FC, Lubchenco LO. A practical classification of newborn infants by weight and gestational age. J Pediatr. 1967;71:159-63.
4. Bernstein IM, Horbar JD, Badger GJ, et al. Morbidity and mortality among very-low-birth-weight neonates with intrauterine growth restriction. The Vermont Oxford Network. Am J Obstet Gynecol. 2000;182:198-206.
5. Schreuder AM, McDonnell M, Gaffney G, et al. Outcome at school age following antenatal detection of absent or reversed end-diastolic flow velocity in the umbilical artery. Arch Dis Child Fetal Neonatal. 2002;86:F108-14.
6. Barker DJ. Fetal growth and adult disease. Br J Obstet Gynaecol. 1992;99:275-6.
7. Aplin J. Maternal influences on placental development. Semin Cell Dev Biol. 2000;11:115-25.
8. Pardi G, Marconi AM, Cetin I. Placental-fetal interrelationship in IUGR fetuses: A review. Placenta. 2002;23(Suppl A): S136-41.
9. Kaufmann P, Scheffen I. Placental development. In: polin RA, Fox WW (Eds). Fetal and neonatal Physiology. Philadelphia, PA: WB Saunders; 1998. pp. 59-70.
10. Cunningham FG, Gant NF, Leveno KJ, et al. Maternal adaptations to pregnancy. In: Williams Obstetrics. New York: McGraw Hill. 2001;167-200.
11. Kingdom JC, Burrell SJ, Kaufmann P. Pathology and clinical implications of abnormal umbilical artery Doppler waveforms. Ultrasound Obstet Gynecol. 1997;9:271-86.
12. Pijnenborg R, Bland JM, Robertson WB, et al. Uteroplacental arterial changes related to interstitial trophoblast migration in early human pregnancy. Placenta. 1983;4:397-413.
13. Castellucci M, Kosanke G, Verdenelli F, et al. Villous sprouting: Fundamental mechanisms of human placental development. Hum Reprod Update. 2000;6:485-94.
14. Maini CL, Rosati P, Galli G, et al. Non-invasive radioisotopic evaluation of placental blood flow. Gynecol Obstet Invest. 1985;19:196-206.
15. Luckhardt M, Leiser R, Kingdom J, et al. Effect of physiologic perfusion fixation on the morphometrically evaluated dimensions of the term placental cotyledon. J Soc Gynecol Investig. 1996;3: 166-71.
16. Meschia G. Placenta respiratory gas exchange and fetal oxygenation. In: Creasy RK, Resnik R (Eds). Maternal Fetal Medicine: Principles and Practice, 1st edition. Philadelphia: WB Saunders; 1987. pp. 274-85.
17. Meschia G, Battaglia FC, Hay WW, et al. Utilization of substrates by the ovine placenta in vivo. Fed et al Proc. 1980;39:245-9.
18. Carter AM. Placental oxygen consumption. Part I: In vivo studies—a review. Placenta. 2000;21:S31-7.
19. Battaglia FC, Regnault TR. Placental transport and metabolism of amino acids. Placenta. 2001;22:145-61.
20. Haggarty P. Placental regulation of fatty acid delivery and its effects on fetal growth – a review. Placenta 2002; 23:S28-38.
21. Illsely NP. Glucose transporters in the human placenta. Placenta. 2000;21:14-22.
22. Sibley CP, Glazier JD, Greenwood SL, et al. Regulation of placental transfer: The Na(+)/H(+) exchanger—a review. Placenta. 2002;23: S39-46.

23. Reece EA, Wiznitzer A, Le E, et al. The relation between human fetal growth and fetal blood levels of insulin-like growth factors I and II, their binding proteins, and receptors. Obstet Gynecol. 1994;84:88-95.

24. Hoggard N, Haggarty P, Thomas L, et al. Leptin expression in placental and fetal tissues: Does leptin have a functional role? Biochem Soc Trans. 2001;29:57-66.

25. Jansson N, Greenwood SL, Johansson BR, et al. Leptin stimulates the activity of the system: a amino acid transporter in human placental villous fragments. J Clin Endocrinol Metab. 2003;88:1205-11.

26. Kiserud T. The ductus venosus. Semin Perinatol. 2001;25:11-20.

27. Rudolph AM. Distribution and regulation of blood flow in the fetal and neonatal lamb. Circ Res. 1985;57:811-21.

28. Guyton AC, Cowley AW Jr, Young DB, et al. Integration and control of circulatory function. Int Rev Physiol. 1976;9:341-85.

29. Bonds DR, Mwape B, Kumar S, et al. Human fetal weight and placental weight growth curves. A mathematical analysis from a population at sea level. Biol Neonate. 1984;45(6):261-74.

30. Molteni RA, Stys SJ, Battaglia FC. Relationship of fetal and placental weight in human beings: fetal/placental weight ratios at various gestational ages and birth weight distributions. J Reprod Med. 1978;21:327-34.

31. Heinonen S, Taipale P, Saarikoski S. Weights of placentae from small-for-gestational age infants revisited. Placenta. 2001;22: 399-404.

32. Herrera E, Amusquivar E. Lipid metabolism in the fetus and the newborn. Diabetes Metab Res Rev. 2000;16:202-10.

33. Sparks JW, Girard JR, Battaglia FC. An estimate of the caloric requirements of the human fetus. Biol Neonate. 1980;38(3-4):113-9.

34. White DR, Widdowson EM, Woodard HQ, et al. The composition of body tissues (II). Fetus to young adult. Br J Radiol. 1991;64:149-59.

35. Ziegler EE, O'Donnell AM, Nelson SE, et al. Body composition of the reference fetus. Growth. 1976;40:329-41.

36. Kingdom J, Huppertz B, Seaward G, et al. Development of the placental villous tree and its consequences for fetal growth. Eur J Obstet Gynecol Reprod Biol. 2000;92:35-43.

37. Brosens I, Dixon HG, Robertson WB. Fetal growth retardation and the arteries of the placental bed. Br J Obstet Gynaecol. 1977;84: 656-63.

38. Meekins JW, Pijnenborg R, Hanssens M, et al. A study of placental bed spiral arteries and trophoblast invasion in normal and severe pre-eclamptic pregnancies. Br J Obstet Gynaecol. 1994;101:669-74.

39. Sebire NJ, Talbert D. The role of intraplacental vascular smooth muscle in the dynamic placenta: a conceptual framework for understanding uteroplacental disease. Med Hypotheses. 2002;58:347-51.

40. Aardema MW, Oosterhof H, Timmer A, et al. Uterine artery Doppler flow and uteroplacental vascular pathology in normal pregnancies and pregnancies complicated by pre-eclampsia and small for gestational age fetuses. Placenta. 2001;22:405-11.

41. Ferrazzi E, Bulfamante G, Mezzopane R, et al. Uterine Doppler velocimetry and placental hypoxic-ischemic lesion in pregnancies with fetal intrauterine growth restriction. Placenta. 1999;20:389-94.

42. Kingdom JC, McQueen J, Connell JM, et al. Fetal angiotensin II levels and vascular (type I) angiotensin receptors in pregnancies complicated by intrauterine growth retardation. Br J Obstet Gynaecol 1993;100:47682.

43. Clausson B, Gardosi J, Francis A, et al. Perinatal outcome in SGA births defined by customized versus population-based birthweight standards. BJOG. 2001;108:830-4.

44. Jones CT, Ritchie JW, Walker D. The effects of hypoxia on glucose turnover in the fetal sheep. J Dev Physiol. 1983;5:223-35.

45. Nicolini U, Hubinont C, Santolaya J, Fisk NM, et al. Maternal-fetal glucose gradient in normal pregnancies and in pregnancies complicated by alloimmunization and fetal growth retardation. Am J Obstet Gynecol. 1989;161:924-7.

46. Economides DL, Nicolaides KH. Blood glucose and oxygen tension levels in small-for-gestational-age fetuses. Am J Obstet Gynecol. 1989;160:385-9.

47. Hubinont C, Nicolini U, Fisk NM, et al. Endocrine pancreatic function in growth-retarded fetuses. Obstet Gynecol. 1991;77:541-4.

48. Van Assche FA, Aerts L, DePrins FA. The fetal endocrine pancreas. Eur J Obstet Gynecol Reprod Biol. 1984;18: 267-72.

49. Cetin I, Marconi AM, Corbetta C, et al. Fetal amino acids in normal pregnancies and in pregnancies complicated by intrauterine growth retardation. Early Hum Dev. 1992;29:183-6.

50. Cetin I, Corbetta C, Sereni LP, et al. Umbilical amino acid concentrations in normal and growth-retarded fetuses sampled in utero by cordocentesis. Am J Obstet Gynecol. 1990;162:253-61.

51. Economides DL, Nicolaides KH, Campbell S. Metabolic and endocrine findings in appropriate and small for gestational age fetuses. J Perinat Med. 1991;19:97-105.

52. Vannucci RC, Vannucci SJ. Glucose metabolism in the developing brain. Semin Perinatol. 2000;24:107-15.

53. Fisher DJ, Heymann MA, Rudolph AM. Fetal myocardial oxygen and carbohydrate consumption during acutely induced hypoxemia. Am J Physiol. 1982;242:H657-61.

54. Spahr R, Probst I, Piper HM. Substrate utilization of adult cardiac myocytes. Basic Res Cardiol. 1985;80(Suppl 1):53-6.

55. Soothill PW, Nicolaides KH, Campbell S. Prenatal asphyxia, hyperlacticemia, hypoglycemia, and erythroblastosis in growth retarded fetuses. Br Med J. 1987;294:1051-3.

56. Owens JA, Falconer J, Robinson JS. Effect of restriction of placental growth on fetal uteroplacental metabolism. J Dev Physiol. 1987;9:225-38.

57. Paolini CL, Marconi AM, Ronzoni S, et al. Placental transport of leucine, phenylalanine, glycine, and proline in intrauterine growth-restricted pregnancies. J Clin Endocrinol Metab. 2001;86:5427-32.

58. Wolfe HM, Sokol RJ, Dombrowski MP, et al. Increased neonatal urinary ammonia: A marker for *in utero* caloric deprivation? Am J Perinatol. 1989;6:4-7.

59. Bernstein IM, Silver R, Nair KS, et al. Amniotic fluid glycine-valine ratio and neonatal morbidity in fetal growth restriction. Obstet Gynecol. 1997;90:933-7.

60. Roberts A, Nava S, Bocconi L, et al. Liver function tests and glucose and lipid metabolism in growth-restricted fetuses. Obstet Gynecol. 1999;94:290-4.

61. Battaglia FC. Clinical studies linking fetal velocimetry, blood flow and placental transport in pregnancies complicated by intrauterine growth retardation (IUGR). Trans Am Clin Climatol Assoc. 2003;114:305-13.

62. Spencer JA, Chang TC, Crook D, et al. Third trimester fetal growth and measures of carbohydrate and lipid metabolism in umbilical venous blood at term. Arch Dis Child Fetal Neonatal. 1997;76:F21-5.

63. Fant ME, Weisoly D. Insulin and insulin-like growth factors in human development: Implications for the perinatal period. Semin Perinatol. 2001;25:426-35.

64. Ostlund E, Tally M, Fried G. Transforming growth factor-beta1 in fetal serum correlates with insulin-like growth factor-I and fetal growth. Obstet Gynecol. 2002;100(3):567-73.

65. Nicolini U, Hubinont C, Santolaya J, et al. Effects of fetal intravenous glucose challenge in normal and growth retarded fetuses. Horm Metab Res. 1990;22:426-30.

66. Hubinont C, Nicolini U, Fisk NM, et al. Endocrine pancreatic function in growth-retarded fetuses. Obstet Gynecol. 1991;77:541-4.

67. Goland RS, Jozak S, Warren WB, et al. Elevated levels of umbilical cord plasma corticotropin-releasing hormone in growth-retarded fetuses. J Clin Endocrinol Metab. 1993;77:1174-9.

68. Giles WB, McLean M, Davies JJ, et al. Abnormal umbilical artery Doppler waveforms and cord blood corticotropin-releasing hormone. Obstet Gynecol. 1996;87:107-11.

69. Cianfarani S, Germani D, Rossi L, et al. IGF-I and IGF-binding protein-1 are related to cortisol in human cord blood. Eur J Endocrinol. 1998;138:524-9.

70. Spencer JA, Chang TC, Jones J, et al. Third trimester fetal growth and umbilical venous blood concentrations of IGF-1, IGFBP-1, and growth hormone at term. Arch Dis Child Fetal Neonatal. 1995;73(2):F87-90.

71. Weiner CP, Robillard JE. Atrial natriuretic factor, digoxin-like immunoreactive substance, norepinephrine, epinephrine, and plasma are in activity in human fetuses and their alteration by fetal disease. Am J Obstet Gynecol. 1988;159:1353-60.

72. Greenough A, Nicolaides KH, Lagercrantz H. Human fetal sympathoadrenal responsiveness. Early Hum Dev. 1990;23:9-13.

73. Ville Y, Proudler A, Kuhn P, et al. Aldosterone concentration in normal, growth-retarded, anemic, and hydropic fetuses. Obstet Gynecol. 1994;84:511-4.

74. Thorpe-Beeston JG, Nicolaides KH. Fetal thyroid function. Fetal Diagn Ther. 1993;8:60-72.

75. Thorpe-Beeston JG, Nicolaides KH, Snijders RJ, et al. Relations between the fetal circulation and pituitary-thyroid function. Br J Obstet Gynecol. 1991;98:1163-7.

76. Nieto-Diaz A, Villar J, Matorras-Weinig R, et al. Intrauterine growth retardation at term: association between anthropometric and endocrine parameters. Acta Obstet Gynaecol Scand. 1996;75:127-31.

77. Kilby MD, Gittoes N, McCabe C, et al. Expression of thyroid receptor isoforms in the human fetal central nervous system and the effects of intrauterine growth restriction. Clin Endocrinol (Oxf). 2000;53:469-77.

78. Verhaeghe J, Van Herck E, Bouillon R. Umbilical cord osteocalcin in normal pregnancies and pregnancies complicated by fetal growth retardation or diabetes mellitus. Biol Neonate. 1995;68:377-83.

79. Namgung R, Tsang RC, Specker BL, et al. Reduced serum osteocalcin and 1,25-dihydroxyvitamin D concentrations and low bone mineral content in small for gestational age infants: evidence of decreased bone formation rates. J Pediatr. 1993;122:269-75.

80. Weiner CP, Williamson RA. Evaluation of severe growth retardation using cordocentesis—hematologic and metabolic alterations by etiology. Obstet Gynecol. 1989;73:225-9.

81. Thilaganathan B, Athanasiou S, Ozmen S, et al. Umbilical cord blood erythroblast count as an index of intrauterine hypoxia. Arch Dis Child Fetal Neonatal. 1994;70:F192-4.

82. Maier RF, Gunther A, Vogel M, et al. Umbilical venous erythropoietin and umbilical arterial pH in relation to morphologic placental abnormalities. Obstet Gynecol. 1994;84:81-7.

83. Snijders RJ, Abbas A, Melby O, et al. Fetal plasma erythropoetin concentration in severe growth retardation. Am J Obstet Gynecol. 1993;168:6159.

84. Thilaganathan B, Nicolaides KH. Erythroblastosis in birth asphyxia. Ultrasound Obstet Gynecol. 1992;2:157.

85. Baschat AA, Gembruch U, Reiss I, et al. Neonatal nucleated red blood cell counts in growth-restricted fetuses: relationship to arterial and venous Doppler studies. Am J Obstet Gynecol. 1999;181:190-5.

86. Bernstein PS, Minior VK, Divon MY. Nucleated red blood cell counts in small for gestational age fetuses with abnormal umbilical artery Doppler studies. Am J Obstet Gynecol. 1997;177:1079-84.

87. Baschat AA, Gembruch U, Reiss I, et al. Neonatal nucleated red blood cell count and postpartum complications in growth restricted fetuses. J Perinat Med. 2003;31:323-9.

88. Stallmach T, Karolyi L, Lichtlen P, et al. Fetuses from preeclamptic mothers show reduced hepatic erythropoiesis. Pediatr Res. 1998;43:349-54.

89. Hiett AK, Britton KA, Hague NL, et al. Comparison of hematopoietic progenitor cells in human umbilical cord blood collected from neonatal infants who are small and appropriate for gestational age. Transfusion. 1995;35:587-91.

90. Rondo PH, Abbott R, Rodrigues LC, et al. Vitamin A, folate, and iron concentrations in cord and maternal blood of intrauterine growth retarded and appropriate birth weight babies. Eur J Clin Nutr. 1995;49:391-9.

91. Abbas A, Snijders RJ, Nicolaides KH. Serum ferritin and cobalamin in growth retarded fetuses. Br J Obstet Gynecol. 1994;101:215-9.

92. Ohshige A, Yoshimura T, Maeda T, et al. Increased platelet-activating factor-acetylhydrolase activity in the umbilical venous plasma of growth-restricted fetuses. Obstet Gynaecol. 1999;93:180-3.

93. Trudinger B, Song JZ, Wu ZH, et al. Placental insufficiency is characterized by platelet activation in the fetus. Obstet Gynecol. 2003;101:975-81.

94. Baschat AA, Gembruch U, Reiss I, et al. Absent umbilical artery end-diastolic velocity in growth-restricted fetuses: a risk factor for neonatal thrombocytopenia. Obstet Gynecol. 2000;96:162-6.

95. Van den Hof MC, Nicolaides KH. Platelet count in normal, small, and anemic fetuses. Am J Obstet Gynecol. 1990;162:735-9.

96. Drew JH, Guaran RL, Grauer S, et al. Cord whole blood hyperviscosity: measurement, definition, incidence and clinical features. J Pediatr Child Health. 1991;27: 363-5.

97. Steel SA, Pearce JM, Nash G, et al. Correlation between Doppler flow velocity waveforms and cord blood viscosity. Br J Obstet Gynecol. 1989;96:1168-72.

98. Lemery DJ, Beal V, Vanlieferinghen P, et al. Fetal blood cell membrane fluidity in small for gestational age fetuses. Biol Neonate. 1993;64:7-12.

99. Singh M, Manerikar S, Malaviya AN, et al. Immune status of low birth weight babies. Indian Pediatr. 1978;15:563-7.

100. Davies N, Snijders R, Nicolaides KH. Intrauterine starvation and fetal leucocyte count. Fetal Diagn Ther. 1991;6:107-12.

101. Thilaganathan B, Plachouras N, Makrydimas G, et al. Fetal immunodeficiency: A consequence of placental insufficiency. Br J Obstet Gynecol. 1993;100:1000-4.

102. Harrington K, Carpenter RG, Goldfrad C, et al. Transvaginal Doppler ultrasound of the uteroplacental circulation in the early prediction of pre-eclampsia and intrauterine growth retardation. Br J Obstet Gynecol. 1997;104:674-81.

103. Rigano S, Bozzo M, Ferrazzi E, et al. Early and persistent reduction in umbilical vein blood flow in the growth-restricted fetus: a longitudinal study. Am J Obstet Gynecol. 2001;185:834-8.

104. Morrow RJ, Adamson SL, Bull SB, et al. Effect of placental embolization on the umbilical artery velocity waveform in fetal sheep. Am J Obstet Gynecol. 1989;161:1055-60.

105. Wilcox G, Trudinger B, Cook CM, et al. Reduced fetal platelet counts in pregnancies with abnormal Doppler umbilical flow waveforms. Obstet Gynecol. 1989;73:639-43.

106. Papageorghiou AT, Yu CK, Cicero S, et al. Second-trimester uterine artery Doppler screening in unselected populations: A review. J Matern Fetal Neonatal Med. 2002;12:78-88.

107. Weiner CP. The relationship between the umbilical artery systolic/diastolic ratio and umbilical blood gas measurements in specimens obtained by cordocentesis. Am J Obstet Gynecol. 1990;162:1198-202.

108. Bilardo CM, Nicolaides KH, Campbell S. Doppler measurements of fetal and uteroplacental circulations: relationship with umbilical venous blood gases measured at cordocentesis. Am J Obstet Gynecol. 1990;162:115-20.

109. Ferrazzi E, Bozzo M, Rigano S, et al. Temporal sequence of abnormal Doppler changes in the peripheral and central circulatory systems of the severely growth-restricted fetus. Ultrasound Obstet Gynecol. 2002;19:140-6.

110. Hecher K, Bilardo CM, Stigter RH, et al. Monitoring of fetuses with intrauterine growth restriction: a longitudinal study. Ultrasound Obstet Gynecol. 2001;18:564-70.

111. Rizzo G, Arduini D. Fetal cardiac function in intrauterine growth retardation. Am J Obstet Gynecol. 1991;165:876-82.

112. Reed KL, Anderson CF, Shenker L. Changes in intra cardiac Doppler flow velocities in fetuses with absent umbilical artery diastolic flow. Am J Obstet Gynecol. 1987;157:774-779.

113. Al Ghazali W, Chita SK, Chapman MG, et al. Evidence of redistribution of cardiac output in asymmetrical growth retardation. Br J Obstet Gynecol. 1987;96:697-704.

114. Gramellini D, Folli MC, Raboni S, et al. Cerebralumbilical Doppler ratio as a predictor of adverse perinatal outcome. Obstet Gynecol. 1992;79:416-20.

115. Griffin D, Bilardo K, Masini L. Doppler blood flow waveforms in the descending thoracic aorta of the human fetus. Br J Obstet Gynaecol. 1984;91:997-1006.

116. Akalin-Sel T, Nicolaides KH, Peacock J, et al. Doppler dynamics and their complex interrelation with fetal oxygen pressure, carbon dioxide pressure, and pH in growth-retarded fetuses. Obstet Gynecol. 1994;84:439-44.

117. Wladimiroff JW, Tonge HM, Stewart PA. Doppler ultrasound assessment of cerebral blood flow in the human fetus. Br J Obstet Gynaecol. 1986;93:471-5.

118. Arbeille P, Maulik D, Fignon A, et al. Assessment of the fetal PO_2 changes by cerebral and umbilical Doppler on lamb fetuses during acute hypoxia. Ultrasound Med Biol. 1995;21:861-70.

119. Baschat AA. Integrated fetal testing in growth restriction: combining multivessel Doppler and biophysical parameters. Ultrasound Obstet Gynecol. 2003;21:1-8.

120. Fouron JC, Skoll A, Sonesson SE, et al. Relationship between flow through the fetal aortic isthmus and cerebral oxygenation during acute placental circulatory insufficiency in ovine fetuses. Am J Obstet Gynecol. 1999;181:1102-7.

121. Makikallio K, Jouppila P, Rasanen J. Retrograde net blood flow in the aortic isthmus in relation to human fetal arterial and venous circulations. Ultrasound Obstet Gynecol. 2002;19:147-52.

122. Rizzo G, Capponi A, Chaoui R, et al. Blood flow velocity waveforms from peripheral pulmonary arteries in normally grown and growth-retarded fetuses. Ultrasound Obstet Gynecol. 1996;8:87-92.

123. Gamsu HR, Vyas S, Nicolaides K. Effects of intrauterine growth retardation on postnatal visceral and cerebral blood flow velocity. Arch Dis Child. 1991;66:1115-8.

124. Mari G, Abuhamad AZ, Uerpairojkit B, et al. Blood flow velocity waveforms of the abdominal arteries in appropriate- and small-for-gestational-age fetuses. Ultrasound Obstet Gynecol. 1995;6:15-8.

125. Rhee E, Detti L, Mari G. Superior mesenteric artery flow velocity waveforms in small for gestational age fetuses. J Matern Fetal Med. 1998;7:120-3.

126. Veille JC, Kanaan C. Duplex Doppler ultrasonographic evaluation of the fetal renal artery in normal and abnormal fetuses. Am J Obstet Gynecol. 1989;161:1502-7.

127. Arduini D, Rizzo G. Fetal renal artery velocity waveforms and amniotic fluid volume in growth-retarded and post-term fetuses. Obstet Gynecol. 1991;77:370-3.

128. Mari G. Arterial blood flow velocity waveforms of the pelvis and lower extremities in normal and growth-retarded fetuses. Am J Obstet Gynecol. 1991;165:143-51.

129. Tekay A, Jouppila P. Fetal adrenal artery velocimetry measurements in appropriate-for-gestational age and intrauterine growth-restricted fetuses. Ultrasound Obstet Gynecol. 2000;16:419-24.

130. Abuhamad AZ, Mari G, Bogdan D, et al. Doppler flow velocimetry of the splenic artery in the human fetus: is it a marker of chronic hypoxia? Am J Obstet Gynecol. 1995;172:820-5.

131. Karsdorp VH, Dekker GA, Bast A, et al. Maternal and fetal plasma concentrations of endothelin, lipidhydroperoxides, glutathione peroxidase and fibronectin in relation to abnormal umbilical artery velocimetry. Eur J Obstet Gynecol Reprod Biol. 1998;80:39-44.

132. Harvey-Wilkes KB, Nielsen HC, D'Alton ME. Elevated endothelin levels are associated with increased placental resistance. Am J Obstet Gynecol. 1996;174:1599-604.

133. Rizzo G, Montuschi P, Capponi A, et al. Blood levels of vasoactive intestinal polypeptide in normal and growth retarded fetuses: relationship with acid-base and haemodynamic status. Early Hum Dev. 1995;41:69-77.

134. Saldeen P, Olofsson P, Marsal K. Lack of association between Doppler velocimetry and synthesis of prostacyclin and thromboxane in umbilical cord vessels from growth retarded fetuses. Acta Obstet Gynecol Scand. 1995;74:103-8.

135. Lyall F, Greer IA, Young A, et al. Nitric oxide concentrations are increased in the feto-placental circulation in intrauterine growth restriction. Placenta. 1996;17:165-8.

136. McQeen J, Kingdom JC, Connell JM, et al. Fetal endothelin levels and placental vascular endothelin receptors in intrauterine growth retardation. Obstet Gynecol. 1993;82:992-8.

137. Kingdom JC, McQueen J, Connell JM, et al. Fetal angiotensin II levels and vascular (type I) angiotensin receptors in pregnancies complicated by intrauterine growth retardation. Br J Obstet Gynaecol. 1993;100:476-82.

138. Parboosingh J, Lederis K, Ko D, et al. Vasopressin concentration in cord blood: correlation with method of delivery and cord pH. Obstet Gynecol. 1982;60:179-83.

139. Rizzo G, Capponi A, Rinaldo D, et al. Release of vasoactive agents during cordocentesis: differences between normally grown and growth-restricted fetuses. Am J Obstet Gynecol. 1996;175:563-70.

140. Kilavuz O, Vetter K. Is the liver of the fetus the 4th preferential organ for arterial blood supply besides brain, heart, and adrenal glands? J Perinat Med. 1999;27:103-6.

141. Hecher K, Campbell S. Characteristics of fetal venous blood flow under normal circumstances and during fetal disease. Ultrasound Obstet Gynecol. 1996;7:68-83.

142. Capponi A, Rizzo G, De Angelis C, et al. Atrial natriuretic peptide levels in fetal blood in relation to inferior vena cava velocity wave forms. Obstet Gynecol. 1997;89:242-7.

143. Ville Y, Proudler A, Abbas A, et al. Atrial natriuretic factor concentration in normal, growth-retarded, anemic, and hydropic fetuses. Am J Obstet Gynecol. 1994;171:777-83.

144. Baschat AA, Gembruch U, Reiss I, et al. Demonstration of fetal coronary blood flow by Doppler ultrasound in relation to arterial and venous flow velocity waveforms and perinatal outcome—the 'heart-sparing effect'. Ultrasound Obstet Gynecol. 1997;9:162-72.

145. Arduini D, Rizzo G, Romanini C. Changes of pulsatility index from fetal vessels preceding the onset of late decelerations in growth-retarded fetuses. Obstet Gynecol. 1992;79:605-10.

146. Chaiworapongsa T, Espinoza J, Yoshimatsu J, et al. Subclinical myocardial injury in small-for-gestational-age neonates. J Matern Fetal Neonatal Med. 2002;11:385-90.

147. Gazzolo D, Marinoni E, di Iorio R, et al. Circulating S100beta protein is increased in intrauterine growth-retarded fetuses. Pediatr Res. 2002;51:215-9.

148. Roberts A, Nava S, Bocconi L, et al. Liver function tests and glucose and lipid metabolism in growth-restricted fetuses. Obstet Gynecol. 1999;94:290-4.

149. Hackett GA, Campbell S, Gamsu H, et al. Doppler studies in the growth retarded fetus and prediction of neonatal necrotising enterocolitis, hemorrhage, and neonatal morbidity. Br Med J. 1987; 294:13-6.

150. Rizzo G, Arduini D. Fetal cardiac function in intrauterine growth retardation. Am J Obstet Gynecol. 1991;165:876-82.

151. Rizzo G, Capponi A, Pietropolli A, et al. Fetal cardiac and extracardiac flows preceding intrauterine death. Ultrasound Obstet Gynecol. 1994;4:139-142.

152. Manning FA. Fetal biophysical profile. Obstet Gynecol Clin North Am. 1999;26:557-77.

153. Arduini D, Rizzo G, Romanini C, et al. Computerized analysis of behavioral states in asymmetrical growth retarded fetuses. J Perinat Med. 1988;16:357-63.

154. Arduini D, Rizzo G, Caforio L, et al. Behavioral state transitions in healthy and growth retarded fetuses. Early Hum Dev. 1989;19: 155-65.

155. Nijhuis IJ, ten Hof J, Nijhuis JG, et al. Temporal organization of fetal behavior from 24-weeks of gestation onwards in normal and complicated pregnancies. Dev Psychobiol. 1999;34: 257-68.

156. Vindla S, James D, Sahota D. Computerized analysis of unstimulated and stimulated behavior in fetuses with intrauterine growth restriction. Eur J Obstet Gynecol Reprod Biol. 1999;83:37-45.

157. Romanini C, Valensise H, Ciotti G, et al. Tryptophan availability and fetal behavioral states. Fetal Ther. 1989;4:68-72.

158. Nijhuis IJ, ten Hof J, Mulder EJ, et al. Fetal heart rate in relation to its variation in normal and growth retarded fetuses. Eur J Obstet Gynecol Reprod Biol. 2000;89:27-33.

159. Henson G, Dawes GS, Redman CW. Characterization of the reduced heart rate variation in growth-retarded fetuses. Br J Obstet Gynaecol. 1984;91:751-5.

160. Ribbert LS, Snijders RJ, Nicolaides KH, et al. Relation of fetal blood gases and data from computer-assissted analysis of fetal heart rate patterns in small for gestation fetuses. Br J Obstet Gynaecol. 1991;98:820-3.

161. Smith JH, Anand KJ, Cotes PM, et al. Antenatal fetal heart rate variation in relation to the respiratory and metabolic status of the compromised human fetus. Br J Obstet Gynaecol. 1988;95:980-9.

162. Longo LD, Packianathan S. Hypoxia-ischemia and the developing brain: Hypotheses regarding the pathophysiology of fetal neonatal brain damage. Br J Obstet Gynaecol. 1997;104: 652-62.

163. Ribbert LS, Nicolaides KH, Visser GH. Prediction of fetal acidaemia in intrauterine growth retardation: comparison of quantified fetal activity with biophysical profile score. Br J Obstet Gynecol. 1993;100:653-6.

164. Baschat AA, Gembruch U, Harman CR. The sequence of changes in Doppler and biophysical parameters as severe fetal growth restriction worsens. Ultrasound Obstet Gynecol. 2001;18:571-7.

165. Ribbert LS, Visser GH, Mulder EJ, et al. Changes with time in fetal heart rate variation, movement incidences and haemodynamics in intrauterine growth retarded fetuses: A longitudinal approach to the assessment of fetal well being. Early Hum Dev. 1993;31:195-208.

166. Manning FA, Snijders R, Harman CR, et al. Fetal biophysical profile score. VI. Correlation with antepartum umbilical venous fetal pH. Am J Obstet Gynecol. 1993;169:755-63.

167. Vintzileos AM, Fleming AD, Scorza WE, et al. Relationship between fetal biophysical activities and umbilical cord blood gas values. Am J Obstet Gynecol. 1991;165:707-13.

168. Ribbert LS, Visser GH, Mulder EJ, et al. Changes with time in fetal heart rate variation, movement incidences and hemodynamics in intrauterine growth retarded fetuses: A longitudinal approach to the assessment of fetal well being. Early Hum Dev. 1993;31:195-208.

169. Pillai M, James D. Continuation of normal neurobehavioural development in fetuses with absent umbilical arterial end-diastolic velocities. Br J Obstet Gynaecol. 1991;98:277-81.

170. Rizzo G, Arduini D, Pennestri F, et al. Fetal behavior in growth retardation: its relationship to fetal blood flow. Prenat Diagn. 1987;7:229-38.

171. Arduini D, Rizzo G, Capponi A, et al. Fetal pH value determined by cordocentesis: An independent predictor of the development of antepartum fetal heart rate decelerations in growth retarded fetuses with absent end-diastolic velocity in umbilical artery. J Perinat Med. 1996;24:601-7.

172. Ribbert LS, Snijders RJ, Nicolaides KH, et al. Relationship of fetal biophysical profile and blood gas values at cordocentesis in severely growth-retarded fetuses. Am J Obstet Gynecol. 1990;163:569-71.

173. Zeitlin J, Ancel PY, Saurel-Cubizolles MJ, et al. The relationship between intrauterine growth restriction and preterm delivery: an empirical approach using data from a European case-control study. BJOG. 2000;107:750-8.

174. Ott WJ. Intrauterine growth restriction and Doppler ultrasonography. J Ultrasound Med. 2000;19:661-5.

175. Strigini FA, De Luca G, Lencioni G, et al. Middle cerebral artery velocimetry: different clinical relevance depending on umbilical velocimetry. Obstet Gynecol. 1997;90:953-7.

176. Hecher K, Spernol R, Stettner H, et al. Potential for diagnosing imminent risk for appropriate- and small for gestational fetuses by Doppler examination of umbilical and cerebral arterial blood flow. Ultrasound Obstet Gynecol. 1995;5:247-55.

177. Severi FM, Bocchi C, Visentin A, et al. Uterine and fetal cerebral Doppler predict the outcome of third-trimester small-for-gestational age fetuses with normal umbilical artery Doppler. Ultrasound Obstet Gynecol. 2002;19:225-8.

178. Baschat AA, Towbin J, Bowles NE, et al. Is adenovirus a fetal pathogen? Am J Obstet Gynecol. 2003;189:758-63.

179. Magann EF, Chauhan SP, Barrilleaux PS, et al. Amniotic fluid index and single deepest pocket: weak indicators of abnormal amniotic volumes. Obstet Gynecol. 2000;96:737-40.

180. Chamberlain PF, Manning FA, Morrison I, et al. Ultrasound evaluation of amniotic fluid volume. I. The relationship of marginal and decreased amniotic fluid volumes to perinatal outcome. Am J Obstet Gynecol. 1984;150:245-9.

181. Chauhan SP, Sanderson M, Hendrix NW, et al. Perinatal outcome and amniotic fluid index in the antepartum and intrapartum periods: A meta-analysis. Am J Obstet Gynecol. 1999;181:1473-8.

182. Bukowski R. Fetal growth potential and pregnancy outcome. Semin Perinatol. 2004;28:51-8.

183. Sabbagha RE. Intrauterine growth retardation, In. Sabbagha RE (Ed). Diagnostic Ultrasound applied to Obstetrics and Gynecology, 2nd edition. Philadelphia, PA: JB Lippincott Co; 1987 pp. 112-31.

184. Tamura RK, Sabbagha RE. Percentile ranks of sonar fetal abdominal circumference measurements, Am J Obstet Gynecol. 1980;138:475.

185. Baschat AA, Weiner CP. Umbilical artery Doppler screening for detection of the small fetus in need of antepartum surveillance. Am J Obstet Gynecol. 2000;182:154-8.

186. Divon MY, Chamberlain PF, Sipos L, et al. Identification of the small for gestational age fetus with the use of gestational age-independent indices of fetal growth. Am J Obstet Gynecol. 1986;155:1197-201.

187. Tamura RK, Sabbagha RE, Pan WH, et al. Ultrasonic fetal abdominal circumference: Comparison of direct versus calculated measurement. Obstet Gynecol. 1986;67:833.

188. Weiner CP, Robinson D. The sonographic diagnosis of intrauterine growth retardation using the postnatal ponderal index and the crown heel length as standards of diagnosis. Am J Perinatol. 1989;6:380-3.

189. Hadlock FP, Deter RL, Carpenter RJ, et al. Estimating fetal age: effect of head shape on BPD. Am J Roentgenol. 1981;137:83.

190. Smith PA, Johansson D, Tzannatos C, et al. Prenatal measurement of the fetal cerebellum and cisterna cerebellomedullaris by ultrasound. Prenat Diagn. 1986;6:133.

191. Warsof SL, Cooper DJ, Little D, et al. Routine ultrasound screening for antenatal detection of intrauterine growth retardation. Obstet Gynecol. 1986;67:33.

192. Sarmandal P, Grant JM. Effectiveness of ultrasound determination of fetal abdominal circumference and fetal ponderal index in the diagnosis of asymmetrical growth retardation. Br J Obstet Gynaecol. 1990;97:118.

193. Hadlock FP, Deter RL, Harrist RB, et al. A data-independent predictor of intrauterine growth retardation: femur length/abdominal circumference ratio. AJR. 1983;141:979.

194. McGowan LM, Harding JE, Roberts AB, et al. A pilot randomized controlled trial of two regimens of fetal surveillance for small-for-gestational age fetuses with normal results of umbilical artery Doppler velocimetry. Am J Obstet Gynecol. 2000;182:81-6.

195. Neilson JP, Alfirevic Z. Doppler ultrasound for fetal assessment in high risk pregnancies (Cochrane review). In: The Cochrane Library, Issue 1. Oxford: Update Software. 2002.

196. Westergaard HB, Langhoff-Roos J, Lingman G, et al. A critical appraisal of the use of umbilical artery Doppler ultrasound in high-risk pregnancies: Use of meta-analyses in evidence-based obstetrics. Ultrasound Obstet Gynecol. 2001;17:466-76.

197. Gosling RG, King DH. Ultrasound angiology. In: Marcus AW, Adamson L (Eds). Arteries and Veins, 2nd edition. Edinburgh: Churchill Livingstone; 1975. pp. 61-98.

198. Thompson RS, Trudinger BJ, Cook CM. Doppler ultrasound waveform indices: A/B ratio, pulsatility index and Pourcelot ratio. Br J Obstet Gynaecol. 1988;95:581-8.

199. Hershkovitz R, Kingdom JC, Geary M, et al. Fetal cerebral blood flow redistribution in late gestation: Identification of compromise in small fetuses with normal umbilical artery Doppler. Ultrasound Obstet Gynecol. 2000;15:209-12.

200. Bahado-Singh RO, Kovanci E, Jeffres A, et al. The Doppler cerebroplacental ratio and perinatal outcome in intrauterine growth restriction. Am J Obstet Gynecol. 1999;180:750-6.

201. Baschat AA, Galan HL, Bhide A, et al. Viability in early onset IUGR: Is it time to reconsider intervention thresholds? Am J Obstet Gynecol. 2003;189:S216.

202. Harrington K, Thompson MO, Carpenter RG, et al. Doppler fetal circulation in pregnancies complicated by preeclampsia or delivery of a small for gestational age baby: 2. Longitudinal analysis. Br J Obstet Gynaecol. 1999;106:453-66.

203. Bilardo CM, Wolf H, Stigter RH, et al. Relationship between monitoring parameters and perinatal outcome in severe, early intrauterine growth restriction. Ultrasound Obstet Gynecol. 2004;23:119-25.

204. Baschat AA. Doppler application in the delivery timing of the preterm growth-restricted fetus: another step in the right direction. Ultrasound Obstet Gynecol. 2004;23:111-8.

205. Karsdorp VH, van Vugt JM, van Geijn HP, et al. Clinical significance of absent or reversed end-diastolic velocity waveforms in umbilical artery. Lancet. 1994;344:1664-8.

206. Divon MY, Girz BA, Lieblich R, et al. Clinical management of the fetus with markedly diminished umbilical artery end-diastolic flow. Am J Obstet Gynecol. 1989;161:1523-7.

SECTION 10

Nutrition and Metabolism

PD Gluckman, HN Winn

CHAPTER

87

The Role of Essential Fatty Acids and Antioxidants in Neurovascular Development and Complications of Prematurity

K Ghebremeskel, Y Min, B Thomas

INTRODUCTION

Membrane integrity and function are dependent on the incorporation of appropriate amounts of arachidonic (20:4n-6, AA) and docosahexaenoic (22:6n-3, DHA) acids, and antioxidant protection. AA and DHA are highly unsaturated and therefore must be protected from peroxidative damage. There is an interdependence between membrane AA and DHA, and membrane-bound antioxidant enzymes. Optimum activity of the enzymes is dependent on the physical integrity of the membranes. At the same time, the membrane fatty acids require the antioxidant enzymes for protection. Paradoxically, it has also been shown that n-3 polyunsaturated fatty acids exert protective effects against injury caused by oxidative stress. In the very low birth weight baby, tissue maturation, structural integrity, function and protection are closely intertwined; hence, there is a need to consider both polyunsaturated fatty acids and antioxidants together.

Our proposition is that low AA and DHA, suboptimal antioxidant protection and the immature anatomy in an alien oxygen radical-generating environment predispose the very low birth weight babies to serious disorders often described as the complications of prematurity. This hypothesis of "synergistic insufficiency" brings together the concepts of free-radical damage and structural integrity consistent with the proposition of Saugstad[1] that the various complications of prematurity are "facets of one disease".

ESSENTIAL FATTY ACIDS

The term *essential fatty acids* originated from the discovery that absence of certain fatty acids, which are not synthesized *de novo* by animals, in the diet leads to clinical abnormalities. They are vital for reproduction, normal growth, development and function of all tissues. There are two families of essential fatty acids: namely, the n-3 and n-6 families. Linoleic (18:2n-6, LA) and α-linolenic (18:3n-3, ALA) acids are the parent compounds of the n-6 and the n-3 families, respectively. By convention, the formula for fatty acids is abbreviated as X:Yn-M. X refers to the number of carbon atoms, Y to the number of double bonds, and M the position of the first double bond counting from the terminal methyl (CH_3) group (Fig. 87.1).

Animals cannot synthesize either LA or ALA. However, they can add double bonds and carbon atoms to LA and ALA. This metabolic process produces long-chain derivatives with 20 and 22 carbon atoms, and 3, 4, 5 and 6 double bonds (Fig. 87.2). The two most important members of the n-6 and n-3 families in cell membrane, which often regarded as essential, are AA and DHA.

Dietary Sources of Essential Fatty Acids

Fruits, seeds and vegetable oils such as sunflower, safflower, soybean, cottonseed and corn are the predominant source of LA.[2] ALA is a minor constituent of most vegetable oils except in linseed, soybean and rapeseed oil; it is a major fatty acid in green leafy vegetables.[3,4] Gamma-linolenic acid (18:3n-6, GLA) is found in evening primrose, borage and blackcurrant seed oils. AA is found in eggs, lean meat and offal such as liver, brain and entrails. It is also found in substantial proportions in tropical fish and shellfish.[5-7] Fish, shellfish and fish oils are the main source of eicosapentaenoic acid (20:5n-3, EPA) and DHA. Fish caught in Northern latitudes (> 30° N) have, on average, seven times as much n-3 fatty acids as n-6 fatty acids.[5,7]

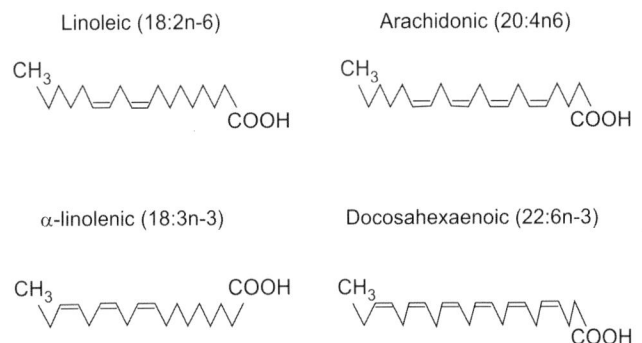

Fig. 87.1: Structural formula of linoleic, α-linolenic, arachidonic and docosahexaenoic acids

N-6 family

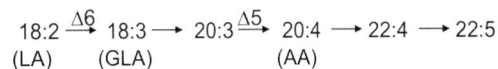

N-3 family

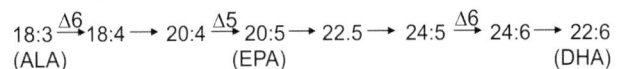

LA, linoleic; GLA, γ-linolenic; AA, arachidonic;
ALA, α-linolenic; EPA, eicosapentaenoic; DHA, docohexaenoic
Δ6, Δ6 desaturation; Δ5, Δ5 desaturation

Fig. 87.2: Metabolic pathway of the synthesis of n-6 and n-3 polyunsaturated fatty acids

Distribution in Tissues and the Brain

Long-chain fatty acids, both of the n-3 and n-6 families, are vital components of cell membrane lipids (Fig. 87.3). AA is present in all biological membranes and represents up to 15% of the total fatty acids in polar phospholipids. DHA is more specifically present at very high levels in the retina, brain, testis and sperm.[3] In the cerebral gray matter, DHA makes up to one-third of the total fatty acid content of ethanolamine and serine phosphoglycerides.[8,9] Among subcellular fractions of brain tissue, the highest levels of DHA are found in synapotosomes, synaptic vesicles, mitochondria and microsomes where there is evidence of selective incorportion.[10] In the photoreceptor outer segments, the level of DHA is as high as 60% of total fatty acids.[11] White matter and its myelin fractions contain low levels of AA and DHA and high levels of saturated and monounsaturated fatty acids.[12]

Essentiality of n-3 and n-6 Fatty Acids

Essential fatty acids are required for the structure and function of membranes.[13-15] They are also converted to eicosanoids, which are regulators and coordinators of local multicellular function. N-6 fatty acids were recognized as essential over 60 years ago.[16,17] However, it is only in the last two decades that the essentiality of the n-3 fatty acid has been conclusively established. Although, AA and DHA can be formed from LA and ALA as described above, $\Delta 6$ desaturase, the enzyme required for the first and last metabolic steps, is rate limiting. In some species such as the cat, the activity of this enzyme is too low to measure hence AA and DHA are essential fatty acids and must be provided in the diet.[18] Fat-free diets or those deficient in n-6 and n-3 polyunsaturated fatty acids produce reproductive failure, retarded growth and abnormal changes in many organs such as the skin, liver and kidney in many species including the human infant.[16,17,19,20]

In experimental animals, membrane structural alterations resulting from changes in the AA and DHA composition leads to loss of cellular integrity and functions.[21-23] Deficits of the essential n-3 fatty acids cause cerebral hemorrhage in chicks,[24] and learning and visual impairment in rats.[25-27] Polydipsia, visual impairment and abnormal electroretinogram are manifested in nonhuman primates deficient in n-3 fatty acids.[20,28]

In addition to their structural and functional properties, some fatty acids, namely, dihommo-γ-linolenic acid (20:3n-6, DHGLA), eicosapentaenoic acid (20:5n-3, EPA) and AA are precursors of hormone-like compounds known as eicosanoids. These are a complex group of highly biologically active compounds, which are involved in the control and regulation of blood flow, intraocular pressure, cell mediated immunity and inflammation, renal function, insulin release and reproduction.[29] Recently, it has been demonstrated that DHA is the precursor of a novel brain protective messenger, 10, 17S-docosatriene, which inhibits ischemia-reperfusion-mediated leucocyte infiltration and proinflammatory gene expression.[30]

Essential Fatty Acids and Pregnancy

During pregnancy, there is a high demand for AA and DHA for the development of fetal brain and other vital tissues. Consequently, in the third trimester the accretion of total n-6 and n-3 fatty acids by the fetal brain increases progressively.[31,32] It is estimated that fetus accumulates about 70 mg/d n-3 long-chain fatty acids, primarily DHA, during the third trimester.[32,33] The fetus has the ability to synthesize AA and DHA from their respective parent compounds LA and ALA.[34] However, the rate of synthesis is not fast enough to meet requirements and hence, these fatty acids are obtained from maternal circulation by placental selection and extraction. This selective transfer is reflected in a significant decrease in the blood level of AA and DHA in healthy pregnant women[35,36] and a concomitant increase in the fetus (Fig. 87.4). Fish-eating populations with a raised intake of long chain n-3 fatty acids have prolonged pregnancies and reduced incidence of both pregnancy-induced hypertension and preterm deliveries.[37] Maternal supplementation

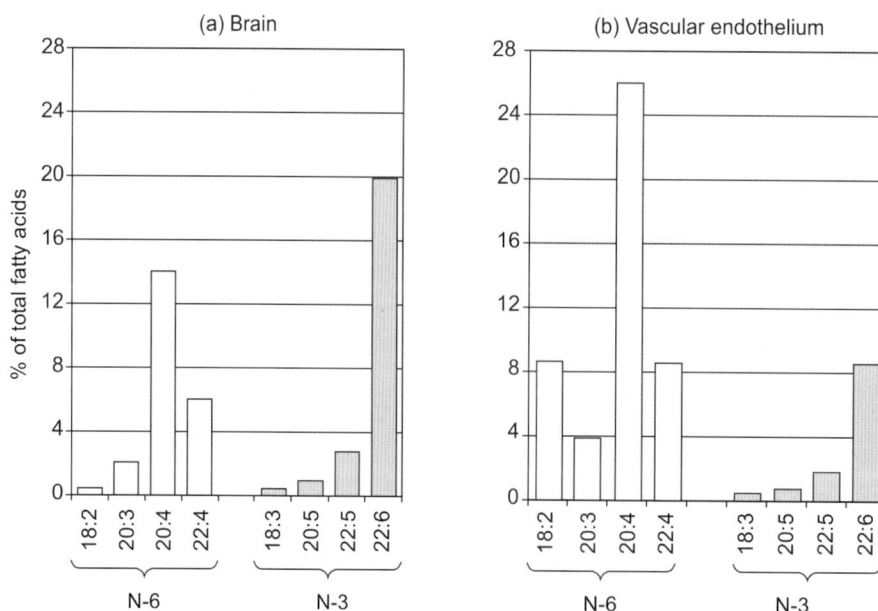

Fig. 87.3: N-6 and N-3 fatty acid composition of the inner cell membrane phospholipid (ethanolamine phosphoglycerides) of the brain and vascular endothelium

with n-3 fatty acids during pregnancy, and pregnancy and lactation are associated with cerebral maturation of the newborn[38] and mental development at 4 years of age,[39] respectively.

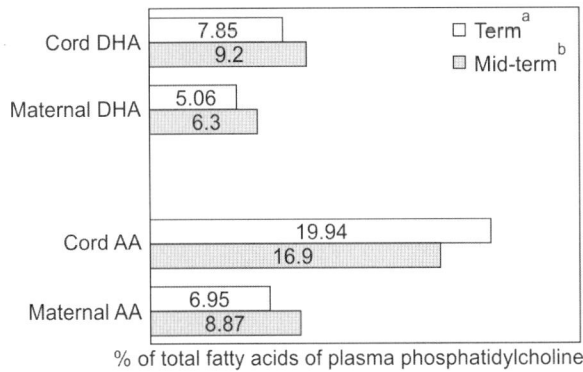

Cord DHA — 7.85 — 9.2
Maternal DHA — 5.06 — 6.3
Cord AA — 19.94 — 16.9
Maternal AA — 6.95 — 8.87

☐ Term[a] ☐ Mid-term[b]

% of total fatty acids of plasma phosphatidylcholine

[a]Term data are from normal deliveries at 39–42 gestation weeks and birth weight >3.0 kg.

[b]Mid-term data are derived from mid-term elective abortion.

Fig. 87.4: Maternal and fetal (cord blood) arachidonic (AA) and docosahexaenoic (DHA) acids in plasma choline phosphoglycerides at mid-term and term

Essential Fatty Acids in the Human Neonates

Appropriately grown term babies of healthy mothers are born with high levels of AA and DHA due to placental enrichment. This selective placental transfer of AA and DHA from the mother to fetus would be reduced if the mothers have chronic disease such as diabetes (Fig. 87.5),[40-42] impaired fatty acid metabolism or placental infarction. Babies born to mothers with marginal or low AA and DHA status because of insufficient intake prior to, and during, pregnancy will also be expected to have depressed levels of these essential fatty acids at birth.

Pre-term and low birth weight babies are born with depressed levels of AA and DHA.[43-45] Our study on maternal and cord blood phosphoglycerides showed that low concentrations of AA and DHA were associated with low birth weight and gestational age, respectively, and low levels of AA and DHA, independently and together, were associated with reduced head circumference.[46,47] A parallel investigation of umbilical arteries over a wide birth weight range demonstrated that the triene/tetraene ratio (20:3n-9/20:4n-6), an index of essential fatty acid deficiency, and the 22:4n-6/22:5n-6 ratio, an index of DHA insufficiency, were abnormal in low birth weight babies.[43] In addition, it has been shown that intrauterine

(a) Plasma and red cell (RBC) choline phosphoglycerides AA and DHA of neonates of nondiabetic (control, n=33) and gestational diabetic (GDM, n=40) women

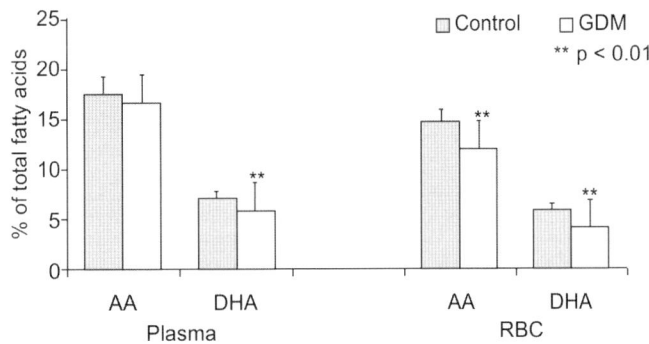

☐ Control ☐ GDM ** $p < 0.01$

% of total fatty acids

AA DHA
Plasma

AA DHA
RBC

(b) Plasma choline phosphoglycerides AA and DHA of neonates of nondiabetics (control n=33), type 1 (n=26) and type 2 (n=15) diabetic women

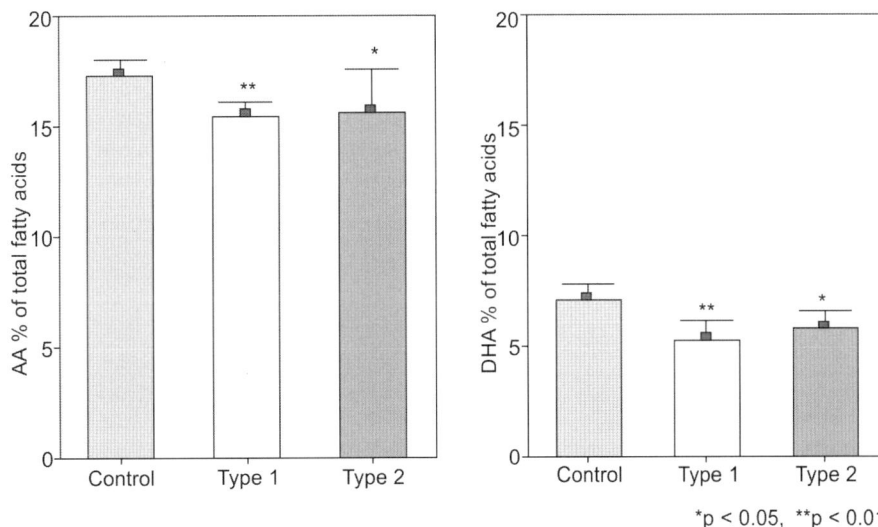

AA % of total fatty acids

Control Type 1 Type 2

DHA % of total fatty acids

Control Type 1 Type 2

*$p < 0.05$, **$p < 0.01$

Fig. 87.5: Neonates of diabetic mothers have reduced blood levels of arachidonic (AA) and docosahexaenoic (DHA) acids

growth restriction is associated with changes in fetal-maternal polyunsaturated fatty acid relationship,[48] and reduced levels of AA and DHA at birth.[49] Moreover, Zhang[50] have demonstrated that treatment with LA and ALA increases biparietal diameter and weight in the intrauterine restricted fetus.

Subsequent to birth, in the human preterm infant, the plasma levels of AA decrease substantially, despite a threefold increase in its precursor LA (Fig. 87.6). A similar fall in DHA is also reported.[45,47] In preterm babies fed formula milk containing LA and ALA but devoid of AA and DHA, the plasma levels of AA and DHA declines by 47 and 23% respectively between birth and postnatal day 15.[51] This indicates that the rate of neonatal synthesis[52,53] is unable to meet the AA and DHA demand for growth and development.[54] Koletzko and colleagues[55] estimated that endogenous synthesis contributed only about 23% of total plasma AA by day 4 in term infants.

Postnatally, a suboptimal nutritional management compounds the prenatal nutrient deficit of AA and DHA when infants are fed on artificial milks devoid of these two nutrients. Predictably, this is reflected in alterations in membrane composition. Term and preterm babies fed on conventional infant formula without AA and DHA, have depressed levels of DHA in the blood[51,56,57] and in brain tissue compared to babies fed on breast milk which does contain AA and DHA.[58,59]

An insufficiency of polyunsaturated fatty acids has a profound impact on neurovisual development in term and preterm infants[60-66] that is shown to be long lasting. Infants fed on formula milk devoid of DHA had lower visual acuity and cognitive scores compared to those fed breast milk. Supplementation of formula with DHA is related with enhanced visual acuity[60-64] and discriminative learning.[67] Bjerve and associates[68] have reported lower psychomotor performance scores associated with low levels of plasma DHA at 1 year of age. At 3 years of age term babies who have been fed on formula milk without DHA, had significantly lowered visual and stereo acuity and letter matching compared to babies fed on breast milk.[61,66] Eight-year-old children previously fed on formula milk as preterm babies had an eight point lower IQ score compared to those fed on breast milk.[69] Lanting and coworkers[70] reported a

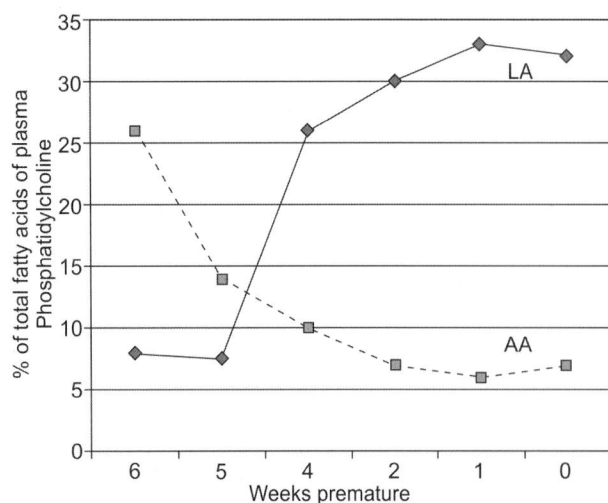

Fig. 87.6: The diagram illustrates the scale and speed of loss of arachidonic acid (AA) from plasma choline phospholgycerides of preterm babies between birth and the expected date of delivery (LA is the precursor of AA)

neurodevelopmental disadvantage in 9-year-old children who had been fed breast milk compared to those fed on formula milks.

Some reports on term infants have demonstrated improved visual acuity with formula milk containing DHA[71] whilst others have not.[72] In the latter study, the range of DHA in human milk is quoted as 0.1–0.9% of the fatty acids and yet the amount of DHA used was 0.02% above the lowest level. Bearing in mind that maternal diet and health will influence milk DHA,[73] one wonders as to the validity of choosing such low levels, which reflect the lowest nutritional status in the range, reported. Unfortunately, few workers select mothers for the study of human milk based on sound evidence of good health and nutritional status.

Human Milk, Lipid and Fatty Acids

In human milk, the lipid fraction provides about 60% of the energy for the infant. It mainly consists of triglycerides, which account for about 96% and phosphoglycerides for about 2–3%. The concentration of lipid in human milk is variable and is influenced by length of gestation (term or preterm), length of lactation, time of day, duration of individual feeds (low in fore and high in hind milk) and most of all maternal diet.[74,75] In contrast to lipid concentration, the fatty acid composition of mature human milk changes little with the duration of the feed, the time of the day and length of lactation.[73,76] Colostrum contains higher levels of AA and DHA than mature milk.[76,77] Similarly, very preterm and preterm human milk contain higher levels of the two fatty acids compared with term milk.[78]

Although, it seems that milk AA and DHA are resistant to dietary change, they do respond to maternal diet, which is the most important determinant of fatty acid composition of human milk. Comparisons of vegetarian and nonvegetarian women show that the milk essential fatty acids reflect the diet.[79] Greenland Eskimos, North Canadian Inuit and Japanese islanders have high intakes of seals, fish and other seafoods. Consequently, breast milk from these communities is high in the n-3 fatty acids, namely, EPA and DHA.[80,81] Mothers from countries where fat provides greater than 35% of the daily energy (high fat intakes) have lower short-chain and higher long-chain fatty acid concentrations. Conversely, those from countries where the habitual diet is relatively low in fat (less than 15% of the energy) have high proportions of short-chain and AA and DHA.[73,82] It is intriguing why breast milk DHA of Western (European and American) women, who are supposed to be "well nourished", is invariably very low (< 0.2%) in contrast to milk of inadequately nourished women from Africa and Asia (> 0.4%). Since plant based foods are the major sources of dietary lipids of the latter group, their intake of saturated fat would be less than 5%, which is well below the amount consumed by Western women (15–25% range). Hence, it is plausible that high total and saturated fat intakes reduce the relative proportions of DHA in breast milk of Western women. This proposition is consistent with our recent experimental study[83] that showed suckling pups born to dams fed high total and saturated fat diet, akin to western foods, during pregnancy and lactation had about 25% lower DHA in liver choline and ethanolamine phosphoglycerides compared with the controls indicating that the metabolism of DHA is adversely influence by saturated fat.

Breast milk and artificial formulations, which simulate breast milk, with respect to DHA, appear to enhance DHA status, cognitive development and visual functions of the preterm baby.

Nevertheless, it is questionable whether these feeds meet the AA and DHA requirement for optimum development of preterm babies. The current AA and DHA recommendation for infants, and the consequential formulation, which is modeled on milk of Western women, is also questionable. It is legitimate to argue that breast milk evolved to support the postnatal development of the term neonate born with appropriate developed and functional systems. The preterm baby, who is born with immature anatomy and metabolic systems, will have to continue its interrupted prenatal development under neonatal conditions. This can only be done if the infant is provided with the appropriate nutrients in the right amounts. What the preterm baby requires in the immediate neonatal period is a surrogate placenta that provides enriched AA, DHA and other essential nutrients rather than mammary glands, which generate breast milk for the normal birth weight term baby.

ANTIOXIDANTS

Membrane integrity and functions are dependent on the incorporation of appropriate amounts of the highly unsaturated fatty acids, AA and DHA, which are susceptible to peroxidation unless protected by antioxidants. There is an interdependence between membrane AA and DHA, and membrane-bound antioxidant enzymes. Optimum activity of the enzymes is dependent on the physical integrity of the membrane. At the same time, the membrane fatty acids require the antioxidant enzymes for protection. It has been shown that the activity of mitocohondrial manganese-superoxide dismutate (Mn-SOD) in influenced by dietary essential fatty acids, while the activity of cystosolic Cu/Zn-SOD remains unaffected.[84]

Reduced competence of the antioxidant defense may lead to damage to the structural membrane of the brain, retina, lungs and other tissues, particularly in a hyperoxic environment. Indeed Saugstad[85] and Sullivan[86] postulated that oxygen radical injury may be a common pathogenic mechanism in the neonatal diseases, bronchopulmonary dysplasia, hemolytic anemia, intraventricular hemorrhage and retinopathy of prematurity.

In the chicken model of intraventricular hemorrhage, we have been able to induce hemorrhage in the cerebellum between 10 days and 28 days after hatching. The window of susceptibility corresponds to the time of rapid growth of the cerebellum and acquisition of long-chain polyunsaturated fatty acids. Provision of vitamin E, or ALA without vitamin E arrests the disease.[24,87] This model illustrates the importance of considering both the membrane structure and its protection together.

Research into the role of antioxidant vitamins and fatty acids in nonhuman primates demonstrates that these nutrients provide protection against oxidative stress. Laboratory-bred mamosets had a high hydrogen peroxide-induced erythrocyte hemolysis in vitro,[88] which correlated negatively with levels of vitamin E and LA.[88,89] The high erythrocyte hemolysis skin lesions and alopecia manifested in these animals were ameliorated by an increased intake of vitamin E and the correction of membrane n-6/n-3 balance.[90] Similarly, other studies[91-94] have reported that dietary n-3 fatty acids exert a protective effect against injury caused by oxidative stress.

Animal studies show reduced activities of the antioxidant enzymes in the lung and kidney of those delivered before term. These studies indicate that functionally protective enzymes are being put in place toward the end of gestation in preparation for a normal term delivery.[95,96] Similarly, the activities of superoxide dismutate, glutathione peroxidase and catalase are low in preterm and low birth weight babies.[97-99]

Preterm and low birth weight infants are born with low circulating and hepatic levels of vitamins A and E.[100-102] Reports suggest a protective effect of vitamin A against bronchopulmonary dysplasia,[103] and of vitamin E against retinopathy of prematurity[104,105] and intra/periventricular hemorrhage.[106-108]

CONCLUSION

All these data show that the preterm baby is born disadvantaged because of the loss of the placental input of structural fatty acids and immature endogenous peroxidative defense systems. Moreover, these premature-birth induced disadvantages persist postnatally. Blood antioxidant protection remains depressed and the proportions of plasma structural fatty acids fall precipitously. These babies are indeed, a mirror of the chicken model of brain hemorrhage caused by a combined deficit of antioxidants and structural fatty acids.

REFERENCES

1. Saugstad OD. Mechanism of tissue injury by oxygen radicals: Implications for neonatal disease. Acta Pediatr. 1996;85:1-4.
2. Gunstone F, Norris FA. Lipids in Foods. Oxford: Pergamon Press; 1983.
3. Tinoco J. Dietary requirements and functions of alphalinolenic acid in animals. Prog Lipid Res. 1982;20:1-45.
4. Budowski P. Omega-3 fatty acids in health and disease. World Rev Nutr Diet. 1988;57:214-74.
5. Ackman RG. Fatty acid composition of fish oils. In: Barlow SM, Stansby ME (Eds). Nutritional Evaluation of Long-chain Fatty Acids in Fish Oils. London: Academic Press: 1982. pp. 25-88.
6. Ackman RG. Unsaturated fatty acids and health. Omega-3 News. 1990;4:1-4.
7. O'Dea K, Sinclair AJ. High arachidonic acid content in Australian fish caught off the coast at 17°S. Am J Clin Nutr. 1982;36:868-72.
8. O'Brian JS, Sampson EL. Fatty acid and fatty acid aldehyde composition of the major brain lipids in normal human gray matter, white matter and myelin J. Lipid Res. 1965;6:545-51.
9. Svennerholm L. Distribution of fatty acid composition of phosphoglycerides in normal human brain. J Lipid Res. 1968;9:570-9.
10. Suzki H, Manable S, Wada O, et al. Rapid incorporation of docosahexaenoic acid from dietary sources into brain microsomal, synaptosomal and mitochondrial membranes in adult mice. Int J Vit Res. 1997;67:272-8.
11. Fliesler SJ, Anderson RE. Chemistry and metabolism of lipids in the vertebrate retina. Prog Lipid Res. 1983;22:79-131.
12. Fleischer S, Rouser G. Lipids of sub-cellular particles. J Am Oil Chem Soc. 1965;42:588-607.
13. Salem N Jr, Kim H-Y, Yergey JA. Docosahexaenoic acid: Membrane function and metabolism. In: Simopoulos AP, Kifer RR, Martin RE (Eds). Healthy Effects of Polyunsaturated Fatty Acids in Seafoods. Orlando, USA: Academic press; 1986. pp. 263-317.
14. Bazan NG. Supply of n-3 polyunsaturated fatty acids and their significance in the central nervous system. In: Wurtman RJ, Wurtman JJ (Eds). Nutrition and the Brain. New York: Raven press; 1990. pp. 1-4.

15. Anderson RE, O'Brian PJ, Weigand RD, et al. Conservation of docosahexaenoic acid in the retina. Adv Exp Med Biol. I992;86: 587-621.

16. Burr GO, Burr MM. A new deficiency disease produced by the rigid exclusion of fat from the diet. J Biol Chem. I929;82:345-67.

17. Holman RT. Essential fatty acid deficiency. Prog Chem Fat. I968;9:275-348.

18. Rivers JP, Sinclair AJ, Crawford MA. Inability of the cat to desaturate essential fatty acids. Nature. I975;258:171-3.

19. Holman RT, Johnson SB, Hatch TG. Human linoleic acid deficiency. Prog Lipid Res. I982;25:29-39.

20. Neuringer M, Anderson GJ, Connor WE. The essentiality of n-3 fatty acids for the development and function of the retina and the brain. Ann Rev Nutr. I988;8:517-41.

21. Clausen J, Moller D. Allergic encephalomyelitis induced by brain antigen after deficiency of polyunsaturated fatty acids during myelination. Acta Neurol Scand. I967;43:375-88.

22. Crawford MA, Sinclair AJ. Nutritional influences in the evolution of mammalian brain. In:Elliot K, Knight J (Eds). Lipids, Malnutrition and the Developing Brain. Ciba Foundation Symposium. Amsterdam: Elsevier; I972. pp. 267-92.

23. Galli C, Socini A. Dietary lipids in pre- and post-natal development. In:Perkins EG, Visek WJ (Eds). Dietary Fats and Health. Proceedings of American Oil Chemists Society Conference. Chicago, USA. 1983;16:278-301.

24. Budowski P, Leighfield MJ, Crawford MA. Nutritional encephalo-malacia in the chick: An exposure of the vulnerable period for cerebellar development and the possible need for both *w*6 and *w*3 fatty acids. Br J Nutr. I987;58:511-20.

25. Wheeler TG, Benolken RM, Anderson RE. Visual membranes: Specificity of fatty acid precursors for the electrical response to illumination. Science. I975;188:13-2.

26. Bourre JM, Marianne FJ, Youyou A, et al The effects of dietary alpha-linolenic acid on the composition of nerve membranes, enzymatic activity, amplitude of electrophysiological parameters, resistance to poisons and electrophysiological parameters, resistance to poisons and performance of learning tasks in rats. J Nutr. I989;19:1880-91.

27. Yamamoto M, Saitoh M, Moriuchi A, et al. Effect of dietary alpha-linolenate/linoleate balance on brain lipid composition and learning ability in rats. J Lipid Res. I987;28:144-51.

28. Connor WE, Neuringer M, Reisbick S. Essential fatty acids: The importance of n-3 fatty acids in the retina and brain. Nutr Rev. 1992;50:21-9.

29. British Nutrition Foundation. The Report of the British Nutrition Foundation's Task Force on Unsaturated Fatty Acids. London, UK: Chapman and Hall; I992.

30. Marcheselli VL, Hong S, Lukiw WJ, et al. Novel docosanoids inhibit brain ischemia-reperfusion-mediated leukocyte infiltration and pro-inflammatory gene expression. J Biol Chem. 2003;278(44):43807-17.

31. Clandinin MT, Chappel JE, Leong S, et al. Intrauterine fatty acid accretion in human brain: Implications for fatty acid requirements. Early Hum Dev. I980;4:120-9.

32. Martinez M. Tissue levels of polyunsaturated fatty acids during early human development. J Pediatr. I992;120: S129-38.

33. Clandinin MT, Chappell JE, Leong S, et al. Intrauterine fatty acid accretion in human brain: Implications for fatty acid requirements. Early Hum Dev. 1980;4:131-8.

34. Chambaz J, Ravel D, Manier MC, et al. Essential fatty acids interconversion in the human fetal liver. Biol Neonate. 1985;47:136-40.

35. Holman RT, Johnson SB, Ogburn PL. Deficiency of essential fatty acids and membrane fluidity during pregnancy and lactation. Proc Natl Acad Sci USA. 1991;88:4835-9.

36. Hornstra G, Al M, Houwelingen AC, et al. Essential fatty acids in pregnancy and early human development. Eur J Obstet Gynecol Reprod Biol. I995;61:57-62.

37. Olsen SF, Sorensen TIA, Secher NJ, et al. Intake of marine fat rich in (n-3) polyunsaturated fatty acids may increase birth-weight by prolonging gestation. Lancet. I986;2:367-9.

38. Helland IB, Saugstad OD, Smith L, et al. Similar effects on infants of n-3 and n-6 fatty acids supplementation to pregnant and lactating women. Pediatr. 2001;108:E82-92.

39. Helland IB, Smith L, Saarem K, et al. Maternal supplementation with very long chain n-3 fatty acids during pregnancy and lactation augments children IQ at 4 years of age. Pediatr. 2003;111:1-10.

40. Ghebremeskel K, Thomas B, Min Y, et al. Fatty acids in pregnant diabetic women and neonates: Implications for pre-natal and post-natal development. Prostaglandins Leukotr Ess Fatty Acids. I997;57:190.

41. Ghebremeskel K, Thomas B, Lowy C, et al. Type 1 diabetes compromises plasma arachidonic and docosahexaenoic acids in newborn babies. Lipids. 2004;39(4):335-42.

42. Min Y, Lowy C, Ghebremeskel K, et al. Fetal erythrocyte membrane lipids modification: Preliminary observation of an early sign of compromised insulin sensitivity in the offspring of gestational diabetics. Diabetic Medicine. 2004;(In print).

43. Crawford MA, Costeloe K, Doyle W, et al. Potential diagnostic value of the umbilical artery as a definition of neural fatty acid status of the fetus during its growth. Biochem Soc Trans. I990;18:761-6.

44. Koletzko B, Martin B. Arachidonic acid and early human growth: Is there a relation? Ann Nutr Metab. I991;35:128-31.

45. Leaf AA, Leighfield MJ, Costeloe KI, et al. Long chain polyunsaturated fatty acids and fetal growth. Early Hum Dev. I992;30:183-91.

46. Crawford MA, Doyle W, Drury PJ, et al. N-6 and n-3 fatty acids during early human development. J Intern Med I989;225(Suppl 1):159-69.

47. Leaf AA, Leighfield MJ, Costeloe KI, et al. Factors affecting long-chain polyunsaturated fatty acid composition of plasma choline phosphoglycerides in preterm infants. J Pediatr Gastroenterol Nutr. I992;14:300-8.

48. Cetin I, Giovanni N, Alvino G, et al. Intrauterine growth restriction is associated with changes in polyunsaturated fatty acid fetal-maternal relationship. Pediatr Res. 2002;52:75-755.

49. Vibergsson G, Wennergreen M, Samsioe G, et al. Essential fatty acids status altered in pregnancy is complicated by intrauterine growth retardation. World Rev Nutr Diet. 1994;76:105-9.

50. Zhang L. The effects of essential fatty acid preparation in the treatment of intrauterine growth retardation. Am J Perinatology. 1997;14:535-7.

51. Ghebremeskel K, Leighfield M, Leaf A, et al. Fatty acid composition of plasma and red cell phospholipids of preterm babies fed on breast milk and formulae. Eur J Pediatr. 1995;154:46-52.

52. Poisson JP, Dupuy RP, Sarda P, et al. Evidence that liver microsomes of human neonates desaturates essential fatty acids. Biochim Biophys Acta. 1993;1167:109-13.

53. Sauerwald TU, Hachey DL, Jensen CL, et al. Intermediates in endogenous synthesis of C22:6 omega-3 and 20:4 omega-6 by term and preterm infants. Pediatr. 1997;41:183-7.

54. Food and Agriculture Organisation/World Health Organisation. The role of dietary fats and oils in human nutrition. Report of a joint expert consultation. Rome: Food and Nutrition; Paper 57, I993.

55. Koletzko B, Decsi T, Demmelmair H. Arachidonic acid supply and metabolism in human infants born at full term. Lipids. I996;31:79-83.

56. Crawford MA, Hassam AG, Williams G, et al. Essential fatty acids and fetal brain growth. Lancet. I976;1:452-3.

57. Carlson SE, Rhodes PG, Ferguson MG. Docosahexaenoic acid status of preterm infants at birth and following feeding with human milk or formula. Am J Clin Nutr. I986;44:798-804.

58. Farquharson J, Cockburn F, Patrick AW, et al. Infant cerebral cortex phospholipid fatty acid composition and diet. Lancet. I992;340:810-3.

59. Makrides M, Neumann MA, Byard RW, et al. Fatty acid composition of brain, retina, and erythrocytes in breast and formula-fed infants. Am J Clin Nutr. l994;60:189-94.

60. Birch EE, Birch DG, Hoffman D, et al. Dietary essential fatty acid supply and visual acuity development. Invest Ophthalmol Vis Sci. l993;33:3242-53.

61. Birch EE, Birch DG, Hoffman D, et al. Breast-feeding and optimal visual development. J Pediatr Opthalmol Strabismus. l993;30:33-8.

62. Carlson SE, Werkman SH, Rhodes PJ, et al. Visual acuity development in healthy preterm infants: effect of marine oil supplementation. Am J Clin Nutr. l993;58:35-42.

63. Carlson SE, Werkman SH, Peeples JM, et al. Arachidonic acid status correlates with first year growth in preterm infants. Proc Natl Acad Sci (USA), 1993;90:901-7.

64. Uauy R, Birch E, Birch D, et al. Visual and brain function measurements in studies of n-3 fatty acid measurements in studies of n-3 fatty acid requirements of infants. J Pediatr. l992;120: S168-80.

65. Vavy R, Peirano P, Hoffman D, et al. Role of essential fatty acids in the function of the developing nervous system. Lipids. l996;31:5167-76.

66. Makrides M, Simmer K, Goggin M, et al. Erythrocyte docosahexaenoic acid correlates with visual response of healthy term infants. Pediatr Res. l993;34:425-7.

67. Wainwright PE. Do essential fatty acids play a role in brain and behavioural development? Neurosci Biobehav Rev. l992;16:193-205.

68. Bjerve KF, Thoresen L, Bonaa K, et al. Clinical studies with alpha-linolenic acid and long chain n-3 fatty acids. Nutrition. l992;8:130-2.

69. Lucas A, Morley R, Cole TJ, et al. Breast milk and subsequent intelligence quotient in children born preterm. Lancet. l992;339:261-4.

70. Lanting CI, Fidler V, Huisman M, et al. Neurological difference between 9-year old children fed breast milk or formula milk as babies. Lancet. l994;344:1319-22.

71. Carlson SE, Ford AJ, Werkman SH, et al. Visual acuity and fatty acid status of term infants fed human milk and formlas with and without docoahexaenoate and arachidonate from egg yolk lecithin. Pediatr Res. l996;30:882-8.

72. Auestad N, Montalto MB, Hall RT, et al. Visual acuity erythrocyte fatty acid composition, and growth in term infants fed formulas with long chain polyunsaturated fatty acids for one year. Ross Pediatr lipid Study. Pediatr Res. l997;41:1-10.

73. Drury P, Crawford MA. Essential fatty acids in human milk. In: Dobbing J, Gracey M, Santerre J (Eds). Clinical Nutrition of the Young Child. Nestec Ltd, New York: Raven Press Ltd; 1990. pp. 289-312.

74. Hall B. Changing composition of human milk and early development of an appetite control. Lancet. l975;1:779-81.

75. Jensen RG. The Lipids of Human Milk. Boca Raton, FL: CRC Press; l989.

76. Gibson RA, Kneebone GM. Fatty acid composition of human colostrum and mature breast milk. Am J Clin Nutr. l981;34:252-7.

77. Crawford MA, Sinclair AJ, Msuya PM, et al. Structural lipids and their polyenoic constituents in human milk. In: Galli C, Jacini G, Pecile A (Eds). Dietary Lipids and Postnatal Development. New York: Raven Press; l973. pp. 41-56.

78. Bitman J, Wood DL, Hamosh M, et al. Comparison of the lipid composition of breast milk from mothers of term and preterm infants. Am J Clin Nutr. l984;38:300-13.

79. Finley DA, Lonnerdal B, Dewy KG, et al. Breast milk composition: Fat content and fatty acid composition of vegetarians and non-vegetarians. Am J Clin Nutr. l985;41:787-800.

80. Innis SM, Kuhnlein HV. Long-chain n-3 fatty acids in breast milk of Inuit women consuming traditional foods. Early Hum Dev. l988;18:185-9.

81. Wang L, Shimizu Y, Kaneko S, et al. Comparison of the fatty acid composition of total lipids and phospholipids in breast milk from Japanese women. Pediatr Int. 2000;42(1):14-20.

82. Crawford MA, Hall B, Laurance BM, et al. Milk lipids and their variability. Curr Med Res Opin. l976;4:33-43.

83. Ghebremeskel K, Bitsanis D, Koukkou E, et al. Maternal diet high in fat reduces docosahexaenoic acid in liver lipids of the newborn and suckling pups. Brit J Nutr. 1999;81:395-404.

84. Phylactos AC, Harbidge LS, Crawford MA. Essential fatty acids alter the activity of manganese-superoxide dismutase in rat heart. Lipids. l994;29:111-5.

85. Saugstad OD. Hypoxanthine as an indicator of hypoxia: Its role in health and diseases through free radical production. Pediatr Res. l988;23:143-50.

86. Sullivan JL. Iron plasma antioxidants, and the 'oxygen radical disease of prematurity'. Am J Dis Child. l988;142:1341-4.

87. Budowski P, Hawkey CM, Crawford MA. The protective effect of alpha-linoleic acid on encephalomalacia in chicks. Ann Nutr Anim. l980;34:389-400 (in French).

88. Ghebremeskel K, Williams G, Harbige L, et al. Plasma vitamins A and E and hydrogen peroxide-induced in vitro erythrocyte hemolysis in common marmosets (Callithrix jacchus). Vet Rec. l990;126:429-31.

89. Harbige LS, Ghebremeskel K, Willliams G, et al. N-3 and n-6 fatty acids in relation to in vitro erythrocyte hemolysis induced by hydrogen peroxide in captive common marmosets (Callithrix jacchus). Comp Biochem Physiol. l990;97B:167-70.

90. Ghebremeskel K, Harbige L, Williams G, et al. The effect of dietary change on in vitro erythrocyte hemolysis, skin lesions and alopecia in common marmosets (Callithrix jacchus), Comp Biochem Physiol. l991;100A:891-6.

91. Lands WE, Miller JF Jr, Rich SM. Influence of dietary fish oil on plasma lipid hydroxperoxides. Adv Prostagl Thrombox Leukotriene Res. 1987;17B;876-9.

92. Sosenko IR, Innis SM, Frank L. Menhaden fish oil n-3 polyunsaturated fatty acids and protection of new born rats from oxygen toxicity. Pediatr Res. l989;25:399-404.

93. Ellis EF, Police RJ, Dodson LY, et al. Effect of dietary n-3 fatty acids on cerebral micro-circulation. Am J Physiol. l992;262: H1379-86.

94. Lehr H-A, Huebner C, Finckh B, et al. Dietary fish oil reduces leukocyte/endothelium interaction following system administration of oxidatively modified low density lipoprotein. Circulation. l991;84:1725-31.

95. Frank L, Sosenko IR. Prenatal development of lung antioxidant enzymes in four species. J Pediatr. l987;110:106-10.

96. Hayashibe H, Assyama K, Dobashi K, et al. Prenatal development of antioxidant enzymes in rat lung, kidney, and heart: Marked increase in immunoreactive superoxide dismutate, glutathione peroxidase and catalase in the kidney. Pediatr Res. l990;27:472-5.

97. Autor AP, Frank L, Roberts RJ. Developmental characteristics of pulmonary superoxide dismutase: A relationship to idiopathic respiratory distress syndrome. Pediatr Res. l976;10:154-8.

98. Ripalda MJ, Rudolph N, Wong SL. Developmental patterns of antioxidant defence mechanisms in human erythrocytes. Paediatr Res. l989;26:366-9.

99. Phylactos AC, Leaf AA, Costeloe K, et al. Erythrocyte cupric/zinc superoxide dismutase exhibits reduced activity in preterm and low birth weight infants at birth. Act Paediatr. l995;84:1421-5.

100. Johnson LH, Schaffer DB, Boggs TR Jr. The premature infant vitamin E deficiency and retrolental fibroplasias. Am J Clin Nutr. l974;27:1158-73.

101. Shenai JP, Chytil F, Jhaveri A, et al. Plasma vitamin A and retinal-binding protein in premature and term neonates. J Pediatr. l981;99:302-5.

102. Ghebremeskel K, Burns, L, Burden TJ, et al. Vitamin A and related essential nutrients in cord blood: relationship with anthropometric measurements at birth. Early Hum Dev. l994;39:177-88.

103. Shenai JP, Kennedy KA, Chytil F, et al. Clinical trial of vitamin A supplementation in infants susceptible to bronchopulmonary dysplasia. J Pediatr. l987;111:269-77.

104. Finer NN, Schindler RF, Grant G, et al. Effect of intramuscular vitamin E on frequency and severity of retrolental fibroplasia. Lancet. l982;1:1087-91.

105. Hittner HM, Godio LB, Speer ME, et al. Retrolental fibroplasia: further clinical evidence and ultrastructural support for efficiency of vitamin E in the preterm infant. Pediatrics. l983;71:423-32.

106. Chiswick ML, Johnson M, Woodhall C, et al. Protective effect of vitamin E (DL-alpha-tocopheral) against intraventricular hemorrhage in premature babies. Br Med J. l983;287:81-4.

107. Chiswick ML, Gladman G, Sinha S, et al. Vitamin E supplementation and periventricular haemorrhage in the newborn. Am J Clin Nutr. l991;53:370S-2S.

108. Speer ME, Blifield C, Rudolph AJ, et al. Intraventricular hemorrhage and vitamin E in the very low-birth-weight infant: Evidence for efficacy of early intramuscular vitamin E administration. Pediatrics. l984;74:1107-12.

88 Maternal Inherited Metabolic Disease

R Floyd, F Cockburn, BJ Clark

INTRODUCTION

Recombinant DNA technology with the mapping of human genome has made possible the localization, identification and isolation of disease-related genes which, in turn, have improved disease diagnosis and prediction, and identified inherited defects underlying many common metabolic disorders affecting adults. Inherited metabolic disease may be diagnosed prenatally, in infancy, or may present as an adult-onset disease, particularly in diseases not generally associated with a detectable chromosome aberration or a clear Mendelian pattern of inheritance. Many of these metabolic disorders have been called polygenic or multifactorial even though it is not usually known how many genetic loci are involved or how they interact with environmental factors. Diabetes mellitus and essential hypertension are examples though the genetics of both of these disease processes are currently being illuminated. There are many perturbations of maternal metabolism which can adversely affect growth and development of the human embryo and fetus. The purpose of this chapter will be to review those maternal inherited metabolic disorders which can result in failure of implantation, early loss of implanted ova, and congenital malformations or metabolic disorder in the newborn infant.

The number of autosomal and X-linked chromosomal disorders identified continues to grow daily, many of which result in metabolic diseases or disorders. The development of management strategies to alleviate or correct these inherited disease processes has encouraged early detection with screening programs. Table 88.1 gives the frequency of some inborn errors of metabolism for which screening tests are available.[1] Although we now have considerable information about phenylketonuria in relation to

Table 88.1: Frequency of some inborn errors of metabolism for which neonatal screening tests are available

Disorder	Average frequency in liveborn infants*
Cystic fibrosis	1 in 2,500
Cystinuria	1 in 6,000
Phenylketonuria	1 in 10,000
αa₁ Antitrypsin deficiency	1 in 8,000
Histidinemia	1 in 10,000
Hartnup disorder	1 in 26,000
Galactosemia	1 in 60,000
Biotinidase deficiency	1 in 60,000
Maple syrup urine disease	1 in 200,000
Homocystinuria	1 in 200,000

*These frequencies vary widely between ethnic groups, e.g. phenylketonuria 1 in 7,000 in Scotland and 1 in 200,000 in Japan.

pregnancy management and outcome there are many other inherited metabolic disorders affecting young women which carry a risk to the developing embryo and fetus.

MATERNAL METABOLIC DISORDERS AND PREGNANCY

Diabetes Mellitus

It has long been known that the infant of the poorly controlled diabetic mother is at increased risk of congenital malformation, fetal overgrowth and neonatal hypoglycemia.[2] With improved care of pregnant diabetic women these complications and perinatal mortality for the infant have been reduced.[3-7] There is a recognized higher prevalence of diabetes mellitus in children born to diabetic parents. A higher incidence of non-insulin-dependent diabetes or gestational diabetes is found in children born to diabetic mothers than when the father is diabetic.[8] There is also a higher incidence of diabetes in offspring from diabetic maternal great-grandmothers but not paternal ones.[9] Genomic imprinting is a possible explanation for these findings.[10-12] In HLA-DR4-positive diabetics, there is evidence of a gene or genes affecting the HLA region on chromosome 6p21 and the region of 11p15 where the genes for insulin and insulin-like growth factor-2 (IGF-2) are located.[13]

A further interesting observation has been that systematic treatment of diabetic mothers during pregnancy, results in a decreased incidence of diabetes in their children.[14,15] This implies that the abnormal intrauterine environment may have as much if not more effect in determining susceptibility to subsequent diabetes in later childhood than do the genetic predisposing factors. Mechanisms for predisposition to diabetes in the infant of a diabetic mother may be related to an intrauterine influence on the effective development of Bislet cells in fetal pancreas or to an alteration in the numbers or sensitivity of insulin receptors in muscle, liver and other body tissues.

Cystic Fibrosis

This is an autosomal recessive condition in which there is an abnormality of transmembrane protein function rather than a defect or deficiency of an enzyme, which characterizes the majority of inherited metabolic disorders. Although there are problems of infertility in both females and males there is no evidence of embryopathy or fetal disorder given an adequate maternal nutritional status during pregnancy.[16]

Histidinemia

Maternal histidinemia is probably benign to the fetus. At least 61 children from 23 histidinemic mothers, most of whom were normal have been reported.[17,18] No adverse outcomes secondary to this disorder have been noted.[17-21]

Hartnup Disorder

Hartnup disease, a disorder of neutral amino acid transport in the intestinal epithelium, is inherited in an autosomal recessive manner. Maternal Hartnup disorder is also probably benign to the fetus. At least 14 children of women with the condition are known and almost all are normal. Therapy requires nicotinamide replacement and a high protein diet. Pregnancy does not appear to have any clinical impact on these families.[22]

Homocystinuria

Homocystinuria is an autosomal recessive disorder that is characterized by increased concentrations of homocystine and methionine in blood and urine, and physical features such as mental retardation, epilepsy, ectopia lentis, osteoporosis, skeletal anomalies, fatty liver and thrombotic vascular disease. These findings are secondary to a deficiency of the enzyme cystathionine β-synthase. The disorder is responsive to B6 cofactor and a low methionine diet in about 50% of patients.[23] Pregnancies have been reported in both pyridoxine responsive and nonresponsive mothers with a normal outcome.[24-26] An adequate intake of pyridoxine should be ensured as treatment with pyridoxine appears to significantly lower the risk of fetal loss.

Heterozygotes are at an increased risk for multiple thromboses, coronary artery disease and other vascular disease.[27] Third trimester complications similar to those with other inherited coagulopathies and postpartum thrombotic deaths have been reported which suggest the use of anticoagulation therapy may be indicated.[28-30]

Folate Metabolism Disorders

A genetic defect in 5,10-methylenetetrahydrofolate reductase in young women has been shown to be a risk factor for neural tube defect.[31-33] This enzyme is involved in the conversion of 5,10-methylenetetrahydrofolate to 5-methyltetrahydrofolate, which is involved in the conversion of homocysteine to methionine. The common mutation of 677CT defect is found in 5–7% of the European population and homozygosity for this mutation results in elevated homocysteine levels, elevated red cell folate and lowered plasma folate concentrations. Periconceptual folate administration reduces neural tube birth prevalence by over 60%.[33-36] Altered folate and vitamin B_{12} metabolism has been found in families with infants having spina bifida.[37] This study did not support a major involvement of methionine synthase in the etiology of neural tube defect but favored the involvement of genetic variation at loci coding for the formation of 5-methyltetrahydrofolate. A relatively mild biochemical defect in folate metabolism, requiring a higher nutritional folate intake, may become of major importance during pregnancy. Whether there would be value in detecting those individuals heterozygous for the known defects is questionable as universal prenatal folate supplementation is so effective. These patients have also been noted to have an increase in complications in the third trimester consistent with those seen in patients with an inherited coagulopathy, and the use of anticoagulation should be considered in those patients with a history of thrombosis or poor pregnancy outcome.

Isovaleric Acidemia

Maternal isolaveric acidemia has minimal impact on pregnancy and vice versa and has no ill effect on the offspring.[38] Treatment of the mother should be instituted prior to conception with protein restriction and additional glycine 0.5 g/day and L-carnitine 1 g/day to reduce the risk of metabolic acidosis in the mother and thus reduce potential hazards to the embryo and fetus. Vomiting in early pregnancy must be actively managed with a high carbohydrate intake, if necessary by nasogastric tube or parenterally, to avoid a catabolic state.

Urea Cycle Defects

The urea cycle defects include citrullinemia, argininosuccinic aciduria (ASLD), ornithine transcarbamylase deficiency (OTC), carbamoylphosphate synthetase deficiency and n-acetyl glutamate synthase deficiency.[39] There are very few reports in the literature as to the effects of these disorders on pregnancy and infants. Heterozygotes for OTC deficiency, the only X-linked disorder of the urea cycle, are known to be at risk for the development of hyperammonemic coma in the peripartum period, possibly due to increased tissue catabolism.[40] It has been reported that woman with carbamoylphosphate synthetase I deficiency developed hyperammonemic coma and died in the postpartum period.[41]

ASLD due to argininosuccinate lyase deficiency usually presents at birth with poor feeding, lethargy, hypotonia, irritability, apnea and death in the neonatal period.[42] More often there is a chronic presentation which involves mental retardation, with or without intermittent episodes of vomiting, lethargy and irritability. Trichorrhexis nodosa is a frequent occurrence, probably because of a relative deficiency of arginine.[39] Early treatment of patients with partial ASLD can result in normal intellectual and psychomotor development and as a result some patients are now surviving into adulthood and considering pregnancy. In females affected with argininosuccinate lyase deficiency careful clinical and biochemical monitoring of pregnancy will minimize the risk of metabolic decompensation in the perinatal period. There is one report of a "successful" pregnancy with no evidence that the argininosuccinate was teratogenic. The mother had been treated with a low protein diet and arginine supplements but her compliance with the arginine supplementation was suboptimal. When reviewed at 3 months of age, the baby was mildly dysmorphic with hypertelorism, a broad nasal bridge and down-slanting palpebral fissures but was developing normally.[43]

In all the urea cycle defects it is essential to ensure an adequate energy intake throughout pregnancy and if vomiting occurs enteral and/or parenteral therapy with carbohydrate should be given immediately.

Glycogen Storage Disorders

The glycogen storage disorders result from an inborn error of glycogen metabolism secondary to mutations in the genes coding for the enzymes involved in glycogen storage. These disorders have a variable age of onset from birth to adulthood and are categorized by number based upon the chronology of recognition of the responsible enzyme defect. Only those with a reasonable likelihood of presence during and potential impact upon pregnancy are discussed.

Glucose-6-phosphate deficiency (Type I glycogen storage disease) is an autosomal recessive disorder involving mutations in the genes for glucose-6-phosphate hydrolase, located at 17q21 (type 1a) and glucose-6-phosphate translocase located at 11q23 (type 1b,c,d). The incidence of specific mutations varies with ethnicity.[44,45] Affected patients typically present in early infancy with hepatomegaly, hypoglycemia and lactic acidosis.[46] The majority of patients will also have hyperuricemia and marked hyperlipidemia.[46] Platelet dysfunction is common and liver adenomas often develop in older children and adults with malignant transformation in approximately 10%.[47] Patients with type 1b also have chronic or intermittent neutropenia and neutrophil dysfunction.

Maintenance of physiologic levels of glucose is the mainstay of therapy. This become markedly more difficult during pregnancy and provision of frequent meals high in carbohydrate content and supplementation with uncooked cornstarch during the day and prior to bedtime can usually accomplish this goal. In some cases the use of continuous infusion of glucose solution via nasogastric tube or additional doses of cornstarch in the early morning hours may be necessary. Multivitamins and calcium should supplement the diet, and fructose and galactose restricted. Intravenous glucose and platelet transfusion may be used for abnormal bleeding; the use of allopurinol and vasopressin during pregnancy are currently prescribed.[48]

Pregnancy outcomes with adequate glucose supplementation appear to be good in most cases. The incidence of growth restriction may be increased and monitoring of the fetus with serial ultrasound measurements in the third trimester should be considered. Patients with type 1b should be monitored for evidence of subclinical infection (upper respiratory, urinary tract) due to the potential for neutrophil dysfunction. Delivery at or near term should be anticipated. The intrapartum glucose levels should be closely monitored and appropriate supplementation provided.[49,50]

Type III glycogen storage disease is inherited as an autosomal recessive trait and is specifically a mutation in the gene that encodes for the debrancher enzyme amyloglucosidase. This gene is located at 1p21 and again, specific mutations vary with ethnic background.[51,52] Clinical features of the disease include liver and muscle involvement with hepatomegaly, hypotonia, weakness and muscle wasting as well as cardiac involvement. Hepatomegaly and liver function typically improve with age and muscle weakness is the primary finding in adults. Involvement of the liver alone occurs in approximately 15% of patients.[53-55]

Case reports of maternal type III glycogen storage disease relate the potential for life-threatening complications specifically cardiac decompensation.[56] Evaluation of cardiac anatomy prior to and during pregnancy (at 28 weeks) and postpartum should be obtained. Management includes supplementation of glucose as described for type I glycogen storage disease.

Type V glycogen storage disease (McArdle Disease) is a disorder caused by mutations in the single gene encoding the muscle isoform of phosphorylase.[57] This gene is located at 11q13.[58] Phosphorylase catalyzes the removal of 1,4 glucosyl residues from the outer branches of the glycogen molecule liberating glucose-1-phosphate. This myophosphorylase deficiency results in accumulation of glycogen in skeletal muscle and reduction in ATP generation. Clinically, this manifests as muscle fatigue and cramping with strenuous exercise. There is no heart or liver involvement. Case reports of pregnancy outcomes relate no deterioration or

exacerbation of symptoms.[59] Limiting activity during pregnancy will control the symptoms associated with the disorder and the only complication of labor reported is that of forearm cramping secondary to the use of an automatic blood pressure cuff.

Hyperglycinemia

Hyperglycinemia is a nonspecific feature of several organic acidurias and is usually associated with intermittent ketosis. Non-ketotic hyperglycinemia is a specific disorder of glycine catabolism caused by a defect in the glycine cleavage system.[60] The disorder usually presents in the first week of life with somnolence, lethargy, and lack of spontaneous movement and apnoeic episodes. There may be seizures and exaggerated reflexes. Milder forms of the disorder are found with nonspecific mental retardation in adult life. The diagnosis is made on the basis of finding hyperglycinemia and hyperglycinuria in the absence of a disorder of organic acid metabolism. The diagnosis is usually confirmed by the finding of high cerebrospinal fluid concentrations of glycine. In the milder forms of the disorder administration of large doses of sodium benzoate has been shown to reduce CSF glycine and the frequency of seizures. The authors have experience of three pregnancies in one nonketotic hyperglycinemic mother managed with oral sodium benzoate. The control of plasma glycine levels in the mother was relatively easy during the pregnancy and indeed was less troublesome than during the nonpregnancy phase. The three infants were normally grown and have thrived with normal subsequent development.

Galactosemia

Galactosemia is the term used to describe disorders of galactose metabolism. The disorder is actually three distinct disorders caused by defects in galactose-1-phosphate uridyltransferase, galactokinase and uridine diphosphate galactose-4-epimerase.[61] The only form discussed here is that caused by defective galactose-1-phosphate uridyltransferase in which conversion of galactose to glucose is impaired. Accumulation of galactose-1-phosphate, galactitol, galactonate, and UDP-galactose is thought to be the cause of the complications of galactose ingestion. In the newborn period ingestion of galactose leads to vomiting and diarrhea with progression to hyperbilirubinemia, hepatomegaly, liver dysfunction and cirrhosis, hemolysis, and sepsis. Cataracts rapidly develop in the first week of life. Despite early therapy these patients still manifest developmental delay, poor growth, mental deficiency and premature ovarian failure. Up to 75% of affected females over 14 years of age will experience ovarian dysfunction. Pregnancies in affected females appear to proceed normally without adverse fetal affects.[62,63] Breastfeeding is contraindicated due to effects on the mother. The production of galactose-1-phosphate from the breakdown of endogenous lactose produced in the mammary glands is problematic leading to accumulation of galactose-1-phosphate, galactitol, galactonate, and UDP-galactose.[64]

Phenylketonuria

Early treatment of phenylketonuria has resulted in a markedly improved outlook for survival with good intellect. In recent years there has been some concern that the withdrawal of dietary therapy in later life may be associated with neurological disorder and gross cerebral changes shown by magnetic resonance imaging.[65]

Charles Dent was probably the first investigator who noted the association of fetal abnormality and maternal phenylketonuria in

1956.[66] Since, that time there have been many reports of fetal abnormalities associated with uncontrolled or poorly controlled maternal phenylketonuria.[67-72] Abnormalities reported in untreated phenylketonuria when the intrapartum maternal plasma phenylalanine concentration exceeded 1.5 mmol/L include mental retardation in 92%, microcephaly in 72%, intrauterine growth delay in 40% and congenital heart malformation in 12% of the offspring.[69] Phenylalanine is transported across the placenta by an active transport process, which results in higher plasma concentrations of phenylalanine in the fetus than in the mother. The ratio of fetal to maternal plasma concentrations of phenylalanine varies throughout pregnancy with a higher ratio in the earlier months. The observed average ratio of fetal to maternal plasma phenylalanine is 1.48 with a range of 1.13–2.91.[73] Any increase in maternal plasma phenylalanine is therefore magnified within the embryonic and fetal tissues. The embryopathy affects the cardiovascular and central nervous systems causing the clinical features described.

Fortunately, fetal defects can be prevented by appropriate maternal dietary management to ensure reasonable plasma concentrations of phenylalanine from before the time of conception.[69-72,74] Two Medical Research Council Working Party reports have summarized the present recommendations for the dietary management of phenylketonuria and expressed the hope that there will be a molecular genetic treatment and prevention program for phenylketonuria.[75,76] Good management of maternal phenylketonuria prevents a variety of dangers and dilemmas for the mother and her medical advisers.[77] Dietary problems are related to the palatability, bulk and osmolality of available amino acid mixtures, and the palatability and nutrient value of the permissible low-protein foods. In spite of the dangers to the developing embryo and fetus there is enormous reward for the families and health care providers for having a healthy baby by achieving good maternal dietary control. Until there is a safe effective method for the substitution of the defective gene or phenylalanine hydroxylase or both in the affected individuals, there continues a need to achieve prenatal and perinatal control of phenylalanine and tyrosine concentrations in mothers with phenylketonuria.

CONCLUSION

Perhaps the most important aspect of maternal inherited metabolic disorders is the need to have clinicians informed and aware of the wide range of maternal disorders, which can predispose to embryonic, fetal and neonatal problems. For optimal pregnancy outcome most of these conditions must be identified and metabolic control achieved preconceptually. This review does not address the effect of abnormal pharmacogenetics on maternal drug metabolism and the potential consequence to the fetus. An inherited predisposition to folate disorder will certainly alter the response to drugs which interfere with folate metabolism and maternal alcoholism is influenced by defects in alcohol dehydrogenases.[78-82] A high degree of clinical awareness and effective management would improve the outcome of infants born to mothers with metabolic disorders.

REFERENCES

1. Scriver CR, Beaudet AL, Sly WS, et al. The Metabolic and Molecular Bases of Inherited Disease, 7th edition. New York: McGraw-Hill; 1995.
2. Farquhar JW. The influence of maternal diabetes in fetus and child. In: Gairdner D (Ed). Recent Advances in Pediatrics, 3rd edition. London: Churchill; 1965.pp.121-53.
3. Fuhrmann K, Reiher H, Semmler K, et al. Prevention of congenital malformations in infants of insulin-dependent diabetic mothers. Diabetes Care. 1983;6:219-23.
4. Damm P, Molsted-Pedersen L. Significant decrease in congenital malformations in newborn infants of an unselected population of diabetic women. Am J Obstet Gynecol. 1989;161:1163-7.
5. Goldman GA, Dickerd D, Feldberg D, et al. Pregnancy outcome in patients with insulin-dependent diabetes mellitus with pre-conceptual diabetic control: A comparative study. Am J Obstet Gynecol. 1986;155:193-7.
6. Steel JM, Johnstone FD, Hepburn DA, et al. Can pre-pregnancy care of diabetic women reduce the risk of abnormal babies? Br Med J. 1990;301:1070-4.
7. Kitzmiller JL, Gavin LA, Gin GD, et al. Pre-conception management of diabetes through early pregnancy prevents the excess of major congenital anomalies of infants of diabetic mothers. J Am Med Assoc. 1991;265:731-6.
8. Martin AO, Simpson JL, Ober C, et al. Frequency of diabetes mellitus in probands with gestational diabetes: possible maternal influence on the predisposition to diabetes. Am J Obstet Gynecol. 1985;151:471-3.
9. Dorner G, Plagemann A, Reinagel H. Familial diabetes aggregation in Type II diabetics: Gestational diabetes as apparent risk factor for increased diabetes susceptibility in the offspring. Exp Clin Endocrinol. 1987;89:84-90.
10. Razin A, Cedar H. DNA methylation and genomic imprinting. Cell. 1994;77:473-6.
11. Efstratiadis A. Parental imprinting of autosomal mammalian genes. Curr Opin Genet Dev. 1994;4:265-80.
12. Barlow DP. Imprinting: A gamete's point of view. Trends Genet. 1994;10:194-9.
13. Julier C, Hyer RN, Davies J, et al. Insulin-IGF2 region on chromosome 11p encodes a gene implicated in HLA-DR4-dependent diabetes susceptibility. Nature. 1991;354:155–9.
14. Dorner G, Steindel E, Thoelke H, et al. Evidence for decreasing prevalence of diabetes mellitus in childhood apparently produced by prevention of hyperinsulinism in the foetus and newborn. Exp Clin Endocrinol. 1984;84:134-42.
15. Pettit DJ, Aleck KA, Baird HR, et al. Congenital susceptibility to NIDDM role of intrauterine environment. Diabetes. 1988;33:622-8.
16. Cohen LF, di Sant'Agenese PA, Friedlander J. Cystic fibrosis and pregnancy. A national study. Lancet. 1980;2:842-4.
17. Lyon IC, Gardner RJ, Veale AM. Maternal histidinemia. Arch Dis Child. 1974;49:581.
18. Neville BG, Harris RF, Stern DJ, et al. Maternal histidinemia. Arch Dis Child. 1971;46:119.
19. Armstrong MD. Maternal histidenemia. Arch Dis Child. 1975;50:830.
20. Matsuda I, Nagata N, Endo F. A family with histidinemic parents. J Pediatr. 1983;103:169.
21. Levy HL, Benjamin R. Maternal histedinemia: Study of families identified by routine cord blood screening. Pediatr Res. 1985;19:210A.
22. Mahon BE, Levy HL. Maternal hartnup disorder. Am J Med Genet. 1986;24:513.
23. Gaull GE, Rassin DK, Struman JA. Pyridoxine dependency in homocystinuria (Letter). Lancet. 1968;2:1302.

24. Bittle AH, Carson NA. Tissue culture techniques as an aid to prenatal diagnosis and genetic counselling in homocystinuria. J Med Genet. 1973;10:120-1.

25. Kurczynski TW, Muir WA, Fleisher LD, et al. Maternal homocystinuria; studies of an untreated mother and fetus. Arch Dis Child. 1980;55:721-3.

26. Rassin DK, Fleisher LD, Muir A, et al. Fetal tissue amino acid concentrations in argininosuccinic aciduria and in maternal homocystinuria. Clin Chim Acta. 1979;94:101-8.

27. Wouters BE, Goers GH, Blom HJ, et al. Hyperhomocystinemia: A risk factor in women with unexplained recurrent early pregnancy loss. Fertil Steril. 1993;60 (5):820.

28. Newman G, Mitchell JR. Homocystinemia presenting as multiple arterial occlusions. W J Med. 1984;210:251.

29. Schulman JD, Mudd SH, Shulman NR, et al. Pregnancy and thrombophlebitis in homocystenimia. Blood. 1980;56:326.

30. Constantine G, Green A. Untreated homocystinemia: A maternal death in a woman with four pregnancies, a case report. Br J Obstet Gynecol. 1987;94:803.

31. Put van der NM, Steegers-Theunissen RP, Frosst P, et al. Mutated methylenetetrahydrofolate reductase as a risk factor for spina bifida. Lancet. 1995;346:1071-2.

32. Whitehead AS, Gallagher P, Mills JL, et al. A genetic defect in 5,10-methylenetetrahydrofolate reductase in neural tube defects. Q J Med. 1995;88:763-6.

33. Smithells RW, Sheppard S, Schorah CJ, et al. Possible prevention of neural-tube defects by periconceptional vitamin supplementation. Lancet. 1980;1:339-40.

34. Smithells RW, Sheppard S, Wild J, et al. Prevention of neural-tube recurrences in Yorkshire, the final report. Lancet. 1989;2:498-9.

35. Medical Research Council Vitamin Study Research Group. Prevention of neural-tube defects; results of the Medical Research Council Vitamin Study. Lancet. 1991;338:131-7.

36. Czeizel AE, Dudas I. Prevention of the first occurrence of neural-tube defects by periconceptional vitamin supplementation. N Engl J Med. 1992;327:1832-5.

37. Put van der NM, Thomas CM, Eskes TK, et al. Altered folate and vitamin B12 metabolism in families with spina bifida offspring. Q J Med. 1997;90:505-10.

38. Simell O. Lysinuric protein intolerance. In: Scriver CR, Beaudet AL, Sly WS (Eds). The Metabolic and Molecular Bases of Inherited Disease, 7th edition. New York: McGraw-Hill; 1995;118:3603-27.

39. Shih VE, Aubrey RH, De Grande G, et al. Maternal isovaleric acidemia. J Pediatr. 1984;105:77.

40. Brusilow SW, Horwich AL. Urea cycle enzymes. In: Scriver CR, Beaudet AL, Sly WS, (Eds). The Metabolic and Molecular Bases of Inherited Disease, 7th edn. New York: McGraw-Hill. 1995;32:1187-232.

41. Arn PH, Hauser ER, Thomas GH, et al. Hyperammoninemia in women with a mutation at the ornithine carbamoyl transferase locus: A cause of postpartum coma. N Engl J Med. 1990;322:1652-5.

42. Wong LJ, Craigen WJ, O'Brien WE. Postpartum coma and death due to carbamoyl-phosphate sythetase I deficiency. Ann Intern Med. 1994;120:216-7.

43. Widhalm K, Koch S, Scheibenreiter S, et al. Long-term follow-up of 12 patients with the late-onset variant of argininosuccinic acid lyase deficiency: No impairment of intellectual and psychomotor development during therapy. Pediatrics. 1992;89:1182-4.

44. Worthington S, Christodoulou J, Wilcken B, et al. Pregnancy and argininosuccinic aciduria. J Inher Metab Dis. 1996;19:621-3.

45. Gerin I, Viega-da-Cunha M, Achouri Y, et al. Sequence of a putative glucose-6-phosphate translocase, mutated in glycogen storage disease type 1b. FEBS Lett. 1997;419: 235.

46. Lei KJ, Chen YT, Chen H, et al, Genetic basis of glycogen storage disease type 1a: Prevalent mutations at glucose-6-phosphatase locus. Am J Hum Genet. 1995;57:766.

47. Matern D, Seydewitz HH, Bali D, et al. Glycogen storage disease type 1: Diagnosis and phenotype/genotype correlation. Eur J Pediatr. 2002;161(Suppl1): S10.

48. Bianchi L. Glycogen storage disease type 1 and hepatocellular tumors. Eur J Pediatr. 1993;152(Suppl1): S63.

49. Johnson MP, Compton A, Drugan A, et al. Metabolic control of von Gierke disease (glycogen storage disease type 1a) in pregnancy: maintenance of euglycemia with cornstarch. Obstet Gynecol. 1990;75:507.

50. Farber M, Knuppel R, Binkiewicz, et al. Pregnancy and von Gierke's disease. Obstet Gynecol. 1976;47:226.

51. Ryan IP, Havel RJ, Laros RK. Three consecutive pregnancies in a patient with glycogen storage disease type 1a (von Gierke's disease). Am J Obstet Gynecol. 1994;170:1687.

52. Yang-Feng T, Zheng K, Yu J, et al. Assignment of the human glycogen debrancher gene to chromosome 1p21. Genomics. 1002;13:931.

53. Bao Y, Denison TL, Chen YT. Human glycogen debranching enzyme gene (AGL): complete structural organization and characterization of the 5' flanking region. Genomics. 1992;38:155.

54. Labrune P, Trioche P, Duvalier I, et al. Hepatocellular adenomas in glycogen storage disease type I and III: a series of 43 patients and review of the literature. J pediatr Gastroenterol nutr. 1997;24:276.

55. Murase T, Ikada H, Muro T, et al. Myopathy associated with type 3 glygenolysis. J neurol Sci. 1973;20:287.

56. Moses S, Gadoth N, Bashan N, et al. Neuromuscular involvement in glycogen storage disease type III. Acta Pediatr Scand. 1986;75:289.

57. Olsen LJ, Reeder GS, Noller KL, et al. Cardiac involvement in glycogen storage disease III: Morphologic and biochemical characterization with endomyocardial biopsy. Am J Cardiol. 1984;59:980.

58. McArdle B. Myopathy due to a defect in muscle glycogen breakdown. Clin Sci. 1951;10:13.

59. Lebo R, Gorin F, Fletterick R, et al. High-resolution chromosome sorting and DNA spot-blot analysis assign McArdle's syndrome in chromosome 11. Science. 1984;225:57.

60. Dinauro S, Breslin N. Phosphorylase deficiency. In: Myology, Engel A, Baker B (Eds). New York, NY: Mcgraw-Hill; 1986.p.1585.

61. Carson NAJ. Selected reviews from the workshop on non-ketotic hyperglycinemia. J Inher Met Dis. 1982;5(Suppl 2):105-28.

62. Bernier FP, Snyder FF, McLeod DR. Deficiency of 5-oxoprolinase in an 8-year old with developmental delay. J Inher Metab Dis. 1996;19:367-8.

63. Komrower GM. Galactosemia – 30 years on. The experience of a generation. J Inher Metab Dis. 1982;5(Suppl 2):96-104.

64. Segal S, Berry G. Disorders of galactose metabolism. In: Scriver CR, (Eds). The Metabolic and Molecular Bases of Inherited Disease, 7th edition. New York, NY: McGraw-Hill; 1995.p.967.

65. Roe T, Hallatt J, Donnell G, et al. Child-bearing by galactosemic women. J Pediatr. 1971;78:1026.

66. Tedesco TA, Marrow G, Mellman WJ. Normal pregnancy and childbirth in a galactosemic woman. J Pediatr. 1972;81:1158.

67. Brivet M, Raymond JP, Konopka P, et al. Effect of lactation in a mother with galactosemia. J Pediatr. 1989;115:280-2.

68. Thompson AJ, Smith I, Brenton D, et al. Neurological deterioration in young adults with phenylketonuria. Lancet. 1990;336:602-5.

69. Dent CE. Report of 23rd Ross Conference. Ross Laboratories, Columbus, Ohio. 1956.

70. Mabry CC, Denniston JC, Nelson TL, et al. Maternal phenylketonuria: A cause of mental retardation in children without the metabolic defect. N Engl J Med. 1963;269:1404-8.

71. Allen JD, Brown JK. Maternal phenylketonuria. In: Holt KS, Coffey VP (Eds). Some Recent Advances in Inborn Errors of Metabolism. Edinburgh: E and S Livingston Ltd; 1968.pp.14-38.

72. Lenke RR, Levy HL. Maternal phenylketonuria and hyperphenylalaninemia. An international survey of untreated and treated pregnancies. N Engl J Med. 1980;303:1202-8.

73. Koch R, Friedman EG, Wenz E, et al. Maternal phenylketonuria. J Inher Metab Dis. 1986;9(Suppl 2):159-68.

74. Drogari E, Beasley M, Smith I, et al. Timing of strict diet in relation to fetal damage in maternal phenylketonuria. Lancet. 1987;2: 927-30.

75. Clark BJ, Cockburn F. Maternal diet in inherited metabolic disease. Acta Pediatr Scand. 1991;373:43-52.

76. Cockburn F, Farquhar JW, Forfar JO, et al. Maternal hyper-phenylalaninaemia in the normal phenylketonuric mother and its influence on maternal plasma and fetal fluid aminoacid concentrations. J Obstet Gynecol Br Commonw. 1972;79: 698-707.

77. Hanley WB, Clarke JT, Schoonkeyt W. Maternal phenylketonuria (PKU) – A review. Clin Biochem. 1987;20:149.

78. Medical Research Council Working Party on Phenylketonuria. Phenylketonuria due to phenylalanine hydroxylase deficiency: an unfolding story. Br Med. 1993;306:115-9.

79. Medical Research Council Working Party on Phenylketonuria. Recommendations on the dietary management of pheny-lketonuria. Arch Dis Child. 1993;68:426-7.

80. Cockburn F, Clark BJ, Byrne A, et al. Maternal phenylketonuria-diet, dangers and dilemmas. Int Pediatr. 1992;7:67-74.

81. Cockburn F. Fetal metabolism. In: Reed GB, Claireaux AE, Cockburn F (Eds). Diseases of the Fetus and Newborn, 2nd edition. London: Chapman and Hall Medical; 1995;81:1267-79.

82. Veghelyi PV. Fetal abnormality and maternal alcohol metabolism. Lancet. 1983;11:53-4.

89

Fetal and Neonatal Nutrition—Lipid and Carbohydrate Requirements and Adaptations to Altered Supply at Birth

H Budge, ME Symonds

INTRODUCTION

The maintenance of a balanced and continuous supply of nutrients from the mother to the conceptus is critical in maintaining both a healthy and viable embryo as well as ensuring fetal growth and development is optimal throughout gestation. In this respect, a deficit in nutrient intake by the mother not only has a detrimental effect on the reproductive process itself but can contribute to long-term ill health in the resulting offspring.[1,2] Even prior to conception, it is important that maternal dietary intake is adequate to ensure normal development of the egg.[3] Inadequate maternal nutrition before ovulation can potentially contribute to a range of clinical conditions including neural tube defects[4] in the fetus and even result in premature labor.[5,6]

There are seven distinct, but inter-related stages, between ovulation and weaning in which inadequate, or an imbalanced supply of nutrition, can have deleterious effects on the conceptus. These can be summarized as follows:

1. Periconceptionally during the time of egg development
2. Fertilization and subsequent period of embryogenesis and elongation
3. Implantation and placental establishment
4. Period of rapid placental growth
5. Period of rapid fetal growth and mammary development
6. Birth and separation of the fetus from the placenta
7. Lactation and the period of postnatal growth.

In order to enable the newborn to establish independent life it undergoes a range of pronounced metabolic, endocrine and functional adaptations at birth.[7,8] These are vital in enabling the infant to commence independent breathing, thermoregulation and nutrient intake. Nutrient supply to the fetus is primarily regulated at the level of the placenta, which effectively acts as the fetal gut. Then, after birth and the onset of breastfeeding, the neonatal bowel takes on this role. There are some similarities between the function of the placenta before birth and the neonatal gut which acts to ensure that nutrient supply is maintained and then increased to meet the much higher postnatal metabolic requirements as growth accelerates.[9]

The fetus grows in a hypoxic environment in which a reduction in supply of both macronutrients, which include oxygen and micronutrients, can have adverse consequences.[10] Fetal arterial blood has a paO_2 of around 2.8 kPa (21 mm Hg) compared with ~12 kPa (90 mm Hg) in the adult. The fetus adapts to this lower paO_2 by maintaining a minimal metabolic rate,[11] ensuring available nutrients can be utilized to promote tissue growth rather than be partitioned toward metabolism. Nevertheless, even when fetal growth rate is maximal, it is usually slower than after birth.[12,13] In conjunction with this relatively low growth rate, cell division, rather than an increase in cell size, primarily contributes to fetal tissue growth. Thereafter, after birth, there is pronounced hypertrophy as nutrient supply is no longer constrained by placental exchange capacity, maternal intake and body stores. One tissue in which this adaptation is most apparent is adipose tissue.[14] Lipid synthesis has a much higher energetic requirement (i.e. 39 MJ/kg) compared with carbohydrate or protein (15–25 MJ/kg), so it is not surprising that fat deposition is normally low in the fetus and is highly dependent on fetal nutrition.[15]

Fetal fat deposition principally occurs over the final third of gestation[16] but, in contrast with all other organs, fat cells can continue increasing in size for the remainder of an individual's life. It is, therefore, not unexpected that in nutritional and environmental conditions of excess feed availability, reduced physical and metabolic activity and raised ambient temperatures, there is an increasing propensity for obesity to occur earlier and in more people.[17] The extent to which predisposition to later obesity is determined by the in utero environment remains an area of significant scientific interest.[18]

In this chapter, we will focus on the acquisition of fat and fatty acids by the fetus and neonate, and consider their roles in brain and adipose tissue development. For the fetus, as in the adult, fat represents a storage site in which excess energy intake is stored to be mobilized in times of later nutrient deficiency.[18] The other major energy storage is glycogen which is deposited in the fetal liver and skeletal muscle.[19] We will, therefore, consider the regulation of carbohydrate metabolism within the fetus as this is the precursor for both stored glycogen and the primary metabolic substrate for fetal lipid synthesis.

COMPARATIVE REQUIREMENTS BETWEEN HUMANS AND OTHER MAMMALIAN SPECIES

The use of other animals has greatly added to our understanding of fetal and neonatal lipid and carbohydrate metabolism, and its impact on brain and fat development. It is, therefore, important to appreciate both the differences and similarities between respective animal models, which have enabled us to make substantial advances in our knowledge of fetal nutrition and physiology that would not be possible within the pronounced limitations of human studies. As a consequence of the substantial differences in length of gestation in various animal species, together with the degree of maturity of the newborn at birth, the impact of compromised placental function, as opposed to poor lactational performance, can have very different outcomes on the resulting offspring.

The most notable difference between human newborn infants and nearly all other mammals is their much higher total fat content

(150 g/kg body tissue) compared with most domestic species and laboratory mammals (<10 g/kg body tissue)[20] except the newborn guinea pig (70 g/kg body tissue). The high fat content of the human fetus reflects the dramatic increase in subcutaneous fat deposition that occurs over the final 10 weeks of gestation. This is largely white fat which has an important insulatory role in the newborn as well as providing a large energy store that can be mobilized over the first few days of neonatal life before lactation is fully established. In the latter respect, the human differs from many other mammalian species in which lactation rapidly commences at birth to ensure survival. For example, in sheep, failure to rapidly establish lactation leads to starvation, hypothermia and death within a few hours of birth.[21]

Newborn sheep, like humans,[22] also possesses brown adipose tissue which is characterized as possessing a unique uncoupling protein (UCP)1 that when maximally activated is able to produce up to 300 watts/kg tissue of heat compared with 1–2 watts/kg tissue by most other tissues.[23] The amount of brown fat, located around the internal organs, in newborn sheep and humans is comparable at about 2% of birth weight.[24,25] This contrasts with rats and mice in which minimal fat is present at birth and in whom brown fat is located in the interscapular region and is recruited postnatally.[26] In contrast, pigs are born with some subcutaneous fat but do not possess any brown fat.[27]

Fetal brain growth relative to adult brain weight is appreciably greater in the human than all other species for which comparable data is available (Fig. 89.1). In addition, its growth rate is normally maintained for the whole of pregnancy so that the weight of the brain in the newborn is ~13% of birth weight.[28] Subsequently, as growth of all other tissues accelerates after birth, brain weight, as a fraction of total body weight, gradually declines to the adult value of ~2%, which is the typical value found in most other large animal species at birth.[29]

These pronounced differences in fetal brain growth are reflected in the ability of nonesterified free fatty acids (NEFA) to cross the placenta. In the chorioallantoic (hemochorial) placenta of humans, although the fetal endothelium and chorionic epithelium separate the maternal and fetal circulations, NEFA can pass relatively freely from mother to fetus.[30] This contrasts with the placentae of species that have a distinct maternal layer (such as the pig and sheep) and are impermeable to NEFA.[31] Small laboratory mammals which have a very short gestation further differ from humans in that the offspring have an immature hypothalamic-pituitary axis at birth with brain and fat growth occurring primarily after birth.[32] This has several major functional consequences, both for organ development and nutritional requirements. The major source of energy in rat milk is lipid and the mother devotes up to 80% of her time suckling the young whose weight doubles in a week.[33] By the time of weaning, brain growth is complete and the neonate has maximized the necessary glucose production necessary to maintain the brain's high metabolic requirements compared to the rest of the body.[34] It is not until weaning that glycogen is laid down as an energy reserve for possible latter food deprivation. This process of events is in marked contrast to long gestation species in which these developments all occur in utero. Not surprisingly, appreciable differences in milk composition between species, likely to reflect the degree of maturity of the offspring at birth, are also apparent. Humans and large mammals, such as the sheep and cow, produce milk with a lower relative fat and protein content compared with that of small mammals, such as rats and mice, that have a lower relative carbohydrate content.[33]

LIPID AND CARBOHYDRATE REQUIREMENTS FOR PLACENTAL AND FETAL GROWTH

Dietary availability, in conjunction with the ability to mobilize maternal body tissue stores determines nutrient supply to the conceptus and, therefore, both placental and fetal growth.[35] A reduction in maternal energy stores either before, or during gestation, can have substantial effects on fetal energy deposition,[15] and these can be exaggerated in the term human infant because it possesses large stores of both lipid and carbohydrate in comparison with most other mammals.[36] Such effects are amplified because the fetus has limited ability to synthesize glucose[37] or essential fatty acids including long-chain (LC) polyunsaturated fatty acids (PUFA).[38] It is, therefore, not surprising that infants with poor energy reserves at birth can have long-term deficits in their metabolic control mechanisms.[39] Indeed, such effects may be compounded by the need to mobilize energy supplies during the sometimes lengthy period of parturition[40] up to the time of full establishment of lactation.[41]

The Placenta—Development and Function as the Site of Nutrient Supply

The human hemochorial placenta is a fetal organ and is regulated by fetal genes. It separates the fetal and maternal circulations by a barrier composed of fetal endothelium and chorionic epithelium. The primary site of nutrient exchange is the chorionic villi which are supported by the syncytiotrophoblast and are surrounded by maternal blood.[42] They act as a lipoidal membrane across which nutrient, dissolved gases, waste products and other substances occur. Like the adult gut, this site of the placenta has a very large surface area which increases from 0.83 m² in week 3 of gestation to peak at ~12.5 m² at term.[42] At the same time, the maternal-fetal diffusion distance decreases from 55 mm to 4.8 mm, thereby facilitating nutrient exchange. The syncytiotrophoblast are also being continuously renewed from the underlying villous cytotrophoblast.

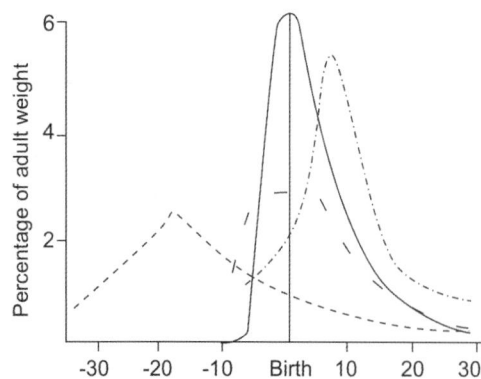

Fig. 89.1: Diagrammatic summary of the rate of fetal and postnatal brain growth (wet weight) in the human compared with other species. Developmental age for each species is represented as follows: human (continuous line) in months; guinea pigs (dotted line) in days; pig (dashed line) in weeks and rat (dotted and dashed line) in days

Source: Adapted from Dickerson[29] with permission

The placenta has a range of transport mechanisms and/or transporters, which can limit or promote uptake of specific nutrients including fatty acids,[38] glucose[43] and amino acids.[44] Their abundances can be developmentally regulated and are normally reduced in placentae of growth-retarded infants. In addition to its role in nutrient transfer, the placenta acts as an important endocrine organ secreting hormones into both the maternal and fetal circulations and, thereby, exerting direct effects on maternal metabolism and nutrient supply to the fetus.[45]

Placental Requirements for Growth and Metabolism

Normal growth and development of the placenta is critical in ensuring that a healthy, appropriately sized fetus is born at term. The placenta grows exponentially during gestation, weighing ~6 g at week 3 of gestation and ~470 g at term. Maximal growth of the placenta precedes that of the fetus[46] but nutritional exchange capacity increases with gestational age in conjunction with structural maturation of the placenta[47] as the fetus grows and its overall metabolic rate rises.[48] At term, placental and fetal weights are positively correlated with placental weight normally being between 10% and 15% of newborn body weight.[49]

Not surprisingly, given the diverse functions of the placenta and its rapid growth, a constant and plentiful source of energy is required. The human placenta derives energy from both glucose[43] and NEFA by glycolysis and β-oxidation,[50] respectively. It utilizes glucose as its major energy source and there are multiple glucose transporters present in the placenta.[43] Enzymes involved in glycolysis and the citric acid cycle are also active within the placenta. Indeed, it has been suggested that adequate glucose supply can prevent NEFA uptake and oxidation within the placenta by inhibiting the enzymes (e.g. carnitine palmitoyltransferase type 1) involved in this process.[51] This is not always the case, as appreciable activities of a number of enzymes involved in β-oxidation (e.g. acyl and hydroxyacyl-CoA dehydrogenases) have been detected although activity decreases with gestational age.[50] The utilization of fatty acids as a metabolic fuel may, therefore, decline as gestation progresses with glucose becoming more important.[52]

As the placenta utilizes both glucose and NEFA, abnormalities in the metabolism of either can be associated with adverse outcomes in pregnancy.[50] Diabetes during pregnancy, in which both the transfer of glucose and NEFA across the placenta are increased, causes placental and fetal macrosomia.[53] Maternal liver diseases of pregnancy may also be the result of a placental defect in NEFA oxidation,[54] with maternal symptoms worsening in late gestation when the higher metabolic demands of the fetus[55] result in increased fat mobilization and a concomitant rise in lipoprotein lipase activity.[54] Defective fatty acid oxidation in the placenta results in placental accumulation of abnormal metabolic precursors (e.g. hydroxy acylcarnitines and dicarboxylic acids),[56] which may further contribute to the intrauterine growth retardation seen in such clinical conditions as preeclampsia.[57]

Fetal Requirements for Brain Growth and Neural Development

As with all fetal organs, the most rapid period of brain cell division is during the period of embryonic growth. Normally, by the end of the second month of gestation, the majority of neurons have migrated within the cerebral cortex forming the gray matter.[58] At this stage of development, approximately 50% of the embryo is made up of the fetal head with the brain utilizing up to 70% of available energy provided by the placenta. The brain has a very high lipid requirement and content of which 60% is structural. The majority (85%) of this is present in the cerebrum. Of the latter, 65% of total lipids are phospholipids with cerebral cortical neuronal membranes being made up of phosphatidylcholine, ethanolamine, serine and inositol.[58]

The structural and metabolic functions of fatty acids in the fetus and placenta are primarily undertaken by PUFA.[59] These fatty acids with double bonds plus three (n-3) or six (n-6) carbons from the n terminus cannot be synthesized in the human body. They must, therefore, be obtained from dietary sources primarily in the form of linoleic, an n-6 fatty acid, or α-linolenic, an n-3 fatty acid.[38] LCPUFAs are also essential for neural, brain and retinal development as they are not only integral components of the membrane but also act as intracellular signals and contribute to triacylglycerol stores. The primary LCPUFAs are arachidonic acid (20 carbons: 4n-6) and docosahexaenoic acid (22 carbons: 6n-3) which are amongst the most metabolically active in the cell. They are not normally limited in the diet but, because of the increased demands by the fetus, their supply may become limited during pregnancy.[60] Interestingly, although the fetal brain has relatively high concentrations of docosahexaenoic acid, the absolute rate of accretion is low (e.g. 50-fold lower than in adipose tissue).[38] Although it is only during late gestation that fetal requirements appear to exceed maternal dietary intake,[38] the amount of fatty acids in the diet may have a significant effect on outcome as a reduced dietary intake has been associated with both intrauterine growth retardation and premature birth.[61]

The precise trigger for parturition remains a matter of debate. In humans, it is determined in part by the size constraints and metabolic demands of the fetal brain.[29] As the greatest period of brain growth occurs in utero there is a definite maternal limitation determined by the dimensions of the pelvic outlet. At the same time, a mismatch between fetal nutrient requirements and placental supply capacity may trigger a centrally coordinated cascade of endocrine signals that initiates parturition.[62]

Fetal Requirements for Adipose Tissue Deposition

Adipose tissue is primarily laid down during the final third of gestation with the majority (~80%) being deposited as subcutaneous fat that can constitute as much as 16% of birth weight in a normally grown term infant.[63] Its major component is lipid which is primarily found in unilocular cells, although internal fat depots which have a high mitochondrial content also possess a large number of multilocular cells[64] in which the brown adipose tissue specific uncoupling protein 1[26] is located. The combination of brown fat plus large lipid stores means that heat production within fat is sufficient to provide up to three quarters of total energy requirements at birth.[19]

Fat is not only transferred directly from the mother to the fetus but is also synthesized in utero primarily from glucose but also from lactate and short-chain volatile fatty acids.[65] An increase in both glucose and fatty acid supply from the mother to the fetus such as during pregnancies complicated with diabetes results in substantially more fetal fat deposition.[66] Conversely, preterm infants, as well as those with intrauterine growth retardation, are born with depleted fat stores. These individuals may, however, have an increased propensity to lay down more fat in later life.[67]

Fetal Deposition of Carbohydrate in the Liver

Glucose is the primary nutrient utilized by the fetus for oxidative metabolism with up to two-thirds of fetal glucose being oxidized to carbon dioxide and the remaining third stored as glycogen.[68] As in the adult, glucose utilization is largely regulated by the pancreatic hormones insulin and glucagon with the adaptation that, because of the higher insulin to glucagon ratio, glycogen synthesis is stimulated whereas glycogenolysis inhibited.[69] Indeed, except under conditions of extreme nutrient deficiency, the fetal liver has minimal capacity to synthesize glucose.[37] At the same, time other counter metabolic hormones, such as growth hormone, do not appear to have a role in glucose homeostasis, as the fetus is normally growth hormone insensitive.[70] The fetus is usually exposed to very high circulating growth hormone concentrations[71] and its growth hormone insensitivity is most likely due to the lack of adult growth hormone receptors in the liver.[72]

Glycogen is stored primarily in the fetal liver, but also in skeletal muscle, and can be utilized to maintain plasma glucose concentrations during periods of reduced nutrient availability.[34] The main factor determining the content of glycogen in fetal tissues is the rate of glucose supply from the mother to the fetus which, in turn, is dependent on the maternal blood concentration.[68] Maternal and fetal blood glucose are usually very closely correlated along a glucose gradient to the fetus with fetal blood glucose being 30% lower than that of the mother.[73] Glycogen accumulation commences from 9 weeks of gestation but, as for adipose tissue, it is primarily synthesized in the last third of gestation.[40]

NUTRIENT SUPPLY TO THE FETUS: MAINTENANCE OF A CONTINUOUS SUPPLY

Lipid Supply from the Mother to the Fetus

As a consequence of their large size and high molecular weight, lipids do not directly cross the placenta.[38] Lipids, carried in the maternal circulation by the carrier protein albumin,[74] must first be hydrolyzed to NEFA before they can be transferred across the placenta. This hydrolysis to NEFAs is performed by the enzyme lipoprotein lipase which is abundant in the human placenta.[75] In addition, intact triacylglycerols and phospholipids can also not be transferred across the placenta.[76] Consequently, as fetal requirements increase with gestation, there is a linear rise in the plasma concentration of triglycerides in maternal blood,[77] whereas plasma NEFAs only rise in late gestation coincident with the mobilization of maternal fat stores.[78]

NEFA Transfer Across the Placenta

The placenta has the capacity to transfer NEFAs both to, or from, the fetus with the net rate of transfer determined by the relative concentrations of NEFAs and their carrier protein, albumin, in the maternal and fetal circulations.[79] Normally, it is the concentration of albumin, which is ~20% higher in fetal than maternal blood, which determines the rate of exchange whereas plasma NEFAs can

be up to three times higher in the maternal compared with fetal circulation.[80] Consequently, the plasma NEFA to albumin ratio is 30% lower in the fetus than mother and this gradient promotes fetal uptake of NEFAs. Conditions which result in an increase in maternal plasma NEFAs such as food deprivation[81] will result in an enhanced transfer of NEFAs to the fetus.

When NEFAs have permeated the microvillus membrane they cross the two lipid bilayers within the syncytiotrophoblast either by simple diffusion[82] or via fatty acid binding proteins.[83] A number of these plasma membrane-associated proteins have been identified including:

- The plasma membrane fatty acid binding protein which functions as an extracellular fatty acid acceptor.
- Fatty acid transfer proteins that span the lipid bylayer and function as such.[84]

Interestingly, the plasma membrane fatty acid binding protein exhibits a hierarchy of binding affinities for the range of LCPUFAs that make up NEFAs in the order of docosahexaenoic acid ≥ arachidonic acid >> linoleic > α-linolenic >> oleic acid.[85] Furthermore, the finding that this hierarchy is only found on the maternal side of the placenta may have the effect of selectively promoting the enrichment of LCPUFAs within the NEFAs that are subsequently taken up into the placental syncytiotrophoblast[86] and then transported across to the placenta.

Glucose Supply from the Mother to the Fetus

As stated earlier, maternal blood glucose concentration is the main determinant of fetal glucose supply.[68] Glucose crosses the placenta by facilitative diffusion across specific glucose transporters (GLUT) with the fetal glucose concentration gradient from the mother increasing in late gestation as fetal demands become maximal.[52] Glucose transporters ensure that the rate of glucose transfer occurs at a greater rate than if its transfer was only dependent on simple diffusion. Two glucose transporters are present in the human placenta, GLUT1 and GLUT3,[87] and their relative abundance can change with gestational age.[43] The peak in GLUT3 abundance in late gestation, in conjunction with its higher affinity for glucose compared to GLUT1, indicates its greater contribution in facilitating placental glucose in late gestation[88] than GLUT1.

CESSATION OF NUTRIENT SUPPLY: THE ENVIRONMENTAL CHALLENGE TO THE NEWBORN AT BIRTH

At birth, in conjunction with separation of the infant from the placenta, there is a rapid transition in metabolic homeostasis. The newborn must rapidly establish independent respiration, thermoregulation and nutrition. At the same time, there is a profound change in the composition of feed supplied to the infant. During fetal life, the primary metabolic nutrient supplied is glucose.[68] In contrast, once the infant commences suckling, it no longer receives a diet in which the main energy source is carbohydrate. Instead, the newborn consumes a diet that is rich in both lipids and carbohydrates, with half of the required energy coming from triacylglycerols and the other half from lactose.[89] As lactation is established, both the concentration and volume of lipid and lactose produced in milk increases in line with the greater demands of the infant. The change

Table 89.1: Summary of the major adaptations at birth within the liver and gut which are necessary to enable the newborn to adapt to separation from the placenta and successfully commence suckling

Tissue	Nutritional influences	Function
Liver	Glycogen synthesis	Energy storage depot that can be mobilized at birth
	Induction of gluco-neogenic enzymes	Initiation of gluconeogenesis at birth
	Protein synthesis	Hormone receptors and binding proteins that promote tissue sensitivity to the postpartum hormones surges at birth
Gut	Maturation of gut morphology	Enables the gut to have maximal digestive capacity after birth
	Induction of digestive enzyme activity	Necessary for the breakdown and absorption of milk after birth
	Onset of digestive capacity	Facilitates the digestion of milk

in nutrient supply and availability is accompanied by the onset of gluconeogenesis within the liver and glucose absorption across the gut.[90] This means that, in addition to the substantial changes in lung function and metabolism[91] around the time of birth, there is also a dramatic change in function of the gut and liver[7] (Table. 89.1) in conjunction with the mobilization and activation of brown and white adipose tissue.[92]

Preparation and Adaptation for Life after Birth

Over the final weeks and days of gestation, there is a gradual process of maturation of the majority of organ systems within the fetus that means it can rapidly and effectively adapt to the extrauterine environment. The gradual increase in fetal plasma cortisol has a primary role in this process, and is important in promoting growth of the gut mucosa,[7] promoting acid secretion, the induction of digestive enzyme activity and hormone secretion by the gut.[93] In the liver, cortisol promotes glycogen deposition, induces the expression of gluconeogenic enzymes,[7] and stimulates hormone and receptor gene expression.[94]

The occurrence of both structural and functional changes within the proximal areas of the gut ensures that ingested nutrients become digested and absorbed soon after birth. It is not uncommon for the intake of milk to be less than requirements for several days after birth.[95] Over this period, energy is largely provided by the mobilization of both fat and glycogen stores which can become greatly depleted. For example, 90% of hepatic and 60% of muscle glycogen stores can be utilized within 24 h of birth.[96] In order to promote these responses, the enzymes essential for glycogenolysis, gluconeogenesis and lipolysis are greatly stimulated. All these processes may be delayed or reduced in preterm infants in which both lipid and glycogen stores are much lower than in term infants. Not unexpectedly, such infants are at much greater risk of hypoglycemia and hypothermia.[97]

The primary role of fat in the newborn relates to protection and maintenance of a normal body temperature.[92] In the infant, this function is achieved both as a result of the production of very large amounts of heat following rapid activation of the brown adipocyte specific uncoupling protein 1 in central fat depots,[98] or by the insulatory properties provided by subcutaneous fat.[99] It is also the main source of a rapidly mobilized energy rich substrate in the form of lipid from which NEFAs are released.[100] The instantaneous activation of thermogenesis at birth, coincident with a near maximal metabolic rate that is seldom matched throughout the rest of the life cycle, is an important example of the very different function of fat in fetal compared with adult life. This adaptation is mediated by the rapid increase in the plasma concentrations of a number of metabolic hormones at birth, including glucocorticoids, thyroid hormones, leptin, catecholamines, insulin, glucagon and growth hormone.[92] These are also important in the range of changes in the lung, gut and liver that are critical for ensuring life after birth (Table. 89.1).

NUTRIENT SUPPLY TO THE NEONATE: ESTABLISHMENT OF LACTATION AND ADAPTATION TO INCREASED SUPPLY

Following birth, the rapid and continuous maintenance of lactation is essential in ensuring that nutrient supply to the newborn does not become limited. Over this period, as nutrient supply increases with requirements, the infant has a greater capacity to meet its full growth potential. The composition of milk and its rate of digestion is very different between breast and bottle fed infants.[101] Type of feeding adopted also leads to substantial differences in waking and sleeping activity cycles that will further impact growth and metabolic requirements.[9] When the infant is fed ad libitum on demand, sleep-wake activity cycles may be limited to 3-4 h at most. Ideally, feeding should be on demand which results in a feeding frequency in the neonate being every 1-2 h compared with longer gaps between feeds in older infants.[102] An environment in which such a pattern of maternal-infant interaction is permitted could be considered to have the greatest beneficial outcome for infant health, growth and mental development.[103] Indeed human breast milk is sufficient as the sole source of energy and nutrients for the infant until around 6 months after birth.[102]

Structure and Function of the Neonatal Gut

As in the adult, the neonatal gut has a range of functions that are all necessary in maintaining metabolic homeostasis as well as regulating appetite. It, therefore, promotes digestion and absorption of nutrients in conjunction with secretory, motility and immunological functions. The neonatal gut is, however, specifically adapted to utilizing a milk diet, the composition of which varies through lactation, over the course of a feed[95] and with maternal diet and health.

As a consequence of the pronounced growth and maturation of the fetal gut during the final third of gestation, it is normally well adapted to absorb the nutrients it receives in milk after birth.[104] Glucose and NEFA are absorbed across the small intestine, whose surface area is substantially increased compared with the remainder of the gut, as a result of substantial number of valvulae conniventes, villi and crypts, together with the microvilli that form the luminal surface of enterocytes.

Gut function in the infant is not only coordinated by counter regulatory hormones secreted by the central and peripheral endocrine glands but possibly by hormones present in milk.[105] In addition, milk contains a range of trophic factors, anti-inflammatory and anti-infective agents, plus digestive enzymes which will enhance gut development and nutrient exchange. One important difference between the transfer of nutrients across the placenta and their transfer across the mammary gland in milk production is the necessity for the nutritional components of milk to be concentrated and packaged so as to survive transfer across the alveoli of the breast and subsequent exposure to the acidic environment of the small intestine.[106]

Fatty Acid Supply and Utilization

The fat content of the milk does not appear to be greatly influenced by maternal diet or fat stores. Fat constitutes 3.9–4.4 g/100 mL of milk.[33] Digestion and absorption of fat in the neonatal gut is similar to adults involving four phases: emulsification, hydrolysis, solubilization and mucosal transfer. The enzymes which digest fat are termed lipases of which three are abundant in the neonatal digestive tract, namely lingual, gastric and pancreatic lipase.[89] Of these, lingual lipase secreted from von Ebner's glands in the tongue is the most important in promoting fat digestion, and its activity decreases with age.[107] In contrast, because of the low concentrations of bile salts in the neonatal duodenum, pancreatic lipase is much less important in fat digestion than in later life.[108] The low activity of pancreatic lipases is partially overcome by the presence of bile-salt stimulated lipase (BSSL) found in milk. This is activated by primary bile salts (cholate and chenodeoxycholate) and amino acids (taurine and glycine) that are present in the small intestine.[109] BSSL completely hydrolyses triacylglycerols to glycerol and NEFAs into micellar forms.[110] These combine with the aggregated bile acids or micelles to form mixed micelles which, subsequently, transport the solubilized lipids to the brush border of the gut lining for uptake into the circulation and, thereafter, uptake and utilization by the liver. This process utilizes a fatty acid binding protein, with triacylglycerol being resynthesized in the endoplasmic reticulum and the formation of chylomicrons.[111]

Not surprisingly, preterm infants in which gut development is immature have a lower rate of fat absorption than term infants.[112] Interestingly, the commercial addition of LCPUFAs to preterm milk formulas can have beneficial effects on long term IQ, suggesting a direct effect on brain development.[113]

Carbohydrate Supply and Utilization

As in the fetus, glucose is a major oxidative fuel for many organs in the infant with the brain having an obligatory requirement. The main sugar in milk is lactose which is hydrolyzed to glucose and galactose by the enzyme lactase that is secreted from the apical membrane of the small intestine.[114] Both of these sugar products are then actively transported across the small intestinal epithelium by glucose transport systems that are similar to those present in the placenta with the principle GLUTs present in the gut being GLUT1, 2, 5 and 12.[115] These transporters are all sodium independent and only GLUT 12 has been shown to be insulin responsive.[116] In contrast, another type of GLUT found in the small intestine forms part of the Na^+-dependent family of transporters.[115] The latter transport sugars by a secondary active transport mechanism rather than by facilitative diffusion. This ensures glucose can be transported into cells across its concentration gradient via the Na^+-electrochemical gradient provided by Na^+–K^+ ATPase pump.[117]

The primary factor which determines glucose supply to the infant is the quality and quantity of milk consumed, which is, in turn, dependent on the nutrient intake and health of the mother.[102] It is not, therefore, surprising that many of the adverse effects of inadequate nutrition in utero can be overcome after birth. These may, however, have much longer term consequences. Infants who have developed a "thrifty phenotype"[118] as an adaptation to an adverse in utero environment may suffer later adverse health effects when exposed to the mismatch of a comparatively plentiful nutrient supply after birth. It must be noted that such adaptations will be in response to a very different nutrient intake from the diet than that to which the fetus is exposed in utero. In this respect, inappropriate accelerated postnatal growth appears to be deleterious with substantial adverse long-term outcomes. By promoting adiposity,[67] inappropriate accelerated postnatal growth compounds cardiovascular risk[119-122] and obesity.[123,124]

REFERENCES

1. Barker DJ. Fetal programming and public health. In: O'brien PM, Wheeler T, Barker DJP (Eds). Fetal programming: Influences on Development and Disease in Later life. London: RCOG Press; 1933. pp.3-11.

2. Rhind SM, Rae MT, Brooks AN. Effects of nutrition and environmental factors on the fetal programming of the reproductive axis. Reproduction. 2001;122:205-14.

3. Symonds ME, Clarke L. Nutrition-environment interactions in pregnancy. Nutrition Research Reviews. 1996;9:135-48.

4. Lumley J, Watson L, Watson M, et al. Periconceptional supplementation with folate and/or multivitamins for preventing neural tube defects. The Cochrane Database of Systematic Reviews, Issue 3. Art. No.: CD001056. DOI: 10.1002/14651858.CD001056. 2001.

5. Edwards LJ, McMillen IC. Impact of maternal undernutrition during the periconceptional period, fetal number, and fetal sex on the development of the hypothalamo-pituitary adrenal axis in sheep during late gestation. Biology of Reproduction. 2002;66:1562-9.

6. Bloomfield FH, Oliver MH, Hawkins P, et al. A periconceptional nutritional origin for noninfectious preterm birth. Science. 2001;300:606.

7. Fowden AL, Li J, Forhead AJ. Glucocorticoids and the preparation for life after birth: Are there long-term consequences of the life insurance? Proceedings of the Nutrition Society. 1998;57:113-22.

8. Symonds ME, Bird JA, Clarke L, et al. Nutrition, temperature and homeostasis during perinatal development. Experimental Physiology. 1995;80:907-40.

9. Symonds ME. The Fetus and Neonate, volume 3. Growth. In: Hanson MA, Spencer JA, Rodeck CH (Eds). Cambridge: Cambridge University Press; 1995.

10. Symonds ME, Budge H, Stephenson T, et al. Fetal endocrinology and development manipulation and adaptation to long term nutritional and environmental challenges. Reproduction. 2001;121:853-62.

11. Hay WW. Nutrient and metabolic needs of the fetus and a very small infant: a comparative approach. Biochemical Society Transactions. 1998;26:75-8.

12. Fry AG, Bernstein IM, Badger GJ. Comparison of fetal growth estimates based on birth weight and ultrasound references. Journal of Maternal-Fetal and Neonatal Medicine. 2002;12:247-52.

13. Freeman JV, TCole TJ, Chinn S, et al. Cross sectional stature and weight reference curves for the UK, 1990. Archives of Disease in Childhood. 1995;73:17-24.

14. Clarke L, Buss DS, Juniper DS, et al. Adipose tissue development during early postnatal life in ewe-reared lambs. Experimental Physiology. 1997;82:1015-7.

15. Symonds ME, Pearce S, Bispham J, et al. Timing of nutrient restriction and programming of fetal adipose tissue development. Proceedings of the Nutrition Society. 2004:63:397-403.

16. Vernon RG. Control and Manipulation of Animal Growth. In: Buttery PJ, Haynes NB, Lindsay DB (Eds). 67-83 London: Butterworths; 1986.pp.67-83.

17. Jolliffe D. Continuous and robust measures of the overweight epidemic: 1971-2000. Demography. 2004;41:303-14.

18. Symonds ME, Gardner DS. In: Developmental Origins of Health and Disease. In: Gluckman PD, Hanson MA (Eds.) Cambridge: Cambridge University Press; 2005.pp.397-403.

19. Mellor DJ, Cockburn FA. Comparison of energy metabolism in the new-born infant, piglet and lamb. Quarterly Journal of Experimental Physiology. 1986;71:361-79.

20. Widdowson EM, Dickerson JW. In: Mineral Metabolism. In: Comar CL, Bronner F (Eds). New York: Academic Press; 1964.pp.1-217.

21. Alexander G. Energy metabolism in the starved newborn lamb. Australian Journal of Agricultural Research. 1961;11:144-64.

22. Lean ME. Brown adipose tissue in humans. Proceedings of the Nutrition Society. 1989;48:243-56.

23. Power G. Biology of temperature: The mammalian fetus. Journal of Developmental Physiology. 1989;12:295-304.

24. Merklin RJ. Growth and distribution of human fetal brown fat. Anatomical Record. 1974;178:637-46.

25. Alexander G, Bell AW. Quantity and calculated oxygen consumption during summit metabolism of brown adipose tissue in newborn lambs. Biology of the Neonate. 1975;26: 214-20.

26. Cannon B, Nedergaard J. Brown adipose tissue: Function and significance. Physiological Reviews. 2004;84:277359.

27. Trayhurn P, Temple NJ, Van Aerde J. Evidence from immunoblotting studies on uncoupling protein that brown adipose tissue is not present in the domestic pig. Canadian Journal of Physiology and Pharmacology. 1989;67.

28. Davison AN, Dobbing J. Myelination as a vulnerable period in brain development. British Medical Bulletin. 1966;22:40-4.

29. Dickerson JW. Nutritional in Early Life: Concepts and Practice. In: Morgan JB, Dickerson JWT (eds). Chichester: Wiley and Sons; 2003. pp.1-38.

30. Hull D, Elphick MC. Evidence for fatty acid transfer across the human placenta. Ciba Foundation Symposium. 1978;63:75-91.

31. Hull D, Elphick MC, Broughton Pipkin F. The transfer of fatty acids across the sheep placenta. Journal of Developmental Physiology. 1979;1:31-45.

32. Symonds ME, Budge H, Stephenson T. Nutritional in Early Life: Concepts and Practice. In: Morgan JB, Dickerson JW (Eds). Chichester: Wiley and Sons; 2003.pp.91-121.

33. Prentice AM, Prentice A. Evolutionary and environmental influences on lactation. Proceedings of the Nutrition Society. 1995;54:391-400.

34. Girard J, Ferre P, Pegorier JP, et al. Adaptations of glucose and fatty acid metabolism during perinatal period and suckling-weaning transition. Physiological Reviews. 1992;72:507-62.

35. Widdowson EM. Nutrition from conception to extreme old age. Food and Nutrition. 1982;8:32-40.

36. Widdowson EM. Chemical composition of newly born animals. Nature. 1950;116:626-8.

37. Sadava D, Frykman P, Harris E, et al. Development of enzymes of glycolysis and gluconeogenesis in human fetal liver. Biology of the Neonate. 1992;62:89-95.

38. Haggarty P. Effect of placental function on fatty acid requirements during pregnancy. European Journal of Clinical Nutrition, (In press) 2004.

39. Eriksson JG, Forsen T, Tuomilehto J, et al. Early growth and coronary heart disease in later life: longitudinal study. British Medical Journal. 2001;322: 949-53.

40. Clarke L, Bryant MJ, Lomax MA, et al. Maternal manipulation of brown adipose tissue and liver development in the ovine fetus during late gestation. British Journal of Nutrition. 1997;77:871-83.

41. Ferre P, Decaux JF, Issad T, et al. Changes in energy metabolism during the suckling and weaning period in the newborn. Reproduction, Nutrition, Developement. 1986;26:619-31.

42. Kaufmann P, Scheffen I. Fetal and Neonatal Physiology. In: Polin RA, Fox F (Eds). New York: Saunders; 1998.pp.47-56.

43. Illsley NP. Glucose transporters in the human placenta. Placenta. 2000;21:14-22.

44. Cetin I. Amino acid interconversions in the fetal-placental unit: the animal model and human studies in vivo. Pediatric Research. 2001;49:148-54.

45. Reitman ML, Bi S, Marcus-Samuels B, et al. Leptin and its role in pregnancy and fetal development. - an overview. Biochemical Society Transactions. 2001;29: 68-72.

46. Heasman L, Clarke L, Dandrea J, et al. Correlation of fetal number with placental mass in sheep. Contemporary Reviews in Obstetrics and Gynaecology. 1998;10:275-80.

47. Stegmann JH. Placental development in sheep. Bijdragen tot de Dierkunde. 1974;44:4-72.

48. Schneider H. Ontogenic changes in the nutritive function of the placenta. Placenta. 1996;17:15-26.

49. Broughton Pipkin F, Hull D, et al. Marshall's Physiology of Reproduction, 4th edition, Volume 3 'Pregnancy and Lactation', Part Two Fetal physiology, Parturition and Lactation. In: Lamming GE (Eds). London: Chapman and Hall; 1994.pp.767-861.

50. Shekhawat P, Bennett MJ, Sadovsky Y, et al. Human placenta metabolizes fatty acids: Implications for fetal fatty acid oxidation disorders and maternal liver diseases. American Journal of Physiology. 2003;284:E1098-E1105.

51. Prip Buss C, Pegorier JP, Duee PH, et al. Evidence that the sensitivity of carnitine palmitoyltransferase I to inhibition by malonyl-CoA is an important site of regulation of hepatic fatty acid oxidation in the fetal and newborn rabbit. Biochemical Journal. 1990;269: 409-15.

52. Molina RD, Meschia G, Battaglia FC, et al. Gestational maturation of placental transfer of glucose. American Journal of Physiology. 1991;261:R697-R704.

53. Evers IM, Nikkels PG, Sikkema JM, et al. Placental pathology in women with type 1 diabetes and in a control group with normal and large-for gestational-age infants. Placenta. 2003;24:819-25.

54. Ibdah JA, Bennett MJ, Rinaldo P, et al. A fetal fatty-acid oxidation disorder as a cause of liver disease in pregnant women. New England Journal of Medicine. 1999;340:1723-31.

55. Herrera E. Metabolic adaptations in pregnancy and their implications for the availability of substrate to the fetus. European Journal of Clinical Nutrition. 2000;54(Suppl) 1:S47-S51.

56. Ibdah JA, Zhao Y, Viola J, et al. Molecular prenatal diagnosis in families with fetal mitochondrial trifunctional protein mutations. Journal of Pediatrics. 2001;138:396-9.

57. Broughton Pipkin F, Roberts JM. Hypertension in pregnancy. Journal of Human Hypertension. 2000;14:705-24.

58. Dobbing J. In: Davis JA, Dobbing J (Eds). Scientific Foundations of Pediatrics, 2nd edition. London: Heinemann; 1981.

59. Crawford MA, Hassam AG, Stevens PA. Essential fatty acid requirements in pregnancy and lactation with special reference to brain development. Progress in Lipid Research. 1981;20:30-40.

60. Clandinin MT, Chappell JE, Heim T, et al. Fatty acid accretion in fetal and neonatal liver. Implications for fatty acid requirements. Early Human Development. 1981;5:355-66.

61. Olsen SF, Secher NJ. Low consumption of seafood in early pregnancy as a risk factor for preterm delivery: Prospective cohort study. BMJ. 2002;324:447.

62. Warnes K, Morris MJ, Symonds ME, et al. Effects of gestation, cortisol and maternal undernutrition on hypothalamic neuropeptide Y mRNA levels in the sheep fetus. J Neuroendocrinol. 1998;10:51-7.

63. Ziegler EE, O'Donnell AM, Nelso SE, et al. Body composition of the reference fetus. Growth. 1976;40:329-41.

64. Yuen BS, Owens PC, Muhlhausler BS, et al. Leptin alters the structural and functional characteristics of adipose tissue before birth. FASEB Journal. 2003;17:1102-4.

65. Vernon RG, Clegg RA, Flint DJ. Aspects of adipose tissue metabolism in foetal lambs. Biochemical Journal. 1981;196:819-24.

66. Greco P, Vimercati A, Hyett J, et al. The ultrasound assessment of adipose tissue deposition in fetuses of "well controlled" insulin-dependent diabetic pregnancies. Diabetic Medicine. 2003;20:858-62.

67. Dietz WH. Critical periods in childhood for the development of obesity. American Journal of Clinical Nutrition. 1994;59:955-9.

68. Hay WW. Current topic: Metabolic interrelationships of placenta and fetus. Placenta. 1995;16:19-30.

69. Jones CT, Rolph TP. Metabolic events associated with the preparation of the fetus for independent life. Ciba Foundation Symposium. 1981;86:214-33.

70. Gluckman PD, Gunn AJ, Cutfield WS, et al. Congenital idiopathic growth hormone deficiency associated with prenatal and early postnatal growth failure. Journal of Pediatrics. 1992;121:920-3.

71. Bauer MK, Breier BH, Harding J, et al. The fetal somatotrophic axis during long term maternal undernutrition in sheep; evidence of nutritional regulation in utero. Endocrinology. 1995;136:1250-7.

72. Li J, Gilmour RS, Saunders JC, et al. Activation of the adult mode of ovine growth hormone receptor gene expression by cortisol during late fetal development. FASEB Journal. 1999;13:545-52.

73. Edwards LJ, Symonds ME, Warnes K, et al. Responses of the fetal pituitary-adrenal axis to acute and chronic hypoglycaemia during late gestation in the sheep. Endocrinol. 2001;142:1778-85.

74. Stephenson TJ, Stammers JP, Hull D. Placental transfer of free fatty acids: importance of fetal albumin concentration and acid base status. Biology of the Neonate. 1993;63:273-80.

75. Mallov S, Alousi AA. Lipoprotein lipase activity of rat and human placenta. Proceedings of the Society for Experimental Biology and Medicine. 1965;119:301-6.

76. Elphick MC, Filshie GM, Hull DT. The passage of fat emulsion across the human placenta. Br J Obstet Gynaecol. 1978;85:610-8.

77. Darmady JM, Postle AD. Lipid metabolism in pregnancy. British Journal of Obstetrics and Gynaecology. 1982;89: 211-5.

78. McDonald RG, Young M, Hytten FE. Changes in plasma non esterified fatty acids and serum glycerol in pregnancy. Br J Obstet Gynaecol. 1975;82:460-6.

79. Lafond J, Simoneau L, Savard R, et al. Linoleic acid transport by human placental syncytiotrophoblast membranes. European Journal of Biochemistry. 1994;226:707-13.

80. Benassyag C, Rigourd V, Mignot TM, et al. Does high polyunsaturated free fatty acid level at the feto-maternal interface alter steroid hormone message during pregnancy? Prostaglandins Leukotrines and Essential Fatty Acids. 1999;60:393-9.

81. Symonds ME, Bryant MJ, Lomax MA. Lipid metabolism in shorn and unshorn pregnant sheep. British Journal of Nutrition. 1989;62:35-49.

82. Kamp F, Zakim D, Zhang F, et al. Fatty acid flip-flop in phospholipid bilayers is extremely fast. Biochemistry. 1995;34:11928-37.

83. Glatz JF, Luiken JJ, vanNieuwenhoven FA, et al. Molecular mechanisms of cellular uptake and intracellular translocation of fatty acids. Prostaglandins Leukotrines and Essential Fatty Acids. 1997;57:3-9.

84. Glatz JF, vanderVusse GJ. Cellular fatty acid-binding proteins: their function and physiological significance. Progress in Lipid Research. 1996;35:243-82.

85. Dutta-Roy AK. Transport mechanisms for long-chain polyunsaturated fatty acids in the human placenta. Am J Clin Nutr. 2000;71:S315-S22.

86. Campell FM, Bush PG, Veerkamp JH, et al. Detection and cellular localization of plasma membrane-associated and cytoplasmic fatty acid-binding proteins in human placenta. Placenta. 1998;19: 409-15.

87. Barros LF, Yudilevich DL, Jarvis SM, et al. Quantitation and immunlocalisation of glucose transporters in the human placenta. Placenta. 1995;16:623-33.

88. Ehrhardt RA, Bell AW. Developmental increases in glucose transporter concentration in the sheep placenta. Am J Physiol.1997;273:R1132-R41.

89. Innis SM. Human milk and formula fatty acids. J Pedi. 1992;120:S56-S61.

90. Shirazi-Beechley SP. Molecular biology of intestinal glucose transport. Nutritional Research Reviews. 1995;8:2741.

91. Symonds ME, Clarke L. Influence of thyroid hormones and temperature on adipose tissue development and lung maturation. Proceedings of the Nutrition Society. 1996;55:567-75.

92. Symonds ME, Mostyn A, Pearce S, et al. Endocrine and nutritional regulation of fetal adipose tissue development. J Endocrinol. 2003;159:293-9.

93. Trahair JF, Sangild P. Systemic and luminal influence on the perinatal development of the gut. Equine Veterinary Journal. 1997;24:S40-S50.

94. McMillen IC, Houghton DC, Phillips ID. Maturation of cytokine-receptors in preparation for birth. Biochemical Society Transactions. 2001;29:63-8.

95. Weaver LT, Prentice A. In: Morgan JB, Dickerson JW (Eds).Nutritional in early life: concepts and practice. Chichester: Wiley and Sons; 2003.pp.205-32.

96. Shelley HJ. Glycogen reserves and changes at birth. Br Med Bulletin. 1961;17:137-43.

97. King C, Harrison M. In: Morgan JB, Dickerson JW. T (eds). Nutritional in early life: concepts and practice. Chichester: Wiley and Sons; 2003.pp.257-90.

98. Clarke L, Heasman L, Firth K, et al. Influence of route of delivery and ambient temperature on thermoregulation in newborn lambs. Am J Physiol. 1997;272:R1931-R9.

99. Symonds ME, Mostyn A, Stephenson T. Cytokines and cytokine-receptors in fetal growth and development. Biochemical Society Transactions. 2001;29:3337.

100. Alexander G, Williams D. Shivering and nonshivering thermogenesis during summit metabolism in young lambs. J Physiol. London. 1968;198:251-76.

101. Sritharan N, Morgan J. In: Morgan JB, Dickerson JW (Eds). Nutritional in Early Life: concepts and Practice. Chichester: Wiley and Sons; 2003;233-56.

102. Lawson M. In:Morgan JB, Dickerson JWT (Eds). Nutritional in Early Life: Concepts and Practice. Chichester: Wiley and Sons; 2003;324-65.

103. McKenna JJ, Mosko S, Dungy C, et al. Sleep and arousal patterns of co-sleeping human mother/infant pairs. A preliminary physiological study with implications for the study of sudden infant death syndrome. American Journal of Physical Anthropology. 1990;83:331-47.

104. Weaver LT. In: Walker WA, Durie PR, Hamilton JR, Walker-Smith JA (Eds). Pediatric Gastrointestinal Disease. Mosby, St Louis; 1996. pp.9-14.

105. Grosvenor CE, Picciano MF, Baumrucker CR. Hormones and growth factors in milk. Endocrine Reviews. 1993;14:710-28.

106. Weaver LT. Egg, placenta, breast and gut: comparative strategies for feeding the young. Endocrine Regulations. 1993;27:95-104.

107. Sarles J, Morean H, Verger R. Human gastric lipase: Ontogeny and variations in children. Acta Paediatrica. 1992;81:511-3.

108. Hamosh M, Scanlon JW, Ganot D, et al. Fat digestion in the newborn. J Clini Invest. 1981;67:838-46.

109. Jensen RG, Clark RM, de Jong FA, et al. The lipolytic triad: Human lingual, breast milk and pancreatic lipases: Physiological implications of their characteristics in digestion of dietary fats. J Pedia Gastroenterol and Nutr. 1982;1:243-55.

110. Hernell O, Blackberg L. Human milk bile salt-stimulated lipase: functional and molecular aspects. J Pedia. 1994;125:S56-S61.

111. Havel RJ. Postprandial lipid metabolism: An overview. Proceedings of the Nutrition Society. 1997;56:659-66.

112. Hamosh M. Digestion in the premature infant: the effects of human milk. Seminars in Perinatology. 1994;18:485-96.

113. Wainwright PE. Dietary essential fatty acids and brain function: a developmental perspective on mechanisms. Proceedings of the Nutrition Society. 2002;61:61-9.

114. Naim HY, Sterchi EE, Levitz MJ. Biosynthesis and maturation of lactase-phlorizin hydrolase in the human small intestinal epithelial cells. Biochemical Journal. 1987;241:427-34.

115. Wood IS, Trayhurn P. Glucose transporters (GLUT and SGLT): Expanded families of sugar transport proteins. Br J Nutr. 2004;89: 3-9.

116. Rogers S, Macheda ML, Docherty SE, et al. Identification of a novel glucose transporter-like protein GLUT-12. Am J Physiol. 2002;282:E733-E8.

117. Joost HG, Thorens B. The extended GLUT-family of sugar/polyl transport fasciators: Nomenclature, sequence characteristics, and potential function of its novel members. Molecular Membrane Biology. 2001;18:247-56.

118. Hales CN, Barker DJP. Type 2 (non-insulin dependent) diabetes mellitus: The thrifty phenotype hypothesis. Diabetologia. 1992;35:595-601.

119. Forsén T, Eriksson JG, Tuomilehto J, et al. Mother's weight in pregnancy and coronary heart disease in a cohort of Finnish men: Follow up study. BMJ. 1997;315:837-40.

120. Cianfarani S, Germani D, Branca F. Low birth weight and adult insulin resistance: the "catch-up growth" hypothesis. Archives of Disease in Childhood. 1999;81: F71-F3.

121. Eriksson JG, Forsen T, Tuomilehto J, et al. Catch-up growth in childhood and death from coronary heart disease: Longitudinal study. BMJ. 1999;318:427-31.

122. Ong KK, Ahmed ML, Emmett PM, et al. Association between postnatal catchup growth and obesity in childhood: Prospective cohort study. BMJ. 2000;320:967-71.

123. Rogers I, Group EB. The influence of birth weight and intrauterine environment on adiposity and fat distribution in later life. Inter J Obesity. 2003;27: 755-77.

124. Parsons TJ, Power C, Manor O. Fetal and early life growth and body mass index from birth to early adulthood in 1958 British cohort: Longitudinal study. BMJ. 2001;323:1331-5.

SECTION 11

Early Pregnancy

LT Merce, S Kupesic

90

Contributions of 3D Ultrasonography to the Study of Embryonic Development

RM Sabatel López, L Martinez-Cortes, JC Prados Salazar

INTRODUCTION

The massive changes a fertilized oocyte undergoes from the time of fertilization up to its transformation into a fetus were hidden from the human eye in vivo for many centuries. Thus, most of our knowledge derived from the microscopic study of anatomical and pathological samples taken from gestating uteruses or aborted specimens.

The evolution of ultrasound imaging and the advent of the transvaginal probe enabled the development of sonoembryology, thus making available to us the development of the embryo in vivo. From the embryological standpoint, this period includes the first 56 days of development.

We have learnt a great deal with conventional diagnostic ultrasound scans, Doppler techniques, and the use of color- and power-Doppler, but the advent of three-dimensional diagnostic ultrasound techniques is changing our understanding tremendously. The opportunity to observe the volumetric morphology of the embryo and its annexa from the very beginning of gestation is clearly of immense importance in understanding the events taking place in this key period of human development.

FIRST TO THIRD WEEK OF EMBRYONIC DEVELOPMENT

Conventional diagnostic ultrasound can detect the gestational sac in the endometrium as a rounded structure with a nonechogenic central area surrounded by a more refringent 2 mm ring (4 weeks and 3 days). Three-dimensional diagnostic ultrasound makes it possible to obtain images much earlier; on the 27th day of the cycle (13 days after fertilization) we can already see the outline of an eccentric structure proximal to the bottom of the endometrium which corresponds to the gestational sac. Four days later we can easily see the yolk sac which is barely 1 mm in size. In a 2D ultrasound scan this can hardly be identified (Figs 90.1A and B).

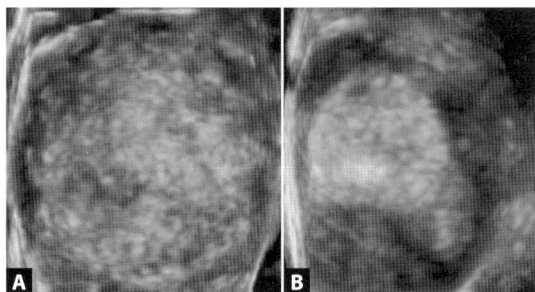

Figs 90.1A and B: (A) Gestational sac on day 13 post-fertilization; (B) Gestational sac with yolk sac in the fourth week and third day

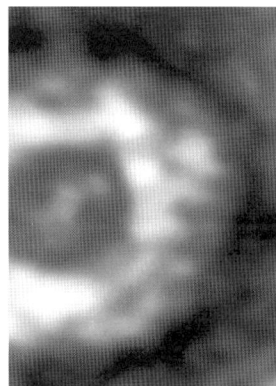

Fig. 90.2: Trophoblast in the fifth week of gestation

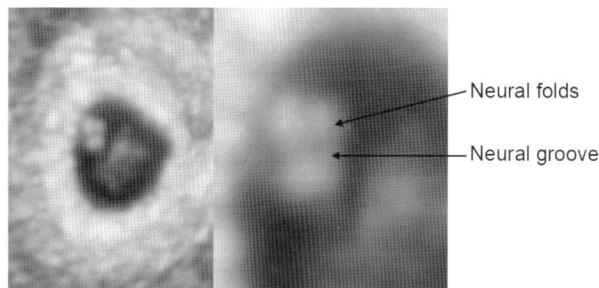

Neural folds

Neural groove

Fig. 90.3: Changes in the shape of the embryo as a consequence of the notochordal process

Placental organogenesis begins on the ninth day postfertilization; villi formation begins on day 13 and on day 21 the intervillous circulation appears. Whereas in 2D diagnostic ultrasound trophoblastic proliferation is identified by the increase in thickness, in 3D ultrasound imaging we can even see the irregularities trophoblastic development confers on the surface of the gestational sac (Fig. 90.2).

In the third week of development, the embryo attains a size of 2 mm and appears sonographically as a hyperrefringent area located on the yolk sac. From an embryological point of view it is a highly complex structure; by the 21st day postfertilization the development of the notochordal process changes its shape from "disc-shaped" to "sandal-shaped". This process, which cannot be visualized with 2D ultrasound scanning, can be seen with 3D ultrasound imaging (Fig. 90.3).

Toward days 21–22 the cardiac tube begins to beat. At this stage, the embryo is actually located between the amniotic cavity and the yolk sac, fixed to the trophoblast by a connecting stalk, which can only beverified with 3D sonography (Fig. 90.4).

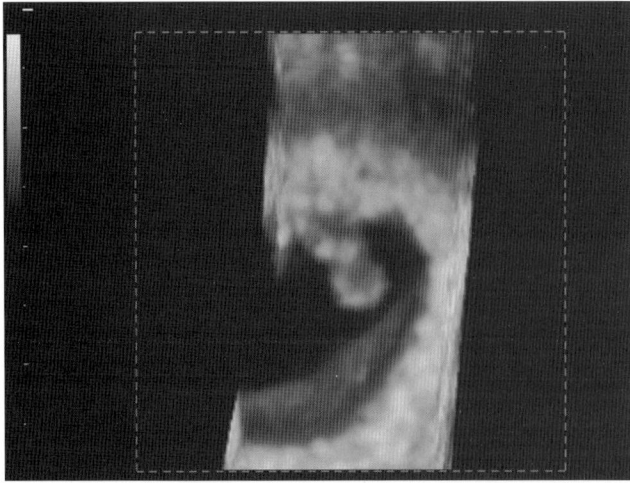

Fig. 90.4: Embryo between amniotic cavity and yolk sac, with visible connecting stalk

FOLDING OF THE EMBRYO

The rapid growth of the nervous system induces and conditions the longitudinal folding of the embryo. At the same time, cross-embryonic growth conditions ventral folding, so that by day 28 the cephalic pole has completely bypassed the cardiac area and by day 35 the embryo has adopted a totally incurved shape.

Embryonic folding is another process that can only be observed in three dimensions: initially, this shows the embryo and the yolk sac in different planes. Subsequently, we can identify the embryonic head and tail, not only in different planes, but joined by a curved nervous system (Figs 90.5A to C).

DEVELOPMENT OF THE LIMBS

The development of limbs is another process unavailable to conventional diagnostic ultrasound techniques but is visible with 3D sonography. Toward days 26–27 postfertilization we see the buds from which the arms will eventually develop, and then later the buds of the lower limbs appear. During the fourth week of development the upper limbs adopt the form of a paddle, due to the appearance of the hand plates whereas the lower limbs look like flippers. By the end of the fifth week the feet plates appear, and in the sixth week the flexure of the elbows. In the seventh week of embryonic development the hand and foot plates are facing each other, and the ridges of the fingers will begin to differentiate, so that by the end of the embryonic phase, the fingers of the hand are visible (Figs 90.6 and 90.7).

DEVELOPMENT OF FACIAL STRUCTURES

Due to the curvature of the ventral area, the changes in facial morphology are not appreciable via three-dimensional diagnostic ultrasound until the sixth week of embryonic development. By looking at the cephalic pole laterally we can see the lens placode,

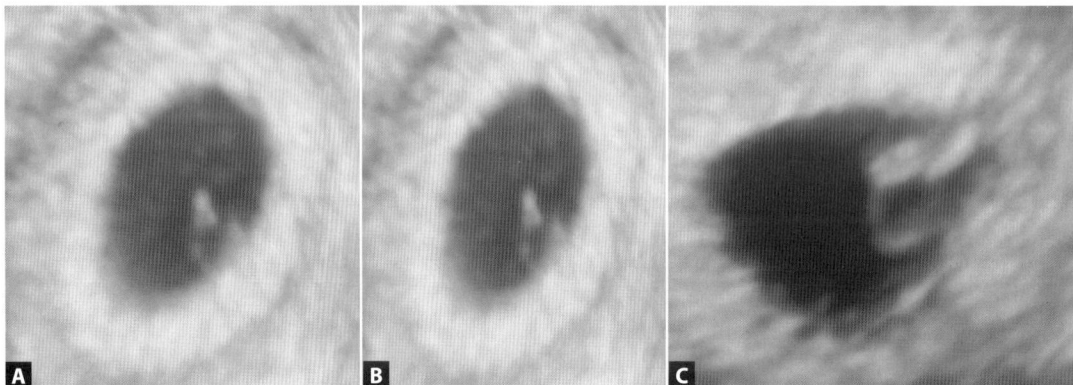

Figs 90.5A to C: Folding of the embryo: (A and C) Longitudinal folding; (B) Ventral folding

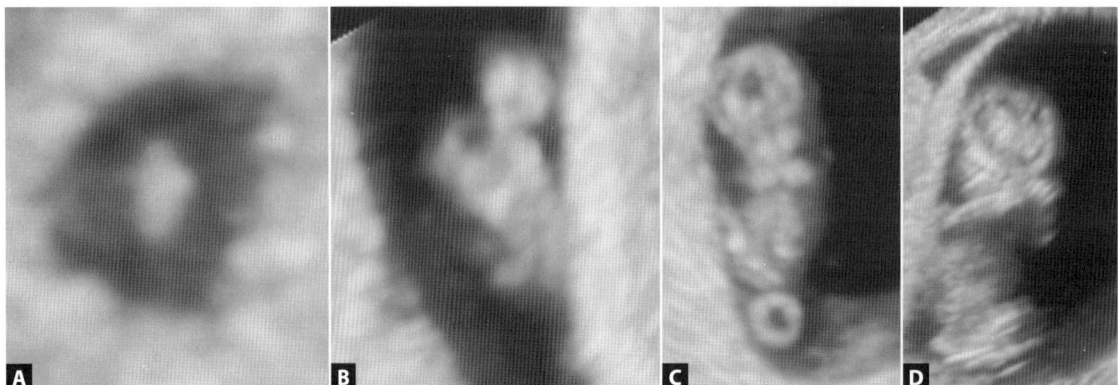

Figs 90.6A to D: Upper limb development: (A) Bud of the arms; (B) Paddle-like arms; (C) The flexure at the elbows permits the placement of the forearm over the thorax; (D) Fingers of the hand at the eighth week of development

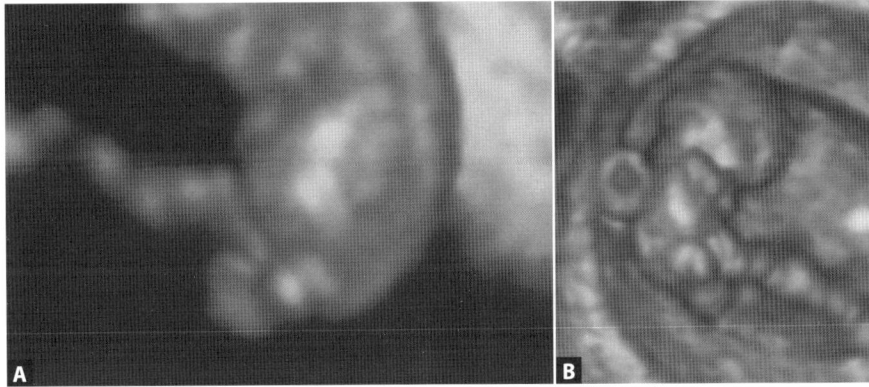

Figs 90.7A and B: 3D view of lower limbs development. (A) In the seventh week the foot plates face each other; (B) Knee and foot plate in the eighth week of development

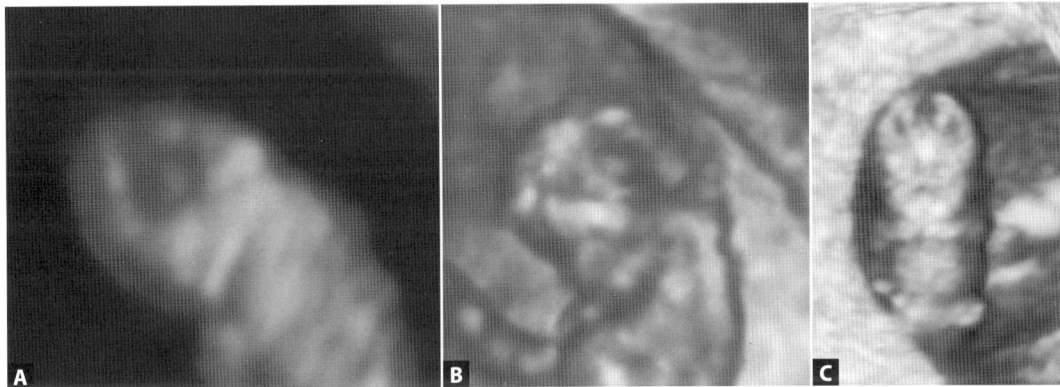

Figs 90.8A to C: Facial structures observed with 3D ultrasound imaging. (A) Lateral view of the face at the sixth week. We can see thelens pits and the prominences of the pharyngeal arches; (B) Frontal view of the face at the sixth week. We can see the mandibular and maxillary prominences as well as the nose pits and the mouth; (C) The frontal view at the eighth week shows the nasal septum, nares and palate

the prominences made by the pharyngeal arches, and the auricular hillocks in whose center we see the exit for the auditory channel. A frontal view shows the mandibular and maxillary prominences of the first pharyngeal arch, the nasal pits, and the wide mouth of the embryo. At the eighth week, the frontal view makes it possible to visualize a completely closed palate and the internal configuration of the nose (Figs 90.8A to C).

ABDOMINAL WALL DEVELOPMENT

The ventral folding of the embryo makes the yolk sac independent and contributes to the progressive closing of the abdominal wall. By the seventh week, the wall is almost closed except for the area corresponding to where the umbilical will attach. This, together with the rapid intestinal development, influences two sonographically visible facts. First, communication between the primitive intestine and yolk sac becomes reduced to a very fine cord, which allows greater separation between the sac and embryo. Second, part of the intestine remains in the proximal side of the umbilical cord and, therefore, is outside the abdominal cavity. This is called the "physiological umbilical hernia", which is visible until the 12–13th week of gestation (Figs 90.9A to C).

THE SPINE DEVELOPMENT

In the fifth week of development the spine presents chondrification centers, visible in 3D at the sixth week of development. Between days 50 and 56 we find three ossification centres in the spine—two lateral centers corresponding to vertebral processes and a central one corresponding to the vertebral body. With 3D ultrasound imaging it is possible to locate the body of the vertebra (greater size) and even the ossification of the vertebral processes of the ribs which have also begun to evolve during this week (Figs 90.10A and B).

DEVELOPMENT OF THE HEART

Toward days 20–21, once the two cardiac tubes fuse into one, the heart begins to beat. At the end of the third week, this single tube bends giving rise to the appearance of the primitive atrium and ventricle, separated by a constriction area: the atrioventricular canal. With 3D PW, we cannot only identify the heart in the fourth week of development, but also its external morphology (Fig. 90.11).

The complex embryology of the heart develops between the 4th week and 5th week. By the end of this stage the septa begins to grow thus separating the atrioventricular canal. Some of the

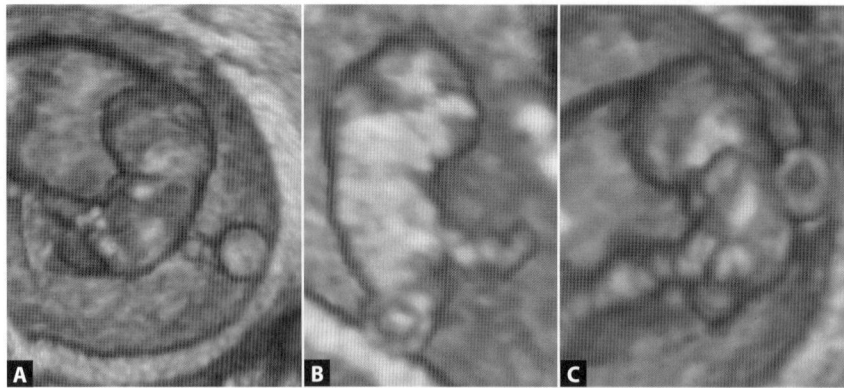

Figs 90.9A to C: Physiological umbilical hernia with 3D sonography

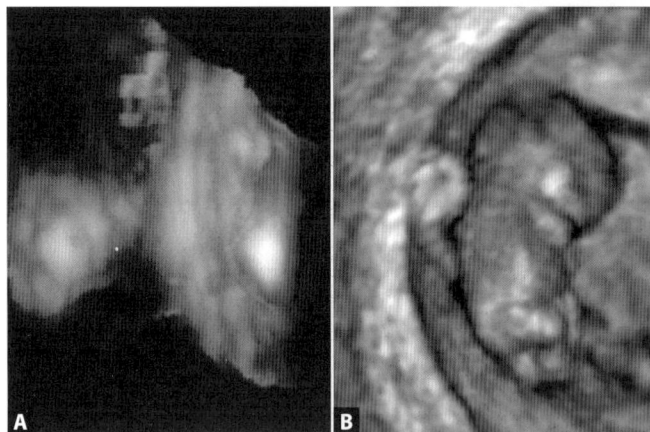

Figs 90.10A and B: The spine (A) in the chondrification phase, sixth week of development; (B) In the ossification phase, eighth week of development

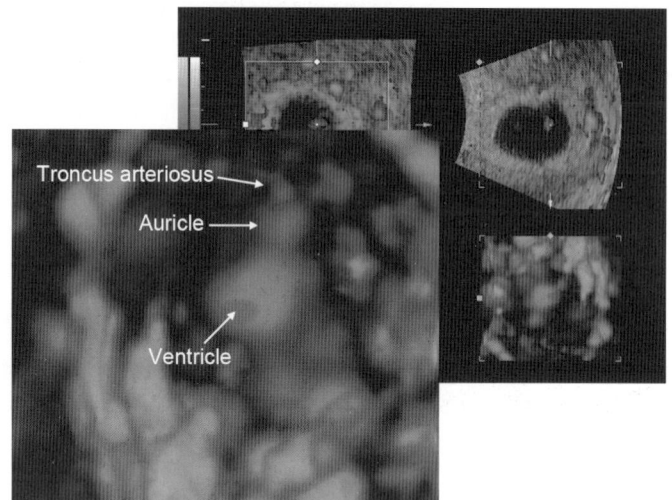

Fig. 90.11: Morphology of the heart at the fourth week of development with 3D PW Doppler

atrioventricular valves also begin to develop. In the heart of an 11 mm embryo it is possible to differentiate the atria from the ventricles. The former are separated by the primum septum and the ventricles are partially separated by the interventricular septum, which still has an orifice for communication between them. In tandem with the process of separation of the four cavities, the aortopulmonary partition undergoes spiral rotation. With 3D color Doppler sonography we can see the four cavities, and with body capture imaging how they rotate (Fig. 90.12).

In the seventh week the ventricles are totally separated because the orifice existing in the previous week is now closed. Using 3D PW doppler, it can be seen that the external morphology is very similar to that of the fetal heart (Fig. 90.13).

We cannot state that the closing of the interventricular partition—and what this implies for the evolution of the heart conduction system—is the cause of a functional change also observed at this time: the peak embryonic heart rate, which takes place at this time. In the ninth week of amenorrhea, seventh week of development, the heart rate curve reaches its highest peak, with an average of 170 beat per minutes, which in some cases can reach nearly 190 beats per minute. From this point onward, the heart

rate decreases until it reaches a plateau by the 14th or 15th week of amenorrhea. These values are maintained during the whole gestation period. This heart rate curve is constant, independent of the number of cases investigated.

DEVELOPMENT OF THE NERVOUS SYSTEM

During the fourth week, the closing of the neural tube has occurred and its differentiation into brain and spinal cord has begun. By the beginning of the fifth week, the three primary vesicles appear (anterior or prosencephalon, middle or mesencephalon and posterior or rhombencephalon) and two flexures (one folding the anterior and middle vesicles, and the cervical flexure). By the end of the week, there are five cerebral vesicles: telencephalon, diencephalon, mesencephalon, telencephalon and myelencephalon. The pontine flexure also appears. The increase in size during the fifth week permits their identification with 3D sonography (Fig. 90.14).

These structures are hollow and each of them bulges to give rise to different ventricles, which by the seventh week are in clear development. By the end of this week, the chorioid plexuses begin to develop inside the lateral ventricles (Figs 90.15A and B).

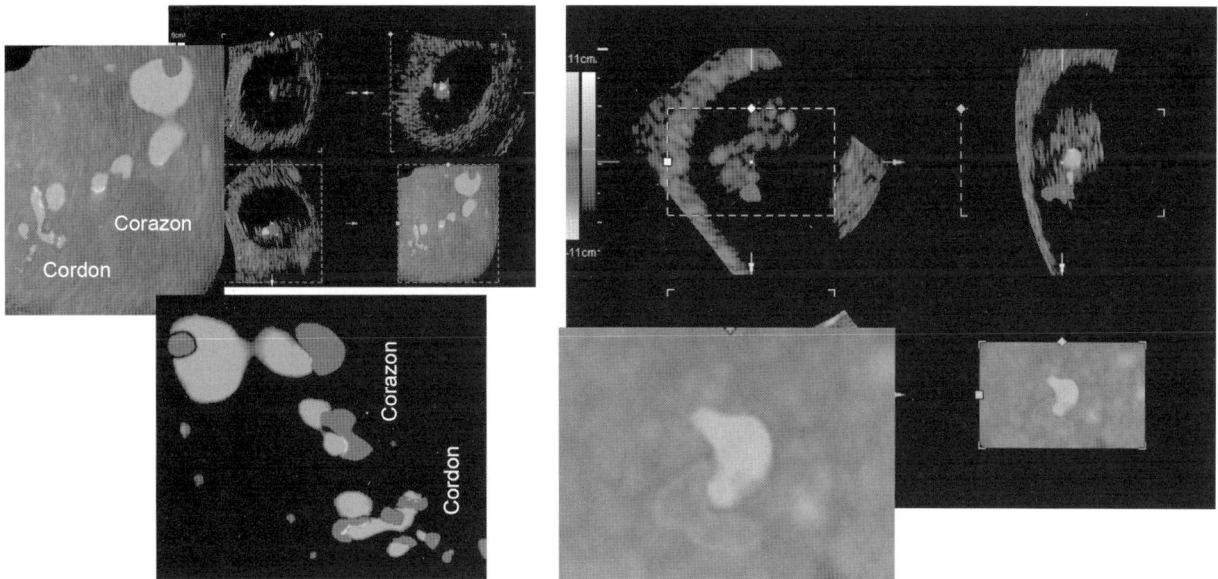

Fig. 90.12: Embryonic heart at the sixth week of development

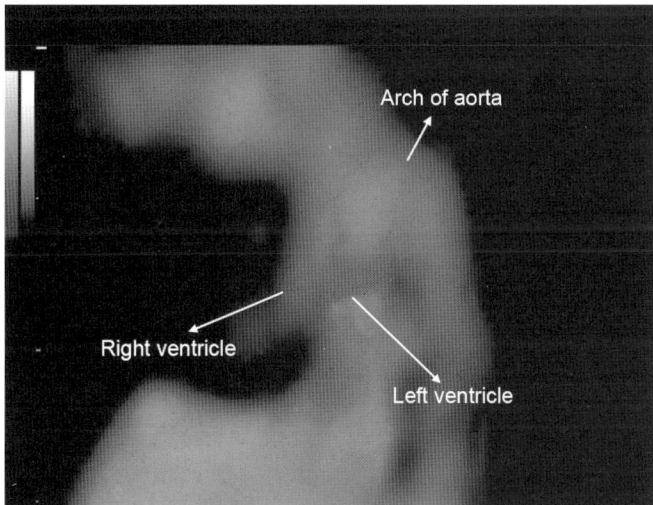

Fig. 90.13: External morphology of the heart at the seventh week of development

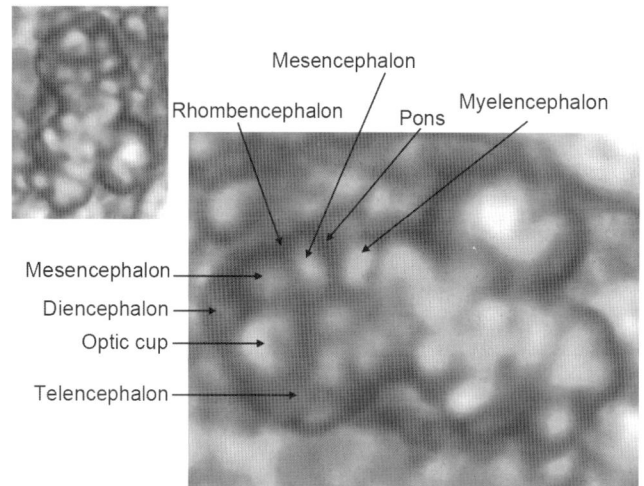

Fig. 90.14: 14-mm embryo cerebral vesicles viewed with 3D sonography

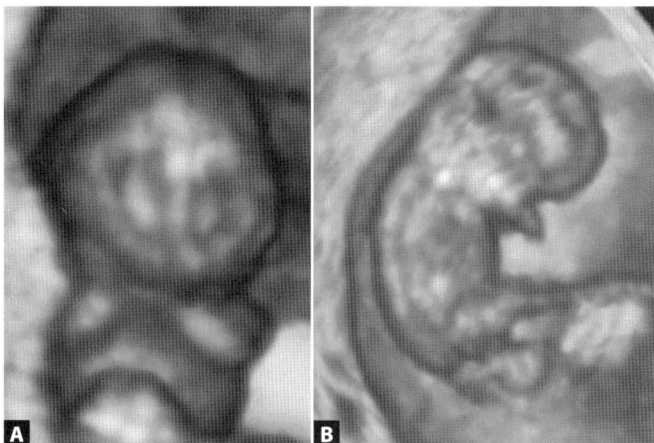

Figs 90.15A and B: Cerebral ventricles at the eighth week of development. (A) Lateral ventricles with chorioid plexuses. (B) Lateral ventricle, third and fourth ventricle

LUNG DEVELOPMENT

In such small embryos, it is practically impossible to follow the development of viscera sonographically due to their small size and the density of the different tissue layers. However, the lungs are different. By the eighth week of development, the bronchial tree is made up of two main bronchi buds (the left and the right, the latter being larger), secondary bronchi and segmentary or tertiary bronchi. From a histological standpoint, the lung is at the pseudoglandular stage. With 3D diagnostic ultrasound, we can identify the embryonic lung, the lobes and even a section of the bronchi (Fig. 90.16).

This review of the first 56 days of development with a 3D ultrasound scanner reveals the real potential of the technique: understanding normal embryological processes which are not visible with 2D sonography and which are clearly necessary to detect early morphological alterations.

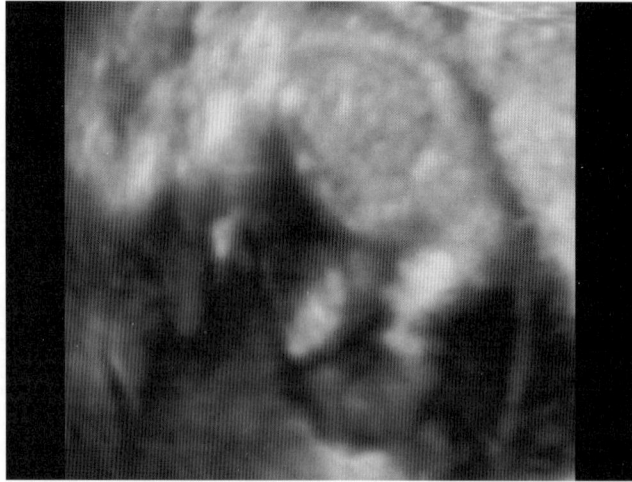

Fig. 90.16: Eighth week of development: right lung views with 3D sonography

BIBLIOGRAPHY

1. Carnegie Institution of Washington. Reports of the Director of the Department of Embryology. Yearbook. Washington, DC: Carnegie Institution; 1926-1947;28, 29, 31, 38, 46.
2. Hertig AT, Rock J. Two human ova of the pre-villous having an ovulation age of about 11-12 days respectively. Carnegie Contrib Embryol. 1941;29:;127-56.
3. Boyd JD, Hamilton WJ. The human placenta. The MacMillan Press LTD; 1975.
4. Timor-Tritsch IE, Farine D, Rosen MG. A close look at early embryonic development with the high-frequency transvaginal transducer. Am J Obstet Gynecol. 1988;159:676-81.
5. Sabatel RM, Galera Martinez R. Diagnostico de gestación precoz mediante la ecografía 3D. Rev Española de Ultrasonidos en Obstey Ginec Vol. 1. 2003.
6. Wilkin P. Pathologie du placenta. Étude clinique et anatomique. Masson et Cie, Editeurs, Paris; 1965.
7. Laing FC, Frates MC. Ultrasound evaluation during the first trimester of pregnancy. In: Pter Callen (Ed). Ultrasonography in Obstetrics and Gynecology, 4th edition, WB Saunders Company; 2000. pp. 105-45.
8. Moore KL, Persaud TV. The Developing Human: Clinically Oriented Embryology, 6th edition. WB Saunders Company; 1998.
9. Genis Galvez JMª. Biologia del desarrollo. Espaxs, Barcelona; 1970.
10. Sabatel RM, Cuadros Lopez JL. Periodo embrionario: Ecografía de las 8 primeras semanas del desarrollo. Aportaciones de la ecografía 3D. Premio Clínica Abril. Real Academia de Medicina del distrito de Granada; 2003.
11. Jiraseck JE. An Atlas of the Human Embryo and Fetus. Parthenon Publishing; 2001.
12. Sadler TW. Lagmann Embriología Médica, 6th edition. Editorial Médica Panamericana; 1993.
13. Hertzberg BS, Mahony BS, Bowie JD. Fisrts trimester fetal cardiac activity: Sonographic documentation of a progressive early rise in heart rate. J Ultrasound Med. 1988;7:573-5.
14. Sabatel RM, Cuadros Lopez JL, Motos MA, et al. Behaviour of the embryonicphoetal Heart rate in the first half of gestation. XIV European Congreso of Gynaecologists and Obstetricians; 1999.

91

2D and 3D Power Doppler Ultrasound from Ovulation to Implantation

LT Merce, MJ Barco, S Kupesic

INTRODUCTION

The ovarian cycle has two main purposes: firstly, the liberation of a mature oocyte through the ovulatory process; secondly, the production of a proper hormonal secretion to prepare the endometrium for the embryo implantation. All these processes require and involve great changes affecting the ovarian and uterine blood flows. The follicular growth, the corpus luteum formation and the endometrial development are physiological processes in which angiogenesis takes place in a natural way, thus providing the blood flow supply.

The uterine and ovarian blood flow changes taking place along the menstrual cycle were known basically from invasive experimental results out of different animal species. Doppler ultrasound examination, especially transvaginal color Doppler, has allowed the noninvasive approach to the importance of the blood flow in natural and artificial human reproduction. Recently, three-dimensional (3D) power Doppler and one sophisticated measurement software make possible to calculate the number of vessels and the blood flowing through them. This technique has greatly increased our knowledge about the uterine and ovarian vascularity.

In the present chapter, the blood flow changes taking place in the ovary and endometrium are analyzed from ovulation to implantation through the different examination techniques previously named. Currently, some of the parameters evaluated are those used in daily practice as oocyte quality and endometrial receptivity markers. Therefore, the different Doppler modalities become an essential technique to investigate the menstrual cycle physiology and a source of diagnostic and prognostic parameters about the outcome of assisted reproductive technologies.

FROM OVULATION

The ovarian and uterine blood flow changes have different physiological and clinical implications during the menstrual cycle, so from a practical point of view, we will separate their study.

Ovarian Blood Flow

Doppler studies have demonstrated the ovarian blood flow participation in the recruitment and selection of the dominant follicle during the *early follicular phase* of the ovarian cycle.[1,2] Our investigations confirm that in the beginning, the intraovarian vascular resistance is correlated with the number of recruited follicles. On the contrary, when a follicle reaches 10 mm of diameter becomes "dominant" and the intraovarian vascular resistance decreases despite the disappearance of the follicles cohort.[3,4] This relationship between the number of follicles and the intraovarian

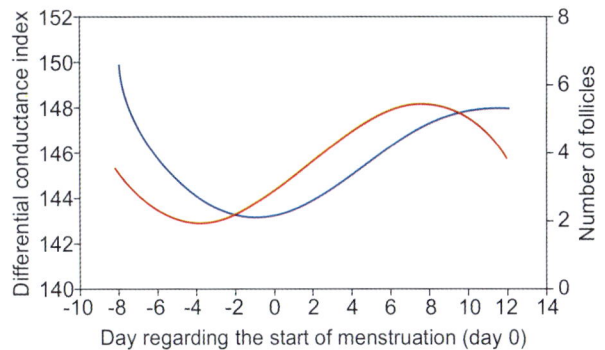

Fig. 91.1: Relationship between the number of recruited follicles (red line) and stromal flow, as assessed by its differential conductance index (blue line), during the transitional luteal-follicular period in 22 normal ovulatory cycles

blood flow supports the utility of these parameters as indicators of the ovarian response to the gonadotropin stimulation treatment (Fig. 91.1).

The number of follicles after pituitary suppression is a better *marker of the ovarian response* than the age of the patient and the ovarian volume.[5] This parameter predicts the number of retrieved oocytes irrespective of age and serum FSH levels.[6] The total number of antral follicles is the best predictor of the ovarian response followed by basal FSH, body mass index and the age of the woman.[7]

The blood flow of the ovarian stroma also predicts the ovarian response. The stromal peak systolic velocity during the early follicular phase is better related to the number of retrieved oocytes than the age of the patient, the basal levels of FSH and the estradiol.[8] A diminished stromal blood flow is responsible of a low ovarian response whereas when it rises over 10 cm/s a high number of oocytes and a better pregnancy rate are achieved (Fig. 91.2A).[9]

Three-dimensions ultrasound and power Doppler angiography make the estimation of the number of antral follicles and the stromal blood flow much easier without disturbing the patients.[10] Kupesic and Kurjak proved that the number of antral follicles and the index of stromal flow are the best predictors of a favorable outcome in vitro fertilization (IVF).[10] An increased or decreased stromal blood flow can explain a high or low response in IVF cycles.[11,12] Nevertheless, some authors believe that 3D Doppler indices do not offer additional information to predict the ovarian response to gonadotrophin stimulation during IVF cycles (Fig. 91.2B).[13]

Our experience in the assessment of 3D power Doppler ultrasound as a marker of the ovarian response comes from a study of 60 patients undergoing their first IVF cycle. A total of 119

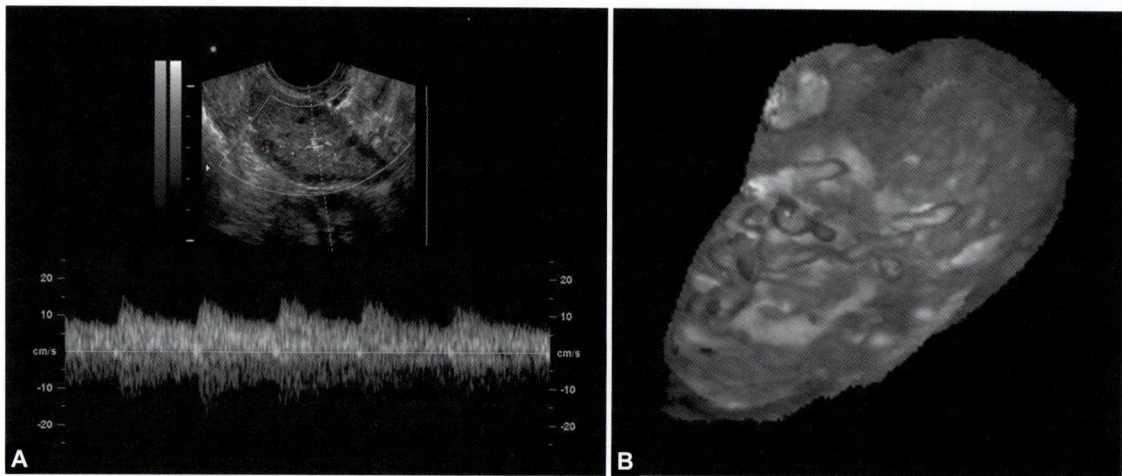

Figs 91.2A and B: Sonographic markers of the ovarian response: (A) recording of the ovarian stromal flow velocity wave (FVW) after pituitary suppression by GnRH analogs. The peak systolic velocity is a good predictor of the number of follicles to grow; (B) 3D ultrasonography and power Doppler angiography allow the assessment of all the sonographic and Doppler parameters involved in the prediction of the ovarian response

Table 91.1: Correlation coefficients of the sonographic parameters and power Doppler indices after pituitary supression, with the number of recruited follicles and the number of retrieved oocytes in 65 IVF cycles

	No. of follicles on hCG day	No. of retrieved oocytes
Ovarian volume	0.46	0.41
Number of follicles	0.52	0.53
Vascularization index	0.36	0.31
Flow index	0.30	0.27
Vascularization flow index	0.34	0.30

Note: All correlation coefficients are significant ($P < 0.01$).

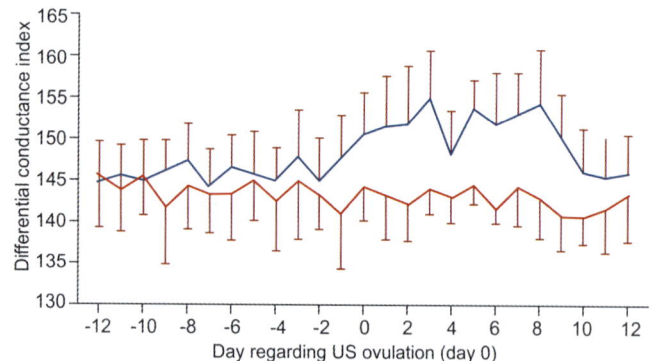

Fig. 91.3: Differential conductance index of the dominant or active ovary (blue line) and the contralateral or inactive ovary (red line) during the ovarian cycle. Luteal values of the dominant ovary are significantly increased compared to those of the follicular phase or those from the luteal phase of the inactive ovary

ovaries have been separately evaluated because hypothetically the ovarian response could be mediated by the local vascular factors. The number of follicles more than or equal to 10 mm the day of human chorionic gonadotropin (hCG) injection and the number of oocytes retrieved are considered as indicators of the ovarian response. A significant correlation (p < 0.01) has been observed between the ovarian volume, the number of antral follicles greater than 2 mm, ovarian vascularization index (VI), ovarian flow index (FI) and ovarian vascularization/flow index (VFI) to the number of recruited follicles and the number of retrieved oocytes (Table 91.1). Nevertheless, when a multiple regression is applied, only the number of follicles and the ovarian volume reach a statistical significance.

During the follicular phase the arterial and venous blood flow increase in the active or dominant ovary.[14-18] The color signal at the wall of the dominant follicle increases progressively to almost encircling it. This is due to the intense angiogenesis produced along with the follicular development. The blood flow also increases progressively at the vessels of the ovarian stroma, the ovarian hilum arteries[16,17] and the venous circulation.[18] Approaching ovulation the blood flow increases significantly compared to the contralateral or inactive ovary (Fig. 91.3).

Several studies of animal experimentation deduce that blood flow increase during the follicular phase is basically due to the growth of the dominant follicle.[5] Our study, along with those of other authors,[19,20] proves this assumption by confirming a significant correlation between the diameter of the dominant follicle and the venous and arterial perifollicular maximum systolic velocity.[21] A high correlation between the dominant follicle size and the serum estradiol is classically acknowledged;[22] nevertheless a significant correlation between the follicular blood flow and the estradiol blood levels has not been proven until now.

The blood flow reaches its maximum values in the *preovulatory follicle* just prior to the follicular rupture. The maximum blood flow velocity increases from 29 hours before the follicular rupture, maintaining a peak until at least 72 hours after the corpus luteum appearance (Fig. 91.4A).[23] The blood flow is similar in every part of the preovulatory follicle before the LH peak. After the LH peak the maximum systolic velocity increases at the base of the follicle and decreases significantly, almost disappearing, at the apical zone.[24] 3D power Doppler shows the preovulatory follicular wall has a number of vessels

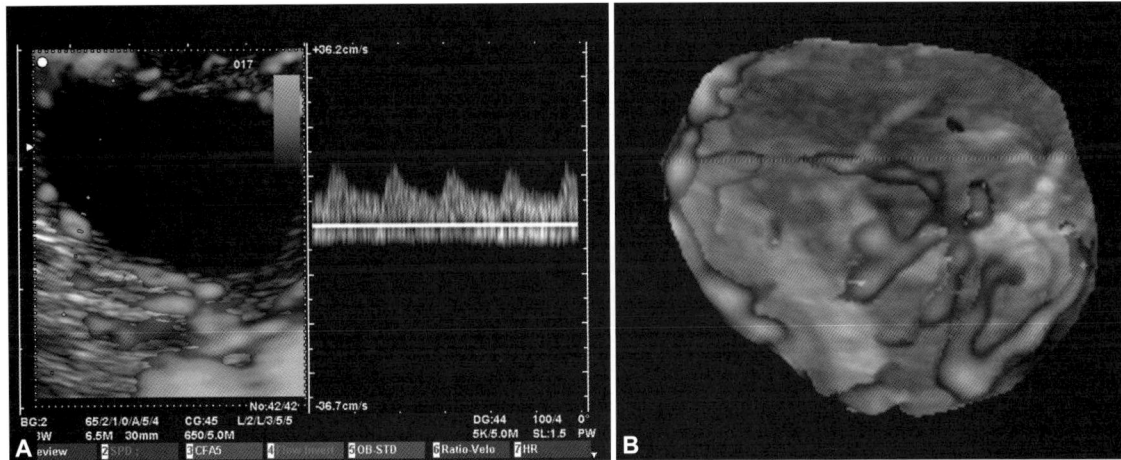

Figs 91.4A and B: Study of the preovulatory follicle blood flow by Doppler technology; (A) Color signal and flow velocity wave (FVW) arterial and venous in the wall of a 20 mm follicle. Look at the absent pulsatility of the venous signal; (B) Vascular network of a preovulatory follicle by 3D power Doppler angiography

(Vascularization Index) and an amount of blood flowing through them (Flow Index) significantly increased as compared with the same ovary (Fig. 91.4B).[25]

Electronic microscopy has shown the preovulatory follicular walls as having a great amount of sinusoidal dilated vessels and avascular zones due to ischemia and arteriovenous shunts.[26] These findings support the vascular mechanism of ovulation and would explain the blood flow velocity increase by the presence of shunts and the apical disappearance of Doppler signals caused by thrombosis and ischemia phenomena.

The process of angiogenesis, development and vasodilatation of the perifollicular vascular network culminates at the *ovulation*. From the follicular rupture onwards, the theca vessels begin the invasion of the granulosa cells showing an intense angiogenesis and wide arteriovenous shunts. Moreover, the growth in size of the ovary leads to a straightening of the spiral arteries which compromise the hemodynamic stability of the whole system producing an increase in the turbulence of the blood flow.[3,4] This flow increase associated with changes in the spectral Doppler signal is named "luteal conversion" and is of great help to the diagnosis of ovulation (Box 91.1). The luteal conversion is independent of the sonographic visualization or appearance of the corpus luteum. In the luteinized unruptured follicle (LUF) syndrome the follicular rupture does not take place so the luteal conversion is not present.[15] Therefore, the luteal conversion is a very reliable parameter of ovulation.

The *corpus luteum* has a greater arterial and venous blood flow than the preovulatory follicle.[3,4,14-18] The helical arteriole of the corpus luteum presents the highest systolic velocities with a small variability.[27]

The luteal vascularity can be depicted with a great accuracy by 3D power Doppler (Figs 91.5A and B). The luteal Vascularization, Flow and Vascularization Flow Indices calculated from 3D are significantly superior to the follicular ones (Table 91.2). During the luteal phase the blood flow increases in the stromal and hilum arteries of the active ovary[16,17] and in the utero-ovarian and ovarian ipsilateral arteries also.[3]

This increase in the amount of blood flow is essentially caused by the development of new vessels in the ovary carrying the corpus luteum but it should be controlled by

Box 91.1: Characteristics of the "luteal conversion" of the intraovarian vascularization

Color signal
- Area increase
- Intensity increase
- Increase of Doppler 3D indices

Spectral signal
- *Velocimetry*
  - Increase of systolic velocity
  - Increase of venous velocity
  - Decrease of resistance
- *Morphology*
  - Intensity increase
  - Dispersion of velocities
  - Superposition of waves
  - Notch absence
  - Easily recorded

local and systemic mediators. An inverse and significant relationship has been proven between the vascular density of the corpus luteum and its pulsatility index.[28] Color Doppler studies confirm that the arterial[17,29,30] and venous[18] blood flow of the corpus luteum is correlated with progesterone secretion.

The cycles with luteal or secretory deficiency show an increase in the luteal vascular resistance[29,30] and a decrease in the venous flow velocity.[18] In the LUF syndrome the blood flow remains unchanged after the LH peak. During the "false" luteal phase, the vascular resistance is similar to that of the follicular phase without detectable differences between them (Figs 91.6A and B).[15,18,31]

Uterine and Endometrial Blood Flow

The blood flow of the uterine arteries and their radial branches does not experiences significant changes during the early and middle follicular phase.[16,30] During the periovulatory period the findings are contradictory. Whereas some authors[32,33] find an increasing uterine and endometrial (uterine, radial and spiral arteries) blood flow from the LH peak onwards, others[16,34,35] find a decreasing blood flow until past ovulation. By means of 3D power Doppler it has been recently proven that the endometrial and sub-endometrial flow and

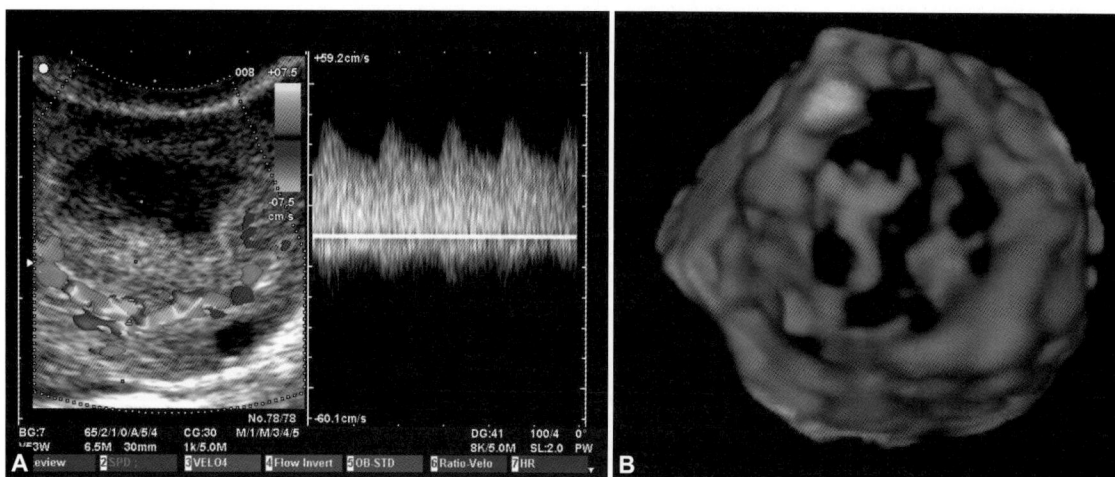

Figs 91.5A and B: Corpus luteum blood flow study by Doppler technology; (A) Color mapping and flow velocity wave (FVW) during the mesoluteal phase of a normal ovulatory cycle. "Luteal conversion" is observed; (B) Vascular network of the corpus luteum assessed by 3D power Doppler angiography

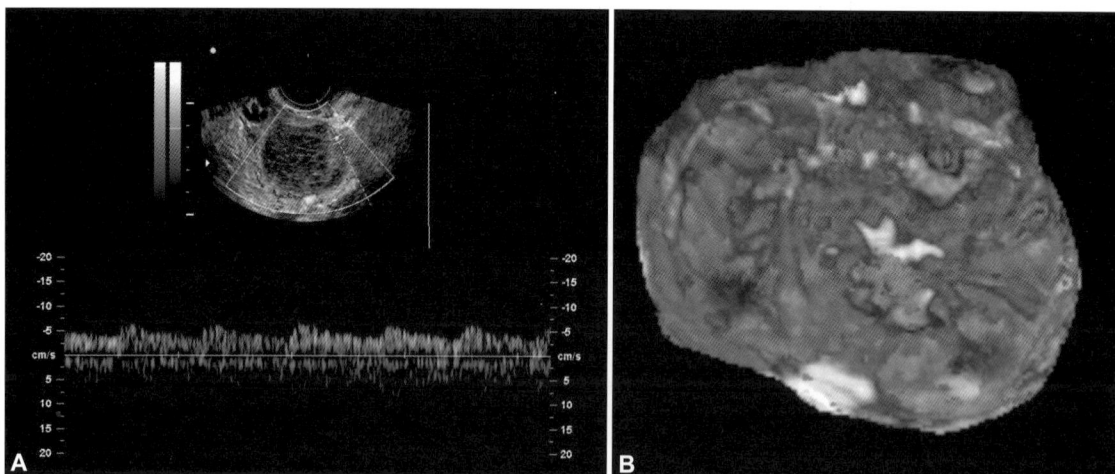

Figs 91.6A and B: Doppler investigation in the LUF; (A) 3D angiographic rendering; (B) Arterial and venous flow velocity wave (FVW). "Luteal conversion" is not present and venous and arterial velocities are very low

Table 91.2: Vascularization index (VI), flow index (FI) and vascularization flow index (VFI) in the preovulatory follicle, corpus luteum and LUF assessed by 3D power Doppler angiography[1]

Parameter	Preovulatory follicle (n = 8)	Corpus luteum (n = 6)	LUF (n = 3)
VI	4.24 ± 2.91	29.91 ± 14.82[2,3]	2.35 ± 1.10[2]
FI	35.46 ± 6.48	47.67 ± 3.98[2,3]	34.00 ± 3.65[2]
VFI	1.59 ± 1.27	14.72 ± 8.17[2,3]	0.83 ± 0.48

1: Mean ± SD; 2: $P < 0.001$ with regard to the preovulatory follicle; 3: $P < 0.005$ regarding to LUF. No significant differences between LUF and preovulatory follicle.
Abbreviation: LUF, luteinized unruptured follicle.

Vascularization indices increase from the middle follicular phase to attain their maximum values 3 days prior to ovulation. After that, these indices decrease until reaching their nadir 5 days after ovulation to increase progressively again during the middle and late luteal phases (Figs 91.7A and B).[36]

During the luteal phase the blood flow in the whole uterine vascular tree, from the uterine arteries to the endometrial spiral arteries, increases significantly compared to that of the follicular phase.[16,32,33] As the menstrual cycle advances but especially during the luteal phase, the color signals from the intramyometrial and endometrial vessels grow in number and intensity.

When no pregnancy is achieved the blood flow in all the utero-ovarian vascular network decreases and menstruation begins a new cycle.

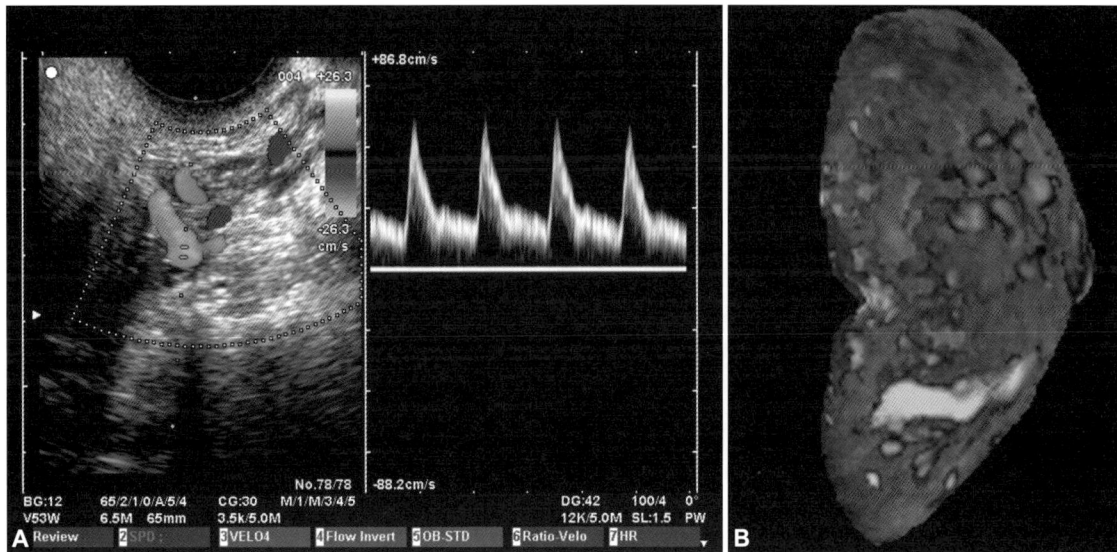

Figs 91.7A and B: Blood flow assessment of the uterine and endometrial circulations; (A) Uterine artery flow velocity wave (FVW); (B) 3D Doppler angiography representation of the endometrial vascularity during the middle luteal phase

TO IMPLANTATION

Implantation is a dynamic process requiring a true dialog between mother and embryo. The assisted reproductive technologies (ART) have demonstrated the success in achieving implantation and a normal ongoing pregnancy depend essentially upon the embryo quality and endometrial receptivity. Since many years ago, sonographic and Doppler parameters have been sought to be used as "implantation markers".[37,38]

The follicular size and perifollicular vascularization have been proposed as ultrasound markers of oocyte quality and competence. The endometrial pattern and thickness have been also evaluated as indicators of endometrial receptivity.

Follicular Blood Flow

The intrafollicular oxygen concentration determines a normal embryo development. Oocytes with cytoplasmatic defects and embryos with multinucleated blastomeres come mainly from follicles with severe hypoxia causing an abnormal arrangement of chromosomes.[39] On the other hand, a defective development of the perifollicular vascular network has been implicated in the origin of intrafollicular hypoxia.[40] The embryonic triploidies rate is significantly raised in the poorly vascularized follicles.[41] On the contrary, the best vascularized follicles are those showing the highest oxygen concentrations.[39] Given that similar size follicles can contain different oxygen concentrations, perifollicular vascularity is an independent marker of the follicular diameter.[42]

The follicular blood flow can be assessed by the maximum systolic velocity in the perifollicular arteries.[43,44] This technique assumes that the blood flow in a single artery represents all the follicular blood flow. The perifollicular color mapping with power Doppler is an easier and reliable technique to assess the follicular blood flow.[41,42,45,46] This procedure assumes that the color signal coming from a single perifollicular vascular plane represents all the follicular blood flow. 3D power Doppler evaluates all the perifollicular vessels and determines the vascularization (number of vessels) and Flow (flow intensity) from the whole follicular

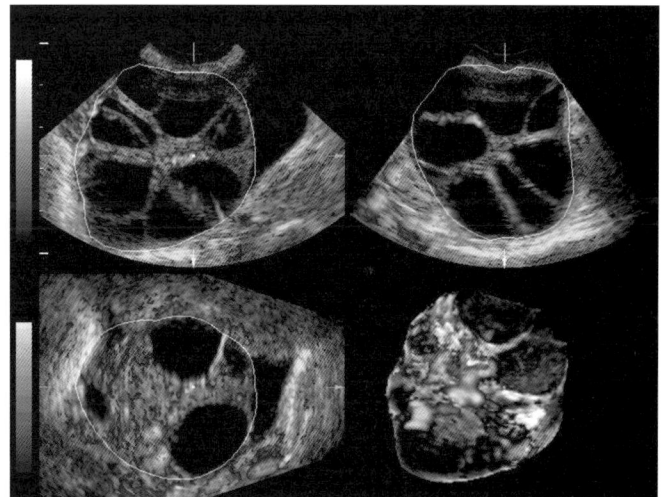

Fig. 91.8: 3D power Doppler angiography rendering of the perifollicular vasculature in an IVF cycle at the day of hCG administration

volume. Therefore, it is the only method directly assessing the entire follicular blood flow (Fig. 91.8).

In accordance to the percentage of color area from the perifollicular power Doppler mapping, follicles have been classified in: Grade 0, when no color can be depicted;[45] Grade I, less than 25% of the follicular circumference; Grade II, between 26% and 50%; Grade III: between 51% and 75% and Grade IV: between 76% and 100% (Figs 91.9A to D).[41,42,46] The number of retrieved oocytes, mature and fertilized is significantly higher from the well vascularized follicles (Grades III and IV) than from those showing poor vascularization (Grades I and II).[41] According to our results, perifollicular vascularization determines especially the maturity and fertilization indices in follicles less than 15 mm, being significantly higher in those well vascularized. The recovery rate is independent from vascularization and shows rates higher than 50% (Table 91.3).

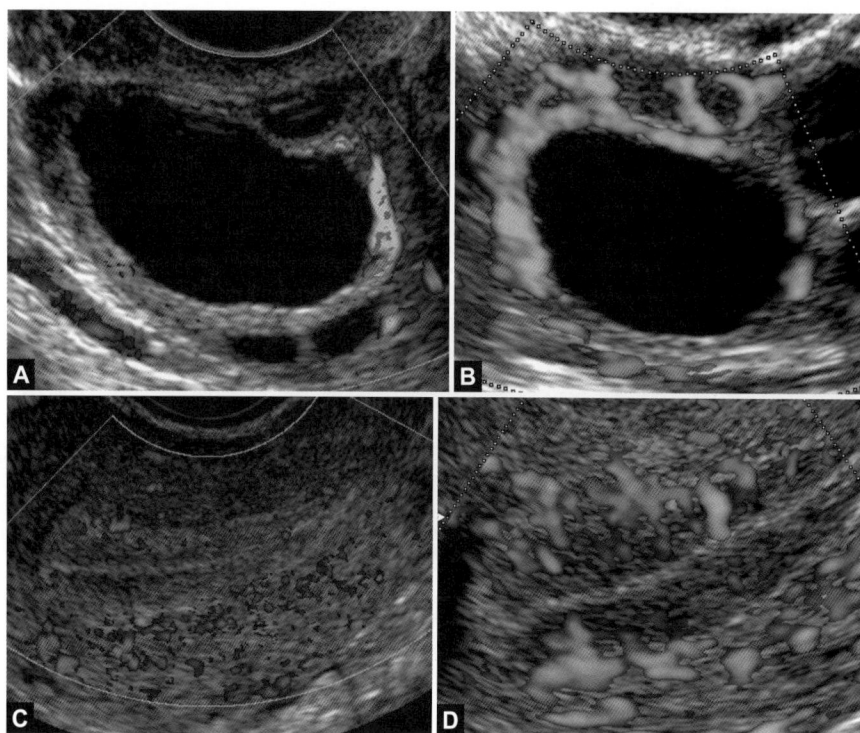

Figs 91.9A to D: Power Doppler mapping of the follicular and endometrial blood flow: (A) Grade I, color mapping encircles less than 25% of the follicular circumference; (B) Grade IV, Doppler signal occupies from 76% to 100% of follicular perimeter; (C) Type I endometrial mapping or peripheral flow, with color signal is visible at myometrium and only reaches outer hyperechogenic endometrial layer; (D) Type III endometrial mapping or central flow, as the color mapping is distributed through the whole endometrial thickness

Table 91.3: Recovery, maturity and oocyte fertilization rates in follicles less than 15 mm according to the percentage of vascularization on day of hCG administration in 32 IVF cycles

Rates	0–25% color		26–50% color		>50% color	
	n	%	n	%	n	%
Recovery[1]	8/13	61.5	12/21	57.1	9/19	47.4
Maturity[2]	2/8	25.0	6/12	50.0	7/9	77.8
Fertilization[3]	1/7	14.3	7/11	63.6	7/7	100.0

1: $cm^2 = 0.708$; $P = 0.702$; 2: $cm^2 = 4.749$; $P = 0.09$; 3: $cm^2 = 10.823$; $P < 0.005$.

We have evaluated 87 IVF cycles by 3D power Doppler. We studied the relationship between the number of follicles more than 10 mm and 3D Doppler indices the day of hCG administration and the laboratory biological parameters (oocyte number, metaphase II oocytes number, fertilized oocytes number, number of embryos, number of Type I embryos, number of multinucleated embryos and embryo score). The vascularization, flow and vascularization flow indices for each ovary and the ratio between follicular volume and these indices have also been evaluated (Table 91.4). The number of follicles and the ratio between the follicular volume and the flow index are the only two variables related to the number of oocytes retrieved, its maturity grade and the possibility of fertilization and developing embryos. On the contrary, the relationship between these variables and the biological quality of embryos do not seem to be clear.

The transfer of an embryo from a well vascularized follicle implies a significantly high pregnancy rate, whereas the pregnancy loss rate is increased when the embryos transferred come from low vascularized follicles.[41,46] The probability of pregnancy has been observed to be higher if at least one follicle shows a peak systolic velocity more than or equal to 10 cm/s.[45] According to our results,[38] the transfer of at least one embryo from one follicle with a vascularity more than or equal to 75% or with a peak systolic velocity more than or equal to 10 cm/s has a positive predictive value of pregnancy greater than 55%. That means that the application of this marker could improve results significantly, almost doubling the pregnancy rate (32% in this series).

Kupesic and Kurjak[10] studied 56 patients with 3D power Doppler after pituitary suppression. When the average stromal flow index from both ovaries was greater than 11, they observed a fertilization rate of 89% and a pregnancy rate of 50%. When this index was between 11 and 13, the fertilization and pregnancy rates were 75.2% and 47.2%, respectively. However, if the average flow index from both ovaries was below 11 the fertilization rate fell to 64.3% and no pregnancy was achieved. Our results are shown on Table 91.5, where significant differences between pregnant and non-pregnant patients for the majority of the IVF laboratory

Table 91.4: Correlation coefficients of the number of follicles and 3D power Doppler indices on day of hCG administration with biological laboratory parameters in 87 IVF cycles

	NO	NOM	NOF	NE	NEI	NEM	SCE
NF	0.87[a]	0.70[a]	0.62[a]	0.62[a]	0.26[a]	0.29[a]	0.46[a]
VI	0.31[a]	0.27[a]	0.20	0.21[a]	0.07	0.18[b]	0.08
FI	0.25[a]	0.21[a]	0.08	0.11	0.09	0.12	0.05
VFI	0.32[a]	0.28[a]	0.21[a]	0.21[a]	0.08	0.18[b]	0.09
FV/VI	0.04	0.00	0.09	0.06	0.08	-0.15	0.06
FV/FI	0.73[a]	0.65[a]	0.62[a]	0.59[a]	0.27[a]	0.20[b]	0.40[a]
FV/VFI	0.00	-0.02	0.06	0.03	0.06	-0.15	0.04

[a]means $P < 0.01$; [b]means $P < 0.05$

Abbreviations: NF, number of follicles >10 mm on day of hCG administration; VI, vascularization index; FI, flow index; VFI, vascularization flow index; FV, follicular volume; NO, number of retrieved oocytes; NOM, number of metaphase II oocytes; NOF, number of fertilized oocytes; NE, number of developed embryos; NEI, number of type I embryos; NEM, number of multinucleated embryos; SCE, score of embryos.

Table 91.5: Comparison of stimulation, 3D power Doppler and biological parameters in 87 IVF cycles according to outcome[1]

Parameter	Pregnancy (n = 31)	No. pregnancy (n = 56)	P
Age, years	33.94 (27–41)	34.63 (27–45)	0.40
E2 on hCG day, pg/mL	3581.52 (943–6000)	2758.54 (285–5223)	0.17
VI	20.83 (5.04–39.33)	19.85 (1.53–42.96)	0.56
FI	64.27 (27.62–76.36)	63.08 (32.87–79.40)	0.31
VFI	7.13 (1.39–14.41)	6.83 (0.37–16.01)	0.67
FV/VI	2.03 (0.68–6.29)	1.98 (0.50–18.12)	0.24
FV/FI	0.56 (0.21–1.15)	0.47 (0.11–1.43)	0.04
FV/VFI	6.23 (1.85–22.77)	6.35 (1.22–76.14)	0.19
NO	10.68 (2–20)	7.50 (0–24)	0.005
NOM	7.55 (1–16)	5.25 (0–20)	0.003
NOF	3.75 (0–18)	5.00 (1–11)	0.02
NE	4.87 (1–11)	3.55 (0–18)	0.01
NEI	2.29 (0–9)	1.23 (0–6)	0.006
NEM	1.23 (0–4)	0.89 (0–4)	0.09
NET	2.08 (1–3)	2.03 (1–3)	0.32
SCE	33.17 (4–104)	23.77 (2–76)	0.01

[1]Numbers represent the value of the mean and the range in brackets.

Abbreviations: VI, vascularization index; FI, flow index; VFI, vascularization flow index; FV, follicular volume; NO, number of retrieved oocytes; NOM, number of metaphase II oocytes; NOF, number of fertilized oocytes; NE, number of developing embryos; NEI, number of type I embryos; NEM, number of multinucleated embryos; NET, number of embryos transferred; SCE, score of transferred embryos.

biological parameters can be appreciated. Although the number of transferred embryos was similar, the biological quality was greater in the pregnant group. The follicular volume/flow index ratio is the only 3D Doppler parameter significantly increased in the pregnant group. When this ratio was between 0.40 and 0.60, the pregnancy rate was 41%. If it was above 0.60, the pregnancy rate of 50% was reached. When it was below 0.40, the rate descended to 18%. The overall pregnancy rate was 35.6%.

Uterine and Endometrial Blood Flow

Goswany, Williams and Steptoe[47] demonstrated that the uterine receptivity improved after increasing the uterine arteries blood flow under hormonal replacement therapy. The optimal uterine receptivity seems to appear when the average pulsatility index from both uterine arteries ranges from 2 to 3.[48-50] The implantation and pregnancy rates decrease significantly when the pulsatility index is greater than 3 or 4[48-56] or when no diastolic flow is registered in the Doppler signal (Table 91.6).[55,56] According to these limits, a diminished blood flow in the uterine arteries would prevent implantation (NPV = 88–100%) but a good uterine perfusion not always will guarantee a pregnancy (PPV = 44–56%).

The endometrial blood flow should reflect more properly the uterine receptivity given that the endometrium is the place for the embryo implantation.[38] In accordance to the color mapping four types of endometrial blood flow can be flow, if the color distinguished:[38,57-59] Type 0 or signal reaches the hyperecogenic negative endometrial *endometrial* border; Type II or intermediate blood flow, when only vessels from the surrounding endometrial

Table 91.6: Cut-off values for the uterine artery pulsatility index in patients undergoing assisted reproduction techniques

Authors	Treatment	Day (d)	Parameter	Limit
Steer et al. 1992[48]	An + CC + hMG	Transfer-d	Mean PI	3
Zaidi et al. 1996[49]	An + hMG	HCG-d	PI	3
Tsai et al. 1996[50]	CC + hMG	HCG-d	Mean PI	3
Coulam et al. 1994[51]	Natural	Ovulation-d	Mean PI	3.3
Coulam et al. 1995[52]	Gn	Retrieval-d + transfer-d	Mean PI	3.3
Bustillo et al. 1995[53]	An + HRT	15-d	Mean PI	3.3
Favre et al. 1993[54]	An + hMG	Transfer-d	PI	3.55
Tekay et al. 1996[55]	?	?	PI	4
Deichert et al. 1996[56]	?	?	PI	4

Abbreviations: hMG, human menopausal gonadotropin; CC, clomiphene citrate; An, gonadotropin releasing hormone analog; HRT, hormone replacement therapy; Natural, nonstimulation treatment; hCG, human chorionic gonadotropin.

blood flow, when the color map myometrium without reaching the endometrium can occupies the external half of the endometrial thickness be depicted; Type I or peripheral endometrial blood and Type III or central endometrial blood flow when vessels come to the endometrial cavity invading the entire endometrial thickness (Figs 91.9A to D). It is more convenient to apply power Doppler to detect the signal from vessels showing low velocity blood flow, thus avoiding the loss of signal due to a perpendicular incidence of the beam, as it occurs with conventional color Doppler.[38]

The absence of a color map at the endometrial and myometrial subendometrial levels implies a complete failure[57] or significant decrease[60,61] of implantation, whereas the pregnancy rate increases when vessels reach the sub-endometrial halo and the endometrium.[57,60] In a study about more than 600 cycles with color Doppler the day of embryo transfer, the implantation and pregnancy rates were 24.2% and 47.8% respectively when endometrial and subendometrial blood flow was detected; 15.8% and 29.7% if there was only subendometrial flow; and 3.5% and 7.5% when no flow was present.[60] Women showing a large endometrial flow area by power Doppler have a greater pregnancy rate, whereas below 5 mm² means that it is very difficult to achieve implantation despite a proper endometrial thickness.[62] Our results from 40 IVF cycles show that the pregnancy rate increases along with vascularity improvement, reaching a 67% when the color signal arrives to the endometrial cavity (Table 91.7).

Ultrasonography and 3D power Doppler have the advantage to assess the endometrial volume and the endometrial and subendometrial blood flow at the same time (Figs 91.10A to C). The subendometrial flow index the day of embryo transfer is greater in the group of patients achieving pregnancy.[63] A subendometrial flow/vascularization index above 0.24 showed a 83.3% sensitivity, a specificity of 88.9%, PPV of 93.8% and NPV of 72.3% to predict gestation when it is evaluated the day of hCG administration in IVF cycles.[64]

Table 91.7: Pregnancy rate according to endometrial blood flow mapping on the hCG administration day in 40 IVF cycles

Endometrial blood flow	No. cases (n%)	Pregnancy rate (n%)
Type 0	5 (12.5)	1 (20)
Type I	17 (42.5)	6 (35)
Type II	12 (30)	5 (42)
Type III	6 (15)	4 (67)

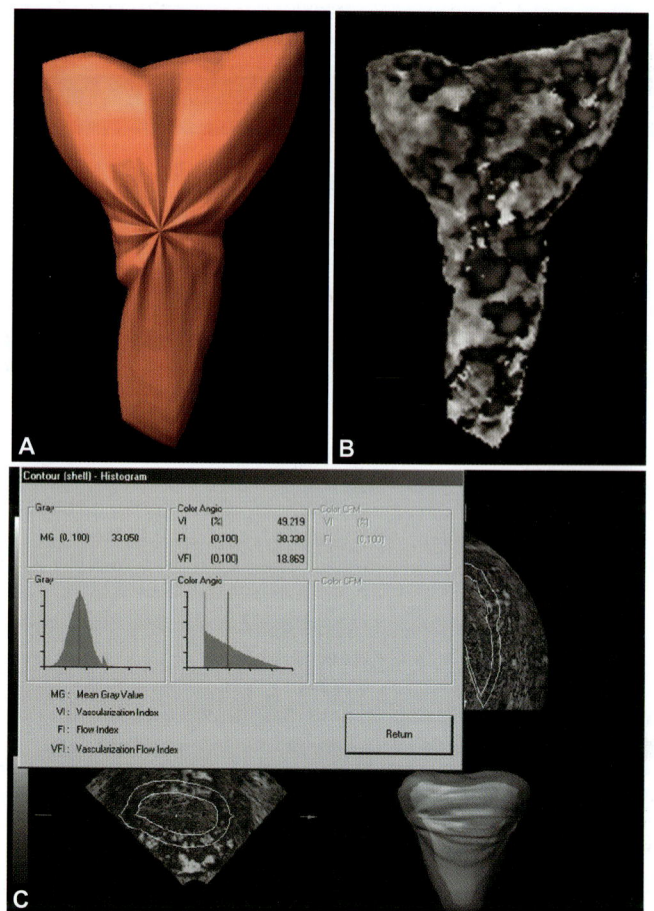

Figs 91.10A to C: 3D ultrasound and power Doppler angiography of the endometrium and its vascularity on the day of hCG administration; (A) Endometrial volume by "skin" rendering; (B) 3D power Doppler mapping of the endometrial vasculature; (C) Technique of "shell" to calculate subendometrial 3D power Doppler vascularity indices

According to our results, an intermediate vascularization, flow and flow vascularization indices are associated to a high pregnancy rate. On the contrary, when the vascularization index is below 10 no pregnancy is achieved. When the blood flow is very high, the pregnancy rate decreases without significant differences (Table 91.8).

Table 91.8: Pregnancy rate according to subendometrial 3D power Doppler indices on the day hCG administration in 40 IVF cycles

Doppler indices		No. case (n%)	Pregnancy rate (n%)
Vascularization	<10	5 (12.5)	0 (0)
	10–35	18 (45)	11 (61.1)
	>35	17 (42.5)	5 (29.4)
Flow	<28	12 (30)	1 (8.3)
	28–34	20 (50)	12 (60)
	>34	8 (20)	3 (37.5)
Vascularization-flow	<6	10 (25)	13 (32.5)
	6–12	17 (42.5)	10 (58.8)
	>12	13 (32.5)	5 (38.5)

REFERENCES

1. Taylor KJW, Burns PN, Wells PNT, et al. Ultrasound Doppler flow studies of the ovarian and uterine arteries. Br J Obstet Gynecol. 1985;92:240-6.
2. Vrtacnik-Bokal E, Meden-Vrtovec H. Utero-ovarian arterial blood flow and hormonal profile in patients with polycystic ovary syndrome. Hum Reprod. 1998;13:815-21.
3. Mercé LT. Velocimetría Doppler durante el ciclo ovárico normal. In: Mercé LT (Ed). Ecografía Doppler en Obstetricia y Ginecología. Madrid: InteramericanaMcGraw-Hill; 1993. pp. 113-28.
4. Mercé LT, Bau S. Velocimetría Doppler del ciclo ovárico. In: Bajo Arenas JM (Ed). Ultrasonografía y reproducción. Barcelona: Prous Science; 1996. pp. 37-66.
5. Tomás C, Nuojua-Huttunen S, Martikainen H. Pretreatment transvaginal ultrasound examination predicts ovarian responsiveness to gonadotrophins in in-vitro fertilization. Hum Reprod. 1997;12:220-3.
6. C hang MY, Chiang CH, Hsieh TT, et al. Use of the antral follicle count to predict the outcome of assisted reproductive technologies. Fertil Steril. 1998;69:505-10.
7. Ng EH, Tang OS, Ho PC. The significance of the number of antral follicles prior to stimulation in predicting ovarian responses in an IVF programme. Hum Reprod. 2000;15:1937-42.
8. Zaidi J, Barber J, Kyei-Mensah A, et al. Relationship of ovarian stromal blood flow at the baseline ultrasound scan to subsequent follicular response in an in vitro fertilization program. Obstet Gynecol. 1996;88:779-84.
9. Engmann L, Sladkevicius P, Agrawal R, et al. Value of ovarian stromal blood flow velocity measurement after pituitary suppression in the prediction of ovarian responsiveness and outcome of in vitro fertilization treatment. Fertil Steril. 1999;71:22-9.
10. Kupesic S, Kurjak A. Predictors of IVF outcome by three-dimensional ultrasound. Hum Reprod. 2002;17:950-5.
11. Pan HA, Wu MH, Cheng YC, et al. Quantification of ovarian Doppler signal in hyperresponders during in vitro fertilization treatment using three-dimensional power Doppler ultrasonography. Ultrasound Med Biol. 2003;29:921-7.
12. Pan HA, Wu MH, Cheng YC, Wu LH, Chang FM. Quantification of ovarian stromal Dopppler signals in poor responders undergoing in vitro fertilization with three-dimensional power Doppler ultrasonography. Am J Obstet Gynecol. 2004;190:338-44.
13. Jarvela IY, Sladkevicius P, Kellly S, et al. Quantification of ovarian power Doppler signal with three-dimensional ultrasonography to predict response during in vitro fertilization. Obstet Gynecol. 2003;102:816-22.
14. Kurjak A, Kupesis-Urek S, Schulman H, et al. Transvaginal color Doppler in the assessment of ovarian and uterine blood flow in infertile women. Fertil Steril. 1991;56:870-3.
15. Mercé LT, Garcés D, Barco MJ, et al. Intraovarian Doppler velocimetry in ovulatory, dysovulatory and anovulatory cycles. Ultrasound Obstet Gynecol. 1992;2:197-202.
16. Sladkevicius P, Valentin L, Marsál K. Blood flow velocity in the uterine and ovarian arteries during the normal menstrual cycle. Ultrasound Obstet Gynecol. 1993;3:199-208.
17. Tan SL, Zaidi J, Campbell S, et al. Blood flow changes in the ovarian and uterine arteries during the normal menstrual cycle. Am J Obstet Gynecol. 1996;175:625-31.
18. Mercé LT, Bau S, Bajo JM. Doppler study of arterial and venous intraovarian blood flow in stimulated cycles. Ultrasound Obstet Gynecol. 2001;18:505-10.
19. Weiner Z, Thaler I, Levron J, et al. Assessment of ovarian and uterine blood flow by transvaginal color Doppler in ovarian-stimulated women: correlation with the number of follicles and steroid hormone levels. Fertil Steril. 1993;59:743-9.
20. Balakier H, Stronell RG. Color Doppler assessment of folliculogenesis in in-vitro fertilization patients. Fertil Steril. 1994;62:1211-6.
21. Mercé LT. Doppler de los cambios ováricos y endometriales preimplantatorios. In: Kurjak A, Carrera JM (Eds). Ecografía en Medicina Materno-Fetal. Barcelona: Masson; 2000. pp. 87-104.
22. Hackelöer BJ, Fleming R, Robinson HP, et al. Correlation of ultrasonic and endocrinologic assessment of human follicular development. Am J Obstet Gynecol. 1979;135:122-8.
23. Campbell S, Bourne TH, Waterstone J, et al. Transvaginal color blood flow imaging of the periovulatory follicle. Fertil Steril. 1993;60:433-8.
24. Brännström M, Zackrisson U, Hagström H-G, et al. Preovulatory changes of blood flow in different regions of the human follicle. Fertil Steril. 1998;69:435-42.
25. Jarvela IY, Sladkevicius P, Kelly S, et al. Three-dimensional sonographic and power Doppler characterization of ovaries in late follicular phase. Ultrasound Obstet Gynecol. 2002;20:281-5.
26. Kitai H, Yoshimura Y, Wright KH, et al. Microvasculature of preovulatory follicles: comparison of in situ and in vitro perfused rabbit ovaries following stimulation of ovulation. Am J Obstet Gynecol. 1985;152:889-95.
27. Parsons AK. Imaging the human corpus luteum. J Ultrasound Med. 2001;20:811-9.
28. Ottander U, Solensten NG, Bergh A, et al. Intraovarian blood flow measured with color Doppler ultrasonography inversely correlates

with vascular density in the human corpus luteum of the menstrual cycle. Fertil Steril. 2004;81:154-9.

29. Gloock JL, Brumsted JR. Color flow pulsed Doppler ultrasound in diagnosing luteal phase defect. Fertil Steril. 1995;64:500-4.

30. Kupesic S, Kurjak A, Vujisic S, et al. Luteal phase defect: comparison between Doppler velocimetry, histological and hormonal markers. Ultrasound Obstet Gynecol. 1997;9:105-12.

31. Kupesic S, Kurjak A. The assessment of normal and abnormal luteal function by transvaginal color Doppler sonography. Eur J Obstet Gynecol Biol Reprod. 1997;72:83-7.

32. Kupesic S, Kurjak A. Uterine and ovarian perfusion during the periovulatory period assessed by transvaginal color Doppler. Fertil Steril. 1993;60:439-43.

33. Bourne TH, Hagström HG, Granberg S, et al. Ultrasound studies of vascular and morphological changes in the human uterus after a positive self-test for the urinary luteinizing hormone surge. Hum Reprod. 1996;11:369-75.

34. Steer CV, Campbell S, Pampiglione JS, et al. Transvaginal color flow imaging of the uterine arteries during the ovarian and menstrual cycles. Hum Reprod. 1990;5:391-5.

35. Hsieh Y-Y, Chang C-C, Tsai H-D. Doppler evaluation of the uterine and spiral arteries from different sampling sites and phases of the menstrual cycle during controlled ovarian hyperstimulation. Ultrasound Obstet Gynecol. 2000;16:192-6.

36. Raine-Fenning NJ, Campbell BK, Kendall NR, et al. Quantifying the changes in endometrial vascularity throughout the normal menstrual cycle with three-dimensional power Doppler angiography. Hum Reprod. 2004;19:330-8.

37. Mercé LT, Kupesic S, Kurjak A. Color Doppler assessment of implantation and early placentation. Prenat Neonat Med. 1999;4:49-112.

38. Mercé LT. Ultrasound markers of implantation. Ultrasound Rev Obstet Gynecol. 2002;2:110-23.

39. Van Blerkom J, Antczak M, Schrader R. The developmental potential of the human oocyte is related to the dissolved oxygen content of follicular fluid: association with vascular endothelial growth factor levels and perifollicular blood flow characteristics. Hum Reprod. 1997;12:1047-55.

40. Gaulden M. Maternal age effect: the enigma of Down syndrome and other trisomic conditions. Mutua Res. 1992;296:69-88.

41. Bhal PS, Pugh ND, Chui DK, et al. The use of transvaginal power Doppler ultrasonography to evaluate the relationship between perifollicular vascularity and outcome in in-vitro fertilization treatment cycles. Hum Reprod. 1999;14:939-45.

42. Chui DKC, Pugh ND, Walker SM, et al. Follicular vascularity—the predictive value of transvaginal power Doppler ultrasonography in an in vitro fertilization programme: a preliminary study. Hum Reprod. 1997;12:191-6.

43. Nargund G, Doyle PE, Bourne TH, et al. Ultrasound derived indices of follicular blood flow before hCG administration and the prediction of oocyte recovery and preimplantation embryo quality. Hum Reprod. 1996;11:2512-7.

44. Ozaki T, Hata K, Xie H, et al. Utility of color Doppler indices of dominant follicular blood flow for prediction of clinical factors in in-vitro fertilization-embryo transfer cycles. Ultrasound Obstet Gynecol. 2002;20:592-6.

45. Coulam CB, Goodman C, Rinehart JS. Color Doppler indices of follicular blood flow as predictors of pregnancy after in vitro fertilization and embryo transfer. Hum Reprod. 1999;14:1979-82.

46. Bhal PS, Pugh ND, Gregory L, et al. Perifollicular vascularity as a potential variable affecting outcome in stimulated intrauterine insemination treatment cycles: a study using transvaginal power Doppler. Hum Reprod. 2001;16:1682-9.

47. Goswany RK, Williams G, Steptoe PC. Decreased uterine perfusion—a cause of infertility. Human Reprod. 1988;8:955-9.

48. Steer CV, Campbell S, Tan SL, et al. The use of transvaginal color flow imaging after in vitro fertilization to identify optimum uterine conditions before embryo transfer. Fertil Steril. 1992;57:372-6.

49. Zaidi J, Pittrof R, Shaker A, et al. Assessment of uterine artery blood flow on the day of human chorionic gonadotropin administration by transvaginal color Doppler ultrasound in an in vitro fertilization program. Fertil Steril. 1996;65:377-81.

50. Tsai Y-C, Chang J-C, Tai M-J, et al. Relationship of uterine perfusion to outcome of intrauterine insemination. J Ultrasound Med. 1996;15:633-6.

51. Coulam CB, Bustillo M, Soenksen DM, et al. Ultrasonographic predictors of implantation after assisted reproduction. Fertil Steril. 1994;62:1004-10.

52. Coulam CB, Stern JJ, Soenksen DM, et al. Comparison of pulsatility indexes on the day of oocyte retrieval and embryo transfer. Hum Reprod. 1995;10:82-4.

53. Bustillo M, Krysa LW, Coulam CB. Uterine receptivity in an oocyte donation programme. Hum Reprod. 1995;10:442-5.

54. Favre R, Bettahar K, Grange G, et al. Predictive value of transvaginal uterine Doppler assessment in an in vitro fertilization program. Ultrasound Obstet Gynecol. 1993;3:350-3.

55. Tekay A, Martikainen H, Jouppila P. The clinical value of transvaginal color Doppler ultrasound in assisted reproductive technology procedures. Hum Reprod. 1996;11:1589-91.

56. Deichert U, Albrand-Thielman C, van de Sandt M. Doppler-sonographic pelvic blood flow measurements and their prognostic value in terms of luteal phase and implantation. Hum Reprod. 1996;11:1591-3.

57. Zaidi J, Campbell S, Pittrof R, et al. Endometrial thickness, morphology, vascular penetration and velocimetry in predicting implantation in an in vitro fertilization program. Ultrasound Obstet Gynecol. 1995;6:191-8.

58. Applebaum M. The Menstrual cycle, menopause, ovulation induction, an in vitro fertilization. In: Copel JA, Reed KL (Eds). Doppler Ultrasound in Obstetrics and Gynecology. New York: Raven Press; 1995. pp. 71-86.

59. Battaglia C, Artini PG, Giulini S, et al. Color Doppler changes and thromboxane production after ovarian stimulation with gonadotrophin-releasing hormone agonist. Human Reprod. 1997;11:2477-82.

60. Chien LW, Au HK, Chen PL, et al. Assessment of uterine receptivity by the endometrial-subendometrial blood flow distribution pattern in women undergoing in vitro fertilization-embryo transfer. Fertil Steril. 2002;78:245-51.

61. Maugey-Laulom B, Commenges-Ducos M, Jullien V, et al. Endometrial vascularity and ongoing pregnancy after IVF. Eur J Obstet Gynecol Reprod Biol. 2002;104:137-43.

62. Yang J-H, Wu M-Y, Chen C-D, et al. Association of endometrial blood flow as determined by a modified color Doppler technique with subsequent outcome of in-vitro fertilization. Hum Reprod. 1999;14:1606-10.

63. Kupesic S, Bekavac I, Bjelos D, et al. Assessment of endometrial receptivity by transvaginal color Doppler and three-dimensional power Doppler ultrasonography in patients undergoing in vitro fertilization procedures. J Ultrasound Med. 2001;20:125-34.

64. Wu HM, Chiang CH, Huang HY, et al. Detection of the subendometrial vascularization blood flow by three-dimensional ultrasound may be useful for predicting the pregnancy rate for patients undergoing in vitro fertilization embryo transfer. Fertil Steril. 2003;79:507-11.

92

Implantation and Yolk Sac

S Kupesic, A Kurjak

INTRODUCTION

Recent advances in perinatal technology increased tremendously our understanding of early human development. This, in turn, has led investigators to ask numerous searching questions on both maternal and fetal placental hemodynamics.

The early beginning of embryonic life is a gestational period of important hemodynamic changes, mainly characterized by establishment of a continuous maternal blood flow in the intervillous space. In this development process, the maternal vascular bed and spiral arterioles form the basis for perfusion of the placenta. Current anatomical knowledge has largely been based upon the classical studies of earlier investigators. In many instances, their theories have been confirmed by new information, but, in others, initial errors in observation or conclusion have been brought to light necessitating revision or replacement of the original concepts.

Many questions are presently directed to the intervillous space, probing in particular its size and form, its source of blood supply, and the mechanism of circulation within it. In 1962, in an excellent review article[1] on circulation in the intervillous space Ramsey wrote: "Old ideas die hard, however, even when their validity has been challenged, and it is well known that they frequently maintain their position in textbooks for some time after they have been discarded by workers in the forefront of the field. Old ideas also have a tendency to leave fragments of themselves, as a complicating legacies, incorporated in the theories which finally replace them".

How little is changed in a period of more than 34 years. We are still learning satisfactory answers to many of the queries on the intervillous circulation. However, a good deal of data is already available especially as the result of recent research on Doppler proofs of the continuous blood flow in intervillous space. In our effort to facilitate a better understanding of present concepts on the intervillous circulation a brief recapitulation of anatomy and embryology will be included in successive sections of this review. It is our intention to synthesize and clear out the chronology and factography of the controversial data and theories about the establishment of the intervillous circulation and yolk sac morphology and function.

THE INTERVILLOUS CIRCULATION

The "Classic" Embryological Concept of the Early Uteroplacental Circulation

The labyrinthine series of cavities which together constitute the intervillous space in the placenta was first identified by William and John Hunter in the 18th century. However, there is still uncertainty concerning many of its features.[2]

The first week of embryonal development is the preimplantation stage. By the end of the day 5, blastocyst is formed consisting of the trophoblast and embryoblast (inner cell mass).[3]

After this period begins the implantation period, the process whereby the blastocyst attaches to and erodes through the endometrial epithelium. One of the earliest modifications of the endometrium after fertilization is an increase in vascular permeability. The other changes of the endometrium include increased vascularity, edema and thickening (i.e. decidual reaction). Trophoblast produces proteolytic enzymes that facilitate the penetration in the endometrium and erodes adjacent maternal capillaries.

By the end of the first week, the blastocyst is superficially implanted in the endometrium. Trophoblast and embryoblast start to develop along different lines.[4,5] In the seventh day after fertilization (Carnegie stage 5a) the trophoblast rapidly differentiates into two layers—an inner layer of mononuclear cytotrophoblastic cells and an outer layer of multinucleated syncytiotrophoblast. The syncytiotrophoblast comes into the direct contact with the endometrial stroma. The endometrial glands in the contact with the trophoblast show degenerative changes, in some instances the glandular epithelium has disappeared and the trophoblast plugs the glandular lumen.[2]

By the eighth day after fertilization, the blastocyst is completely embedded within the endometrial stroma. At the embryonic pole the primitive syncytiotrophoblast on the surface has some deep indentations which contain maternal blood cells.

The ninth day of development (Carnegie stage 5b) is named the lacunar or previllous stage. At this stage the inner cells mass (embryoblast) is differentiated into a bilaminar embryonic disk.[3]

From the eighth day after fertilization intercommunicating fluid-filled spaces of lacunae appear in the rapidly enlarging syncytiotrophoblast. Between the tenth and thirteenth day (Carnegie stage 5c) lacunae convert the syncytiotrophoblast into a sponge-like structure. The lacunae are incompletely separated from each other by trabecular columns of syncytiotrophoblast. The lacunae open into several maternal sinusoids which have probably arisen from endometrial capillaries. The lacunae become confluent. With further extensions of the maternal sinusoids and more dilatation of the endometrial blood vessels, the supply of blood to the lacunae comes largely from venous sinusoids. The lacunae rapidly become filled with a combination of maternal blood and secretion from eroded endometrial glands.[6] At this stage, there is no evidence for direct arterial communication with the lacunae. It would seem that the earliest maternal blood which enters the developing lacunae is not arterial but is derived from the capillaries and venules which

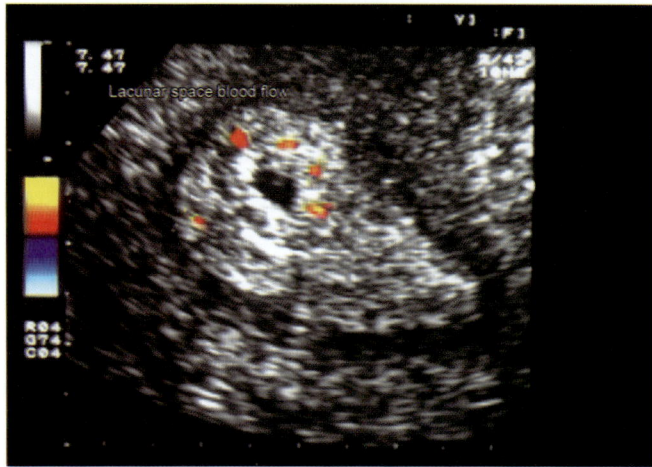

Fig. 92.1: Lacunar space blood flow at the periphery of an early gestational sac as seen by color Doppler ultrasound

dilate to form sinusoids.[2] Using transvaginal color Doppler venous signals are clearly obtainable from these spaces (Fig. 92.1)

With continuing trophoblastic invasion the maternal vessels disappear progressively back to the level of the spiral arteries and their venules permitting a true circulation. The trabeculae are called "primary villous stems". They are not true villi but serve as the framework from which villi later develop. They are arranged radially and divide lacunae into a labyrinth at the fourteenth day after fertilization. The placenta in this stage of development is a labyrinthine rather than a villous organ.[7]

Primary chorionic villi develop between 13 and 15 days of development (Carnegie stages 6a and 6b). The trabeculae have a central cellular core produced by proliferation of the cytotrophoblastic cells. At the same time, the formation of the first blood vessels starts in the extraembryonic mesoderm of the yolk sac, the connecting stalk and the chorion. The cytotrophoblastic cells extent distally toward the attachment of the syncytiotrophoblast to the endometrium. These cells from the villous tips break through syncytiotrophoblast and expand laterally to fuse with adjacent columns to form a cytotrophoblastic shell. The shell is completed by the fifteenth day after fertilization. Villi which are attached to the maternal tissue via the cytotrophoblastic shell are "stem" or "anchoring villi". The villi which grow from the sides of the stem villi are "branch villi".

Days 15–21 are a period of intensive trophoblastic growth. By the fifteenth day the maternal circulation becomes fully functional, when the syncytial lacunae become confluent and connected with endometrial capillaries.[8] The trabeculae, which are at first unoriented, gradually become more regularly arranged. The number of initial villi is determined by the number of trabeculae which are invaded by proliferating cytotrophoblast. In the sixteenth day, the extraembryonal mesenchime appears and extends toward villous distal end. Primary chorionic villi gradually convert into secondary villi.[3] By the eighteenth day the villous mesenchymal cells begin to differentiate into blood capillaries forming an arteriocapillary venous network which is completed by 20 days after fertilization. The villi are called "tertiary villi". The villous vessels become connected with the embryonic heart tube via vessels differentiated in the chorion and the connecting stalk.[6]

The establishment of the trophoblastic shell allows rapid circumferential growth of the developing placenta. This leads to the expansion of the intervillous space into which sprouts extend from the primary villous stems. The placenta is by the twenty-first day of gestation a vascularized villous organ.[7] The extensive system of venous sinusoids around the implantation site constitutes venous connections between the intervillous space and the maternal circulation.

In the fourth week of development, the cytotrophoblastic shell is thinner than in the earlier stages. At the junctions of the shell with the decidua there are many clefts and spaces. Some of them open into the adjacent intervillous space. The twenty-first day after fertilization (Carnegie stage 10) the primitive embryonal heart begins to beat, and embryonal blood circulates through villous capillaries.[6] The communications with the terminal branches of the spiral arteries have not yet been completely established.[2] There are 6–8 endometrial spiral arteries opening directly to the decidua basalis. They possess a wide lumen. The media of the vascular wall becomes attenuated and finally disappears completely. The linning endothelium is surrounded only by a layer of reticular and collagen fibers. As a result of these changes, it is often difficult to identify the spiral arteries and to establish their relationship to the intervillous space. From this region several narrow clefts penetrate the shell to enter to the intervillous space.

There are two types of nonvillous migratory trophoblast: (1) the interstitial or stromal trophoblast which invades decidua and myometrium, and (2) the endovascular trophoblast which migrates into spiral arteries and modifies them into uteroplacental arteries. The endovascular trophoblast is closely linked to the development of the trophoblastic shell.[9] It is the key factor for physiological modifications of spiral arteries. These gestational changes are needed for development of hemochorial placentation.

Migrating trophoblast penetrates the uterine wall and invades venous sinusoids of increasing size and superficial arterioles during the fourth week. The extravillous cytotrophoblastic cells expand from the tips of the anchoring villi into the lumina of the spiral arteries. They convert the thick-walled muscular arteries into flaccid sac-like uteroplacental vessels which can passively dilate to accommodate the greatly increased maternal blood flow required for fetal oxygenation and growth.[10]

Trophoblastic cells can be found within the spiral arteries in about the sixth week after fertilization. The trophoblastic disruption of the muscular cells and elastic fibers of the spiral arteries has two effects. Increasing blood flow causes progressive distension of these arteries into the uteroplacental arteries capable of accommodation the increasing blood supply. Uteroplacental arteries are not responsive to change within the autonomic nervous system.[6]

In the second lunar month as the result of the extensive branching villi the intervillous space increase. During the second month, many terminal parts of spiral arteries near the intervillous space contain plugs of cytotrophoblastic cells. By the end of this period of development centrally placed communications between the decidual veins are numerous and large. After 40 days (crown-rump length 15 mm) numerous spiral arteries show direct openings into the intervillous space.[2]

The cytotrophoblastic cells appear within the lumina of the spiral arteries. The maternal blood reaches the intervillous space through the gaps between the cells of the endovascular trophoblast.

The persistence of the cytotrophoblastic plugs in the lumina of the spiral arteries suggest that the blood pressure in them is not very high, otherwise the plugs would be dislodged.[2] Maximal trophoblastic activity occurs at the center of the placental bed and then extends centrifugally toward its periphery.

During the third month of gestation in the lumina of the terminal segments of most of the spiral arteries, the cytotrophoblastic plugs are always present. None of spiral arteries open freely into the intervillous space. Later in this period of development the plugs are more loosely arranged and they are probably then less able to impede maternal blood flow into the intervillous space.[2]

Up to the end of the fourth month of gestation the chorion frondosum develops into the definitive placenta. The chorionic villi associated with the decidua capsularis degenerate and the associated intervillous space disappears. The smooth avascular chorion laeve forms.[6] There is regression in the trophoblastic shell where the cytotrophoblastic cell columns degenerate. The trophoblastic infiltration of the myometrium occurs between 8 and 18 weeks of development.[10] The endovascular cytotrophoblast partially replaces the endothelium and invades the muscular cells of the myometrial vessels. The result is a progressive distension of these myometrial vessels.

The uteroplacental circulatory system is a low-pressure one because of progressive increase in the diameter of the vessels as they approach their entry into the intervillous space. There is a considerable drop in pressure from the proximal non-dilated portions of the uteroplacental arterioles to the distal dilated portions and full arterial pressure is not transmitted to the intervillous space.[7]

The "Heretic" Concept of Separation of Villous Tissue from the Maternal Circulation

This classic concept of establishment of the intervillous circulation was challenged in 1987 and 1988 by the experiments of Hustin and Shaaps.[11,12] They examined slice radiographs of hysterectomy specimens with pregnancy in situ collected at 7, 8 and 9 weeks of gestation and found no contrast medium in the intervillous space. When the examination was performed at 13 weeks of gestation, the placenta was rapidly filled with contrast medium. Histological examination of these hysterectomy specimens showed occlusion of the uteroplacental arteries by trophoblastic cells up to 12 weeks of gestation. Reconstruction of serial spiral arterial sections was also suggestive of the absence of the intervillous circulation before 12 weeks of gestation. At 13 weeks, on the other hand, the uteroplacental arteries were free of trophoblastic plugs, and contrast medium was found in the intervillous space, encircling the chorionic villi. This was partially confirmed in vivo by means of hysteroscopy, examination of chorionic villous sampling material and transvaginal sonography. These results suggest that early placenta is bathed predominantly by fluid derived from maternal plasma and uterine gland secretions. The authors believed that blood flow in the intervillous space is absent or incompletely developed before 12 weeks of gestation. Transformation of spiral arteries continues during the first trimester, when they widen progressively. Around 12 weeks of gestation all trophoblastic plugs are eventually loosened and dislocated. This allows free entry of maternal blood to the intervillous space and establishment of a fully developed placental circulation.

Further support has been supplied by more recent study[13] using a polarographic oxygen electrode inserted under ultrasound guidance demonstrated that between 8 and 10 weeks of gestation placental pO_2 levels were significantly lower compared with endometrial pO_2 levels, while between 12 and 13 weeks, the levels were similar. Intraplacental pO_2 levels increased significantly from 8–10 to 12–13 weeks of gestation. These results suggest that the increase of placental pO_2 may be related to the establishment of continuous maternal blood flow in the intervillous space at the end of the first trimester.

The advent and development of transvaginal color Doppler has enabled in vivo hemodynamic investigation of almost all segments embryonic/fetal and uteroplacental circulation.[14-21]

In 1991 and 1992, Jauniaux et al.[22,23] and Jaffe et al.[24] were unable to detect "intraplacental" flow before 12 weeks of gestation using the transvaginal color Doppler. They found the appearance of intraplacental flow at around 14 weeks of gestation to coincide with the appearance of pandiastolic flow in the umbilical artery and with an abrupt increase in uterine artery peak systolic velocity. In agreement with the theories of Hustin and Shaaps,[11,12] they hypothesized that the simultaneous appearance of intraplacental flow, pandiastolic umbilical artery flow, and abrupt increase in uterine artery blood flow velocity was to be explained by sudden loosening and disappearance of the trophoblastic plugs in the spiral arteries. By this time Kurjak et al.[25] were unable to demonstrate an abrupt change in the uteroplacental circulation between 12 and 14 weeks of gestation.

HI-TECH EVIDENCES OF THE "CLASSIC" THEORY: THE CIRCLE IS CLOSED

It must be emphasized that color Doppler measurements in studies mentioned above were performed on devices of relatively moderate capability in detection of low velocities. After the introduction of the new generation of far more sensitive color Doppler devices in last few years, several authors reported a positive finding of intervillous circulation during first trimester of pregnancy (Figs 92.2 and 92.3).

In 1995, Kurjak et al.[26] presented the first report on a combined Doppler and morphopathological study of intervillous circulation. Using a transvaginal color Doppler continuous intervillous flow of two types was detected in all examined patients: pulsatile arterial-like (Fig. 92.2) and continuous venous-like flow (Fig. 92.3). Parallel

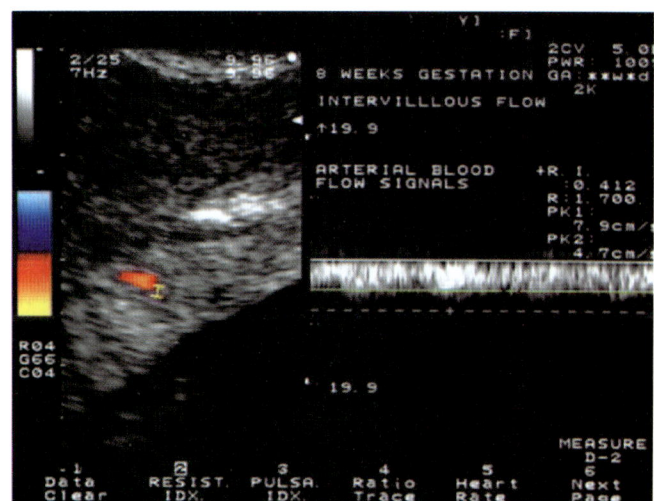

Fig. 92.2: Arterial blood flow velocity waveforms from the intervillous space at 10 weeks of gestation demonstrate low impedance (RI = 0.41). Note typical spiky outline of the arterial signal

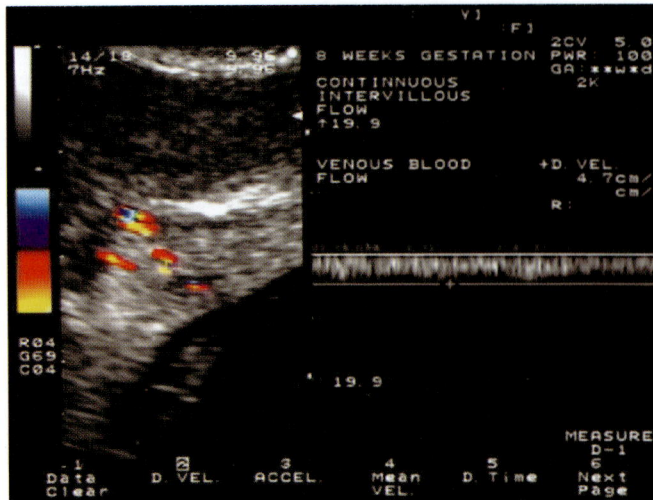

Fig. 92.3: Continuous flow of a venous type in the same patient as in Figure 92.2; venous blood flow is easily detectable from the intervillous space

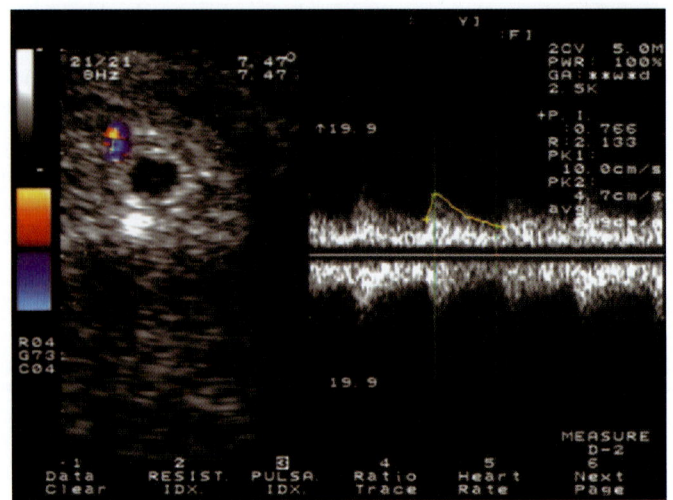

Fig. 92.4: Transvaginal power Doppler imaging of a gestational sac at 5/6 weeks of gestation. This technique easily depicts blood flow surrounding the gestational sac

histological study has shown that the lumen of spiral arteries was never completely obstructed by the trophoblastic plugs. These data indicate that establishment of the intervillous circulation is a continuous process rather than an abrupt event at the end of the first trimester. One should note that arterial-like blood flow signals have shown lower resistance and pulsatility index values than those obtained in spiral arteries.

Shortly after, several other groups of authors reported similar findings. Valentin et al.[27] performed a combined study of uteroplacental and luteal flow with pathomorphologic analysis. Color Doppler measurements revealed positive finding of intervillous circulation from the sixth week of normal pregnancy onward. The same two types of Doppler signals, the pulsatile and continuous, were detected and measured with a visualization rate of more than 90% on 64 pregnancies from 5 to 11 weeks of gestation. Authors stated that high blood velocities recorded from the subchorionic arteries were not compatible with these arteries being completely occluded by trophoblastic plugs. At the pathomorphologic analysis trophoblast plugging of the spiral arteries was incomplete, allowing passage of red blood cells. Authors concluded that the intervillous circulation was present as early as the first trimester.

Merce et al.[28] reported similar results on the group of 108 normal singleton pregnancies of 4–15 gestational weeks. They were able to detect intervillous flow from 5 weeks 6 days of gestation (Fig. 92.4). It was a slightly undulating venous-like signal with tendency of increasing velocity throughout the first trimester. They also recorded arterial signals in retrochorionic segments of uteroplacental vasculature. The conclusion was that their results were in accordance with the classic embryological concept of establishment of the intervillous flow from fourth to seventh weeks of gestation. By Merce et al.[28] uteroplacental circulation is the earliest to be affected in pregnancy, with pronounced changes from week 4 onward. Intervillous circulation and primitive umbilical blood flow was identified from week 5 on.

In more recent publications Kurjak et al.[29,30] studied a group of 60 normal pregnancies of gestational age from 6 to 12 weeks of pregnancy and, for the first time, a group of 34 pathological early pregnancies: 22 cases of missed abortion

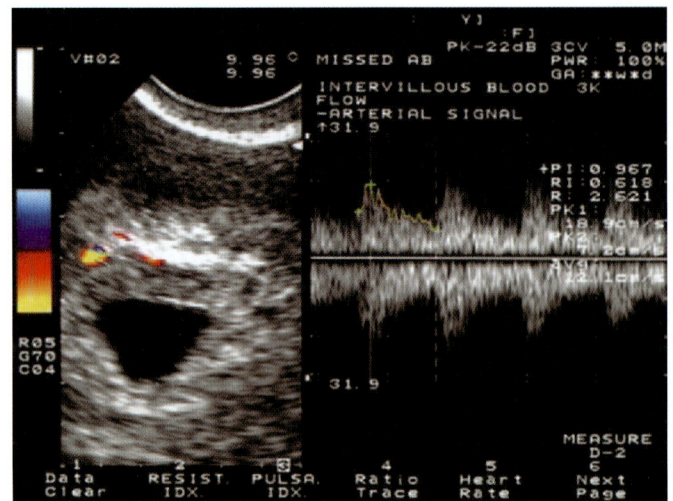

Fig. 92.5: A transvaginal scan of the missed abortion at 12 weeks of gestation. Note increased RI value (0.62) of the arterial-like signal from the intervillous space

(Fig. 92.5) and 12 cases of anembryonic pregnancy (Fig. 92.6) between 7 and 12 weeks of gestation. The same Doppler features were detected in the intervillous space of all pregnancies; pulsatile arterial-like signals with characteristic spiky outline, and venous-like continuous signals. There was no difference in Doppler parameters between the group with missed abortion and group of normal pregnancy. However, lower impedance (measured in resistance and pulsatility indices) was detected in the group with anembryonic pregnancies. These results are significantly different from those published by Jauniaux et al.[31] who found increased intervillous blood flow in 70% of abnormal pregnancies before 12 weeks of gestation. In these cases, a histopathologic examination showed that the trophoblastic shell was discontinuous and thinner, and that the intervillous space had been massively infiltrated by maternal blood. Authors hypothesized that trophoblast plugs in the spiral arteries restrict the maternal blood to flow in the intervillous space, protecting vulnerable villi from high pressure of arterial

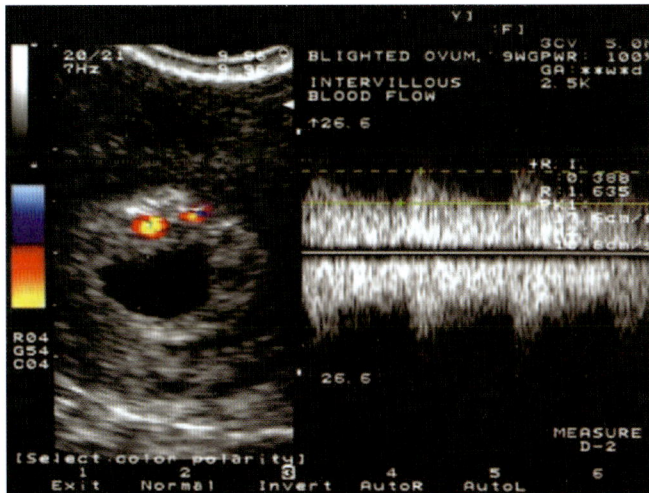

Fig. 92.6: The transvaginal scan demonstrates anembryonic pregnancy. Note spiky outline and low vascular resistance (RI 0.39) of the arterial-like signals obtained from the intervillous space of an anembryonic pregnancy

blood. By this concept the premature entry of maternal blood in the intervillous space can disrupt the maternoembryonic interface, causing the separation of early placenta and, eventually, abortion.

In the research of placental development and formation of the uteroplacental circulation of crucial importance was experimental work with animal models, particularly with non-human primates, mostly with Macaca species. The classical work by Elisabeth Ramsey on the circulation in the intervillous space of the primate placenta is the base for all contemporary research in this field.[1,32] Recently Nimrod et al.[33,34] reported about the assessment of the early uteroplacental circulation in cynomolgus monkey (Macaca fascicularis) by color Doppler technique. They were able to detect the intervillous circulation from the 18 days post conception. Regardless the known differences in the depth of trophoblastic invasion of the spiral arteries between human and monkey, this finding can be considered as an additional evidence of early establishment of intervillous circulation in all primate placentas, although the "argument by analogy" must be used with caution.

Publication of similar, if not the same, results obtained by few independent groups and published in prestigious journals usually produces a respectful attention of the scientific community. However, a recent editorial by Jauniaux,[35] repeating most of the facts known from his previous papers, did not appreciate enough the early reports on continuous intervillous flow. Although Jauniaux admitted that using a new equipment he was able to detect flow in some areas of intervillous space during the first trimester of pregnancy, his concern was whether these signals were originated the intervillous space of the definitive placenta or from the chorion laeve area, because very often the areas of detectable color and spectral Doppler signals were visible near the margins of the placenta. From our own experience, we do support this observation; however, there are also signals obtained from below the center of early placenta that are, by no means, signals belonging to the area of chorion laeve. One can speculate that these signals could be from the tips of spiral arteries in the decidua under the early placenta or chorion frondosum. It is our opinion, and it is in concordance with papers by Valentin et al.[27] and Merce et al.[28] that the relatively high velocities of blood flow detected in these vessels or vascular spaces

are not compatible with complete occlusion by trophoblastic plugs unless there are arteriovenous shunts in the decidual portion of the choriodecidual junction. Their existence in the myometrium is still controversial. Hustin et al.[12] found some evidence while Laurini has not (personal communication). Hustin et al.[36] are postulating that myometrial arteriovenous shunts exist and are functional, serving to limit considerably the entry of maternal blood in the intervillous space. Even more, he is postulating without further explanation, that the pressure in the intervillous space is temporarily higher than at the uteroplacental artery level, and thus maintains the intravascular trophoblastic plugs in place. This statement can be an objective for further investigation.

Jauniaux speculated that the finding of focal intervillous flow in the first trimester was a sign of consecutive formation of echo-poor areas as an early sign of pregnancy complications.[37,38] If this is true, how could one explain the high rate of visualization of these signals in normal pregnancies reported by our group[30,39,40] and Malmo group.[27] It is hard to believe that all these pregnancies were destined to fail. According to Jauniaux et al.[31] continuous flow in the intervillous space during the first trimester is a highly pathologic event, causing the disruption of the maternoembryonic interface by high pressure blood flow and consequent spontaneous abortion. In his opinion,[35] this fact is the most striking evidence in favor of Hustin's concept.[11] In fact, we also do believe that the high pressure of arterial blood can disrupt the maternoembryonic interface and cause spontaneous abortion. However, this fact is not opposite to the finding of a continuous intervillous flow during the first trimester of pregnancy. This means that there are some areas where trophoblastic plugs in spiral arteries are loosened allowing the intervillous circulation of blood. In the beginning there are only few areas of such a flow giving enough oxygen and nutrients for the progression of pregnancy. At this stage, the intervillous space is not undisrupted like in the mature placenta. There are parts with active continuous intervillous flow and parts in which such a flow has not yet been established and nutrients and oxygen diffuse through the intercellular fluid. The number of areas with the established intervillous flow is increasing with embryonic and placental growth in order to keep a state of metabolic balance. This process ends with a fully formed intervillous space under the mature placenta. Such a hypothesis can be in concordance with findings of lower oxygen levels in the placental tissue than in the endometrium between 8 and 10 weeks of pregnancy.[13]

Also, it can be in concordance with the fact that in cases of inappropriate trophoblastic plugging of spiral arteries the uncontrolled pressure of arterial blood can mechanically disrupt the maternoembryonic interface.

Merce et al.[28] recently reported that the abnormal Doppler patterns, such as the increase of retrochorial vascular resistance and the presence of intervillous flow in pregnancies with gestational sac measuring less than 12 mm has greater incidence of miscarriage. However, intervillous flow was also detectable in pregnancies with normal outcome but in smaller proportion than in those ending with miscarriage (11% vs 53%). This finding confirms that intervillous circulation does exist throughout early pregnancy, but in the same time limitation of the amount and pressure of incoming maternal blood seems to be of essential importance for normal pregnancy development.

There are numerous data provided by histological and color Doppler studies proving that the intervillous circulation begins early in normal pregnancy, which is in accordance with classical

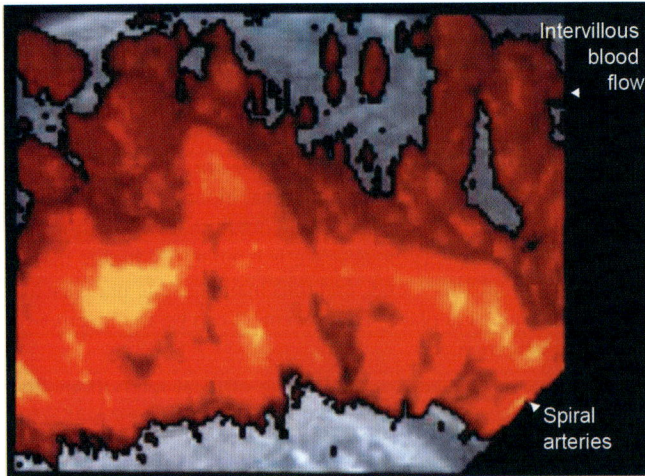

Fig. 92.7: Demonstration of the intervillous circulation by three-dimensional power Doppler

embryological theories. This is possible because the trophoblastic invasion is a progressive process and although some of the spiral arteries are totally occluded, the majority of them are opened or only partially occluded. In this way, the inflow of the blood in the intervillous space is controlled and increased progressively during the first trimester. These changes are complementary to the progressive loss of the endovascular trophoblast and coherently explain the increase in blood flow within the vascular territory of the uteroplacental arteries, a universal finding in all Doppler studies and very difficult to explain if these arterial lumens are plugged up with the trophoblast. It is probable that changes occurring in the trophoblast in spontaneous abortions can alter the blood perfusion in both the uteroplacental arteries and intervillous space. However, the importance of these findings in the genesis or in the mechanism of miscarriage has not yet been sufficiently documented. Furthermore, recent ultrasound technology in terms of three-dimensional power Doppler angiography offers numerous advantages in the evaluation of the intervillous space (Fig. 92.7), which have to be clinically tested in the future.

YOLK SAC

Yolk Sac Development

The embryonic vascular system includes the heart, the blood and lymphatic vessels. It is the first functional organ system in the body which pumps blood through the embryonic and extraembryonic vessels to provide nutritions for rapid growth and removal of the waste products.[53] Circulatory system of an embryo is much larger relative to body size which considers its important role during the early embryonic development.

Development of the vascular system begins in the mesoderm of the yolk sac close to endoderm, at about 17 days after fertilization.[53] It is believed that there are some endodermally produced factors which stimulates mesoderm to differentiate in this way. The first evident form of vascular system are aggregations of cells called blood islands. The central cells will differentiate into red blood cells and the outer cells into flattened endothelial layer. These elements of vascular system are perceptible as red spots in the mesoderm of the yolk sac wall. The blood islands fuse to form primitive vascular network.

Precursors of the heart and the major paired blood vessels are formed in the mesoderm of intraembryonic coelom. Course of events is analogous with those happening in the mesoderm of the yolk sac. Very similar process of creating vascular system occurs in the chorionic mesoderm. Blood vessels formed in this way are dorsal aortae, cardinal veins and the major umbilical arteries and veins.

At first, blood washes back and forth in this primitive network of blood vessels, but eventually it takes on a patterned flow. It seems that these dynamic fluid effects are very important because they stimulate primitive blood vessels to differentiate further and to take their own definitive form. If there is an obstruction to the blood flow, it bypasses blocked vessel and passes through the surrounding small vessels. In time one of these vessels will become major blood vessel and will overtake the role of blocked one. This sometimes vitally needed ability survives in the adult and leads to anastomoses.

Vitelline Blood Vessels

The heart begins to beat at about 21 days after fertilization. It pumps blood dorsally through blood vessels called branchial arches.[53] Blood enters the dorsal aortae (paired at this stage) from which the precursors of the internal carotid artery separate and run forward to supply the head. The main direction of blood in the dorsal aortae is toward the tail. It runs through the intersegmental arteries which are branches of dorsal aortae and are situated between the developing somites. Furthermore, at the level of the gut, there is an arterial complex of branches separating from dorsal aortae and running toward the site of blood formation in the yolk sac wall. By the time, this arterial complex of branches will represent vitelline arteries. Toward the tail dorsal aortae form a plexus from which one single blood vessel branches off and runs in the connecting stalk to the chorionic wall where placenta is developing. This single blood vessel is umbilical artery.

Toward the tail dorsal aortae form a plexus from which one single blood vessel branches off and runs in the connecting stalk to the chorionic wall where placenta is umbilical artery.

Blood returns from the placenta through the paired umbilical veins which also pick up blood from the yolk sac. Connection between yolk sac vascular network and umbilical veins is venous complex of branches which are going to be vitelline veins. The head veins, which lie just lateral to the neural tube, pick up blood from the head region. Finally, blood enters the sinus venosus and reaches the heart. This is the moment when the circle of the blood consider around the embryonal body is closed.

The vitelline and umbilical veins have very important role in further embryonal development. Initially the liver bud lies between the vitelline veins. Since it enlarges it comes to incorporate the vitelline and umbilical veins. These blood vessels form common plexus of sinusoid vessel running through the liver. In time the vitelline veins and left umbilical vein are converted into the hepatic portal vein. The right umbilical vein decreases in size and forms ductus venosus which carries the blood to the right side of the heart.[53]

Hematopoiesis in human embryos begins in the yolk sac at about the middle of the third week of embryogenesis. Later, it appears in the liver and bone marrow at fourth to fifth week and the eighth week respectively.[54,55] At about the tenth to twelfth week, hematopoietic tissues are found distributed evenly in the bone marrow through the body.[55-57] Maturation of blood cells is considered to take place extravascular. With occasional exceptions, the blood cells in the endodermal layers are the most immature and maturation appears to proceed as the cells migrate to the mesenhymal layers and further into the blood vessels.

Color Doppler Studies of Yolk SAC and Vitelline Duct

Circulation in Normal Pregnancy

Little is known about a transitory subject such as the yolk sac, an organ only active during the first few weeks of embryonic life. The description of formation of the human yolk sac has proven surprisingly controversial over the years.

Recently, interesting results have been published on the assessment of yolk sac vascularization in normal pregnancy. Kurjak et al.[21] performed transvaginal color Doppler study on 105 patients whose gestational age ranged from 6 to 10 weeks from the last menstrual period. Transvaginal color and pulsed Doppler examination was performed before the termination of pregnancy for psychosocial reasons.

The first color and pulsed signals from yolk sac were obtained between 5 and 6 weeks of gestation. The visualization rate of the yolk sac vessels in sixth week of gestation was 33.33%, and it increased to a value of 85.71% during the seventh and eighth weeks of gestation. As the functional activity of the yolk sac progressively declined the visualization rate of 78.26% for 9 weeks of gestation and 61.11% for 10 weeks of gestation paralleled this process (Table 92.1). The overall visualization rate for yolk sac vessels was 72.38%. The highest visualization rates were obtained in seventh and eighth weeks of gestation reaching the values of 85.71%. A characteristic waveform profile included: low velocity (5.8 ± 1.7 cm/s) and absence of diastolic flow (Figs 92.8 and 92.9). The PI showed the mean value of 3.24 ± 0.94 without significant changes between subgroups ($p > 0.05$). The distribution of mean PI values for yolk sac vascularity is shown in Table 92.2.

Vitelline stalk vessels (Fig. 92.10) showed similar PSV (5.4 ± 1.8 cm/s) and PI values (3.14 ± 0.91) ($p > 0.05$) to that obtained from the yolk sac (Figs 92.8 and 92.9). The distribution of the vitelline artery PI values is demonstrated on Table 92.3. The overall visualization rate for vitelline arteries was 66.67%. Color and pulsed Doppler signals could be obtained from the vitelline duct during the seventh week of gestation in 85.71% of patients. The peak of visualization (89.28%) occurred during the eighth week of gestation (Table 92.3). The process of the elongation of the vitelline duct together with the removal of the yolk sac from the body wall is paralleled with decrease rate of vitelline duct visualization during the ninth (73.91%) and tenth (55.55%) week of gestation. Furthermore, progressive decrease of the yolk sac vascularity at the end of the first trimester coincides with visualization of more prominent blood flow within the intervillous space.[58]

All of these findings will surely help in better understanding the early development of both blood cells and blood vessels.

Vascularization of Yolk Sac in Abnormal Pregnancies

Kurjak et al.[21,58] recently performed a research analyzing the vascularization of yolk sac in abnormal pregnancies. The authors

Table 92.1: Resistance index (RI), pulsatility index (PI), peak systolic velocity (PSV), end-diastolic velocity (EDV) and temporal averaged maximum velocity (TAMV) obtained from the intervillous space and in the spiral arteries in different gestational age groups

Gestational weeks	Intervillous blood flow					Spiral artery blood flow				
	RI (SD)	PI (SD)	PSV (SD)	EDV (SD)	TAMV (SD)	RI (SD)	PI (SD)	PSV (SD)	EDV (SD)	TAMV (SD)
7–9	0.48	0.71	28	18	25	0.58	0.88	31	22	26
	(0.05)	(0.09)	(10)	(7)	(9)	(0.06)	(0.11)	(16)	(12)	(15)
10–12	0.41	0.61	28	21	26	0.51	0.73	36	20	31
	(0.06)	(0.11)	(12)	(9)	(10)	(0.07)	(0.09)	(14)	(16)	(15)
13–15	0.34	0.43	35	22	30	0.43	0.55	41	26	37
	(0.07)	(0.08)	(14)	(10)	(15)	(0.05)	(0.11)	(21)	(15)	(15)
16–22	0.29*	0.34*	40	35	37	0.41*	0.55*	37	23	32
	(0.06)	(0.09)	(19)	(17)	(19)	(0.06)	(0.12)	(16)	(15)	(15)
23–28	0.30	0.36	36	30	32	0.40	0.52	42	26	34
	(0.07)	(0.10)	(20)	(14)	(16)	(0.06)	(0.11)	(15)	(11)	(13)
29–36	0.25	0.29	36	26	32	0.34	0.42	31	21	26
	(0.06)	(0.08)	(12)	(9)	(10)	(0.07)	(0.10)	(9)	(6)	(7)
37–42	0.27	0.31	32+	23**	27+	0.37	0.48	30+	19	25+
	(0.06)	(0.09)	(14)	(10)	(12)	(0.09)	(0.15)	(12)	(9)	(11)

*$p < 0.01$
**$p < 0.05$
+$p < 0.07$
Abbreviation: SD, standard deviation.
Source: With permission from Reference 41.

Table 92.2: Visualization rate of yolk sac vascularity between 6 and 10 weeks of gestation

Gestational age (weeks)	N	Visualization rate		PI ± SD
		No.	%	
6	15	5	33.33	3.42 ± 0.58
7	21	18	85.71	3.14 ± 0.82
8	28	24	85.71	3.10 ± 0.94
9	23	18	78.26	3.12 ± 0.85
10	18	11	61.11	3.45 ± 0.72
Total	**105**	**76**	**72.38**	**3.24 ± 0.94**

Source: With permission from Reference 21.

Table 92.3: Visualization rate of the vitelline duct vascularity between 6 and 10 weeks of gestation

Gestational age (weeks)	N	Visualization rate		PI ± SD
		No	%	
6	15	–	–	3.02 ± 0.92
7	21	18	85.71	3.05 ± 0.89
8	28	25	89.28	3.08 ± 0.91
9	23	17	73.91	3.38 ± 0.82
10	18	10	55.55	3.14 ± 0.92
Total	**105**	**70**	**66.67**	**3.24 ± 0.94**

Source: With permission from Reference 21.

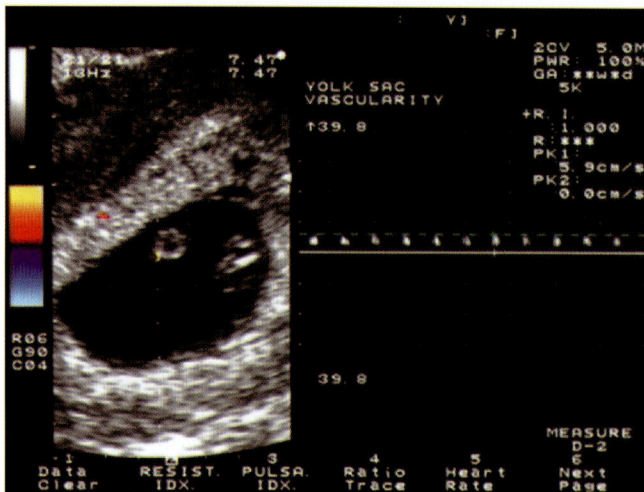

Fig. 92.8: A transvaginal sonogram of a gestational sac at sixth week of gestation. Note regular contours of the yolk sac. Pulsed Doppler signals obtained from the wall of the yolk sac demonstrate low velocity and absence of diastole (RI = 1.0)

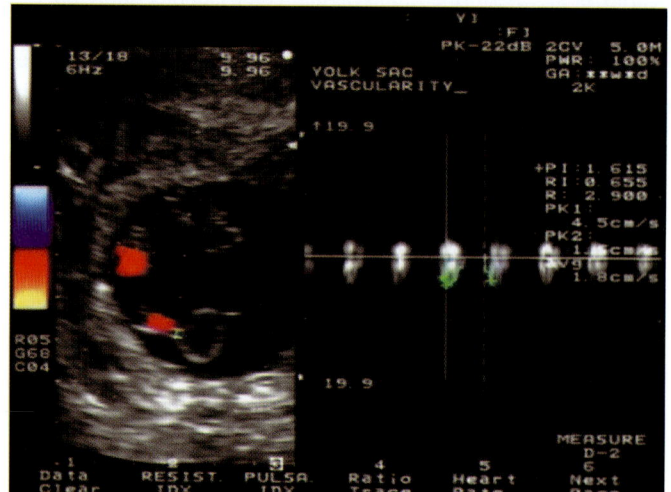

Fig. 92.9: A color image of the yolk sat at 7 weeks of gestation. Pulsed Doppler signals isolated from the connection of the yolk sac and vitelline duct show absence of diastolic flow

analyzed 48 patients with missed abortion between 6 and 12 weeks of gestation. Yolk sac blood flow was detected in 18.54% of missed abortions. They obtained three types of abnormal vascular signals from the yolk sac in these patients: irregular blood flow (Fig. 92.11), permanent diastolic flow (Fig. 92.12) and venous blood flow signals (Figs 92.13 and 92.14).

Changes in vascularization of the yolk sac noticed in missed abortions in this study are probably a consequence of embryonic death and resorption of the embryo through the vitelline duct. Abnormal patterns of the yolk sac vascularity can be related to decreased vitelline blood flow, which may cause progressive accumulation of nutritive secretions not utilized by the embryo. This process ends with enlargement of the yolk sac indicative of an early pregnancy failure. Indeed, we were able to detect yolk sac vascularity in 28.57% (6/21) of missed abortions with large diameter of the yolk sac (Fig. 92.14), and 20% (3/15) of those with normal yolk sac diameter. Sometimes, a careful ultasonographer can visualize double yolk sac (Fig. 92.15) and color Doppler ultrasound may observe abnormal Doppler patterns in these cases.

Cases with echogenic yolk sac walls (N = 7) were characterized by absence of blood flow. Yolk sac calcification was reported to result

from the typical dystrophic changes that occur in non-viable cellular material.[59] Since studies in lower animals demonstrated that yolk sac endoderm bounds calcium, one can postulate that a derangement in the calcium transport mechanism may lead to accumulation of calcium in the yolk sac cells in humans as well. Therefore, recognition of a calcified yolk sac without blood flow signals suggests longstanding demise in the first trimester, which directs the clinician for further diagnostic workup (Figs 92.16 and 92.17).

These data indicate that there is an interaction between the yolk sac vascularity and intervillous circulation in patients with missed abortion. In patients with long standing demise vascular signals could not have been extracted from the hyperechoic walls of the yolk sac. Parallel assessment of the intervillous circulation in this subgroup (N = 7) demonstrated numerous color-coded areas within the intervillous space indicating low mesenchymal turgor and progressive disruption of the maternoembryonic interface. Therefore, the changes in the intervillous circulation noticed in some missed abortions are rather the consequence of embryonic death and inadequate drainage than being the primary cause of early pregnancy failure. This is contrary to the statement of Jaffe, et al.[60] and Jauniaux et al.[61] who found that increased continuous intervillous flow during the first trimester of pregnancy is associated

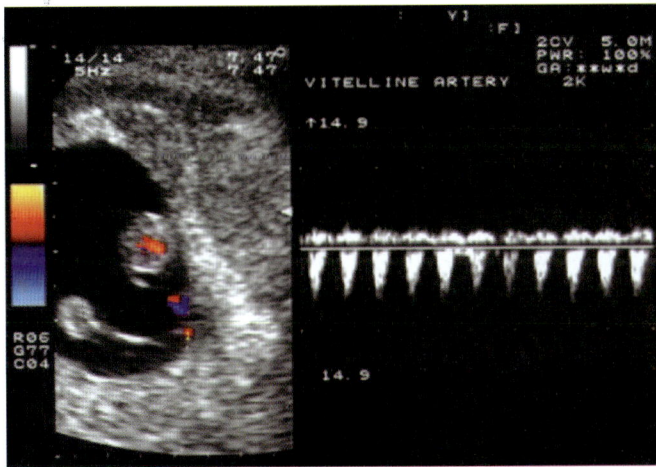

Fig. 92.10: Color Doppler signals are easily obtainable from the vitelline stalk

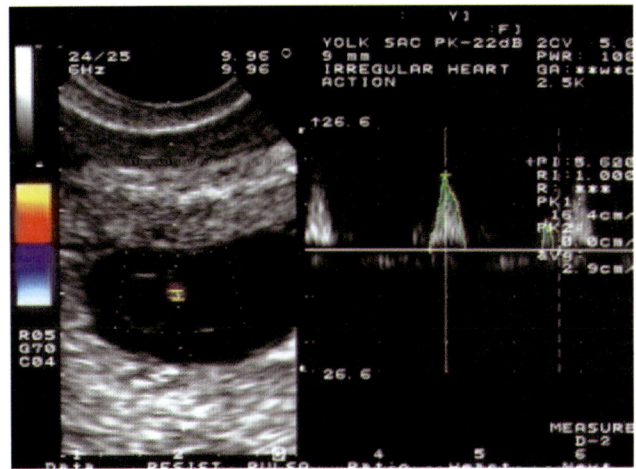

Fig. 92.11: Pulsed Doppler signals derived from the yolk sac in a patient with missed abortion. Note larger diameter (7 mm) of the yolk sac and irregular blood flow signals at its periphery

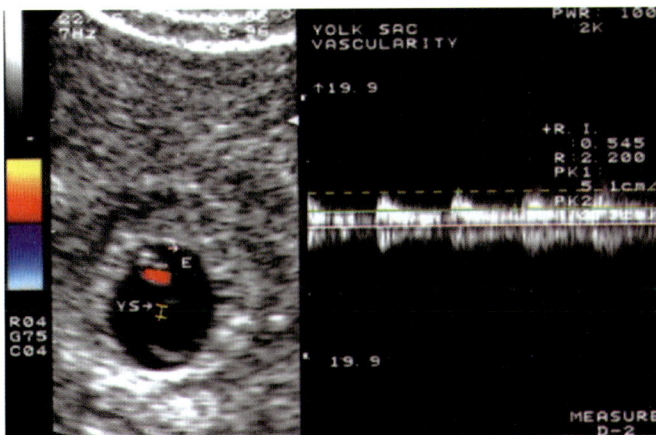

Fig. 92.12: The transvaginal scan of a 9 weeks of gestation, complicated by bleeding. The pulsed Doppler waveform analysis indicates continuous blood flow. Few days after examination was completed spontaneous abortion occurred

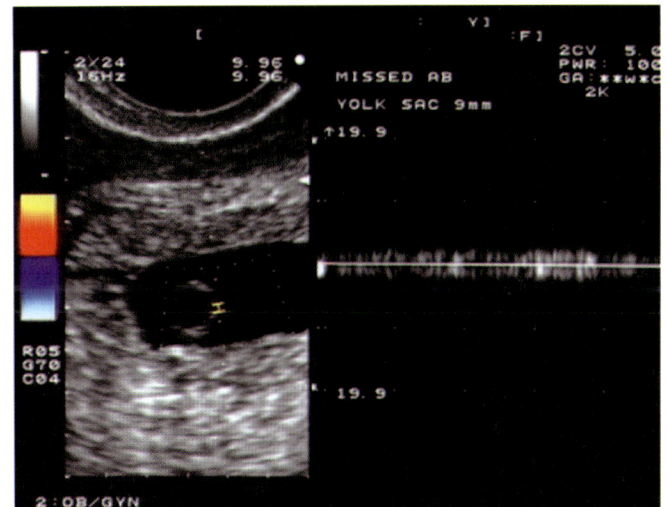

Fig. 92.13: Venous blood flow signals obtained from the yolk sac at 8 weeks of gestation in a patient with missed abortion

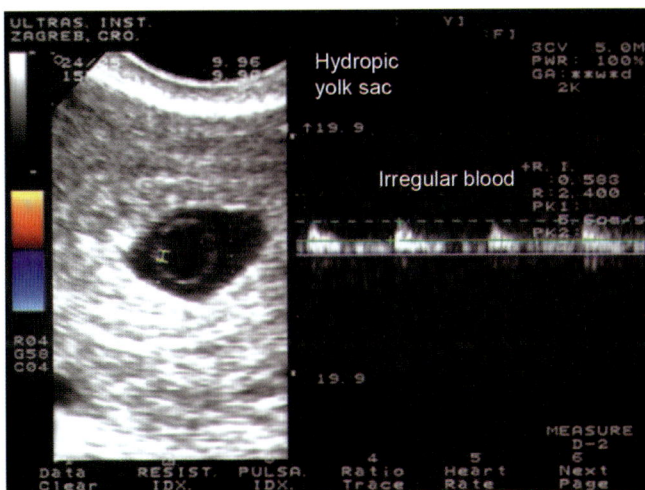

Fig. 92.14: A transvaginal sonogram of a hydropic yolk sac at 6 weeks of pregnancy. Continuous diastolic flow is easily obtained from the hydropic yolk sac (RI = 0.58). Patient aborted in 1 week and karyotyping of the residual products of conception revealed trisomy 21

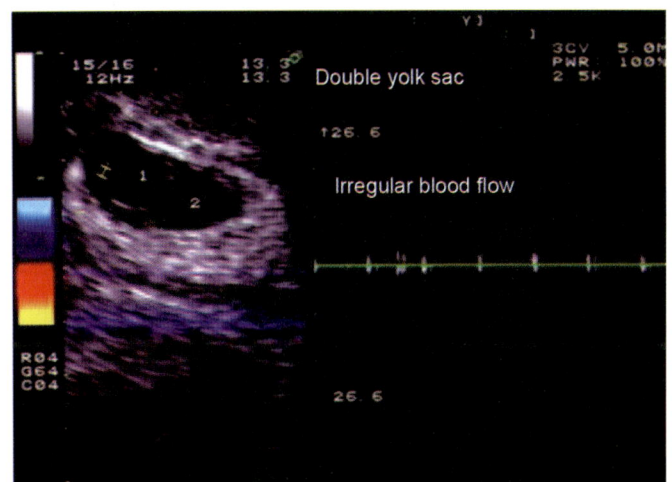

Fig. 92.15: A transvaginal color Doppler scan of a gestational sac containing double yolk sac with irregular blood flow signals

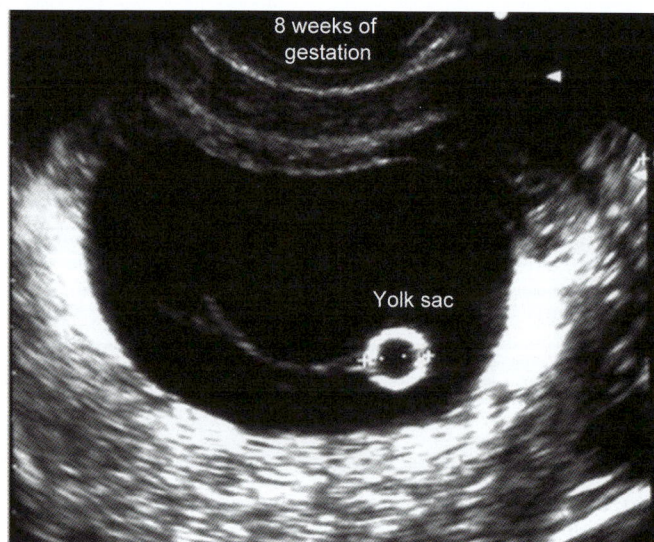

Fig. 92.16: Transvaginal two-dimensional image of the hyperechogenic yolk sac

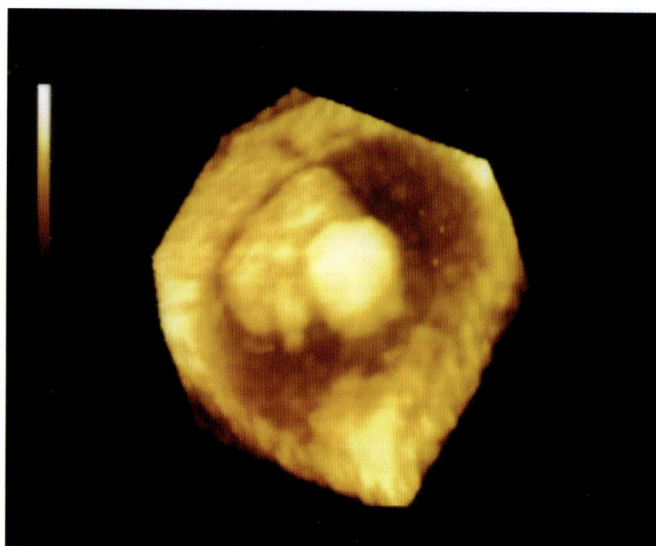

Fig. 92.17: Three-dimensional scan of the hyperechogenic yolk sac

with adverse pregnancy outcome. According to their results increased flow pressure in the spiral arteries may dislocate the thin trophoblastic shell causing the loose of villi to forceful arterial flow which may result in miscarriage.[62] However, independent Doppler studies from three institutions using sensitive conventional and power Doppler velocimetry found that continuous and pulsatile blood flow can be extracted from intervillous space in both normal pregnancies and those with adverse outcome.[17-21,63,64]

Data presented in this study support the concept that establishment of the intervillous circulation is a progressive process during the first trimester of pregnancy. Between the sixth and tenth week of gestation relatively slow blood flow in the intervillous space is detected. Simultaneously clear blood flow signals are derived from the walls of the yolk sac supporting the hypothesis that this fragile structure is responsible for optimal delivery of nutrients and oxygen to developing embryo up to 10 weeks of gestation. Progressive decrease of the yolk sac vascularity coincides with visualization of more prominent color-coded areas within the intervillous space demonstrating increased metabolical needs of the developing pregnancy.

Volume of the Yolk Sac: Correlation with Blood Flow Studies

It is well known that the prognostic significance of the yolk sac diameter as determined by ultrasound is not clearly established. Most of abnormal pregnancies were demonstrated to have normal yolk sac measurements,[65-67] while only a minority of abnormal early pregnancies was presenting either "too small" or "too big" yolk sac dimensions.[68,69]

Recently we performed a study on eighty women with uncomplicated singleton pregnancy (between 5 and 12 weeks gestation).[70] The volumes of the gestational and yolk sacs were measured by three-dimensional ultrasound (Voluson 530, Kretztechnik, Austria). Regression analysis revealed exponential growth of the gestational sac volume. The yolk sac volume was found to increase gradually from 5 to 10 weeks of gestation. However, when the yolk sac reaches its maximum size and volume at around 10 weeks it has already started to degenerate (Fig. 92.18), which can be proved by a significant reduction in visualization rates of the yolk sac vascularity (Fig. 92.19). This suggests that the evaluation of the biological function of the yolk sac by measuring the diameter and/or the volume is limited. Therefore, the combination of functional and volumetric studies is necessary to point out some of the important moments during the early pregnancy:[71]

1. Simultaneous beginning of yolk sac angiogenesis and vascular development of the embryo.
2. Noninvasive evaluation of the functional capacity of the yolk sac.
3. Definition of the shift from embryo-vitelline to embryo-placental circulation.[7]
4. Three-dimensional ultrasound studies of the direct connection between the yolk sac and the embryonic gut.
5. Evaluation of the yolk sac degeneration and location by 3D ultrasound at the end of the first trimester.

The fact that blood vessels first develop in the secondary yolk sac may be related to the important role of this structure in the process of early embryonic nutrition. Further Doppler studies analyzing large cohort of patients with both normal and abnormal pregnancies will probably answer some of the numerous questions on the role of yolk sac vascularity in early embryonic development. The introduction of 3D ultrasound coupled with power Doppler imaging has produced more accurate information on implantation and yolk sac and we look forward to the future developments in this field.

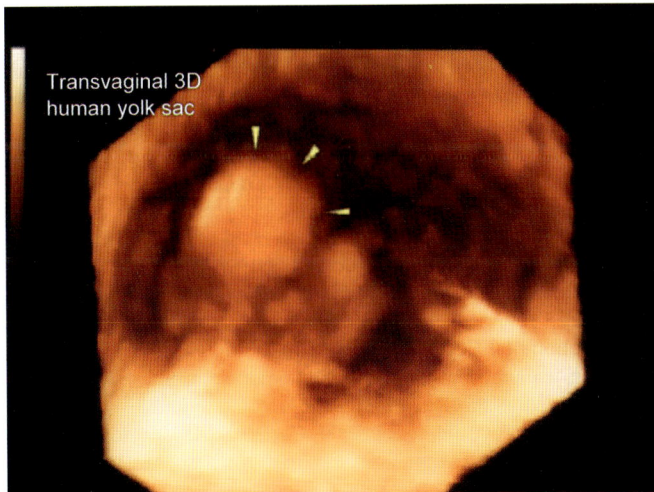

Fig. 92.18: Three-dimensional scan of the yolk sac at 8 weeks of gestation. Note the regular echogenicity and contours of the yolk sac

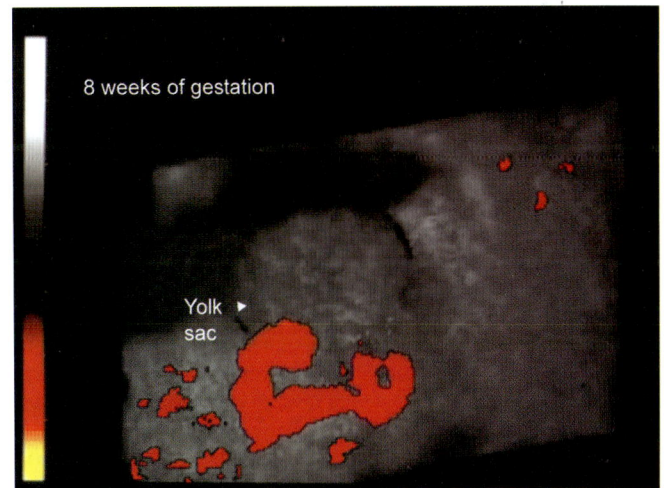

Fig. 92.19: Three-dimensional power Doppler demonstrates turgescent blood vessels above the surface of the yolk sac

REFERENCES

1. Ramsey EM. Circulation in the intervillous space of the primate placenta. Am J Obstet Gynecol. 1962;84:1649-63.
2. Boyd JD, Hamilton WJ. The Human Placenta. Cambridge: Heffer and Sons; 1970.
3. Sadler TW. Langman's Medical Embryology, 7th edition. Baltimore: Williams and Wilkins; 1995.
4. O'Rahilly R. Developmental stages in human embryos. Part A: Embryos of the first three weeks (Stages 1 to 9). Carnegie Inst Wash Publ. 1973;631.
5. Gasser RF. Atlas of Human Embryos. New York, Evanston, San Francisco, London: Harper and Row; 1975.
6. Khong TY, Pearce JM. Development and investigation of the placenta and its blood supply. In: Lavery JP (Ed). The Human Placenta. Clinical Perspectives, Rockville: Aspen Publishers; 1987. pp. 25-45.
7. Fox H. Pathology of the Placenta. London, Philadelphia, Toronto: W.B. Saunders Company; 1978.
8. Padykula HA. The human placenta. In: Weiss L (Ed). Cell and Tissue Biology, 6th edition. Baltimore, München: Urbanand Schwarzenberg; 1983. pp. 901-27.
9. Bulmer JN, Johnson PM. Antigen expression by trophoblast populations in the human placenta and their possible immunobiological relevance. Placenta. 1985;6:127-40.
10. Fox H. Current topic: trophoblastic pathology. Placenta. 1991;12:479-86.
11. Hustin J, Shaaps JP. Echographic and anatomic studies of the maternotrophoblastic border during the first trimester of pregnancy. Am J Obstet Gynecol. 1987;157:162-8.
12. Hustin J, Shaaps JP, Lambotte R. Anatomical studies of the uteroplacental vascularization in the first trimester of pregnancy. Troph Res. 1988;3:49-60.
13. Rodesch F, Simon P, Donner C, et al. Oxygen measurements in endometrial and trophoblastic tissues during early pregnancy. Obstet Gynecol. 1992;80:28-35.
14. Kurjak A, Zalud I, Salihagic A, et al. Transvaginal color Doppler in the assessment of abnormal early pregnancy. J Perinat Med. 1991;19:155-65.
15. Kurjak A, Predanic M, Kupesic S, et al. Transvaginal color Doppler in the study of early normal pregnancies and pregnancies associated with uterine fibroids. J Matern Fetal Invest. 1992;3:81-5.
16. Kurjak A, Kupesic S, Predanic M, et al. Transvaginal color Doppler assessment of the uteroplacental circulation in normal and abnormal early pregnancy. Early Hum Dev. 1992;29:385-9.
17. Kurjak A, Predanic M, Kupesic S, et al. Transvaginal color Doppler study of middle cerebral artery blood flow in early normal and abnormal pregnancy. Ultrasound Obstet Gyneco. 1992;2:424-8.
18. Kurjak A, Zudenigo D, Funduk-Kurjak B, et al. Transvaginal color Doppler in the assessment of the uteroplacental circulation in normal early pregnancy. J Perinat Med. 1993;21:25-34.
19. Kurjak A, Zudenigo D, Predanic M, et al. Recent advances in the Doppler study of early fetomaternal circulation. J Perinat Med. 1994;22:419-39.
20. Kurjak A, Zudenigo D, Predanic M, et al. Transvaginal color Doppler study of fetomaternal circulation in threatened abortion. Fetal Diagn Ther. 1994;9:341-7.
21. Kurjak A, Kupesic S, Kostovic LJ. Vascularization of yolk sac and vitelline duct in normal pregnancies studied by transvaginal color Doppler. J Perinat Med. 1994;22:433-40.
22. Jauniaux E, Jurkovic D, Campbell S. In vivo investigations of anatomy and physiology of early human placental circulations. Ultrasound Obstet Gynecol. 1991;1:435-45.
23. Jauniaux E, Jurkovic D, Campbell S, et al. Doppler ultrasonographic features of the developing placental circulation: correlation with anatomic findings. Am J Obstet Gynecol. 1992;166:585-7.
24. Jaffe R, Warsof SL. Transvaginal color Doppler imaging in the assessment of uteroplacental blood flow in the normal first trimester pregnancy. Am J Obstet Gynecol. 1991;164:781-5.
25. Kurjak A, Predanic M, Kupesic-Urek S. Transvaginal color Doppler in the assessment of placental blood flow. Eur J Obstet Gynecol Reprod Biol. 1993;49:29-32.
26. Kurjak A, Laurini R, Kupesic S, et al. A combined Doppler and morphopathological study of intervillous circulation. Ultrasound Obstet Gynecol. 1995;6(Suppl. 2):116.
27. Valentin L, Sladkevicius P, Laurini R, Sodeberg H, Marsal K. Uteroplacental and luteal circulation in normal first trimester pregnancies: Doppler ultrasonographic and morphologic study. Am J Obstet Gynecol. 1996;174:768-5.
28. Merce LT, Barco MJ, Bau S. Color Doppler sonographic assessment of placental circulation in the first trimester of normal pregnancy. J Ultrasound Med. 1996;15:135-42.

29. Kurjak A, Kupesic S, Kos M, Latin V, Zudenigo D. Early hemodynamics studied by transvaginal color Doppler. Prenat Neonat Med. 1996;1:38-49.

30. Kurjak A, Kupesic S. Doppler assessment of the intervillous blood flow in normal and abnormal early pregnancy. Obstet Gynecol. 1997;89:252-6.

31. Jauniaux E, Zaidi J, Jurkovic D, et al. Comparison of color Doppler features and pathohistological finding in complicated early pregnancy. Hum Reprod. 1994;9:2432-7.

32. Ramsey EM, Chez RA, Doppman JL. Radioangiographic measurement of the internal diameters of the uteroplacental arteries in Rhesus monkeys. Am J Obstet Gynecol. 1979;135(2):247-51.

33. Nimrod C, Simpson N, De Vermette R, et al. Placental and early fetal haemodynamics: the suitability of the monkey model. The Fetus as a Patient, XII International Congress, 23-25 May, Grado, Italy. Book of Abstracts. 1996;68.

34. Nimrod C, Simpson N, Hafner T, et al. Assessment of early placental development in the cynomolgus monkey (Macaca fascicularis) using color and pulsed wave Doppler sonography. J Med Primatol. 1996;25:106-11.

35. Jauniaux E. Intervillous circulation in the first trimester: the phantom of the color Doppler obstetric opera (editorial). Ultrasound Obstet Gynecol. 1996;8:73-6.

36. Hustin J, Kadri R, Jauniaux E. Spontaneous and habitual abortion—a pathologists point of view. Biol Med. 1996;2:85-9.

37. Jaffe R, Dorgan A, Abramowicz A. Color Doppler imaging of uteroplacental circulation in the first trimester: value in predicting pregnancy failure or complication. Am J Roentgenol. 1995;164:1255-8.

38. Jauniaux E, Nicolaides KH. Placental lakes, absent umbilical artery diastolic flow and poor fetal growth in early pregnancy. Ultrasound Obstet Gynecol. 1996;7:141-4.

39. Kurjak A, Kupesic S. Doppler proof of the presence of intervillous circulation (letter). Ultrasound Obstet Gynecol. 1996;7:463-4.

40. Kurjak A, Kupesic S, Hafner T, et al. Conflicting data on intervillous circulation in early pregnancy. J Perinat Med. 1997;25:225-36.

41. Kurjak A, Dudenhausen JW, Hafner T, et al. Intervillous circulation in all three trimesters of normal pregnancy assessed by color Doppler. J Perinat Med. 1997;25:373-80.

42. Kurjak A, Kupesic S, Hafner T, et al. Intervillous blood flow in patients with missed abortion. Croatian Med J. 1998;39:41-4.

43. Burchell RC. Arterial blood flow into the human intervillous space. Am J Obstet Gynecol. 1967;98:303-11.

44. Karimu AL, Burton GJ. Star volume estimates of the intervillous clefts in the human placenta: how changes in umbilical arterial pressure might influence the maternal placental circulation. J Dev Physiol. 1993;19:137-42.

45. Salafia CM, Minor VK, Pezzullo JC, et al. Intrauterine growth restriction in infants of less than thirty two weeks gestation: associated placental pathologic features. Am J Obstet Gynecol. 1995;173:1049-57.

46. Jackson MR, Walsh AJ, Morrow RJ, et al. Reduced placental villous tree elaboration in small-for-gestational-age pregnancies: relationship with umbilical artery Doppler waveforms. Am J Obstet Gynecol. 1995;172:518-25.

47. Arabin B, Jimenez E, Vogel M, et al. Relationship of utero- and fetoplacental blood flow velocity waveforms with pathomorphological placental findings. Fetal Diagn Ther. 1992;7:173-9.

48. Harris JWS, Ramsey EM. The morphology of human uteroplacental vasculature. Contrib Embryol. 1966;38:43-58.

49. Brosens I, Robertson WB, Dixon HG. The role of the spiral arteries in the pathogenesis of pre-eclampsia. Obstet Gynecol Annu. 1972;1:177-91.

50. Khong TY, DeWolf F, Robertson WB, et al. Inadequate maternal vascular response to placentation in pregnancies complicated by pre-eclampsia and small-for-gestational age infants. Br J Obstet Gynaecol. 1986;93:1049-59.

51. Boyd PA, Scott A. Quantitative structural studies on human placentas associated with pre-eclampsia, essential hypertension and intrauterine growth retardation. Br J Obstet Gynaecol. 1985;92:714-21.

52. Fleischer A, Schulman H, Farmakides G, et al. Uterine artery Doppler velocimetry in pregnant women with hypertension. Am J Obstet Gynecol. 1986;154:806-13.

53. Mc Lachlan. The vascular system. Medical Embryology. New York: Addison-Wesley Publishing Company; 1994. pp. 105-15.

54. Fukuda T. Fetal hemopoiesis-electronic microscopic studies on human yolk sac hemopoiesis. Virchows Arch. 1973;14:197-213.

55. Zamboni L. Electronic microscopic studies of human blood embryogenesis in human. II. The hemopoietic activity in the fetal liver. J Ultrastruct Res. 1965;12:525-41.

56. Fukuda T. Fetal hemopoiesis. II. Electron microscopic studies on human hepatic hemopoiesis. Virchow Arch. 1974;16:249-70.

57. Fukuda T. Ultrastructure of fetal hemopoiesis. Acta Haematol Jpn. 1978;41:1204.

58. Kurjak A, Kupesic S. Parallel Doppler assessment of yolk sac and intervillous circulation in normal pregnancy and missed abortion. Placenta. 1988;196:19-23.

59. Harris RD, Vincent LM, Askin FB. Yolk sac calcification: a sonographic finding associated with intrauterine embryonic demise in the first trimester. Radiology. 1988;166:109-16.

60. Jaffe R, Warsof SL. Color Doppler imaging in the assessment of uteroplacental blood flow in abnormal first trimester intrauterine pregnancies: an attempt to define etiologic mechanisms. J Ultrasound Med. 1992;11:41-4.

61. Jauniaux E, Zaidi J, Jurkovic D, et al. Comparison of color Doppler features and pathologic findings in complicated early pregnancy. Hum Reprod. 1994;9:2432-7.

62. Jaffe R, Jauniaux E, Hustin J. Maternal circulation in the first trimester human placenta—Myth or reality? Am J Obstet Gynecol. 1997;176:695-705.

63. Valentin L, Sladkevicius P, Laurini R, et al. Uteroplacental and luteal circulation in normal first-trimester pregnancies: Doppler ultrasonographic and morphologic study. Am J Obstet Gynecol. 1996;174:768-75.

64. Merce LT, Barco MJ, Bau S. Color Doppler sonographic assessment of placental circulation in the first trimester of normal pregnancy. J Ultrasound Med. 1996;15:135-42.

65. Crooij MJ, Westhuis M, Schoemaker J, et al. Ultrasonographic measurements of the yolk sac. Br J Obstet Gynaecol. 1982;89:931-4.

66. Reece EA, Sciosca AL, Pinter E, et al. Prognostic significance of the human yolk sac assessed by ultrasonography. Am J Obstet Gynecol. 1988;159:1191-4.

67. Goldstein SR, Kerenyi T, Scher J, et al. Correlation between karyotype and ultrasound findings in patients with failed early pregnancy. Ultrasound Obstet Gynecol. 1996;8:314-7.

68. Jauniaux E, Jurkovic D, Henriet Y, et al. Development of the secondary human yolk sac. Correlation of sonographic and anatomical features. Hum Reprod. 1991;6:1160-6.

69. Lindsay DJ, Lyons EA, Levi CS, et al. Endovaginal appearance of the yolk sac in early pregnancy: normal growth and usefulness as a predictor of abnormal pregnancy outcome. Radiology. 1992;83:115-22.

70. Kupesic S, Kurjak A. Volume and vascularity of the yolk sac studied by three-dimensional ultrasound and color Doppler. J Perinat Med. 1999;27:91-6.

71. Kurjak A, Azumendi G, Solak M. Clinical application of four dimensional sonography in perinatal medicine. In: Kurjak A, Jackson D (Eds). Boca Raton, USA: Taylor and Francis; 2004. pp. 127-46.

93 First Trimester Ultrasound

N Montenegro, A Matias

INTRODUCTION

In obstetrics, ultrasound has been used for many years and since the beginning, investigators have been interested in changes in the uterus and its contents in early pregnancy.[1]

Moreover, in recent years, the introduction of higher-resolution equipment and transvaginal endosonography has brought new possibilities for the study of early gestational events.[2-4]

Nowadays, ultrasound is increasingly used in early pregnancy, either as a routine procedure or selectively for specific clinical indications. Routine ultrasonography during the first trimester is used for accurate pregnancy dating, early diagnosis of major malformations, characterization of multiple pregnancy and screening of chromosomal anomalies.[5-18]

Although the quality of images obtained during the first trimester seems to be superior when using the transvaginal approach, transabdominal ultrasonography is still widely used in this period of gestation for cultural and practical reasons.[19,20]

The use of diagnostic ultrasound during pregnancy is considered to be safe for both mother and fetus. Even in critical periods of development and using high-frequency transvaginal transducers, no adverse bioeffects have been demonstrated.[21-23] The benefits to patients exposed to the ultrasound intensities used at present outweigh the risks, if any.

This chapter will review the main applications of ultrasound examination during early pregnancy, relying on the experience of the authors together with that reported in the literature. Special emphasis will be placed on embryonic development during the first weeks of gestational age determination, characterization of multiple pregnancy and screening and diagnosis of fetal anomalies. In the text, gestational age will be expressed as complete weeks from last menses.

EMBRYONIC DEVELOPMENT: ULTRASOUND FINDINGS

The decidual thickening is the first indirect sign of pregnancy that can be disclosed by ultrasound.[24,25] Although it is seen more often in the early phases of an intrauterine pregnancy, this hyperechogenic mantle filling the uterine cavity can also coexist with an ectopic pregnancy. As the same pattern can be found in the late luteal-phase endometrium, it should be considered as a non-specific sign.

A few days before the expected menses, a typical image of a hyperechogenic ring inside the uterine cavity can be identified by transvaginal ultrasound. This corresponds to the gestational sac, the echogenic ring being the chorionic villi surrounding the chorionic cavity. At this time, the mean level of the β-subunit of human chorionic gonadotropin (β-hCG) is found to be about 500 mIU/mL

(2nd reference standard).[26] Thereby, the diagnosis of intrauterine pregnancy can be confirmed and a chorionic sac internal diameter of 2–6 mm will be found, corresponding to 4 weeks' menstrual age.

During the fifth week, the chorionic sac measures 7–10 mm. When this diameter reaches 9 mm, the yolk sac can always be identified as a round, fluid-filled and eccentric structure with a diameter of 3 mm. In the present author's experience, this 9–10 mm diameter of the chorionic sac represents an early discriminatory value for the diagnosis of a blighted ovum. At some time during the end of the fifth week, pulsations can be visualized on real-time imaging, close to the wall of the yolk sac and within a 2–3 mm echogenic line corresponding to the embryo. After this time, the heart rate can be measured using simultaneous M-mode.

At 6 weeks, the echogenic line corresponding to the developing embryo is always close to the yolk sac and measures 4–6 mm. Cardiac motion can be clearly seen and the mean heart rate at this gestational week is about 118 bpm.[26] The amnion is not yet clearly seen, so the embryo and the yolk sac are apparently free-floating in the chorionic cavity, although eccentrically fixed by the connecting body stalk.

During the seventh week, the embryonic length is 7–12 mm and the yolk sac, with a diameter of 5 mm, separates from the embryo, probably owing to the growth of the vitelline duct. At this time, the cephalic pole becomes distinguishable and an apparent single hypoechoic cavity can be seen, corresponding to a part of the primitive cerebral ventricle in the rhombencephalic area, probably the future fourth ventricle.[20-24]

At 8 weeks, the embryonic length is 12–18 mm and the upper and lower limb buds are now visible. The folding of the hypoechoic cerebral vesicle limits the lateral recesses of the rhombencephalic cavity.[27-30] The placental site can even be identified, following the umbilical cord from the abdominal wall of the embryo. Discrete undulating body movements can be sporadically seen on real-time imaging at the end of the eighth week.

During the ninth week, the embryo assumes a typical C-shaped curvature and the crown-rump length (CRL) will be more than 2 cm (21–31 mm).[31] As landmarks, the head represents one-third of the entire body and inside the head, the hyperechoic falx and choroid plexuses and a hypoechoic heart-shaped structure corresponding to the cerebral peduncles are visible. The physiological midgut herniation, which can be identified close to the anterior abdominal wall, will persist until the end of the 11th week. Body movements are now more frequently seen.

Between 8 weeks and 10 weeks, the amnion surrounding the embryo is always clearly seen, the yolk sac being outside in the exocoelomic/chorionic cavity.[26,32]

At 10 weeks of gestation (Carnegie stages 20–23), the CRL is 32–41 mm and the embryo is slightly more curved. The choroid plexuses fill the lateral ventricles completely, and are the most prominent structures in the cephalic pole (Fig. 93.1). In the posterior fossa, the cisterna magna and cerebellum can be identified, though the development process of the posterior fossa will only be concluded by 16 weeks.

In the trunk, the cardiac valvular apparatus can sometimes be distinguished inside the heart by the end of the 10th week, although more accurately from the 11th week onwards. Also at the end of the 10th week, the stomach filled with a small amount of liquid, can sometimes be identified in the abdomen.

The three segments of the upper and lower limbs are clearly identified with both hands and feet in the midline. The first trimester of pregnancy is the best occasion to assess the number of fingers as normally the hands are wide open. Abduction of the lower limbs with lateral rotation of the hips is typically encountered between 10 weeks and 13 weeks (Fig. 93.2).

Body and even isolated limb movements are often identified on real-time imaging.

At 11 weeks, the fetus (no longer the embryo) acquires a human appearance and the CRL will be greater than 42 mm, reaching 76

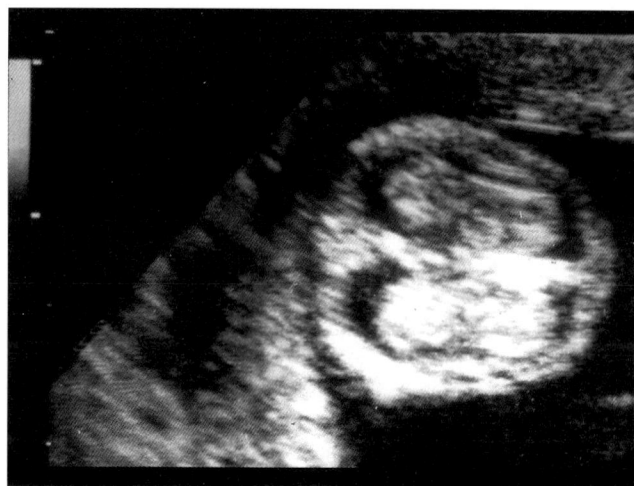

Fig. 93.1: Lateral ventricles and choroid plexuses in a 10-week embryo

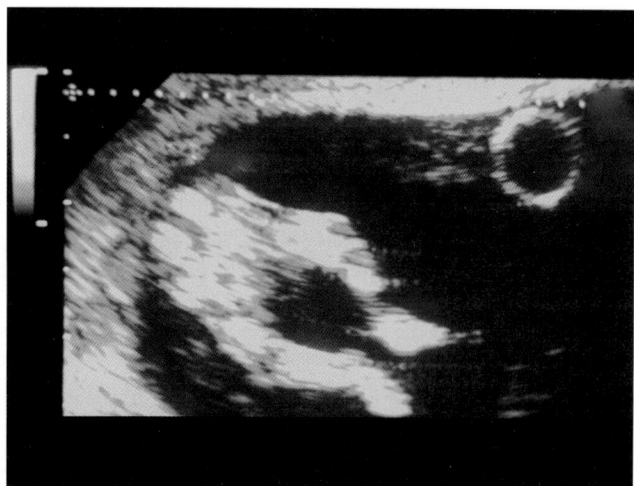

Fig. 93.2: Upper and lower limbs at 11 weeks. Note the abduction of lower limbs

mm at 13 weeks. From now on, a more detailed anatomical survey can be obtained, including the cerebral and cardiovascular systems and the digestive and urinary tracts.[33] The midgut is no longer herniated and can be seen as a hyperechoic round image inside the coelomic cavity and situated in the median region of the lower abdomen.

Between 11 weeks and 14 weeks of gestation, that is, between 45 mm and 84 mm CRL, a subcutaneous translucency behind the neck region can be disclosed in a sagittal section of the fetus. The maximum thickness between the skin and the soft tissue overlying the cervical spine can be measured, and was called nuchal translucency (NT).[13] Initially, the normal values have been reported as less than 3 mm. After the prospective study of 100,000 pregnancies from Snijders and co-workers (1998) increased NT has been defined as the value higher than the 95th centile for gestational age.[34] Increased NT has been found in association with major chromosomal anomalies and cardiac defects, and proposed, together with maternal age, as an efficacious screening procedure during the first trimester of pregnancy.[34]

More recently, the first reports on the use of three-dimensional ultrasound in the first trimester of pregnancy suggest its potential for early-pregnancy anatomic survey.[35]

GESTATIONAL AGE DETERMINATION

Gestational age assignment is one of the most important issues in perinatal medicine for both clinical and research purposes. In addition to an indication of medical problems, it could result in serious personal and social implications for the parents.

Even today, worldwide, the last menstrual period (LMP) is still the basis for calculation of gestational age and expected day of confinement. Nevertheless, in clinical practice, health professionals are frequently confronted by difficulties concerning the exact estimation of the LMP, incorrect reporting, cycle irregularities and the recent use of oral contraceptives. It has been estimated that about one-third of women attending antenatal care fall into one of these categories.[11]

Even in the population of women with certain dates and regular cycles, reliable biological correspondence between LMP and ovulation or fertilization is still difficult to obtain. In addition to long-available information about this phenomenon, recent studies in this field provide the confirmation that conception can occur within a 6-day period from intercourse ending at the day of ovulation.[36]

In very early pregnancies, gestational age determination by ultrasound scan is a little inaccurate, and is based on chorionic sac mean or maximum diameters. At the beginning of the 4th week, the diameter is 2–3 mm, reaching 9–10 mm when the yolk sac can be identified.[25] Once the embryo is visible, embryonic length should be measured.

As reported by Goldstein, before 10 weeks of gestation, it is really the embryonic length rather than the CRL that is being measured.[31] On the other hand, operator errors are more frequent below than above 10 weeks.[37]

A large number of reference tables for CRL measurements are available, all showing identical mean values to those originally reported in the literature, despite variations in ultrasound machines, ethnic groups and methodological aspects (Fig. 93.3).[31,38-42] However, in a trisomy-18 fetus or in a fetus with triploidy, the CRL is smaller than normal, while in other major chromosomal anomalies, the CRL is not significantly different from normal.[43]

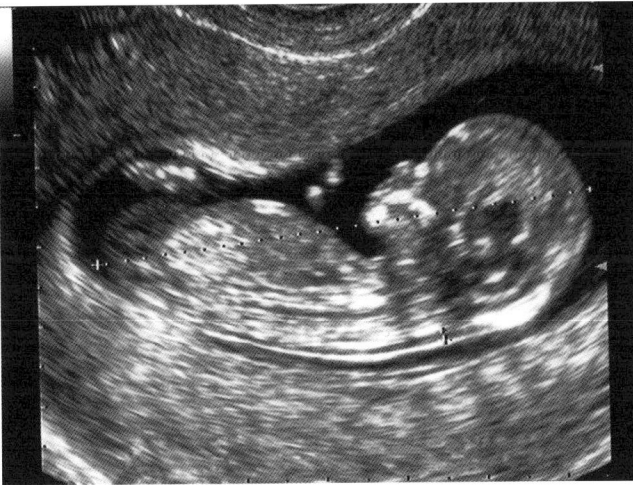

Fig. 93.3: Crown-rump length, the gold standard for dating pregnancy

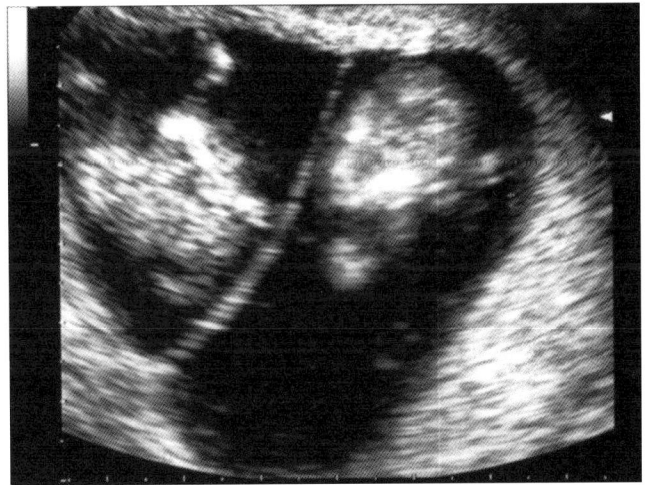

Fig. 93.4: Monochorionic diamniotic twin pregnancy with the T-sign

Furthermore, several studies have been reported dealing with the validity and benefits of routine ultrasound examination in the first half of pregnancy, having as end-points reduced perinatal morbidity and mortality.[44,45] One of the major goals was improving the determination of gestational age. The ultrasonographic measurement of CRL before 13 weeks' or the biparietal and transverse cerebellar diameters between 14 weeks and 22 weeks of gestation, respectively, have been widely used for this since the beginning of the 1970s.[37-50]

When comparing the accuracy of menstrual dates and ultrasonography in the first half of pregnancy, for calculating the expected date of delivery, dating by ultrasonographic biometry was more predictive than the former or even the combination of both methods.[12,46] Therefore, even with known menstrual dates, most authors would rather use ultrasound biometry, namely measurement of the CRL and biparietal diameter (BPD), than the LMP for estimation of gestational age or expected date of confinement.

Clinical and ethical considerations support the medical value of routine ultrasonography in the first half of pregnancy as a standard of obstetric care.[49] If there is a tendency towards an ideal policy in such a field, some of the above quoted reasons point to the late first trimester as the best gestational age period for a routine ultrasound examination.

MULTIPLE PREGNANCY

Today, mainly as a result of the expanded use of assisted reproductive methods, multiple pregnancy is more frequently found in antenatal clinics all over the world. In the United States, over the past 20 years, births of twins have increased at twice the rate, and multiple births of triplets or more have increased seven-fold faster than births of singletons.[51]

Meanwhile, higher perinatal morbidity and mortality in such pregnancies can be reduced by accurate pregnancy dating, by avoiding unnecessary prolongation of gestation and from determination of chorionicity.[52,53] It is chorionicity rather than zygosity that determines several aspects of antenatal management

and perinatal outcome. Antepartum death of one twin is three times more frequent in monochorionic than in dichorionic gestation.[54]

Today, management protocols in multiple pregnancies include successful intrauterine treatments and single invasive diagnostic tests for monozygotic twins, and multifetal reduction in higher-order gestations.[55-58]

Antenatal determination of chorionicity by ultrasound is much easier in the early first trimester when two or more separate gestational sacs and embryos are identified. It is also accurate to perform an ultrasound scan between 10 weeks and 14 weeks, relying on the demonstration of the lambda sign[47] for dichorionic (with a positive predictive value of 100% for dichorionicity), or the T-sign (Fig. 93.4) for monochorionic twin pregnancies. In the second or third trimesters of pregnancy, dividing membranes can be seen.[53] Other criteria such as number of placentas and fetal gender are unreliable, as fused placentas and identical sex are often found in dichorionic twins.

For all these reasons, it seems relevant to advise a routine ultrasound scan at 10–14 weeks of gestation. An earlier examination, although eventually more reliable for the determination of chorionicity, will be less accurate for pregnancy dating.[38] Furthermore, at 10–14 weeks, it will encompass the common event of the vanishing twin, either in spontaneous or in *in vitro* fertilization pregnancies.[58]

FETAL ANOMALIES: SCREENING AND DIAGNOSIS

The ultrasonographic fetal examination in the late first trimester is useful for both screening and diagnostic purposes.

Concerning chromosomal defects, NT thickness determination between 11 weeks and 14 weeks of gestation was the first marker to be incorporated in first-trimester routine ultrasound examination as a screening procedure.[13,34] Increased NT has been found in association with major chromosomal defects (Fig. 93.5), namely trisomies 13, 18 and 21, Turner syndrome and triploidy as with cardiac defects, other malformations and genetic syndromes.[59,60]

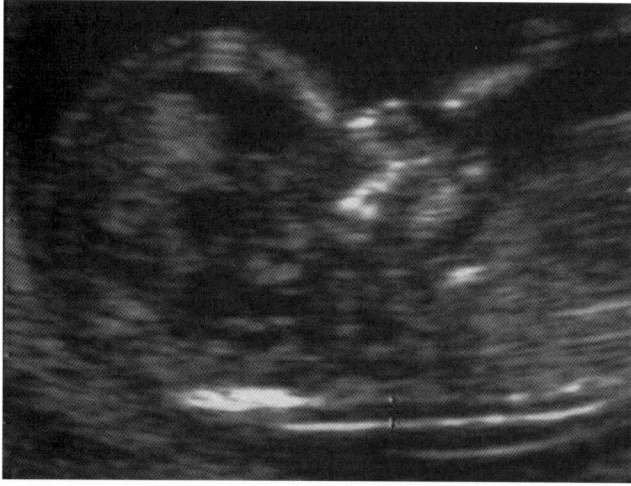

Fig. 93.5: Sagittal plane of a 12-week fetus showing the adequate plane for measuring nuchal translucency. Increased nuchal translucency (NT = 4 mm) in a 12-week fetus with Down's syndrome

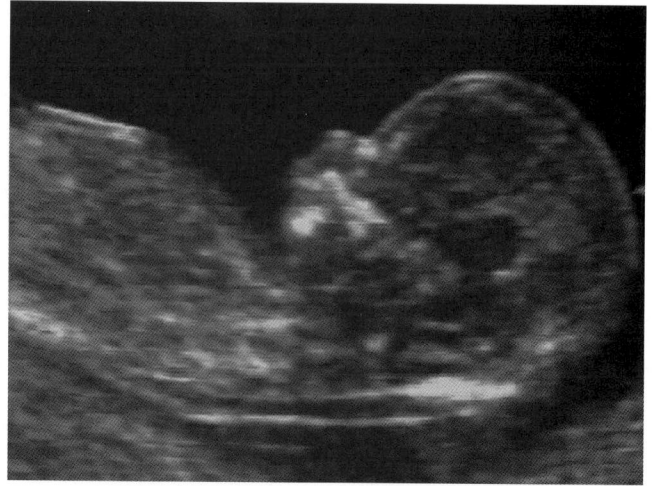

Fig. 93.7: Ultrasound image off nasal bones in a 12-week fetus with normal karyotype

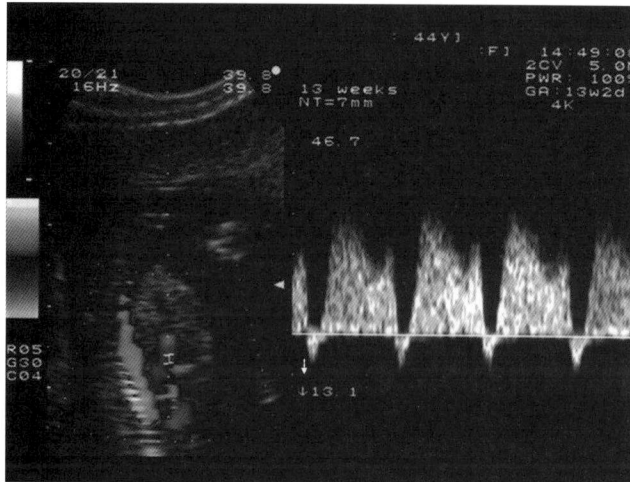

Fig. 93.6: Abnormal ductus venosus blood flow in a 12-week fetus with trisomy 21

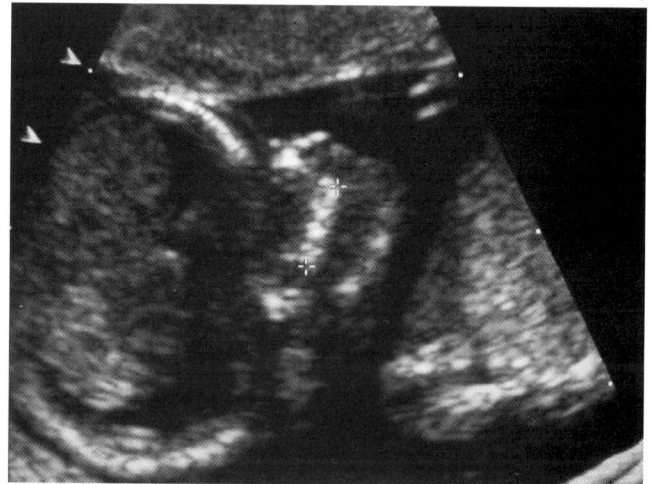

Fig. 93.8: Ultrasound image of a 12-week fetus demonstrating the measurement of the maxillary bone measurement in a normal fetus

If increased NT is combined with maternal age and factors concerning trisomy 21, the detection rate for chromosomal anomalies will be 80% with false positive rate of 5%. When fetal heart rate or maternal serum free β-h-CG and pregnancy-associated plasma protein A (PAPP-A) (OSCAR clinic) were also incorporated at 11–14 weeks, detection rates will be 83% and 90%, respectively.[61,62]

The pathogenic basis of increased NT is still obscure, in spite of published work reporting an association of such an increase with cardiac defects/dysfunction.[63-66] Investigational work from our group clearly demonstrated abnormal ductus venosus (DV) blood flow in the majority of fetuses with increased NT and abnormal karyotype[15] and/or cardiac defects.[16] The combination of maternal age, NT and DV evaluation yielded a similar detection rate of NT alone, but decreased significantly the invasive testing rate.[15]

Still emphasizing the importance of ultrasound screening in the first trimester, when we adopt the same sagittal plane used for NT, other sonographic markers can be obtained and have recently been proposed to improve the detection rate for trisomy 21: ductus blood flow evaluation[15,16,63-69] (Fig. 93.6), fetal nasal bones[17] (Fig. 93.7) and maxillary bone length[18] (Fig. 93.8). Preliminary data suggest that combining sonographic and biochemical markers in the first trimester of pregnancy could result in a detection rate of 97% for a false-positive rate of 5%, or a detection of 95% for a false-positive rate of 2%.[62]

Detailed assessment of fetal anatomy in the late first trimester is possible using either transabdominal or higher-resolution transvaginal sonography.[27,70] Therefore, potentially, the antenatal diagnosis of the majority of structural anomalies in this period of gestation can be carried out. Good examples of first trimester diagnosis of major malformations are exencephaly/acrania (Figs 93.9A and B), omphalocele (Figs 93.10A and B) and osteochondrodysplasia (Fig. 93.11).

After the first report of an early ultrasonic diagnosis of anencephaly in the 1970s,[71] many case reports have been published in the literature.

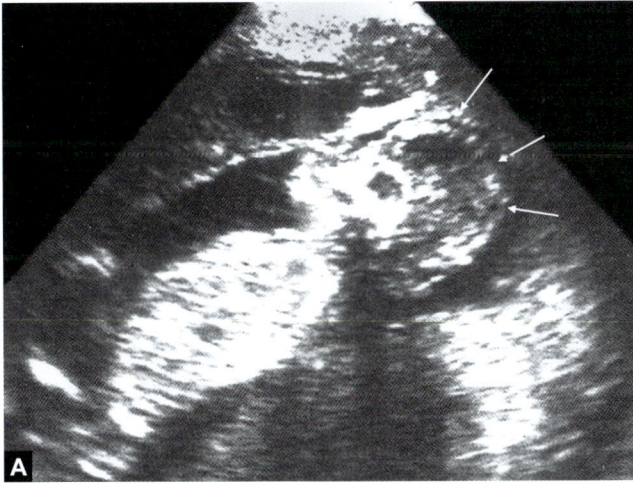

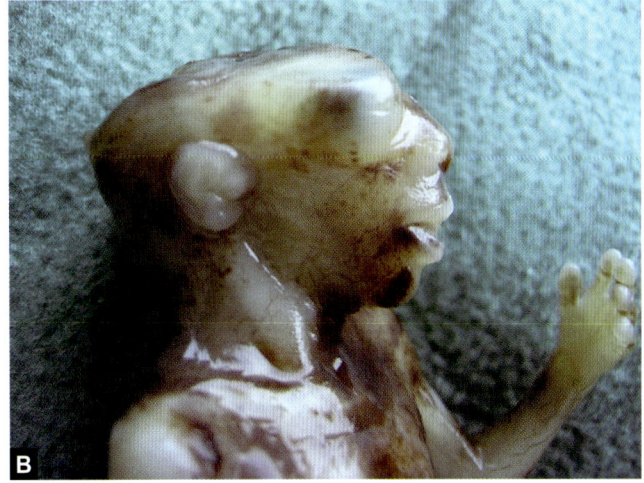

Figs 93.9A and B: (A) Ultrasound image of an exencephaly/acrania detected at 13 weeks of gestation, showing the the absence of cranial bones; (B) necropsic specimen of the same fetus after termination of pregnancy, confirming the prenatal diagnosis

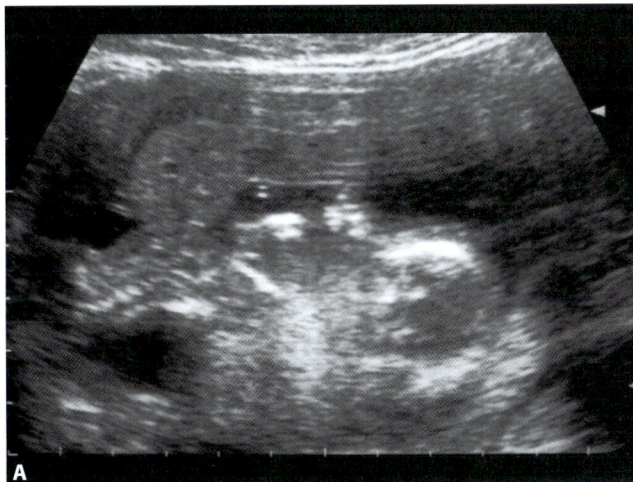

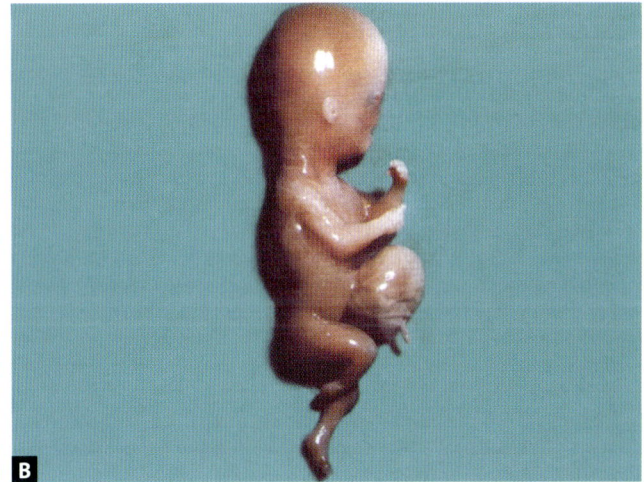

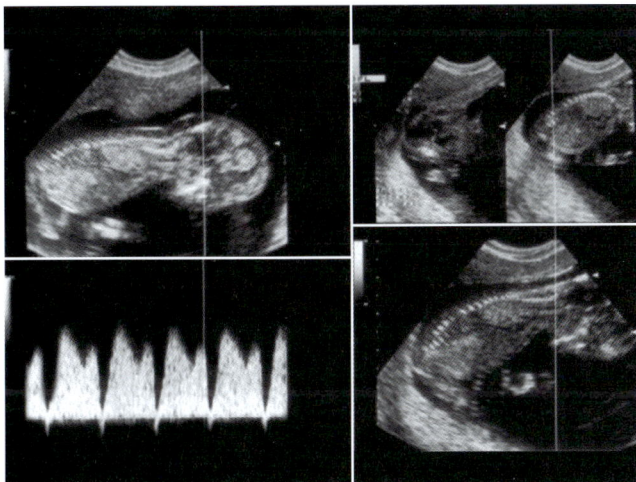

Figs 93.10A and B: (A) Ultrasound image of an omphalocele detected at 12 weeks of gestation, showing the outbulging liver and a pronounced lordosis; (B) necropsic specimen of the same fetus after termination of pregnancy, confirming the prenatal diagnosis

Fig. 93.11: Sonographic aspects of a osteochondrodysplasia diagnosed at 12 weeks of gestation, showing short limbs, increased nuchal translucency and abnormal flow in the ductus venosus

Following the "natural history of fetal anomalies", the IRON-FAN registry has been able to demonstrate how early anomalies can be diagnosed, in particular those which are potentially lethal, such, as those occurring in the central nervous and cardiovascular systems, urinary tract and abdominal wall.[72] To date, more than 2,000 anomalies, diagnosed between 9 weeks and 15 weeks' of gestation, have been reported.

We consider that the policy of routine ultrasound examination in the second trimester will be reviewed within the next few years, once most, if not all, the lethal defects are able to be diagnosed and managed earlier in pregnancy. Furthermore, late first-trimester scan has other advantages, already discussed above, as a more accurate method of gestational age determination and for sufficiently early characterization of multiple pregnancy.

CONCLUSION

During recent years, interest in first trimester pregnancy has been reinforced by the achievement of detailed imaging of early human intrauterine life using high-resolution ultrasound equipment, namely transvaginal ultrasonography.

It is now possible to look at intrauterine events from the beginning of pregnancy, close to the time of implantation.

Acquired experience of first-trimester ultrasound examination either as a routine procedure or complementary to clinical evaluation demonstrates its essential role in obstetrical care.

Accurate gestational age determination, sufficiently early characterization of multiple pregnancy, early diagnosis of lethal anomalies and screening of chromosomal defects are important end points to be taken into account by health authorities and to recommend routine ultrasound examination in the late first trimester of pregnancy.

REFERENCES

1. Donald I. Diagnostic uses of sonar in obstetrics and gynaecology. J Obstet Gynecol Br Commonw. 1965;72:907-19.
2. Timor-Tritsch IE, Farine D, Mortimore GR. A close look at early embryonic development with the high-frequency transvaginal transducer. Am J Obstet Gynecol. 1988;159:676-81.
3. Fossum GT, Davayan V, Keltzky OA. Early detection of pregnancy with transvaginal ultrasound. Fertil Steril. 1988;49: 788-91.
4. De Crespigny LC. Early diagnosis of pregnancy failure with transvaginal ultrasound. Am J Obstet Gynecol. 1988;159:408–9.
5. Persson PH, Kullander S. Long-term experience of general ultrasound screening in pregnancy. Am J Obstet Gynecol. 1983;146:942-6.
6. Eik-Nes SH, Okland O, Aure JC. Ultrasound screening in pregnancy: A randomized controlled trial. Lancet. 1984; 1:1347.
7. Cochlin D. Effect of two ultrasound scanning regimens on the management of pregnancy. Br J Obstet Gynecol. 1984;91: 885-8.
8. Lilford R, Chard T. The routine use of ultrasound. Br J Obstet Gynecol 1985;92:434-7.
9. Neilson J, Grant A. Ultrasound in pregnancy. In: Enkin M, Keirse MJN, Chalmers I (Eds). A Guide to Effective Care in Pregnancy and Childbirth. New York: Oxford University Press 1989:48-56.
10. Belfrage P, Fernstrom I, Hallenberg G. Routine or selective ultrasound examinations in early pregnancy. Obstet Gynecol. 1991;69:747-81.
11. Geirsson RT. Ultrasound instead of last menstrual period as the basis of gestational age assignment. Ultrasound Obstet Gynecol. 1991;1:212-19.
12. Todros T, Ronco G, Lombardo D, et al. The length of pregnancy: An echographic reappraisal. J Clin Ultrasound. 1991;19:11-14.
13. Nicolaides KH, Azar G, Byrne D, et al. Fetal nuchal translucency: Ultrasound screening for chromosomal defects in first trimester pregnancy. Br Med J. 1992;304:435-9.
14. Achiron R, Tadmor O. Screening for fetal anomalies during the first trimester of pregnancy: Transvaginal versus transabdominal sonography. Ultrasound Obstet Gynecol. 1991;1:186-91.
15. Matias A, Gomes C, Flack N, et al. Screening for chromosomal abnormalities at 10-14 weeks: The role of ductus venosus blood flow. Ultrasound Obstet Gynecol. 1998;12:380-4.
16. Matias A, Huggon I, Areias JA, et al. Cardiac defects in chromosomally normal fetuses with abnormal ductus venosus blood flow at 10-14 weeks. Ultrasound Obstet Gynecol. 1999;14:307-10.
17. Cicero S, Curcio P, Papageorghiou, et al. Absence o f nasal bone in fetuses with trisomy 21 at 11-14 weeks of gestation: An observational study. Lancet. 2001;358:1665-7.
18. Cicero S, Curcio P, Rembouskos G, et al. Maxillary length at 11-14 weeks of gestation in fetuses with trisomy 21. Ultrasound Obstet Gynecol. 2004;24:19-22.
19. Kossof G, Griffiths KA, Dixon CE. Is the quality of transvaginal images superior to transabdominal ones under matched conditions? Ultrasound Obstet Gynecol. 1991;1:29-35.
20. Pennell RG, Needleman L, Pajak T. Prospective comparison of vaginal and abdominal sonography in normal early pregnancy. J Ultrasound Med. 1991;10: 63-7.
21. Gershoni-Baruch R, Scher A, Itskovitz J, et al. The physical and psychomotor development of children conceived by IVF and exposed to high-frequency vaginal ultrasonography (6.5 MHz) in the first trimester of pregnancy. Ultrasound Obstet Gynecol. 1991;1:21-8.
22. Kossof G. Contentious issues in safety of diagnostic ultrasound: Editorial. Ultrasound Obstet Gynecol. 1997;10: 151-5.
23. EFSUMB (Clinical Safety Statement for Diagnostic Ultrasound). efsumb@compuser.co. 1998.
24. Montenegro N. First trimester ultrasound. Presented at the Euro-Team Early Pregnancy 2nd Post-Graduate Course, Porto, Portugal. 1993.
25. Gruboeck K, Zosmer N, Jurkovic D. Ultrasound features of early pregnancy development. In Jurkovic D, Jauniaux E (Eds). Ultrasound and Early Pregnancy. New York: Parthenon Publishing. 1996. pp. 41-52.
26. Montenegro N, Beires J, Campos I, et al. The human development along the first trimester of intra-uterine life. The contribution of transvaginal endosonography. Prog Diagn Prenat. 1994;6:24-44.
27. O'Rahilly R, Muller F. Ventricular system and choroid plexuses of the human brain during the embryonic period proper. Am J Anat. 1990;189:285-302.
28. Larsen WJ. Human Embryology. New York: Churchill Livingstone. 1993:375-418.
29. Achiron R, Achiron A. Transvaginal ultrasonic assessment of the early fetal brain. Ultrasound Obstet Gynecol. 1991;1:336-44.
30. Blaas HG, Eik-Nes SH, Kiserud T, et al. Early development of the hindbrain: A longitudinal ultrasound study from 7–12 weeks of gestation. Ultrasound Obstet Gynecol. 1995;5:151-60.
31. Goldstein SR. Embryonic ultrasonographic measurements: Crown–rump length revisited. Am J Obstet Gynecol. 1991;165:497-501.
32. Exalto N. Early human nutrition. Eur J Obstet Gynecol Reprod Med. 1995;61:3-6.
33. Braithwaite JM, Amstrong MA, Economides L. Assessment of fetal anatomy at 12 to 13 weeks of gestation by trans-abdominal and transvaginal sonography. Br J Obstet Gynaecol. 1996;103:82-5.
34. Snijders RJM, Noble P, Sebire N, et al. UK multicentre project on assessment of risk of trisomy 21 by maternal age and fetal nuchal translucency thckness at 10-14 weeks of gestation. Lancet. 1998;351:343-6.
35. Bonilla-Musoles F. Three-dimensional visualization of the human embryo: A potential revolution in prenatal diagnosis. Ultrasound Obstet Gynecol. 1996;7:393-7.
36. Wilcox AJ, Weinberg CR, Baird DD. Timing of sexual intercourse in relation to ovulation. N Engl J Med. 1995;333:1517-21.
37. Vollebergh JHA, Jongsma HW, van Dongen PWJ. The accuracy of ultrasonic measurement of fetal crown–rump length. Eur J Obstet Gynecol Reprod Med. 1989;30:253-6.
38. Robinson HP, Fleming JEE. A critical evaluation of sonar crown–rump length measurements. Br J Obstet Gynaecol. 1975;82: 702-10.
39. Lasser DM, Peisner DB, Vollebergh JHA, et al. First trimester fetal biometry using transvaginal sonography. Ultrasound Obstet Gynecol. 1993;3:104-8.

40. Daya S. Accuracy of gestational age estimation by means of fetal crown–rump length measurement. Am J Obstet Gynecol. 1993;168:903-8.

41. Parker AJ, Davies P, Newton JR. Assessment of gestational age of the Asian fetus by the sonar measurement of crown–rump length and biparietal diameter. Br J Obstet Gynaecol. 1982;89:836-8.

42. Wisser J, Dirschedl P, Krone S. Estimation of gestational age by transvaginal sonographic measurement of greatest embryonic length in dated human embryos. Ultrasound Obstet Gynecol. 1994;4:457-62.

43. Kuhn P, Brizot ML, Pandya PP, et al. Crown–rump length in chromosomally abnormal fetus at 10 to 13 weeks' gestation. Am J Obstet Gynecol. 1995;172:32-5.

44. Eik-Nes SH, Okland O, Aure JC, et al. Ultrasound screening in pregnancy: A randomized controlled trial. Lancet. 1984;1:347-54.

45. Gomez KJ, Copel JA. Routine ultrasound screening. Curr Opin Obstet Gynecol. 1994;6:426-9.

46. Mongelli M, Wilcox M, Gardosi J. Estimating the date of confinement: ultrasonographic biometry versus certain menstrual dates. Am J Obstet Gynecol. 1996;174:278-81.

47. Campbell S, Newman GB. Growth of the fetal biparietal diameter during normal pregnancy. J Obstet Gynaecol Br Commonw. 1971;78:513-9.

48. Levi S, Smets P. Intrauterine fetal growth studied by ultrasonic biparietal measurements. Acta Obstet Gynecol Scand. 1973; 52:193-8.

49. Skupski DW, Chervenak FA, McCullough LB. A clinical and ethical evaluation of routine obstetric ultrasound. Curr Opin Obstet Gynecol. 1994;6:435-9.

50. Montenegro N, Pereira Leite L. Fetal cerebellar measurements in second trimester ultrasonography—clinical value. J Perinat Med. 1989;17:365-9.

51. Luke B. The changing pattern of multiple births in the United States: maternal and infant characteristics, 1973 and 1990. Obstet Gynecol. 1994;84:101-6.

52. Minakami H, Sato I. Reestimating date of delivery in multifetal pregnancies. J Am Med Assoc. 1996;275:1432-4.

53. Sepulveda W, Sebire NJ, Hughes K, et al. The lambda sign at 10–14 weeks of gestation as a predictor of chorionicity in twin pregnancies. Ultrasound Obstet Gynecol. 1996;7:421-3.

54. Embom JA. Twin pregnancy with intrauterine death of one twin. Am J Obstet Gynecol. 1985;152:424-8.

55. Nicolaides KH, Pettersen H. Fetal therapy. Curr Opin Obstet Gynecol. 1994,6:468-71.

56. Evans MI, Dommergues M, Johnson MP, et al. Multifetal pregnancy reduction and selective termination. Curr Opin Obstet Gynecol. 1995;7:126-9

57. D'Alton ME, Dudley DK. The ultrasonographic prediction of chorionicity in twin gestation. Am J Obstet Gynecol. 1989;160:557-61.

58. Sampson A, de Crespigny LC. Vanishing twins: The frequency of spontaneous fetal reduction of a twin pregnancy. Ultrasound Obstet Gynecol. 1992;2:107-9.

59. Souka A, Snijders RJM, Novakov A, et al. Defects and syndromes in chromosomally normal fetuses with increased nuchal tarslucency at 10-14 weeks of gestation. Ultrasound Obstet Gynecol. 1998;11:391-400.

60. Hyett JA, Noble PL, Snijders RJM, et al. Fetal heart rate in trisomy 21 and other chromosomal abnormalities at 10–14 weeks of gestation. Ultrasound Obstet Gynecol. 1996;7:239-44.

61. Bindra R, Heath V, Liao A, et al. One-stop clinic for assessment of risk of trisomy 21 at 11-14 weeks: A prospective study of 15030 pregnancies. Ultrasound Obstet Gynecol. 2002;20:219-25.

62. Nicolaides KH. Nuchal translucency and other first-trimester sonographic markers of chromosomal abnormalities. Am J Obstet Gynecol. 2004;191:45-67.

63. Hyett JA, Moscoso G, Papapanagiotou G, et al. Abnormalities of the heart and great arteries in chromosomally normal fetuses with increased nuchal translucency thickness at 11–13 weeks of gestation. Ultrasound Obstet Gynecol. 1996;7:245-50.

64. Montenegro N, Matias A, Areias JC, et al. Ductus venosus revisited: A Doppler blood flow evaluation in the first trimester of pregnancy. Ultrasound Med Biol. 1997;23:171-6.

65. Montenegro N, Matias A, Areias JC, et al. Early cardiac failure as a putative pathogenic mechanism for increased nuchal translucency. Ultrasound Obstet Gynecol. 1996;8(Suppl. 1):111.

66. Montenegro N, Matias A, Areias JC, et al. Increased fetal nuchal translucency: Possible involvement of early cardiac failure. Ultrasound Obstet Gynecol. 1997;10:265-8.

67. Murta CG, Moron AF, Avila MA, et al. Application of ductus venosus Doppler velocimetry for the detection of fetal aneuploidy in the frist trimester of pregnancy. Fetal Diagn Ther. 2002;17: 308-14

68. Zoppi MA, Putzolu M, Ibba RM, et al. First trimester ductus venosus velocimetryin relation to nuchal translucency thickness and fetal karyotype. Fetal Diagn Ther. 2002;17:52-7.

69. Toyama JM, Brizot ML, Liao AW, et al. Ductus venosus blood fow assessment at 11 to 14 weeks of gestation and fetal outcome. Ultrasound Obstet Gynecol. 2004;23:341-5.

70. Timor-Tritsch IE, Monteagudo A, Peisner DB. High-frequency transvaginal sonographic examination for the potential malformation assessment of the 9-week to 14-week fetus. J Clin Ultrasound. 1992;20:231-8.

71. Campbell S, Johnstone FD, Holt EM, et al. Anencephaly: early ultrasonic diagnosis and active management. Lancet. 1972;2: 1226-7.

72. Rottem S. IRONFAN—a sonographic window into the natural history of fetal anomalies. Ultrasound Obstet Gynecol. 1995;5:361-3.

94

Hemodynamic Assessment of Early Pregnancy

LT Merce, MJ Barco, S Kupesic

INTRODUCTION

Under the title "hemodynamic assessment of early pregnancy" we wish to refer to the study of the changes in the uteroplacental, intervillous, fetal-placental, embryo-fetal and luteal ovarian circulations during the first trimester of normal pregnancies.

Although several invasive methods have been applied to experimental animal models to the study of early gestation hemodynamics, in the human species it has only been possible since the arrival of Doppler examination. This method has experienced great technological improvements from the continuous and pulsed Doppler to the 3D power Doppler angiography.

The transvaginal color Doppler has proven to be a highly efficient technique to the assessment of the placental, embryo-fetal and luteal circulations during the first trimester. Nevertheless, the theoretical risk of adverse biological effects on the embryo has restricted significantly its use during this pregnancy period. The 3D Doppler angiography represents a new technological advance that applies the ALARA principle, being minimal the acquisition time of the angiographic volumes. Moreover, it is a proceeding only available in high technological level equipments that fulfill precisely all the international regulations about ultrasound safety. Therefore, it seems necessary to have at our disposal new reports that guarantee the possibility of a careful but more liberal use of this new method during the early pregnancy.

UTEROPLACENTAL BLOOD FLOW

The uteroplacental circulation is composed by the uterine vessels and their intramyometrial branches: arcuate, radial and spiral endometrial arteries. The spiral arteries will become uteroplacental arteries under the trophoblastic invasion process along the first-half of pregnancy.

The uteroplacental blood flow increases progressively during the first trimester of normal gestations to accomplish the great demands imposed during the organogenesis period.[1] The invasion of the radial and spiral arteries by the cytotrophoblast is the mechanism to secure the progressive increase of the utero-placental perfusion. These arteries loose their autoregulation ability and increase their diameters to become the uteroplacental arteries.[2]

The spiral and radial arteries are those showing the greatest and significant changes under Doppler examination as they are the target vessels of the trophoblastic invasion.[3-7] From the ultrasonographic detection of the gestational sac it is possible to depict a color signal coming out it and getting inside the myometrium that was named the "comet sign" (Figs 94.1A and B).[5-7] The flow velocity waveform (FVW) of these arteries shows a low vascular resistance and usually the protodiastolic notch is absent.

The proximity of the spiral and radial arteries in the placental basal plate rends its differentiation impossible. For that reason we call them retrochorionic arteries. Other authors use the term of subchorionic and peritrophoblastic arteries.[8,9] Out of the placental site the radial arteries are placed at the myometrial internal third. The arcuate arteries run along the myometrial external third near the serosa. From the seventh week onwards it is possible to identify through transvaginal color Doppler the spiral, radial and arcuate signals in the 100% of the examinations.[10,11] The uterine arteries can be explored on both sides of the cervical isthmus. The FVW of the uterine arteries shows a high resistance with a protodiastolic notch usually present (Figs 94.2A to D).

The retrochorionic arteries blood flow experiences a gradual increase during the normal first trimester of gestation. The resistance index diminishes from 0.52 ± 0.03 at the 4th week until 0.31 ± 0.05 at the 15th week (Fig. 94.3), whereas the systolic and diastolic velocities increase progressively.[5,6] Changes at the placental vascular bed will affect in a retrograde way the entire uteroplacental vascular tree. The blood flow will also increase in the radial, arcuate and uterine arteries. The vascular resistance decreases gradually in all the uteroplacental vessels during the normal first trimester of pregnancy, but it increases along with the distance from the chorionic implantation site[8-15] (Figs 94.2 A to D). The average resistance index of the uterine arteries falls from 0.94 ± 0.08 at the 5th week until 0.76 ± 0.09 at the 12th week, while the maximum systolic velocity increases from 43.67 ± 16.72 cm/s until 79.13 ± 26.33 cm/s in the same period of time (Fig. 94.4).[3,4] The protodiastolic notch is always present at the beginning but it will disappear in the second trimester.

The uteroplacental blood flow, as evaluated by the retrochorionic vascular resistance, increases to a 36% during the first trimester of normal pregnancies. This percentage is greater than the 30% observed during all the remaining pregnancy and doubles the 16% attributed to the second trophoblastic wave between the 15th and 20th weeks (Fig. 94.5).[16] This fact demonstrates the importance of the vascular changes taking place in this gestational period and its unquestionable value for a successful pregnancy outcome.

INTERVILLOUS BLOOD FLOW

From an embryological point of view, the intervillous circulation seems to be initiated around the 12th day of embryo development, when the maternal blood flows inside the syncytiotrophoblastic lacunae.[17] Nonetheless, Doppler studies have produced conflicting results.

Jauniaux et al.[18,19] and Jaffe and Woods.[20] using transvaginal color Doppler did not find intervillous blood flow before 12 gestational weeks. Trophoblastic plugs would occlude the spiral arteries lumen[21,22] to maintain a relatively hypoxic environment to

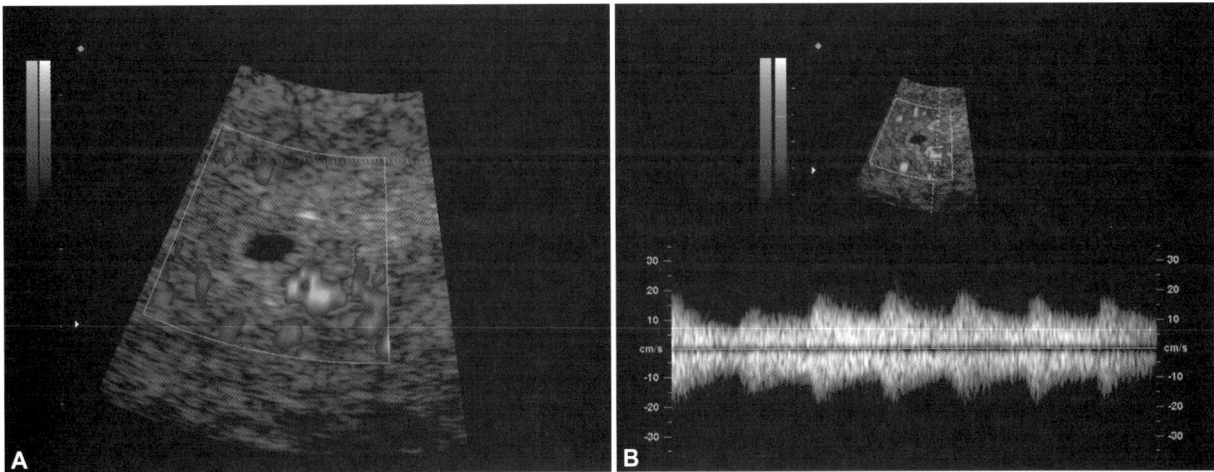

Figs 94.1A and B: (A) Color map of the retrochorionic circulation of a gestational sac of 4 mm. The blood flow increase in the spiral and radial arteries depicts the "comet sign"; (B) FVW of the retrochorionic circulation in the same gestational sac

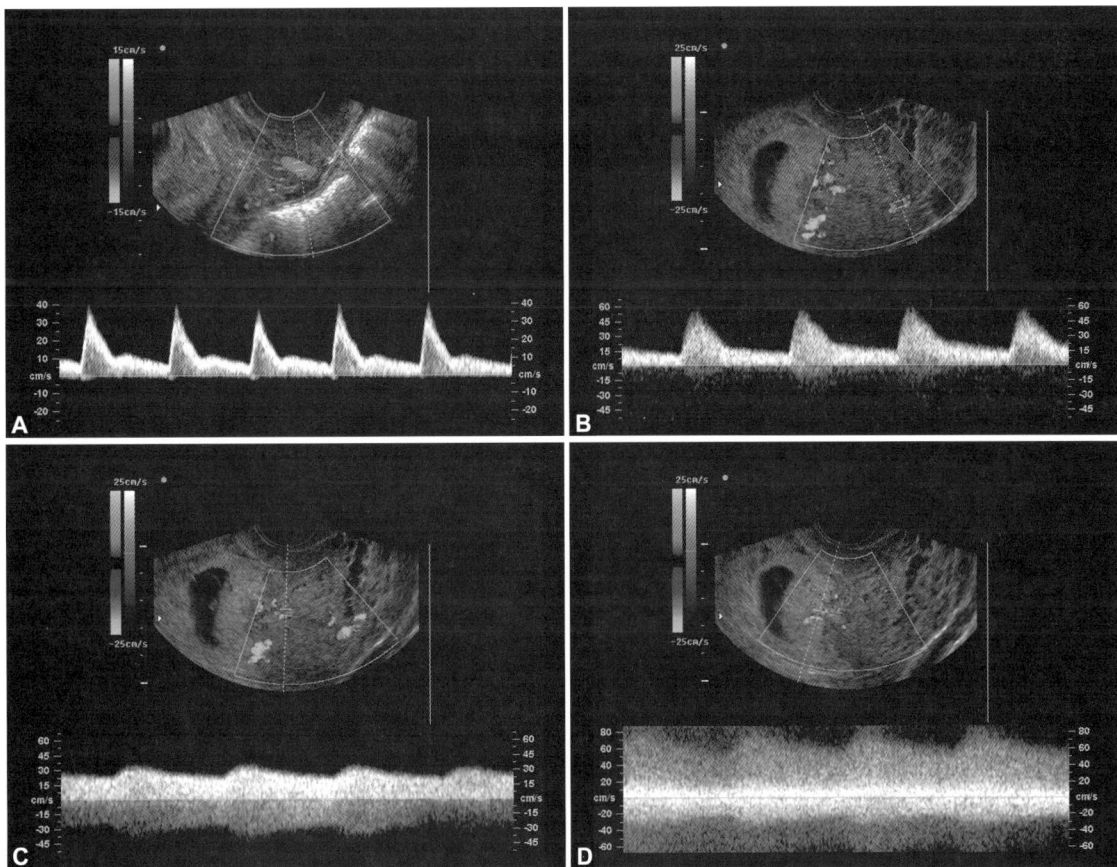

Figs 94.2A to D: FVW of the uterine artery in a normal gestation of 8 weeks of amenorrhea. (A) arcuate artery; (B) radial artery; (C) and spiral or uteroplacental arteries; (D) The vascular resistance increases as the distance from the placental insertion site increases

favor the embryo development.[23] The intervillous blood flow was only present in miscarriages.[24,25]

Kurjak and Kupesic.[26] Valentin et al.[14] and Mercé et al.[5,6] using a similar technology were capable to detect the intervillous blood flow from the 6th normal pregnancy week onwards. Two patterns of flow have been registered: A continuous venous type and a pulsatile arterial type, this last one probably next to the uteroplacental arteries entrance (Figs 94.6A and B).

The maximum venous velocities in the intervillous space (IVS) are low and increase gradually during all the first trimester from 2 ± 0.77 cm/s at 6 weeks to 5.12 ± 2.23 at 12 weeks (Figs 94.6A and B).[5,6] For some authors[27] that increase from the 10th week

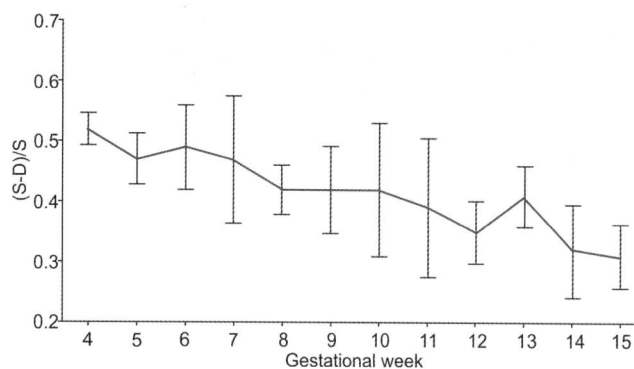

Fig. 94.3: Resistance index of the retrochorionic arteries (spiral–radial) during early gestation (mean ± SD)

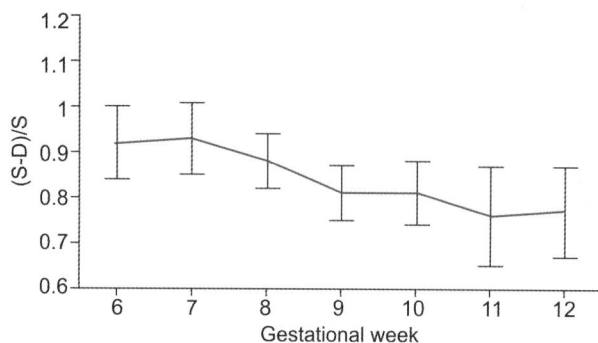

Fig. 94.4: Average resistance index from both uterine arteries during the early pregnancy (mean ± SD)

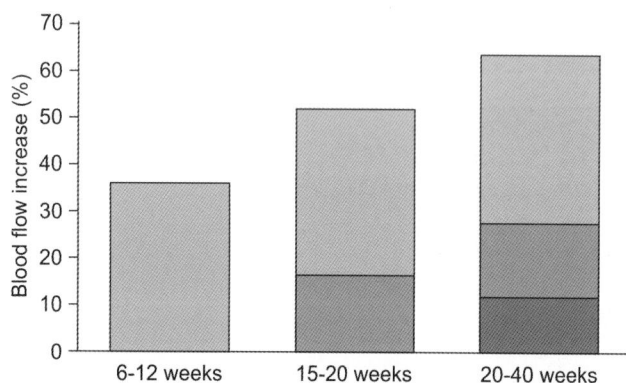

Fig. 94.5: Percentage of blood flow increase at the placental site at different stages of normal pregnancy. During the first trimester a decrease in the vascular resistance takes place, which is greater than the rest of gestation

Figs 94.6A and B: Doppler signal from the intervillous circulation of arterial type: (A) On seventh week, and venous type; (B) On ninth week

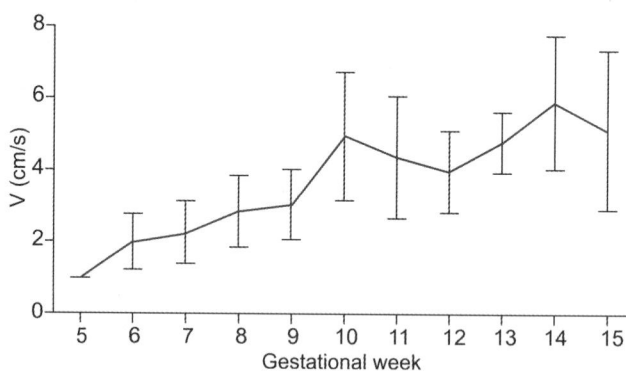

Fig. 94.7: Venous maximum velocity of the intervillous circulation during the normal early pregnancy (mean ± SD)

occurs simultaneously with the vitelline circulation decline (Fig. 94.7). The arterial FVW in the IVS does not experience significant changes during the first trimester.[14,26,27]

Our recent experience with 3D PDA confirms our previous results with transvaginal color Doppler. The VOCAL (Virtual Organ Computer Aided Analysis) technology allows the differentiation of the IVS and retrochorionic circulations and their independent assessment (Figs 94.8A to D). We have observed a progressive and significant increase in the vascularization, flow and vascularization flow indices between the 6th week and 12th week in normal pregnancies (Figs 94.9A to C).

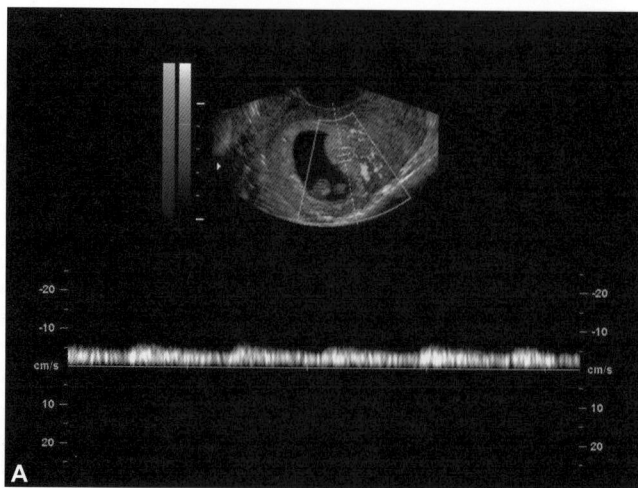

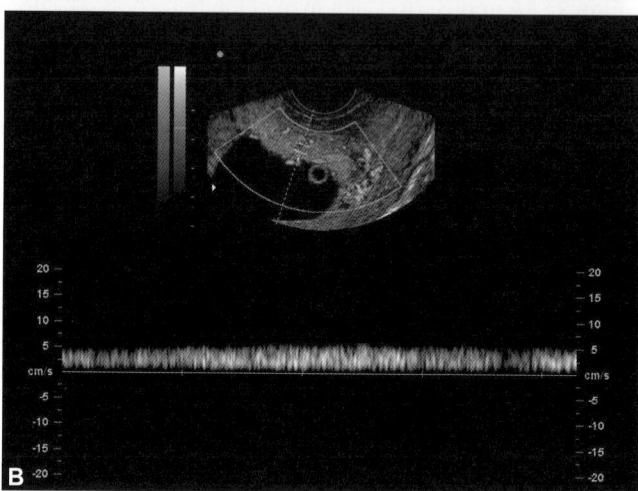

These findings are in accordance with a gradual disappearance of the trophoblastic plugs from the spiral arteries during the first trimester. That would produce an increase in the Doppler signals at the chorion frondosum (vascularization index) and an increase in their intensity (flow index) that constitute the increase in the IVS blood flow in this period. Jauniaux et al.[28] in their last publication seem to admit this possibility that we are defending for more than 10 years.

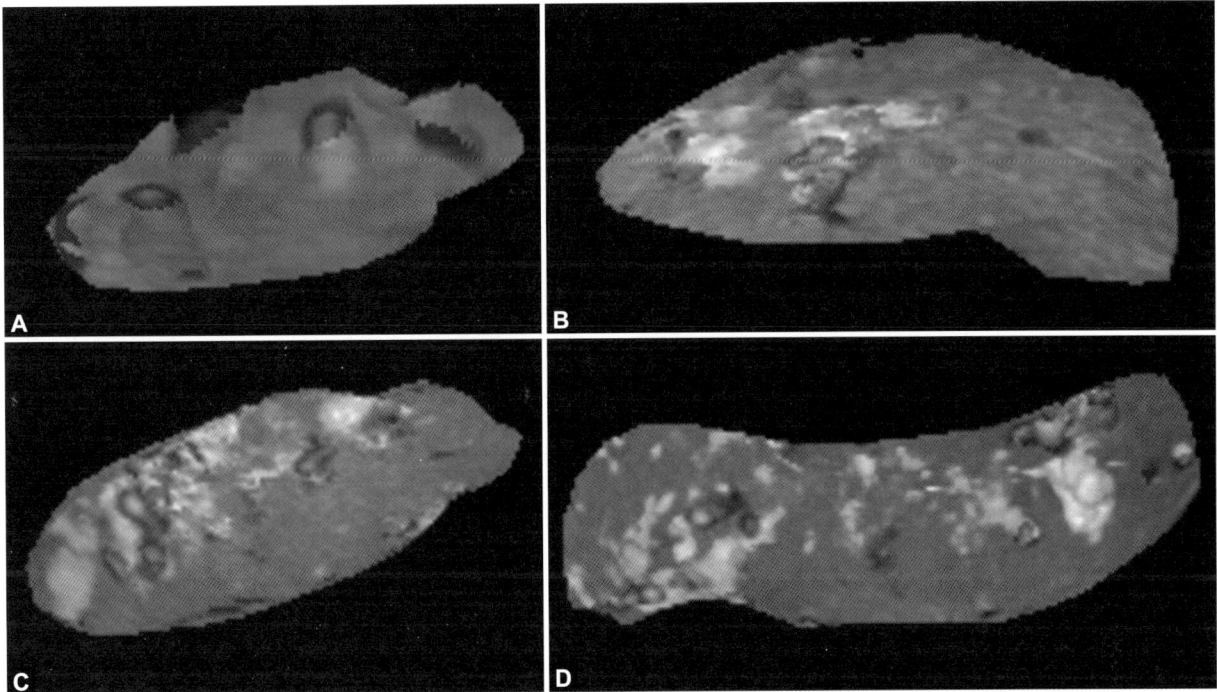

Figs 94.8A to D: 3D power Doppler angiography of the intervillous flow at 6 weeks: (A) 8 weeks; (B) 10 weeks; (C) and 12 weeks; (D) of normal pregnancies

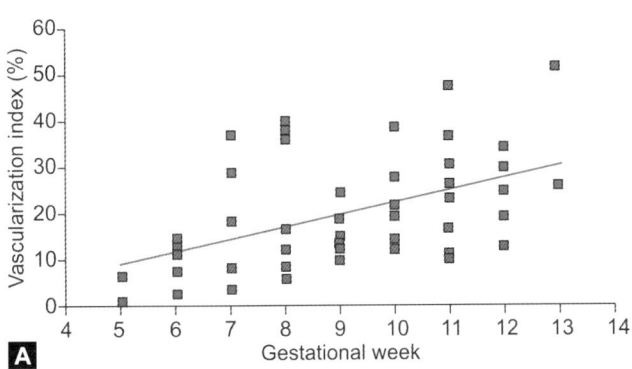

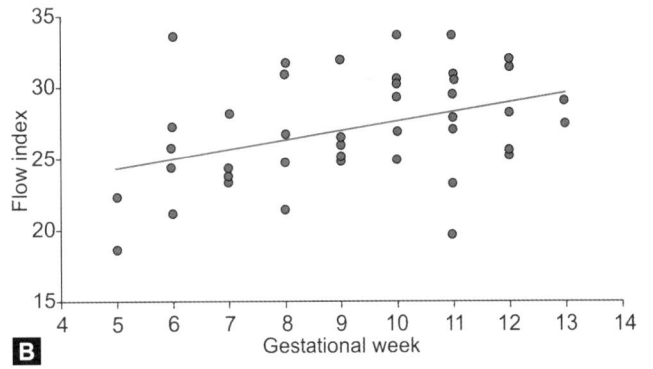

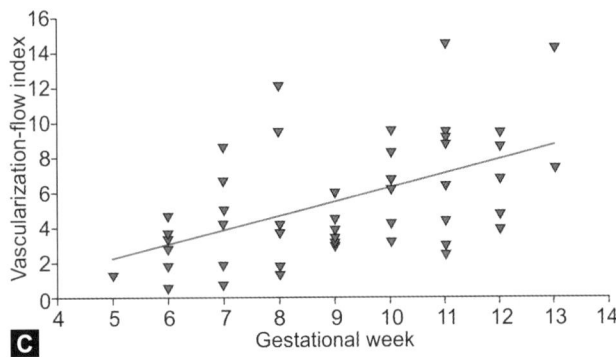

Figs 94.9A to C: Vascularization index. (A) flow index; (B) and vascularization-flow index; (C) of the intervillous circulation during the normal first trimester of pregnancy

BLOOD FLOW OF THE YOLK SAC

The circulation of the yolk sac precedes the fetal-placental or umbilical circulations in the embryonic development.[17]

The yolk sac circulation can be detected by Doppler from the 5th week of amenorrhea onwards.[29-31] It is feasible to integrate the Doppler signal in the 44%[3] to 67%[27] of normal gestations. During the sixth week it could be difficult to differentiate from the initial umbilical signal.[30] Its FVW is ofarterial type without diastolic flow (Fig. 94.10). The blood flow of the yolk sac is characterized by low velocities (between 3 cm/s and 7 cm/s) and a pulsatility index ranging from 2.19 to 4.78.[30] The yolk sac blood flow diminishes from the 10th week onwards, together with the size of the sac and coincides with the blood flow increase to the IVS.[27]

FETAL-PLACENTAL BLOOD FLOW

The fetal-placental or umbilical circulation links the villous vascular system with the embryo-fetal vascular system. The umbilical artery Doppler signal is detected at the end of the 5th or the beginning of the 6th weeks of amenorrhea, when the embryo starts to be sonographically detectable. The umbilical artery FVW is characterized by not showing a diastolic component until the 10th week of amenorrhea. The umbilical diastolic flow appears in a small percentage of cases from the 11th week onwards and will be constantly present from the 14th week onwards (Figs 94.11A and B).[5,6,8,30,32-34]

From the 7th week onwards it is possible to register the umbilical vein signal. The umbilical venous blood flow shows a characteristically undulated profile during the first trimester (Fig. 94.11). The umbilical vein pulsations are physiological in this period of pregnancy and will disappear from the 11th week onwards.[35,36]

The umbilical artery blood flow increases significantly alongside the entire first trimester of normal gestations.[5,6,8,30,32-34] Between the 6th week and 14th week the maximum systolic velocity is increased from 5.63 ± 2.26 cm/s at 6 weeks to 21.28 ± 4.6 cm/s at 14 weeks, whereas the pulsatility index falls from 4.4 ± 1.1 to 1.38 ± 0.34 (Fig. 94.12).

The decrease in the umbilical artery resistance during the first 12 weeks of gestation is essentially due to the maturation of the villous vascular tree. The appearance of diastolic velocities would explain this fact. The beginning of the fetal period will lead to increasing demands of oxygen and nutrients that will be supplied by an improvement in the villous transfer.

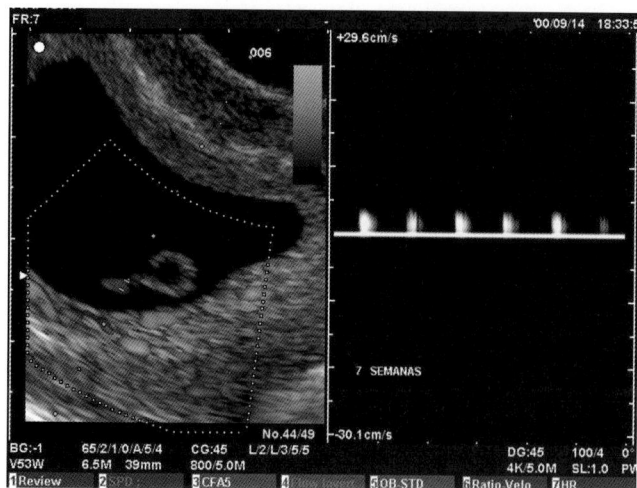

Fig. 94.10: Doppler signal from the yolk sac circulation on the 7th pregnancy weeks

EMBRYO-FETAL BLOOD FLOW

Transvaginal color Doppler allows the evaluation of the whole intraembryonic circulation, but only the blood flow in the aorta, cerebral arteries and ductus venosus have been studied.

The trajectory of the aorta can be clearly visualized from the seventh gestational week onwards. As it occurs to the umbilical artery, its Doppler signal is characterized by the absence of diastolic velocities, that begin to appear around the 13th week, being always present at the 14th and 15th weeks (Fig. 94.13).[8,30,33,34] The aortic blood flow increases progressively during the whole first trimester, as it is proven by the augment of systolic velocity and the reduction of the pulsatility index (Fig. 94.14).[8,30,33,34]

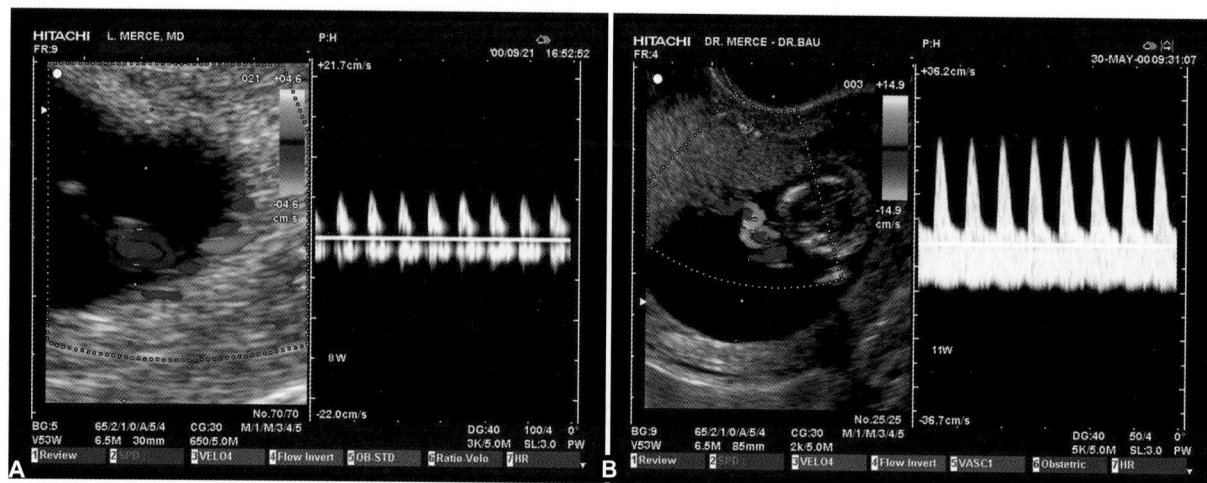

Figs 94.11A and B: Umbilical artery Doppler on 8th (A) and 11th (B) gestational weeks. At the inferior channel, the undulating profile of the umbilical venous signal can be appreciated

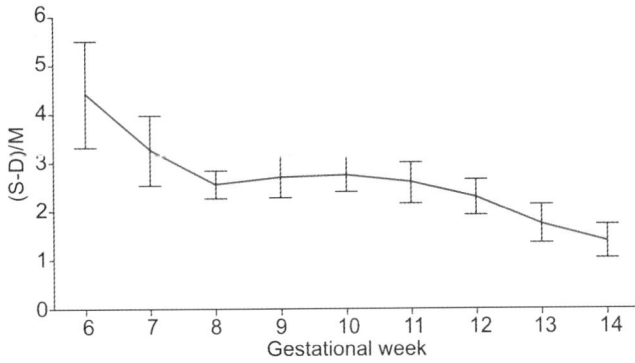

Fig. 94.12: Umbilical artery pulsatility index during early pregnancy (mean ± SD)

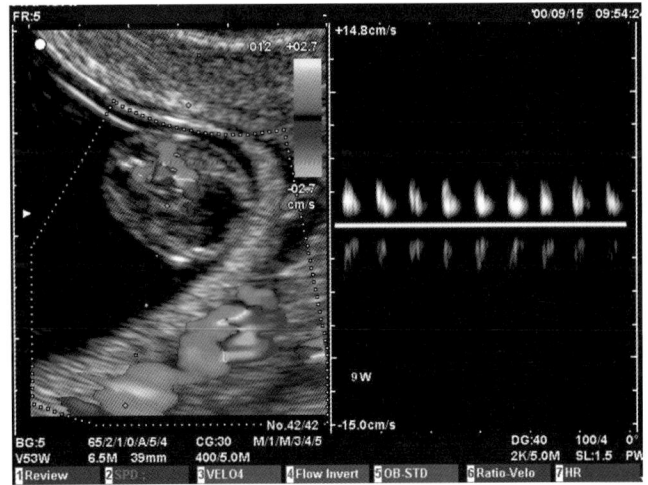

Fig. 94.15: Mean cerebral artery FVW in a normal pregnancy of 9 weeks

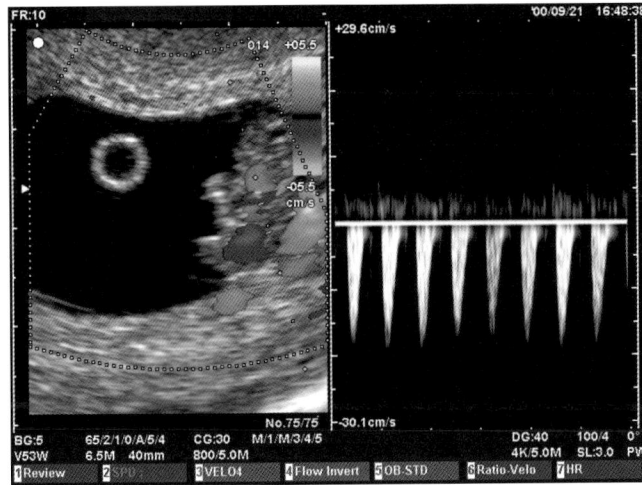

Fig. 94.13: Color signal and FVW of the embryonic aorta in the ninth gestational week

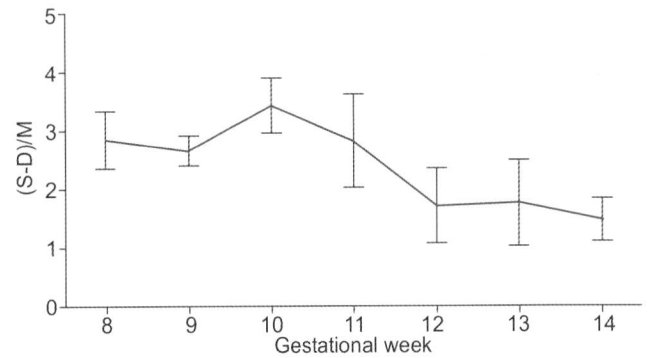

Fig. 94.16: Pulsatility index of the mean cerebral artery during normal early pregnancy (mean ± SD)

decreases steadily from 2.86 ± 0.49 at the 8th week to 1.49 ± 0.37 at the 14th week (Fig. 94.16).

The cerebral arteries show diastolic velocities from the 11th week onwards, in contrast to their absence in the umbilical and aorta arteries. The ratio between the umbilical and cerebral pulsatility indices is usually inferior to 1 during the first trimester.[37] These data suggest that the cerebral blood flow is independent from the vascular changes taking place in the aorta and the villous network. This auto regulation mechanism of the cerebral circulation during the early pregnancy should be aiming to secure a proper blood supply to the growing fetal brain.

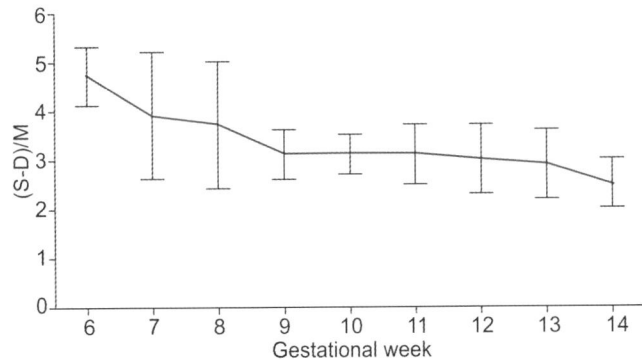

Fig. 94.14: Pulsatility index of the embryonic aorta during normal first trimester of pregnancy

Intracerebral signals can be registered by transvaginal color Doppler in the eighth week of amenorrhea. However, the centrifuge trajectory of the mean cerebral arteries can be depicted only from the 10th week. The cerebral blood flow increases between the 8th and 14th pregnancy weeks. Systolic velocities are present from the 11th week onwards. They are visible in an 80% of the 12th week registers and are constantly present during the following weeks (Fig. 94.15). The maximum systolic velocity is 4.97 cm/s at the 8th week, rising to 19.08 ± 5.21 at the 14th. The Pulsatility Index

The ductus venosus is a circulatory shunt connecting the umbilical vein with the inferior cava vein. The Doppler signal shows a forward flow and triphasic morphology with three components: (1) ventricular systole; (2) early diastole with passive ventricular filling; and (3) late diastole with a nadir in the signal that reflects the active ventricular filling due to the atrial contraction. Although all three components of the ductus venosus FVW can be identified from the 9th week onwards, its visualization is more constant from the 12th week to 15th week onwards (Fig. 94.17).[38] The blood flow increases progressively in the ductus from the 9th week all along the entire pregnancy. Blood flow velocities increase as the vascular resistance decreases.[39,40]

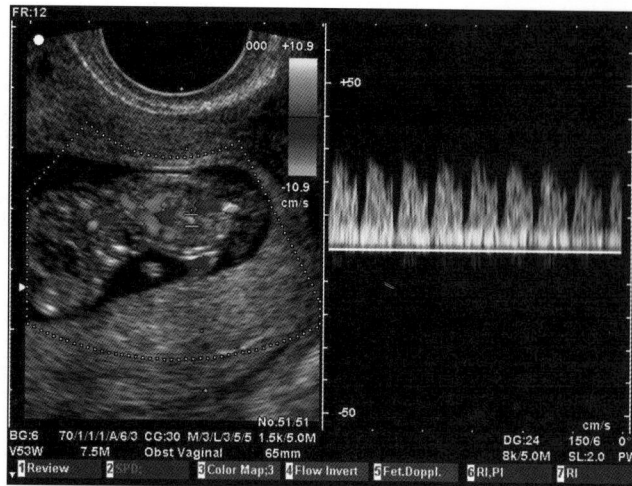

Fig. 94.17: Normal Doppler recording of the ductus venosus on 11th week

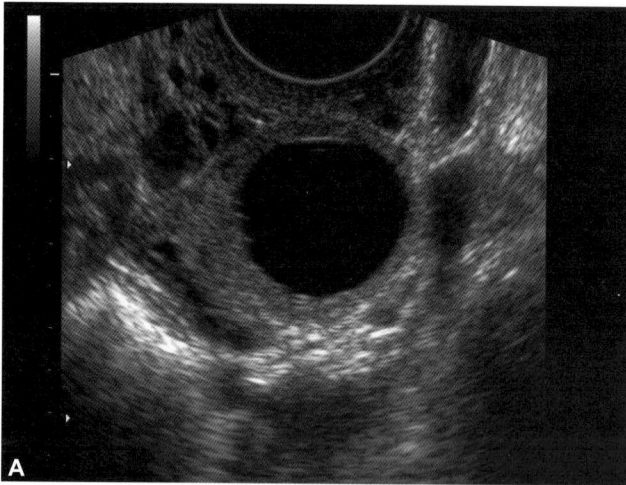

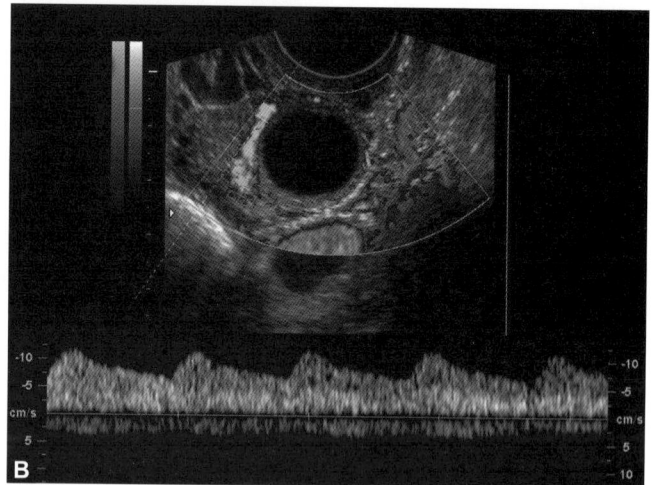

Figs 94.18A and B: Sonolucent corpus luteum image (A) and color signal and FVW; (B) in a normal 5th week gestation

The pulsatility increase in the ductus venosus at the end of the first trimester could indicate the presence of a fetal chromosomal anomaly associated or not to a congenital cardiac malformation.[41,42] It has been suggested as a marker for chromosomal abnormalities independent of the nuchal translucency,[43] and associated with this one it could increase the specificity by maintaining an adequate detection rate.[44]

LUTEAL OVARIAN BLOOD FLOW

The luteal function is essential during the early gestation, given that its hormonal secretion sustains the pregnancy until the functional take over of the placenta. Along the first twelve gestational weeks the luteal blood flow can be easily evaluated by transvaginal color Doppler.

The corpus luteum is visualized from 66%[37] up to 100% of pregnancies.[45] In the majority of cases it has an anechogenic appearance (77%) which can hinder the differential diagnosis with a persistent follicle.[37] The Doppler examination confirms the gestational corpus luteum when it shows a "luteal conversion" of the FVW, quite similar to that of the second half of the ovarian cycle (Figs 94.18A and B).[16]

The luteal blood flow during the early pregnancy is similar to that of the luteal phase of the ovarian cycle and there are no significant differences in the velocimetric parameters.[16,46,47] Maximum systolic

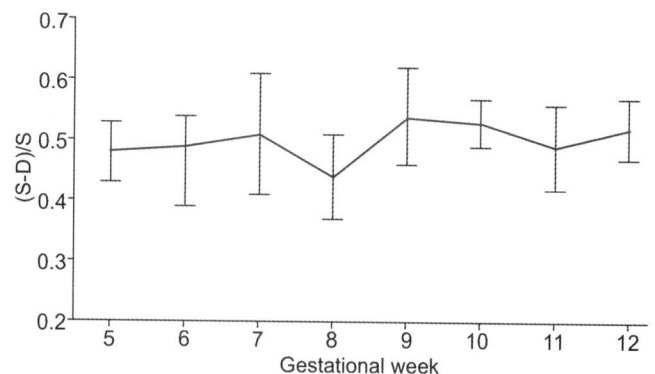

Fig. 94.19: Resistance index of the normal corpus luteum vascularity during the first trimester of normal gestations (mean ± 5D)

velocities are usually high.[46-48] The helical or nutricia artery shows the highest systolic velocities and a low variability. The resistance index ranges from 0.48 ± 0.05 at the 5th week to 0.52 ± 0.05 at the 12th week, with a slight tendency to the increase of the intraovarian vascular resistance (Fig. 94.19).[16]

Recently, the 3D power Doppler angiography allows the representation of the luteal angiogenesis and the study of the blood flow in a more real and precise way (Figs 94.20A and B).

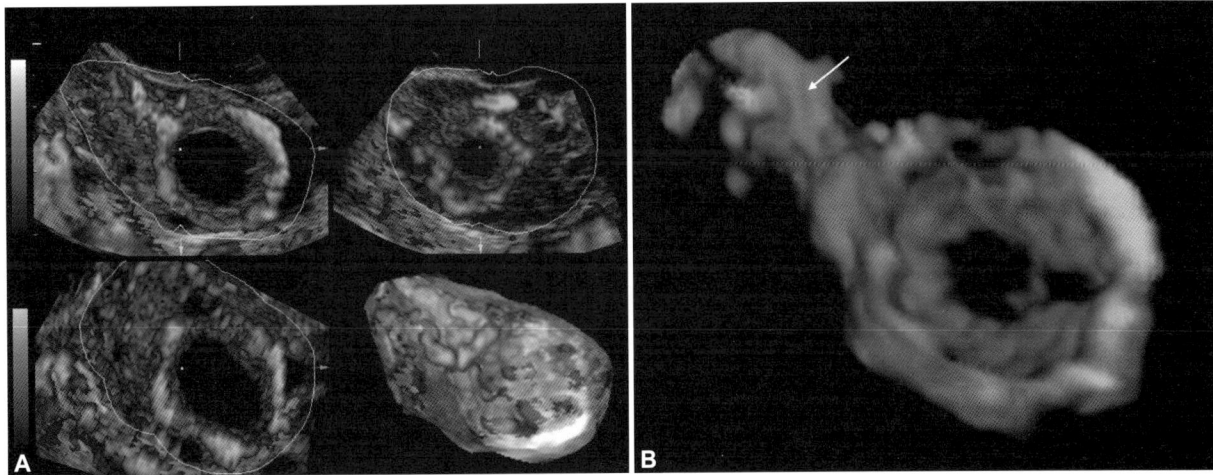

Figs 94.20A and B: Luteal circulation assessment during the early pregnancy by 3D power Doppler angiography. (A) Acquisition technique applying the VOCAL software; (B) Three-dimensional angiographic rendering of the vascular network in a gestational corpus lluteum. The arrow points to the helical artery

REFERENCES

1. Greiss FC Jr, Anderson SG. Uterine blood flow during early ovine pregnancy. Am J Obstet Gynecol. 1970;106:30-8.
2. Reynolds SRM. Gestation mechanisms. Ann NY Acad Sci. 1959;75:691-9.
3. Mercé LT, Barco MJ, de la Fuente F. Doppler velocimetry measured in retrochorionic space and uterine arteries during early human pregnancy. Acta Obstet Gynecol Scand. 1989;8:603-7.
4. Mercé LT. Velocimetría Doppler en la gestación precoz normal y patológica: Estudio del proceso de placentación. En: Carrera JM y cols (eds). Doppler en Obstetricia. Hemodinamia perinatal. Barcelona: Masson-Salvat Medicina. 1992;127-45.
5. Mercé LT, Bau S, García del Real E. Estudio Doppler en el diagnóstico prenatal precoz. Progr Diag Pren. 1994;6:63-77.
6. Mercé LT, Barco MJ, Bau S. Color Doppler sonographic assessment of placental circulation in the first trimester of normal pregnancy. J Ultrasound Med. 1996;15:135-42.
7. Mercé LT, Kupesic S, Kurjak A. Color Doppler assessment of implantation and early placentation. Prenat Neonat Med. 1999;4:94-112.
8. Kurjak A, Crvenkovic G, Salihagic A, et al. The assessment of normal early pregnancy by transvaginal color Doppler ultrasonography. J Clin Ultrasound. 1993;21:3-8.
9. Jaffe R, Woods JR. Color Doppler imaging and in vivo assessment of the anatomy and physilogy of the early uteroplacental circulation. Fertil Steril. 1993;60:293-7.
10. Predanic M, Zudenigo D, Funduk-Kurjak B, et al. Assessment of early normal pregnancy. In: Kurjak A (ed). An Atlas of transvaginal color Doppler. London: The Parthenon Publishing Group. 1994;5169.
11. Kurjak A, Zudenigo D. Circulación maternofetal incipiente visualizada mediante Doppler color transvaginal. En: Carrera JM, Kurjak A, eds. Medicina del embrión. Barcelona: Masson, 1997;77-84.
12. Jurkovic D, Jauniaux E, Kurjak A, et al. Transvaginal color Doppler assessment of the uteroplacental circulation in early pregnancy. Obstet Gynecol. 1991;77:365-9.
13. Coppens M, Loquet P, Kollen M, et al. Longitudinal evaluation of uteroplacental and umbilical blood flow changes in normal early pregnancy. Ultrasound Obstet Gynecol. 1996;7:114-21.
14. Valentín L, Sladkevicius P, Laurini R, et al. Uteroplacental and luteal circulation in normal first trimester pregnancies: Doppler ultrasonographic and morphologic study. Am J Obstet Gynecol. 1996;174:768-75.
15. Makikallio K, Tekay A, Jouppila P. Uteroplacental hemodynamics during early human pregnancy. Gynecol Obstet Invest. 2004;58:49-54.
16. Mercé LT. Velocimetría Doppler durante la gestación precoz. En: Mercé LT (ed). Ecografía Doppler en Obstetricia y Ginecología. Madrid: Interamericana McGraw-Hill. 1993;145-60.
17. Sadler TW. Langman: Embriología Médica, 7th ed. Madrid: Panamericana/Williams and Wilkins, 1996.
18. Jauniaux E, Jurkovic D, Campbell S. In vivo investigations of the anatomy and the physiology of early human circulation. Ultrasound Obstet Gynecol. 1991;1:435-45.
19. Jauniaux E, Jurkovic D, Campbell S, et al. Doppler ultrasonographic features of the developing placental circulation: Correlation with anatomic findings. Am J Obstet Gynecol. 1992;166:585-7.
20. Jaffe R, Woods JR. Color Doppler imaging and in vivo assessment of the anatomy and physiology of the early uteroplacental circulation. Fertil Steril. 1993;60:293-7.
21. Hustin J, Schaaps JP. Echocardiographic and anatomic studies of the maternotrophoblastic border during the first trimester of pregnancy. Am J Obstet Gynecol. 1987;157:162-8.
22. Hustin J, Schaaps JP, Lambotte R. Anatomical studies of the uteroplacental vascularization in the first trimester of pregnancy. Trophoblast Res. 1988;3:49-60.
23. Rodesch F, Simon P, Donner C, et al. Oxygen measurements in endometrial and trophoblastic tissues during early pregnancy. Obstet Gynecol. 1992;80:283-5.
24. Jauniaux E, Zaidi J, Jurkovic D, et al. Comparison of color Doppler features and pathological findings in complicated early pregnancy. Human Reprod. 1994;9:2432-7.
25. Jaffe R, Dorgan A, Abramowicz JS. Color Doppler imaging of the uteroplacental circulation in the first trimester: Value in predicting pregnancy failure or complication. AJR. 1995;164: 1255-8.
26. Kurjak A, Kupesic S. Doppler assessment of the intervillous blood flow in normal and abnormal early pregnancy. Obstet Gynecol. 1997;89:252-6.
27. Kurjak A, Kupesic S. Parallel Doppler assessment of yolk sac and intervillous circulation in normal pregnancy and missed abortion. Placenta. 1998;19:619-23.
28. Jauniaux E, Greenwold N, Hempstock J, et al. Comparison of ultrasonographyic and Doppler mapping of the intervillous circulation in normal and abnormal early pregnancies. Fertil Steril. 2003;79:100-6.

29. Kurjak A, Kupesic S, Kostovic L. Vascularization of yolk sac and vitelline duct in normal pregnancies studied by transvaginal color and pulsed Doppler. J Perinat Med. 1994;12:433-40.

30. Van Zalen-SprocK MM, van Vugt JMG, Colenbrander GJ, et al. First trimester uteroplacental and fetal blood flow velocity waveforms in normally developing fetuses: A longitudinal study. Ultrasound Obstet Gynecol. 1994;4:284-8.

31. Makikallio K, Tekay A, Jouppila P. Yolk sac and umbilicoplacental hemohynamics during early human embryonic development. Ultrasound Obstet Gynecol. 1999; 14:175-9.

32. Arduini D, Rizzo G. Umbilical artery velocity waveforms in early pregnancy: A transvaginal color Doppler study. J Clin Ultrasound. 1991;19:335-9.

33. Huisman TWA, Stewart PA, Wladimiroff JW. Doppler assessment of the normal early fetal circulation. Ultrasound Obstet Gynecol. 1992;2:300-5.

34. Alcázar JL, Laparte C, López-García G. Estudio de la circulación embrio-fetal en la gestación precoz normal mediante Doppler pulsado transvaginal. Progr Diag Pren. 1997;9:456-66.

35. Rizzo G, Arduini D, Romanini C. Umbilical vein pulsations: A physiologic finding in early gestation. Am J Obstet Gynecol. 1992;166:675-7.

36. Van Splunder P, Huisman TWA, De Ridder MAJ, et al. Fetal venous and arterial flow velocity waveforms between eight and twenty weeks of gestation. Pediatr Res. 1996;40:158-62.

37. Mercé LT. Estudio Doppler durante la gestación precoz. En: Kurjak A, Carrera JM (Eds). Ecografía en Medicina Materno-Fetal. Barcelona: Masson. 2000;199-212.

38. Huisman TWA, Steward PA, Wladimiroff JW, et al. Flow velocity waveforms in the ductus venosus, umbilical vein and inferior vena cava in normal fetuses at 12-15 weeks of gestation. Ultrasound Med Biol. 1993;19:441-5.

39. Kiserud T, Eik-Ness SH, Hellevik LR, et al. Ductus venosus: A longitudinal Doppler velocimetric study of the human fetus. J Matern Fetal Invest. 1992;2:5-11.

40. Huisman TWA, Stewart PA, Wladimiroff JW. Ductus venosus flow velocity waveforms in the human fetus: A Doppler study. Ultrasound Med Biol. 1992;18:33-7.

41. Montenegro N, Matias A, Areias JC, et al. Increased fetal nuchal translucency: Possible involvement of early cardiac failure. Ultrasound Obstet Gynecol. 1997;10: 265-8.

42. Matias A, Gomes C, Flack N, et al. Screening for chromosomal abnormalities at 10-14 weeks: The role of ductus venosus blood flow. Ultrasound Obstet Gynecol. 1998;12:380-4.

43. Borrell A, Antolín E, Costa D, et al. Abnormal ductus venosus blood flow in trisomy 21 fetuses during early pregnancy. Am J Obstet Gynecol. 1998;179:1612-7.

44. Antolín E, Comas C, Torrents M, et al. The role of ductus venosus blood flow assessment in screening for chromosomal abnormalities at 10-16 weeks of gestation. Ultrasound Obstet Gynecol. 2001;17(4):295-300.

45. Durfee SM, Frates MC. Sonographic spectrum of the corpus luteum in early pregnancy: Gray-scale, color, and pulsed Doppler appearance. J Clin Ultrasound. 1999;27:55-9.

46. Zalud I, Kurjak A. The assessment of luteal blood flow in pregnant and non-pregnant women by transvaginal color Doppler. J Perinat Med. 1990;18:215-21.

47. Alcázar JL, Acosta MJ, Laparte C, et al. Assessment of luteal blood flow in normal early pregnancy. J Ultrasound Med. 1996;15:53-6.

48. Parsons AK. Imaging the human corpus luteum. J Ultrasound Med. 2001;20:811-9.

CHAPTER

95

Ultrasonographic Signs of Miscarriage

JM Bajo Arenas, T Perez-Medina

INTRODUCTION

The recent advances in ultrasonographic technology along with the availability of high-frequency transvaginal transducers allows, every day more precisely, to emit precise diagnosis. For every sonographist, the decision of informing the sonographic exploration performed to a patient as corresponding to an interrupted pregnancy or embryonic demise represents a challenge. As more is the experience, more precociously can be confirmed that a pregnancy is actually not viable. It is not sensible to emit a diagnosis of miscarriage if any doubt exist, when most of the patients allows to wait without risk for their health. Nonetheless, it is good practice to write the diagnosis of suspicion in the clinical history to avoid unpleasant situations in the following sonographic exploration. Is it preferable to repeat the scan a few days later to inform the pregnancy like "not viable" if the diagnosis is not absolutely straightforward?

The problems for the sonographists, especially for the less experienced ones, arise when they are required to reach definitive conclusions in the presence of signs corresponding to a pregnancy of less time than expected for the last menstrual period (LMP) without the aid of a previous sonographic exploration. It should be interpreted if it is a pregnancy of less time or an abortion. Some of the data that can be obtained will help to emit a diagnosis, and in other situations, already in this first sonographic exploration should exist enough information to reach a definitive diagnosis, that is to say that does not require confirmation with a posterior sonographic exploration. Repetition of the sonographic exploration, 7–10 days later, should allow, in most of the cases, to reach a definitive diagnosis.

NORMAL DEVELOPMENT OF THE PREGNANCY IN THE FIRST TRIMESTER

Knowing the chronology of appearance of the visible embryonic structures with the sonography and its variations is relevant to know when the pregnancy is correctly evolving or not.

When findings that do not correspond to the gestational age are detected, the first thing to do should be to value the probability that an error exists in the LMP or that ovulation has not been produced in the 14th day of the cycle. In this situation, when the embryo is alive (positive heartbeat) the only responsibility is to correctly date the pregnancy in most of the cases. According to the crown-rump length (CRL) size, the LMP is calculated for sonography, and the date of the conception and the probable date of the childbirth is obtained. This is specially true when the pregnancy is of more time than the correspondent for the LMP referred by the patient. When the data of the sonographic exploration correspond to a pregnancy of less time, that is to say, retarded ovulation, the approach is different, since the fact of finding a smaller embryo that the one expected already supposes a risk factor for poor pregnancy outcome.

A useful tool to adjunct to the ultrasonography is the plasmatic determination of the β-hCG hormone (mIU/mL) between the fourth and eighth weeks of pregnancy. This determination is, among all those that can be performed in this period, the one that better clinical diffusion has obtained. Its behavior, although with wide variations from a pregnancy to another, presents some peculiarities that make it very useful in concrete cases. The normal course pregnancies duplicate the β-hCG levels in a period from 2 days to 3 days, while abnormal pregnancies (ectopic or interrupted) usually show levels of irregular ascent or, even, descend. The simultaneity of the biochemical and sonographic data permit to outline an useful perspective to know the expected outcome in normal pregnancies. Essentially, it is necessary to know the β-hCG system of measure performed in each own laboratory and adapt it to our medium.

Based on the sonographic capacity of prediction of the actual gestational age of different structures (the diameter of the gestational sac, the yolk sac and the CRL) with 1 week margin, the diameter and growth of each structure with the interval of confidence from the moment of appearance are reflected in many tables by different authors. Generally, gestational sacs of 3–4 mm of diameter average can usually be seen (Fig. 95.1) yolk sacs of 2–3 mm (Fig. 95.2) and embryos with CRL of 2–4 mm (Fig. 95.3). The amniotic vesicle is usually identified at the same time that the yolk sac, known as the double-bubble sign (Fig. 95.4). The heartbeat can be detected starting from a CRL of 3–4 mm in most of the cases (Fig. 95.5), being frequently detected before the embryonic echoes. Goldstein[1] states that the heartbeat is present in the embryo a few days before we are able to detect it with the sonographic exploration.

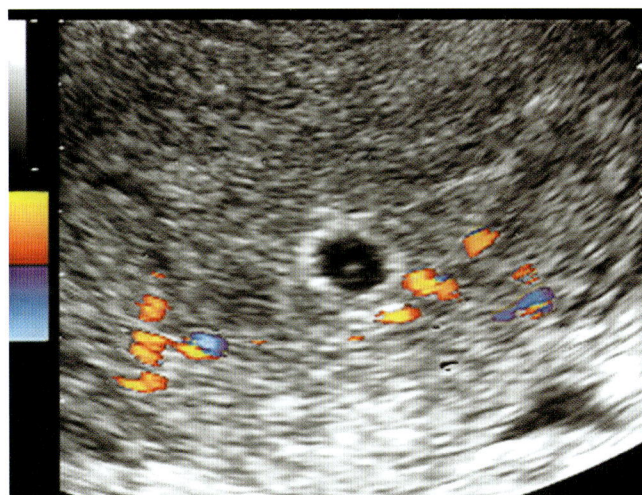

Fig. 95.1: Gestational sacs above 3–4 mm of diameter can usually be seen

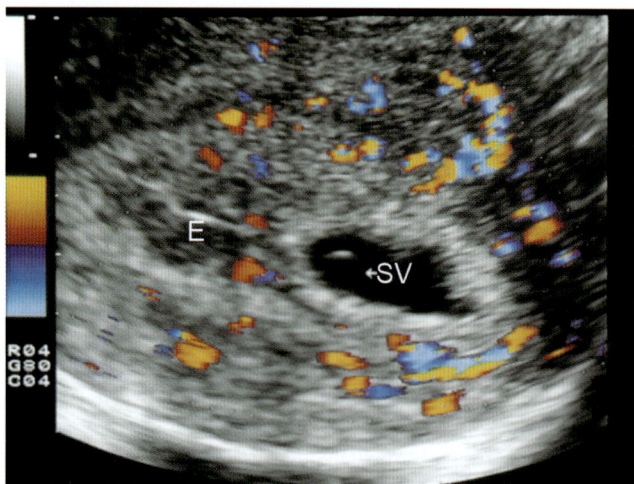

Fig. 95.2: The yolk sac can be observed when measures 2–3 mm

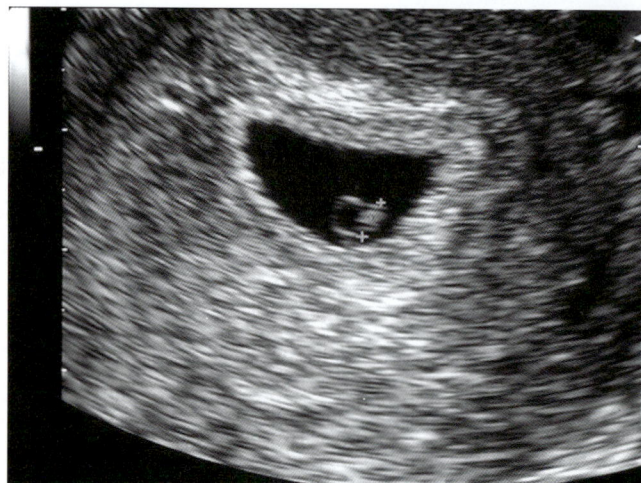

Fig. 95.3: A 2–4 mm CRL embryo must be seen in the exploration

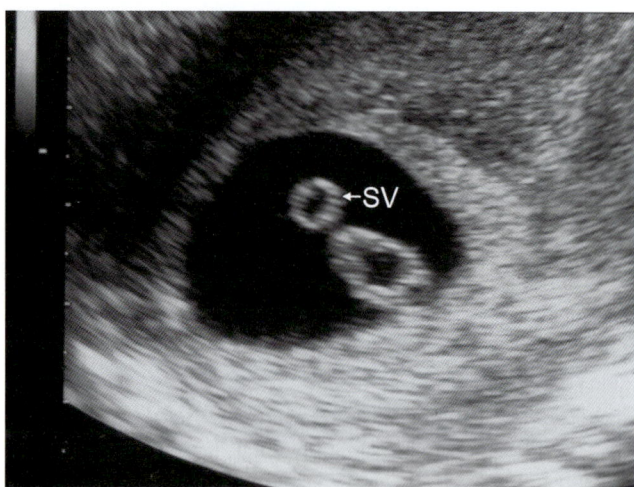

Fig. 95.4: The amniotic vesicle is usually observed at the same time that the yolk sac (double-bubble sign)

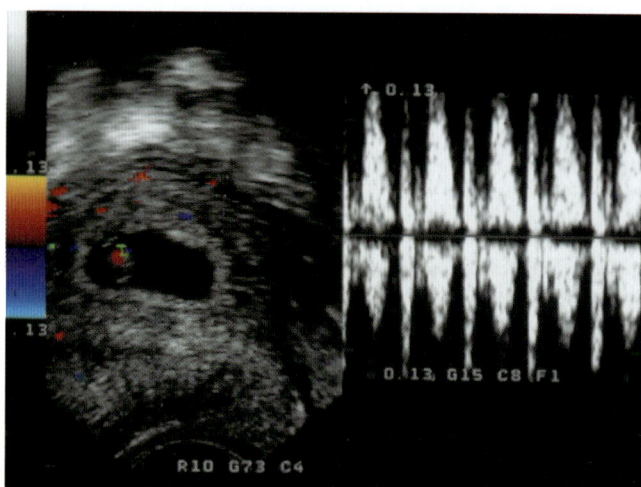

Fig. 95.5: The heart motion can be detected in most of the cases starting from a 3 mm to 4 mm CRL embryo

All the exposed data correspond to what is possible to visualize in each moment in normal pregnancies in patients in which conception began 14 days after the LMP. The normal pregnancies that have begun before or after this moment, will have a difference with regard to the prospective findings, but the rhythm of change among successive sonographic explorations will be the same described. So, after two sonographic explorations with at least 1 week of difference, starting from the moment in which has been visualized as minimum a gestational sac of 5–10 mm of diameter, the definitive diagnosis for the viability of the pregnancy will be obtained.

More than 80% of the sonographic explorations performed in the first trimester of the pregnancy, in asymptomatic women without risk factors, will be strictly normal. Anyway, as more precociously, the first sonographic exploration is performed, higher will be the probability that we find abnormal data or not rigorously diagnoses, and with more probability the repetition of the sonographic exploration should confirm the normality. A pregnancy of 2 weeks less, in the 10th week will allow to see a normal sac and an alive embryo of 16 mm of CRL, but if the sonographic exploration is performed in the 7th week, a small gestational sac of 8 or 10 mm of

diameter will probably be the only finding. The confirmation that a pregnancy evolves correctly and with a prediction of good outcome (low abortion probability) is only obtained when a live embryo is visualized and history of associate risks does not exist. On the other hand, the confirmation that a pregnancy has been interrupted, can only be made when an embryo is visualized with a certain size without heartbeat. When there is not embryo, except in cases when the gestational sac has reached a big size, another sonographic exploration 7–10 days later is to be performed.

SPONTANEOUS INTERRUPTIONS OF THE DEVELOPMENT OF THE CONCEPTION'S PRODUCT, FREQUENCY OF THE SPONTANEOUS ABORTION, CAUSES OF MISCARRIAGE

The frequency of spontaneous interruptions of the development of the reproductive process is very high, mainly when is considered from the most initial stages. It is calculated that considering the shortcoming of the fecundation, of each 100 potential pregnancies, only 31 will arrive to term with a live fetus.[2,3] The frequency of the miscarriage, considering this as the spontaneous interruption of the pregnancy before the fetus has reached the viability depends therefore on the approach that we use to define that pregnancy exists. When only considering the pregnancies reaching implantation (biochemical pregnancy), the miscarriage frequency is from the 30% to 40%.[4,5] Reached the clinical diagnosis of pregnancy, the frequency descends to 10–15%. If the pregnancy progresses until reaching the 12th week, the probability of abortion descends to the 3–4%. When the embryo is alive in the 12th week, the abortion rate until the 20th week is only 2%.[6]

Siddiqi[7] reports that in pregnancies under 12 weeks, the controls have 5.2% of miscarriages, while the cases that presented bleeding had 16.4%. Also, when patient is older than 34 years, the frequency ascended to 11.1%, in comparison with those patients under 35 years, with only 4.4%. Levi[8] finds a 24% rate of abortions when positive heartbeat exists, but the embryo has a CRL smaller than 5 mm.

Goldstein and colleague[9] present their data with great clinical applicability allowing to know the probability of miscarriage in function of the sonographic findings, as is shown in the Table 95.1.

Choong[10] in a series of 322 pregnant women concludes that the most discriminatory test for predict spontaneous miscarriage in live embryo is an personalized multivariate analysis model, constructed with the LMP, CRL, embryonic heart rate, mean sac diameter and maternal age as variables, for an area under the curve in his ROC curve of 0.87.

The embryonic and fetal causes, basically chromosomal anomalies, are the most frequent causes of miscarriage.[11] The different rates reported depend on the approaches used (if only clinical pregnancies are considered or not). In the first weeks, they can overcome 80–90% of the cases. Above the 12th week, the chromosomal anomalies and the malformations are less relevant, although they continue being an important cause. From this moment on, the maternal and environmental causes acquire more importance.

The frequency of the spontaneous miscarriage when is considered from their very beginning, along with the theoretical knowledge of the causes of the abortion, should provide a perspective to the obstetrician who performing a sonographic exploration, finds discoveries not corresponding to those characteristics in a normal pregnancy. The precocity of the realization sonographic explorations in the pregnancy will allow to diagnose many more cases of spontaneous interruptions of the development of pregnancy.

Table 95.1: Probability of spontaneous abortion according to the sonographic findings (Goldstein SR, 1994)

Structure visualized	Probability of abortion (%)
Yolk sac	8.5
Embryo CRL < 5 mm	7.2
Embryo CRL 6–10 mm	3.3
Embryo CRL > 10 mm	0.5

POOR PROGNOSIS OF PREGNANCY: SONOGRAPHIC FINDINGS (TABLE 95.2)

There exist some circumstances that, when present in a sonographic exploration performed in the first trimester of the pregnancy, hampers the prognosis, although they do not allow the definitive diagnosis of "interruption of the development", they determine that the prognosis for normal outcome is reduced. In the previous days to the detention of the development, some phenomenons are usually detected. However, none of them is sufficiently reliable as to emit definitive diagnoses. To be able to diagnose an abortion, or embryonic death, it is necessary to check the existence of an embryo of 5 mm CRL like minimum in which heartbeat is lacking it.

Anomalies of the Gestational Sac

The gestational sac and the CRL develop simultaneously. It is possible to check how between the 6th and the 10th week, the difference usually overcomes the 15–20 mm. Other authors[12,13] communicates that when the difference between the diameter of the gestational sac and CRL is less than 5 mm (precocious oligoamnion), the miscarriage occurred in 95% of the cases (Fig. 95.6). Dickey[14] reports that when the difference among these two measures was less than 5 mm, the miscarriage occurred in 80% of the cases; when the difference was between 5 mm and 7.9 mm, the miscarriage occurred in 26.5% of the cases, and when overcame the 8 mm, occurred in only 10.6% of the cases.

Anomalies of the Heart Frequency Interpreted as a Function of the Gestational Age or CRL

Bradycardia or Relative Bradycardia

It is characteristic the ascent of the fetal heart rate (FHR) until the 10th week, from 90 bpm in the first weeks of visualization up to 180–190 bpm in the 12th week. From this moment, FHR diminishes progressively until reaching the 140–150 bpm in the 20th week. However, important variations exist in the frequency in every week of pregnancy among the different authors. Merchiers[15] gives importance

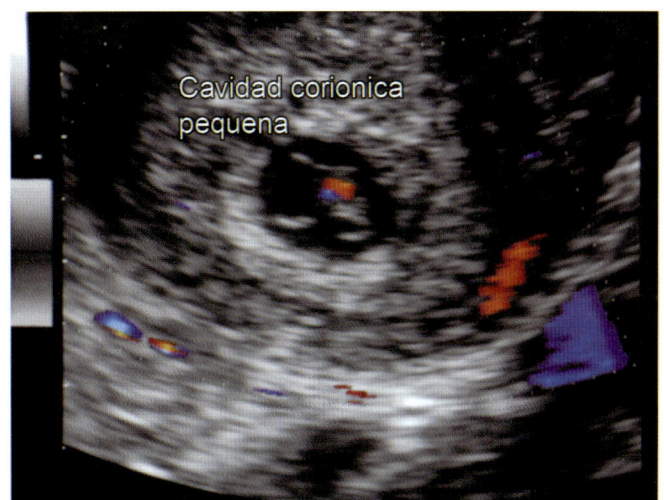

Fig. 95.6: Gestational sac showing precocious oligoamnion, good predictor for abortion

Table 95.2: Ultrasonographic signs of poor prognosis for embryonic viability

Anomalies of the gestational sac	Precocious oligoamnion: When the difference between the diameter average of the gestational sac and the CRL is smaller to 5 mm, poor prognosis Very thin decidual reaction (mm) for the corresponding gestational age (weeks) (>3 difference) Low implantation, distorted aspect
Alterations of the heart frequency	Bradycardia is always sign of poor prognosis. It should be interpreted in function of the gestational age. Frequencies under 85 bpm until the 7th week and under 100 bpm from this moment on, poor diagnosis
Small live embryo for the LMP	Especially in women with regular cycles, the visualization of a CRL smaller in at least 1 week to the corresponding for the LMP, increases the risk for abortion
Anomalies of the yolk sac	Alterations in the size (big vesicles, more than 6 mm of diameter) increases the risk, alterations in the structure (hyperechogenic vesicle) poor prognosis
Reverse implantation	Risk for abortion increased
Intrauterine bleeding (hematomas)	Big hematomas, mainly retrochorionic, maximum risk Subchorionic hematomas located in corpus or fundus more risk that next to the uterine cervix If no vaginal bleeding or small size of hematoma, low risk
Fetal movements	Absence of fetal movements, starting from the 8th week
Doppler	Poor color map around the gestational sac Values of Doppler flow in uterine, radial, arcuata, spiral, retrochorial and intervillous arteries, as well as the umbilical artery in the first trimester of pregnancy have limited clinical applicability
Other factors	Existence of associated pathology: myomas, malformations Uterine hemorrhage, maternal age over 35 years. Antecedent of 1 or more abortions (as more abortions, more risk). Serial hormonal determinations. Two β-hCG determinations separate 2–3 days

to that a decrease of the heart frequency takes place successive sonographic explorations between two. For Laboda,[16] a FHR under 85 bpm comports very poor prognosis, since in its series, all the embryos that presented this finding, finished miscarrying. May[17] also finds poor prognosis in this finding: 6 out of 11 cases with FHR under 85 bpm between the 4.5th and the 7.3rd weeks miscarried.

Benson[18] sets the limit in 90 bpm for the whole 1st trimester to affirm that a poor prognosis exists. In his series, all the cases that a FHR under 70 bpm ended in abortion. Between 70 bpm and 79 bpm, 91% of abortions, and between 80 bpm and 89 bpm, 70% of abortions. Doubilet[19] suggests that a FHR more than 100 bpm until the 6.2nd week and superior to 120 bpm between the 6.3rd and the 7th week, are signs of good prognosis. When he observes among the 7th and 8th week an inferior FHR to 110 bpm, considers it a sign of poor prognosis. Stefos[20] presents in his series that, when exist a FHR under 85 bpm between the 6th and 8th week, any fetus survive. For this author, when between the 6th and the 7th week the FHR is between 116 bpm and 125 bpm, the prognosis is good, as is when the FHR is more than 146 bpm between the 8th and the 9th week. Anyway, any finding except the absence of heartbeat is able to diagnose the embryonic death definitively. However, the scientific evidence allows to be possible to emit more and more precise diagnosis. In general, heart frequencies under 80–90 bpm until the 7th week and under 100 bpm from this moment on, is associated with an adverse result, and high abortion probability.

Anomalies of the Yolk Sac (Size, Shape, Echogenicity)

The yolk sac is the first extraembryonic structure that appears and is visible practically in all the pregnancies between the 5th and the 12th week. The yolk sac can be observed initially when the diameter of the gestational sac reaches 3.7 mm, in the 36th day from the LMP and is reliably observed when the diameter is from 6.7 mm, in the 40th day of amenorrhea. Even more, for Levi[9] the yolk sac should always be observed when the diameter of the gestational sac is of more than 8 mm (corresponding to 33 days), so that its absence would suppose for him an approach bigger than loss gestational sac.

The interest that the knowledge of the visibility of the yolk sac has for the echographists resides in that is the first identifiable structure in the gestational sac, preceding 4–7 days to the visualization of the embryo. Their aspect is an echogenic circle that defines a sonolucent area inside the chorionic cavity, extra-amniotically located.

Some anomalies are described in their initial development as the shape and volume alterations.[21,22]

As a general idea, it is difficult to make important clinical decisions (as diagnosing a pregnancy interruption) based on findings related to the yolk sac. This is a structure with important variations as for their size and dimensions. The visualization is not also absolutely safe, even in pregnancies of normal course. The alterations at their level are usually late, and it is believed that they are consequence of the process that determines the miscarriage, not the cause. However, multiple publications have been in charge of their measure, of the valuation of their characteristics, and of the epidemic analysis of their association with a poor outcome of the pregnancy.

Lindsay[23] refers that the existence of a yolk sac of more than 2 standard deviations above those expected for the gestational age supposes a poor prognosis. Any case evolved favorably with a yolk sac bigger than 5.6 mm under the 10th week in his series (Figs 95.7 to 95.9). This agrees with the data from Kupesic,[24] who informs of a poor prognosis in yolk sacs with abnormal size and abnormal Doppler vascularization. Iniesta and col[25] inform that the alterations in the yolk sac as for their size, the shape or the echogenicity are parameters that guide on the normal or pathological development of the pregnancy. Of the 100 patients in their series, 87 (87%) had a normal development and evolved correctly until the end of the first trimester (control group).[13] 13% had an abnormal course of the

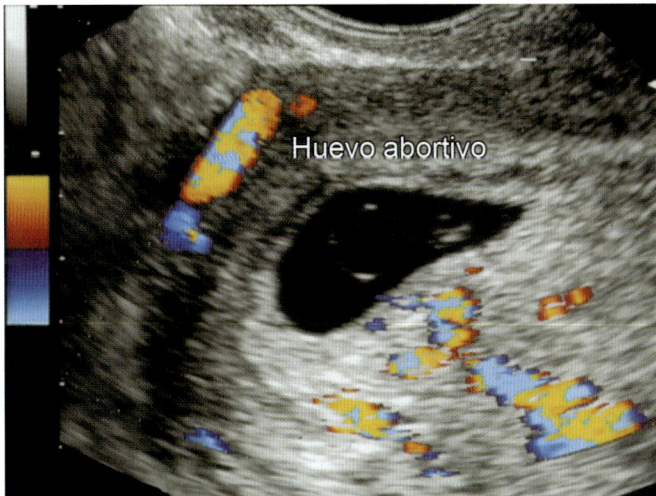

Fig. 95.7: Yolk sac of 8 mm (more than 2 standard deviations for the gestational age)

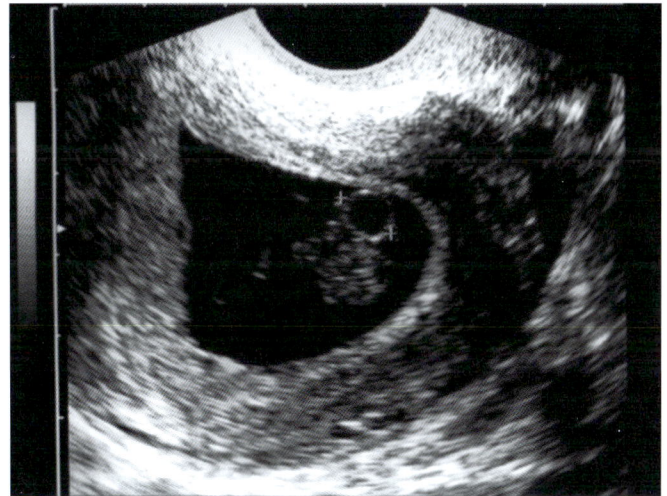

Fig. 95.8: Giant yolk sac, sign that is rapidly and easily appreciated in the sonographic exploration

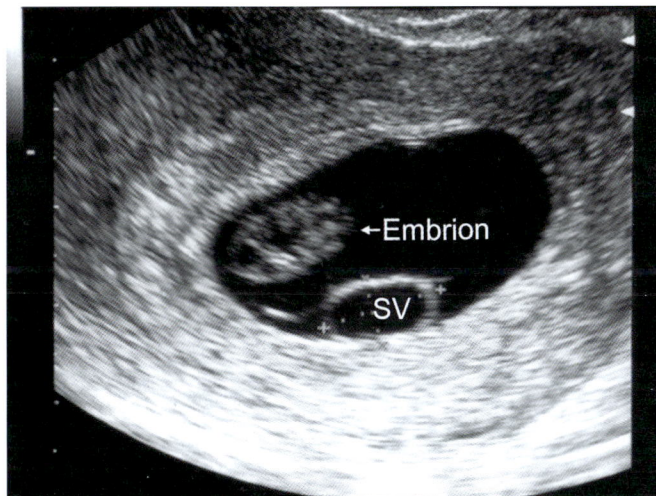

Fig. 95.9: Gestational sac of 9 mm. This is a very sensitive marker for abortion

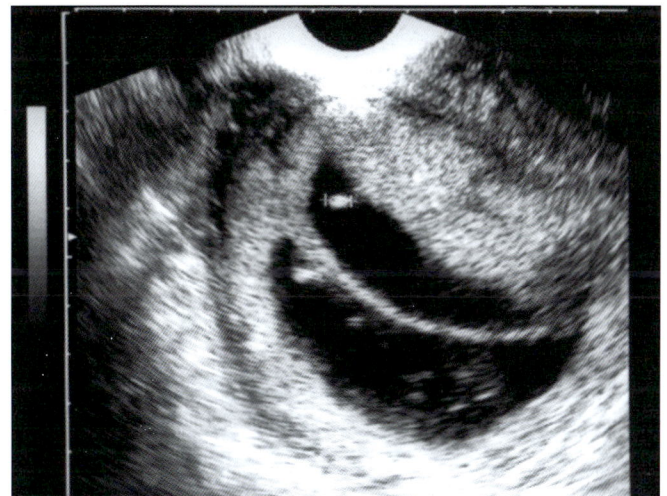

Fig. 95.10: The regressive yolk sac is observed by a progressive increase of the internal refrigency as seen in both yolk sacs of this double pregnancy

pregnancy (study group). Of the 87 patients with correct development, 3 had a diameter of yolk sac of more than 1 SD. Of the 13 patients with abnormal course, 6 had a diameter of yolk sac bigger than 1 SD. They conclude that the sensitivity of the size of the yolk sac to predict an abnormal course of the pregnancy is 92.3%, the specificity 66.6% the VPP 96.5% and the VPN 46% and when some of these anomalies appears, is necessary to closely follow the pregnancy.

The regressive yolk sac is sonographically observed by a progressive increase of the refrigency until the more extreme form that would be the calcification of the sac (Fig. 95.10).

Trophoblastic Thickness at the Embryonic Implantation Site

Bajo and cols[26] describe the trophoblastic thickness at the embryonic implantation site in a prospective, observational study in 592 normal pregnancies in whom serial ultrasound scans were performed from 5th to 12th weeks of pregnancy. Trophoblastic thickness was measured at the embryonic implantation site to determine the

significance of the difference between the gestational age in weeks and the trophoblastic thickness in millimeters. A difference of more than 3 was highly predictive for poor pregnancy outcome (Fig. 95.11). The sensitivity of this sign in the prediction of spontaneous abortion was 82%, the specificity was 93%, the positive predictive value was 63% and the negative predictive value was 97%.

Intrauterine Bleeding: Subchorionic and Retroplacental Hematomas

The existence of liquid collections, mainly in subchorionic situation, is a relatively frequent finding in the sonographic explorations performed during the first trimester of the pregnancy (Fig. 95.12). Some of these images are evident, they have a great size and they coincide with clinical symptomatology (vaginal bleeding), while others are casual findings in asymptomatic women and have a minimum volume. Discrepancies exist as for the risk that suppose and their association with abortion in function of the approaches used for the diagnosis of intrauterine hemorrhage. Dickey[27]

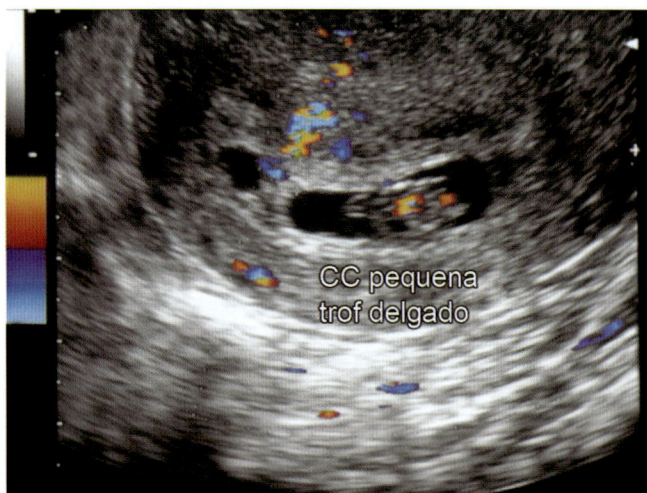

Fig. 95.11: A thin trophoblast is observed. A difference of more than 3 between gestational age (weeks) and the trophoblastic thickness (mm) is highly predictive for poor pregnancy outcome

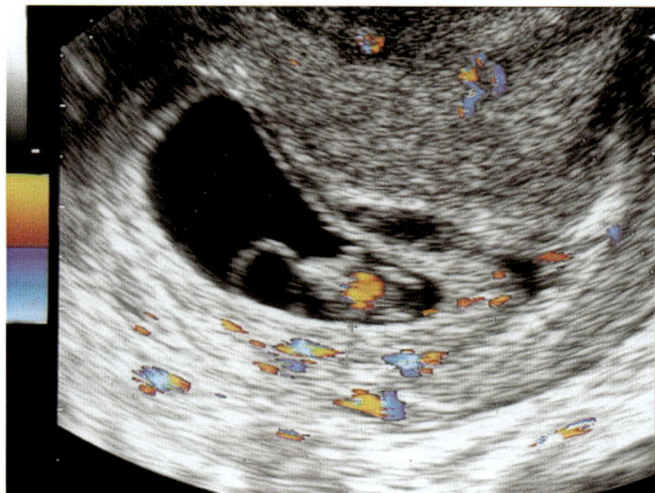

Fig. 95.12: The existence of liquid collections in subchorionic situation is a frequent finding in the explorations performed in the first trimester

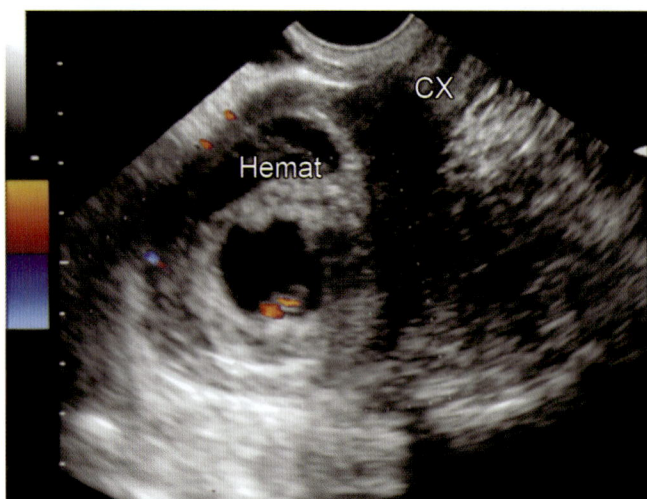

Fig. 95.13: The retrochorionic or subplacental localization have worse prognosis than the subchorionic localization

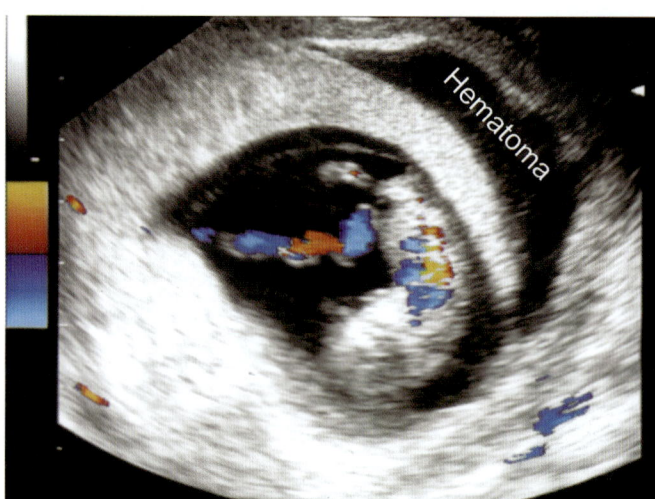

Fig. 95.14: Hematomas located in uterine corpus or fundus have worse prognosis than those located near the uterine cervix

demonstrated with Doppler color that in 37% of the sonographic explorations in the first trimester subchorionic bleeding exists, and that in 47% of the cases, subchorionic liquid is detected so concludes that the liquid and the subchorionic bleeding are frequent discoveries in the early pregnancy and they are not associated to embryonic deaths unless accompanied of vaginal bleeding. Stabile[28] states that the existence of small subchorionic hematomas (less than 16 mL) in women with genital bleeding does not increase the risk for miscarriage in comparison to women with bleeding without hematoma.

With regard to the meaning diagnosis that has the size and the localization of the hematoma, Glavind[29] does not find relationship between the size of the hematoma and the week of pregnancy in which was diagnosed with the outcome of the pregnancy. For this author, the retrochorionic or subplacental localization have worse prognosis that the subchorionic localization (Fig. 95.13). For Kurjak[30] the subchorionic hematomas influences in the abortion frequency (17% in study group versus 6.5% in the control group).

Neither influences the size of the hematoma a lot, being transcendent the localization. The hematomas in uterine corpus or fundus have worse prognosis than those located near the uterine cervix (Fig. 95.14). Again Kurjak[31] finds a higher RI (resistance index) of the spiral arteries in the cases with retrochorionic hematoma that in the controls, due to the mechanism of compression of the hematoma.

For Ball,[32] it is not clear that the subchorionic bleeding is the cause or simply an underlying process that is the one that produces the negative effects. He presents an interesting study in which divides the patients in three groups: the first is formed by women that present with subchorionic bleeding; the second is a control group of women without hematoma; the third is another control group without hematoma but with vaginal bleeding. When he performs comparisons with controls without bleeding, an odds ratio (OR) 2.8 is obtained for abortion, 4.5 for stillbirth, 11.2 for abruptio placentae and 2.6 for preterm birth. When comparing with controls with bleeding all the ORs increase except the corresponding for abortion. The weight at birth is diminished when comparing it with the two control groups. The genital bleeding by itself is able to increase the risk of miscarriage. Bennet[33] compares the abortion frequency in women with genital bleeding and subchorionic hemorrhage. When the hematoma is big, the frequency of abortions is 18.8%, if medium 9.2%, and 7.7% if small. When the woman is older than 35 years, the abortion rate is 13.8%, in comparison with 7.3% in women younger than 35 years. When the bleeding appeared before the 8th week, the frequency was 13.7%, while if appeared later than the 8th week, the rate is reduced to 5.9%.

The presence of scarce quantity of retrochorial liquid has less implications, when is observed as an isolated finding and in the context of a rigorously normal sonographic exploration in a pregnancy of normal course. The existence of a subchorionic hemorrhage, especially when associated to vaginal bleeding, increases the abortion risk and demands to perform another sonographic explorations a few days later. New sonographic explorations are justified when small or moderate hemorrhage exist. The worst prognosis are the big size hematomas (more than 40–50 mL), especially if located next to uterine neck, in uterine corpus or fundus. The retrochorionic or subplacental hematomas, especially if moderate or big always carry a poor diagnosis. The frequency of visualization of these images is low, probably because a rapid chorial detachment develops leading to the miscarriage, with bleeding and expulsion of remnants. Another uncommon type of hematoma or intrauterine bleeding is the preplacental that appears after the realization of invasive techniques that need the introduction of a needle in the uterine cavity. In general, they are moderate and evolve favorably although threatened miscarriage in the first trimester is associated with an increased incidence of adverse pregnancy outcome, independently of the presence of an intrauterine hematoma.[34] Nagy compared perinatal outcome in 187 pregnant women with intrauterine hematoma and 6,488 controls in whom hematomas were not detected at first trimester. He concludes that the sonographic presence of an intrauterine hematoma during the first trimester identifies a population of patients at increased risk for adverse pregnancy outcome.[35] In other occasions, they reach such a volume that cause an effect of occupation of the chorionic cavity, with effect of fetal death because the compression (Fig. 95.15).

Small CRL for the Gestational Age

In general, when a small for gestational age CRL with positive heartbeat embryo is observed, a pregnancy of less time is the first diagnosis to approach. This is frequent in women with long or irregular cycles. However, sometimes may be observed in normal cycling women. First of all, the date of conception should be corrected, but data that allow to associate this alteration with a higher risk of poor pregnancy outcome exist (Fig. 95.16).

Koornstra[36] informs that 22.7% of the embryos from regular cycling women have CRL inferior in 1 week or more than the expected from the LMP. Analyzing the results observes that among these embryos a rate of abortions of 16% existed, in comparison with only 5% in the embryos with a LMP correct size.

Leelapatana[37] communicates that a small CRL for gestational age in comparison with the prospective one during the first trimester of pregnancy could be associated to triploidy, but not to the 18 and 21 trisomies. Later, Besso[38] communicated that fetuses finishing in miscarriage had a quotient measured CRL/expected CRL of 0.74, in comparison with the 0.98 observed in fetuses that did not miscarry. This author does not find differences in the quotient among chromosomally normal and abnormal fetuses. The information has also been confirmed in the series from Coulam[39] who finds no differences in the frequency of blighted ovum and small CRL for gestational age among chromosomally normal and abnormal fetuses.

Pattern of Fetal Movements

Along the sonographic chronology of findings in a normal pregnancy, the existence and verification of fetal movements should be observed.

In a classic publication by Anderson,[40] the results presented were obtained in a series of 149 cases of threaten abortion and more than 7 weeks of gestational age. Only 2 of 65 pregnancies that later aborted presented fetal movements. On the other hand, 64 of 72 normal pregnancies presented fetal movements. So the absence of fetal movements after a relatively long period of sonographic exploration, especially above the 8th week, should also be considered as a sign of poor prognosis.

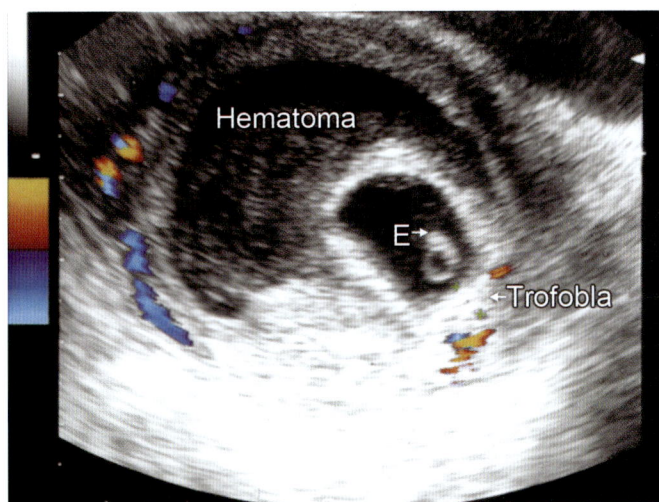

Fig. 95.15: Large hematoma causing distortion in the gestational sac

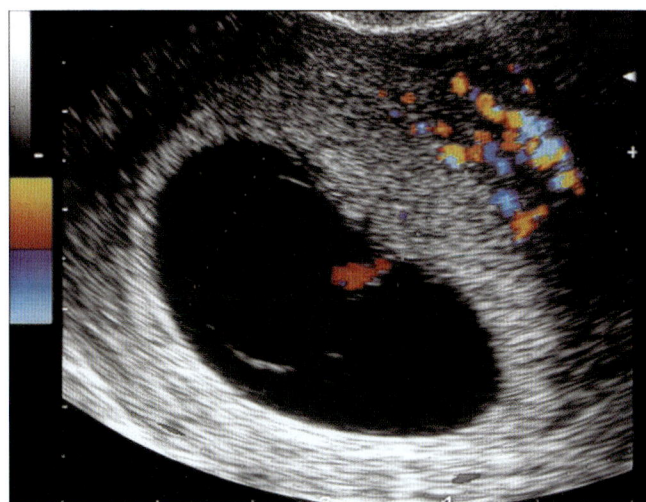

Fig. 95.16: Small CRL for the gestational age, as referred to gestational sac

Doppler Flow Alterations

The number of publications during the last years regarding the Doppler velocimetry in the first stadiums of the normal and pathological pregnancies is profuse. The knowledge of the data that the investigators contribute has an enormous interest to improve our knowledge on the phenomenon that exist in the placentation process and development of the embryo from their beginning. Kurjak[41] refers that the process of trophoblastic invasion of the decidua is progressive, mediated by the action of proteolytic enzymes that facilitate the penetration and maternal erosion of the capillary arteries and the formation of lagoons. That is why exist variations of the flows that can be measured in the uterine, retrochorionic and intervillous arteries during the first trimester of pregnancy (Fig. 95.17). This is the reason why the PI (pulsatility index) and high RI in the first trimester should not be interpreted as of bad result, like it would be made in the second trimester as Jaffe informs.[42] This author explains[43] how the intervillous circulation persists until the late first trimester. In complicated pregnancies, analyzed precociously, the uteroplacental circulation is different to that of normal pregnancies. In these abnormal pregnancies the intervillous flow is increased. The hypothesis that is based on other studies establishes that the embryo of a pregnancy of normal course favors an atmosphere with a low concentration of tisular oxygen in placental tissues. Martin[44] explains that the increased impedance to flow in the uterine arteries in the first trimester is associated with the development of preeclampsia and intrauterine growth retardation (likelihood ratio of 5 and 2 respectively).

Mercé[45] measured the velocity of systolic peak, PI and RI in retrochorionic arteries and fetal umbilical artery in 108 pregnancies between 4th and 15th week. The most precocious sign in retrochorionic circulation was obtained in the 4.5th week, and the most precocious of umbilical artery at the end of the 5th week. Their results indicate that as gestational age increases, the systolic peak of the retrochorionic, intervillous and umbilical arteries increase, while PI and RI diminish. Kurjak[46] again assessed yolk sac morphology and vascularity and intervillous blood flow in normal early pregnancy and missed abortion in a prospective analysis of 87 normal pregnancies and 48 missed abortions between 6 and 12 weeks of gestation. He concludes that progressive decrease of yolk sac vascularity coincides with visualization of more prominent color-coded areas within the intervillous space. In patients with missed abortion, such changes do not occur.

In general, most of the authors does not find differences in the Doppler indexes among normal outcome pregnancies and those ending in miscarriage. Jauniaux[47] compares 30 confirmed abortions with 30 normal pregnancies. The PI of the uterine artery was higher in the abortions than in the normal pregnancies. Differences were not observed in RI and systolic peak of the uterine artery neither in PI or RI of spiral arteries among abortions and normal pregnancies. This author concludes that the velocity of abnormal flow found in some complicated pregnancies with embryonic death would be related to a defective placentation and "dislocation" of the trophoblastic wall, to which the embryonic death follows. The premature access of maternal blood to the intervillous space would break the embryonic-maternal interface, and would be the cause that probably determines the miscarriage (Fig. 95.18). Alcazar[48] communicates that no apparent alteration occurs in the early uteroplacental circulation in patients with threatened abortion with a living embryo so the use of transvaginal color Doppler ultrasound is not helpful for predicting pregnancy outcome in cases of threaten abortion (Fig. 95.19).

Salim[49] measures PI and RI at the level of the corpus luteum. The pregnancies with threaten abortion or ending in abortion show higher values that normal pregnancies. However, he does not observe differences when comparing data of ectopic pregnancies, hydatidiform moles, or anembryonic pregnancies. Alcazar[50] measures the flows at the level of the corpus luteum, not finding differences among controls, threaten abortion or blighted ovum. In pregnancies with confirmed miscarriage, the values of RI are higher.

Other Factors to Consider (Clinical Nature)

- Maternal age: superior to 35–40 years
- Presence of uterine bleeding
- Moment of beginning of the uterine bleeding
- Hormonal dynamics determination (β-hCG)
- Reproductive antecedents (one or more previous miscarriages)
- Existence of associate pathology (multiple myomas or submucosas, uterine malformations).

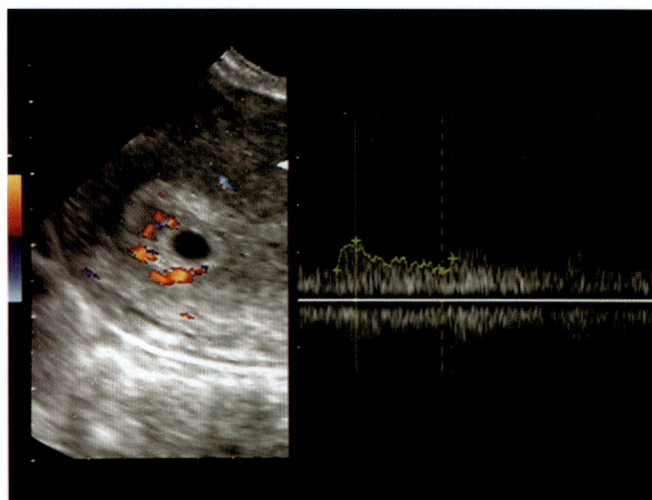

Fig. 95.17: Doppler flows can be obtained in the retrochorionic and intervillous arteries in the first trimester of pregnancy

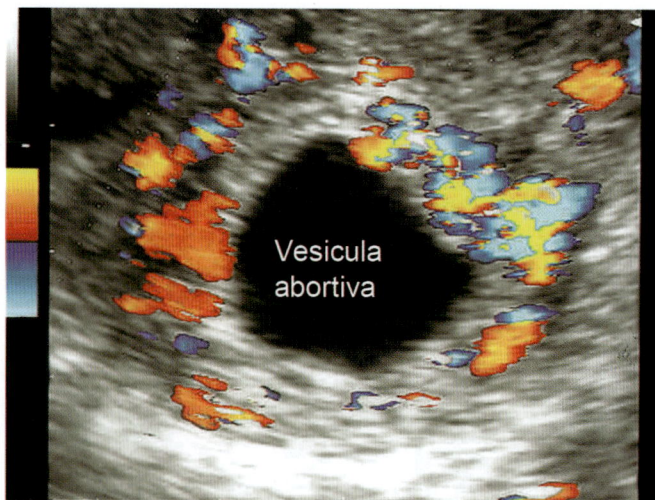

Vesicula abortiva

Fig. 95.18: The premature access of maternal blood to the intervillous space has broken the embryonic-maternal interface, probably the cause that determines the abortion

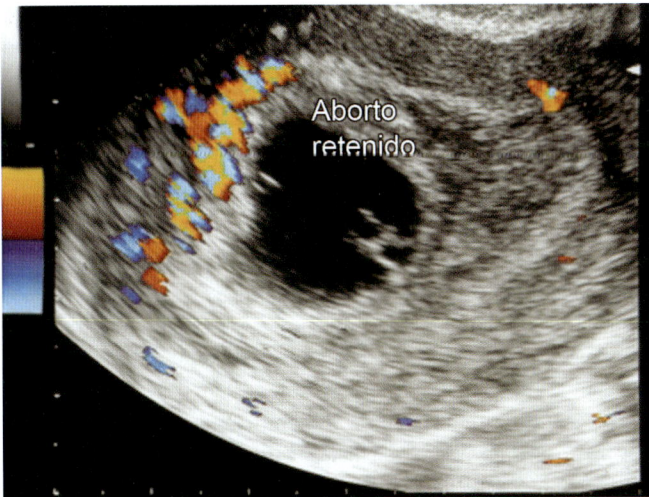

Fig. 95.19: The use of transvaginal color Doppler is not helpful for predicting pregnancy outcome in cases of living embryos

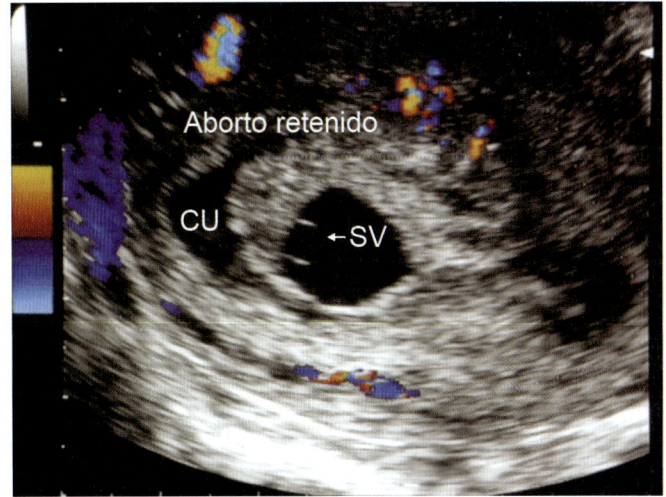

Fig. 95.20: Differed abortion

SONOGRAPHIC FINDINGS TO DIAGNOSE AN INTERRUPTED PREGNANCY (TABLE 95.3)

The two types of spontaneous interruptions of pregnancy in patients without bleeding are, from a practical point of view, the differed or missed abortions, and the blighted ovum or anembryonic pregnancies. Academically the *differed* abortions were considered as those in which the measured CRL corresponded to 6 weeks less than the expected in an embryo lacking heartbeat (Fig. 95.20). Nowadays, due to the better accessibility of women to the initial sonographic exploration, is infrequent to reach so much time without diagnosis, so this kind of miscarriage, when the interruption is recent and bleeding has not begun, are called *missed* abortions. With regard to the anembryonic pregnancies, their frequency is much lower of what is thought from a clinical point of view. It would be pregnancies initially with embryo, that was dead precociously and was reabsorbed, so is not sonographically visualized. All the gestational sacs in which an amniotic or a yolk sac is observed, although embryo is not seen, do not correspond to anembryonic pregnancies, since these structures require the development of an embryo to appear (Fig. 95.21).

The false positive diagnoses, the really important mistakes, are of two types. The first is when the sonographist is not able to detect the heartbeat in an embryo that actually has heart motion, and would be motivated by a small size of the embryo, inadequate or obsolete team, or suboptimal visualization due to patient's characteristics. The other type of error would be to consider that before a certain size

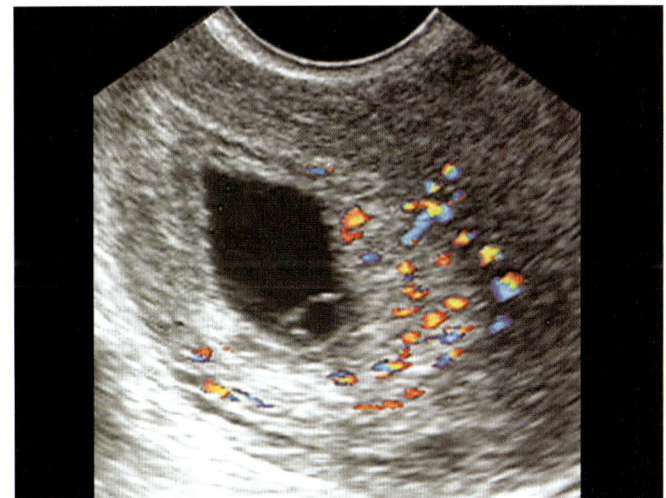

Fig. 95.21: A gestational sac with a yolk sac but lacking embryo corresponding to a missed abortion

of gestational sac an embryo must be seen. The error is motivated by the selection of a low level from which we already diagnose anembryonic pregnancy, and that this level could correspond to the highest range in the normality. In the first case it would suppose that after 1 week, for instance, in an embryo of 4–5 mm in the one that had not seen heartbeat, saw it and it measured 9–10 mm. In the second case, in a 21 mm diameter vesicle, in which the embryo was not seen, after one week a 5–6 mm CRL and positive heartbeat

Table 95.3: Ultrasonographic signs in the interrupted pregnancy

Embryonic death (differed or missed miscarriage)	Absence of heartbeat in embryo of 5 mm CRL as minimum (even in first sonographic exploration)
Blighted ovum or pregnancy anembryonic	Gestational sac of 25 mm or more without embryo (even in first sonographic examination). For some authors, gestational sac of 20 mm or more without yolk sac. Gestational sac of 16 mm or more with yolk sac and amniotic vesicle without embryo ("empty amnion").
Interrupted pregnancy	Successive sonographic examinations: Absence of significant changes in two sonographic examinations separate 7–10 days when in the first sonographic examinations a gestational sac of 15–20 mm as minimum has been visualized

embryo will be observed. According to Daya[51] an embryo is not seen until the gestational sac measures 8.3 mm diameter, coincident with the 41st of amenorrhea. However, always is to be observed when the gestational sac reaches 14 mm diameter, in the 46th day of amenorrhea (6 weeks and 4 days). Goldstein[52] informs that when the pregnancy is correctly developing, the gestational sac is reliably observed in the 5th week. When the sac measures 20 mm diameter, the embryo is observed in 100% of the cases. In the 6 weeks and 4 days (46th day amenorrhea) heartbeat is observed in 100% of the cases, and when the diameter is 30 mm, in 100% of the normal cases, even embryonic movements are already presents (8 weeks).

Norwitz[53] confirms the importance of exploration at the very beginning of the pregnancy. To confirm the diagnosis of "embryonic death" at the first sonographic exploration, the CRL should be higher than 10 mm. Levi[8] considers "not viable" to all gestational sacs of more than 8 mm of diameter without yolk sac and of 16 mm or more without embryo. He diagnoses embryonic death when the embryo is between 4 mm and 5 mm CRL. Several cases with CRL smaller than 4 mm in those that heartbeat was not detected, evolved correctly in his series.

Brown[54] recommends to wait until 5 mm CRL to confirm embryonic demise if heartbeat is not detected. Bernard[55] in the differentiation among blighted ovum and "viable precocious pregnancy", considers that although the visualization of sacs with 20 mm or more without embryo is a sign of poor prognosis, definitive signs do not exist, so recommends to repeat the sonographic exploration after 1–2 weeks. Nyberg[56] waits to observe a gestational sac of more than 20 mm of diameter without yolk sac or a sac of 25 mm in diameter with distorted aspect without embryo to consider a pregnancy as not viable.

McKenna[57] reports that between the 6th and the 10th week, the amniotic cavity is similar to the size of the embryo, and the visualization of an amniotic cavity without embryo corresponded to an "empty amnion" and diagnoses interrupted pregnancy. This author communicates that before gestational sac reaches 16 mm or more, when the yolk sac is identified and embryo neither nor heartbeat are detected, and an empty amniotic sac is seen, an interrupted pregnancy can be diagnosed.

In conclusion, to diagnose the embryonic death, is essential to wait to see an embryo with a 5 mm CRL minimum lacking heartbeat. For the diagnosis of blighted ovum or anembryonic pregnancy in a first sonographic exploration, seems reasonable to wait a 25-mm gestational sac, equivalent to 7 weeks pregnancy with conception the 14th day of the cycle. This corresponds to a pregnancy in which in 100% of the cases an alive embryo would be visualized if correctly develops. In all other cases, the sonographic exploration must be repeated after 7–10 days. In the great majority of the cases, the second sonography will allow us to confirm the diagnosis of normal or interrupted pregnancy.

REFERENCES

1. Goldstein MR. Significance of cardiac activity on endovaginal ultrasound in very early embryos. Obstet Gynecol. 1992;80:670-2.
2. Barri PN. Pérdidas embrionarias preimplantatorias. In: Carrera JM, Kurjak A (Eds). Medicina del embrión. Barcelona: Masson. 1996;143-8.
3. Leridon H. Human Fertility. Chicago: Chicago Press; 1977.
4. De la Fuente P. Aborto espontáneo. In: Fabre E (Ed). Manual de Asistencia a la Patología Obstétrica. Zaragoza INO Reproducciones. 1997;73-87.
5. Knudsen UB, Hansen V, Juul S, et al. Prognosis to new pregnancy following previous spontaneous miscarriages. Eur J Obstet Gynecol Reprod Biol. 1991;39:31-6.
6. Cashner KA, Christopher CR, Dysert GA. Spontaneous fetal loss after demonstration of to live fetus in the first trimester. Obstet Gynecol. 1987;70:827-30.
7. Siddiqi TA, Caligaris JT, Miodovnik M, et al. Rate of spontaneous abortion after first trimester sonographic demonstration of fetal cardiac activity. Am J Perinatol. 1988;5:1-4.
8. Levi CS, Lyons EA, Zheng XH, et al. Endovaginal US: Demonstration of cardiac activity in embryos of less than 5.0 mm in crown-rump length. Radiology. 1990;176:71-4.
9. Goldstein MR. Embryonic death in early pregnancy: a new look at the first trimester. Obstet Gynecol. 1994;84:294-7.
10. Choong S, Rombauts L, Ugoni A, et al. Ultrasound prediction of risk of spontaneous miscarriage in live embryos from assisted conceptions. Ultrasound Obstet Gynecol. 2003;22:571-7.
11. Phillip T, Phillip K, Reiner A, et al. Embryoscopic and cytogenetic analysis of 233 missed abortions: Factors involved in the pathogenesis of developmental defects of early failed pregnancies. Hum Reprod. 2003;18:1724-32.
12. Bromley B, Harlow BL, Laboda LA, et al. Small sac size in the first trimester: A predictor of poor fetal outcome. Radiology. 1991;178:375-7.
13. Paspulati RM, Bhatt S, Nour S. Sonographic evaluation of first trimester bleeding. Radiol Clin North Am. 2004;42:297-314.
14. Dickey RP, Olar TT, Taylor SN, et al. Relationship of small gestational sac and crown-rump length differences to abortion and abortus karyotypes. Obstet Gynecol. 1992;79:554-7.
15. Merchiers EH, Dhont M, De Sutter PA, et al. Predictive valued of early embryonic cardiac activity for pregnancy outcome. Am J Obstet Gynecol. 1991;165:11-4.
16. Laboda LA, Estroff JA, Benacerraf BR. First trimester bradycardia. A sign of impending fetal loss. J Ultrasound Med. 1989;8:561-3.
17. May DA, Sturtevant NV. Embryonal heart rate ace to predictor of pregnancy outcome: A prospective analysis. J Ultrasound Med. 1991;10:591-3.
18. Benson S. Slow embryonic heart rate in early first trimester: Indicator of poor pregnancy outcome. Radiology. 1994;192:343-4.
19. Doubilet PM, Benson CB. Embryonic heart rate in the early first trimester: What rate normal is? J Ultrasound Med. 1995;14:431-4.
20. Stefos TI, Lolis OF, Sotiriadis AJ, et al. Embryonic heart rate in early pregnancy. J Clin Ultrasound. 1998;26:33-6.
21. Kücük T, Duru NK, Yenen MC, et al. Yolk sac size and shape are predictors of poor pregnancy outcome. J Perinat Med. 1999;27:316-20.
22. Stampone C, Nicotra M, Muttinelli C, et al. Transvaginal sonography of the yolk sac in normal and abnormal pregnancy. J Clin Ultrasound. 1996;24:3-9.
23. Lindsay DJ, Lovett IS, Lyons EA, et al. Yolk sac diameter and shape at endovaginal US: Predictors of pregnancy outcome in the first trimester. Radiology. 1992;183:115-8.
24. Kupesic S, Kurjak A. Volume and vascularity of the yolk sac assessed by three-dimensional and power doppler ultrasound. Early Pregnancy. 2001;5:40-1.

25. Iniesta S, Pérez-Medina T, Redondo T, et al. Alteración ecográfica del saco vitelino como predictor de mal pronóstico de la gestación. Toko Gin Prakt. 2004;674:151-4.

26. Bajo J, Moreno-Calvo FJ, Martinez-Cortés L, et al. Is trophoblastic thickness at the embryonic implantation site to new sign of negative outcome in first trimester pregnancy? Hum Reprod. 2000;15:1629-31.

27. Dickey RP, Olar TT, Curole DN, et al. Relationship of first trimester subchorionic bleeding detected by color Doppler ultrasound to subchorionic flows, clinical bleeding, and pregnancy outcome. Obstet Gynecol. 1992;80:415-20.

28. Stabile I, Campbell S, Grudzinskas JG. Threatened miscarriage and intrauterine hematomas. Sonographic and biochemical studies. J Ultrasound Med. 1989;8: 289-92.

29. Glavind K, Nohr S, Nielsen PH, et al. Intrauterine hematoma in Pregnancy. Eur J Obstet Gynecol Reprod Biol. 1991;40:7-10.

30. Kurjak A, Schulman H, Zudenigo D, et al. Subchorionic hematomas in early pregnancy: Clinical outcome and blood flow patterns. J Fetal Matern Med. 1996;5:41-4.

31. Kurjak A, Zalud I, Predanic M, et al. Transvaginal color and pulsed Doppler study of uterine blood flow in the first and early second trimesters of pregnancy: Normal versus abnormal. J Ultrasound Med. 1994;13: 43-7.

32. Ball RH, Ade CM, Schoenborn JA, et al. The clinical significance of ultrasonographically detected subchorionic hemorrhages. Am J Obstet Gynecol. 1996;174:996-1002.

33. Bennett GL, Bromley B, Lieberman Y, et al. Subchorionic bleeding in first trimester pregnancies: Prediction of pregnancy outcome with sonography Radiology. 1996;200:803-6.

34. Johns J, Hyett J, Jauniaux E. Obstetric outcome after threatened miscarriage with and without a hematoma on ultrasound. Obstet Gynecol. 2003;102:483-7.

35. Nagy S, Bush M, Stone J, et al. Clinical significance of subchorionic and retroplacental hematomas detected in the first trimester of pregnancy. Obstet Gynecol. 2003;102:94-100.

36. Koornstra G, I Exalt N. Echography in the first pregnancy trimester has prognostic value. Ned Tijdschr Geneeskd. 1991;135:2231-5.

37. Leelapatana P, Garrett WJ, Warren PS. Early growth retardation in the first trimester: Is it characteristic of the chromosomally abnormal fetus? Aust N Z J Obstet Gynecol. 1992;32:95-7.

38. Bessho T, Sakamoto H, Shiotani T, et al. Fetal loss in the first trimester after demonstration of cardiac activity: Relation of cytogenetic and ultrasound findings. Hum Reprod. 1995;10:2696-9.

39. Coulam CB, Goodman C, Dorfmann A. Comparison of ultrasonographic findings in spontaneous abortions with normal and abnormal karyotypes. Hum Reprod. 1997;12:823-6.

40. Anderson SG. Management of threatened abortion with real-cheats sonography. Obstet Gynecol. 1980;55:259-2.

41. Kurjak A, Kupesic S. Doppler assessment of the intervillous blood flow in normal and abnormal early pregnancy. Obstet Gynecol. 1997;89:252-6.

42. Jaffe R, Jauniaux AND, Hustin J. Maternal circulation in the first trimester human placenta—myth or reality? Am J Obstet Gynecol. 1997;176:695-705.

43. Jaffe R, Woods JR. Doppler velocimetry of intraplacental fetal vessels in the second trimester: Improving the prediction of pregnancy complications in high-risk patients. Ultrasound Obstet Gynecol. 1996; 8:262-6.

44. Martin AM, Bindra R, Curcio P. Screening for pre-eclampsia and fetal growth restriction by uterine artery Doppler at 11-14 weeks of gestation. Ultrasound Obstet Gynecol. 2001;18:583-6.

45. Kurjak A, Kupesic S. Parallel Doppler assessment of yolk sac and intervillous circulation in normal pregnancy and missed abortion. Placenta. 1998;19:619-23.

46. Mercé LT, Barco MJ, Bau S. Color Doppler sonographic assessment of placental circulation in the first trimester of normal pregnancy. J Ultrasound Med. 1996;15:135-42.

47. Jauniaux AND, Johnson MR, Jurkovic D, et al. The role of relaxin in the development of the uteroplacental circulation in early pregnancy. Obstet Gynecol. 1994;84:338-42.

48. Alcazar JL, Ruiz-Perez ML. Uteroplacental circulation in patients with first trimester threatened abortion. Fertil Steril. 2000;73:130-5.

49. Salim A, Zalud I, Farmakides G, et al. Corpus luteum blood flow in normal and abnormal early pregnancy: Evaluation with transvaginal color and pulsed Doppler sonography. J Ultrasound Med. 1994;13:971-5.

50. Alcazar JL, Laparte C, Lopez-Garcia G. Corpus luteum blood flow in abnormal early pregnancy. J Ultrasound Med. 1996;15:645-9.

51. Daya S, Woods S, Ward S, et al. Early pregnancy assessment with transvaginal ultrasound scanning. CMAJ. 1991;144:441-6.

52. Goldstein I, Zimmer EA, Tamir A, et al. Evaluation of normal gestational sac growth: Appearance of embryonic heartbeat and embryo body movements using the transvaginal technique. Obstet Gynecol. 1991;77:885-8.

53. Norwitz ER, Scust DJ, Fisher SJ. Implantation and the survival of early pregnancy. N Eng J Med. 2001;345:1400-8.

54. Brown DL, Emerson DS, Felker RE, et al. Diagnosis of early embryonic demise by endovaginal sonography. J Ultrasound Med. 1990;9:631-6.

55. Bernard KG, Cooperberg PL. Sonographic differentiation between blighted ovum and early viable pregnancy. Am J Roentgenol. 1985;144:597-602.

56. Nyberg DA, Mack THE, Laing FC, et al. Distinguishing normal from abnormal gestational sac growth in early pregnancy. J Ultrasound Med. 1987;6:23-7.

57. McKenna KM, Feldstein VA, Goldstein RB, et al. The empty amnion: The sign of early pregnancy failure. J Ultrasound Med. 1995;14:117-21.

96

2D and 3D Doppler Assessment of Abnormal Early Intrauterine Pregnancy

JL Alcazar, LT Merce, M Garcia-Manero

INTRODUCTION

The introduction of transvaginal ultrasound allowed assessing in vivo and non-invasively, until then, a non-explored territory: the early gestation. This technique revolutionized the evaluation and management of many clinical situations during this period of pregnancy. The advent of color and power Doppler ultrasound, as a further step, allowed the assessment of early pregnancy hemodynamics. Traditionally, two-dimensional (2D) color and pulsed Doppler has been applied to evaluate early human pregnancy hemodynamics during the last 15 years.[1] In recent years, a new technological advancement has been introduced: three-dimensional (3D) power Doppler ultrasonography. This new technique allows a more objective and global assessment of organ vasculature.[2]

The scope of the present chapter is to address the assessment of ovarian, uteroplacental, yolk sac and embryo-fetal hemodynamic changes in abnormal early intrauterine pregnancy by means of 2D and 3D transvaginal color and power Doppler ultrasonography. We shall review missed abortion and anembryonic pregnancy, threatened abortion and complete/incomplete abortion.

Hemodynamic changes in normally developing pregnancy have been dealt in another chapter in this book, so we have addressed specifically what happens in abnormal early pregnancy.

ABNORMAL EARLY PREGNANCY

Missed Abortion and Anembryonic Pregnancy

Luteal Circulation

Three studies have found that luteal blood flow resistance was increased in missed abortion.[3-5] This finding may be a consequence rather a cause for missed abortion, because missed abortion consists of a failure of early pregnancy to develop, in which the production of human chorionic gonadotropin is impaired, which in turn could have a negative effect on luteal function. However, Frates and coworkers did not find any difference among missed abortions and normal pregnancies.[6]

Regarding anembryonic pregnancies, Alcázar and colleagues[3] and Salim and coworkers[4] did not find any differences in luteal blood flow as compared with normal developing pregnancies. This could be explained by the fact that in anembryonic pregnancy trophoblastic activity continues during a time without the presence of the embryo. Furthermore, some studies have demonstrated that luteal activity in anembryonic pregnancy, as assessed by progesterone serum levels, does not differ from normal pregnancies but it is impaired in missed abortions.[7]

Uteroplacental Circulation

Several authors have investigated uteroplacental circulation in abnormal early pregnancies. In the case of missed abortion and anembryonic pregnancy most studies did not find significant differences as compared with normal pregnancies in uterine, arcuate, radial and spiral arteries or retrochorionic arteries.[8-13]

Regarding intervillous flow conflicting data have been reported. According to embryological studies, uteroplacental circulation is established around day 12 of the embryo development, when maternal blood flows into the syncytiotrophoblast lacunae. Therefore, actual blood flow in the intervillous space begins around days 14–15 of the embryonic development (4th week of amenorrhea) and never later than day 40 (7 weeks + 5 days).[14,15]

However, Hustin and Schaaps challenged this concept and brought a new theory up.[16] They stated that intervillous blood flow does not actually exist until the 12th week. Their theory was based on the findings from in vitro studies using four placentas perfused with barium sulfate and hysteroscopic studies in ten patients. Using transvaginal color Doppler, Jauniaux and colleagues,[17] Jaffe and Woods[18] and Coppens and coworkers[19] supported this theory, because they did not detect intervillous flow until the 12th week.

However, several studies have reported that intervillous flow can be detected from the 6th week onwards in normal early pregnancy.[20-23] This is also our findings (Alcázar, data not published) (Figs 96.1 and 96.2). We agree with Mercé et al.[20] and Kurjak et al.[21] that two types of intervillous flow can be found: one pulsating arterial-type (Fig. 96.3) and other continuous venous-type (Fig. 96.4).

In abnormal pregnancies, Jauniaux et al. found that 70% of complicated pregnancies showed intervillous flow as compared with 0% in normal developing pregnancy.[24] However, a more recent study from this group showed that intervillous flow may be detected in around 60% of normally developing pregnancies between the 7th and 13th weeks,[25] being a progressive phenomenon (36% at 8–9 weeks, 60% at 10–11 weeks and 90% at 12–13 weeks). They found that in abnormal pregnancy, the cases in which intervilluos flow could be detected were higher than in normal pregnancies at 8–9 and 10–11 weeks, but not later. They did not discriminate between missed abortions and anembryonic pregnancies. They speculated that a premature entry of maternal blood in the intervillous space disrupts the materno-embryonic interface and is probably the final mechanism causing abortion. Similar findings have been reported by Jaffe et al.[26] Kurjak et al found that a significant increase of venous peak velocity in the intervillous flow occurs in normal pregnancies from the 11th week onwards. This change does not occur in missed abortion or anembryonic pregnancy.[21] These authors did not find differences in arterial intervillous flow between normal and abnormal pregnancies.[21,27]

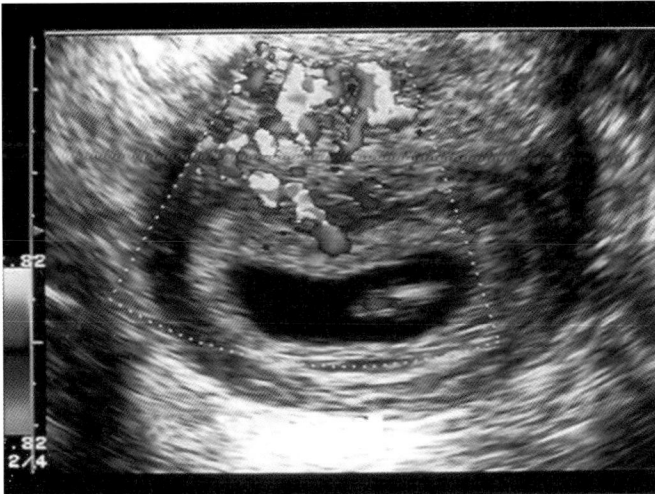

Fig. 96.1: Intervillous blood flow in early pregnancy. It can be clearly seen vessels penetrating the chorion

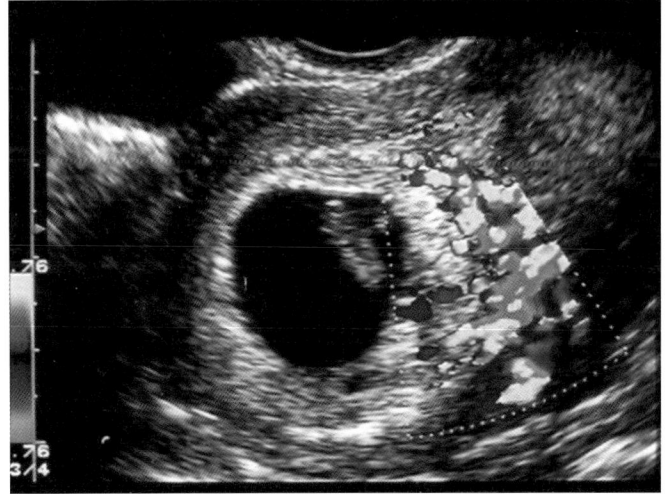

Fig. 96.2: Intervillous flow in early pregnancy

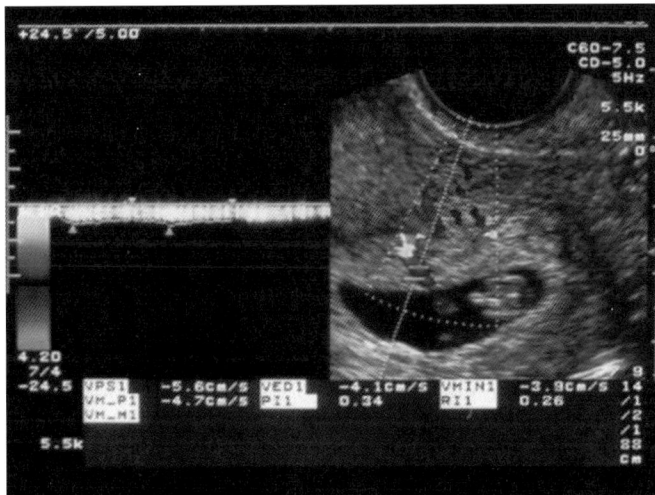

Fig. 96.3: Arterial-like flow velocity waveform from intervillous space

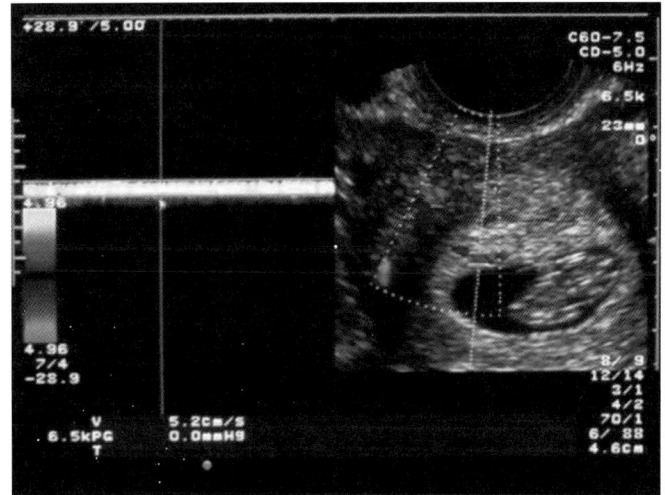

Fig. 96.4: Venous-like flow velocity waveform from intervillous space

Yolk Sac Circulation

Analyzing yolk sac hemodynamics, Kurjak et al. reported that yolk sac blood flow was detected only in 19% of patients with missed abortion as compared with 67% in normal pregnancies.[27]

Threatened Abortion

Those studies addressing hemodynamics changes in missed abortion or anembryonic pregnancy are interesting from a pathophysiologic point of view but may not be relevant to clinical practice because diagnosis can be made with B-mode ultrasound and assessment of the uteroplacental circulation does not add clinical or prognostic information. However, this situation is different in patients with threatened abortion, even more if a living embryo is identified.

Luteal Circulation

Salim and coworkers analyzing luteal blood flow found a significantly higher mean RI (resistance index) in threatened

abortion.[4] However, we did not find any differences in luteal blood flow in threatened abortion as compared with normal developing pregnancies.[3] This difference regarding our results might be explained by the fact that all cases of threatened abortion in our study had an uneventful outcome, indicating that luteal function might be normal. Frates and coworkers reported similar findings to ours. They did not find any relationship between luteal blood flow and first trimester pregnancy outcome.[6]

Uteroplacental Circulation

Most studies assessing uteroplacental blood flow in threatened abortion conclude that Doppler assessment does not provide prognostic information because no significant differences between pregnancies with normal outcome and those that ended in abortion were found.[28-31]

Some authors have evaluated the predictive value for abnormal outcome of uteroplacental blood flow assessment in early pregnancy. Jaffe et al. found that an abnormally high RI (cut-off RI

= 0.55) in the spiral arteries was associated with a higher probability of spontaneous abortion.[32] Leible et al. showed that a discordant uterine artery (pulsatility index > 1.1) would predict a subsequent miscarriage in otherwise normally developing pregnancies during first trimester (odd ratio: 29, 95% CIS: 1.5–5.8).[33]

On the other hand, uteroplacental blood flow assessment seems to be useless to predict pregnancy outcome in women with recurrent spontaneous abortion.[34]

Regarding intervilluos flow, Mercé et al. observed an increase in venous velocity in 64% of spontaneous abortion before embryo death.[35]

We have evaluated the role of 3D power Doppler ultrasound in assessing intervilluos flow in normal pregnancy (Figs 96.5 to 96.7). This technique has been show to be reproducible,[2] overcoming one of the main problems of 2D color or power Doppler ultrasound and allowing an assessment of the entire chorion and early placenta. We found that Flow Index was significantly higher in pregnancies that ended in spontaneous abortion as compared with those that had normal outcome (Fig. 96.8). No differences were found in Vascularity and Vascularity-Flow indexes (Figs 96.9 and 96.10). This finding is very interesting because the Flow Index reflects flow velocity, thus confirming the previous finding from Mercé et al.[35]

Yolk Sac Circulation

Makikallio et al. have reported that yolk sac hemodynamics is not affected in cases of threatened abortion with or without retrochorionic hematoma.[36]

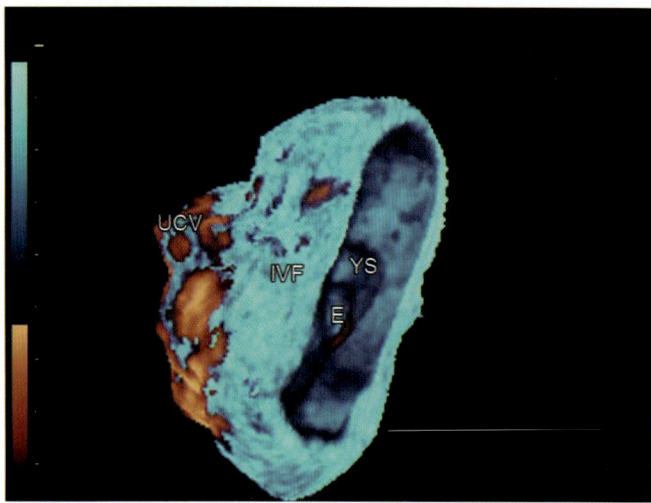

Fig. 96.5: Rendering of utero-chorionic vessels (UCV) and intervillous blood flow (IVF) by power Doppler three-dimensional angiography in a 7 weeks normal pregnancy

Abbreviations: YS, yolk sac; E, embryo

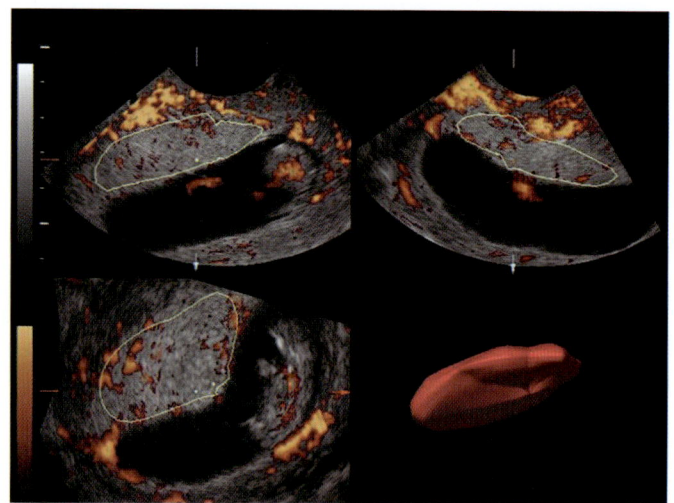

Fig. 96.6: Intervillous blood flow assessment by VOCAL software during early pregnancy

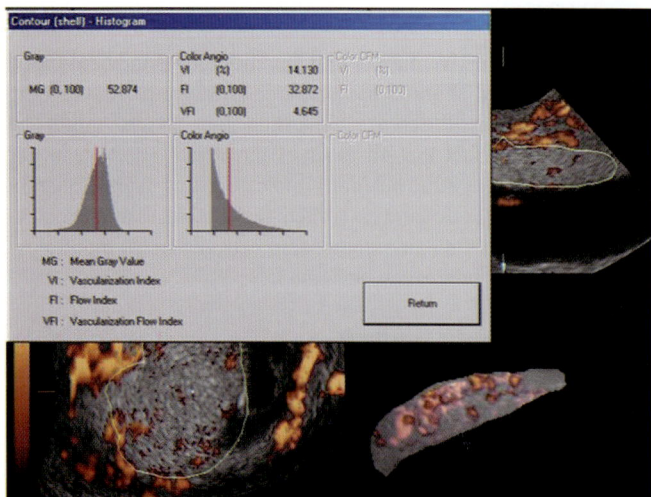

Fig. 96.7: Vascularization index (VI), flow index (FI) and vascularization-flow index (VFI) are useful to evaluate intervillous blood flow during normal and abnormal early pregnancy

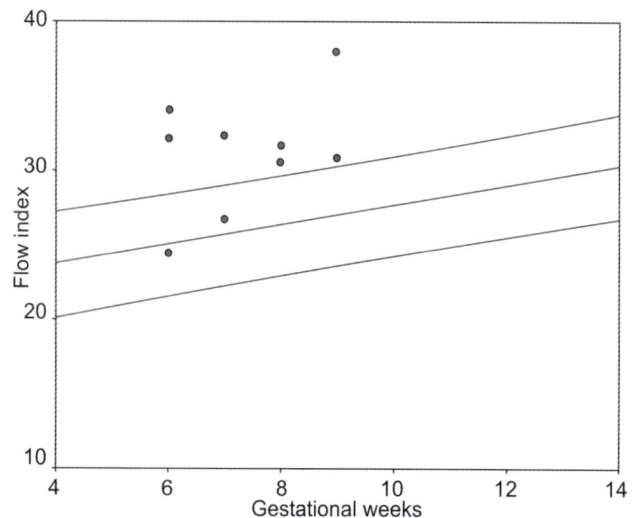

Fig. 96.8: Flow index in cases of spontaneous abortion (closed circles). Regression line for normal pregnancies [y = 21.050 + 0.659 (gestational age), R^2 = 0.16]. It can be seen how most cases of spontaneous abortion are outside normal range

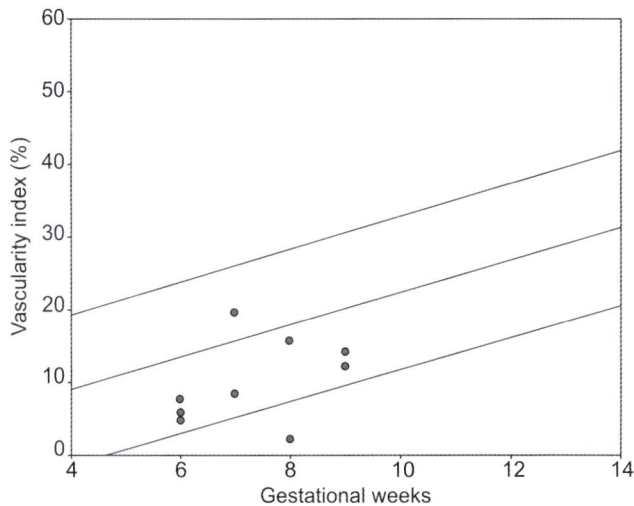

Fig. 96.9: Vascularity index in cases of spontaneous abortion (closed circles). Regression line for normal pregnancies [y = 7.018 + 2.892 (gestational age), R^2 = 0.28]. It can be seen how most cases of spontaneous abortion are within normal range

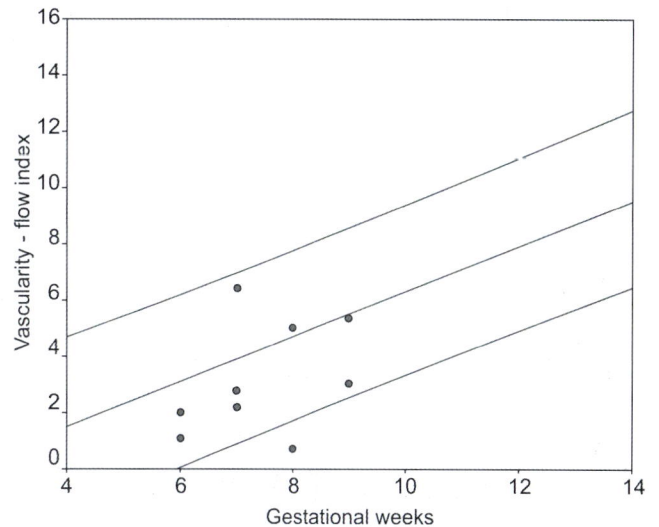

Fig. 96.10: Vascularity-flow index in cases of spontaneous abortion (closed circles). Regression line for normal pregnancies [y = –2.383 + 0.859 (gestational age), R^2 = 0.29]. It can be seen how most cases of spontaneous abortion are within normal range

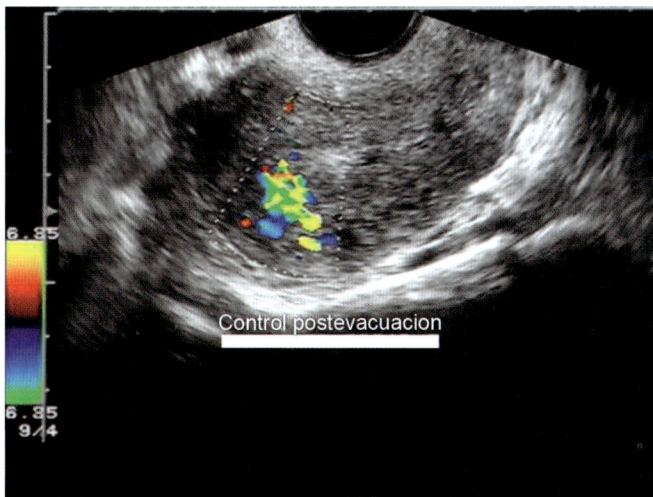

Fig. 96.11: Transvaginal color ultrasound after D&C (dilation and curettage) and persistent spotting. This figure shows a focal area of vascularization at the level of fundus and posterior myometrium. Retained tissue was found after D&C

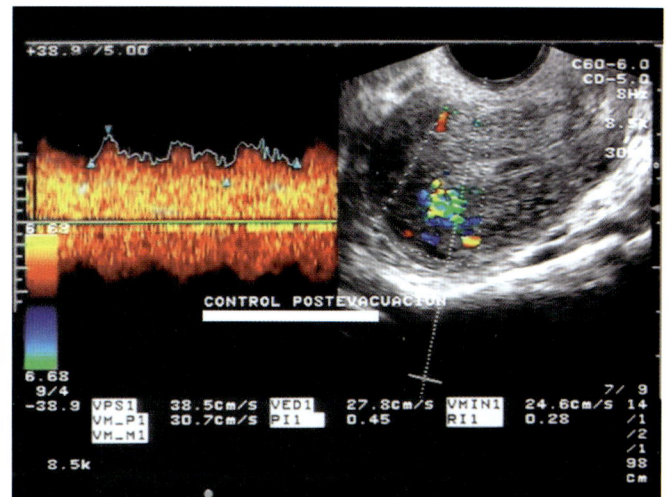

Fig. 96.12: Same patient as in Figure 96.11. A low resistance and high velocity vascularity-flow index, suggestive of trophoblastic flow is clearly found

Embryo-fetal Circulation

The assessment of embryo-fetal circulation in abnormal early pregnancy is unique to threatened abortion with a living embryo. Assessment of embryo-fetal circulation has been focused in three arterial vessels: umbilical artery, abdominal and cerebral vessels.

Some authors have evaluated the role of fetal hemodynamics assessment for predicting pregnancy outcome in cases of threatened abortion with retrochorionic hematoma. All studies concluded that fetal circulation assessment is not useful to predict pregnancy outcome.[29,37,38]

Complete and Incomplete Abortion

Differentiate between incomplete and complete spontaneous abortion is one of the most difficult tasks, which a clinician could

deal with. Management may be quite different if the presence of retained tissue can be ruled out.

The use of transvaginal color Doppler ultrasonography for detecting retained products of conception after spontaneous first trimester abortion has not been extensively evaluated to date. In our experience, this technique can be useful to detect retained trophoblastic tissue in patients with suspected incomplete abortion.[39] The presence of focal areas highly vascularized within myometrium just beneath the endometrium, or even within the endometrium (Fig. 96.11) with flow velocity waveforms characterized by high peak systolic velocity and low impedance (Fig. 96.12) was associated with presence of retained tissue in the vast majority of the cases. On the contrary, the absence of color signals or presence of scanty color signals (Fig. 96.13) with high resistance blood flow

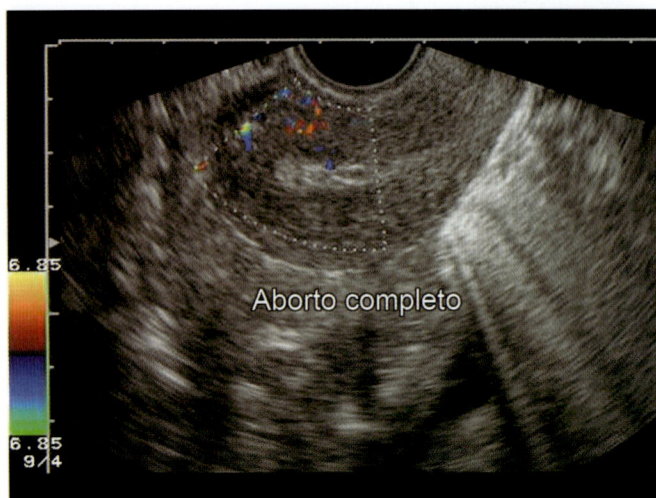

Fig. 96.13: Transvaginal color Doppler ultrasound after heavy vaginal bleeding in first trimester. Scanty flow was found, suggestive of no retained tissue

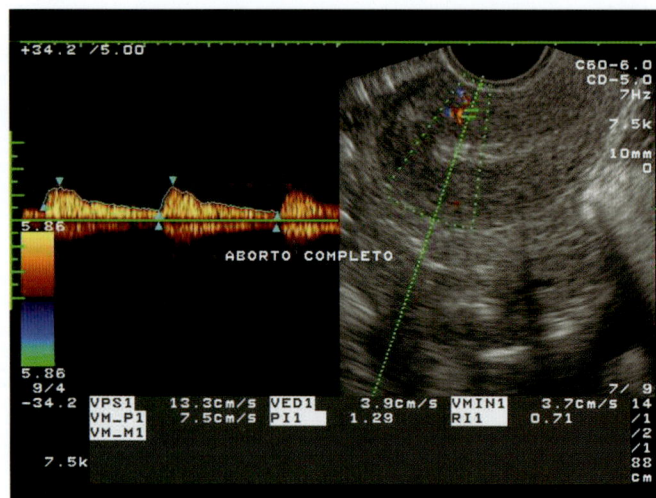

Fig. 96.14: FVW from an arterial vessel in the case of Figure 96.13. High velocity and high resistance flow was found. Typical in no retained tissue

(Fig. 96.14) was associated with absence of retained tissue. In our study, the sensitivity and specificity for color Doppler ultrasound to detect retained tissue was 93.3% and 96%, respectively. We have evaluated prospectively the role of transvaginal color Doppler ultrasonography in the management of first trimester spontaneous abortion, and we found this technique quite useful to rule out retained trophoblastic tissue.[40] Similar results have been reported by other authors.[41]

CONCLUSION

Transvaginal color and power Doppler allows the assessment of abnormal early pregnancy hemodynamics. The results of most published studies reveal that 2D Doppler assessment of luteal, uteroplacental and yolk sac circulations are conflicting or conclude that this assessment has a low clinical value, except for discriminating complete from incomplete abortion.

Three-dimensional power Doppler ultrasonography provides promising results and opens a formidable new research field.

REFERENCES

1. Mercé LT, Barco MJ, de la Fuente F. Doppler velocimetry measured in retrochorionic space and uterine arteries during early human pregnancy. Acta Obstet Gynecol Scand. 1989;68:603-7.
2. Mercé LT, Barco MJ, Bau S. Reproducibility of the study of placental vascularization by three-dimensional power Doppler. J Perinat Med. 2004;32:228-33.
3. Alcázar JL, Laparte C, López García G. Corpus luteum blood flow in abnormal early pregnancy. J Ultrasound Med. 1996;15:645-9.
4. Salim A, Zalud I, Farmakides G, et al. Corpus luteum blood flow in normal and abnormal early pregnancy: Evaluation with transvaginal color and pulsed Doppler sonography. J Ultrasound Med. 1994;13:971-5.
5. Kurjak A, Zudeningo D, Predanic M, et al. Recent advances in the Doppler study of early fetomaternal circulation. J Perinat Med. 1994;22:419-39.
6. Frates MC, Doubilet PM, Durfee SM, et al. Sonographic and Doppler characteristics of the corpus luteum: Can they predict pregnancy outcome? J Ultrasound Med. 2001;20:821-7.
7. Al-Sebai MAH, Kingsland CR, Diver M. The role of a single progesterone measurement in the diagnosis of early pregnancy failure and prognosis of fetal viability. Br J Obstet Gynecol. 1995;102:364-7.
8. Alfirevic Z, Kurjak A. Transvaginal colour doppler ultrasound in normal and abnormal early pregnancy. J Perinat. Med. 1990;18:173-80.
9. Kurjak A, Zalud I, Crvenkovic G, et al. Transvaginal color Doppler in the assessment of abnormal early pregnancy. J Perinat Med. 1991;19:155-65.
10. Kurjak A, Kupesic-Urek S, Predanic M, et al. Transvaginal color Doppler assessment of uteroplacental circulation in normal and abnormal early pregnancy. Early Hum Dev. 1992;29:385-9.
11. Jaffe R. Investigations of abnormal first trimester gestations by color Doppler imaging. J Clin Ultrasound. 1993;21:521-6.
12. Kurjak A, Zalud I, Predanic M, et al. Transvaginal color Doppler study of uterine blood flow in the first and early second trimesters of pregnancy: Normal versus Abnormal. J Ultrasound Med. 1994;13:43-7.
13. Giacobbe M, Zeferino LZ, Franzin C, et al. Uteroplacental circulation during the first trimester of normal and abnormal pregnancy. Reprod Biomed Online. 2001;4:605.
14. Haufmann P. Entwicklung der plazenta. In: Becker V, Schiebler TH, Kubli F (eds). Die Plazenta des Menschen. Stuttgart: Georg Thieme Verlag. 1981;37-64.
15. Mercé LT, Kupesic S, Kurjak A. Color Doppler assessment of implantation and early placentation. Prenat Neonat Med. 1999;4:94-112.
16. Hustin J, Schaaps JP. Echographic and anatomic studies of the maternotrophoblastic border during the first trimester of pregnancy. Am J Obstet Gynecol. 1987;157:162-8.

17. Jauniaux E. Intervillous circulation in the first trimester: The phantom of The color Doppler obstetric opera. Ultrasound Obstet Gynecol. 1996;8:73-6.

18. Jaffe R, Woods JR. Color Doppler imaging and in vivo assessment of the anatomy and physilogy of the early uteroplacental circulation. Fertil Steril. 1993;60:293-7.

19. Coppens M, Loquet P, Kollen M, et al. Longitudinal evaluation of uteroplacental and umbilical blood flow changes in normal early pregnancy. Ultrasound Obstet Gynecol. 1996;7:114-21.

20. Mercé LT, Barco MJ, Bau S. Color Doppler sonographic assessment of placental circulation in the first trimester of normal pregnancy. J Ultrasound Med. 1996;15:135-42.

21. Kurjak A, Kupesic S. Doppler assessment of the intervillous blood flow in normal and abnormal early pregnancy. Obstet Gynecol. 1997;89:252-6.

22. Alouini S, Carbillon L, Perrot N, et al. Intervillous and spiral artery flows in normal pregnancies between 5 and 10 weeks of amenorrhea using color Doppler ultrasonography. Fetal Diagn Ther. 2002;17:163-6.

23. Makikallio K, Tekay A, Jouppila P. Uteroplacental hemodynamics during early human pregnancy. Gynecol Obstet Invest. 2004;58:49-54.

24. Jauniaux E, Zaidi J, Jurkovic D, et al. Comparison of colour Doppler features and pathological findings in complicated early pregnancy. Hum Reprod. 1994;9:2432-7.

25. Jauniaux E, Greenwold N, Hempstock J, et al. Comparison of ultrasonographic and Doppler mapping of the intervillous circulation in normal and abnormal early pregnancies. Fertil Steril. 2003;79:100-6.

26. Jaffe R, Warsoff SL. Color Doppler imaging in the assessment of uteroplacental bood flow in abnormal first trimester intrauterine pregnancies: An attempt to define etiologic mechanisms. J Ultrasound Med. 1992;11:41-4.

27. Kurjak A, Kupesic S. Parallel Doppler assessment of yolk sac and intervillous circulation in normal and missed abortion. Placenta. 1998;19:619-23.

28. Kurjak A, Schulman H, Zudenigo D, et al. Subchorionic hematomas in early pregnancy: Clinical outcome and blood flow patterns. J Mat Fet Med. 1996;5:41-4.

29. Kurjak A, Zudenigo D, Predanic M, et al. Assessment of fetomaternal circulation in threatened abortion by transvaginal color Doppler. Fetal Diagn Ther. 1994;9:341-7.

30. Alcázar JL, Ruiz-Pérez ML. Uteroplacental circulation in patients with first trimester threatened abortion. Fertil Steril. 2000;73:130-5.

31. Pellizzari P, Pozzan C, Marchiori S, et al. Assessment of uterine artery blood flow in normal first-trimester pregnancies and in those complicated by uterine bleeding. Ultrasound Obstet Gynecol. 2002;19:366-70.

32. Jaffe R, Dorgan A, Abramowicz JS. Color Doppler imaging of the uteroplacental circulation in the first trimester: Value in predicting pregnancy failure or complication. Am J Roentgenol. 1995;164:1255-8.

33. Leible S, Cumsille F, Walton R, et al. Discordant uterine artery velocity waveforms as a predictor of subsequent miscarriage in early viable pregnancies. Am J Obstet Gynecol. 1998;179:1587-93.

34. Frates MC, Doubilet PM, Brown DL, et al. Role of Doppler ultrasonography in the prediction of pregnancy outcome in women with recurrent spontaneous abortion. J Ultrasound Med. 1996;15:557-62.

35. Mercé LT, Barco MJ, Bau S. Color Doppler sonography of the retrochorionic and intervellous circulation: Predictive value in small gestational sacs. Med Imag Internat. 1997;7:16-9.

36. Makikallio K, Tekay A, Jouppila P. Effects of bleeding on uteroplacental, umbilicoplacental and yolk-sac hemodynamics in early pregnancy. Ultrasound Obstet Gynecol. 2001;18:352-6.

37. Rizzo G, Capponi A, Seregaroli M, et al. Early fetal circulation in pregnancies complicated by retroplacental hematoma. J Clin Ultrasound. 1995;23:525-9.

38. Alcázar JL. Assessment of fetal circulation in patients with retrochorionic hematoma during the first trimester of pregnancy. Prenat Neonat Med. 1998;3:458-63.

39. Alcázar JL. Transvaginal ultrasonography combined with color velocity imaging and pulsed Doppler to detect residual trophoblastic tissue. Ultrasound Obstet Gynecol. 1998;11:54-8.

40. Alcázar JL, Ortiz C. Transvaginal color Doppler ultrasonography in the management of first trimester spontaneous abortion. Eur J Obstet Gynecol Reprod Biol. 2002;102:83-7.

41. Zalel Y, Gamzu R, Lidor A, et al. Color Doppler imaging in the sonohysterographic diagnosis of residual trophoblastic tissue. J Clin Ultrasound. 2002;30:222-5.

97 Ultrasonography of Ectopic Pregnancy

S Iniesta, F Salazar, JM Bajo

DEFINITION

The term *ectopic pregnancy* is applied to pregnancy following implantation of the fertilized ovum on any tissue other than the uterus endometrium.

The tubal presentation is the most common one, especially if it is in its distal third portion or in the middle third one (both of them are nearly 95–97% of all ectopic pregnancies). Occasionally, it can appear in the interstitial portion (cornual pregnancy, 2–5%) and exceptionally in the ovary (0.5–1%), in the cervix (0.10–15%) or inside the abdomen (1.4%).[1,2]

The common denominator in this group of patients is delay in transport of the ovum fertilized in the ampulla of the tube to the normal implantation site in the uterus.

INCIDENCE

The incidence of ectopic pregnancy is increasing during the last years.[3,5] Although it is difficult to calculate, it is nearly 0.94–2.6% of all pregnancies. This increased incidence can be explained by the use of reproduction treatments, the use of some contraceptive methods and because of the pelvic inflammatory disease.

Day by day, with vaginal ultrasound development and with the earlier detection of beta-subunit human chorionic gonadotropin by radioimmunoassay (β-hCG), the diagnosis of ectopic pregnancies is getting better, and it is possible to recognize an ectopic pregnancy at earlier stages (some days or weeks earlier) than some years ago, including some cases that before happened unnoticed.

ETIOLOGY

Although the ectopic pregnancy etiology is still unknown, there are several risk factors that can be associated to ectopic pregnancy:[3,6]

- Previous pelvic inflammatory disease.[7] It increases by four the incidence of ectopic pregnancy (it is the most important cause of it). The only presence of circulating Chlamydia antibodies increases its incidence by two.[8]
- Previous tubal surgery (for infertility, because of previous ectopic pregnancies, bipolar tubal coagulation in sterilization context, etc.) or any other kind of surgery in the inferior hemiabdomen that may cause tubal adhesions as well.
- Other organic tubal alterations: tubal tumors, endometriosis, peritubal adhesions, etc.
- Reproduction treatments (TRA, ovulation induction treatments, etc.).[9]
- Contraception failures. *Intrauterine devices* do not increase these incidence of ectopic pregnancy by themselves, but once the pregnancy is established, the possibility of it being an ectopic one is much higher. The lowest ectopic pregnancy rates are observed with the high cooper dose intrauterine devices, instead of the ones with low cooper dose or the ones that release progesterone, that the highest ectopic pregnancies rate. Nevertheless, the levonorgestrel intrauterine devices show a low rate, similar to those of high dose copper loads.[10] Failures of tubal coagulation techniques also increase the risk of ectopic pregnancies, because they may cause tubal fistulas:[11]
- Previous ectopic pregnancies.
- Tobacco.
- Infertility.

All these factors could be involved in the transportation of the fertilized ovum to the uterus, although there are also some embryonic factors that can be responsible for ectopic pregnancy, and more or less, a third of them have chromosomal abnormalities.

SYMPTOMS AND SIGNS

Physical findings are quite variable, and the clinical presentation has changed considerably over the last years because of its earlier diagnosis. Although the incidence of ectopic pregnancy has increased, the frequency of its complications (such as ectopic pregnancy rupture, tubal abortion, etc.) is decreasing at a very important rate, because the greater exactitude of the diagnosis methods allows to detect ectopic pregnancies in asymptomatic women and in precocious phases of the process.[12,13]

This has also allowed to develop different protocols for non-surgical treatment of ectopic pregnancy, as well as less invasive surgical procedures.

CLINICAL SITUATIONS OF ECTOPIC PREGNANCY

- Asymptomatic women.
- Vague abdominal pain, without any specific findings, in unruptured cases. Sometimes we can find vaginal bleeding, usually in scanty amounts. The classic clinical triad of ectopic pregnancy is pain, vaginal bleeding and amenorrhea, although the amenorrhea is sometimes difficult to value because of the vaginal bleeding.
- Acute hemorrhagical accident, generally caused by tubal rupture or by tubal abortion with peritoneal hemorrhage. In this case, patients will present all the symptoms and signs of acute abdomen (positive blumberg, peritoneal defense) and hypovolemic signs (extreme pallor of the skin and mucous membranes, tachycardia, hypotension, etc.).

The first symptom noticed by patients is likely to be a 1 or 2 weeks delay in menstruation, followed by slight bleeding which persists, with perhaps only a scant show of blood, almost everyday. Although this spotting type of bleeding is rather characteristic, not infrequently the bleeding may be somewhat free, but it is rarely so profuse as with an incomplete abortion. Instead of the menstrual period being delayed, there may be an apparent anticipation of the flow by a few days.

Pain is an early symptom, although it is sometimes very slight. At the beginning, there may be only a vague tenderness in the affected side of the pelvis, but often the patient complains of sharp colicky pain occurring from time to time. When rupture or tubal abortion takes place, the pain may be very severe, and it may be associated with faintness or actual syncope and often nausea and vomiting. These symptoms are the result of the peritoneal reaction produced by the escape of blood of the tube.

DIAGNOSIS

The clinical image of ectopic pregnancy is so typical in many cases that diagnosis is very easy, but many errors can be made, so we always have to keep in mind the ectopic pregnancy if we do not want to make mistakes.[14,15]

The diagnosis is actually based on:

- Anamnesis, insisting on the classic clinical triad and on the investigation of ectopic pregnancy risk factors.
- Abdominal and pelvic examination.
- Pregnancy test.
- Ultrasonography.

If we have a positive pregnancy test and any gestational vesicle within the uterine cavity is observed in transvaginal ultrasonography, it is necessary to determinate the beta-subunit human chorionic gonadotropin (β-hCG) levels in maternal serum.[16]

The hCG is a glucoprotein composed by two subunits, alpha and beta, united by non-covalent unions by disulfide bonds. The alpha-subunit is composed by 92 amino acids and the beta-subunit by 145 amino acids. This last one is responsible for the biological activity and it is the one that allows the production of some high specific antibodies highly important for the radioimmunoassay detection.

The hCG is produced in the syncytiotrophoblast and its detection in maternal serum is possible 1 day after the blastocyst implantation.

In a normal gestation (non-ectopic one), the circulating β-hCG levels at the time of the first delay of menstruation is, approximately, 100 UI/L, and it reaches its maximum level (50,000–100,000 UI/L) between eighth and tenth gestational weeks. Later, its value decreases, being around 10,000–20,000 UI/L at eighteenth to twentieth week and it remains more or less constant until the end of pregnancy.[17]

On the other hand, the β-hCG levels in an ectopic pregnancy can be very variable; cases of ectopic pregnancies with β-hCG levels as low as 14 UI/L have been documented, as well as others with 100,000 UI/L. Thus, the value of a single determination of β-hCG is often of little use for the ectopic pregnancy diagnosis. Nevertheless, the consecutive determinations of β-hCG levels allow to differentiate between a normal gestation and an ectopic one, since the increase of the β-hCG levels is different in both of them.

In an intrauterine pregnancy of normal course, the serum β-hCG concentration follows a linear pattern in the first 6 weeks and duplicated in 2 days when its level is lower than 10,000 UI/L.

The trophoblast tissue in an ectopic pregnancy usually produces less hCG than the one of an intrauterine pregnancy, and therefore, its increase in the same period of time is usually smaller.

Nevertheless, some cases of ectopic pregnancy with the same increased levels of β-hCG as intrauterine ones have been described (nearly 13%), at least during a period of time. In addition, 10% of the normal intrauterine pregnancies can present alterations in the increase of the β-hCG.

Some studies, during the last years, have tried to predict the tubal rupture, the possibility of resolution or the possibility of hemorrhage by using β-hCG levels.[18,19] Although some authors have found good results having used the β-hCG levels to predict tubal rupture,[20] considering that this one is not probable with values lower than 2,000 UI/L, with a predictive value of 80%, other authors have observed this complication with levels as low as 100 UI/L and even smaller.[21-24] Therefore, the hemorrhage is not probable, though it is not impossible, with low levels of β-hCG and its decreasing levels do not guarantee that rupture cannot take place. However, most of the authors find a statistically significant difference between the values of β-hCG between ruptured and non-ruptured ectopic pregnancies.

The decreasing levels of β-hCG combined with ultrasonography findings allows to avoid the surgical treatment in non-ruptured cases, although a very careful following is needed because, as we exposed before, the possibility of rupture exists even with decreasing levels of β-hCG. This situation can be explained if the trophoblast is separated of the tubal wall, which may cause an intratubal bleeding with accumulation of intratubal clots, that increase the pressure, and may cause distension and necrosis.

With transvaginal ultrasound an intrauterine gestational sac can be identified with 1,000 UI/L of β-hCG ("discriminatory level"),[25] that is usually observed after 1 week of delay of the menstruation. In a twin gestation this discriminatory level can be slightly higher and an ultrasonography control must be carried out within 2 or 3 days to try to find the gestational vesicle.

Once we have determinate the β-hCG levels, if we do not find any gestational vesicle, we must differentiate two situations: the first one takes place when we find a β-hCG level below 1,000 UI/L, and the second one when it is higher than 1,000 UI/L.

β-hCG Less than 1,000 UI/L without Intrauterine Gestational Sac

In asymptomatic patients or with light symptoms, a new ultrasonography must be repeated in 1 week, as well as a new β-hCG determination. At this time, it will be possible to find a β-hCG level higher than 1,000 UI/L and also to see an intrauterine gestational sac.[26]

Nevertheless, it is necessary to keep in mind that ectopic pregnancies produce in the endometrium some changes very similar to the ones induced by normal intrauterine pregnancies.[27]

- In 50% of ectopic pregnancies, it is possible to observe a deciduate endometrium, that appears ultrasonographically as a thickened and hyperrefringent endometrium (Fig. 97.1).
- In 10–20% of ectopic pregnancies, it is possible to observe a gestational pseudosac[28] (Fig. 97.2), which appears like a sonoluscence image, located centrally in the endometrium and surrounded by a single echogenic ring. This image really corresponds to the presence of liquid in the decidua

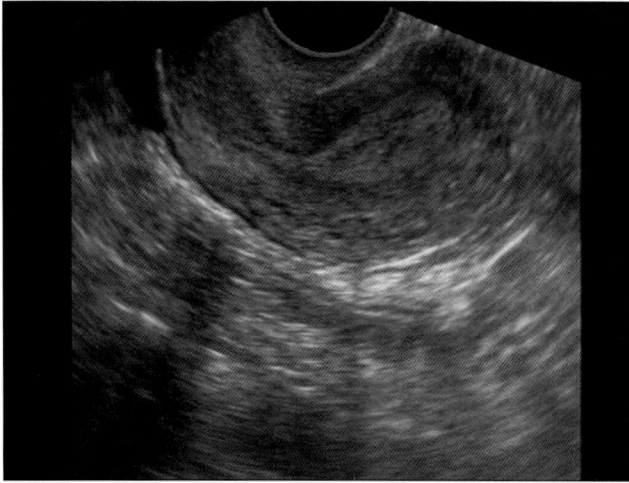

Fig. 97.1: Decidual reaction of the endometrium. Positive β-hCG. Ectopic pregnancy with a tubal gestational sac

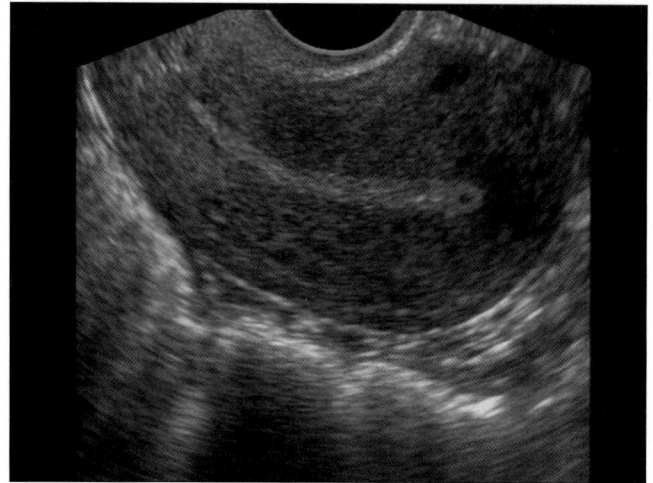

Fig. 97.2: Pseudosac image inside the endometrium

endometrium. In a real gestational sac, it is seen a double echogenic ring, composed by the vera decidua and the capsularis decidua, that form two concentric rings around the gestational sac (double decidua sign). This sign can be observed between fifth and ninth gestational weeks and its presence makes easier the differential diagnosis.

- The color Doppler can contribute also to the diagnosis. An intrauterine gestational sac shows peritrophoblast vascular signals with low resistance index (0.40–0.45). The pseudosac does not present increase of the local flow and its resistance index may be higher (> 0.55).[29-32]

Another common problem when making the diagnosis is to differentiated the ectopic pregnancy with a complete or incomplete abortion. In this last case, ultrasonography shows a hyperechogenic image inside the uterine cavity that correspond to clots or retained abortion rests. These findings can delay diagnosis in nearly 21% of the patients.

Also the possibility of differentiating an ectopic pregnancy from a spontaneous abortion according to the reduction form of β-hCG levels in a period of time more than 48 hours has been investigated. Some authors diagnose a complete abortion when the average life of the β-hCG is less than 1.4 days, whilst if it is more than 7 days, the ectopic pregnancy diagnosis is much more probable. Similarly, a plateau level of β-hCG (that has been defined as a duplication of its levels equal or higher in 7 days) is very suggestive of ectopic pregnancy.

The simultaneous presence of an intrauterine pregnancy and an ectopic one (heterotopic gestation) is not frequent at all, although its incidence is higher in pregnancies obtained by reproductive techniques. It occurs nearly in one of each 100 of these pregnancies, which supposes a much higher frequency than the one referred historically (one of each 30,000).[33,34]

β-hCG More than 1,000 UI/L without Intrauterine Gestational Sac

In this situation a high suspicion of ectopic pregnancy exists, and the gestational sac must be search outside the uterus, considering

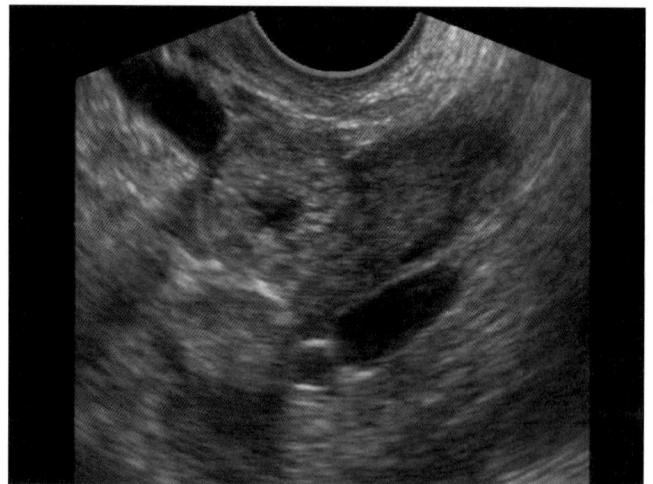

Fig. 97.3: Ectopic pregnancy with ultrasound findings type 1. Outside the uterus and inside the tube, it is visible an anechoic formation of 3 mm, corresponding to the gestational vesicle

that the most common location is the tube. Ultrasound findings can be systematized, depending on the visible structures, in five types.

Ultrasound Image Type 1

A vesicle within the tube is visualized (Fig. 97.3). The yolk sac and the embryo are not visible. The size of the gestational sac is over 3 mm (ultrasound resolution limit). It appears as a cleared formation, in parauterine region, with a central echogenic area surrounded by a hyperechogenic ring (Figs 97.4 and 97.5) that corresponds to the trophoblastic tissue which presents an abundant color map because of its important retrochorionic vascularization proliferation (Fig. 97.6). The Doppler signals show low and medium resistance index (Fig. 97.7), very different to the ones found in normal tube walls that show a high resistance. It is usual to find an average decrease of 15.5% in the ectopic pregnancy side with respect to the contralateral one. This ultrasound image is not easy to find and sometimes the gestational vesicle has less relevance than the corpus luteum that appears close to it, which we have to differentiate (Fig. 97.8).

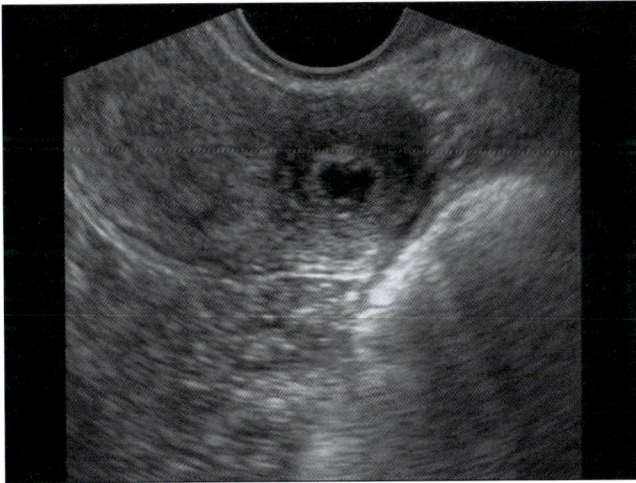

Fig. 97.4: Ectopic pregnancy with ultrasound findings type 1. The vesicle inside the tube and also the tube wall as a ring around the anechoic vesicle are visible

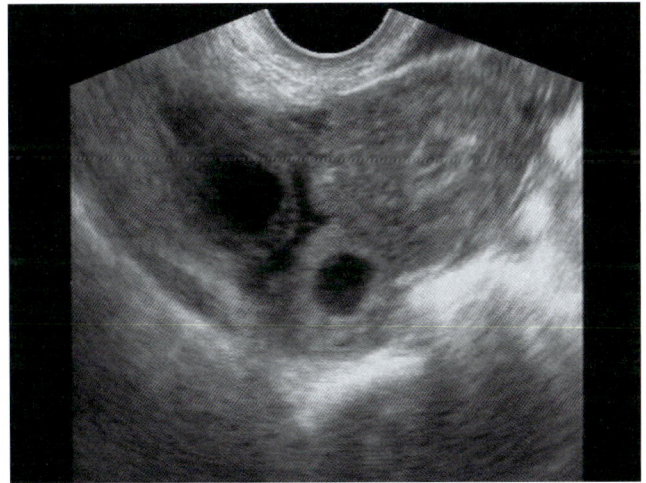

Fig. 97.5: Ectopic pregnancy with ultrasound findings type 1. The corpus luteum close to the gestational vesicle and the tube wall are visible

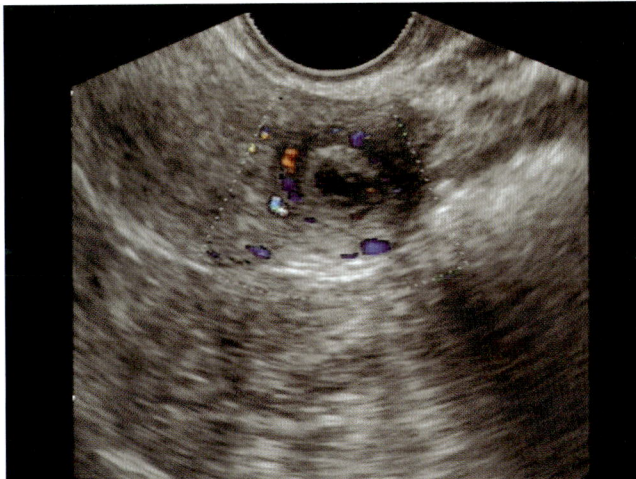

Fig. 97.6: Ectopic pregnancy with ultrasound findings type 1. There is an important vascularization around the gestational coat that corresponds to the trophoblast

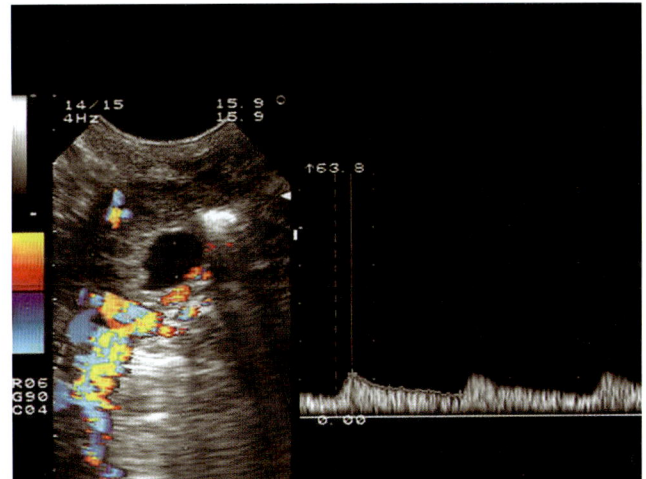

Fig. 97.7: Blood flow inside the gestational sac in an ectopic pregnancy type 1

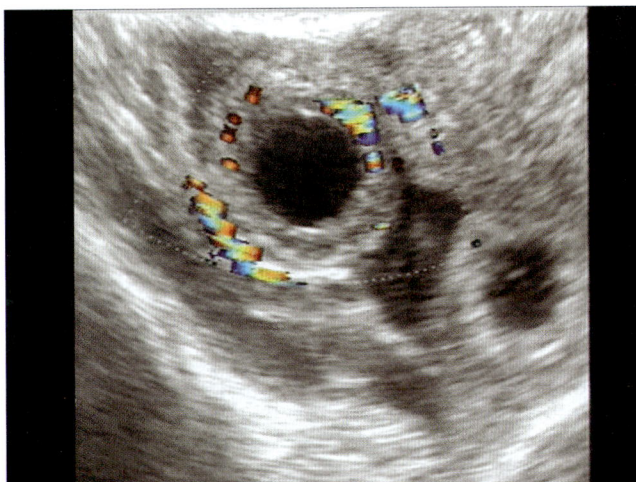

Fig. 97.8: Ectopic pregnancy with ultrasound findings type 1. The anechoic ring is the gestational sac, and there is a corpus luteum close to it with its typical ring fire

Ultrasound Image Type 2

It is possible to see the same findings that in the previous type, but inside the gestational vesicle the yolk sac can be visualized (Figs 97.9 and 97.10). The yolk sac finding is not a trivial question because it makes easier the diagnosis, because it makes impossible to characterize the gestational vesicle that is very difficult to see mainly when it is small. The only presence of the yolk sac clarifies everything (Figs 97.11 and 97.12), and there is now no doubt of the presence of an ectopic pregnancy. The fact that the embryo cannot be seen does not mean that it has not existed, because we know that is the embryo the one that induces the yolk sac formation. In the yolk sac surroundings, it is possible to find blood flows with abundant Doppler signal and low resistance index, as well as in type 1 (Fig. 97.13).

Ultrasound Image Type 3

It is possible to visualize the gestational vesicle, the yolk sac and also the embryo, but not its heart beating (Figs 97.14 and 97.15). The embryo size usually is not very big (Figs 97.16 and 97.17).

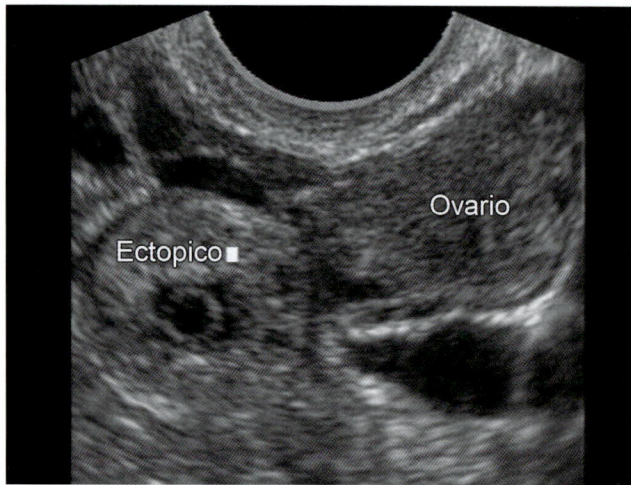

Fig. 97.9: Ectopic pregnancy with ultrasound findings type 2. The gestational sac has inside the yolk sac

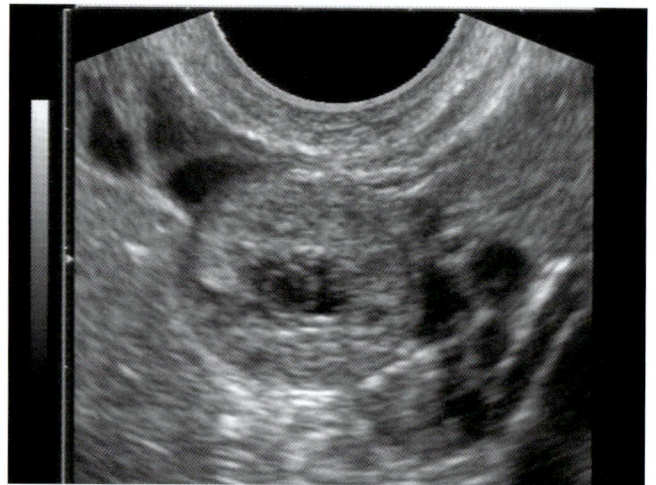

Fig. 97.10: Ectopic pregnancy with ultrasound findings type 2. It is possible to see the yolk sac. The trophoblastic vascularization is also visible

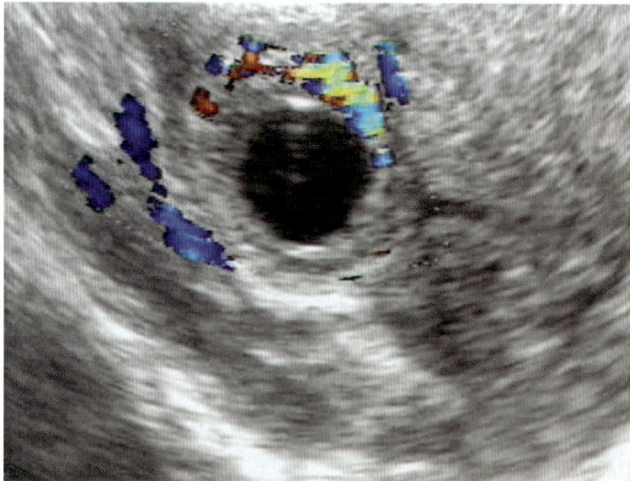

Fig. 97.11: Ectopic pregnancy with ultrasound findings type 2. The yolk sac is inside the gestational sac. It is visible an adjacent image probably originated by the corpus luteum

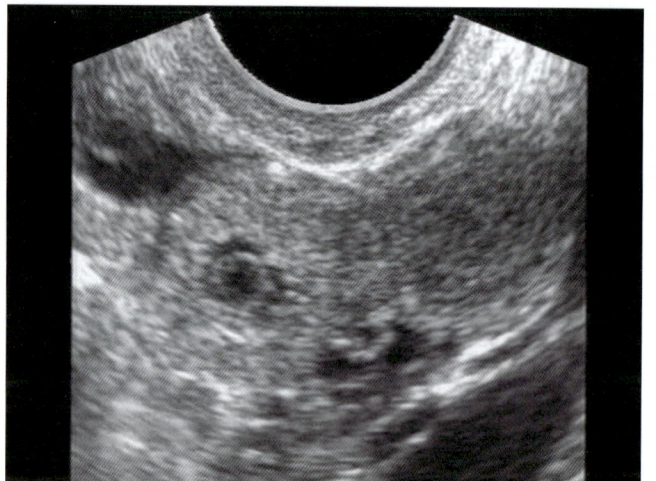

Fig. 97.12: Ectopic pregnancy with ultrasound findings type 2. It is possible to see the yolk sac inside the gestational vesicle and the trophoblastic vascularization with the blood flow

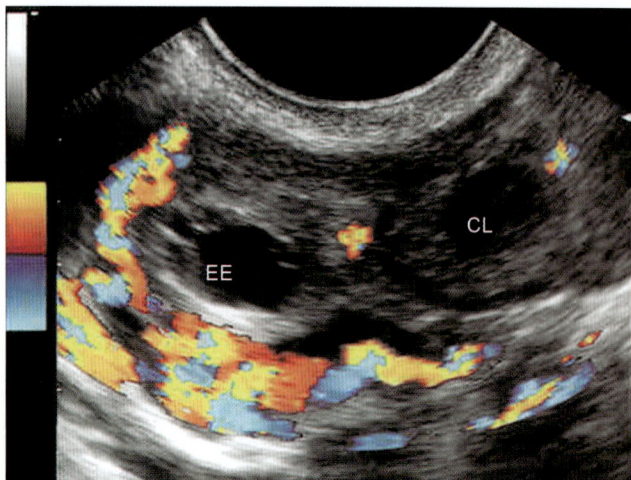

Fig. 97.13: Ectopic pregnancy with ultrasound findings type 3. The tube is pointed. Inside the gestational sac, the yolk sac and also an embryo with no visible heart activity are visible

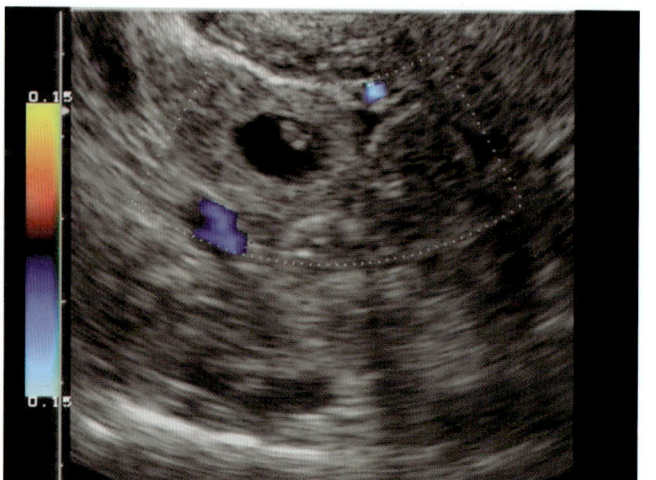

Fig. 97.14: Ectopic pregnancy with ultrasound findings type 3. Gestational sac with the yolk sac and an embryo of very small size in which beat is still not seen

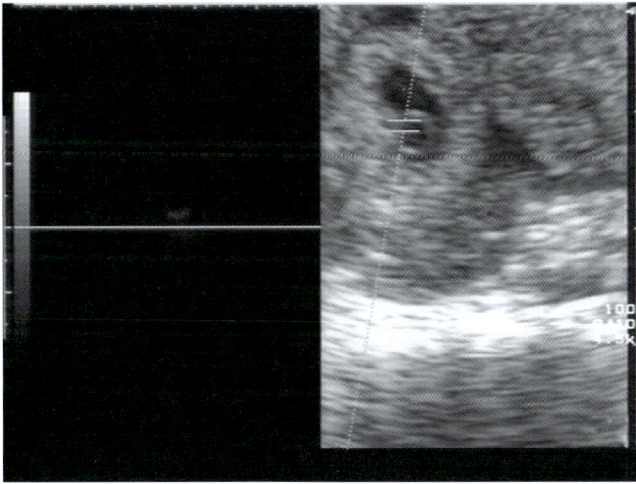

Fig. 97.15: Ectopic pregnancy with ultrasound findings type 3. Inside the gestational sac, the yolk sac and also an embryo with not visible heart activity are visible

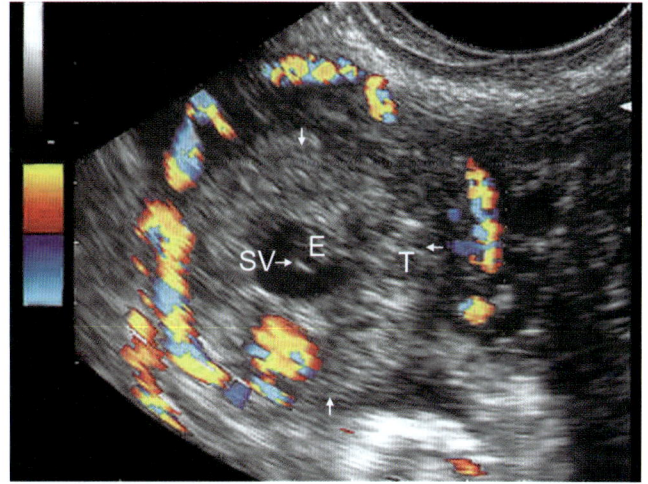

Fig. 97.16: Ectopic pregnancy with ultrasound findings type 3. Inside the gestational sac, it is visible the yolk sac and also an embryo with no visible heart activity. The Doppler signal is captured on the peritubal trophoblast

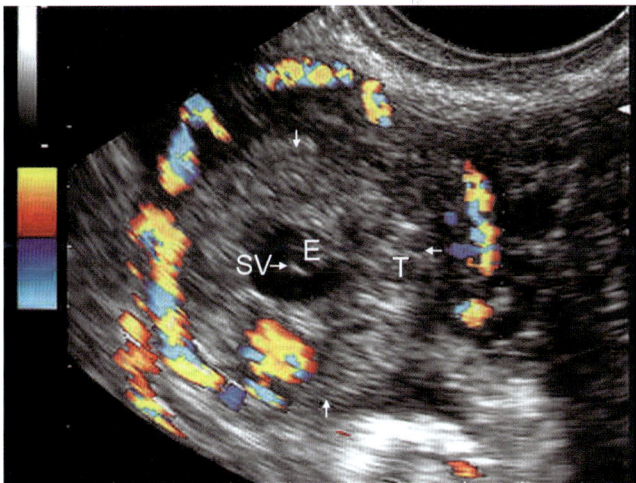

Fig. 97.17: Ectopic pregnancy with ultrasound findings type 4. Inside the gestational sac, it is visible the yolk sac and also an alive embryo, which heart activity is seen by using the color signal

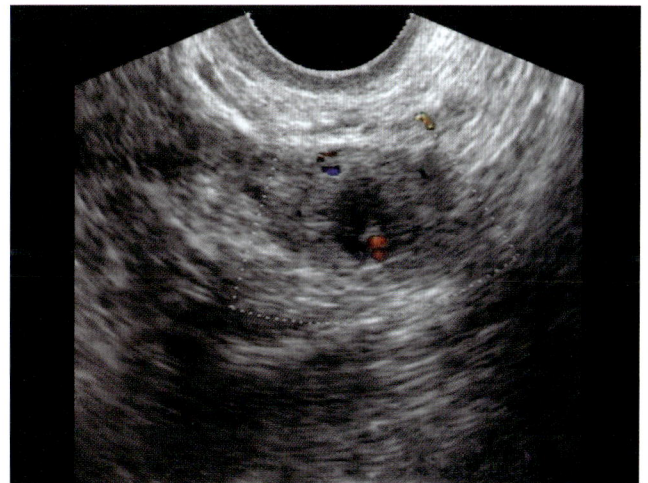

Fig. 97.18: Ectopic pregnancy with ultrasound findings type 4. Inside the gestational sac the yolk sac and also an alive embryo, which heart activity is seen by using the color signal can be seen

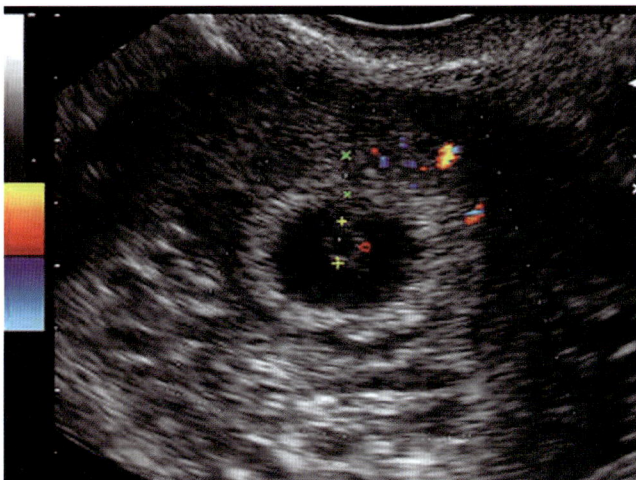

Fig. 97.19: Ectopic pregnancy with ultrasound findings type 4. Inside the gestational sac, it is visible the yolk sac and also an alive embryo with its heart beating

It seems like it is going to start a reabsorption process and soon it disappears or it is confused with the gestational sac.

Ultrasound Image Type 4

The typical image of a gestational vesicle with the yolk sac and the embryo is visualized, but this time with visible cardiac beat inside the embryo. It is very easy to see the beat by using color map (Figs 97.18 and 97.19) or the flow wave (Figs 97.20 and 97.21). When this finding appears, the diagnosis of ectopic pregnancy is made. With an abdominal probe, it is possible to visualize this image only in 10% of all the cases, but with the transvaginal one in 21% of all the ectopic pregnancies.

Ultrasound Image Type 5

This image corresponds with the tubal rupture or with the tubal abortion. In these cases, the acute accident is present and the symptoms and signs are usually important. The most important

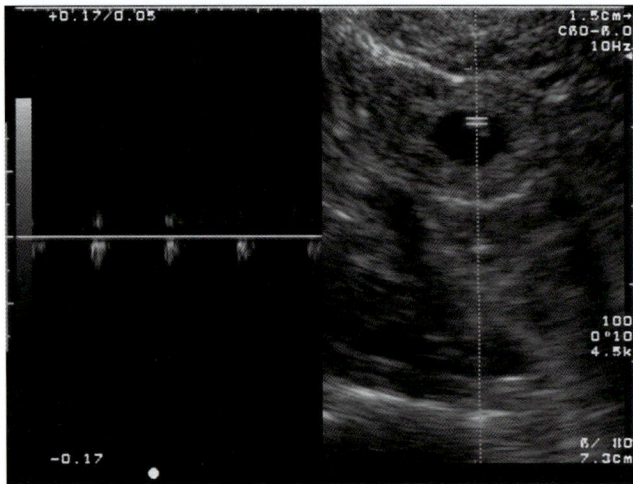

Fig. 97.20: Ectopic pregnancy with ultrasound findings type 4. Inside the gestational sac the yolk sac and also an alive embryo, which heart activity is seen by using the color signal are visible

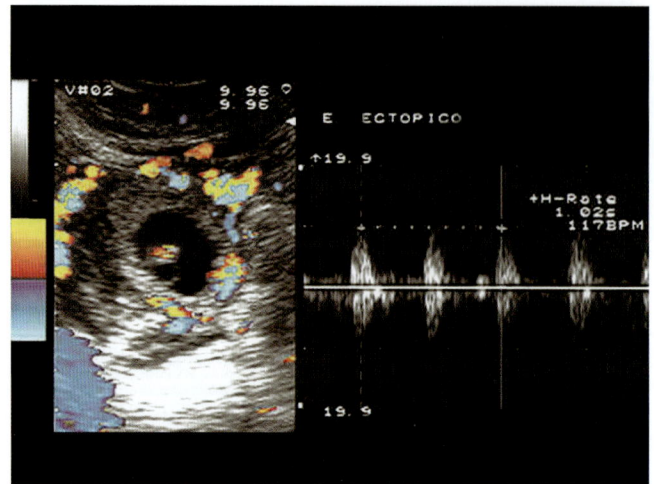

Fig. 97.21: Rupture of an ectopic pregnancy (ultrasound findings type 5). An important hemoperitoneum is visible, with clots

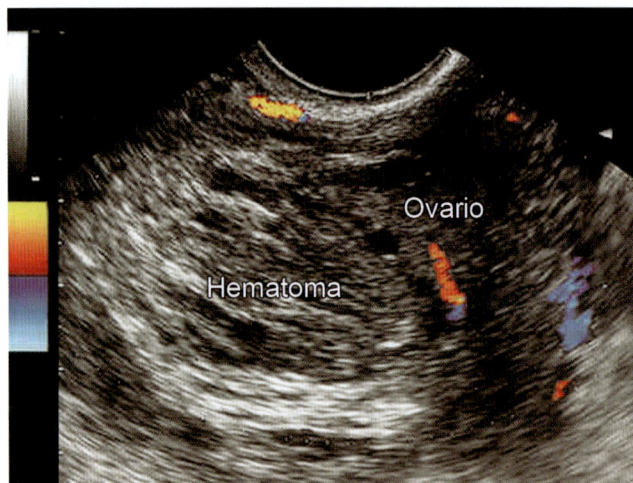

Fig. 97.22: Ruptured tubal ectopic pregnancy, type 5. Hemoperitoneum is around the tube, and neither the embryo nor the gestational sac are visible

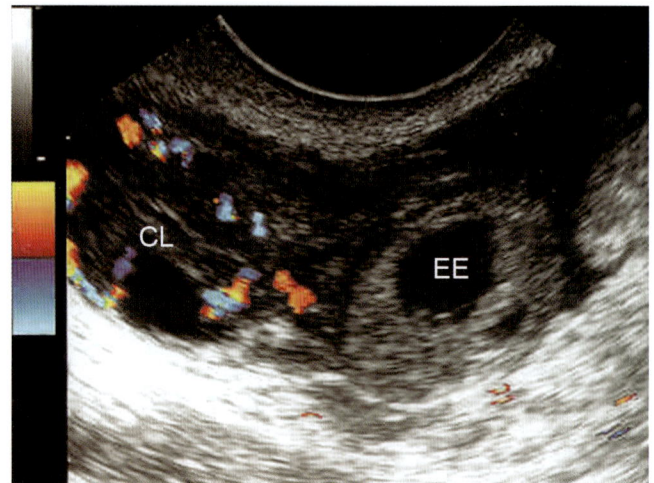

Fig. 97.23: Ruptured ectopic pregnancy, type 5. Inside the blood, the tube surrounded by multiple clots is visible

sign is the hemoperitoneum (Figs 97.22 and 97.23), and the patient may present hypotension and anemia. A large amount of fluid may be visible in the abdomen, in the flanks and in the cul-de-sac if a tubal rupture is present. These fluid collections may be presented as free fluid or as organized blood clots in the cul-de-sac lateral and cranial to the uterus. The clots exhibit the sonographic features of solid masses, appearing homogeneous and contrasting poorly with surrounding tissues. The tube appears refringent ultrasonographically (Fig. 97.24), thickened, or included in a mass of blood clots (Fig. 97.25). In some cases, the tube appears normal, and the blood located around it draws it, showing its shape and the fimbrias.

The mere presence of fluid in the cul-de-sac is not a specific sign of ectopic pregnancy.[35] It is present in nearly 40–83% of all ectopic pregnancies but small collections of free fluid may be seen under normal conditions in the nongravid patients, especially during the periovulatory period, and also in 20% of intrauterine pregnancies and in some other pathologies.

The total absence of ultrasonographic findings in the adnexal area does not exclude the ectopic pregnancy diagnosis. In these cases, it is necessary to repeat the β-hCG levels, to establish its

decreasing or increasing profile, and to repeat the ultrasonography to look for the gestational vesicle in any location. If the patient is stable, we should not undertake the laparoscopy so fast, since very initial phases of ectopic pregnancies have been described with absolutely normal laparocopy.

Generally, in all previous assumptions, the existence of a corpus luteum can be observed. It is visualized as a round hypoechogenic structure, surrounded by a ring of ovarian tissue. It can appear in the contralateral ovary in 13–23% of the cases. The transvaginal ultrasound sensitivity for the ectopic pregnancy diagnosis is very high, nearly 99%, with 98% of specificity, 98% of positive predictive value and 99% of negative predictive value.

ULTRASONOGRAPHY AID TO CONSERVATIVE TREATMENT

Ultrasound is useful as a diagnostic tool in the evaluation of a gestational sac inside or outside the uterus.

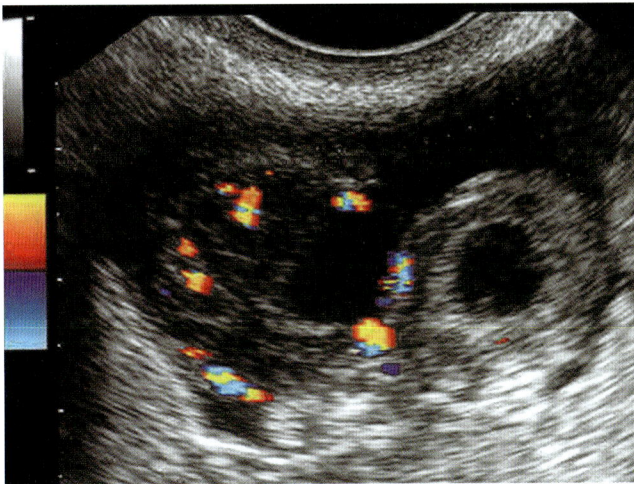

Fig. 97.24: Ruptured ectopic pregnancy, type 5. Inside the blood, there are some refringent masses that may correspond to the tube and to multiple clots

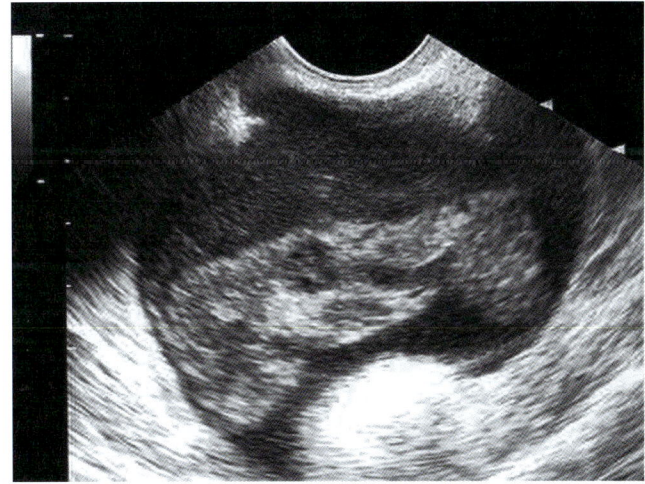

Fig. 97.25: Ectopic pregnancy. Tubal abortion. Hemoperitoneum with blood delimiting the tube in which fimbriae are seen

At the moment, the precocious diagnosis of ectopic pregnancy allows other treatment possibilities different to surgical boarding, that was the only option considered classically.[36-38] These treatment possibilities are:

- Expectant handling.
- Systemic methotrexate administration.
- Local methotrexate administration.

The surgical handling can be performed by laparoscopy or by laparotomy.

Expectant Handling

With a precocious diagnosis of the ectopic pregnancy, before symptoms appear, and adopting more conservative attitudes, it has been possible to see that the spontaneous regression of the tubal ectopic pregnancy is a phenomenon much more common that we thought previously. This fact means that there is a high percentage of ectopic pregnancies that are solved with no need of treatment, and that is why the expectant handling has a place on the ectopic pregnancy management.[39,40]

The main advantages that present the expectant handling are that it avoids the surgery risks, the general anesthesia and the potential indirect effects of the drugs used in the treatment of the ectopic pregnancy.

The greater difficulty of the expectant handling is to select the suitable patients for it. The selection criteria used differ for different authors, but in most cases there are some common aspects; the most outstanding ones are:

- Asymptomatic patient, clinically stable.
- Size: maximum diameter of the ectopic pregnancy of 2–4 cm, according to the authors.
- Absence of embryonic cardiac beat (ultrasonography findings type 1, 2 or 3).
- Decreasing values of β-hCG levels (also variable according to the authors, but at least a decrease of 2% in two determinations with a delay of at least 24 hours).
- Little amount of free fluid in cul-de-sac.

Patients will have to be under periodic ambulatory controls with multiple determinations of β-hCG levels and with an ultrasound following, three times a week at the beginning, and later once a week, according to the different protocols.[41] The signs that oriente to a reabsorption and therefore to a spontaneous resolution of the problem are:

- β-hCG decreasing levels: the typical evolution of a normal curve of β-hCG levels. It is important to be aware that sometimes 70 days are needed to get the β-hCG negative because of the trophoblast persistence.[42]
- The gestational vesicle, the yolk sac and all the embryonic structures happen through a reabsorption process, becoming increaslingly small, refringent (Figs 97.26 and 97.27) and disappearing, not being able to see inside a solid complex image (Fig. 97.28).
- The color map inside the trophoblast is smaller each time (Figs 97.29 and 97.30), with a slight Doppler signal, which is sometimes very difficult to find.
- The resistance and pulsatility index inside the trophoblastic vessels is increased and, at the end, it is impossible to specify anything objectively (Fig. 97.31).[43]

Systemic Methotrexate Administration

The most common drug used in the ectopic pregnancy treatment is the methotrexate, that interferes in trophoblastic development.

Methotrexate acts inhibiting the reduction of folic acid to tetrahydrofolic acid. Because tetrahydrofolic acid is essential in the transfer of one-carbon fragments in the synthesis of DNA, methotrexate effectively blocks DNA synthesis, inhibiting cell replication.

In the 1960s, methotrexate was used for the treatment of persistent trophoblastic tissues after an abdominal pregnancy. In 1982, it was used, for the first time, in the ectopic pregnancy treatment.

As we did with expectant handling, it has to be a patient's profile to administrate methotrexate. The selection criteria are different for several authors, but most of them agree in using methotrexate

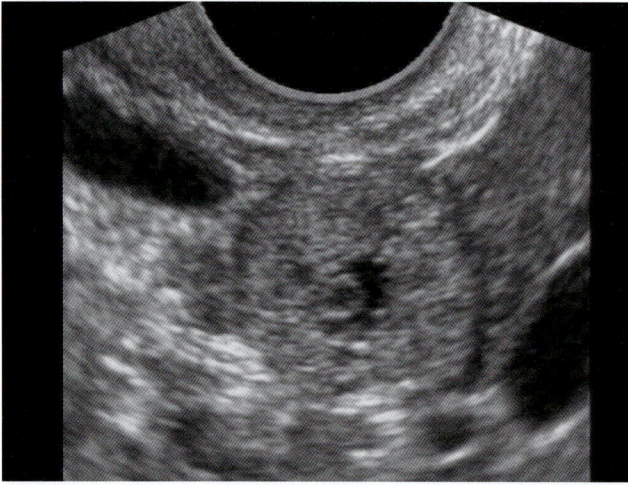

Fig. 97.26: Ectopic pregnancy with spontaneous reabsorption. A yolk sac smaller every time and a refringent ring around it are visible

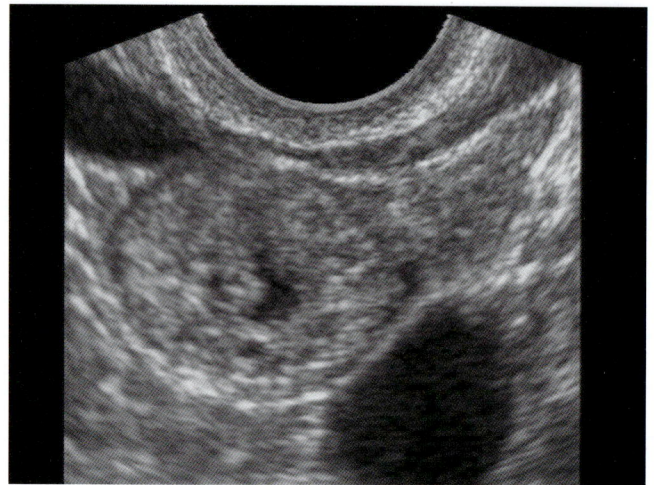

Fig. 97.27: Ectopic pregnancy with spontaneous reabsorption. The refringent ring is each time bigger, as the size of the yolk sac decreases

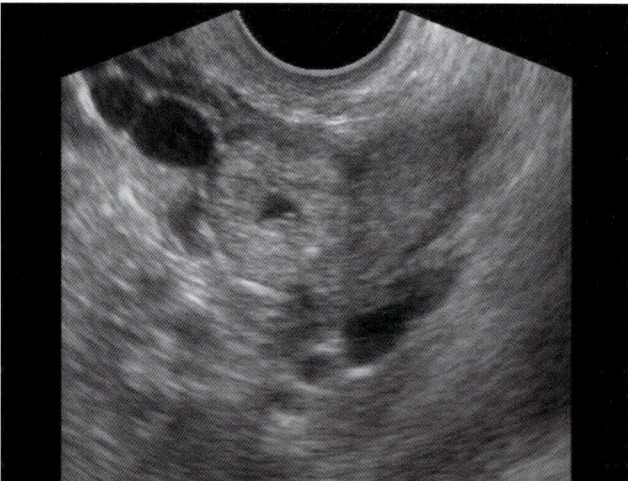

Fig. 97.28: Ectopic pregnancy with spontaneous reabsorption. Yolk sac is nearly disappeared

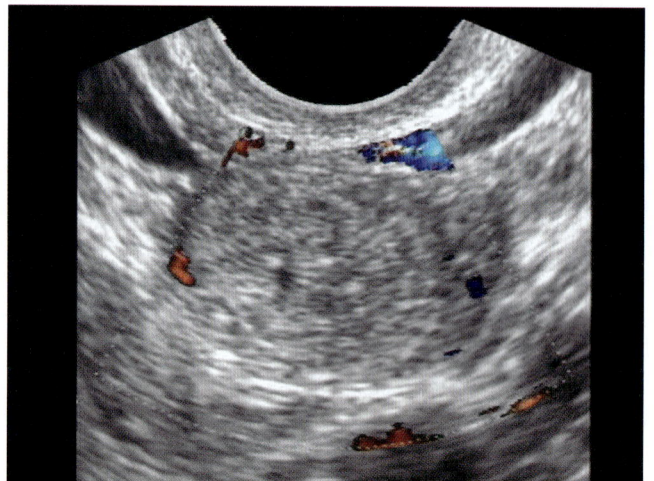

Fig. 97.29: Ectopic pregnancy with spontaneous reabsorption. The yolk sac has disappeared and has been replaced by a refringent area that shows the tube more compact

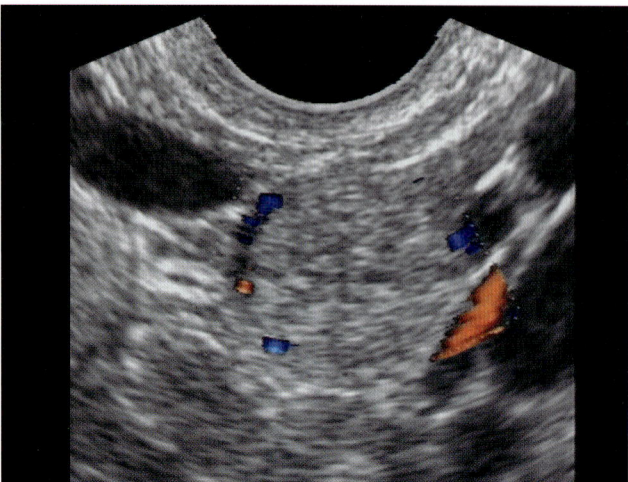

Fig. 97.30: Ectopic pregnancy with spontaneous reabsorption. Color map of the detectable trophoblast

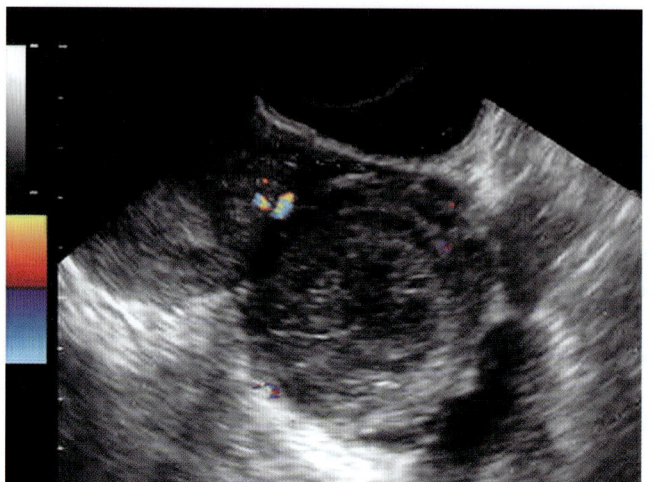

Fig. 97.31: Ectopic pregnancy with spontaneous reabsorption. Color map progressively fades away

in hemodynamic stable patients, with a non-ruptured ectopic pregnancy, with a little amount of liquid on Douglas sac and with less than 4 cm diameter of tubal affection, with ultrasonography findings types 1, 2 or 3.

The presence of embryonic heart movements is for some authors an absolute contraindication for this kind of treatment, because results in these cases are worse and it would be better to indicate a surgical treatment.

Before methotrexate administration, a complete hemogram (including platelet count), and some biochemical values to be sure that hepatic and renal functions are normal are needed.

The doses of methotrexate that have been used in different studies are quite variable. The most usual dose is 1 mg/kg, intramuscularly, each 48 hours, until a total of four doses are completed or until a reduction of β-hCG levels in two consecutive days is observed. Methotrexate is usually combined with folinic acid (0.1 mg/kg) in alternating days.

At the moment, a single dose of 50 mg/m^2 of methotrexate has been used, and has proved to be as effective as the multiple dose therapy. This model does not need the folinic acid combined, and it has less secondary effects.

The β-hCG levels can increase during the first 3 days after the treatment, but they must be less on the seventh day. If this reduction is smaller than 15%, it is necessary to repeat the methotrexate administration (which is necessary in nearly 8% of the cases).

The oral administration has also been used, but its results are not as good as with intramuscularly administration.

Toxicity to methotrexate frequently involves mucous membranes, with stomatitis, esophagitis, vaginitis and, occasionally, gastrointestinal ulcerations, but they are not very common, and are dose-dependent. Bone marrow suppression with granulocytopenia and thrombocytopenia is common, but generally not severe. Skin rashes and alopecia are uncommon, but they do occur; nephrotoxicity, hepatotoxicity and pulmonary fibrosis are very rare.

After 3 or 4 days of methotrexate administration, the presence of an abdominal pain of variable intensity is common, described in 60% of the patients. It is usually a side effect that disappears spontaneously in 1 or 2 days although sometimes hospitable entrance is needed to discard hemodynamic instability and the possible rupture.

The success rate is 83–100% according to different studies.

Periodical ultrasonography and β-hCG levels controls are needed after the conservative treatment. The ultrasonography image of the ectopic pregnancy can continue being observed when the β-hCG levels are negative. The persistence of this sign does not have to be interpreted as a treatment failure and it can even take months to disappear.[44]

Asymptomatic Tube Ectopic Pregnancy with Alive Embryo

If the gestational sac is visualized inside the tube and we can see an embryo with positive heart movements, there are two treatment options: the first one is the laparoscopic extirpation, and the other one is the transvaginal puncture with methotrexate injection inside the gestational sac, that it is used only in selected cases.[45]

One of the most important indications for local methotrexate administration is the presence of embryo heart activity. In these cases, with the local puncture, we have the methotrexate action and the blast effect of the needle. With this direct administration, it is possible to reduce the dose of the drug, diminishing therefore its side effects.

The gestational sac puncture has to be guided by transvaginal ultrasonography or carried out by laparoscopy. After the puncture, the first thing that we have to do is to aspirate the sac content and after that to inject the methotrexate. The methotrexate dose used is variable in different studies, but it is around 10–50 mg.

After the puncture, it is visible a very refringent image (Figs 97.32 to 97.37) that changes very slowly in some cases, as we described before, during its reabsorption.

The success rate is nearly 85–100%, according to different authors.

Some other substances have been used for local administration instead of methotrexate (such as prostaglandins, potassium chloride, hyperosmotic glucose, etc.) for the ectopic pregnancy treatment, but they have been used no more because of their important secondary effects and because of their minor action.

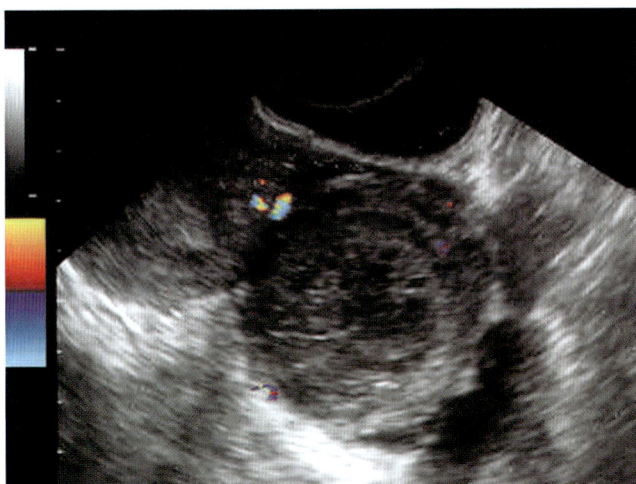

Fig. 97.32: Ectopic pregnancy with spontaneous reabsorption. Neither color map inside the tube and nor trophoblastic color signal are visible

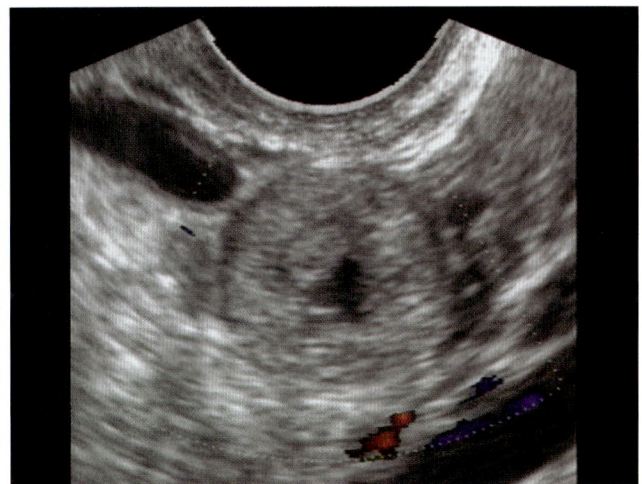

Fig. 97.33: Ectopic pregnancy with no color signal. It is not possible to measure the resistance index

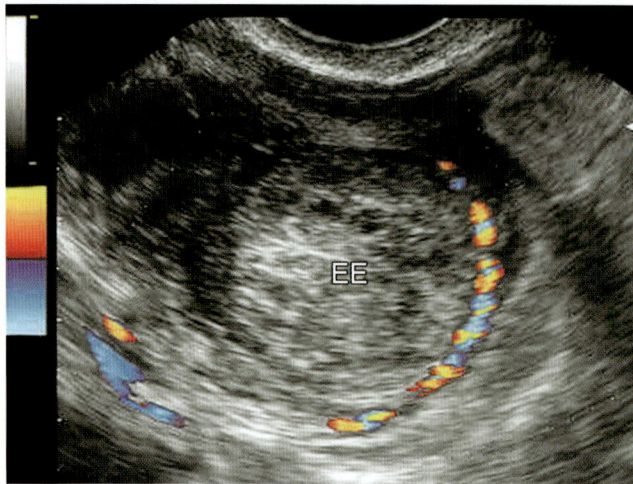

Fig. 97.34: Ectopic pregnancy in reabsorption process. It appears very refringent

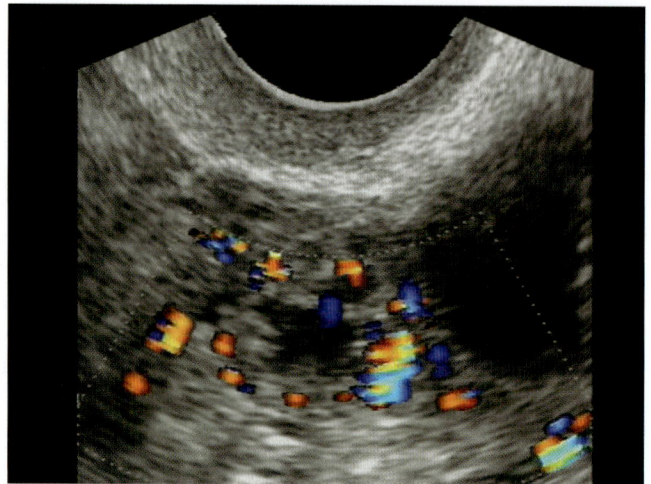

97.35: Ectopic pregnancy treated with methotrexate successfully. It is visible the reabsorption process of the tubal formation

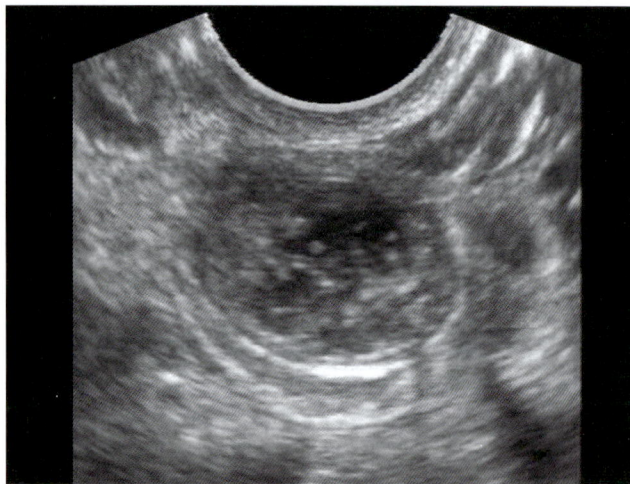

Fig. 97.36: Ectopic pregnancy treated with methotrexate successfully. The refringent formation is still visible

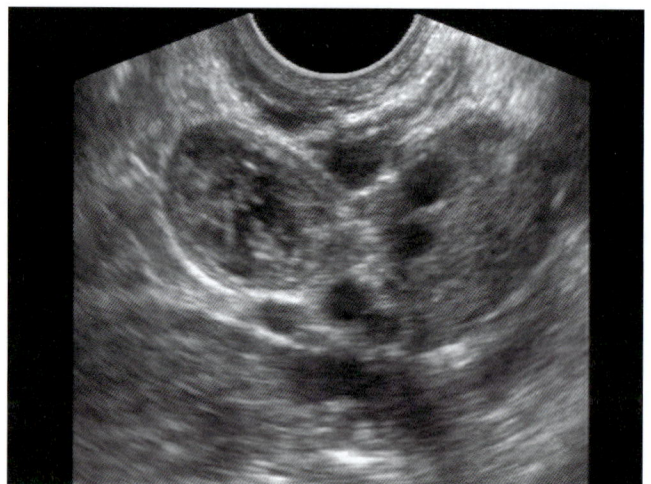

Fig. 97.37: Ectopic pregnancy after intra-sac methotrexate injection. Both the gestational vesicle and embryo have been transformed into a refringent structure that will initiate the same process of reabsorption when it does spontaneously

The local or systemic methotrexate administration is also indicated in cornual or cervical ectopic pregnancies, to avoid surgical treatments, in attempt to preserve fertility.

If the tube has not been blown apart by rupture, preservation of the tube can be obtained by making a longitudinal incision along the antimesenteric border of the tube and suturing the incision with fine material.

ACUTE RUPTURE OF TUBAL ECTOPIC PREGNANCY TREATMENT

If the intraperitoneal bleeding is very profuse, symptoms of shock occur and it is obvious that surgical attention is required.

The treatment in this case consists of evacuating the hemoperitoneum and excising the ectopic pregnancy by laparoscopy or laparotomy, once the patient is on an stable state.

ABDOMINAL ECTOPIC PREGNANCY TREATMENT

The treatment in these cases consists of evacuating the fetus outside the abdominal cavity with ligation of the umbilical cord. It is not necessary to remove the placenta, which may be firmly fixed to the mesentery and the abdominal viscera. Profuse hemorrhage can occur on manipulation, and the placenta, if left in situ, resorbs without sequelae in most instances.

In these cases, it is also possible to use the methotrexate intramuscularly and to do ultrasonography and β-hCG levels controls after it. Some authors have suggested the methotrexate use to facilitate devascularization and absortion of any unremoved placenta.

Ultrasonography makes possible to monitor the placenta left in situ after removing the fetus,[46] whose image persists inside the abdomen during a long time.

REFERENCES

1. Speroff L, Glass RH, Kase NG. Ectopic pregnancy. In: Speroff L, Glass RH, Kase NG (Eds). Clinical Gynecologic Endocrinology and Infertility. London: Williams and Wilkins; 1999. pp. 1149-67.
2. Bouyer J, Coste J, Fernandez H, et al. Sites of ectopic pregnancy: a 10 year population-based study of 1800 cases. Hum Reprod. 2002;17:3224-30.
3. Coste J, Bouyer J, Ughetto S, et al. Ectopic pregnancy is again on the increase. Recent trends in the incidence of ectopic pregnancies in France (1992–2002). Hum Reprod. 2004;19:2014-8.
4. Boufous S, Quartararo M, Mohsin M, et al. Trends in the incidence of ectopic pregnancy in New South Wales between 1990–1998. Aust N Z J Obstet Gynaecol. 2001;41:436-8.
5. Rajkhowa M, Glass MR, Rutherford AJ, et al. Trends in the incidence of ectopic pregnancy in England and Wales from 1966 to 1996. BJOG. 2000;107:369-74.
6. Strandell A, Thorburn J, Hamberger L. Risk factors for ectopic pregnancy in assisted reproduction. Fertil Steril. 1999;2:282-6.
7. Kamwendo F, Forslin L, Bodin L, et al. Epidemiology of ectopic pregnancy during a 28 year period and the role of pelvic inflammatory disease. Sex Transm Infect. 2000;76:28-32.
8. Barlow RE, Cooke ID, Odukoya O, et al. The prevalence of Chlamydia Trachomatis in fresh tissue specimens from patients with ectopic pregnancy or tubal factor infertility as determined by PCR and in situ hybridization. J Med Microbiol. 2001;50:902-8.
9. Jun SH, Milki AA. Assisted hatching is associated with a higher ectopic pregnancy rate. Fertil Steril. 2004;81:1701-3.
10. Bouyer J, Rachou E, Germain E, et al. Risk factors for extrauterine pregnancy in women using an intrauterine device. Fertil Steril. 2000;74:899-908.
11. Dahiya K, Khosla AH. Ectopic pregnancy after sterilization. Trop Doct. 2004;34(4):255.
12. Wong E, Suat SO. Ectopic pregnancy—a diagnostic challenge in the emergency department. Eur J Emerg Med. 2000;7:189-94.
13. Shalev E, Yaron I, Bustan M, et al. Transvaginal sonography as the ultimate diagnosis tool for the management of ectopic pregnancy: experience with 840 cases. Fertil Steril. 1998;69:62-5.
14. Hertzberg BS, Kliewer MA. Ectopic pregnancy: ultrasound diagnosis and interpretive pitfalls. South Med J. 1995;88:1191-8.
15. Chan LY, Fok WY, Yuen PM. Pitfalls in diagnosis of interstitial pregnancy. Acta Obstet Gynecol Scand. 2003;82:867-70.
16. Mueller MD, Raio L, Spoerri S, et al. Novel placental and nonplacental serum markers in ectopic versus normal intrauterine pregnancy. Fertil Steril. 2004;81:1106-11.
17. Shepherd RW, Patton PE, Novy MJ, et al. Serial beta-hCG measurements in the early detection of ectopic pregnancy. Obstet Gynecol. 1990;75:417-20.
18. Roussos D, Panidis D, Matalliotakis I, et al. Factors that may predispose to rupture of tubal ectopic pregnancy. Eur J Obstet Gynecol Reprod Biol. 2000;89:15-7.
19. da Costa Soares R, Elito J Jr, Han KK, et al. Endometrial thickness as an orienting factor for the medical treatment of unruptured tubal pregnancy. Acta Obstet Gynecol Scand. 2004;83:289-92.
20. Laurie S, Insler V. Can the serum bega hCG level reliably predict likelihood of a ruptured tubal pregnancy? Isr J Obstet Gynecol. 1992;3:152-544.
21. Bozoklu S, Bozoklu E, Ciftci A, et al. Ruptured ectopic pregnancy with indetectable beta-hCG levels coexisting with acute appendicitis. Acta Obstet Gynecol Reprod Scand. 1997;76:181-2.
22. Lurie S, Katz Z, Weissman A, et al. Declining beta-human chorionic gonadotropin level may provide false security that tubal pregnancy will not rupture. Eur J Obstet Gynecol Reprod Biol. 1994;53:72-3.
23. Tulandi T, Hemmings R, Khalifa F. Rupture of ectopic pregnancy in women with low and declining serum beta-human chorionic gonadotropin concentrations. Fertil Steril. 1991;56:786-7.
24. Weston G, Kashyap R. Failed conservative management of cervical pregnancy despite failing beta-hCG. Aust N Z J Obstet Gynaecol. 2001;41:346-7.
25. Peisner DB, Timor-Tritsch IE. The discriminatory zone of beta hCG for vaginal probes. J Clin Ultrasound. 1990;18:280-5.
26. Counselman FL, Shoar S, Heller RA, et al. Quantitative pregnancy: pelvic ultrasound still useful. J Emerg med. 1998;16:699-703.
27. Albayram F, Hamper UM. First-trimester obstetric emergencies: spectrum of sonographic findings. J Clin Ultrasound. 2002;30:161-77.
28. Hill LM, Kislak S, Martin JG. Transvaginal sonographic detection of the pseudogestational sac associated with ectopic pregnancy. Obstet Gynecol. 1990;75:986-8.
29. Jurkovic D, Bourne TH, Jauniaux E, et al. Transvaginal color Doppler study of blood flow in ectopic pregnancies. Fertil Steril. 1992;57:68-73.
30. Dillon EH, Feyock AL, Taylor KJW. Pseudogestational sacs: Doppler US differentiation from normal or abnormal intrauterine pregnancies. Radiology. 1990;176:359-64.
31. Tekay A, Jouppila P. Color Doppler flow as an indicator of trophoblastic activity in tubal pregnancies detected by transvaginal ultrasound. Obstet Gynecol. 1992;80:995-9.
32. Wherry KL, Dubinsky TJ, Waitches GM, et al. Low resistance endometrial arterial flow in the exclusion of ectopic pregnancy revisited. J Ultrasound Med. 2001;20:335-42.
33. Breyer MJ, Constantino TG. Heterotopic gestation: another possibility for the emergency bedside ultrasonographer to consider. J Emerg Med. 2004;26:81-4.
34. Kumor S, Vimala N, Dadhwal V, et al. Heterotopic cervical and intrauterine pregnancy in a spontaneous cycle. Eur J Obstet Gynecol Reprod Biol. 2004;112:217-20.
35. Dart R, McLean SA, Dart L. Isolated fluid in the cul-de-sac. How well does it predict ectopic pregnancy? Am J Emerg Med. 2002;20(1):1-4.
36. Yao M, Tulandi T. Current status of surgical and non-surgical management of ectopic pregnancy. Fertil Steril. 1997;67:421-33.
37. Tulandi T, Sammour A. Evidence-based management of ectopic pregnancy. Curr Opin Obstet Gynecol. 2000;12:289-92.
38. Canis M, Savary D, Pouly JL, et al. Ectopic pregnancy: criteria to decide between medical and conservative surgical treatment? J Gynecol Obstet Biol Reprod. 2003;32:54-63.
39. Atri M, Chow CM, Kintzaen G, et al. Expectant treatment of ectopic pregnancies: clinical and sonographic predictors. AJR Am J Roentgenol. 2001;176:123-7.
40. Atri M, Bret PM, Tulandi T. Spontaneous resolution of ectopic pregnancy: initial appearance and evolution at transvaginal US. Radiology. 1993;186:83-6.
41. Ylostalo P, Cacciatore B, Sjoberg J, et al. Expectant management of ectopic pregnancy. Obstet Gynecol. 1992;80:345-8.
42. Thompson GR, O'Shea RT, Harding A. Beta hCG levels after conservative treatment of ectopic pregnancy: is a plateau normal? Aust N Z J Obstet Gynaecol. 1994;34:96-8.
43. Turan C, Ugur M, Dogan M, et al. Transvaginal sonographic findings of chronic ectopic pregnancy. Eur J Obstet Gynecol Reprod Biol. 1996;67:115-9.
44. Tekay A, Martikainen H, Heikkinen H, et al. Disappearance of the trophoblastic blood flow in tubal pregnancy after methotrexate injection. J Ultrasound Med. 1993;12:615-8.
45. Venezia R, Zangara C, Comparetto G, et al. Conservative treatment of ectopic pregnancy using a single echo-guided injection of methotrexate into the gestational sac. Ultrasound Obstet Gynecol. 1991;1:132-5.
46. Bajo JM, Garcia FA, Huertas MA. Sonographic follow-up of a placenta left in situ after delivery of the fetus in abdominal pregnancy. Ultrasound Obstet Gynecol. 1996;7:285-8